Brief Contents

Become a better student
and an
EFFECTIVE NURSE

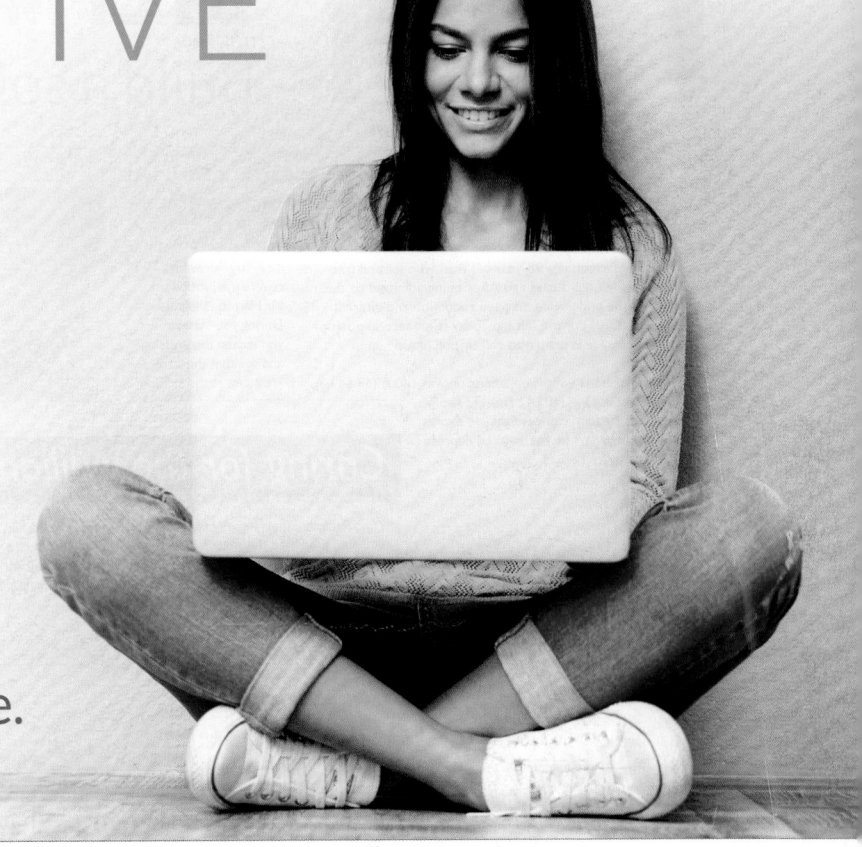

Davis Advantage is a personalized, interactive learning platform with proven results to help you succeed in your course.

94%
of students said Advantage improved their test scores.

"My grades have improved; my understanding about topics is much clearer; and overall, it has been the total package for what a nursing student needs to succeed."

— Hannah, Student, Judson University

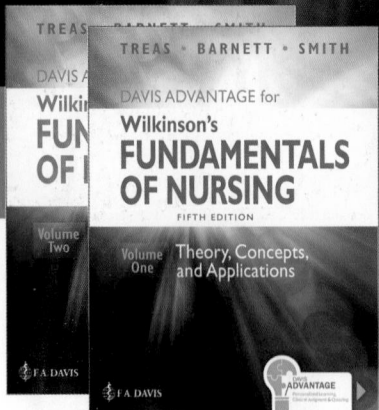

STEP #1
Build a solid foundation.

Meet Your Patient

William Harmon is a 78-year-old man who fell and fractured his left hip 3 days ago. After being admitted to the hospital, he underwent an open reduction and internal fixation (ORIF) of the left hip. Today is his second postoperative day. He is unable to roll or pull himself up in the bed.

Mr. Harmon's weight on admission was 140 lb (63.64 kg). His height is 73 in (185.42 cm). His family [...] has been steadily losing weight. He express[...] in eating and says he has suffered depressi[...] died last year.

A large dressing covers the incision on Mr. Harmon's left hip. During your assessment, you loosen the dressing and see that the staples are intact at the incision [...]

Two types of **case studies** bring concepts to life, connecting what you read to what you will see and do in practice.

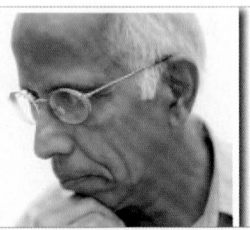

Caring for the Williams Family

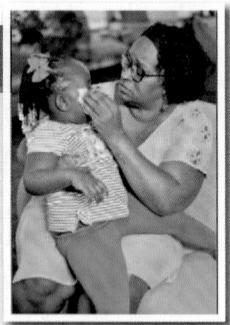

Kayla Robinson, Stanley and Nadine Williams' 3-year-old grandchild, fell at the neighborhood playground. She has abrasions on her knees, a deep puncture wound on her left hand, and a laceration on her scalp. Mr. and Mrs. Williams bring her to the clinic for assessment. She is crying loudly and moving all extremities. No treatment has been given.

▲ Think**Like a Nurse** 32-2:
Clinical Judgment **in Action**

Recall the case of Mr. Harmon (Meet Your Patient). What form of wound healing (primary, secondary, or tertiary) is he undergoing? How long would you expect it to take before his wounds heal?

iCare highlights the role of caring in nursing by modeling behaviors and conversations that demonstrate how to provide compassionate care.

Think Like a Nurse: Clinical Judgment in Action questions put you in the nurse's role to develop your clinical judgment skills from day one.

▼ iCare 32-1

Skin Integrity and Wound Healing

- *Scenario 1*—Mary is caring for Mrs. Skylar, a 62-year-old patient with diabetes and venous stasis ulcers on her legs. Since developing these venous stasis ulcers, Mrs. Skylar has become very self-conscious and embarrassed about her legs. When taking Mrs. Skylar to x-ray, Mary covers Mrs. Skylar's legs with a bath blanket for comfort and privacy. Mary was not only providing comfort and protecting privacy. She was also aware of Mrs. Skylar's feelings and cared enough to respond to them.
- *Scenario 2*—Mr. Robert Brown is an 18-year-old paraplegic who has developed a stage 4 sacral pressure ulcer with a foul odor. He is expecting some of his friends from school for a visit. Ken, his nurse, while nonchalantly cleaning up the room, makes sure to remove the garbage liner with the old dressings in it. He also brings in some fresh-cut flowers and a cup of wet coffee grounds. Both the flowers and the coffee grounds are natural odor eliminators. Mr. Brown has a great visit with his friends from school.

 Social Determinants of Health 8-1

Economic Stability

- Employment
- Food insecurity
- Housing instability
- Poverty

> - **Contact burns** may occur from contact with metal surfaces and vinyl seats when cars are parked in the sun. The risk of contact burns in all age-groups is greater in the presence of such heating devices as kerosene heaters, wood-burning stoves, and home sauna heating elements. People may use these as heat

Social Determinants of Health boxes and icons help you to think about the many conditions that affect health.

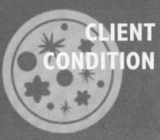

CLIENT CONDITION

Key Point: *Like domestic violence, elder abuse is seen in all cultures and socio-economic groups.*

Abuse Types

Abuse takes many forms:
Physical   Emotional
Sexual   Financial
Neglect   Abandonment

Risk Factors

Key Point: *The risk of abuse is higher for women and those with physical and cognitive vulnerabilities.*
Advanced age
Physical, functional, or cognitive impairment

Risk Factors

Mental illness
Alcoholism or drug abuse in patient or caregiver
Dependence on others
Past history of abusive relationships
Depression
Low self-esteem
Poor health of patient or caregiver
Caregiver stressed or frustrated with difficult caregiving tasks

Social Determinants of health:

Ageism
Social isolation or poor social network
Low-income status

RECOGNIZING CUES

Key Point: *If an older adult presents with subdural hematomas, pe... ity injuries, along with ... was inflicted.* Elder abuse ...

Example Client Conditions graphically illustrate the key concepts and need-to-know information in each chapter and reflect the cognitive skills of the NCSBN Clinical Judgment Measurement Model.

CLINICALREASONING
Applying the Full-Spectrum Nursing Model

PATIENT SITUATION

Tio Santos is a 66-year-old man with obesity, diabetes, and hypertension. He is being seen for a wound on his right foot that doesn't seem to be healing. He injured his foot when repairing drywall at home. He is otherwise relatively sedentary at home. The wound is oozing, swollen, tender, and warm to the touch. Mr. Santos is now running a low-grade fever of 100.4°F (38°C) at home. He tells you his foot is very painful, especially with any weight bearing, and throbs when he is sitting or lying still. You measure the wound bed to be 6 cm x 4 cm and note purulent exudate at the distal edge. He is referred to an outpatient wound care center for treatment.

THINKING

1. *Theoretical Knowledge:*

   a. What is the Braden scale and why might it be used for Mr. Santos?

   b. What risk factors for de...

2. *Critical Thinking (Consideri...*

   a. To care for Mr. Santos' ... Explain your thinking.

DOING

3. *Practical Knowledge (Assess...*

   a. What symptoms of infe...

   b. To be certain the wound...

CARING

Critical Thinking and Clinical Judgment

1. You are caring for a 22-year-old man with paralysis from the waist down secondary to a motor vehicle accident. He has been admitted to the hospital with a urinary tract infection manifested by a fever of 102°F (39°C) and lethargy. His family reports he has been withdrawn and sits in his wheelchair looking at his phone all day.

   a. What risk factors does this patient have for skin breakdown?

   b. What locations of his body should you be most concerned for the formation of pressure injury?

   c. What actions should you take to decrease the risk of pressure injury for your patient? What further information do you need?

2. A 63-year-old male patient is admitted to your unit after an emergency appendectomy. His appendix was ruptured, and the surgeon has left the wound open to heal by secondary intention. A Jackson–Pratt drain is in place in the wound bed. A moderate amount of purosanguineous drainage is visible in the drain. The surgeon has ordered saline-moistened gauze packing every 4 hours.

   a. What actions should you take as you prepare to do the first dressing change?

   b. How will you secure the dressing?

Applying the Full-Spectrum Nursing Model and **Critical Thinking and Clinical Judgment** exercises guide you in applying your critical-thinking and clinical-reasoning skills to real-world patient scenarios.

Procedure 32-13 ■ Shortening a Wound Drain

➤ For steps to follow in *all* procedures, refer to the Universal Steps for All Procedures on the inside back cover.

Equipment
■ Nonsterile gloves
■ Sterile gloves
■ Sterile scissors
■ Two safety pins or other clips (sterile)
■ Sterile gauze

Delegation

Assessment of the incision line or wound and the drain is a registered nurse's responsibility and cannot be delegated. This procedure should not be delegated to a UAP. The risk for accidently losing the drain into the body or pulling it out of the wound is too high.

Preprocedure Assessment

■ Inspect the site around the drain, noting skin excoriation, tenderness, erythema, warmth to the touch, and drainage seeping from the wound.
Could indicate a wound infection or irritation of the drain at the skin site. Excoriation can be the result of seeping drainage around

the tube (e.g., if the tube diameter is not sufficient size to handle drainage output) or, more likely, an obstruction within the tubing.

■ Assess the characteristics of the drainage, including color, volume of drainage, presence of blood, odor, pus, and any change in the type or amount of drainage through the tubing.
A sudden decrease in drainage might indicate a blocked drain. Presence of fresh blood might be a sign of irritation within the wound. Pus and odor in the drainage could indicate wound infection.

■ Check the suction apparatus to be sure it is functioning properly.
A self-suction apparatus might need to be recompressed from time to time to maintain effective vacuum. Electric suction units can fail, delivering too much suction, which can lead to injury. Too little suction can contribute to insufficient drainage, which can lead to pressure on sutures if present, or cause the wound to become infected or heal more slowly.

➤ When performing the procedure, always identify your patient according to agency policy, using two identifiers, and be attentive to standard precautions, hand hygiene, patient safety and privacy, body mechanics, and documentation.

Procedure Steps

1. **Perform hand hygiene** and don nonsterile gloves. Remove wound dressings.

2. **Remove soiled gloves** and discard in a moisture-proof biohazard collection container. Perform hand hygiene.

3. **Open sterile supplies** (scissors, etc.).

4. **Don sterile gloves;** use sterile scissors to cut halfway through a sterile

The pin or clamp keeps the drain from disappearing into the wound. ▼

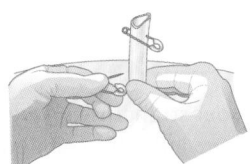

9. **Cleanse the wound,** using sterile gauze swabs and the prescribed cleaning solution. In some situations, you may use sterile forceps to manipulate the swabs.

10. **Apply precut sterile gauze** around the drain; then redress the wound. ▼

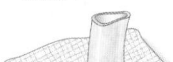

Over 230 step-by-step procedures with rationales teach you how to perform and master essential nursing skills.

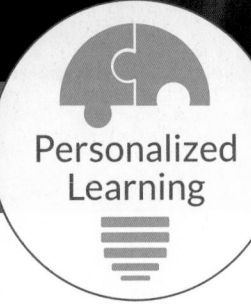

LEARN

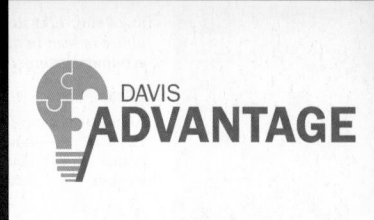

DAVIS ADVANTAGE

STEP #2

Make the connections to key topics.

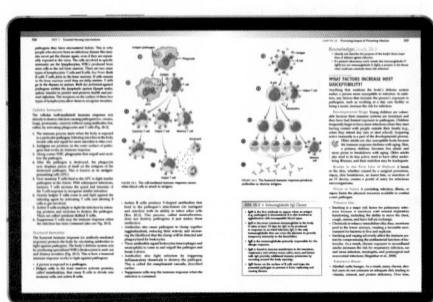

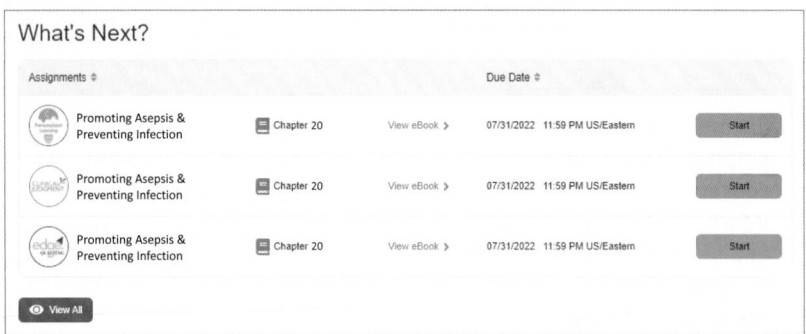

What's Next?

Assignments ⇕				Due Date ⇕		
	Promoting Asepsis & Preventing Infection	Chapter 20	View eBook >	07/31/2022 11:59 PM US/Eastern		Start
	Promoting Asepsis & Preventing Infection	Chapter 20	View eBook >	07/31/2022 11:59 PM US/Eastern		Start
	Promoting Asepsis & Preventing Infection	Chapter 20	View eBook >	07/31/2022 11:59 PM US/Eastern		Start

👁 View All

Assignments in Davis Advantage correspond to key topics in your book. Begin by reading from your printed text or click the ebook button to be taken to the **FREE, integrated ebook.**

Following your reading, take a **Pre-Assessment** to evaluate your understanding of the content. Questions feature single answer, multiple-choice, and select-all-that-apply formats.

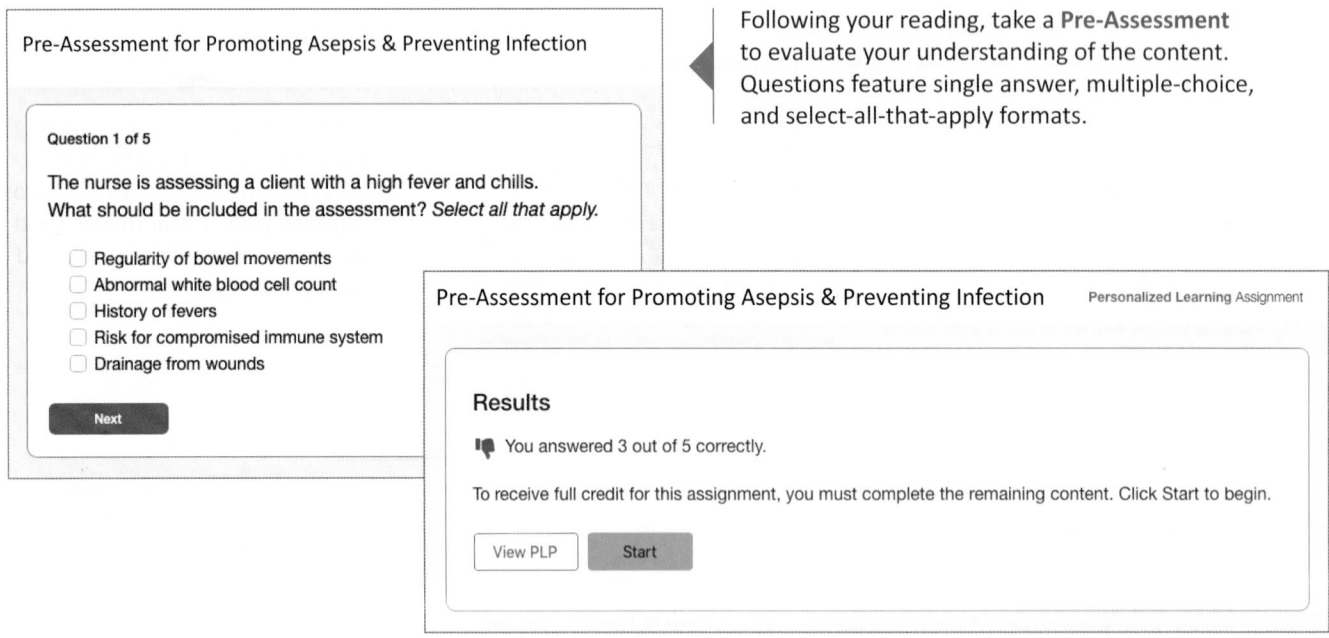

Pre-Assessment for Promoting Asepsis & Preventing Infection

Question 1 of 5

The nurse is assessing a client with a high fever and chills.
What should be included in the assessment? *Select all that apply.*

☐ Regularity of bowel movements
☐ Abnormal white blood cell count
☐ History of fevers
☐ Risk for compromised immune system
☐ Drainage from wounds

Next

Pre-Assessment for Promoting Asepsis & Preventing Infection   Personalized Learning Assignment

Results

👎 You answered 3 out of 5 correctly.

To receive full credit for this assignment, you must complete the remaining content. Click Start to begin.

View PLP   Start

Immediate feedback identifies your strengths and weaknesses using a thumbs up, thumbs down approach. *Thumbs up* indicates competency, while *thumbs down* signals an area of weakness that requires further study.

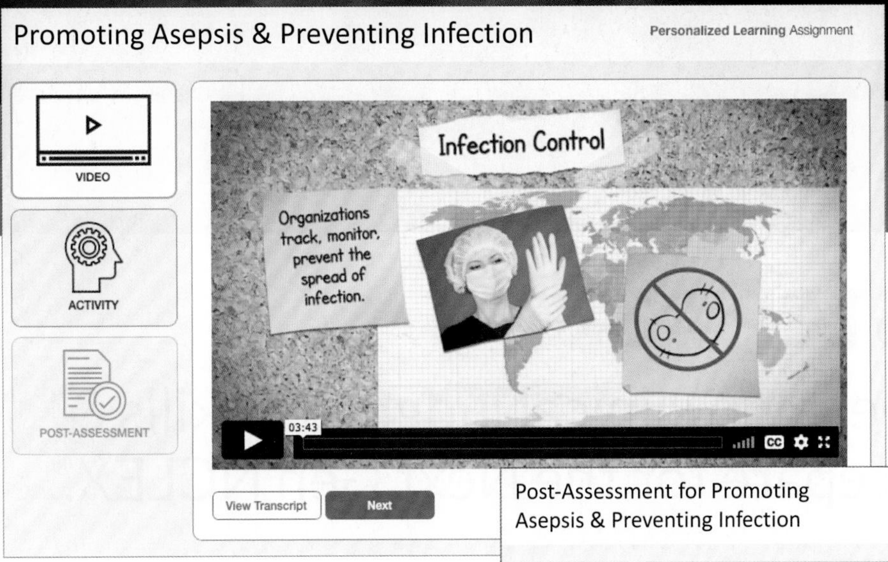

Promoting Asepsis & Preventing Infection

VIDEO

ACTIVITY

POST-ASSESSMENT

Infection Control

Organizations track, monitor, prevent the spread of infection.

03:43

View Transcript | Next

After working through the video and activity, a **Post-Assessment** tests your mastery.

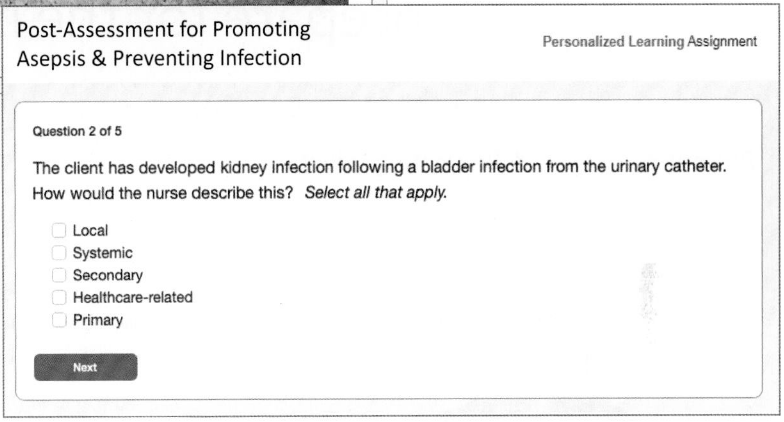

Animated mini-lecture videos make key concepts easier to understand, while **interactive learning activities** allow you to expand your knowledge and make the connections to important topics.

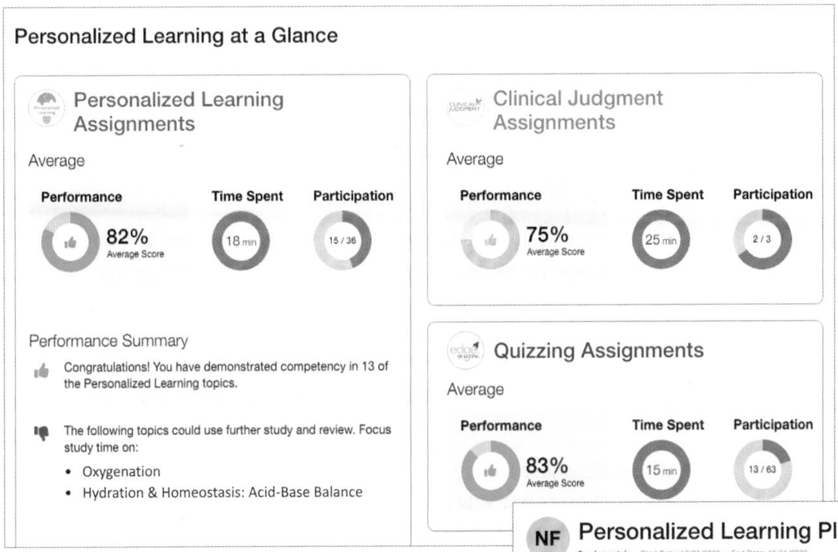

Post-Assessment for Promoting Asepsis & Preventing Infection

Personalized Learning Assignment

Question 2 of 5

The client has developed kidney infection following a bladder infection from the urinary catheter. How would the nurse describe this? *Select all that apply.*

- [ ] Local
- [ ] Systemic
- [ ] Secondary
- [ ] Healthcare-related
- [ ] Primary

Next

Personalized Learning at a Glance

Personalized Learning Assignments

Average

Performance	Time Spent	Participation
82% Average Score	18 min	15 / 36

Clinical Judgment Assignments

Average

Performance	Time Spent	Participation
75% Average Score	25 min	2 / 3

Performance Summary

👍 Congratulations! You have demonstrated competency in 13 of the Personalized Learning topics.

👎 The following topics could use further study and review. Focus study time on:
- Oxygenation
- Hydration & Homeostasis: Acid-Base Balance

Quizzing Assignments

Average

Performance	Time Spent	Participation
83% Average Score	15 min	13 / 63

Your **Dashboard** provides an at-a-glance snapshot of your performance as you work through your assignments.

Your **Personalized Learning Plan** is tailored to your individual needs and tracks your progress **across all your assignments**, helping you to identify the specific areas that require additional study.

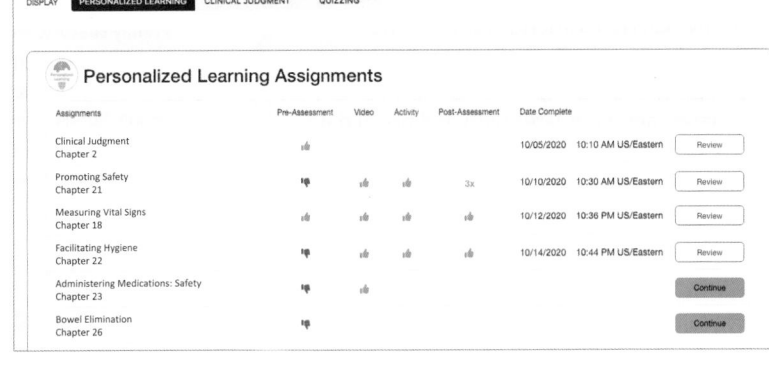

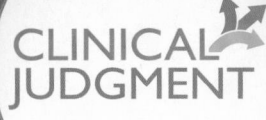

APPLY

STEP #3
Develop clinical judgment skills & prepare for the Next Gen NCLEX.®

Promoting Asepsis & Preventing Infection

Promoting Asepsis & Preventing Infection

The nurse is admitting a 42-year-old female with a fever and cough during a pandemic virus outbreak.

This case consists of six clinical judgment questions. Read each question carefully and select the best answer(s). Use the chart to help answer the question. The chart is dynamic and may change as the case progresses.

Next

Real-world cases mirror the complex clinical challenges you will encounter in a variety of health care settings. Each **case study** begins with a patient photograph and a brief introduction to the scenario.

The **Patient Chart** displays tabs for History & Physical Assessment, Nurses' Notes, Vital Signs, and Laboratory Results. As you progress through the case, the chart expands and populates with additional data.

Scenario

The nurse is admitting a 42-year-old female with a fever and cough during a pandemic virus outbreak. Use the chart to answer the questions. *The chart may update as the scenario progresses.*

History and Physical Assessment	Nurses' Notes	Vital Signs	Laboratory Results

Medical/Surgical history: Otherwise healthy female developed fever and cough 24 hours ago. Attended a large social event recently without wearing a mask or following social distancing during a pandemic virus outbreak.

Social history: Denies use of drugs, alcohol, and tobacco. Avid distance runner. Married with 4 children.

Family History: Mother and father alive and healthy.

Assessment: Alert and oriented but tired looking in appearance. Skin warm to touch, face flushed. No signs of respiratory distress but occasional dry cough. Lungs clear. States things "smell and taste" different. CV, GI, GU assessments all within the normal limits. States feeling "weak and tired."

Medications: None

Promoting Asepsis & Preventing Infection

Scenario

The nurse is admitting a 42-year-old female with a fever and cough during a pandemic virus outbreak. Use the chart to answer the questions. *The chart may update as the scenario progresses.*

History and Physical Assessment	Nurses' Notes	Vital Signs	Laboratory Results

Medical/Surgical history: Otherwise healthy female developed fever and cough 24 hours ago. Attended a large social event recently without wearing a mask or following social distancing during a pandemic virus outbreak.
Social history: Denies use of drugs, alcohol, and tobacco. Avid distance runner. Married with 4 children.
Family History: Mother and father alive and healthy.
Assessment: Alert and oriented but tired looking in appearance. Skin warm to touch, face flushed. No signs of respiratory distress but occasional dry cough. Lungs clear. States things "smell and taste" different. CV, GI, GU assessments all within the normal limits. States feeling "weak and tired."
Medications: None

Question 1 of 6

The nurse reviews the medical record. *Select and highlight the findings that justify the need for infection precautions.*

Medical/Surgical history: Otherwise healthy female developed fever and cough 24 hours ago. Attended a large social event recently without wearing a mask or following social distancing during a pandemic virus outbreak.
4/20/XX
1010
Temp. 100.6°F (38.1°C)
HR 108 bpm
RR 20 breaths/min
SpO$_2$ 95% on room air
BP 117/62 mm Hg

Next

Promoting Asepsis & Preventing Infection

Results

 You answered 2 out of 6 questions correctly.

Review the questions, answers and rationales below to improve your understanding. Identify which questions you answered correctly (indicated by a green check mark) and incorrectly (identified by a red x). Remember, you must choose all correct options and only the correct options to get a question correct. Expand the questions to review your individual answer choices, the correct answers (indicated by green shading), and complete rationales.

[Hide All Details ▲]   [Return to Assignments]

⊗ **Question 1 of 6**   Hide ▲

The nurse reviews the medical record. *Select and highlight the findings that justify the need for infection precautions.*

Medical/Surgical history: Otherwise healthy female developed <u>fever and cough 24 hours ago</u>. Attended a large social event recently without wearing a mask or following social distancing during a pandemic virus outbreak.
4/20/XX
1010
Temp. 100.6°F (38.1°C)
HR 108 bpm
RR 20 breaths/min
SpO$_2$ 95% on room air
BP 117/62 mm Hg

Rationale

During a virus outbreak (including both pandemic or seasonal viruses), any person with minimal symptoms should be considered contagious and appropriately quarantined to protect healthcare workers and other patients and visitors. This client has a history of possible exposure and symptoms of infection including fever and cough. The respiratory rate and SpO2 are normal.

Clinical Judgment Cognitive Skill: **Recognize Cues, Analyze Cues**	Page Reference: **pp. 520–521**

💬 **Test-Taking Tip**   Identify those symptoms that best answer the question asked.

NGN format questions that align with the cognitive areas of the **NCSBN Clinical Judgment Measurement Model** require careful analysis, synthesis of the data, and multi-step thinking.

Immediate feedback with **detailed rationales** identifies the cognitive skills practiced according to the NCSBN Clinical Judgment Measurement Model and includes page references to the text for further remediation.

Test-taking tips provide important context and strategies for how to consider the structure of each question type when answering.

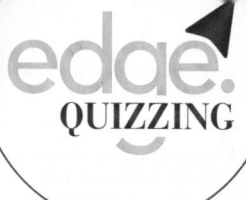

edge. QUIZZING

ASSESS

STEP #4

Improve scores and build confidence with NCLEX®-style questions

High-quality questions, including Next Gen NCLEX® bowtie and trend, test your knowledge and challenge you to think critically.

Quizzing: Assignment

Question 4 of 4

The nurse is caring for a 52-year-old client coming to the emergency department with peripheral edema, periorbital edema, flank pain, and shortness of breath. The nurse is preparing to notify the provider of the client's status. Complete the below using the dropdown choices.

The nurse's priority concern is the change in
[Vital Signs ▾] because of the client's hydration status.
The nurse should request an order for [antihypertensive ▾]
minimize the risk for complications.

[Next]

Client Data

Nurses' Notes
03/12/XX
11:20
A 52-year-old client came to the emergency department with shortness of breath and swelling of the legs, hands, and face that has increased over the last week. Flank pain is present and described as "a nagging ache that does not go away" and "feels like another kidney infection." States pain is 6 on a 1 to 10 scale. States "I have not been going to the bathroom much." History of steroid dependent rheumatoid arthritis, poorly controlled diabetes mellitus, and reoccurring urinary tract infections (UTIs). Alert and oriented, swan-neck deformities of hands. Lungs with fine crackles, bilaterally, mild shortness of breath. S1, S2 heart sounds with a murmur. 3+ radial and pedal pulses, bounding. 4+ edema of the lower legs, ankles, and feet, 2+ edema of the fingers and hands,

Feedback

👍 **You answered 3 out of 4 correctly.**
Review the questions, answers and rationales below.

[Hide All Details ▲]   [Return to Assignments]

✓ Question 4 of 4

The nurse is caring for a 52-year-old client coming to the emergency department with edema, periorbital edema, flank pain, and shortness of breath. The nurse is preparing to notify the provider of the client's status. Complete the below using the dropdown choices.

Client Data

Nurses' Notes
03/12/XX
11:20
A 52-year-old client came to the emergency department with shortness of breath and swelling of the legs, hands, and face that has increased over the last week. Flank pain is present and described as "a nagging ache that does not go away" and "feels like another kidney infection." States pain is 6 on a 1 to 10 scale. States "I have not been going to the bathroom much." History of steroid dependent rheumatoid arthritis, poorly controlled diabetes mellitus, and reoccurring urinary tract infections (UTIs). Alert and oriented, swan-neck deformities of hands. Lungs with fine crackles, bilaterally, mild shortness of breath. S1, S2 heart sounds with a murmur. 3+ radial and pedal pulses, bounding. 4+ edema of the lower legs, ankles, and feet, 2+ edema of the fingers and hands, periorbital edema present. Head of bed elevated for shortness of breath

Question ID:
MED52-RDC-16
Course Topic:
Renal Disorders
Concept:
Clinical Judgment, Elimination, Fluid and Electrolytes, Oxygenation Perfusion
Cognitive:
Evaluation [Evaluating]
Difficulty Level:
Difficult
Client Need:
Physiological Integrity
Chapter:
Chapter 62: Coordinating Care for Patients with Renal Disorders
Page Reference:
pp. 1452-1459

The nurse's priority concern is the change in [Vital Signs] because of the client's hydration status. The nurse should request an order for [antihypertensive] minimize the risk for complications.

Rationale: The client is demonstrating signs of acute kidney injury, oliguric phase. This is identified by low urine output, edema, shortness of breath, hypertension, hyperkalemia, elevated BUN/creatinine, anemia, and hyperkalemia. It is anticipated that this client has a compromised GFR due to risk factors of poorly controlled diabetes and reoccurring UTIs. The risks for developing acute kidney injury include infection and medications. Fever, elevated WBCs, flank pain are signs of a kidney infection, and extended to excessive use of NSAIDS will impair kidney function, leading to injury. In evaluating the client data, the nurse should be most concerned about the changing vital signs, including a rising temperature, heart rate, respiratory rate, and blood pressure, as the SpO2 decreases. This indicates a deterioration of oxygenation and perfusion. Priority medical management is the delivery of oxygen and an antihypertensive to prevent tissue hypoxia and stroke. The nurse should also notify the provider about the hyperkalemia, hyperglycemia, anemia, renal impairment shown in the lab results, and the assessment findings of oliguria, edema, crackles, and bounding pulses.

💬 **Test-Taking Tip**   Navigate the EHR trends by looking at how the cues presented relate to each other. Make the connection between the information to reach priority conclusions.

Immediate Feedback with **comprehensive rationales** explains why your responses are correct or incorrect. **Page-specific references** direct you to the relevant content in your text, while **Test-Taking Tips** improve your test-taking skills.

Practice Quizzes   [Create Practice Quiz]

You may generate their own practice quizzes (NCLEX®-style assessments) to test or expand your understanding of topics).

Assignments		Competency	Percent Correct	Date Complete	
Health Assessment	15 Questions	👍	85%	09/11/2020 10:40 PM US/Eastern	[Review]
Clinical Judgment	15 Questions	👍	79%	09/25/2020 10:45 PM US/Eastern	[Review]

[👁 View All]   KEY: 👍 80% ~ 100% 👍 70% ~ 79% 👎 ≤ 69%

Create your own practice quizzes to focus on topic areas where you are struggling, or to use as a study tool to review for an upcoming exam.

GET STARTED TODAY!

Use the access code on the inside front cover to unlock Davis Advantage for Wilkinson's Fundamentals of Nursing!

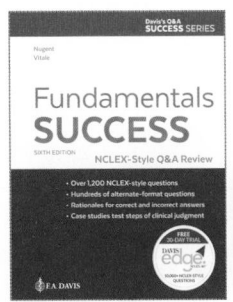 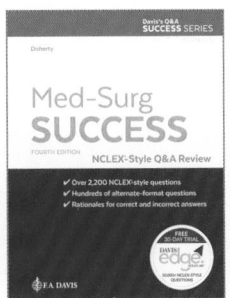 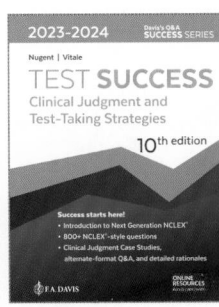 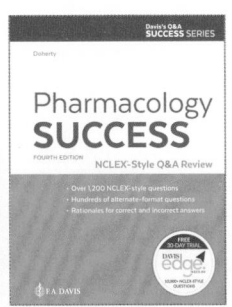 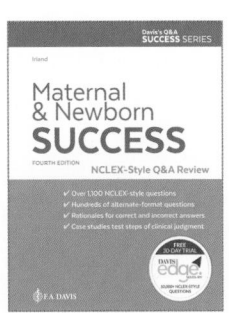 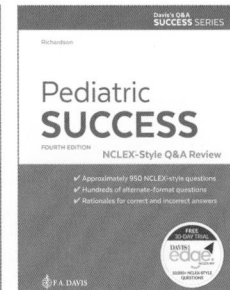
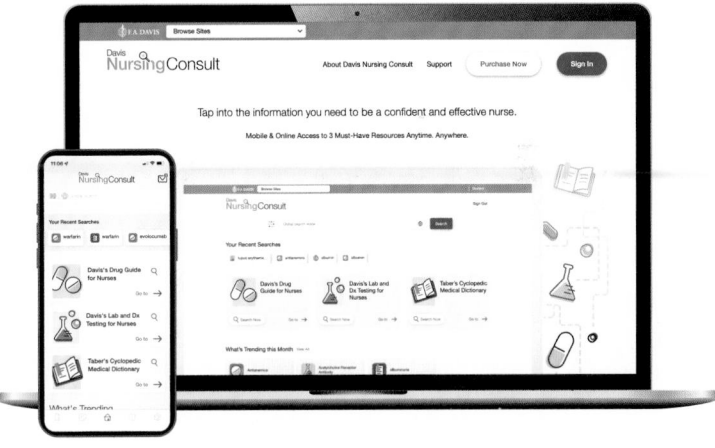

DAVIS ADVANTAGE for

Wilkinson's
FUNDAMENTALS
OF NURSING
Theory, Concepts, and Applications

FIFTH EDITION

Volume One

Leslie S. Treas, PhD, RN, CPNP-PC, NNP-BC

Karen L. Barnett, DNP, RN

Mable H. Smith, PhD, JD, MN, NEA-BC

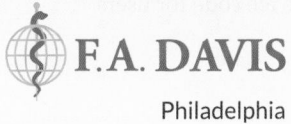

F.A. DAVIS

Philadelphia

F. A. Davis Company
1915 Arch Street
Philadelphia, PA 19103
www.fadavis.com

Printed in China

Last digit indicates print number: 10 9 8 7 6 5 4 3 2 1

Senior Acquisitions Editor: Jacalyn Sharp
Senior Content Project Manager: Amy M. Romano
Design and Illustrations Manager: Carolyn O'Brien

ISBN: 978-1-7196-4797-7

As new scientific information becomes available through basic and clinical research, recommended treatments and drug therapies undergo changes. The author(s) and publisher have done everything possible to make this book accurate, up to date, and in accord with accepted standards at the time of publication. The author(s), editors, and publisher are not responsible for errors or omissions or for consequences from application of the book, and make no warranty, expressed or implied, in regard to the contents of the book. Any practice described in this book should be applied by the reader in accordance with professional standards of care used in regard to the unique circumstances that may apply in each situation. The reader is advised always to check product information (package inserts) for changes and new information regarding dose and contraindications before administering any drug. Caution is especially urged when using new or infrequently ordered drugs.

Library of Congress Cataloging-in-Publication Data

Names: Treas, Leslie S., author. | Barnett, Karen L., author. | Smith,
  Mable H., author. | Wilkinson, Judith M., 1946- Davis advantage for
  fundamentals of nursing.
Title: Davis advantage for Wilkinson's fundamentals of nursing : theory,
  concepts, and applications / Leslie S. Treas, Karen L. Barnett, Mable H.
  Smith.
Other titles: Advantage for Wilkinson's fundamentals of nursing
Description: Fifth edition. | Philadelphia, PA : F.A. Davis Company, [2024]
  | Preceded by Davis advantage for fundamentals of nursing / Judith M.
  Wilkinson, Leslie S. Treas, Karen L. Barnett, Mable H. Smith. Fourth
  edition. [2020]. | Includes bibliographical references and index.
Identifiers: LCCN 2023015270 (print) | LCCN 2023015271 (ebook) | ISBN
  9781719647977 (v. 1 ; hardcover) | ISBN 9781719647984 (v. 2 ; paperback)
  | ISBN 9781719650540 (ebook)
Subjects: MESH: Nursing Process | Nursing Care | Nursing Theory
Classification: LCC RT49 (print) | LCC RT49 (ebook) | NLM WY 100.1 | DDC
  610.73—dc23/eng/20230516
LC record available at https://lccn.loc.gov/2023015270
LC ebook record available at https://lccn.loc.gov/2023015271

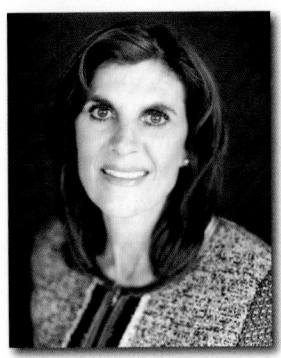

Leslie S. Treas, PhD, RN, CPNP-PC, NNP-BC

Dr. Leslie Treas, one of the founders and former vice president of research and development for Assessment Technologies Institute, LLC (ATI), demonstrated leadership and expertise in forecasting and directing the design and development of ATI product testing and educational product line in the formation and development of the company. In this role, Dr. Treas planned and implemented norming, test validation, and standard-setting studies to support data-driven product development, constructing tests with sound psychometric properties. Under her management, she produced a series of NCLEX-review books and nursing skills videos. She conducted clinical and educational research, publishing in peer-reviewed journals of health and education. Dr. Treas was also involved in the start-up of a continuing education company for nurses, physicians, and allied health professionals, serving as director of Education and Accreditation at Acamedic Institute, LLC.

Dr. Treas earned a BSN from Pennsylvania State University and an MSN degree with emphasis in maternal–child health at the University of Kansas. She obtained a PhD from the University of Kansas in the Educational Psychology and Research Department, with dual areas of study of testing and measurement and nursing education.

Her primary area of clinical expertise is the care of sick newborns in the neonatal intensive care unit (NICU) and labor and delivery settings in the clinical role of a neonatal nurse practitioner for 17 years. Dr. Treas obtained dual pediatric and neonatal nurse practitioner certifications at the Cleveland Metropolitan General Hospital, an affiliate of Case Western University.

Journal and textbook publications have featured clinical topics ranging from the fundamentals of nursing to the care of neonatal patients. Other publications are in education-based areas related to nursing licensure preparation and prediction, critical thinking, and others. Dr. Treas has also written articles geared toward new graduate readers, addressing contemporary issues involving role change, employment, and communication. Dr. Treas has presented at annual conferences for Sigma Theta Tau, the National Association of Associate Degree Nurses, the National Association of Neonatal Nurses, the American Association of Colleges of Nursing, the National Conference on Professional Nursing Education and Development, and the Association for the Advancement of Educational Research, to name a few. She served as an item writer for the National Certification Examination for Pediatric Nurse Practitioners and Nurses as well as the National Certification Corporation for Neonatal Nurse Practitioner Exam.

—*Leslie S. Treas*

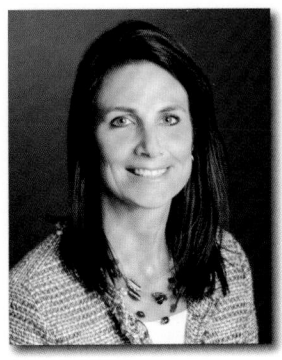

Karen L. Barnett, DNP, RN

Karen Barnett has been a nurse for more than 25 years and has held various positions in nursing, including the areas of patient care, administration, and education. Currently, Dr. Barnett serves as assistant dean of undergraduate studies for the College of Nursing and Health Sciences at the University of Massachusetts Dartmouth. Before that, she was the dean of health sciences at St. Vincent's College in Bridgeport, Connecticut. She has served as tenured faculty at Southern Connecticut State University and Norwalk Community College. Dr. Barnett's areas of clinical expertise are critical care, medical–surgical, and cardiac-telemetry. Dr. Barnett earned a BS in nursing from Southern Connecticut State University and an MSN degree with a focus in nursing administration from Sacred Heart University. She earned a DNP, Educational Leadership track, from the Francis Payne Bolton School of Nursing at Case Western Reserve University. Dr. Barnett is a member of the American Nurses Association, Massachusetts/Rhode Island League for Nursing, National League for Nursing, and Sigma Theta Tau International Nursing Honor Society. She was honored with a Nightingale Award for Excellence in Nursing in 2013. Research interests include student learning outcomes, simulation as a learning tool, and critical thinking/clinical judgment. Dr. Barnett has contributed to chapters in several textbooks and authored other ancillary materials, including test banks and concept maps.

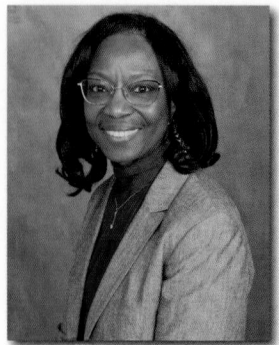

Mable H. Smith, PhD, JD, MN, NEA-BC

Dr. Mable Smith has an extensive background in academia, administration, and clinical practice. She is currently the senior vice president of academic affairs and provost of Arizona College of Nursing. Dr. Smith was also the dean of the College of Nursing and Public Health at South University and the founding dean of the Colleges of Nursing at Roseman University of Health Sciences, Nevada and Utah. She has been in the field of education for more than 25 years and has taught at all academic levels, including undergraduate courses in professional nursing, leadership and management, role transition, legal/ethical aspects of practice, healthcare policies, and adult health/critical care nursing. She has developed and taught graduate-level courses in theoretical foundations, research, healthcare finance, trends and issues, and the role of the nurse educator. She has published and presented in numerous arenas on legal and ethical issues in nursing education and in nursing/healthcare. Her publications have appeared in leading refereed journals, and she authored the book *The Legal, Professional, and Ethical Dimensions of Education in Nursing*, currently in its second edition.

In addition to the academic environment, Dr. Smith is a colonel in the U.S. Air Force Reserves. She is an Individual Mobilization Augmentee (IMA) to the Surgeon General Chair, Air University, at Maxwell Air Force Base, Alabama.

Dr. Smith earned a BSN from Florida State University (FSU) and an MN from Emory University, with an emphasis in education. She obtained a PhD in higher education administration and a JD from FSU. Dr. Smith has served on the faculties of Florida A&M University, Old Dominion University, and the University of South Mississippi. Her primary area of clinical expertise is adult health/medical–surgical nursing. Dr. Smith is a member of the American Nurses Association, the Georgia Nurses Association, and the American Association of Nurse Attorneys. She was honored by the National Association of Women Business Owners as a Woman of Distinction for her contributions to the education field in southern Nevada and was named a Healthcare Headliner by *In Business Las Vegas*, one of southern Nevada's premier business publications. She is also a Robert Wood Johnson Executive Nurse Fellow Alumna.

Dedication

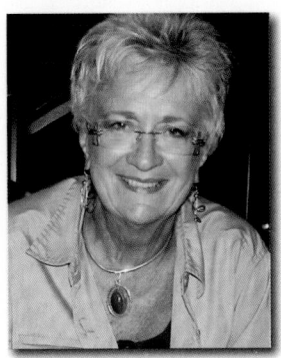

Judith M. Wilkinson, PhD, ARNP

This book is dedicated to Dr. Judith Wilkinson, our most respected and endeared mentor, teacher, leader, colleague, role model, and friend. It was her inspiration and tireless efforts that laid the foundation for the first edition of the textbook and subsequent editions. As an experienced nurse educator, Judith understood what kind of tools educators need to teach in this ever-changing world. And with keen insight into how students of today learn best, she committed to creating this book using a "say it direct, say it clear, say it well" approach. At the same time, Judith's sentinel work with the nursing process focused the content on the application of knowledge and the development of critical-thinking skills.

With a genuine love for students and educators, Judith truly exemplifies to learners and educators alike what it means to be a "thinking, doing, and caring nurse." In addition to attending to all details, great and small, she also had a way of adding levity to this arduous work. Perhaps the strongest expression of Judith's commitment to perfection, precision, and excellence is her signature line, "Good is the enemy of great." It was our pleasure and our deepest honor to work with one of today's great thinkers, Dr. Judith Wilkinson.

We dedicate this book to:

■ Creative, dedicated nurse educators, who give so much of themselves to help prepare their students to provide quality care across the full spectrum of nursing

■ Nursing students, as they strive to acquire the knowledge, skills, and attitudes that they must transfer to their imminent practice

■ Practicing nurses, who struggle with daily realities to promote and maintain health and to provide comfort and care during illness and at the end of life

The health of the nation depends on all of us.

—Leslie S. Treas

Preface

We carefully chose the word *fundamentals* for the title of this text because it is truly that: the foundation for all that follows. This basic content teaches essential functions that nurses will use throughout their careers, and in that sense, we believe it is of central importance. It is—or should be—the most important course students take. We want them to say, "Everything I need to know, I learned in fundamentals—all I needed to know about how to think, what to do, and how to be as a nurse" (at least at a basic level). Moreover, in the subtitles of both volumes, *theory, concepts, application, thinking, doing,* and *caring* reflect our belief that excellent nursing requires a mix of clinical judgment, concern, and kindness. Even so, the skillful performance of tasks, coupled with nursing wisdom and caring, is essential to fulfillment of the nursing role.

The thoroughly revised and updated fifth edition preserves the same open, user-friendly, easy-to-read style that students have been telling us they love.

ORGANIZATION

We have organized the learning package into two volumes to make it easier for on-the-go students to have at hand the material they need in either the classroom or the clinical setting. Volume 1 contains all the theoretical and conceptual material (the why behind the what) typically present in a fundamentals text, and it is primarily, but not exclusively, used in classroom teaching. Volume 2 is designed primarily, but not exclusively, for use in the skills laboratory and clinical setting. It contains nursing procedures and learning activities to promote critical thinking and clinical judgment in the application of Volume 1 content.

Chapters are self-contained, with plenty of cross-references, so that educators and students can use them in any order that best fits their needs. The cross-references assist them in seeing the relationships between Volumes 1 and 2 and among the chapters, as well as in navigating easily between the two volumes.

Within-Chapter Organization—Content within each chapter is generally organized into two major sections: Theoretical Knowledge (Knowing Why) and Practical Knowledge (Knowing How). There is some overlap in these concepts because the two types of knowledge are interdependent. We have made this general distinction because many nursing programs integrate knowledge from prerequisite classes into theoretical knowledge

to explain the rationale for nursing actions and activities (practical knowledge). The distinction also affords more flexibility in teaching fundamentals. For example, it is useful to educators who believe students are more motivated when they first present the concrete (practical knowledge) and then the conceptual material (theoretical knowledge); it is equally useful for those who teach from the theoretical to the practical.

Procedures (Nursing Skills) and Clinical Insights—Procedures are presented in Volume 2, primarily: (1) so that they do not interrupt the logical flow of content when the student is studying the learning materials, (2) so that they can be easily located when the student is looking for a particular procedure, and (3) so that students will not usually need to carry Volume 2 to classes that are intended primarily for theoretical and conceptual instruction and information.

CLINICAL JUDGMENT

It will come as no surprise to you that the National Council of State Boards of Nursing (NCSBN) Clinical Judgment Measurement Model (CJMM) figures prominently in NCLEX testing. Clinical judgment is an essential competency for registered nurses that enables them to provide safe, effective nursing care. It also enables them to apply a systematic process (identify and solve problems), synthesize knowledge and past experience, and sometimes reason intuitively to make decisions that support quality care and safety.

We conceptualize the more abstract **critical-thinking** and **clinical reasoning** processes as the foundation for implementing the more concrete and action-oriented **nursing process** and **clinical judgment** processes. Each of those four broad concepts comprises several discrete skills, identified in different ways by different authors. Moreover, the four processes "overlap"—that is, they are used simultaneously. For example, *cue recognition* is an important part of both the nursing process and clinical judgment, and *problem identification and problem-solving* require critical thinking. As you can see, teaching or fostering clinical judgment is a complex undertaking because it requires a variety of skills and processes. As you also know, a complex skill such as clinical judgment cannot be taught as a whole, especially to novices. We must break it down into smaller chunks (e.g., cue recognition, problem identification, choosing evidence-based interventions), using logic to identify strengths and weaknesses of alternative solutions.

- The development of **clinical judgment** depends on deep thinking that builds on theoretical nursing knowledge, practical nursing knowledge, self-knowledge, and ethical knowledge. You may recognize these concepts in our **full-spectrum nursing model.**
- **The goals of such deep thinking and knowledge** are to observe and assess presenting situations, identify a prioritized client problem, and generate the best possible evidence-based solutions to deliver safe client care. You may recognize those activities as aspects of the **nursing process** as well as of the **CJMM.**

You can be assured that *Fundamentals of Nursing* will support your students in attaining the essential knowledge and thinking skills they need to begin developing clinical judgment. The NCSBN describes **clinical judgment** as the observed outcome of two unobserved mental processes, **critical thinking** and **decision making.** Others describe **clinical judgment** as the observed outcome of two underlying thinking processes: **critical thinking** and **problem-solving.** Throughout this text, students develop thinking skills that are used for the broader processes of critical thinking, problem-solving, clinical decision making, and clinical judgment. Almost every activity and theme in this textbook provides a small building block for **clinical reasoning** and **clinical judgment.** Excellent educators will nurture students' **clinical judgment** as they guide them through the activities we have provided.

FEATURES

The chapters have numerous pedagogical features to facilitate student learning:

- *Interactive Approach*—The text is written in an engaging style that speaks directly to the student. Knowledge checks and critical-thinking questions are integrated throughout the content to break chapters up into small, manageable segments and guide students' development of clinical judgment. Skill development is also guided by the clinical reasoning and clinical judgment exercises in each chapter and in other activities on Davis Advantage.
- *Learning Outcomes and Main Points in the Chapter*— These focus the student's study and provide repetition to facilitate retention of material.
- *Example Client Conditions*—These are graphic-driven, content-rich examples of client conditions that are tied to key concepts within the chapter. The need-to-know information is attractively displayed, with an easy-to-use and easy-to-remember format.
- *Knowledge Checks*—These questions encourage students to test their recall of a section of content

immediately after they read it. Answers are provided on Davis Advantage.

- *Clinical Judgment Activities*—Thought-provoking questions in both volumes facilitate critical thinking and clinical reasoning, building blocks for clinical judgment. They also allow the student to synthesize content and explore personal beliefs, supporting self-knowledge. Suggested responses are found on Davis Advantage.
- *Key Concept Lists and Concept Maps*—In the chapter opener, we have listed the key concepts to help students begin to use concepts to organize content in their memory. An explanation of the key concepts (About the Key Concepts) is found at the beginning of the Theoretical Knowledge section. A Concept Map on Davis Advantage illustrates the relationships among the key concepts and subconcepts in each chapter.
- *Meet Your Patient*—This chapter-opening feature in Volume 1 introduces one or more patients, as you might see in "real-life" nursing. The scenario is used throughout the chapter to illustrate theoretical points and make the content come alive. These patients are often followed in the clinical reasoning and clinical judgment activities in Volume 2, as well. This facilitates contextualizing information rather than learning facts in isolation.
- *More Key Points*—We know students skim the content, so we have made visible the many points we want to be certain they see and remember.
- *More Bullet Lists*—These help students organize data in memory, as well as scan the content for review.
- *Care Plans*—These are found in Volume 1 and on Davis Advantage. They are based on case studies and allow students to see the nursing process in action. Evidence-based rationales support interventions.
- *Care Maps*—For each care plan, a care map allows visual learners to grasp the connection between the phases of the nursing process by illustrating an alternative method of care planning.
- *Highlights of Procedures Boxes*—These features in Volume 1 contain the highlights of all chapter procedures presented in Volume 2. These boxes serve as a reference when studying the practical knowledge content in Volume 1 and may also be used as a quick review just before performing a procedure in the clinical area.
- *Caring for the Williams Family*—This ongoing case study begins every chapter of Volume 2. It allows students to become familiar with a single family and experience the continuity of care they may encounter in outpatient settings. As with all exercises in the two volumes, suggested responses are provided on Davis Advantage. This feature supports clinical judgment, for example, by providing context and opportunities for problem identification and the use of logic to identify the strengths and weaknesses of alternative solutions.

- *Clinical Judgment Section: Applying the Full-Spectrum Nursing Model*—In Volume 2, these clinically based exercises help students to safely apply their clinical reasoning and judgment skills to chapter content and, at the same time, reinforce the full-spectrum model concepts of thinking, doing, and caring introduced in Volume 1 and integrated throughout the learning package.
- *Critical Thinking and Clinical Judgment*—This set of clinically based exercises (in Volume 2) guides students to safely practice critical thinking in preparation for exercising clinical judgment in the clinical area. Frequently, these clinical exercises make use of material related to the Meet Your Patient scenario in Volume 1, thereby reinforcing the application and retention of content.
- *Safe, Effective Nursing Care Competencies*—These competencies for nurses focus on providing safe, effective patient and family care. To illustrate practical knowledge, many of the chapters have a Safe, Effective Nursing Care box, providing an example of how a competency is expressed in practice.
- *Social Determinants of Health*—As the *Future of Nursing 2020-2030: Charting a Path to Achieve Health Equity* points out, nurses are well prepared to address Social Determinants of Health (SDoH) in a variety of roles and across settings (National Academies of Sciences, Engineering, and Medicine [NASEM], 2021). Helping nursing students understand that conditions in which people are born, grow, live, work, and age, combine together to affect the health of individuals and communities. Nursing students can address SDoH starting with the first step of the nursing process, assessment, and continue to utilize their knowledge and skills throughout the nursing process to reduce the impact of SDOH on health outcomes.
- *Thinking About the Procedure*—These procedures in Volume 2 include a cross-reference to the Davis's Nursing Skills Videos Web site on FADavis.com for exercises that require students to watch the associated Davis's Nursing Skills Videos to answer the questions. Questions and suggested responses are provided on FADavis.com.
- *What If . . .*—Volume 2 procedures include a section to aid students in knowing what to do in special situations that require decisions during a procedure. What If features are placed after the procedure steps so that they will not distract from the steps while the student learns the procedure. This feature is valuable in developing clinical judgment.
- *Toward Evidenced-Based Practice Boxes*—In every chapter, we describe research related to the chapter topic and pose critical-thinking exercises for students to examine these findings. The concept of evidence-based practice is introduced in Chapter 3 (The Steps of the Nursing Process), further explained in Chapter 4 (Evidence-Based Practice: Theory & Research), and appears in other chapters as well.
- *Diagnostic Testing Boxes*—These are found in Volume 2 in applicable chapters. We believe it is more meaningful to place the diagnostic test information near the related content rather than in an isolated chapter. If students need a more comprehensive reference, we recommend a diagnostic testing book.
- *Knowledge Maps*—These are maps showing the relationships among the various topics covered in the chapter and can be found on Davis Advantage for each chapter.
- *Concept Maps*—These visually demonstrate the relationship among chapter key concepts and subconcepts and are found at the end of each chapter in the book. This feature is especially useful to visual learners.
- *PICOT Boxes*—We have added this feature to most chapters to facilitate the skill of inquiry, especially as it relates to evidence-based practice.
- *End-of-Chapter Box*—This is another navigation tool in Volume 1: a list of features to remind students and help them benefit from using Davis Advantage. In Volume 2, the box is in the chapter opener.

THEMES

The following themes are stressed throughout—some of them in every chapter:

- *Clinical Judgment, Critical Thinking, Clinical Reasoning, and the Full-Spectrum Model of Nursing.* In addition to the critical-thinking questions and exercises integrated throughout every chapter in Volumes 1 and 2, we promote critical thinking and clinical judgment in various ways, often using an inductive manner, such as by posing a question (e.g., "What would happen if . . .?"). **The full-spectrum model of nursing** (presented in Chapter 2) is a comprehensive approach to care that uses critical thinking in all aspects of care. Because students cannot focus on everything at once, different model parts are stressed at different times. Sometimes the discussion asks, "What theoretical knowledge do you need to . . .?" In other instances, the question posed might be, "What biases do you have that might interfere with . . .?" These types of questions help frame the problem or situation so that students can begin to make decisions and develop clinical judgment.
- *Nursing Process.* The nursing process is a common framework for nursing thinking and is a type of problem-solving identified with clinical judgment. Chapter 2 explains the relationships among the nursing process, critical thinking, clinical reasoning, and clinical judgment. Chapter 3 is a comprehensive presentation of the nursing process, which is presented as multifaceted rather than linear. The Practical Knowledge sections of Volume 1 are organized according to the phases of the clinical judgment model and nursing process; the procedures in Volume 2 all have assessment and evaluation components.

- **Safety.** Safety is a central focus in nursing and health-care. To emphasize and help students remember important aspects of safe care, we have key safety points marked with shading and an icon to make them visible and memorable. This book also includes an entire chapter on safety, Chapter 21, Promoting Safety.

- **Caring.** Caring is an important dimension of nursing that matters to patients and families. The iCare feature offers concrete ways that nurses can show compassion in patient care. Additionally, caring passages in the text are highlighted with an icon to call attention to the integration of caring into nursing practice. Caring is introduced in Chapter 1 with historical examples of nursing as a caring profession. Chapter 4 describes the important caring theories. All full-spectrum nursing model features offer questions involving caring.

- **Inquiry and Evidence-Based Practice.** The concept of evidence-based practice is introduced in Chapter 3 (The Steps of the Nursing Process), further explained in Chapter 4 (Evidence-Based Practice: Theory & Research), and mentioned frequently in other chapters as well. The following boxes are examples:

- **Gerontology.** To allow for an in-depth discussion of aging and gerontology, provided by an expert on this topic, Chapter 7 is entirely devoted to the older adult (e.g., developmental stage, assessments, and interventions). Throughout the book, you will find content specific to older adults is marked with a distinctive icon and shading. You will also find that many features and exercises feature an older adult as the patient.

- **Diversity and Multiculturism.** Multiculturalism is highlighted throughout the text in clinical scenarios, illustrations, and theoretical discussions. Chapter 12 focuses on providing care to patients in multicultural healthcare environments, with an emphasis on culturally sensitive nursing care. The Caring for the Williams feature, an ongoing case study throughout Volume 2, features an extended family; culturally based variations are described in procedures, as applicable.

- **Standardized Nursing Language.** Because consistent terminology is important for electronic health records, this book includes a thorough discussion of nursing taxonomies (e.g., Clinical Care Classification, NANDA-I, etc.) in the nursing process and other chapters. Nursing Outcomes Classification (NOC) outcomes and Nursing Interventions Classification (NIC) interventions are included in clinical chapters in Volume 1.

- **Wellness.** Many examples and scenarios in this text refer to people who are not ill. Chapter 8 emphasizes health and the nurse's role in health promotion.

- **Spirituality.** Chapter 13 is one of the most extensive presentations of spiritual care available in a fundamentals text. Spirituality is also integrated within various chapters in scenarios, examples, and exercises.

- **Documentation.** All chapters include reference to documentation, where relevant. The procedures in Volume 2 all have guidelines for and examples of how to document the procedure. Chapter 17 contains a thorough presentation of documentation and reporting as the essential tool for professional communication of patient care.

- **Delegation.** Delegation is introduced early in the book and is a thread in most Volume 1 chapters. Chapter 40, Leading & Managing, presents a more detailed discussion of delegation. In Volume 2, all procedures have guidelines for delegating.

- **American Nurses Association (ANA) Standards.** Nursing and other healthcare standards (e.g., The Joint Commission, Medicare) are frequently referenced. We provide links to pertinent Web sites so that students can keep up with changes to standards.

- **Life Span/Developmental Stages.** Chapter 6 is entirely devoted to growth and development, from conception through middle age; Chapter 7 thoroughly discusses the life-span considerations of older adults. The Theoretical Knowledge section in most chapters devotes a portion to the discussion of the effects of the life span on the chapter topic. In Volume 2, the procedures include variations for children and older adults.

- **Ethics.** In addition to the comprehensive treatment in Chapter 5, ethical knowledge is an aspect of our full-spectrum nursing model. As such, many of the critical-thinking exercises ask students to grapple with ethical issues. In Volume 2, good examples are found in Chapter 3 and in the Applying the Full-Spectrum Nursing Model feature in every chapter. Ethical knowledge is one type of nursing knowledge and is therefore important in making clinical judgments.

- **Legal Issues.** Chapter 39 is devoted to legal issues that nurses face in their practice. Legal issues are integrated into many other chapters as well (e.g., licensing in Chapter 1; end-of-life legal considerations in Chapter 14).

- **Nursing Informatics.** Chapter 38 is an excellent introduction to nursing informatics. Standardized language and electronic care planning and documentation are interspersed throughout the book. We also emphasize electronic documentation in Chapter 17 and in our illustrations for documenting some procedures in Volume 2. We further encourage the use of technology by providing students with links to other Web sites related to the chapter topic.

- **Community and Home Health Nursing.** Chapter 37 is devoted exclusively to these topics. In other chapters, clinical scenarios and examples involve nurses in these settings. The procedures in Volume 2 have sections for adapting skills to home care, where applicable. Volume 1 includes special feature boxes:
  - **Home Care Boxes**—These provide guidelines for safely modifying care for delivery in the home.
  - **Teaching: Self-Care Boxes**—Teaching: Self-Care boxes appear throughout Volume 1. They are similar to the

traditional "teaching boxes" but focus on equipping patients to perform self-care.

- **Complementary Therapies.** Nursing is presented as holistic throughout. Several chapters in Volume 1 (e.g., Chapter 12, Caring in Multicultural Healthcare Environments) contain material related to this topic. Others present research concerning a particular complementary therapy as one form of holistic healthcare.
- **Contemporary Issues.** In Chapter 20, we include extensive information about bioterrorism, multi-drug-resistant organisms, emerging infectious diseases, and healthcare-related infections. These topics are also included in Chapter 37 in relation to community nursing, as well as in the Meet Your Nurse Role Model scenario in the informatics chapter. The safety chapter includes ways to assess for and cope with violence in the healthcare setting.

THE TEXT AS A RESPONSE TO CHANGE

This learning package was developed to address the needs of today's nursing students and in response to the following changes in nursing education and practice.

Changes in Students

- **Nontraditional Students.** Students range from traditional, younger students just out of high school to older, second-career students. Many have responsibilities that compete with the time and attention needed for classes and studying. To address this change, we have followed three principles of adult learning: that learning must be relevant, efficient, and meaningful to the person.
  - *Efficiency:* Volume 1 is intended for classroom use, whereas Volume 2 is for clinical use.
  - *Technology:* Learning activities on Davis Advantage deliver enhancements to the printed text, developed with the knowledge that highly motivated students will welcome the chance to use technologies to maximize their learning.
  - *Meaningfulness/Relevance:* Because learning improves when content is meaningful to the learner, each chapter opens with a patient scenario or story of a practicing nurse. This story is woven throughout the chapter to provide context for factual information and to show how concepts are applied and how nurses think.
  - *Practical Application:* Adults learn and retain information best when the content is important and relevant to real-life circumstances. This book uses a case study, called *Caring for the Williams Family,* in every chapter of Volume 2; this feature provides practical clinical scenarios and questions for learners so that they can apply chapter concepts to common clinical situations.
- **Variety in Learning Styles.** Students learn in different ways. To assist visual learners, we have used

more than 1,400 photos and many diagrams, concept maps, care maps, and graphic displays for the Example Client Conditions. To teach psychomotor skills, we have—in addition to step-by-step procedures—skills videos and checklists that students can print out for practicing procedures or for educators to use in evaluations.

- **Reading Comprehension.** Because the learners of today take in information in ways that are less focused on reading long passages of text, we addressed this change by writing in an informal style, addressing the student directly ("you will . . ."). With this adaptation of the content to be more inviting and user-friendly, learners have a better opportunity to be successful in reading and retaining important information. Our motto is to say what's important, say it clearly, and say it so that it's memorable. For terms that are unfamiliar to students, we define their first use in each chapter.
- **The Technology Generation.** The current generations of students are accustomed to using technology and multitasking. To hold their attention, in addition to our easy-to-read style, we present information in an interactive manner and in relatively short segments interspersed with review questions and critical-thinking questions. For this same reason, the text frequently directs students to find related information on Davis Advantage and on the Internet.

The e-Book of *Wilkinson's Fundamentals of Nursing* lets students access their textbook from wherever they have Internet access without needing to lug around heavy books. Also available from the same authors is a set of skills videos that can be purchased on FADavis.com.

Changes in Nursing Curricula

- **Concept-based learning is emphasized.** Even if a curriculum is not entirely concept based, there is a trend toward teaching and learning in a more concept-based manner. We believe that all fundamentals books are, by nature, concept based. That is, each chapter consists of the explication of one or two basic concepts. To assist educators and students in adopting a more concept-based approach, in each chapter, we have listed the key concepts, included an explanation of their use, made use of Example Client Conditions graphics (e.g., Urinary Retention in Chapter 25), and added a Concept Map to illustrate the relationships among the key concepts and subconcepts in the chapter. These are available in the Student Resources on Davis Advantage.
- **Educators often say they do not have enough time to "cover the content."** A concept-based approach is one way to limit the amount of content that must be presented. See the preceding discussion. Another way to address this problem is to not reteach material students have had in other classes. We provide, for example, just enough anatomy and physiology

(A&P) in each chapter to aid students who need to review A&P or who are taking A&P concurrently with nursing courses. You should not need to reteach it in class.

- **Understanding and retention continue to be a problem.** To aid in retention, we have interspersed knowledge checks and critical-thinking questions throughout Volume 1 to allow students to check and reinforce their recall and understanding of the content as they progress through the chapters. Recognizing that repetition aids retention, we provide Learning Outcomes at the beginning of each chapter in Volume 1. In addition, chapters in Volume 2 include a list titled *What Are the Main Points in This Chapter?* and a full-page Knowledge Map of the chapter content.

- **Some curricula have de-emphasized mental health.** Mental health may be taught in other clinical areas (e.g., medical–surgical), without a separate mental health course in the curriculum. In response to pleas from educators, we include expanded mental health content and tools for psychosocial assessment. In addition to the usual concepts of self-concept and self-esteem, Chapter 10 includes basic assessments and interventions for client conditions pertaining to anxiety and depression, which students will commonly encounter in all areas, not just on mental health units. In Chapter 15, the communication chapter, we have practical content pertaining to the nurse–patient relationship and communication techniques that mental health professionals find so essential. Chapter 9, Stress & Adaptation, includes information about defense mechanisms.

- **The curriculum does not include separate pharmacology, nutrition, ethics, nursing process, or leadership courses.** Because all nurses need grounding in these topics, we have provided extensive coverage of them. The medications chapter provides in-depth pharmacology information. Chapter 24, Nutrition, provides a foundational understanding of patients' nutritional needs. Chapter 40 is a thorough presentation of leadership. Chapter 5 is a comprehensive look at nursing ethics. We have, arguably, the most useful and thorough presentation of the nursing process available in a fundamentals text. These chapters, as well as most others, will be a valuable reference for students when they take other clinical nursing courses.

Changes in Nursing and Healthcare

- *The nursing role is increasingly complex, requiring management, decision-making, delegation, and supervision skills early in the career.*
  To address this change, the critical-thinking and clinical decision-making exercises, as well as the Williams feature, help students to develop clinical judgment. Delegation is presented early on,
in the nursing process chapter, and emphasized in the rest of the chapters in Volume 1, as applicable. Each clinical procedure in Volume 2 contains a section on delegation.

- *Healthcare has moved increasingly from the hospital to the home and community.*
  To address this change, Chapter 1 discusses the history of nursing and the contemporary healthcare delivery system. In addition, Chapter 38 discusses community and home nursing, and those concepts are integrated throughout Volume 1 (e.g., *Healthy People 2030* goals are cited where relevant). The procedures in Volume 2 include home care adaptations, as well as patient-teaching points that enable patients and caregivers to assume more responsibility for self-care.

- *Nurses need to be critical thinkers and lifelong learners.*
  To address this change, the text is organized around a model of full-spectrum nursing, a comprehensive approach to care that uses critical thinking in all aspects of care. The model of nurses' thinking, doing, and caring is reinforced in each chapter of Volume 2 in the feature Applying the Full-Spectrum Nursing Model. Critical thinking is integrated throughout both volumes of the text, both in discussion and in the Think Like a Nurse: Clinical Judgment in Action exercises (in Volume 1). Discussion of this model follows.

THE FULL-SPECTRUM MODEL OF NURSING

We believe that nursing knowledge is a fusion of theoretical knowledge, practical knowledge, self-knowledge, and ethical knowledge. To function at the highest level, nurses use critical thinking and the nursing process to blend thinking and doing to put caring into action. We refer to this blend as **full-spectrum nursing.** We have organized our learning package to reflect this philosophy. This model includes the major concepts of thinking, doing, caring, patient situation, and patient outcomes. It is presented in Chapter 2 and referred to and used throughout the text. The concepts in the full-spectrum nursing model support concepts in the CJMM of the NCSBN.

THE TEACHING AND LEARNING PACKAGE

This is a well-integrated and cross-referenced package containing a two-volume text and student and instructor resources provided on Davis Advantage. Although both volumes can be used in either the classroom or clinical settings, Volume 1 will usually be used in the classroom setting, whereas Volume 2 will usually be used in the clinical setting or learning laboratory. Also available from the same authors, for purchase to expand the learning package, are a comprehensive set of skills videos and a small *Pocket Nursing Skills* book (a handy review of skills to be used in the clinical setting).

Davis Advantage

How students learn is evolving. In this digital age, learners take in information in various ways. Online, information is offered in bite-sized, dynamic, and memorable chunks.

To meet the needs of today's learners, the way educators teach is also evolving. Classroom time is valuable for active learning. This approach makes students responsible for the key concepts, allowing educators to focus on clinical application. Relying on the textbook alone to support an active classroom leaves a gap. *Davis Advantage* fills that gap with the following resources:

- **A Strong Core Textbook** that provides the foundation of knowledge that today's nursing students need to pass the NCLEX and enter practice prepared for success.
- **An Online Solution** that provides resources for each step of the learning cycle: learn, apply, assess.
  - **Personalized Learning** assignments are the core of the product and are designed to prepare students for classroom (live or online) discussion. They provide directed learning based on needs. After completing text reading assignments, students take a preassessment for each *topic.* Their results feed into their *Personalized Learning Plan.* If students do not pass the preassessment, they are required to complete further work within the topic: watch an animated mini-lecture, work through an activity, and take the postassessment.

    The personalized learning content is designed to connect students with the foundational information about a given topic or concept. It provides the gateway to helping make the content accessible to all students and complements different learning styles.
  - **Clinical Judgment** assignments are case based and build off key Personalized Learning Plan topics. These cases help students develop clinical judgment skills through exploratory learning. Students will link their knowledge base (developed through the text and personalized learning) to new data and patient situations. Cases include dynamic charts that expand as the case progresses and use complex question types that require students to analyze data, synthesize conclusions, and make judgments. Each case will end with comprehensive feedback, which provides detailed rationales for the correct and incorrect answers.
  - **Quizzing** assignments build off Personalized Learning Plan topics (and are included for every topic) and help assess students' understanding of the broader scope and increased depth of that topic. The quizzes use NCLEX-style questions to assess understanding and synthesis of content. Quiz results include comprehensive feedback for correct and incorrect answers to help students understand why their answer choices were right or wrong.
- **Online Instructor Resources** create a dynamic learning experience that relies heavily on interactive participation and is tailored to students' needs. Results from the postassessments are available to faculty, in aggregate or by student, and inform a **Personalized Teaching Plan** that faculty can use to deliver a targeted classroom experience. Faculty will know students' strengths and weaknesses before they come to class and can spend class time focusing on where students are struggling. Suggested in-class activities are provided to help create an interactive, hands-on learning environment that helps students connect more deeply with the content. NCLEX-style questions from the **Instructor Test Bank** and **PowerPoint slides** that correspond to the textbook chapters are referenced in the Personalized Teaching Plans. Also included are Next Generation NCLEX (NGN)-style questions to help familiarize students with the alternative style questions on the NGN.

The Textbook

Volume 1

Volume 1 contains all the theoretical and conceptual material typically present in a fundamentals text, presented in a clinically focused, user-friendly manner and incorporating many examples. This presentation allows students to see how the content will be useful to them. The nursing process is used as the model to organize the Practical Knowledge section in most chapters.

Unit 1 focuses on how nurses think. It begins by showing how nursing history relates to our present healthcare system. Chapter 2 is Clinical Judgment and includes a thorough discussion of NCSBN's CJMM. This unit prepares students to follow the organization of subsequent chapters and provides the thinking tools and processes they need to apply the content of the other chapters. Chapter 4 contains an overview of the processes of theory building, nursing research, and evidence-based practice as they relate to the nurse in practice. Chapter 5 provides in-depth coverage of ethics and values that nurses encounter in practice.

Unit 2 is about the internal and external factors that affect an individual's health (e.g., family, culture, spirituality, and life stage). Internal factors are personal beliefs or attributes that influence how the client views health, healthcare, and nursing. Chapter 8 describes the health–illness–wellness continuum in an experiential way, encouraging self-knowledge, personal growth, and effective learning of that content.

Unit 3 examines essential nursing interventions. We consider these skills "essential" because nurses use some or all of these skills in *all* areas of nursing, regardless of setting or patient diagnosis. The unit begins with documentation and includes communication, teaching, taking vital signs, health assessment, asepsis, safety, hygiene, and medication administration.

Unit 4 concentrates on nursing care that supports physiological function. We examine broad categories of physiological function (e.g., nutrition, elimination, oxygenation) and discuss related nursing care. Most of these chapters make use of Example Client Conditions to help students focus on concept-based learning and the importance of nursing problems and interventions.

Unit 5 looks at the context of nurses' work. This includes chapters covering community and home care, as well as the legal context for nursing work. We believe that a fundamentals book, overall, provides all concepts needed for a holistic view of the patient—just scan our chapter titles to see what we mean by that. This unit also explores diverse nursing functions, such as ways nurses lead, advocate, and manage the many challenges in the healthcare setting. We introduce the use of technology and informatics in a more thorough introduction to informatics than you will usually find in a fundamentals text.

Volume 2

Volume 2 is designed primarily, but not exclusively, for use in the skills laboratory and clinical setting. Critical-thinking and clinical judgment activities require students to use their thinking skills and the clinical judgment model to apply theoretical knowledge and specific concepts to specific patient situations. Clinical procedures, assessment tools, clinical forms, diagnostic testing information, and standardized language tables make up the Practical Knowledge sections. Throughout Volume 2, students have access to a simulated experience known as *Caring for the Williams Family,* an ongoing case study through which they learn about the nursing role, the healthcare system, and the real-world application of the content in Volume 1.

Contributors for this Edition

Dawn Carson, MSN, CRNP, CWOCN, NHA
Co-Director of LaSalle University WOCN Education Program
Philadelphia, Pennsylvania
Skin Integrity & Wound Healing chapter

Megan Treas Clary, BSN, RN, FNE
Forensic Nursing Services Coordinator—Emergency
    Department
Hutchinson Regional Medical Center
Maternal–Fetal Transport
Wesley Medical Center
Wichita, Kansas
Communicating & Therapeutic Relationships chapter

Teri Rada, NMD, MSN-Ed, RN
Arizona College of Nursing
Director of Curriculum and Instruction
Phoenix, Arizona
Interprofessional Partnerships: Documenting & Reporting chapter

Reviewers for this Edition

Lyn Behnke, DNP, FNP-BC, PMHNPBC, CAFCI, CHFN
Assistant Professor of Nursing
University of Michigan–Flint
Tawas City, Michigan

Dawn Carson, MSN, CRNP, CWOCN, NHA
Co-Director of LaSalle University WOCN Education Program
LaSalle University
Philadelphia, Pennsylvania

Victoria Haynes, DNP, APRN, PMHNP-BC, FNP-C
Tenured Professor of Nursing
Coordinator of Diversity & Cultural Competency
MidAmerica Nazarene University
Olathe, Kansas

Kesa Herlihy, PhD, RN, CNE
Clinical Associate Professor
University of Kansas School of Nursing
Kansas City, Kansas

Kim Pickett, PhD, FNP-BC, BC-ADM
Assistant Professor
Associate for Research on Health Disparities
Clemson University
Greenville, South Carolina

Hiba Whebe-Alamah, PhD, RN, FNP-BC, CTN-A, FAAN, FTNSS
Professor
University of Michigan–Flint
Flint, Michigan

Contributors to Previous Editions

The following people contributed material that was used in creating this learning package. We are grateful for their assistance.

Julia Aucoin, RN, DNS, BC, CNE
Clinical consultant and literature reviews

Karen Barnett, DNP, RN
Concept Maps

Linda Blazovich, RN, MSN
Procedure checklists

Diane Bligh, RN, MS, CNS
Knowledge Maps, Instructor's Guide, Lecture Outlines, Care Planning Exercises

Diane Breckenridge, RN, PhD, MSN
Assessment and Diagnosis chapter content

Stephanie Scovill Bronsky, RN, MSN-Ed
PICOT feature

Patricia-Ann Calarco, RN, MSN
Item writer, teacher test bank

Dr. Lindsey Carlson, MSN, FNP-BC
Skin Integrity & Wound Healing chapter

Lu Ann Connor, RN, BSN, MBA
Community & Home Health Nursing chapter

Leanne Cowin, RN, PhD
Literature searches

Lisa Culliton, MSN, CPN
Literature searches

Debbie Ellison, RN, MSN
Nursing care plans; oxygenation procedures

Garrett Fardon
Clerical assistance

Rebecca Flynn, RN, APRN, CPNP-PC
Skin Integrity & Wound Healing chapter

Mary Gant, APN, ACNS-BC, RRT
Oxygenation procedures

Susan J. Garbutt, DNP, RN, CIC, CNE
Promoting Asepsis & Preventing Infection chapter

Susan Goncalves, PhD, DNP, MS, RN-BC
iCare feature

Kathie Hayes, DNSc
Test bank items

Tracey Hopkins, RN, BSN
QSEN boxes

Dr. Cherie Howk, PhD, FNP-BC
Sexual Health chapter

Kia Skrine Jeffers, PhD, RN, PHN
Caring in Multicultural Health Environments chapter

Kathleen C. Jones, RN, MSN
Wounds & Skin Integrity chapter

Patricia A. Koral, RN, MSN, CNE
QSEN feature

Karen LoCascio, RN-BC, MSN
Urinary Elimination chapter

Lisa Lyons, RN, BSN
Procedures for sensory perception, pain management, activity and exercise, and skin integrity chapters

Elaine F. Martin, PhD, RNC, FNP, PNP
Active Caring: Patient Experiences in Fundamentals of Nursing, *3rd edition*

Jacqueline Patton Mayer, RN, MSN
QSEN feature

Denise M. McEnroe-Petitte, PhD, MSN, BSN, AS, RN
Urinary Elimination chapter

Debra S. McKinney, RN, MSN/MBA/HCA
Item writer, teacher test bank

Lisa LaMothe Melo, RN, BSN
Procedures for sensory perception, pain management, activity and exercise, and skin integrity chapters

Mary N. Meyer, MSN, ARNP-BC
Procedures for Safety and Bowel Elimination chapters

Alice C. Murr, BSN, RN (retired)
Nursing Process chapters

Rose M. Nieves, PhD, ARNP, FNP-C, CNE, RN
Caring in Multicultural Healthcare Environments chapter

Amando Okolo, JD, BSN, RN
Legal Accountability chapter

Lori Ormsby, MSN, GCNS-BC, APRN, CWOCN
Skin integrity content

Pamela Owen, BSN
Healthcare in Canada

Jessica Pedersen, ARNP, FNP-C
Nutrition procedures

Cynthia Pivec, BS
Procedure checklists

Phyllis Puckett, RN, MS
Contributor, instructor lecture notes

Linda Puetz, RN, BA, BSN, MEd
Documentation chapter content

Veronica Rempusheski, RN, FAAN, PhD
Older adults, expanded discussion

Elizabeth Richmond, BSN, MEd
Hygiene procedures

Sarah Kennedy Roland, RN, MSN
Documentation exercises, sample nurses' notes, test bank items

L. Jane Rosati, EdD, MSN, RN
Instructor's guide contributor, classroom enrichment strategies

Pennie Sessler Branden, PhD, CNM, RN
Item writer, teacher test bank

Susan Simmons, ARNP-BC, PhD
Clinical consultant, literature reviews

Melanie H. Simpson, PhD, RN-BC, OCN, CHPN
Pain chapter

Mable H. Smith, BSN, MN, JD, PhD
Legal issues chapter content

Darlene Sperlazza-Anthony, PhD, DNP, MSN, APRN, FNP-BC
Spirituality chapter

Lynne Sullivan, RN, MS
Procedures for sensory perception, pain management, activity and exercise, and skin integrity chapters

Mary Pat Szutenbach, RN, CNS, PhD
Nutrition chapter content

Janet Terra, RN, MSN
Hygiene procedures

Cynthia Thompson, RN, BSN
Hygiene procedures

Diana Tilton, RN, MSN
Asepsis procedures

Lisa Watkins, RN, MS
Urinary elimination procedures

Janis Watts, RN, MSN
Nursing informatics content

Michelle Williams, RN, MSN
Nursing care plans

Ashleigh Woods, EdD, RN, CNE
Skin Integrity & Wound Healing chapter

Reviewers of Previous Editions

Jocelyn Amberg, MSN, RN
Albuquerque, New Mexico

Elizabeth M. Andal, PhD, PMHCNS-BC, FAAN
Bakersfield, California

Deborah A. Andris, MSN, APNP
Milwaukee, Wisconsin

Patrice Balkcom, RN, MSN
Milledgeville, Georgia

Barbara Bonenberger, RN, MNEd, CNE
Pittsburgh, Pennsylvania

Wanda Bonnel, PhD, RN
Kansas City, Kansas

Jean Byrd, DNP, RN, MSN, CNE
Philadelphia, Pennsylvania

Valerie Cline, MSN, RN
Vancouver, Washington

Ann Curtis, DNP, RN
Lewiston, Maine

Martha Desmond, DNS
Troy, New York

Colette Dieujuste, RNC, MS
Boston, Massachusetts

Joyce Arlene Ennis, RN, MSN, ANP-BC
Waukesha, Wisconsin

Sally Flesch, BSN, MS, EdS, PhD
Moline, Illinois

Deborah L. Galante, RN, MSN, CNOR
Newark, Delaware

Deborah B. Hadley, RN, MSN, CNOR
Natchez, Mississippi

Linda K. Heitman, PhD, RN, ACNS-BC
Cape Girardeau, Missouri

Gladys L. Husted, RN, PhD, CNE
Pittsburgh, Pennsylvania

Jeanie Krause-Bachand, EdD, MSN, RN
York, Pennsylvania

Janice Garrison Lanham, RN, MS, CCNS, FNP
Seneca, South Carolina

Dawn LaPorte, BSN, RN, CRRN
Salem, New Hampshire

Maureen McDonald, RN, MS
Brockton, Massachusetts

Laura Smith McKenna, DNSc, RN
Concord, California

Pamela S. Miller, MS, RN
Columbus, Ohio

Jodi Noga, MSN, RN, CHPN
Grand Junction, Colorado

Christine Ouellette, MS, NP
Quincy, Massachusetts

Linda Pasto, MS, RN, CNE
Dryden, New York

Carla E. Randall, RN, PhD
Lewiston, Maine

Debra L. Renna, MSN, CCRN
North Miami, Florida

Patsy M. Spratling, MSN, RN
Ridgeland, Mississippi

Lynn M. Stover, RN, BC, DSN, SANE
Morrow, Georgia

Marcy Tanner, RN, MSN
Weatherford, Oklahoma

Barbara Timmons, RN, MSN
Appleton, Wisconsin

Geraldine Tyrell, DNP, RN, CNE
North Newton, Kansas

Pamela K. Weinberg, RN, MSN
Sumter, South Carolina

Acknowledgments

We wish to extend sincere gratitude to the exceptional team that helped us create this learning package, and especially to the following people:

- **Lisa Houck,** Publisher, Nursing Department, for her vision and forward thinking for the needs and style of today's learners, starting with the first edition, and for her vision, wisdom, and continued support throughout subsequent revisions. She sparks and supports our creativity while challenging our author team to think outside the box to develop a learning product that is more relevant and more effective than ever before.
- **Amy Romano,** Senior Content Project Manager, deserves extraordinary thanks. She has grasped and managed the many interlocking details of this complex project and worked tirelessly to keep it on track. Her efforts and attention to detail enabled us to better focus on content and didactic issues.
- **Julia Curcio,** Content Project Manager, for her skill in organizing and retrieving information and files, all the while churning out a mountain of work. She made our lives easier and kept the process moving smoothly.
- **Beth LoGiudice,** Developmental Editor, for her keen eye for detail and amazing attitude, making this project an enjoyable endeavor.
- **Cathy Carroll,** Project Manager and eProject Manager, for her continued support of the fundamentals projects.

Contents

CHAPTER **4**

Evidence-Based Practice: Theory & Research 92

Unit 3

Essential Nursing Interventions   371

CHAPTER **20**

Promoting Asepsis & Preventing Infection   514

CHAPTER **21**

Promoting Safety   544

Unit 4
Supporting Physiological Function   663

CHAPTER 24

Nutrition 665

CHAPTER 25

Urinary Elimination 716

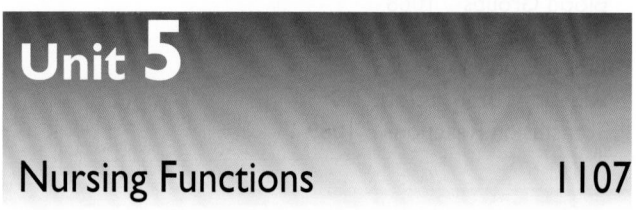

Unit 5

Nursing Functions　1107

CHAPTER 37

Community & Home Health Nursing　1109

CHAPTER 38

Nursing Informatics　1137

CHAPTER 39

Legal Accountability   1155

CHAPTER 40

Leading & Managing   1180

How Nurses Think

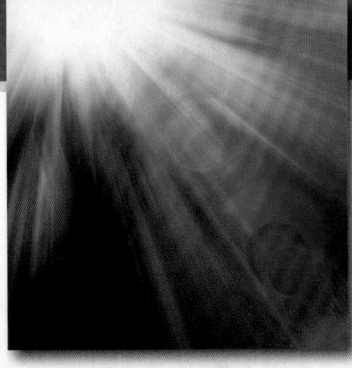

Evolution of Nursing Thought & Action

Learning Outcomes

After completing this chapter, you should be able to:

➤ Define *nursing* in your own words.
➤ Describe how person-centered care is the foundation of professional nursing.
➤ Discuss the transitions that nursing education has undergone in the last century.
➤ Differentiate among the various forms of nursing education.
➤ Explain how nursing practice is regulated.
➤ Give four examples of influential nursing organizations.

➤ Name and recognize the four purposes of nursing care.
➤ Describe the healthcare delivery system in the United States, including sites for care, types of workers, regulations, and financing of healthcare.
➤ Name nine expanded roles for nursing.
➤ Discuss issues related to healthcare reform.
➤ Delineate the forces and trends affecting contemporary nursing practice.

Key Concepts

Contemporary nursing education
Contemporary nursing practice
Healthcare delivery system
Nursing
Nursing history

Related Concepts

See the Concept Map on Davis Advantage.

Nurses Make a Difference . . .

Then & Now

Time: 1854, the Crimean Conflict (Russia). Place: Üsküdar (Scutari), Turkey, across the Bosporus Strait from Constantinople (Istanbul).

The hospital in Scutari is several days' journey by ship from the battle in Crimea. The injured and dying lie on cots or on crowded floors covered with filth. There are few blankets; soldiers arrive muddy from battle and covered with crusted blood. Outside, the air is crisp, yet the barrack reeks of disease and death. For several weeks, the army physicians refuse to allow Florence Nightingale and her staff of 38 nurses to do any real nursing work. Meanwhile, the nurses review environmental conditions and note the health problems of the soldiers and the available supplies and equipment. They open windows to clear the fetid air, scrub all surfaces from ceiling to floor, prepare nutritious meals, bathe the wounded, sew bedclothes, and fashion bandages. As they prove their usefulness, they are allowed to dress wounds, feed the injured, and comfort those who

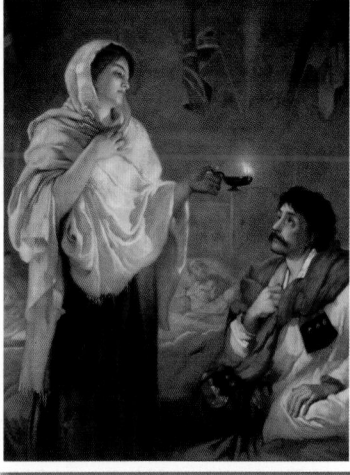

are in pain or dying. They offer encouragement and emotional care to soldiers and help them write letters home. Within a few months, the mortality rate drops from 47% to 2%, and morale improves immeasurably.

Time: 2023. Place: Your Local Hospital.

While standing at the bedside verifying medications, Susan listens to the ventilator cycle. She notes that her client has begun to trigger breaths on his own. In the background, she hears the cardiac monitor sounds, which have become more irregular over the past hour. She mentally runs through her client assessment. "Why is his heart so irritable?" she wonders. She checks the results of the blood work on the computer.

(Continued)

Nurses Make a Difference . . . (continued)

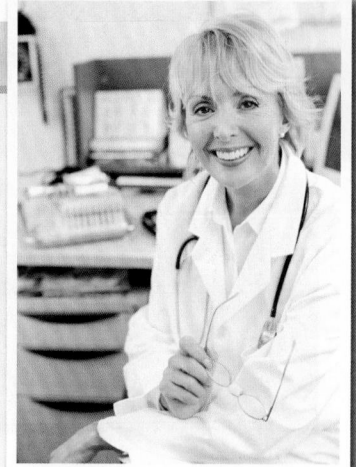

Susan notes that the potassium level is low (2.9 mEq/L). She notifies the provider of the laboratory results and the client's cardiac irritability, adding, "The client's potassium is low from the diarrhea he's had since we began the antibiotics." Together, they develop a plan to administer IV potassium to raise the client's potassium level and to check it every 8 hours. Several hours later, Susan documents in the electronic health record (EHR) that the *ectopy* (irregular heartbeat) has decreased to fewer than 2 beats/min.

Time: 2050. Place: A Local Home.

Yesterday, Mr. Samuels underwent robotic cardiac surgery. He was discharged to his home this morning and is now under your care. Since discharge, he has been monitored remotely via implanted technology. As a home health nurse, you have been reviewing and analyzing his physiological and biochemical data and adherence to provider guidelines (e.g., medication, dietary, and activity compliance). The provider has reviewed the networked data and guided you to focus on activity compliance and assessment of several incidences of spikes indicating anxiety or discomfort. Mrs. Samuels greets you at the front door. She tells you that her husband is reluctant to move for fear of pain. She looks frightened as she says, "I am not comfortable with the telemonitoring. I prefer to have the 'human touch' as my parents had many years ago." You explain that changes in technology and the healthcare system allow you to take care of clients in their own homes who would previously have been in the hospital. As you begin your assessments, you tell Mrs. Samuels, "Your husband's networked data are constantly evaluated. Any indication of problems will trigger emergency personnel immediately. We have 24/7 monitoring." You further explain that the data show that Mr. Samuels has not complied with the activity prescription that is important to prevent cardiac and respiratory complications. "We want you to feel comfortable with the

technologies and the plan of care."

In each of these scenarios, the nurses engaged in *full-spectrum nursing;* that is, they used their minds and their hands to improve the client's comfort and condition. Their actions exemplify caring.

As the scenarios illustrate, nursing roles have changed over time, yet nursing remains a profession dedicated to care of the client. The actions of Florence Nightingale and her team exemplified person-centered care of the soldiers. They demonstrated compassion, respect, and individualized care. A plan of care was developed based on their assessment of the environment and needs of the soldiers, with interventions prioritized to promote optimal outcomes. Florence Nightingale communicated with key stakeholders (e.g., physicians, politicians) to obtain needed support and resources. Her meticulous notes and analysis of data became the foundation of evidence-based practice, as she continuously correlated interventions with outcomes.

In addition to evidence, person-centered care incorporates clinical judgment. Florence Nightingale used clinical judgment to improve the care of wounded soldiers. She immediately assessed environmental conditions and the soldiers' needs to make decisions to promote safe, effective quality care. Similarly, Susan used her applied knowledge of cardiac dysrhythmias and laboratory data to obtain essential nursing care for the client. The home health nurse used advanced technologies in the care of her client. All of these scenarios highlight the need for a sound knowledge base to make safe clinical decisions.

▲ ThinkLike a Nurse 1-1: Clinical Judgment in Action

The Institute of Medicine (IOM; now the National Academy of Medicine) identified core competencies for healthcare providers (Greiner & Knebel, 2003; see the accompanying Safe, Effective Nursing Care [SENC] box, "What Is Safe, Effective Nursing Care [SENC]?"). These competencies are the basis for the SENC competencies. You will see them used throughout this text. Which of these competencies did Florence Nightingale demonstrate? Explain your thinking.

ABOUT THE KEY CONCEPTS

The overarching concept for this chapter is **nursing**. As you come to understand other key concepts (i.e., **nursing history, contemporary nursing education, contemporary**

nursing practice, healthcare delivery system), you will grasp how nursing has evolved into today's contemporary nursing practice.

HISTORICAL LEADERS WHO ADVANCED THE PROFESSION OF NURSING

Key Point: *An understanding of how the actions of others have advanced the profession of nursing demonstrates how your actions and advocacy can make a difference.*

Florence Nightingale (Fig. 1-1) Historically, the military and religions have had positive impacts on the advancement of the nursing profession. Many individuals answered the call to promote quality

Safe, Effective Nursing Care

What Is Safe, Effective Nursing Care (SENC)?

Competencies: This table contains the competencies of the Institute of Medicine (IOM; now the National Academy of Medicine) and their parallels to safe, effective nursing care that a graduate nurse should be able to provide within the framework of the full-spectrum nursing model (see Chapter 2). To implement full-spectrum nursing, a nurse must demonstrate the model concepts (thinking, doing, and caring) that are aspects of every competency.

National Academy of Medicine* Core Competencies	Safe, Effective Nursing Care (Thinking, Doing, Caring)
Provide patient-centered care ➤ Respect clients' differences, values, preferences, and expressed needs ➤ Relieve pain and suffering ➤ Coordinate continuous care ➤ Communicate and provide client education ➤ Focus on health promotion and illness prevention	**Provide goal-directed, patient-centered care** ➤ Establish mutual goals with clients ➤ Show respect for client values, religious beliefs, needs, and preferences ➤ Implement interventions to promote client comfort, promote health, prevent illness, or transition to a peaceful death ➤ Provide client education to foster informed decisions and involvement in care and to facilitate postdischarge health
Work on interprofessional teams ➤ Collaborate, communicate, and jointly implement client care	**Collaborate with the interprofessional healthcare team** ➤ Function as an essential member of the healthcare team ➤ Develop a comprehensive plan of client care that includes members of the interprofessional healthcare team ➤ Evaluate client care from a holistic, interprofessional approach
Employ evidence-based practice ➤ Integrate research with clinical expertise and client values for optimal care ➤ Maintain knowledge of current research	**Validate evidence-based research to incorporate into practice** ➤ Incorporate evidence-based findings into client care ➤ Evaluate client outcomes using valid and reliable research tools ➤ Utilize data/findings to generate research questions
Apply quality improvement ➤ Identify and avoid care errors ➤ Design a framework that includes structure, process, and outcomes in relation to client and community needs ➤ Evaluate the framework	**Provide safe, quality client care** ➤ Evaluate and use techniques/processes to avoid medical/nursing errors in the delivery of client care ➤ Design a "Thinking, Doing, Caring" framework that incorporates a holistic approach to client care ➤ Evaluate the framework, incorporating the structure, process, and outcomes components of quality improvement approaches ➤ Use data to foster improvements and implement innovative processes
Utilize informatics ➤ Communicate, manage knowledge, mitigate error, and support decision making using information technology	**Embrace/incorporate technological advances** ➤ Use technology to deliver safe, effective care ➤ Remain current in information technology ➤ Communicate with technology support systems to ensure optimal client outcomes ➤ Maintain accurate and comprehensive electronic health records

*Formerly Institute of Medicine (IOM).
Source: Greiner, A., & Knebel, E. (Eds.). (2003). *Health professions education: A bridge to quality.* Institute of Medicine (US) Committee on the Health Professions Education Summit.

healthcare for soldiers and wounded warriors. The most notable individual and advocate for quality healthcare is Florence Nightingale, also known as the "Founder of Modern Nursing." She transformed nursing into a widely respected profession. Her diligent efforts provided the foundation for research, evidence-based practice, and interprofessional communications.

The wounded soldiers in the hospital in Scutari were dying due to poor environmental conditions, poor nutrition, and lack of quality care. In spite of resistance from the medical community, Florence Nightingale persisted in her determination to provide and promote quality care to soldiers. Her primary focus was ensuring that she and her team of nurses addressed the care needs of the soldiers. Using a lantern for light, she would visit

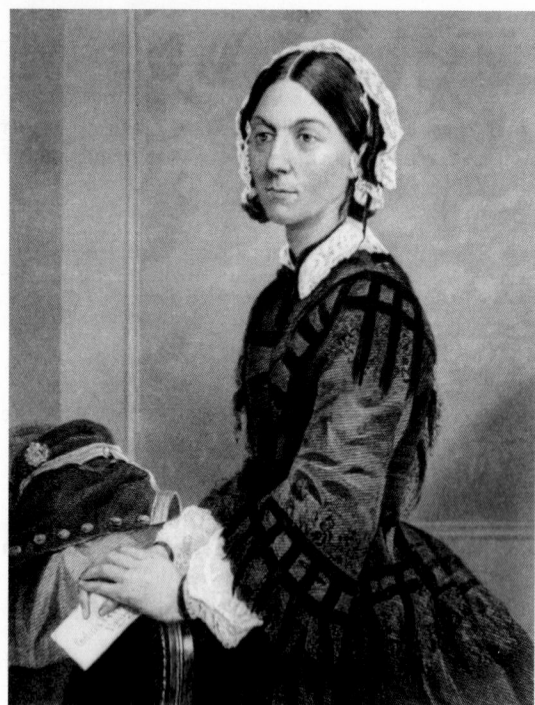

FIGURE 1-1 Florence Nightingale (1820–1910).

soldiers at night, earning her the name "Lady With the Lamp." She kept meticulous notes and statistics that were used to advocate for and obtain changes in healthcare. She used her clinical judgment, political connections, and social standing to ensure that nursing was recognized as a respectable profession. The Nightingale Home and Training School for Nurses was opened in 1860 and is considered the first official nursing program.

In her *Notes on Hospitals* (1863), Nightingale stated that air, light, nutrition, and adequate ventilation and space were essential for soldiers to recuperate. The hospitals she designed incorporated these ideas, which decreased mortality rates, lengths of hospital stays, and rates of nosocomial infection (infection associated with a healthcare facility, now more commonly called *healthcare-associated infection*).

Other Leaders Nursing presence on the battlefield became more common during the Civil War when the U.S. government established the Army Nursing Service to organize nurses and hospitals and coordinate supplies for the soldiers. Thousands of laypersons also volunteered, including the following:

- **Dorothea Dix** served as superintendent of the U.S. Army Nurses.
- **Clara Barton** provided care in tents set up close to the fighting. When the war was over, Barton continued this universal care through the establishment of the **American Red Cross.**

Other nurses who were instrumental in developing the roles of nursing as we now know it—promoting

health, providing care, preventing illness, and advancing the profession—include the following:

- **Lillian Wald and Mary Brewster,** the pioneers of public health nursing, founded the Henry Street Settlement in New York to fight the spread of diseases among poor immigrants.
- **Edward Lyon** was the first male nurse to receive a commission as a reserve officer.
- **Mary Mahoney,** the first African American graduate nurse in the United States, cofounded the National Association of Colored Graduates in 1908, which eventually merged with the American Nurses Association (ANA).
- **Lavinia Dock,** a nurse, feminist, and social activist, compiled the first manual of drugs for nurses in 1890. She was a contributing editor to the *American Journal of Nursing* and helped establish the American Society of Superintendents of Training Schools for Nurses of the United States and Canada, now the National League for Nursing (NLN).
- **Linda Richards,** the first professionally trained nurse in America, created the first system for keeping individual medical records and promoted mental health nursing.

Nursing Today: Full-Spectrum Nursing

Nurses today are highly trained, well-educated, caring, and competent professionals. They are essential members of the healthcare team. The complexity of healthcare delivery requires that nurses use clinical judgment, communication, organizational, leadership, advocacy, and technical skills to ensure that clients receive safe and effective care.

Safe, Effective Nursing Care Nursing education emphasizes quality and safety so that students will be able to deliver safe, effective nursing care in their practice after graduation.

- *Nursing Practice.* The IOM (now the National Academies of Sciences, Engineering, and Medicine) has identified quality and safety competencies that all health professionals are expected to demonstrate in their practice (Greiner & Knebel, 2003; see the SENC box "Quality Improvement Competency" later in this chapter).
- *Nursing Education.* The Quality and Safety Education for Nurses (QSEN) project is one of the organizations that has identified competencies that students are expected to acquire before graduation (Cronenwett et al., 2007). Others include the American Association of Colleges of Nursing (AACN) in the publication *The Essentials: Core Competencies for Professional Nursing Education* (2021) and the NLN Practical/Vocational Curriculum guidelines.
- *Full-Spectrum Nursing and Safe, Effective Nursing Care.* To implement quality care using the full-spectrum

nursing model (Chapter 2), we will refer to "safe, effective nursing care" competencies (see the SENC boxes that appear in almost all chapters in this book).

Application of Knowledge, Skill, and Caring Key Point: *Nurses apply knowledge from the arts and sciences in their various roles to provide person-centered care (Table 1-1).* Nurses use clinical judgment, critical thinking, and problem-solving as they care for clients. (You will learn more about full-spectrum nursing in the section titled What Is Full-Spectrum Nursing? in Chapter 2.)

To be safe providers, nurses must carefully consider their actions and think carefully about the client, the treatment plan, the healthcare environment, the client's support system, the nurse's support system and resources, and safety.

- **Clinical judgment** requires a strong, solid knowledge base. It involves a process that consists of recognizing

Table 1-1 ➤ Roles and Functions of the Nurse

ROLE	FUNCTION	EXAMPLES
Direct care provider	Addressing the physical, emotional, social, and spiritual needs of the client	Listening to lung sounds Giving medications Client teaching
Communicator	Using interpersonal and therapeutic communication skills to address the needs of the client, facilitate communication in the healthcare team, and advise the community about health promotion and disease prevention	Counseling a client Discussing staffing needs at a unit meeting Collaborating with the provider about a client's condition
Client/family educator	Assessing and diagnosing the teaching needs of the client, group, family, or community. Once the diagnosis is made, nurses plan how to meet these needs, implement the teaching plan, and evaluate its effectiveness.	Preoperative teaching Prenatal education for siblings Community classes on nutrition
Client advocate	Supporting clients' right to make healthcare decisions when they are able to voice their opinions and protecting clients from harm when they are unable to make decisions	Helping a client explain to their family that they do not want to have further chemotherapy
Counselor	Using therapeutic communication skills to advise clients about health-related issues	Counseling a client on weight-loss strategies
Change agent	Advocating for change on an individual, family, group, community, or societal level that enhances health. The nurse may use counseling, communication, and educator skills to accomplish this role.	Working to improve the nutritional quality of the lunch program at a preschool
Leader	Inspiring others by setting an example of positive health, assertive communication, and willingness to improve	Florence Nightingale Walt Whitman Harriet Tubman Malala Yousafzai
Manager	Coordinating and managing the activities of all members of the team	Charge nurse on a hospital unit (e.g., assigns clients to staff nurses)
Case manager	Coordinating the care delivered to a client	Coordinator of services for clients with mobility challenges
Research consumer	Applying evidence-based practice to provide the most appropriate care, identify clinical problems that warrant research, and protect the rights of research subjects	Reading journal articles Attending continuing education; seeking additional education

and analyzing the cues, prioritizing hypotheses, generating solutions, taking actions, and evaluating outcomes of the client's condition to determine whether change has occurred. It also involves careful consideration of the client's condition, medications, and treatment in the evaluation of their health status. Consider how clinical judgment was evident in each of the three scenarios. The nurses analyzed the cues present in each situation to implement actions to promote quality client care. The use of the nursing process, discussed in Chapter 3 and in each of the clinically focused chapters, facilitates the development of clinical judgment.

- **Critical thinking** is a reflective thinking process that involves collecting information, analyzing the adequacy and accuracy of the information, and carefully considering options for action. Nurses use critical thinking in every aspect of nursing care. Critical thinking is discussed at length in Chapter 2 and applied in every chapter in this text.
- **Problem-solving** is a process by which nurses consider an issue and attempt to find a satisfactory solution to achieve the best outcomes. You will often use problem-solving in your professional life. The nursing process (see Chapter 3) is one type of problem-solving process.

Core Competencies for Professional Nursing. The AACN identified 10 domains that are essential to the practice of nursing (AACN, 2021). Integrated within various domains are concepts that reflect essential knowledge for professional nursing. You have already learned about some of these concepts (e.g., clinical judgment) and will gain knowledge of the others as you progress in your nursing courses. For example, you will be introduced to the concept of social determinants of health as you individualize care and consider how the environment in which patients live, work, play, and learn affect health risks and outcomes.

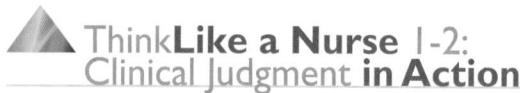

ThinkLike a Nurse 1-2: Clinical Judgment in Action

In the three scenarios of Nurses Make a Difference . . . Then & Now, describe how clinical judgment has evolved over time.

CONTEMPORARY NURSING: EDUCATION, REGULATION, AND PRACTICE

As a student about to enter your new professional life, you need a realistic grasp of the nature and demands of your chosen career. To help better acquaint you with nursing today, the remainder of this chapter discusses the current state of nursing, discusses nursing education, presents the trends affecting nursing, and provides an overview of the healthcare delivery system.

How Is Nursing Defined?

Based on historical and television depictions, many individuals have different images of nurses. That makes it difficult for the public to understand the reality of nursing. In addition, the various levels of nurses and their associated roles can be confusing to the public and to other members of the healthcare team. In addition, the constantly changing nature of nursing, healthcare, and society further complicates the definition of *nursing*. **Key Point:** *It is important for nurses to articulate clearly, for themselves and for the public, what nursing is and what nurses do.* The following sections articulate the views of two important nursing organizations in answer to the question, "What is nursing?"

International Council of Nurses Definition

The International Council of Nurses (ICN), an organization that represents nurses throughout the world, defined nursing in accordance with theorist Virginia Henderson as follows:

> The unique function of the nurse is to assist the individual, sick or well, in the performance of those activities contributing to health or its recovery (or to peaceful death) that he would perform unaided if he had the necessary strength, will or knowledge. (Henderson, 1966, p. 15)

In the decades since the adoption of that definition, nursing throughout the world has changed. Advances in healthcare have altered the type of care required by clients, and nurses have taken on expanded roles. To reflect these changes, the ICN has revised its definition of nursing, as follows:

> Nursing encompasses autonomous and collaborative care of individuals of all ages, families, groups and communities, sick or well and in all settings. Nursing includes the promotion of health, prevention of illness, and the care of ill, disabled and dying people. Advocacy, promotion of a safe environment, research, participation in shaping health policy and in patient and health systems management, and education are also key nursing roles. (ICN, n.d.)

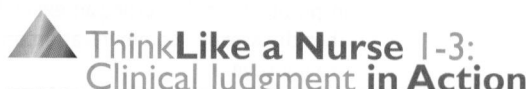

ThinkLike a Nurse 1-3: Clinical Judgment in Action

Look at the three scenarios of Nurses Make a Difference . . . Then & Now. What nursing actions did the nurses perform that are represented in the ICN definition of nursing?

American Nursing Association Definition

You can see similar changes in the approach of the ANA. In 1980, the ANA defined nursing as "the diagnosis and treatment of human responses to actual and potential health problems" (p. 2). Attempts to refine this definition have been difficult. Nurses are a widely varied group of people with varying skills. They perform activities designed to provide care ranging from basic to complex in numerous healthcare environments. Therefore, it is not easy to describe the boundaries of the profession.

In 2010, the ANA acknowledged five characteristics of registered nursing:

- Nursing practice is individualized.
- Nurses coordinate care by establishing partnerships (with persons, families, support systems, and other providers).
- Caring is central to the practice of the registered nurse.
- Registered nurses use the nursing process to plan and provide individualized care to their healthcare consumers.
- A strong link exists between the professional work environment and the registered nurse's ability to provide quality healthcare and achieve optimal outcomes. (ANA, 2010, pp. 4–5)

The ANA now defines professional nursing as follows:

Nursing is the protection, promotion, and optimization of health and abilities, prevention of illness and injury, facilitation of healing, alleviation of suffering through the diagnosis and treatment of human response, and advocacy in the care of individuals, families, groups, communities, and populations. (ANA, 2015a, p. 1)

Why Is a Definition Important?

Nursing organizations and leaders have pushed for accurate definitions to (1) help the public understand the value of nursing, (2) describe what activities and roles belong to nursing versus other health professions, and (3) help students and practicing nurses understand what is expected of them within their role as nurses. From history, you can tell that nursing has undergone tremendous change, from a role limited to providing kindness and support to full-spectrum nursing, which is based in science but still focuses on care and nurturing. Box 1-1 lists several additional definitions of nursing for you to consider.

As a student entering nursing, you can use definitions and descriptions to understand what is expected of you. To aid you in this task, refer to Table 1-1 and review the essential components of the nursing role. While in the clinical setting, you will observe nurses functioning in each of these capacities and identify the qualities listed in Box 1-2 that are essential for safe nursing practice.

KnowledgeCheck 1-1
- What factors make it difficult to define the term *nursing*?
- Based on the ICN definition of nursing, what does a nurse do?
- What is clinical judgment? Critical thinking?

Is Nursing a Profession, Discipline, or Occupation?

One strategy used to describe a field of work is to categorize it as a profession, a discipline, or an occupation.

BOX 1-1 ■ What Is Nursing?

I use the word *nursing*, for want of a better. It has been limited to signify little more than the administration of medicines and the application of poultices. It ought to signify the proper use of fresh air, light, warmth, cleanliness, quiet, and the proper choosing and giving of diet—all at the least expense of vital power to the patient. (Nightingale, 1876, p. 5)

Events that give rise to higher degrees of consideration for those who are helpless or oppressed, kindliness and sympathy for the unfortunate and for those who suffer, tolerance for those of differing religion, race, color, etc.—all tend to promote activities like nursing which are primarily humanitarian. (Dock & Stewart, 1938, p. 3)

Nursing has been called the oldest of the arts and the youngest of the professions. As such, it has gone through many stages and has been an integral part of societal movements. Nursing has been involved in the existing culture—shaped by it and yet helping to develop it. (Donahue, 1985, p. 3)

Nurses provide care for people in the midst of health, pain, loss, fear, disfigurement, death, grieving, challenge, growth, birth, and transition on an intimate front-line basis. Expert nurses call this the privileged place of nursing. (Benner & Wrubel, 1989, p. xi)

Nurses provide and coordinate patient care, educate patients and the public about various health conditions, and provide advice and emotional support to patients and their family members. (U.S. Bureau of Labor Statistics, 2021b)

Profession Although the term *profession* is freely used, a group must meet certain criteria to be considered a **profession** (see Table 1-2). Nursing appears to meet all criteria of a profession as defined by Starr (1982) and Miller et al. (1993).

Discipline To be considered a **discipline,** a profession must have a domain of knowledge that has both theoretical and practical boundaries. The **theoretical boundaries** of a profession are the questions that arise from clinical practice and are then investigated through research. The **practical boundaries** are the current state of knowledge and research in the field—the facts that dictate safe practice (Meleis, 1991). A case can be made that nursing is both a profession and a discipline:

- It is a scientifically based and self-governed *profession* that focuses on the ethical care of others.
- It is a *discipline,* driven by aspects of theory and practice. It demands mastery of both theoretical knowledge and clinical skills.

Occupation In spite of meeting criteria for both designations (profession and discipline), nursing is often described as an **occupation,** or job. Most physicians are in control of their practice environment, working conditions, and schedule. In contrast, most nurses are hourly wage earners. The employer, not the nurse, decides the conditions of practice and the nature of the work. Nevertheless, nurse practice acts do not prevent nurses from functioning more autonomously.

BOX 1-2 ■ Important Qualities for Nurses

Critical-Thinking Skills

Required Action: Monitor the client, note changes, and take actions to ensure safe and effective care.

Example: Call the provider to obtain a stronger pain medication for a client who, 2 hours after receiving pain medication, rates their pain as 7 out of 10.

Caring and Compassion

Required Action: Show kindness, concern, and sincerity that convey to clients that you care about their well-being.

Example: Sit with and hold the hand of a client who has just been told that they have a terminal illness.

Detail Oriented

Required Action: Pay attention to details to prevent and identify potentially harmful errors in care.

Example: Seek clarification and correct a dosage that is written as "7 mg" that should be "0.7 mg."

Organizational Skills

Required Action: Prioritize and meet the needs of the most critical clients first.

Example: Care for the postoperative client with difficulty breathing before performing a dressing change.

Speaking Skills

Required Action: Communicate correct and pertinent information to clients and members of the healthcare team.

Example: Teach the client how to perform a dressing change at home after discharge from the hospital.

Listening Skills

Required Action: Listen to clients' concerns and feedback from the interprofessional healthcare team.

Example: The interprofessional team is having a conference discussing the needs of your client after discharge.

Patience

Required Action: In stressful situations in the work environment, think clearly and take the correct actions.

Example: Remain calm when a client's condition deteriorates, provide the needed care, and transfer the client to the intensive care unit.

Competence

Required Action: Obtain the knowledge and skills to ensure safe, quality client outcomes.

Example: Recognize that the correct dose for the drug is 0.10 mg rather than 10 mg.

Emotional Stability

Required Action: Develop the ability to cope with human suffering, emergencies, and other stresses.

Example: Provide care to a client accused of child abuse and to the child who suffered severe head injuries.

Physical Stamina

Required Action: Perform physical tasks and endure long hours walking and standing.

Example: Assist another nurse in lifting a 300-lb client after working 10 hours of a 12-hour shift.

Source: Adapted from U.S. Bureau of Labor Statistics, U.S. Department of Labor (2021b). Registered nurses. In *Occupational outlook handbook.* https://www.bls.gov/ooh/healthcare/registered-nurses.htm

---

Key Point: *The following actions can strengthen nursing's classification as a profession:*

- *Standardize the educational requirements for entry into practice.*
- *Enact uniform continuing education requirements.*
- *Encourage the participation of more nurses in professional organizations.*
- *Educate the public about the true nature of nursing practice.*

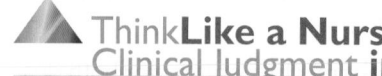

ThinkLike a Nurse 1-4: Clinical Judgment in Action

Evaluate the status of nursing. Is nursing a respected profession? Give examples to support your opinion.

How Do Nurses' Educational Paths Differ?

The transition into the nursing profession involves the concepts of formal and informal processes. **Formal education** consists of completing the initial and continuing education required for licensure. **Informal education** involves a gradual progression in skill and clinical judgment that allows the nurse to advance in the profession.

Formal Education

When the client calls out "Nurse," who can respond? To legally use the title *nurse,* a person must be a graduate of an accredited nursing education program and have successfully passed the National Council Licensure Examination (NCLEX®). Other personnel might respond to the client's call, but they cannot legally be considered nurses. Students may enter nursing through two paths: as a practical nurse or as a registered nurse.

Practical and Vocational Nursing Education

Practical nursing education prepares nurses to provide basic care to clients under the direction of a registered nurse (RN) or primary care provider. Practical nurses are known as licensed practical nurses (LPNs) or licensed vocational nurses (LVNs). Educational programs for LPNs/LVNs offer both classroom and clinical

Table 1-2 ➤ Nursing: Is It a Profession?

STARR CRITERION	EXAMPLES IN NURSING
The knowledge of the group must be based on technical and scientific knowledge.	Entry-level nursing education requires coursework in basic and social sciences, as well as humanities, arts, and general education. Nursing education and practice are increasingly based on research from nursing and related fields.
The knowledge and competence of members of the group must be evaluated by a community of peers.	State regulatory bodies define the criteria that nurses must meet to practice and monitor members for adherence to standards.
The group must have a service orientation and a code of ethics.	Nursing is clearly focused on providing service to others. The major professional organizations have developed ethical guidelines to guide the practice of nursing.

Source: Starr, P. (1982). *The social transformation of American medicine.* Basic Books.

teaching and usually last 1 year. After completing the practical nursing education program, the graduate must pass the NCLEX-PN® examination to become licensed. LPNs/LVNs usually work in nursing and residential facilities, providers' offices, home healthcare, and hospitals. Employment growth is expected to increase 9% between 2020 and 2030 (U.S. Bureau of Labor Statistics, 2021a).

Registered Nursing Entry Education

Currently, various educational pathways lead to licensure as an RN. Graduates of all these programs must successfully complete the NCLEX-RN® examination to practice as RNs. Their job growth is expected to grow 9% between 2020 and 2030, based on the increased growth of the aging population (U.S. Bureau of Labor Statistics, 2021b).

- **Diploma programs.** Hospital-based programs, modeled after Nightingale's school of nursing apprenticeship style of learning, were the mainstay of nursing education until the 1960s. The typical program lasts 3 years and focuses on clinical experience in direct client care. Since the 1960s, the number of diploma programs has steadily decreased to less than 10% of RN programs (AACN, 2019a).
- **Associate's degree.** This type of program, conceptualized by Mildred Montag, emerged during the nursing shortage after World War II. Associate's degree (AD) programs are primarily offered in community colleges. Although the nursing component typically lasts two years, students are required to take numerous other courses in liberal arts and the sciences. Nurses with an associate's degree in nursing (ADN) are prepared to provide direct client care.
- **Baccalaureate degree.** The course of study in prelicensure bachelor of science in nursing (BSN) programs lasts at least eight semesters. Graduates are prepared to assume administrative responsibilities, address complex clinical situations, oversee and provide direct client care, work in community care, apply research findings, and enter graduate education. The IOM (2011), now the National Academy of Medicine, established a goal to increase the proportion of baccalaureate-prepared nurses to 80% by 2020. Of first-time U.S.-educated candidates taking the NCLEX-RN® in 2020, those with BSN degrees exceeded those with ADN degrees by 2,127 test-takers (National Council of State Boards of Nursing [NCSBN], 2021). The AACN recognizes the baccalaureate degree as the minimum education for professional-level nursing practice (2019). However, the AACN acknowledges support of licensure at the ADN level and is an advocate for educational advancement.
- **RN to BSN.** Graduates from ADN programs are increasingly enrolling in RN-to-BSN programs to obtain the BSN degree, in alignment with the IOM recommendation for an 80% baccalaureate-prepared workforce. Currently there are over 775 RN-to-BSN completion programs (AACN, 2019b). Within 4 to 6 months after graduation, 93% of entry-level nurses with BSN degrees had job offers; this trend is expected to continue because the AACN has embraced the RN-to-BSN articulation model, and employers show a preference for hiring BSN-prepared nurses (AACN, 2021).
- **Accelerated BSN.** This prelicensure program is designed for students who have a baccalaureate degree in another field and want to get a degree in nursing. The didactic component is usually online, but students must complete traditional skills laboratory and clinical rotations that are consistent with traditional prelicensure programs.
- **Direct-entry master's degree.** The typical student in these programs has a baccalaureate degree in another field and has entered nursing as a second career. Programs usually are completed in 3 years of full-time study, with the first year devoted to basic nursing content. At the program's completion, the student is eligible to take the NCLEX-RN and is awarded a master's degree in nursing.
- **Direct-entry doctorate.** A direct-entry doctoral program is usually designed for students who have a baccalaureate degree in another field and seek an accelerated path to the doctorate degree. Students take the NCLEX-RN while enrolled in the program.

Some offer a nurse practitioner program of study that prepares students to take the certification examination to become licensed as an advanced practice registered nurse (APRN).

Graduate Nursing Education

Graduate education prepares the RN for advanced practice and an expanded role in other areas (e.g., research). A baccalaureate degree is required to enter a traditional master's program.

- **Master's degree programs** prepare RNs to function in a more independent and autonomous role, such as nurse practitioner, clinical specialist, nurse educator, nursing informatics, or nurse administrator. It typically takes 2 years to complete the master's degree.
- **Doctoral programs** in nursing offer professional degrees. A master's degree is required to enter a traditional doctoral program. Doctoral degree programs in nursing offer one of the following:
  - Doctor of nursing practice (DNP)—a practice degree
  - Doctor of philosophy (PhD)—a degree focused on scholarly research and knowledge generation

Other Forms of Formal Education

Advances in healthcare have a strong influence on nursing practice. You will become familiar with the concept of "nurses as lifelong learners" as the means to keep current in your practice. You will be expected to engage in continuing education to enhance your intellectual and practical knowledge throughout your nursing career.

- **Continuing education** (CE) is designed to help you stay current in your theoretical and clinical knowledge after graduation. CE programs are offered at work sites, in educational settings, at professional conferences, on the Internet, and in professional journals. In many states, renewal of the nursing license requires successful completion of a specified number—and in some cases, type of—CE courses. When you apply for your license, the state board of nursing will notify you about CE requirements (if any) that you must complete to receive, or later renew, your license. You should also know your state requirements.
- **In-service education** is another form of ongoing education. It is offered at the work site and usually does not count toward meeting the CE requirement for license renewal. In-service education is typically institution specific (e.g., change in policies) or product specific (e.g., use of new equipment). It is designed to enhance your continuing competence in knowledge, skills, and attitudes.

Informal Education

Socialization is the informal education that occurs as you move into your new profession. It is the knowledge gained from direct experience, real-world observations, and informal discussion with peers and colleagues.

Key Point: *Professional socialization begins when you enter the educational program and continues as you gain expertise throughout your career.* Informal education complements formal education to create clinical competence and professional growth.

Benner's Model

Nursing theorist Patricia Benner (1984) described the process by which a nurse acquires clinical skills and judgment. Benner's model notes that expertise is a personal integration of knowledge that requires technical skill, thoughtful application, and insight. **Key Point:** *That is what we mean in this text when we use the term* full-spectrum nursing *it involves thinking, doing, and caring.* Benner's model has five stages:

- *Stage 1: Novice.* This phase begins with the onset of education. The novice has little clinical experience, is task oriented, and is focused on learning the rules and following the written sequential process. For example, when performing a sterile dressing change, the nurse may be so concerned with following the steps in the skills checklist that they forget to assess the client's reaction to the procedure.
- *Stage 2: Advanced beginner.* A new graduate usually functions at this level. An advanced beginner begins to focus on more aspects of a clinical situation and applies more facts. The nurse can distinguish abnormal findings but cannot readily understand their significance. For example, a new graduate assesses that the postoperative client's blood pressure has decreased, their pulse rate has increased, and they have become more restless during the last 2 hours. However, the nurse probably will not recognize that these signs/symptoms may indicate early blood loss. Through repeated experiences or mentoring, the nurse begins to readily attach meanings to findings.
- *Stage 3: Competence.* Nurses achieve competence after 2 to 3 years of nursing practice in the same area. Competent performers have gained additional experience and are able to handle their client load, deal with complexity, and prioritize situations while providing compassionate care. In the previous scenario, the competent nurse would immediately connect the changes in the vital signs with the surgical procedure, recognize possible early signs of shock, and conduct a more in-depth assessment.
- *Stage 4: Proficient.* The proficient nurse is able to quickly take in all aspects of a situation and immediately give meaning to the cluster of assessment data. Proficient nurses are able to see the "big picture" and can coordinate services and forecast needs. They are much more flexible and fluent within their role and able to adapt to the nuances of various client situations.
- *Stage 5: Expert.* Expert nurses understand what needs to be achieved and how to do it. They trust in and use their intuition while operating with a deep understanding of a situation, often recognizing a problem in the absence of its classic signs and symptoms. They

have highly competent skills and are often consulted when others need advice or assistance.

Benner's model deals with the development of clinical wisdom and competence. Keep in mind that this progression is not automatic. Nurses do not simply move through the stages as they gain experience. Instead, this model assumes that to improve in skill and judgment, you must also be attuned to each clinical situation. This requires the ability to process information from a variety of sources and notice subtle variations to guide decision making. Although expertise (stage 5) is a goal, not everyone can achieve this level.

Nursing Organization Guidelines

The ANA and other organizations are also involved in helping nurses to improve their practice by setting standards and articulating nursing values. For example, in the *Code of Ethics for Nurses*, the ANA provides guidelines, including acceptable and unacceptable behaviors, for how nurses should conduct themselves in their day-to-day practice (ANA, 2015b). Box 1-3 presents values and behaviors essential to nursing practice. See Chapter 5, Ethics & Values, for further discussion of nursing values and the ANA *Code of Ethics for Nurses*.

KnowledgeCheck 1-2
- Compare and contrast formal and informal education.
- Name and describe five educational pathways leading to licensure as an RN.

How Is Nursing Practice Regulated?
Laws, standards of practice, and guidelines from professional organizations regulate the practice of nursing.

Nurse Practice Acts In the United States, each state enacts its own nurse practice act, which is a compilation of laws that govern the practice of nursing and empower a state board of nursing to oversee and regulate nursing practice. Although there are minor variations, each board of nursing is responsible for the following:

- Defining the practice of professional nursing. This definition usually includes the scope of practice (i.e.,

activities that nurses are expected to perform and, by implication, those they may not).
- Approving nursing education programs
- Establishing criteria that allow a person to be licensed as an APRN, RN, or LPN/LVN
- Developing rules and regulations to provide guidance to nurses
- Enforcing the rules that govern the education of nursing and nursing practice

Key Point: *To practice nursing, you must be licensed as a nurse by the state board of nursing.* All states require graduation from an approved nursing program and successful completion of the NCLEX. To receive licensure in another state, the nurse simply applies for licensure by endorsement (reciprocity) or follows the guidance of the mutual recognition model. For further details about licensing and the regulation of nursing practice, see Chapter 39, Legal Accountability.

Standards of Practice Nursing is also guided by **standards of practice,** which "describe a competent level of nursing care as demonstrated by the critical thinking model known as the nursing process" (ANA, 2015a, p. 4). Standards are "authoritative statements of the duties that all registered nurses, regardless of role, population, or specialty, are expected to perform competently" (ANA, 2015a, p. 3). They provide a guide to the knowledge, skills, and attitudes (KSAs) that nurses must incorporate into their practice to provide safe, quality care.

- **As a student nurse,** you will use the ANA standards to better define your nursing practice.
- **Practicing nurses** use the standards to judge their own performance, develop an improvement plan, and understand employers' expectations.
- **Employers** may incorporate the standards into annual employee evaluation tools.
- **Professional organizations** use the standards to educate the public about nursing, to plan for continuing education programs for nurses, and to guide their efforts at lobbying and other advocacy activities for nurses.
- **Other professionals** read the standards of practice to examine the boundaries between nursing and their professions.

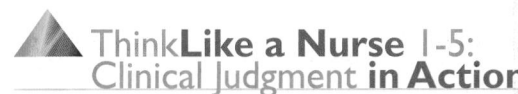 ThinkLike a Nurse 1-5: Clinical Judgment in Action

What do you see as the relationship between the nurse practice acts and nursing values and behaviors (see Box 1-3)?

What Are Some Important Nursing Organizations?
Numerous organizations are involved in the profession of nursing. Some of the most influential are discussed here.

BOX 1-3 ■ Nursing Values and Behaviors

The nurse's primary concern is the good of the client.

Nurses should maintain professional competency.

Nurses demonstrate a strong commitment to service.

Nurses believe in the dignity and worth of each person.

Nurses constantly strive to improve their profession.

Nurses work collaboratively within the profession.

Nurses adhere to a professional code of ethics.

Nurses commit to lifelong learning and professional development.

American Nurses Association

The ANA is the official professional organization for nurses in the United States. The ANA was formed in 1911 from an organization previously known as the Nurses' Associated Alumnae of the United States and Canada. Originally this organization focused on (1) establishing standards of nursing to promote high-quality care and (2) working toward licensure as a means of ensuring adherence to the standards.

The ANA continues to promote the interests of the nursing profession and update its standards. Representatives are elected from the local branches of the state organizations to bring their concerns to the national level. Local representatives

- Track healthcare legislation
- Serve as liaisons with national government representatives
- Communicate the impact of enacted legislation on nursing in their area
- Develop and sponsor legislation expected to have a positive effect on nursing and client care

Additionally, the ANA publishes educational materials on nursing news, issues, and standards. The official publication is *The American Nurse.*

National League for Nursing

Originally founded as the American Society of Superintendents of Training Schools for Nurses in 1893, the National League for Nursing (NLN) was the first nursing organization with a goal to establish and maintain a universal standard of education. The NLN

- Sets standards for all types of nursing education programs
- Studies the nursing workforce
- Lobbies and participates with other major healthcare organizations to set policies for the nursing workforce
- Aids faculty development
- Funds research on nursing education
- Publishes the journal *Nursing Education Perspectives*

International Council of Nurses

The ICN represents more than 27 million nurses on a global scale. It is composed of a federation of national nursing organizations from more than 130 nations. The ICN aims to ensure quality nursing care for all by

- Supporting global health policies that advance nursing and improve worldwide health
- Promoting knowledgeable and respected professionals
- Fostering a competent, satisfied workforce worldwide

National Student Nurses' Association

The National Student Nurses' Association (NSNA) represents nursing students in the United States. It is the student counterpart of the ANA. Like the ANA, this association comprises elected volunteers who advocate on behalf of student nurses. Local chapters are usually organized at individual schools. The official magazine of NSNA, *Imprint,* is dedicated to nursing student issues.

Sigma Theta Tau International

Sigma Theta Tau International (STTI) is the international honor society of nursing. Membership includes the clinical, education, and nursing research communities and senior-level baccalaureate and graduate programs. The goal of STTI is to foster nursing scholarship, leadership, service, and research to improve health worldwide. The official publication of STTI is the *Journal of Nursing Scholarship.*

Specialty Organizations

Numerous specialty organizations have developed around clinical specialties, group identification, or similarly held values. The following are some examples:

- *Clinical specialty*—Association of periOperative Registered Nurses (AORN), Academy of Medical-Surgical Nursing (AMSN), Emergency Nurses Association (ENA)
- *Group identification*—National Association of Hispanic Nurses (NAHN), American Association for Men in Nursing (AAMN), The American Association of Nurse Attorneys (TAANA), National American Arab Nurses Association (NAANA)
- *Similar values*—Nurses Christian Fellowship (NCF), Nursing Ethics Network (NEN)

Nursing Practice: Caring for Clients

Look again at the definitions of the term *nursing* in this chapter (e.g., see Box 1-1). Notice that they all agree that nursing is about caring for clients. **Key Point: *Research trends show that staffing and the educational preparation of the nurse are related to client outcomes.***

- **Hospitals with a higher percentage of baccalaureate-prepared RNs reported lower client complications** (e.g., lower levels of pressure ulcers, client falls, urinary tract infections), shortened length of stays, and better-overall-quality client care (Djukic et al., 2019; Lasater et al., 2021).
- **Smaller nurse-to-client ratios (i.e., when each nurse cared for fewer clients) were also related to positive client outcomes,** lower client mortality, less nurse burnout, and higher job satisfaction for nurses (Ball et al., 2018; Halm, 2019; Hill, 2017).

Nurses also use research results to guide their interventions in planning and implementing evidenced-based practice.

Who Are the Recipients of Nursing Care?

The recipients of nursing care may be individuals, groups, families, or communities. They can be referred to as *patients, clients,* or *persons.*

- **Direct care** involves personal interaction between the nurse and clients (e.g., giving medications or teaching a client about a treatment).

Toward Evidence-Based Practice

Falls among hospitalized patients are a major safety concern. Current nursing practice on fall prevention is grounded in evidence-based research findings that have evolved over time from a single to a multifactorial approach, as demonstrated in the studies that follow.

Brush, B. L., & Capezuti, E. (2001). Historical analysis of siderail use in American hospitals. *Journal of Nursing Scholarship, 33*(4), 381–385. https://doi.org/10.1111/j.1547-5069.2001.00381.x

Siderails became a permanent fixture of the hospital bed as a way to decrease patient falls. Although research identified their negative effects (e.g., siderail-induced injuries, negative physical and emotional consequences of sustained bedrest), siderail use remained the norm in promoting patient safety.

Spoelstra, S. L., Given, B. A., & Given, C. W. (2012). Fall prevention in hospitals: An integrative review. *Clinical Nursing Research, 21*(1), 92–112. https://doi.org/10.1177/1054773811418106

This study found that intervention programs that included a multiple-intervention approach to preventing client falls were more effective than relying on a single intervention. Fall-prevention programs should include staff education, fall-risk assessments, environmental assessments and modifications, alarm systems, and client assistance with transferring and toileting.

Chu, R. (2017). Preventing in-patient falls: The nurse's pivotal role. *Nursing2017, 47*(3), 24–30. https://doi.org/10.1097/01.NURSE.0000512872.83762.69

Evidence-based interventions for fall prevention include an integrated plan that includes identification of high-risk patients (e.g., impaired gait, weak, poor vision); hourly rounding; communication to the team (e.g., report, color-coded bracelets, door signs), to the client (e.g., reinforce use of call device, nurses' role in providing assistance), and to the family (e.g., request assistance from nursing staff); bed in low position; bed alarms;

and low nurse-to-patient ratios. In addition, centralized video monitoring decreased falls and is cost-effective.

Turner, K., Staggs, V. S., Potter, C., Cramer, E., Shorr, R. I., & Mion, L. C. (2022). Fall prevention practices and implementation strategies: Examining consistency across hospital units. *Journal of Patient Safety, 18*(1), e236–e242. https://doi.org/10.1097/PTS.0000000000000758.

Researchers investigated the consistency of fall-prevention practices and implementation strategies among medical and medical-surgical units across U.S. hospitals. The results revealed that resource-intensive strategies (hourly rounding, scheduled toileting, staying with patient in the bathroom) were used less consistently than less nonintensive ones (signage, patient bracelet, room door open). Among patient safety practices, nonskid socks and an accessible call light were used more consistently than having ambulatory aids accessible and ensuring a clutter-free floor. Maintaining the bed in a locked, lowered position, with an alarm and bedside commode, took precedence over a specialty low bed and bedside floor mat. The most-used quality management strategy was to increase awareness (posting fall rates, using dashboards), in contrast to feedback strategies (post-fall huddles among nurses and the interdisciplinary team, conduction of post-fall audits). Equipment (specialty low beds, bed/chair alarms) was more commonly used than people (sitters, replacement nursing personnel) to support fall-prevention efforts. Although the value of a multicomponent approach is recognized, considerable variations in the implementation of fall-prevention practices and implementation strategies exist among hospitals.

1. What current trends and factors might influence whether siderail use, as a fall-prevention strategy, will change in the near future?

2. What strategies would you include in a fall-prevention program?

3. What should be the focus of future research to decrease falls in hospitalized patients?

- **Indirect care** is working on behalf of clients to improve their health status (e.g., ordering unit supplies or serving on an ethics committee).

A nurse may use independent judgment to determine the care needed or may work under the direct order of a primary care provider. As a nurse, you should view clients as active recipients of care. **Key Point:** *Your role is to encourage clients to actively participate in decisions about their care and to collaborate with members of their healthcare teams.*

What Are the Purposes of Nursing Care?
Nurses provide care to achieve the goals of health promotion, illness prevention, health restoration, and end-of-life care. Together, these aspects of care represent a

range of services that cover the health spectrum from complete well-being to death. Nurses

- Plan to ensure consistency of client care over time.
- Individualize care according to client needs.
- Ensure that holistic care is provided.
- Collaborate with the interprofessional health team for optimal client outcomes.

Where Do Nurses Work?
As a nurse, you will have the opportunity to work in a variety of settings. As a student, you will have assignments in many settings and environments that will allow you to see some of the options available to you after you obtain your nursing license. Approximately 61% of nurses work in hospitals. Others work in extended

care facilities, providers' offices, ambulatory care, home health, correctional facilities, public health, the military, or schools (U.S. Bureau of Labor Statistics, 2021b).

What Models of Care Are Used to Provide Nursing Care?

Nursing care is structured in various ways. The organization of the nursing team reflects the philosophy and beliefs of the facility, as well as its prevailing views on nursing. The structure of the team is often referred to as the *model of care.* The most common models include the following:

Case Method This is also called *total care.* **Case method** is one-to-one care; one nurse provides all aspects of care for one client during a single shift. In this method, the nurse and client work more closely together, the client's needs are quickly met, and the nurse has a greater degree of autonomy. Although satisfying for clients and nurses, the high costs limit its widespread use. The case method is used mainly in intensive care units (ICUs), labor and delivery, and private-duty care.

Functional Nursing This requires a clear understanding of what tasks each member may perform (scope of practice). In **functional nursing,** care is compartmentalized, with each task assigned to a staff member with the appropriate knowledge and skills. For example, the RN is in charge and performs complex treatments, the LPN/LVN may distribute medications, and the nursing assistant may give bed baths and make beds. Although this approach is economical and efficient, it can make it difficult for the nurse to have the "whole picture" of the client and may result in fragmentation of care.

Team Nursing This approach is efficient. It maintains the cost savings of functional nursing while limiting fragmentation. In **team nursing,** a licensed nurse (RN or LPN/LVN) is paired with an unlicensed assistive personnel (UAP). The team is then assigned to a group of clients. Teams led by RNs are assigned to high-acuity clients. Team nursing maximizes the contributions of each team member to provide safe, high-quality client care (Parreira et al., 2021). The team model, with its focus on levels of nursing proficiency, provided the foundation for establishing a pyramid staffing model to meet the needs of ICU patients during the COVID-19 hospitalization surge (Perlstein et al., 2021).

Primary Nursing With this method, one nurse manages care for a group of clients. Primary nurses assess the client, develop a plan of care, and provide care while at work. Associate nurses deliver care and implement the plan developed by the primary nurse when the primary nurse is not available.

Differentiated Practice A variation of primary care, differentiated practice recognizes that education and experience lead to differences in the care delivered by nurses. Each unit identifies the type of expertise needed by the clients and the nursing competencies required to deliver that care. Individual nurses develop a portfolio of their competencies and are assigned to clients who need those particular competencies.

THE HEALTHCARE DELIVERY SYSTEM

The healthcare delivery system in the United States is a complex collection of clients, providers, facilities, vendors, and rules. The rest of this chapter is designed to help you gain a beginner's understanding of this system. You will need to know the components of the system to understand the continuum of healthcare that clients receive, the providers involved in that care, and the factors that influence the type and amount of care that clients receive.

What Types of Care Are Provided?

Clients can receive acute care or long-term support services.

- **Acute care** is defined as the services used to "treat active sudden, often unexpected, urgent or emergent episodes of injury and illness that can lead to death or disability without rapid intervention (Hirshon et al., 2013, pg 386)." The six domains of acute care are (1) trauma care and acute care surgery, (2) emergency care, (3) urgent care, (4) short-term stabilization, (5) prehospital care, and (6) critical care. The goal is to prevent deterioration and restore health (Hirshon et al., 2013).
- **Long-term support services** (LTSSs) is an array of services provided to individuals with long-term chronic conditions, disabilities, or frailty and encompasses "human assistance, assistive technologies and devices, environmental modifications, care and service coordination (Nguyen, 2017)" on a regular or intermittent basis (Hado et al., 2019; Nguyen, 2017). LTSSs are provided in a variety of nonhospital settings, such as extended care facilities, ambulatory care centers, and home healthcare agencies.

Clients are classified based on their admission status:

- **Inpatient** refers to a client who has been admitted to a healthcare facility. The length of stay is limited to the amount of time that the client requires 24-hour care.
- **Outpatient** refers to a client who receives treatment at a healthcare facility but does not stay overnight.

Where Is Care Provided?

The client's medical condition determines where care is provided. Acute care is provided in hospitals. Once stabilized, the client is discharged to home or, if further care is needed, to an extended care facility. The various types of care facilities are discussed next.

Hospitals

Hospitals are the most expensive and the most frequently used site for care. They provide a broad range of services to treat various injuries and disease processes (Fig. 1-2). Hospitals vary in size, ownership, and the services provided. Smaller hospitals offer basic services, whereas larger medical centers usually have an emergency department, diagnostic centers, and other units, such as intensive care, medical, surgical, pediatrics, and maternal/newborn. Hospitals employ a variety of healthcare providers (e.g., nurses, allied health therapists, hospitalists, case managers, pharmacists) to meet the around-the-clock needs of acute care clients.

Extended Care Facilities

- **Extended care facilities** provide long-term care and support that can range from a few months to a lifetime. As the length of stay in hospitals continues to decline, extended care facilities deliver services that were previously provided in hospitals. **Key Point: *The distinction among extended care facilities is based primarily on whether they provide skilled or custodial care.***
- **Skilled care** includes the services of trained professionals that are needed for a limited period of time after an injury or illness (e.g., wound care, IV infusions). Clients are expected to improve with these treatments.
- **Custodial care,** in contrast, consists of help with activities of daily living: bathing, dressing, eating, grooming, ambulation, toileting, and other care that people typically do for themselves (e.g., taking medications, monitoring blood glucose levels).

The use of extended care facilities will continue to increase because of the aging population and increased longevity of clients with traumatic injuries and chronic diseases (Nguyen, 2017). Residents in extended care facilities are commonly older adults, but clients of any age who require assistance with self-care activities may live in these facilities. Extended care is delivered in nursing homes, skilled nursing facilities (also known as *convalescent hospitals*), and rehabilitation facilities.

Nursing Homes These facilities provide custodial care for people who cannot live on their own but are not sick enough to require hospitalization. They may be permanent homes for people who require continual supervision to ensure their safety. Various services are offered to residents, such as recreational activities and salon services.

Rehabilitation Centers These facilities provide extended care and treatment for clients with physical and mental illness. Rehabilitation involves an interprofessional, collaborative approach, with weekly team and family conferences to discuss the treatment plan. Types of services include alcohol and drug rehabilitation, physical rehabilitation services for clients who have experienced traumatic injuries, and rehabilitation of clients after stroke or heart attack. Nurses have an ongoing relationship with their clients due to the lengthy time of treatment.

Assisted Living Facilities These were designed to bridge the gap between independence and institutionalization for older adults who have a decline in health status and cannot live independently. Residents of these facilities are able to perform self-care activities but require assistance with meals, housekeeping, or medications. Nurses have a limited presence at assisted living sites because skilled care is usually not required.

Ambulatory Care Centers

Ambulatory (or outpatient) care centers offer cost-effective healthcare to clients who are able to come and go from the facility for same-day or special services (e.g., chemotherapy, dialysis, surgery). Ambulatory care sites include medical offices, urgent care clinics, retail clinics, outpatient therapy centers, and hospitals (Fig. 1-3).

Home Healthcare Agencies

After hospitalization, **home healthcare agencies** provide continuing care to clients in their homes. Services

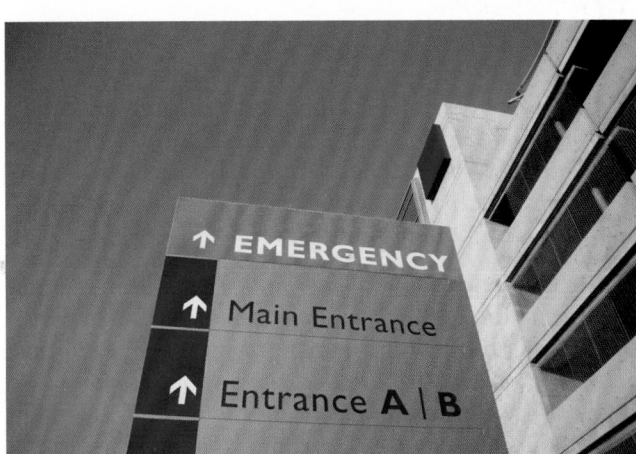

FIGURE I-2 Emergency departments may be the primary source of healthcare for many individuals.

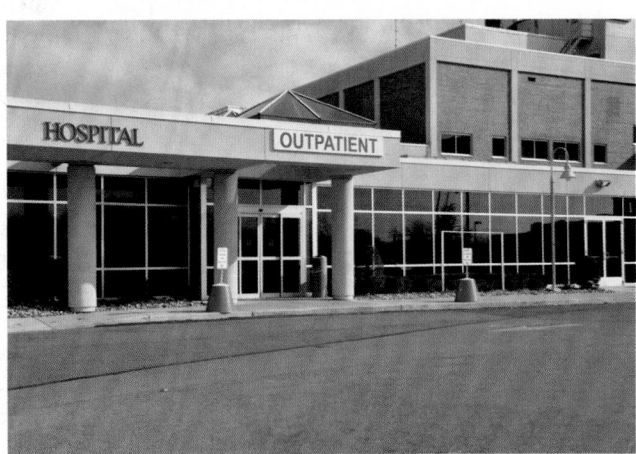

FIGURE I-3 The shift to outpatient care is a cost-saving strategy.

are usually coordinated by a home health or visiting nurse service and include nursing care as well as various therapies (e.g., physical, respiratory) and home assistance programs. Chapter 38, Community and Home Health Nursing, provides further discussion on home health nursing.

Community/Public Health Centers

Community or public health centers are community-based centers that provide care for the community at large. Community health nurses provide services to at-risk populations and devise strategies to improve the health status of the surrounding community (e.g., school-based pregnancy reduction programs, healthcare for the homeless). Community care is provided to client groups at various sites, such as churches, schools, shelters, workplaces, and public clinics. Chapter 38 provides further discussion of community healthcare.

Independent Living Facilities

Also known as *retirement homes,* **independent living facilities** are designed for seniors 55 years or older who (1) are independent in all aspects and (2) want to live in a community with other senior citizens. Services usually include a peer support network that provides socialization opportunities, structured recreational activities, transportation arrangements, fitness centers, pools, and quiet environments. Living facilities range from apartment-style homes to smaller separate residential homes. Nurses may provide periodic health screening and health information.

How Is Healthcare Categorized?

Because the boundaries of care have become fluid, it is useful to look at the system in a different light. **Key Point:** *The complexity of care is no longer a predictor of where care will be delivered. Instead, regulators, finances, and the client's support system dictate where a client will be located in the system.* On a basic level, healthcare is categorized as primary, secondary, and tertiary based on the complexity and the type of services needed.

Primary Services

Nursing and Health Promotion In 1948, the World Health Organization (WHO) defined health as "a state of complete physical, mental, and social well-being and not merely the absence of disease or infirmity." The definition has not been amended since that time (WHO, 2006). Health-promotion activities foster the highest state of well-being of the recipient of the activities. The following are examples:

- *Individual level*—Counseling a pregnant client about the importance of adequate prenatal nutrition to promote health for the client and baby

- *Group and family level*—Teaching about nutrition during pregnancy in family education programs
- *Community level*—Advocating for prominent billboards highlighting the importance of prenatal care and nutrition; posting signs in grocery stores recommending the best foods for pregnant women
- *Societal level*—Working with international partners to establish worldwide prenatal nutrition standards

Nursing and Illness Prevention The focus of illness prevention is the avoidance of disease, infection, and other comorbidities. Activities are targeted to minimize the risk of development of or exposure to disease. For example, pneumonia causes many deaths every year. It affects society's most vulnerable: the very young, the very old, and the very ill. Some nursing activities to decrease the risk of pneumonia include the following:

- Teaching the importance of hand hygiene
- Advocating for and administering pneumonia immunizations, especially to those at high risk
- Promoting smoking cessation
- Promoting adequate nutrition, including a diet high in vitamin C, to increase the person's resistance to the disease should exposure occur

Secondary Services

Secondary services are directed toward early diagnosis and treatment of illness, disease, and injury. Increasingly, these services are being performed in surgery centers, offices, and outpatient centers. The trend away from the hospital is related to containing costs, increasing specialization of hospitals, and growing evidence that hospitals often harbor medication-resistant infectious organisms.

Nursing and Health Restoration Health-restoration activities foster a return to health for those already ill. The nurse provides direct care to ill individuals, groups, families, or communities to restore their health. The nursing role includes addressing the physical, mental, spiritual, and social dimensions of client care.

Tertiary Services

Tertiary services refer to long-term rehabilitation services and care for the dying. Historically, these services were provided in extended care facilities. Now, however, many tertiary care services are provided in the home or in outpatient settings.

Nursing and End-of-Life Care Death is an inevitable destination on the journey of life. Nurses work with dying individuals, their family members and support persons, and organizations (hospice) that focus on the needs of the terminally ill to promote comfort, maintain quality of life, provide culturally relevant spiritual care, maintain dignity, and ease the emotional burden of death (see Chapter 14).

KnowledgeCheck 1-3

Recall the last time that you had a cold. Identify health-promotion, illness-prevention, and health-restoration activities for individuals, families, groups, and communities in relation to the common cold.

Who Are the Members of the Interprofessional Healthcare Team?

As a nurse, you will be part of an interprofessional healthcare team consisting of numerous professionals whose primary role is to ensure quality client outcomes (Fig. 1-4). The composition of the team varies depending on the healthcare needs of the client. Each provider's role in the health team is covered in the discussion that follows.

- **Physicians** are licensed as medical doctors (MDs) or doctors of osteopathy (DOs). Their primary role is to diagnose and treat disease and illness through medical and surgical services. A physician may work independently, as part of a medical group, as an employee of a health facility, or as a hospitalist who leads the medical team to coordinate care for inpatients.
- **Nurse practitioners (NPs)** are independent practitioners with advanced education and training and are licensed to provide a broad range of medical and nursing care based on their specialty area. NPs engage in activities ranging from health promotion to caring for clients with acute or chronic healthcare problems. They can practice independently or in collaboration with a provider.
- **Physician assistants (PAs)** practice under the supervision of a physician to diagnose and prescribe treatments and medications to treat certain diseases and injuries. As an extension of the physician, nurses are permitted to follow a PA's prescriptions, unless this is prohibited by the state's nurse practice act or policies and procedures.

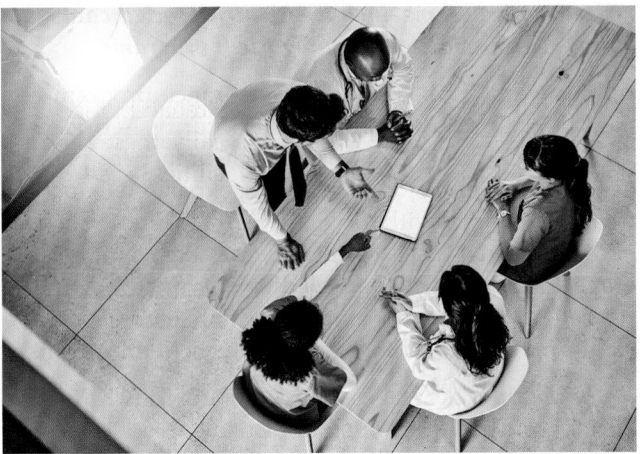

FIGURE 1-4 Quality client outcomes require the collaboration of the entire healthcare team.

- **RNs** assess clients, administer treatments and medications, provide education, and modify nursing care plans based on client responses to treatment. They have the most direct contact with clients and provide holistic, continuous, and comprehensive nursing care.
- **LPNs** work under the supervision of the RN to provide noncomplex care, administer certain medications, and communicate client responses.
- **UAP** is a broad term that covers nursing assistants, aides, and technicians. UAPs provide custodial care under the direction of nurses and providers in a variety of settings. **Key Point:** *Some UAPs introduce themselves to clients by stating, "I'm your nurse." Because they are not licensed nurses, they are making a false claim. Be sure to clarify your role and the UAP's role with all of your clients.*
- **Pharmacists** prepare and dispense medications and therapeutic solutions in various health settings. They function as the leaders in pharmacological therapy. Pharmacists provide information about medication contraindications, side effects and adverse reactions, dosage, and administration tips. They also collaborate with nurses, providers, and other health-team members to ensure the selection of safe and effective medications in the treatment plan. Pharmacy assistants serve as support personnel for pharmacists.
- **Therapists** focus on a variety of rehabilitative needs of the client. The goal of the rehabilitative team is to treat and maximize functioning and/or assist the client in adapting to limitations and achieving optimal outcomes. Types of therapists include the following:
  - *Physiatrists* function as the rehabilitative team leaders to improve mobility and strength and teach motor skills.
  - *Physical therapists* (PTs) focus on the rehabilitation of muscles and bones to help clients use assistive devices and gain self-care skills for activities of daily living.
  - *Occupational therapists* (OTs) work closely with PTs to help clients regain function and independence in everyday activities (e.g., work, school, social skills).
  - *Respiratory therapists* (RTs) provide prescribed treatments for effective respiration and ventilation (e.g., oxygen therapy, mechanical ventilation).
  - *Speech and language therapists* (SLTs) provide assistance to clients experiencing swallowing and speech disturbances from developmental or neurological impairment.
  - *Recreational therapists* use leisure activities to promote the physical, social, and emotional well-being of clients.
  - *Marriage and family therapists* provide counseling services to individuals, families, and groups.
- **Technologists** perform selected activities in hospitals, diagnostic centers, and emergency care facilities (e.g., laboratory technologists, radiology technologists).
- **Registered dietitians/licensed nutritionists** apply specialized knowledge of nutrition science to plan

food treatments and goals to promote client health and treat illnesses.

- **Social workers** throughout healthcare systems provide psychosocial support and client services and coordinate continuity of care for clients after discharge.
- **Spiritual care providers** offer organized religious services, client visits, and family and staff support, particularly with serious illness or at the end of life.
- **Alternative care providers,** such as chiropractors, naturopaths, and herbalists, offer health services that are primarily outside the traditional healthcare system.

How Is Healthcare Financed?

Payers for healthcare in the United States include individuals, individual private insurance, employment-based group private insurance, the government, and charitable sources.

Individuals

Individuals are responsible for the costs of their healthcare services. We refer to payments made directly by individuals as *direct payment of services* and *out-of-pocket expenses*. Individuals with private or government insurance pay for services through cost sharing in the form of *insurance deductibles, copayments,* and coinsurance. **Key Point: *Individuals with and without insurance sometimes avoid or delay services because they cannot afford to pay the direct cost of services or the high cost-sharing out-of-pocket expenses.***

Individual Private Insurance

Insurance is intended to protect persons from "medical bankruptcy" associated with the costs incurred by a major medical event (Fig. 1-5). It protects individuals from having to pay the entire costs associated with illness and hospitalization. A person with private insurance pays premiums to an insurance company. The insurance company then contracts with healthcare

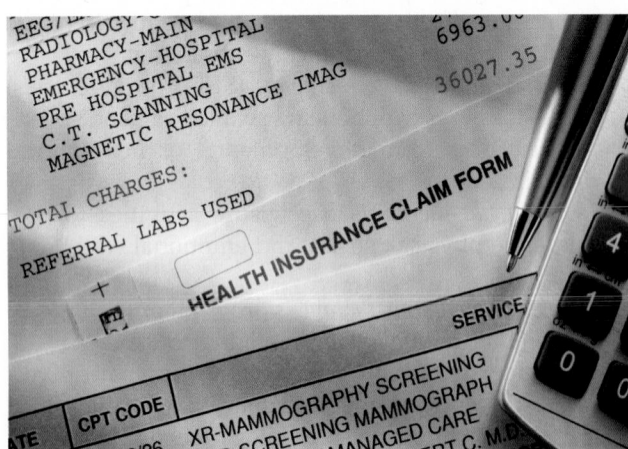

FIGURE I-5 The high cost of healthcare is a barrier to early screening and prevention.

providers to deliver care to insured members at prearranged rates. Insured individuals are encouraged to obtain routine care from their provider to prevent additional out-of-pocket expenses. The costs associated with seeking nonemergency care at an emergency room can be 15 times higher than those for seeking treatment at the provider's office or at an urgent care facility (UHG, 2017).

Employment-Based Private Insurance

Most private insurance in the United States is employment based, meaning the employer pays all or a portion of the costs (e.g., premiums) under a group plan that lowers costs. Because payment of employment-based insurance premiums is a major-cost fringe-benefit expense for employers, more costs are being shifted to employees. In the United States, the average annual total premium per enrolled employee was $7,149, with the employer paying $5,617 (79%) and the employee paying $1,532 (21%; Kaiser Foundation, 2021). The cost of family coverage is much higher. The employer can deduct the costs of health insurance premiums as a business expense. In addition, healthy employees benefit employers because of reduced sick time and a full workforce to maintain productivity.

Organization or Association Group Insurance

Individuals can also obtain group insurance through organizations or associations. The AARP (formerly the American Association of Retired Persons) is an example of a group whose members share the cost of health insurance. Many of these organizations or associations contract with a third-party insurance vendor to offer their members health insurance. Having more members who pay premiums helps to lower the overall cost of individual premiums.

Government (Public) Financing

Key Point: *Government-funded programs are paid for with revenue from federal, state, and local taxes on the citizenry. Programs include Medicare; Medicaid; and children's, specialty, and categorical programs.*

Medicare This is a federal insurance program created by Title XVIII of the Social Security Act of 1965. This act was designed to provide insurance for persons aged 65 years and older. It was later expanded to include younger people with permanent disabilities, such as end-stage renal disease, but provides only limited coverage for long-term care. Medicare is financed from a payroll tax levied on employers and employees and from premiums paid by Medicare subscribers (clients).

Medicaid This was developed under Title XIX of the Social Security Act of 1965 to provide access to healthcare services for individuals with low incomes and minimal resources. Medicaid is a joint federal and state program; therefore, the eligibility criteria for Medicaid and the range of medical services offered vary from state to state. Medicaid offers a fairly comprehensive set of benefits, including prescription drugs, skilled care, and long-term care.

Children's Health Insurance Program (CHIP) CHIP is a joint federal and state program. It provides health insurance to millions of children whose families have income levels that exceed Medicaid eligibility criteria but who cannot afford private insurance and whose children are not covered under a parent's policy. CHIP's goal is to ensure that children have health insurance and can access healthcare, either through an expansion of Medicaid or the development of a separate program. The continuation of CHIP is not guaranteed because it is based on federal and state funding that is subject to budgetary allocations.

Specialty and Categorical Programs Categorical programs are designated by federal laws to provide access to healthcare for certain categories of people, such as immigrants or children in Head Start programs. *Specialty programs* target certain populations (e.g., Indian Health Service, military personnel and dependents).

KnowledgeCheck 1-4
- Compare and contrast private and government-funded health insurance.
- How might being uninsured affect a person's health status?

Charitable Organizations
Charitable organizations are an increasingly important funding source for healthcare. Community agencies that are funded through networks such as the United Way, Salvation Army, and Red Cross provide important resources to children, poor families, the aged, and vulnerable populations (e.g., the homeless, mentally ill, and victims of violence). Charitable organizations provide direct services and cover the costs for some traditional health services.

How Are Supplies and Equipment Provided?
Suppliers are the companies and corporations that bring goods to the healthcare industry. Pharmaceutical companies and medical equipment suppliers are the largest suppliers. The costs associated with the research, development, and testing of pharmaceuticals and medical equipment are passed on to consumers in the form of higher prices, rising insurance premiums, and increased out-of-pocket expenses.

How Is Healthcare Regulated?
Regulators are governing bodies that exert influence or control over the healthcare system or preparation of healthcare providers. They include accrediting agencies (e.g., Accreditation Commission for Education in Nursing, Commission on Collegiate Nursing Education, Commission for Nursing Education Accreditation), licensing agencies (boards of nursing), and legislators. The most prominent regulating body in the healthcare system is The Joint Commission, which establishes standards for hospitals to promote client safety. Legislators also affect the healthcare system by redefining eligibility criteria for government-funded health plans or establishing minimum nurse–client ratios in acute care hospitals.

How Have Healthcare Reform Efforts Affected Care?
Healthcare reform has affected not only access to care but also reimbursement rates for providers. The following are examples.

Affordable Care Act (ACA)
The Affordable Care Act (ACA), implemented in 2010, had a major impact in providing access to health insurance and thus healthcare. The number of uninsured people reached a historical low of 26.7 million in 2016 compared with 44.2 million in 2013 (Garfield et al., 2019). The number of people obtaining health coverage under ACA programs reached a record 31 million in 2021 (U.S. Department of Health and Human Services [USDHHS], 2021). People with insurance are more likely to seek essential primary care, such as screenings, chronic illness follow-ups, and prenatal care.

Medicare and Public Policy
When Medicare was initially created, health services were reimbursed using a **retrospective system** that paid hospitals based on the actual cost of providing services to individuals. With no cap on expenses, Medicare payments made to hospitals increased from $3 billion in the early years of the program to $37 billion by 1983.

To slow the rising costs of healthcare, a **prospective reimbursement system** was created under the Social Security Amendments of 1983. Hospitals were reimbursed on a per-case, flat-rate basis determined by client groups having similar needs. These groups were called **diagnostic-related groups (DRGs).** If the client's hospital costs were greater than the reimbursed ("set") amounts, the hospital lost money. If the costs were less than the rate set by Medicare, the hospital made a profit. Private insurance companies, following the lead of Medicare, reimbursed in the same manner.

The introduction of DRGs forced hospitals to consider new ways of delivering care and created a number of changes in client care, such as the following:

- *The length of stay in hospitals decreased dramatically* as care moved away from hospitals and out into the community and home.
- *The cost of delivering nursing care became an expenditure.* As a result, team nursing with UAPs replaced the

comprehensive care provided by RNs at the bedside, even though research consistently supports fewer adverse client outcomes with a higher proportion of RNs on staff.

- *Fewer choices for care resulted from corporate mergers and acquisitions* in large regional facilities (e.g., fewer hospitals and nursing homes in a community).
- *Reduced staffing and higher client acuity produced a more stressful work environment for nurses.*
- *Insurance premiums and cost-sharing increased, whereas availability of services decreased.* This led to a growing number of people who could not afford needed care.

Managed Care

Managed care, designed to control healthcare costs, is a competitive approach to healthcare pricing. A managed care organization (MCO) contracts with medical providers to provide services at discounted rates or based on a predetermined fixed payment per individual covered under the plan (capitation). An employer contracts with the MCO and selects a type of health plan for its employees. The most common types of managed care plans are described next.

Health Maintenance Organizations (HMOs) HMOs are a model of care based on **capitated** (per head) costs. Each HMO primary care provider receives a predetermined, fixed amount each month, regardless of whether the client receives healthcare services or not. The primary care provider coordinates all care, including referrals to specialists. Providers often choose to be part of an HMO because of the steady income it offers. HMOs are the least costly plans available, but the HMO will pay only for specified services and only if the client uses a provider on the HMO list ("in the network").

Preferred Provider Organizations (PPOs) The PPO has many of the features of an HMO, such as a network of providers who will provide healthcare at the established contracted rate. Compared with HMOs, the client pays more in premiums, deductibles, and coinsurance; however, the client has greater choice among in-network providers (including specialists), medications, and devices. Clients pay higher costs for out-of-network providers.

Point of Service (POS) POS combines features from HMOs and PPOs. The client selects a physician from a list of network physicians who will be the POS for treatment and referrals to in-network specialists. There is limited out-of-network coverage, with higher coinsurance and copay rates.

Integrated Delivery Networks (IDNs) IDNs are a consolidation of services into one healthcare system. Providers see only IDN clients, in IDN facilities, using IDN services and IDN-approved pharmaceuticals. The system is designed to promote a culture of collaboration, safety, and teamwork among the providers and limit barriers to services for clients (Feinberg et al., 2018).

What Are the Issues Related to Healthcare Reform?

The profound changes created by the transition of the healthcare system from a retrospective to a prospective fixed-rate payment system have created unprecedented leadership opportunities for nurse executives.

ANA Principles for Health System Transformation

In 2016, the ANA outlined several principles for transforming the health system:

- The need to ensure universal access to a standard package of essential healthcare services for all
- Provision of an adequate supply of skilled workers to provide quality healthcare services
- Promotion of ways to stimulate economical use of healthcare services that supports individuals who have limited resources to share in costs
- Optimization of primary, community-based, and preventive services that integrate the economical use of innovative, technology-driven, acute, hospital-based services

Work Redesign

Work redesign involves looking at the level of care required and the mix of personnel necessary to achieve the best client outcomes. The following concepts emerged:

- **Critical pathways** is an interprofessional approach that outlines the direction of client care. Based on scientific evidence, critical pathways allow the interprofessional team to implement best practices that yield the desired outcomes in the quickest manner to reduce the client's length of stay (Stark, 2019). (See Chapter 3 for more information on critical pathways.)
- **Case management** is the coordination of care across the healthcare system. Case managers assess clients, develop care goals, identify resources, and manage outcomes. Many hospitals, home health agencies, and insurance companies employ nurse case managers to ensure that a client receives efficient, quality care using the most cost-effective resources while hospitalized and after discharge.

Is Healthcare a Right or a Privilege?

Underlying all healthcare reform is the fundamental question of whether healthcare is a right or a privilege. This question raises more questions. For example, if healthcare is a right of all citizens, should noncitizens be offered coverage? Moreover, what responsibility does an individual have to preserve their own health through lifestyle changes (e.g., diet, exercise)? Should extensive and/or expensive therapies be offered if they have little likelihood of success? Finally, if you believe that healthcare should be affordable for all, are you willing to limit your salary and benefits to help control the costs of care? Are you willing to pay higher taxes? These fundamental questions will continue to emerge as debates on universal healthcare continue to evolve.

KnowledgeCheck 1-5

- Do you agree with the ANA's principle that a healthcare system "must ensure access to a standard package of essential healthcare services for all citizens and residents" (ANA, 2016)?
- What factors influence your answer to the previous question? (Draw on your self-knowledge to answer this question.)

How Do Providers and Facilities Ensure Quality Care?

As you learned previously, a number of accrediting bodies inspect healthcare organizations to ensure that clients receive safe, quality care. To promote safety, regulators establish a minimum competency level that must be met to receive accreditation. However, most healthcare organizations and professionals identify a goal of *excellent* care rather than merely meeting minimum standards.

Continuous Quality Improvement Programs

Continuous quality improvement (CQI) programs, used interchangeably with *total quality management* (TQM), focus on quality (excellent) care as an ongoing goal through an evaluation process that identifies problems, develops solutions, implements corrective plans, and evaluates effectiveness. Although CQI is a system-level approach, different methods are used at the unit level to promote quality improvement:

- **Process reviews** look at issues related to guidelines, policies, or procedures related to the delivery of care. For example, a CQI committee wants to reduce the time it takes nurses to implement all fall precautions based on the client's risk level. The committee may recommend a new process and evaluate the outcomes to determine whether it was efficient and cost-effective.
- **Outcome reviews** are conducted to determine whether the desired outcome was achieved and the influence of environmental or system factors. For example, a unit may set a goal that 100% of nurses' notes will state the reason why medication was not administered. If a retrospective audit of those records indicates the goal was not met, the evaluation process is initiated.
- **Structure reviews** investigate the adequacy, availability, and quality of resources (e.g., nursing personnel, supplies, bed capacity) and their effect on processes and outcomes.

For more information on the quality improvement process, see the accompanying SENC box, Quality Improvement Competency.

Quality Improvement Competency

Chapter Key Concept: Healthcare Delivery System

Competency: Provide Safe, Quality Client Care

Question. Based on work done by the Institute of Medicine (now the National Academy of Medicine), this textbook identifies quality improvement (QI) as a competency you should achieve during your nursing education. QI includes the ability to "evaluate and use techniques/processes to avoid medical/nursing errors" and to evaluate the framework used for care delivery, incorporating structure, process, and outcomes of the care. How do you think the staffing mix in a hospital might affect care quality?

Research. Recent research shows that when the proportion of registered nurses (RNs) increases in an agency, the quality of care rises, and rates of death, falls, missed nursing care, and infection drop. Consider the following examples from various research findings (Aiken et al., 2017; Lasater et al., 2021; Leary et al., 2016; Livanos, 2018; Shang et al., 2019):

- Replacing six support workers with RNs on high-fall units significantly reduced patient falls.
- Higher client mortality rates, falls, and medication administration errors were associated with lower nursing staffing levels.
- The risk of mortality significantly increased with high bed occupancies and client transfers; however, an increase in the number of nurses decreased this risk. In addition, higher workloads were associated with increased client mortality.
- Hospitals with a higher proportion of RNs on staff performed better on a variety of performance measures, including decreased patient infections and shorter lengths of stay.
- An increase in the number of temporary RN staff members was associated with an increased rate of client falls and injuries.

Think about it: How does the SENC competency of quality improvement relate to the chapter's key concept: healthcare delivery system?

FACTORS THAT INFLUENCE CONTEMPORARY NURSING PRACTICE

Factors that influence nursing practice include societal factors at large as well as factors within nursing and healthcare.

What Are Some Trends in Society?

In addition to our historical roots, nursing is influenced by trends in the economy—the growing number of older adults, increased consumer knowledge, legislation, the women's movement, and collective bargaining.

The National Economy

The national economy has a tremendous impact on nursing. Consider the following examples:

- *Historically, in the United States, health insurance coverage has been linked to full-time employment with health insurance benefits.* When the unemployment rate increases, the number of people without health insurance also increases. Uninsured people often delay seeking treatment or use the emergency department for healthcare. The ACA, which expanded health insurance coverage for unemployed persons, resulted in a greater demand for care and for more advanced practice nurses.

- *Recessions can affect the nursing workforce.* During recessions, many nurses at retirement age often remain employed, thus decreasing available positions for new nurse graduates. As the economy improves, these nurses retire, which can create a shortage of registered nurses.

- *The healthcare system employs an enormous number and variety of people.* In 2021, registered nurses numbered 5.1 million (NCSBN, 2022); physicians and surgeons, 1 million (Michas, 2021); pharmacists, 315,470 (Mikulic, 2021); and APRNs, 325,000 (American Association of Nurse Practitioners [AANP], 2021). Looking at these numbers, you begin to understand how large the healthcare system is when all other providers are added to the count.

The Growing Proportion of Older Adults in the United States

In 2019, 54.1 million individuals were 65 years and older (Centers for Disease Control and Prevention [CDC], 2022). This number is expected to increase to 80.8 million in 2040 and to 94.7 million in 2060. By 2030, baby boomers will have reached age 65 years and older, and by 2034, they will outnumber children under the age of 18 years for the first time in U.S. history (U.S. Census Bureau, 2019). The ratio of retired to working adults will have significant implications for the federal and state revenues used to fund healthcare programs and the healthcare system.

Changes in Healthcare Consumers

Historically, clients relied on the knowledge and decision making of the healthcare team. Now, however, consumers are demanding greater choice in the decisions that affect their health.

- *Clients have access to vast amounts of health and medical information, particularly through the Internet.* Informed consumers tend to be active participants in discussions about their health problems and therapy options. Clients need to be taught which sites are valid for finding information.

- *Direct-to-consumer marketing is another form of health information* in which corporations advertise medications and therapies, with ads directed at potential users (e.g., Internet, magazines, television). You need to educate and present balanced information to clients, particularly as it is appropriate for their conditions. **Key Point: *You must also be comfortable with your knowledge and not be unduly persuaded by consumers who may be relying on the latest fads. Your knowledge, standards of nursing practice, and communications with the healthcare team should be the foundation for making client-related decisions.***

Legislation

Consumer interest sometimes generates legislation that affects nursing care. Legislation directed at the confidentiality of client records, treating clients who need emergency care (Emergency Medical Treatment and Labor Act [EMTALA]), the client's right to know (informed consent), and the client's right to a dignified death (living will/advance directives) all govern the care that nurses render to clients. Such legislation is discussed further in Chapters 5 and 39.

Gender Diversity in Nursing

Traditionally, nursing was one of the few career options available to women. Over the centuries, changes in societal norms and beliefs expanded career opportunities for both women and men. As occupations became open to all people, men entered the nursing profession, with men currently comprising 13% of licensed nurses (Fig. 1-6).

Collective Bargaining

Collective bargaining, a form of negotiating conducted by unions or organizations, has resulted in significant improvements in wages, benefits, and working conditions for nurses as a group, as well as safer conditions for clients. These improvements have made nursing more attractive as a career choice. Not all states have collective-bargaining groups for nursing.

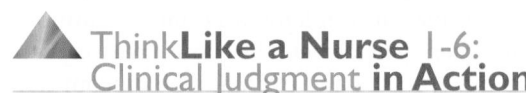

ThinkLike a Nurse 1-6: Clinical Judgment in Action

How do you think changes in healthcare consumers may affect your interactions with clients?

What Are Some Trends in Nursing and Healthcare?

In addition to societal factors, trends in nursing and healthcare also affect contemporary practice. We discuss some of those trends here.

Increased Use of Complementary and Alternative Medicine

Treatments or services outside the traditional healthcare system are known as **complementary and alternative medicine (CAM).** They include medical systems, such

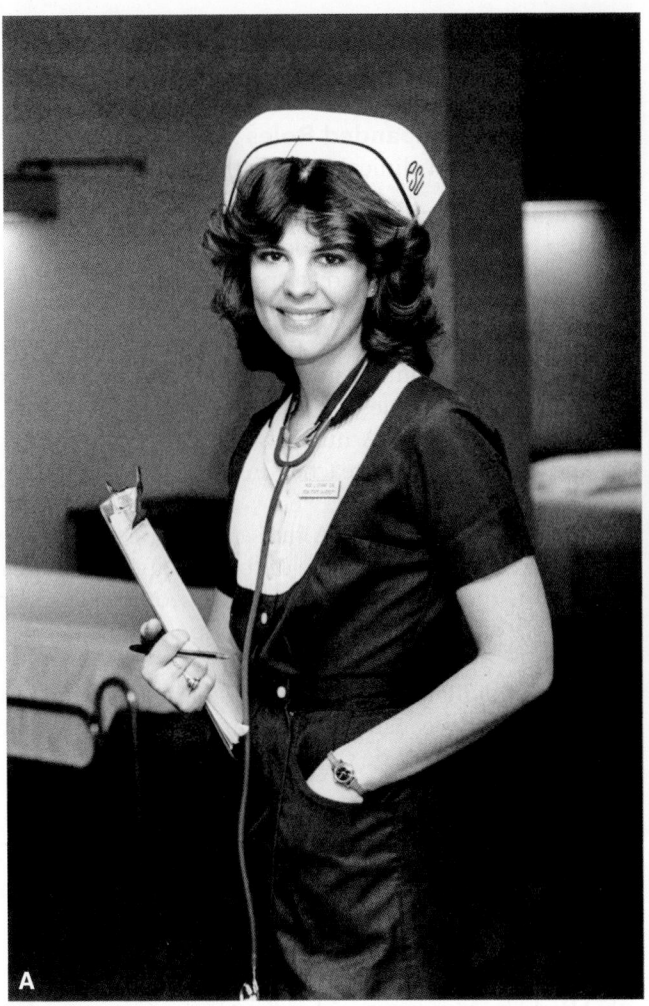
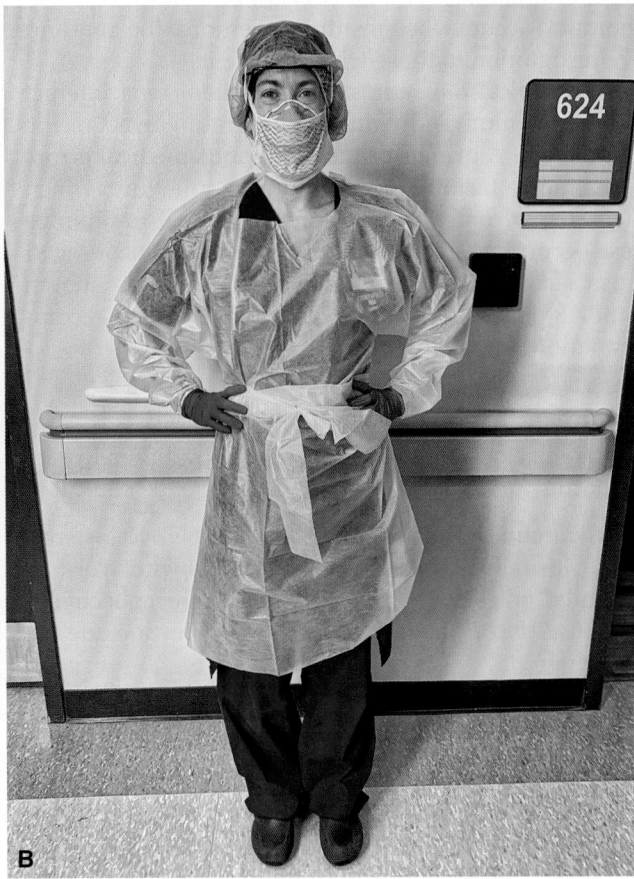

FIGURE I-6AB Nursing students. (A) Then. (B) Now.

as homeopathy, naturopathy, chiropractic, and traditional Chinese medicine, as well as specific treatments, such as herbal medications, dietary changes, massage therapy, yoga, aromatherapy, prayer, and hypnotism. There is growing interest in CAM for various reasons, including the costs of traditional care and increasing cultural diversity in the population.

Expanded Variety of Settings for Care

Nearly 39% of RNs now work outside the hospital setting (U.S. Bureau of Labor Statistics, 2021b). As this trend continues, nurses must be prepared to function in alternative settings. In the hospital, you have access to support personnel, consultation with other nurses and healthcare providers, equipment, and diagnostic testing services. As more care is delivered in outpatient, community, or home settings, you must be prepared to function more autonomously and become more proficient in interprofessional communications.

Telehealth nursing is practiced in a variety of settings, including rural clinics, home healthcare, corrective facilities, and providers' offices, using mobile medical tools and communication devices, such as the videophone or

two-way video technology. As telehealth nursing continues to evolve, you will need to combine the use of technology with your nursing knowledge to safely care for clients remotely.

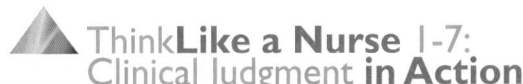

ThinkLike a Nurse I-7:
Clinical Judgment in Action

What is your nursing program doing to prepare you to work outside of the hospital environment?

Interest in Interdisciplinary Collaboration

Nursing has changed from a largely supportive role to one of increasing responsibility. This is due, in part, to the growing role of nursing in outpatient settings, the increasing complexity of care, consumer demands, and the increased use of technology. Healthcare leaders are finding that interprofessional teamwork is essential to achieving safe, high-quality client outcomes.

Interdisciplinary collaboration is defined as "when multiple health workers from different professional backgrounds work together with patients, families, carers [caregivers], and communities to deliver the highest quality of care" (Vega & Bernard, 2017). Although providers, nurses, therapists, and other team members place different emphases on their aspects of client care, communications among all foster collaboration, sharing, coordination, and quality client outcomes. True collaboration occurs when institutions enforce the goal and give recognition to those who practice it.

On a typical day, a hospitalized client may interact with six or more individuals who are involved in the plan of care. A primary cause of serious medical errors in healthcare facilities is communication failure, which often stems from a lack of collaboration. To minimize these occurrences, healthcare providers are encouraged to use a standardized system of communication known as *SBAR* (situation, background, assessment, recommendation; see Chapter 17).

Expanded Career Roles for Nurses

Numerous expanded roles extend the traditional practice of the nurse. The roles may or may not be clinical.

Advanced Practice Nurses (APNs) Registered nurses, usually with a master's degree, who work in expanded roles with a clinical focus are collectively termed *advanced practice nurses (APNs).* They include the following:

- **Clinical nurse specialist (CNS)**—A nurse with advanced education and theoretical and practical expertise in an area of clinical specialization (e.g., cardiovascular, pulmonary, orthopedics). The CNS may provide direct client care; consult on client care; engage in client, family, community, or staff teaching; and/or conduct research.
- **Nurse practitioner (NP)**—A nurse with advanced education focused on providing primary care (comprehensive healthcare) to an age group or within a specialty area. NPs assess, diagnose, and treat diseases and illnesses and prescribe medications and treatments independently or in practice with a provider.
- **Certified registered nurse anesthetist (CRNA)**—A nurse with advanced education focused on providing anesthesia. Nurse anesthetists conduct preoperative screening and evaluation of clients, administer anesthesia during surgery, and evaluate clients' responses to anesthesia in the postoperative period.
- **Certified nurse midwife (CNM)**—A nurse with advanced education focused on women's health, pregnancy, and delivery. A CNM administers Pap tests; performs breast examinations; and provides prenatal care, performs uncomplicated deliveries, and provides postpartum care.

Professional and public reports demonstrate high client satisfaction with APNs, comparable and sometimes superior client outcomes over physician-provided care, better understanding of and compliance with treatment regimens, higher staff nurse satisfaction, fewer hospitalizations, and greater cost-effectiveness compared with physician providers (Aiken et al., 2021; Kippenbrock et al., 2019). This positive reaction to APNs has resulted in increased acceptance and demand.

Non-APN Expanded Roles Expanded roles with a focus other than clinical include the following:

- **Nurse researcher**—A nurse with advanced education at the master's or doctoral level who engages in research related to clinical practice, the discipline, or nursing education.
- **Nurse administrator**—A nurse whose practice focuses on the management and administration of nursing care, health facilities, or health resources.
- **Nurse educator**—A nurse with advanced education and expertise who teaches in a clinical or academic setting.
- **Nurse informaticist**—A nurse with specialized education focused on the use of technology in healthcare and the incorporation of standardized languages and classifications into nursing practice.
- **Nurse entrepreneur**—A nurse who has created an independent or innovative business. Entrepreneurs may serve as consultants, administer a health-related business, or provide educational services.

KnowledgeCheck 1-6

Compare and contrast advanced practice clinical roles for nurses.

Increased Use of Assistive Personnel

UAPs help nurses provide client care. Common UAP roles include nurse aide, assistant, orderly, and technician. UAPs may perform simple nursing tasks (e.g., bathing, taking vital signs) under the direction of the licensed nurse. Some institutions even train UAPs to perform more complex tasks traditionally reserved for licensed nurses (e.g., inserting urinary catheters, administering certain medications). This redistribution of workload has prompted controversy about safety and quality of care.

Although it may be appropriate to allow the UAP to assume simple tasks, this distances the licensed nurse from many aspects of direct client care. **Key Point:** *The nurse retains ultimate responsibility for the client; therefore, they should not base important client care decisions solely on information obtained by the UAP. The nurse is expected to use a higher level of critical thinking and a greater depth of knowledge to gather more in-depth client data.*

As you progress through your program, you will notice that nurses often gather different information from a client than does someone without nursing experience. For example, after bathing an older adult, a UAP will be able to tell the nurse that there are no open areas on the skin. However, a nurse performing the same task would assess the client's level of cognition (orientation to surroundings and self), tolerance for activity, breath sounds, heart sounds, bowel sounds, and condition of the skin. The nurse might also use the time during the bath to teach the client or gather information for discharge planning.

Influence of Nurses on Health Policy
Professional nursing organizations are actively involved in local, state, and national politics. For example:

- Major professional organizations actively lobby and educate government officials about the role of nursing in healthcare.
- Nursing organizations sponsor legislation that promotes the interest of the profession and supports changes that positively influence health outcomes (e.g., safe staffing in hospitals, funding for nursing education, client access to care).

As individuals, nurses should vote, lobby their elected representatives, and run for political office. Together, nurses represent the largest health professional group (more than 5.1 million); thus, when united as a voting bloc, they have strong political power. Many nurses organize local nursing groups to support candidates or legislation or run successful campaigns at local, state, and national levels.

Nurses also influence policy by serving on federal or state advisory panels. For example, nurse leaders serve on the National Advisory Council for Healthcare Research and Quality to provide a nursing voice on issues related to healthcare quality, safety, and evidence-based practice. You should consider all of these political activities as you move into the profession.

Divergence Between High-Tech and High-Touch
Advances in clinical knowledge and technology have contributed to improved care and a longer life for many clients who are critically ill (e.g., premature newborns; clients with advanced cardiovascular, pulmonary, or renal disease; COVID-19 patients). This trend is in contrast to the concurrent trend toward holism and high-touch therapies, which often avoid technology. One of the responsibilities in healthcare is integrating these two divergent trends.

To explore learning resources for this chapter,

Go to Davis Advantage and find:

Answers and Suggested Responses for all questions in this chapter
Concept Map
Knowledge Map
References and Bibliography

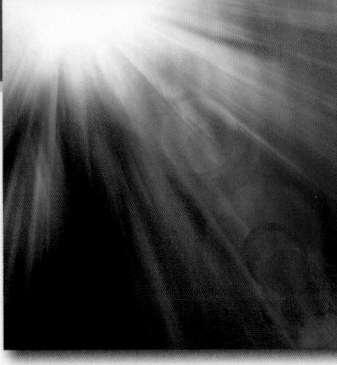

Clinical Judgment

Learning Outcomes

After completing this chapter, you should be able to:

➤ Give one definition and one example of clinical judgment.

➤ List and describe at least one clinical judgment model.

➤ List the four types of nursing knowledge.

➤ Discuss the relationship between critical thinking and clinical judgment.

➤ Discuss the relationship between clinical reasoning and clinical judgment.

➤ Explain ways in which nurses use clinical judgment.

➤ Name and describe the main concepts of the full-spectrum nursing model.

➤ Explain how nursing knowledge, clinical reasoning, critical thinking, nursing process, and clinical judgment work together in full-spectrum nursing.

➤ Relate clinical judgment to person-centered care.

Key Concepts

Clinical judgment
Clinical reasoning
Critical thinking
Full-spectrum nursing
Nursing knowledge

Related Concepts

See the Concept Map on Davis Advantage.

Explore Your Nursing Role

Jan graduated from nursing school 8 months ago and has worked on the medical-surgical unit for 3 months. She completed orientation 6 weeks ago and is on the 1900-to-0700 shift. She has five clients. At 2045, Jan received an admission from the postanesthesia care unit (PACU) and was given the following report: Mr. Anderson, 72-year-old patient, had a colon resection several hours earlier. He is accompanied by his wife, Lilly. Mr. Anderson had an uneventful recovery. Vital signs stable (VSS) at 2025: blood pressure (BP) 158/82, pulse (P) 78, respirations (R) 14, temperature (T) 98.9. Oxygen saturation 99% on room air, IV fluid (IVF) intake 500 mL, urinary output via Foley catheter, 200 mL, clean and yellow. Abdominal dressing clean, dry, and intact. Nasogastric tube patent with 100 mL of gastric drainage.

Jan did not have any questions and documented the following information in the nurses' notes:

2100: Admission vital signs (VS), BP 160/84, P 82, R 16, and T 99.1. Abdominal dressing clean, dry, and intact. Drowsy, oriented. Skin warm and dry. Rated

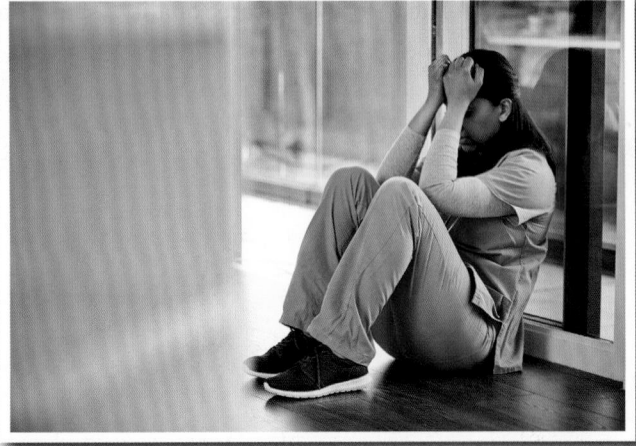

his pain as 2 on a 10-point scale (2/10). IVF infusing at 125 mL/hour. History positive for non–insulin-dependent diabetes (type 2), high blood pressure, and early-stage Alzheimer disease. The nursing plan of care discussed with the Andersons. No questions asked. —Jan Watsone, RN

2200: VS stable at BP 150/78, P 90, R 20, T 99.5. He rates his pain as 4/10 but refuses pain medication. He is drowsy, sleepy. His wife says he has been sleeping since admission. —Jan Watsone, RN

Explore Your Nursing Role (continued)

2400: Mr. Anderson appears lethargic. States that he is on his boat fishing and asks if I see the fish he has caught. VSS: BP 138/68, P 102, R 24, T 100. Skin cool, moist. Abdominal dressing dry and intact. The surgeon notified of client's confusion. Prescriptions received for pain medication and hourly vital signs. He explains that Mr. Anderson is experiencing sundowning, which is late-evening or late-night confusion in clients with dementia. —Jan Watsone, RN

Feeling uncomfortable, Jan discusses Mr. Anderson with the charge nurse, Lisa, who immediately conducts an assessment and notifies the hospitalist. Mr. Anderson is transferred to the intensive care unit (ICU) with a diagnosis of shock from abdominal bleeding.

As Jan completes her documentation, she wonders, "Lisa has been a nurse for 10 years—how did she know something was wrong? Should I be a nurse? Did I miss anything? What went wrong?" You will be asked to apply full-spectrum thinking to Jan's case throughout the chapter as you learn the major concepts associated with the development of clinical judgment.

KEY CONCEPTS

Keep the key concepts in mind as you read this chapter. They will give you the "hooks" on which you can "hang" the other details in the chapter. As you gain an understanding of **clinical judgment, critical reasoning, critical thinking, nursing knowledge,** and the **nursing process,** you will begin to see how they all work together in **full-spectrum nursing.**

WHAT DOES NURSING INVOLVE?

Chapter 1 introduced you to nursing roles, responsibilities, and activities and to the profession of nursing. Throughout this text, you will learn that nurses need to have technical skills; a sound knowledge base; and skills in therapeutic communication, critical thinking, and critical reasoning to develop sound clinical judgment. Much of nursing emphasis is on *thinking,* which is the foundation of being activity oriented *(doing),* and now more than ever, the importance of *caring.* So, another way to describe nursing is to say that *nursing involves thinking, doing,* and *caring.* Thus, your view of the essential roles nurses have in the care of their clients will expand as you progress in your studies. To track your progress, you can later compare your developing view with the baseline you will establish in the exercises in this chapter.

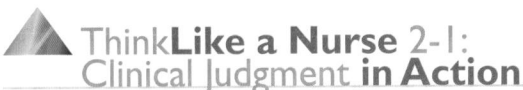

ThinkLike a Nurse 2-1: Clinical Judgment in Action

What are your thoughts about Jan as a nurse? What strengths do you see, and in which areas, if any, is improvement needed?

TheoreticalKnowledge knowing why

Nursing practice has increased in complexity as a result of sicker clients, shortened hospital stays, and increasing demands. This requires that in the context of multiple responsibilities (e.g., interacting with different healthcare providers; administering numerous medications; performing various treatments; documenting in the electronic health record; admitting, transferring, and discharging clients; addressing client and family issues and concerns), you will need to multitask, prioritize, delegate, and make decisions to safely address client care needs (Manetti, 2019). As a new nurse, you must use sound clinical judgment to ensure safe client care and outcomes.

WHAT IS CLINICAL JUDGMENT?

Common factors in definitions of clinical judgment are processes that promote safe client care decisions and outcomes.

- The National Council of State Boards of Nursing (NCSBN, 2019) acknowledges that clinical judgment integrates critical thinking and decision making. Nurses must apply nursing knowledge "to observe and access presenting situations, identify a prioritized client concern, and generate the best possible evidence-based solutions in order to deliver safe client care" (p. 2).
- Tanner (2006) defines clinical judgment as the "interpretation or conclusion about a patient's needs, concerns, or health problems, and/or the decision to take action

(or not), use or modify standard approaches, or improvise new ones as deemed appropriate by the patient's response" (p. 204). This definition emphasizes the importance of understanding the disease process, pathophysiology, diagnostic aspects, and impact of the illness experience for the client and family.

- Benner et al. (2009) note that clinical judgment is the "ways in which nurses come to understand the problems, issues, or concerns of client and patients, to attend to salient information, and to respond in concerned and involved ways" (p. 201). This definition includes the processes of acquiring, analyzing, and using information to address client needs.

Inherent in each of these definitions is the requirement to use processes to achieve desired client outcomes. They require nurses to assess/recognize evidence of client problems, interpret the problems, prioritize a response, take action, evaluate outcomes, and modify actions to ensure the client's needs are met. You must also consider the context of practice, which includes environmental factors in clinical activities (e.g., staffing, resources, client/family roles) and individual factors (e.g., skill level, knowledge, prior experience).

WHAT ARE THE DIFFERENT KINDS OF NURSING KNOWLEDGE?

Theoretical knowledge—*knowing why*—consists of information, facts, principles, and evidence-based theories in nursing and related disciplines (e.g., physiology, psychology). It includes research findings and rationally constructed explanations of phenomena. It also includes an understanding of the pathophysiology of the disease process, medical treatment (e.g., dietary, medications, activity), surgical treatment and perioperative care, and client and family factors. You will use it to describe your clients, understand their health status, explain your reasoning for choosing interventions, and predict client responses to interventions and treatments.

Practical knowledge—*knowing what to do and how to do it*—is an aspect of nursing expertise. It consists of processes (e.g., the decision process, nursing process) and procedures (e.g., how to give an injection). Practical knowledge requires an understanding of the "how and why" of correctly performing nursing skills.

Self-knowledge is self-understanding. Clinical judgment requires you to be aware of your beliefs, values, and cultural and religious biases. You can gain self-knowledge by developing personal awareness—by reflecting (asking yourself), "Why did I do that?" or "How did I come to think that?"

Ethical knowledge is knowledge of obligation, or right and wrong. Ethical knowledge consists of information about moral principles and processes for making moral decisions. Ethical knowledge helps you to

fulfill your ethical obligations to clients and colleagues. Chapter 5 will help expand your ethical knowledge.

Key Point: *Sound clinical judgment requires the nurse to integrate various types of knowledge (e.g., theoretical, practical, ethical, self-knowledge).* Refer to the scenario in Explore Your Nursing Role. As you probably realize, knowledge is essential in nursing practice. Let's examine some of the theoretical and practical knowledge Jan needed to identify signs of a deteriorating client condition and initiate appropriate interventions for Mr. Anderson.

Foundational Knowledge Required:

- Handoff report (SBAR)
- Care of the general postoperative client
- Care of postoperative client after abdominal surgery
- IV fluids: types, infusion rates, indicators of complication, size and type of access device
- Care of client with drains (nasogastric tube, Foley, wound; type, drainage, patency)
- Care of surgical wounds
- Pain management
- Diabetes and its management
- Types and management of dementia
- Role and responsibilities of members of the interprofessional team
- Complications (potential, signs and symptoms)

As you can see, the care of one client may require you to synthesize lots of areas. You will obtain this knowledge and more in your nursing program. You will learn how to put it all together. As you cover topics in your courses, always ask yourself, "How will I apply this knowledge to provide safe, quality care to my clients?

KnowledgeCheck 2-1

- Define the term *clinical judgment* in your own words.
- What is the difference between theoretical and practical knowledge?

What Are Models of Clinical Judgment?

A **model** is a set of interrelated concepts that represents a way of thinking about something—much in the same way that the shape of a lens affects what you see. For example, you would look through a telescope to view a distant star. Looking at the star through reading glasses or a magnifying glass would give a different view. You will learn more about models in Chapter 4.

The clinical judgment models used throughout this book provide ways of making sense of the concept of clinical judgment. They define the processes involved in arriving at sound client care decisions.

Tanner Model of Clinical Judgment

This model describes the four aspects of the clinical judgment process used by experienced nurses. The critical-reasoning processes that nurses use to foster clinical judgment are noticing, interpreting, responding, and reflecting (Tanner, 2006).

Noticing entails forming an impression of the client situation based on the nurse's expectations, knowledge of the client, past experiences with similar clients, theoretical or textbook knowledge, and work environment (e.g., unit culture, patterns of care). For example, a nurse caring for an elderly client with pneumonia will look for certain signs and symptoms based on information learned from textbooks, past experiences with both elderly adults and clients with pneumonia, unit guidelines on the care of clients with respiratory illnesses, and knowledge of the client.

Interpreting is the reasoning processes nurses use to make sense of the initial clinical situation.

- Analytical reasoning would be used by a new nurse who probably relies heavily on information from textbooks and limited client encounters. The nurse would develop several diagnoses and use the assessment data to select the most favorable one. Interventions are selected based on their likelihood of producing the desired outcome.
- Intuitive reasoning is used by experienced nurses and is based on their in-depth knowledge to intuitively grasp the situation and know how to respond.
- Narrative reasoning helps the nurse to use the information obtained to understand the meaning of the client's illness experience, coping abilities, and vision of the future to develop person-centered plans of care.

Responding is the course of action taken by the nurse.

Reflection is a powerful tool that involves examining the actions implemented for validation or modification, and it can foster personal and professional growth. **Reflection-in-action** is used during the implementation process to evaluate results and determine whether a different course of action is needed. **Reflection-on-action** involves a self-evaluation process to learn and refocus actions in future situations. Reflection is essential for the development and expansion of intellectual and professional growth.

KnowledgeCheck 2-2

- Define *reflection*.
- Why is reflection an important process for nurses?
- What are the two types of reflection?

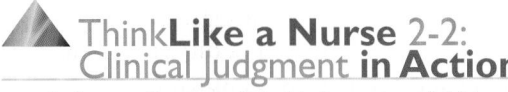

ThinkLike a Nurse 2-2: Clinical Judgment in Action

- Reflect on Tanner's clinical judgment model. How do errors or weaknesses in the noticing phase affect client outcomes?
- Jan asked herself, "Lisa (the charge nurse) has been a nurse for 10 years—how did she know something was wrong?" How would you answer this question?

Lasater Clinical Judgment Rubric (LCJR)

The LCJR identifies 11 dimensions that are used to measure each of the four aspects of Tanner's clinical judgment model (Table 2-1).

Table 2-1 ➤ Model of Clinical Judgment With Corresponding Dimensions	
ASPECTS OF CLINICAL JUDGMENT (TANNER, 2006)	**MEASUREMENT DIMENSIONS (LASATER, 2007)**
Noticing— understanding the situation or scenario	Focused observation—a perceptual understanding of the situation
	Recognizing deviations from expectations
	Information seeking
Interpreting—based on the use of evidence to form understanding	Prioritization of data
	Making sense of data
Responding—selecting the best course of action	Manner of response— expectation of a calm, rational, purposeful, confident response
	Concise, clear, comprehensive communication
	Well planned, executed, safe; appropriate actions (skillful)
Reflection—focusing on the outcomes	Reflection-in-action and reflection-on-action

Sources: Data from Tanner (2006) and Lasater (2007).

The LCRJ measures and categorizes the progressive development of clinical judgment in each dimension as *beginning, developing, accomplished,* and *exemplary.* The rubric assigns a ranking of 1 to 4 to each of the 11 dimensions as the student performs the simulation-based scenario or actual clinical experience. Participants' development of clinical nursing judgment is scored as beginning (1 to 11), developing (12 to 22), accomplished (23 to 33), and exemplary (34 to 44; Lasater, 2007).

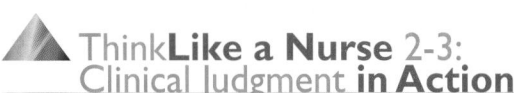

ThinkLike a Nurse 2-3: Clinical Judgment in Action

Using the LCJR, how would you categorize Jan's level of clinical nursing judgment?

National Council of State Boards of Nursing (NCSBN) Clinical Judgment Measurement (CJM) Model

Why Is the CJM Model Important? (Fig. 2-1) Research revealed that many new graduate nurses enter the work setting with a "preparation-to-practice" gap (Kavanagh & Szweda, 2017). Most new nurses

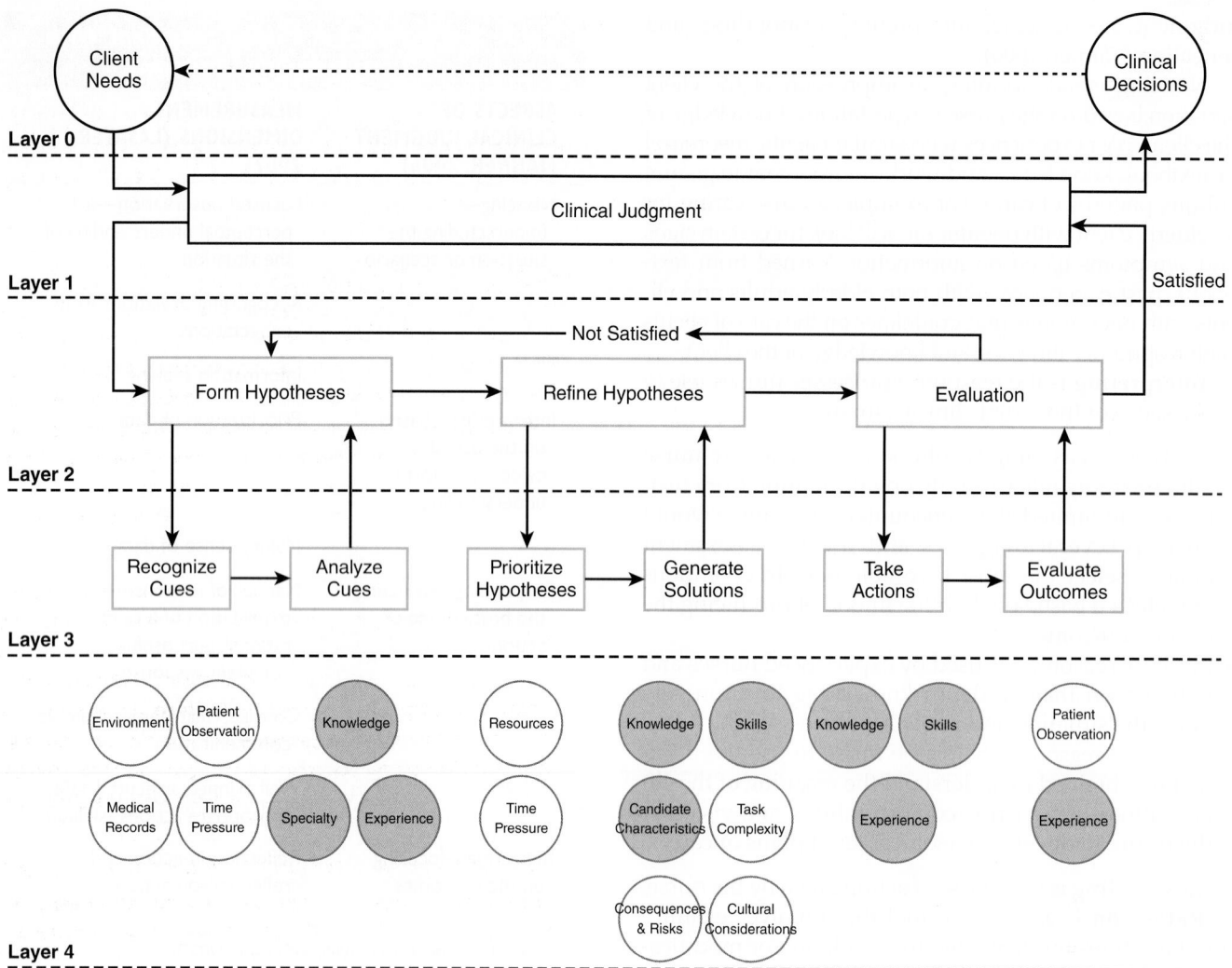

FIGURE 2-1 National Council of State Boards of Nursing (NCSBN) clinical judgment model.

do not possess the competencies necessary for entry-level practice in complex healthcare environments. They do not have the high level of clinical judgment that characterizes more experienced nurses, who use their experience to readily anticipate a client's needs. Less experienced nurses are unable to detect the subtle changes in client cues that indicate a change in condition. Your program of study will include activities (e.g., critical-thinking activities, simulation, direct client care, testing) that are designed to foster your development of clinical judgment.

The NCSBN CJM model measures whether a test-taker has the established degree of clinical judgment and decision-making abilities to be a safe practitioner. The model helps you to recognize, analyze, organize, prioritize, and use your knowledge to make safe client care decisions. This process will be important in preparation for the licensure examination (NCLEX) to become a registered nurse after graduation. Using this process now and throughout your nursing program of study will facilitate your readiness for the examination. The

NCLEX assesses and measures your abilities to be a safe practitioner.

Key Point: *To make sound clinical nursing judgment, nurses need the theoretical knowledge and practical competencies to recognize and analyze cues, formulate hypotheses, generate solutions, implement interventions, and appropriately evaluate client outcomes.* In addition, the context (environmental and individual factors, e.g., time constraints, resources, risks, support) of the situation or scenario should be considered. The CJM model defines and assesses clinical judgment. Therefore, you should be familiar with the framework for how you should develop and use your nursing knowledge.

The CJM model has five layers, 0 to 4, with the formulation of clinical decisions to meet the client's needs as layer 0 (Dickison et al., 2018):

- **Layer 4**, the context layer, identifies the individual and environmental factors that can affect the nurse's reasoning or cognitive processes. Examples of individual factors include one's knowledge base, skill level, and the type and number of prior experiences. For example, a novice nurse with a limited knowledge base and little to no patient experience will encounter difficulty in analyzing essential cues of a deterioration in a client's condition. This nurse should be working with a preceptor or seek assistance to ensure safe client care. In contrast, environmental factors identify influences, such as the physical environment, available resources, time constraints, task complexity, and cultural considerations. For example, a nurse who has never changed a central line dressing (a complex task) may not understand the importance of or may deviate from infection-prevention measures. This nurse should be mentored throughout the process.

- **Layer 3** requires you to have a solid knowledge base to recognize patterns, understand connections between cues, examine pathophysiological processes, organize data, and relate data back to the client's problems. It involves an independent recurring and repetitive processes of **recognizing and analyzing cues** from different sources (e.g., signs and symptoms, medical history) to form and refine hypotheses in layer 2. The nurse then prioritizes the hypotheses and generates solutions by determining desired outcomes and the best interventions to achieve them. Next, actions are implemented, and finally, outcomes are evaluated. When actual outcomes deviate from those expected, the process will restart. **Key Point:** *The failure to recognize cues is a major detriment to making sound clinical decisions because significant factors are omitted from the subsequent processes (e.g., analyzing cues,*

formulating hypotheses). The nurse's professional and personal experience can influence what cues are recognized; thus, self-knowledge is important.

- **Layer 2** involves forming, refining, prioritizing, and evaluating hypotheses to achieve the desired outcomes. This may involve repeated cycles, depending on one's experience level. Novice or new nurses may have multiple cycles, whereas experienced nurses may immediately formulate the more appropriate hypothesis. Layer 2 requires a refined scientific, theoretical, and practical knowledge base.
- **Layer 1** comprises the outcome, which is clinical judgment.
- **Layer 0** is the clinical decisions made by the nurse to address the client's needs.

With continued clinical experiences, you will recognize patterns and more easily make connections between cues, theoretical knowledge, and client care decisions. As you gain more clinical experience, your abilities in layers 2 and 3 will become less deliberate and analytical and more intuitive. You will become more confident and accurate in your abilities to recognize and analyze cues; form, refine, and evaluate hypotheses; and generate solutions to address your clients' needs. Let's examine how use of the model would have been beneficial to Jan in the care of Mr. Anderson (Explore Your Nursing Role; see Table 2-2). Jan would need to have the knowledge to engage in the essential tasks in layer 3 to facilitate clinical decisions to meet the needs of Mr. Anderson.

Table 2-2 ➤ National Council of State Boards of Nursing (NCSBN) Clinical Judgment Model (CJM) Application

NCSBN CJM LAYER 3	KNOWLEDGE AND CONTEXT FACTORS	EXPECTED BEHAVIORS/ACTIONS
Contextual factors	▪ Novice nurse, newly admitted postoperative client, medical-surgical unit, 5 other patients, family member present	▪ Self-knowledge (recognize competency level; deficits in knowledge; time pressures, prior experiences, client presentation) ▪ Know available resources
Recognize cues	▪ Postoperative abdominal patient ▪ Drains (nasogastric tube, wound, Foley) ▪ IV fluids ▪ Changes in vital signs ▪ Comorbidities (diabetes, Alzheimer, obesity, hypertension) ▪ Changes in skin color and moisture ▪ Changes in level of consciousness ▪ Laboratory values ▪ Handoff report	▪ Recognize changes in vital signs as abnormal ▪ Recognize signs and symptoms of shock ▪ Identify diabetes, obesity, dementia condition ▪ Identify effective handoff report (SBAR)

(Continued)

Table 2-2 ➤ National Council of State Boards of Nursing (NCSBN) Clinical Judgment Model (CJM) Application—cont'd

NCSBN CJM LAYER 3	KNOWLEDGE AND CONTEXT FACTORS	EXPECTED BEHAVIORS/ACTIONS
Analyze cues	■ Requires theoretical knowledge—care of general postoperative client and client with abdominal surgery, shock, diabetes symptoms, abnormal vital signs ■ Requires practical knowledge (skill levels, management of drains, prior experiences)	■ Relate client observations to potential postoperative complications ■ Describe patterns in data ■ Explore gaps in evidence (present; needed) to form and prioritize hypotheses
Prioritize hypotheses	■ Explain observations, data collected ■ Fluid and electrolyte imbalances ■ Pain ■ Loss of blood volume ■ Expected postoperative presentation ■ Expected presentation with dementia diagnoses ■ Blood glucose alterations ■ Oxygen saturation values	■ Prioritize the most life-threatening—loss of blood volume
Generate solutions	■ Requires knowledge of life-threatening nature of shock ■ Requires knowledge of shock management ■ Requires knowledge of provider's role	■ Fluid replacement ■ Obtain additional assistance ■ Client needs care beyond what is available on the medical-surgical unit
Take action	■ Fluid resuscitation ■ Obtain oxygen saturation value ■ Determine patency of drainage tubes ■ Determine intake and output ■ Determine amount of blood loss (nasogastric drainage) ■ Determine renal status (output in relation to intake) ■ Collaborate with providers ■ Educate family member on situation ■ Establish another IV site with large-gauge needle ■ Type and crossmatch for blood administration ■ Delegate responsibilities for care of other clients	■ Administer IV fluids at specified rate ■ Administer oxygen at prescribed rate ■ Transfer to a higher level of care
Evaluate outcomes	■ Status of client at time of transfer	■ Stability in vital signs ■ Urinary output present ■ Level of conscious ■ Skin color, temperature, turgor

Table 2-2 ➤ National Council of State Boards of Nursing (NCSBN) Clinical Judgment Model (CJM) Application—cont'd

NURSING ACTIONS FOR POSTOPERATIVE CLIENT

1. Analysis of vital signs
2. Assessment and analysis of intake and output
3. Maintain respiratory status
   a. Oxygen saturation value
   b. Turn, cough, and deep breathe; incentive spirometry
   c. Ambulation
4. Maintain circulatory status
   a. Monitor intake and output
   b. Monitor skin color, temperature, moisture, turgor
5. Maintain skin integrity
   a. Positioning
   b. Wound care
6. Monitor laboratory results
   a. Hemoglobin and hematocrit
   b. White blood cells
7. Maintain safety
   a. Fall-risk assessment and appropriate follow-up measures
   b. Education on safety measures (use of call bell, assistance getting out of bed)
8. Pain management
9. Patient/family education
10. Discharge planning
    a. Postdischarge interventions
    b. Available resources
    c. Follow-up care

KnowledgeCheck 2-3

Identify the tasks in each layer of the NCSBN CJM.

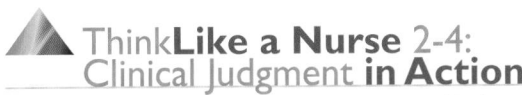

ThinkLike a Nurse 2-4: Clinical Judgment in Action

- How could factors in layer 4 have affected Jan's performance?
- Evaluate Jan's strengths and areas for improvement in layer 3.

What Is Clinical Reasoning?

Clinical reasoning and critical thinking are essential components of clinical judgment. Because both concepts are important to developing sound clinical judgment, we will discuss each separately.

Clinical reasoning is the process of synthesizing knowledge and information from numerous sources and incorporating experience to develop a plan of care for a particular client or case scenario. It requires a reliance on your knowledge and experience to form a conceptual image of a client's problem and its effective management. The nurse uses this conceptual problem to guide additional data collection, then reevaluates and revises the problem until the nurse reaches a level of confidence in the diagnosis and the best approach to care (Gruppen, 2017). In essence, clinical reasoning is the application of knowledge, information from various sources, and experience to a client situation to make judgments, generate alternatives, evaluate them based on evidence, and select the most appropriate action. Tools to develop and

Toward Evidence-Based Practice

Manetti, W. (2018). Evaluating the clinical judgment of prelicensure nursing students in the clinical setting. *Nurse Educator, 43*(5), 272–276. https://doi.org/10.1097/NNE.0000000000000489

This study used the Lasater Clinical Judgment Rubric (LCJR) to measure the clinical judgment of junior and senior baccalaureate nursing students, using the scales of *beginning, developing, accomplished,* and *exemplary* to describe Tanner's performance levels. Findings revealed that junior nursing students demonstrated a clinical judgment performance level of accomplished on all 11 dimensions. In contrast, senior nursing students demonstrated an exemplary performance level in all areas, except for interpreting, which was at the accomplished level. In addition, students who had previous knowledge and experience in healthcare environments had higher total clinical judgment scores. The latter is consistent with the finding by Sterner et al. (2021) that students with previous experience in healthcare before nursing education were better able to prioritize interventions.

Dix, S., Morphet, J., Jones, T., Kiprillisa, N., O'Hallorana, M., Piperac, K., & Innes, K. (2021). Perceptions of final year nursing students transfer to clinical judgment skills from simulation to clinical practice: A qualitative study. *Nurse Educator in Practice, 56*(2021), 103218. https://doi.org/10.1016/j.nepr.2021.103218

Researchers investigated the transfer of clinical judgment skills into clinical practice. Undergraduate students in their final clinical course participated in two simulated clinical scenarios, followed by 160 hours of clinical practice. The findings indicated that students transferred learning from simulation to clinical practice. In addition, students with a solid knowledge of normal values and anatomy and physiology displayed good clinical judgment. Although sound foundational knowledge is essential for understanding and interpreting data and using those data to make decisions, the volume of data in acute situations can be overwhelming to novice nurses who are not exposed to making complex clinical decisions as students.

Sterner, A., Ramstrand, N., Palmér, L., & Hagiwara, M. A. (2021). A study of factors that predict novice nurses' perceived ability to provide care in acute care situations. *Nursing Open, 8*(4), 1958–1969. https://doi.org/10.1002/nop2.871

Working in acute care facilities can be intimidating and fearful for novice nurses because their level of competence is perceived as unequal to that of experienced nurses. This study investigated factors that influenced the novice nurses' perception of readiness to provide safe, quality patient care. The findings revealed the following regarding novice nurses:

- Trust in their abilities was influenced by experience in acute care facilities during nursing education.
- Their ability to exercise clinical judgment (noticing, interpreting, responding) in acute situations was positively associated with experience during nursing education, postgraduate experience in acute care, and duration of experience.
- Their ability to prioritize interventions was associated with experience in healthcare before nursing education, duration of work experience, and acute care experience.
- Their ability to act independently was influenced by duration of work experience.
- Their ability to determine the most appropriate intervention was associated with a longer duration of work experience and postgraduation experience in acute situations.

This study identifies several factors important to the development of clinical judgment.

1. What do the studies reveal about the knowledge, level, and experience of nursing students and the development of clinical judgment?

2. What is the importance of clinical rotations as a student nurse and in postgraduate experience?

3. What is the role of simulation in nursing education?

refine clinical reasoning include the use of algorithms, reflective journaling, thinking aloud (Victor-Chmil, 2013), simulation, and case studies.

The practice of professional nursing requires strong clinical reasoning skills because of the rapidly changing healthcare environment, technological advances, the complexity of client problems, and shortened hospital stays. Research has indicated that ineffective clinical reasoning is a major factor in the failure of nurses to respond appropriately to deteriorating client conditions (Liaw et al., 2018). Each client presents with a different problem and background, different contextual factors, and different needs and goals. You will need to use your knowledge and experience to assess the client and make decisions on the treatment plan or the need to obtain additional information. Clinical reasoning skills are important for safe client care. It is necessary to detect and appropriately respond to a client's worsening condition. Your clinical faculty will help you to focus your learning experiences and client assignments to enhance your clinical reasoning skills.

KnowledgeCheck 2-4

- Define *clinical reasoning*.
- Why is clinical reasoning important in nursing practice?
- What evidence exists that Jan used clinical reasoning?

WHAT IS CRITICAL THINKING?

Unlike clinical reasoning, critical thinking does not require a client situation or scenario. Yet, critical thinking is needed for clinical reasoning, and both clinical reasoning and critical thinking are essential to the development of clinical judgment (Manetti, 2019).

Any situation that requires critical thinking is likely to have more than one so-called right answer. For example, you do not need critical thinking to add 2 + 2 and come up with the answer. You simply need to know and follow the rules of addition. However, you *do* need critical thinking to work through important decisions and those in which the best answer is not so clear (e.g., "Should I buy a new car or a used one?").

- **Critical thinking is a complex concept, and people think about it in different ways.** As applied to nursing, it can be defined as a cognitive process that uses intellectual standards based on evidence and science to approach a subject, content, or problem (Victor-Chmil, 2013). Another closely related definition is, "critical thinking is the ability to apply higher-order cognitive skills (conceptualization, analysis, evaluation) and the disposition to be deliberate about thinking (being open-minded or intellectually honest) that lead to action that is logical and appropriate" (Papp et al., 2014, p. 716). **Key Point: *Critical thinking is an analysis process. It is a combination of reasoned thinking, openness to alternatives, an ability to reflect, and a desire to seek truth.*** There are many definitions of critical thinking because it is a complex concept and people think about it in different ways.
- **Critical thinking is linked to evidence-based practice**, which is a research-based method for judging and using nursing interventions. An important aspect of critical thinking is the process of identifying and checking your assumptions—and this process is also an important part of the research process.
- **Critical thinkers are flexible, nonjudgmental, inquisitive, honest, and interested in seeking the truth.** They possess intellectual skills that allow them to use their curiosity to their advantage, and they have critical attitudes that motivate them to use those skills responsibly. They continually critically reflect on their assumptions to continue to develop their critical-thinking skills.

What Are Critical-Thinking Skills?

Skills in critical thinking refer to the cognitive (intellectual) processes used in complex thinking operations such as problem-solving and decision making. In this example, the skills are italicized, and the complex thinking processes are in bold type:

> When planning nursing care, *nurses gather information* about the client and then ***draw tentative conclusions about the meaning of the information*** to identify the client's problems. Then they think of several different actions they might take to help **solve or relieve the problem**.

The following are a few examples of critical-thinking skills:

- Objectively gathering information on a problem or issue
- Recognizing the need for more information
- Evaluating the credibility and usefulness of sources of information
- Recognizing gaps in one's own knowledge
- Recognizing differences and similarities among things or situations
- Listening carefully; reading thoughtfully
- Separating relevant from irrelevant data and important from unimportant data
- Organizing or grouping information in meaningful ways
- Making inferences (tentative conclusions) about the meaning of the information
- Integrating new information with prior knowledge
- Visualizing potential solutions to a problem
- Exploring the advantages, disadvantages, and consequences of each potential action

What Are Critical-Thinking Attitudes?

Attitudes consist of beliefs, feelings, and views toward something or someone. Your attitudes and character determine whether you will use your thinking skills fairly and with an open mind. Without a critical attitude, people tend to use thinking skills to justify narrow-mindedness and prejudice and to benefit themselves rather than others. The following are some critical-thinking attitudes (Paul, 1990; Paul & Elder, 2010; Papathanasiou et al., 2014):

- **Intellectual autonomy.** Critical thinkers do not believe everything they are told; they listen to what others think, and they learn from new ideas. They do not accept or reject an idea before they understand it.
- **Intellectual curiosity.** Critical thinkers love to learn new things. They show an attitude of curiosity and inquiry, and they frequently think or ask, "What if ...?"; "How could we do this differently?"; "How does this work?"; or "Why did that happen?"
- **Intellectual humility.** Critical thinkers ask for help when they don't know; seek the wisdom of mentors with knowledge, skill, and ability; and reevaluate their conclusions or actions in light of new information.
- **Intellectual empathy.** Critical thinkers try to understand the feelings and perceptions of others. They try to see a situation as the other person sees it.
- **Intellectual courage.** Critical thinkers consider and examine fairly their own values and beliefs, as well as the beliefs of others, even when this is uncomfortable. They are willing to rethink, and even reject, previously ill-justified beliefs.
- **Intellectual perseverance.** Critical thinkers don't jump to conclusions or settle for the quick, obvious answer. They explore effective solutions even when it takes a great deal of effort and time.

- **Fair-mindedness.** Critical thinkers try to make impartial judgments, realizing that personal biases, customs, and social pressures can influence their thinking.
- **Confidence in reasoning.** Critical thinkers rely on inductive and deductive processes to have confidence in their own reasoning.

Critical thinking can be used in all aspects of your life. Whenever you are trying to reach an important decision, reasoned action (critical thinking) is called for. Everyday uses of critical thinking might include deciding where you should live or which job offer to accept. The rest of this chapter shows you why critical thinking is important to you in your chosen profession, nursing.

Knowledge Check 2-5

- Define *critical thinking* in your own words.
- List five skills or attitudes that reflect critical thinking.

WHY IS CRITICAL THINKING IMPORTANT FOR NURSES?

Critical thinking helps you to know what is important about each client's situation. Nurses use complex critical-thinking processes (e.g., problem-solving, decision making, clinical reasoning, and clinical judgment) in every aspect of their work. Because nurses care for a variety of clients with a multitude of concerns, a client's response to therapy may not always be apparent. **Key Point:** *You constantly assess your clients to determine how they are responding to nursing interventions and medical treatments.* Reasoning and reflection are required to determine what interventions to use and whether they worked—and if not, figure out why.

Nurses Deal With Complex Situations

Critical thinking is important for nurses because they deal with complicated situations. One such situation is that of caring for clients with **comorbidities** (more than one health problem occurring at the same time). Consider the following situations:

- **A healthy 9-year-old who fell and fractured their right arm; they have no comorbidities**. They would experience pain and discomfort, but with proper casting and time to heal, the child would recover. While recovering, they may have to limit the use of their injured arm and use their left hand to eat. The child would likely be discharged home from the urgent setting in the care of their parent(s) or guardian(s). The nurse's primary interventions would be to teach the and recognize signs of complications.

  - **An older adult who has fractured their right arm; they are also recovering from a stroke that limits the use of their left arm.** Their experience would be quite different from that of the 9-year-old. A right-arm fracture would severely affect this person's ability to provide self-care. The nurse

would need to evaluate whether the adult requires care in the hospital or in a skilled care facility and what support services they will need as they convalesce. In the inpatient setting, nursing interventions might initially include assisting the client with eating, bathing, and toileting.

Clients Are Unique

Critical thinking is important because each client is unique. This means that the response to therapy may vary from client to client. Their differences (e.g., type of illness, comorbidities, culture, and age) make it impossible to provide rigid rules for all client care.

Individual Differences Research-based care plans and protocols identify guidelines for providing care; however, nurses must evaluate and modify these guidelines to be appropriate for each client. Consider the following example: You may have been told to drink plenty of fluids when you have a cough, to keep the secretions moist. Now imagine you are caring for a client with renal failure. Your client no longer urinates and may need dialysis. When they develop a persistent cough, should you encourage them to drink as much fluid as possible? Do you see how you could cause harm to a client by unthinkingly doing as you have been told or what has worked well for another client? **Key Point:** *Nurses must always think, "How will that work in this instance?" and "How is this similar or different from other client situations?"*

Client's Personal Beliefs Ethnic, cultural, and spiritual background affect a person's view of health and the healthcare system, as well as their responses to health problems. Personal beliefs influence how people define sickness, at what point they seek healthcare, what type of healthcare provider they see, and the type of treatment they consider acceptable. Critical thinking enables the nurse to assess the client's and family's beliefs and adapt care so that it is culturally sensitive and responsive to their needs.

Client's Roles A person's roles influence when, how, and why they seek healthcare. A single parent with young children may ask to be discharged from the hospital early to meet the needs of their family. Clients with extensive support from family or friends may be willing to take more time to convalesce when ill. Nurses take these things into consideration, for example, when determining whether a nursing intervention is appropriate or why it was (or was not) successful.

Other Factors The following factors may also influence how a person responds to illness or to healthcare intervention:

- *Age.* Each of us was raised with a set of beliefs, values, and knowledge that was strongly influenced by the prevailing views of our times.

- *Personal bias.* Clients may have fixed beliefs about health and illness.
- *Personality.* Individuals have unique personalities. This means every person is different; all have individual ways of responding to stress, fear, illness, and pain. Some are hardy and show an attitude of strength, endurance, and a high threshold for pain. Others are less tolerant and may outwardly express pain or other emotions associated with illness, hospitalization, and death.
- *Previous experience.* Clients are often affected by previous problems with healthcare. For example, a boy who has experienced a painful injection in the past may be terrified when he sees the nurse approaching with a syringe.

Nurses Apply Knowledge to Provide Holistic Care

In addition to the need to individualize care for each client, there are some aspects of nursing itself that require the nurse to be a critical thinker:

- *Nursing is an applied discipline.* Nurses deal with complex, ill-defined, and sometimes confusing problems—client problems may not be well defined and straightforward. **Key Point: *This means that you must analyze client cues and apply your knowledge and skills and not just try to memorize and regurgitate facts from the textbook.***
- *Nursing uses knowledge from other fields.* Nurses integrate knowledge from chemistry, physiology, psychology, social sciences, and other disciplines into the practice of nursing to identify and plan interventions for client problems. Nurses collaborate with members of the interdisciplinary healthcare team to provide a multifaceted approach to client care.
- *Nursing is fast-paced.* Nurses often deal with demanding situations in a complex healthcare environment. A client's condition may change from hour to hour or even minute to minute, so knowing the routine may not be adequate. You will need to respond appropriately and quickly under stress.
- *The scientific basis for client care changes constantly.* Therefore, you must constantly update your knowledge and skills throughout your career. You will need to continuously expand and refine your critical-thinking skills as well.
- *Critical thinking is linked to evidence-based practice,* which you will learn more about later in this book. **Evidence-based practice** is a research-based method for judging and choosing nursing interventions.

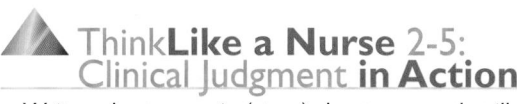
ThinkLike a Nurse 2-5: Clinical Judgment in Action

Write a short scenario (story) about a nurse that illustrates one of the reasons why nurses need to be critical thinkers.

A MODEL FOR CRITICAL THINKING

You will recall that a **model** is a set of interrelated concepts that represents a way of thinking about something. The critical-thinking model used throughout this book organizes critical thinking into five major categories. Box 2-1 defines each category and provides questions to help you focus your thinking during clinical reasoning. You can use some of the questions when deciding what to think about and do; you can use others when analyzing a situation after it happens (reflecting). Figure 2-2 is a simpler representation of the model, relating it to the nursing process, which is introduced later in this chapter.

Use the model as a guide when faced with clinical decisions or unfamiliar situations. The questions can help you to "think about your thinking" as you apply principles and knowledge from various sources to a problem. This should help you to achieve good outcomes for your clients. Only ask yourself the questions that are relevant to the situation. The processes do not occur "sequentially," so you may jump back and forth among them. As you advance in your nursing program, these questions will become more intuitive.

Applying the Model: An Example

Let's apply the model to a situation faced by all nursing students. Soon you will begin your clinical rotations, if you have not already done so.

How could you use the five points of the critical-thinking star (see Fig. 2-2) to approach your first clinical day so that you will be well prepared and able to function safely?

Contextual Awareness One of the first things you need to consider is your usual response to new experiences. Consider several questions that will help you address the star point of contextual awareness: How do you react to change? What other tasks or assignments do you have that will dictate the timing of your preparation? What previous experiences will aid or hamper you in your preparation? What beliefs and assumptions will affect the way you prepare for your first day of client care?

Using Credible Sources You need to use *credible sources* of data to prepare for the clinical experience. Until you gain more experience, you can:

- Ask your instructor for guidance on how to best prepare.
- Consult a student who has successfully completed the same course.

You will also need accurate information about the clients assigned to you. Use only *knowledgeable, reliable sources* of information, such as the following:

- The client's medical records
- Credible Internet sites—your instructor can provide guidance.
- Nursing texts and scholarly journals

BOX 2-1 ■ Critical-Thinking Model

Contextual Awareness

- Deciding what to observe and consider
- An awareness of what's happening in the total situation, including values, cultural issues, interpersonal relationships, and environmental influences

Questions for Focusing Thinking

- What is going on in the situation that may influence the outcome?
- What factors may influence my behavior and that of others in this situation (e.g., culture, roles, relationships, economic status)?
- What about this situation have I seen before? What is different? What is new?
- Who should be involved to improve the outcome?
- What else was happening at the same time that affected me in this situation?
- What happened just before this incident that made a difference?
- What emotional responses influenced how I reacted in this situation?
- What changes in behavior alerted me that something was wrong?

Inquiry

- Based on credible sources
- Applying standards of good reasoning to your thinking when analyzing a situation and evaluating your actions

Questions for Focusing Thinking

- How do I go about getting the information I need?
- What framework should I use to organize my information?
- Do I have enough knowledge to decide? If not, what do I need to know?
- Have I used a valid, reliable source of information (e.g., client, other professionals, references)?
- Did I (do I need to) validate the data (e.g., with the client)?
- What else do I need to know? What information is missing?
- Are the data accurate? Precise?
- What's important and what's not important in this situation?
- Did I consider professional, ethical, and legal standards?
- Have I jumped to conclusions?

Considering Alternatives

- Exploring and imagining as many alternatives as you can think of for the situation

Questions for Focusing Thinking

- What is one possible explanation for what is happening or what happened?
- What are other explanations for what is happening? What is one thing I could do in this situation?
- What are two more possibilities/alternatives?

- Are there others who might help me develop more alternatives?
- Of the possible actions I am considering, which one is most reasonable? Why are the others not as reasonable?
- Of the possible actions that I am considering, which one is most likely to achieve the desired outcomes?

Analyzing Assumptions

- Recognizing and analyzing assumptions you are making about the situation and examining the beliefs that underlie your choices

Questions for Focusing Thinking

- What have I (or others) taken for granted in this situation?
- Which beliefs/values are shaping my assumptions?
- What assumptions contributed to the problem in this situation?
- What rationale supports my assumptions?
- How will I know my assumption is correct?
- What biases do I have that may affect my thinking and my decisions in this situation?

Reflecting Skeptically and Deciding What to Do

- Questioning, analyzing, and reflecting on the rationale for your decisions

Questions for Focusing Thinking

- What aspects of this situation require the most careful attention?
- What else might work in this situation?
- Am I sure of my interpretation of this situation?
- Why is (was) it important to intervene?
- What rationale do I have for my decisions?
- In priority order, what should I do in this situation and why?
- Having decided what was wrong/happening, what is the best response?
- What might I delegate in this situation?
- What got me started taking action?
- What priorities were missed?
- What was done? Why was it done?
- What would I do differently after reflecting on this situation?

Source: Model based on Brookfield, S. D. (1991). *Developing critical thinkers.* Jossey-Bass; McDonald, M. E. (2002). *Systematic assessment of learning outcomes: Developing multiple-choice exams.* Jones & Bartlett Publishers; Paul, R. W. (1993). *Critical thinking: What every person needs to survive in a rapidly changing world* (3rd ed.). Foundation for Critical Thinking; Raingruber, B., & Haffer, A. (2001). *Using your head to land on your feet.* F. A. Davis; Wilkinson, J. M. (2012). *Nursing process and critical thinking* (5th ed.). Prentice Hall; Victor-Chmil, J. (2013). Critical thinking versus clinical reasoning versus clinical judgment: Differential diagnosis. *Nurse Educator,* 38(1), 34–36. https://doi.org/10.1097/NNE.0b013e318276dfbe; Von Colln-Appling, C., & Giuliano, D. (2017). A concept analysis of critical thinking: A guide for nurse educators. *Nurse Education Today, 49,* 106–109. https://doi.org/10.1016/j.nedt.2016.11.007

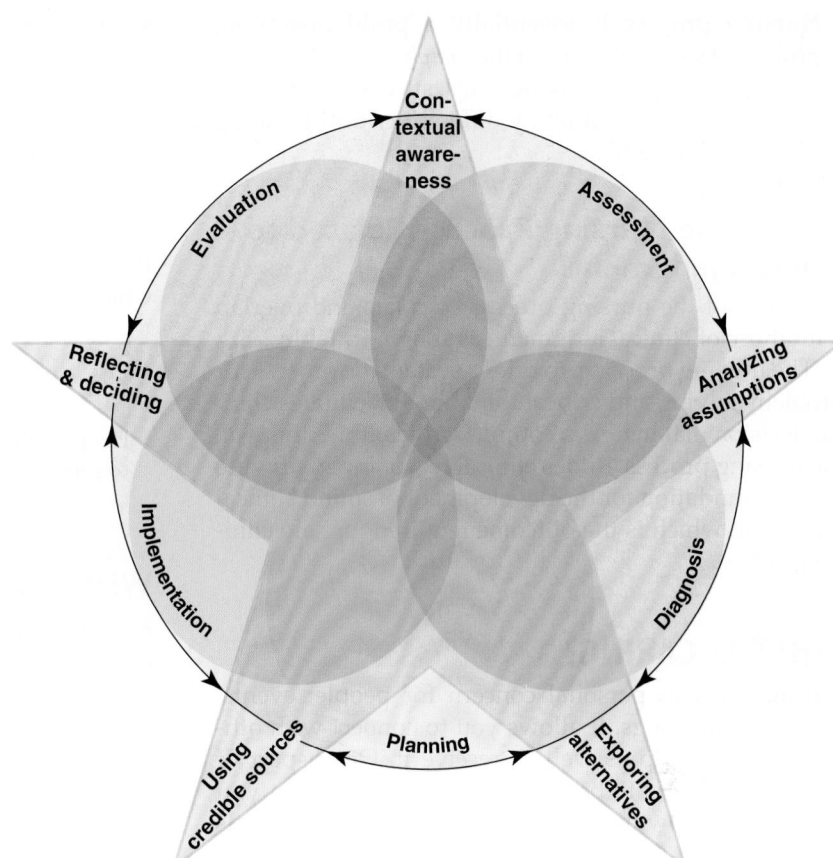

FIGURE 2-2 Model of critical thinking and the nursing process.

As you gain more information, go back and analyze your response to the situation. Use reflection. You may find that you are already feeling less anxious! All of this is a part of *inquiry*.

Exploring Alternatives and Analyzing Assumptions Now that you know something about the clinical experience, you can plan your day. You need to consider alternatives and analyze your assumptions about the experience:

- What is expected of you?
- What do you expect from the experience?
- How should you approach your client?
- How will you introduce yourself?
- How will you apply your skills in caring for your client?

Reflecting and Deciding After you feel that you have addressed these concerns, you need to quickly review your preparation (*reflective skepticism*):

- Have you gathered enough information to feel comfortable in the situation?
- Do you need more information? What are the gaps in the information?

This was a demonstration of how you might apply the critical-thinking model to a real experience. In this example, you also used various types of knowledge discussed earlier (e.g., theoretical, practical, personal, and ethical knowledge).

KnowledgeCheck 2-6

Think about the preceding discussion of applying the five points of the critical-thinking model, and identify the actions that demonstrate the use of each of the four types of knowledge.

PracticalKnowledge
knowing **how**

HOW IS THE NURSING PROCESS RELATED TO CRITICAL THINKING?

The **nursing process** is a multistep, systematic problem-solving process that guides all nursing actions. It is the type of "thinking and doing" nurses use in their practice. For detailed information on the nursing process, see Chapter 3. **Key Point: *Critical thinking and the nursing process are interrelated but not identical.*** The nursing process is a tool to foster critical thinking.

- **Nurses use critical thinking for decisions other than direct client care** (e.g., to decide how many nurses are needed to staff the unit).
- **Some nursing activities do not always require reflective critical thinking** (e.g., applying a cardiac monitor, inserting a urinary catheter), although they must be done skillfully.

- **Nursing process is essentially a problem-solving process.** As such, it is one of the *complex critical-thinking processes.* Complex thinking skills, such as the nursing process, make use of many different critical-thinking skills (see Fig. 2-2).

How Is the Nursing Process Related to Clinical Judgment?

The steps of the nursing process correlate and overlap with those of clinical judgment, as shown in Table 2-3.

The nursing process provides a systematic process for problem-solving and critical thinking. It facilitates clinical decision making. As a complex critical-thinking tool, the nursing process guides clinical reasoning to provide a solid foundation for the development of sound clinical judgment, which is the outcome required for safe clinical practice.

WHAT IS CARING?

Caring involves personal concern for people, events, projects, and things. It allows you to connect with others and give help as well as receive it. One aspect of self-knowledge is to be aware of what and whom you care about. Knowing what the client cares about reveals what the client considers stressful because only things that matter can create stress. Caring also enables you to notice which interventions are effective.

- *Caring is always specific and relational for each nurse–person encounter.* A caring perspective highlights each person as unique and valued.
- *Caring is not an abstraction.* That is, you don't just care for "suffering humankind," but you respond compassionately to this client's needs right now, in the moment, even if you are busy and tired.

Table 2-3 ➤ Comparison of Nursing Process With Clinical Judgment Model	
NURSING PROCESS STEPS	**NURSING CLINICAL JUDGMENT MODEL LAYER 3**
Assessment	Recognize and analyze cues
Analysis/Diagnosis	Analyze cues and begin to prioritize hypotheses
Planning (outcomes and interventions)	Prioritize hypotheses and generate solutions
Implementation	Take action on solutions generated
Evaluation	Evaluate implementation and outcomes

Source: Adapted from Dickison et al. (2018); Next Generation NCLEX News (2019); Wilkinson et al. (2020).

- *Caring involves thinking and acting in ways that preserve human dignity and humanity.* It does not treat people as objects. A caring nurse's actions are never routine or impersonal. For example, a caring nurse drapes a client for privacy when inserting a urinary catheter.

Caring has at least five components (see Table 2-4). Caring is the central concept in several nursing theories. You will learn more about the caring theories in Chapter 4.

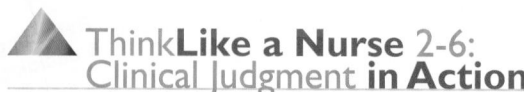

ThinkLike a Nurse 2-6: Clinical Judgment **in Action**

Using the five components of caring, how can you show caring to your client?

WHAT IS FULL-SPECTRUM NURSING?

Key Point: *Full-spectrum nursing is a unique blend of thinking, doing, and caring.* It is performed by nurses who fully develop and apply nursing knowledge, critical thinking, clinical reasoning, and the nursing process to client situations to make sound clinical judgments. The purpose of full-spectrum nursing is to practice safe, effective care and achieve good client outcomes.

What Concepts Are Used in Full-Spectrum Nursing?

Recall that when we put concepts (ideas) together to explain something, it is called a **model.** You will learn more about concepts in Chapter 4; for now, think of them as ideas. The four main concepts that describe full-spectrum nursing are *thinking, doing, caring,* and *client situation* (or *context;* Table 2-5).

When nurses think, they use the nursing knowledge that they have stored in their memory and the experiences that they have had. In addition, they think about the client situation, which they understand through the use of the nursing process. **Situation,** or **context,** refers to the context for care: the client's environment outside the care setting, relationships, resources available for client care, and so on. Figure 2-3 is a simple visual model of full-spectrum nursing. You can see that the concept's full model involves everything you have learned about in this chapter—clinical judgment, clinical reasoning, critical thinking, nursing knowledge, and nursing process—but organized under the simple concepts of thinking, doing, caring, and client situation.

Let's see how the model concepts work together for a full-spectrum nurse. They are all interrelated and overlapping, but we divide them into simple categories to help you understand and remember them. You can see that a full-spectrum nurse needs excellent clinical judgment, clinical reasoning, and critical-thinking skills because there is so much to think *about* and much to *do* in the complex healthcare environment.

Table 2-4 ➤ Five Components of Caring

CARING COMPONENT	DEFINITION	EXAMPLES
Knowing	Striving to understand what an event means in the life of the client	Illness A new baby Loss of loved one
Being With	Being emotionally present for the client	Making eye contact Active listening
Doing For	Doing what clients would do for themselves if they were able	Bathing Feeding Calling the client's pastor
Enabling	Supporting the client through coping with life changes and unfamiliar events	Hospitalization Birth of a premature infant
Maintaining Belief	Having faith in the client's ability to get through the change or event and to find fulfillment and meaning (Swanson, 1990)	Adapting to a new colostomy Adapting to loss of a limb Cardiac rehabilitation

Table 2-5 ➤ Full-Spectrum Nursing Concepts

THINKING	DOING	CARING	CLIENT SITUATION
Critical Thinking Enables you to fully use your knowledge and skills Clinical Reasoning Enables you to synthesize knowledge, experience, and information from various sources to develop an effective plan of care for a client Clinical Judgment Enables you to make the sound clinical decision for action. It is the outcome of critical thinking and clinical reasoning.	Practical Knowledge Skills, procedures, and processes (including the nursing process)	Self-Knowledge Awareness of your values, beliefs, and biases	Client Data Physical, psychosocial, spiritual
THEORETICAL KNOWLEDGE	**NURSING PROCESS**	**ETHICAL KNOWLEDGE**	**CLIENT PREFERENCES AND CONTEXT**
Principles, facts, theories; what you have to think *with*	**Assessment and Evaluation:** Everything you know about the client, including context ***Planning and Implementation:*** ***What you do for the client***	Understanding your obligations; sense of right and wrong	Context for care includes individual and environmental factors (e.g., time pressures, support, relationships, culture, resources)

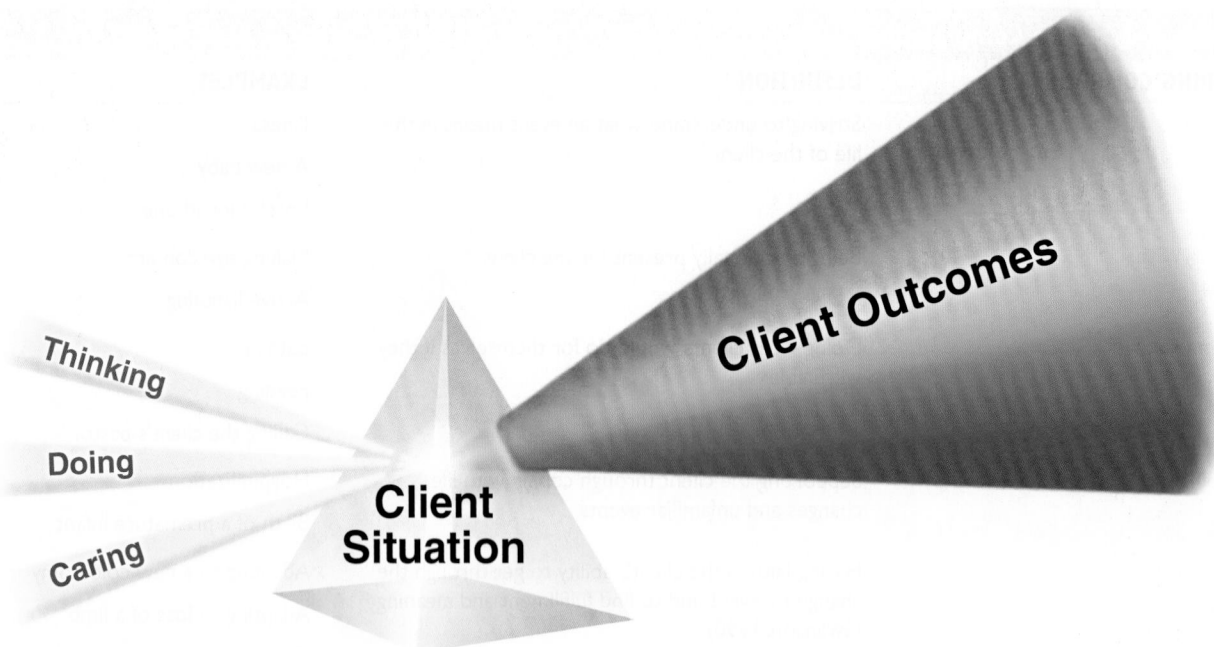

FIGURE 2-3 Model of full-spectrum nursing.

KnowledgeCheck 2-7

- What are the four main concepts of the full-spectrum model of nursing?
- Where do the four types of nursing knowledge fit into the full-spectrum model?
- What is the ultimate purpose of full-spectrum nursing?

How Does the Model Work?

The full-spectrum nursing model is used throughout this text, so it is important that you understand how it works.

- Nurses use *clinical reasoning, critical thinking,* and *the nursing process* to make sound clinical decisions. They also apply these competencies to the four kinds of *nursing knowledge.*
- When they are *doing* for the client, *caring* motivates and facilitates the *thinking* and *doing.*
- The goal of *thinking, doing, and caring* is to have a positive effect on a client's *health outcomes.*

The following client situation illustrates how the four main dimensions of full-spectrum nursing work together. As you read, notice how the concepts overlap. Also, notice how the nurse uses clinical reasoning and critical thinking with nursing knowledge and the nursing process.

Client Situation

When taking a client's oral temperature, a nurse sees a glass of ice water on the over-the-bed table. Realizing that a cold drink can reduce the accuracy of the temperature reading, she asks the client, "How long since you've taken a drink of water?" The client tells the nurse

it was just a minute ago. The nurse is busy and tired, but she returns to retake the client's temperature later, when it will be accurate.

Thinking

- *Theoretical knowledge.* The nurse realized that a cold drink can lower the temperature reading. The nurse used interviewing principles to get more information from the client.
- *Recognize cues.* The class of ice water on the bedside table is a relevant cue for a temperature reading.
- *Analyze cues.* The nurse used theoretical knowledge to link the effect of cold water on the temperature value.
- *Clinical reasoning.* The nurse synthesized knowledge and information from textbooks and experience to alter the plan of care for the client based on the information obtained.
- *Critical thinking.* The nurse recognized relevant information and identified the need for more information. She used the client's answer to decide what to do.
- *Context.* Being aware of context is important to decision making. The context in this scenario includes ice water within the client's reach and that the client was physically capable of reaching it. The context also includes the nurse's other responsibilities.
- *Prioritize hypotheses.* Select the hypotheses that best explain the client's cues and can be used to generate possible solutions.

Doing

- *Practical knowledge.* The nurse used a psychomotor skill when she measured the client's temperature to acquire more vital sign data and a communication process to question the client.

- *Nursing process. (Assessment)* The nurse observed the glass of ice water on the table. The nurse asked, "How long since you've taken a drink of water?" The nurse also observed the environmental data (e.g., ice water at the bedside). *(Implementation/Take Action)* The nurse returned later and took the client's temperature.

Caring

The scenario does not say this, but a caring nurse, even a very busy one, would not be annoyed with the client for the inconvenience of having to come back again to take the temperature.

- *Self-knowledge* might include the nurse's awareness that she is tired and feeling irritable.
- *Ethical knowledge* would tell her that she has an obligation to get an accurate temperature from the client rather than thinking, "Oh, I'll just record the reading a degree or two higher, as it doesn't matter that much."

As a full-spectrum nurse, you will apply thinking, doing, and caring to client situations to achieve good outcomes.

Clinical Judgment

The nurse's actions presented under the dimensions of the full-spectrum nurse incorporated critical thinking and decision making to facilitate the development of clinical judgment. Each bullet shows the synthesis process the nurse used to decide on the safe action for the client. The full-spectrum nurse integrates a comprehensive and systematic approach that fosters clinical reasoning to make and prioritize decisions regarding the appropriate actions to promote quality care and client safety. As you progress through your nursing program, you will develop and expand your clinical judgment.

To explore learning resources for this chapter,

Go to Davis Advantage and find:

Answers and Suggested Responses for all questions in this chapter
Concept Map
Knowledge Map
References and Bibliography

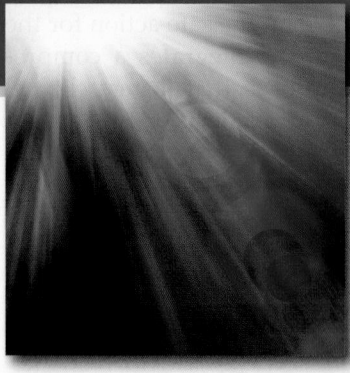

CHAPTER 3

The Steps of the Nursing Process

Learning Outcomes

After completing this chapter, you should be able to:

➤ List the steps of the nursing process and describe features common to each phase.

➤ Explain how each of the steps (assessment, diagnosis, planning, interventions, and evaluation) is related to each of the other steps of the nursing process.

➤ Differentiate among four sources of data: subjective, objective, primary sources, secondary sources.

➤ Describe and differentiate among initial, ongoing, comprehensive, focused, and special needs assessment.

➤ Discuss how to prepare for and conduct an interview.

➤ Describe instances when you should validate data.

➤ Describe the diagnostic process.

➤ Explain the relationship between nursing diagnoses and goals/interventions.

➤ Differentiate between nursing diagnoses, medical diagnoses, and collaborative problems.

➤ Describe the information contained in a comprehensive patient care plan.

➤ Describe a process for writing an individualized care plan, making use of available standardized care-planning documents.

➤ Explain how a goal is derived from a nursing diagnosis.

➤ Explain how nursing interventions are determined by problem status (i.e., as actual or potential problems).

➤ Write complete, detailed nursing orders, in correct format, for the patient.

➤ Define *implementation,* including a description of the three broad phases (doing, delegating, recording).

➤ Identify and describe the "five rights" of delegation.

➤ Describe a process for evaluating client health status (outcomes) after interventions.

➤ Describe a process for evaluating the effectiveness of the nursing care plan.

➤ List variables that may influence the effectiveness of a nursing care plan; state which ones the nurse can and cannot control.

Key Concepts

Assessment

Nursing diagnosis

Planning outcomes

Planning interventions

Implementation

Evaluation

Related Concepts

See the Concept Map on Davis Advantage.

Meet Your Patient

You will be admitting a patient, Todd, from the emergency department (ED). According to the ED report, Todd's admitting medical diagnosis is chronic renal failure. He is married, 58 years old, and employed, and he has a long-standing history of type 2 diabetes mellitus (DM). During the past 3 days, he reports that he has developed swelling and decreased sensation in his legs and difficulty walking, which he describes as "slight loss of mobility." You have many questions concerning Todd's immediate and long-term needs, which include the following:

His medication regimen

His compliance with his diabetes treatment plan

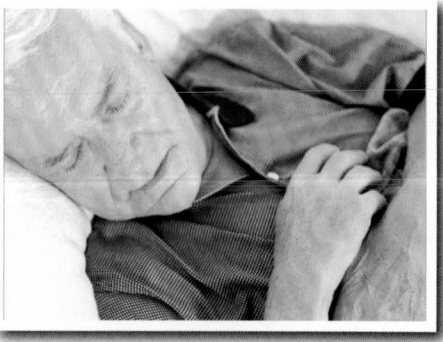

Meet Your Patient (continued)

The extent to which his family is involved
What laboratory tests have been completed
How severe his renal dysfunction has become
His safety needs

After you obtain the necessary data, you need to organize and analyze them to form some initial impressions about what they mean. Diabetes and renal failure require a complex treatment regimen and self-care. Is Todd managing his therapy effectively? If not, what is preventing him from managing it?

Admitting diagnosis is chronic renal failure.

You rank the following nursing diagnoses as the highest priority:

1. Fluid balance excess secondary to chronic renal failure
2. Impaired Mobility secondary to decreased sensation in lower extremities

You write the following desired outcomes (goals) on the care plan:

Goal for Diagnosis 1

Pt will weigh 200 lb by discharge.
Pt will have no evidence of edema in lower extremities within 48 hours of hospitalization.

Goal for Diagnosis 2

Patient performs physical activity independently or within limits of disease by discharge.
Patient uses safety measures to minimize potential for injury continually during hospitalization.
Patient is free from complications of immobility, as evidenced by intact skin, absence of thrombophlebitis, normal bowel pattern, and clear breath sounds by discharge.

These goals will guide you in choosing nursing interventions for relieving Todd's fluid volume excess and preventing complications related to his impaired mobility.

ABOUT THE KEY CONCEPTS

The nursing process is the five-step problem-solving process that nurses use to guide their professional actions. An easy way to remember the steps of the nursing process is through the use of the mnemonic ADPIE:

Assessment: involves gathering **data** about the patient and the patient's health status.
Diagnosis: using critical-thinking skills, the nurse analyzes the assessment data to identify patterns in the data and draw conclusions about the client's health status, including strengths, problems, and factors contributing to the problems.
Planning: encompasses identifying **goals** and **outcomes,** choosing **interventions,** and creating **nursing care plans.**
Implementation: involves performing or delegating planned interventions; this is the step in which you carry out the care plan.
Evaluation: occurs as the last step of the process and involves making judgments about the client's progress toward desired health outcomes, the effectiveness of the nursing care plan, and the quality of nursing care in the healthcare setting.

One important aspect of the nursing process to remember is that even though there are steps, it is not a linear process. One step does not rigidly follow another. Instead, it is a cyclical process that follows a logical progression. You will find that you go back and forth between the steps, especially as you gain nursing experience.

ASSESSMENT: THE FIRST STEP OF THE NURSING PROCESS

Assessment is the systematic gathering of information related to the physiological, psychological, sociocultural, developmental, and spiritual status of an individual, group, or community. The purpose of assessment is to obtain data to allow you to help the patient. Data must be accurate and complete because the remainder of the nursing process rests on this foundation. Assessment:

- Provides contextual information that becomes a part of the **patient database**
- Supplies the data necessary for diagnosis
- Reveals information about motivation and resources that help formulate outcomes
- Helps guide the choice of effective interventions and how to best implement them
- Acts as a guidepost for reassessment in the evaluation step that may determine changes in the care plan

Types and Sources of Data

Assessment data can be categorized as either subjective or objective according to their source. **Subjective data,** also called *covert data* or *symptoms data,* are data the nurse receives via direct communication with the client, family, or community. Subjective data:

- **Reveal the perspective of the person giving the data** and include thoughts, feelings, beliefs, and sensations.
- **Can be used to clarify objective data** (e.g., "How did you get this scar?").

Some people (e.g., infants, adults with mental illness) are unable to provide subjective data. Others can give subjective data, but their accuracy may be in question. For example, how trustworthy is a patient's response that they follow their diet and medication regimen when the results of their blood work are markedly abnormal? For a given situation, the data you obtain from two or more people may not be the same. For example, people with insomnia often report getting much less sleep than their sleep partner says they do.

On the other side of subjective data are **objective data,** also called *overt data* or *signs data*.

Objective data:

- **Are gathered by physical assessment and from laboratory or diagnostic tests**.
- **Can be measured or observed by the nurse or other healthcare providers** (e.g., vital signs, urine output).
- **May be used to validate (check) or verify (confirm) subjective data.** For example, if you think a patient's report of dietary intake and exercise is inaccurate, you would measure the patient's weight and ask for a dietary journal.

Data can also be classified as either primary or secondary (Table 3-1). **Primary data** are data, either subjective or objective in nature, that are obtained directly from the client, either through what the client says or what you observe yourself. **Secondary data** are obtained secondhand, for example, from the medical record or from another caregiver.

Table 3-1 ➤ Examples of Data Types and Sources

Data Types

SUBJECTIVE DATA	OBJECTIVE DATA
"My throat hurts when I swallow."	White patches noted at the back of the throat, and tonsillar area reddened and swollen.
"Our children have no place to go after football games. That is why they get into so much trouble."	In a windshield survey, no public facility was open after football games to allow young people to socialize under supervision.

Data Sources

PRIMARY SOURCE (CLIENT)	SECONDARY SOURCES (EVERYTHING ELSE)
Pulse rate 100 beats/min	From chart: WBC count 14,000/mm^3
States feeling short of breath	In transfer report, nurse states that the surgical dressing is dry.

KnowledgeCheck 3-1

During an appointment at the women's clinic, a client informs the nurse that her menstrual flow is very heavy and that she experiences severe abdominal cramping during menstruation. The client's breast examination is normal. When the nurse sees the laboratory results (i.e., Pap smear result is normal, but hemoglobin level is low), they suspect that the heavy flow may be causing anemia. According to clinic protocol, birth control pills (hormone therapy) are prescribed to control the heavy, painful periods and to provide contraception. Ongoing assessment will include visits every 6 months to evaluate the client's response to hormone therapy and to monitor the anemia. State whether the following data are primary or secondary, subjective or objective:

- You see in the client's health record that the breast examination was normal.
- The client tells the nurse that she experiences cramping with her menstrual cycle.
- The nurse tells you that the client is anemic.
- You check the result of the Pap smear in the electronic health record and see that it is normal.

Nursing Assessment Skills

Nurses collect data using all their senses. Whether assessment is initial or ongoing, comprehensive or focused, you will use the skills of observation, physical examination, and interviewing.

Observation refers to the deliberate use of all of your senses to gather and interpret patient and environmental data. Try to use the same sequence of observation at each patient contact. By making systematic observations each time you are with a patient, you are less likely to miss an assessment area. The mnemonic (memory aid) in Box 3-1 may help.

Physical Assessment or *physical examination* produces primarily objective data and makes use of the following techniques: inspection (visual examination), palpation (touch), percussion (tapping a body surface), direct auscultation (listening with the unaided ear), and indirect auscultation (listening with a stethoscope). All of these are described in detail in Chapter 19.

BOX 3-1 ■ Mnemonic for Systematic Observing

Use the first letter of each word to help you observe systematically as you enter a patient's room.

HELP!

Help. First, observe signs that the patient may be in distress (e.g., pain, pallor, labored breathing)

Environment and equipment. Next, look for safety hazards; look at machines and lines (electrocardiogram monitor, IV). Check that equipment is working (e.g., oxygen, catheter drainage)

Look. Examine the patient thoroughly (i.e., appearance, breathing, dressings, odors)

People. Who are the people in the room? Family? Other caregivers? What are they doing?

The **Nursing Interview** is purposeful, structured communication in which you question the patient in order to gather subjective data for the nursing database. The admission interview is planned, but during ongoing assessment, the interview may be informal, brief, and narrowly focused. Your interview will go more smoothly if you take time to prepare yourself, your patient, and the interview space before you begin asking questions. To learn how to do that, and for tips on conducting and closing an interview,

 Go to **Chapter 3, Clinical Insights 3-1, 3-2, and 3-3,** in Volume 2.

KnowledgeCheck 3-2

Give at least two more examples of data you might obtain with each of the following senses. One example is provided for each.

- Touch (e.g., bladder distention)
- Vision (e.g., facial expression of pain)
- Smell (e.g., fecal odor)
- Hearing (e.g., bowel sounds)

Types of Assessment

Key Point: *Assessment can be broad and general or specific. The type of assessment you do depends on the client's status.* In acute care settings, such as the ED, the assessments are rapid and focused on the presenting problem. In inpatient settings, you may perform an initial comprehensive assessment at admission and other, more focused assessments over time, according to the client's needs.

Initial and Ongoing Assessments

Assessments are said to be "initial" or "ongoing," depending on the time they are performed (e.g., one time on initial patient contact or repeated at intervals). For a comparison of initial assessment and ongoing assessment, see Table 3-2.

Comprehensive Assessments

A comprehensive assessment (also called a *global assessment, patient database,* or *nursing database*):

- Provides holistic information about the client's overall health status.
- Enables you to identify client problems and strengths.
- Enhances your sensitivity to a patient's culture, values, beliefs, and economic situation.
- Uses the nursing skills of observation, physical assessment, and interviewing.

Focused Assessments

A focused assessment is performed to obtain data about an actual, potential, or possible problem that has been identified or is suspected. It focuses on a particular topic, body part, or functional ability rather than on overall health status (e.g., focused assessments of pain or nutrition).

 ThinkLike a Nurse 3-1: Clinical Judgment in Action

Give examples of each type of assessment (initial, ongoing, comprehensive, focused) using patients you have observed or cared for or your own personal experiences as a patient. See Table 3-2.

Suppose you are the triage nurse at the acute care facility in the Meet Your Patient scenario. Explain the kind of assessment you might perform (initial, ongoing, comprehensive, focused).

Special Needs Assessments

A **special needs assessment** is a type of focused assessment that provides in-depth information about a particular area of client functioning. It often involves using a specially designed form. Accrediting agency standards may require certain special needs assessments (e.g., nutrition status, pain) for all clients. You should perform

Table 3-2 ➤ Initial Versus Ongoing Assessment		
	INITIAL ASSESSMENT	**ONGOING ASSESSMENT**
When Performed	Completed when the client first comes to the healthcare agency.	Performed as needed, at any time after the initial database is completed.
Purpose of Data	*Data points:* ■ Are related to the person's reason for seeking nursing or medical assistance ■ Provide guidance for care ■ Help determine need for further assessment	*Data points:* ■ Help identify new problems ■ Follow up on previously identified problems
Discussion	A comprehensive assessment can be completed as the client's condition permits.	The data points reflect the ever-changing state of the client; for example, vital signs may change rapidly, which is an important indicator of developing or resolving health problems.

a special needs assessment any time assessment cues suggest risk factors or problems for the patient. The following are some special needs assessments:

- **Nutritional assessment.** Perform a nutritional assessment when warranted by the patient's needs or condition (i.e., malnourishment or new diabetes diagnosis). In addition to information about food intake, it includes information related to personal, psychosocial, and economic problems that may affect nutrition. See Chapter 24 for more information about nutritional assessments.

- **Pain assessment.** Good nursing care and some accrediting agency standards require you to perform a thorough pain assessment (The Joint Commission, 2022) for all patients during initial and ongoing assessments. For more information on pain assessments, see Chapter 28.

- **Cultural assessment.** Awareness of cultural influences should guide your assessment and nursing care. For the content included in a cultural assessment, see Chapter 12.

- **Spiritual health assessment.** Spiritual health assessment provides insight into how a client's spirituality is affected by current life events and health status—far more than merely asking about the client's religious preference. See Chapter 13 for more detailed information on assessing spiritual health.

- **Psychosocial assessment.** A psychosocial assessment typically includes data about family, lifestyle, usual coping patterns, understanding of the current illness, personality style, previous psychiatric disorders, recent stressors, major issues related to the illness, and mental status. See Chapters 9 and 19 for more details.

- **Wellness assessment.** A wellness assessment includes data about spiritual health, social support, nutrition, physical fitness, health beliefs, and lifestyle, as well as a life-stress review. See Chapter 8 for a more detailed discussion of assessing wellness.

- **Family assessment.** A family assessment provides a better understanding of the client's family-related health values, beliefs, and behaviors. Refer to Chapter 11 for a discussion of family assessment.

- **Community assessment.** A community assessment provides information about community demographics; health concerns; environmental risks; and community resources, norms and values, and points of referral. See Chapter 37 for more information on community assessments.

- **Functional ability assessment.** A functional ability assessment evaluates functional status. Health problems and normal aging changes often bring a decline in functional status. Future rehabilitation needs are derived from initial and ongoing functional ability assessments.

 Go to **Chapter 3, Assessment Guidelines and Tools,** Functional Ability Assessment, in Volume 2.

▲ ThinkLike a Nurse 3-2: Clinical Judgment in Action

Based on the data you have so far about Todd (Meet Your Patient), consider the need to perform any of the special-purpose assessments. What is your rationale for using or not using a special needs assessment for your patient?

PracticalKnowledge knowing how

In this chapter, practical knowledge involves your skill in using structured and unstructured methods of data collection and validating, organizing, and documenting your assessment findings.

INTERVIEWING TO OBTAIN A NURSING HEALTH HISTORY

Imagine an older man is admitted to the hospital with a fractured hip. The physician is interested in the cause of the fracture, the extent of the injury, and any preexisting medical problems that suggest the client is a poor surgical risk. As the nurse, you, too, would ask about the cause of the injury. However, you would also want to (1) know what effect the injury has on the man's ability to perform his everyday activities and (2) identify his supports and strengths to begin planning for his eventual discharge and self-care. **Key Point: *So you see, the nursing health history covers some of the same topics as the medical history, but the reason for the questions is different.***

Health history forms vary among agencies and according to purpose (e.g., inpatient, clinic, surgery, medical, ED), but most include questions about the following components:

- Biographical data
- Chief complaint (reason for seeking healthcare)
- History of present illness
- Client's perception of health status and expectations for care
- Past health history (sometimes called *medical history*)
- Family health history
- Social history
- Medication history and device use
- Complementary/alternative modalities (CAM) used
- Review of body systems and associated functional abilities

Types of Interviews

Interviews may be directive or nondirective (see Table 3-3). A successful interviewer uses a combination of closed and open-ended questions.

- **Closed questions** are those that can be answered with "yes," "no," or other short, factual answers. They usually begin with *who, when, where, what, do (did, does),* and *is (are, were).*

Table 3-3 ➤ Comparison of Directive and Nondirective Interviews

	DIRECTIVE INTERVIEW	NONDIRECTIVE INTERVIEW
Characteristics	Nurse controls the topics Uses mostly **closed questions**	Patient controls subject matter Nurse clarifies, summarizes, and questions Uses mostly **open-ended questions**
Uses	Obtain factual, easily categorized information In emergency situation	Promote communication Facilitate thought Build rapport Help patient to express feelings

■ **Open-ended questions** specify a topic to be explored but phrase it broadly to encourage the patient to elaborate. Use such questions when you want to obtain subjective data. From the answers to the broad questions, you can decide which topics to clarify or follow up with using specific and closed questions.

Preparing for an Interview

While you are learning, you may feel uncomfortable interviewing patients. You may be concerned that:

■ **You are imposing on the patient, who clearly needs rest more than you need information.** This feeling may be because you believe a "real nurse" has already obtained the information or because you don't have a clear idea of how the information will be used to help the patient.
■ **The patient won't be receptive to answering personal questions from a stranger (you).** To help set the tone for the interview, be sure to tell your patients that the information given will be kept confidential and that the patient is free to choose what to tell and what to withhold from you. Also, be aware that the patient may have been feeling the need to talk about something, has not known how to bring it up, and is actually relieved that you have introduced the topic.
■ **Some of your questions will upset the patient—the person might cry or become angry.** Remember that patients usually feel better after releasing their emotions. Expressions of strong emotion may cause you discomfort, but you must learn to accept them. You will have large gaps in your data if you avoid difficult topics, and your patients will not get the help they need.

Your interviews will go more smoothly if you take time to prepare yourself, your patient, and the interview space before you begin asking questions. To learn how to do that, and for tips on conducting and closing an interview,

 Go to Chapter 3, **Clinical Insights 3-1, 3-2, and 3-3,** in Volume 2.

How and When Should I Validate Data?

Suppose a patient has told you that they have never had high blood pressure (BP), but you obtain an abnormal BP reading of 180/98 mm Hg. Would you record the 180/98 mm Hg reading, or would you:

■ Ask the patient some more questions, such as, "What do you mean when you say you have never had high blood pressure?" or "What have you been doing in the last 15 minutes?"
■ Check the BP in the patient's other arm?
■ Wait a few minutes and take the reading again in the same arm?
■ Retake the BP using a different sphygmomanometer?
■ Compare the reading to previous entries in the chart?
■ Ask another nurse to double-check your findings?

All of these are ways to **validate** (double-check) your data. Validating data helps to ensure information is accurate, complete, and factual and that you have not jumped to conclusions. Not all data must be validated; you should validate data under the following circumstances (Wilkinson, 2017):

■ **Subjective and objective data do not agree or do not make sense together.**
  Example: In the preceding situation, the subjective data item "never had high BP" does not agree with the objective data item, BP 180/98 mm Hg, a high reading.
■ **The patient's statements differ at different times in the interview.**
  Example: A patient tells you that they follow a low-cholesterol diet. However, when describing their usual daily food pattern, they mention that they eat eggs, cheese sandwiches, and hamburgers.
■ **The data fall far outside the normal range.**
  Example: A patient has no symptoms of infection or high fever, but you obtain an elevated oral temperature reading of 104°F (40°C). (Hint: Ask the patient whether they have just had something warm to drink.)

- **Factors are present that interfere with accurate measurement.**
  Example: The patient has very large arms, and there are no appropriately sized BP cuffs available. Therefore, because the BP will probably not be accurate, you should measure it again after you are able to obtain the appropriate equipment .

HOW CAN I ORGANIZE DATA?

Professional standards require systematic data collection (American Nurses Association [ANA], 2021; National Council of State Boards of Nursing [NCSBN], 2017, revised August 2021; The Joint Commission, 2022). This means you collect and record data in predetermined categories, not just at random. The data in most initial assessments are already categorized by the agency's data-collection form. Many agency assessment forms use a **body systems (medical) framework.** This model is useful for identifying medical problems, but it needs to be combined with other models to provide the holistic data you need to identify both nursing and medical problems.

Maslow's Hierarchy of Needs (Maslow, 1970; Maslow & Lowery, 1998) groups data according to human needs. It states that the basic needs must be met before higher needs can be addressed. Maslow's hierarchy of needs provides another way to organize data. This framework is useful in setting priorities when planning nursing care. See Chapter 4 for an in-depth discussion of Maslow's model.

HOW SHOULD I DOCUMENT DATA

The ANA's *Scope and Standards of Practice* (2021) and The Joint Commission's *Hospital Accreditation Standards* (2021) emphasize the importance of complete, accurate, and timely patient records. Documentation of all assessment findings benefits both patients and nurses:

- It benefits patients by providing the basis for planning effective nursing care.
- It protects nurses by establishing that you actually performed the needed assessments. The nursing database is a permanent part of the client's record (a legal document). Malpractice suits are not unusual in our society, and a malpractice suit may be filed years after you care for a patient. The assumption in malpractice cases is "If it isn't documented, it wasn't done."

Guidelines for Recording Assessment Data

Follow these guidelines when recording assessment data:

- **Document as soon as possible** after you perform the assessment.
- **Write neatly, legibly, and in black ink,** or record data electronically.

- **Use proper spelling and grammar.**
- **Use acronyms sparingly,** using only agency-approved abbreviations.
- **Write the patient's own words, when possible,** in quotation marks. If the comments are too long, summarize what the patient says (e.g., "Patient states they are sleepy").
- **Record only the most important patient words.** If you record everything the patient says, your notes will contain irrelevant data and be too long. For example, write, "Patient states, 'I hardly slept at all last night,'" even though what they actually said was, "I hardly slept at all last night. People kept waking me up, then I had to get up to go to the bathroom, and my wife called early this morning."
- **Use concrete, specific information** rather than vague generalities such as *normal, adequate, good,* and *tolerated well.*
- **Record cues, not inferences. Cues** are what the client says and what you observe. **Inferences** are judgments and interpretations about what the cues mean. When recording cues, you do not need to use words such as *appears* and *seems* (e.g., "incision seems red" or "edges appear separated").

Cues	Inferences
Incision red, draining pus, edges separated.	Incision is infected.
Tearful. States that father died of a heart attack. Trembling.	Anxious about scheduled cardiac catheterization.
States, "I hate my mother. I wish I was dead."	Angry and suicidal.

Tools for Recording Assessment Data

Each organization has its own forms and formats for documenting initial and ongoing assessments. You will record data on a variety of documents, including the following:

- **Graphic flow sheet.** Includes vital signs such as blood pressure, pulse, respirations, and temperature so that trends over time can be seen clearly (Fig. 3-1).
- **Intake and output (I&O) sheet.** May be on the graphic flow sheet, as in Figures 3-1 and 3-2, or separate document. This form records all intake (e.g., oral, intravenous, and tube feedings) and all output (e.g., urine, fluid from drainage tubes, wound drainage, and emesis).
- **Nursing admission assessment.** Forms may differ among organizations, but all collect similar data as specified by accrediting agencies for standards for initial assessment.
- **Nursing discharge summary.** This may be a part of the initial assessment form because data obtained at admission are used for discharge planning.
- **Special-purpose forms.** Includes diabetic flow sheets and medication administration forms, along with many others.
- **Electronic documentation.** In most facilities, initial data and ongoing assessment data are entered into a computer program for organization, shared communication, and easy retrieval (Fig. 3-2).

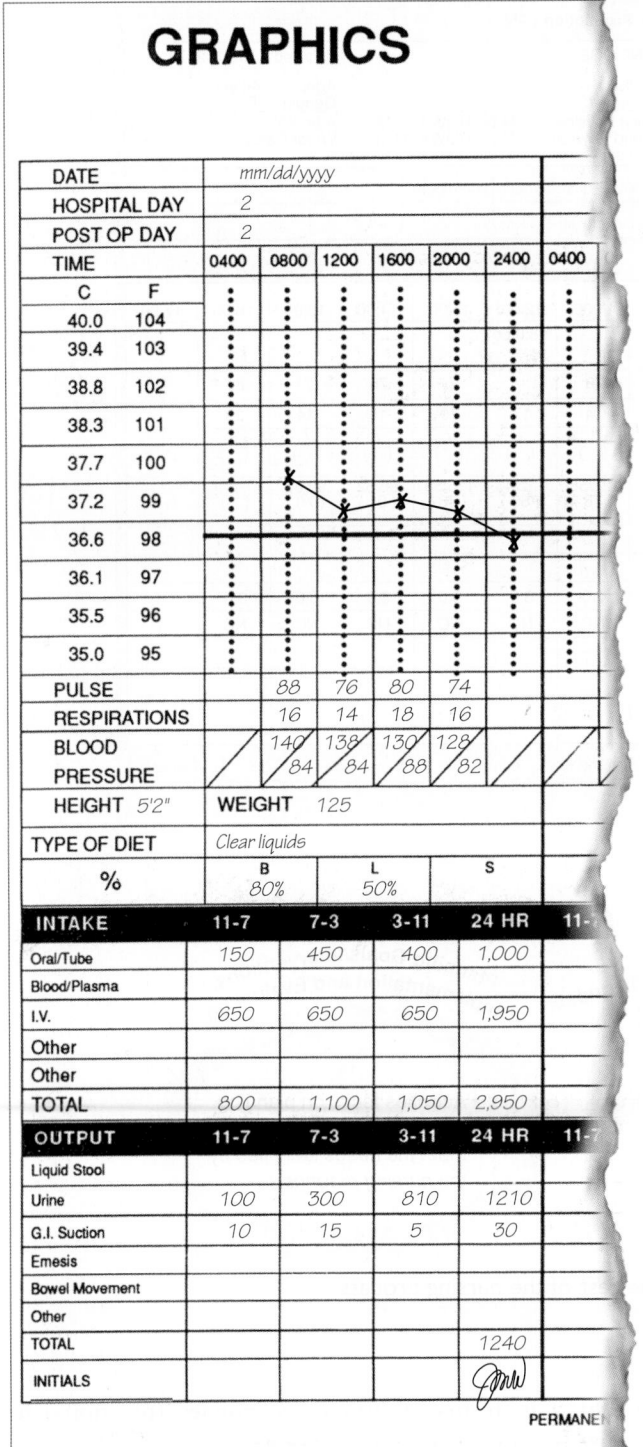

GRAPHICS

DATE	mm/dd/yyyy						
HOSPITAL DAY	2						
POST OP DAY	2						
TIME	0400	0800	1200	1600	2000	2400	0400

C	F
40.0	104
39.4	103
38.8	102
38.3	101
37.7	100
37.2	99
36.6	98
36.1	97
35.5	96
35.0	95

PULSE	88	76	80	74	
RESPIRATIONS	16	14	18	16	
BLOOD PRESSURE	140/84	138/84	130/88	128/82	
HEIGHT 5'2"	WEIGHT	125			
TYPE OF DIET	Clear liquids				
%	B 80%	L 50%	S		

INTAKE	11-7	7-3	3-11	24 HR	11-
Oral/Tube	150	450	400	1,000	
Blood/Plasma					
I.V.	650	650	650	1,950	
Other					
Other					
TOTAL	800	1,100	1,050	2,950	

OUTPUT	11-7	7-3	3-11	24 HR	11-7
Liquid Stool					
Urine	100	300	810	1210	
G.I. Suction	10	15	5	30	
Emesis					
Bowel Movement					
Other					
TOTAL				1240	
INITIALS					

PERMANE

FIGURE 3-1. Graphic flow sheet.

ANALYSIS/DIAGNOSIS: THE SECOND STEP OF THE NURSING PROCESS

Diagnosis (or analysis) is the phase in which you use your critical-thinking skills to analyze the assessment cues. In analyzing, you identify patterns in the data and draw conclusions about the client's health status, including strengths, problems, and factors contributing to problems. As in all phases of the nursing process, involve the patient and family as much as possible.

Most nurses begin diagnostic reasoning during the assessment phase. For example, if a client has a medical diagnosis of chronic renal failure, you would immediately consider the nursing diagnosis of Risk for Imbalanced Fluid Volume. However, you would obtain more data before confirming and recording that as a nursing diagnosis; your tentative diagnostic conclusion leads you to identify more cues: *Is the client still producing urine? What is the client's oral intake? Does the client demonstrate edema?* Do you see how you would move back and forth between assessment and diagnosis?

Diagnosis is critical because it links the assessment step, which precedes it, to all the steps that follow it (Fig. 3-3). Assessment data must be complete and accurate for you to make an accurate nursing diagnosis. **Key Point:** *The purpose of diagnosing is to identify the client's health status. Accuracy is essential because the diagnosis is the basis for planning client-centered goals and interventions.*

What Are the Origins of Nursing Diagnosis?

Until the early 1970s, nursing diagnosis was not widely used in nursing practice, but two major events in 1973 spurred change:

- The First National Conference on the Classification of Nursing Diagnoses was held (Gebbie & Lavin, 1975). A national task force was formed to begin developing a language to describe the health problems treated by nurses.
- The ANA's *Nursing Scope and Standards of Nursing Practice* included nursing diagnosis as an expectation of professional nurses.

In 1980, the ANA published *Nursing's Social Policy Statement,* which characterized nursing as "the diagnosis and treatment of human response to actual or potential health problems" (ANA, 1980). **Key Point:** *The formal list of nursing diagnostic labels describes health problems that can be addressed by independent nursing actions and, in that sense, forms the body of knowledge that is unique to nursing.*

Since the first conference, the nursing diagnosis group has continued to meet every 2 years and is now known as NANDA International, Inc. (NANDA-I). NANDA-I continues the work of refining diagnostic labels and reviewing nursing diagnoses submitted by individuals or nursing organizations. Diagnoses on the official list are approved for clinical use and further study. They do not represent a finished product because many of the diagnoses are only partially substantiated by research.

KnowledgeCheck 3-3

- Why is the diagnosis step so critical to the other phases of the nursing process?
- Which two nursing organizations have been responsible for making diagnosis a part of the professional nursing role?

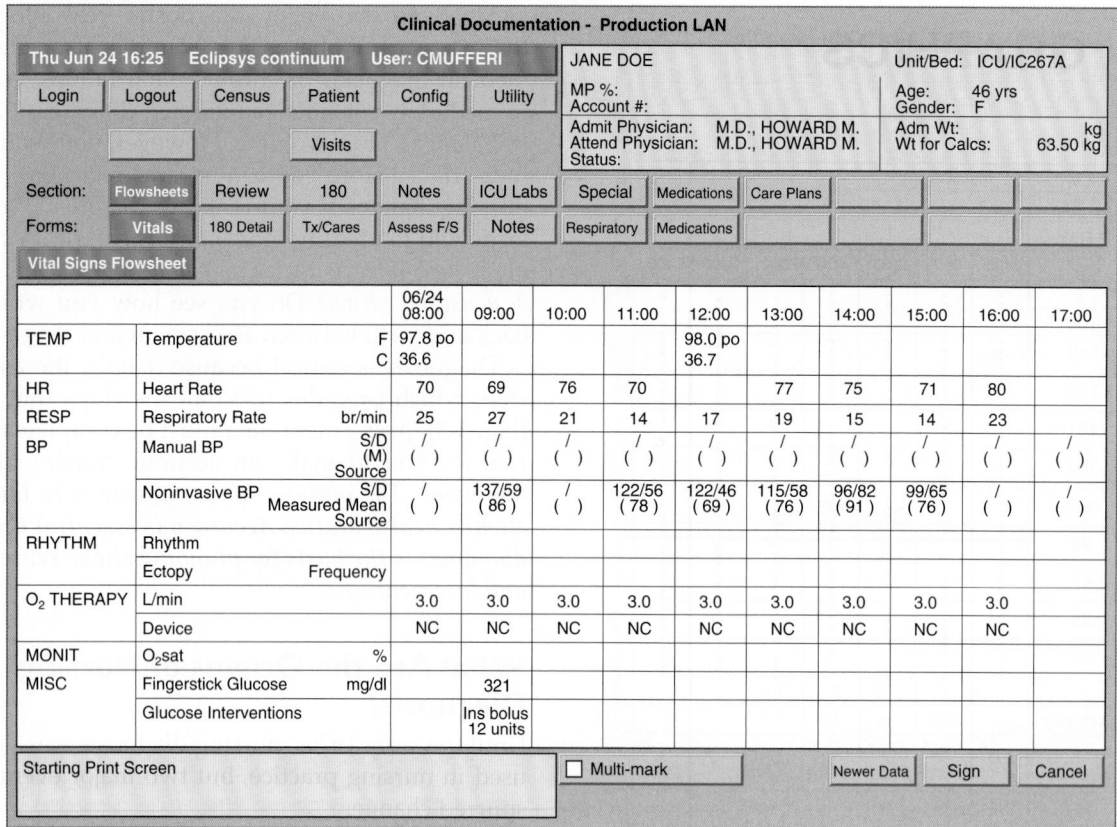

FIGURE 3-2. Computer screen capture: Assessment data.

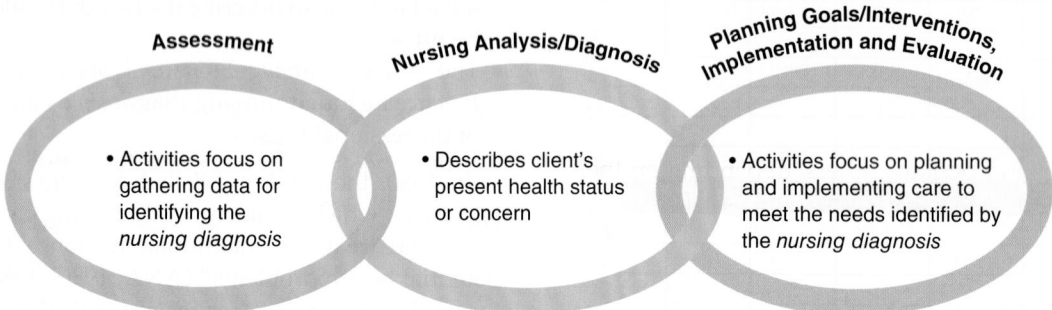

FIGURE 3-3. Diagnosis links the assessment phase to the rest of the nursing process.

Recognizing When to Use Nursing Diagnoses

A **health problem** is any condition that requires intervention to promote wellness or to prevent or treat disease or illness. After you identify a health problem, you must decide how to treat it—independently or in collaboration with other health professionals. **Key Point:** *The answer determines whether it is a nursing diagnosis, a medical diagnosis, or a collaborative problem.* Knowing how to differentiate among these is an important part of nursing care.

A **nursing diagnosis** is:

■ A statement of client health status that nurses can identify, prevent, or treat independently.

■ Stated in terms of **human responses** (reactions) to disease, injury, or other stressors.

■ A human response that can be biological, emotional, interpersonal, social, or spiritual and can be either a problem or a strength. For example, a *physical* response to renal failure might be excess fluid volume; an *emotional* response might be anxiety or fear.

A **medical diagnosis** describes a disease, illness, or injury. Its purpose is to identify a pathology so that appropriate treatment can be given to cure the condition. Todd (Meet Your Patient) has two medical diagnoses: chronic renal failure and type 2 DM.

Key Point: *Except for advanced practice nurses, nurses cannot legally diagnose or treat medical problems.*

Your assessment data can, however, be helpful in identifying disease states and in evaluating the effects of medical therapies (e.g., whether a medication relieves a patient's pain). The following are differences between medical and nursing diagnoses:

- **A medical diagnosis is more narrowly focused than a nursing diagnosis.**
- **A medical diagnosis, disease, or pathological condition can have any number of nursing diagnoses associated with it.** In the Meet Your Patient scenario, Todd's medical diagnosis of type 2 DM will not change because his body's ability to properly utilize glucose will not change. A *nursing diagnosis* is different in that respect. Nursing diagnoses are human responses, complex and unique to each person. For example, suppose Todd has a nursing diagnosis of "Nonadherence to diabetic diet r/t (related to) lack of knowledge about food groups." If he learns about the foods and begins following his diet, he will no longer have a diagnosis of nonadherence, even though his medical diagnosis (type 2 DM) has not changed.
- **A medical diagnosis, disease, or pathological condition can have any number of nursing diagnoses associated with it.** For example, in response to his type 2 DM, Todd might have nursing diagnoses of Lack of Knowledge, Risk for Impaired Skin Integrity, and Nonadherence.
- **Clients with the same medical diagnosis may have different nursing diagnoses.** Another client with type 2 DM may not have a diagnosis of Nonadherence but instead may have a diagnosis of Denial because they simply cannot accept that they truly have diabetes. Other patients with type 2 DM might have diagnoses of Anxiety, Ineffective Health Management, Negative Body Image, and perhaps others, depending on their unique responses to the stressor, type 2 DM.

Recognizing Collaborative Problems

Collaborative problems are "certain physiological complications that nurses monitor to detect onset or changes in status"; nurses manage collaborative problems using physician-prescribed and nursing-prescribed interventions to minimize the complications of the events (Carpenito, 2016, p. 8). Collaborative problems have the following characteristics:

- **All patients who have a certain disease or medical treatment are at risk for developing the same complications.** That is, the collaborative problems (complications) are determined by the medical diagnosis or pathology. Use your knowledge of anatomy, physiology, microbiology, pathophysiology, and other subjects as the basis for identifying the complications associated with a particular disease or treatment. Consider these examples:
  - Because Todd has type 2 DM, he has the collaborative problem Potential Complication of type 2 DM: hyperglycemia and/or hypoglycemia. All other patients with type 2 DM also have those potential complications.

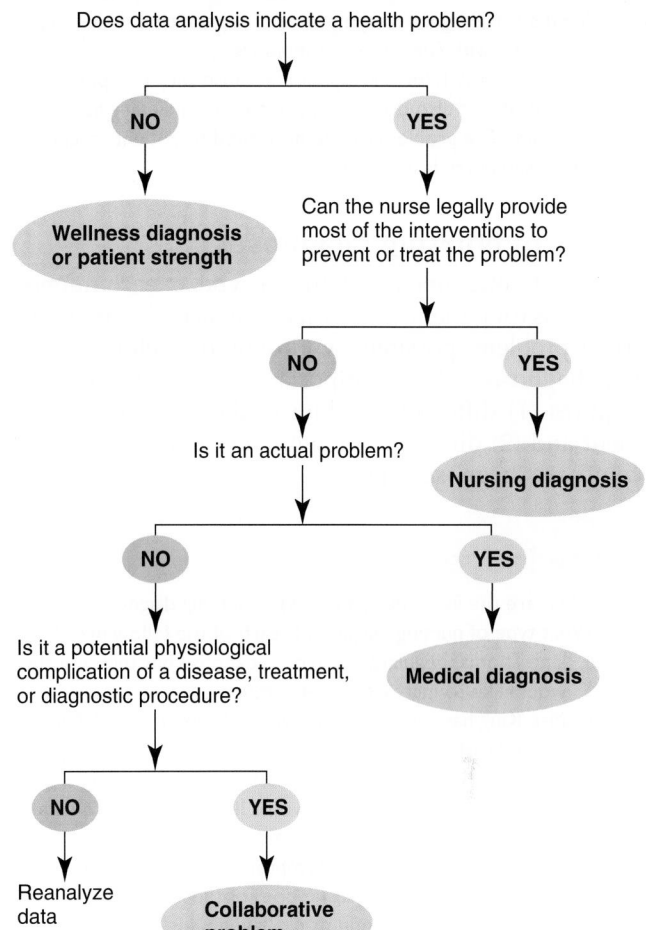

FIGURE 3-4. Algorithm for distinguishing among nursing, medical, and collaborative problems.

- All patients having surgery have the collaborative problem Potential Complication of surgery: infection.
- **A collaborative problem is always a *potential* problem.** If it becomes *actual*, then it is a medical diagnosis requiring interventions by a healthcare provider. Consider what would be needed if a risk for infection became an *actual* infection of a surgical incision. Could a nurse treat that independently?
- **If you can prevent the complication with independent nursing interventions alone, it is not a collaborative problem.** The purpose of independent nursing interventions is primarily to monitor for onset of the complication, although nurses can provide some independent preventive measures.

See Figure 3-4 for an algorithm to help you differentiate nursing diagnoses from medical diagnoses and collaborative problems.

KnowledgeCheck 3-4

State whether each of the following represents a nursing diagnosis, medical diagnosis, or collaborative problem:

- After giving birth, all patients are at risk for developing postpartum hemorrhage.

- A patient has signs and symptoms of appendicitis, which must be treated with surgery and antibiotics.
- A client is at risk for constipation because they postpone defecation and also do not consume enough dietary fiber and fluids. The problem can be prevented by patient teaching, which the nurse is licensed to do.

Types of Nursing Diagnoses

You must determine the status, or type, of each nursing diagnosis (or patient concern). Is it an actual or potential (risk) problem, possible, syndrome, or wellness nursing diagnosis? This is important because each status requires (1) different wording in the diagnostic statement and (2) different nursing interventions. Table 3-4 compares diagnosis types.

KnowledgeCheck 3-5

- What are the five types (statuses) of nursing diagnoses?
- What type of nursing diagnosis is each of the following?
  a. Jane Thomas regularly engages in exercise but tells you she would like to increase her endurance.
  b. Mrs. King has several of the signs and symptoms (defining characteristics) of the nursing diagnosis Ineffective Coping.
  c. Alicia Hernandez seems anxious, but you are not sure whether she actually is. You would like to have more data in order to diagnose or rule out a diagnosis of Anxiety.
  d. Charles Oberfeldt has no symptoms of constipation. However, he reports that he does not include many fiber-rich foods in his diet and drinks few liquids. In addition, he is now fairly inactive because of a back injury. These are all risk factors for a diagnosis of Constipation.

WHAT IS DIAGNOSTIC REASONING

Key Point: *Diagnostic reasoning is the thinking process that enables you to make sense of data gathered during a comprehensive patient assessment. It is also known as analysis or the diagnostic process.* This text presents diagnostic reasoning in separate steps so that it is easier to learn, but that is not the way it really occurs (Fig. 3-5). Just as you move back and forth between assessing and diagnosing, you will soon find yourself moving back and forth among the steps of diagnostic reasoning.

In diagnostic reasoning, you will think critically to analyze and interpret data, draw conclusions about the patient's health status, verify problems with the patient, prioritize the problems, and record the diagnostic statements.

Analyze and Interpret Data

As you analyze and interpret the data (also called *cues*), you will gradually narrow the field of data to significant points and patterns, and you will note the need for new information and further assessment. To analyze and interpret data, follow three steps: (1) identify significant cues, (2) cluster cues, and (3) identify data gaps and inconsistencies.

Step 1. Identify Significant Cues
Significant cues:

- Usually are unhealthy responses.
- Draw on your theoretical knowledge (e.g., of anatomy, physiology, psychology).
- May be related—one cue should alert you to look for others that might be related to it (forming a pattern).
- Influence your conclusions about the client's health status.

Pay special attention to deviations from population norms, changes in usual behaviors in roles or relationships, and behavior (either recent or long-standing) that is nonproductive or dysfunctional.

> *Example:* Suppose you have noted that a woman's pulse rate is 110 beats/min. Is this an unhealthy response—a cue? Compare the rate with your theoretical knowledge—for example, the normal range for an adult pulse is 60 to 100 beats/min. This woman is a longtime cigarette smoker who also drinks a lot of coffee. These habits increase pulse rate, so 110 beats/min may be a normal finding for this client.

See Box 3-2 for indicators that help you recognize clues.

KnowledgeCheck 3-6

- What is a cue?
- What are four ways you can recognize a cue?

Step 2. Cluster Cues

A **cluster** is a group of cues that are related to each other in some way. The cluster may suggest a health problem. **Key Point:** *To help ensure accuracy, you should always derive a nursing diagnosis from data clusters rather than from a single cue.*

> *Example:* Alma was transferred to the hospital from a long-term care facility. Because of a cerebrovascular accident (CVA), or stroke, Alma can make sounds but cannot speak; because of joint contractures, she cannot use her hands and arms. Alma is frequently incontinent of urine, so the nurses have diagnosed *Total Urinary Incontinence* and are resigned to the idea that Alma will not be able to control her urine. When a nursing student is assigned to care for Alma, the student looks for additional cues.

- The student notices that Alma is often incontinent after loud vocalizing.
- The student observes that Alma is incontinent, cannot use her hands and arms, and cannot communicate in words but is vocalizing.
- Seeing a pattern in the cues, the student changes the nursing diagnosis to *Toileting Self-Care Deficit* related to immobility and inability to communicate the need to void.
- After the student provides a call device that fits under the arm, Alma is able to press the device and call the nurse when she needs to void. She is no longer incontinent.

Table 3-4 ➤ Differentiating Problem Types: Medical, Collaborative, and Nursing Diagnoses

DIAGNOSIS TYPE	DEFINITION AND CHARACTERISTICS	EXAMPLES
Medical Diagnosis	Describes a disease, illness, or injury. Its purpose is to identify a pathology so that appropriate treatment can be given.	Examples: Chronic renal failure, type 2 diabetes (T2D)
Collaborative Problem	Determined by medical diagnosis or pathology and is a potential event that nurses monitor to detect onset or changes in status. Managed by physician-prescribed and nursing-prescribed interventions to minimize the complications.	Example: A patient with T2D has the collaborative problem Potential Complication of T2D: hyperglycemia and/or hypoglycemia. All other patients with T2D also have those potential complications.
Actual Nursing Diagnosis: *Problem Is Present*	A problem response that exists at the time of the assessment. Cues (signs and symptoms) that are present.	A patient with T2D may have an actual nursing diagnosis of Impaired Walking or perhaps Impaired Physical Mobility, related to lack of peripheral sensation
Risk (Potential) Nursing Diagnosis: *Problem May Occur*	A problem response that is likely to develop in a vulnerable patient if the nurse and patient do not intervene to prevent it. No cues of the problem, but risk factors are present that increase the patient's vulnerability. The patient is more susceptible to the problem than others in the same or a comparable setting (e.g., one who is undernourished or who has a compromised immune system).	*Examples:* 1. A patient with loss of lower-limb sensation might have a risk, or potential, diagnosis of Risk for Falls even though they have no history of falling. 2. All surgical patients have at least some risk for developing infection, so it is logical to write *Potential Complication of surgery: infection (incision and systemic)* on every surgical care plan.
Possible Nursing Diagnosis: *Problem May Be Present*	Use when your intuition and experience direct you to suspect that a diagnosis is present, but you do not have enough cues to support the diagnosis. The main reason for including this type of diagnosis on a care plan is to alert other nurses to continue to collect data to confirm or rule out the problem.	A patient has the symptom "slight difficulty walking." This could indicate the diagnosis Impaired Physical Mobility, Impaired Walking, or Risk for Falls. You need more data about the difficulty walking to decide which mobility nursing diagnosis is appropriate.
Syndrome Nursing Diagnosis: *Several Related Problems Are Present*	Represents a collection of nursing diagnoses that usually occur together. Use when you notice that the patient has more than one nursing diagnosis with the same etiology (cause, contributing factors).	Example: The NANDA-I label Risk for Disuse Syndrome is used to represent all the complications that can occur as a result of immobility (e.g., pressure injury, constipation, stasis of pulmonary secretions, thrombosis, body image disturbance).
Patient Strengths	Data include history and observations obtained during assessment. Noticing the patient's strengths (what and who matters to the patient) helps support recovery and healing.	A patient might mention their marital status, family involvement, religious activities, and steady employment
Wellness Nursing Diagnosis: *No Problem Is Present*	Describes health status but does not describe a problem; can apply to an individual, family, group, or community. Use when the patient is in transition from one level of wellness to a higher level. Two conditions must be present: 1. The patient's present level of wellness is effective. 2. The patient wants to move to a higher level of wellness.	Suppose that a patient tells you that they pray, participate in religious activities, and trust in God, but they would like to feel even closer to God. They ask to meet with the minister from their church. You might make a diagnosis of Readiness for Enhanced Spiritual Well-Being.

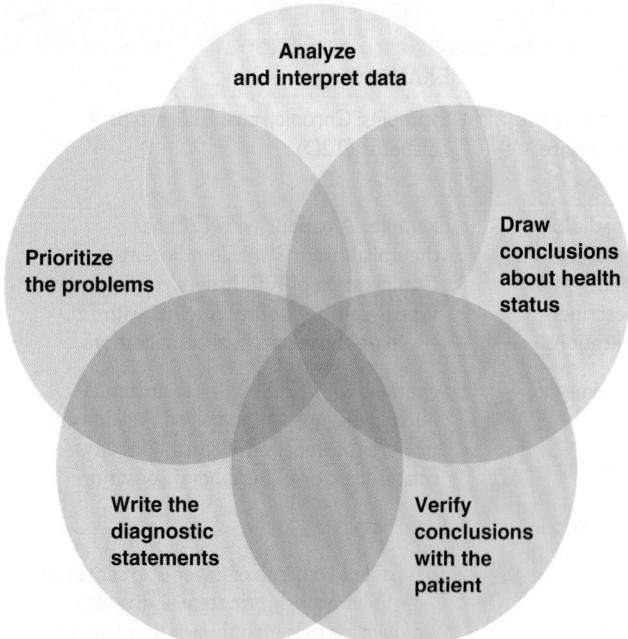

FIGURE 3-5. The process of diagnostic reasoning.

BOX 3-2 ■ Focused Ability Assessment

Questions that may be part of a focused ability assessment include the following:

Does the client require devices such as a cane or crutches for support? (Mobility)

Can the client get in and out of bed or chair without assistance? (Transfer)

Can the client feed self without assistance? (Feeding)

Can the client bathe self without help? (Bathing)

Can the client get all necessary clothing from drawers and closets and get dressed without help? (Dressing)

Can the client go to the bathroom, use the toilet, clean self, and rearrange clothing without help? (Toileting)

Does the client independently control urination and bowel movements? Does the client require an indwelling urinary catheter? (Continence)

If the client is unable to provide self-care for any of these issues, determine the type of assistance they require.

 Think**Like a Nurse** 3-3:
Clinical Judgment **in Action**

For each of the following cue clusters, decide whether the cues represent a pattern; that is, are all the cues related in some way? If so, explain how they are related. If not, state which cue does not fit. If you do not have enough theoretical knowledge to know for sure, draw on your past experiences and discuss the clusters with other students.

a. Dry skin; abnormal skin turgor (more than 4 seconds); thirst; and scanty, dark-yellow urine
b. Pain and limited range of motion in knees, uses walker, medical diagnosis of osteoarthritis
c. Hard, painful bowel movement about every 3 days; does not exercise regularly; eats very little dietary fiber; skin is dry

Step 3. Identify Data Gaps and Inconsistencies

As you cluster cues and think about relationships among them, you will identify the need for data that were not previously gathered.

Data Gaps Data gaps are missing pieces of the diagnostic puzzle. As an example, look again at Todd's data (Meet Your Patient). Except for medical diagnoses, there are very few pieces of data. The following data gaps exist:

■ His admitting diagnosis, chronic renal failure, suggests the possibility of fluid imbalance; however, the data needed to support that are decreased intake and output, dark urine, skin turgor, and complaints of thirst.
■ Admission to the ED could cause anxiety. To pursue that line of thinking, observe for physical and verbal symptoms of anxiety.
■ Decreased sensation in his lower extremities could create mobility or safety problems. You would need to know the degree of sensation loss and the exact meaning of "slight loss of mobility" to confirm a diagnosis.

Inconsistencies in Data Inconsistencies occur when subjective and objective data do not align or when a client's statement of the problem changes in significant ways. Suppose a woman tells you, "I really don't eat much." However, she is 5 feet tall and weighs 190 pounds. The client's statement and the data appear inconsistent. Your theoretical knowledge tells you that obesity is usually caused by excessive intake of calories, although there may be other factors contributing to the condition. You need more specific data, such as what she actually eats, whether she has any medical problems that might contribute to obesity (e.g., hypothyroidism), and whether she lacks knowledge about the calorie content in various foods.

Draw Conclusions About Health Status

After clustering cues and collecting any missing data, the next step is to begin drawing conclusions about the patient's health status—strengths as well as problems. You will need to make inferences and identify problem etiologies, as well as decide which type of problem the cue cluster represents.

Step I. Make Inferences

Making inferences is a critical-thinking skill. Recall that cues are facts (or data), whereas inferences are conclusions (judgments, interpretations) that are based on the data. An inference is not a fact because you cannot directly check its truth or accuracy, for example:

Fact: Patient is crying. (You can observe that directly.)
          Patient is trembling. (You can observe that directly.)
Inference: Patient is anxious. (You cannot observe anxiety, but you know that crying and trembling may be signs of anxiety.)

Checking inferences for accuracy is always a good idea. Suppose you say to the patient, "You seem upset. Can you tell me what's going on?" The patient replies, "So much has been happening. I guess I'm just anxious about everything." Now you have enough data to support your inference, and you can be reasonably sure that it is accurate (valid).

Key Point: *Nursing diagnoses are inferences—and are only your reasoned judgment about a patient's health status. Try not to think of a diagnosis as being right or wrong but instead as more accurate or less accurate. You can never construct a perfect diagnosis, but you must strive to make your diagnostic statements as accurate as possible to ensure that care is effective.*

KnowledgeCheck 3-7

- What are the possible conclusions you can draw about a client's health status (e.g., that no problem exists)?
- What is the difference between a cue and an inference?

Step 2. Identify Problem Etiologies

An **etiology** consists of the factors that are causing or contributing to a problem. Etiologies may be pathophysiological, treatment related, situational, social, spiritual, developmental, or environmental. It is important to correctly identify the etiology because it directs the nursing interventions. Consider this nursing diagnosis:

Constipation related to inadequate intake of dietary fiber

The etiology suggests that you encourage the client to eat more high-fiber foods. But what if that etiology is incomplete? What if you overlooked the fact that the client does not drink enough fluids? Or that they get very little exercise? In that case, your efforts to increase the intake of high-fiber foods would probably not help relieve the client's constipation.

To identify the etiology of a health problem, use theoretical knowledge (e.g., of psychology, physiology, disease processes) to answer questions such as the following:

- What factors are known to cause this problem?
- What cues are present that may be contributing to this problem?
- How likely is it that these factors are contributing to the problem?
- Are these cues *causing* the problem, or are they merely *symptoms* of the problem?

Key Point: *An etiology is always an inference because you can never actually observe the "link" between etiology and problem.* For example, in the preceding Constipation diagnosis, you could measure (observe) the person's fiber intake. You could also observe infrequent, hard stools. But you cannot observe that the lack of fiber is the cause of the constipation. You have to infer that link based on your knowledge of normal elimination and your experiences with other patients.

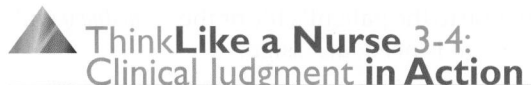

ThinkLike a Nurse 3-4:
Clinical Judgment in Action

How would your nursing interventions be different for the following diagnoses?

a. Constipation related to lack of knowledge about laxative use
b. Constipation related to weak abdominal muscles secondary to long-term immobility

Verify Problems With the Patient

After identifying problems and etiologies, verify them with the patient. A diagnostic statement is an interpretation of the data, and the patient's interpretations may differ from yours. For example, if you have diagnosed Ineffective Breastfeeding related to a lack of knowledge about breastfeeding techniques, you might verify it by saying, "It seems to me you are not sure how to position him and get him to latch onto your breast. Is that accurate?" The patient might confirm your diagnosis, or they might say, "No. I *do* know how to do it; I am just tired and a little nervous with you watching me." **Key Point:** *Think of nursing diagnoses as tentative, and be open to changing them based on new data or insights from the patient.*

Prioritize Problems

Key Point: *Clients often have more than one problem, so you must use nursing judgment to decide which to address first and which are safe to address later. This is prioritizing.*

Prioritizing puts the problems in order of importance, but it does not mean you must resolve one problem before attending to another.

You will usually prioritize problems as you are recording them.

Problem priority is largely determined by the theoretical framework that you use (i.e., whether your criteria are human needs, problem urgency, future consequences, or patient preference). You can indicate the priority by designating each problem as high, medium, or low priority or by ranking all the problems in order from highest to lowest (e.g., 1, 2, 3, 4).

Labeling Each Problem	*Ranking the Problems*
Pain (high)	1—Risk for falls
Falls risk (high)	2—Pain
Chronic low self-esteem disturbance (low)	3—Nutrition deficit
Nutrition deficit (medium)	4—Chronic low self-esteem

Many nurses use Maslow's hierarchy to prioritize nursing diagnoses. For further information on Maslow's theory, see Chapter 4.

Problem Urgency

If you use problem urgency as your ranking criterion, you would rank problems according to the *degree of threat* they pose to the patient's life or the *immediacy* with which treatment is needed. Assign:

High priority to problems that are life threatening (e.g., ineffective airway clearance) or that could have a destructive effect on the client (e.g., substance abuse)

Medium priority to problems that do not pose a direct threat to life but that may cause destructive physical or emotional changes (e.g., denial of illness, unilateral neglect)

Low priority to problems that require minimal supportive nursing intervention (e.g., altered role performance, mild anxiety)

Future Consequences

When assigning priorities, also consider the possible future effects of a problem. Even if a problem is not life threatening at the moment, it may result in harmful future consequences for the patient. For example, suppose that Todd's (Meet Your Patient) provider prescribes a renal diet and insulin (instead of his previous oral medications) to treat the diabetes underlying his renal failure. Todd announces that he would like to go home to his job and family as soon as possible. He resists being taught about his medicines and how to administer his insulin. He admits neglecting to take his medication as prescribed in the past. You suspect that he has not been taking his medicines because he is in denial about his health problems. Clearly, his denial may lead to further problems with his treatment plan. You would assign high priority to this problem and address it before attempting to provide teaching for his nursing diagnosis of Deficient Knowledge (insulin).

Patient Preference

Give high priority to problems the patient thinks are most important, provided that this does not conflict with basic/survival needs or medical treatments.

- Patients cooperate more fully with interventions they consider important.
- Patients may be more motivated to work on other health problems after their own priorities are addressed.

    Example: Mr. Amani has had major surgery within the past 24 hours. He refuses to turn, deep-breathe, and cough (TDBC) because doing so causes pain. However, as his nurse, you realize that these activities are essential for preventing *Ineffective Airway Clearance* (high priority), so you cannot safely support Mr. Amani's refusal. You should provide pain medication before helping him TDBC. You would explain that airway clearance is a high priority and emphasize the importance of TDBC but also acknowledge the patient's need for pain relief.

Key Point: *When you explain the importance of your priorities, patients often come to agree with them and cooperate more fully with interventions.*

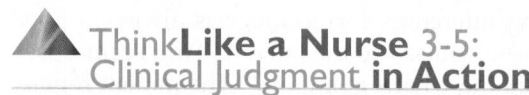

ThinkLike a Nurse 3-5: Clinical Judgment in Action

Suppose that on Todd's transfer from the ED (Meet Your Patient), you made the following nursing diagnoses for him. Using problem urgency as your criterion, assign each of these diagnoses a low, medium, or high priority.

- Fluid Volume Excess secondary to renal failure
- Risk for Falls related to decreased sensation and mobility in legs
- Lack of Knowledge (renal disease process) r/t new diagnosis of renal involvement secondary to type 2 DM

Computer-Assisted Diagnosing

Many institutions use computers for planning and documenting patient care. Some systems allow you to enter assessment data, and the computer program will then generate a list of possible problems. After you choose a problem label, the computer will provide a screen with the definition and defining characteristics of the problem so that you can compare them with the actual patient data. After you "accept" the diagnostic label, you complete the problem statement by choosing etiologies from the next computer screen.

REFLECTING CRITICALLY ON YOUR DIAGNOSTIC REASONING

Diagnostic reasoning is complex and vulnerable to error. Therefore, after prioritizing your list of problems, you need to evaluate the list for accuracy. Take time to apply critical thinking to your theoretical and self-knowledge and your overall use of the diagnostic process.

Think About Your Theoretical Knowledge

The better your knowledge base is, the better your diagnostic reasoning. Ask yourself the following questions:

- Is this diagnosis based on sound knowledge (e.g., of pathophysiology, psychology, nutrition, and other related disciplines)?
- Do I have sound knowledge about the cues associated with various nursing diagnoses?
- Do I feel reasonably sure I have interpreted the data correctly?
- Have I identified the problem type correctly—that is, can this problem be treated primarily by nursing interventions?

To avoid diagnostic error, build a good knowledge base and learn from your clinical experiences. These will help you to (1) recognize cues and patterns, (2) associate patterns with the correct problem, (3) gain confidence in your ability to reason, and (4) keep you from relying too much on authority figures (Wilkinson, 2017).

Think About Your Self-Knowledge

Realize that your beliefs, values, and experiences affect your thinking and can be misleading. For example, a nurse working in a labor and delivery unit believes it is important to be strong and uncomplaining even when experiencing pain. When this nurse cares for a patient in early labor who cries out and complains of pain, the nurse sees it as a problem of either anxiety or ineffective coping, not as a problem of pain. Can you see how that changes the focus of the nurse's care? To reflect on your self-knowledge, ask yourself the following questions (Wilkinson, 2017):

What Biases and Stereotypes May Have Influenced My Interpretation of the Data?

- A **bias** is the tendency to slant your judgment based on personal opinion or unfounded beliefs, as the nurse did in the preceding example.
- **Stereotypes** are judgments and expectations about an individual based on personal beliefs you have about a group (e.g., all men are unemotional; all teenagers are irresponsible). You form stereotypes by making flawed assumptions when you have had little experience with a person or group.

Did I Rely Too Much on Past Experiences? This is like stereotyping in that you draw conclusions about an individual based on what you know about people in similar situations.

Did I Rely Too Much on the Client's Medical Diagnosis, the Setting, or What Others Say About the Client Instead of on the Data? Medical diagnoses and statements from others can help you to think of possible explanations for your data, but they can also bias your thinking and prevent you from gathering your own data.

Think About Your Thinking

After reflecting on your knowledge, think about how you used the diagnostic process. Be sure your analysis of the data was thorough, that you have accurately identified the patient's problems, and that the problems are logically linked to the etiologies. Refresh your critiquing process by reviewing Box 3-3.

STANDARDIZED NURSING LANGUAGES

A **standardized language** is one in which the terms are carefully defined and mean the same thing to all who use them. One example is the periodic table of chemical elements. When a chemist in the United States writes *Fe*, chemists throughout the world know that notation means "iron." There is no confusion.

Nurses also need clear, precise, consistent terminology in their practice when referring to the same clinical problems and treatments. A **standardized nursing language** can do the following:

- Support electronic health records.
- Define, communicate, and expand nursing knowledge.

BOX 3-3 ■ Critiquing Your Diagnostic Reasoning Process

Data Analysis

Did you:

- Identify all the significant data (cues)?
- Omit any important cues from the cluster?
- Include unnecessary cues that may have confused your interpretation?
- Try more than one way of grouping the cues?
- Consider the patient's social, cultural, and spiritual beliefs and needs?
- Identify all the data gaps and inconsistencies?

Drawing Inferences and Interpretations of the Data

Did you consider all the possible explanations for the cue cluster?

Is this the best explanation for the cue cluster?

Did you have enough data to make that inference?

Did you look at patterns, not single cues?

Did you look at behavior over time, not just isolated incidents?

Did you jump to conclusions? Or did you take the time to carefully analyze and synthesize the data?

Critiquing the Diagnostic Statement (Problem + Etiology)

Is the diagnosis relevant, and does it reflect the data?

Does the diagnostic statement give a clear and accurate picture of the patient's problem or strength?

When identifying the problem and etiology, did you look beyond medical diagnoses and consider human responses?

Did you consider strengths and wellness diagnoses?

Can you explain how the etiology relates to the problem—that is, how it would produce the problem response?

Does the complete list of problems fully describe the patient's overall health status?

Verifying the Diagnosis

Did the patient verify this diagnosis?

When you verified the diagnosis, were you certain the patient understood your description of his health status?

Did you obtain feedback from the patient, or did you merely assume that the patient agreed?

Did you keep an open mind, realizing all diagnoses are tentative and subject to change as you acquire more data?

Prioritizing

Considering the whole situation, what are the most important problems?

What aspects of the situation require immediate attention?

Did you consider patient preferences when setting priorities? If not, was there a good reason?

- Increase visibility and awareness of nursing interventions.
- Facilitate research to demonstrate the contribution of nurses to healthcare and influence health policy decisions (Mushta et al., 2018).
- Improve patient care by providing better communication between nurses and other healthcare providers and facilitating the testing of nursing interventions.

Classification Systems Used in Healthcare

The following classification systems are widely used in healthcare:

- The American Psychiatric Association (APA) *Diagnostic and Statistical Manual of Mental Disorders, Fifth Edition* (*DSM-5*) describes mental disorders (APA, 2015).
- The *International Statistical Classification of Diseases and Related Health Problems* (ICD-10) names and classifies medical conditions (World Health Organization, 1993).
- The Current Procedural Terminology (CPT) codes are used for reimbursement of physician services; they name and define medical services and procedures. CPT code updates are ongoing (American Medical Association [AMA], 2022).

The following are classification systems that the ANA has recognized for describing nursing diagnoses (some describe outcomes and interventions as well).

- The NANDA-I classification is based on the identification of client problems and strengths obtained during assessment. The current taxonomy includes more diagnostic labels, domains, and classes (NANDA-I, 2021) with etiologies, risk factors, and defining characteristics.
- The Clinical Care Classification (CCC) uses a framework of care components to classify healthcare patterns (e.g., diagnoses and interventions). Specifically designed for clinical information systems, the CCC system facilitates nursing documentation at the point of care. See Chapter 37 for more information about CCC.
- The Omaha System consists of three interrelated components: the Problem Classification Scheme, the Intervention Scheme, and the Problem Rating Scale for Outcomes. It contains nursing diagnosis concepts, interventions, and outcomes. The Omaha System was designed to be computer compatible from the outset and is used across the continuum of healthcare settings. Refer to Chapter 37 for more information about the Omaha System.
- The Perioperative Nursing Data Set (PNDS) is designed for use only in perioperative nursing (Petersen, 2011). Nursing diagnoses are focused on risk identification and safety within the perioperative environment (safety, physiological responses, behavioral responses, and health system factors). See Chapter 36 for more information about the PNDS.

- The International Classification for Nursing Practice (ICNP) includes diagnoses, outcomes, and nursing actions. The ICNP intends to provide a common language and comparison of nursing data across clinical populations, settings, geographic areas, and time (International Council of Nurses, 2022).

NANDA-I Diagnostic Classification System

Because NANDA-I was the earliest taxonomy of nursing diagnoses, we will use that in this chapter to explain taxonomies and standardized language. The NANDA-I diagnostic classification system provides a **standardized terminology,** or standardized language, to use when describing human responses. You can see the complete taxonomy by referring to the most recent NANDA-I *Nursing Diagnoses Definitions and Classification* (2021) or a nursing diagnosis handbook.

What Are the Components of a NANDA-I Nursing Diagnosis?

Each nursing diagnosis in the NANDA-I system has the following parts: diagnostic label, definition, defining characteristics, and either related factors or risk factors. You must consider all four parts when formulating a nursing diagnosis. Table 3-5 describes the diagnosis components.

WRITING DIAGNOSTIC STATEMENTS

Key Point: *A diagnostic statement consists of a problem and an etiology linked by a connecting phrase. If you do use NANDA-I terminology, you must pay attention to their definitions and defining characteristics in order to use their diagnoses accurately.*

Problem

- **Describes the client's health status** (or a human response to a health problem)
- **Identifies a response that needs to be changed**

Use a NANDA-I, CCC, Omaha System, or other standardized label when possible, including descriptors (e.g., *acute, imbalanced, impaired, ineffective, deficient, disturbed, risk-prone*).

In alphabetical lists, you will see diagnosis labels arranged with the descriptor after the main word (e.g., Physical Mobility, Impaired). However, you should record diagnosis statements as you would say them, for example:

> *Incorrect:* Physical Mobility, Impaired r/t pain in left knee
>
> *Correct:* Impaired Physical Mobility r/t pain in left knee

Etiology

- **Contains one or more factors that cause, contribute to, or create a risk for the problem.** Factors may include a NANDA-I label, defining characteristics, related factors, or risk factors.

Table 3-5 ➤ Components of a NANDA-I Nursing Diagnosis

DEFINITION AND CHARACTERISTICS	EXAMPLES
Component: DIAGNOSTIC LABEL (title or name)	
A word or phrase that provides a name for the diagnosis	Disturbed Body Image
Represents a pattern of related cues and describes a problem or wellness response	Readiness for Enhanced Nutrition
Note: Some labels include modifiers (also called *descriptors*) for time, age, and other factors	Acute, chronic, complicated, compromised, decreased, deficient, delayed, disturbed, effective, excess, impaired, ineffective
Component: DEFINITION	
Explains the meaning of the label	For a patient with a sleep problem, would you label the problem Sleep Deprivation or Disturbed Sleep Pattern? The following definitions can help you to decide:
Distinguishes it from similar nursing diagnoses	Sleep Deprivation: Prolonged periods of time without sleep
	Disturbed Sleep Pattern: Prolonged periods of time without sustained natural, periodic suspension of relative consciousness that provides rest
Component: DEFINING CHARACTERISTICS	
Cues (signs and symptoms) that allow you to identify a problem or wellness diagnosis	For the diagnosis Sleep Deprivation—Agitation, anxiety, fatigue, perceptual disorders
A cluster of defining characteristics must be present in the patient data to use the problem label appropriately.	For example, you cannot decide to use the Sleep Deprivation label merely by reading the definition. You must be sure the patient actually has some of the defining characteristics (previous examples).
Component: RELATED FACTORS	
Related factors are the cues, conditions, or circumstances that cause, precede, influence, contribute to, or in some way show a patterned relationship with the problem (label).	For Sleep Deprivation—Age-related sleep stage shifts, narcolepsy, overstimulating environment, prolonged discomfort
Related factors can be pathophysiological, psychological, social, treatment related, situational, maturational, and so forth.	
The list of related factors is not exhaustive. Factors other than those listed by NANDA-I could also be associated with the problem.	For example, imagine the vast number of factors that might cause someone to have a diagnosis of Chronic Low Self-Esteem.
The problem may have more than one related factor. Human beings are complex, and their problems rarely have a single cause.	
An individual patient's etiology will not include all the related factors that NANDA-I lists.	
Component: RISK FACTORS	
Risk factors function as the defining characteristics in potential (risk) diagnoses.	For the diagnosis Constipation—
They are events, circumstances, or conditions that increase the vulnerability of a person or group to a health problem.	Habitually ignores the urge to defecate
	Abdominal muscle weakness
They can be environmental, physiological, psychological, genetic, or chemical.	Obesity
	Pregnancy
Must be present to make the diagnosis, and they almost always form at least a part of the etiology of the diagnostic statement.	
Key Point: *To help you remember:* *Related factors are similar to signs and symptoms (of actual problems).* *Risk factors are similar to etiologies (of potential problems).*	

- **Helps you individualize nursing care because etiologies are unique to the individual.** Suppose two patients have the following nursing diagnoses:

  John: Anxiety r/t lack of knowledge of the treatment procedure

  Janet: Anxiety r/t prior negative experiences and lack of trust in health professionals

  The problem, Anxiety, has the same definition for both patients. They may share some of the defining characteristics, and you would use some of the same nursing interventions. However, to prevent anxiety from occurring or recurring, you would need to treat its cause.

  To relieve John's anxiety, you would teach the patient what to expect from the impending procedure.

  For Janet, you would need to (1) spend time building a relationship that demonstrates you can be trusted and (2) encourage the patient to talk about fears and feelings.
- **The etiology directs the nursing interventions,** so include only those factors that are influenced by nursing interventions.
- **Avoid using a medical diagnosis or treatment as an etiology** because you cannot write nursing interventions to change it.

Connecting Phrase (Related to)

- **Most nurses use *related to (r/t)* to connect the problem and etiology,** believing that the phrase *due to* implies a direct causal relationship.
- **Because humans are complex, there are usually many factors that combine to "cause" a problem,** so it is nearly impossible to prove an exact cause. In fact, even if you eliminate the etiological factors, the problem might remain. For example, even if Janet begins to trust health professionals, she may become anxious for another reason.

Formats for Diagnostic Statements

The format of a diagnostic statement varies depending on the type of problem you are describing.

One-Part Statement

Certain kinds of diagnostic statements need no etiology:

- **Syndrome diagnosis**—A label that represents a collection of several nursing diagnoses

  Example: Disuse Syndrome
- **Wellness diagnosis**—As a rule, this is a one-part statement beginning with the phrase "Readiness for Enhanced." A wellness label does not describe a problem, so there is no etiology.

  Example: Readiness for Enhanced Nutrition
- **Very specific NANDA-I labels**—Some labels are so specific that they imply the etiology. *Example: Latex Allergic Reaction*

It would be redundant to write *Latex Allergic Reaction r/t sensitivity to latex.*

Basic Two-Part Statement

Two-part statements can be used for actual, risk, and possible diagnoses. The format is: Problem (standardized label)_r/t Etiology (related factors)

- **Actual** diagnoses—The etiology consists of related factors (*e.g., Nausea r/t anxiety*).
- **Risk** diagnoses—The etiology consists of risk factors (*e.g., Risk for Deficient Fluid Volume r/t excessive vomiting*).
- **Possible** diagnoses—The etiology consists of the patient's cues, which are not complete enough to diagnose (*e.g., Possible Constipation r/t patient's statement of no BM for 2 days*).

Basic Three-Part Statement

This is also called the **PES format** (problem, etiology, and symptom format). Primarily for students, this method helps ensure there are enough data to support the problem identified.

- The format is:

  Problem r/t etiology as manifested by (AMB) signs or symptoms
- The connecting phrase can be either *as evidenced by (AEB)* or *AMB*. After the connector (AMB), this format adds the patient signs or symptoms that confirm or support the diagnosis.

  *Constipation r/t inadequate intake of fluids and fiber-rich foods **AMB painful, hard stool and bowel movement every 3 or 4 days***
- You cannot use the PES format for risk nursing diagnoses because patients "at risk" do not yet have symptoms.

Other Format Variations

"Secondary to" (add to the Etiology) When the defining characteristics are vague (e.g., *Self-Care Deficit*), you may need to add a second part to the etiology, usually a disease or pathophysiology. Use "secondary to" (symbolized as 2°) only if it adds to the understanding of your diagnostic statement.

Example: Impaired walking r/t stiffness and pain 2° rheumatoid arthritis.

Two-Part NANDA-I Label The first part describes a general response; the second part, after a colon, makes it more specific.

Example: Imbalanced Nutrition: Less Than Body Requirements *r/t . . .*

Adding Words to the NANDA-I Label Key Point: *The "rule" for adding words is first to try to make the statement specific or descriptive by writing a good etiology, using the PES format, or adding "secondary to." If that does not fully describe the health status, add descriptive words to the problem label.* Does "Impaired Bed Mobility" mean that the patient cannot roll from side to side or that they cannot move at all? You would need to add your own words to the label to make it more descriptive.

Example: Impaired Bed Mobility: Inability to turn self in bed r/t weakness, secondary to low sodium level.

Decide whether the clarifying words belong in the problem or in the etiology. For example, you may see a diagnosis of Acute Pain r/t surgical incision. However, surgical incision is a medical treatment and should not be used as the etiology. It would be better to write:

Example: Acute pain (abdominal incision) r/t turning and moving 2º abdominal surgery.

Unknown Etiology Sometimes you will not be able to identify the etiology. For example, you might diagnose a patient's Parental Role Conflict, but you may need more information to determine the cause. In this case, you could write *Parental Role Conflict r/t unknown etiology.* Later, when you obtain more data, you will be able to complete the etiology.

Complex Etiology Some problems have too many etiological factors to list, or the etiology is too complex to explain in a brief diagnostic statement. Imagine the number of factors that might contribute to problems such as Disabled Family Coping. For such problems, you can replace the etiology with the phrase *complex factors* (e.g., *Disabled Family Coping r/t complex factors*).

Collaborative Problems

Key Point: *A collaborative problem is always a potential problem (e.g., a complication of a disease, test, or medical treatment).* The disease, test, or treatment is actually the etiology of the problem. You cannot treat the etiology with independent nursing interventions, so the focus of your interventions is monitoring for and preventing the complication. The word(s) after the colon represent the problem you are monitoring and trying to prevent.

Example: Potential Complication of thrombophlebitis: Pulmonary embolism

KnowledgeCheck 3-8

Write an example of each of the following diagnostic statement formats, using the listed components—mix and match:

Problem labels: Anxiety, Pain (lower back)
Etiologies: Unknown outcome of surgery; muscle strain and tissue inflammation
Cues: Exhibits physical manifestations of anxiety (e.g., hands shaking); states pain is 9 on a scale of 1 to 10.
- Basic two-part statement
- Basic three-part statement
- Basic two-part statement, using "secondary to" (create your own disease/pathology)
- Statement with unknown etiology
- Possible nursing diagnosis
- Risk nursing diagnosis

How Do the Nursing Diagnoses Relate to Outcomes and Interventions?

Key Point: *As a general rule, the problem suggests goals, and the etiology suggests interventions.* Keep in mind that there are exceptions to this rule.

The Problem Suggests Goals

The problem describes a health status that needs to be changed. The problem guides you in determining the patient outcomes for measuring this change. Consider the following diagnostic statement: *Risk for Impaired Skin Integrity r/t complete immobility 2° spinal cord injury.*

- **The goal, or outcome, is the opposite of the unhealthy response:** Skin will remain intact and healthy.
- **The goals suggest assessments** that are actually a type of nursing intervention. For example, the diagnosis *Risk for Impaired Skin Integrity* tells you to monitor the patient's skin condition.
- **If the problem is not an accurate statement of health status, then your goals and resulting assessments will be wrong.** If you incorrectly identified the problem as *Impaired Physical Mobility 2° spinal cord injury,* then the goal would suggest that you monitor the patient's mobility. That nursing action would not improve the mobility and might cause you to miss a developing skin problem.

The Etiology Suggests Interventions

Key Point: *The aim of the nursing interventions is to remove or alter the factors contributing to the problem.* In the previous example, nursing care cannot cure the spinal cord injury or restore the patient's ability to move about. However, you could provide some mobility by turning and repositioning the patient frequently. This would help prevent Impaired Skin Integrity.

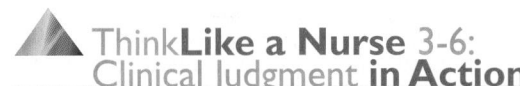 ThinkLike a Nurse 3-6: Clinical Judgment in Action

Rewrite the following diagnostic statement so that it contains no legally questionable language. Use imaginary etiological factors if you need to: **Risk for Falls r/t lack of staff to assist with ambulation.**

PLANNING: THE NEXT STEP OF THE NURSING PROCESS

The professional nurse is responsible for care planning and cannot delegate it. Planning may occur in one of two ways: it can be formal and occur as a conscious, deliberate activity involving decision making, critical thinking, and creativity (Wilkinson, 2017), or it can be informal and occur as the nurse is performing other nursing process steps. Regardless of how it occurs, the end product of planning is a holistic plan of care that addresses the patient's unique problems and strengths.

To develop a plan of care with realistic goals and effective nursing interventions, you:

- Must have accurate, complete *assessment* data.
- Need correctly identified and prioritized *nursing diagnoses.*
- Must recognize that *goals/desired outcomes* flow logically from the nursing diagnoses.
- Should understand that by stating what is to be achieved, the goals suggest nursing interventions (written as nursing orders).

Types of Planning

There are three different types of planning:

Initial Planning Begins With the First Patient Contact. It refers to the development of the initial comprehensive care plan, which should be written as soon as possible after the initial assessment. Sometimes, the patient may require emergency care before assessment is complete. In such a situation, make a preliminary plan with whatever information you have. You can complete and refine the plan when you are able to perform a more detailed assessment.

Ongoing Planning Refers to Changes Made in the Plan as You: (1) Evaluate the patient's responses to care [*Evaluation* step of the nursing process] or (2) obtain new data and make new nursing diagnoses. This allows you to decide which problems to focus on each day that you care for the patient.

Discharge Planning is the process of planning for self-care and continuity of care after the patient leaves a healthcare setting. The purpose of discharge planning is to (1) promote the patient's progress toward health or disease management outside of facility care and (2) reduce early readmissions to hospital care.

Comprehensive discharge planning involves collaboration. Ideally, it is done *with,* not *for,* the patient. In addition, a patient's postdischarge needs often call for the services of an interprofessional team as well as members of the patient's family.

To learn more about the process of discharging patients from an institution, refer to the section Maintain Trust During Transitions in Chapter 8.

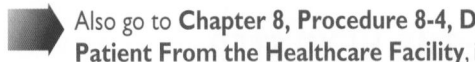 Also go to **Chapter 8, Procedure 8-4, Discharging a Patient From the Healthcare Facility**, in Volume 2.

Discharge Planning Begins at Initial Assessment

Because patient stays in the hospital or surgery center are typically short, discharge planning must begin at the initial assessment and should include the following patient data:

- Estimated date of discharge
- Physical condition and functional and self-care limitations
- Emotional stability and ability to learn

- Financial resources (e.g., personal finances, community resources such as nutrition assistance programs, Medicaid)
- Family or other caregivers available
- Caregiving responsibilities the patient may have for others
- Environment, both home and community (e.g., stairs, space for supplies and equipment, availability of transportation to healthcare services)
- Use of community services before admission

Written Discharge Plans

All patients need discharge planning, but you will not always need a separate written discharge plan. Sometimes the discharge planning can be included as nursing interventions on the patient's comprehensive care plan. For example, a middle-aged patient who has been hospitalized for deep vein thrombosis (a blood clot in a major vein) will be able to care for themselves independently when they go home. For this patient, you could simply write a nursing order to teach them about the side effects of the anticoagulant that they will be taking at home. In contrast, you will probably need a written, comprehensive discharge plan if the patient is an older adult or is likely to have one or more of the following (Fox, 2016; Henke et al., 2017; Saunier, 2017):

- **Personal characteristics that interfere with self-care,** such as difficulty learning or a memory deficit, emotional or mental illness, poor mobility, self-care deficits (e.g., dressing, feeding, bathing, toileting), and incontinence
- **Disease or treatment characteristics or coexisting illness,** such as terminal illness, complicated major surgery, complex treatment regimen (including more than three medications to continue at home), an illness with an expected long period of recovery, a newly diagnosed problem or multiple chronic health problems (e.g., diabetes, chronic pain), preexisting wound, and malnutrition
- **Social or family factors,** including inadequate services available in the community, inadequate financial resources, and no family or significant others to help provide care. For an example of a discharge planning form,

 Go to **Chapter 3, Discharge Planning Form** in Volume 2.

Discharge Planning for Older Adults

Older adults tend to have complex needs when discharged. Therefore, it is especially important to start discharge planning at the initial admission assessment. Functional abilities, cognition, vision, hearing, social support, and psychological well-being must be a part of the initial assessment so that you can identify needed services at discharge.

A comprehensive discharge process for older adults should help to achieve the following objectives:

- Maintain functional ability.
- Lengthen the time between rehospitalizations.
- Involve all concerned parties in decision making.
- Improve interagency communication (e.g., hospital to nursing home).
- Emphasize client and family involvement and inter-professional collaboration.

PATIENT CARE PLANS

The **comprehensive nursing care plan** (a type of *patient care plan*) is the central source of information needed to guide holistic, goal-oriented care to address each patient's unique needs. It specifies dependent, interdependent, and independent nursing actions necessary for a specific patient.

A well-written comprehensive care plan benefits the patient and the healthcare institution by:

- Ensuring that care is complete
- Providing continuity of care
- Promoting efficient use of nursing efforts
- Providing a guide for assessments and charting
- Meeting the requirements of accrediting

Comprehensive care plans include directions for four kinds of care and include both medical and nursing interventions:

- Basic needs and activities of daily living (ADLs)
- Medical/interprofessional treatment
- Nursing diagnoses and collaborative problems (nursing diagnosis care plan)
- Special discharge needs or teaching needs

Standardized Plans

In most healthcare organizations, caregivers use pre-printed, standardized plans that can be adapted to meet individual needs. **Key Point: *Some essential client data either do not change or are used or updated often. This includes the client's profile (e.g., age, providers), basic needs (e.g., for hygiene and elimination), and diagnostic tests and treatments (e.g., laboratory tests, radiology procedures). To provide quick and easy access, such information is usually recorded on a standardized form and not organized according to medical or nursing diagnoses.***
Standardized plans:

- Save nursing time.
- Promote consistency of care.
- Help ensure that nurses do not overlook important interventions.
- May contain nursing or multidisciplinary interventions.
- May prescribe care for one or more nursing diagnoses or medical conditions.

The following are examples of standardized, preprinted instructions for care.

Policies and Procedures are similar to rules and regulations. When a situation occurs frequently or requires a consistent response regardless of who handles it, management develops a policy to govern how it is to be handled. You should consider individual needs and use critical thinking to interpret policies in a caring manner.

Protocols cover the specific actions usually required for a clinical problem unique to a subgroup of patients. Protocols may be written for a particular medical diagnosis (e.g., seizure), treatment (e.g., administration of oxytocin to induce labor), or diagnostic test (e.g., barium enema). They contain both medical prescriptions and nursing interventions (written as nursing orders).

Unit Standards of Care describe the care that nurses are expected to provide for all patients in defined situations (e.g., all patients admitted to a labor unit or all patients admitted to a critical care unit). Unit standards of care differ from nursing care plans in the following ways:

- They describe the *minimum* level of care rather than *ideal* care.
- They describe the care that nurses are expected to achieve, given the institution's resources and the client population.
- They are not usually organized according to nursing diagnoses.
- They resemble a list of "things to do" (e.g., complete comprehensive assessment within 2 hours of admission) rather than detailed instructions for care.

Standardized (Model) Nursing Care Plans detail the nursing care that is usually needed for a particular nursing diagnosis or for all nursing diagnoses that commonly occur with a medical condition. Figure 3-6 is a standardized care plan for a single nursing diagnosis. Although similar to unit standards of care, model care plans are different in that they usually:

- Provide more detailed interventions than do unit standards of care.
- Are organized by nursing diagnosis.
- Include specific patient goals and nursing interventions (written as nursing orders).
- Become a part of the permanent record.
- Describe ideal rather than minimum nursing care.
- Allow you to incorporate addendum care plans.
- Include checklists, blank lines, or empty spaces so that you can individualize goals and interventions.

Key Point: *Model care plans can be used as guides, but they do not address a client's individual, specific needs. For this reason, they may lead you to focus on the common, predictable problems and overlook an unusual—and perhaps more important—problem that the person is experiencing.*

PATIENT PLAN OF CARE - GENESIS MEDICAL CENTER - Davenport, Iowa

PAIN, ACUTE: Experience of an unpleasant sensory and emotional sensation for a duration of less than 6 months.
SIGNS & SYMPTOMS: Observed or reported (select at least 2)

☐ Change in BP   ☐ Restlessness   ☐ Grimacing   ☐ Crying
☐ Patient's self-report of pain ☐ Diaphoresis   ☐ Increased muscle tension   ☐ Change in pulse rate
☐ Change in respiratory pattern ☐ Whimpering   ☐ Whining

OUTCOME SCORING

RELATED FACTORS	OUTCOMES	ADM			DC	INTERVENTIONS
☐ Physical injuring agent ☐ Psychological injuring agent	`4` Pain-control behavior – Recognizes causal factors – Uses non-analgesic relief measures – Uses analgesics appropriately – Reports pain controlled `3` Pain level – Oral/facial expressions of pain – Change in respiratory rate, heart rate, BP – Restlessness – Reported pain `3` Comfort level – Reported satisfaction with symptom control – Expressed satisfaction with pain control – Reported physical well-being					☐ Pain management ☐ Analgesic administration ☐ Patient-controlled analgesic (PCA) assistance ☐ Analgesic administration: Intraspinal ☐ Environmental management: comfort ☐ Anxiety reduction ☐ Transcutaneous electrical nerve stimulation (TENS) ☐ Heat/cold application ☐ Distraction ☐ Simple relaxation therapy ☐ Simple massage ☐ Developmental care ☐ Preparatory sensory information ☐ Positioning

Definition of scoring scales	1	2	3	4	5
Pain control — Personal actions to control pain	Never demonstrated	Rarely demonstrated	Sometimes demonstrated	Often demonstrated	Consistently demonstrated
Pain level — Severity of reported pain	Severe	Substantial	Moderate	Slight	None
Comfort level — Extent of physical and psychological ease	None	Limited	Moderate	Substantial	Extensive

Diagnosis _____

Date Initiated _____ RN Initials _____

Date Resolved _____

FIGURE 3-6. Computer printout of a standardized care plan for a single nursing diagnosis.

Critical Pathways Critical pathways are outcomes-based, interprofessional plans that sequence patient care according to case type. They specify predicted patient outcomes for each day or, in some situations, for each hour (see Fig. 3-7). They describe the minimal standard of care required to meet the recommended length of stay for patients with a particular condition or *diagnosis-related group (DRG)* (e.g., postpartum, myocardial infarction).

Key Point: *An agency usually develops critical pathways for its most frequent case types or for situations in which standardized care can produce predictable outcomes.*

Integrated Plans of Care (IPOCs) are standardized plans that function as both care plan and documentation form. Many critical pathways are designed as IPOCs; however, IPOCs do not necessarily (1) organize care according to diagnosis, (2) describe minimal standards of care, or (3) specify a timeline for interventions and outcomes.

ThinkLike a Nurse 3-7:
Clinical Judgment in Action

- Think of some other "defined situations" for which unit standards of care might be useful.
- Suggest some other subgroups for which a protocol might be appropriate.

Individualized Nursing Care Plans

Nurses use individualized care plans to address nursing diagnoses unique to a particular client. These care plans reflect the independent component of nursing practice and, therefore, best demonstrate the nurse's critical thinking and clinical expertise.

You may sometimes include medical prescriptions in a nursing diagnosis or collaborative problem care plan. For example, for Todd (Meet Your Patient), a patient with a nursing diagnosis of Fluid Volume Excess, you might list the medical prescription for intravenously administered medication in the Nursing Orders column:

Nursing Diagnosis	**Nursing Orders**
Excess Fluid Volume r/t renal insufficiency	
	Monitor vital signs q4hr Monitor urine output . . . ***Medical Prescriptions*** Administer IV diuretics as prescribed

Special Discharge or Teaching Plans

A nursing plan of care may also contain one or more discharge or teaching plans. These are sometimes referred to as *special-purpose* or *addendum* care plans. You can address routine discharge planning and teaching needs by using standardized plans or by including teaching as part of the nursing orders on an individualized care plan.

Chapter 16 shows an example of a teaching plan for the diagnosis Deficient Knowledge.

Computer Plans of Care

Most healthcare organizations use electronic health records (EHRs), including *computer-generated care plans.* The computer stores standardized plans (e.g., for nursing diagnoses, medical diagnoses, or DRGs). When you enter a diagnosis or a desired outcome, the computer generates a list of suggested interventions from which to choose. You can individualize them by choosing from checklists or typing in your own interventions and strategies. Computer prompts help ensure that you consider a variety of actions and do not overlook common and important interventions. Standardized nursing care plans serve multiple purposes, such as collecting data on a patient's health condition or illness for planning and evaluating care, communication among healthcare professionals, research, public health management, norms and standards development, and providing evidence for legal issues (Zaman et al., 2021).

KnowledgeCheck 3-9

- In addition to care related to the patient's basic needs, what other types of information does a comprehensive care plan contain?
- How are critical pathways different from other standardized care plans?
- Can you think of a disadvantage of using computerized and standardized care plans?

ThinkLike a Nurse 3-8:
Clinical Judgment in Action

Suppose a nurse sees one of your student care plans and says to you, "You're wasting your time writing those things. We never use the nursing process in the real world." Take a few minutes to write how you might respond.

Student Care Plans

You may have noticed that the care plans you see in clinical settings look different from the ones you create as part of your clinical preparation. This is because student care plans are designed to help you learn and apply concepts from the nursing process, physiology, and psychopathology. For this reason, they may contain more detailed nursing orders as well as other information the instructor may require. Some instructors may ask you to write rationales and cite references to support them. **Rationales** state the scientific principles or research that supports nursing interventions. Writing rationales helps ensure that you understand the reasons for the interventions. For an example of a student care plan,

Go to Davis Advantage, Resources, **Chapter 3, Student Care Plan Example, and Care Map of Student Care Plan Example.**

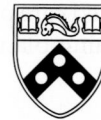

HOSPITAL OF THE UNIVERSITY OF PENNSYLVANIA

TOTAL LOWER JOINT (HIP/KNEE)
CLINICAL PATHWAY

ELIGIBILITY CRITERIA: All primary unilateral total hip or total knee
replacements

EXPECTED LOS: 3 Days   ADDRESSOGRAPH

CLINICAL KEYS:

1.	Pain managed midpoint on pain scale
2.	Transfer to chair/commode with assistance POD 1; Ambulate in room, bathroom POD2
3.	DVT precautions
4.	Discharge plan completed by POD2
5.	Patient verbalizes knowledge of hip or knee precautions
6.	Knee motion 10 to 70 or better (TKA patients only)

	PACU	IMMED. POST- OP	POD 1	POD 2	POD 3-4
ASSESSMENTS	• NV checks with VS q1h × 4 • Pain • Effects of narcotics/tolerance • 1 & 0 × 24hr • Pulse Ox q8 if on O2	• NV check / VS q 4hr → → • S/S DVT →	→ → → → • Pulse Ox × 1 on RA • Dsg/wound status q4	• NV check / VS q 8hr → → → • D/C pulse ox if O2 D/C • Dsg/wound status q8	→ → → → →
CONSULTS		• PT • PMR	→ (If not done already) → (If not done already)		
TESTS	• A/P hip X-ray (THA) • A/P knee X-ray (TKA)		• CBC	→ • INR (if on warfarin)	• A/P hip X-ray →
TREATMENTS	• O2	• D/C O2 if sat 94% • Incentive spirometry • Order walker (hip chair, elevated commode if needed) • Pneumatic compression device (ankle for knees, calf for hips)	→ → • D/C Foley • Dressing change (1st dsg change by MD) →	→ → • Dressing change q day and pm	→ → →
MEDICATIONS	• PCA or epidural	→ • Anticoagulation	• IV heplock → • Consider conversion to oral pain meds	• D/C heplock → • D/C PCA/PCEA • PO pain meds	→
ACTIVITY	• Bedrest • Hip precautions if THA • CPM for total knee	→ → →	• OOB to chair BID → → • Weight bear per order • Ambulate with assistive device	• OOB TID → → → → • PT × 2	→ → → → → →
NUTRITION	• NPO	• NPO → ice → advance to full as tolerated	• Regular	→	→
EDUCATION / D/C PLANNING	• Deep breathing exercises	• Pain management • Initiate d/c plan	→ • Home vs rehab decision • Anticoagulation if indicated	→ • S/S wound infection • Medications • Activity level • D/C plan in place	→ → → • Car transfer

Transfer to rehab when:	Discharge to home when:
1. Able to participate in care 2. Tolerating 2 physical therapy sessions 3. Not requiring IV pain medicine 4. Blood values are stable 5. Motivation is commensurate with projected functional status	1. Mobility and ADL's appropriate for degree of assistance at home and home environment 2. Appropriate assistive device and necessary adaptive equipment is used 3. Independent with hip/knee precautions 4. Independent with home exercise program or ongoing PT in the home or outpatient **IF D/C TO HOME, ENSURE APPROPRIATE CONSULTS TO ARRANGE HOME CARE FOLLOW-UP AND EQUIPMENT

FIGURE 3-7. Portion of a critical pathway.

Mind-Mapping Student Care Plans

Mind-mapping is a technique for showing relationships between ideas and concepts in a graphical, or pictorial, way. A mind-mapped care plan uses shapes and pictures to represent the steps of the nursing process, as well as the patient's pathophysiology and other pertinent information. For an example of a care map, refer to the care plan and care map in Chapter 30.

WHAT IS THE PROCESS FOR WRITING AN INDIVIDUALIZED NURSING CARE PLAN?

Writing an individualized nursing care plan follows in natural sequence from the assessment and diagnosis phases of the nursing process:

1. **Make a working problem list. Suppose that after assessment, you prioritize Todd's (Meet Your Patient) problems as follows:**
   Examples:
   A. Fluid Volume Excess
   B. Immobility r/t decreased sensation in lower extremities.
   C. Self-Care Deficit (Total) r/t immobility secondary lower-extremity edema
   D. Risk for Impaired Skin and Tissue Integrity r/t impaired circulation secondary to Diabetes Mellitus
2. **Determine which problems can be managed with standardized care plans or critical pathways.**
   Example: Suppose that the hospital has a critical pathway for "Fluid Volume Excess." It should contain assessments, outcomes/goals, and interventions for problems.
3. **Individualize the standardized plan as needed.**
   Example: If the plan reads, "Perform skin integrity checks q_____," you would fill in the frequency of the skin checks according to the client's needs.
4. **Transcribe medical prescriptions to appropriate documents.**
   Example: You might write prescriptions for pain medications on a special medication administration record.
5. **Write ADLs and basic care needs in the patient care summary.**
   Example: In the patient care summary, you might note that the patient requires a complete bed bath and help with ambulating.
6. **Develop individualized care plans for problems not addressed by standardized documents.**
   Example 1: The critical pathway probably contains some outcomes and basic interventions for problem A (Fluid Volume Excess), but you might need to individualize them to make them more effective. If your unit had a routine protocol for vital signs, you would add it to the care plan. If not, you

would write goals and interventions for the Fluid Volume Excess diagnosis or choose them on the interactive page of the electronic record.
   Example 2: Problem C, Self-Care Deficit, would be partially addressed in the basic care section of the patient care summary, but the patient will need teaching and therapy to increase his ability to care for himself. You would need to write a plan for this nursing diagnosis.

KnowledgeCheck 3-10

Briefly describe a process for creating a comprehensive, individualized care plan that incorporates collaborative care and standardized planning documents.

PLANNING PATIENT GOALS/OUTCOMES

After assessment and diagnosis, the next step in individualized care planning is to formulate goals for improving or maintaining the patient's health status. **Key Point:** *Goals (also called* **expected outcomes,** **desired outcomes,** *or* **predicted outcomes)** *describe the changes in patient health status that you hope to achieve.* Although critical pathways describe the expected outcomes of interprofessional care, they do not provide a way to judge *nursing* effectiveness. **Nurse-sensitive outcomes** are those that can be influenced by nursing interventions.

The purposes of precise, descriptive, clearly stated goals/expected outcomes are to:

- Provide a guide for selecting nursing interventions by describing what you wish to achieve.
- Motivate the client and the nurse by providing a sense of achievement when the goals are met.
- Form the criteria you will use in the evaluation phase of the nursing process.

How Should I Use the Terms Goals and Outcomes?

- **Key Point:** *When goals are stated as broad, nonspecific statements, you must include both goals and expected outcomes on the care plan because a broad goal does not provide enough guidance for evaluating patient responses to care.*
- **Key Point:** *You must include expected outcomes on the care plan; however, the use of broad goals is optional.*

In this text, we usually use the Nursing Outcomes Classification (NOC) terminology:

- The word *outcome,* used alone, means *any* patient response (positive or negative) to interventions (e.g., pain could become better or worse; both are outcomes).
- We use *goals, expected outcomes, desired outcomes,* or *predicted outcomes* when referring to desired (positive) patient responses.

- You can combine the broad goal and specific expected outcome into a single statement by writing *as evidenced by*, as in the following example:

Broad statement (goal)	Constipation relieved
Specific expected outcome (evaluation criteria)	Will have soft, formed bowel movement within 24 hours
Combined statement (goal + outcome)	Constipation will be relieved *as evidenced by* soft, formed bowel movement within 24 hours

How Do I Distinguish Between Short-Term and Long-Term Goals?

Short-term goals are those you expect the patient to achieve within a few hours or days. **Long-term goals** are changes in health status that you wish to achieve over a longer period—perhaps a week, a month, or longer. Short-term goals are most relevant in settings such as acute care and clinics, whereas long-term goals are more likely to be utilized in home healthcare, extended care, and rehabilitation centers.

What Are the Components of a Goal Statement?

Every expected outcome/goal statement must have the following parts:

- **Subject.** The subject is understood to be the client, but it can also be a function (e.g., lung sounds) or part of the client. Assume the client is the subject; specify only if the client is not the subject.
- **Action verb.** Use an action verb to indicate what activity the client will perform: what the client will learn, do, or say (e.g., Will *walk* to the doorway). Use verbs that describe actions you can observe or measure.
- **Performance criteria.** These describe the extent to which you expect to see the action or behavior, using concrete, observable terms. Specify how, what, when, or where something is to be done, along with the amount, quality, accuracy, speed, distance, and so forth, as applicable.

♥ iCare 3-1

The caring nurse formulates patient-focused goals.

Benefiting the patient is a priority of the caring nurse.

Remember that outcomes should state patient behaviors, not nursing activities.

Example: If a patient outcome is to walk 10 feet unassisted with a walker by the end of the day, you might ask, "At what time of the day do you like to walk?" or "At what time of day is it easier for you to walk?"

You should involve the patient as much as possible in goal setting because goal achievement is more likely if the goals are realistic and important to the client.

- **Target time.** This is the realistic date or time by which the client should achieve the performance or behavior.
  Example: Will walk to the doorway with the help of one person *within 24 hours.*

For risk (potential) nursing diagnoses, the desired outcome is that the problem will never occur. You can assume that the desired response should occur "at all times," but you may wish to schedule times for evaluating the outcome. For example:

Nursing diagnosis: Risk for Constipation r/t inadequate fluid intake
Expected outcome: Bowel movements will be of normal frequency and consistency.
Target time: At all times
Evaluate: Daily

- **Special conditions.** These describe the amount of assistance or resources needed or the experiences/treatments the client should have to perform the behavior. Include special conditions when it is important for other nurses to know them.

KnowledgeCheck 3-11

In the following predicted outcomes, identify the subject, action verb, performance criterion, target time, and special conditions (if any). State which components are assumed, if any.

- Will walk to the doorway with the help of one person within 24 hours.
- After two teaching sessions, by discharge [patient] will be able to identify foods to avoid on a low-fat diet.
- Bowel movements will be soft and formed and of usual frequency.
- Lungs will be clear to auscultation at all times.

How Do Goals Relate to Nursing Diagnoses?

Expected outcomes are derived directly from the nursing diagnosis. Therefore, they will be appropriate only if you identify the nursing diagnosis correctly. The problem clause of a nursing diagnosis describes the response or health status you wish to change. A desired outcome states the *opposite* of the problem and implies this response is what the interventions are intended to achieve.

▲ ThinkLike a Nurse 3-9: Clinical Judgment in Action

Answer the following questions for Todd's (Meet Your Patient) nursing diagnosis of Impaired Mobility secondary to decreased sensation in the lower extremities:

- What would be the opposite, healthy response to his problem?
- If the problem is prevented or solved, how will Todd look or behave? What will you be able to observe?
- What should Todd be able to do to demonstrate a positive change? How well, or how soon, should he be able to do it?

Essential Versus Nonessential Goals

Essential patient goals flow from the problem side of the nursing diagnosis because the problem side describes the unhealthy response you intend to change.

Example: Suppose that for a patient with Ineffective Airway Clearance, you had written the following goals:

- Coughs forcefully/effectively
- Rates pain as less than 3 on a 1 to 10 scale
- Splints incision while coughing

If the patient achieves all three goals, you might think you could discontinue the interventions for Ineffective Airway Clearance. However, even a client who demonstrates all three of those responses still might not be coughing productively enough to clear the airways and still might not have clear lung sounds.

Key Point: *For every nursing diagnosis, you must state one goal that, if achieved, would demonstrate resolution or improvement of the problem.*

Goals for Actual, Risk, and Possible Nursing Diagnoses

You will develop expected outcomes to promote, maintain, or restore health, depending on the status of the nursing diagnosis. See Table 3-6 for explanations and examples.

Goals for Collaborative Problems

Collaborative problems are physiological complications of diseases or medical treatments that nurses monitor to detect onset or changes in status. The desired outcome is always that the complication will not develop. Consider the following example:

Collaborative problem: Potential Complication of abdominal surgery: Paralytic ileus (paralysis of the ileum of the small intestine)
Goal: Patient will not develop paralytic ileus.

Suppose that 36 hours after surgery, the patient's bowel sounds are absent, their abdomen is distended and painful, and they begin vomiting. Can the nurse

Table 3-6 ➤ Expected Outcomes for Various Problem Types

TYPE OF PROBLEM	EXAMPLE OF DIAGNOSIS	EXPLANATION OF DIAGNOSIS	EXAMPLE OF EXPECTED PATIENT OUTCOME	PURPOSE OF NURSING INTERVENTIONS
Actual Nursing Diagnosis	Constipation r/t inadequate dietary fiber and fluids	Symptoms of constipation present (e.g., no bowel movement [BM] 3 days)	Will have normal, formed BM within 24 hr after receiving stool softener.	Resolution or reduction of problem; prevention of complications.
Risk (Potential) Nursing Diagnosis	Risk for Constipation r/t inadequate dietary fiber and fluids	Risk factors present (e.g., not drinking enough or eating adequate fiber)	Will have bowel function within normal limits for patient (e.g., daily BM with no need for stool softener or laxative).	Prevention and early detection of problem.
Possible Nursing Diagnosis	Possible Constipation r/t suspected inadequate intake of dietary fiber and fluids	Not enough data (e.g., no BM for 2 days, but no data on intake or on the patient's usual bowel habits)	No patient goal. The *nursing* goal is "Confirm or rule out the problem."	Confirm or rule out problem.
Collaborative Problem	Potential Complication of abdominal surgery: ileus	Medical treatment creates risk for complication that is prevented by collaborative care.	None. Patient responses depend on collaborative care. The broad nursing goal is early identification of the problem.	Primarily detection; prevention is collaborative.
Wellness Diagnosis	Readiness for Enhanced Bowel Elimination	Bowel habits and dietary intake within normal limits, but fiber content and fluid intake can be improved.	Reports increased intake of dietary fiber and fluids; reports bowel functioning within normal limits.	Maintain or promote higher level of health.

relieve the ileus and bring about the return of peristalsis? Actually, there is very little that the nurse could do. The primary interventions are medical and, if there is obstruction, probably surgical. Therefore, it is not appropriate to include a goal for this problem on a nursing care plan.

Collaborative goals are appropriate on multidisciplinary care plans and critical pathways. For collaborative problems, you might wish to write a *nursing goal,* such as "Early detection of complication, should it occur."

How Do I Use Standardized Terminology for Outcomes?

The ANA has approved several standardized vocabularies for describing client outcomes. The one used throughout most of this book is the *NOC.*

Components of an NOC Outcome

Each NOC outcome consists of an outcome label, indicators, and a measurement scale.

- The **outcome label** (referred to as *the outcome*) is broadly stated (e.g., Decision Making, Concentration). It is neutral to allow for positive, negative, or no change in patient health status. Because NOC outcomes are linked to NANDA-I nursing diagnoses, you can use the NANDA-I/NIC/NOC "linkages" book to look up a nursing diagnosis and see the list of outcomes suggested for it (Johnson et al., 2012).
- **Indicators** are the behaviors and states that you can use to evaluate patient status. The indicator "Identifies relevant information" means that Decision Making (the broad outcome) was achieved. For each outcome, select the indicators that are appropriate to the patient. You can add to the list of indicators if necessary.
- NOC has a **measurement scale** for describing patient status for each indicator, with 1 being least desirable and 5 being the most desirable. During your initial assessment, you assigned the number that represents the patient's present health status. To form the "goal," you assign the scale number that the patient can realistically achieve after the interventions.
  Example:
  - (NOC Outcome) **Decision Making**
  - *Goals (Indicators + Measurement scale)*
  - Identifies relevant information (4, mildly compromised)
  - Identifies alternatives (4, mildly **compromised**)
  - Identifies potential consequences of each alternative (5, not compromised)

KnowledgeCheck 3-12

Figure 3-6, a patient plan of care for Acute Pain, uses NOC language.
- What outcomes did the nurse choose for this patient?
- List two indicators for each of the outcomes.

- For which outcome does the nurse expect the highest level of functioning to occur after interventions? (Note that in this care plan, the measuring scale has been applied to the outcomes rather than to the indicators.)

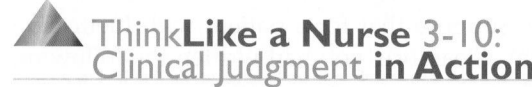
ThinkLike a Nurse 3-10: Clinical Judgment in Action

In Figure 3-6, what do you think the nurse expects to happen? Why do you think the nurse ranked the outcomes this way?

Using NOC With Computerized Care Plans

Standardized language is especially useful in computerized care systems. For example, the nurse could choose Circulation Status as a patient outcome; the program would then provide the definition and NOC indicators for Circulation Status. The nurse needs only to check the indicators that apply to the patient.

Key Point: *The computer does not think for you. You are responsible for deciding which outcomes and indicators to use for each patient and for identifying a target time.*

How Do I Write Goals for Wellness Diagnoses?

Expected outcomes for wellness diagnoses describe behaviors or responses that demonstrate health maintenance or achievement of a higher level of health—for example, "Over the next year, will continue to eat a balanced diet with more emphasis on including whole grains and fiber." You can use the NOC to write wellness outcomes. For example:

> *Nursing diagnosis:* Readiness for Enhanced Nutrition
> *Expected outcome:* Nutritional Status: (5) Not compromised

In addition, many NOC outcomes can be used with other diagnoses (e.g., Activity Tolerance, Child Development, Growth, Nutritional Status). See Chapter 37 or go to the NOC Web site for a complete list of wellness outcomes.

PLANNING NURSING INTERVENTIONS

Key Point: *Nursing interventions are actions based on clinical judgment and nursing knowledge that nurses perform to achieve client outcomes.* They can either be direct-care interventions or indirect-care interventions.

- **Direct-care interventions** are performed through interaction with the client(s) (e.g., physical care, emotional support, and patient teaching).
- **Indirect-care interventions** are performed away from the client but on behalf of a client or group of clients (e.g., advocacy, managing the environment, consulting with other members of the healthcare team, and making referrals).

Interventions may also be independent, dependent, or interdependent (collaborative).

Independent Interventions are those that registered nurses (RNs) are **accountable** for and are licensed to prescribe, perform, or delegate based on their knowledge and skills. They do not require a provider's prescription. Knowing how, when, and why to perform an activity makes the action **autonomous** (independent). Nurses prescribe and perform independent interventions in response to a nursing diagnosis. **Key Point:** *As a nurse, you are accountable (answerable) for your decisions and actions with regard to nursing diagnoses and independent interventions.*

Dependent Interventions are those prescribed by a physician or advanced practice nurse but carried out by the nurse. Dependent interventions are usually prescriptions for diagnostic tests, medications, treatments, IV therapy, diet, and activity. In addition to carrying out medical prescriptions, you will be responsible for assessing the need for the prescription, explaining the activities to the patient, and evaluating the effectiveness of the prescription.

Collaborative (Interdependent) Interventions are exactly what they sound like: interventions carried out in collaboration with other health team members (e.g., physical therapists, physicians). Because nurses care for the whole person, their responsibilities often overlap with those of other healthcare team members.

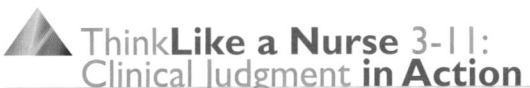 Think**Like a Nurse** 3-11:
   Clinical Judgment **in Action**

- Can you think of an example of a direct-care intervention?
- Can you think of an example of an indirect-care intervention?

HOW DO I DECIDE WHICH INTERVENTIONS TO USE?

Key Point: *As a nurse, you will be responsible for choosing nursing interventions. You cannot delegate this responsibility to unlicensed assistive personnel.* As a rule, licensed practical/vocational nurses (LPN/LVNs) give care according to a plan created by the RN. The LPN/LVN contributes to the plan by providing data or by giving feedback about the effectiveness of the interventions. For more information about delegation, see Chapter 39.

How Does Nursing Research Influence My Choice of Interventions?

Although much nursing and medical practice is based on tradition, experience, and professional opinion, this is not an ideal basis for choosing an intervention. Ideally, a nurse should choose an intervention because of firm evidence that it is the best possible approach for the patient. Such interventions would be those that were developed from a sound body of scientific research.

What Is Evidence-Based Practice?

Evidence-based practice (EBP) is an approach that uses firm scientific data rather than anecdote, tradition, intuition, or folklore in making decisions about medical and nursing practice. In nursing, EBP includes blending clinical judgment and expertise, the best available research evidence, patient characteristics, and patient preferences. **Key Point:** *The goal of EBP is to identify the most effective and cost-efficient treatments for a particular disease, condition, or problem.* For more discussion on the importance of research and evidence-based nursing practice, see Chapter 4.

Types of Research-Based Support

Research-based support for an intervention includes single studies, critical pathways and protocols, clinical practice guidelines, systematic reviews of the literature, and evidence reports.

Single Studies Individual studies can give you an idea of the effectiveness of an intervention. Keep in mind that single studies may not be reliable when choosing an intervention because of the following limitations:

- Not all interventions have been included in the study.
- There may be only one or two studies of an intervention.
- The available studies may have included only a small number of patients.

Critical Pathways and Protocols Also called *clinical pathways* and *collaborative care plans,* critical pathways and protocols are standardized plans of care for the following situations:

- Frequently occurring conditions (e.g., total hip replacement) in the healthcare agency.
- Similar outcomes and interventions are appropriate for all patients who have the condition.

Critical pathways:

- Are tools developed by an organization for its own use.
- Are intended to guide best practice only at the local level.
- May not be based on research.

Evidence Reports Evidence reports are systematic reviews of clinical topics for the purpose of providing evidence for practice guidelines, quality improvement, and funding decisions. Evidence reports are usually developed by scientists rather than by clinicians, patients, and advocacy groups. One source of such reports is the Evidence-Based Practice Center (EPC) program of the federal Agency for Healthcare Research and Quality (AHRQ). The EPC uses explicit grading

Toward Evidence-Based Practice

de Freitas Luzia, M., Vidor, I. D., da Silva, A. C. F. E., & de Fátima Lucena, A. (2020). Fall prevention in hospitalized patients: Evaluation through the nursing outcomes classification /NOC. *Applied Nursing Research, 54,* 151273.

This cross-sectional study of 68 hospitalized adult patients evaluated five standardized nursing outcomes (NOC) of patients at high risk for falls: Knowledge: Fall Prevention (1828), Fall Prevention Behavior (1909), Vital Signs (0802), Medication Response (2301), and Safe Health Care Environment (1934). Each outcome had its own indicators that were assessed using a 5-point Likert scale (1 = worst score and 5 = most desirable).

Patients received three assessments, each 24 hours apart, during the time that the nurses performed nursing intervention prescriptions based on NIC (Risk for Falls). Statistical differences were found between the first and last assessment, indicating improvement in several of the indicators and outcomes, including the following:

- Knowledge: Fall Prevention—showed that patients have a limited level of knowledge, but over the three assessments, the patients' knowledge of the indicators significantly increased from none to limited.

- Fall Prevention Behavior was rarely demonstrated by patients, but a significant change in behavior level was observed in two of the six indicators assessed: Uses grab bars and Adjusts bed height.
- Vital Signs, Medication Response, and Safe Health Care Environment had high initial scores and no significant difference over the three assessments, indicating that patient monitoring and the healthcare environment were safe and adequate.

Conclusions: The results of this study indicated that fall-prevention nursing interventions may have contributed to improved knowledge and preventive behavior for hospitalized patients at high risk for falls. The researchers concluded that the evaluation of patient outcomes supported by a standardized classification system, such as the NOC, highlights the importance of care planning and nursing interventions that lead to effective and safe practice.

Based on this study, can you think of at least two more conclusions in addition to those listed here?

systems to review studies and rank the strength of their evidence. For free access to online reviews:

 Go to the AHRQ Web site at **https://www.ahrq.gov/ research/findings/evidence-based-reports/index.html**

Clinical Practice Guidelines Clinical practice guidelines, such as the Joanna Briggs Institute (JBI) Database of Systemic Reviews and Implementation Reports and the National Guideline Clearinghouse (NCG), are systematically developed statements to assist practitioners and patients in making decisions about appropriate healthcare for a particular disease or procedure. They are typically developed by clinicians, patients, and advocacy groups and are published by specialty organizations, universities, and government agencies. They form the basis for nursing interventions.

KnowledgeCheck 3-13

- Explain how theory influences your choice of nursing interventions.
- Why does a clinical practice guideline provide better support for an intervention than does a single study?
- Why does a clinical practice guideline provide better support for an intervention than does an agency's critical pathway?

How Does Problem Status Influence Nursing Interventions?

Nursing interventions include activities for observation/assessment, prevention, treatment, and health promotion. As you can see in Table 3-7, the problem status

determines which types of activities are required. **Key Point: *A nursing intervention can be a preventive measure in one situation and a treatment in another.*** For example, you might write the nursing order, "Teach the importance of adequate fluids."

- For a patient with an actual diagnosis of Constipation, that is treatment.
- For a patient with a diagnosis of Risk for Constipation, that is prevention.

What Process Can I Use for Generating and Selecting Interventions?

Several nursing measures might be effective for any one problem. The idea, of course, is to select those most likely to achieve the desired goals. In doing that, you must consider the patient's abilities and preferences; the education, experience, and capabilities of the nursing staff; the resources available (e.g., time, equipment); medical prescriptions; and institutional policies and procedures. Generating interventions requires you to use critical thinking skills. A full-spectrum nurse takes the following into account before choosing an intervention.

1. Review the Nursing Diagnosis

Choose strategies you expect will reduce or remove the etiological factors that contribute to actual problems (unhealthy responses) or that will reduce or remove risk factors for potential problems.

- ***When it is not possible to change the etiology,*** choose strategies to treat the patient's symptoms (the AMB/

Table 3-7 ➤ Relationship of Problem Status to Intervention Type

Intervention Type

PROBLEM STATUS	OBSERVATION INTERVENTION	PREVENTION INTERVENTION	TREATMENT INTERVENTION	HEALTH PROMOTION INTERVENTION
Actual Nursing Diagnosis	To detect change in status (improvement, exacerbation of problem)	To help keep the problem from becoming worse	To relieve symptoms and resolve etiologies (contributing factors)	
Potential (Risk) Nursing Diagnosis	To detect (1) progression to an actual problem or (2) an increase or decrease in risk factors	To remove or reduce risk factors in an effort to keep the problem from developing		
Possible Nursing Diagnosis	To obtain more data to confirm or rule out a suspected nursing diagnosis			
Collaborative Problem	To detect onset of a complication for early physician notification	To implement nursing orders and medical prescriptions to help prevent the development of a complication	To implement nursing orders and medical prescriptions for relieving or eliminating the underlying condition for which complications may develop	
Wellness Diagnosis	To assess a client's wellness practices	To prevent specific diseases (e.g., giving immunizations)	Clients usually manage their own wellness treatment	To support a client's health promotion efforts and achieve a higher level of wellness

AEB part of a diagnosis). For example, if the cause of pain is a surgical incision, you cannot "cure" the incision. Your nursing actions should focus on measures to relieve the pain.

- **When you do not know the etiology of the problem.** Some interventions may relieve a problem regardless of its cause. For example, when a client is anxious, it is helpful to approach them calmly, regardless of the cause.

Key Point: *As a rule, standardized interventions (care common to all patients with a particular condition) flow from the problem side of a nursing diagnosis; individualized interventions flow from the etiology.*

2. Review the Desired Patient Outcomes

Desired outcomes (goals) suggest nursing strategies that are specific to the individual patient (Table 3-8). For each goal on the care plan, ask the question, "What intervention(s) will help to produce this patient response?" There may be one or more interventions for each goal, and a single intervention may help to achieve more than one goal.

3. Identify Several Interventions or Actions

The next step is to think of several nursing activities that might achieve the desired outcomes. Do not try to narrow your list at this point; include unusual and creative ideas. To get started, ask yourself: for this nursing diagnosis, (1) What assessments/observations do I need to make? and (2) What do I need to do for the patient? Include both dependent and independent activities as appropriate.

You can refer to a standardized list of interventions or choose interventions from standardized care plans and agency protocols. Alternatively, you can generate the interventions yourself based on your knowledge and experience and the use of nursing texts, journal articles, practice guidelines, and professional nurses.

4. Choose the Best Interventions for the Patient

The best interventions are those you expect to be most effective in helping to achieve client goals. When possible, choose interventions based on research and scientific principles. Use critical-thinking questions from the full-spectrum nursing model to help you determine the best actions (Box 3-4).

5. Individualize Standardized Interventions

Practice guidelines, protocols, critical pathways, and even textbooks describe interventions that are appropriate for most people. However, they cannot take into account all the factors that contribute to a problem or

Table 3-8 ➤ Interventions Flow From Desired Outcomes

OUTCOMES	INTERVENTIONS
1. **Will have bowel movement within 12 hours after receiving stool softener and laxative.**	A. **Administer prescribed stool softener and laxative at bedtime today.**
2. Will have daily soft, formed bowel movement during rest of hospital stay.	B. Instruct in and encourage high-fiber diet.
	C. Encourage increased fluid intake.
3. Within 24 hours, will need narcotics to manage pain less than 2×/day.	D. Use nonpharmacological measures (e.g., distraction) to minimize need for narcotics.
4. Calls nurse when urge to defecate is felt; does not delay defecation.	E. Encourage Mr. Ivanos to summon the nurse when he feels the urge to defecate.
	F. Provide privacy (e.g., pull the bed curtain, turn on the TV, leave room).

Discussion:

Strategy A would help to achieve goal 1, but because the effects of these medications are short-lived, it would do nothing to achieve goals 2 through 4.

Strategies B and C both help to achieve goal 2.

Strategy D (minimize narcotics), in contrast, directly addresses goal 3 and indirectly helps to achieve goal 2.

Strategies E and F both directly address goal 4 and indirectly address goal 2.

Note: Dotted lines indicate indirect contribution to goal.

---

that might affect the effectiveness of an intervention. You must always consider how an intervention can be used with a particular person. **Key Point: *Each person has unique needs and responds in unique ways.***

Computer-Generated Interventions

Most electronic care planning programs will generate a list of suggested interventions when you enter either a problem (nursing diagnosis, medical, collaborative) or an outcome. You then choose the interventions appropriate for the patient or type in nursing actions on your own. Computer prompts provide a wide range of interventions for your consideration. However, always look for other, perhaps more effective, strategies based on the patient data. Always think, "Are there other interventions I have overlooked? How should I adapt this for this patient?"

HOW CAN I USE STANDARDIZED LANGUAGE TO PLAN INTERVENTIONS?

Recall that standardized nursing terminologies are important for EHRs; for research; and for clear, precise, consistent communication among nurses and with other disciplines.

The Nursing Interventions Classification (NIC) was the first comprehensive standardized classification of nursing interventions (McCloskey & Bulechek, 1992). The NIC (Butcher et al., 2018) describes more than 500 direct- and indirect-care activities performed by nurses.

The NIC (pronounced "nick") is versatile and appropriate for use in all specialty and practice areas, including home health and community nursing.

Each NIC intervention consists of a label, a definition, and a list of the specific **activities** nurses perform in carrying out the intervention (Box 3-5). The **label,** usually consisting of two or three words, is the standardized terminology. The **definition** explains the meaning of the label. You are free to word the activities any way you choose in a care plan or client record.

Locating Appropriate NIC Interventions and Activities

NIC interventions are linked to NANDA-I nursing diagnoses and NOC outcome labels in a "linkages" book, *NOC and NIC Linkages to NANDA-I and Clinical Conditions,* referred to by most nurses as the *NNN linkages book* (Johnson et al., 2012). In this book, you can look up a nursing diagnosis to see the list of outcomes suggested for it and the interventions for achieving each outcome.

Once you have chosen the interventions (based on your knowledge and judgment), you then choose the appropriate activities to carry out the intervention. Choose the best ones to fit the situation, the client, and the resources (e.g., supplies, equipment). As you might guess from looking at Box 3-5, you will probably never need to perform all the activities for a client. Choose the best ones for the situation, the client, and the available resources (e.g., supplies, equipment).

BOX 3-4 ■ Questions to Ask When Choosing Interventions

The following critical-thinking questions can help you determine the best actions.

Contextual Awareness

Is this intervention acceptable to the patient (e.g., congruent with the patient's culture, values, and wishes)?

Is this intervention culturally sensitive?

What is going on in the patient's life (e.g., family, work) and health status (e.g., knowledge, abilities, resources, severity of illness) that could affect the success of the intervention?

Credible Sources

Have I used valid, reliable sources of information to identify this intervention (e.g., other professionals, best practice resources)?

Did I consider professional, ethical, and legal standards?

What is the research basis for this intervention, if any?

Considering Alternatives

Is there adequate rationale for this intervention (e.g., principles, theory, facts)?

Which action(s) is (are) most likely to achieve stated goals?

Analyzing Assumptions

What beliefs, values, or biases do I have that may affect my thinking and choices?

Do I feel any discomfort with this intervention?

Reflecting Skeptically

Are there other interventions I have overlooked?

What might be the consequences of this intervention? Does it have any potential ill effects? If so, how will we manage them?

Is this intervention feasible? For example, is it cost effective; can the patient or family manage it at home?

How will the intervention interact with medical prescriptions? For example, you cannot order "elevate head of bed" to facilitate breathing if there is a medical prescription to keep the patient flat.

Do I have the knowledge and skills needed for the intervention, or do I need to consult with someone more qualified in this area?

In priority order, what should I do in this situation, and why?

Using NIC in Electronic Care Plans

Standardized language is especially useful in computerized care systems. For any NIC intervention, the program will also list the more specific nursing activities, which you can individualize as nursing orders. **Key Point:** *Remember that you, not the computer, are responsible for choosing which interventions to use for each patient, when to use them, and which activities to write as specific nursing orders.* You can reject all the suggested interventions if they

BOX 3-5 ■ NIC Intervention: Bathing

Definition

Cleaning of the body for the purposes of relaxation, cleanliness, and healing

Activities

Assist with chair shower, tub bath, bedside bath, standing shower, or sitz bath, as appropriate or desired.

Wash hair, as needed and desired.

Bathe in water of a comfortable temperature.

Use fun bathing techniques with children (e.g., wash dolls or toys; pretend a boat is a submarine; punch holes in bottom of plastic cup, fill with water, and let it "rain" on child).

Assist with perineal care, as needed.

Assist with hygiene measures (e.g., use of deodorant or perfume).

Administer foot soaks, as needed.

Shave patient, as indicated.

Apply lubricating ointment and cream to dry skin areas.

Offer handwashing after toileting and before meals.

Apply drying powders to deep skin folds.

Monitor skin condition while bathing.

Monitor functional ability while bathing.

Source: Butcher, H., Bulechek, G., Dochterman, J., & Wagner, C. (2018). *Nursing interventions classification (NIC)* (7th ed.). Mosby.

do not fit the patient's unique needs, and in many systems, you can type or write in your own interventions and activities.

Standardized Languages for Home Health and Community Care

The NIC includes interventions applicable in all settings, including home health and community nursing. However, the following taxonomies were created specifically for community-based practice:

■ **The Clinical Care Classification (CCC),** previously called the *Home Healthcare Classification,* was developed for use in home healthcare (Saba, 1995, 2012). For a complete description of the CCC system, see the nursing process section of Chapter 37 and

 go to the CCC Web site at **http://www.sabacare.com.**

■ **The Omaha System** was developed for community health nurses to use in caring for individuals, families, and **aggregates** (community groups or entire communities) (Martin, 2005; Monsen et al., 2017). For a complete description of the Omaha System, see the nursing process section of Chapter 37 and

 go to the Omaha system Web site at **http://www. omahasystem.org.**

KnowledgeCheck 3-14

- Name and describe three standardized intervention vocabularies recognized by the ANA.
- In the NIC system, what is the difference between interventions and activities?

Does Standardized Language Interfere With Holistic Care?

Some nurses have criticized standardized terminologies for focusing on illness and physical interventions. However, NIC, Omaha, and CCC include interventions to address health promotion and cultural and spiritual needs. Using a common language should help rather than hinder your choice of interventions and make clear in health records that holistic techniques are appropriate as nursing interventions.

Wellness Interventions When you are caring for a healthy client, you will function mainly as a teacher and health counselor. Frequently, the nursing orders outline lifestyle modification or behavioral changes the client wants to make, along with self-rewards to reinforce the behaviors. For example,

> *Specific behavior change:* I will consume fewer than 1,400 calories per day for the next week.
> *Self-reward:* I will reward myself with an evening out to hear my favorite band.

For more information on using standardized languages to describe wellness interventions, see Chapter 8.

Spiritual Care Interventions NIC, CCC, and the Omaha System all include terminology to describe spiritual interventions. The following are just a few examples:

NIC: Spiritual Growth Facilitation, Religious Ritual Enhancement
CCC: Spiritual Care, Coping Skills
Omaha: Spiritual Support, Bereavement Support

Chapter 13 provides a full discussion of standardized nursing interventions to address spiritual needs. You could also use most of those interventions (e.g., Coping Skills) for problems that are not spiritual in nature.

Culturally Sensitive Care Except for the NIC Culture Brokerage intervention, there are no standardized interventions that are unique to culturally based needs. All standardized interventions will result in culturally sensitive care if they are delivered by a culturally competent nurse.

WHAT ARE NURSING ORDERS, AND HOW DO I USE THEM?

Nursing orders are instructions that describe how and when nursing interventions are to be implemented. They are usually written on a nursing care plan. Other nurses and unlicensed assistive personnel (UAP) are responsible and accountable for implementing nursing orders.

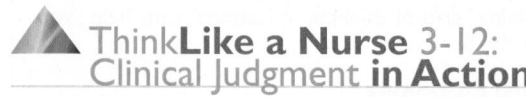

ThinkLike a Nurse 3-12: Clinical Judgment in Action

Suppose you are caring for a patient 24 hours after a major surgery. You see the following order on the nursing care plan: Ambulate 24 hours postoperatively.

- When you care for the patient, how will you go about implementing this nursing order?
- What else do you need to know to effectively carry out this order?

Components of a Nursing Order

Did you have trouble answering the previous questions? Even experienced nurses would because this nursing order is incomplete. As you see from this example, nursing orders must be specific and detailed because many caregivers will use the care plan, and they all need to be able to interpret the orders correctly. A well-written nursing order contains the following components:

- **Date.** Indicate the date the order was written. Change the date each time you review or revise the order.
- **Subject.** Nursing orders are instructions to nurses, so they are written in terms of *nurse* behaviors. It is understood that the subject of the order is "the nurse," just as the subject of a goal statement is understood to be "the patient." **Key Point:** *Goals state patient behaviors; nursing orders state nurse behaviors.*

Goal/Expected Outcome	*Nursing Order*
[Patient will] Drink 100 mL fluid per hour during the day	[Nurse will] Offer 100 mL fluids (water or juice) per hour on the day shift

- **Action verb.** This tells the nurse what action to take—what to do. Examples of action verbs are *assist, assess, auscultate, bathe, change, demonstrate, explain, give, teach,* and *turn.*
- **Times and limits.** State when (e.g., which shift, what day), how often, and how long the activity is to be done. Consider the unit routines (e.g., visiting hours, mealtimes), the patient's usual rest times, scheduled tests and procedures (e.g., x-ray studies), and treatments (e.g., physical therapy). Specify exact times when needed. The following nursing orders show times and limits:
  - Teach the components of a healthy diet *on 9/13, day shift.*
  - Offer 100 mL water *every hour between 0700 and 1900.*
  - Administer acetaminophen 500 mg orally *at least 30 min before dressing change.*
- **Signature.** The nurse who writes the order should sign it, followed by their credentials. For example, include *RN* or *BSN.* A signature indicates that you

accept legal and ethical accountability for your orders and allows others to know whom to contact if they have questions or comments. An electronic signature is legally equivalent to an actual signature.

IMPLEMENTATION: THE ACTION PHASE OF THE NURSING PROCESS

Implementation involves action and thinking, but the emphasis is on doing.

- During implementation, you perform or delegate planned interventions—that is, carry out the care plan.
- This phase ends when you document the nursing actions.
- Implementation evolves into evaluation as you document the resulting client responses.

   Key Point: *In short, implementation is doing, delegating, and documenting.* It is intricately tied into every other step of the nursing process:

- **Implementation overlaps with assessment.** Nurses use assessment data to individualize interventions. Implementation provides the opportunity to assess your patient at every contact. When performing an ongoing assessment, you are both implementing and assessing.
- **Implementation overlaps with diagnosis.** Nurses use data discovered during implementation to identify new diagnoses or to revise existing ones.
- **Implementation overlaps with planning outcomes and interventions.** As you care for a patient, you begin to know them better, and their unique needs become more apparent.
- **Implementation overlaps with evaluation.** When evaluating patient health status and progress toward goals (next step in the nursing process), you will compare the responses you observe during implementation with the existing goals (which were written in the planning outcomes phase).

Preparing for Implementation

Implementation involves some preparation. Although the care plan will already have been developed in the planning stages of the nursing process, you should do some more planning just before implementing the plan, as described in the following steps. Notice how important critical thinking and nursing knowledge are to this "doing" phase of the nursing process.

Check Your Knowledge and Abilities

Before you begin a nursing activity, review the care plan and reflect critically on the nursing and medical prescriptions.

- **Clarify orders.** As a nurse, you are obligated, ethically and legally, to clarify or question prescriptions that you believe to be unclear, incorrect, or inappropriate.
- **Be sure you are qualified/authorized.** Is the action allowed by your state's nurse practice act, your facility's policies and procedures, and your job description? Is it allowed by your instructor or supervisor? Do you have the required knowledge, skill, and experience? Can you accept accountability for the outcomes of your action?
- **Be sure the action is safe, reasonable, and prudent.** Assess the patient to see whether the action is still indicated. Have you checked for contraindications, identified possible harmful patient responses, and minimized risks? Do you have a plan for what to do if something does not go as planned? Have you planned for safety, privacy, and comfort? Have you considered whether the action is ethical (Alfaro-Le-Fevre, 2008)?

   Key Point: *If the answer to any of the preceding questions is no, then you must get help or advice from your instructor or supervisor.*

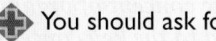 You should ask for help when:

- You do not have the knowledge or skill needed to implement a provider prescription (e.g., when administering an unfamiliar medication).
- You cannot perform the activity safely alone (e.g., helping patient who is weak and has obesity to ambulate).
- Performing the activity alone would cause undue stress for the patient (e.g., giving back care to a patient with multiple fractures).

Organize Your Work

You must work efficiently to control healthcare costs and to make the most of every patient contact. Think ahead and plan interventions you can perform at the same time. For example, while changing a dressing, you might teach the patient about wound care at home. Many institutions have forms for scheduling your work, or you may need to write your own list of "things to do" in the order you need to do them. For example, you could make a form with a column for tasks you must accomplish and a column for each of your patients. In column 1, include information such as the following:

Room #
Name patient prefers
Admitting diagnosis
Significant others
Current health status (from report); does care plan
   need to be modified?
Basic care needs (e.g., hygiene, elimination, feeding,
   dressing, other)
Safety precautions
Medications
IVs
Tests and treatments today

Prioritized nursing diagnoses
Interventions that must be done today
New medical orders to implement
Teaching and counseling for today

Establishing Feedback Points You cannot assume you will be able to carry out a nursing order in exactly the way it was written.

Example: *Suppose the nursing order states, "Help to ambulate in the hall b.i.d [twice a day]." When you help the patient to stand, he becomes pale, dizzy, diaphoretic, and short of breath. Would you still carry out the order?*

You must always be ready to alter the activity on the spot as the patient's responses demand. This means that you observe how the patient is responding to the activity as you perform care. Because this evaluation is done before the intervention is complete, we call it **feedback.** Feedback could be verbal, or it could be a change in vital signs, skin color, or level of consciousness, as in the preceding example. When organizing your work, identify points in each intervention where you want to pause for feedback. **Key Point:** *Notice how the concept of feedback relates to the concept of organization and how they both are related to the key concept, implementation.*

Prepare Supplies and Equipment Gather all the supplies and equipment you need before going to the patient's room. This allows you to work efficiently by eliminating the need to leave the room to obtain items you have overlooked.

Prepare the Patient

Before performing a nursing activity, identify and reassess the patient to make sure the activity is still necessary and the patient is physically and psychologically ready for the intervention.

Check Your Assumptions Don't assume that an intervention is still needed simply because it is written on the care plan.

Example: *On postoperative day 6 after Jeannette Wu's surgery, the UAP is preparing to give her a bed bath, as instructed on the care plan. However, Mrs. Wu has regained some of her strength and is able to sit in a chair. Based on this, the nurse and the assistant agree that, with help, Mrs. Wu can bathe at the sink instead of requiring a complete bed bath.*

Assess the Patient's Readiness To obtain the most benefit from an intervention, a client must be physically and psychologically ready.

Example: *The hospital's critical pathway for hip fractures recommended a "help bath" on postoperative day 3 for Mrs. Wu. However, her physical condition indicated that she needed a bed bath on day 3. The nurse did not assume Mrs. Wu was ready to progress just because the critical pathway dictated it.*

Explain What You Will Do and What the Patient Will Feel Many interventions require the patient's participation or cooperation. ♥ **iCare** Caring nurses take time to explain because they want to motivate the patient and provide the necessary information needed to participate. Knowing what to expect helps to relieve anxiety, enables the patient to cope with unpleasant or painful sensations, and promotes a trusting relationship.

Provide Privacy This helps to assure psychological readiness and respects the patient's dignity.

KnowledgeCheck 3-15

- Why is it important to organize your work before implementing care?
- In addition to organizing your work, what other preparations should you make before implementing care?

Implementing the Plan: Doing or Delegating

After both you and the patient are prepared, it is time to act.

- Nursing actions include both those you do yourself and those you delegate.
- Interventions may be *collaborative, independent,* or *dependent.*
- During implementation, you will coordinate and carry out both the nursing orders on the nursing care plan and the medical prescriptions that relate to the patient's medical treatment.

During implementation, you can expect to use all types of knowledge—theoretical, practical, personal, and ethical—as well as knowledge about the patient situation. You will also use various combinations of cognitive, psychomotor, and interpersonal skills to perform nursing activities (thinking, doing, caring).

Example: *When you are inserting an IV catheter, you need cognitive knowledge of sterile procedure, interpersonal skills to reassure the patient, and psychomotor skills to apply the tourniquet and insert the IV catheter.*

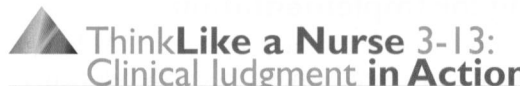 **ThinkLike a Nurse** 3-13:
Clinical Judgment **in Action**

Use the examples provided in the preceding paragraph to help you write a definition for each of the following terms:

- Cognitive skills
- Interpersonal skills
- Psychomotor skills

How Can I Promote Client Participation and Adherence?

Different interventions require differing levels of participation. However, even a nurse-initiated intervention, such as inserting a urinary catheter, goes more smoothly if the patient participates, at least to the extent of holding still while you perform the procedure. When promoting participation and adherence, remember:

- **Many interventions depend almost entirely on the patient's adherence to the therapy.**
- **People fail to follow therapeutic regimens for various reasons,** such as lack of understanding, cultural or religious objections, embarrassment, or hesitation to ask questions.
- **People need access to information that they can understand,** including knowledge of medical words, how their healthcare system works, and how to manage their disease.

Box 3-6 provides tips for promoting client cooperation.

What Should I Know About Collaborating and Coordinating Care?

For successful implementation, you need the skills of collaboration and coordination.

Collaborating As you have learned, *collaboration* simply means working with patients and other caregivers (e.g., physicians, respiratory therapists) to plan, make decisions, or perform interventions. Unlike delegated activities, true collaboration requires shared decision making. One of the competencies you must acquire in school is the ability to function on an interprofessional team. This means, in part, that you will learn to be assertive in discussions about patient care. At the same time, you need to recognize the differences in authority and power that exist on interprofessional teams and then choose your communication style carefully.

Coordination Coordinating care includes scheduling treatments and activities with other departments (e.g., laboratory, physical therapy, radiology). But it is more than that. Nurses are the professionals who have the most frequent and continuous contact with the patient, so they have the most complete picture of the person. You will be expected to read reports of other professionals, help interpret the results for the patient and family, and make sure that everyone sees the whole picture.

BOX 3-6 ■ Tips for Promoting Client Cooperation

You can promote client cooperation with treatments and therapies by following these guidelines.

Provide Teaching

Assess the client's understanding of his illness and treatments.

Provide essential and desired information in plain language.

Keep instructions simple, clear, and as specific as possible.

Ask the client to state in their own words the key concepts about the current health issues, decisions, and instructions you just discussed.

Supply a written copy of instructions to the client and/or caregiver, taking into account cognitive abilities and readiness for additional information.

Utilize pictures and other visual aids relevant to the client's medical condition and needs.

Assess the Client's Supports and Resources

People may not have enough money for treatments or medicine, even if they wish to follow the therapy.

Some people cannot read or understand printed instructions.

Some do not have family or friends to help with their care at home.

The patient may not have transportation to the healthcare facility.

Be Sensitive to the Client's Cultural, Spiritual, and Other Needs

Keep in mind that shared decision making is a way to reach a goal, and the goal in patient care is to achieve outcomes that (1) matter most to the patient and (2) promote the patient's health.

Modify interventions as much as possible to reflect client preferences and beliefs.

Incorporate benign alternative practices and preferences into client's care plan (e.g., food preference and preparation, folk remedies, family presence and decision making, use of significant spiritual rituals).

Realize and Accept That Some Attitudes Cannot Be Changed

Information alone will not change a person's behavior. For example, regardless of the effects of obesity on blood pressure, a client will not lose weight simply because you tell the client it is important. The client must *want* to lose weight.

Determine the Client's Main Concerns

A client's main concern may be different from that of the client's healthcare providers. For example, you may be concerned that lack of exercise makes it difficult to regulate a client's blood sugar; the client's main concern may be that exercise makes their joints hurt.

Help the Client Set Realistic Goals

Clients usually more readily accept small, rather than drastic, behavioral or lifestyle changes. For example, perhaps a client with a child who has asthma cannot even imagine that they could stop smoking. But you may be able to convince them that it would be better for the child if they smoke outdoors rather than in the house or in the car.

Talk Openly and Regularly About Adherence

Let the client know you understand how difficult treatment can be and that others struggle with adherence as well.

Offer information about support groups/resources that might be helpful.

What Should I Know About Delegation and Supervision?

Delegation Delegation takes place when the RN, who holds the *authority* for nursing care delivery, transfers *responsibility* for the performance of a task to UAP while retaining *accountability* for a safe outcome (ANA, 2012; Wagner, 2018). When the UAP accepts the responsibility for the delegated task, they have the authority to complete it as directed. As an RN, you will frequently delegate patient care activities to licensed vocational (or practical) nurses (LVN/LPNs) and UAPs.

Delegating Is Not the Same as Assigning You may *assign* tasks to other RNs (e.g., the charge nurse makes unit assignments for the day). However, this is not delegation because those RNs are accountable for the outcome of their activities. Remember, you can only delegate down in the chain of command. For specific activities that can be safely delegated,

 Go to **Chapter 3 Delegation Decision-Making Grid,** in Volume 2.

You Cannot Delegate Nursing Care Decisions
You can delegate only the responsibility for performing a defined activity in a particular situation.

Example: Even though the nurse has delegated the task of turning a client every 2 hours to a UAP, it is *the nurse* who must assess the client's skin condition and take action if it does not improve.

Five Rights of Delegation
When deciding whether to delegate tasks, you should think critically about the five critical elements, or "five rights," of delegating. For a checklist to help with your decision, see Box 3-7.

KnowledgeCheck 3-16
- List the "five rights" of delegation.
- As an RN, how could you establish that a UAP is competent to perform a task?
- List at least three ways to help ensure that the UAP will clearly understand what they need to do when you delegate a task.
- List at least three things you should do when providing supervision to an unlicensed caregiver.

Documenting: The Final Step of Implementation

After giving care, record the nursing activities and the patient's responses. **Documentation** is a mode of communication among the members of the health team, and it provides the information you need to evaluate the patient's health status and the nursing care plan. For a thorough discussion of documenting, refer to Chapter 17.

Reflecting Critically About Implementation

During the implementation phase, perhaps more than at any other time, nurses combine thinking and doing. You should always be prepared to modify the activity based on the patient's responses. Afterward, when you have some time to reflect, you can think critically about what happened and why. Use the following questions or refer to the critical-thinking model:

- What was done? Why was it done? What were the patient's responses?
- Did I forget to do anything?
- What was going on in the situation that may have influenced the outcome?
- What factors influenced my behavior (or others' behavior) in this situation?
- What assumptions or biases (mine or the patient's) contributed to the problem in this situation?
- Did I communicate clearly to the patient?
- Did I convey respect and caring?
- What could I have delegated? What did I delegate that I should not have? Why?
- After reflecting on it, what would I do differently in this situation?

The following is an example of how reflection questions might be used in a clinical situation:

Example: The nursing order read, "Assist to ambulate to the end of the hall . . ." However, the patient was able to walk only half that distance before becoming too weak to stand.
Question for Reflection: What was going on in the situation that may have influenced the outcome?
What Might Have Happened: Perhaps the patient was weak because they had not slept well the night before, or perhaps they had just completed a long, tiring session of physical therapy.

EVALUATION: THE FINAL STEP OF THE NURSING PROCESS

Evaluation is a planned, ongoing, systematic activity in which you will make judgments about:

- The client's progress toward desired health outcomes
- The effectiveness of the nursing care plan
- The quality of nursing care in the healthcare setting

How Is Evaluation Related to Other Steps of the Nursing Process? Patient outcomes related to the *planning outcomes* stage must be concrete, observable, and appropriate for the patient in order to be useful as evaluation criteria. Appropriate outcomes, in turn, depend on complete and accurate *assessment* data and *nursing diagnoses*. You will observe and evaluate client responses during *implementation* in order to make on-the-spot changes in activity. And of course, *interventions* must be *planned* and *implemented* to produce the patient

BOX 3-7 ■ The Five Rights of Delegation: Checklist

Right Task (Can I delegate it?)

As a rule, you should delegate an activity only if it meets *all* of the following criteria:

Delegable for a specific patient

Within the licensed nurse's scope of practice and the delegatee's job description

Permitted by the state's nurse practice act

Permitted by the agency's policies

Is performed according to an established sequence of steps and requires little or no modification from one situation to another

Does *not* require independent, specialized nursing knowledge, skills, or judgment

Is *not* health teaching or counseling

Does not endanger a client's life or well-being

Right Circumstance (Should I delegate it?)

Before delegating, assess the patient to be certain that their needs match the abilities of the UAP or LPN. Consider patient safety:

Is the patient setting appropriate?

Is the patient's condition relatively stable?

Can the patient perform self-care activities without extensive help?

Are adequate resources available?

Are there other factors to maintain safety?

Right Person (Who is best prepared to do it?)

The right person:

Is delegating the task (the nurse must be competent to delegate).

Will be performing the task (the UAP must be competent to do the task).

Will receive the care (i.e., the severity of the patient's illness is considered).

Has performed the task often or has worked with patients with similar diagnoses.

Has a workload that allows time to do the task properly.

The facility:

Has documented proof that the person has demonstrated competence. If evidence is lacking, you need to establish the UAP's competence (e.g., observe and evaluate their performance or ask the UAP, "How many times have you done this procedure?").

Right Direction/Communication (What does the UAP need to know?)

Explain exactly what the task is. For example, "Empty the catheter bag, and measure the amount of urine using the clear, marked plastic container"—not just "Measure the urine."

Include specific times and methods for reporting. For example, "Come tell me the patient's temperature every hour."

Explain the purpose or objective of the task. For example, "Change the patient's position every 2 hours to prevent bedsores; they are not able to turn by themselves."

Describe the expected results or potential complications. For example, "I have given the patient their medications, so their temperature should be below 100°F by 0900. If not, let me know immediately."

Be specific in your instructions. For example, "Let me know whether Ms. Reynolds has any more red spots or broken skin areas when you turn her," not "Tell me what her skin looks like."

Be certain the delegatee (UAP) understands the communication and that they cannot **modify the task** without first consulting the nurse.

Right Supervision/Evaluation (How will I follow up?)

As the RN, you are responsible for providing supervision and evaluating the outcomes. This includes the following:

Monitoring the UAP/LVN's work. Does it comply with standards of practice and agency policy and procedures?

Intervening as needed. Some UAPs receive little training, so you may need to demonstrate and receive return demonstrations of the UAP's ability to perform some activities.

Obtaining feedback from the patient. Evaluate both the patient's responses to the UAP interventions and the relationship with the UAP.

Obtaining feedback from the delegatee. Provide both positive and negative feedback. If performance is not acceptable, speak privately with the UAP to explain the specific mistakes. Listen to the UAP's view of the situation.

Evaluating client outcomes.

Ensuring proper documentation of the delegatee's actions. Some agencies permit UAPs to record vital signs and other patient data. However, the RN is still responsible for seeing that all necessary data are recorded and that they are accurate.

Sources: American Nurses Association. (2012). *ANA's principles for delegation by registered nurses to unlicensed assistive personnel (UAP)*; American Nurses Association (ANA) and the National Council of State Boards of Nursing (NCSBN). (2006). *Joint statement on delegation.* https://www.ncsbn.org/Delegation_joint_statement_NCSBN-ANA. pdf; National Council of State Boards of Nursing. (2016). National guidelines for nursing delegation. *Journal of Nursing Regulation, 7*(1), 5–14. http://dx.doi.org/10.1016/S2155-8256(16)31035-3

behaviors that you evaluate. **Key Point: *Evaluation and assessment both involve data collection. The difference is in when you collect and how you use the data.***

- **Assessment data** are collected before interventions are performed to determine initial or baseline health status and to make nursing diagnoses.
- **Evaluation data** are collected after interventions are performed to determine whether client goals were achieved.

Why Is Evaluation Essential to Full-Spectrum Nursing?

The following are a few reasons:

- The patient is the nurse's first priority. The aim of all nursing activity is to achieve positive outcomes for patients. Evaluation lets you know whether your interventions are helping the patient as intended and guides your next actions.

- Evaluation helps nurses to conserve scarce resources. Nursing time must be used wisely and efficiently. Evaluation allows you to discard interventions that are not working well and focus on more effective ones.
- The ANA *Code of Ethics* requires evaluation. "Nurses have a responsibility to define, implement, and maintain standards of professional practice. Nurses must plan, establish, implement, and evaluate review mechanisms to safe-guard patients, nurses, colleagues, and the environment" (ANA, 2021, Provision 4.3, p. 15).
- The Joint Commission and other professional standards-review organizations require evaluation. These organizations use outcomes and performance measures to evaluate the quality of care in healthcare institutions. They conceptualize quality of care as the degree to which health services increase the likelihood of desired health outcomes.
- Evaluation helps ensure nursing's survival. Linking nursing interventions to the achievement of client outcomes demonstrates the value of nursing. In today's competitive healthcare market, that is essential for ensuring continued funding for nursing services, education, and research.

♥ **iCare** Evaluation demonstrates caring and responsibility. Without evaluation, you would not know whether your care was effective. Examining outcomes implies that you care about how your activities affect your clients.

How Are Standards and Criteria Used in Evaluation?

In a broad sense, evaluation is the systematic process of judging the quality or value of something (e.g., a car, a movie) by comparing it with one or more standards or criteria. **Key Point:** *For formal evaluation, however, you must decide in advance which standards and criteria you will use.* In nursing, standards are used to describe quality nursing care.

- **The ANA's standards of practice** are a good example of *broadly written standards.*
- **Criteria and competencies.** Criteria are measurable or observable characteristics, properties, attributes, or qualities. They describe the specific skills, knowledge, behaviors, and attitudes that are desired or expected. The ANA standards (ANA, 2021) include a set of measurement criteria, called *competencies,* to help describe the standard.
- **Patient goals and outcomes** are also examples of criteria. As you learned, criteria should be concrete and specific enough to serve as guides for collecting evaluation data. In addition, they should be reliable and valid.

Reliability A criterion is **reliable** if it yields the same results every time, regardless of who uses it. For example, suppose you measure a patient's temperature by (1) using an oral thermometer and (2) placing the back of your hand on the patient's forehead. Which method would probably give the same (or nearly the same) results every time? As you probably concluded, the oral thermometer is more reliable.

Validity A criterion is **valid** if it is really measuring what it was intended to measure. For example, fever is often used as a criterion for concluding that a person has an infection. However, if used alone, it is not a valid indicator because (1) other conditions, such as dehydration, can cause a fever, and (2) elevated temperature is not present in all infections. The validity of that criterion is increased when you use additional criteria (e.g., elevated white blood cell count, presence of signs of infection such as redness and pus).

ThinkLike a Nurse 3-14: Clinical Judgment in Action

- The outcome "Patient will not complain of pain" by itself is not a valid criterion for measuring pain. Why? What would be a more valid criterion for pain?
- A criterion reads, "Measures client vital signs once per shift, or as prescribed." For which of the following standards would it be valid (that is, which conclusion could you draw if you knew that a nurse measured the vital signs once per shift, or as prescribed)?
  - Follows unit policies.
  - Performs skills accurately.

What Are the Types of Evaluation?

Evaluation is categorized according to (1) what is being evaluated (structures, processes, or outcomes) and (2) frequency and time of evaluation.

Evaluation of Structures, Processes, and Outcomes

Structures, processes, and outcomes all work together to affect care. However, each requires different criteria and methods of evaluation.

Structure Evaluation

- Focuses on the setting in which care is provided
- Explores the effect of organizational characteristics on the quality of care
- Requires standards and data about policies, procedures, fiscal resources, physical facilities and equipment, and number and qualifications of personnel

The following are examples of criteria for structure evaluation:

- At least one RN is present on each unit at all times.
- A resuscitation cart is available on each unit.

Process Evaluation

- Focuses on the manner in which care is given—the activities performed. As a rule, it does not describe the *results* of your activities.
  Example: Your instructor uses process evaluation to assess your clinical performance—that is, what you did and how well you did it.

- Explores whether the care was relevant to patient needs, appropriate, complete, and timely.
  Examples: Protects patient's privacy when performing procedures.
  Washes hands before each patient contact.

Outcomes Evaluation

- Focuses on observable or measurable changes in the patient's health status that result from the care given.
- Although structure and process are important to quality, the most important aspect is improvement in patient health status.
- Used in the evaluation step of the nursing process.
  Examples:
  - Patient will walk, assisted, to the end of the hall by postoperative day 3.
  - Patient reports pain of less than 4 on a scale of 1 to 10 within 1 hour after analgesic administration.
- Also used when evaluating the quality of care in an organization. When used for that purpose, the criteria also state the percentage of clients expected to have the outcome when care is satisfactory.
  Example: Postcatheterization urinary tract infection does not occur.
  Expected compliance: 100% (Criterion would be met only if no patients developed a urinary tract infection after being catheterized.)

Ongoing, Intermittent, and Terminal Evaluation

Evaluation begins as soon as you have completed the first nursing activity and continues during each client contact until all goals are achieved or the client is discharged from nursing care. The client's status determines how often you evaluate.

Examples:
- After a patient undergoes surgery, you may measure vital signs every 15 minutes; as the patient nears discharge, you may evaluate once a day.
- In long-term care settings, residents often have chronic health problems that require evaluation over an extended period of time. Care providers may participate in weekly care conferences to evaluate the resident's response to the current plan of care.
- Ongoing evaluation is performed while implementing care, immediately after an intervention, and at each patient contact.
- Intermittent evaluation, in contrast, is performed at specified times.
  Examples:
  - Will rate pain as less than 3 on a scale of 1 to 10 within 1 hour after medication.
  - Will lose 1 lb per week until a weight of 125 lb is achieved.
- **Terminal evaluation** describes the client's health status and progress toward goals at the time of discharge. Most institutions have special discharge forms for terminal evaluation that also include instructions about medications, treatments, and follow-up care.

Key Point: *As the nurse, you are responsible for drawing evaluative conclusions; however, you should use input from the patient, the family, UAPs, and other caregivers.*

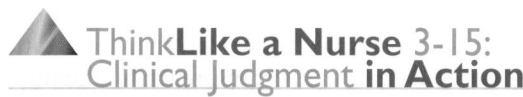

ThinkLike a Nurse 3-15: Clinical Judgment in Action

For each of the following goals, when or how often should the nurse collect evaluation data?

- Will rate pain as less than 3 on a scale of 1 to 10 within 1 hour after medication.
- By the second home visit, patient will demonstrate proper techniques for breastfeeding.

KnowledgeCheck 3-17

- Explain what is evaluated in each of the following types of evaluation (i.e., the focus of each type of evaluation): structure, process, and outcomes.
- Identify what is evaluated using the following criteria: structure, process, or outcomes.
  1. In the ED, the time from patient sign-in to assessment by a healthcare worker will be less than 15 minutes.
  2. A fire extinguisher is located in an accessible spot on each unit.
  3. No patients with indwelling urinary catheters will develop a urinary tract infection.

How Do I Evaluate Patient Progress?

Evaluation does not "end" the nursing process. It merely provides the information you need to begin another cycle. After giving care, you compare patient responses to the desired outcomes (goals) and use that information to reflect critically on (1) the care plan and (2) each step of the nursing process as it applies to that patient. When evaluating patient progress, you review the desired outcomes, collect reassessment data, judge whether goals have been met, and record the evaluative statement.

Review Outcomes

The goals and indicators identified in the planning outcomes phase serve two purposes in evaluation:

- Suggest the kind of assessments you need to make
- Provide criteria by which to judge the data

Collect Reassessment Data

Assess client responses to the current interventions. To minimize confusion, assessments made for the purpose of evaluation are called *reassessments*. Reassessments are always focused assessments. As in the assessment phase, you will collect data from the client, family, friends, and health team members, as well as from the client's chart.

Example: The nursing care plan for Todd (Meet Your Patient) lists the following goal: "By 8/24/XXXX, will walk, unassisted, to the end of the hall without pallor or shortness of breath." What kind of assessments would you make to know whether this goal has been met?

Answer: You would observe the patient's skin color as he walked, count his respirations, and ask him whether he felt short of breath. You must question to clarify—for example, "Were you short of breath at any time? Were you short of breath by the time the walk was finished?"

Key Point: *The RN is responsible for evaluating goal achievement, even though someone else may have supplied the data.*

For a checklist to use for evaluation,

 Go to **Chapter 3, Evaluation Checklist,** in Volume 2.

Judge Goal Achievement

Compare the reassessment data with the patient's goals. As always, get the patient's input: for example, do they think the goals have been achieved? Goals or outcomes can be judged to be one of the following:

- **Achieved.** The actual responses are the same as the desired outcome.
- **Partially achieved.** Some, but not all, of the desired behaviors were observed, or the desired response occurs only some of the time (e.g., the desired heart rate is less than 100 beats/min, a goal that is achieved except for one or two episodes a day when it is 120 beats/min).
- **Not achieved.** The desired response did not occur.

Record the Evaluative Statement

Professional standards require that you record your evaluations (ANA, 2021). You may write an evaluative summary in the nursing notes or on the care plan, depending on agency procedures. An evaluative statement should include the following:

- The conclusion about whether the goal was achieved
- Reassessment data to support the judgment
  Example: An evaluative statement for a pain goal of "By 8/24/XXXX will notify nurse as soon as pain begins" might be the following:
  8/25/XXXX, 0100. Goal not met. Has not used call light at all this a.m. Restless and grimacing with movement during a.m. care. When asked, described pain as 8 on a scale of 1 to 10.

When using standardized outcomes or electronic care plans, your evaluative statements may be different. In the NOC system, each outcome has a scale and indicators, numbered 1 through 5, that you can use to write goals.

Example: A patient with a problem of decreased peripheral circulation might have this goal: "Circulation status not compromised."

Using standardized language from the NOC, you might write a goal (*desired* status) of:

Goal: Circulation Status: *5* (5 means "no deviation from normal range" in the NOC scale).

Each of the indicators could also be made into a goal by adding the desired scale numbers, as follows:

Systolic BP in expected range: 5
Diastolic BP in expected range: 5
Mean BP in expected range: 5

Evaluation statements are written the same as goals are written, but the scale number describes the patient's *actual* status.

Example: If on reassessment, the patient's blood pressure is quite low and he has orthostatic hypotension, the evaluative statement might be:
Evaluative Statement: Circulation Status: *3* (3 means "moderately compromised" on this NOC scale).

Figure 3-8 shows a computer screen displaying the NOC outcome of Acceptance: Health Status. The Initial Scale shows the initial assessment, the Expected Scale is the goal, and the Outcome Scale is the evaluative statement after intervention and reassessment. Did the interventions achieve the desired effect?

KnowledgeCheck 3-18

Using the following outcomes and reassessment data, determine whether each goal has been met, partially met, or not met.

1. *Goal:* By 8/24/XXXX, will walk, unassisted, to the end of the hall without pallor or shortness of breath.

Reassessment data: 8/24/XXXX. Walked, unassisted, to end of hall; states no shortness of breath, but skin color was noticeably pale.

2. *Goal:* By 8/24/XXXX, will walk, unassisted, to the end of the hall without pallor or shortness of breath.

Reassessment data: 8/24/XXXX. Walked, unassisted, to end of hall. Skin color pink; respirations 14/min; no dyspnea observed; states no shortness of breath.

3. *Goal:* By 8/24/XXXX, will walk, unassisted, to the end of the hall without pallor or shortness of breath.

Reassessment data: 8/24/XXXX Walked halfway to end of hall before becoming pale and short of breath.

Evaluate Collaborative Problems

Because collaborative problems are the responsibility of the entire healthcare team, goals for collaborative problems are not included on the care plan, and the evaluation process is slightly different. The desired outcome for all collaborative problems is that no complication will occur. To evaluate, you will compare the reassessment data with established norms and determine whether data are within an acceptable range.

- **If the reassessment data are within normal limits,** this does not mean that the collaborative problem is resolved—only that the complication has not

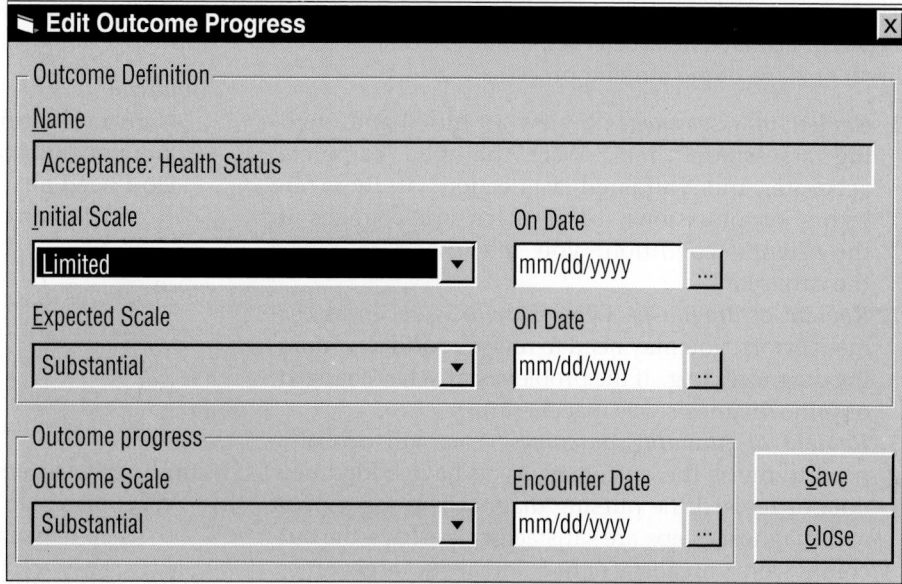

FIGURE 3-8. Computer screen showing outcome progress, using NOC.

Explanation of Figure

Computer field	Nursing process terminology	Represents	Status recorded on computer
Initial scale	Initial assessment	*Actual* status *before* intervention	Limited acceptance of health status
Expected scale	Goal	*Desired* status *after* intervention	Substantial acceptance of health status
Outcome scale	Evaluative statement	*Actual* status *after* intervention	Substantial acceptance of health status

occurred. As long as the patient has the medical condition (e.g., myocardial infarction), the collaborative problem (e.g., congestive heart failure) still exists.

- **If the data indicate the client's condition is worsening,** notify the primary healthcare provider.

Evaluating and Revising the Care Plan

After evaluating patient progress, you will use your conclusions about goal achievement to decide whether to continue, modify, or discontinue the care plan.

Relate Outcomes to Interventions

Even when goals have been met, you cannot assume that the patient outcomes were a result of the nursing interventions. You need to use critical reflection to identify factors that might have supported or interfered with the effectiveness of an intervention. The following are variables that can affect the ability of an intervention to produce the desired outcome:

- The client's ability and motivation to follow directions for treatment
- Availability and support from family and significant others
- Treatments and therapies performed by other healthcare team members
- Client failure to provide complete information during assessment

- Client's lack of experience, knowledge, or ability
- Staffing in the institution (ratio of licensed to unlicensed caregivers; number of patients for whom a nurse is responsible)
- Nurse's physical and mental well-being

Identifying these factors allows you to reinforce or change them. Remember, though, that you cannot control all the variables that might affect the success of an intervention.

Draw Conclusions About Problem Status

Whether you retain or remove a nursing diagnosis from the care plan depends on whether goals were met, as follows:

Goals met: If all goals for a nursing diagnosis have been met, you can **discontinue the care plan** for that diagnosis.

Goals partially met: If some outcomes are met and others are not, you may **revise the care plan** for that problem.

Goals not met: You should **examine the entire plan and review all steps** of the nursing process to decide whether to revise the care plan.

Revise the Care Plan

To decide how to revise the care plan, you must review each step of the nursing process. You cannot merely discontinue the ineffective interventions and try new ones.

The interventions may not need to be changed at all. When goals have not been met, it may be due to errors in other steps of the nursing process.

1. *Review of assessment.* Review all initial and ongoing assessment data. Were the data complete, accurate, and validated as needed? If there are errors or omissions, or if there are changes in the client's condition, you may need to revise the care plan.
2. *Review of diagnosis.* Even if there were no assessment errors, you may need to revise or add new nursing diagnoses (e.g., if the problem status has changed, or if the diagnosis was inaccurate).
3. *Review of planning outcomes.* You will probably need to revise the outcomes if you have added new data or revised the nursing diagnosis. If assessment and diagnosis steps are satisfactory, perhaps the outcomes were unrealistic or had unrealistic target times.
4. *Review of planning interventions.* You will probably need to modify nursing orders (a) if you determine that interventions were not effective (e.g., they were unclear, incomplete, or not specific) or (b) if you have revised nursing diagnoses or outcomes.
5. *Review of implementation.* It could be that goals were not met because of a failure to implement the nursing orders or because of the manner in which they were implemented. Get input from the client, significant others, other caregivers, and the client records to find out what went wrong.

Reflecting Critically About Evaluation

After evaluating the patient's health status and the nursing care plan, reflect on your thinking during the evaluation process. That's right: Think about your thinking, not just about your actions.

Inquiring
Is my evaluation statement clearly stated?
Were my information sources reliable?
Do I need any other data to validate my conclusion?

Noticing context
What was going on either before or during evaluation that might have influenced my ability to gather data or draw conclusions?
What emotional responses influenced my conclusions about goal achievement?

Analyzing assumptions
What biases do I have that may have affected my ability to reassess or evaluate goal achievement?

Reflecting skeptically
Did I make evaluating a priority?
Did I schedule time for it, the same as I do for interventions?

Key Point: *The most common errors of evaluation are failing to:*

- *Evaluate systematically.*
- *Record the results.*
- *Use the reassessment data to examine and modify the care plan.*

It is relatively easy for most nurses to make a plan and take action. However, you will need determined effort to make the time to observe regularly and systematically and document the patient's responses and include them in your actions. Only in that way can you be sure the care has met the client's needs.

Safe, Effective Nursing Care (SENC)

The SENC model of safe, quality care requires the nurse to:

➤ **Evaluate and use techniques/process to avoid nursing errors in the delivery of client care.**

Example: You suspect that the incidence of central line infections has increased on your pediatric unit. Before you can obtain a positive outcome, you must first be able to quantify the poor outcomes and then determine the cause of that outcome.

➤ **Design a "Thinking, Doing, Caring" framework that incorporates a holistic approach to client care.**

Example of thinking: You have noticed a lot of variation in how different nurses provide central line care. Knowing that variation in treatment often leads to negative variations in outcomes, what data do you need to support your suspicions? What outcome must you measure? What root cause should be assessed? Now, how can you obtain data about those two factors?

Example of doing and caring: Suppose you identified the rate of central line infections as the poor outcome and how central line dressing changes are performed as the problem in nursing practice. Your next steps would be to develop and implement an action plan that improves on the manner in which you are performing central line dressing care. Tracking the changes in nursing interventions and client responses is an essential part of doing and caring.

➤ **Evaluate the framework, incorporating the structure, processes, and outcomes components of quality improvement issues.**

Example: Improving the quality of care is possible only by evaluating goals with clear measurements. Evaluations and reevaluations provide insight and provide a baseline against which practice changes and patient outcomes can be judged.

Source: Draper, D., Felland, L., Liebhaber, A., & Melichar, L. (2008). *The role of nurses in hospital quality improvement* (HSC Research Brief No. 3). http://www.hschange.org/CONTENT/972/

Evaluating the Quality of Care in a Healthcare Setting

As a nurse, you will be involved in evaluating and improving the overall quality of nursing care in an organization or a geographic area. Applying quality improvement in healthcare is a core competency of all health professionals (ANA, 2021; Cronenwett et al., 2007, 2009; Institute of Medicine, 2011). At a minimum, your documentation will provide data that regulatory agencies use to determine whether nursing care meets nursing standards.

Quality Assurance Programs These are specially designed programs to promote excellence in nursing. Variations of quality assurance are *quality improvement, continuous quality improvement, total quality management,* and *persistent quality improvement.* Whatever the approach, the goal is to evaluate and improve the care provided in an agency or for a group of patients.

To explore learning resources for this chapter,

Go to Davis Advantage and find:

Answers and Suggested Responses for all questions in this chapter

Concept Map

Knowledge Map

References and Bibliography

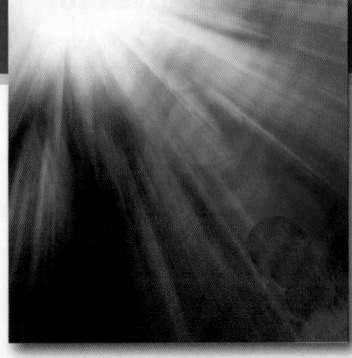

CHAPTER 4

Evidence-Based Practice: Theory & Research

Learning Outcomes

After completing this chapter, you should be able to:

➤ Define *nursing theory.*

➤ Explain how the four building blocks (components) are used in developing a theory.

➤ List the four essential concepts in a *nursing* theory.

➤ List three ways in which you can use nursing theory.

➤ Discuss two prominent nurses who proposed theories of caring.

➤ Describe three nonnursing theories and their contributions to nursing.

➤ Discuss the significance of evidence-based nursing practice.

➤ Compare and contrast quantitative and qualitative nursing research.

➤ Identify three components of the research process and explain their importance.

➤ Name three priorities in the process of protecting research participants.

➤ Apply the PICOT method to formulate a question for guiding a literature search.

➤ Discuss the process of analytic reading and explain its significance to the appraisal of research.

➤ Discuss how you might integrate nursing research into your nursing practice.

Key Concepts

Evidence-Based practice
Nursing research
Nursing theory
Theory

Related Concepts

See the Concept Map on Davis Advantage.

Meet Your Patient

Imagine you are the home health nurse providing care to an older, frail man in his home. Mr. Khatri is visibly upset and is grabbing at the belt around his waist as he sits in the chair. He is crying out to his deceased mother to come take him to her. What are you going to do to address this situation, and why do you think it will help? Don't be concerned if you don't think you know enough to answer this question. Before you read on, try to answer it based on the knowledge and experience that you *do* have.

There are two general ways to approach this problem. One way is to firmly explain to the resident that his behavior is not acceptable and that he must stay in his chair. Another possibility is to talk quietly to Mr. Khatri and gently guide his hands to his lap, not rushing him. While you are talking to him, you might ask, "Tell me more about your memories of your mother. What does she look like? Do you miss her?" By the time you lead him to his room,

you might realize he is exhibiting stage II dementia and is confused as to place and time.

If you chose the first approach in the scenario, you were demonstrating **mechanistic nursing,** which is based on getting the tasks done. If you chose the second solution, you based your behavior on **holistic nursing,** which addresses meeting the needs of the whole person using person-centered care. This scenario demonstrates the powerful impact of nursing theory and research on your daily practice as a nurse.

ABOUT THE KEY CONCEPTS

The overall goal of this chapter is that you will understand the concepts of **nursing theory, nursing research,** and **evidence-based practice** well enough to see how they are related and how they form the foundations for patient care. You will learn about a related concept, *caring,* which is central to some theories and to the full-spectrum nursing model introduced in Chapter 2.

Theoretical Knowledge
knowing why

This chapter introduces you to nursing theory and research and looks at them as the foundations for patient care. It emphasizes caring theory; however, in later chapters you will find other theories that pertain to specific aspects of practice. For example, Chapters 6 and 7 use developmental theories, Chapter 10 uses theories of self-esteem, and Chapter 11 makes use of family theories.

Think of full-spectrum nursing as a jigsaw puzzle (Fig. 4-1).

- *Practice, the first puzzle piece*—Initially, a nurse has an idea, which is usually based on experiences in

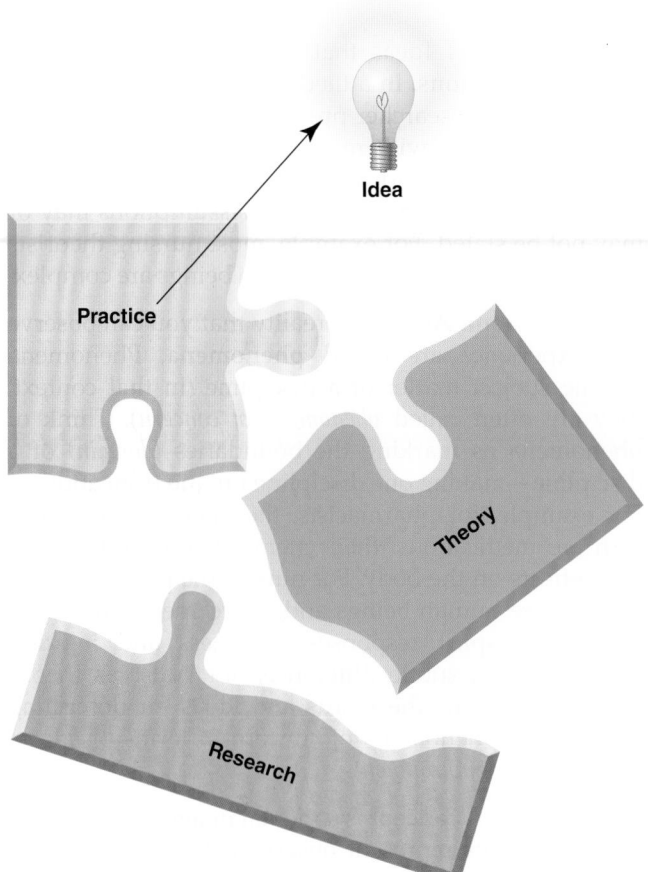

FIGURE 4-1 Practice, theory, and research are interrelated. A nurse has an idea, conducts research to test the idea, and finally develops a theory.

practice and a need for an improvement of some kind. Perhaps the idea is something simple, such as, "How can I spend more time with the patients' families in ways that would help the patient and family to cope with the stress of illness?"

- *Research, the second puzzle piece*—After considering the idea, the nurse may decide it is worth investigating with *research.* The research question might be, "How does spending more time with family members affect the perceived quality of care the patient receives?"

- *Theory, the third puzzle piece*—If the research supports the nurse's idea, the nurse could then use the research findings to develop a *theory.* The nurse might even take the research results to nursing administrators to determine whether the theory could be put into practice in the organization—perhaps as a policy or in a standardized care plan. That would be the beginning of what is called a **clinical practice theory,** a theory that is immediately applicable in the clinical setting.

THE IMPORTANCE OF NURSING THEORY AND RESEARCH

Following are three classic examples that demonstrate how important theory and research are to the foundations for patient care.

The Framingham Studies The Framingham studies are a longitudinal, multidisciplinary research project (*longitudinal* means "done over a long period of time"). They consist of several studies carried out over 50 years (from 1948 to 1998) to identify the health and healthcare practices of one community: Framingham, Massachusetts. The results of the various Framingham studies have influenced healthcare practices for diabetes mellitus, breast cancer, heart disease, osteoarthritis in older adults, and other disease and client conditions. For example, there was a time when mammography was considered unreliable and unimportant in screening for breast cancer. The Framingham project changed that attitude and, as a result, improved the healthcare of women (Boston University and the National Heart, Lung, and Blood Institute, n.d).

♥ **iCare**   **Watson's Science of Human Caring** Dr. Jean Watson developed a nursing theory called the **Science of Human Caring** (Watson, 1988). This theory describes what *caring* means from a nursing perspective. It may not seem that nurses need to be taught how to care, but Dr. Watson and other nursing theorists found that they did. Before the "caring theorists," nurses were somewhat mechanistic in the work they did, much like the first alternative for dealing with Mr. Khatri (Meet Your Patient). A mechanistic nurse has a list of things to do, completes the list, and does nothing more. The "something more" often consists of caring behaviors, such as singing to a frightened child or taking the time to teach a new mother for the second time how to bathe her baby.

This is not to say that nurses didn't care about their patients before Watson. The point is that a *theory* can change the *focus* of nursing. Certainly, Nightingale must have cared about the soldiers who were her patients. But what she wrote about and what she taught the nurses was a set of things to do. Nurses were valued for the tasks they performed in patient care. Caring theories demonstrate the value of the non–task-oriented aspects of nursing.

Benner's Novice to Expert (Fig 4-2) Dr. Patricia Benner, in her work entitled *From Novice to Expert* (1984), proposed a theory that should be of special interest to you. This theory, which is explained in Chapter 1, describes the progression of a beginning nurse to increasing levels of expertise. You are a **novice,** or a beginning nurse, simply because you are new to the nursing profession and have limited experience and judgment as a nurse. Benner's theory provides the information necessary to understand how you learn and perform your nursing responsibilities and advance your role as a professional nurse. Benner's theory of caring is discussed later in this chapter.

KnowledgeCheck 4-1

- Compare mechanistic and holistic nursing. Select one of these concepts and describe a scenario in which it is used.
- Briefly describe the Framingham studies and list three diseases for which these studies influenced care.

NURSING THEORIES

Florence Nightingale (1859/1992) stated that nursing theories describe and explain what is and what is not nursing. That makes it helpful to learn them at the beginning of your nursing education. Before focusing on nursing theory, though, you need to learn a little more about theory in general. Exactly what *is* a theory? And how is a theory created?

A **theory** is an organized set of related ideas and concepts that helps us:

- Find meaning in our experiences (such as nursing).
- Organize our thinking around an idea (such as caring).
- Develop new ideas and insights into the work we do.

Simply put, a theory answers the questions, What is this? And how does it work? Although a theory is based on observations of facts, the theory itself is *not* a fact. A theory is merely a way of viewing phenomena (reality); it defines and illustrates concepts and explains how they are related or linked. **Key Point:** *Theories can be, and usually are, revised.*

What Are the Components of a Theory?

Theories are made up of assumptions, phenomena, concepts, definitions, and statements (or propositions). You can think of these as the building blocks of a theory.

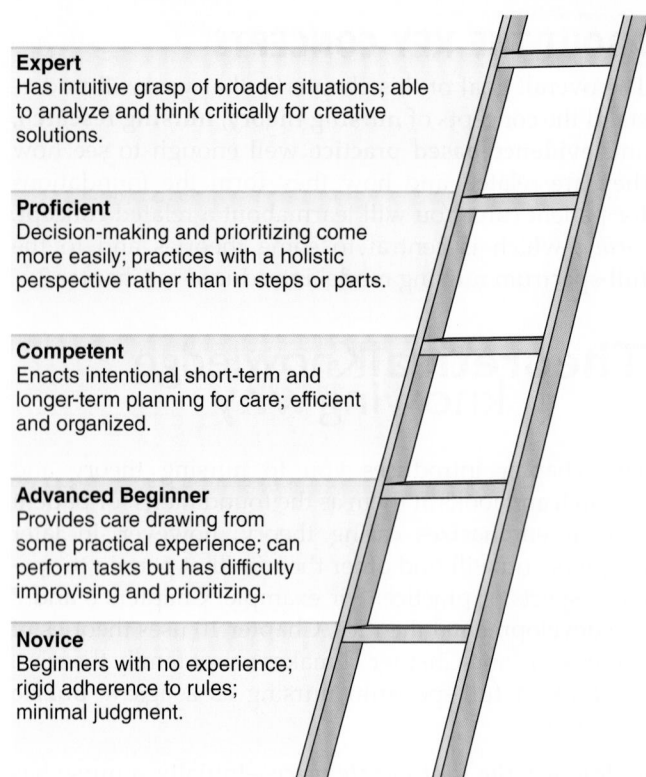

Expert
Has intuitive grasp of broader situations; able to analyze and think critically for creative solutions.

Proficient
Decision-making and prioritizing come more easily; practices with a holistic perspective rather than in steps or parts.

Competent
Enacts intentional short-term and longer-term planning for care; efficient and organized.

Advanced Beginner
Provides care drawing from some practical experience; can perform tasks but has difficulty improvising and prioritizing.

Novice
Beginners with no experience; rigid adherence to rules; minimal judgment.

FIGURE 4-2 Benner's nursing model: From novice to expert.

Assumptions Ideas that we take for granted are called **assumptions.** In a theory, they are the ideas that the theorist or researcher presumes to be true and does not intend to test with research. For example, Watson assumed nursing had its own professional concepts and that one of them was caring. Assumptions may or may not be stated. For example, most nursing theorists assume but do not state that human beings are complex.

Phenomena Aspects of reality that you can observe and experience are called **phenomena.** Phenomena are the subject matter of a discipline (in that context, they are often called *phenomena of concern*). Think of phenomena as marking the boundaries *(domain)* of a discipline—making one discipline unique from another. For example, for pharmacists, the phenomena of concern are medications: their chemical composition and their effects on the body. For nurses, the phenomena of concern are human beings and, more specifically, their body–mind–spirit responses to illness and injuries. It may seem a subtle difference, but Watson's theory of caring gave us the words and ideas for describing the nursing phenomena of concern in terms of *human beings in their environments.*

Concepts A **concept** is a mental image of a phenomenon. Concepts represent observations or experiences. They are typically used to draw similarities, make distinctions among, organize, and categorize information, objects, or like ideas. For example, what does the word *fever* bring to mind? From your own experience with fever, you know the subjective feeling of discomfort that fever produces. You have the theoretical knowledge that fever is an elevated body temperature; you know the physiology of temperature regulation, so you understand what is going on in the body to fight infection. You may have the visual image of a thermometer or someone who is warm to the touch and possibly sweating (diaphoretic). The word *fever* is a symbol for all of those ideas and images. It is a concept.

Concepts range from simple to complex and from concrete to abstract. Simple, concrete concepts are those you can observe directly (e.g., height, weight). More abstract and complex concepts are those you observe indirectly (e.g., hematocrit, brain activity, nutritional status). Abstract concepts are those you must infer from many direct and indirect observations (e.g., self-esteem, wellness).

A theory usually contains several concepts. For example, Watson includes 10 "caring processes" in her original theory (Box 4-1).

Definitions A **definition** is a statement of the meaning of a term or concept that sets forth the concept's characteristics or indicators—that is, the things that allow you to identify the concept. A definition may be general or specific.

- A **theoretical definition** refers to the conceptual meaning of a term (e.g., *pain*).
  Example: Pain is an unpleasant sensory and emotional experience associated with actual or potential tissue damage.
- An **operational definition** specifies how you would observe or measure the concept (e.g., when doing research on pain).
  Example: Pain is the patient's verbal statement that he is in pain.

BOX 4-1 ■ Watson's 10 Caring Processes

1. Forming a humanistic–altruistic system of values
2. Instilling faith and hope
3. Cultivating sensitivity to self and others
4. Forming helping and trusting relationships
5. Conveying and accepting the expression of positive and negative feelings
6. Systematically using the scientific problem-solving method that involves the caring process
7. Promoting transpersonal teaching–learning
8. Providing for a supportive, protective, and corrective mental, physical, sociocultural, and spiritual environment
9. Assisting with gratification of human needs
10. Sensitivity to existential–phenomenological forces

Source: Watson, J. (1988). *Nursing: Human science and human care. A theory of nursing* (NLN Publication No. 15-2236). National League for Nursing Press.

Statements Also called **propositions, statements** systematically describe the linkages and interactions among the concepts of a theory. The statements, taken as a whole, make up the theory. In Maslow's theory, for example, two concepts are *physiological needs* and *self-esteem needs.* An example of a statement in that theory would be the following: "*Physiological needs* must be met to an acceptable degree before a person can attempt to meet their *self-esteem needs.*"

Paradigm, Framework, Model, or Theory?

In any discussion of nursing knowledge, you may hear the terms *paradigm, framework, model,* or *theory.* It may be difficult to differentiate between these terms because (1) they are abstract, (2) they are defined differently by theorists, and (3) they are often used interchangeably in general conversation among nurses. As you progress in your career and education, you will need to pay careful attention to the similarities and differences among these terms. For now, you can use the following basic definitions (*theory* was defined earlier).

A **paradigm** is the worldview or ideology of a discipline. It is the broadest, most global conceptual framework of a discipline. For example, the medical paradigm views a person through a lens that focuses on identifying and treating disease. This lens causes you to look in depth at the person's "parts" (e.g., cells, organs). The nursing paradigm views the person through a lens that focuses more broadly on the entire person and how they respond to isolated changes in their cells and organs. **Key Point: *Paradigms are not theories; they are just "how we see things."***

A **conceptual framework** (also referred to as a *theoretical framework*) is a set of concepts that are related to form a whole or pattern. As a rule, frameworks are not developed using research processes and have not been tested in practice. Frameworks and models are broader and more philosophical than theories. Don't be concerned if you can't tell the difference between a theory and a theoretical framework. Experts don't always agree, either. Many theorists, for example, classify the early nursing theories (e.g., those presented in this chapter) as conceptual frameworks; others classify them as theories.

A **model** is a symbolic representation of a framework or concepts—a diagram, graph, picture, drawing, or physical model. The plastic body parts you have seen in anatomy class are three-dimensional models of the real human body. Figure 4-1 is a graphic model of the relationships between nursing practice, theory, and research. Some models are more complex.

A **conceptual model** (often used interchangeably with *conceptual framework*) is a model that is expressed in language—the symbols are words. In one sense, all models are "conceptual" because they all represent ideas. The full-spectrum model (see Fig. 2-3) is a conceptual model or framework.

For now, it is enough for you to remember that:

1. **Key Point: *The terms theory, model, and framework all refer to a group of related concepts.***
2. *The terms differ in meaning, depending on the extent to which the set of concepts has been used and tested in practice and on the level of detail and organization of the concepts.*
3. *A theory has a higher level of research, detail, and organization of concepts compared to models and frameworks.*

KnowledgeCheck 4-2

- Name the five building blocks of a theory.
- How is a paradigm different from a theory?

How Are Theories Developed?

As you learned in Figure 4-1, a theorist begins a theory with an idea that seems worth exploring. Then evidence is collected to verify whether the ideas make sense. Validated ideas are used to develop the theory.

Theories are developed through a specific way of thinking called *logical reasoning* (Alligood, 2018). Generally, you can think of **reasoning** as connecting ideas in a way that makes sense. The purpose of **logical reasoning** is to develop an argument or statement based on evidence that will result in a logical conclusion. The most commonly used types of logical reasoning are inductive and deductive reasoning.

- **Inductive reasoning** is making an inference based on an observation. For example, if you walk into a patient's room and note that the patient's temperature is 101°F (38°C), pulse is 104 beats/min, and respiration rate is 20 breaths/min, you could reasonably *induce* (conclude) that the person is ill. **Key Point: *Induction moves from the specific to the general.*** You gathered separate pieces of information, recognized a pattern, and formed a generalization. Remember induction by thinking, "IN-duction: I have specific data 'out there,' and I bring the data 'IN' to make the generalization" (Fig. 4-3).

- **Deductive reasoning** is the opposite of inductive reasoning. It is making an inference based on widely accepted facts. Suppose you receive a call from the emergency department stating they will be receiving a new patient with acute pyelonephritis (kidney infection). Because you know what is involved in the general premise (pyelonephritis), you deduce that the patient will probably have a fever and back pain. **Key Point: *Deduction starts with a general premise and moves to a specific deduction. You have the "big picture" about what is true in general, and from that, you can figure out logically what is likely to be true for a particular individual.***

Understanding logical thinking, even on this basic level, will help you understand the thinking that goes into both nursing theory and nursing research.

ThinkLike a Nurse 4-1: Clinical Judgment in Action

- Your patient is grimacing, groaning, and holding their hands over their abdominal incision. You induce that the patient is having incision pain. How could you be sure your induction is factual (true)?
- Earlier, you deduced that your emergency department patient with pyelonephritis will have an elevated temperature and back pain. How confident are you that this is actually so? How could you be more certain your deduction is correct?

The preceding exercise should demonstrate that inductions and deductions are not facts or truth; rather, they point you in the direction to go in seeking truth (reality).

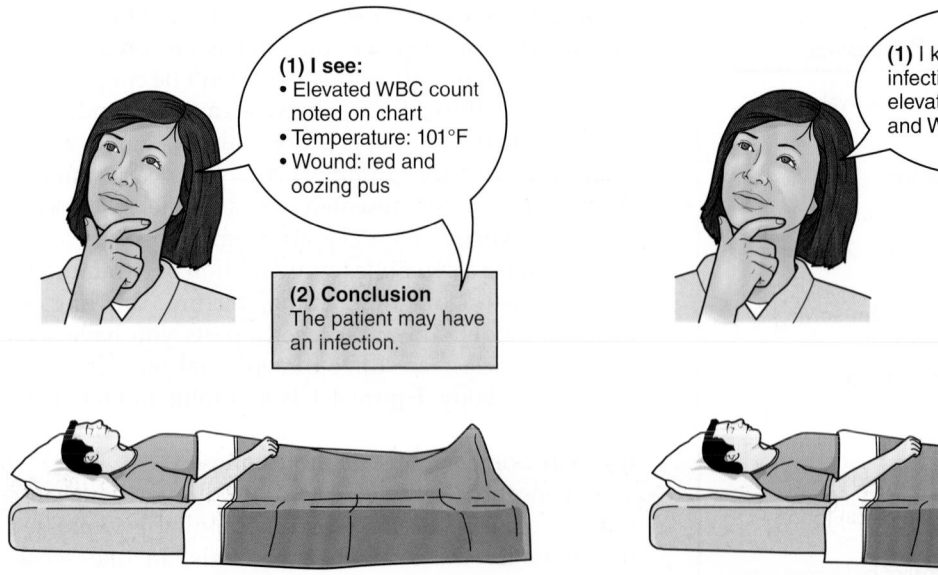

Inductive reasoning

(1) I see:
- Elevated WBC count noted on chart
- Temperature: 101°F
- Wound: red and oozing pus

(2) Conclusion
The patient may have an infection.

Deductive reasoning

(1) I know that infection causes elevated temperature and WBC count.

(2) This patient has a diagnosis of kidney infection.

(3) Conclusion
I will monitor his temperature and WBC count.

FIGURE 4-3 A comparison of inductive and deductive reasoning. Theorists and nurses use both types of reasoning in practice.

Induction and deduction allow you to make connections between ideas when you are developing a theory. The more information you have to support your conclusions, the more confident you can be that they are correct.

What Are the Essential Concepts of a *Nursing* Theory?

Any nursing theory should address four basic concepts: **person, environment, health,** and **nursing** (Yura & Torres, 1975). These concepts are said to represent phenomena of concern for nursing. Notice that this further divides the puzzle piece for nursing theory into four more pieces (Fig. 4-4).

A meaningful nursing theory defines those four puzzle pieces and explains how they are related to one another. Consider a theory that does not include the concept of person. Such a theory would not deal with the person's reaction to their health or lack of health. As a result, the person's learning needs, fears, family concerns, or discharge arrangements would not be considered. That sounds mechanistic, doesn't it?

Watson (1988) focused on the following basic concepts:

- *Caring* as it relates to the person, environment, health, and nursing.

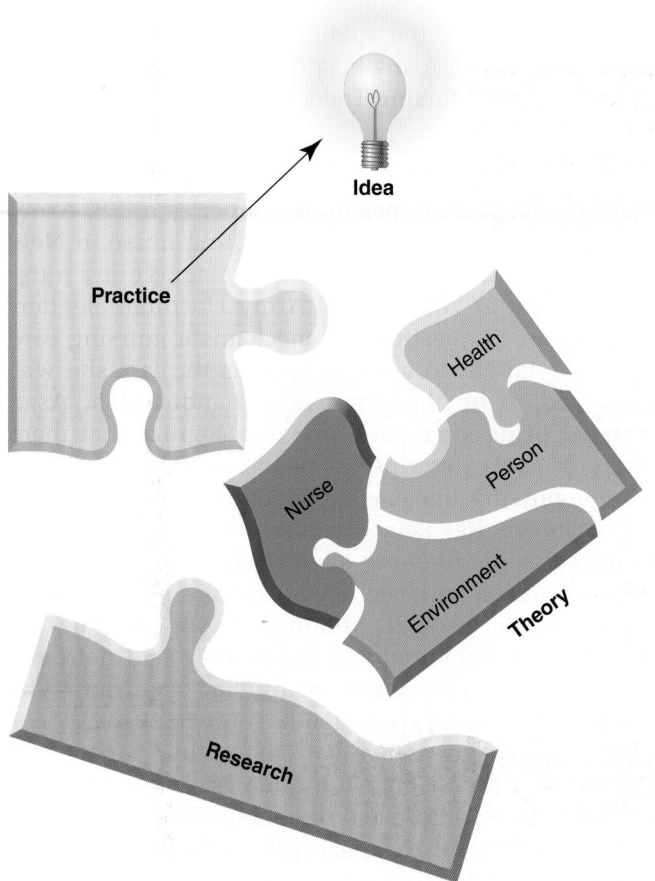

FIGURE 4-4 The four components of a nursing theory are person, nurse, health, and environment.

- The *person* and the *nurse*
- Transpersonal caring moments that exist between the nurse and person (patient)
  - ♥ **iCare** ▪ The *environment* as another way to show caring. For example, Watson described how keeping the patient's surroundings clean, colorful, or quiet or including whatever promotes health for the person is caring behavior.

All of the caring behaviors (see Box 4-1) listed in Watson's theory focus on improving the *health* of the person.

Observing nursing situations within the framework of the four components of nursing theory will help you understand the importance of each. This is very important because the finished puzzle reflects excellent (full-spectrum) nursing care.

▲ Think Like a Nurse 4-2: Clinical Judgment in Action

Think of an experience you have had in clinical. Perhaps it was taking vital signs or bathing a confused patient. Describe how each of the four components of a nursing theory occurred in your clinical situation. Share your thinking with a classmate or coworker.

- Who was the *person(s)* involved (*person* refers to the patient or resident or the family and support persons)?
- What was the *environment?* A community center? A bathing room in a skilled nursing facility? The person's bedside in a hospital?
- What was the *health* condition of the person? For example, was the person seeking information for self-care? Critical? In pain? Ready for discharge?
- How was *nursing* involved? For example, was the nurse compassionate? Angry? Efficient? A novice or an expert?

Knowledge Check 4-3

- What are the four essential concepts in a nursing theory?
- What is the title of Dr. Watson's theory?
- Caring processes are critical to Watson's theory. What is the purpose of the caring processes?

How Do Nurses Use Theories?

Nursing theories try to describe, explain, and predict human behavior. The case of Mr. Khatri (Meet Your Patient) shows how the use of a certain theory might guide the nurse to more compassionate care. Think of a theory as a lens. You can see the stars more clearly if you look at them through a telescope than you can by using binoculars. Theories offer a way of looking at nursing, and in this way, they affect your entire perspective. The theory you use influences what you look for, what you notice, what you perceive as a problem, what outcomes you hope to achieve, and what interventions you will choose.

In Nursing Practice

Nursing theories serve as a guide for assessment, problem identification, and nursing interventions. They help nurses communicate to others what it is that makes nurses unique and important to the interdisciplinary team.

Clinical practice theories very specifically guide what you do each day. They are limited in scope—that is, they do not attempt to explain all of nursing. A theory on human interaction can direct nurse–client communication; another theory provides a guide for teaching people how to be self-reliant. The following are other examples:

- **Nightingale's** theory emphasized the importance of the environment in the care of patients. Her work affected the design and building of hospitals for decades.
- **Dr. Imogene Rigdon** had an idea and developed a theory about bereavement in older women after studying how older women handled grief differently from men and younger women (Rigdon et al., 1987). Hospice organizations now use this theory to work with older women who have lost a significant other.
- **Nola Pender's** theory (Murdaugh et al., 2019) on health promotion (see Chapter 8) is the basis for most health-promotion teaching done by nurses.
- **Dr. Katharine Kolcaba** (1994) developed a theory of holistic comfort in nursing that provides a more holistic view than earlier theories of pain and anxiety.

In Nursing Education

The theories used to guide program and curriculum planning in schools of nursing are frequently grand theories, such as Watson's theory of caring or Rogers' science of unitary human beings.

- **Grand theory** covers broad areas of concern within a discipline. It is usually abstract and does not outline specific nursing interventions. Instead, it tends to deal with the relationships among nurse, person, health, and environment. Theories used to guide program and curriculum planning in schools of nursing are frequently grand theories, such as Watson's theory of caring or Rogers' science of unitary human beings.
- **Midrange (or practice) theory** is narrower and more specific and can be used to create nursing protocols and procedures and design educational programs. For instance, an in-service education director in a residential care facility may choose a midrange theory about comfort.
- **Practice theory** focuses on a particular situation, defining explicit goals and interventions to address the situation.

In Nursing Research

Researchers use theories and models as a framework for structuring a study. Theories provide a systematic way to define the questions to study, identify the variables to measure, and interpret the findings. For example, Kolcaba tested her statement that comfort interventions, as defined in her theory, would improve the health of the whole person.

Who Are Some Important Nurse Theorists?

As an educated nurse, you should have at least a basic understanding of the nurse theorists who have influenced nursing practice. The following three theorists, along with the caring theorists, are presented because of their historical significance. Their theories are simple and applicable to what you do every day as a nurse.

Florence Nightingale

As you learned in Chapter 1, Florence Nightingale, considered the "mother of modern nursing," transformed nursing. In the hospital in Scutari during the Crimean War, **Key Point:** *Nightingale's "idea" was that more soldiers would survive if they had a clean and healthy environment and nutritious food (so that the body could heal itself).* That may not seem remarkable to you, but consider that the germ theory of infectious disease had not yet been identified.

Nightingale is considered the first nurse-scientist. After establishing a theory supporting the relationship between humans and the environment and the influence on health, she postulated that a clean environment would improve the health of patients. Nightingale tested that theory through meticulous data collection and recording of observations and patients' responses to nursing action (Smith & Gullett, 2020). Because of her scientific approach, Nightingale dramatically reduced the death rate of the soldiers and changed the way the entire British Army hospital system was managed (Dossey, 1999; Nursing Theory, 2016).

Virginia Henderson

Virginia Henderson began her career as a U.S. Army nurse in 1918. She also was a visiting nurse in New York City and then a teacher of nursing. While a nursing student at Walter Reed Army Hospital, Henderson began to question the mechanistic nursing care she was taught to give, as well as the fact she was expected to be the physicians' handmaiden. As a teacher of nursing, she came to recognize that there were no clear descriptions of the purpose and function of nursing. She was the first nurse to identify that as a concern. **Key Point:** *Henderson's "idea" was that nurses deserve to know what it means to be a nurse.* She identified 14 basic needs that are addressed by nursing care (Box 4-2). Although the simple things on that list are commonplace today, they had not been identified as components of nursing care until Virginia Henderson did so. Henderson's (1966, p. 3) definition of nursing states that "the unique function of the nurse is to assist the individual, sick or well, in the performance of those activities contributing to health or its recovery (or to a peaceful death) that he would perform unaided if he had the necessary strength, will or knowledge. And do this in such a way as to help him gain independence as rapidly as possible."

BOX 4-2 ■ Virginia Henderson's List of Basic Needs

1. Breathe normally.
2. Eat and drink adequately.
3. Eliminate body waste.
4. Move and maintain desirable posture.
5. Sleep and rest.
6. Select suitable clothes—dress and undress.
7. Maintain body temperature within normal range by adjusting clothing and modifying the environment.
8. Keep the body clean and well groomed; protect the integument.
9. Avoid dangers in the environment and avoid injuring others.
10. Communicate with others in expressing emotions, needs, fears, or opinions.
11. Worship according to one's faith.
12. Work in such a way that there is a sense of accomplishment.
13. Play or participate in various forms of recreation.
14. Learn, discover, or satisfy the curiosity that leads to normal development and health and use of the available health facilities.

Source: Alligood, M. R. (2018). *Nursing theorists and their work* (9th ed.). Elsevier.

Through her work, Henderson defined nursing in the 20th century.

Hildegard Peplau

Hildegard E. Peplau was a psychiatric nurse from the early 20th century who influenced the advancement of standards in nursing education, promoted self-regulation in nursing through credentialing, and was a strong advocate for advanced nursing practice.

Key Point: *Dr. Peplau's idea was that health could be improved for psychiatric patients if there were a more effective way to communicate with them.* Again, you may feel this is an unnecessary theory because nurses communicate with patients all the time. But remember that in the early 1900s, talking to and developing a personal relationship with patients with psychiatric illnesses simply were not done. Patients with psychiatric issues did not have the benefit of psychotropic drugs, so they were often agitated and extremely difficult to communicate with.

Peplau's research showed that developing a relationship with patients with mental health issues does make their treatment more effective. She developed the theory of interpersonal relations that focuses on the relationship a nurse has with the patient. This theory that interpersonal communication can improve mental health is one that you use every day without even knowing about Peplau's psychodynamic theory.

The Caring Theorists

♥ **iCare** It could be argued that the three leading caring theorists in nursing are Dr. Jean Watson, Dr. Patricia Benner, and Dr. Madeleine Leininger. We have been using Watson's ideas to illustrate principles and concepts of theory. In this section, we discuss Benner and Leininger.

Patricia Benner

♥ **iCare** *Caring* is the central concept in Benner and Wrubel's *primacy of caring model*. **Key Point: *Their idea was that the nurse's caring helps the client cope.*** Moreover, it offers an opportunity for the nurse to connect with others and to receive as well as give help (Benner & Wrubel, 1989). Caring involves personal concern for persons, events, projects, and things. Therefore, it reveals what is stressful for a person (because if something does not matter to a person, it will not create stress) and provides motivation. Caring also makes the nurse notice which interventions are effective. This theory stresses that each person is unique, so caring is always specific and relational for each nurse–person encounter.

In Chapter 1, we discussed another of Benner's theories.

Key Point: *Benner's idea was to find out what makes an expert nurse. In this case, the idea took the form of a question.* For Benner, who was an intensive care unit (ICU) nurse, an example of an expert nurse was an ICU nurse who "knew" intuitively when it was time to intubate a critical patient. Benner wanted to know what makes a nurse expert enough to know that and other critical information. She therefore interviewed ICU nurses and, from her research, identified five stages of knowledge development and acquisition of nursing skills. As you may recall, the first level is that of a novice nurse (you). The others are advanced beginner, competent, proficient, and expert nurse (see Chapter 1 if you need to review).

Benner's theory meets the criteria of the four components of a theory, although some are emphasized more than others. Differences in emphasis are typical of theories.

- ***Person and nurse*** are clearly points of focus. Knowing the *nurse's* skill level (novice, advanced beginner, competent, proficient, or expert) provides a logical way to match the nurse's skill with the patient's (*person*) acuity. This is the basis of the theory.
- ***Health*** as a criterion is met because the nurse contributes to the person's *health* according to their skill level.
- ***Environment*** is clearly stated as the ICU.

Madeleine Leininger

Leininger is the founder of transcultural nursing and was the first nurse in the United States to earn a doctoral degree in cultural and social anthropology. Her theory focuses on caring as **cultural competence** (using knowledge of cultures and of nursing to provide culturally congruent and responsible care). Her approach to nursing care came from working with children from diverse cultures who were under her care in a psychiatric hospital: *Would psychotherapy for children be more effective if delivered within the framework of the child's culture?* (See Marriner-Tomey & Raile-Alligood, 2018.)

Leininger conducted qualitative research to confirm her idea that culturally competent care made a difference, and then she developed her theory. The theory includes all the puzzle pieces referred to throughout this chapter.

- **Person**—an individual with cultural beliefs that are specific to themselves and that may differ from the beliefs of others. All human beings can feel concern for others, but ways of caring vary across cultures.
- **Nurse**—the professional who values the cultural diversity of the person and is willing to make cultural accommodations for the health benefit of the person. This requires specialized cultural knowledge.
- **Environment**—wherever the *nurse* and the *person* are together in the healthcare system.
- **Health**—defined by the *person* and may be culturally specific in its definition.

You will learn more about Leininger's theory in Chapter 12. You may be thinking, "This is all about culture; what does that have to do with caring?" Leininger's theory brings together the cultures of the *person*, the *nurse*, and the *healthcare system* to improve healthcare delivery and its effectiveness.

A nurse tells this true culture-care story. It is an example of applying a theory directly to the needs of an ill person:

As a young nurse, I was caring for a patient who was a monk. He had just had surgery, and he would not take any pain medication. He wanted to "offer the pain up to God." This conflicted with my beliefs that the patient was jeopardizing his health, yet respected his right to live his cultural beliefs. We worked out a compromise. The monk agreed to take pain medication every 8 hours (instead of the prescribed every 3 to 4 hours), and I made sure to support his ambulation, hygiene, and other needs during the times the medication was in effect.

Other Selected Nurse Theorists

You will find a list of selected nurse theorists and a brief description of their theories in Table 4-1.

KnowledgeCheck 4-4

Define in a brief conceptual form or title the nursing theory of each of the following theorists:
- Florence Nightingale
- Virginia Henderson
- Hildegard Peplau

How Do Nurses Use Theories From Other Disciplines?

Theory development is relatively new in nursing. Except for Nightingale (1859/1992), it was not until the mid-1950s that nursing leaders began to publish their theories about nursing. The profession relied heavily on the theories of other disciplines (you may hear these referred to as "borrowed" theories). Nurses still use knowledge from other disciplines as a part of their scientific knowledge base. The following are a few of the many theories used by other disciplines that, nevertheless, apply to nursing.

Maslow's Hierarchy of Basic Human Needs

One classic theory still used in most nursing education and practice settings is Maslow's hierarchy of needs (1943). Maslow observed that certain human needs are common to all people, but some needs are more basic than others. **Key Point:** *The lower-level (e.g., physiological) needs must be met to some degree before the higher needs (e.g., self-esteem) can be achieved (Fig. 4-5).* For example, as a student, if you sit down to study but the room is cold, you will likely decide to put on a sweater or turn up the heat before you can start studying. Nevertheless, a person may consciously choose to ignore a lower-level need in order to achieve a higher need. For example, the first responders in Las Vegas after the mass shooting at a country music festival ignored their own need for safety and security to help others (transcendence of self). In daily life, most people are partially satisfied and partially unsatisfied at each level.

Key Point: *Everyone has a dominant need, but it varies among individuals.* For example, a teenager may have a self-esteem need to be accepted by a group. A tobacco addict needs to satisfy their cravings for nicotine and will be less concerned with the long-term effects on health. The following are the needs in Maslow's hierarchy:

- **Physiological needs**, the most basic, are those that must be met to maintain life. They include the needs for food, air, water, temperature regulation, elimination, rest, sex, and physical activity. Most healthy adults meet their physiological needs through self-care. However, many of your nursing interventions will support patients' physiological needs.
- **Safety needs** are the next priority. Safety needs may refer to either health, physical, emotional, or financial security needs.
  Health, defined as the physical, mental, and social well-being and not merely the absence of disease and infirmity," is necessary for feelings of safety (World Health Organization, 1958).
  Physical safety means protection from physical harm (e.g., falls, violence, infection, effects of medications) and having adequate shelter (e.g., housing with sanitation, heat) and economic security to meet basic needs.
  Emotional safety and security involve freedom from fear and anxiety—feeling safe in the physical environment as well as in relationships. We need the security of a home and family. In an abusive home, for example, the spouse will likely spend most of their time and energy trying not to trigger episodes of violence or abuse. This leaves little energy for

Table 4-1 ➤ Selected Nurse Theorists

CATEGORY	THEORIST	THEORY
Needs Theories Based on helping individuals to fulfill their physical and psychosocial needs	Faye G. Abdellah	Twenty-one **nursing problems;** deliver care to the whole person. Concepts of health are related to nursing problems and problem-solving.
	Virginia Henderson	Fourteen **basic needs** addressed by nursing care; definition of nursing; do for the patient what they cannot do for themselves.
	Dorothea Orem	The **self-care deficit nursing theory** explains what nursing care is required when people are not able to care for themselves. Goal is to help client attain total self-care.
Caring/Humanistic Theories Centered on the person and capacity for achieving health, growth, and self-actualization	Patricia Benner and J. Wrubel	Nursing practice is a **caring art** based on ethics. Caring helps the client cope with stressors of illness. The acquisition of nursing knowledge, skills, and intuition is progressive and gained through experience.
	Madeline M. Leininger	Considered the founder of **transcultural nursing.** Caring is universal and varies among cultures; must consider cultural values.
	Carl Rogers	A **person-centered model** of psychotherapy that recognizes each client as a unique individual.
	Jean Watson	Nursing is an **interpersonal process.** Caring promotes health and individual/family growth; involves accepting the person not only as they are now but what they may become.
Interaction/Interpersonal Theories Revolve around the relationships that nurses form with individuals and groups	Imogene King	**Theory of goal attainment** focuses on mutual goal setting between a nurse and patient and the process for meeting the goals. Nurse–client interactions can promote growth and development.
	Betty Neuman	Based on **general system theory** that reflects on the total person as an open system with physiological, psychological, sociocultural, spiritual, and developmental subsystems. Internal and external environment influence the system.
	Margaret Newman	Theory of health where nurses help patients recognize their own pattern of **interacting with the environment** and use the power from within to achieve higher level of self and health. Humans cannot be divided into parts.
	Hildegard E. Peplau	**Interpersonal communication** can improve mental health. Focus on the therapeutic relationship using communication and collaboration.
	Ernestine Wiedenbach	The purpose of nursing is to meet patients' **needs for help.**
Outcomes Theories Nurse as the change agent for promoting health and coping with illness	Dorothy Johnson	The **behavioral system model:** Incorporates five principles of systems thinking to establish a balance or equilibrium (adaptation) in the person. The patient is a behavioral system consisting of subsystems.
	Myra Levine	**Conservation model** is designed to promote adaptation of the person while maintaining wholeness, or health.
	Ida Jean Orlando	Nurses are in tune with **verbal and nonverbal expressions** to meet patient needs to alleviate distress. Nurses use the nursing process to improve patient outcomes.
	Rosemarie Rizzo Parse	**Theory of human becoming** focuses on the client's ability to reach their potential. Quality of life is central.
	Nola Pender	**Health belief model** focuses on promoting optimum health through disease prevention, identifying patient's risk for illness, and removing obstacles for patients to comply with plan for care.
	Martha Rogers	**Science of unitary human beings** focuses on the betterment of humankind through new and innovative modalities. Maintaining an environment free of negative energy is important.
	Sr. Callista Roy	**Adaptation model** was inspired by the strength and resiliency of children. The model relates to the choices people make as they adapt to illness and wellness.

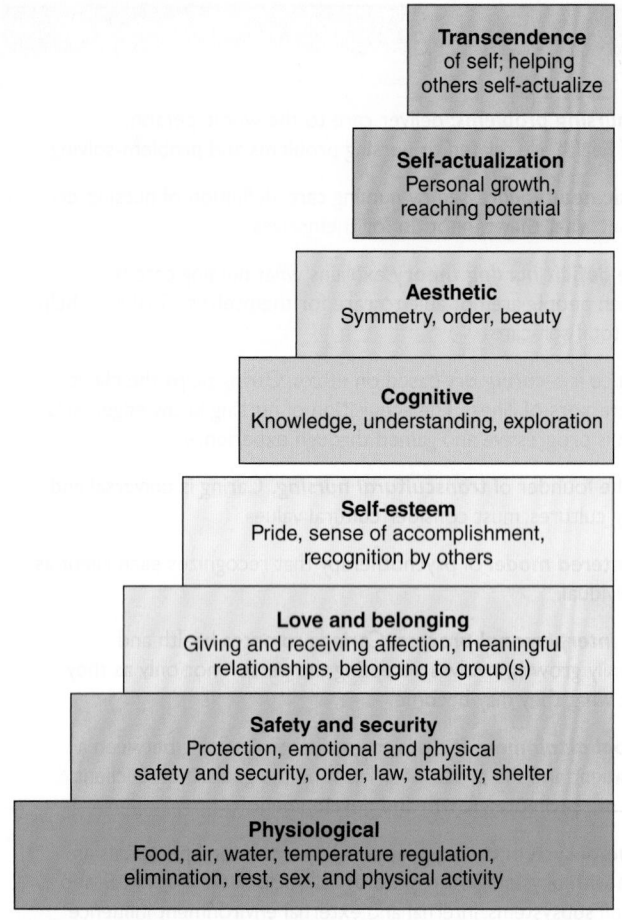

FIGURE 4-5 Maslow's hierarchy of human needs is a theory nurses use every day.

meeting their own needs and establishing healthy self-esteem.

Financial security refers to having income or other resources to support the basic needs of self and dependents. The inadequacy of financial income leads to vulnerability and threatens well-being.

- **Love and Belonging Needs.** People have a basic need to love and be loved, give and receive affection, and have a feeling of belonging (e.g., in a family, peer group, or community). Friendship, intimacy, trust, and acceptance are key to fulfilling social or affiliation needs. When these needs are not met, a person may feel isolated and lonely and may withdraw or become demanding and critical. The person attempting to meet needs for love and belonging will strive to establish meaningful relationships with others.

- **Self-Esteem Needs.** Self-esteem reflects a person's overall sense of their value or worth. The state is a result of a sense of accomplishment and recognition from others (prestige) and yields confidence and independence. As we discuss in Chapter 9, illness can affect self-esteem by causing role changes (e.g., inability to perform one's job) or a change in body image (e.g., loss of a body part or rapid weight gain). When recognition cannot be obtained through positive behaviors, the person may resort to disruptive or irresponsible actions.

- **Self-Actualization Needs.** The highest level on Maslow's original hierarchy, *self-actualization* refers to the need to reach your full potential and to act unselfishly. At this level, a person develops wisdom and knows what to do in a variety of situations. In his later work, Maslow identified two growth needs that must be met before reaching self-actualization (Maslow & Lowery, 1998):
  Cognitive needs to know, understand, and explore
  Aesthetic needs for symmetry, order, and beauty

- **Transcendence of Self.** Later research led Maslow to identify another, even higher need (Maslow, 1971): the need for *transcendence of self.* This is the drive to connect to something beyond oneself and to help others realize their potential. Some people include spirituality at this level, which is also the basis for acts of self-sacrifice (e.g., donating a kidney so that another person can live).

- **Applying Maslow's Theory.** The following example illustrates how you might use Maslow's theory when teaching patients. Suppose you are assigned to teach your patient about how to care for a colostomy before discharge. Because the patient speaks little English, you obtain materials in their primary language and arrange for an interpreter in case they have some questions you can't understand or answer. As you enter the room to begin teaching, you observe that they appear to be in a great deal of pain. What will you do?

Maslow's hierarchy of needs tells you that until the pain (a physiological need) is controlled, your patient cannot learn. (Maslow considered the pursuit of knowledge a self-actualization need.) You arrange for pain medication to be administered and reschedule the teaching session. If you had gone ahead with the patient education, the experience would be for the sole purpose of crossing it off your list (remember mechanistic nursing?) rather than effective teaching.

Validation Theory

Validation theory (Feil, 2015) arises from social work and provides a way to communicate with older people with dementia. The theory asks the caregiver to *go where the person with confusion is in their own mind.* For example, Mr. Khatri (Meet Your Patient) is talking about his mother, who died many years ago. Learning of his mother's death would be a traumatic experience. So instead of telling him that she is gone, you would *go where Mr. Khatri is in his own mind* by asking him, for example, about the color of his mother's eyes, what songs she sings to him, or other personal questions that will likely stimulate meaningful conversation and positive memories about his mother.

Stress and Adaptation Theory

Hans Selye (1993) developed the stress and adaptation theory. His was the forerunner of the many existing theories about stress. Selye's theory states that a certain amount of stress is good for people; it keeps them motivated and alert. However, too much stress, called *distress,* results in physiological symptoms and eventual illness. Does that happen to you at the end of the semester when you are distressed over the number of papers due and the difficulty of the tests for which you are studying? Generally, the human body will respond to distress with an illness, such as a cold, that will force the body to slow down or simply go to bed. Selye's theory is discussed more in Chapters 8 and 9.

Developmental Theories

Developmental theories look at stages through which individuals, groups, families, and communities progress over time. The following are some important examples:

- Erickson's psychosocial developmental theory (discussed in Chapter 6)
- Theories of family development (discussed in Chapter 11)
- Kohlberg's and Gilligan's theories of moral development (discussed in Chapters 5 and 6)

These theories are useful in nursing practice because they identify norms and expectations at various stages of development and help you identify actions that are appropriate for your client.

System Theory

Ludwig von Bertalanffy created system theory in the 1940s (von Bertalanffy, 1976). He intended it to be abstract enough to use for theory and research in any discipline. Today, the understanding of systems has evolved to the point that many of the concepts are a part of our everyday language (e.g., healthcare system, body systems, information systems, family systems).

Key Point: *One of the premises of systems theory is that all complex phenomena, regardless of their type, have some principles, laws, and organization in common.* A **system** is made up of separate components (or **subsystems**), which constantly interact with one another and with other systems. For example, the cardiovascular and renal systems are subsystems of the body; the cells are subsystems of those systems. Those systems and subsystems exchange processes and information with one another and with systems outside the body.

A system maintains some organization even though it is constantly facing internal and external changes. All systems have some common elements. For example, the **goal** (purpose) of any system is to process **input** (the energy, information, or materials that enter the system) for use within the system or in the **environment** (everything outside the system) or both. Other common elements include the following:

- **Throughput** consists of the processes the system uses to convert input (raw materials) into output (products). Examples of throughput are thinking, planning, sorting, meeting in groups, sterilizing, hammering, and cutting.

- **Output** is the product or service that results from the system's throughput. Examples of output are documents, money, cars, and nursing diagnoses.
- **Feedback** is information about some aspect of the processing that is used to monitor the system and make its performance more effective (e.g., evaluation in the nursing process: how the patient responded to nursing actions).
- **Open systems** exchange information and energy freely with the environment. Open systems are capable of growth, development, and adaptation. Examples of open systems include people, body systems, hospitals, and businesses.
- **Closed systems** have fixed, automatic relationships among their components and little give-and-take with the environment. One example is a rock. A nursing example is a family that is isolated from the community and resists outside influences.

Several nursing theories have been built on system theory, for example, Johnson's (1968, 1980) behavioral system model, King's (1971) interacting systems framework and King's theory of goal attainment (1981, 1997, 2001), the Neuman systems model (Neuman & Young, 1972), Roy's adaptation model (1976), and Orem's self-care theory (1971).

KnowledgeCheck 4-5

- Name four theories that nurses "borrow" from other disciplines.
- What are the five original levels of Maslow's basic human needs (not including cognitive needs, aesthetic needs, and transcendence)?

PracticalKnowledge
knowing **how**

Practical knowledge about theory means using theories to guide you in your use of the nursing process. Recall the lens metaphor.

- **Assessment**. In this step of the nursing process, you apply nursing theory to the clinical judgment process. When *recognizing cues* about your client's condition, your theory, concepts, and principles tell you what to assess and provide the rationale for the assessments. The theory's major concepts serve as categories for organizing the data.
- **Diagnosis.** Nursing theory combined with clinical judgment guides you in defining client problems by *clustering your client's clinical cues and analyzing* them. You then form your hypotheses about your client's condition and prioritize them for developing nursing actions for client conditions.
- **Outcomes and Interventions**. After generating appropriate, achievable client outcomes, you *take action* to deliver safe and effective client care.

To show you how, this section applies caring theory to the planning of nursing interventions. Of course, you can use *any* theory for this purpose. We use caring theory because of the powerful and positive impact it can have on your nursing care. In reading this chapter, you should have become familiar with two well-known caring theories. Test your recall by writing the theorists' names and basic ideas. If you have difficulty, be sure to review the information about caring theorists before proceeding.

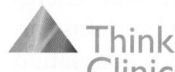

ThinkLike a Nurse 4-3:
Clinical Judgment in Action

Write a paragraph describing a clinical experience in which you applied or observed one or both of the caring theories. Record your thinking on a piece of paper and be prepared to share it with your classmates. You may title it "My Experience in Caring."

Planning Theory-Based Interventions/ Implementation

The Nursing Interventions Classification, or NIC (Butcher, 2018), introduced in Chapter 3, is theory development in an early stage. Each of the standardized intervention labels (e.g., Exercise Promotion, Infection Control) is a concept, and defining or describing concepts is an important step in theory development.

♥ **iCare** In this section, we use nine key concepts of Watson's caring theory to describe how a theory might influence your choice of nursing activities and approaches.

1. **Holistic Nursing Care.** Nurses assess the complete person and their context when making healthcare decisions. This goes beyond just giving the medication or dressing a wound. Physical care is important, but try to see nursing as providing person-centered care and all that this entails (e.g., fears, cultural beliefs, loved ones).
2. **Honoring Personhood.** Caring theorists believe patients deserve to be honored for their individuality in behavior as well as needs. If you accept that belief, you will learn the names of the people in your care and what makes them unique individuals. Refer to them by name instead of "Room 331" or "the kidney infection down the hall." Honoring personhood requires you to control the fast pace of nursing and take time with your patients. You need to look at, talk to, and touch the person to understand their personhood.
3. **Transpersonal Caring Moments.** The concept of transpersonal caring is a moral ideal rather than a task-oriented behavior. Such moments occur when an actual caring occasion or caring relationship exists between the nurse and the person. This can be a challenge! The current healthcare environment moves people rapidly through the system. Challenge yourself to find the time to develop authentic caring relationships. The first step is to make a commitment to be a caring nurse: to go to work with the thought, "Today I will be authentic [genuine, real] with the people in my care." Or you might think, "I will focus on creating a caring environment instead of rushed and harried interactions." As a student, you might think, "Today I will practice changing dressings or starting intravenous solutions." However, developing the ability to have transpersonal caring moments is just as important. Think back to Mr. Khatri (Meet Your Patient at the beginning of the chapter). Where did opportunities arise for transpersonal caring moments with him?

4. **Personal Presence.** Another phrase for being authentic and in the moment is *personal presence*. The concept of presence suggests that you, the nurse, are emotionally and physically *with* the person for the time you are there. You are not thinking about a medication you need to give or nursing actions you need to perform. If the patient in the bed is fearful, you should be fully present, recognize the fear, and support the person experiencing it. Your support may take the form of answering simple questions or providing more in-depth education. It may simply be staying with your patients for a few minutes while quietly listening. As your psychomotor and nursing process skills become second nature to you, you will find it easier to remain in the moment.
5. **Comfort.** Some nurses think of comfort as the relief of pain, but it is much more. In Kolcaba's (1994) theory, comfort occurs in four contexts: physical, psychospiritual, social, and environmental. For example, is the person comfortable with you as the caregiver? Some women may be uncomfortable with male nurses as their caregivers. You must know and respect the person's cultural values. Other aspects to consider for a complex picture of comfort are whether
   - The patient's modesty is being respected.
   - There is the right amount of environmental stimuli.
   - The room temperature is not too cold nor too warm.
   - The patient needs more rest periods in order to heal.
   - The patient needs someone to spend a transpersonal caring moment with them so that they can express fears and anxiety.
6. **Listening.** Active listening requires you to quiet your mind and truly listen with your mind and heart. The caring theorists also talk about listening from within yourself. Some call that *intuition*. Benner believes it is intuition that allows nurses to advance to expert-level practice.
7. **Spiritual Care.** Spiritual care is a critical aspect of holistic nursing care. You need to know what an individual's spiritual needs are and make appropriate plans to meet them. If the person does not want to talk about or deal with their spirituality, you will listen and follow their instructions. However, the opposite is generally true. People who are ill often want to talk about their spiritual needs, but they may be uncomfortable doing so. Helping someone to meet spiritual needs may be as simple as offering to call a clergy member or praying with the person who is sick. Chapter 13 provides more information about spiritual care.
9. **Caring for the Family.** Nurses who base their practice on caring theories recognize the importance of including the family of the person who is receiving care, regardless of family structure, age, race, culture, religion, health status, socioeconomic status, personality, and other individual factors. You will find more information about family care in Chapter 11.
10. **Cultural Competence.** This was discussed in the explanation of Leininger's cultural care theory. Also see Chapter 12 if you want more information.

Do you see the value of each of these nine abstract concepts? From them flow very real, concrete nursing actions that make a difference in the lives of patients. Understanding nursing theories and applying them throughout your career is essential to full-spectrum nursing care. To perform the essential clinical tasks of nursing within the framework of caring is the highest possible performance of the profession.

KnowledgeCheck 4-6

List and explain three ways to incorporate caring theory into your nursing care.

NURSING RESEARCH

You now have a good beginning (novice) grasp of the concepts in nursing theory. Remember the puzzle pieces (see Fig. 4-3)? A nurse has an idea, does research to determine whether the idea is a valid one, and then develops a nursing theory. It is now time to study the research piece of the puzzle.

TheoreticalKnowledge knowingwhy

Were you aware of the research done in the field of caring before reading this chapter? Most novice nurses would not be. Remember the Framingham studies, which changed medical and nursing practice? Had you heard of that before you read about it in this book? Many people, including some nurses, do not realize that nurses do research. They think of nurses primarily as healthcare providers who work in hospitals, wear scrubs, and carry a stethoscope. To be an effective professional nurse in the 21st century, you need to understand the basic principles of nursing research and their powerful impact on healthcare and the nursing profession. This section of the chapter is designed to show you what research is and how to incorporate it into your practice.

Definition of Nursing Research Although there are many definitions of nursing research, this chapter defines **nursing research** as the systematic, objective process of analyzing phenomena of importance to nursing (Nieswiadomy, 2012). Its purpose is to develop knowledge about issues that are important in nursing. Nursing research encompasses all clinical practice, nursing education, and nursing administration.

Evidence-Based Practice Example Nurse researchers are currently making important contributions to the evidence-based practice necessary for professional nursing. Consider this example: When you are in the clinical setting, you will notice that when a nurse discontinues an IV fluid infusion, they sometimes replace it with a lock to maintain a route for IV medications, even though the patient no longer needs the fluids. Not many years ago, the nurse would periodically flush the plug with heparin to keep blood from clotting and blocking the IV catheter. But heparin is a drug, and it has side effects. Nurses and other professionals performed several studies to see whether saline (which has no side effects) would work just as well. Goode and colleagues

(1996) performed a meta-analysis of those studies showing that saline was indeed just as effective, and it is now the standard of care in most institutions. (A **meta-analysis** combines and analyzes the data from several different studies.)

Why Should I Learn About Research?

The best reason for learning about research, of course, is that the ability to read and use nursing research enhances your ability to give quality patient care. Like theory, research affects you every day you are a nurse. Full-spectrum nurses participate in research by doing the following:

- Identifying ideas that should be examined through the research process
- Designing a qualitative or quantitative research study, collecting data, analyzing research findings
- Applying research findings to clinical practice

ANA Standards

The position of the American Nurses Association (ANA) is that all nurses share a commitment to the advancement and ethical conduct of nursing science (ANA, 2021). The registered nurse integrates evidence and research findings into practice. Competencies of the ANA Standards of Professional Performance, Standard 13, Evidence-Based Practice and Research, include the following:

- "Identifies questions in the healthcare setting and practice that can be answered by nursing research.
- Promotes ethical principles of research in practice and the healthcare setting.
- Uses current evidence-based nursing knowledge, including research findings, to guide practice decisions.
- Incorporates evidence when initiating changes in nursing practice.
- Participates in the formulation of evidence-based practice through research.
- Shares peer-reviewed research findings with colleagues to integrate into nursing practice" (ANA, 2021, p. 77).

Educational Competencies

QSEN Recall that the Quality and Safety Education for Nurses (QSEN) project has identified quality and safety competencies for nurses. One important competency is evidence-based practice: the ability to "integrate the best current evidence with clinical expertise and patient/family preferences and values for delivery of optimal healthcare" (Cronenwett, Sherwood, Barnsteiner, et al., 2007, pp. 122–131).

Institute of Medicine The National Academy of Medicine (NAM) core competencies for health providers are the basis for the Safe, Effective Nursing

Care (SENC) competencies used in this text. See Chapter 1. The competencies related to research include the following:

NAM—Employ evidence-based practice.
SENC—Validate evidence-based research to incorporate in practice:
- Incorporate evidence-based findings into client care.
- Evaluate client outcomes using valid and reliable research tools.

What Is the History of Nursing Research?

The records Florence Nightingale kept while nursing soldiers in the Crimean War were the beginning of formalized nursing research. As she developed schools of nursing throughout Britain and the United States, Nightingale urged her students to conduct clinical research. Yet because she had passed on to them the authoritarian tradition of her time, they were usually not prepared to perform it. Authority-style education does not promote intellectual inquiry or critical thinking, two characteristics essential for research. This is one reason nursing research was slow to develop, although this is rapidly changing now as a result of nursing's professional commitment to evidence-based practice.

Nursing research is supported by federal funds and private grants, and the results are reported in a growing number of nursing (and other) research journals. Nurses present their research at national and international conferences and publish their results in national and international journals. The preparation of doctoral-level nurses with a strong background in research has enhanced the quality and diversity of nursing research.

How Are Priorities for Nursing Research Developed?

Nursing research provides evidence on which to base nursing care. Ideally, all nursing interventions should be validated through research to show their safety and effectiveness. Professional organizations, such as the ANA and specialty organizations (e.g., the Oncology Nursing Society), have established research priorities that will assist nursing in building a strong knowledge base in areas of importance to society. The National Institute of Nursing Research (NINR), a federally funded agency that is a part of the National Institutes of Health (NIH), periodically identifies research themes and priorities for funding, including:

1. **Wellness**—promoting health and preventing illness
2. **Self-management**—improving quality of life for individuals with chronic conditions
3. **End-of-life and palliative care**—the science of compassion
4. **Promotion of innovation**—technology to improve health (NINR, 2016)

KnowledgeCheck 4-7
- Define *nursing research*.
- According to the text, why has nursing research been slow to develop?

What Educational Preparation Does a Researcher Need?

At each level of educational preparation, nurses function in different roles in the research process.

Associate Degree and Diploma Nursing At this educational level, there are four basic research roles for Associate's degree and diploma nurses to fulfill:

- Being aware of the importance of research to evidence-based practice.
- Identifying problem areas in clinical care.
- Assisting with the collection of data with a more experienced nurse researcher.
- Implementing evidence-based practice when planning nursing actions.

Baccalaureate Degree in Nursing If you are a baccalaureate-educated nurse, you should be able to:

- Critique research for application to clinical practice.
- Identify nursing research problems and participate in the planning and implementation of research studies.
- Apply research findings to establish sound, evidence-based clinical practice.

Master's Degree in Nursing Nurses with graduate degrees should be able to:

- Identify and analyze problems so that appropriately designed research can be used to solve the problem.
- Through clinical expertise, apply evidence-based practice to nursing care situations.
- Provide support to ongoing research projects.
- Plan and conduct research for the purpose of assuring quality nursing care.

Doctoral Degree in Nursing or Related Field Doctoral prepared nurses are specifically educated to be nurse researchers. They are qualified to:

- Plan and conduct nursing research.
- Serve as leaders in applying research results to the clinical arena.
- Develop ways to monitor the quality of nursing care being administered by nurses (adapted from ANA, 1981).
- Disseminate their research findings via publications and conferences.

PracticalKnowledge
knowing **how**

No one expects you to have an in-depth understanding of the research process at this point in your nursing career. However, you do need some basic practical knowledge, including information about the scientific method, types of research designs, the research process, how to find practice-related research articles, how to identify researchable problems, and how to critique research reports.

How Do We Gain Knowledge?

Recall that in Chapter 2, you learned about the different kinds of nursing knowledge: theoretical, practical, ethical, and self-knowledge. There are also various ways to *acquire* knowledge.

Trial and Error Plus Common Sense Suppose a patient has been medicated but is still in pain. You might try repositioning the patient. If that doesn't help, you might try distraction, visualization techniques, and perhaps various other measures. If visualization provides some relief, you would likely try that technique first when a similar situation occurs with another patient.

Authority and Tradition This means relying on an expert or doing what has always been done. For the patient with unrelieved pain, this would mean you might ask a more experienced nurse what to do. Or you could consult a procedure manual.

Intuition and Inspiration Intuition is a feeling about something—an inner sense. Nurses say, "I just had a feeling something was wrong with the patient, but I can't explain why." For the patient in pain, you might have a feeling that a complication is developing, that the pain is due to more than just ineffective pain medication. However, as a novice, you should always check with a more experienced nurse before acting on your intuition.

Logical Reasoning Using your knowledge and the facts available, you form conclusions (refer to the section How Are Theories Developed?). For the patient in pain, you might think, "My patient has class 3 obesity [body mass index (BMI) 42], yet I administered only the standard dose of analgesic medication. Likely they need a higher dose to achieve relief."

Scientific Method Research uses the scientific method (or scientific inquiry). The **scientific method** is the process in which the researcher, through use of the senses, systematically collects observable, verifiable data to describe, explain, or predict events. The goals of scientific inquiry are to find solutions to problems and to develop explanations (theories). The scientific method has two unique characteristics that the other ways of gaining knowledge do not:

Objectivity, or self-correction. This means the researcher uses techniques to keep their personal beliefs, values, and attitudes separate from the research process.

The use of empirical data. Researchers use their senses to gather empirical data *through* observation. They attempt to verify the information gathered through a variety of methods so that the research conclusions are based on objective data rather than on the researcher's personal beliefs, biases, or opinions.

Box 4-3 summarizes the characteristics of the scientific method.

What Are Two Approaches to Research?

The scientific method makes use of a variety of procedures and study designs intended to help ensure that the data collected will be reliable, relevant, and unbiased. You should recognize the two major categories of research design: *quantitative* and *qualitative*. Each category has within it several specific types of research methodologies; however, for now, you need to understand only the basic differences (Table 4-2).

Quantitative Research

Key Point: *The main purpose of* **quantitative research** *is to gather data from enough* **subjects** *(people being studied), using sound sampling methods, to be able to generalize the results to a similar* **population.** **Generalizing results** means that you think, "What I found to be so for this sample group of people will probably be the same for all people who are similar" (e.g., "My findings for this group of women over age 60 in the United States will probably be useful for *all* women over age 60 in the United States"). In quantitative research, researchers carefully control data collection and are careful to maintain the objectivity of the process.

Quantitative data are reported as numbers, for example, weight in kilograms, length in centimeters, or temperature in Fahrenheit degrees. Quantitative data can also be measured in categories, such as race, gender, or selection of a particular answer on a test. Tools for collecting quantitative data include surveys and **closed-ended questionnaires** (selection from specified choices), rating scales, standardized tests, checklists, and biophysical measures. Statistical procedures (e.g., chi-square or regression analyses) analyze quantitative data. The Framingham studies are a classic example of

---

BOX 4-3 ■ Characteristics of the Scientific Method

Begins with an identified problem or need to be studied

Uses theories, models, and conceptual themes that have been empirically tested

Involves systematic, orderly methods to acquire empirical evidence to test theories

Uses methods of control for ruling out other variables that might affect the relationships among the variables they are studying

Avoids explanations that cannot be empirically tested

Prefers to generalize the findings (knowledge) so that they can be applied in cases other than those in the study

Uses built-in mechanisms for self-correction

Source: Adapted from Wilson, H. S. (1992). *Introducing research in nursing* (2nd ed.). Addison-Wesley Nursing.

Table 4-2 ➤ Comparison of Quantitative and Qualitative Research

	QUANTITATIVE RESEARCH	QUALITATIVE RESEARCH
Data	Numerical data, such as questionnaires, number of incidents, or reactions to a medication	Nonnumerical data; data may consist of words from interviews, observations, written documents, and even art or photos
Persons studied	Large numbers of *subjects* so that results can be generalized to other similar populations	Often uses small numbers of *participants;* is not designed with the intent to generalize
Hypothesis	Has a hypothesis	No hypothesis because it is the research of the "lived experience" of the person or persons being studied; study may be guided by research questions
Environment	Can be a laboratory setting; needs to be a controlled environment	Is often done in a "natural" setting (i.e., the person's home or work site)
Analysis	Objective data, tested with statistical methods	Subjective data; identify themes; sometimes converted to numerical data (e.g., by counting categories)

a quantitative study—actually of several quantitative studies.

Another example of **quantitative** nursing research is the Conduct and Utilization of Research in Nursing (CURN) project, which was intended to increase the use of research by direct-care nurses (Horsley et al., 1983). Many of the protocols (procedures) developed from these studies are currently used with some modifications. The following are some CURN protocol examples:

Clean intermittent catheterization
Intravenous cannula change
Distress reduction through sensory preparation
Preventing decubitus ulcers

Qualitative Research

Key Point: *The purpose of qualitative research is not to generalize the data but to share specific experiences of those involved in the study.* Qualitative research is conducted to gain an understanding of a phenomenon or concept or to explain behavior, perceptions, or ideas. This is generally done with interviews; focus groups; journals; observations; and discussions through audio, video, and Internet formats. Interviews may be highly structured, guided by **open-ended questions** (descriptive answers to questions), or less structured, using a conversational style (Bengtsson, 2016).

The Nun Study, a long-term, multidisciplinary project, was designed to study aging and disability caused by Alzheimer disease. Qualitative data included interviews with Catholic nuns, 75 to 102 years old, in a convent in Minnesota. Researchers also examined samples of writing from the nuns' diaries, reports, and letters.

KnowledgeCheck 4-8

- Define *quantitative research.*
- Define *qualitative research.*

What Are the Phases of the Research Process?

At the novice level, you will be reading and applying evidence-based findings to your clinical practice even though you are not yet conducting original research. But to implement the research, you should understand the steps for conducting valid, reliable research. The research process is a problem-solving process, similar to but not the same as the nursing process. In general, the steps include the following five phases:

1. Select and define the problem.
2. Select a research design.
3. Collect data.
4. Analyze data.
5. Use the research findings.

ThinkLike a Nurse 4-4: Clinical Judgment in Action

Take 10 minutes to sit quietly and think about nursing research. Do you have an idea or a patient problem you would like to see investigated with a research project? Is there a nursing procedure that could be performed more effectively or efficiently? Record your thoughts and share them with your instructor and other students.

- What would you like to have more information about in nursing? Explain why it is a problem or what brought about your idea.
- If you were the research assistant on a nursing research project on your topic, what one-sentence problem statement would you write regarding your research idea?
- What is the purpose of doing this research project? Why should it be done?

You may struggle with this assignment and wonder about its value to you, yet one of the most important things that nurses do is identify problems. Here is your chance to practice.

What Are the Rights of Research Participants?

Key Point: *Every nurse has a moral and legal responsibility to protect research participants from being harmed during the research process.* Although research is crucial to the development of the profession, it should never be held in higher regard than the rights of the individuals being studied. The U.S. government, through the Department of Health and Human Services (USDHHS), has a complex set of standards that all researchers must follow.

Informed Consent

As a rule, **informed consent** must be obtained from every participant in a study. Consent is obtained by discussing what is expected of the participant, providing written information about the project to the participant, providing ample opportunity for questions, and obtaining the participant's written consent to be a subject. **Key Point:** *Most importantly, any and every potential subject has the right to refuse participation without consequences of any kind.*

The following critical concepts are part of the informed consent:

- **Right to not be harmed**. The information given to the participant outlines the safety protocols of the study. If preliminary data indicate potential harm to the participant, the study must be stopped immediately.
- **Right to full disclosure.** Participants have a right to answers to such questions as, What is the purpose of this research? What risks are there? Are there any benefits? Would I be paid? What happens if I get sick or feel worse? Whom do I contact with questions and concerns? What is involved with participation or the procedures that will be implemented? Are there alternatives to participation?
- **Right to self-determination**. This refers to the right to say no. At any time in a study, the participant has the right to stop participating, for any reason.
- **Rights of privacy and confidentiality**. All research participants have the right to have their identity protected. Generally, they are assigned a participant identifier rather than being referred to by name. Once the study is completed and the data are analyzed, the researcher is responsible for protecting the raw data (such as questionnaires and interviews).

A written consent serves as documentation of the subject's agreement to participate in the study. The investigator, subject, and witness will sign the consent form. The subject's signature indicates they understand the requirements and consent to participation. A copy of the signed consent is provided to the subject to use as reference for the terms of the participation. The investigator's signature indicates the subject meets all study inclusion criteria and has provided complete and informed consent.

Institutional Review Boards

The mechanism for overseeing the ethical standards established by the USDHHS is the institutional review board (IRB). Every federally funded hospital, university, or other healthcare facility has an IRB. It consists of healthcare professionals and people from the community who are willing to review and critique research proposals. The two main responsibilities of the IRB are to (1) protect the research participants from harm and (2) ensure that the research is of value.

KnowledgeCheck 4-9

- List the phases of the research process.
- List four critical concepts that make up informed consent.

How Can I Base My Practice on the Best Evidence?

Experts and professional groups evaluate the quality of the research reports and translate them into guidelines for practice. In your own evidence-based practice, you should use research findings and practice guidelines when they are available. When they are not, you will need to rely on the research reports themselves. Similar to the phases of research, the following steps should assist you in finding the best evidence for your own nursing action.

Identify a Clinical Nursing Problem

Even as a novice nurse, you should be prepared to identify clinical problems for research by being alert and interested in what you are doing each day in your clinical setting. How do you think the temporal thermometer came into clinical use? Someone became frustrated with the discomfort patients experienced when temperatures were taken rectally. At the same time, there was a great deal of concern over the inaccuracy of axillary temperatures. Someone noticed the problem and wondered, "Is there a better way to do this?"

Common sources of clinical problems are experience, social issues, theories, ideas from others, and the nursing literature (Polit & Beck, 2021). Most of these sources are relevant whether you are identifying a problem for a research study or doing a literature search.

Experience As you go about your work, you will notice interventions that require a great deal of effort for the minimal good they do. You will wonder, "How could we do this better?" Or you may notice that outcomes for clients with a particular health problem are often not good. You will wonder, "How could we improve the care so that the patient's health improves?" Another question might be, "Why do we do this procedure this way?" If you are curious about why things are done and about what might happen if changes were made, you will find plenty of problems—for example, problems in staffing, equipment, nursing interventions, or coordination among health professionals.

Social Issues You may be concerned about broader social issues that affect or require nursing care, such as issues of gender equity, sexual harassment, and domestic violence. You may be concerned about patients who do not have access to healthcare or about the health problems of a particular group or subculture.

Theories Recall that theories must be tested in order to be useful in nursing practice. You might want to suggest research to test a theory in which you are interested. If the theory is accurate, what behaviors would you expect to find, or what evidence would you need to support the theory?

Ideas from Others Your instructor may suggest a topic to research, or perhaps you might brainstorm with nurses or other students about a better way to provide care to your patients. Agencies and organizations that fund research often ask for proposals on certain topics (e.g., the American Nurses Association and the National Institute of Nursing Research).

Nursing Literature You may identify clinical problems by reading articles and research reports in nursing journals.

- An article may stimulate your thoughts and interest in a topic.
- You may notice a discrepancy in what staff nurses are doing and what is supported in scientific research articles and authority source guidelines.
- You may detect inconsistencies in the findings of two different studies on the same topic.
- You may read a study on a topic of interest to you (e.g., a technique for measuring blood pressure) and wonder whether the results would be the same if the study had been done in a different setting (e.g., a clinic instead of a hospital) or with a different population (e.g., healthy instead of ill people).

Formulate a Searchable Question

When you have found a topic of interest, the next step is to state it in such a way that you can find it in the vast amount of nursing literature that is published. Stated too broadly, the search may yield an excess of irrelevant results. Stated too narrowly, you may get limited results that fail to address your topic of interest. Using the acronym PICOT enables you to search efficiently by asking focused questions. The acronym stands for

Patient or problem
Intervention
Comparison interventions
Outcomes
Time

You may not always need a comparison intervention (C) or a time (T). (See PICOT box.)

Search the Literature

Once you have stated your guiding question, the next step is to look for research articles related to the question (or problem statement). You may be thinking, "Where do I look for research articles?" Evidence reports and practice guidelines may already exist for your clinical problem, so look for those first. Then proceed to search for your topic in research reports in scientific and interdisciplinary journals.

Indexes and Databases

Online search engines and databases or onsite library services will help you search scholarly literature for evidence-based health information (Table 4-3). A **database** is an electronic bibliographic file that can be accessed online. One of the best databases for you as a novice nurse is the Cumulative Index to Nursing and Allied Health Literature (CINAHL). Once you have access to CINAHL, select words that relate to your topic (e.g., *dementia* or *nursing ethics*). The index or database will list journal articles related to the keywords. Sometimes you will get a large number of articles that contain that word or phrase. A PICOT question should help you narrow your search.

KnowledgeCheck 4-10
Where can you go to use CINAHL?

Journals
- **Why use refereed journals?** You will find the highest-quality research articles published in refereed journals. **Refereed journals** are scholarly journals (not popular magazines, such as *Men's Health* or *Fitness*) in which professionals with expertise in the topic review each article and then recommend whether it should be published. The easiest way to identify a refereed journal is to see whether it has an extensive editorial board listed in the front of the journal. Refereed journals have a high standard for publication, which makes the information you read more credible (and therefore more useful to your work). Two examples of refereed nursing research journals are *Advances in Nursing Science* and *Nursing Research.*
- **How to identify a research article.** Simply look for the steps in the research process described earlier in this chapter. For example, does the article have a problem statement and a purpose? Is there a section on the sample and site of the research?
- **Specialty journals.** If your focus is clinical practice, you should not overlook specialty journals, such as *Geriatric Nursing* or the *Journal of Gerontological Nursing* if you are looking for information about older adults with dementia, for example. They are not research journals, but they often have one or two research-style articles in each issue.
- **General-interest journals.** If you do not have a specialty interest, review the *American Journal of Nursing, Nursing,* or *RN* for articles of general interest.

PICOT

Skin Care for Pressure Injury in Frail, Older Woman

Situation: An older, frail resident in a skilled nursing care facility experiences urinary incontinence. Her skin is reddened and beginning to break down at pressure points on her sacrum. Knowing that urine is harsh on the skin and that moisture, pressure, friction, and shear can lead to skin breakdown, the nurse is concerned that the woman may be developing a pressure injury. She searches the literature for an evidence-based intervention that would be most effective.

	Sample Questions	Example
P—Patient, population, or problem	▸ What is the medical diagnosis, nursing diagnosis, patient problem, symptom, situation, or need that requires an intervention? ▸ How would you describe a group of similar patients?	For patients with Impaired Skin Integrity (sacrum, perineum) related to urinary incontinence
I—Intervention, treatment, cause, contributing factor	▸ Which intervention are you considering? Specifically, what might help the problem (improve the situation, etc.)?	Would applying a hydrocolloid dressing help?
C—Comparison intervention	▸ What other interventions are being considered or used?	Compared with applying a gauze dressing after incontinent episodes
O—Outcome	▸ What effect could the intervention realistically have? What do you hope to achieve?	To prevent or reduce sacral excoriation? Are there any undesired effects associated with the intervention?
T—Time	▸ How often or when will the outcome be measured? How often or for how long will the intervention or treatment be administered?	After incontinent episodes

Searchable Question: Do (P) who receive (I) as compared to (C) demonstrate (O) after (T)?

Example of Evidence: The American College of Physicians (Qaseem et al., 2015) published practice guidelines for risk assessment, prevention, and treatment of pressure injuries. Among other interventions, guidelines recommend using hydrocolloid dressings in patients with pressure injuries to promote healing by absorbing wound exudate and forming a protective surface around the wound. The evidence showed that hydrocolloid dressings are better than gauze for reducing wound size.

Practice Change: The nurse verified knowledge of skin care, including cleansing and applying barrier cream for the prevention and early treatment of pressure injuries in a woman at risk for skin breakdown.

Source: Adapted from Qaseem, A., Humphrey, L. L., Forciea, M. A., Starkey, M., & Denberg, T. D. (2015, March 3). Treatment of pressure ulcers: A clinical practice guideline from the American College of Physicians. *Annals of Internal Medicine, 162*(5), 370–379. https://doi.org/10.7326/M14-1568; Wound, Ostomy and Continence Nurses Society. (2016). *Guideline for prevention and management of pressure ulcers (injuries);* University of North Carolina, Health Sciences Library. (2022, January 18). *Forming focused questions with PICO: About PICO.* http://guides.lib.unc.edu/pico; Strauss, S. E., Glasziou, P., Sacket, D., Richardson, W. S., Rosenberg, W., & Haynes, R. B. (2019). *Evidence-based medicine: How to practice and teach EBM* (5th ed.). Churchill Livingstone; Stilwell, S., Fineout-Overholt, E., Melnyk, B. M., & Williamson, K. M. (2010). Evidence-based practice, step by step: Asking the clinical question: A key step in evidence-based practice. *American Journal of Nursing, 110*(3), 58–61. https://doi.org/10.1097/01.NAJ.0000368959.11129.79

Evaluate the Quality of the Research

If you find clinical practice guidelines related to your topic, the related research should have a notation about the level of evidence supporting the guideline. Additionally, you will need to critically consider the quality of the individual research articles you find.

Analytic Reading

You cannot expect to do a complex critique of a research report at this early stage of your education or perhaps even on graduation from your basic education. However, you need to know enough to help you decide which articles are worthy of using in your practice. You will make that decision after you have examined the research to determine whether it is well done and meaningful to your work. Begin this process by learning to read analytically. **Analytic reading** occurs when you "begin asking questions of what you are reading so that you can truly understand it" (Wilson, 1992, p. 25). For questions to use when reading analytically, see Box 4-4. For questions to ask when researching health topics, refer to Box 38-4, How to Evaluate Health Information on the Internet.

Table 4-3 ➤ Selected Databases for Health Literature

DATABASE	DESCRIPTION
CINAHL (Cumulative Index to Nursing and Allied Health Literature)	Covers nursing, allied health, biomedical, and consumer health journals; publications of the American Nursing Association; and publications of the National League for Nursing. Updated monthly.
Cochrane Library	A collection of six evidence-based medicine databases, including systematic reviews, reviews of effectiveness, and a controlled-trials register to inform healthcare decision-making.
Digital Commons Network™	Free, full-text, scholarly articles from peer-reviewed journals, book chapters, dissertations, conference proceedings, and other original works worldwide.
DOAJ (Directory of open Access Journals)	Database with an extensive index of open-access, peer-reviewed, scholarly journals of various disciplines, languages, and geographic locations.
Google Scholar	Provides a platform for searching scholarly literature across many disciplines. Resources include articles, theses, books, abstracts, court opinions from universities, academic publishers, professional organizations, and other authority sources.
MEDLINE	Produced by the U.S. National Library of Medicine, MEDLINE is the world's largest medical library in all areas of biomedicine and healthcare.
PLOS	Nonprofit, open-access platform for researchers to share their work. PLOS publishes research from more than 200 scientific communities, such as immunology, biology, infectious diseases, neuroscience, cancer research and treatment.
PubMed®	PubMed is an Internet-based database with free and unlimited access to more than 30 million references of biomedical literature from approximately 7,000 journals.
APA PsycInfo®	Covers worldwide literature in psychology and related disciplines, such as psychiatry, sociology, anthropology, education, linguistics, and pharmacology. Journal articles, technical reports, and dissertations are included. Updated weekly.

Research Appraisal

Key Point: *Not all research is good research.* Some published studies contain serious flaws in design, sampling method, data collection, or analysis of findings. You need to be able to recognize them. An effective strategy for conducting a research appraisal is to read the research article using the four analytic reading questions in Box 4-4 and make note of questions you have. Then go back and evaluate the article section by section, thinking critically about each (Wilson, 1992).

BOX 4-4 ■ Reading Analytically

When reading analytically, ask yourself the following questions:

1. **What is the book, journal, or article about as a whole?** That is, what is the topic, and how is it developed?

2. **What is being said in detail, and how?** What are the author's main ideas, claims, and arguments? In a research article, you will find this mainly in the abstract and the conclusions.

3. **Is the book, journal, or article factual in whole or part?** You must decide this for yourself. The discussion may reveal limitations of the study or flaws in research design or sampling.

4. **What of it?** Is it of any significance? How can you apply the information to improve patient care or enhance other areas of the nursing profession?

- **Researcher qualifications** are an easy place to start. Is the researcher qualified as an expert on the study topic? Try to determine whether the author's credentials and background fit with the topic.
- The **title** should be concise and clear. Keywords in the title should indicate the topic of the research topic.
- The **abstract** typically summarizes the purpose, methods, sample, and findings of the study.
- The **introduction** may contain the *review of the literature, theoretical (conceptual) framework, assumptions,* and *limitations.* At this stage of your expertise, you should primarily check that these are present; however, some explanation is as follows:
  - The **review of the literature** should be thorough and relevant. The references should logically pertain to the study topic and methods and consist primarily of research and theory articles. The references should support the researcher's variable definitions, methodology, and choices of data-collection tools and present background work on the topic being studied.
  - **Study assumptions** are beliefs that you take for granted as true but that have not been proven. For

example, you assume that when people eat, they are hungry; and you assume that study participants answer the researcher's questions truthfully. Assumptions should be clearly stated to avoid confusion regarding the study.

- **Limitations of the study**. Every study has limitations or weaknesses. The author should clearly identify the factors or conditions that could not be controlled. For example, a nurse researcher may test a population of people that would not generalize to other populations (e.g., testing only Hispanic students instead of testing a variety of students who represent the ethnic diversity of the university).

- The **purpose** should state the reasons for doing the study. Ask the following to help you judge it: Will the study (1) solve a problem relevant to nursing, (2) present facts that are useful to nursing, or (3) contribute to nursing knowledge?

- The **problem statement** should appear early in the report, and it should be researchable; that is, it (1) is stated as a question, (2) involves the relationship between two or more variables, and (3) can be answered by collecting empirical data.

- **Definition of terms** is essential in a formal research report. However, definitions are often not included in a published article because of the lack of space.

- **The research design** indicates the plan for collecting data. As a novice, you may not be ready to judge the adequacy of the design, but you should be sure the researcher names and describes it and discusses its strengths and weakness. **Key Point:** *The researcher should include an explanation of what was done to enhance the validity and reliability of the study.* To say it simply, **validity** means the study measures the concept it intends to measure. **Reliability** refers to the accuracy, consistency, and precision of a measure. That is, if someone else repeated the study using the same design, would they obtain similar results? For example, if you weighed the same item on a scale each day and obtained the same weight each time, you could say the scale is reliable—but a scale would not give you a valid height.

- **Setting, population, and sample**. The researcher should clearly identify the type of setting where the data were collected, describe the population and sample, and state the criteria that were used for choosing study participants. This section may also contain information about how informed consent was obtained.

- **Data-collection methods** answer the basic questions of what, how, who, where, and when. Data-collection instruments are the tools used to gather the data (e.g., questionnaires or a laboratory instrument). The researcher should provide evidence (pilot tests, literature) that the tools used were reliable and valid.

- **Data analysis**. Statistical methods for analyzing data differ depending on the type of data collected. A *quantitative* report would include statistical analyses of the data, frequently in the form of tables and graphs. A *qualitative* report would include a narrative summary of findings, including direct quotes from the participants.

- The **discussion of findings** and **conclusion** are the sections of a research report that you may find most interesting. They are the "What was learned?" and "What it means" sections. The researcher should present all findings objectively and compare them with information found in the literature. Errors you may recognize with your present knowledge level are that the researcher:

1. Generalizes beyond the data or the sample. For example, the sample may have been young adult women in a clinic setting, but the researcher might have suggested that the same intervention be used for all women in the clinic, regardless of age, or women who are not like those included in the study sample.
2. Does not mention limitations that might have influenced the results.
3. Does not present findings in a clear, logical manner (i.e., you have trouble figuring out what the findings are).

- **Implications and recommendations** are the final pieces of the research critique. The implications are the "shoulds" of the research. In essence, the researcher says, "Now we know this fact; therefore, nurses should . . ." For example, "The research should be replicated with another population," or "The instrument should be revised and retested," or "This is how nurses could use the study intervention in their practice."

When you read a research article, examine it for each of the preceding items. Although you have limited knowledge and experience, every time you review an article thoroughly, you will learn more about the research process. As you learn, you will be better able to determine the quality of research you will accept as a basis for changing your nursing practice.

KnowledgeCheck 4-11
- Explain the difference between analytic reading and research appraisal.
- What are the parts of a PICOT question?

Integrate the Research Into Your Practice
Evidence-based practice requires that after discovering and critiquing the best available evidence, nursing expertise must be applied to see how the recommended interventions fit into the practice setting and whether they are compatible with patient preferences. The nurse researcher must consider costs, barriers to change, facilitators for change, and staff education before deciding to implement the clinical practice guideline in the unit or hospital.

Research is more than just a project that nurses conduct in order to earn master's and doctoral degrees. The ultimate reason for conducting research is to establish an evidence-based practice, improve patient care, or gain a greater understanding of a phenomenon. This means that nurses have a responsibility to find and use the credible scientific research that others do. Remember the discussion of authority-based practice during Florence Nightingale's era? Even in current times, much nursing practice is still based on authority and tradition. However, today's full-spectrum, professional nurses have reasons for what they do in clinical practice that are based on sound scientific evidence.

To explore learning resources for this chapter,

Go to Davis Advantage and find:

Answers and Suggested Responses for all questions in this chapter
Concept Map
Knowledge Map
References and Bibliography

CHAPTER 5

Ethics & Values

Learning Outcomes

After completing this chapter, you should be able to:

➤ Differentiate among *morals, ethics, bioethics,* and *nursing ethics.*

➤ Discuss what is meant by *ethical agency.*

➤ Identify at least four factors that contribute to the frequency of nurses' moral problems.

➤ Differentiate personal values and morality from professional values.

➤ Explain how developmental stages, values, ethical frameworks, professional guidelines, and ethical principles affect moral decisions.

➤ Describe five major ethical principles that are used in reasoning about healthcare.

➤ Compare and contrast four ethical frameworks: consequentialism (e.g.,

utilitarianism), deontology, an ethics of care, and feminist ethics.

➤ Identify the ethical issues and principles involved in a given ethical situation.

➤ Describe a systematic approach to resolving ethical dilemmas.

➤ Discuss the concept of an integrity-producing compromise.

➤ Describe the nurse's obligations in ethical decisions.

➤ Discuss the role of the nurse as client advocate in ethical situations.

➤ Apply the steps identified in the MORAL model to make ethical decisions.

Key Concepts

Morals

Nursing ethics

Values

Related Concepts

See the Concept Map on Davis Advantage.

Example Client Conditions

Moral Distress

Whistleblowing

Meet Your Patients

Angie and Edward Frese and their two teenage children are a close and loving family with a large network of family and friends. Their son, Alan, 15 years old, has just been severely injured in a high school soccer game. At the hospital, Angie and Edward are told that Alan has multiple bone fractures and active internal bleeding.

The surgeon informs the distressed parents that Alan will need a blood transfusion to survive. Although genuinely devastated, the parents adamantly refuse to consent to a lifesaving blood transfusion, stating they are Jehovah's Witnesses and that receiving blood is against their religious beliefs. The surgeon asks you, Alan's nurse, to convince the parents to change their minds right away. You talk with the couple, but they continue to refuse a blood

transfusion. You immediately contact your charge nurse. Try to answer the following critical-thinking questions about Alan and his parents. You may not have the experience or theoretical

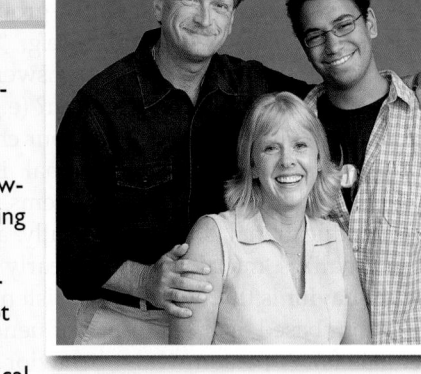

knowledge to answer them all—you will acquire that in this chapter and in Chapter 39—but do your best based on the background you have.

ThinkLike a Nurse 5-1:
Clinical Judgment in Action

- Do Alan's parents have the right to refuse a blood transfusion based on their religious beliefs?
- Do you think the fact that Alan is a minor (age less than 18 years) may make a difference in this situation?
- What actions do you think the charge nurse should take?
- Can an ethical conflict such as this be resolved to everyone's satisfaction?

Theoretical Knowledge
knowing why

The theoretical knowledge you will need to begin professional practice includes an understanding of the nature of morals and ethics (and especially nursing ethics) and basic information about factors that affect moral decisions (i.e., values, moral frameworks, professional guidelines, and ethical principles).

ABOUT THE KEY CONCEPTS

Nursing ethics, morals, and **values** are key concepts in this chapter because everything in the chapter is related to those concepts in some way—as you will discover. The subconcepts of *advocacy* and *compromise*, for example, are intimately integrated into the implementation of nursing ethics in clinical practice. Remember to use the key concepts to help you organize chapter content in your mind. As you read, try to understand how each subconcept you encounter relates to nursing ethics, morals, and values.

ETHICS AND MORALS

The terms *ethics* and *morals* have similar meanings, but they are different concepts. In modern theory, the term **morals** refers to private, personal, or group standards of what is good or bad, right or wrong (e.g., "In general, it is wrong to steal"). In contrast, **ethics** answers the question, What should I do in a given situation? (e.g., "Is it wrong to steal if you have to do it to feed your children?").

Morals are learned from external influences and communicated through various systems (e.g., religious, political, educational, societal). Usually, a person learns and internalizes moral standards early in childhood. **Moral behavior** is that which is consistent with customs or traditions based on the external influence (such as religious beliefs). A person whose behavior is inconsistent with traditional notions of right and wrong is labeled as immoral. Consider the following conversation between two nurses discussing a teenager who assaulted and robbed a 92-year-old woman who was in a wheelchair:

Nurse A: "I cannot believe someone would be so heartless as to attack an innocent, helpless older woman."

Nurse B: "I agree—that person is immoral. Absolutely no morals."

You may agree with this because you were taught to respect and protect older adults. Morals are linked to a person's character and often determine how we treat others. Another example is the "Golden Rule," which states that you should treat others as you wish to be treated.

- Can you think of another example of moral behavior that you may have learned as a child?
- Can you identify any morals that are evident in the scenario about Alan at the beginning of the chapter?
- How do his parents' morals influence Alan's care?

Ethics is the study of a system of moral principles and standards, or the process of using them to decide your conduct and actions. Ethics helps us to decide what is right or wrong and what actions should be taken in certain circumstances, using a set of well-defined principles and rules. Although a nurse's *moral code* would find the act of "driving under the influence" thoughtless and reprehensible, their *ethics* as a nurse would require them to provide care to the driver for the injuries received in the motor vehicle accident. In the case of Alan and his family (Meet Your Patients), the ethical decision making is quite different from the moral perspective of Alan's parents. The parents believe a blood transfusion is morally wrong; this fits with their religious beliefs. The surgeon and the nurse, however, believe withholding blood from Alan would be unethical.

Ethics and the Law How are laws related to ethics and morals? In some situations, there is a fine line between law and ethics. Think about the following:

- *Law:* It is illegal to drive faster than the speed limit.
  Situation: A child is bleeding profusely and may have cut an artery. The driver drives very fast and even drives through a red light.
  Question: Was that illegal? Was it immoral?
- *Law:* In the United States, it is legal in certain situations to have an abortion.
  Fact: Although everyone would have to agree that the act is legal, people are about evenly divided as to whether they believe it is moral.

The adage "Courts are ill equipped to deal with ethical issues" reflects the difficulty of trying to decide a case on a continuum of right and wrong (ethics) versus applying strict legal principles (law). Although ethics is rooted in the religious values, political values, customs, and other values of a society, you should now be able to see that ethics is not the same as law, religion, institutional practices, or customs. An action that is legal or customary may not be morally right or ethically justifiable. The same holds true of religion. You cannot assume that an accepted practice of a certain religion is an ethical practice in every situation.

What Is Nursing Ethics?

- **Bioethics** refers to the application of ethical principles to every aspect of healthcare. Bioethics is concerned with every area of healthcare, including direct care of patients, allocation of resources, utilization of staff, and medical and nursing research.
- **Nursing ethics** is a subset of bioethics. It refers to ethical questions that arise out of nursing practice. The first things to come to your mind may be the dramatic questions, such as, "Should we turn off the ventilator and allow this patient to die?" or "Should this baby have surgery even though their quality of life will probably never be good?"

In reality, you may have some input, but the patient, provider, and family will make the final decision in such ♥ **iCare** situations. As a nurse, you are responsible for deciding the nature and extent of your own participation in each situation to protect your emotional well-being, and you must support patients who are making ethical decisions or perhaps coping with the results of decisions made by others. Consider the following true story paraphrased from Curtin and Flaherty (1982, pp. 3–4):

A woman took her 6-year-old son to the emergency department (ED) to have a scalp laceration sutured. On the way to the hospital, she tried to calm him by telling him that the doctors would "numb" him and "no one would hurt him" on purpose. On arrival, they were placed in a cubicle next to another little boy who was awaiting treatment for a similar laceration. His father was also trying to reassure his son.

In the cubicle of the father and son, a nurse roughly cleansed the cut with no explanation or words of comfort. The provider came and sutured the laceration without a word and without waiting for the local anesthetic to take effect. The boy screamed in pain and terror the whole time. The woman was horrified, and her son was scared. But when the same nurse approached the woman and her son, she was kind and gentle. The same provider carefully injected a local anesthetic and waited for it to take effect before suturing.

Why do you think there was such a difference in the treatment? Was it because the man and boy appeared to be of lower socioeconomic status? Was it the presence of a father rather than a mother? Was it because the father and son were from a minority group and the woman and son were not? It may have been all of these reasons or none of them. Regardless of why it happened, what makes this case important? After all, both boys received medical treatment; both incisions will heal; no one's life or health was threatened; no life-and-death decisions were made. But notice that the first child's humanity and dignity were violated, and the actions were not fair. **Key Point:** *This case is a perfect example of nursing ethics: questions that have to do with the nurse's actions, not the actions of others. The nurse did not need a medical prescription or permission from hospital administration to act ethically.*

In the Meet Your Patients scenario, you, as the nurse, are not responsible for deciding the broad questions: "Is blood transfusion right or wrong?"; "Do the parents have a right to refuse blood transfusion?" *Your* decision is "What should *I* do? Should I try to persuade the parents to change their minds, as the surgeon directs, or not?" That is the *nursing ethics* question. And in that scenario, you will need to deal with the effects of the final decision on Alan. He may be frightened; he may be angry; he may die. The nurse is there for patient's most human and vulnerable moments.

Why Should Nurses Study Ethics?

This section will help you understand why nurses should study ethics.

- **You will encounter ethical problems frequently in your work.** You will be prepared to make an informed decision and knowledgeable of the ethical issues involved. A consciously made, informed decision will be better than one made without awareness of the ethical issues involved. As a nurse, you will deal with important human events, such as birth, death, and suffering. You will be at the bedside, where critical decisions are made about the best way to treat clients and solve healthcare problems. Many ethical issues surround these sensitive areas. The most difficult question you will face as a nurse will not be "How do I do this?" but "Should I do this?"
- **Ethics is central to nursing.** Commitment to caring for other human beings supports the claim that nursing is a moral art (Butts & Rich, 2020). Caring for the sick, promoting health, and practicing with care and compassion are central values in nursing.
- **Interprofessional input is important.** Many healthcare facilities have an ethics committee to address complex ethical issues. The committee is composed of providers, nurses, clergy, social workers, therapists, case managers, attorneys, and so on, depending on the issues. Interprofessional input becomes increasingly important to adequately evaluate the complex ethical issues.
- **Ethical knowledge is necessary for professional competence.** Being a professional includes being accountable to others in the profession for the ethical conduct of your work. Using professional expertise for social good is one hallmark of a profession. Therefore, to conduct our work well and have it stand the test of public scrutiny, we need to be clear about the ethics of our work.
- **Ethical reasoning is necessary for nursing credibility among other disciplines.** For your opinion to be valued by others, you must be able to clearly express your moral position in a logical way. To be an accountable practitioner, you must be able to (1) understand your own values as they relate to basic

morality and (2) use ethical reasoning to articulate your moral position.

- **Ethical proficiency is essential for providing holistic care.** Nurses care for the whole person—that includes providing support for spiritual and moral concerns.
- **Nurses have a responsibility to be advocates for patients.** Advocacy is the communication and defense of the rights and interests of another. Since the 1960s, schools have socialized nurses to include patient advocacy in their role conceptions. Currently, the American Nurses Association (ANA) *Code of Ethics for Nurses* (2015, p. 9), provision 3, states: "The nurse promotes, advocates for and strives to protect the health, safety and rights of the patient."

Advocacy includes protecting patients' legal or moral rights (e.g., taking appropriate action when the actions of a healthcare team member jeopardize the patient's rights or best interests). You can also advocate for patients in everyday practice, for example, by contacting a primary provider to request a new prescription when a pain medication is not effective. **Key Point:** *To advocate for patients in ethical situations, you must be able to identify the ethical issues, know your resources, and communicate the patient's wishes.*

- **Studying ethics will help you to make better decisions.** Most ethical nursing problems have more than one acceptable answer. Each situation is unique in its details—for example, the people involved differ in how they evaluate what is and is not beneficial for themselves. The study of ethics prepares you to analyze ethical dilemmas from multiple perspectives rather than relying entirely on your personal values, intuition, and emotions. Practice in analyzing ethical dilemmas will help you to become an informed decision maker, capable of understanding the perspectives of all the people in each situation—to understand, for example, why the Freses (Meet Your Patients) are refusing a blood transfusion.

Ethical Scenario: Advocacy

Ms. Wyatte, a 70-year-old, was hospitalized for a kidney infection. During the admission assessment, you observe numerous bruises on her extremities and shoulders. In response to your questions, Ms. Wyatte says they are skin tears associated with aging. You ask if she is being abused. She becomes very distressed and begs you to keep it a secret because she can't afford for her son to lose his job. Ms. Wyatte also tells you that he is usually wonderful until he starts drinking alcohol. Reflect on what you would do. Discuss with your peers.

KnowledgeCheck 5-1

- Define *morals* and give an example from your textbook.
- Define *ethics* and give an example from your textbook.
- How is bioethics different from ethics?
- Why do nurses need to study ethics?

What Is Ethical Agency?

Moral agency or **ethical agency** for nurses is the ability to base their practice on professional standards of ethical conduct and participate in ethical decision making. Simply stated, it means that nurses have choices and are responsible for their actions. An ethical agent must be able to:

- Perceive the difference between right and wrong.
- Understand abstract ethical principles.
- Reason and apply ethical principles to make decisions, weigh alternatives, and plan sound ways to achieve goals.
- Decide and choose freely.
- Act according to choice (this assumes both the power and the capability to act).

External and internal factors that prevent nurses from implementing their ethical decisions are as follows:

External constraints
- *Providers.* Nurses express fear that the provider would be angry, have them fired, retaliate, or make their job difficult.
- *Laws or lawsuits.* Nurses seem to have an exaggerated fear of losing their nursing license and of being sued. In addition, they express the need to protect the healthcare organization from lawsuits.
- *Nursing administration.* Nurses may view nurse administrators more as a source of punishment than support and may fear being punished, reprimanded, or fired.
- *Other nurses.* Nurses do not view other staff nurses as being supportive on ethical issues. They express the need to keep the peace and not cause problems in work relationships.
- *Clients and families.* Nurses say that they sometimes fail to do what they view as the "right thing" out of concern for the effect it might have on the client's family or out of fear that the family would tell the provider that the nurse interfered.

Internal constraints
- Nursing students are socialized to follow orders, not to question.
- Some say that it is useless to try to do the right thing because the outcome for the client would be the same anyway. They believe that taking a stand would make no difference.
- Some nurses fail to act ethically because they doubt their knowledge or motivation: "I think, maybe I'm biased. What if I'm wrong?"
- Others mention a lack of courage, concern for reputation, and hope for a miracle.

Moral Distress

When situational constraints prevent nurses from acting on their moral decisions, **moral distress** may occur (Fig. 5-1). Said another way, moral distress can occur when nurses are unable to act as moral agents.

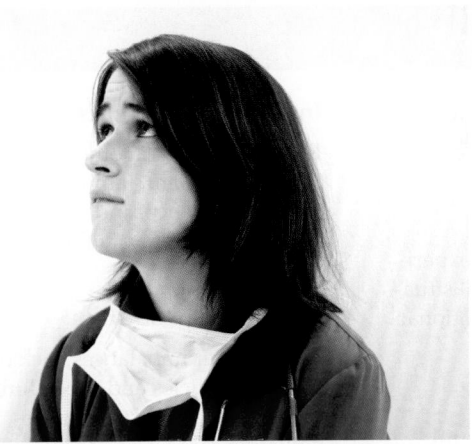

FIGURE 5-1 Ethical problems can create moral distress.

Ethical Scenario: Moral Distress

The family of a 94-year-old patient who is on a ventilator and has Alzheimer disease, congestive heart failure, diabetes, and sepsis refused to sign a do not attempt resuscitation (DNAR) status for him. The patient's wishes were unknown, although the family indicated that he would want to have full-code status. The nurses providing care experienced outrage because they felt the family was putting the patient through unnecessary suffering by prolonging his life. An unsuccessful full code was implemented 2 weeks later when the patient experienced cardiac arrest. Reflect on your feelings. Would you do everything possible to preserve life? Did the family make the right decision? Discuss with your peers.

For more information, see the Example Client Condition: Moral Distress.

Whistleblowing

Providers experience **moral outrage** when they perceive that others are behaving immorally (Wilkinson, 1987/1988). Moral outrage is similar to moral distress, except that in cases of moral outrage, nurses do not participate in the act. Therefore, they do not believe that they are responsible for doing wrong but that they are powerless to prevent others from doing so (Davidson et al., 2020). Driven by moral outrage, individuals become whistleblowers, making public the unsafe, illegal, or fraudulent behaviors of others (Cypher, 2021). The following scenarios provide examples of whistleblowing.

Ethical Scenario: Moral Distress

Example 1. A nonemployee provider claimed a hospital retaliated against him for reporting improper patient transfers in violation of the Emergency Medical Treatment & Labor Act (EMTALA). The provider's refusal to authorize (accept) the patient transfers from the other hospital was ignored. Ruling in favor of the whistleblower, the court held that EMTALA is designed to prevent patient dumping, and its whistleblower provision protects individuals who are in positions to observe and report violations (*Muzaffar v. Aurora Health Care Southern Lakes, Inc.,* 2013).

Example 2. A nurse filed a report with the peer-review committee outlining his perception of poor care that led to a patient's death. Within days of receiving the complaint, the reporting nurse was written up for several infractions and later terminated. The court upheld his claim of retaliation and wrongful discharge (*Landin v. Healthsource Saginaw, Inc.,* 2014).

These two examples show that nurses or other providers who advocate for quality patient care can experience repercussions for "blowing the whistle" (see Example Problem: Whistleblowing).

Impaired Nursing Practice

Impaired nursing practice occurs when the nurse's ability to perform the essential nursing functions is diminished by chemical dependence on drugs or alcohol or by mental illness. Impairment is a threat to clients, and the impaired nurse may have difficulty being accountable for their own actions or assessing their self-competence. Nurses are required to report impaired nurses to their nursing leadership. The *Code of Ethics for Nurses* (ANA, 2015a) guides that advocacy includes supporting nurses who return to practice after receiving the appropriate assistance and treatment for substance abuse.

KnowledgeCheck 5-2

- Define *ethical agency.*
- What five abilities must be present for ethical agency to exist?
- List at least three constraints that can keep nurses from carrying out their ethical decisions.

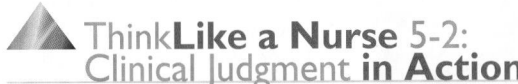

ThinkLike a Nurse 5-2: Clinical Judgment in Action

Consider the five components of ethical agency. To what extent do you believe nurses possess those abilities? Explain your thinking.

What Are Some Sources of Ethical Problems for Nurses?

Factors that contribute to the frequency of nurses' ethical problems include societal factors, the nature of nursing work, and the nature of the nursing profession itself.

Societal Factors

This section discusses how some ethical problems for nurses are created by the ever-changing nature of our dynamic, multicultural society.

Increased Consumer Awareness Historically, sick people sought the advice of a physician without

EXAMPLE PROBLEM: Moral Distress

THEORETICAL KNOWLEDGE

Definition: Response to the inability to carry out one's chosen ethical/moral decision or action

Defining Characteristics

Mental anguish and/or physical pain experienced based on involvement in a moral situation. Feelings of frustration, anger, emotional exhaustion.

Etiology

Nurse feels morally responsible for an outcome or client and identifies an acceptable course of action but is unable to implement the chosen intervention, based on real or perceived constraints (Altaker et al., 2018; Rushton et al., 2017; Wilkinson, 1987/1988). It is a compromise of one's values or moral agency.

Internal Constraints

Relationships with others (e.g., providers, colleagues, client, family members); lack of skills, confidence, and courage; fear; concerns about perceptions of others; perception of poor ethical climate

External Constraints

Time, power imbalances, lack of institutional support, policies and procedures, threat of lawsuits, regulatory directives, integrated palliative care teams, degree of empowerment (Sirilla et al., 2017).

ANALYZING CUES/ DIAGNOSING

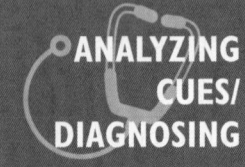

Moral Distress

Response to the inability to carry out one's chosen ethical/moral decision or action.

Note: Nurses were primarily the subjects of moral distress research; NANDA-I has accepted a nursing diagnosis for use with patients.

EVALUATING OUTCOMES

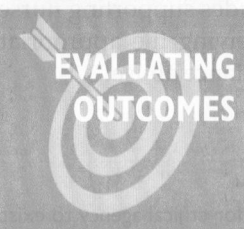

- Decreased anxiety level
- Lack of fear
- Psychospiritual comfort status
- Spiritual health

- Preservation of personal autonomy and integrity
- Relief from frustration and anger
- Quality communications
- Caring behaviors

TAKING ACTION

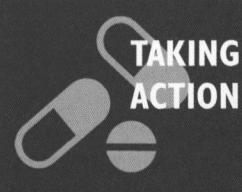

Note: These interventions focus on nurses experiencing moral distress.
- Recognize the source of the moral distress.
- Understand your values, thoughts, and beliefs.
- Reflect on your values that are threatened in the situation. Are these personal or professional values?
- Engage in values clarification.
- Self-manage emotions; discuss with a mentor if you are having difficulty.
- Make decisions based on reasoned choices.
- Discuss the basis for your decision with members of the interprofessional team, client, and family members. Be sure to express it logically and clearly and with controlled emotions.
- View the situation from the other perspective. Identify reasons that support this perspective. This helps to ensure that you have a comprehensive knowledge of the factors that led to the other person's decision.

- Engage with personal and professional resources to resolve intrapersonal conflicts that occur when decisions are made that are contrary to your selected choice.
- Consult with a nurse ethicist.
- Accept that clients have the right to make decisions that they feel best adhere to their values and beliefs. Treat them with kindness and respect, and show compassion. The client is also experiencing some type of loss in these situations.
- Make a commitment to care for self.
- Acknowledge your feelings and seek support sources; separate personal from professional.
- Engage in self-care activities (e.g., exercise, meditation, reflection, recreational activities, adequate sleep, balanced diet).
- Seek spiritual guidance and support.
- Develop a network of supportive interprofessional colleagues.
- Seek counseling for unresolved feelings or development of moral outrage (anger directed toward others).

EXAMPLE PROBLEM: Whistleblowing

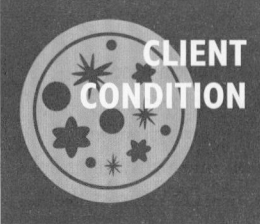

THEORETICAL KNOWLEDGE

Definition

A **whistleblower** is a person who reveals information about practices of others that are perceived as wrong, fraudulent, corrupt, illegal, or a detriment to the health, safety, and welfare of the clients they serve.

Risks and Consequences

- Nurses must carefully weigh their ethical obligations to advocate for clients against their obligations to the employer.
- Whistleblowing can have harmful and long-lasting effects on nurses' personal and professional lives. The impact can include loss of employment, fear of physical violence, and rejection by colleagues (Berry 2015; Dungan et al., 2019).

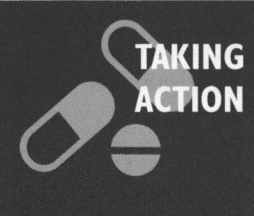

CLIENT CONDITION

- **Moral outrage** occurs when unresolved moral distress leads to anger, disgust, and powerlessness (Rushton, 2013). The anger or outrage is directed toward individuals or groups perceived as responsible for the wrongdoings or acts.

- Policies that created the threat to one's personal and/or professional integrity, values, or beliefs (Altaker et al., 2018; Rushton et al., 2017; Wilkinson, 1987/1988).
- A nurse may respond to moral outrage by becoming a whistleblower.

TAKING ACTION

Actions

To determine whether to **ACT** or **THINK:** assess the nature of the action, the likelihood of immediate harm, and the accuracy and completeness of your data.
- In some situations, you will **ACT** by immediately reporting situations that involve an immediate threat to the health, safety, and well-being of others.
- In other situations, **THINK.**
  Talk with an attorney or other legal representative. Whistleblowing laws must be strictly followed.
  Have concrete and credible evidence of the violation or wrongdoing.
  Institute a survival plan if your job is put in jeopardy or you are fired.
  Note the nature and consequences of the problem—its type, severity, and potential impact. Weigh the risks against the benefits.
  Know your reporting options and support systems that can correct the problems.

Rationale

The ANA *Code of Ethics*, provision 3.5, **Protection of Patient Health and Safety by Acting on Questionable Practice,** guides the need to support nurses who become whistleblowers:
All nurses have a responsibility to assist whistleblowers who identify potentially questionable practices that are factually supported in order to reduce the risk of reprisal against the reporting nurse (ANA, 2015, p. 12).

---

question. Now, the Internet has increased consumer awareness and the availability of information. People are more actively involved in healthcare decisions. Providers are now expected to share knowledge with clients, defend treatment choices different from those found on the Internet, and obtain truly informed consent for treatments.

Technological Advances New technology creates new ethical issues. For example, in vitro fertilization and embryo transfer methods raise questions about the ownership of embryos not implanted into a uterus. If implanted without the father's consent, what child support obligations exist? Other ethical questions include the right to a late-term abortion when amniocentesis reveals fetal defects, human embryonic stem cell research, costs versus quality of life for ventilator-dependent patients, and security of electronic healthcare records.

Multicultural Population We live in a multicultural, multifaith society. You cannot assume that your values and beliefs are similar to those of your patients, other providers, and colleagues. You will need to respect a variety of belief systems and serve as a patient advocate even when the patient's value system is strikingly different from your own. There are nursing theories that can help you recognize various cultural values, for example, Leininger's (2002) theory of cultural care diversity and universality (for a review, see Chapters 4 and 12).

Toward Evidence-Based Practice

Nicholls, A., Fairs, L. R. W., Toner, J., Jones, J., Mantis, C., Barkou-kis, V., Perry, J. L., Micle, A. V., Theodorou, N. C., Shakhverdieva, S., Stoicescu, M., Vesic, M. V., Dikic, N., Andjelkovic, M., García Grimau, E., Amigo, J. A., & and Schomöller, A. (2021). Snitches get stitches and end up in ditches: A systematic review of the factors associated with whistleblowing intentions. *Frontiers in Psychology, 5.* https://doi.org/10.3389/fpsyg.2021.631538

Researchers examined the association of numerous factors and the likelihood of individuals to engage in whistleblowing activities. Several factors related to morality had positive associations, indicating a high likelihood of blowing the whistle on wrongdoings. These included moral reasoning, moral competence, moral perception, moral conviction, and moral development. Individuals with favorable attitudes toward policies and whistleblowing, an aversion to wrongdoing, and who did not have a close relationship with the wrongdoer were more likely to engage in the act of whistleblowing. In addition, the intent to blow the whistle on wrongdoing was positively associated with the severity and duration of the wrongdoing.

Dungan, J., Young, L., & Waytzc, A. (2019). The power of moral concerns in predicting whistleblowing decisions. *Journal of Experimental Social Psychology, 85,* 103848. https://doi.org/10.1016/j.jesp.2019.103848

The literature shows that often whistleblowers must balance organizational loyalties with concerns of fairness and justice to others. Researchers examined the role that moral concerns played in predicting the decision to become a whistleblower. The results supported the hypothesis of a strong association between moral concerns and whistleblowing decisions. Individuals with a high organizational loyalty were less likely to blow the whistle, whereas those with a high concern for public well-being (fairness and justice) were more likely to engage in the act of whistleblowing. In addition, organizational factors played a significant role in whether whistleblowers used internal or external channels. Whistleblowers who perceived their organization to be fair and reported that the organization educated them on their rights were more likely to use internal channels to report unethical or unfair activities.

Stephen, S., & Welch, K. (2018). Research: Whistleblowers are a sign of healthy companies. *Harvard Business Review.* https://hbr.org/2018/11/research-whistleblowers-are-a-sign-of-healthy-companies

Researchers analyzed a database of over 1.2 million records of internal whistleblowing reports made by employees. They concluded that having an internal reporting system for employees is a sign of a healthy organization. Internal systems are a means of open communication for employees to express their concerns to administrative leaders. In addition, early reporting of issues allowed for immediate handling of issues. Results revealed 6.9% fewer lawsuits and 20.4% less in monetary settlements over a 3-year period. The lack of an internal system pushes whistleblowers to use external systems of reporting.

1. What implications does the research by Dungan et al. have for organizational policies and practices?

2. What are the benefits of an internal reporting system for whistleblowers?

3. What do you view as alternatives to whistleblowing?

Cost Containment The emphasis on reducing healthcare costs creates many ethically questionable situations. For example:

- **Clients are being sent home from the hospital while they still require considerable nursing care.** During discharge planning, clients may discover that insurance payments are limited for services outside the hospital, including specialists, home care, and medical supplies (e.g., bandages, walkers).
- **To contain costs, healthcare agencies have increased the number of clients assigned to each nurse.** You will undoubtedly find yourself in situations in which fewer nurses are available than clients' acuity requires. You will have to decide how far you will stretch your own resources to maintain clients' safety.

The Nature of Nursing Work

Ethical problems exist in all kinds of work. However, the nature of nursing work itself can create unique ethical problems.

Nurses' Ethical Problems Nurses' ethical problems are immediate, serious, and frequent. In the classroom, you have the luxury of leaving questions unsettled. In the real world, you must always decide: either you take action or you do not. **Key Point: *For a nurse, deciding not to act is, in effect, an act.*** For example, suppose the family wishes a patient to have aggressive resuscitation efforts (code). However, you know the patient does not wish to be "coded." When the patient's heart stops, whether or not you know the "right" thing to do, you must decide immediately to carry out or not carry out the code. If you wait too long to ponder the ethical issues, the patient may die before you decide. If you do not decide, the effect is the same as though you had decided it was wrong to code.

Nurses' Unique Position in Healthcare Organizations Nurses have multiple obligations and relationships, and sometimes they have conflicting loyalties.

- They are *employees* (with a relationship with the agency) as well as *professionals* (with a special relationship with patients).

- Nurses are expected to follow the provider's prescriptions for client care, although the provider is not the nurse's employer.
- At most organizations, the providers are higher on the power and status hierarchy than are nurses.

Ethical dilemmas arise when nurses experience conflicts among their loyalties to patients, families, providers, employers, and other nurses. Consider the following example: A patient wants to know their test results, but the provider is reluctant to tell the patient that information. What are the conflicting loyalties? Should the nurse give the patient the information or not? There are two options:

Tell. By providing the test results, the nurse would honor the principle of autonomy and their obligation to the patient. But this might harm the patient's relationship with the provider, which is important to the patient's well-being. Furthermore, if the nurse tells the patient the test results, it may create problems between the provider and the employer (e.g., the hospital) and between the provider and the nurse. In addition, this action may in some instances violate hospital policies and therefore harm the nurse's relationship with the hospital.

Don't tell. The nurse could preserve the patient–provider relationship by withholding the test results from the patient. This choice does not honor their relationship with the patient. Also, if the nurse does not tell the patient their test results, the patient may find out anyway and be angry with the hospital, the provider, and the nurse.

Ethical Scenario: Conflict

Your best friend since childhood is also a nursing student. She confides in you that her registered nurse makes her sign narcotic wastes, stating that no one checks names, only that there are two signatures. This is against both hospital and school policies. The school has zero tolerance for violation of clinical policies, and you know that your friend will fail the course if this becomes known. What would you do in this situation? Is your loyalty to your friend, the school, or the hospital? What are the broader implications? Discuss with your peers.

According to professional ethics, your first allegiance is to the patient. However, the patient's needs often conflict with institutional policies, family desires, or even the laws of the state. There may also be conflicts in your relationships with the patient and their family. You can see an example of this in the Meet Your Patients scenario, wherein the nurse finds it impossible to honor the parents' autonomy and at the same time advocate for Alan. You may also encounter this type of conflict when a patient does not want any heroic measures and wishes only to die peacefully, but the family members have not yet been able to accept the imminent death and are insisting on full resuscitation.

The Nature of the Nursing Profession

Ethical problems may arise because of value conflicts and a lack of clarity within the nursing profession. We have unresolved questions about the nature, scope, and goals of our practice, as well as our professional values. In most of the following examples, we value both of the opposites. We would not wish to give up either one, but specific situations require us to choose between them, which can be a source of discomfort.

- *Caring versus time spent with patients.* Nursing values caring, humanistic care, and nurse–patient relationships—but nurses now spend less time at the bedside than ever before. One reason is understaffing and heavier patient loads, but there are other factors: the use of technology; the need for careful documentation; and the emphasis on leading, managing, and delegating instead of hands-on patient care.
- *Autonomy versus escaping hard choices.* On the one hand, we believe nurses should have an equal status with other healthcare professionals; on the other hand, many nurses want to escape hard choices by "letting the provider decide."
- *Higher pay versus cost-effectiveness.* Most nurses believe we deserve higher pay—yet, we claim nurses are cost effective because we work less expensively than the primary providers.
- *Professionalism versus caring.* We claim the nurse is a professional, citing critical thinking, knowledge, and management skills—but on the other hand, we emphasize caring, with the nurse at the bedside offering comfort and doing hands-on tasks.

WHAT FACTORS AFFECT MORAL DECISIONS?

By now, you should have an idea of the nature of morals and ethics and of the need to study nursing ethics. We turn our focus now to some basic theoretical knowledge about factors that are involved in making ethical decisions: developmental stages, values, ethical frameworks, ethical principles, and professional guidelines. As you learn about these concepts, consider how each affects moral decision making.

Developmental Stage

A person's stage of moral development affects the way they reason about moral issues. We learn and internalize our morals throughout the life span, beginning in childhood.

Kohlberg Kohlberg's research (1968, 1981) led him to conclude that children go through a sequence of moral reasoning ability, proceeding through several stages (see the section "Moral Development Theory: Kohlberg" in Chapter 6 for an in-depth description of the stages).

- Stage I—Moral reasoning is based on personal interest and avoiding punishment.
- Stage II—Moral principles focus on pleasing others and following rules.
- Stage III—Moral principles are based on universal and impartial principles of justice. This is the final level; it occurs in adulthood.

The stages overlap. Kohlberg found that more than half of a person's thinking reflects the stage they are in, and the remainder reflects the stage they are leaving or the stage into which they are moving. Some people never achieve Kohlberg's highest levels, yet progression through the stages is always forward, never backward, except in extreme trauma; people do not skip stages.

Gilligan Gilligan (1993) challenged Kohlberg's perspective of moral development, citing it as male biased. Gilligan found through her research that girls develop morally by paying attention to community and to relationships, whereas boys tend to process dilemmas through more abstract ideals or principles. If you need a review of Gilligan's three stages—caring for oneself, caring for others, and caring for self and others—refer to Chapter 6.

Values, Attitudes, and Beliefs

Your values are entangled in all ethical situations because they influence what you think and do. This is important to know because your values unconsciously influence your moral judgment. If asked, could you identify your values and explain how they affect your views about right and wrong in a given situation? If so, that's a great beginning. If not, you will learn more as you move through this section.

What Are Values? A **value** is a belief about the worth of something; it serves as a principle or a standard that influences decision making.

- **Values are ideals, beliefs, customs, modes of conduct, qualities, or goals that are highly prized or preferred by individuals, groups, or society.** You can value an idea, a person, a way of doing things, or even an object (e.g., money).
- **People express their values through behaviors, feelings, knowledge, and decisions.** For example, the nurse who values compassion will interact with patients in a sensitive, caring manner.
- Your *value* set is your "list" of values. It gives direction for your life and forms a basis for behavior.
- Your *value system* is your value set ranked from the most to the least important value. Your value system begins to emerge shortly after birth and continues throughout your life as various sources (parents, teachers, religious figures, peers, and so on) influence your values.

- **The total number of values a person has is rather small.** The number of significant ones is even smaller, but they have a consistent and predictable impact on your actions (e.g., love, freedom, responsibility).
- **Values are highly individualized.**
- **Values can vary and change** with new experiences and thoughtful consideration. As you progress through your study of nursing, you will incorporate the professional values associated with the practice of a nurse (e.g., caring, compassion, human dignity). You will experience role conflict when your values are different from practice expectations.

KnowledgeCheck 5-3
- What are values?
- What are three characteristics of values?

ThinkLike a Nurse 5-3: Clinical Judgment in Action
- Think about what you value personally in your own life. What are the five ideals, principles, or things that are most important to you?
- Now refer to the previous bullet, where you were asked to list five ideals, principles, or things that were most important to you. What did you list? Do you anticipate that your list will change once you have gained more clinical experience and theoretical knowledge?

What Are Attitudes? **Attitudes** are mental dispositions or feelings toward a person, object, or idea. They can be cognitive (thinking), affective (feeling), and behavioral (doing). Attitudes are our way of responding to situations or things. For example, you might have a positive *attitude* about cleanliness—that is, you may think it is a good thing (e.g., "The floor is clean—that's nice"). But if you *value* cleanliness, you would be willing to scrub the floor. You would also wash your hands at appropriate times, bathe regularly, and teach others about hygiene.

What Are Beliefs? A **belief** is something that one accepts as true (e.g., "I believe that germs cause disease and that by washing my hands, I remove germs").

- Beliefs are sometimes based on faith and sometimes on facts.
- A belief may or may not be true.
- **Our beliefs can be altered by acquiring knowledge and experiences.** Research shows that nursing students' attitudes toward and beliefs about older adults changed when they spent quality time with older adults through team and interprofessional experiences (Neils-Strunjas et al., 2020).
- **Beliefs may or may not involve values.** Consider the following statements of belief.
  "I believe the Earth is round." (Does not involve a value)
  "Working hard to achieve goals is important to me; therefore, I believe that I must work during the summer to save money for college." (Involves a value)

How Are Values and Ethics Related? Values and morals are learned in conscious and unconscious ways and become a part of your makeup. When we evaluate right and wrong, or good and bad, we are using moral judgment. Therefore, our individual preferences (values) of right or wrong become our moral values. Whether or not you are aware of it, your values shape the manner in which you make ethical decisions in your nursing practice (Butts & Rich, 2020). **Key Point:** *It is important to clarify the influence of your values each time you enter into a situation in which you are called on to be objective in your decision making.*

ThinkLike a Nurse 5-4: Clinical Judgment in Action

- Think about Alan and his family (Meet Your Patients). What do you think were the values of Alan's parents that influenced their behavior at the hospital? First, identify their behaviors specifically. Then speculate about the values underlying each behavior.
- How do you think values can influence health?

KnowledgeCheck 5-4

- Define *belief*; give a new example.
- Define *attitude*; give a new example

Professional Versus Personal Values

Your **personal value system** is a set of values that you have reflected on and chosen that will help you to lead a good life (Doherty & Purtilo, 2021). You have internalized some *societal values* and have come to perceive them as your own (e.g., good manners, such as saying "please" and "thank you"). In addition, you probably have some *personal values* (e.g., friendship, fairness, creativity) that are important to you but may or may not be important to society at large.

As you move forward in your profession, you will integrate what you learn and experience to form **professional values,** such as those identified by the American Association of Colleges of Nursing (AACN). Many of these will simply expand your personal values (e.g., caring, veracity). **Personal and professional values are not always congruent.** Consider the situation in the following ethical scenario.

Ethical Scenario: Personal and Professional Values

Alexandra Jensen is a 17-year-old pregnant female patient who comes into your ambulatory surgical center for a voluntary termination of an early pregnancy. You are assigned to complete her preoperative care. Imagine that your personal value is that you do not believe patients should have an abortion. Yet, your professional value is guided by the ANA standards of professional practice, which require that the nurse provides holistic care that incorporate the "norms and values, health and illness perspectives and practices, customs, behaviors, and beliefs of the healthcare consumer (ANA, 2021).

How might you feel in this situation?

Do you think that your personal and professional values need to be compatible for you to be a competent nurse?

Do you think that you should have the absolute right to refuse to participate in a situation (such as the one involving Alexandra) that may violate your personal values?

How Are Values Transmitted?

Think about how values are transmitted to children (e.g., modeling, rewards, punishment). Table 5-1 outlines the methods of value transmission. Research supports the reciprocal transmission of values between parents and child, which is enhanced in the presence of a motivated, receptive, and supportive parent (Barni et al. 2017). Another study found that parents transmitted work values to their children during midadolescence to early adulthood. A strong association of extrinsic work values with those of the parents was found when the children were in their late 30s and when navigating career uncertainties (Johnson et al., 2019).

Nursing students develop professional values through education and clinical experiences. Research found that nursing students' top values were protecting patients' confidentiality and safeguarding their right to privacy. Other important values, such as confronting practitioners with inappropriate or questionable practices rank much lower (20 out of 26). Researchers concluded that the rules of clinical practice are the focus of undergraduate students (Poorchangizi et al., 2019). The importance of other professional values will emerge with experience and practice.

What Is Value Neutrality?

You have probably been taught that nurses need to be nonjudgmental in working with their patients. As a nurse, you do have a duty to provide the best care to patients. You should not assume that your personal values are right, and you should not judge patients' values as right or wrong on the basis of whether they agree with your value system. Think back to the ethical scenario regarding Alexandra, who was seeking to terminate her pregnancy. A nurse who does not believe that patients should have abortions could still provide competent nursing care to Alexandra even though their personal values are antiabortion.

Value neutrality means that we attempt to understand our own values regarding an issue and to know when to put them aside, if necessary, to become nonjudgmental when providing care to clients. However, many ethicists and some healthcare providers believe it is not possible to achieve value neutrality. Further, healthcare providers must acknowledge their own deepest moral

Table 5-1 ➤ Modes of Value Transmission

MODE	DESCRIPTION	RESULTS
Modeling	Children learn values from a variety of role models (parents, peers, rock stars, significant others) by observation.	Modeling can lead to socially acceptable or unacceptable behaviors.
Moralizing	"This way is the only way." Children are taught a complete set of values in an authoritarian approach. If the child does not conform, the parent may inflict guilt and fear on them.	This approach by parents, teachers, church leaders, and other authority figures may make it difficult for young people to make independent choices because they have no experience selecting values that are good for them.
Laissez-faire	"Doing your own thing." Children are allowed to explore differing sets of values on their own, with little guidance or discipline.	This may lead to conflict and confusion on the part of the child.
Reward and punishment	The child's behavior is controlled by offering rewards for certain valued behaviors and punishing the child who fails to comply.	Rewards can strengthen behavior, whereas physical punishment may teach that violence is an acceptable behavior.
Responsible choice	A balance of freedom and restriction allows children to select values, explore new behaviors, and experience the consequences.	Having choices can result in personal satisfaction and parental support.

and religious beliefs in delivering patient-centered professional care (Kørup et al., 2020). Highly controversial issues can decrease the degree of value neutrality (Lynöe et al., 2017); thus, you must recognize the impact on you to minimize ethical dilemmas. It requires significant insight to recognize how your value-laden perspective affects your perceptions and thus conclusion about a situation.

 Think**Like a Nurse** 5-5:
    Clinical Judgment **in Action**

- Name some examples of societal values.
- What groups and social experiences have helped to form your values?
- Examine your personal values to see whether they match the AACN's professional values.
  - Which of those values, if any, do you not share? Explain your thinking.
  - Name a few of your personal values that are not on this list of professional values.

KnowledgeCheck 5-5

- What is the difference between personal and professional values?
- What is an example of professional values?
- What are some other types of values?
- What are some ways that values can be transmitted?
- What is value neutrality?

Ethical Frameworks

Ethical (or **moral**) **frameworks** are systems of thought (theories) can explain the differing perspectives people have in ethical situations. Many of these frameworks are rooted in ancient works, for example, those of the Greek philosophers Plato and Aristotle.

There is no single "best" theory that will provide the one "true" answer to an ethical problem because each provides a different perspective. Using more than one framework to analyze a situation enables you to perform a more comprehensive analysis of the problem. **Key Point:** *No matter how well you know the theories, they will not provide the "right" answers for what to do in a specific patient situation. They merely offer a lens through which you can examine an ethical problem.* See Chapter 4 to review the purposes and use of theories.

What Is Consequentialism?

In **consequentialist** theories, the rightness or wrongness of an action depends on the consequences of the act rather than on the act itself. **Utilitarianism,** the most familiar consequentialist theory, asserts that the value of an action determines its usefulness. The **principle of utility** states that an act must result in the greatest good (positive benefit) for the greatest number of people. Any act can then become the ethical choice if it delivers "good" results. In healthcare, the principle of "first, do no harm" is consequentialist in nature. Because of this principle, we are concerned with weighing the risks and benefits of our care (e.g., a medication may kill cancer cells, but side effects may harm the patient's quality of life).

Using utilitarianism to address an ethical problem requires you to engage in a **risk–benefit analysis.**

- **Evaluate every alternative action** for its potential outcomes, both positive (pros) and negative (cons)—similar to a technique you may already use when making other decisions.

- **Then select the action that results in the most benefits** for the greatest number of people involved in the situation.

The following is an example of utilitarian reasoning: The practice of triage is used in a disaster when emergency workers sort patients to determine who will be treated first or who will receive the limited resources (e.g., oxygen or intravenous therapy). If a victim has little potential for survival, they may receive comfort care, or their treatment may be postponed, allowing the healthcare team to treat those victims with the greatest potential to survive (i.e., "benefit the greatest number").

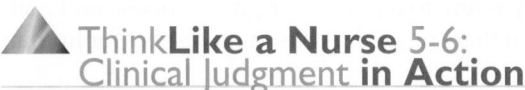

ThinkLike a Nurse 5-6: Clinical Judgment in Action

- Describe a time in your life when you used consequentialism to resolve a difficult situation.
- What types of clinical dilemmas might be best resolved using this theory?

What Is Deontology?

Unlike the utilitarian theory, **deontology** uses rules, principles, and standards to determine whether an action is right or wrong. The consequences of the act are not the major considerations. Many of the deontological theories share similar principles:

Rights and Duties Major concepts derived from deontological frameworks are rights (e.g., the right to freedom, the right of self-determination) and duties (obligations). Nurses have a duty to help others and accept the patient's decision, even if it produces some undesirable consequences. Think back to the possible outcome if Alan Frese (Meet Your Patients) does not receive a blood transfusion.

Treat People as Ends and Never as Means This means that the person is more important than the goal you may be trying to accomplish. Can you imagine the ethical concerns created if research subjects were exposed to intolerable risk (e.g., a new surgical procedure) to find a drug or treatment that will benefit many other people?

Ethical Rules and Principles An analysis of a situation to determine which actions are right or wrong uses ethical rules and principles, such as justice, autonomy, doing good, and doing no harm. These principles come from universal values that underlie all major religions and are regarded as unchanging and absolute.

The Categorical Imperative This principle, established by the philosopher Immanuel Kant (1724–1804), states that one should act only if the action is based on a principle that is universal—or in other words, if you believe that everyone should act in the same way in a similar situation.

Additional Considerations The following are two issues that may arise when using a deontology framework:

- **Conflict of Universal Principles.** Sometimes you must choose between conflicting universal principles. It is not always clear which principle to honor. Allowing Alan's parents (Meet Your Patients) to refuse to provide him with blood honors the principle of autonomy, but their decision may interfere with a right: Alan's right to life. Can you see that it might be difficult to decide the appropriate principle to honor?
- **Evaluating Motives.** In deontology, it is important to consider motives. It is one thing for Alan's parents to refuse a blood transfusion because they are honoring a religious principle; it would be quite another thing if they refused the transfusion because they stood to inherit a large trust fund left to Alan by his grandfather. Motives may place more weight on one of the conflicting universal principles than the other, which makes a decision clearer. Unfortunately, it is sometimes hard to recognize your own motives, much less to be sure about the motives of others.

Key Point: *As a nurse, you will always need to consider the consequences of your actions; you will almost never be able to decide based only on principles and rules.*

KnowledgeCheck 5-6

- Describe utilitarianism.
- Define *deontology*.

What Is Feminist Ethics?

Feminist ethics encompass the belief that traditional ethical models provide a mostly masculine perspective that devalues the moral experience of women (Butts & Rich, 2020). Virtues such as love, relationships, caring, nurturing, and sympathy are more relevant but usually omitted in traditional theories that focus on abstract principles such as fairness, justice, and rights. Feminist ethical reasoning uses relationships and stories rather than universal principles. Advocates of this theory argue that the influence of relationships is positive and should not be lessened by an attempt at objectivity, which is seen as impossible to achieve.

Feminist theories contain principles and consequences, but they also ask you to look at gendered, cultural, and socially diverse issues in the ethical situation, especially those involving women (Morley et al., 2019; Pullen & Vachhani, 2021). The point is to address issues of gender inequality within each situation. This example shows how the issue of gender influences the reasoning process:

A group is deciding whether to allocate federally funded healthcare resources to younger people or to older adults. Feminist reasoning might say that, all other considerations being equal:

- *In the United States, older women outnumber older men.*
- *Older women tend to be poorer and are more likely to be alone than are older men.*

- Therefore, if healthcare for older adults were to be rationed, it would negatively affect women more than men.
- Thus, more healthcare resources should be allocated to older adults, especially women.

♥ iCare What Is Ethics of Care?

An **ethics-of-care** nursing philosophy directs attention to the specific situations of individual patients, viewed within the context of their life narrative. You would ask, "What is the story of this person's life? What is going on right now in their life? And what does that have to do with the morality of the action I'm considering?" Care theories (which grew out of feminist ethics) integrate the notion that caring is a natural human quality with the commitment and responsibility that you assume by entering into a helping profession (Leget et al., 2019; Schuchter & Heller, 2017). Care is not viewed as an obligation (deontology, utilitarianism) but as a responsibility based on your relationship with the person. An ethics of care emphasizes the role of feelings (the art of nursing) but also includes some of the principles that are part of traditional ethics, such as *autonomy* (self-determination) or *beneficence* (doing good), responsibility, and commitment.

Using an ethics-of-care perspective, you would ask the question, "How do I best care for this client?" Consider the guidance provided by the ANA *Code of Ethics* as you plan your care. Some aspects of care include the ability and duty to appreciate, understand, and even share the client's pain or condition. The following guidance is derived from an ethics-of-care philosophy (Leget et al., 2019; Schuchter & Heller, 2017):

- Caring is viewed as a central responsibility for nurses.
- Knowing the client's story promotes dignity and respect for the client as a person.
- Your relationship and professional competence allow you to meet the client's needs.
- You should cultivate a habit of care that includes virtues such as kindness, attentiveness, empathy, compassion, and reliability.

The following is a question that reflects this model of reasoning: Should we provide free medical care to the homeless? A person with an ethics-of-care perspective would probably say yes, even though that might not, for example, provide the greatest good for the greatest number of people. Ethics-of-care models provide a refreshingly new perspective on ethical situations. As you gain more clinical experience, revisit these philosophies and reflect on how they apply to your nursing practice.

KnowledgeCheck 5-7

- How does feminist ethics affect ethical decision making?
- What do ethics-of-care philosophies emphasize?

Ethical Concepts and Principles

Remember from Chapter 4 that concepts and principles make up theories. The same is true for ethical theories. Ethical concepts and principles are useful in patient care discussions because they provide a common language for healthcare professionals to identify the issues. **Key Point:** *Even if people disagree about which action is right in a situation, they can agree on which principles apply. Agreement "in principle" can provide common ground for a compromise or other resolution of the problem.* The following ethical principles are used in healthcare.

Autonomy

Autonomy refers to a person's right to choose and ability to act on that choice. It is based on respect for human dignity.

- You demonstrate respect for autonomy when you:
  - Treat clients with consideration.
  - Believe clients' stories about the course and symptoms of their illnesses.
  - Protect those who are unable to decide for themselves.
  - Protect privacy and confidentiality.
- You honor autonomy when you respect the client's or surrogate decision maker's right to decide, without judgment, even when you believe those choices are not in the client's best interest.

In the Meet Your Patients scenario, if you believed autonomy to be the most important principle in the situation, you would respect Alan's parents' decision to refuse blood products for their son. If respect for autonomy were not your dominant ethical principle, you would probably try to persuade them to change their minds.

Informed Consent The principle of autonomy incorporates informed consent—the right of competent patients to decide whether to agree to a proposed treatment. **Key Point:** *Remember this general nursing principle: "Every competent adult has the right to accept or refuse treatment and should be provided all the information needed to make an informed decision."*

To ensure truly informed consent, patients need to know the diagnosis and related information, the recommended treatment, alternative treatment options, the risks and benefits associated with each, and the providers involved in the treatment regimen. The nurse's role is to verify that the patient understands and to obtain their signature. **Key Point:** *The nurse should notify the provider if the patient does not understand the treatment, before obtaining their signature.* To promote autonomy, you should educate clients and encourage them to formulate advance directives to ensure they have a voice in their long-term treatment. Advance directives (e.g., living will, durable power of attorney for healthcare) allow adults, while they are competent, to make decisions about their healthcare that will guide their care when they are no longer able to do so on their own.

Ethical Scenario: Autonomy

The surgeon explained the surgical procedure to Mr. Epkey, who then signed the consent form. You are aware that the surgeon omitted essential information about the risks and postoperative care. In response to your concerns, the supervisor says, "Don't worry about it. He is extremely paternalistic and doesn't want his patients to worry. Besides, he always has excellent outcomes." What would you do in this situation? If unsure, what information would you need to determine a course of action?

Privacy and Confidentiality The principles of **privacy** and **confidentiality** are also partly derived from the principle of autonomy. An autonomous person has control over the collection of, use of, and access to their personal information. Clients share sensitive information with nurses that they would not share with others based on the nurse–client relationship. To maintain that trust, you should:

- **Discuss information relevant to client care in approved areas** (conference rooms, bedside) and not in areas where others can overhear you (e.g., hallways, cafeterias, elevators).
- **Share information with team members who have a need to know** based on their involvement in client care.
- **Obtain the client's consent** before providing information to family members or friends.
- **Never post pictures of clients on social media sites.** Even inadvertently capturing patients in photographs has led to harsh disciplinary actions against the nurse.

Key Point: *A person who knowingly violates the privacy and confidentiality requirements of the Health Insurance Portability and Accountability Act (HIPAA) can incur civil penalties of $50,000 per violation up to a maximum of $1.5 million per violation category per year and criminal penalties of up to 1 year in prison or more based on the extent of the violation (Alder, 2021).*

If you would like more information about privacy and confidentiality, see Chapters 17 and 39.

Nonmaleficence

The principle of **nonmaleficence** is the twofold duty to (1) do no harm and (2) prevent harm. It encompasses actual harm, risk of harm, and intentional and unintentional harm. Both the physicians' Hippocratic Oath and the nurses' Nightingale Pledge state that care providers have a duty to cause no harm to patients.

> *When you are careful to prevent medication errors or use an ambulation belt for assisting patients to walk, you honor the nonmaleficence principle.*

It is rare in nursing to find intentional harm, but unintentional harm does occur, primarily from failure to follow the rights of medication administration.

Key Point: *Nonmaleficence requires that you think critically and identify the potential risks and benefits of the treatment plan. You should then analyze whether the treatment causes more harm than good.*

- **Risk of harm is not always clear.** Suppose you are about to get a patient out of bed for the first time after surgery to prevent postoperative complications such as pneumonia and thrombophlebitis. However, the risks, in terms of excessive pain or unintentional damage to the operative site, may be less clear.
- **Weighing risks and benefits is a value-laden exercise.** Who determines whether pain is excessive—you or the patient? To honor the principle of nonmaleficence in this situation, you would need to have theoretical knowledge of the potential postoperative complications, be sure to premedicate the patient, and carefully assess their status during ambulation.

Respect for dignity refers to the nurse's respect for the intrinsic worth of each person, without respect to age, race, religion, medical condition, gender identification, or any other factors. This is an essential value in nursing. You must recognize that patients are vulnerable and not exploit that vulnerability for personal gain. Avoid inappropriate sexual or romantic relationships or other breaches of professional boundaries. To learn more about professional boundaries, search online for the National Council of State Boards of Nursing Web site, look for the publication *A Nurse's Guide to Professional Boundaries,* or

 Go to https://www.ncsbn.org/ProfessionalBoundaries_Complete.pdf

Think**Like a Nurse** 5-7: Clinical Judgment **in Action**

Think about the Meet Your Patients scenario in terms of nonmaleficence. The parents refuse to allow a blood transfusion. You, the nurse, have tried to persuade them to change their minds. You do not need to decide what you ought to do—just analyze the situation in terms of the risks.

- What is it that creates the risk of harm to Alan?
- What is the risk of harm to Alan's parents because of the nurse's actions?

Beneficence

Beneficence is the duty to do or promote good. You can think of this principle as being on a continuum with nonmaleficence. At one end of the continuum is beneficence, the duty to bring about positive good; at the other end is the duty to do no harm. The following examples illustrate the duties in priority order:

- **Do no harm.** (Do not administer the wrong medication to a patient.)
- **Prevent harm when you can.** (If you notice a nurse violating the rights of administration, warn them that this can result in a medication error.)

- **Remove harm** when it is being inflicted. (Remove unattended medications left at the patient's bedside.)
- **Bring about positive good.** (Follow up with the patient's nurse to ensure the patient receives their medication.)

When weighing the risks and benefits of an action, you are actually balancing nonmaleficence with beneficence. Keep in mind that clients, family members, and other professionals may identify benefits and harms differently. A benefit to one may represent a burden to another. For example, in the Meet Your Patients scenario, you may see a blood transfusion as a benefit to Alan, but to the parents, it may represent harm. Doing good very much depends on the context and the rights of the person for whom the action is being taken.

Paternalism Although viewed by some as beneficence, **paternalism** (treating others like children) can have negative consequences. For example, you will lose the client's trust if you coerce the client to act based on what you think you know is best rather than what the client wishes. Saying, "Trust us; we know what is best for you to do in this situation," may seem to be beneficent because you are trying to support the client and relieve anxiety. However, this paternalistic behavior lacks respect for the patient's autonomy (and therefore represents harm) (Fig. 5-2).

Fidelity

Fidelity (faithfulness) is the duty to keep promises. It is a basic part of every nurse–client relationship. Sometimes the promises are of major significance, such as promising not to share certain information with other members of the healthcare team. At other times it may be only a promise to come back to provide a requested item or check the effectiveness of a pain medication.

In practice, you will often find that competing tasks prevent you from being able to deliver something exactly as you have promised. Instead of "I'll be right back with your medication," you might say, "I'll get back with your medication as quickly as I can," or "I

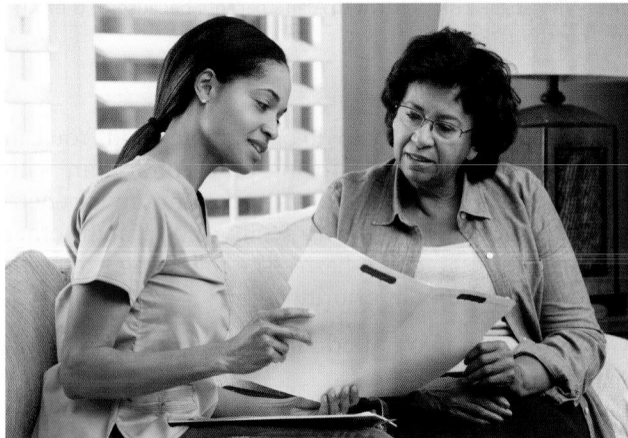

FIGURE 5-2 Nurse involves the patient in her plan of care.

must go help another client, but I'll get here with your medication as quickly as I can."

Key Point: *The duty to keep a promise is the same regardless of its level of importance. Make promises in a thoughtful, careful manner to maximize the likelihood that you can keep them.*

Veracity

Veracity is the duty to tell the truth. This seems straightforward, and most nurses would agree that it is not hard to tell the truth. However, there are times when veracity presents a challenge, and it may be very hard to determine how *much* of the truth to tell.

Example. Healthcare professionals may feel uncomfortable giving families "bad news." So instead of saying, "Your father has a fatal illness and is unlikely to live for more than a month," they may say, "Your father is very ill, but we will do everything we possibly can for him."

In this, as in most situations, the risk of losing patient trust outweighs any benefit of withholding the truth.

Although you always presume the value of telling the truth, there may be times when you are justified to withhold information. The dominant culture of the United States tends to place a high value on autonomy. However, some families go to great lengths to protect a dying patient from the harsh truth of their prognosis, and the patient may not wish to know. In such a situation, you need to be culturally sensitive so that your care incorporates the family's personal values and not the dominant cultural values. **Key Point:** *Always consider the context.*

Ethical Scenario: Veracity

Mr. Chung, 89 years old, had a stroke during hip surgery 2 days ago. His prognosis is poor, and the family made him a DNAR. His two sons and daughter visit daily from breakfast to after dinner. They explain that their father has sacrificed so much for them, and it is important to them that they are present when he passes. Mr. Chung's condition starts to deteriorate at 0200, and you notify the family. They ask you to remain with their father until they arrive. When you return to the room after checking on another patient, Mr. Chung has died. The family arrives 15 minutes later and is grief-stricken. When asked if he died alone, you tell them that you were present and holding his hand. They are very relieved, knowing that you were there. What would you have done in this situation? Would you tell the truth when you know that it would cause distress to the family? Is there an alternate approach?

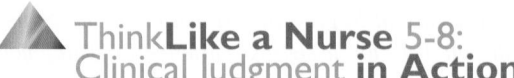

ThinkLike a Nurse 5-8: Clinical Judgment in Action

Review the Meet Your Patients scenario. Alan will not survive without a blood transfusion, yet the parents refuse to allow one. He asks the nurse, "Am I going to die?" You do not need to decide which response is best; just write an example that illustrates each of the following. What would you say in each of these scenarios?

- Tell Alan the truth.
- Withhold or partially disclose the truth.
- Answer with an untruth.

Justice

Justice is the obligation to be fair. It implies equal treatment of all patients. Questions of justice will become a part of your everyday experience in patient care, from deciding how to allocate your time among patients to larger decisions, such as how to allocate limited healthcare resources. Justice can be distributive, compensatory, or procedural in focus.

Distributive Justice Distributive justice requires a fair distribution of both benefits and burdens (Butts & Rich, 2020). It is especially relevant to healthcare, as in the following issues:

- **Allocating Resources**. Distributive justice questions come up when more than one person or group competes for the same resources (e.g., human organ for transplantation). How do we decide which patient should receive an available organ? Is an 18-year-old more deserving of a kidney than a 75-year-old? Is a person with liver disease due to alcoholism less deserving of a liver than someone with liver disease caused by a birth defect? The decision of who should live and who may die is never an easy decision. In the United States, a national committee sets criteria for who receives organs, so the standard of justice is considered.
- **Fair Access to Care**. Access to care is a specific kind of healthcare resource. The principle of distributive justice holds that we should provide equal access to healthcare for all. As nurses from the baby boomer generation retire, there may be fewer nurses to care for more aging patients at a time of decreasing national healthcare dollars. How will the nation decide where to spend the limited dollars? How will nurse managers decide how to provide adequate care if they do not have enough staff nurses? The ability to develop sound criteria on which to allocate resources is the challenge of distributive justice.

Compensatory Justice Compensatory justice focuses on making amends for wrongs that have been done to individuals or groups. Malpractice lawsuits consider this type of justice when they decide how much money to award a victim for the harm incurred. The goal is to make the person "whole."

Procedural Justice Procedural justice is important in processes that require ranking or ordering (Dunham et al., 2018). For example, written institutional policies are to ensure that the same procedures apply to all clients or employees in the same way (e.g., visiting hours, working on holidays, sick leave). Can you think of an example of procedural justice that you have experienced during your nursing education?

ThinkLike a Nurse 5-9: Clinical Judgment in Action

Look again at the emergency department situation described in What Is Nursing Ethics? at the beginning of this chapter. In this scenario, two little boys received treatment for lacerations. Which principle of justice was violated: distributive, compensatory, or procedural? Explain your thinking.

KnowledgeCheck 5-8

Define each of the six ethical principles.

Professional Guidelines

You should consult professional guidelines when making ethical decisions. Healthcare professionals have an obligation to society to be competent in their field, to allow only qualified persons entry into the profession, to discipline members of the profession who do not practice at an acceptable level, to do no harm, and to use high moral and ethical standards to resolve dilemmas (Forte et al., 2018; Husted et al., 2015). You can find ethical standards for nurses in codes of ethics, standards of practice, statements of patients' rights, and various laws.

Nursing Codes of Ethics

Professional codes of ethics are formal statements of a group's expectations and standards for professional behavior generally accepted by members of the profession. Codes of ethics set forth ideal behaviors, but they are only as effective as the behaviors of the nurses who live up to the codes.

The purposes of the nursing codes of ethics are to:

- Inform the public about the profession's minimum standards.
- Demonstrate nursing's commitment to the public it serves.
- Outline major ethical considerations of nursing.
- Provide general guidelines for professional behavior.
- Guide the profession's self-regulating functions.
- Remind us of the special responsibility we assume in caring for the sick.

Nursing codes are not legally binding. However, they often exceed legal obligations. In most states, the state board of nursing uses the nursing code of ethics as the standard against which to evaluate a nurse's ethical behavior. The board has the legal authority to censure or reprimand the nurse who does not practice within the boundaries of ethical practice. The following nursing organizations have had long-standing codes to guide nurses' ethical decision-making. The codes differ in specific details but have similar principles.

International Council of Nurses The International Council of Nurses (ICN) adopted its *Code of Ethics for Nurses* as "a guide for action based on social values and needs" (ICN, revised 2012). It serves as the standard for nurses worldwide. It stresses respect for human rights, including cultural rights; the right to life and choice; the right to dignity; and the right to be treated with respect. The *Code of Ethics* guides nurses in everyday choices and supports their refusal to participate in activities that conflict with caring and healing. If you wish to see the revised code, you can search for *The ICN Code of Ethics for Nurses,* or

 Go to the ICN Web site at https://www.icn.ch/sites/ default/files/inline-files/2012_ICN_Codeofethicsfornurses_ %20eng.pdf

The American Nurses Association The ANA's *Code of Ethics for Nurses* "establishes the ethical standard for the profession" and serves as a "guide for nurses to use in ethical analysis and decision making" (2015, p. vii). The code has nine provisions, followed by interpretive statements to explain each provision. If you would like more information about the ANA *Code,*

 Go to the ANA Web site at https://www.nursingworld.org/ coe-view-only

ANA Standards of Care

In addition to its *Code of Ethics*, the ANA sets standards for all aspects of clinical practice. In *Nursing: Scope and Standards of Practice* (2021), standard 7 focuses on ethical practice. This standard directs nurses to practice within the parameters described in the *Code of Ethics for Nurses*. Standard 7 speaks to the nurse's responsibilities to patients and directs nurses to contribute to the establishment and maintenance of an ethical environment.

The Patient Care Partnership

When admitted to hospitals or to extended care facilities, patients are entitled to specific rights in terms of their treatment—the right to:

- Make their own decisions.
- Be active partners in the treatment process.
- Be treated with dignity and respect.

Because rights are rooted in values, and values are derived from culture, patient rights are different throughout the world. The American Hospital Association (AHA) published *The Patient Care Partnership* (2003). Instead of using "rights" language, this document focuses on patient expectations and responsibilities. *The Patient Care Partnership* encourages healthcare providers to be more aware of the need to treat patients in an ethical manner and to protect their rights (Box 5-1).

The Joint Commission Accreditation Standards

The Joint Commission standards contain sections on organizational ethics and individual rights. The section on organizational ethics requires ethical behavior in care, treatment, services, and business practices. Consider the

---

BOX 5-1 ■ American Hospital Association: *The Patient Care Partnership*

Patients, when hospitalized, should expect the following:

- High-quality care, including the right to know the identity of caregivers
- A clean, safe environment, including safety, freedom from abuse and neglect, and discussion of any changes in care
- Respect for healthcare goals, values, and spiritual beliefs
- To be involved in making decisions about their care and treatment. This includes receiving information about:

  Health condition and treatments

  The benefits and risks of treatments and whether a treatment is experimental or part of a research study

  What the patient and family will need to do regarding treatment follow-up after leaving the hospital

- Information about the right to make decisions and the right to refuse care, including advance directives and counselors or chaplains available to help with decision making
- Protection of privacy and confidentiality
- Help reviewing the bill and filing insurance claims
- Preparation and information when leaving the hospital, including:

  Identification of sources for follow-up care and whether the hospital has a financial interest in any of the referrals

  Coordination of hospital activities with caregivers outside the hospital

  Information and training about the self-care the person will need at home

Source: Excerpted and adapted from American Hospital Association. (2003). *The patient care partnership: Understanding expectations, rights and responsibilities.* Chicago: Author.

---

patient's values, preferences, need for information, and other factors that promote autonomy in the plan of care. You must initiate actions to meet the patient's needs before transfers or referrals. Always consider the organization's legal responsibility to patients.

KnowledgeCheck 5-9

- How would you use a professional guideline or code of ethics to assist in the ethical decision-making process?
- What are some examples of such resources?

ETHICAL ISSUES IN HEALTHCARE

As a nurse, you are likely to encounter several ethical issues that occur in healthcare. For example, ethical questions arise in the following situations:

Abortion
Advance directives
Allocation of healthcare goods and services

Compelling unwanted treatment

Confidentiality and privacy (e.g., reporting gunshot wounds and child abuse)

DNAR/allow natural death (AND) prescriptions

Medical aid in dying/continuous palliative sedation

Organ transplantation

Withdrawing or withholding life-sustaining treatments (e.g., ventilators, artificial nutrition, and hydration)

Refer to an ethics text or ethics course for an extended discussion of these and other ethical issues. They are beyond the scope of a fundamentals text.

PracticalKnowledge
knowing how

To fulfill your professional obligations for ethical practice, you will need practical knowledge of the processes of values clarification, ethical decision making, patient advocacy, and integrity-producing compromise.

ASSESSMENT/ANALYSIS/DIAGNOSIS NP

A holistic, comprehensive patient assessment will help you establish the context for making ethical decisions. For patients struggling with ethical issues, the following diagnoses may apply:

- **Decisional Conflict**—Use this label when the patient is uncertain about which course of action to take. The patient may verbalize distress and uncertainty, may delay decision-making, may show physical signs of distress (e.g., increased heart rate), and may question moral rules and values and personal beliefs.
- **Moral Distress**—Use this label when the patient has made a moral decision but is unable to carry out the chosen action. Cues include expressions of powerlessness, guilt, frustration, anxiety, self-doubt, and fear.

NANDA-I also lists other diagnoses in the Value/Belief/Action Congruence class, including the following: Impaired Religiosity, Readiness for Enhanced Religiosity, Risk for Impaired Religiosity, Powerlessness, Risk for Powerlessness, Spiritual Distress, Risk for Spiritual Distress, and Readiness for Enhanced Spiritual Well-Being.

VALUES CLARIFICATION

Values clarification refers to the process of becoming conscious of and naming one's values (Witteman et al., 2021). If you are clear about your values, you will be better able to make good decisions and avoid imposing your values on others. Because each person has a unique values set, it is important that you appreciate how others' values influence their decisions. Clarifying values should be a positive process of growth that results in more awareness, empathy, and insight (Good Therapy,

2019). **Key Point:** *A values-clarification process does not tell you what your values ought to be; it merely helps you discover what they are.* Values change over time, so you may need to repeat the process more than once in your lifetime.

How Can I Clarify My Values?

As a nurse, you will need to examine your values regarding life, death, wellness, and illness. A good place to start is to think about situations in which you may be uncomfortable, such as caring for a patient who molested a 5-year-old child; an unwed adolescent mother pregnant for the second time in 11 months; or parents such as the Freses (Meet Your Patients), who refuse treatment for a child because of religious beliefs. Ask yourself questions such as:

- Could I take care of this person?
- Does this bother me?
- What would I do if confronted with such a situation?
- Could I provide the same quality care as for my other patients?

How Can I Help Patients to Clarify Their Values?

Some clients may exhibit behaviors that indicate that their values are not clear. Consider the following scenario.

Ethical Scenario: Clarifying Values

Jon White is the chief executive officer of a large healthcare facility. Jon has had two myocardial infarctions (heart attacks) in the past 5 years. He also has hypercholesterolemia (high cholesterol) and hypertension (high blood pressure). Jon's provider has prescribed a heart medicine, low-dose aspirin, and medications to control his hypertension and cholesterol. Jon previously had several educational sessions about his diet, medications, and activity. He insists he is compliant. Jon's wife tells you that he has stopped exercising and is eating whatever he wants, including saturated fats. Jon tells her it is okay to eat what he wants because he is taking a "cholesterol-buster" pill. What are your immediate feelings about Jon? Do you think he values health?

The following behaviors may indicate that a patient needs values clarification:

- Ignoring the advice of a health professional
- Patient's words not consistent with their actions
- Numerous admissions for the same problem
- Uncertainty or confusion about which action to take

Which of those behaviors did Jon exhibit? To help Jon clarify his values, you might ask him to list the three things that are most important to him in life. You can also help him work through the steps in Table 5-2 (choosing, prizing, and acting).

Table 5-2 ➤ Values Clarification

STEP AND DESCRIPTION	QUESTIONS TO ASK YOUR PATIENT
Choosing (cognitive)	
Beliefs are chosen: Freely (allows you to cherish your choice) From alternatives After considering all consequences (ensures that the alternative is right for you)	▪ Do (did) you have any choice about what you do? ▪ Do you have any control over what happens? ▪ What have you decided to do? ▪ Can you list some alternative actions? ▪ What are your options? ▪ What could you do instead of ...? ▪ What do you think will happen if you do that? ▪ What will you gain by doing that? ▪ What is the disadvantage of doing that?
Prizing (affective)	
Beliefs and behaviors that are chosen are prized: With pride (feeling good about your choice) With public affirmation	▪ How do you feel about your decision? ▪ People sometimes feel good after making such a decision. Others feel pressured. How is it for you? ▪ How do you intend to tell your family (friends) about this decision? ▪ What will you say to your spouse (friends, family)? ▪ When will you announce your decision to ...?
Acting (behavioral)	
Beliefs are acted on: By incorporating the choice into one's own behavior With consistency and repetition	Try to determine whether the client will act on the decision: ▪ How do you think your spouse (significant other) will react when you do that? ▪ When will you actually carry out this decision? ▪ Try to predict consistent behavior by asking: ▪ How many times in the past have you ...? ▪ What kind of schedule have you worked out? ▪ How often and when will you ...?

Source: Adapted from Raths, L. E., Harmin, M., & Simon, S. B. (1978). *Values and teaching: Working with values in the classroom.* Merrill; Good Therapy. (2019). *Values clarification.* https://www.goodtherapy.org/learn-about-therapy/issues/values-clarification

KnowledgeCheck 5-10

▪ What does the term *values clarification* mean?
▪ What are the steps in values clarification?

ETHICAL DECISION MAKING

Decision models used in bioethics do not offer easy decisions, but they do provide a guiding structure to help you arrive at the best answer in specific situations. Decision models can help you decide on a course of action even if they do not tell you absolutely that the action is right or wrong.

How Can I Recognize Ethical Issues? We have said it is important to be aware of the ethical issues in patient care situations, but how will you recognize them? **Key Point:** *The key is that one or more of the following conflicts exists:*

▪ About the right action to take
▪ Among the duties and obligations of healthcare professionals (or they are unclear)

- Between the needs and interests of an individual and a group of clients
- Between what the family wants and what the client wants or needs
- Between the family and health professionals
- Among ethical principles or values (e.g., autonomy versus nonmaleficence, as in the Meet Your Patients scenario)

Problem or Dilemma?

In the best of all possible worlds, you could easily apply ethical principles and decide what to do. However, in situations involving morals, one ethical principle often conflicts with another equally important principle. It is also possible for a philosophical framework to produce more than one acceptable option. An **ethical dilemma** is a situation in which a choice is required between two equally undesirable actions. There is no clearly right or wrong option.

Such situations are emotionally painful for everyone involved, as you can see from the Meet Your Patients scenario at the beginning of this chapter. If you support Alan's parents' right to refuse a blood transfusion, you honor the principle of autonomy, but at the expense of the principle of nonmaleficence, which says we should prevent harm to Alan.

Fortunately, not all ethical problems are dilemmas, nor are they all complex and difficult. You may only occasionally confront a true dilemma and are more likely to encounter ethical questions or problems. For example, you can easily answer this question: "Should I take the patient's morphine to relieve my back pain?" Only problems that pose a question between competing and equally valuable interests are true dilemmas.

Key Point: *Ethical behavior and decision making do not deal only with dilemmas. They really involve choosing to be ethical in the everyday aspects of your practice.* For example, ethical actions include treating colleagues and patients with respect, not passing by a room when you see a patient crying, helping out a new graduate who is frustrated and anxious, and adhering to your commitment to the employer.

Ethical Scenario: Ethical Behavior

Your nursing unit is extremely short-staffed due to unexpected retirements and resignations. You had planned to request four additional days after your scheduled time off to spend six days at an inclusive resort with your fiancé before he goes on an extended deployment. The chief nursing officer has denied all PTO requests, explaining that ensuring adequate staff is a top priority. Your physician friend has offered to write you a sick note to cover the four days. What would you do in this situation? What is the ethical action?

How Do I Work Through an Ethical Problem?

Once you have identified an ethical problem, a decision model can help you logically decide the best action to take. Still, in the case of a true ethical dilemma, you will probably not be comfortable with any course of action, no matter how logically you think it through.

Ethical decision-making models will help you carefully consider several perspectives, guide your reasoning, and explain the reasons for your final action. Each approach may produce a different solution. One of the easiest to remember and use is the MORAL model. This model has been credited to two different authors: Thiroux (1977) and Crisham (1985). The letters in *MORAL* will remind you of the steps in this model, which is described in the following section. To use the model in clinical settings,

 Go to Chapter 5, Clinical Insight 5-1: Using the MORAL Model for Ethical Decision Making, in Volume 2.

First, Use Problem-Solving

As a first step in ethical decision making, use a systematic approach, such as the nursing process, to describe the problem and alternative approaches:

- **Assessment—What are the relevant facts?** Alan needs a blood transfusion to survive. Both you and the surgeon have tried to persuade the parents to consent, but they still refuse. The parents' religion prohibits blood transfusions. Alan is 15 years old (a minor), so you cannot administer a transfusion without his parents' consent.
- **Analysis/Diagnosis—Identify the problem; state the conflict.** There is a values conflict: the healthcare professionals value preserving physical life; the parents place more value on preserving the soul. There is an ethical dilemma, as well: if no transfusion is given, you violate the principle of nonmaleficence (harm to Alan); if you somehow coerce the parents to consent, you have violated the principle of autonomy (respect for their values and their freedom to choose). Therefore, the decision is whether to (1) follow the parents' wishes, (2) find a legal way to transfuse without their consent, or (3) find some compromise that will work.

Next, Use the MORAL Model

Now use the MORAL model to come up with alternative solutions for the Frese family.

M—MASSAGE THE DILEMMA

1. **First identify and define the issues in the dilemma, and consider the values and options of all the major players:** Mr. and Mrs. Frese, Alan, the surgeon, you (the nurse), and possibly a member of the clergy or a legal counselor. You have already

identified the values in the problem-solving approach: physical life versus spiritual life. You and the surgeon also value the principles of autonomy and nonmaleficence.

2. **Then identify the information gaps.** In massaging the situation, you should ask yourself:

   - Do I fully understand the situation that is causing the need for blood?
   - How much time is available to make this decision— is there time for the parents to consult with their congregational elders?
   - Does the surgeon have alternative treatment options available to stabilize Alan while the parents discuss the situation?
   - Does the surgeon know that the family members are Jehovah's Witnesses?
   - Do Alan's parents fully understand the nature of Alan's physical emergency?
   - In the Freses' religious view, what is the consequence of receiving blood?
   - Do they understand the consequences if blood is not administered?
   - Has Alan discussed in the past how he feels about blood transfusions? Have they ever had family discussions when other young Jehovah's Witnesses faced such a decision? Where did Alan stand in those discussions?
   - How is this situation like other situations they have experienced in their lives?
   - Have they thought about their opposing duties: the duty to uphold their religious values and the duty to protect their son from harm?
   - Has everyone voiced their opinions?
   - Have the parents contacted their congregational elders and discussed the situation?
   - What emotions are coming into play in this situation?
   - How is this decision affecting the parents as individuals? Are they in agreement on the issue, or is there dissension? If there is dissension, are both sides supported fairly?
   - Is there some common ground between what the surgeon wants and what the parents feel they need to do to uphold their religious convictions?

O—OUTLINE THE OPTIONS

At this step in the MORAL model, you or others (e.g., charge nurse, ethics committee member) should outline the options to all parties, including those that are less realistic and conflicting. You might ask a member of the ethics committee or the hospital chaplain to help the family and the doctor understand the opposing viewpoints.

The surgeon needs to outline the state of emergency that exists for Alan and explain what the limited medical options are: to transfuse blood or, if no blood is given, what other treatments are available (e.g., volume enhancers). The surgeon will need to inform the parents of the consequences of each action and the time frame for a decision based on Alan's condition.

The family (or the congregational elders) should explain to the surgeon and nurse the basis for their refusal to consent and what they believe are the consequences of blood administration.

R—RESOLVE THE DILEMMA

Now carefully review the issues and options. Apply basic ethical principles. If you can, also look at the situation using alternate ethical frameworks.

- **Autonomy.** By their refusing to give consent, the Freses are exercising their *autonomy*. How far will we go to honor their autonomy?
- **Beneficence and Nonmaleficence.** How are we defining "good" (*beneficence*) and "harm" (*nonmaleficence*) in this situation? The surgeon defines "good" as Alan receiving the needed blood. He defines "harm" as the outcome for Alan without the blood, even if he uses a less effective alternative. Alan's parents would define "good" as following their religious mandates and making sure their son will remain pure in the eyes of God. They might explain that a Jehovah's Witness who willingly accepts a blood transfusion might forfeit their eternal life. The Freses might believe the taking of blood to be more harmful than death because they believe that would affect Alan's eternal life, not just his physical life.
- **Fidelity.** The surgeon is being loyal (exhibiting *fidelity*) to the principles of medicine and evidence-based practice, which mandate the administration of the blood. To the parents, their loyalty to their religious principles to ensure that Alan has eternal life may be more important than the loss of the physical life itself.
- **Veracity.** The principle of *veracity* holds that the surgeon should not exaggerate the need for the blood, and he should be honest with the parents in terms of the consequences of the alternative actions. Another question of veracity involves the parents: Are they being honest with each other regarding their feelings?

Your role as a nurse is to be an advocate for the patient and the family. Talk with the family and their religious representative, if available, about what they are thinking about their opposing duties: the duty to uphold their religious values and the duty to protect their son from physical harm. Explain to the surgeon the reasoned position of Alan's parents, if you can do so.

Key Point: *Ensure that everyone's viewpoint is respected and considered. This may be as important as the final decision reached. In this and other difficult situations, always look for the opportunity for a good compromise (discussed later in this chapter).*

A—ACT BY APPLYING THE CHOSEN OPTION

This is the first step that actually requires action. The hospital is bound to follow the parents' decision because

Alan is a minor. However, if there is time, administrators might refer this situation to the hospital ethics committee. The hospital might also ask a legal court authority to resolve the situation. If an emergency requires an immediate decision, the only *legal* action is to follow the parents' decision, whether or not you consider it the best moral action.

♥ **iCare** Whatever happens, Alan's parents will need emotional support. If they decide to refuse the blood transfusion, you must remain nonjudgmental in supporting them, even if you do not agree with their decision. If they, or the courts, decide on blood administration, they may need even more support. They may feel overwhelming guilt, and they may fear that Alan will have long-lasting guilt at the realization that they violated church doctrine with the medical care. If their family is not present, you could volunteer to call in extended family, friends, and church members if the parents wish. They will need a quiet, private place to await the outcome of the treatment.

L—LOOK BACK AND EVALUATE

This phase calls for evaluation of the entire process, not just the consequence of the decided action.

- **How well did the process work?** Were processes in place to discuss the dilemma respectfully without undue delay in treatment?
- **Were all parties' expectations realistic?**
- **How are all of the affected parties feeling now** (surgeon, parents, family, Alan, you)? Do all involved feel respected? Were their voices heard, regardless of the final decision?
- **How well did you do in the situation?** Did you act as an effective advocate for the rights of Alan and his parents? Did the power and authority of the provider or hospital in the situation unduly influence you?
- **Were policies and procedures in place to guide you** in the process of working out this situation?
- **Has anything changed since the dilemma emerged?** Can you identify a greater good applicable to future situations? Has any aspect of this ethical decision become a universal policy at the institution?
- **Are further actions required** in terms of this or similar situations?

Look for a Good Compromise

Even if you believe you know the right thing to do, others may not agree with you, or there may be constraints that prevent you from doing it. For example, in the case of Alan, even if you decided the right thing to do is give him a blood transfusion, (1) his parents do not agree with you, and (2) the law says you cannot do so without his parents' consent or a legal mandate. This will happen often—much more often than a true dilemma, in which you cannot *decide* the right thing to do. No matter how well we work together, there will

always be ethical problems and disagreements. Many cases are full of complexity and uncertainty, and sometimes the price of acting on your beliefs is extremely high. For example, what might have happened if the surgeon had infused blood without the Freses' consent? What might have happened if you had refused to talk to the parents as the surgeon asked you?

Many times, it will be possible to reach a "good" compromise. A **good compromise** is one that preserves the integrity of all parties. This means that:

- **The discussions are carried out in a spirit of mutual respect**—all viewpoints are respected and considered.
- **The compromise solution itself is ethically sound;** that is, you should be able to provide a principles-based rationale for the compromise, as well as for each of the opposing positions. In the case of Alan and his parents, there probably is no compromise position between "give blood" and "don't give blood." Perhaps the parents would agree to one, but no more than one, transfusion, but that is hard to justify ethically. If one transfusion is acceptable (to honor nonmaleficence), why not two or three? If two transfusions are against their religious beliefs, why would one be acceptable? Nevertheless, in many cases, compromise is possible.

So how do you compromise without losing moral integrity? First, realize there is more at stake than the issue itself ("Is a blood transfusion right or wrong?"). Some things are inherently good in compromising.

- **First, it is never good to settle things by force** (as you would if you got a court order to transfuse Alan without his parents' consent). You have probably heard the old saying "Might doesn't make right." A compromise can preserve the rights of the less powerful party in a disagreement.
- **Keeping peace on a nursing unit is good for both the nurses and patients.** When there is upheaval and moral suffering, care quality throughout the unit can suffer. A compromise can bring peace.
- **There is intrinsic good in taking part in a process in which we try to see things from others' points of view.** It may make us more open-minded, more creative, and less judgmental.
- **Keep in mind that most issues do contain room for reasonable differences of opinion.** In the Meet Your Patients scenario, can you see that people on each side of the dilemma have ethical reasons to justify their opinions?
- **A compromise may achieve mutual respect.** It is a significant thing to reach a settlement in which each party feels assured of the other's respect for its seriousness and sincerity.

Given all those ideas, a person of goodwill might want to reexamine and back away from a very strong opinion. Remember, sometimes your position is not that strong, and the other position is not that weak (as in the case of Alan). There is also always the chance that you may have made an error in your reasoning or have not completely understood some facts of the case. Ethical disputes can be settled only if you are willing to engage in discussions and admit that the other people might have a point. There may be cases in which you cannot compromise (perhaps Alan's case is one), but do not listen to people who say, "You can never reach agreement on ethical issues. They are too complex." It is possible to achieve integrity-producing compromises, and in nursing, it is often necessary.

What Are My Obligations in Ethical Situations?

As you can see, in making ethical decisions, nurses rarely act alone. Usually, you will be one of several healthcare professionals and family members who will jointly arrive at the best decision. Your role when an ethical decision is needed includes the following:

- *Be aware of and sensitive to issues* so that you can identify them when they arise. Educate yourself—attend workshops, read, and talk to other nurses.
- *Assume responsibility for your own ethical actions.* Even if you do not have the "last word" about what happens to a patient or about what others do, you are always responsible for your own actions in every situation.
- *Function as a team member* when ethical problems arise. Realize that you should have input—no one profession has full ethical expertise—and realize that your input can be valuable.
- *Support the patient and family members* while they are making the decision and afterward. Listen. Ask questions. Provide unbiased information. Be helpful without being too directive or judgmental.
- *Support clients who cannot decide for themselves.* For example, in the Meet Your Patients scenario, you would want to be sure Alan's wishes were considered, if possible. However, if the parents insist on deciding for him, against his wishes, he may need a great deal of emotional support.
- *Use and participate in institutional ethics committees* if you are given the opportunity.
- *Most important, advocate for your client.* You may need to balance your client's autonomy with the wishes of family members or the responsibilities of other healthcare professionals to the patient. As an advocate, you may find yourself in conflict with other team members or family members who have different ethical perspectives.
- *Continually strive to improve your ethical decision making.*

Use and Participate in Institutional Ethics Committees

There is no easy way to decide which principle should outrank another principle or which person's values are best in a given situation. For this reason, many healthcare institutions have ethics committees. These interprofessional committees typically include nurses, doctors, clergy, ethicists, a legal counselor, and lay representatives. Ethics committees develop guidelines and policies and provide education and counseling. In the case of ethical dilemmas, they review the case and provide a forum for the expression of the diverse perspectives of those involved. Ethics committees usually follow one of three models when discussing a dilemma: the autonomy model, the patient benefit model, and the social justice model.

Autonomy Model The **autonomy model** is useful when the patient is competent to decide and emphasizes patient autonomy and choice. For example, if this committee knew Alan's (Meet Your Patients) wishes, they might be inclined to try to persuade his parents to do as Alan wants.

Patient Benefit Model The **patient benefit model** assists in decision making for the incompetent patient by using substituted judgment (i.e., what the patient would want for himself if he were capable of making his wishes known). If Alan is unconscious and cannot say what he wants, this committee would probably ask Alan's parents, family, and friends, "What do you think Alan would want? Have you ever heard him talk about a situation such as this?"

Social Justice Model The **social justice model** focuses more on broad social issues involving the entire institution rather than on a single client issue (Yoder-Wise, 2019). Such a committee might consider whether, in general, an institution ought ever to seek a legal order to act against the wishes of the parents. Or they might discuss whether supporting parents' religious beliefs in this instance might have implications for supporting other types of religious beliefs in future cases.

KnowledgeCheck 5-11

- Define *ethical dilemma*.
- How can you recognize an ethical problem?
- What is an integrity-producing compromise?
- What are the functions of an ethics committee?
- What does the mnemonic MORAL stand for?

Be a Patient Advocate

The role of advocates is to safeguard patients against abuse and violation of their rights. When you think of the rights and values described, for example, in *The Patient Care Partnership* and codes of ethics for nurses, you can see the importance of this role. Be aware that advocacy in everyday clinical practice is less about the patient's legal rights and ethical theory and more about such seemingly "routine" measures, such as obtaining a new prescription when an analgesic is ineffective, even if it means telephoning the prescriber for the third time on your shift. The advocacy role requires you to be respectful, considerate, courageous, persistent, and concerned with justice.

Why do you think advocacy is so important? Why can't patients do these things for themselves? The following are some of the reasons.

You Have Special Knowledge That the Patient Does Not Have Diseases, treatments, and the healthcare system are so complex that when patients become ill, they may not have the energy to deal with the complexity, even if they do have the necessary knowledge. You may need to help them navigate the system to get what they need. When others deny patients' rights or when patients do not have the ability to exert their rights, nurses have a responsibility to step in. Advocacy is essential in ensuring patients' rights are protected.

Your Professional Role Includes Defending Patients' Autonomous Decisions Recall that the ANA *Code of Ethics* requires you to be a patient advocate. That means you must defend your patients' autonomous decisions, even if you do not agree with them and even if they conflict with the opinions of other healthcare providers. You may find yourself the sole supporter of a patient's right to choose the direction of their care.

You Have a Special Relationship With Patients You may find that you are able to obtain information about a patient that is not available to other professionals. In general, nurses interact with patients over longer time intervals and are involved in very personal activities, especially in inpatient settings. They often become the most trusted caregivers. Details about family life, coping styles, personal preferences, fears, and insecurities are all more likely to be discussed during the time involved in nursing interventions than in the brief minutes of interaction when a provider makes rounds.

In addition, patients may perceive less social distance between themselves and the nurse and, therefore, feel freer to confide in them. The nurses' point of view can be a valuable asset to resolving an ethical problem satisfactorily. Of course, many providers have long-standing relationships with their patients; however, this does not negate the importance of the nurse's input, which may provide a different perspective.

Your Role as an Advocate Is to Inform, Support, and Communicate You should inform patients of their rights and provide the information they need to make informed decisions, if they can do so. Then you must remain objective and support them in the decisions they make. If others are not respecting patient choices, you will need to intervene. This may be a matter of simply conveying information and clarifying the patient's wishes to family or healthcare professionals (e.g., "I know how hard it is for you to let him go, but

your dad says he has made peace and is ready to die. His treatments make him feel even more ill, and he simply does not want to fight anymore."). Advocacy may require you to arrange for the patient to consult with a religious leader or an attorney for advice and support or may require you to consult an institutional ethics committee.

You Should Inform Patients About Advance Directives Advocacy includes asking clients whether they have an advance directive and educating them on their significance. Kossman (2014) found that completion of advance directives increased when providers asked culturally sensitive questions and educated clients on advance directives. However, detailed advance directives ensure adherence to patients' wishes. Even people who have an advance directive may not understand the statements they have checked in the boxes on the form. Take the time to review the form with your clients. See Chapters 14 and 39 if you need further discussion on advance directives.

For guidelines that will help you to function effectively as an advocate,

 Go to Chapter 5, Clinical Insight 5-2: Guidelines for Advocacy, in Volume 2.

Ethical Scenario: Advocacy Dilemma?

Joane is a 16-year-old immature female who is 7 months pregnant. Her parents plan to put the baby up for adoption. Joane confides in you that she wants to keep her baby and has found a couple on the Internet who will take care of her and the baby. The couple plans to pick Joane up after school in 3 weeks. What are your ethical obligations? Who is your patient? How would you advocate for Joane?

Improve Your Ethical Decision Making

Research has shown that when faced with ethical dilemmas, nurses tend to base their moral reasoning on their values and beliefs. In addition, nurses use professional relationships and ethical frameworks in making decisions (Barlow et al., 2017; Sari et al. 2018). A full-spectrum nurse must continuously apply their knowledge, advocacy skills, and professional relationships to address ethical dilemmas. The following suggestions can provide guidance:

- **Use Theoretical Knowledge.** Review nursing and other literature for discussions of cases and the experiences of other nurses. This will give you a broader view of the problems you may confront and the strategies for managing them. Become familiar with the various codes of ethics, *The Patient Care Partnership*, and ethical frameworks and principles.
- **Use Self-Knowledge.** Examine your personal value system. Explore the influences of your religion, cultural beliefs, and personal experiences. This will help you to recognize your comfort zone with specific ethical issues.

- **Use Practical Knowledge.** While still a student, you should ask to attend either ethical rounds or an ethics committee meeting. As a graduate nurse, to gain insight into ethical situations at your institution, volunteer to serve on the ethics committee or participate in nursing ethics rounds.
- **Consult Reliable Sources.** Attend ethics education programs and discuss issues with healthcare providers, attorneys, ethicists, and clergy to obtain the perspectives of others.
- **Share.** Regularly engage in discussions with the staff on your unit to determine differences in value systems and collaborate proactively to work out methods to resolve ethical dilemmas effectively. When faced with a difficult ethical decision, seek guidance and support from peers, coworkers, and teachers.
- **Evaluate.** After the situation is resolved, evaluate your decision and the effects of your actions. You should be able to learn from even the worst decision. And when everything goes well, you can file your strategies away to use in future similar situations.

KnowledgeCheck 5-12

- What are three reasons why patients may need a nurse advocate?
- Briefly describe the nurse's role as a patient advocate.

To explore learning resources for this chapter,

Go to Davis Advantage and find:

Answers and Suggested Responses for all questions in this chapter

Concept Map

Knowledge Map

References and Bibliography

Factors Affecting Health

CHAPTER 6

Life Span: Infancy Through Middle Adulthood

Learning Outcomes

After completing this chapter, you should be able to:

➤ Discuss the principles of growth and development.

➤ Compare and contrast developmental task theory, psychoanalytic theory, cognitive theory, and the psychosocial theory of growth and development.

➤ Outline the major principles involved in moral and spiritual development.

➤ Identify conditions that influence growth and development at all ages.

➤ Discuss the cognitive and psychosocial challenges for each age-group, infant through middle age.

➤ Identify common health problems seen in each stage of development.

➤ Describe special assessments unique to each age-group.

➤ Discuss age-appropriate interventions for each age-group.

➤ Incorporate developmental principles into nursing care.

Key Concepts

Growth

Development

Stages

Related Concepts

See the Concept Map on Davis Advantage.

Example Client Conditions

Abuse, Neglect, and Violence

Substance Abuse

Meet Your Patient

At the end of your first clinical day on the pediatric unit, you reflect on your experiences. You provided care for three children who were diagnosed with pneumonia:

■ Tamika, a 3-year-old, lives with her grandparents. Her grandmother is present only during afternoon visiting hours because she must care for her husband, who suffers from numerous health problems.

■ Miguel, a 2-month-old, lives with his mother. Since his admission yesterday, Miguel's mother has stayed at his bedside and provided most of her son's care. Miguel's mother is 17 years old and is very concerned about her son's condition.

■ Carrie, a 13-year-old, lives with her parents. Both parents are able to visit only during evening visiting hours, when they leave work.

You think back to another clinical day when you were assigned to care for Ms. Lowenstein, a middle-aged patient

with pneumonia who lives alone.

Each of these patients is unique. Although they share the same medical diagnosis, their needs and your nursing care differ dramatically. These differences stem from a variety of factors, one of the most significant of which is each patient's developmental stage. Throughout the life span, human beings are in a constant process of physical, cognitive, and emotional change, whether or not it is visible to the eye.

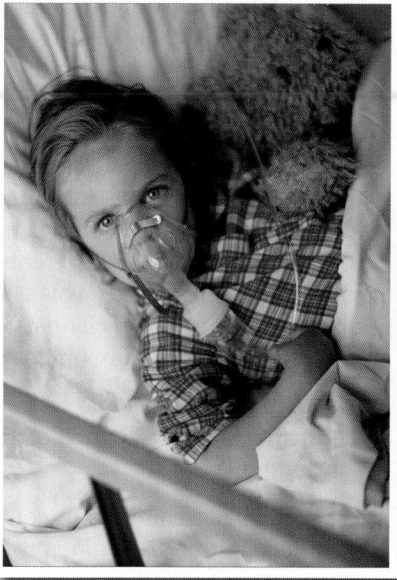

TheoreticalKnowledge
knowing why

In this chapter, you will learn principles and theories of growth and development that can form the foundation for planning and delivering effective patient care. You will also find a discussion of normal growth and development across the life span. A fundamentals course or textbook can provide only a basic foundation covering infant and child development. For situations in which you need more in-depth or specialized knowledge, refer to a child development or pediatric nursing textbook.

ABOUT THE KEY CONCEPTS

- **Development**—the process of adapting to one's body and environment over time through skill progression and increasing complexity of function, for example, a child who comes to recognize right from wrong, an adolescent who decides on a vocation, and an older adult who recognizes the nearness of death.
- **Growth**—physical changes that occur over time (e.g., increases in height, sexual maturation, or gains in weight and muscle tone). Growth is the physical aspect of development; the rest is behavioral.
- **Stages**—As you read this chapter, you will see how the key concept of **stages** interrelates with the concepts of growth and development.

HOW DOES DEVELOPMENT OCCUR?

The Greek philosopher Heraclitus said, "Nothing is permanent but change." We readily see this truth in the dramatic physical, cognitive, and emotional growth that children undergo from one month to another, but it is also true for adults. **Key Point:** *Change is constant throughout the life span.*

What has been the most important force in your becoming the person you are now: characteristics that you inherited from your parents or the environment in which you were raised? This is not an easy question to answer. For centuries, scientists have debated the effects of nature versus nurture on growth and development.

- **Nature** refers to genetic endowment.
- **Nurture** is the influence of the environment on the individual.

The birth of a child can be compared with the planting of a tulip. Within the bulb is nearly everything it needs to sprout, but whether it grows into a flowering plant also depends on the environment (e.g., the soil, water, sunshine). Similarly, the ovum and sperm join to form chromosomes, which determine appearance and characteristics and affect how the child will grow and develop. However, environmental factors, such as access to food, love, affection, and education, also affect how the child develops and thrives throughout the life span.

Principles of Growth and Development

Important principles of growth and development include the following:

- **Growth and development usually follow an orderly, predictable pattern.** However, the timing, rate of change, and response to change are unique for each individual. For example, children learn to sit before they walk. One child may learn to sit at 6 months of age and walk at 10 months; another child may first sit at 7 months and not walk until 15 months. Each of these children is developing in the same pattern and progressing within a normal time frame.
- **Growth and development follow a cephalocaudal pattern,** beginning at the head and progressing down to the chest, trunk, and lower extremities. The following are examples:

    Cephalocaudal growth—When an infant is born, the head is the largest portion of the body. In the first year, the head, chest, and trunk gain in size, yet the legs remain short. Growth of the legs is readily apparent in the second year.

    Cephalocaudal development—This is the tendency of infants to use their arms before their legs.
- **Growth and development proceed in a proximodistal pattern,** beginning at the center of the body and moving outward.

    Proximodistal growth—This occurs in utero, for example, when the baby's central body is formed before the limbs.

    Proximodistal development—Infants first begin to focus their eyes, then lift the head, and later push up and roll over. As infants gain strength and coordination distally, they will crawl and later walk.
- **Simple skills develop separately and independently.** Later, they are integrated into more complex skills. Many complex skills actually represent a compilation of simple skills. For example, feeding yourself requires the ability to find your mouth, grasp an object, control movement of that object, coordinate movement of the hand from the plate to the mouth, and swallow solid food.
- **Each body system grows at its own rate.** This principle is readily apparent in fetal development and at the onset of puberty. In the years leading up to puberty, the cardiovascular, respiratory, and nervous systems grow and develop dramatically, yet the reproductive system changes very little. Puberty is a series of changes that leads to full development of the reproductive system and also triggers growth in the musculoskeletal system.
- **Body system functions become increasingly differentiated over time.** Have you ever seen a newborn respond to a loud noise? The newborn's startle response involves the whole body. With maturity, the response becomes more focused, for example, covering the ears. An adult is often able to state the location of the sound and distinguish the origin of the sound.

Theories of Development

Theories of development describe and explain patterns of development common to all people. Such theories provide a basis for your nursing interventions and clinical decision making. The needs of a 6-year-old differ greatly from those of a 25-year-old or a 65-year-old, even though they all may have the same medical diagnosis (e.g., asthma) or even the same nursing diagnosis (e.g., Anxiety). Understanding the tasks associated with a person's developmental stage assists you in assessing whether behaviors are as expected or whether they need further assessment. Knowledge of development also suggests specific interventions to support and encourage the person's developmental progress and health outcomes.

Key Point: *Developmental theories divide the life span into stages.* Each stage represents a period of time that shares common characteristics. Most theories also identify tasks that are usually accomplished in each stage. An understanding of the following key developmental theories is essential to full-spectrum nursing practice.

Developmental Task Theory

Robert Havighurst theorized that:

- Learning is a lifelong process.
- A person moves through six life stages, each associated with a number of tasks that must be learned.

- Conceptually, a **developmental task** is "midway between an individual need and societal demand. It assumes an active learner interacting with an active social environment" (1971, p. vi).
- Failure to master a task leads to difficulty mastering future tasks and interacting with others.

Table 6-1 presents the tasks associated with each stage of life. It is easy to evaluate a client's completion of Havighurst's broadly written tasks, but the nonspecific time frame limits the theory's usefulness for assessing individuals for appropriate development.

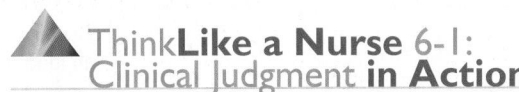

ThinkLike a Nurse 6-1: Clinical Judgment in Action

Which stage in Havighurst's developmental task theory contains the most complex tasks and would be the most difficult to master? Why?

Psychoanalytic Theory

Sigmund Freud was a pioneer in the science of human development. Psychoanalytic theory became the foremost theoretical foundation of early 20th-century psychotherapy. Freud developed his theory in the Victorian era, when societal norms were strict; sexual repression and male dominance over female behavior were the cultural standard. Because of this, many of today's social

Table 6-1 ➤ Havighurst's Developmental Task Theory	
STAGE	**TASKS**
Infants and Toddlers	
Physical Development	**Cognitive and Social Development**
▪ Walking	▪ Acquiring psychological stability
▪ Taking solid foods	▪ Forming concepts; learning language
▪ Talking	▪ Getting ready to read
▪ Controlling bowel and bladder elimination	
▪ Learning sex differences and sexual modesty	
Preschool and School Age	
Physical Development	**Cognitive and Social Development**
▪ Learning physical skills necessary for ordinary games	▪ Building wholesome attitudes toward oneself as a growing organism
	▪ Learning to get along with age-mates
	▪ Learning masculine or feminine social role
	▪ Acquiring fundamental skills in reading, writing, and calculating
	▪ Developing concepts necessary for everyday living
	▪ Developing a conscience, morality, and a scale of values
	▪ Achieving personal independence
	▪ Acquiring attitudes toward social groups and institutions

(Continued)

Table 6-1 ➤ Havighurst's Developmental Task Theory—cont'd

STAGE	TASKS
Adolescents	
Physical Development	**Cognitive and Social Development**
■ Accepting one's physique and using the body effectively	■ Achieving new and more mature relations with age-mates of both sexes
	■ Achieving a masculine or feminine social role
	■ Developing emotional independence from parents and other adults
	■ Preparing for future marriage and family life
	■ Preparing for a career
	■ Acquiring a set of values and an ethical system to guide behavior; developing an ideology
	■ Aspiring to and achieving socially responsible behavior
Young Adults	
	Cognitive and Social Development
	■ Choosing a mate
	■ Achieving a masculine or feminine social role
	■ Learning to live with a partner
	■ Rearing children
	■ Managing a home
	■ Establishing an occupation
	■ Taking on community responsibilities
	■ Finding a compatible social group
Middle Adults	
Physical Development	**Cognitive and Social Development**
■ Adjusting to the physiological changes of middle age	■ Assisting teenage children to become responsible and happy adults
	■ Achieving adult civic and social responsibility
	■ Reaching and maintaining satisfactory performance in one's occupational career
	■ Developing adult leisure-time activities
	■ Relating oneself to one's spouse as a person
Older Adults, refer to Chapter 7.	

Source: Havighurst, R. J. (1971). *Developmental tasks and education* (3rd ed.). Longman.

scientists question whether his theory should be applied to life in the 21st century.

Key Point: *Freud's psychoanalytic theory focuses on the motivation for human behavior and personality development.* He believed human development is maintained by instinctual drives, such as libido (sexual instinct), aggression, and survival (Table 6-2) (Sadock & Sadock, 2021). Different drives predominate, depending on the age of the individual.

In Freud's theory, the personality consists of the id, ego, and superego—different "parts" that develop at different life stages. Each factor, or force, has a unique function:

■ The **id** represents instinctual urges, pleasure, and gratification, such as hunger, procreation, pleasure, and aggression. We are born with our id. It is dominant in infants and young children, as well as in older children and adults who cannot control their urges.

■ The **ego** begins to develop around 4 to 6 months of age and is thought to represent reality. It strives to balance

STAGE AND AGE	DESCRIPTION
Oral Birth–18 months	The infant's primary needs are centered on the oral zone: lips, tongue, mouth. Hunger and the need for pleasure are satisfied through the oral zone. Trust is developed through the meeting of needs. When needs are not met, aggression can manifest itself in the form of biting, spitting, or crying.
Anal 18 months–3 years	Neuromuscular control over the anal sphincter allows the child to have control over expulsion or retention of feces. This coincides with the child's struggle for separation and independence from caregivers. Successful completion of this stage yields a child who is self-directed, cooperative, and without shame. Conversely, the anal child will exhibit wilfulness, stubbornness, and a need for orderliness.
Phallic 3–6 years	The focus is on the genital organs. This coincides with the development of gender identity. Unconscious sexual feelings toward the parent of the opposite sex are common. Children emerge from this stage with a sense of sexual curiosity and a mastery of their instinctual impulses.
Latency 6–12 years	Ego functioning matures, and sexual urges diminish. The child focuses their energy on same-sex relationships and mastery of their world, including relationships with significant others (teachers, coaches).
Genital 13–20 years	Puberty causes an intensification of instinctual drives, particularly sexual. The focus of this stage is the resolution of previous conflicts and the development of a mature identity and the ability to form adult relationships.

Table 6-2 ➤ Freud's Stages of Psychosexual Development

Source: Freud, A. (1966). *The ego and the mechanisms of defense.* International Universities Press.

what is *wanted* (id) and what is *possible* to obtain or achieve.

- The **superego** is sometimes referred to as the *conscience*. This force develops in early childhood (age 5–6) as a result of the internalization of primary caregiver responses to environmental events.
- The **unconscious mind** is composed of thoughts and memories that are not readily recalled but unconsciously influence behavior.

In the mid-1950s, Freud's daughter, the psychologist Anna Freud, identified a number of **defense mechanisms,** which she described as thought patterns or behaviors that the ego makes use of in the face of threats to biological or psychological integrity (Townsend, 2018). These defense mechanisms protect us from excess anxiety. All people use defense mechanisms to varying degrees. For a comprehensive discussion of defense mechanisms, see Chapter 9 and Table 9-1.

KnowledgeCheck 6-1

- According to Freud, which motivator of personality is based in reality?
- Which personality factor is referred to as our conscience?
- What is the purpose of defense mechanisms?

Cognitive Development Theory

Swiss psychologist Jean Piaget studied his own children to understand how humans develop **cognitive abilities** (i.e., the ability to think, reason, and use language).

According to Piaget, cognitive development requires three core competencies.

- **Adaptation** is the ability to adjust to and interact with one's environment. To be able to adapt, one must assimilate and accommodate.
- **Assimilation** is the integration of new experiences with one's own system of knowledge.
- **Accommodation** is the change in one's system of knowledge that results from processing new information. For example, an infant is born with an innate ability to suck. Presented with the mother's nipple, the infant is able to assimilate the nipple to the behavior of sucking. If given a bottle, the infant can learn to accommodate the artificial nipple.

Key Point: *According to Piaget, cognitive development occurs from birth through adolescence in a sequence of four stages: sensorimotor, preoperational thought, concrete operations, and formal operations* (Table 6-3). A child must complete each stage before moving to the next. The rate at which a child moves through the stages is determined by the inherited intellect and the influence of the environment. Piaget does not address cognitive development after adolescence.

KnowledgeCheck 6-2

- According to Piaget, what core competencies are necessary for cognitive development?
- During which stage is the child the most egocentric?
- When does abstract thinking develop?

Table 6-3 ➤ Piaget's Stages of Cognitive Development

STAGE AND AGE	CHARACTERISTICS OF DEVELOPMENT
Sensorimotor Birth–2 years	■ Learns the world through the senses. ■ Displays curiosity. ■ Shows intentional behavior. ■ Begins to see that objects exist apart from self. ■ Begins to see objects as separate from self.
Preoperational 2–7 years	■ Uses symbols and language. ■ Sees self as the center of the universe: egocentric. ■ Thought based on perception rather than logic.
Concrete operations 7–11 years	■ Operates and reacts to the concrete: what is perceived is actual. ■ Egocentricity diminishes, can see from others' viewpoints. ■ Able to use logic and reason in thinking. ■ Able to conserve: to see that objects may change but recognizes them as the same (e.g., water may change to ice, or a tower of blocks is the same as a long fence of blocks).
Formal operations 11–adolescence	■ Develops the ability to think abstractly: to reason, deduce, and define concepts in a logical manner. ■ Some individuals do not develop the ability to think abstractly.

Source: Piaget, J. (1952). *The origins of intelligence in children.* International Universities Press.

Psychosocial Development Theory

Erickson's theory of psychosocial development was introduced in the 1950s and is widely used in nursing and healthcare. He was strongly influenced by Freud but believed that personality continues to evolve throughout the life span. **Key Point: *Erickson hypothesized that individuals must negotiate eight stages as they progress through the life span. Most people successfully move from stage to stage; however, a person can regress to earlier stages during times of stress or be forced to face tasks of later stages because of unforeseen life events (e.g., terminal illness).*** Failure to successfully master a stage leads to maladjustment. Erikson's eight stages include the following:

Stage 1: Trust versus mistrust (birth to about 18 months)
Stage 2: Autonomy versus shame and doubt (about 18 months to 3 years)
Stage 3: Initiative versus guilt (3 to 5 years)
Stage 4: Industry versus inferiority (6 to 11 years)
Stage 5: Identity versus role confusion (11 to 21 years)
Stage 6: Intimacy versus isolation (21 to 40 years)
Stage 7: Generativity versus stagnation (40 to 65 years)
Stage 8: Ego integrity versus despair (over 65 years)

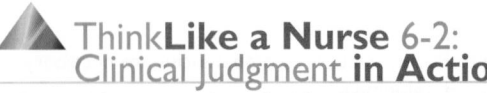

ThinkLike a Nurse 6-2: Clinical Judgment in Action

Review the case study in the Meet Your Patients section of the chapter. On the basis of what you know about the theories of development, what kind of behavior would you anticipate from Carrie?

Moral Development Theory: Kohlberg

Lawrence Kohlberg (1968) studied the responses to moral dilemmas of 84 boys whose development he followed for a period of 20 years. From the data, **Key Point: *Kohlberg hypothesized that a person's level of moral development can be identified by analyzing the rationale they give for action in a moral dilemma.***

In this theory, moral reasoning appears to be somewhat age-related, and moral development is based on one's ability to think at progressively higher levels. Increased maturity provides some degree of higher-level thinking but does not guarantee the ability to function at the highest level. Kohlberg described the following levels; each has two stages (Kohlberg, 1968, 1981; Waugh, 1978):

Level I. Preconventional

Stage 1—punishment–obedience orientation (right action is that which avoids punishment)
Stage 2—personal interest orientation (right action is that which satisfies personal needs)

Level II. Conventional

Stage 3—"good boy–nice girl" orientation (right actions are those that please others)
Stage 4—law-and-order orientation (right action is following the rules)

Level III. Postconventional, Autonomous, or Principled

Stage 5—legalistic, social contract orientation (right action is decided in terms of individual rights and standards agreed upon by the whole society)

Stage 6—universal ethical principles orientation (right action is determined by conscience and abstract principles, such as the Golden Rule)

Moral Development Theory: Gilligan

Although all of his research subjects were male, Kohlberg claimed that his sequence of stages applies equally to everyone. The validity of his theory for women has been sharply criticized, most prominently by Carol Gilligan (1982, 1993). **Key Point:** *To address the moral development of women, Gilligan proposed an alternative theory that incorporates the concepts of caring, interpersonal relationships, and responsibility. She described a three-stage approach to moral development.*

- **Stage 1: Caring for Oneself.** In this stage, the focus is on providing for oneself and surviving. The individual is egocentric in thought and does not consider the needs of others. When concerns about being selfish begin to emerge, the individual is signaling a readiness to move to stage 2.
- **Stage 2: Caring for Others.** At this level, an individual recognizes the importance of relationships with others. The person is willing to make sacrifices to help others, often at the expense of their own needs. When they recognize the conflict between caring for oneself and caring for others, the individual is ready to move to stage 3.
- **Stage 3: Caring for Self and Others.** This represents the highest stage of moral development. In this stage, care is the focus of decision making. The individual carefully balances their own needs against the needs of others to decide on a course of action.

Spiritual Development Theory

James Fowler, a minister, defined faith as a universal human concern and as a process of growing in trust. He noticed that his congregants had very different approaches to faith, depending on their age. Basing his studies on the work of Piaget, Erikson, and Kohlberg, he developed a theory of faith development, which includes a prestage (stage 0) and six stages of faith (Fowler, 1981).

- *Stages 0, 1, and 2* are closely associated with evolving cognitive abilities. In these stages, faith depends largely on the views expressed by the parents, caregivers, and those who have a significant influence on the life of the person.
- *Stage 3* coincides with the ability to use **logic** and **hypothetical thinking** to construct and evaluate ideas. At this point, faith is largely a collection of conventional, unexamined beliefs. Fowler's studies demonstrated that approximately one-fourth of all adults function at this level or lower.

- *Stages 4, 5, and 6* represent increasing levels of refinement of faith. With each increase in level, there is a decreasing likelihood that an individual can attain this stage of development. Fowler found that very few people achieve stage 6.

The rest of this chapter describes the human life span as a series of developmental stages: physical, cognitive, and psychosocial. Development and common health problems are discussed for each stage. To simplify organization, you will find nursing assessments and interventions included with each stage rather than together in a single Practical Knowledge section.

THE GESTATIONAL PERIOD: CONCEPTION TO BIRTH

The time between conception and birth is called the **gestational period.** Human gestation (pregnancy) is calculated from the first day of the patient's last menstrual period and lasts approximately 40 weeks, or 280 days. Full discussions of pregnancy and childbirth are beyond the scope of a fundamentals text. If you need more information, refer to a maternal health textbook.

Fetal Development During Gestation

Pregnancy is usually divided into three trimesters, each lasting about 13 weeks.

First Trimester The first 8 weeks is known as the **embryonic phase.** It begins when an egg released from an ovary unites with a sperm cell, usually in one of the fallopian tubes. This is called **fertilization** (or conception).

- *First 7 days.* Continual cell division leads to the development of a tiny ball of cells called the **morula,** which travels toward the uterus for a period of about 7 days before implanting in the uterus.
- *Upon implantation,* three primary germ layers begin to differentiate, and the **embryo** begins to resemble a tiny organism with a head and tail.
- *By week 4,* the brain, heart, and liver have begun to form, and tiny limb buds are present.
- *As early as 6 to 7 weeks,* you can hear the fetal heartbeat with a fetal ultrasound Doppler.
- *By the end of week 8,* all organs are formed, and the embryo is then called a *fetus.*

Second Trimester Rapid fetal growth and further development of the body systems characterize the second trimester. At about 16 to 20 weeks of pregnancy, fetal movement is usually felt, a sensation called **quickening.** At the end of the second trimester, the fetus has all organs and body parts intact, and organs become more efficient during the last trimester. For example:

- *The kidneys are intact and begin to produce urine,* although they do not effectively concentrate it until late in the third trimester.

- *The lungs are formed*, although they do not contain enough of the substance to keep air sacs open after birth until late in the third trimester.

Third Trimester The fetus continues to grow in size and add subcutaneous fat. Body systems mature in preparation for extrauterine life. If born prematurely during this trimester, the newborn may be able to survive with intensive care (National Child and Maternal Health Education Program, n.d.).

- *The fetus is considered* **early term** *from 37 weeks through 38 weeks and 6 days.*
- *The fetus is considered* **full term** *at 39 weeks. A normal full-term baby weighs, on average, 5 lb 8 oz to 8 lb 13 oz (2.5 to 4.9 kg) and is 20 in. (50 cm) long.*
- *At 41 weeks, the baby is considered* **late term**.
- *At 42 weeks and beyond, the baby is considered* **post-term**
  For more information on fetal development:

 Go to Chapter 6, Assessment Guidelines & Tools, Fetal Development, in Volume 2

Maternal Changes During Pregnancy

A patient's health during pregnancy is essential for healthy, sustained growth and development of the fetus. It is important to develop good health practices well before conception, including exercise, a balanced diet, smoking cessation, avoidance of alcohol, and regular dental checkups.

Key Point: *The growing fetus depends entirely on the placenta for oxygen and nutrition. Therefore, many of the physical changes experienced during pregnancy are for the purpose of increasing blood flow through the placenta to the baby.*

- The heart typically enlarges slightly.
- Cardiac output increases significantly.
- The chest wall expands, so the respiratory rate increases significantly.
- Normal blood flow increases by about 30% by the 35th week of pregnancy.

First Trimester Menses typically cease. Hormone shifts occur, primarily in progesterone and estrogen. These cause morning sickness, fullness in the pelvic area, breast enlargement and tenderness, urinary frequency, and fatigue.

Second Trimester The uterus enlarges, and hyperpigmentation of the skin occurs, often creating a dark line from the umbilicus to the symphysis pubis and causing the nipples to darken. Other common changes include mottling of the cheeks and forehead, swelling and bleeding of the gums, and "stuffiness" from swelling in the mucous membranes in the nose. The patient begins to feel the fetus moving and may experience mild contractions called *Braxton Hicks*.

Third Trimester Fetal movement is the predominant feature of the latter period of pregnancy. The breasts begin to produce and secrete colostrum in preparation for lactation. Pressure from the enlarged fetus may cause shortness of breath and urinary frequency.

Psychosocial Challenges Because the birth of a child is a life-changing condition, it is normal for the patient to feel ambivalent about pregnancy at first. However, these feelings usually resolve in the second trimester. The pregnant patient must adapt to changes in body image and role and expectations, concerns about sexuality and whether their partner is sexually satisfied, fears about labor and delivery, concern for the baby's health and safety, planning for care of the child after delivery, financial pressures, and stresses involving employment during pregnancy.

Common Health Problems During Gestation

Blood circulating through the placenta carries nutrients and oxygen to the fetus and toxins and metabolic wastes away from the fetus. Other substances also cross the placenta—for example, **teratogens.**

Teratogens Teratogens are substances that interfere with normal growth and development.

Key Point: *Because the brain and other vital organs develop rapidly during the first trimester, this is the time when the fetus is most vulnerable to teratogens, including the following:*

- *Alcohol* can cause birth defects, growth retardation, developmental delay, and impaired intellectual development. Babies exposed to alcohol in the womb can develop **fetal alcohol spectrum disorders (FASDs)**. These disorders include a wide range of physical, behavioral, and learning problems. The most severe type of FASD is **fetal alcohol syndrome** *(FAS).*
- *Nicotine* interferes with the transport of oxygen to the fetus, contributing to premature birth, low birth weight, and learning disabilities.
- *Morphine, heroin, methadone, and other narcotics,* when used during pregnancy, cause the newborn to suffer from withdrawal at birth. Symptoms include tremors, restlessness, hyperactive reflexes, poor temperature control, vomiting and diarrhea, high-pitched cries, seizures, and sometimes death.
- *Cocaine, including crack, and methamphetamines* are highly addictive and potentially harmful to the fetus. Infants born to users of cocaine and crack are more likely to suffer from growth retardation and to have sleep disturbances, hyperactive reflexes, irritability, feeding difficulties, attention and behavioral disorders, and learning disabilities at school age. These infants are also more likely to die of **sudden infant death syndrome (SIDS)**, the sudden, unexplained death of an infant (discussed in more detail in the section about infancy).

- ✚ *Medications*, both prescribed and over the counter (OTC), can have teratogenic effects. Examples include the acne medication isotretinoin (Accutane), tetracycline (Achromycin), phenytoin (Dilantin), and lithium (Lithobid). Pregnant women should check with their primary care provider before taking any medications or herbal remedies.

Effects of Maternal Age

- *Adolescence.* The risk for preterm birth, low birth weight, and fetal death is higher for infants born to adolescent mothers.
- *Over Age 40.* The risk of fetal death is also higher in pregnancies with mothers over age 40 (Ely & Driscoll, 2019).
- *Down syndrome.* The risk of conceiving a child with Down syndrome (trisomy 21) and other congenital anomalies increases for each year the mother is over 35 years of age but dramatically after 42 years of age.

Effects of Maternal Health

- *Maternal diseases, such as rubella, syphilis, and gonorrhea,* although not common, can cause fetal blindness, fetal deafness, or fetal loss.
- *Cytomegalovirus (CMV)* is a common, flu-like viral infection in adults. If CMV is acquired during pregnancy, the fetus can suffer intrauterine growth retardation, poor brain growth, enlarged liver (hepatomegaly) with jaundice, irritation of the lung (pneumonitis), and bleeding problems.
- *Toxoplasmosis* can be transmitted to the unborn fetus through the handling of contaminated cat litter.
- *Genital herpes* can be passed to the infant during delivery if the mother experiences an outbreak of genital herpes at that time.
- *Maternal diabetes* can result in low blood sugar after birth and can also have lasting effects on the fetus. Poor glucose control during pregnancy may lead to neural tube and heart defects, as well as **macrosomia** (large body size).

Effects of Maternal Nutrition Appropriate healthy weight management before conception contributes to fetal and maternal health. During pregnancy, appropriate maternal weight gain contributes to appropriate fetal development and weight and reduces the risk of fetal illness and infections (Fig. 6-1).

- *The recommended average weight gain* for a pregnancy is 25 to 35 pounds. The expected weight gain is higher for underweight patients and lower for overweight patients.
- ✚ *Folic acid deficiency is a risk factor for neural tube defects,* especially in the first weeks of pregnancy, before the patient even knows they are pregnant. Neural tube defects (e.g., spina bifida) occur during the first weeks of fetal development.

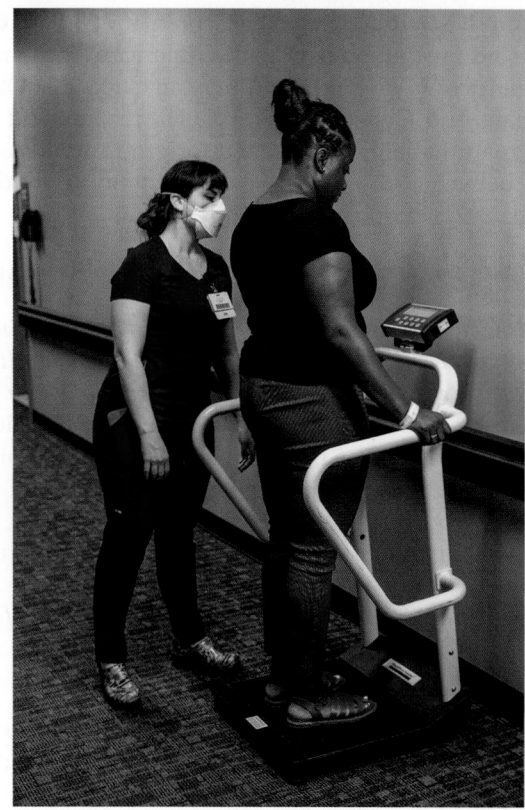

FIGURE 6-1 After establishing a baseline weight in early pregnancy, monitor for appropriate gain at each prenatal visit.

ASSESSMENT/RECOGNIZING CUES (PRENATAL)

Routine prenatal visits and screenings usually take place monthly until 28 weeks, then every 2 weeks until 36 weeks, then weekly until birth. In addition to vital signs, weight, fetal heart tones, nutritional status, and other measures of maternal–fetal well-being, the following should be assessed at each visit:

- **Common discomforts associated with pregnancy,** such as nausea, fatigue, and back pain.
- **Preexisting conditions** (e.g., heart disease).
- **Medication use,** including OTC drugs, the use of alternative therapies, and other substances.

Screening is also done for complications of pregnancy, such as the following:

- **Birth defects.** Patients who are at higher risk for a fetus with a birth defect are those with advanced maternal age (over age 40), a family history of congenital anomalies, maternal diabetes with insulin use, viral infection during pregnancy, and exposure to high levels of radiation. Blood markers and ultrasound screening are done to detect neural tube defects, abdominal wall defects, trisomy 21 (Down syndrome), and trisomy 18.
- **Gestational diabetes.** Screening for gestational diabetes is most often done between 24 and 28 weeks' gestation—earlier if there is a history of gestational diabetes with a previous pregnancy.

- **Group B** *Streptococcus.* The Centers for Disease Control and Prevention (CDC), the American Academy of Pediatrics (AAP), and the American College of Obstetricians and Gynecologists (ACOG) recommend that pregnant patients be screened for group B *Streptococcus* between 36 and 38 weeks' gestation (Dhudasia et al., 2021; Puopolo et al., 2019).

IMPLEMENTATION/TAKING ACTION (PRENATAL)

Key Point: *One of the most important nursing interventions for promoting maternal and fetal health is to facilitate and teach the importance of early and continuing prenatal care.* Early prenatal care can identify complications of pregnancy, prevent some of the effects of maternal diseases such as diabetes, and provide an opportunity for patient education. Each prenatal visit is an opportunity for patient education, for example:

Key Point: *Maternal nutrition is important for a healthy baby. The mother's food intake should be well balanced.*

- *Vitamins and minerals.* The recommended dietary allowances of vitamins and minerals for the pregnant patient range from 25% to 50% higher than those for the nonpregnant patient.
- *Calories.* For most normal-weight pregnant patients, the right number of calories is:
  - first trimester—1,800 calories per day;
  - second trimester—2,200 calories per day;
  - third trimester—2,400 calories per day
- *Protein.* Daily protein intake increases from 45 to 71 g, and inadequate protein affects the formation of the placenta and fetal brain development.
- *Folic acid.* Increasing folic acid (also called *folate*) intake to 0.4 to 0.8 mg (400 to 800 mcg) daily reduces the risk of neural tube defects.

Persons who are of childbearing age and wish to become pregnant should follow these guidelines even before pregnancy. This will help achieve a national goal for the year 2030 of reducing the incidence of neural tube defects (U.S. Preventive Services Task Force, 2017a). You can find this goal and other national goals for 2030 on the *Healthy People 2030* Web site,

 http://www.healthypeople.gov/

Other teaching topics include the following:

Information regarding sexually transmitted infections (STIs) and vaginal infections
Information about urinary tract infections
Exercise patterns
Childcare
Fetal growth and development
Hazardous substances to avoid
Avoiding the use of OTC medication without approval from the supervising provider

Self-care measures for common discomforts of pregnancy
Danger signs that alert the woman to call her care provider
Signs of impending labor; when to go to the birthing unit

KnowledgeCheck 6-3

- What are the most common health concerns to monitor for in the gestational period?
- Identify at least four important topics for health teaching with the expectant mother.
- Why is early prenatal care so important?

THE NEONATAL PERIOD: BIRTH TO 28 DAYS

During the **neonatal period** (the first month of life), the newborn's primary task is to stabilize the body's major organ systems and adapt to life outside the uterus. Behaviors are primarily reflexive.

Physical Development of the Neonate

Growth The following are characteristics of the normal full-term newborn:

- *Weight.* 5 lb 8 oz to 8 lb 13 oz (2.5 to 4.0 kg). Lower birth weights are seen with prematurity; higher birth weights are associated with gestational diabetes.
- *Length.* Between 18 and 22 in. (46 and 56 cm) (Fig. 6-2). The arms are slightly longer than the legs.
- *Head and skull.* At birth, the head is one-fourth the total body length, with a head circumference of 13 to 14 in. (33 to 35 cm). The head may appear asymmetrical for a few days because of molding during vaginal birth. The skull consists of six soft bones separated by sutures composed of cartilage (Fig. 6-3), with anterior and posterior **fontanels** (soft spots). These spaces allow room to accommodate the rapid growth of the infant's brain during the first months of life.

Respirations Key Point: *At birth, the most critical adaptation is the establishment of respirations.* Pressure on the baby's chest during vaginal birth helps

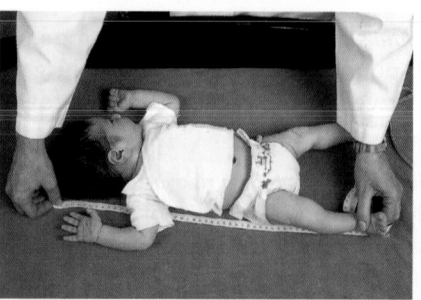

FIGURE 6-2 Measuring the length of a newborn.

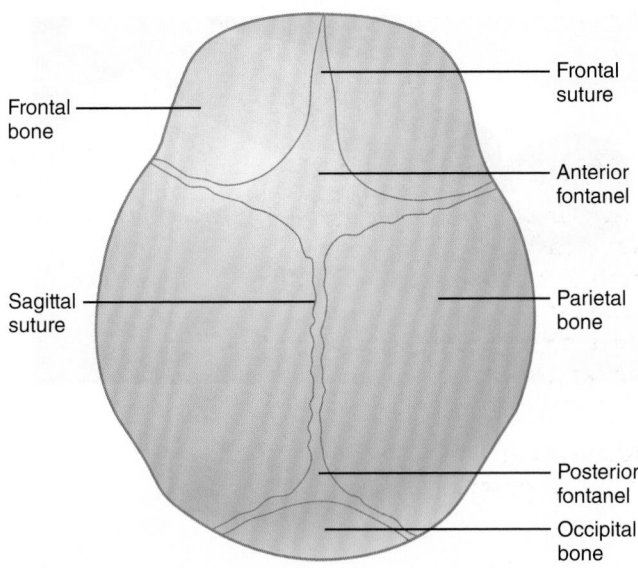

Frontal bone

Frontal suture

Anterior fontanel

Sagittal suture

Parietal bone

Posterior fontanel

Occipital bone

FIGURE 6-3 Sutures and fontanel of the newborn's skull.

remove amniotic fluid from the lungs in preparation for breathing. A normal newborn's respirations are:

Irregular
Shallow
30 to 50 breaths/min

It is normal to have brief episodes of **periodic breathing** (pauses in breathing).

Cardiovascular System The cardiovascular system must also adapt to the change from placental blood flow and convert to independent circulation. The average heart rate of a newborn is 120 to 140 beats/min, with slightly lower rates at rest and higher rates with activity or crying. Poor peripheral circulation causes a bluish coloration of the hands and feet; this is normal and usually disappears within a few hours of birth.

Thermoregulation The normal newborn's temperature is close to that of an adult. Maintaining a normal body temperature is a critical task at birth because the newborn chills easily. The newborn can produce adequate heat but cannot protect against heat loss. Heat may be lost by exposure to cool air temperatures, by contact with cooler solid surfaces, or by evaporation of moisture from the skin. **Key Point: *To facilitate thermoregulation, it is important to keep the newborn warm and dry, with a cap covering the head.***

Elimination The following are normal characteristics:

- *Kidneys.* At birth, the kidneys produce 15 to 60 mL of urine per kilogram of body weight per day. During the first 24 hours, the newborn voids 5 to 25 times. Newborns have limited ability to concentrate urine.
- *Bowel.* At birth, the newborn's lower intestine is filled with **meconium,** a sticky, greenish-black substance formed from amniotic fluid and intestinal secretions. Meconium is usually passed within 12 hours of birth, and the stool progressively changes in color to yellow.

- *Gastrointestinal system.* The full-term infant is able to swallow, digest, metabolize, and absorb proteins and simple carbohydrates. Stomach capacity varies from 30 to 90 mL, depending on the infant's weight. Normal colonic bacteria are established within a week of birth.

Epidermis and Dermis The epidermis and dermis are very thin at birth and can be easily damaged. Infants are born with varying features that present no health dangers and disappear spontaneously:

- **Vernix caseosa**—a cheese-like protective covering for the skin
- **Milia**—tiny white spots present on the newborn's face
- **Congenital dermal melanocytosis**—a darkly pigmented area, typically on the buttocks or lower back.

Neuromuscular System The neuromuscular system is not completely developed at birth. However, the following **reflexes** (automatic responses) are present at birth. Selected reflexes are illustrated in Figure 6-4.

- **Rooting.** Rooting is elicited by stroking the infant's cheek with the nipple or finger. In response, the newborn turns their head toward the stimulus, opens their mouth, takes hold, and sucks. This reflex disappears by 3 to 4 months of age.
- **Sucking Reflex.** The sucking reflex is elicited by touching the infant's lips.
- **Swallowing Reflex.** The swallowing reflex is coordinated with sucking and usually occurs without gagging, coughing, or vomiting. This response is weak with prematurity or neurological defect.
- **Grasp Reflex.** The grasp reflex is triggered by placing a finger in the palm of the infant's hand (palmar) or at the base of the toes (plantar). The infant's fingers curl around the examiner's fingers, or the toes curl downward. The palmar reflex lessens by 3 to 4 months, and the plantar reflex lessens by 8 months.
- **Tonic Neck or Fencing Reflex.** The tonic neck, or fencing, reflex is elicited by rotating the infant's head to the left with the left arm and leg extended and the right arm and leg flexed. Turn the head to the right, and the extremities assume the opposite posture. The response disappears by 3 to 4 months.
- **Moro or Startle Reflex.** This reflex is elicited by placing the infant on a flat surface and striking the surface to startle the infant. Symmetrical abduction and extension of the arms are expected as an indicator of overall neurological health. The fingers fan out and form a C with the thumb and forefinger. This response is absent by 6 months.
- **Stepping Reflex.** Elicit the stepping reflex by holding the infant vertically, allowing one foot to touch a surface (e.g., tabletop). The infant will simulate walking by alternating flexion and extension of the feet during the 3 to 4 weeks of life.
- **Crawling Reflex.** The crawling reflex is noted by placing the infant on their abdomen. The newborn makes

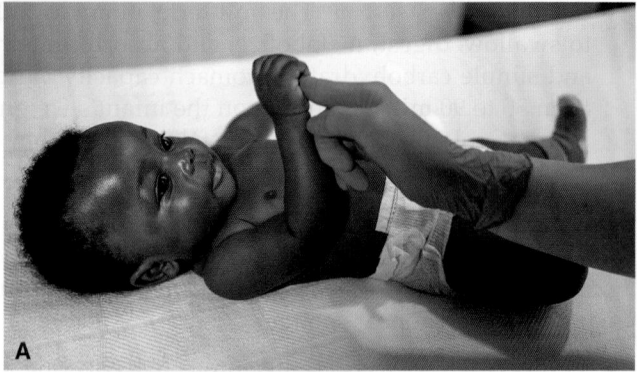

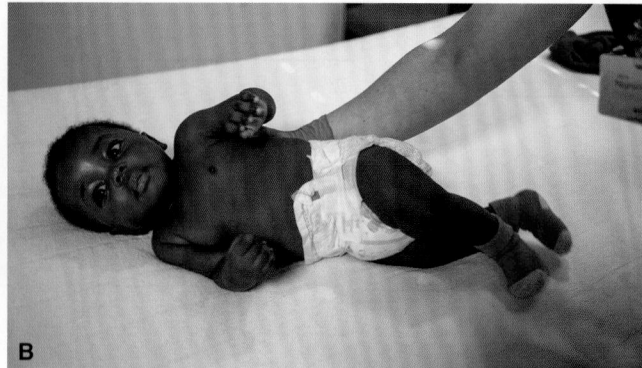

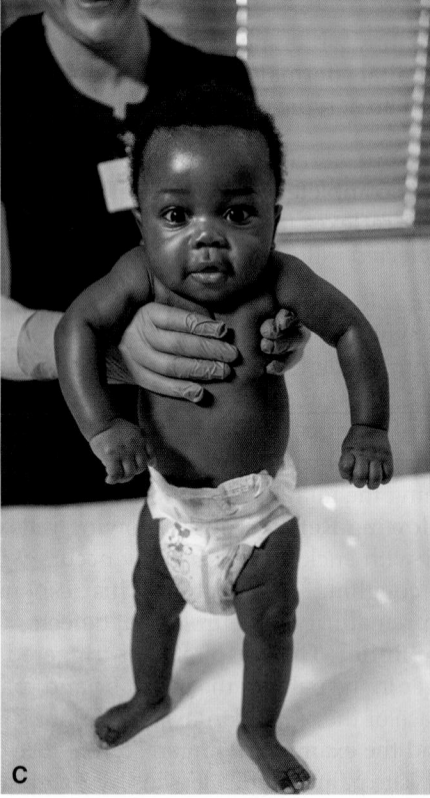

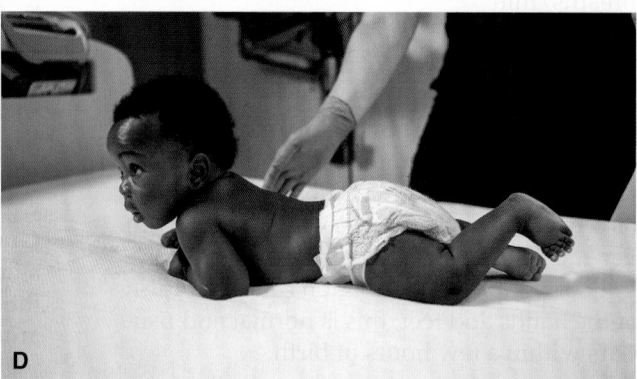

FIGURE 6-4 Several infant reflexes: *A,* the palmar grasp reflex; *B,* tonic neck reflex; *C,* stepping reflex; and *D,* crawling reflex.

crawling movements with their arms and legs. This response should disappear by 6 weeks of age.
- **Babinski Reflex.** The Babinski reflex is elicited by stroking upward along the lateral aspect of the sole. A positive response occurs when the toes hyperextend and the great toe dorsiflexes. An infant who does not respond in this manner should undergo a neurological evaluation. This reflex disappears as the infant begins to walk or between 12 and 18 months.

Cognitive Development of the Neonate

In the first month of life, the neonate responds to stimuli in a reflexive manner. Piaget described this as the *sensorimotor phase.* Despite the newborn's limited voluntary abilities, the sensory functions are well developed.

Vision At birth, the eyes are treated with antibiotics to prevent blindness caused by a mother infected with

gonorrhea or chlamydia. After the ointment has been absorbed, the newborn begins to fixate on an object. During the first few weeks of life, the infant focuses on objects, following from side to side with their gaze.

- The infant has visual preferences for the human face, black-and-white contrasting patterns, and large objects.
- Some newborns appear cross-eyed because of undeveloped ocular muscle control; this normally resolves in 3 to 4 months.
- Eye color varies from dark brown to slate gray to pale blue.
- Because the lacrimal apparatus is not fully developed, the newborn does not produce tears until at least week 4 of life.

Hearing and Smell Once the amniotic fluid drains from the ears, hearing is equivalent to that of an adult.

Newborns react strongly to pungent odors by turning the head away from a smell and are able to distinguish their own mother's breast milk from other breast milk. They will cry for their mother when her breasts are engorged and leaking.

Touch The newborn has a highly developed sense of touch, and their tactile sensation is surprisingly sophisticated, especially around the mouth, hands, and feet.

Psychosocial Development of the Neonate

The neonate calms when held or with other pacifying measures, such as a warm blanket, pacifier, and swaddling. Crying is the principal method for communicating a need or displeasure. Sometimes crying occurs simply because the neurological system is immature. Erikson identified the central developmental task of the first 18 months of life as developing a sense of trust. The neonate is completely dependent on their caretakers for all needs. Prompt responses to cries of discomfort create security and trust and promote **attachment,** or emotional bonding between parent and child.

Common Health Problems of the Neonate

Respiratory Distress Respiratory distress is one of the most serious problems facing newborns. It occurs most commonly in infants born before the lungs mature but can also be caused by aspiration of meconium during the birthing process. Symptoms are pale or mottled skin, labored respirations, hypothermia, and flaccid muscle tone.

Birth Injuries Injuries may occur at the time of the birthing process. The following are three examples:

- **Caput succedaneum,** edema of the scalp that crosses the suture lines, results from head compression against the cervix during labor. The fluid is reabsorbed in 1 to 3 days.
- **Fracture of the clavicle** occurs with breech presentation or as a result of difficulty delivering a large baby whose shoulder gets stuck behind the pelvic bones. Often no intervention is needed except for careful handling and support of the affected bone.
- **Birth asphyxia** is a serious and potentially permanent injury resulting from perinatal events, such as a *cord prolapse* (compression of the umbilical cord), *placental abruption* (bleeding secondary to tear of the placenta), other interruptions of the blood supply between the baby and placenta, or a delay in infant respiration after birth.

Congenital Anomalies Congenital anomalies (birth defects) may be visible at birth or may become apparent in the neonatal period. Treatment may be initiated, if appropriate. Congenital heart defects, fistulas, cleft lip and palate, and inborn metabolic problems are some common birth defects.

Infectious Microorganisms Infectious microorganisms that do not cause illness in older babies can cause sepsis in newborns, especially those born prematurely. Pregnant patients should be screened prenatally for STIs, and treatment should be initiated, if possible. Newborns exposed to infections during the gestational period should be tested as soon as possible after birth.

Jaundice Within 48 to 72 hours after birth, the newborn's red blood cell (RBC) count normally begins to decrease. One by-product of RBC destruction is **bilirubin,** a yellowish pigment. If the newborn is not successful in eliminating the excess bilirubin, jaundice develops, giving the newborn's skin a yellowish cast. If the bilirubin level becomes too high, the newborn can suffer neurological consequences as the pigment enters the brain. Sunlight breaks down bilirubin; thus, phototherapy is a treatment of choice for jaundice.

Effects of Maternal Substance Abuse. See Example Client Condition: Substance Abuse.

ASSESSMENT/RECOGNIZING CUES (NEONATE)

Physical assessment begins at birth.

Apgar Scoring. The initial assessment tool is the **Apgar scoring system.** The score is based on heart rate, respiratory effort, muscle tone, reflex irritability, and skin color. Each category is scored at 1 and 5 minutes after birth.

- The 1-minute score indicates how well the baby tolerated the birthing process.
- The 5-minute score indicates how well the baby is adapting to their new environment.
- A high score indicates fetal well-being.
- Factors that can lower the score are prematurity, neuromuscular disease, and maternal sedation during the birthing process

  For a table with Apgar scoring,

 Go to Chapter 6, **Assessment Guidelines & Tools, Apgar Scoring,** in Volume 2.

Transition to Extrauterine Life. During the first 24 hours after birth, the nurse assesses the infant's transition to extrauterine life:

- *First 8 hours.* The infant alternately cries and appears interested in the environment.
- *Sleep Stage.* The infant then enters the sleep stage, which lasts 2 to 4 hours. The heart and respiratory rates decrease, and the infant is in a state of calm.
- *Alert Stage.* After the sleep phase, the infant is alert and responsive. The heart and respiratory rates again increase.

Screening. Shortly after birth, newborns are screened for a variety of genetic disorders. Most states require screening for phenylketonuria (an inborn error of metabolism), hypothyroidism, galactosemia, and sickle cell disease.

Other You will also need to assess the following parameters:

Vital signs
Elimination (first urine and meconium)
Presence of congenital anomalies
Reflexes
Ability to breastfeed or take formula from a bottle
Skin integrity
Parent–infant attachment

IMPLEMENTATION/TAKING ACTION (NEONATE)

The neonatal period is a time of transition. Feeding concerns and uncertainty about appropriate care are the primary reasons parents seek healthcare advice. Nursing interventions for the neonate are designed to smooth the transition to extrauterine life and help the neonate adjust to their new environment. Activities include the following:

■ ✛ Thoroughly dry the neonate at birth and after bathing to prevent heat loss via evaporation. Also, wrap the neonate in blankets, and place them in their mother's arms or in a warmed crib.

■ Assist the mother with breastfeeding or formula feeding. Assistance is often needed with the first few feedings as the newborn learns to latch on to the nipple.

■ Teach parents the importance of providing warmth, nutrition, and a clean environment to prevent infection.

■ Teach the caregivers about expected behavior, including crying, eating, and elimination.

■ Provide circumcision care. **Circumcision** is the surgical removal of the foreskin of the penis. Parental consent is required for this procedure. Many male infants are circumcised a day or two after birth, although there is controversy over risks and benefits. The main reason most parents elect circumcision for their infant is social, so their child looks like other family members and peers. Care of the site depends on the procedure used. Whatever the procedure, regularly observe and teach parents to observe for hemorrhage, swelling, or oozing (signs of infection).

INFANCY: 1 MONTH TO 1 YEAR OF AGE

The remainder of the first year is known as **infancy.** This is a time associated with rapid and dramatic physical changes and the acquisition of numerous skills.

Physical Development of the Infant

Growth

The full-term newborn:

■ Loses approximately 8% to 10% of birth weight in the first days of life but will regain it by 2 weeks of age.
■ Gains about 1.5 pounds per month for the first 3 months.

■ Doubles birth weight by 5 months of age and triples by 1 year.
■ Increases in length approximately 1 inch per month until 6 months of age; it then slows to 1 inch over the next 6 months.
■ Increases in head circumference by about 33% in the first year.

Eruption of Primary Teeth Eruption of teeth varies among children, but there is a distinct, predictable pattern.

■ The first tooth typically appears between 6 and 8 months of age.
■ First to appear are the lower central incisors, followed by the upper central incisors.

Feeding Infants typically consume about 30 oz of breast milk or formula per day by 4 months of age. Breastfeeding is recommended because it is considered the most complete nutritional source for infants up to 6 months of age. However, if breastfeeding is not possible or acceptable to the parents, the nurse should support the parents' choice of method.

■ **Key Point:** *Breastfed infants have a lower incidence of food allergies, gastroenteritis, ear infections, and overweight in childhood, adolescence, and adulthood (Yasmeen et al., 2019).*
■ **Key Point:** *Breast milk supplies immunoglobulins that help the infant to resist infection.*

Most infants are physiologically ready to take solid foods between 4 and 6 months of age, but adequate nutrition can be maintained with breast milk or formula for a full year. The choices of when to begin introducing solid foods and when to wean are often culturally determined.

Sleep Patterns Generally by 3 to 4 months, the infant has developed a night pattern of sleeping and can sleep approximately 10 hours. Infants vary in the number and length of naps they take, but the total number of hours they sleep per day is about 15.

Motor Development Motor development follows a predictable pattern. Box 6-1 lists typical milestones.

Cognitive Development of the Infant

Piaget describes the infancy phase of cognitive development as the *sensorimotor phase:*

■ Whereas the neonate responds in a reflexive manner, the infant makes major strides in motor development and is able to vocally interact with caregivers.
■ An infant's visual acuity and color discrimination allow them to see and explore the environment.
■ Hearing is becoming more discriminating, and infants please themselves by vocalizing with cooing, laughing, and repeating sounds they find pleasurable.
■ By the 12th month, the infant is able to imitate sounds and understand simple words and may have a vocabulary of four or five simple words, such as *da-da.*

BOX 6-1 ■ Milestones of Infant Development

- By the age of 3 months, infants can smile.
- By 5 months, rolls from abdomen to back.
- By 6 months, turns from back to abdomen.
- At 7 months, most can sit alone.
- At about 9 months, crawls on hands and knees.
- By 10 months, pincer grasp is well enough developed to pick up finger foods and can move from a prone to sitting position.
- At 11 months, can "cruise"—walk while holding on to furniture.
- By 12 months, many infants attempt their first independent steps.
- By 12 months, many can pick up objects and let them go, put objects into a container, and take them out again. Typically, can also find an object that has been hidden and are beginning to use objects, such as cups and combs, correctly, as when "combing dolly's hair."
- By 12 months, typically responds to simple verbal requests and commands, such as "Stop!" or "No." May also use simple gestures, such as waving bye-bye or shaking their head no, and they may try to imitate adults' words.
- Psychosocial milestones include testing of caregivers to see what response is elicited by crying or refusals, for example; anxiety with strangers; and strong preference for the primary caregiver (usually the mother).

- At this stage, infants learn by doing. They develop a simple sense of cause and effect, delighting in the fact that squeezing a ball, for example, causes it to squeak and repeating their experiment over and over again.

Psychosocial Development of the Infant

Key Point: *In infancy the central task remains the development of trust.* The response of the caregivers in the neonatal phase has set the tone for ongoing interaction between caregivers and child. Continued prompt responses to discomfort, cuddling, and stimulating interaction provide the infant with a sense of trust in the world.

Freud refers to infancy as the *oral stage.*

- The infant receives pleasure in sucking and learns to quiet themself by oral stimulation, such as eating, sucking on a pacifier, or placing a hand in the mouth.
- At 2 or 3 months of age, infants begin to smile in response to others.
- At about 9 months, they interact more with their environment and socialize with others. They enjoy simple games such as peek-a-boo and patty-cake.

Common Health Problems of the Infant

Common problems that cause distress for infants and their caregivers include the following.

Crying and Colic

Crying often alarms parents, but it is a form of communication for the normal infant, as well as a normal reaction to discomfort, cold, or hunger. A healthy infant will have "fussy" periods each day that may last up to 1 to 2 hours.

Extended crying may be a sign of **colic,** a term used to describe frequent episodes of abdominal pain. The infant is often inconsolable during these episodes. The cause is unknown, although you may hear several theories. Colic typically disappears at about 3 months of age.

Failure to Thrive

Infants depend on their caregivers for food, water, warmth, comfort, and love. An infant who is deprived of a comforting, responsive relationship with a mother or caregiver will not thrive even if supplied with adequate nutrition. The infant will fail to gain weight, be unable to meet age-appropriate developmental tasks, be malnourished, and may have difficulty interacting with others. This syndrome, known as **failure to thrive,** is exhibited, for example, in infants born into families with inadequate support or understanding of infant needs and who may not provide the right kinds or amounts of food. Erikson believed the syndrome was proof of the essential nature of the trust-versus-mistrust stage. **Key Point:** *Notice, however, that failure to thrive can also stem from organic causes, such as disease or drug withdrawal.*

Dental Caries

Dental caries (tooth decay) can develop even by the end of the first year in infants allowed to sleep with a bottle containing anything other than water. Caries are caused by pooling in the back of the mouth of fluids containing sugar, such as breast milk, formula, or juice. If you need more information about dental problems, see Chapter 22.

Unintentional Injury

- Automobile accidents are a major cause of death in infants, often because the child was not properly restrained.
- Falls, burns, choking, and drowning are other common causes of accidental injury and death in infants. As infants mature, they may attempt to climb from cribs onto chairs or tables, or up or down ungated stairs.
- Their tendency to explore things with their mouths may lead to choking on small objects, such as bottle caps, buttons, and parts of toys.

If you require more information about infant safety, refer to Chapter 21.

Sudden Infant Death Syndrome (SIDS)

SIDS is the sudden death of a previously healthy infant with no explainable cause.

- Although the cause is unknown, evidence indicates that SIDS may be associated with defects in the portion of an infant's brain that controls breathing and arousal from sleep. Researchers have identified measures that can protect an infant from SIDS. Perhaps the most important is placing the baby on their back to sleep. The peak incidence is usually around 3 to 4 months of age, although it may occur up to 12 months of age.

- An increased incidence is associated with prematurity, low birth weight, male gender, African American/Black race, smoking in the household, swaddling, and putting an infant to sleep in the prone position.

- Breastfeeding and offering a pacifier at naptime and bedtime are thought to be preventive measures (Horne, 2019).

Example Client Condition: Abuse, Neglect, and Violence

Abuse and neglect are a classic example of a problem of development. For more information, refer to the accompanying Example Client Condition: Abuse, Neglect, and Violence.

EXAMPLE CLIENT CONDITION: Abuse, Neglect, and Violence

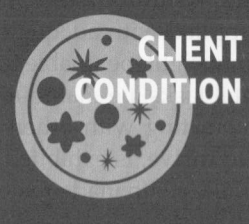
CLIENT CONDITION

Client Condition

Abuse, neglect, and violence are common problems that occur in all developmental stages and in all ethnic and socioeconomic groups. Abuse may be physical, emotional, or sexual; neglect is also a form of abuse. **Domestic violence** (or intimate partner violence [IPV]) is the abuse of power and control within an intimate relationship, most often between spouses or domestic partners. However, the abuser may be another family member. The Centers for Disease Control and Prevention (CDC) recognizes four categories of IPV:

- Physical violence
- Sexual violence
- Threat of physical or sexual violence
- Psychological or emotional abuse.

Incidence

Globally, 1 in every 3 women has been assaulted, coerced into sex, or otherwise abused at some point in her life (UN Women, 2016). Many victims do not report the abuse, so survey results vary.

Social determinants of health, including poverty, parental educational attainment, housing instability, food insecurity, and lack of health insurance, are associated with abuse, neglect, and violence.

- Approximately one in seven o women have experienced severe physical violence from an intimate partner. These numbers do not reflect the impact of the COVID-19 pandemic, which has increased risk factors for violence against women (WHO, 2021).
- Data from National Intimate Partner and Sexual Violence Survey (CDC, 2015) also show that nearly 1 in 11 women (8.8%) has been raped by a current or former intimate partner.
- Approximately 9.2% of women and 2.5% of men have been stalked by an intimate partner (Breiding, et al., 2015).

Factors Contributing to Domestic Partner Violence

Factors associated with intimate partner violence include young age, low-income status, pregnancy, young maternal age, low maternal education, large family size, mental health problems, alcohol or substance abuse by victims or perpetrators, separated or divorced status, single-parent household, and history of childhood sexual or physical abuse (Fraze et al., 2019).

Developmental Considerations

Infants

Abusive head trauma (formerly shaken-baby syndrome) caused by violent shaking of an infant; it can cause severe brain injury.

Toddlers, Preschoolers

- Often detected in this stage as children come in contact with more people outside the home.
- The youngest children are the most vulnerable to maltreatment. In the United States more than one-quarter (27.3%) of victims were younger than 3 years. The rate was highest for children younger than 1 year (Peterson et al., 2018).

Adolescents

Dating violence is widespread. It has serious short- and long-term effects. Many teens do not report it because they are afraid or embarrassed to tell friends and family. Females 6 to 24 years of age are the most vulnerable to nonfatal violence.

Young Adulthood

- Each year, more than 10 million women and men in the United States experience physical violence by a current or former intimate partner.
- In the United States, women are 7 to 14 times more likely to be abused than are men. About 31% of female murder victims are killed by an intimate partner, compared with 3% of male victims.

EXAMPLE CLIENT CONDITION: Abuse, Neglect, and Violence—cont'd

- The U.S. Preventive Services Task Force (2018d) recommends that clinicians screen women of childbearing age for abuse or domestic violence and provide or refer women who screen positive to intervention services.

Middle Adulthood
- *Intimate murder*—Women aged 30 to 49 are the most vulnerable.
- *Intimate violence*—Occurs more often in younger women.

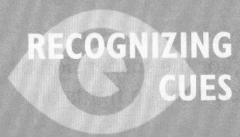

RECOGNIZING CUES

- Use a nonjudgmental approach. Do not make assumptions.
- Screen for risk factors associated with domestic abuse.
- Take a health history, assessing for physical, sexual, and psychological abuse.
- Perform a physical assessment; ensure the integrity of evidence that may be needed for criminal prosecution.
- Assess whether injuries are consistent with history and with the description of cause.
- Observe for signs of neglect.

Recognizing Cues of Child Violence

The following are a few of the cues you may look for:

Parental Characteristics
The parent or caregiver:
- Was abused as a child
- Has unrealistic expectations of the child
- Has unmet emotional needs
- Exhibits immaturity or lack of parenting knowledge
- Has issues of difficulty in relationships
- Is addicted to alcohol or drugs

Characteristics of the Child
- Has special needs that increase caregiver stress (e.g., disabilities, mental health issues, and chronic physical illnesses
- Is less than age 4 years

Recognizing Situational Cues
- The living space is crowded for the number of people it holds.
- There are the usual stresses of childcare to contend with.
- The parents face employment pressures or unemployment.
- The family must cope with poor housing and frequent household moves.

Also refer to the accompanying Safe, Effective Nursing Care box and

 Go to Chapter 6, Procedure 6-1, Assessing for Violence, in Volume 2

- ✚ Be aware of factors that increase the risk for child abuse and screen families for social determinants of health.

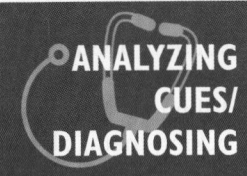

ANALYZING CUES/ DIAGNOSING

Self-esteem disturbance related to feeling guilty, deserving of abuse, and responsible for being a victim.

(continued)

EXAMPLE CLIENT CONDITION: Abuse, Neglect, and Violence—cont'd

GENERATE SOLUTIONS AND TAKE ACTION

- Refer to Procedure 6-1 in Volume 2.
- Federal funds support a variety of home-visit programs directed at high-risk mothers (identified on the basis of risk factors).
- Provide confidential information regarding domestic violence shelters.
- Based on social determinants of health, refer family to appropriate resources and monitor use of community resources.

- *Infants:* Teach parents the dangers of shaking a baby or picking a baby up by an arm or leg.

- *School-Age.* School violence can be addressed through psychological counseling, weapon-screening devices, school-wide educational programs, and policies calling for the suspension or expulsion of students who are caught intimidating other children or participating in fights on school property.
- **Key Point:** *If you suspect abuse, you are legally responsible for reporting your observations. As a beginning student, it is best to discuss your concerns with your instructor or the nurse assigned to the client before you make a report.*

- *Adults.* If the patient discloses domestic violence, act immediately. Ask the patient whether they would like you to contact the agency's domestic violence advocate (if there is one). If not, provide contact information for community domestic violence programs. Patients are often fearful, isolated, and in real danger, but they may refuse help the first time it is offered.

EVALUATING OUTCOMES

The patient will:
- Verbalize improved personal judgment of self-worth.
- Recognize an abusive relationship.
- Have evidence of healing of physical and psychological injuries.
- Demonstrate improved self-esteem.

ASSESSMENT/RECOGNIZING CUES (INFANT)

The infant typically has regular appointments with the pediatrician or primary care provider until at least 6 months of age. **Key Point:** *Visits are timed to coincide with the immunization schedule at 2, 4, 6, and 12 months.* At each visit:

- Measure the infant's growth and development and compare against standards for height, weight, head circumference, and gross and fine motor skills.
- The Denver Developmental Screening Test (Denver II) is a frequently used standardized test to assess development. The Denver II evaluates four major areas: personal-social, fine motor skills, language, and gross motor skills. It requires specialized training to administer and evaluate.

- Be aware of factors that increase the risk for child abuse. Assess for abuse anytime there is an injury that is not well explained by the parent's account of how it occurred.

- To assess for abuse and neglect, see the Example Client Condition: Abuse, Neglect, and Violence. Also refer to the accompanying Highlights of Procedures box and the Safe, Effective Nursing Care Box.

IMPLEMENTATION/TAKING ACTION (INFANT)

Key Point: *Nursing interventions for the infant focus on health promotion, safety, and growth and development.*

- **Nutrition.** Teach parents about adequate nutrition, adding foods to the diet, and expected elimination patterns. If breastfeeding is not possible or is not the parents' method of choice, commercially prepared formulas fortified with vitamins and minerals are acceptable. Cow's milk should not be used during the first year of life because infants have difficulty digesting the fat, and cow's milk is low in iron.
- ♥ **iCare** ▪ **Colic.** Provide information about using warmth, motion, and security to relieve colic. For example, parents might try swaddling the baby, cuddling them close to their body, rocking them, placing them in a "kangaroo" pouch or a back pack, or placing them in a swinging chair, which are all interventions that may provide relief.

- **Sudden Infant Death Syndrome (SIDS).** In accordance with recommendations in *Healthy People 2030*, teach parents to place infants on their backs to sleep (Fig. 6-5). Research shows that this greatly decreases the risk of SIDS. Additional interventions are discussed in Chapter 21.

Safe, Effective Nursing Care (SENC)

Detecting and Preventing Abuse

Chapter-Related Concepts: Age-Specific Assessments/Cue Recognition, Age-Specific Nursing Actions

Competency: Thinking, Doing, Caring

Thinking: Detection and prevention of abuse require collaborative efforts of the healthcare team. The goal of the collaborative approach is to reduce trauma to the victims during the investigation and assessment of the patient.

Doing: The team (comprising members from the Department of Child and Family Services [DCFS], law enforcement, state attorney's office, medical personnel, and mental health counselors) employs a multidisciplinary approach in dealing with issues of child abuse.

Caring: The team approach decreases the number of interviews and invasive procedures a child must endure, thereby reducing the trauma that children face when they have been victims of sexual or physical abuse.

Think about it

Do you see how teamwork and collaboration relate to the key concepts of development and stage?

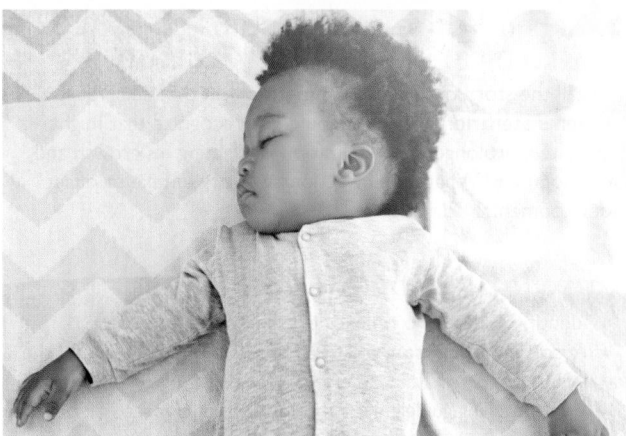

FIGURE 6-5 The "Back to Sleep" campaign teaches parents to place the infant in the supine position for sleeping.

 Car Seats. Stress the importance of car seats. Under federal law, infants must be secured in an approved car seat (in the back seat) every time they are in a vehicle. Because of poorly developed musculoskeletal head support, infants should be placed in a rear-facing position until 2 years of age and until they reach the height and weight recommended by the seat manufacturer (Durbin & Hoffman, 2018). For more information about car-seat restraints, refer to Chapter 21 in this book and

> Go to the American Academy of Pediatrics Web site at https://www.healthychildren.org/English/safety-prevention/on-the-go/Pages/Car-Safety-Seats-Information-for-Families.aspx

Immunizations. Immunizations are a major aspect of health promotion for the infant. The infant receives immunizations at 2, 4, 6, and 12 months. The immunization schedule and the catch-up immunization schedule have been approved by the AAP, the American Academy of Family Physicians (AAFP), and the ACOG. To see the CDC's optimal immunization schedule for children up to 6 years of age,

> Go to the CDC Web site at https://www.cdc.gov/vaccines/schedules/easy-to-read/child.html

 Unintentional Injury. Stress the importance of constant supervision. As the infant gains greater mobility, potential dangers (e.g., drowning, falls, and burns) increase. To prevent drowning, infants should never be left unattended in sinks, shallow baths, and plastic wading pools, even for a few seconds. To prevent scalding, caregivers should not drink or carry hot foods or fluids while holding the baby.

Play. Encourage sensory stimulation for the infant through parental interaction and age-appropriate toys.

Abuse, Neglect, and Violence. For interventions, see the preceding Example Client Condition: Abuse, Neglect, and Violence.

Highlights of Procedures 6-1

For steps to follow in all procedures, refer to the Universal Steps for All Procedures found on the inside back cover of Volume 2. Go to the full procedures in Volume 2 to practice and learn the skill. Use these Procedure Highlights later to help you review key steps.

Procedure 6-1: Assessing for Abuse

➤ Use a nonjudgmental approach. Do not make assumptions.

➤ Take a health history, identifying cues for physical, sexual, and psychological abuse.

➤ Perform a physical assessment; ensure the integrity of evidence that may be needed for criminal prosecution.

➤ Assess whether injuries are consistent with history.

➤ Observe for signs of neglect.

➤ If appropriate, refer for help in escaping the abusive situation.

➤ If appropriate, refer parent, caregiver, or partner involved in abuse to hotlines or agencies focused on stopping the abuse.

➤ Report abuse according to agency and state guidelines.

ThinkLike a Nurse 6-3:
Clinical Judgment in Action

Recall the story of Miguel, a 2-month-old, in the Meet Your Patients scenario. What cues could you recognize that might indicate a prolonged hospitalization is affecting his growth and development? What nursing actions would you take to offset developmental delays?

KnowledgeCheck 6-4

- Identify at least two reflexes present in the neonate.
- According to Erikson, what is the developmental stage of the infant?
- What teaching guideline is important in reducing the risk of SIDS?

TODDLERHOOD: AGES 1 TO 3 YEARS

Toddlerhood is a period of increased mobility, independence, and exploration. It is also the time of temper tantrums and negative behavior stemming from a toddler's desire to gain autonomy.

Physical Development of the Toddler

- **Key Point:** *The growth rate for toddlers is much slower than it is in infancy.*

   Weight. The average toddler gains 5 lb (2.3 kg) per year. By the second birthday, the typical toddler weighs 27 lb (12.25 kg).

   Height. By the second birthday, the typical toddler is 34 in. (86 cm) tall. Length is added mainly in the legs.

   Head Circumference. Head circumference is equal to the chest circumference. Between 12 and 18 months, the anterior fontanel closes (see Fig. 6-3).

- **Respirations and heart rate** slow in comparison with infancy, but blood pressure increases.

- **The stomach** increases in size to accommodate larger portions. Toddlers typically eat about 6 times a day, in relatively small portions, and join the family at mealtimes. Most toddlers enjoy picking up food with their hands to feed themselves.

- **The physical ability to control the anal and urethral sphincters develops** between 18 and 24 months. However, the child is ready when they can signal that their diaper is wet or soiled or is able to say that they would like to go to the toilet. This usually occurs at about 18 to 24 months of age, but it is not uncommon for a child to be in diapers until 3 years of age (AAP, n.d.).

- **Gross motor skills continue to be refined** during toddlerhood.

   By 10 to 15 months—Can walk using a wide stance.

   At 24 months—Many can walk up and down stairs one step at a time.

   At 30 months—Can jump using both feet.

   Before age 3—Can stand on one foot and climb steps with alternating feet.

- **Fine motor skills also continue to be refined.** The toddler uses their new motor skills and all five senses to explore their environment, and safety continues to be an important concern.

   By 15 months—Can grab and release small objects.

   By 18 months—Can throw a ball overhand (Fig. 6-6).

- **Visual acuity improves to 20/40** by the end of the toddler stage, and **strabismus** (crossed eyes) may still be seen transiently.

- **Hearing should be fully developed by toddlerhood.**

   Developmental milestones of toddlerhood are listed in Box 6-2.

Cognitive Development of the Toddler

During toddlerhood, the child completes Piaget's *sensorimotor phase* and moves into the *preconceptual phase*. This is a time of rapid language development and increasing curiosity. The toddler is able to name many things and begins to recognize that different objects (such as a ball, a block, and a puzzle) may be named the same thing (toys). This is the beginning of categorization and concept development. The child abandons trial and error and begins to solve problems by thinking. However, reasoning and judgment lag far behind. This discrepancy places the child at risk for accidents and injuries.

Psychosocial Development of the Toddler

- **The most important psychosocial developmental task for the toddler is to initiate more independence, control, and autonomy.** Erikson refers to this stage as

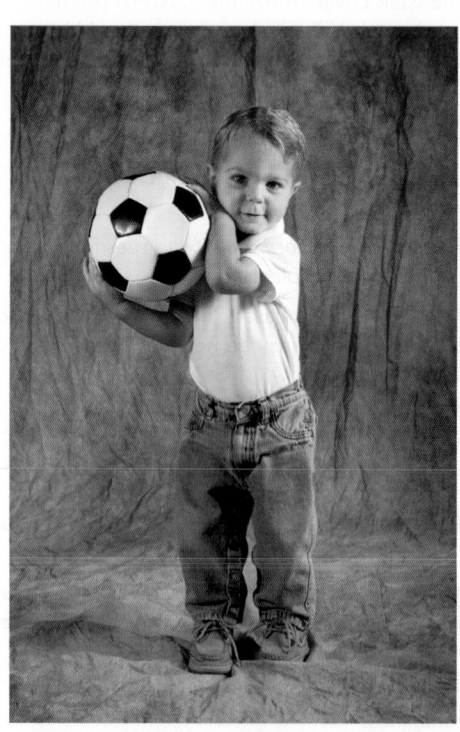

FIGURE 6-6 By 18 months, the toddler can throw a ball overhand.

BOX 6-2 ■ Milestones of Toddlerhood

- Can ride a tricycle, put simple puzzles together, build a tower of six to eight blocks, turn knobs, and open lids.
- Most can copy a circle or a vertical line.
- Can find an object that has been hidden in their view and can actively search for and find a hidden object.
- By age 3 years, most are toilet-trained. However, it is not abnormal for toddlers to continue to experience toileting problems well into the preschool period.
- Most can play matching games, sorting games, and simple mechanical games.
- Most have only a limited understanding of jokes and hyperbole; thus, if teased, "That balloon is so big, it might fly away with you," the child may become frightened and try to give the balloon away.
- Many can speak sentences of four or five words. However, some perfectly healthy toddlers do not yet speak, whereas others can speak in sentences of 10 or 11 words in length and even tell complex stories. If the toddler does speak, enunciation is good enough by the end of this period that strangers can usually understand what is said.
- *Psychosocial milestones* include the following: tolerates short separations from the primary caregiver, feels possessive of personal property, and openly expresses affection.
- Most object vehemently to changes in routine and may suffer regression after a move, change of school, or other upset.
- The toddler imitates adults, peers, and characters seen on television and videos and enjoys pretending to cook, iron, or repair something broken and mimicking other familiar adult tasks.
- In shared play, they can understand the concept of "taking turns" and wait a short period of time for their turn.

autonomy versus shame and doubt. To successfully negotiate this stage, the child must:

Learn to see themself as separate from caregiver.
Tolerate separation from the parents.
Withstand delayed gratification.
Learn to control anal and urinary sphincters.
Begin to communicate verbally and interact with others

- **Toddlers exert their independence by saying no to parental requests or actions or by "throwing a tantrum"** to protest a parental decision they don't like. This behavior is best understood as a necessary attempt to define boundaries and test parental limits; it may be far more challenging to parents who view it as stubbornness or naughtiness. A firm but calm parental response to such "misbehavior" allows toddlers to feel secure while exploring their boundaries.
- **Freud defined this phase as the** *anal stage.* To Freud, a successful toilet-training experience accompanied by praise is necessary to becoming a well-functioning adult; difficulty in this phase leads to obsessive-compulsive behavior in adulthood.

Common Health Problems of Toddlers

Unintentional Injury Drowning is the leading cause of accidental death in this age-group (Dellinger & Gilchrist, 2019). Most drowning accidents are due to unsupervised access to swimming pools or other water sources (bathtubs). Other common causes of injuries to toddlers are falls, motor vehicle accidents, burns and scalds, and choking. As toddlers gain increasing mobility, poisoning from household medications and toxic cleansers becomes a concern, as does access to knives, guns, and other dangers. For further discussion of safety concerns for toddlers, see Chapter 21.

Infections The most common infections are colds, ear infections, and tonsillitis. Other common infections include parasitic diseases, such as lice and tapeworms. The shorter and wider eustachian tube in infants and toddlers increases their risk for multiple ear infections, which in turn increases the risk for hearing loss. Upper respiratory infections are common among toddlers for the following reasons:

- Toddlers no longer have the passive immunity acquired in utero.
- Because breastfeeding usually ends before the first birthday, most toddlers no longer receive maternal antibodies in breast milk.
- As toddlers enter into more public and social settings, they are exposed to more children. Those in day care and those who have school-age siblings are particularly at risk.

Immunizations Key Point: *The CDC (2022a) recommendations for immunization are designed to protect infants and children early in life, when they are most vulnerable and before they are exposed to potentially life-threatening diseases.* Vaccines should be administered at the recommended age, but if not done, a vaccine can be administered at a later well-child visit. Catch-up schedules and minimum intervals between doses for children whose vaccinations have been delayed are included in the recommendations.

The CDC updates the immunization schedules periodically. To see the CDC's optimal immunization schedule for children up to 6 years of age,

> Go to the CDC Web site at https://www.cdc.gov/vaccines/schedules/index.html

The CDC (2022a) immunization schedule for toddlers includes the following vaccines:

Hepatitis A	Pneumococcal pneumonia
Hepatitis B	(PCV)
Haemophilus	Influenza vaccine (yearly)
influenza (Hib)	Inactivated poliovirus
Tetanus and diphtheria	(IPV)
toxoids and acellular	Measles/mumps/
pertussis (TdaP)	rubella (MMR)
Varicella	

Delayed Toilet Training Although not strictly speaking a "health" problem, many parents are concerned about what they perceive as delayed toilet training. Physiologically, most children develop sphincter and neurological control by age 2, but more is involved in successful toileting. Toddlers must learn to unfasten their clothing and pull down their pants, use toilet paper effectively, dress again, and wash their hands before they are completely independent. The child also must be able to sense the need to go to the bathroom, even when preoccupied with play activities, before it is "too late." Accidents are frequent, and parents should expect them.

ASSESSMENT/RECOGNIZING CUES (TODDLERHOOD)

♥ **iCare Children of this age are generally fearful of strangers.** Thus, before beginning your assessment, you will need to establish rapport. To do so, you might engage the child in play—for example, by playing catch with a soft ball or asking the child to introduce you to the stuffed animal they may have brought along. This is also a nonthreatening way to assess language skills and motor development. Encourage parents to relieve their child's stress and anxiety by holding the child during the examination and speaking to them in a calm and reassuring voice.

Toddlers Need Regular Physical Examinations At each office visit, evaluate the child's weight, height, growth, and development against standard growth charts and by comparing their skills against age-appropriate norms. Beginning at age 3, blood pressure should be checked at least once yearly, and the results should be recorded with age, gender, and height percentiles and reviewed with parents. Children with obesity, renal disease, diabetes, or underlying cardiac disease and those who are taking medications known to increase blood pressure should have their blood pressure measured at every office visit (Flynn et al., 2017).

IMPLEMENTATION/TAKING ACTION (TODDLERHOOD)

Health Teaching You cannot stress safety strongly enough to parents. Teach them:

- How to childproof the environment. Emphasize that increasing motor skills and dexterity allow the toddler to find many dangers, including stairways, windows, and electrical outlets.
- To provide constant supervision to prevent injury or death from such hazards.
- To use consistent, firm limits to help the toddler remain safe.
- To be vigilant about the toys they buy for their children in light of recent toy recalls because they contained lead and other toxic substances. Toys should be larger than the diameter of the trachea in order to avoid choking accidents.
- About basic first aid and the choking rescue maneuver. Encourage parents to enroll in a basic life-support class.

You will find the choking rescue maneuver and a detailed list of safety measures for toddlers in Chapter 21.

Health-Promotion Interventions At each wellness visit, reinforce the need for hand washing, tooth brushing, regular dental examinations, and a balanced diet. This is also a time for additional immunizations and boosters. Oral health teaching should include information on brushing, fluoride, nonnutritive oral habits, and dental injury prevention and recommend that children have a dental visit by 1 year of age (Davidson et al., 2021).

Methicillin-Resistant *Staphylococcus aureus* **(MRSA) and Vancomycin-Resistant Enterococci (VRE)** These organisms have put a spotlight on the threat posed by drug-resistant bacteria. **Key Point:** *Teach parents that antibiotics should not be used for simple colds and "flu." Explain the importance of taking the entire prescription when an antibiotic must be prescribed, even if the child's symptoms resolve before all the medication has been taken.* These actions help prevent the development of drug-resistant strains of bacteria.

Remind parents that many OTC cough and cold medicines are not safe for and may not have been approved for use in children, regardless of how they are marketed. Parents should be certain that any OTC medicines are truly safe for children.

KnowledgeCheck 6-5
- According to Erikson, what is the developmental stage of the toddler?
- What is the leading cause of accidental death in toddlers?

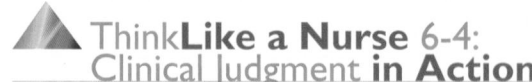

ThinkLike a Nurse 6-4: Clinical Judgment in Action
Recall Tamika, a 3-year-old girl, in the Meet Your Patients scenario. Her grandmother, who is also caring for her ill husband, is raising Tamika. What concerns does that raise about the home environment?

PRESCHOOL STAGE: AGES 4 AND 5 YEARS
The preschooler is growing increasingly verbal and independent and is refining gross and fine motor skills. They are able to maintain separation from parents, use language to communicate needs, control bodily functions, and cooperate with children as well as adults. These skills prepare the child to enter school.

Physical Development of the Preschooler
Growth
- By 4 years of age, the average preschooler weighs about 36 lb (16.3 kg) and is 40 in. (1 m) tall.

- By age 5, the preschooler has gained an additional 5 lb (2.3 kg) and grown 3 more in. (7.6 cm) in height.
- The proportions of head to trunk are somewhat closer.
- The "potbelly" and exaggerated lumbar curve of toddlerhood gradually disappear.
- The average pulse rate is 90 to 100 beats/min.
- Respirations are 22 to 25 breaths/min.

Sensorimotor Development The preschooler has mature depth and color perception and 20/20 vision. Hearing is also mature. The preschooler continues to develop eye–hand coordination. Improvement in fine motor skills is most evident in artwork. Drawings become much more precise and detailed. Developmental milestones for preschoolers are listed in Box 6-3.

Cognitive Development of Preschoolers

According to Piaget, the preschooler has entered the phase of *intuitive thought.* In general:

- They are able to classify objects and continue to form concepts.
- They still use trial and error as a way to solve problems but increasingly use thought to reason them out.

BOX 6-3 ■ Milestones of Preschool Development

- By age 5 years, most children can stand on one foot for 10 sec, skip, jump, hop on one foot or both feet together, climb play structures with ease, repeat simple dance steps, and begin to learn to skate.
- Most preschoolers can copy a triangle, square, and stick figure; print at least some letters; and use a fork and spoon.
- Most can dress and use the bathroom without assistance.
- Language abilities continue to be variable, but most preschoolers can tell stories, recall parts of a story told to them, and speak in sentences of more than five words. Most can state their name, age, and address, and many can repeat their home phone number. A toddler who is not speaking intelligibly by age 4 years requires evaluation.
- Preschoolers can count 10 or more objects, such as buttons or coins, and may be able to name several colors and shapes. They can compare big and small, long and short, and so on, and often delight in completing simple mazes and "connect the dots" games.
- Preschoolers become increasingly aware of sex organ differences and curious about sexuality.
- Preschoolers may begin to ask about God, death, how babies are born, and other questions of a philosophical or scientific nature.
- Preschoolers typically can distinguish fantasy from reality and enjoy jokes and simple riddles.
- Psychosocial milestones include assertion of independence; pride in showing off skills, new toys and clothes, and prize possessions to friends; and a strong desire to socialize with peers.

- Verbal skills expand dramatically during this phase, allowing the child to interact with more people.
- Preschool children are interested in books, learning to read, and counting.
- Preschoolers lack the ability to reason formally and are unable to understand that two objects that appear different may in fact be the same (e.g., two balls of clay in two different shapes).
- They have a limited ability to tell time or understand the passage of time, and they may say "yesterday" in describing an event of several months ago.
- Preschoolers retain a strong belief in magic, monsters, and mythic figures, such as Santa Claus.
- Preschoolers often have irrational fears—for example, of tigers lurking in the basement. Their fascination with powerful figures, such as dinosaurs and superheroes, is one way of coping with their feelings of powerlessness.

Psychosocial Development of Preschoolers

- **The preschooler is in Erikson's stage of** *initiative versus guilt.* In this stage, the child develops a conscience and readily recognizes right from wrong. The child becomes socially aware of others and develops the ability to consider other people's viewpoints. At this age, play is often used to teach life experiences.
- **The preschool child begins to fully express their personality and develop a self-concept** (see Chapter 10 if you need to learn more about self-concept). They readily express likes and dislikes. Encouraging the child to participate in their favorite activities helps foster a positive self-concept (Fig. 6-7). Preschool children enjoy playing in small groups and use their language skills to facilitate imaginative play. Elaborate stories, improvised costumes, and role-playing often become part of the play experience. Many preschoolers have a best friend.
- **Freud identified the preschool years as the** *phallic stage* of development. The child is aware of gender

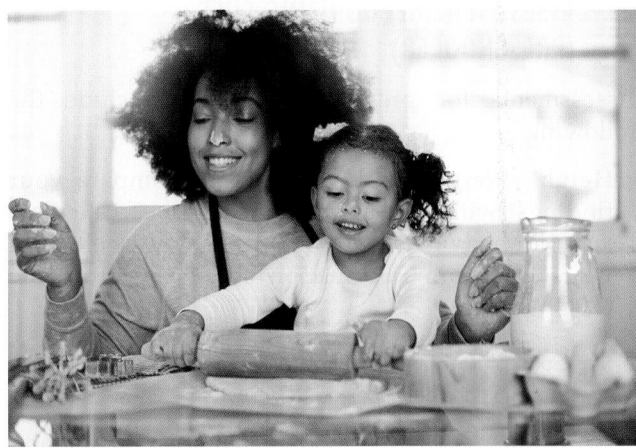

FIGURE 6-7 Preschoolers typically enjoy helping a parent in the kitchen.

differences and often imitates the same-sex parent. The child also develops an attraction to the opposite-sex parent and may feel jealousy toward the same-sex parent.

Common Health Problems of Preschoolers

The preschooler experiences health problems similar to those of the toddler.

Communicable Diseases Communicable diseases (e.g., respiratory infections, intestinal viruses, and parasitic infections such as scabies and lice) remain a major health issue, especially as preschoolers start to come into contact with more children in play and structured preschool experiences. They interact more with playmates and are hands-on, so they tend to readily transmit viruses through direct contact and airborne vectors.

Poisoning Poisoning remains a significant risk for preschoolers. They use imitation as a way to learn about new things. They may be predisposed to ingesting substances used by the adults in the house (prescription medicines and alcohol, or substances that appear similar).

Enuresis Parents of preschoolers may report a concern about bed-wetting (**enuresis**), especially in males. The causes of enuresis are not fully understood, but it is known that in some children, the bladder is simply unable to hold a full night's output of urine until later in childhood, whereas other children lack the neurological ability to waken in response to a full bladder. Most cases resolve spontaneously, with only very occasional episodes past age 6. In contrast, daytime wetting or soiling (**encopresis**) requires evaluation.

Example Client Condition: Child Abuse, Neglect, and Violence For information on child abuse, see the preceding Example Client Condition: Abuse, Neglect, and Violence.

ASSESSMENT/RECOGNIZING CUES (PRESCHOOLER)

Assessments for preschoolers should include the following:

- **Height, Weight, and Vital Signs.** Compare your findings with age-appropriate norms. Calculate and plot body mass index (BMI) at every well-child visit. To obtain information about this from the CDC Web site,

  Go to BMI—Body Mass Index at http://www.cdc.gov/nccdphp/dnpa/bmi/index.htm

- **Nutrition.** Assess for food preferences, habits, and amount eaten. The preschool child often has strong food preferences.

- **Sleep Habits.** Assess the number of hours slept, bedtime rituals, and problems with night awakenings. Preschoolers are generally very active but require adequate rest. This is also the stage when children stop taking afternoon naps.
- **Vision Screening.** The U.S. Preventive Services Task Force (USPSTF) (2017b) recommends vision screening for all children at least once between the ages of 3 and 5 years to detect the presence of amblyopia (lazy eye) or its risk factors.
- **Dental Hygiene.** During the preschool years, all deciduous teeth have erupted. Therefore, dental hygiene is very important. At each visit, ask the child about toothbrushing habits. If possible, have the child demonstrate how they brush. The child should already have made at least one visit to a dentist by age 3. *Healthy People 2030* oral health goals include prevention and control of oral and craniofacial diseases by providing access for all school-age children to fluoridated water, tooth sealants, and preventive oral care. For more information,

  Go to the *HealthyPeople 2030* Web site at health.gov

- **Safety Risks** Assess for parent and child knowledge of hazards and precautions. Because the preschool child is mobile and involved in active play (riding a tricycle, crossing streets), accidents increase.

- **School Readiness.** A physical examination is required before the child enters school. This examination should include an *assessment for readiness*—whether the child has acquired skills such as the ability to converse with adults, follow instructions, hold a pencil, and perform a variety of motor skills, such as jumping, hopping, and walking a straight line.

  Also *review the immunization record.* Several boosters and immunizations are due at this time, and any that are missed must be administered before the child enters school. To see the CDC's Catch-Up Immunization Schedule,

  Go to the CDC Web site at https://www.cdc.gov/vaccines/schedules/hcp/child-adolescent.html

- For other information, refer to Common Health Problems of Toddlers earlier in this chapter.

IMPLEMENTATION/TAKING ACTION (PRESCHOOLER)

The preschool child is interactive and curious. Speak directly to the child, and include the child in your teaching sessions. Teaching topics include the following:

- *Frequent hand washing to prevent the spread of disease.* Teach the child hand-washing technique, and encourage parents to model frequent hand washing.
- *Proper brushing and flossing of teeth.* Most preschoolers still need supervision while brushing their teeth.

- *Essentials of a balanced diet.* Encourage parents to offer a well-balanced diet and instill healthy eating habits. By age 5, most children are willing to try new foods and are better able to sit during an entire meal. Generally, preschoolers eat half of the food portion of an adult.
- *Importance of adequate rest.* The average preschooler requires at least 12 hours of sleep each night.
- ✚ *Hazard of stranger danger.* Increasing independence and mobility place the preschool child at risk for abduction. Teach the child to avoid talking to strangers and to never enter a stranger's home or car. This topic is explored in depth once the child is in school.
- ✚ *Importance of seat belts and car seats.* Current recommendations are to use a booster seat for children weighing between 40 and 80 lb and to continue using the seat until the child is at least 4 feet 9 inches tall.

KnowledgeCheck 6-6

- According to Erikson, what is the developmental stage of the preschooler?
- Identify at least two important assessments to make when providing care to a preschooler.

SCHOOL-AGE: AGES 6 TO 12 YEARS

The school-age child becomes more independent and confident and places more importance on relationships outside the immediate family. Developmental milestones of the school-age period are summarized in Box 6-4.

BOX 6-4 ■ Milestones of School-Age Development

- By age 7 years, most children can tie their own shoelaces, print their names, and perform self-care, such as bathing and feeding themselves. Many can even prepare simple meals.
- By age 8 years, improved fine motor skills allow the child to begin to write, learn to knit or crochet, and/or take up a musical instrument.
- By age 9 years, motor development approaches that of an adult.
- School-age children understand the concept of payment for work and the value of money.
- Fears of ghosts and monsters may continue through age 7 years but give way to more realistic fears, such as of school failure or divorce of parents, by age 8 or 9 years.
- By age 6 years, the child has a vocabulary of 3,000 words and usually can read. By the end of the school-age period, the child can write complex compositions with appropriate grammar, spelling, and accurate description.
- Psychosocial development includes team play, peer friendships, and the ability to look beyond family members for social support.

Physical Development of the School-Age Child

Growth During the school-age years, the child grows about 2 in. (5 cm) taller and gains 4 to 7 lb (2.3 to 3 kg) per year. The child takes on a slimmer appearance, with longer legs and a lower center of gravity.

- *Musculoskeletal.* Muscle mass rapidly increases, and ossification of bones continues throughout this stage. Strength and physical abilities rapidly improve, and the child gains more poise and coordination.
- *Brain and skull.* The brain and skull grow slowly, and facial characteristics mature.
- *GI system.* The gastrointestinal system matures and stomach capacity increases, although caloric demands decrease.
- *Immune system.* As the immune system develops, the school-age child begins to produce antibodies and antigens.
- *Biological sex comparisons.* Initially, males and females vary little in size. Toward the end of this phase, marked differences become apparent. Girls grow rapidly in the latter school-age years as puberty begins. They experience the onset of puberty about 2 years before boys do.

Visual Acuity Visual acuity improves with age. By 6 years of age, distance visual acuity should be at least 20/30 in each eye, with less than two lines' difference between the two eyes. Any child not meeting these criteria should be referred for a complete eye examination.

Dentition School-age children begin to lose their primary teeth (baby teeth) at about age 6 or 7, and the permanent teeth appear soon after. Their large size in relation to the remaining primary teeth and the child's jaw, as well as the gaps left by teeth not yet replaced, can make even the most beautiful children look somewhat awkward at this stage.

Cognitive Development of the School-Age Child

Key Point: *School-age children use their thought processes to experience actions and events. Piaget describes this as concrete operations.*

- Concrete and systematic
- Magical beliefs gradually replaced with a passion to understand how things really are
- Can see another person's point of view and develops an understanding of relationships
- Learns to classify objects according to similarities
- Enjoys learning by handling and manipulating objects
- Learns to tell time and gains an experiential understanding of the length of days, months, and years
- Reads independently; does numerical calculations without representative objects such as fingers or beads

■ By the end of this stage, is able to think through a task and understand it without actually performing the task

Psychosocial Development of the School-Age Child

Erikson describes this stage as a time of industry versus inferiority. During this stage, the child is able to work on more complex projects independently. Through participation in school, they are recognized for achievements and accomplishments. For the child to progress through this stage, the parent must also provide praise for accomplishments. This recognition builds self-confidence. The child will develop a sense of inferiority and lack of self-worth if their accomplishments are met with a negative response.

Peers take on increasing importance, influencing the child's choices of what to eat, wear, and do. Friendships during the school-age years are usually with children of the same gender and may be intense but short-lived (Fig. 6-8). However, some children have one best friend throughout their childhood. In the later school-age years, friendships become more reciprocal, with each child recognizing the unique qualities of the other.

Common Health Problems of School-Age Children

School-age children are at risk for problems similar to those of preschoolers, including upper respiratory tract infections, parasitic infections such as scabies and lice, and dental caries. Although violence, bullying, smoking, and experimentation with alcohol, drugs, and sex are more common among adolescents, these problems are also seen toward the end of the school-age years. The presence of a gun in the home significantly increases the risk of accidental death, even in the school-age population.

Childhood Obesity

■ **Obesity is a growing health problem for the school-age child.** According to the CDC (2021c),

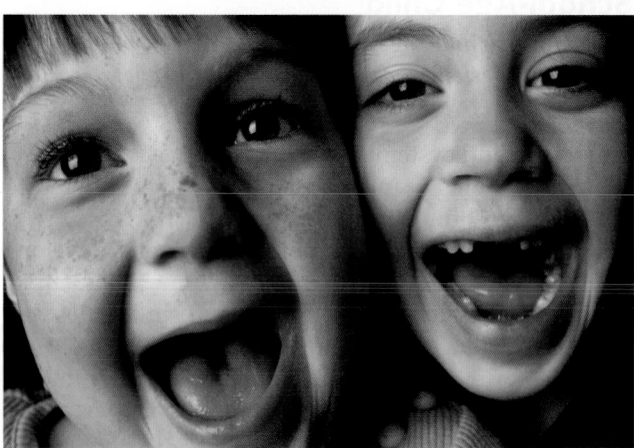

FIGURE 6-8 Same-gender friendships are important to school-age children.

the percentage of children with obesity in the United States has more than tripled over the past 5 decades. Today, about one in five school-age children (ages 6–19 years) has obesity.

■ **Nutrition and lifestyle are primarily responsible for this epidemic.** Children spend more time in sedentary activities (e.g., watching television, playing video games, texting, using social media) and less time participating in more physical activities. They consume more fast food and bigger portions and eat fewer vegetables. Fifty percent of all meals are taken outside the home, and fast food contributes to 30% of overall calorie intake (Saksena et al., 2018).

■ **Children with obesity are at higher risk for chronic health conditions and diseases,** such as asthma, sleep apnea, and type 2 diabetes mellitus (DM), and are at higher risk for heart disease.

■ **Children with obesity experience bullying** more than their normal-weight peers and may experience social isolation, depression, and lower self-esteem.

■ **Childhood obesity also is associated with having obesity as an adult.**

Childhood Asthma

■ *Asthma,* **a chronic inflammatory disorder of the airways, is one of the most common chronic disorders in childhood,** currently affecting an estimated 5.1 million children under 18 years. Of those, 2.2 million suffered from an asthma attack or episode in 2020 (CDC, 2020a).

■ **Asthma is the leading cause of school absenteeism and the third-leading cause of hospitalization** of children under the age of 15 years.

■ **Social problems may occur; for example, children may be teased and stigmatized** as being "wheezers" or "lazy." Even in children who do not require emergency care, asthma can decrease attention span in school and make participation in school activities difficult.

■ **Asthma has complex causes, including a strong genetic component,** but poverty appears to play at least some role. Recent research has focused on indoor air allergens, such as pet dander, dust mites, fungi or mold, and the decomposing corpses of cockroaches, as significant triggers.

Unintentional Injuries in School-Age Children

School-age children experience fewer injuries than preschoolers because of their increased coordination and improved reasoning abilities. Nevertheless, they have a high incidence rate of fractures, sprains, strains, cuts, and abrasions. Falls are the most common form of nonfatal injury for children ages 6 to 12 years, whereas the leading cause of unintentional injury death is motor vehicle and traffic injury (National Center for Health Statistics, 2021).

Concussions are one of the most commonly reported injuries in children and adolescents who participate in sports and recreation activities. Although many concussions may be considered mild, they can result in health consequences such as impaired thinking, memory problems, and emotional or behavioral changes (Halstead et al., 2018). If you would like more information about unintentional injuries, see Chapter 21.

ASSESSMENT/RECOGNIZING CUES (SCHOOL-AGE)

The school-age child should have a routine health maintenance visit every 1 or 2 years. Annual physical examinations are scheduled for those who participate in sports. Allow time to meet with the child alone as well as time with the caregiver present. School-age children often have questions about puberty and the changes their bodies are undergoing. Private time with the child will allow you to explore these concerns in a private manner.

Nursing Interview The nursing interview should address the following topics:

- **Nutrition.** Assess the child's nutrition, including intake of key nutrients such as calcium, vitamin D, and iron.
- **Allergies.** Ask the child whether they ever experience difficulty breathing or feel too tired to play. Ask about symptoms, such as clear nasal discharge, frequent sneezing, or watery eyes. Listen to breath sounds and observe for allergy symptoms.
- **Visual Acuity.** Ask about any eye screenings. Because children do not complain about visual difficulties, the AAP recommends that children aged older than 5 years be screened every 1 to 2 years (Donahue et al., 2016).
- **Dental Hygiene.** Interview the child to determine their knowledge of dental hygiene. Inspect the mouth for secondary teeth eruption according to expected patterns and for tooth decay and gum disease.
- **Sleep Pattern.** Assess the child's sleep pattern. To remain healthy and function well at school, the school-age child needs 9 to 10 hours of sleep each night.
- **Safety.** Determine the child's awareness of safety. Be sure to assess risk-taking behavior:
  Smoking—Has the child tried smoking or vaping? Do they have friends who are smoking or vaping?
  Substances—What is the child's experience with alcohol and drugs? Have they tried them? What does their peer group think about drinking and drugs?
  Sexual activity—Have they ever been sexually active? Do they have friends who are sexually active?
  Violence—Has the child engaged in fistfights or fights with knives or other weapons?
  Weapons—Is there a gun in the home? Does the child have access to it?

Although these concerns are seen with greater frequency in adolescence, you should assess for them among school-age children.

BMI At each visit, assess the child's vital signs, height, weight, and developmental skills. After weighing the child, correlate your measurements with growth charts. The American Heart Association (2013) BMI classifications are as follows:

Overweight	At 85th percentile
Obese	At or above the 95th percentile—obese

Visual Acuity Visual acuity should be at least 20/30 in each eye, with less than two lines' difference between the two eyes. Any child not meeting these criteria should be referred for a complete eye examination.

Scoliosis Screening Scoliosis is an abnormal spinal curvature that primarily affects females. Screening is done in the preadolescent period, usually in the sixth grade. Refer to an orthopedic surgeon for evaluation and follow-up if an abnormal curvature is discovered.

Immunizations Review the immunization record. Although immunization against hepatitis B is recommended in infancy, parents may skip these immunizations. Several states require students to complete the hepatitis B series before entry into seventh grade. The child must begin the series at or before 12 years of age to complete it in time for seventh grade. The CDC (2022a) recommends the following vaccines for school-age children: human papillomavirus; meningococcal; pneumococcal; influenza; hepatitis A; hepatitis B; inactivated poliovirus; measles, mumps, and rubella; varicella; and tetanus, diphtheria, and pertussis booster. Other vaccinations may be required if the child is catching up on missed vaccines. To see this schedule,

 Go to the CDC, 2021 Recommended Immunizations for Persons Aged 0 Through 18 Years https://www.cdc.gov/vaccines/schedules/hcp/imz/child-adolescent.html

Also refer to the previous section, Common Health Problems of School-Age Children.

IMPLEMENTATION/TAKING ACTION (SCHOOL-AGE)

The *Healthy People 2030* campaign focuses on reducing fatal and nonfatal injury rather than on treating illness. Your efforts in patient teaching will help promote the national *Healthy People 2030* population objectives. Use age-appropriate teaching materials and methods.

Teaching for Safety

To help prevent injury in the school-age child:

- Educate the child and parents on safety and the proper use of equipment and gear.
- Teach them to wear seat belts at all times in a vehicle.
- Encourage parents to be firm about the use of helmets for bicycle safety.
- Stress that head injury is a common cause of death in this group.
- For those who play sports, stress the importance of warming

up before playing, using safety equipment that is properly fitted, and avoiding overtraining.

Teaching About Nutrition and Exercise for Weight Loss

Counsel overweight and obese children about nutrition for weight loss and the importance of daily physical activity.

Teaching About Nutrition

- Encourage children to develop good eating habits by choosing nutritious foods and snacks. For example, encourage them to avoid junk foods, such as sodas, and to choose water instead.
- Focus on making small but permanent changes. If the diet is severely restrictive, and if it has none of the child's favorite foods, it is likely to fail.
- Refer for further counseling, if indicated.

Teaching About Exercise

- *Recommend at least 60 minutes of enjoyable, moderate-intensity physical activities every day* that are developmentally appropriate and varied (American Heart Association, 2018a). If children do not have a full 60-minute activity break every day, encourage at least two 30-minute periods or four 15-minute periods.
- **Key Point:** *Explain how important exercise is to weight loss—diet alone will not achieve it for them.*
- *Exercise does not necessarily need to be structured.* For example, it might consist of family walks in the community, bike riding, skateboarding, or swimming in a neighborhood pool. Even table tennis requires more activity than watching television. The American Heart Association (2018a, 2018b) recommends the following:
  - Limit screen time, including watching television, playing video games, and using a digital device.
  - Provide kids with opportunities to be active (e.g., bikes, skateboards, roller skates, scooters, jump ropes).
  - Start slowly and increase the amount and intensity of activity gradually.
- Teach children about self-regulation of impulse control, decision-making skills, and social competence. Making more informed choices could help reduce calorie intake and establish good physical activity habits early.
- **Key Point:** *The most effective programs for preventing obesity focus on children rather than their parents. However, management of obesity does involve the whole family.* A child cannot make lifestyle changes if their environment remains the same. Parents can help by modeling healthy eating.
- Recommend group-based or family-based counseling. Many parents do not perceive that their child is overweight; they must come to recognize this if they are to cooperate with needed changes.
- Work with the community to involve the schools in obesity prevention. Many schools have removed soda from campuses and are now offering healthy menus in their cafeterias. In addition, physical education in public schools has been mandated in many U.S. states.

Teaching About Diabetes

The parents and child must understand that diabetes involves dietary changes, weight loss, and exercise. Medications are required if the lifestyle changes are not sufficient to control blood sugar, but they cannot be relied on. You may need to refer the family to a nutritionist or diabetes counselor.

Teaching About Asthma

- *Teach parents and children about indoor environmental asthma triggers.* Examples are mold, cockroaches, pets, and nitrogen dioxide (a gas that is a by-product of indoor fuel-burning appliances such as gas stoves, fireplaces, or wood stoves) (U.S. Environmental Protection Agency, last updated 2022).
- *Provide and help fill out, as necessary, an asthma action plan* for the child to carry when away from home. An action plan should include (1) the child's asthma triggers, (2) instructions for asthma medicines, (3) what to do if the child has an attack, (4) when to call the doctor, and (5) emergency telephone numbers.

Teaching About Violence and Risk-Taking Behaviors

At the community health level, school violence can be addressed through psychological counseling, weapon-screening devices, school-wide educational programs, and policies calling for the suspension or expulsion of students who are caught intimidating other children or participating in fights on school property. The school-age period also offers many opportunities to educate children about the hazards of smoking, drinking, and using drugs, which often contribute to violence.

Helping the Hospitalized Child

Help children express their fears and respond to specific needs. Hospitalized children may fear the unknown, the strange environment, and strange professionals. They are afraid of tests and treatments (e.g., operations, needles), pain, and dying. They miss the comforts of home: their mother's cooking, their own room, and so on. They are bothered by separation from family and friends and by the loss of control over their personal needs. You can help them in the following ways:

- Maximize their contact with outside friends and school.
- Minimize the adverse aspects of the hospital environment.
- Offer choices, when possible, to restore some sense of control (e.g., whether to have a tub or shower bath or what they prefer to eat for meals).

- Encourage parents to bring familiar items from home to personalize their space.
- Involve parents in their child's care, and provide them with accurate information so that they can relieve children's anxieties.

KnowledgeCheck 6-7

- What important physical changes occur in the school-age group?
- According to Piaget, what is the cognitive developmental stage of the school-age child?

ADOLESCENCE: AGES 12 TO 18 YEARS

Adolescence marks the transition from child to adult. **Puberty** refers to the beginning of reproductive abilities. In this period, the child experiences progressive physical, cognitive, and psychological change.

Physical Development of Adolescents

Physical and hormonal changes are readily apparent during the adolescent years. Developmental milestones of adolescence are summarized in Box 6-5.

Growth

- *Females* undergo a growth spurt between 9 and 14 years of age. Height increases 2 to 8 in. (5.1 to 7.6 cm), and weight gain varies from 15 to 55 lb (6.8to 24.9 kg). By the onset of menstruation, females have attained 90% of their adult height.
- *Males* undergo a growth spurt between the ages of 10 and 16 years. Height increases by 4 to 12 in. (10.2 to 30.5 cm), and weight increases by 15 to 65 lb (6.8 to 29.5 kg). Males continue to grow until 18 to 20 years of age. Bone mass continues to accumulate until about age 20.
- *In both males and females,* the blood pressure and the size and strength of the heart increase. The pulse rate

decreases. By the end of adolescence, blood values are that of the adult. Respiratory rate, volume, and capacity also reach the adult rates. By the end of the adolescent period, all vital organs reach adult size.

Onset of Puberty The onset of puberty varies widely, but the sequences of these changes are standard (Tanner, 1962).

- *In females*, the time from the first appearance of breast tissue to full sexual maturation is 2 to 6 years. **Menarche** (first menstruation) occurs approximately 2 years after the beginning of puberty. The average age of menarche is 12 years, depending on race and body mass.
- *In males*, the onset of puberty occurs between 9 and 14 years of age. Throughout puberty, boys become more muscular, the voice deepens, and facial hair begins to grow and coarsen. It may take 2 to 5 years for the genitalia to reach adult size.
- *In both males and females*, hormonal changes are accompanied by increased activity of the sweat (apocrine) glands, and heavy perspiration may occur for the first time. For the same reason, the sebaceous glands become active, and the adolescent may experience acne.

For more information about the changes in secondary sexual characteristics associated with puberty for males and females,

 Go to Procedures 19-17 and 19-18, respectively, in Volume 2

Cognitive Development of Adolescents

Piaget referred to adolescence as the period of formal operations. The adolescent develops the ability to think abstractly and is receptive to more detailed information. This opens the door to scientific reasoning and logic. An adolescent can now imagine what may occur in the future as well as the consequences of their own decisions. Although the adolescent has more refined cognitive abilities, adolescents may still lack judgment and common sense. These develop later through life experiences.

Psychosocial Development of Adolescents

The major psychosocial task of the adolescent is to develop a personal identity. Teenagers shift emotional attachment away from their parents and create close bonds among their peers (Fig. 6-9). This helps teenagers to further characterize the differences between themselves and their parents. The adolescent often takes on a new style of dress, dance, music, or hairstyle; develops personal values; and begins to make choices about career and further education.

Group Acceptance One of the strongest needs for teens is to feel accepted within a group of their own choosing. Acceptance onto a sports team, into a club, or

---

BOX 6-5 ■ Milestones of Adolescent Development

- The adolescent reaches adult height and about 90% of peak bone density by the end of this stage.
- Menarche occurs by age 14 years in most female individuals, who develop adult primary and secondary sex characteristics by about age 16 years.
- Male individuals have developed adult primary and secondary sex characteristics by about ages 17 to 19 years.
- Motor development is equal to that of adults.
- Maturation of the central nervous system allows formal operational thought processes, logic, and abstract reasoning.
- Psychosocial development includes the teen's increasing reliance on peers, ambivalent feelings toward family, anxiety over and/or preoccupation with sex and sexuality, and determination of sexual orientation.

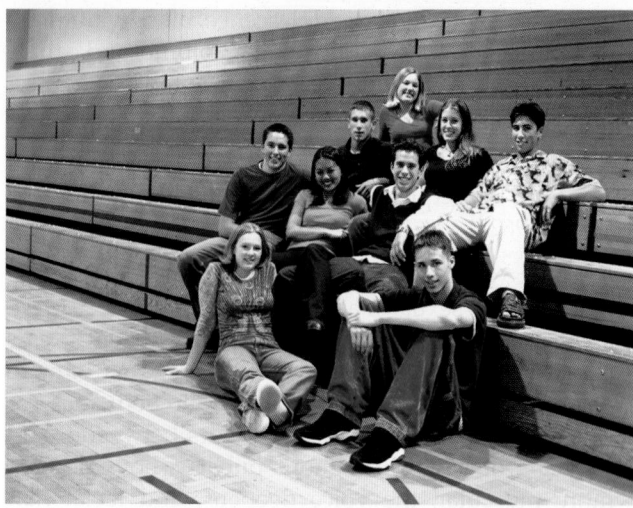

FIGURE 6-9 Teenagers create close bonds among their peers.

into a clique or gang increases the teen's sense of self-esteem. In contrast, unpopular teens feel alienated and resentful, experience loneliness, and may react with violence directed at themselves or others (Danneel et al., 2019).

Tattoos and Piercings Adolescents may engage in the trend of body art and piercings for a number of reasons, including a desire for social bonding, a desire to look like their peers, and the wish to commemorate a friend or loved one. In the past, body modification was often socially associated with adolescent high-risk behaviors; current data have not consistently reported this association (Beal, 2018). Among adolescents 12 years and older:

- Tattooing ranged from 10% to 23%.
- Body piercing (other than the earlobe) ranged from 27% to 42%.
- Rates of tattooing and body piercing were higher among girls than boys.

Both tattoos and piercings can cause skin infections and bloodborne diseases such as HIV and hepatitis.

Emerging Sexual Orientation Most adolescents have a sense of their emerging sexual orientation. Nationwide, 84.4% of students (grades 9–12) identified as heterosexual, 2.5% identified as gay or lesbian, 8.7% identified as bisexual, and 4.5% were not sure of their sexual identity (Kann et al., 2018). A higher percentage report having had same-sex intercourse at least once but consider themselves heterosexual.

Common Health Problems of Adolescents

Illnesses are responsible for less than one-fourth of deaths; cancer and heart disease are the most common. In the United States, 70% of all deaths among young people ages 15 to 24 result from four causes:

Motor vehicle crashes (20.2%)
Suicide (by firearm) (19.9%)

Homicide (firearm) (16%)
Drug-induced deaths (14.5%)

Many adolescents engage in behaviors that increase their likelihood of death or injury from these four causes:

Distracted driving (texting, eating)
Driving under the influence of alcohol or drugs
Carrying a weapon
Using alcohol or drugs

Example Client Condition: Substance Abuse

> Substance abuse is a major concern because it is widespread and because of the physical, mental, and spiritual toll it takes on teens, families, and communities. See the accompanying Example Client Condition: Substance Abuse. Also see Substance Abuse and Mental Illness in Chapter 10, as needed.

Depression

- *Incidence:* Depression affects up to 17% of adolescents in the United States and is more common among the following groups (National Institute of Mental Health, 2022):
  - Adolescent females (29.2%) compared with males (9.2%)
  - Adolescents reporting two or more races (29.9%)
- *Risk factors* for adolescent depression include female sex, family history of depression, negative family environment, physical illness, bullying, trauma exposure, substance abuse, and low self-esteem (Wahid et al., 2021).
- If you would like more information about depression, see Chapter 10.

Suicide

- *Incidence:* Among students in grades 9 through 12 in the United States in 2019 (CDC, 2020b):
  - 19.0% of students reported seriously considering suicide in the previous 12 months (24.1% of females and 13.3% of males).
  - 15.7% of students made a plan about how they would attempt suicide.
  - Boys tend to use more irreversible methods, such as guns and hanging; they are more likely to die of the attempt.
- *Risk factors* include mood disorders, family history of psychiatric illness, history of abuse, availability of a gun, and past suicide attempt.

Eating Disorders

Key Point: *Although anorexia and bulimia create nutritional problems and manifest as eating disorders, they are psychiatric disorders that require medical and psychiatric intervention.*

Anorexia Nervosa A person with **anorexia nervosa** dramatically restricts food intake and may exercise excessively in an attempt to lose weight. Anorexia is

EXAMPLE CLIENT CONDITION: Substance Abuse

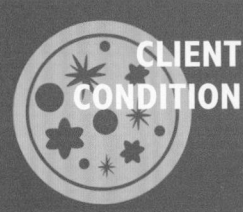

CLIENT CONDITION

Problem

Substance abuse is the regular use of drugs or other substances for purposes other than medical use that causes physical or psychological harm to the person.

- A major concern because of the physical, mental, and spiritual toll it takes on teens, families, and the community
- Associated with risk-taking behaviors resulting in injury and death (e.g., car accidents, suicide)

Incidence

- **Marijuana**—In 2019, about 18% (48.2 million) of Americans reported using marijuana at least once. Recreational marijuana is legal in some states, but it is illegal for anyone under age 21 years to purchase or possess marijuana for recreational use. Despite that, 36% of high school seniors said they had used marijuana in the past year, and 20% reported being current users.
- **Tobacco (cigarettes, cigars, smokeless tobacco or electronic vapor products)**—It is illegal to sell tobacco to minors, yet 7.4% of middle school students and 36.5% of high school students currently use some form of tobacco (Centers for Disease Control and Prevention, 2020c).
- **Opioids**—In 2020, 3.4% (9.5 million) of people age 12 years or older misused opioids. Of those 9.5 million people, 9.3 million misused prescription pain medications, and 900,000 people used heroin (Substance Abuse and Mental Health Services Administration [SAMSHA], 2022). The CDC reports that an average of 128 Americans die every day as a result of opioid overdose.
- **Other drugs**—Cocaine, crack, methamphetamine, and the "designer drugs" (ecstasy, bath salts, and others) may be abused.

Community Health Efforts

The overall percentage of people aged 16 or older who drove under the influence of alcohol, illicit drugs, or a combination of alcohol and drugs has been decreasing among men and young adults—the gender and age-group that have higher rates of driving while impaired. This suggests that prevention messages may be having an effect (Heron, 2021; SAMHSA, 2022). However, the results of a recent study indicate that driving while impaired remains a problem in the United States.

Possible Consequences

Tobacco

Tobacco use is associated with alcohol use and acts as a "gateway drug" to using illegal drugs.

- Cigarette use causes an increase in the frequency and severity of respiratory illness, and decreased physical fitness.
- Smoking during childhood often forms an addiction that persists into adulthood.
- Increased risks of cancer, high blood pressure, cirrhosis, epilepsy, and homicide

Other Consequences

- Violence, sexual assault, rape, and alcohol/drug overdose
- Associated with risk-taking behaviors resulting in injury and death (e.g., automobile accidents, falls, drowning, suicide)
- Persons diagnosed with drug disorders are roughly twice as likely to have mood or anxiety disorders.
- Newborns born to women who abuse substances during pregnancy are at risk for respiratory distress, behavioral abnormalities, and birth defects, as well as drug withdrawal.
- *Fetal alcohol syndrome* may occur in infants of pregnant women addicted to alcohol. It is characterized by irregular facial features and cognitive deficits.
- Every year, 599,000 people are unintentionally injured while under the influence.
- **And more than 10,000 die.**

(continued)

EXAMPLE CLIENT CONDITION: Substance Abuse—cont'd

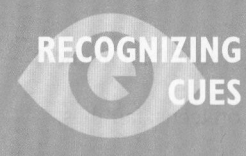

RECOGNIZING CUES

- Assess for risk factors.
- Ask about drug, alcohol, and tobacco use.
- Recognize signs and symptoms of addiction
- Client observation cues
- Medical record cues

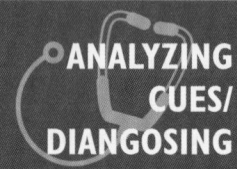

ANALYZING CUES/ DIANGOSING

- **Risk-Prone Health Behavior** r/t excessive alcohol, smoking, drug use
- **Ineffective Parenting** r/t alcohol abuse
- **Inadequate Social Interaction** r/t substance abuse
- **Impaired Role Performance** r/t changes in mental status secondary to substance abuse
- **Risk for Suicide** r/t to feelings of powerlessness

GENERATE SOLUTIONS

Teaching

- Discuss the effects of drugs, alcohol, and tobacco and the hazards associated with their use.
- Remind teens that the earlier a person begins using tobacco, the harder it is to break the addiction.
- Stress the unattractive physical effects, such as bad breath, stained teeth and fingers, and a long-term cough.
- Stress the expense and inconvenience of purchasing cigarettes and smokeless tobacco.
- Correct misinformation that smokeless tobacco products are safer than smoking.
- See the Collaborating category, following.

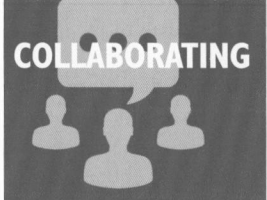

COLLABORATING

- Make appropriate referrals or provide information on cessation programs.
- Discuss and plan for risk-reduction activities in collaboration with individual or group.
- If your assessment identifies drug or alcohol use, make appropriate referrals.
- Participate in community health efforts and messaging to prevent impaired driving.

EVALUATION

- Patient will:
  - Implement healthy lifestyle behaviors to promote alcohol/drug/tobacco elimination:
    - Identifies emotional state that precipitates substance abuse.
    - Uses available support groups and community resources.
    - Commits to alcohol/drug and/or tobacco abstinence.
- The overall percentage of people aged 16 or older who drive under the influence of alcohol, illicit drugs, or a combination of alcohol and drugs will decrease in the following year.

---

characterized by a distorted body image; often, the person sees themselves as fat despite being markedly thin.

- *Incidence*—It occurs predominantly in, but is not limited to, high-achieving adolescent girls from upper-middle-class backgrounds.
- *Physical consequences* include amenorrhea, bradycardia, low white blood cell count, anemia, infertility, and bone loss.
- *Mortality*—Eating disorders have the highest mortality of any mental illness: 5% to 10% of patients die within 10 years of developing anorexia nervosa.

Bulimia Bulimia is an eating disorder characterized by binge eating followed by inappropriate mechanisms to remove the food that was consumed (usually by inducing vomiting, using laxatives, or engaging in excessive exercise). Binge eating may occur every few days or as often as several times a day.

- *Incidence*—Bulimia is seen in adolescent girls (1%) and boys (0.1%).
- *Physical consequences*—Electrolyte imbalances, decayed teeth (from gastric acid exposure), or abdominal pain (from gastric overload or laxative use).

Overweight and Obesity

Overweight and obesity continue to be a concern during adolescence, partly because the incidence is so high. Moreover, overweight children are more likely to be overweight adults. Consider these facts:

- *Today, about 1 in 3 American teens is overweight or obese,* nearly triple the rate in 1971 (Fryar et al., 2020).

- *Causes of teen obesity are similar to those of childhood obesity:* sedentary lifestyles; eating larger portions; eating fast foods; and substituting high-calorie, nutrient-poor snacks for balanced meals. Even school vending machines contain so-called junk foods such as soda, snack cakes, candy, and chips, although this is changing in some areas.
- *One-third of American children aged 4 to 19 years eat fast food daily.* The percentage is undoubtedly higher for adolescents, who eat fewer meals at home and have more freedom to choose their own foods. Food preferences are influenced by television and marketing strategies in other media; on children's television shows, most of the advertising is for foods of poor nutritional value.
- *Type 2 DM, hypertension, high cholesterol, and heart disease are occurring with increasing frequency* in adolescents, now that so many are affected by obesity. These diseases were previously seen mostly in adults.

Also refer to Chapter 8 for more information.

Risky Sexual Behaviors

Although rates have decreased slightly in the past few years, sexual activity is common among teenagers. By age 13, 3.4% of all students, including 3.0% of heterosexual students; 6.1% of gay, lesbian, and bisexual students; and 4.1% of students who are unsure of their sexuality, report having had sexual intercourse. This tends to increase with age, with 39.5% of students in grades 9 to 12 being sexually active. About 10% of students report having had sexual intercourse with four or more persons (CDC, 2020c).

Condom Use A little less than half of sexually active high school students reported that they did not use a condom during their most recent sexual intercourse. Unprotected sexual intercourse was:

- Higher among gay, lesbian or bisexual students (60.1%) than heterosexual students (43.9%).
- Higher among heterosexual female students (50.4%) than heterosexual male students (38.2%) (CDC, 2020c).

Through its *Healthy People 2030* initiative, the federal government has set a national goal of increasing effective condom use among sexually active adolescents ages 15 to 19 years, with the goal of preventing pregnancy and providing barrier protection against disease.

Oral Sex Many adolescents engage in sexual behaviors other than vaginal intercourse. Between 2015 and 2019, 52% of males and 54% of females aged 15 to 19 years reported that they had engaged in oral sex with an opposite-sex partner. This often occurs before initiating sexual intercourse (Lindberg et al., 2021). **Key Point:** *Oral sex does not put adolescents at risk of pregnancy; however, unless barrier precautions are taken, it can put them at increased risk of STIs.*

Social Media Social media may have a significant impact on the social and sexual well-being of adolescents. In many adolescents, self-regulation and judgment skills are not yet fully mature. This often leads to risky behaviors, especially on social network sites.

- **Online disinhibition effect.** This means that people more readily release personal and private information into the public domain than they would in face-to-face interactions. Adolescents can easily fall prey to this effect because of the anonymity social network sites provide.
- **Social network sites provide an attractive outlet for adolescents** during a time in development in which self-expression and validation are important. This expression may then translate into risky social and sexual behaviors.
- **"Sexting."** Adolescents may not directly reference sexual behavior but may partake in a practice known as "sexting": sending, receiving, or forwarding sexually explicit messages, photographs, images, or videos via the Internet, a cell phone, or another digital device. One survey found that 30% of adolescents between 13 and 19 years old have received sexts, and 16% have sent sexts (Burén & Lunde, 2018).
- **Risky behaviors and sexual wellness.** Risky sexual behaviors, including having concurrent sexual partners, multiple sexual partners, and a lack of consistent condom use, put adolescents in the highest-risk group for contracting an STI. Experts believe that social media may lead to an increase in risky sexual behaviors and a decrease in overall social and sexual wellness in adolescents (Vannucci et al., 2020).

Sexually Transmitted Infections Approximately 1 in 4 U.S. teens has an STI. STIs, including HIV/AIDS, are a major health consequence associated with sexual activity, especially with unprotected sexual activity. **Key Point:** *A majority of adolescents believe that sex without a condom is not worth the risk, but most also mistakenly believe that condoms are a foolproof method of preventing STIs and HIV/AIDS.* Trichomonal and monilial infections and human papillomavirus (HPV) are common. Those and other infections occur in both males and females and can have serious complications.

AIDS is a major cause of death worldwide, reaching epidemic proportions in some countries. It is transmitted primarily through genital, oral, or anal sexual activities, but it can be transmitted in other ways (e.g., by sharing needles with an infected person).

According to the CDC (2021a), in 2019:

- Adolescents and young adults aged 13 to 24 years accounted for 21% (7,648) of all new HIV diagnoses, with gay and bisexual young men accounting for 83% (6,385).
- Black/African American males and females accounted for 42% (15,340) of all new HIV diagnoses, with adolescent and young adult Black/African American gay and bisexual men representing 50% (3,209) of the total.

- Hispanic/Latino people accounted for 29% (10,502) of all new HIV diagnoses.

For more information about STIs, see Chapter 30.

Adolescent Pregnancy The birth rate for this age-group is 16.7 per 1,000 females. This is a record low for the United States and a drop of 4% from 2018. Birth rates fell by 7% for females aged 15 to 17 years and by 4% for females aged 18 to 19 years. Still, the teen pregnancy rate in the United States is substantially higher than it is in other Western industrialized nations (CDC, 2021b). A similar percentage of teens are sexually active in the United States; however, the rates of consistency and effectiveness of condom use are lower. Social determinants of health, including lack of education and low family income levels, may contribute to high birth rates. Adolescents in certain settings are at higher risk of teen pregnancy and birth than other groups, such as young women living in foster care.

Pregnant adolescents are at higher risk for complications of pregnancy and having a low-birth-weight infant. They also face physiological and psychosocial risks, such as:

- bone density loss,
- iron deficiency anemia,
- interruption of progress in their own developmental tasks, and
- loss of educational opportunities.

Teen mothers are more likely to live in poverty than other teens and less likely to complete high school. Compared with older mothers, they are less likely to:

- be married,
- receive prenatal care, and
- gain appropriate weight.

ASSESSMENT/RECOGNIZING CUES (ADOLESCENTS)

Adolescents should have a general health examination every 2 years. Communicating with adolescents can be challenging because they may feel the need to resist "authority" and may be hesitant to share information with adults. Attempt to establish rapport and reassure the teenager that you will maintain confidentiality. At these visits, you should assess for the common problems of adolescence, including abuse and neglect (see Procedure 6-1 in Volume 2).

Obtain a Thorough Health History Obtain information in the following areas:

- **Medications and other drugs.** Be sure to ask about the use of prescription and over-the-counter medications, tobacco, e-cigarettes or vaping, and recreational drugs. If any are being used, find out what, how much, and for how long.
- **Psychosocial profile.** Obtain a psychosocial profile focusing on health practices and behaviors. Assess the adolescent's ability to cope with stressors. **Key Point:** *A change in academic performance or a lack*

Toward Evidence-Based Practice

Hu, P., Samuels, S., Maciejewski, K. R., Li, F., Aloe, C., Name, M. V., Savoye, M., & Sharifi, M. (2022). Changes in weight-related health behaviors and social determinants of health among youth with overweight/obesity during the COVID-19 pandemic. *Childhood Obesity, 18*(6), 369–382. https://doi.org/10.1089/chi.2021.0196

A total of 129 caregivers and 34 adolescents with overweight/obesity during the COVID-19 pandemic completed surveys to determine weight-related health behaviors (physical activity, screen time, sleep, and diet) and social determinants of health (food insecurity, income/childcare, and caregivers' perceived stress) before and during the pandemic. Compared with prepandemic, caregivers reported a significant decrease in physical activity and a significant increase in recreational screen time. Researchers also found that fewer adolescents had regular bedtimes, and more ate most meals while watching television. Food insecurity increased from 27% to 43%, 45% reported reduced household income, and caregivers experienced more stress.

Neshteruk, C. D., Zizzi, A., Suarez, L., Erickson, E., Kraus, W. E., Li, J. S., Skinner, A. C., Story, M., Zucker, N., & Armstrong, S. C. (2021). Weight-related behaviors of children with obesity during the COVID-19 pandemic. *Childhood Obesity, 17*(6), 371–378.

Fifty-one parents of children with obesity participated in semistructured interviews during the time frame of the COVID-19 pandemic. Parents were asked to describe their experience during the COVID-19 pandemic with their children's diet, physical activity, sleep, and screen-time behaviors. Researchers identified themes around changes in children's weight-related behaviors, including dietary changes (increased snacking and more meals prepared and consumed at home), a shift in sleep schedules, with children going to bed and waking up later, and an increase in leisure-based screen time. Parents played a role in promoting activity and managing children's screen time.

1. What similarities do you see in the first and second studies?

2. What implications do the findings from the research studies have on how you might provide healthy lifestyle teaching to children?

of interest in school may indicate a problem such as depression. Young adolescents may have difficulty identifying and describing their emotional or mood states. Instead of saying how bad they feel, they may be irritable or act out by disobeying or misbehaving; they may sulk, be negative or grouchy, feel misunderstood, and get into trouble at school.

- **Peer relationships.** Assess the quality of the adolescent's peer relationships to assess the risk for social isolation and to determine the risk for school-related and/or gang-related violence.

- **Nutrition and body image.** Ask questions about body image in relation to the adolescent's nutritional status. Assess both overeating and undereating patterns, as well as intake of key nutrients, such as protein, iron, calcium, and vitamin D.

- **Tattoos and piercings.** The tattoo or piercing may be in a concealed location, so ask about tattoos and piercings and ask to look at them during the visit. Discuss the risks of body art and modification.

- **Activity and exercise patterns.** If the adolescent engages in activities that increase the risk for injuries, ask about the use of protective equipment, such as helmets, mouth guards, and padding. If the adolescent reports no regular physical activity, assess their understanding of the benefits of exercise.

- **Sleep patterns.** Teens often get little sleep during school days and sleep late on weekends. Ask whether the teen feels refreshed after a night's sleep.

- ✛ **Safety.** Determine whether the adolescent wears a seat belt. Determine whether they are aware of the hazards of driving under the influence of drugs and alcohol and while texting or talking on the phone. Such distractions, including other teens in the car, can compete with the attention and focus needed for traffic and driving safely.

- **Sexual activity.** Determine whether the adolescent is sexually active. If so, ask about condom use.

- **Review all body systems.** While doing so, keep in mind changes or problems that are specific to the adolescent.

Perform a General Survey Complete a general survey after you have gathered the subjective data.

- Include vital signs, height, and weight. Follow with a head-to-toe physical examination.
- If you identify any problems in the course of the history and physical examination, actively involve the adolescent and the parents in a plan of care.
- Calculate the BMI using a BMI calculator and BMI-for-age percentiles for children and teens. Adult calculators will not give accurate results for teens. The following are the CDC weight status categories:

Underweight	Less than 5th percentile
Healthy weight	5th to less than 85th percentile
At risk of overweight	85th to less than 95th percentile
Overweight	95th percentile or greater

To use the CDC BMI Calculator for Child and Teen,

 Go to the CDC Web site at https://www.cdc.gov/healthyweight/bmi/calculator.html

To see the CDC BIM-for-age percentile charts for girls and boys aged 2 to 20 years,

 Go to the CDC website at https://www.cdc.gov/growthcharts/

IMPLEMENTATION/TAKING ACTION (ADOLESCENTS)

When working with adolescents, your goal is to help the adolescent make informed decisions. Avoid scare tactics, and encourage open discussion. A teenager will often feel more comfortable asking a nurse or other health professional about sensitive topics than asking a parent. **Key Point: *Reassure the adolescent that you will maintain confidentiality. However, if there is concern about suicide, explain to the adolescent that you are required to share this information with others. Provide mental health referrals immediately when an adolescent contemplates suicide.*** Focus your age-specific interventions on educating the teenager about common health problems and avoidance of injury and disease. Include the following topics.

Preventing and Treating Obesity

Help the patient to make small but permanent changes in eating and exercise. These usually work better than a series of extreme short-term diets and exercise plans that cannot be sustained. Gradual weight loss is the healthiest approach. Even for teens, parental involvement is important, primarily to model healthy eating and physical activity.

Caloric Intake Reducing caloric intake is usually the easiest change to make. As a rule, avoid highly restrictive diets that forbid favorite foods. It is important to encourage strong support from parents and others involved in buying and preparing food. Teach the teen to:

- Choose highly nutritious foods at home and school
- Replace junk foods with fruit and other healthy snacks
- Limit fruit juices and sodas

Physical Activity Stress the importance of regular physical activity. Suggest walking to school instead of driving or taking a bus. If this is not practical, involve the family in planning regular physical activities (e.g., a long walk after dinner). Even mild exercise, such as shooting hoops or swimming, provides more activity than watching television or playing computer games. You might start with the following goals:

- *Limit television and video game use* to 1 or 2 hours a day. Discourage use before school, during homework, and late at night. Keep the television off during family mealtimes.

■ *Engage in 30 minutes of outdoor activity every day,* no matter how mild the activity. Work in up to an hour a day of more strenuous exercise.

Preventing Pregnancy and STIs

One of the *Healthy People 2030* national goals is to increase the percentage of adolescents who either abstain from sex or use condoms with hormonal or intrauterine contraception. To see the *Healthy People 2030* objectives,

 Go to the *Healthy People 2030* Web site at https://www. healthypeople.gov/

Abstinence is the only 100% effective way to prevent pregnancy and STIs. However, if the adolescent is sexually active, explain that using condoms can greatly reduce, although not eliminate, those risks. Be sure adolescents understand that STIs can be transmitted orally and anally, as well as vaginally, so it is important that they use a condom, regardless of the type of sexual activity.

Current recommendations are that schools make condoms available for adolescents and, with community involvement, develop a comprehensive sequential sexuality education program as a part of a K–12 health education program. Some parents may worry that sex education and condom availability encourage teenage sex, but data show that making condoms available does not increase the rate of sexual activity (Hogan, 2018; Maziarz, 2018).

Breast Self-Examination

It is important to promote breast self-awareness, which educates patients about the normal feel and appearance of their breasts. For many patients, breast self-awareness also may include performing breast self-examinations. **Breast self-examination (BSE)** is a step-by-step approach that a woman can use to look at and feel her breasts. Although BSE has the potential to alert patients to changes in the breast, many guidelines no longer recommend BSE as a screening tool for breast cancer. Although it seemed promising when it was first introduced, studies have shown that BSE does not offer the early detection and survival benefits of other screening tests (U.S. Preventive Services Task Force, January, 2016c).

For information on how to perform a BSE,

 Go to The National Breast Cancer Foundation Website at: http://www.nationalbreastcancer.org/breast-self-exam

Testicular Self-Examination

Guidelines regarding testicular self-examination (TSE) include:

■ The USPSTF (July 2016a) recommends against routine screening of asymptomatic patients, stating that outcomes are not sufficiently improved to merit routine TSE.

■ The American Cancer Society (ACS, 2018a) recommends that men be aware of testicular cancer risk and consult a doctor if they find a lump in a testicle. The ACS does not recommend for or against routine screening for testicular cancer.

■ Nevertheless, some doctors recommend that all men examine their testicles monthly after puberty.

If your patient chooses to perform TSE, advise them to perform the examination after a warm bath or shower (heat relaxes the scrotum, making it easier to find abnormalities). To learn how to do a TSE:

 Go to the Testicular Cancer Resource Center Web site at http://tcrc.acor.org/tcexam.html

Immunizations

Although most children get the recommended vaccines, some U.S. communities have low vaccination coverage that puts them at risk for outbreaks. Strategies to make sure more adolescents get vaccinated include using vaccination information systems, sending patient reminders, and starting vaccination programs in schools.

Key Point: *Currently, the HPV vaccine is recommended for both males and females at age 11 to 12 years (Advisory Committee on Immunization Practices, 2014) so that they are protected before ever being exposed to the virus.* HPV is a common virus that affects nearly 80 million people. Specific strains of HPV can cause cervical, vaginal, and vulvar cancers in female persons; penile cancer in male persons; and anal cancer and mouth/throat (oropharyngeal) cancer, as well as genital warts, in all persons. Since HPV vaccination was first recommended in 2006, infections with the HPV strains that cause most HPV cancers and genital warts have dropped 88% among adolescent girls and 81% among young adult women.

To see the national goals for 2030,

 Go to the *Healthy People 2030* Web site at https://www. healthypeople.gov

For the recommended immunization schedule for adolescents,

 Go to the CDC Web site at https://www.cdc.gov/vaccines/ schedules/easy-to-read/preteen-teen.html

Other Health Promotion Activities

Other nursing activities include promoting adolescent health and safety.

■ **Rest.** Explain the importance of adequate rest. Teens need 8 hours of sleep a night for maximum performance in academics and sports.

■ **Nutrition.** Stress the importance of adequate nutrition, including intake of 1,300 mg of calcium and 400 IU of vitamin D daily to reach maximum bone density during this critical period of rapid increase in growth and bone mass. Teach teens how to choose foods that include fruits, vegetables, cereal and grains, lean meats, chicken, fish, and low-fat dairy products in their diet and to avoid foods and drinks that are high in sugar, fat, or caffeine.

■ **Dental hygiene.** Advise parents that the adolescent should have a preventive dental care visit at least once a year. Teach the teen to brush twice a day with a soft toothbrush and to floss daily.

■ **Safety.** Remind teens to wear a seat belt when riding in the car and avoid distractions while driving (e.g., talking or texting on a cell phone, changing a radio station). Ask them never to drive under the influence of alcohol or drugs. Remind them to wear a helmet and protective gear for activities such as bicycling, inline skating, and skateboarding. Teach the importance of sun safety (e.g., applying sunscreen of at least SPF 15, avoiding tanning beds, wearing sunglasses when in the sun).

KnowledgeCheck 6-8

■ According to Erikson, what is the developmental stage of the adolescent?
■ Name two common health problems of adolescents.

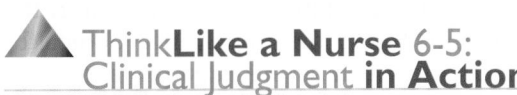

ThinkLike a Nurse 6-5: Clinical Judgment in Action

Recall Carrie, a 13-year-old, in the Meet Your Patients scenario. Carrie is hospitalized for pneumonia. What cues might indicate that the hospitalization is having an effect on her behavior? As her nurse, how might you intervene?

YOUNG ADULTHOOD: AGES 19 TO 40 YEARS

Young adulthood is the time of transition to independence and responsibility. This is usually the healthiest stage of a person's life.

Physical Development of Young Adults

■ Maturation of the body systems is complete.
■ Peak bone density is achieved for both females and males by age 25 years.
■ Vision and hearing are typically acute.
■ For female individuals, the ages between 20 and 30 years are the optimal years for childbearing.
■ For male individuals, hormone levels that surged in adolescence begin to slowly decrease and stabilize around age 24 years.

Cognitive Development of Young Adults

Key Point: *According to Piaget, learning continues throughout life, but patterns of thinking do not alter after adolescence.* In the *formal operations* phase, young adults are able to think rationally, predict outcomes, and hypothesize about the future. At this point, thought processes and mental abilities are well established; the young adult is able to think rationally, predict outcomes, and hypothesize about the future.

Key Point: *Contemporary psychologists have proposed an additional and more complex stage of cognitive development called postformal operations.* In this phase, the young adult is able to accept contradictions and fine points in thinking. For example, the postformal thinker recognizes that their opinion on a social controversy has aspects of two opposing viewpoints. They see merit in both parts of the argument and are comfortable with the discrepancy.

Psychosocial Development of Young Adults

The transition to adulthood involves important life events, such as graduating from high school, entering college or starting a career, and leaving home and becoming self-sufficient. Young adults begin to explore options for intimate relationships, marriage or alternative relationships, and careers. Around age 30 years, most young adults experience a period of self-evaluation. This often results in job, career, or relationship changes.

■ **Key Point:** *Erikson describes this period as the stage of intimacy versus isolation.* Successful completion of this phase requires the establishment of lasting friendships and associations.
■ **Freud described this phase of life as the** *genital stage.* He believed that young adults are instinctively driven to form a sexually intimate relationship.

Common Health Problems of Young Adults

Young adults are generally active and in good physical health. Frequently seen health problems may include STIs, unplanned pregnancies, traumatic injury, suicide attempts, substance abuse, domestic violence, obesity, diabetes, and hypertension. Unintentional injury is the leading cause of death in young adults (Heron, 2021).

Sexually Transmitted Infections

Sexual experimentation often continues in this stage.

■ Among those 15 to 44 years of age, nearly all have had penile-vaginal intercourse, and most have had oral sex with an opposite-sex partner.
■ The CDC (2021c) estimates that 1 in 5 people in the United States had an STI in 2018, accounting for about 68 million infections. Nearly half (46%) of all new STIs in the United States in 2018 occurred in young adults aged 15 to 24 years. Social determinants of health, such as poverty, lack of stable housing, substance use, lack of medical insurance or access to healthcare providers, and a high burden of STIs in the community, put some individuals at higher risk of STI.

Some common STIs include chlamydia, genital warts (condyloma acuminata), gonorrhea, genital herpes,

HPV, and HIV. Some activities that can put young adults at increased risk for both STIs and HIV include:

- Having anal, vaginal, or oral sex without a condom
- Having multiple sex partners
- Having anonymous sex partners
- Having sex while under the influence of drugs or alcohol (associated with lower inhibitions and greater sexual risk taking)

For more information about STIs, see Chapter 30.

Substance Abuse and Violence

Drug abuse is commonly thought of as an adolescent problem; however, alcohol and marijuana are commonly abused by young adults. The National Institute on Drug Abuse (2016) reports that young adults are the highest abusers of prescription opioid pain relievers, attention deficit–hyperactivity disorder (ADHD) stimulants, and antianxiety drugs. In the young adult years, there is a strong emphasis on "getting ahead," establishing a career and family, and becoming independent. These tasks are emotionally difficult. See Example Problem: Substance Abuse, earlier in the chapter.

Obesity

Obesity rates have increased to crisis levels in the United States. In 2020, non-Hispanic Black adults had the highest prevalence of self-reported obesity (40.7%), followed by Hispanic adults (35.2%), White adults (30.3%), and Asian adults (11.6%) (CDC, 2022b). The racial and ethnic disparities in obesity highlight the importance of addressing social determinants of health, such as poverty, education, and housing, to remove barriers to health that lead to obesity. With the increase in obesity, the incidence of type 2 DM and hypertension has grown dramatically among young adults. Additionally, ethnic groups with a higher prevalence of obesity are more likely to suffer worse outcomes from emerging diseases, such as COVID-19.

ASSESSMENT/RECOGNIZING CUES (YOUNG ADULTS)

Young adults should have an annual physical examination, including assessment of physical health, mental health, and lifestyle. Be sure to assess nutrition, exercise, and sleep, as well as the use of tobacco, alcohol, and drugs. For female patients, the examination should include a pelvic examination.

Screening Screening for diabetes and hypertension is very important in the young adult years, especially for those who are overweight or who have a family history of cardiac disease.

- *Breast examinations.* The ACS recommends a clinical breast examination at least once every 3 years.

- *Testicular examinations.* The USPSTF (2016a) no longer recommends clinical testicular examinations or monthly TSE. The ACS (2018) recommends a discussion with the healthcare provider to determine whether a testicular examination should be part of a routine cancer-related checkup.

Violence Screening Intimate partner violence (IPV) is common but often remains undetected, so screening should be a part of every examination. If there is any reason to suspect abuse, conduct a thorough assessment. For further information on assessing and reporting abuse, see Procedure 6-1 in Volume 2. Also see the Example Client Condition: Abuse, Neglect, and Violence in this chapter and Mandatory Reporting Laws in Chapter 39.

IMPLEMENTATION/TAKING ACTION (YOUNG ADULTS)

Nursing actions for the young adult are similar to those for the adolescent. As a newly independent person, the young adult is establishing health patterns, including how they will interact with healthcare providers. Reinforce the teaching that was begun in the earlier age-group. Stress the importance of health-promotion activities such as the Papanicolaou (Pap) test (to screen for cervical cancer) every 3 years for female patients between the ages of 21 and 29 (USPSTF, 2018a).

Breast Cancer Prevention Breast cancer prevention starts with healthy habits.

- **Teach for risk reduction.** Teach patients what they can do to reduce their breast cancer risk (e.g., limit alcohol, stay physically active).
- **Promote breast self-awareness.** Tell patients to be vigilant about breast cancer detection. If a patient notices any changes in their breasts, such as a new lump or skin changes, instruct them to consult a doctor.
- **Advise about mammograms.** Patients younger than 40 years who have risk factors should ask their healthcare provider whether they need mammograms. Risk factors include personal and family history of breast cancer, having the first child late in the childbearing cycle, having the first menstrual period before age 12, and certain breast changes (e.g., cells that look abnormal under a microscope). Studies have shown no link between abortion or miscarriage and breast cancer.

Exercise Recommend that adults engage in 2.5 hours a week of moderate-intensity, or 75 minutes a week of vigorous-intensity, aerobic physical activity. Increasing exercise to 300 minutes a week provides even more health benefits. They should also do muscle-strengthening activities that involve all major muscle groups performed on two or more days per week (U.S. Department of Health and Human Services, n.d.).

KnowledgeCheck 6-9

- According to Erikson, what is the developmental stage of the young adult?
- What is the leading cause of death for this age-group?
- What sex-specific assessments should be emphasized with this age-group?

MIDDLE ADULTHOOD: AGES 40 TO 64 YEARS

The middle-adult years are a time when people realize the difference between their early aspirations and their actual achievements.

Physical Development of Middle Adults

Physiological changes that occur during the middle-adult years include graying or thinning of hair; decreases in the elasticity of the blood vessels; and decreases in muscle tone, skin moisture and turgor, and gastrointestinal (GI) motility. A decrease in bone mass often causes a slight loss of height.

Menopause One of the principal changes that middle-adult female individuals experience is **menopause,** the cessation of menstrual periods for at least 12 months. The ovaries no longer produce eggs on a cyclical basis, and reproductive ability is lost (although some people do become pregnant after not having menses for a year). The average age of menopause is 52 years. Most individuals experience a transition that takes place over several years.

Perimenopausal symptoms are related to a decline in estrogen levels and may precede menopause by as much as 5 to 7 years. These symptoms include hot flashes, a decrease in breast size, changes in the length of the menstrual cycle and menstrual flow, vaginal dryness, night-time awakenings, and moodiness.

Andropause Men do not experience such a clear-cut transition, but many men do experience a transitional period known as andropause. **Andropause** is characterized by a decline in testosterone production, a lower sperm count, and a need for more time to achieve an erection. Andropause does not result in an inability to reproduce but does limit reproductive abilities.

Cognitive Development of Middle Adults

Piaget theorizes that the middle adult moves freely between formal operations, concrete operations, and problem-solving as the task demands. Middle adults are able to reflect on the past and anticipate the future. Creativity may reach its peak during this stage. Memory is intact, but reaction time begins to diminish because of diminishing nerve impulses.

Psychosocial Development of Middle Adults

Key Point: *Erikson describes middle adulthood as a stage of generativity versus stagnation.*

- **Generativity** is the process of guiding the next generation or improving the whole of society.
- **Stagnation** occurs when development ceases: a stagnant middle adult cannot guide the next generation or contribute to society.

Erikson believed that an inability to meet the developmental tasks of the middle adult years results in a lack of preparedness for the final life stage of old age.

Middle adulthood is a time of transition. This is often a time when children mature and leave the home. As a result, many middle adults and their children feel a need to redefine family roles.

Middle adults often complain of declining energy and competing demands as they raise children, care for aging parents, and work at the peak of their career (Fig. 6-10). These stressors, in combination with visible signs of aging, may produce a **midlife crisis**—a recognition that youth is over and that life is limited. Coping skills learned in earlier years are important predictors of how the middle adult reacts to these changes.

Common Health Problems of Middle Adults

In the middle-adult years, chronic diseases emerge as a major health problem. The most common chronic diseases are cancer, obesity, diabetes, hypertension, and cardiovascular disease. Many interventions for younger age-groups are directed at preventing the development of these disorders.

Cancer Key Point: *The majority of cancer diagnoses occur in the middle- and older-adult years.*

- **Lung cancer** is the leading cause of cancer death among both men and women, causing approximately 25% of all cancer deaths.

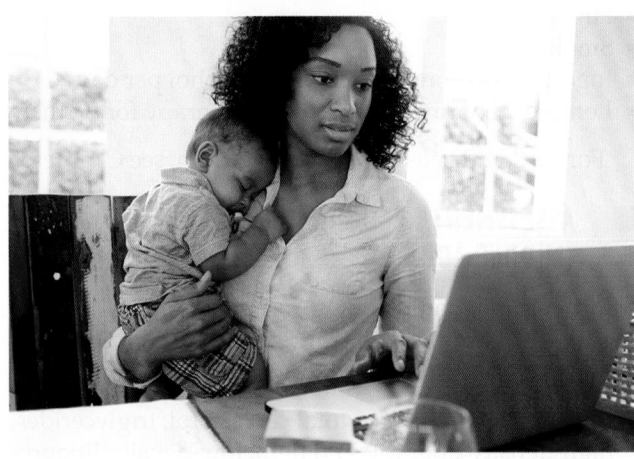

FIGURE 6-10 Middle adulthood is a time of competing demands.

- **Female breast and colorectal cancer rates** have each declined slightly in recent years, but the number of deaths attributed to each has remained stable, with an average of approximately 44,000 and 53,000 annual deaths, respectively (ACS, 2021).
- **Prostate cancer risk** increases with age. Nearly 65% of prostate cancer occurs after the age of 65. Other factors that increase the risk of prostate cancer are family history, race (African American/Black men have the highest rate), and possibly diet. There is some evidence that a diet high in animal fat may increase the risk.

Obesity As you have learned, obesity is a major health problem in all age-groups. It often triggers the development of type 2 DM, hypertension, joint pain, and cardiovascular diseases, such as coronary artery disease, atherosclerosis, and venous insufficiency. Diet and exercise must be consistently used together to combat obesity. Ironically, obesity leads to a variety of problems that make it even harder to exercise.

Cardiovascular Disease (CVD) CVD is among the leading causes of death in the middle-adult years. Atherosclerotic plaque can develop in the peripheral vascular system, the heart, major vessels, or any combination of these areas. CVD may result from:

- Inadequately treated hypertension
- Ongoing weight gain or obesity
- Poorly controlled type 2 DM
- A sedentary lifestyle

Hypertension (high blood pressure) is a complex disorder. As the elasticity of the vascular system declines with each passing year, the incidence of hypertension increases. If there is a strong family history of hypertension, the likelihood of needing treatment escalates sharply.

Except for age and family history, factors that increase the risk of hypertension are under the patient's control. They include:

- Excess weight
- Sedentary lifestyle
- High sodium intake
- High fat intake
- Smoking
- Ingestion of more than 1.5 oz of alcohol per day
- Long-term hormone replacement therapy for women

For further discussion of hypertension, see Chapter 8.

ASSESSMENT/RECOGNIZING CUES (MIDDLE ADULTS)

Middle adults should undergo an annual physical examination. In addition to height, weight, BMI, and vital signs, the examination should include the following:

- **Lipid panel screening:** total cholesterol, triglycerides, high-density lipoprotein (HDL), low-density lipoprotein (LDL), and ratios.
- **Blood glucose screening.**
- **Clinical breast and pelvic examination** for female clients. The American College of Obstetricians and Gynaecologists (2017, reaffirmed 2021) recommend clinical breast examination every 1 to 3 years for women aged 25 to 39 years and annually for women beginning at age 40 years. Female clients older than 30 should have a Pap test every 3 to 5 years based on health history and discussion with their primary care provider.
- **Annual or biannual mammogram** for women. The recommended age for average-risk female clients to begin mammography differs among the consensus guidelines groups in the United States. The USPSTF recommends starting at age 50 years; the American Cancer Society recommends that high-risk individuals should have the opportunity to begin screening at age 40 years, whereas regular screening should begin at age 45 years. The National Comprehensive Cancer Network and the ACOG recommend annual screening mammograms starting at age 40 years for all average-risk female clients. Screening should begin after shared decision making between the client and their care provider. Discussion should include the benefits and harms of annual and biennial screening and incorporate patient values and preferences (ACOG, 2017, reaffirmed 2021).
- **Digital rectal examination for prostate evaluation** in male clients should be offered but not routinely done (ACS, 2018b). An enlarged prostate can indicate either benign prostatic hypertrophy or prostate cancer. The serum prostate-specific antigen (PSA) level is a sensitive indicator of prostate disorders. Recommendations vary. Some caution against routine screening; however, the ACS suggest that patients talk with their healthcare provider about the uncertainties, risks, and potential benefits of testing. Social determinants such as poverty, low education level, immigration status, lack of social support, and social isolation have been associated with prostate cancer stage at diagnosis and poorer outcomes (Coughlin, 2020). African American/Black men and men with close family members (father, brother, son) who had prostate cancer before age 65 are at high risk.
- **Annual eye examination.** Visual changes are common in this age-group and include the development of presbyopia (far-sightedness) and the onset of glaucoma and cataracts.
- **Colorectal cancer screening.** Regular screening, beginning at age 50, is the key to preventing colorectal cancer. The USPSTF (2021) recommends screening for colorectal cancer using stool for occult blood testing, as well as sigmoidoscopy or colonoscopy beginning at age 50 years (or at age 40 for high-risk patients) and continuing until age 75 years. The frequency of repeat examinations depends on the findings. African American/Black adults across all age-groups, including those younger than 50 years, have a higher incidence of and mortality from colorectal cancer than White adults.

- **Osteoporosis screening** at or before menopause for at-risk clients who elect it. Most guidelines recommend assessing all adults age 50 years and older for risk factors (e.g., smoking, low body weight) with bone density measurement (e.g., a DXA test) based on the risk profile (USPSTF, 2018b).

IMPLEMENTATION/TAKING ACTION (MIDDLE ADULTS)

Care for middle adults focuses on identifying risk factors and promoting a healthy lifestyle. At each annual examination and at periodic health visits, you should discuss the hazards of alcohol and tobacco use, the importance of regular exercise, stress-management techniques, safety, and the benefits of balanced nutritional intake. You will also need to add teaching interventions if any chronic problem is discovered.

Nutrition For menopausal clients, encourage daily intake of 1,200 mg of calcium and 600 IU of vitamin D, as well as regular weight-bearing exercise, to promote optimal bone density. There is a growing consensus that even this amount may be too low. Many clinicians are prescribing higher doses, especially in cases of known deficiency.

Hormone Replacement Therapy (HRT) HRT was used extensively in the past, but multiple studies have raised questions about the safety of hormone therapy to treat a naturally occurring phenomenon. HRT can relieve symptoms such as hot flashes and vaginal dryness. It may also protect against osteoporosis and age-linked eye disease. Some studies show that it may help prevent dementia; others show that it does not. However, the risks of HRT include heart disease, breast cancer, stroke, and blood clots.

The National Institutes of Health (2007) concluded that the risks of long-term combination hormone (estrogen and progestin) therapy outweigh the benefits for postmenopausal women. Advise women to consult their primary care provider about estrogen-alone therapy, bioidentical therapies, and certain natural remedies that can provide symptom relief.

Exercise Although the usual recommendation is for 60 minutes of exercise daily, and that amount brings the most health benefits, researchers now suggest that even smaller amounts of exercise can improve the quality of life for sedentary, overweight, or obese postmenopausal women. Even just 10 to 30 minutes a day can improve social functioning and decrease limitations in work and other activities due to physical or emotional problems (U.S. Department of Health and Human Services, n.d.).

Immunizations Review the patient's immunization record regularly. Middle adults often require periodic boosters (e.g., pertussis). Teach patients that annual influenza vaccination is recommended for all persons aged 6 months and older who do not have

contraindications. Strongly encourage clients with respiratory problems to receive a pneumonia vaccination as well. The CDC recommends that people aged 60 years and older get two doses of the shingles vaccine. To see the CDC immunization schedule,

 Go to the CDC Web site at https://www.cdc.gov/vaccines/ schedules/hcp/adult.html

KnowledgeCheck 6-10

- According to Erikson, what is the developmental stage associated with middle adulthood?
- Identify at least five appropriate topics for health teaching during middle adulthood.

PracticalKnowledge knowing **how**

NURSING DIAGNOSIS/ANALYZING CUES

Most NANDA-I diagnoses can be used for any age-group; however, the following discussion of growth and development nursing diagnoses applies to patients in all age-groups. Age-specific assessments and interventions were discussed within each of the developmental stages in the Theoretical Knowledge section of this chapter. Risk for Delayed Development diagnoses for older adults are found in Chapter 7.

- **An example of a diagnosis you might write for a child** is *Risk for Delayed Development r/t inadequate stimulation secondary to parental substance abuse.*
- **Short-term illness does not usually lead to delays in growth and development.** Such delays are more likely to be caused by family dysfunction, inadequate nutrition, or severe or long-term illness. Of course, patients you see for other problems may also be growth or developmentally delayed.
- **Growth and development diagnoses can, instead of being the problem focus, be defining characteristics or risk factors** for other diagnoses. For example: *Impaired Parenting r/t mother's chronic disability and evidenced by child's delayed growth.*
- **Only one NANDA-I diagnosis specifically addresses growth and development**; however, other NANDA-I diagnoses do address age-specific problems (e.g., Ineffective Breastfeeding, Parental Role Conflict).

PRIORITIZING HYPOTHESES/GENERATING SOLUTIONS

Individualized goals/outcomes and interventions for growth and development might include the following examples:

Diagnosis: Risk for Delayed Development
- *Goal:* The child will continue to meet developmental cognitive milestones as measured at the next well-child check.

- *Intervention (example):* Teach parent(s) three techniques they can use to stimulate the child's cognition.

PUTTING IT ALL TOGETHER

Recall the case of 3-year-old Tamika, who is being raised by her grandmother and has been hospitalized with pneumonia (Meet Your Patients scenario). Imagine that Tamika has been abandoned by her mother, who is addicted to heroin. You observe that Tamika is small for her age. You could write the following *diagnostic statement:*

> *Delayed Growth and Development r/t abandonment by mother, recent change in living status, and gestational heroin exposure as evidenced by short stature.*

To address Tamika's diagnosis, you might use the following *outcomes:*

NOC outcome: Child Development: 3 Years
Individualized goal: Tamika will achieve developmental milestones as demonstrated by (1) specified weight gain at next visit, (2) showing affection and bonding with grandmother, and (3) grandmother's report of adequate nutrition.

Because Tamika's grandmother is also caring for her ill husband, you may need to refer this family to community support services for ongoing help in the home and for nutritional services.

 To explore learning resources for this chapter,

 Go to Davis Advantage **and find:**

Answers and Suggested Responses for all questions in this chapter
Concept Map
Knowledge Map
References and Bibliography

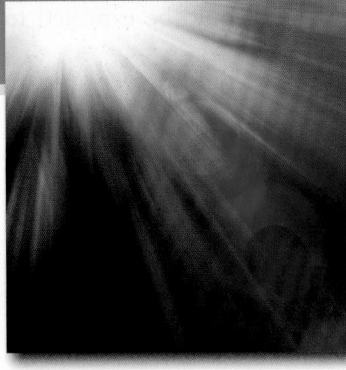

CHAPTER 7

Life Span: Older Adults

Learning Outcomes

After completing this chapter, you should be able to:

➤ Discuss the relationship between life expectancy and livable communities.

➤ Discuss the developmental challenges for each older adult age-group.

➤ Identify common health problems seen in each group and for all older adults.

➤ Describe any special assessments unique to each group of older adults.

➤ Discuss age-appropriate interventions for older adults and for each group.

➤ Incorporate developmental principles of aging into nursing care.

Key Concepts

Developmental changes

Functional status

Older adulthood

Related Concepts

See the Concept Map on Davis Advantage.

Example Client Conditions

Dementia

Elder abuse

Frail elderly

Meet Your Patient

Ethel Higginbotham, an 80-year-old woman, is in the hospital with pneumonia. She lives alone. Her son tells you that she began to lose weight rapidly, complains of no appetite, and became withdrawn after the death of her husband. At a recent visit to her home, he found his mother confused, with a productive cough, and with small open lesions on her lower legs. This led to her hospitalization. Even though she is no longer receiving oxygen, you observe that she is very thin and weak, sleeps most of the time, and refuses to eat. "I just want to die," she tells you.

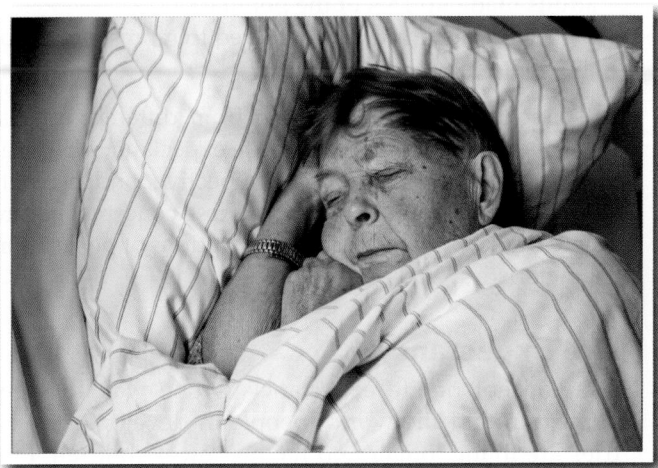

TheoreticalKnowledge
knowing why

Why should you learn about older adults? One very important reason is that most of your patients are likely to be older adults. Half of all hospitalized patients are older adults. Moreover, because older adults are more likely to have disabilities and chronic health problems, they will make up a sizable number of the patients you see in clinics, home care, and other settings, as well. This chapter presents the most important topics and issues about aging and the development of older adults.

ABOUT THE KEY CONCEPTS

You may have thought of **developmental stages** as something that applies mostly to children. However, as you learned in Chapter 6, **developmental changes** occur throughout life, even in **older adulthood.** Many normal changes occur in older adulthood. You will learn how normal changes, as well as illness, can affect **functional status**—a major focus in caring for older adults.

PERSPECTIVES ON AGING

Older adults constitute the fastest-growing age-group in developed nations. To understand this, you will need to look at some statistics from the U.S. Census Bureau (2021).

- In 1900, a mere 4.1% of the U.S. population was 65 or older.
- By 2014, life expectancy had increased, and older adults made up 15% of the population
- By 2060, older adults are expected to represent 24% of the population.

This chapter examines aging from different angles. We will discuss the concepts of life expectancy, distribution of age-groups, life-span perspective, and percentage of the total population. All of these concepts require you to think about numerical descriptions of population characteristics.

Life Expectancy

The concept of life expectancy is one way to view aging. Around the world, people in developed countries are living longer and having fewer children. Life expectancy can be calculated in one of two ways: life expectancy at birth or life expectancy measured at age 65. The following data from the U.S. Department of Health and Human Services (2018) illustrate these two methods:

- **Life expectancy at birth** has risen dramatically in the United States.
    In 1900, the average life expectancy at birth was 49.2 years.
    In 2017, the average life expectancy at birth was 79.7 years.

- **Life expectancy measured at age 65** has also risen, as the following two statements show:
    In 1960, a 65-year-old person could be expected to live 14.3 more years.
    In 2017, a 65-year-old person could be expected to live 19.9 more years.

This means that a baby born in 2017 could expect to live for nearly 79.7 years, whereas a person who was 65 years old in 2017 could expect to live another 19.9 years, to age 85. Those numbers reflect the average life expectancy for both sexes and all ethnic/racial groups. However, differences in life expectancy emerge when you examine sex and ethnic group data.

Gender- and Sex-Based Disparities The following differences emerge when taking gender and sex into account:

- **Life expectancy at birth.** For infants born in 2017, the average total life expectancy at birth is:
    For females, 82 years
    For males, 77.3 years
    This difference is especially noticeable in the 85-years-and-older population, in which women greatly outnumber men.
- **Life expectancy measured at age 65** was nearly the same for men and women in 1900; however, women had a lead of about 4 years over men in 2017, narrowing the gap as men age. So, the longer men live, the longer they *will* live.

Racial Disparities In 1900, race defined U.S. life expectancy at birth. As of 2015, the picture was less clear (as you can see in the following data from National Center for Health Statistics [2017]):

- **Life expectancy at birth:** Hispanic populations had the longest life expectancy at birth, and non-Hispanic Black populations had the shortest:
    Hispanic females, 84.5 years
    Non-Hispanic Black females, 78 years
    Hispanic males, 79.8 years
    Non-Hispanic Black males, 73.2 years
    In 2017, the life expectancy at birth for Black people was less than that for White people:
    White males, 77.7 years
    Black males, 73.2 years
    White females, 82.2 years
    Black females, 79 years
- **Life expectancy at age 65:**
    - Hispanic women led in life expectancy, with 22.7 more years, followed closely by White women, at 21.2 more years, and Hispanic men, at 20 more years.
    - Black men at age 65 had the lowest life expectancy (16.7 more years).
    - Notice, though, that the gap for ethnicity decreases as a person ages.
    A Black male baby born in 2017 could expect to live to about age 73.
    A Black man at age 65 in 2017 could expect to live another 16.7 years, to age 82.

The future population of older adults will be more ethnically and racially diverse, with all groups except the non-Hispanic, single-race White population expected to represent 56% of the population in 2060. The non-Hispanic White population is currently the "majority" group in the United States; it is both the largest racial and ethnic group and accounts for greater than 50% of the nation's total population. However, by 2060, this group is projected to be just 44% of the population. The Hispanic population and Black population are projected to compose 29% and 14% of the total population, respectively, in 2060 (U.S. Census Bureau, 2021).

Migration and Distribution of Age-Groups

In addition to life expectancy, in-migration and out-migration within and between countries or states contribute to the distribution of age-groups and the median age of a population. From 2013 to 2014, only 3% of older persons moved, as opposed to 13% of the under-65 population. Most older movers (60%) stayed in the same county, and 81% remained in the same state. Only 19% of the movers moved from out of state or abroad. In 2021, the median age (years):

Of the U.S. population	was	38.3
Of the state of Maine	was	44.1
Of the state of Utah	was	31.2

The median age of the population in the United States is increasing. By 2034, people aged 65 and older are projected to outnumber children under the age of 18, and by 2060, nearly 1 in 4 Americans will be at least 65 years old.

Percentage of Total Population

Yet another way to view aging is by the *percentage of the total population* each age-group represents. In the United States, older adults comprised approximately:

4.1% of the population in 1900
15% of the population in 2014

By 2060, it is projected that they will compose 24% of the population (U.S. Census Bureau, 2021).

The age distribution of a population is often illustrated in a pyramid, with the youngest age-group (0–4) at the base and the oldest age-group (85+) at the peak, with men on the left of the figure and women on the right. The shape of a population pyramid changes to that of a rectangle in developed countries with fewer births and increased life expectancy.

To view a population pyramid that illustrates the projected age distribution of the U.S. population in 2010, 2030, and 2050, see Figure 7-1. To see an animated pyramid,

 Go to the Web site **http://www.pewresearch.org/next-america/age-pyramid/**

Notice also that the percentage of centenarians almost doubles from 2030 to 2050. The U.S. Census Bureau

reports the following total numbers of centenarians (U.S. Census Bureau, 2018):

82,000 centenarians—actual total number in 2016
589,000 centenarians—projected total number in 2060

 ThinkLike a Nurse 7-1: Clinical Judgment **in Action**

- What factors do you think account for the overall increase in life expectancy?
- What effect will the distribution of the population by age within your state have on your nursing practice?
- Refer to Figure 7-1 to answer the following three questions:
  In the 85-to-89 age-group in the 2030 data, what percentage of the population is male? What percentage is female?
  In the 85-to-89 age-group in the 2050 data, what percentage of the population is male? What percentage is female?
  In the 85-to-89 age-group, which group increases the most between 2030 and 2050: female or male?

Life-Span Perspective

Another way to view aging is from a *life-span perspective*. In this perspective, *genes* inherited at conception; *behaviors* expressed throughout a lifetime; and the *environments* within which a person lives, works, and plays interact with each other over time. The cumulative effect of these interactions is seen in older adulthood.

Think of the *genetic–behavior–environment interaction* as a survival mechanism of aging. Attending to healthy behaviors (e.g., daily exercise) and avoiding unhealthy behaviors (e.g., tobacco use) is a lifelong process. A lifetime of positive health behaviors interacting with a healthful environment has the potential to shift the effects of a harmful genetic trait—that is, a person may have the genetic trait for a particular disease but never show signs of the disease.

Remember the nun study discussed in Chapter 4? Some of the nuns demonstrated no symptoms of Alzheimer disease during their lifetime, yet upon autopsy, scientists discovered the typical neurological changes associated with Alzheimer disease (Snowdon, 2003). The results of the nun study illustrate strong evidence of the power of behaviors and the environment over genes, resulting in centenarians who are cognitively intact and asymptomatic for Alzheimer disease.

 ThinkLike a Nurse 7-2: Clinical Judgment **in Action**

Plot your birth year on a timeline that extends in 10-year increments through your 65th and 100th year. What is the projected distribution of age and gender when you are an older adult? What genetic, environmental, and behavioral attributes will influence your life expectancy and state of health as an older adult?

AGING IN PLACE AND ALTERNATIVES

Key Point: *Contrary to popular belief, most older adults live independently (Roy et al., 2018).* **Aging in place** means that as they age, persons live in their own

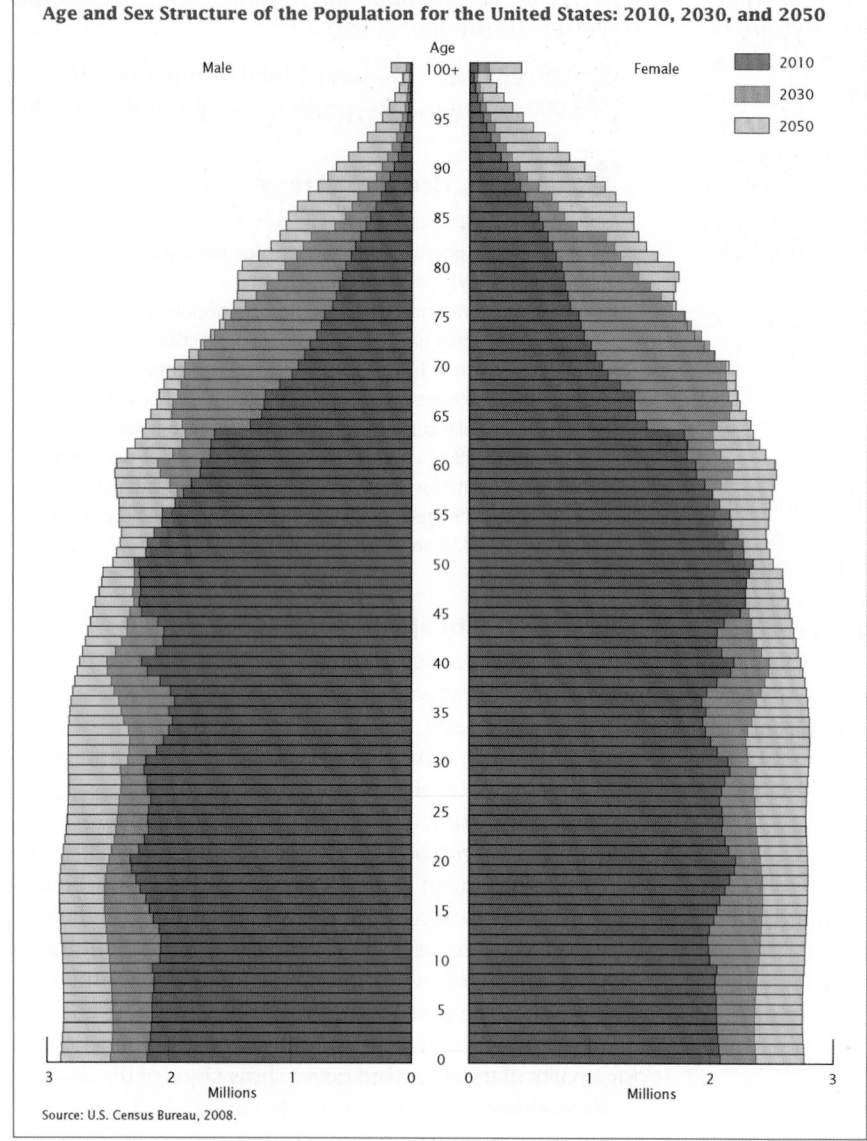

Age and Sex Structure of the Population for the United States: 2010, 2030, and 2050

Source: U.S. Census Bureau, 2008.

FIGURE 7-1 Age and sex structure of the population for the United States: 2010, 2030, and 2050.

residences and receive supportive services for their changing needs, rather than moving to another type of housing. Aging in place requires an elder-friendly residence and an elder-friendly or livable community that provides maximum accessibility, minimal barriers, and adequate resources and services to maintain independence for as long as possible.

Age-Friendly Residences Among the considerations for a safe and *age-friendly residence* are the following:

- Ground-level entry or no-step entry
- One-level living area
- Wide doorways to allow for assistive devices such as walkers and wheelchairs
- Lever-style door and faucet handles for easy grasp
- Grab bars, shower seats, and elevated toilet seat in bathrooms
- Kitchen appliances, cabinets, and surfaces no higher than 48 inches above the floor

- Shelves no more than 10 inches deep for easy accessibility
- Adequate light in all areas, both inside and outside
- Walking areas free of clutter, including area rugs

Age-Friendly Communities Livable communities (also referred to as *age-friendly*) emphasize older people's continuing participation in social, economic, cultural, spiritual, and civic affairs (Buffel & Phillipson, 2018). To illustrate the need for age-friendly communities, consider these facts about older adults in 2015 (U.S. Department of Health and Human Services, 2018):

- Ten million (19.6 %) Americans age 65 and over were in the labor force.
- Over 4.5 million people age 65 and over (9.2%) were below the poverty level, and another 2.5 million, or 4.9% of older adults, were classified as "near poor" (between the poverty level and 125% of poverty level).
- Twenty-nine percent held a bachelor's degree or higher.

- Of people who are aging in place and are age 65 and older, 46% assessed their health as excellent or very good.
- Many older adults spent about one-third of their income on housing. This includes:
  - 30% (approximately) of older adults who owned their own homes
  - 65% of older adults who were renters

Livable communities offer the following:

- Housing that is affordable and appropriate for all ages
- Supportive services and features
- Dependable and affordable transportation and housing
- Resources that facilitate individual independence and socialization of residents (AARP, 2017)
- Affordable and accessible healthcare
- Safe, low-crime environment
- Community engagement

Naturally Occurring Retirement Communities

When persons "age in place" within a specific apartment building or a community/street of single-family homes, that area is referred to as a **naturally occurring retirement community (NORC).** Persons within a NORC have aged together. More often than not, they have, over the years, developed access to services needed to maintain the highest quality of life for all within the NORC. When one neighbor needs assistance, others pitch in to help or to obtain help. The U.S. Administration on Aging provides competitive funding to support the development and maintenance of services within a NORC.

Retirement Communities

Some housing developments are planned specifically as **retirement communities.** They are planned to provide age-friendly dwellings and environments for independent living and allow older adults to "downsize" into a house that has less than 2,000 square feet in single-level, livable space. The purchase of a home in a retirement community usually includes, for an annual association fee, services such as home maintenance and repair, lawn care and trash removal, some home utilities, security, home fire and theft insurance, recreational amenities (e.g., pool, golf), and planned activities. They usually have a minimum age restriction of 55, 60, or 62 for residents. Age restriction may be problematic if grandparents become the primary care providers for a grandchild.

Continuing Care Retirement Communities

Continuing care retirement communities (CCRCs), or *life care communities,* offer a wide range of living accommodations, from residential living (e.g., cottages, cluster homes, apartments) to assisted living, skilled nursing care, rehabilitation, and dementia care, on a large, campus-like setting. CCRCs include many amenities, ranging from golf courses, pools, and indoor sports facilities to a full range of hobby rooms, clubrooms, and personal services. A CCRC is an example of aging in place, except that an older adult must first move to it. So, in that sense, it is not a NORC.

Entrance requirements include physical, mental, and financial health evaluations. Contracts may include lifetime care, time-specified care, or fee-for-service care. CCRCs are usually expensive, requiring a contract, an entrance fee, and monthly fees that may increase with annual cost-of-living estimates. Depending on the contract, monthly fees may cover a set number of meals per month, transportation, housekeeping, unit maintenance, laundry service, health monitoring, some utilities, coordinated social activities, emergency call monitoring, and round-the-clock security. A health clinic is usually located on-site. Healthcare providers may include a registered nurse, nurse practitioner, physician, dentist, and physical therapist.

CCRCs vary by their affiliation (e.g., ethnic or religious group, university, corporation) and whether the living space is rented or purchased. University-affiliated CCRCs incorporate all aspects of academic life into the lives of residents and provide opportunities for cross-generation interactions on the CCRC and university campuses.

Assisted-Living Facilities

Assisted-living facilities (ALFs) are congregate residential settings that provide or coordinate personal services, 24-hour supervision and assistance (scheduled and unscheduled), activities, and health-related services. ALFs are *not* aging-in-place environments. State regulations and the level of services provided do not allow residents to stay in an ALF when their needs become greater than the resources and services provided. ALFs are designed to:

- Minimize the need to move
- Accommodate individual residents' changing needs and preferences
- Maximize residents' dignity, autonomy, privacy, independence, and safety
- Encourage family and community involvement

ALFs have multiple definitions and goals; they have no physical size, design, or model in common. ALFs might be self-standing or housed within a CCRC as one level of housing and service. Each ALF has its own culture, rules, norms, values, and rituals that are created by the residents. An ALF may have limitations, such as reduced consumer choice, little flexibility, and an illusion of certainty.

Nursing Care Facilities (Nursing Homes)

Nursing care facilities, or **nursing homes,** provide skilled and unskilled nursing care for older adults and adults with disabilities. To understand the scope of nursing care facilities in the overall picture of aging, consider the following facts. In 2018:

- About 1.3 million residents lived in more than 16,000 U.S. nursing facilities.
- Only 1% of persons age 65+ lived in nursing facilities; however, this rises to 9% for people over 85 years.
- Nearly half of the residents of nursing homes had dementia, and one-fifth had other psychological diagnoses.
- Women comprised more than 65% of the nursing home population (National Center for Health Statistics, 2019).
- Medicaid is the primary source of payment for most (62%) of the residents; Medicare pays for about 13%, primarily for short stays, and individual long-term care insurance or private sources pay for 22%.

KnowledgeCheck 7-1

- Approximately what percentage of people over age 65 live in nursing facilities?
- What percentage of people over 85 years old live in nursing facilities?
- Who has the longer life expectancy, women or men?

KnowledgeCheck 7-2

What is the difference between a retirement community and a CCRC?

 ThinkLike a Nurse 7-3:
   Clinical Judgment **in Action**

How age-friendly is the community in which you live? What cues did you identify to help you determine your answer?

THEORIES OF AGING

There is no single explanation for how the body ages, but four groups of physiological theories predominate. **Key Point:** *Despite wide debate on these theories, most scientists consider aging to be a combination of factors, including inherited traits and the cell's response to environmental stressors.*

   Wear-and-tear theory proposes that repeated insults and the accumulation of metabolic wastes eventually cause cells to wear out and cease functioning.

   Genetic theories of aging propose that cells have a preprogrammed, finite number of cell divisions. Therefore, the time of death is determined at birth. The genetic messages within the various body cells specify how many times the cell can reproduce, thus defining the life of that cell.

   Cellular malfunction hypothesizes that a malfunction in the cell causes changes in cellular DNA, leading to problems with cell replication. The cellular malfunction can be the result of:

- A chemical reaction with the DNA (cross-linking theory)

- An abundance of free radicals that damage cells and impair their ability to function normally (free-radical theory)
- A buildup of toxins over time that causes cell death (toxin theory)

   Autoimmune reaction hypothesizes that cells change with age. Over time, the changes cause the immune system to perceive some cells as foreign substances, thus triggering an immune response to destroy the cells.

STAGES OF OLDER ADULTHOOD

Most references use 65 years as the age when older adulthood begins. The stages of older adulthood are typically referred to as the *young-old* (age 65 to 74), *middle-old* (age 75 to 84), and *oldest-old* (age 85 and older). **Key Point:** *The fastest-growing segment of older adults is the oldest-old, some of whom are the frail elderly and centenarians (people older than 100 years).* For more in-depth information about aging and older adults, refer to a life-span development or gerontology resource.

Young-Old: Age 65 to 74

Physical and psychological adaptations to retirement are paramount in this age-group. At retirement, a person's usual social contacts and structure for daily activities may change markedly. A newly retired older adult may be searching for new interests outside of the previous work environment.

   One key indicator of well-being is the use of leisure time. On an average day, young-old persons spend most of their time (61%) watching television, with smaller amounts devoted to solitary activities of reading (8.6%) or relaxing and thinking (5.9%); socializing and communicating (9.3%); and participating in sports, exercise, and recreation (4%), with the remaining time spent engaging in other activities, including travel (Federal Interagency Forum on Aging-Related Statistics, 2020).

   By the time they reach age 65, many young-old persons are experiencing the effects of chronic illnesses that began in middle adulthood, along with the effects of a lack of time for self-care because of the demands and stressors of work during middle adulthood. Retirement frees up time for the young-old to make up for these effects and focus on health-promoting behaviors to help prevent the decline of health as they age. However, young-old persons face barriers to health, such as the following:

- A lack of supplemental insurance for health screening or physicals that are not covered under Medicare
- Perceptions of self as "getting old"
- Changes in physical activity
- Being in a deconditioned state as a result of not participating in exercise before retirement

   There is some evidence that physical activity declines as early as age 63 for some and by age 70 for most people.

Middle-Old: Age 75 to 84

The developmental challenge of middle-old persons is an increasingly solitary, sedentary lifestyle. This age-group spends one-fourth of their leisure time in solitary activities of reading, relaxing, and thinking—more than their younger cohort. They spend only 3% of their time participating in sports, exercise, and recreation—less than their younger cohort (Federal Interagency Forum on Aging-Related Statistics, 2020). Without physical activity, the risk of disability associated with chronic conditions increases during the middle-old years.

Adapted Physical Activity (APA) APA programs are group exercise programs designed for persons with chronic conditions. APA programs are aimed at correcting a sedentary lifestyle and preventing disability secondary to the chronic condition. **Key Point:** *The focus of APA programs is on functional ability rather than treating existing disability, and they are beneficial throughout the older adult years.* Adopting a lifestyle that includes physical activity contributes to better health and a higher quality of life among community-dwelling older adults (Song & Doris, 2019).

Senior centers are beginning to offer APA opportunities as they update their programs for the active baby-boomer generation. Some health and fitness facilities may also offer senior health programs and books that illustrate adapted strategies for lifelong walkers and marathon runners. Although physical activity declines in the middle-old group overall, older adults represent the fastest-growing segment of participants in competitive sports, with a rise in the 80-plus-year-old finishers at road races such as the New York City Marathon.

Oldest-Old: Age 85 and Older

The developmental challenges of the oldest-old are sensory impairments, oral health, inadequate nutritional intake, and functional limitations. The following examples are from the Federal Interagency Forum on Aging-Related Statistics (2020):

- *Hearing.* Many older adults reported difficulty hearing. This was higher for the 85+ age-group (13.4%) than it was for the young-old and the middle-old (6.7%).
- *Vision.* Of the 85+ age-group, 6.6% reported trouble seeing, even while wearing glasses.
- *Edentulism.* Of those over 85 years old, 31% reported **edentulism** (having no natural teeth). This tends to be income related: 42% of older adults below the poverty line reported edentulism, whereas for those above the poverty line, the incidence was only 23%.
- *Nutrition.* Edentulism compromises the already inadequate nutritional intake of older adults and fosters a diet of "soft" foods that may be higher in fats, carbohydrates, and calories. For the oldest-old, this occurs at a time when they need to decrease the intake of these foods to combat obesity and counter decreased activity levels.

- *Functional limitations.* Ability to stoop/kneel, reach overhead, walk two or three blocks, and lift 10 pounds are common parameters for determining the functional abilities of older adults. More than half of men and about 60% of women in that group were unable to perform at least one activity. There were minimal to no differences across ethnic and racial groups.

Centenarians People aged 100 years and older **(centenarians)** are a subgroup of the oldest-old. It appears that surviving to an extreme old age is the result of favorable interactions between genetic composition, environment, and lifestyle (behaviors). The most significant factor may be the presence of a loved one in the life of the older adult. Their commitment to the community is also linked to their longevity. One genetic variation of centenarians has been linked with longevity, but mapping the centenarian genome is essential to determine whether they do, in fact, carry a so-called longevity gene (Perls, 2006; Perls et al., 1999). Among the characteristics of centenarians are that 12% live independently, and 90% are cognitively intact into their 90s.

Example Client Condition: Frail Elderly This category of older adults is characterized by health status rather than age. See the Example Client Condition: Frail Elderly.

KnowledgeCheck 7-3

- Name and give the age ranges for the four stages of older adulthood.
- Name and briefly describe four theories of aging.

DEVELOPMENTAL CHANGES OF OLDER ADULTS

Although not all people age at the same pace, there are predictable patterns of physical, cognitive, and psychosocial change. Older adults also have several, often chronic, health problems in common.

Physical Development of Older Adults

Although there is variation among individuals, patterns of change can be predicted in each body system. Table 7-1 presents an overview of changes seen with aging, as well as corresponding areas for assessment.

Cognitive Development of Older Adults

Older adults learn new material more slowly because:

Reaction time slows.
Short-term memory declines.
Response time to a stimulus becomes longer
Ability to process incoming information becomes slower.

Key Point: *However, there is no loss of intelligence as a person ages.*

EXAMPLE CLIENT CONDITION: Frail Elderly

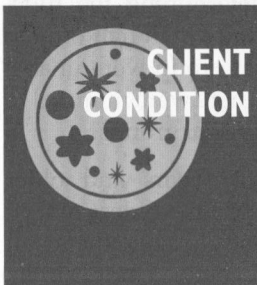
CLIENT CONDITION

Definition of Frailty

As humans age, they are gradually less able to adapt to internal challenges (e.g., disease) and external environments (e.g., injury). Multiple systems are usually involved.

- **Frailty** is a syndrome (set of characteristics) that describes a heightened state of vulnerability for developing adverse health outcomes.

- **Frailty** is the point at which the human organism is believed to have its least capacity for survival and will fail in response to a minor internal or external insult.

  Example: A frail older adult might die merely as a result of an upper respiratory infection (such as a cold).

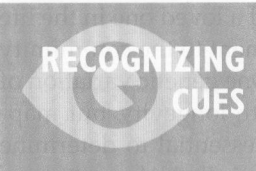
RECOGNIZING CUES

Assess for:
- Weakness
- Ability to live independently, assistance needed to perform activities of daily living (ADLs)
- Impaired mental abilities
- Medical problems
- Psychosocial and behavioral factors (e.g., depression, caregiver problems, housing)
- Other risk factors (e.g., smoking, underweight)

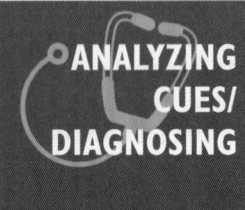
ANALYZING CUES/ DIAGNOSING

Psychosocial and behavioral factors (e.g., depression, caregiver problems, housing) are important to a person's interactions with the environment and are believed to predict vulnerability (frailty) and ability to survive.

To be considered frail, a person must have three or more of the following characteristics:
- Low physical activity
- Muscle weakness
- Slowed performance
- Fatigue or poor endurance

PRIORITIZING HYPOTHESIS

- **Perceived Powerlessness** related to dependence on others
- **Injury Risk** related to poor balance, confusion
- **Reduced Self-Care Ability** related to loss of mobility, fatigue, mental status changes

GENERATING SOLUTIONS

- Fall-preventive (moderate-intensity) group (Martínez-Velilla et al., 2019)
- For the obese and frail, combined weight loss and exercise therapy (Xu et al., 2019)
- Internet access may maintain physical and cognitive status (Macdonald & Hülür, 2021).
- Teach and assist to keep the mind active (socializing, reading, puzzles, games).
- Arrange for care as needed, and teach caregivers how and when to seek profession help.
- Recognize and treat depression and other medical problems.
- Facilitate good nutritional status (Kurkcu et al., 2018).

Advise caregivers and older adults to take the following measures to prevent or slow the progression of frailty:
- Engage in daily physical activity to the extent possible: walking and weights to build aerobic fitness, build muscle, and improve joint stiffness and pain.
- Eat a balanced diet, including enough protein, fiber, and fluids.
- If you smoke, stop.
- Get regular checkups.
- Keep the mind active by socializing, working puzzles, reading, or playing games.

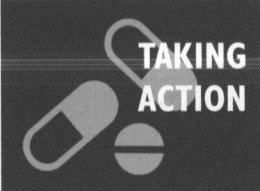
TAKING ACTION

Monitor for positive changes in functional ability and level of independence.

Evaluate changes in mobility, fatigue, or mental status.

EXAMPLE CLIENT CONDITION: Frail Elderly—cont'd

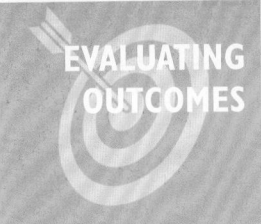

EVALUATING OUTCOMES

- Identifies normal changes, adapts routine, and reports alterations in ADLs and instrumental activities of daily living (IADLs) that are outside expected change for age
- Maintains independence longer and delays the aging process

Table 7-1 ➤ Age-Related Changes and Areas for Assessment

	NORMAL AGING CHANGE	AREAS FOR ASSESSMENT
Musculoskeletal	Decreased muscle strength, body mass, bone mass, joint mobility Increased fat deposits	▪ Activity/exercise tolerance ▪ Joint pain, range of motion ▪ Gait, balance, posture, change in height ▪ Susceptibility to falls ▪ Ability to perform activities of daily living
Cardiovascular	Decreased cardiac output Increased peripheral resistance, systolic blood pressure	▪ Activity tolerance ▪ Blood pressure ▪ Orthostatic hypotension ▪ Arrhythmia
Respiratory	Decreased elasticity of chest wall, intercostals muscle strength, cough reflex Increased anteroposterior diameter of chest, rigidity of lung tissue	▪ Cough reflex ▪ Use of accessory muscles ▪ Gas exchange ▪ Mouth breathing
Gastrointestinal	Decreased saliva production, gastrointestinal motility, gastric acid production	▪ Ability to chew ▪ Dentition ▪ Pattern of elimination ▪ Frequency/size of meals
Integument	Decreased skin elasticity, nail growth Increased dryness of skin, thinning of skin layers, nail thickening, hair thinning	▪ Susceptibility to hypo/hyperthermia ▪ Intact skin, bruising ▪ Dry skin ▪ Bathing pattern
Genitourinary	Decreased glomerular filtration rate, blood flow to kidneys, bladder capacity, vaginal lubrication, hardness of erection	▪ Continence ▪ Urgency, frequency, nocturia ▪ Hydration status ▪ Drug levels ▪ Sexual pattern
Nervous	Decreased nerve cells, neurotransmitters, rapid eye movement (REM) sleep, blood flow to central nervous system	▪ Diminished reflexes ▪ Sleep pattern ▪ Depression

(Continued)

Table 7-1 ➤ Age-Related Changes and Areas for Assessment—cont'd

	NORMAL AGING CHANGE	AREAS FOR ASSESSMENT
Endocrine	Decreased insulin release, thyroid function, estrogen and testosterone	▪ Change in weight ▪ Libido ▪ Energy level
Sensory	Decreased visual acuity (presbyopia, or impaired near vision) and depth perception, tear production, pupil size, accommodation, acuity of smell and taste, hearing of high-frequency sound, sense of balance changes in pain sensation Increased glare sensitivity, thickening of lens of the eye, changes in pain sensation Macular degeneration causing loss of central vision (not a normal change, but a common one)	▪ Adequate lighting ▪ Cerumen buildup ▪ Home safety ▪ Pain sensation ▪ Driving ability ▪ Environmental stimulation
Cognition	Decreased short-term memory Increased reaction time, information-processing time	▪ Memory changes ▪ Learning barriers ▪ Adaptive coping
Personality	Increased cautiousness Retirement, widowhood, grandparenthood	▪ Sources of social support ▪ Social network

Memory The loss of short-term memory is more common than the loss of long-term memory; thus, older adults may remember incidents from many years ago but may have trouble recalling what they did earlier in the day.

▪ Physical health problems or medications may affect memory.
▪ An active social life with complete engagement and participation in the community delays memory loss with aging (Kotwal et al., 2016).
▪ Regular mental exercises (e.g., crossword puzzles, conversation) appear to stimulate the brain and enhance memory.
▪ Other factors that slow memory loss are adequate sleep and rest, a nourishing diet, and avoidance of drugs and alcohol.

Psychosocial Development of Older Adults

Rather than explaining how the body ages, psychosocial theories of aging attempt to explain the psychological and social adjustments associated with aging.

Disengagement Theory (1961)

Cumming and Henry (1961) hypothesized that the older adult and society gradually and mutually withdraw or disengage from each other. Mandatory retirement, chronic illness, the deaths of relatives and friends, and poverty are among the factors that may contribute to this phenomenon. As the interaction between a person and their world decreases, there is (1) more time for reflection and (2) freedom from societal roles. Power transfers

to younger members of society as the older adult withdraws. **Key Point:** *Disengagement is not the norm for the current generation of older adults in America, nor is it universally true for cultures that value older adults' advice as essential for family decision making.*

Activity Theory (1963)

Activity theory posits that the individual should stay as active and engaged as possible to enjoy the highest life satisfaction (Fig. 7-2). On retirement, another activity, such as travel, sports, hobbies, or volunteering, replaces time spent at work. Havighurst's theory (1963) is the counterpart of disengagement theory. According to Havighurst (1971), the following are physical, cognitive, and social developmental tasks of older adults:

Adjusting to decreasing physical strength and health
Adjusting to retirement
Adjusting to a lower income
Adjusting to the death of a spouse
Establishing an open affiliation with one's age-group
Adopting and adapting flexible social roles
Establishing satisfactory physical living arrangements

Psychosocial Development Theory (1963)

Erikson's developmental theory (1963) identifies *ego integrity versus despair* as the task of the older adult. This stage of development has as its cornerstone the acceptance that one's life has had meaning and that death is a part of the continuum of life. This outlook allows a person to accept the inevitable changes in health and life circumstances. The basic virtue gained at this stage is wisdom. Recall that Erikson's theory is discussed in Chapter 6.

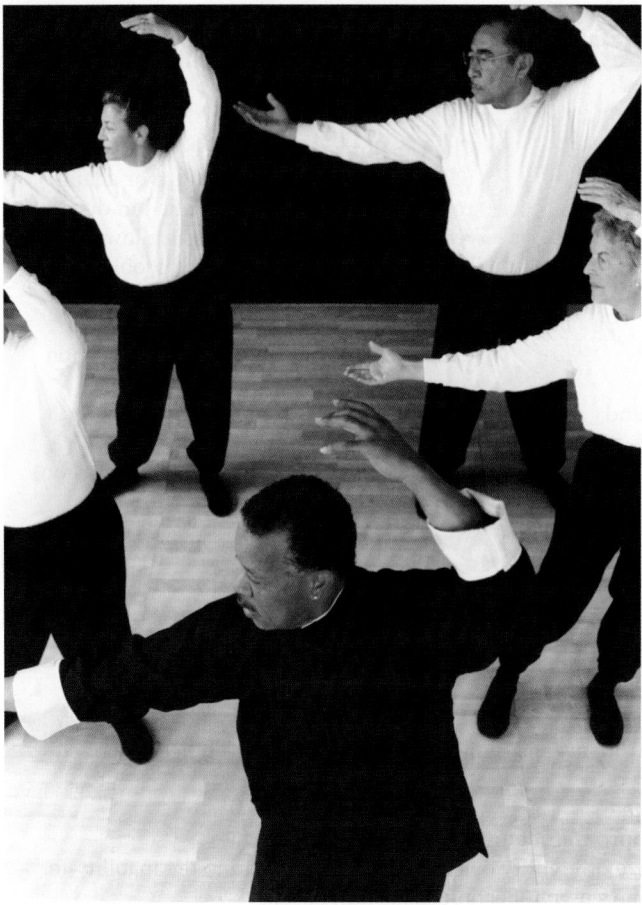

FIGURE 7-2 Many older adults are able to remain active and engaged well into their later years.

BOX 7-1 ■ Leading Causes of Death for Older Americans

The leading causes of death for older Americans are as follows:

1. Heart disease
2. Cancer
3. Chronic lower respiratory diseases
4. Stroke
5. Alzheimer disease
6. Diabetes mellitus
7. Influenza and pneumonia

Source: Federal Interagency Forum on Aging-Related Statistics. (2020). _Older Americans 2020: Key indicators of well-being 2020._ https://agingstats.gov/docs/LatestReport/OA20_508_10142020.pdf

Psychosocial changes in this age-group are many and significant. The older adult must face multiple losses, such as the following:

■ Death of a spouse or partner, family members, and friends
■ Challenges to health and youthful vitality
■ Loss of independence and the ability to live without assistance

Cumulative losses often have a negative psychological effect on the older adult. Loss is discussed in detail in Chapter 14.

Common Health Problems of Older Adults

The leading causes of death for older Americans are found in Box 7-1.

Chronic Diseases

Key Point: _Six of the seven leading causes of death among older adults are chronic diseases._

■ _The prevalence of chronic conditions differs by race and ethnicity._ For example, compared with the non-Hispanic White population, the prevalence of diagnosed and undiagnosed diabetes was higher among populations of Asian heritage, non-Hispanic Black populations, and Hispanic populations (Centers for Disease Control and Prevention, 2021a).
■ _**Heart disease, cancer, stroke, and diabetes**_ are among the most common and costly chronic health conditions. These are long-term illnesses that are rarely cured, but many can be prevented or modified with therapeutic lifestyle changes.

Osteoporosis

Osteoporosis, a loss in bone mineral density that increases the risk of fracture, affects an estimated 10 million Americans. In advanced cases, the bones become so porous that they fracture spontaneously, merely from the stress of bearing the person's weight. The risk of osteoporosis is increased:

■ With age
■ For females (1) because of their normal bone density is less than that of males and (2) because of hormonal changes at menopause and inadequate calcium intake
■ By cigarette smoking
■ By moderate to heavy alcohol consumption
■ By lack of weight-bearing exercise

Dementia

For an overview, see Example Client Condition: Dementia. To learn about distinguishing dementia from normal aging, see Table 7-2.

Polypharmacy

Polypharmacy, the use of multiple medications, is a risk factor for acute confusion, delirium, and depression in older adults. Continued growth in knowledge about the human genome has accelerated the field of **pharmacogenomics** (the discipline that blends pharmacology with genomic capabilities). Pharmacogenomics

EXAMPLE CLIENT CONDITION: Dementia

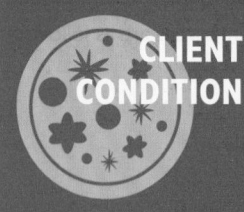

CLIENT CONDITION

Definition

Irreversible progressive decline in mental abilities; affects about 1 in 5 adults older than 70 years. **Key Point: *Dementia is not a normal result of aging—common, but not normal.***

Alzheimer Disease

- The primary form of dementia
- Considered progressive
- Affects about half of adults aged 85 and older

  The National Institute on Aging, among others, is working on a blood test for a specific brain protein that can be definitively used to diagnose Alzheimer before symptoms appear. Tests are still in the early stages of development, and more research will be needed before the test can be used clinically (Loewenstein et al., 2019).

Screening and Identification

- The U.S. Preventive Services Task Force (2020) does not recommend for or against routine screening for dementia but does recognize that early diagnosis allows clinicians to anticipate future problems the patients may have.
- Some dementias may be treatable—for example, those resulting from medication toxicity, sensory deficits, and some physiological problems. For this reason, it is important to differentiate such dementias from delirium (acute confusion) and depression (see Chapter 10).

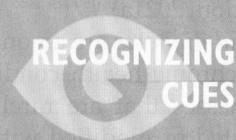

RECOGNIZING CUES

Dementia involves both memory impairments and a disturbance in at least one other area of cognition, such as the following:

- **Aphasia** (loss of ability to communicate)
- **Apraxia** (loss of ability to carry out purposeful movements)
- **Agnosia** (impaired ability to recognize or identify objects). Agnosia can lead to the inability to recognize family members or even one's own reflection in the mirror.
- **Disturbance in executive functioning** (ability to organize, manage, and make decisions)

  Dementia makes it progressively difficult for older adults to remember things, think clearly, communicate with others, or take care of themselves. In addition, dementia can cause mood swings and even change a person's personality and behavior.

ANALYZING CUES

- **For a step-by-step procedure for assessing mental status**, see Procedure 19-16, Assessing the Sensory-Neurological System.
- **Assess for risk factors,** including old age, family history, cardiovascular disease, and environmental factors such as a head injury or alcohol abuse.
- **Differentiate dementia from normal changes of aging.** See Table 7-2.
- **Assessment tools for dementia.** Use one or more of the following mental status examinations:
  - **The "Sweet 16"**
    Correlates highly with MMSE
    16 oral questions; easy to use
    Tests for orientation, registration, sustained attention, and short-term memory (Fong et al., 2010)
  - **Mini Mental State Examination (MMSE):** Tests a number of different mental abilities, including a person's memory, attention, and language.
  - **Ultrabrief screening:** Ask patient to recite the months of the year backward; then ask the day of the week (Fick et al., 2015).

PRIORITIZE HYPOTHESIS

- **Impaired Verbal Communication** related to irreversible, progressive decline in mental abilities
- **Fear** related to difficulty speaking and understanding

EXAMPLE CLIENT CONDITION: Dementia—cont'd

GENERATE SOLUTIONS AND TAKE ACTION	**Key Point:** *Realize that the patient's reality is distorted and they are behaving in the only way they are able.*
	• Provide a safe environment.
	• To facilitate communication:
	  Use simple, short sentences containing one idea each.
	  Avoid vague comments.
	  If the patient doesn't understand, repeat your words *exactly*.
	  Also see Communicating With Persons With Cognitive Deficit in this chapter.
	• Promote cognitive function: Provide activities and materials that are engaging and involve some degree of cognitive processing (e.g., reading, playing board games, playing a musical instrument, dancing).
	• Activities should be person-centered and appropriate for age-group.
	• Orient the patient to reality.
	• Use life review and reminiscence.
	• Provide supervision (sometimes 24 hours a day) and management of difficult behavior.
	• Assist with activities of daily living (ADLs), such as bathing, eating, getting out of bed to a chair or wheelchair, toileting, and other personal care.
	• Provide caregiver support.
	• Emphasize and support social activities.

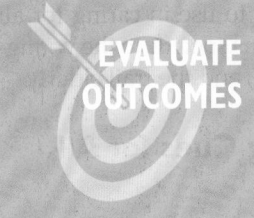 **EVALUATE OUTCOMES**	• Will not be fearful • Carries out simple 2- and 3-word commands. • Will be free from harm

---

Table 7-2 ➤ Distinguishing the Changes of Typical Aging From Dementia

TYPICAL AGING	DEMENTIA
Independence in daily activities preserved	Dependent on others for key independent-living activities
Complains of memory loss but able to provide considerable detail regarding incidents of forgetfulness	May complain of memory problems only if specifically asked; unable to recall instances in which memory loss was noticed
Is more concerned about forgetfulness than are close family members	Close family members much more concerned about incidents of memory loss than patient
Recent memory for important events, affairs, conversations is intact	Significant decline in memory for recent events and ability to engage in conversation
Occasional word-finding difficulties	Often has difficulty finding words; uses many pauses and substitutions
In familiar territory, may have to pause momentarily to remember way, but doesn't get lost	Gets lost in familiar territory while walking or driving; sometimes taking hours to eventually return home
Unwilling to learn how to operate new devices but is able to operate common and familiar appliances	Unable to operate common and even familiar appliances; cannot learn to operate even simple new appliances
Maintains prior level of interpersonal social skills	Shows loss of interest in social activities; behaves inappropriately in social situations
Performs normally on mental status examinations, taking into account education and culture	Abnormal performance on mental status examinations; performance not explained by education or cultural factors

Source: Adapted from Agency for Healthcare Research and Quality. (1996, November). *Clinical practice guidelines.* No. 19. Publication #97-0702. U.S. Department of Health and Human Services.

will aid in improving the selection of a particular drug treatment and allow for the tailoring of the dose and dosing schedule to the patient's genetic profile. For older adult patients with comorbidities and a risk of polypharmacy, this technology is expected to increase the efficiency of the drug industry and result in cheaper, more effective drug therapies.

Depression

Medical problems can cause depression in older adults, either directly or as a psychological reaction to the illness. Any chronic medical condition, particularly if it is painful, disabling, or life threatening, can lead to depression or make depression symptoms worse. In 2018, 13% of older women reported depressive symptoms, compared with 9% of older men, numbers that have remained fairly stable for nearly a decade and may be related to appropriate antidepressant drug treatment for older adults (Federal Interagency Forum on Aging-Related Statistics, 2020).

Depression not only affects mood but also affects energy, sleep, appetite, and physical health. Many of the symptoms of depression are similar to those of dementia (memory problems, sluggish speech and movements, and low motivation), so it may be difficult to tell the two apart. **Key Point: *Symptoms of depression can also be the side effect of many commonly prescribed drugs, especially if the person is taking multiple medications. Older adults are more sensitive to mood-related side effects of prescription medication because as they age, their bodies become less efficient at metabolizing and processing drugs.***

Elder Abuse

Be alert for patterns of injury in older adults because there is a strong possibility of abuse in this population. **Key Point: *If you suspect abuse, your first priority is to ensure the client is safe and cared for.*** Next, you must report the abuse. To learn about elder abuse, see the Example Client Condition: Elder Abuse.

Ageism

Ageism is age-based discrimination. Ageism is recognized as a social determinant of health and can lead to various harms, including age-based health inequities and poorer health outcomes. Negative expectations for older adults can cloud nursing assessments, planning, and interventions. According to the World Health Organization (2021), ageism:

- Shortens the life span
- Worsens physical and mental health
- Hinders recovery from disability
- Accelerates cognitive decline
- Exacerbates social isolation and loneliness
- Reduces access to employment, education, and healthcare

KnowledgeCheck 7-4

- Name two age-related changes seen in older adults.
- According to Erikson, what is the developmental stage of the older adult?
- What are the top-two causes of death among older adults?

PracticalKnowledge
knowing **how**

You would expect differences in functioning in older adults who are relatively healthy and those who have one or more illnesses. You will, of course, base nursing care on individual needs, not on a person's age category. However, in general, you would expect a patient's needs to be different at age 65 than they would be at age 85. **Key Point: *Remember, though, that an individual's health status and needs are affected by many more variables than just their age (e.g., chronic illness, stressors).***

■ ASSESSMENT/RECOGNIZING CUES

This section presents information to use in caring for all older adults, as well as interventions specific to the young-old, the middle-old, the oldest-old, and the frail elderly.

Assessment/Recognizing Cues for All Older Adults

Recommend to older adults that they have an annual physical and dental examination. The *complete physical examination* should include the same categories as in middle adulthood (see Chapter 6), as well as *screening examinations* for mood, cognition, ability to perform activities of daily living (ADLs; e.g., bathing and dressing), and instrumental activities of daily living (IADLs; e.g., shopping, doing laundry). **Key Point: *Expect frequent changes to recommendations for screening examinations (e.g., for breast, cervical, and colon cancer).***

Table 7-1 identifies the areas for physical assessment related to the aging process. For a focused assessment for all older adults,

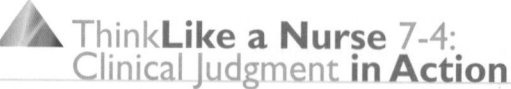 Go to **Focused Assessment Box, Assessment for All Older Adults,** in Volume 2.

▲ Think**Like a Nurse** 7-4:
Clinical Judgment **in Action**

To determine whether Mrs. Higginbotham's pneumonia is resolving (Meet Your Patient), you are monitoring her vital signs. Her oral temperature is 98.9°F (37.2°C). What do you need to keep in mind when evaluating the meaning of this reading? Do you think this represents a fever?

Assessing Cognitive Status

The U.S. Preventive Services Task Force (2014) recommends that although evidence on routine cognitive screening is insufficient, healthcare providers should

EXAMPLE CLIENT CONDITION: Elder Abuse

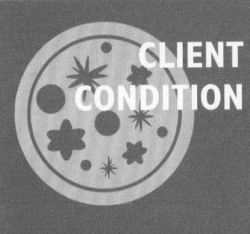

CLIENT CONDITION

Key Point: *Like domestic violence, elder abuse is seen in all cultures and socio-economic groups.*

Abuse Types

Abuse takes many forms:

Physical	Emotional
Sexual	Financial
Neglect	Abandonment

Risk Factors

Key Point: *The risk of abuse is higher for women and those with physical and cognitive vulnerabilities.*
Advanced age
Physical, functional, or cognitive impairment

Risk Factors

Mental illness
Alcoholism or drug abuse in patient or caregiver
Dependence on others
Past history of abusive relationships
Depression
Low self-esteem
Poor health of patient or caregiver
Caregiver stressed or frustrated with difficult caregiving tasks

Social Determinants of Health:

Ageism
Social isolation or poor social network
Low-income status
Financial or other family problems (of patient or caregiver)
Inadequate or unsafe housing
Lack of health insurance

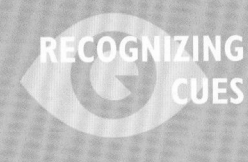

RECOGNIZING CUES

Key Point: *If an older adult has an injury such as maxillofacial trauma, dental trauma, subdural hematomas, periorbital and laryngeal trauma, rib fractures, or upper extremity injuries, along with a wasted and unkempt appearance, it is possible that the injury was inflicted.* Elder abuse takes many forms, including the following:

- Battering
- Inappropriate use of drugs and physical restraints
- Force-feeding, physical punishment
- Nonconsensual sexual contact
- Treating an older person like an infant, including infantilizing communication (also referred to as *elderspeak*)
- Giving an older person the "silent treatment"
- Enforced social isolation
- Demeaning an older adult
- Neglect
- Abandonment
- Financial or material exploitation, such as illegal or improper use of an older adult's funds, property, assets, or Social Security checks

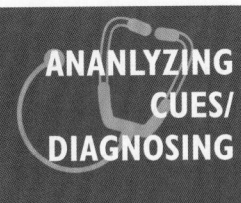

ANANLYZING CUES/ DIAGNOSING

- Assess older adults for abuse anytime there is a possibility that an injury may have been inflicted rather than accidental.
- Assess for social determinants, risk factors, and etiology of the abuse.
- For a screening tool and a procedure to aid you in assessing for abuse,

 Go to **Procedure 6-1** in Volume 2.

PRIORITIZING HYPOTHESES

- **Low Self-esteem** related to physical abuse and demeaning communication
- **Risk for Injury** related to physical or psychological abuse

(continued)

EXAMPLE CLIENT CONDITION: Elder Abuse—cont'd

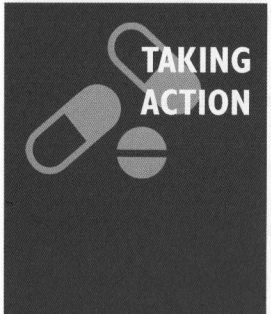

GENERATING SOLUTIONS

Key Point: *Prevention is key: listen, intervene, educate.*

Prevention Measures

- Screen for social determinants and risk factors associated with elder abuse.
- Observe for injuries indicative of elder abuse.
- Determine congruence of injury and the description of cause.
- Remove patient from dangerous situation.
- Notify appropriate authorities of suspected abuse.

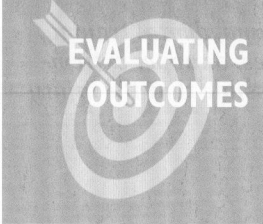

TAKING ACTION

Stop Elder Abuse: REPORT IT.

- *Suspicion of elder abuse must be reported* to adult protective services and/or the authority designated by law in each state to investigate and prosecute elder abuse.
- *Call the police or 9-1-1 immediately if someone you know is in immediate, life-threatening danger.*

Elder Abuse Resources

- The National Center on Elder Abuse (NCEA) **(https://ncea.acl.gov/)**
- Clearinghouse on Abuse and Neglect of the Elderly (CANE) **(https://www.nsvrc.org/organizations/133)**

EVALUATING OUTCOMES

- Remains safe and free from physical and/or psychological harm
- Maintains dignity
- Verbalizes positive self-worth

---

remain alert to early signs or symptoms of cognitive impairment (for example, problems with memory or language) and evaluate as appropriate. Assessing the mental status of older adults can help guide decisions about when it may be appropriate to screen for cognitive impairment in the primary care setting.

Also see the Example Client Condition: Dementia.

For a step-by-step procedure for a complete assessment of mental status,

 Go to **Procedure 19-16, Assessing the Sensory-Neurological System,** in Volume 2.

Assessing Functional Status

Functional status is the ability to perform self-care and other ADLs and IADLs.

- **Activities of Daily Living.** You can use the Katz Index of Independence in Activities of Daily Living to rate a client's independence in bathing, dressing, toileting, transferring, continence, and feeding (Katz et al., 1970; Katz Index, 2007). To use the Katz assessment tool,

 Go to **https://hign.org/consultgeri/try-this-series/katz-index-independence-activities-daily-living-adl**

- **Instrumental Activities of Daily Living. IADLs** are the activities needed to maintain one's immediate environment, for example, shopping, using the telephone, housekeeping, managing money, preparing food, and managing one's medications. Loss of ability to perform IADLs frequently marks a need for assisted living, nursing home placement, or the aid of family or homemaker services to allow an older adult to age in place.

Assessing for Depression

For more information about depression in older adults, see the box Example Client Condition: Depression in Chapter 10. To assess for depression, you may wish to use the Geriatric Depression Scale (GDS), a 30-item questionnaire that screens for depression. It is tailored to the concerns that older adults face. To learn more:

 Go the The Geriatric Depression Scale (GDS): **http://www.stanford.edu/~yesavage/GDS.html**

Assessment/Recognizing Cues (Young-Old)

Your assessments of young-old patients should also include the following:

- *Daily routines, social interactions, and short- and long-term goals:* This helps to identify cues about the degree to which the person has adapted to retirement.

- *Level of fitness and the level of effort for physical activity:* This and the following point are essential to identify cues needed to determine a program of routine exercise.
- *Chronic conditions:* The cues that indicate how a chronic condition affects the client's ability to do regular physical activities safely, and to what extent.
- *Barriers to exercise*
- *Client's self-confidence in their ability to maintain an exercise program*

Assessment/Recognizing Cues (Middle-Old)

It is critical for you to assess the function, support system, social network, and mental health of the middle-old client. ✚ Observe for cues that the client is entering a **spiral of vulnerability.** For example, a decrease in an older adult's mobility and the use of an assistive device such as a cane may be cues of prolonged inactivity associated with physiological changes. These may be associated with an unsteady or slow gait and slower response and reaction times—all resulting in deliberate, slow actions.

Thus begins a spiral of vulnerability: The older adult may become a victim of abuse, suffer a fall, or sustain an injury; the injury may require hospitalization, giving rise to the potential complications of infection and pressure ulcers and the need for rehabilitation. The impact of this spiral of vulnerability is felt in psychological and financial costs to the client and society, as well as loss of client independence. It is easier to intervene and stop the spiral if cues are found early (Fig. 7-3).

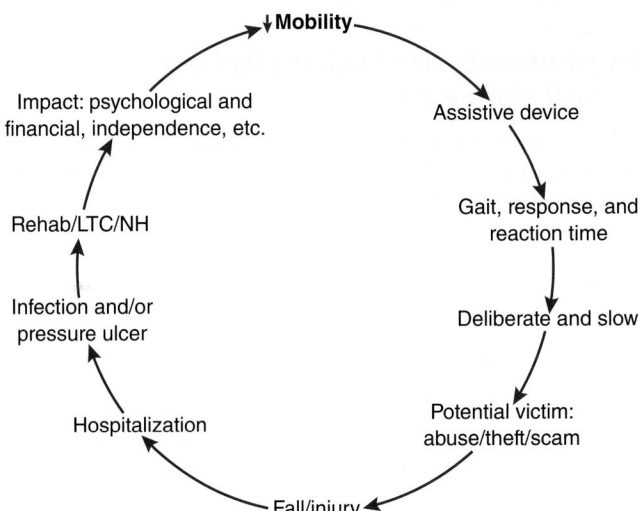

Assessment of the Middle-Old
Spiral of Vulnerability Example

FIGURE 7-3 A seemingly small event for a middle-old adult may trigger a spiral of vulnerability.

Assessment/Recognizing Cues (Oldest-Old)

The oldest-old need similar assessments as the middle-old. Keep in mind that assessment of physical, psychosocial, and cognitive abilities; social engagement; and living conditions are crucial for the oldest-old. Psychosocial and environmental factors may be the cues for frailty when subtle physiological changes are not obvious.

NURSING DIAGNOSIS/ANALYZING CUES (ALL OLDER ADULTS)

Frail Elderly Syndrome
Risk for Frail Elderly Syndrome
Nutrition Deficit: Less than Body Requirements
Risk for Impaired Growth and Development

An understanding of age-related changes can help older adults identify normal changes, adapt their routine, and report alterations in ADLs and IADLs that are outside the expected changes for their age. Many such changes signal conditions that are treatable. Consider these examples:

- *Frequent falls and loss of balance* are not the result of normal age-related changes but could signal neuropathology, such as Parkinson disease or early symptoms of dementia, and should be reported to a healthcare provider.
- *Urinary incontinence* is not the result of usual age-related changes. It may signal a urinary tract infection, a prostate problem, excessive urogenital drying, or the need for in-home assistance.

PLANNING/PRIORITIZING HYPOTHESIS AND GENERATING SOLUTIONS (ALL OLDER ADULTS)

Nursing goals for all older adults should be to maintain the person's ability to function independently for as long as possible, arrange for appropriate care, and teach clients and caregivers how and when to call for professional help.

IMPLEMENTATION/TAKING ACTION

As you already know, the actions you take depend on the nursing diagnoses that you identify for each individual. This section presents actions specific to each of the older-adult age-groups, as well as actions that apply to all older adults. Also refer to Example Client Conditions for Frail Elderly, Dementia, and Elder Abuse.

Implementation/Taking Action (Young-Old)

Young-old adults may need support for positive retirement, identifying and overcoming barriers to health promotion, evaluating methods for introducing health promotion for positive long-term change, and describing short- and long-term benefits of health promotion (Baxter et al., 2016). Providing resources for social and civic engagement will help a new retiree reestablish a satisfying and rewarding retirement.

Physical Activity It is also important to teach and help the client plan for physical exercise. A sedentary lifestyle increases the risk of aging-related diseases and premature death. DNA changes occur partly because of stress and oxidative damage to cells. By reducing stress, exercise may slow some of these oxidative changes and, thereby, the aging process (Amer & Rasheedy, 2018). More research is needed in this area.

The Centers for Disease Control and Prevention (2021b) recommends the following activities for older adults:

- **Regular aerobic physical activity**. Engage in 150 minutes a week of moderate-intensity aerobic exercise. Alternatively, engage in 75 minutes a week of vigorous-intensity activity. Each episode of activity should last for at least 10 minutes, and the client should spread the exercise throughout the week. Additional benefits can be obtained by gradually increasing the amount of exercise (perhaps up to 300 minutes a week).
- **Muscle-strengthening activities.** Perform moderate- or high-intensity muscle-strengthening activities on 2 or more days a week. The weight-bearing and toning exercises should involve all major muscle groups.
- **Balance-promoting activities.** These are especially important for older adults at risk for falls.
- **Adapted physical activities.** Older adults with chronic conditions should be as physically active as abilities and conditions allow. (The nurse should help them to make adaptations that allow them to do so, or refer them to an exercise therapist.)

Key Point: *Some activity is better than none, and more is even better.* Remind clients that doing some activity at least 3 days a week produces health benefits and helps avoid excessive fatigue. Some practical suggestions for exercising include the following:

- **A brisk 15-minute walk twice a day,** every day of the week, would easily meet the minimum guidelines for aerobic activity.
- **Muscle-strengthening activities** at least 2 days a week can include the use of exercise bands, handheld weights, digging, lifting, and carrying as part of gardening, carrying groceries, and some yoga and tai chi exercises.
- **Inactive older adults or those with a very low level of fitness** should begin with 10 minutes of walking and increase minutes and intensity slowly with subsequent walks.

You can provide support for the client's exercise regimen by suggesting a range of choices and a list of community resources (e.g., parks, organizations, recreation centers). Also, teach the client how to walk, as

needed, and safety considerations. Help the young-old adult institute self-monitoring methods to help them see their progress (e.g., a graph, a chart, a step counter), and reinforce personal progress, such as weight loss and decreased fatigue.

Implementation/Taking Action (Middle-Old)

Older adults who have maintained healthy behaviors throughout their lifetime are likely to remain vital and actively engaged. However, the occurrence of a health crisis and even a short period of restrictive activity will lead to decreased functional ability and the need for encouragement, support, and a planned program of limited activity progressing to optimal function for clients in this age-group.

Implementation/Taking Action (Oldest-Old)

The goal of interventions for the oldest-old is to ensure independence for as long as possible by maximizing function and preventing disability or loss of function. Broad interventions important for the oldest-old include the following:

- **Supportive environments** and conditions allow a person to function.
- **Modified adapted activity** is especially important for this age-group and may include walking, flexibility exercises, yoga, tai chi, and water aerobics.
- **Nutrition** is an important focus, as well. Whole grains, dark green and orange vegetables and legumes, all types of fruits and vegetables, and fat-free and low-fat dairy products are among the food groups most needing inclusion in this age-group to combat obesity and inactivity.

For interventions for the frail elderly, see the Example Client Condition: Frail Elderly.

Implementation/Taking Action for All Older Adults

♥ **iCare** For all interventions and interactions, always ask yourself, "Does this promote the client's dignity and self-esteem?"

Promoting Independence and Maintaining Functional Ability

Key Point: *The overall goals of nursing care of older adults are to maximize independent activity and enhance function.* Often this will involve helping clients to adapt and develop new skills so that they can continue to take part in the activities they enjoy.

- **Focus on preserving the patient's functional abilities,** including both the ability and motivation to function in their environment. Consider any environmental

Physical Activity and Well-Being of Older Adults

PICOT

Situation

While caring for patients in the rehab unit, the nurse notes that there is a wide range of health among older adult clients and that not all 75-year-old clients heal at the same rate.

PICOT Components

P	Population/patient	=	Older adults
I	Intervention/indicator	=	Regular exercise and physical activity
C	Comparator/control	=	No regular exercise, sedentary
O	Outcome	=	Improved well-being into aging
T	Time	=	None

Searchable Question

Do _____ (P) who receive/are exposed to _____ (I) demonstrate _____ (O) compared with _____ (C) _____ (T)?

Example of Evidence

Advances in healthcare have increased the life span as well as the quality of life for many people. Physical fitness as a younger adult may improve physical and emotional well-being later in life. One of the specific goals of *Healthy People 2030* is to increase physical activity, with the expectation that it will slow the decline in physical functioning associated with age. This should help to improve the quality of life in later adulthood, promote faster recovery time, and therefore help decrease the dollars spent each year on medical care.

Practice Change

The nurse emphasizes to all their patients the importance of regular exercise and helps them think of ways they might incorporate more activity into their present routines. They also discuss with the unit manager the possibility of incorporating this nursing action into unit routines.

Reference: O'Brien, E. L., Hess, T. M., Kornadt, A. E., Rothermund, K., Fung, H., & Voss, P. (2017). Context influences on the subjective experience of aging: The impact of culture and domains of functioning. *The Gerontologist, 57*(Suppl. 2), S127–S137. https://doi.org/10.1093/geront/gnx015

modifications that might aid independence, including assistive technology.

- **Electronic technology is increasingly being used to deliver care "remotely"** and support older adults in their own homes. Telehealth technologies include electronic reminder systems, videoconference visiting, and remotely controlled security sensors and have been found to be effective in improving self-care skills, self-monitoring behaviors, and clinical outcomes among older adults with chronic condition(s) (Greenwald et al., 2018; Guo & Albright, 2017).
- **Look for simple things you can do to promote better functioning.** For example, if the patient cannot see to sort their medications, you might try turning on more lights or having a brighter light installed.
- **Facilitate and encourage physical exercise** in order to help improve continence and help prevent further loss of mobility. Exercise also improves strength, balance, and endurance and aids in fall prevention. Older adults who engage in progressive aerobic training can maintain their independence longer, improve health, and reduce morbidity (Amireault et al., 2019).
- **Facilitate empowerment.** Many older adults are Internet savvy. You can empower them by suggesting Web sites that offer resources to help them understand and cope with the unknowns of their situation.

Promoting Cognitive Function

The National Institute for Health and Care Excellence (2018) identified a link between improving cognitive symptoms and the ability to maintain day-to-day functioning for interventions to promote cognitive function; refer to the box Example Client Condition: Dementia.

Teaching for Safety

Teach older adults about age-related changes and what these changes mean for their daily routine. For example, age-related changes diminish stamina, conditioning, reflexes, and the speed of processing information. Therefore, when multitasking and performing seemingly nonthinking physical activities, older adults need to be very purposeful in their actions and pay attention to the details of the task or activity. Failing to do so could result in missteps, injury, or exhaustion.

Illness Prevention

Although the risks of disease and disability increase with age, poor health need not always occur. Known prevention measures can help older adults avoid many illnesses and disabilities associated with chronic diseases.

- **Healthy lifestyle.** Stress the importance of a healthy lifestyle (e.g., healthy eating; regular physical activity; avoiding tobacco use; and screening for breast, cervical, and colorectal cancers).
- **Immunizations.** Health-promotion activities include teaching and facilitating immunizations for varicella, influenza, pneumonia, herpes zoster (shingles), and

tetanus/diphtheria/pertussis. To see the Recommended Adult Immunization Schedule,

 Go to Recommended Adult Immunization Schedule, United States, 2022, at **https://www.cdc.gov/vaccines/schedules/hcp/imz/adult.html**

Communicating With Older Adults

Many normal changes of aging affect communication. For example, older adults tend to process information more slowly, so speak slowly and allow time for the patient to form an answer. See the iCare box regarding personhood and dignity, in addition to the following:

- *Check for sensory deficits at the beginning of your interaction.* Until you know there is no hearing deficit, look at the patient as you speak to allow for lip reading. But do not assume that all older adults are deaf or that they do not understand the meaning of your communication.
- *You will need to rely on body language more than usual.* Notice nonverbal communication, such as fidgeting, hand-wringing, tearfulness, or quivering lips. Memory deficits make it difficult for some older adults to find the words to express what they mean.
- *Appropriate speech may be accompanied by inappropriate affect.* For instance, a client may speak coherently and make sense while telling you that they were able to walk to the bathroom today, then begin crying for no apparent reason. Nevertheless, the information about their ambulation may be credible.
- *Conversely, inappropriate affect and incoherent speech do not always indicate a lack of understanding.* For example, a client may laugh appropriately at something funny but not be able to speak clearly or find the words to ask you what time it is.
- *Be aware that some older adults are confused at one time and not another.* A client may begin by giving

you credible information, but as the conversation progresses, they may lose track of the topic or talk about something irrelevant. When a client seems confused, use focused assessment to determine their mental status. If you conclude that their ability to communicate is unreliable, you can always finish the talk later, when they are less confused.

- **Key Point:** *The ability to speak does not always reflect the person's ability to understand, and what the patient says may or may not match what they are feeling.*

Communicating With Persons With Cognitive Deficits

In addition to the normal changes of aging, many older adults have more severe problems with memory and at least one other cognitive ability (e.g., judgment, thinking, language, or coordination). Because of their decline in mental abilities, people with dementia have difficulty speaking and understanding. In addition to the general approaches for all older adults, the following are some ideas to help you communicate with people with cognitive deficits:

- *Use simple, short sentences with one idea at a time.* Ask, "Where does it hurt?" rather than, "Please describe the quality and location of your pain."
- *Avoid vague comments* (e.g., "I see," "Um-hmm," "Yes, yes, okay"). The patient will not be able to interpret these responses. Instead, echo the patient's comment and state your response directly and simply: "You are hungry. I will bring your lunch."
- *Repeat your words exactly if the patient doesn't understand what you say.* Under other circumstances, you usually rephrase your sentences when someone doesn't understand, but for patients with dementia, giving new information just adds to their confusion.

♥ iCare 7-1

Caring Is Respecting Personhood and Dignity

There are several ways you can demonstrate caring in patient interactions:

- *Never call a person "sweetie" or "honey" or "dear."* This sends a message that you think the person is not your equal.
- *Ask,* "What is your name?" *and* "How would you like to be addressed?"
- *Provide eyeglasses,* hearing aids, and dentures before engaging in conversation.
- *Get to know the patient as a person.* (What work did they do? What are their likes/dislikes?)
- *Encourage storytelling* and reminiscing.
- *Pull up a chair and sit down* to speak with the person at eye level.
- *Be present.* Do not check your phone or take notes while conversing. Focus on what the person is saying.
- *Try to respond to the person's feelings* instead of the content of their words. This helps to reassure them. For example,

if a patient is constantly searching for their husband, don't say, "Your husband is not here." Instead, say, "You must miss your husband," or "Tell me about your husband."
- *Approach unhurriedly;* do not rush an older adult, and do not speak too rapidly.
- *Allow the patient time to speak* and express their concerns.
- *If the person has difficulty finding the right word,* supply it unless doing so upsets the person. This helps control frustration levels.
- *If you do not understand what the patient is trying to say,* ask them to point to it or describe it (e.g., "What does [the unknown entity] look like?").
- *Avoid providing care standing up,* and especially with your back to the person.
- *Provide privacy* during bath time or when in the bathroom.
- *Gently hold or pat the person's hand,* offering comfort and reassurance.

- *Try to understand that the patient's reality is distorted* and they are behaving in the only way they are able. When the patient is conversing superficially and seems comfortable, it may seem they are competent.

Providing Caregiver Support

A diagnosis of dementia or a debilitating physical condition can be traumatic and devastating. Family members are often the primary caregivers (either through choice or necessity). Caregivers of any patient are more likely than noncaregivers to be at risk for depression, heart disease, high blood pressure, and other chronic illnesses, even death. Caring for a person with dementia puts them at even higher risk.

Most caregivers of those suffering from dementia are also older adults who themselves have special needs. It is not uncommon for the caregiver to feel abandoned and unsupported, not only by services but also by family and friends. Exhaustion and despair can quickly follow.

♥ **iCare** Supportive interventions such as the following can contribute to physical and psychological well-being, help maintain hope, and reduce caregiver burden (Chiao et al., 2015):

- Education about dementia
- Supportive counseling
- Psychotherapy
- Rapid support in a crisis
- Support from other caregivers (respite)
- Faith-based spiritual assistance

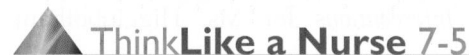

ThinkLike a Nurse 7-5

What factors contribute to a community of functionally active older adults?

PUTTING IT ALL TOGETHER

Recall Ethel Higginbotham from the Meet Your Patient scenario. She is very thin and frail and refuses to eat. She says, "I just want to die." Do you feel ready to plan her nursing care now?

- You might *diagnose* Ms. Higginbotham with Frail Elderly Syndrome.
- An appropriate *NOC outcome* would be Will to Live.
- An *individualized goal* might be "Ms. Higginbotham will gain 1 pound and participate in at least one daily group activity by the first of next month." Interventions depend on the diagnosis and its etiology.

Ms. Higginbotham will need care that helps her adjust to widowhood, provides adequate nutrition, and offers activities that provide interaction with others.

- *NIC interventions* appropriate for Ms. Higginbotham are as follows:
    Coping Enhancement
    Hope Inspiration
    Self-Care Assistance
    Spiritual Support

Toward Evidence-Based Practice

Thomas, K. S., Parikh, R. B., Zullo, A. R., & Dosa, D. (2018). Home-delivered meals and risk of self-reported falls: Results from a randomized trial. *Journal of Applied Gerontology, 37*(1), 41–57. https://doi.org/10.1177/0733464816675421

This study evaluated whether home-delivered meals and the frequency of delivery reduced self-reported falls among homebound older adults. Three hundred seventy-one older adults on Meals on Wheels programs' waiting lists were randomized to receive (a) daily meal delivery; (b) once-weekly frozen meal delivery; or (c) control, remain on the waiting list for meals. At follow-up, 33 (23.7%) of those in the group receiving daily delivered meals, 29 (27.4%) of those in the group receiving once-weekly delivered meals, and 36 (28.6%) of those in the control group reported a fall. The research suggests that daily delivered meals may reduce the risk of falls.

Li, F., Harmer, P., Voit, J., & Chou, L. S. (2021). Implementing an online virtual falls prevention intervention during a public health pandemic for older adults with mild cognitive impairment: A feasibility trial. *Clinical Interventions in Aging, 16*, 973.

Community-dwelling older adults with mild cognitive impairment (MCI) were randomly assigned to either an intervention group (*n* = 15) or a control group (*n* = 15). The intervention group participated in Tai Ji Quan exercise with a trained instructor, and the control group participated in stretching with a trained instructor. Each group included 60-minute virtual exercise sessions, via Zoom, twice weekly for 24 weeks (total of 48 sessions).

Compared with the control group (stretching exercise), the intervention (Tai Ji Quan exercise) did not reduce falls or the number of fallers by the end of the study. The Tai Ji Quan group, however, performed consistently better than the stretching group in balance, 30-second chair stands, and Timed Up and Go and dual-task conditions (participant was asked to walk while performing an arithmetic task).

1. Based on the articles, what suggestions might you make to an older adult living at home or their caregiver to prevent falls?

2. Based on your reading, what other health-promotion activities can you recommend to help older adults remain safe at home?

- *Individualized interventions* for Ms. Higginbotham include:
    Grief counseling
    Nutritional support
    Working with her and her family to determine whether it is appropriate for her to continue to live independently

As a full-spectrum nurse, you should assess the developmental stage of each of your clients. In maternity and pediatric care, this is a routine part of nursing care. However, growth and development continue to be important throughout the life span. To assess growth and development, you must gather data such as the client's age, height, and weight; activities the client engages in; and the client's communication skills. You should also perform age-specific assessments, such as those discussed in previous sections.

To explore learning resources for this chapter,

Go to Davis Advantage **and find:**

Answers and Suggested Responses for all questions in this chapter

Concept Map

Knowledge Map

References and Bibliography

CHAPTER 8

Promoting Wellness: Health & Illness

Learning Outcomes

After completing this chapter, you should be able to:

➤ Explore the concepts of wellness, health, and illness from a holistic perspective.

➤ Define *health, health promotion,* and *health protection.*

➤ Identify health-protection activities and categorize them as primary, secondary, or tertiary levels of prevention.

➤ Compare and contrast models of wellness, health, and illness.

➤ Describe the various ways that people experience health and illness.

➤ Identify social determinants that disrupt health.

➤ Describe the five stages of illness behavior.

➤ Differentiate between acute and chronic illness.

➤ Apply Pender's Health Promotion Model to plan activities designed to change unhealthy behavior.

➤ Identify Prochaska and DiClemente's four stages of change.

➤ Identify factors that influence individuals' responses to illness.

➤ Discuss the *Healthy People 2030* report in relation to the leading causes of death and health-promotion strategies: nutrition, exercise, lifestyle, and environment.

➤ Identify specific health-promotion strategies (including immunizations and screenings) across the life span.

➤ Discuss nurses' roles in health promotion, and list health-promotion activities that a nurse may conduct in acute care facilities, the workplace, local communities, and schools.

Key Concepts

Health
Health experience
Health promotion
Health protection
Illness
Illness experience
Illness prevention
Wellness

Related Concepts

See the Concept Map on Davis Advantage.

Meet Your Patient

Evelyn is 87 years old and has lived in a long-term care facility for the last 5 years. She suffers from congestive heart failure, hypertension, diabetes, macular degeneration resulting in near blindness, a severe hearing deficit, urinary incontinence, and immobility resulting from a hip fracture.

Evelyn was married nearly 60 years to Lloyd, who died 6 years ago. Evelyn has 5 children, 17 grandchildren, and 14 great-grandchildren. In these last few years, she has experienced the loss of her husband, home, vision, hearing, mobility, and bladder control. Despite these limitations, she keeps current on the lives of all of her extended family and friends.

She is the confidante of the facility staff and knows about their children and their romances and the gossip around the institution. She is an avid Minnesota Twins fan and also keeps track of the televised high school basketball tournaments. Whenever there is an election, she makes sure that she votes. She

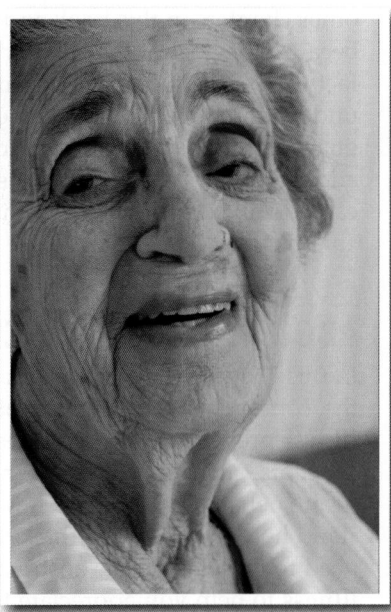

(Continued)

Meet Your Patient (continued)

"reads" every audiobook she can get her hands on. Recently, Evelyn was admitted to the hospital in severe congestive heart failure. She told her pastor, "I don't want to die yet. I'm having too much fun!"

Evelyn's situation is a far cry from what most people would picture as good health. However, as you consider the ideas of health and wellness presented in this chapter, you might conclude that in many ways, she is experiencing wellness and is a reasonably healthy person.

TheoreticalKnowledge
knowingwhy

Every day, there is something in the news about well-ness, health, or illness. Politicians talk about their desire to improve our health and reorganize healthcare. Schools want students to eat healthy foods, exercise, and receive regular immunizations. In an attempt to reduce health insurance claims, employers open on-site fitness centers and employ nurses and counselors to work with employees to focus on wellness. Everyone says they want to be healthy.

As a nursing student, you have probably already cared for clients in various stages of wellness, health, and illness. But have you ever considered what those terms mean? Our understanding of wellness, health, and illness is influenced by our family, culture, health history, and a host of other factors. As you evolve as a nurse, you'll find that your understanding of these concepts evolves, too. We will examine some ways that you and your clients might define *wellness, health,* and *illness* and some ways that full-spectrum nurses have come to understand these terms through their thinking, doing, and caring.

You may find this chapter a little different from other chapters in this book and other textbooks. That is because the goal of the chapter is not to help you learn facts about wellness, health, and illness but for you to understand how people experience them. Even the language of the chapter is designed for that purpose. Relax and flow with the chapter. Instead of agonizing over each detail, read it in a way that will help you see the "big picture."

ABOUT THE KEY CONCEPTS

In this chapter, the emphasis is on strategies to support the concepts of **health promotion, health protection, illness prevention,** and **wellness.** As you study various concepts, such as health screening, role modeling, and health behaviors (to name a few examples), try to under-stand how they relate to the key concepts. You will also need to understand the abstract concepts of **health** and **illness** to help you appreciate the **experience of health and illness** as lived by real, not abstract, people. Strive for an overview of factors that are disruptive to health and factors that nourish health. Understand the subcon-cepts of **hardiness** as it relates to patients and **healing presence** as it relates to your work as a nurse.

HOW DO WE UNDERSTAND WELLNESS, HEALTH, AND ILLNESS?

First let's examine the key concepts of *health* and *wellness.* We will use the following definitions to synthesize a meaning.

World Health Organization The World Health Organization (WHO, 1948) defines health as "a state of complete physical, mental and social well-being and not merely the absence of disease or infirmity." At the first conference for health promotion, the WHO defined **health promotion** as the process of equipping people to have control over and improve their physical, emo-tional, and social health (WHO, 1986).

Jean Watson This nursing theorist proposed that health consists of three elements: (1) a high level of over-all physical, mental, and social functioning; (2) a general adaptive-maintenance level of daily functioning; and (3) the absence of illness (or the presence of efforts that lead to its absence). She also refers to health as being a state of mind, the perception of the individual. Individ-uals may have a terminal illness and yet consider them-selves healthy (Watson, 1979).

Betty Neuman This nursing theorist describes health as an expression of living energy available to an individual. The energy is displayed as a continuum, with high energy (wellness) at one end and low energy (illness) at the opposite end. Individuals have varying levels of energy at various stages of life. When more energy is generated than expended, there is wellness. When more energy is expended than is generated, there is illness, possibly death (Neuman, 1995).

Myers, Sweeney, and Witmer In 2000, these the-orists defined *wellness* as "a way of life oriented toward optimal health and well-being in which body, mind, and spirit are integrated by the individual to live more fully within the human and natural community" (p. 252). This definition includes lifestyles and habits as components of health and permits people who have been diagnosed with disease to be considered healthy.

Synthesis Applying aspects of these definitions of wellness, health, and **health promotion** means finding ways to help individuals develop a state of physical, spiritual, and mental well-being. Health-promotion activities are useful to all individuals, whether well or sick, because they encourage optimal function. How does this compare with the WHO definition of health promotion you read earlier?

What is your image of health? Here are some ideas.

- **The "body beautiful."** Being a "picture of health" can depend on whether you were born in the right era—or in the right country. Styles of beautiful bodies come and go. For instance, much Indian, African, Greek, and European art portrays ideal women as well-rounded creatures. The perfect-body view of health also denies the possibility of health to people who use wheelchairs, prosthetics, or even eyeglasses and hearing aids. Yet many full-spectrum nurses working with disabled clients would indeed describe their clients as healthy.
- **Not having illness.** In describing healthy people, would you disqualify someone with a cold, dandruff, or athlete's foot? What about diabetes, heart disease, or cancer? Doing so would reflect another view of health—that is, not having illness. This view may be unfair because it restricts health to those who do not have some kind of physical impairment.
- **Something you can buy.** Another popular view is that health is something you can buy: exercise equipment, membership in a health club, medicine, liposuction, a coronary artery bypass, and so on. In this view, health does not come from within. It's something "out there" that is available if you have enough money or insurance.
- **Ideal physical and mental well-being.** Health can also be described as an ideal state of physical and mental well-being: something to strive for but never to attain. Good health is never actually reached because there is always something more to be achieved. Health is the goal itself, the end instead of one of the means to fulfilling life's purposes.

The Ability of the Soul to Cope Theologian Jürgen Moltmann (1983) described health in a different way: "True health is the strength to live, the strength to suffer, and the strength to die. Health is not a condition of my body; it is the power of my soul to cope with the varying condition of that body" (p. 142). Similarly, author Robert Louis Stevenson (1878) wrote of health, "It is not a matter of holding good cards, it's playing a poor hand well."

Nurses Understand Wellness, Health, and Illness as Individual Experiences

If you were the nurse caring for Evelyn (Meet Your Patient), would you understand health as a perfect body or the absence of disease? Probably not. **Key Point:** *Nurses*

understand wellness, health, and illness as individual experiences, emerging from each patient's unique responses. The person with an illness rarely perceives the experience as a medical diagnosis. Instead, people describe their illness in terms of how it makes them feel.

Think back to the last time you were ill. How did you feel? Did you feel pain, sadness, fatigue, loss? Did you feel overwhelmed? These responses are **disruptions** to health and, as such, constitute the lived experience of illness. **Lived experience** is unique to each patient: Just as Evelyn might describe herself as "raring to go," another patient who is 10 years younger and on half as many medications may describe themselves as "exhausted all the time" and "just waiting to die." In short, nurses honor the client's understanding of their state of being.

For many years nurses have recognized that, like Evelyn, some clients strive to maintain a state of optimal health even when coping with chronic or even terminal disease. Many experience this state as wellness: "a way of life oriented toward optimal health and well-being in which body, mind, and spirit are integrated by the individual to live more fully within the human and natural community" (Myers et al., 2000, p. 252). This perspective acknowledges the influence of attitude and lifestyle choices on the client's state of being. It also implies that nursing interventions in support of wellness are important for clients who are illness-free but also for those who are experiencing disease or even facing death.

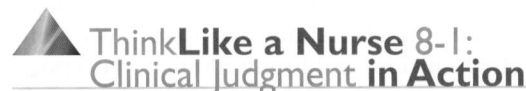
ThinkLike a Nurse 8-1: Clinical Judgment in Action

What qualities are essential to your own personal definition of *health*? How do you define *illness*?

KnowledgeCheck 8-1

- Provide at least two common definitions of *health*.
- Explain how full-spectrum nurses define *health* and *illness*.
- Define *wellness* in your own words.

Nurses Use Conceptual Models to Understand Health and Illness

You can use a variety of models to understand health and illness. Each emphasizes somewhat different aspects of these experiences. Nurses have found the following models particularly useful.

The Health–Illness Continuum

Most of us recognize that our health status changes frequently. For example, "Although today I feel pretty good and yesterday I was exhausted, I believe I was healthy on both of those days. I know that my exhaustion was related to staying up late, enjoying the company of good friends. My medical record states that I have diabetes and hypertension, but I keep both diseases in control. I take multiple medications, read food labels, exercise aerobically 5 days a week, and lift weights 3 days a week. Am I healthy, ill, or a health nut?"

The preceding example illustrates the complex and dynamic nature of human health. In an effort to describe this complex state, many theorists speak of a **health–illness continuum;** that is, they see health and illness as a graduated spectrum that cannot be divided—except arbitrarily—into parts. A person's position moves back and forth on the continuum with physiological changes, lifestyle choices, and the results of various therapies. As shown in Figure 8-1, the number 1 represents a state of being gravely ill, and 10 represents excellent health, or a person in peak form. Notice, however, that a client such as Evelyn (Meet Your Patient) may view herself as being at various points on this continuum according to how she feels on any particular day. In other words, the continuum is personal and dynamic. Health changes over the course of time.

Dunn's Health Grid

Dunn (1959) created a health grid that plots a person's status on the health–illness continuum against environmental conditions (Fig. 8-2). Many nurses use this grid to help them predict the likelihood that a client will experience a change in health status. For example, Evelyn (Meet Your Patient) has several health problems. On a scale of 1 to 10, an observer who does not know Evelyn well might rate her health as a 3. However, Evelyn has a positive outlook and tells her pastor, "I don't want to die yet. I'm having too much fun!" She also has excellent support from her friends, family, and the facility staff. Clearly, Evelyn is in a favorable environment. This positive setting protects her from harm and provides a good quality of life. On Dunn's grid, Evelyn would probably fall in the area of "protected poor health."

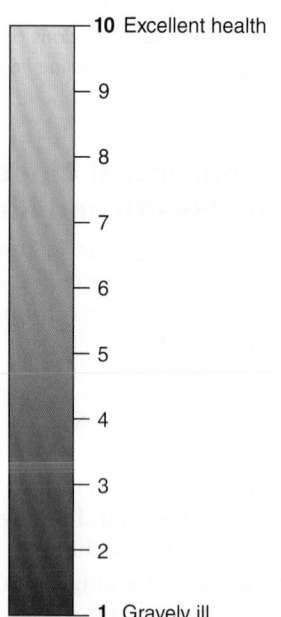

FIGURE 8-1 Over a lifetime, an individual moves up and down on the health–illness continuum.

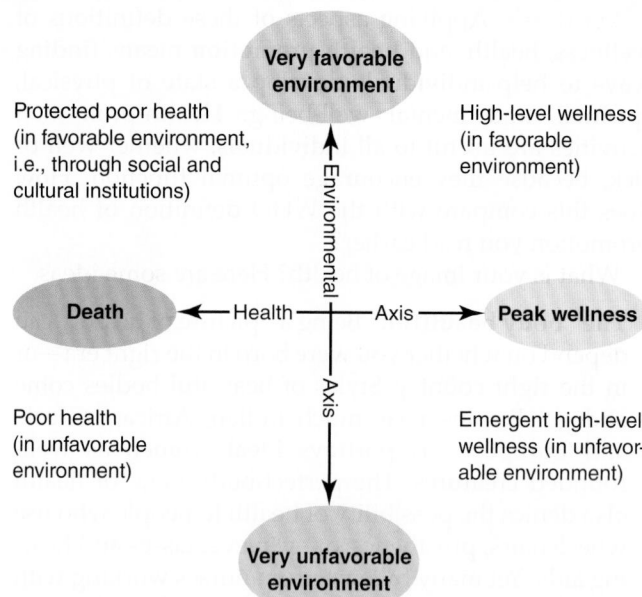

FIGURE 8-2 Dunn's health grid: Health is affected by an individual's status on the health–illness continuum as well as environmental conditions.

Neuman's Continuum

Nursing theorist Betty Neuman (2002) views health as an expression of living energy available to an individual. The energy is displayed as a continuum, with high energy (wellness) at one end and low energy (illness) at the opposite end (Fig. 8-3). The person is said to have varying levels of energy at various stages of life. When more energy is generated than is expended, there is wellness. When more energy is expended than is generated, there is illness—possibly death. Although Evelyn (Meet Your Patient) has several clearly identified health problems, she is engaged in life and active with her family, friends, and long-term care facility staff. We might not all agree on where to place her on Neuman's continuum, but certainly her activity and energy counterbalance her physical frailty.

What Are Social Determinants of Health?

Healthy behaviors start in our homes, schools, workplaces, neighborhoods, and communities. Activities like following a nutritious diet and getting regular physical activity, not smoking or drinking an excessive amount of alcohol, getting the recommended immunizations and screening tests, and seeking healthcare when needed all influence health and illness. Although access to healthcare is important, health is also driven by many other factors, such as safety within workplaces and communities and access to clean water, healthy food, quality education, and reliable transportation (National Academies of Sciences, Engineering, and Medicine [NASEM], 2019a).

General living conditions and lifestyle partly explain why some people are healthier than others and why

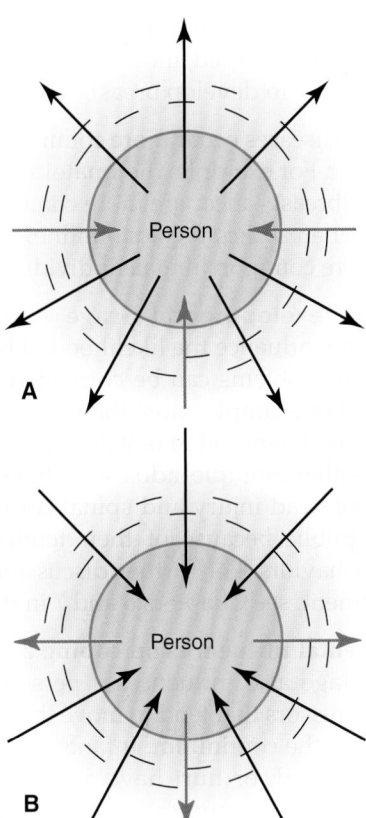

FIGURE 8-3 Neuman's continuum: A balance of input and output. *A*, When energy output exceeds input, illness results. *B*, Wellness occurs when more energy is generated than is expended.

Social Determinants of Health

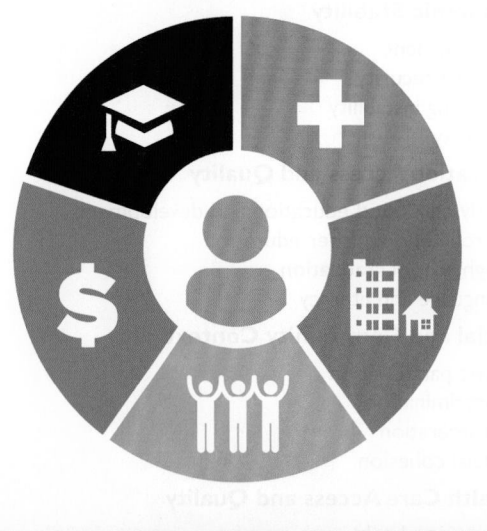

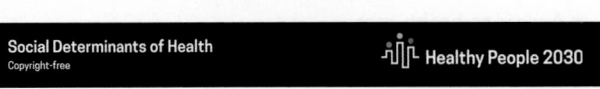

FIGURE 8-4 Social Determinants of Health. (*Source*: U.S. Department of Health and Human Services, Office of Disease Prevention and Health Promotion. [n.d.]. *Healthy People 2030*. https://health.gov/healthypeople/objectives-and-data/social-determinants-health)

many are not as healthy as they could be. For a variety of reasons, low-income individuals, people of color (POC), and residents of rural areas in the United States experience a greater burden of disease and lower life expectancy (NASEM, 2019b), and this gap continues to widen (Escarce, 2019). For more information about life expectancy, please refer to Chapter 7.

All people deserve an equal opportunity to make the choices that lead to good health (*Healthy People 2030*). **Social determinants of health (SDOH)** are "the conditions in the environments where people are born, live, learn, work, play, worship, and age that affect a wide range of health, functioning, and quality-of-life outcomes and risks" (*Healthy People 2030*; Fig. 8-4).

SDOH can be protective of good health. Those who live in neighborhoods with safe, walkable parks and clean air are likely to take advantage of opportunities to be physically active outdoors. However, many people live in environments with overcrowding; excessive noise; poor air and water quality; radiation in the workplace; racism, discrimination, and violence; and low language and literacy—all of which have a profound effect on health and well-being (Hood, 2005).

One goal of *Healthy People 2030* is to improve access to fresh produce and nutritious food. **Food insecurity** is the physical feeling of hunger and anxiety about access to food. **Food deserts** are areas in which the

population resides more than 1 mile from a supermarket or large grocery store (≥10 miles in rural populations; U.S. Department of Agriculture [USDA], 2021). Proximity to grocery stores may be a determinant of body mass index, and better access to fresh food is associated with a reduced risk for obesity and diabetes (American Public Health Association, 2015; Seligman, n.d.).

The U.S. Department of Health and Human Services defines SDOH in five areas: economic stability, education, social and community context, health and health care, and neighborhood and built environment (*Healthy People 2030*; Box 8-1).

As you will see, many of these factors are interrelated.

Health Equity Health equity is having access to resources that everyone else has access to so that people can live a healthy life. Resources include transportation to get to a provider office, access to therapies and supportive equipment after being ill, and having insurance that will pay enough so that people don't have to decide between buying medication or purchasing food. In the absence of health equity, we have health disparities.

Health Disparities Health disparities are systematic health differences that negatively affect certain groups of people. The differences among groups vary, and this leads to unfair and preventable differences in health outcomes relative to care, treatment, suffering, and longevity. Differences can be based on racial or ethnic group, religion, socioeconomic status, gender, mental health, cognitive or physical disability, or other characteristics that are historically linked to discrimination or exclusion.

Social Determinants of Health 8-1

Economic Stability

- Employment
- Food insecurity
- Housing instability
- Poverty

Education Access and Quality

- Early childhood education and development
- Enrollment in higher education
- High school graduation
- Language and literacy

Social and Community Context

- Civic participation
- Discrimination
- Incarceration
- Social cohesion

Health Care Access and Quality

- Access to health care
- Access to primary care
- Health literacy

Neighborhood and Built Environment

- Access to foods that support healthy eating patterns
- Crime and violence
- Environmental conditions
- Quality of housing

Source: U.S. Department of Health and Human Services, Office of Disease Prevention and Health Promotion. n.d. *Healthy People 2030*, https://health.gov/healthypeople/objectives-and-data/social-determinants-health

HOW DO PEOPLE EXPERIENCE WELLNESS, HEALTH, AND ILLNESS?

In envisioning health and illness as a continuum, full-spectrum nurses promote wellness regardless of the circumstances a client faces now or in the future. This approach requires the holistic understanding that health is multidimensional. The following are some of the many dimensions of health that we experience along the health–illness continuum. An understanding of these dimensions should broaden your concept of health.

Biological Factors

Although biological factors are not entirely within our control, most people consider them when they describe themselves as "well" or "ill." A healthy genetic makeup and freedom from debilitating age-related changes are certainly desired states, and along with gender, they tip the scale toward the wellness end of the health–illness continuum.

Genetic Makeup For example, the risk of breast cancer increases dramatically in women who have a family history of a mother, sister, or daughter with breast cancer. A genetic marker for this type of breast cancer has been discovered, indicating that some people inherit a tendency to develop breast cancer.

Sex Many diseases occur more commonly in one sex than in another. For example, rheumatoid arthritis, osteoporosis, and breast cancer are more common in female individuals, whereas ulcers, color blindness, and bladder cancer are more common in male individuals.

Age and Developmental Stage Age and developmental stage influence the likelihood of becoming ill. Certain health problems can be correlated to developmental stage. For example, more than 75% of new breast cancer cases are diagnosed in female patients older than age 50. As another example, adolescent boys have much higher rates of head injury and spinal cord injury than the general public because of their tendency toward risk-taking behaviors. For further discussion of growth and development, see Chapters 6 and 7 in this book.

- **Developmental influences on coping ability.** Developmental stage also influences a person's ability to cope with stressors that tend to move them toward the illness end of the continuum. Infants or children who are ill, frightened, or hurt have a limited repertoire of experiences, communication ability, and understanding to help them in their responses. As we progress through the stages of development, we develop understanding and skills to help us deal with illness.
- **Developmental influences on perceptions.** When disease, loss, or other disruptions occur at a younger age than expected, they change our perception of the event and may present a greater challenge to our coping skills than disruptions that are expected. For example, a child's death may seem more tragic than that of an older adult. It is important, though, not to discount the impact of disruptions that occur during the period of a person's life when they might be expected.

 For example, the death of a spouse is no less traumatic for an older adult than it would be for a young spouse. Losing someone with whom one has spent most of one's life is an incredible loss, whether or not it is "expected" at that stage of life.

Nutrition

Health requires nourishment, and the most obvious form of nourishment is food. The influence of diet on human health is undeniable: nutrient-deficiency diseases, such as scurvy and night blindness, are unknown in people who consume a nutritious diet. In addition, many chronic diseases, such as type 2 diabetes mellitus and heart disease, are influenced by our diets. Nutrition appears to play at least a moderate role in a variety of other diseases, such as osteoporosis and some forms of cancer (Thompson & Manore, 2017). As more studies look at the protective properties of some foods (e.g., antioxidants) and the hazards of others (e.g., refined carbohydrates, *trans*-fatty acids), the phrase "You are what you eat" seems more accurate each day. Chapter 24 discusses nutrition in greater detail.

Physical Activity

Healthy people are usually active people. When they are unable to maintain previous levels of activity, they may perceive themselves as less healthy. Studies support the benefit of moderate physical activity in reducing the risk of chronic disease and promoting longevity (Thompson & Manore, 2017). As little as 30 minutes of gardening or 15 minutes of jogging on most days of the week can lead to these benefits. In addition, certain types of exercise have been shown to reduce the risk of specific diseases, such as osteoporosis and heart disease. For example, weight training has been shown to increase bone density and reduce the risk of osteoporosis in women older than age 40, and aerobic activity, such as walking, decreases the risk of heart disease. Physical activity is discussed more fully in Chapter 29.

Sleep and Rest

Sleep nourishes health. Most of the body's growth hormone, which assists in tissue regeneration, synthesis of bone, and formation of red blood cells, is released during sleep. Sleep is also important to mental health because it provides time for the mind to slow down and rejuvenate. In controlled studies, people kept awake for 24 hours experienced difficulty concentrating and performing routine tasks. With increasing levels of sleep deprivation, sensory deficits and mood disturbances occurred. Outside the laboratory, mild but chronic sleep deprivation is common, particularly among students, mothers of infants and young children, and people in pain. Sleep and rest are discussed in more detail in Chapter 31.

Meaningful Work

Many people find that work is a healthy way to cope with stressors. Psychologist Victor Frankl, who survived internment in a Nazi concentration camp, observed in *Man's Search for Meaning* (1959, 1962, 1984, 2004) that engaging in meaningful work promotes health and, even in the midst of horrific stressors, can defend against physical and mental breakdown. The definition of meaningful work varies, but many share the view offered by Morrie Schwartz in *Tuesdays With Morrie:* "You know what really gives you satisfaction? Offering others what you have to give. . . . [D]evote yourself to your community around you, and . . . to creating something that gives you purpose and meaning. You notice, there's nothing in there about a salary" (Albom, 1997).

People also experience meaningful work as a determinant of wellness. For many people, volunteering, pursuing hobbies, and engaging in pleasurable activities can be forms of meaningful work. For example, some find that singing, playing a musical instrument, or listening to music is particularly healing. For others, it may be reading, painting, playing basketball, knitting, gardening, hiking in the wilderness, or even shopping. Being healthy is not all about denying yourself the pleasure of ice cream and French fries. Healthful activities can be fun, too. By supporting clients' life work, hobbies, and personal interests, you help them nourish their health in their unique way.

Lifestyle Choices

People who consider themselves healthy are usually those who make healthy lifestyle choices. They are aware of the threats to health created by cigarette smoking, consuming alcohol, abusing drugs, engaging in unprotected sex, and other risky behaviors. Consider the following examples:

- **Smoking.** Nicotine is the primary agent in both regular cigarettes and e-cigarettes (vaping devices), and it is highly addictive. Nicotine is a toxic substance. It raises blood pressure and spikes adrenaline, which increases heart rate and the likelihood of having a heart attack. Traditional tobacco use (i.e., cigarette smoking) is known to increase recovery time from illnesses, injuries, and surgery. Tobacco use also increases the risk of cancer, respiratory diseases, diabetes, infertility, low-birth-weight babies, and perinatal death. There are many unknowns with the use of e-cigarettes (vaping), but emerging data suggest links to chronic lung disease and asthma, and vaping of nicotine at a young age can negatively affect concentration and memory (Selekman, 2019; Walley et al., 2019).
- **Alcohol.** Studies indicate that drinking a glass of red wine each day can reduce the risk of heart disease and slow bone loss. In contrast, excessive alcohol consumption damages the brain, liver, pancreas, intestines, and neurological system and can lead to malnutrition. It has also been implicated in several forms of cancer and in fetal alcohol syndrome in newborns. **Key Point:** *Excessive alcohol consumption is implicated in about half of all motor vehicle accidents, falls, and other injuries.*
- **Other substances.** Substance abuse is a risk factor in many diseases. For example, people who inject drugs and share needles are at increased risk of hepatitis and HIV. Even prescription drugs can be abused. Abuse of alcohol and illicit drugs can lead to deterioration in health, functioning, and relationships.

Personal Relationships

Living in a healthy family is an important determinant of wellness. Moreover, the family influences a person's view of themselves as well or ill. Of the five pairs of families listed in Table 8-1, which family in each pair would you expect to experience a higher level of wellness?

Many people deal with challenges and dangers that are out of their control, such as discrimination, an unsafe neighborhood, or issues with affording the basics

Table 8-1 ➤ Family Personal Relationships

Which family would likely experience a higher level of wellness?

Family A: Places a high priority on health promotion	OR	**Family B:** Responds to health issues only in times of serious illness
Family C: Encourages adventure and risk taking	OR	**Family D:** Emphasizes caution in new situations
Family E: Is very open about expressing feelings and disagreements	OR	**Family F:** Squelches personal feelings to avoid conflict in the family
Family G: Views the family as capable and successful	OR	**Family H:** Views them as powerless victims
Family I: Teaches good negotiation skills and builds a network of family support while encouraging the development of independence	OR	**Family J:** Parents do not have a large repertoire of coping and communication skills to share with their children

they need. Healthy relationships within the home, in the community, and at work can provide support to meet these challenges. But some people, like children whose parents are in jail or adolescents who are bullied, may not get the support they need.

When illness occurs, some people prefer to be totally independent, priding themselves on never asking for or accepting help. But the reality is that during times of disruption, support from others (e.g., family, friends, coworkers, pastors, counselors) is crucial. Weeks before his death from amyotrophic lateral sclerosis, a neurological disease, sociologist Morrie Schwartz stated, "It's become quite clear to me as I've been sick. If you don't have the support and love and caring and concern that you get from a family, you don't have much at all" (Albom, 1997). You will learn more about the role of the family in human health in Chapter 11. Knowing that support is available, and being willing to accept the support, can determine a person's response to disruptions.

Culture

The healthcare culture has traditionally responded to illness with specific therapies aimed at treating a biophysical disorder, whereas nursing, as part of the culture of holism, responds to the physical, emotional, mental, and spiritual dimensions of illness. The culture of a region, a neighborhood, a school or work environment, or a religious group is a social determinant of individual and family health. Culture affects the experience of illness in the following ways:

- **It influences health decisions, behaviors, perceptions, and view of self as well or ill.** For example, the cultural group may share health-promoting values, such as a nutritious diet or regular physical activity. This is not to say that individuals can be "defined" by their culture. Some, either consciously or unconsciously, decide to break away from culturally conditioned responses.
- **It influences responses to illness.** For example, people who belong to certain religions may interpret illness as a punishment from God and may bear their

symptoms stoically (i.e., hide their symptoms) to try to pay for their sins (retribution), whereas some members of other religions may believe that illness is a lesson we give ourselves to teach us something we need to learn for our spiritual evolution. If you need more information about the influence of culture on health and illness, see Chapter 12.

Religion and Spirituality

Clients' religious beliefs and practices can influence their healthcare choices. For example, some people believe that spiritual beliefs influence the mind–body connection to promote wellness and healing. A dramatic example is seemingly spontaneous recovery after a religious rite, such as when a person who can't walk undergoes a special rite or ceremony and then recovers enough to walk across the room. When healing is not possible because of terminal illness or external circumstances beyond our control, spiritual reserves can help maintain our view of ourselves as "well." You will learn more about the influence of spirituality on health in Chapter 13.

Environmental Factors

- **The environment can nourish wellness.** For institutionalized clients, establishing a little corner of the room that is uniquely "theirs," with photos and other mementos, can be healing. Other clients may be soothed by the quiet of a chapel, a walk in the park, or even a trip to a shopping mall. Spending time in any place where they feel harmony and peace and draw strength can promote clients' health.
- **Environmental pollutants are also a common cause of illness.** For example, exposure to secondhand smoke causes an estimated 7,300 deaths from lung cancer among American adults each year (Centers for Disease Control and Prevention [CDC], 2020). Carbon monoxide and lead poisoning, mold, radon, chemicals (e.g., insecticides), and other pollutants also cause serious disease. Families who are considered low-income families or are part of racial and

ethnic minority groups are more likely to live in high-risk areas. See Chapter 21 for more information about environmental pollutants.

Finances

It is often said that money doesn't buy happiness. Certainly this is true. However, money does buy healthcare choices and access and thus is a social determinant of wellness. In the United States:

- One in 10 people in the United States lives in poverty. Many can't afford healthy food, healthcare, or housing.
- Although stable employment is linked to healthy behaviors, some who have secure jobs may not make enough money to afford the things they need to stay healthy, including health insurance, which is often tied to employment or income level.
- Health insurance dictates which providers a person has access to and what services are available to each person.

Even in countries with national health programs, such as Canada and some European countries, the standard care available may not include all the services or medications that a person desires. The same is true in the United States with Medicare.

People often do not take advantage of services that are available to them. Healthcare professionals may wonder why patients let things go so long before seeking help—or why they do not follow up with recommended treatment plans. **Key Point:** *A client's apparent lack of concern or lack of compliance to a treatment regimen may be, in reality, a problem of access to healthcare. One or more social determinants of health may keep individuals and families from getting the help that they need (e.g., distance from the resources, knowledge of available resources, trust in the available resources, financial status, and lifestyle adjustments such as a change in employment).*

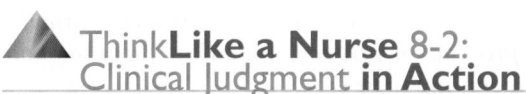

ThinkLike a Nurse 8-2: Clinical Judgment in Action

- In what ways could you improve your eating, exercise, and sleep habits?
- How might a hospitalized patient get away from the routine and find peace and harmony?

WHAT FACTORS DISRUPT HEALTH?

We spend much of our lives trying to maintain good health—eating, sleeping, keeping our bodies at a comfortable temperature—in general, tending to our high-maintenance bodily needs. It's a continual process because of the many disruptions to health we face. Not all disruptions are incapacitating, but all challenge our ability to function and enjoy our everyday lives, and they tend to move us toward the illness end of the health–illness continuum. What are **health disruptions?** Let's explore the concept by learning about some specific examples.

Physical Disease

Disease disrupts our lives in so many ways:

- It may reduce our ability to perform our life roles effectively or to engage in activities we enjoyed before the illness.
- The diagnosis of a chronic or life-threatening disease may bring shock, fear, anxiety, anger, or grief: Will I become disabled? How will I support my family? What did I do to deserve this?
- Physical illness may also cause clients to question the meaning and purpose of their lives, to become more inwardly focused, or to embrace life even more fully.

When she first learned of her diagnosis of breast cancer at age 36, Treya Killam Wilber wrote, "Strange things happen to the mind when catastrophe strikes. . . . I was so stunned that it was as if absolutely nothing had happened. A tremendous strength descended on me, the strength of being both totally jolted and totally stupefied. I was clear, present, and very determined. (Wilber, 2000)

Injury

Although injury can cause the same symptoms and emotions as disease, perhaps its most disruptive aspect is its suddenness. In *Still Me*, actor Christopher Reeve described his thoughts in the first days after he recovered consciousness following his cervical spinal cord injury: "The thought that kept going through my mind was: I've ruined my life. I've ruined my life, and you only get one. There's no counter you can go up to and say, 'I dropped my ice cream cone; could I please have another one?'. . . . Why isn't there a higher authority you can go to and say, 'Wait a minute, you didn't mean for this to happen to *me*'?" (Reeve, 1998).

Mental Illness

Mental illness causes clients and their families to experience a level of pain, suffering, and chronic sorrow that is difficult for healthy people to fully appreciate (Foster & Isobel, 2018; Zeighami et al., 2018). In addition, if the illness affects work ability, they experience loss of income and altered role relationships, accompanied by the costs of various therapies.

Mental illness carries with it a stigma that may be diminishing slowly but is highly visible to those who suffer from its effects. This stigmatization can also disrupt the health of family members. Families must adjust to a major upheaval in their lives as they experience the pain associated with the loss of a once-promising child or relative to the spiral of mental illness (Townsend, 2017). Family members may also live in constant fear that their loved one may hurt themselves or die by suicide.

Chronic Illness and Self-Management Through Telehealth

Chapter Key Concepts: Health, Illness

Competency: Embrace/Incorporate Technological Advances

Background. Telehealth encourages patients to be in more control of their health and to take ownership of their condition (Kaminski, 2016). Healthcare is transitioning to a focus on patient self-management. Telecommunication provides a strategy for self-management by empowering patients and helping them feel more secure in monitoring and managing their care. In chronic conditions, there is a window of opportunity for remote monitoring to detect health changes sooner and to initiate earlier interventions (Foster & Sethares, 2014).

Scenario. A patient with long-standing chronic obstructive pulmonary disease (COPD) frequently experiences exacerbations requiring hospital admission. Because the patient lives in a remote rural area, he often delays seeking healthcare. At the last clinic visit, the nurse provided the patient with home-monitoring devices that connected him to telehealth services.

Think about it:

➤ What advantages can telehealth provide for a patient with chronic illness?

➤ How might telehealth increase the patient's self-care management of COPD?

➤ Discuss how informatics (specifically telehealth) can affect an individual's position on the health–illness continuum.

Pain

Whether mild or severe, temporary or long lasting, pain is a disruption. It's not that we can't live with pain—many people do, every day of their lives. However, pain disrupts the smooth operation of our lives; it can change personality, erode coping skills, and interfere with healthy communication. It's hard to concentrate on what we are trying to accomplish when pain is competing for our attention.

Pain that is easily remedied with over-the-counter medications or that is short-lived serves only as a minor disruption in our lives. However, pain that is all-encompassing permeates a person's entire existence. Sometimes that pain is physical, sometimes psychological. One young mother of a 14-year-old girl with profound intellectual disabilities spoke of "hurting so bad that my bones hurt."

As you know, some of our nursing interventions inflict pain. We ask patients to turn, deep-breathe, and cough after surgery, even though it hurts—a *lot*! We put needles in them, catheterize them, and get them out of bed when they would rather sleep. We pull off tape. We invade their personal physical space. We ask them questions about personal things, such as their bowel movements. It is a challenge to be a comforting, healing presence when we have to do things that cause discomfort.

Loss

Loss is a disruption that cuts to the core of who we are—whether the loss of a job; the end of a romantic relationship; the death of a loved one; or the loss of youth, beauty, functioning, or identity. Most of us cling to a unique identity, which usually does *not* include gaining weight or getting wrinkles and gray hair, let alone being a "patient" or losing major bodily functions. When such a loss occurs, the resulting period of significant disintegration may continue until the person either finds a way to cope with the loss or succeeds in reinterpreting the loss in a meaningful way. Toward the end of her battle with cancer, Treya Killam Wilber lost her near vision. One way she coped with this loss was by replacing her passion for reading with sitting at her window, contemplating the mountains beyond (Wilber, 2000).

Loss of Sense of Self Many have written about the indignities people suffered in concentration camps, including nakedness, exposure to human excrement, and being treated like children, incapable of thoughtful judgment (Bettelheim, 1979; Frankl, 1959, 1962, 1984, 2004; Valladares, 2001). Those three indignities are crucial threats to a person's sense of self. Sadly, patients in healthcare institutions may also suffer those indignities.

Think how patients feel when they have to don a hospital gown and allow their bodies to be exposed for various tests or procedures, or how it feels to lose control of bladder or bowel function. One woman who was paralyzed as a result of a lesion on her spine indicated that one of the toughest things she had to deal with was having her daughter give her enemas and clean her up as if she were a baby.

♥ **iCare** *As healthcare providers, we may easily forget how humiliating such "routine procedures" may be for the patient. You can help relieve the disruption of disease and injury when you respect patients' dignity, provide for privacy, and allow them to make choices regarding their care.*

Permanent Loss If temporary losses are difficult, what about those that are permanent? C. S. Lewis (1961) wrote about his response to the death of his wife: "I know that the thing I want is exactly the thing I can never get. The old life, the jokes, the drinks, the arguments, the love-making, the tiny, heartbreaking commonplace" (p. 22).

♥ **iCare** As nurses, we would like to "fix" everything. Although we can't "fix" the holes that are left when a person suffers a loss, we can be open and sensitive to their heart's cry.

Impending Death

It is easy for most of us to ignore that we have a 100% chance of dying, and we live as though death were only a remote possibility. Lifton and Olson (1974) state that during middle age, even without the presence of life-threatening illness, people tend to become more aware of the compelling reality of death: "One's life is suddenly felt to be limited. . . . It also becomes apparent that . . . there will not be time for all one's projects" (p. 63).

As a nurse, you will care for clients who are living in the disruption of the shadow of death. Some may be aware of their condition; others may choose to deny it, ignore it, or "fight it to the end" by trying a series of conventional and alternative therapies. Caring for dying clients makes us painfully aware of our own frailty and is one of the most difficult experiences you will face as a nurse. Chapter 14 provides further discussion of loss, grieving, and dying.

Competing Demands

Even in the normal flow of life, there are many competing demands. Taken independently, they may be easy to handle. Taken together, the cumulative effect wears us down.

In times of illness, the other competing demands continue. Children need to be cared for. Aging parents may need care. Bills still need to be paid. Job responsibilities press in. One man with depression reported, "[T]he whole thing bundled together—one caused the other which caused more and it was just a degenerative loop. . . . [O]ne thing feeds another which feeds another and so forth until you just constantly go down" (Smith, 1992, p. 104).

Sometimes people ignore health issues because the competing demands are too great. Symptoms may even go unnoticed because attention is scattered in so many directions, and there are not enough time and energy to research one's symptoms, schedule a doctor's appointment, or follow through with treatments.

When an illness is acute, such as a broken bone, the stress is usually bearable because it usually lasts for a set amount of time. Bettleheim (1979) states: "The worst calamity becomes bearable if one believes its end is in sight" (pp. 3–4).

But when the illness is chronic, the competing demands can take a heavy toll. One woman who took care of her husband who lived at home, his breathing assisted by a ventilator, recounted the overwhelming burden she felt when, after 2 years, he was "no better and no worse. This could go on forever!" Although people came in to help, she felt she had to maintain constant alertness in case something went wrong with his ventilator, and she still had to meet many other demands and challenges each day.

As nurses, we sometimes find it easy to criticize how people deal with their situations. But it is so important to realize that the short amount of time that you spend with someone in a hospital or clinic or in a home visit is only one tiny fragment of the cumulative experience that patients and their families experience, sometimes unrelentingly for years on end.

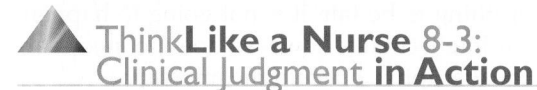

ThinkLike a Nurse 8-3: Clinical Judgment in Action

How might you assist your patient to maintain normalcy in spite of illness?

The Unknown

The following are examples of unknowns that patients experience:

- **Normal life changes.** Even normal life changes present challenges. For example, most parents bringing their first baby home from the hospital are in for plenty of surprises.
- **Anticipated life changes.** With some unknowns, there is time to investigate the potential problem and prepare. For example, if an expectant couple learns via amniocentesis (a prenatal test) that their child has a genetic defect, then during the remaining months of pregnancy, they can read about the disorder and meet with other parents who have had children similarly affected.
- **Unexpected/sudden life changes.** However, injuries and illnesses can happen abruptly, with no chance to prepare for new realities. A woman described her experience of finding out she had cancer of the lung with metastasis: "It was on a . . . Friday—I got to feeling kind of bad—kind of like you had the flu or something, you know? . . . so I went to the doctor. . . . And . . . they started doin' tests on me—all kinds of tests—and found out I had cancer" (Smith, 1992, p. 107).

Imbalance

Our sense of justice tells us that when we are good, good things should happen. When we are bad, bad things should happen. The Buddhist concept of *karma* suggests that there is a fair balance between what one gives to life and what one receives. Thus, when we perceive that life has violated this rule, we experience that as a disruption, as in these examples:

- **Death of a child.** Our sense of balance is perhaps most dramatically disturbed by the death of children. Such deaths are sometimes referred to as "out of order" because children (of any age) "should not" die before their parents.
- **Treatment failure.** Balance is also disrupted when patients, expecting that their painful and harrowing treatments "should" help them get better, do not get better. One young woman under treatment for advanced cancer described it like this: "It's just—you've been working hard . . . . you're doin' what you're supposed to be doin' and focusing and all this and that—and your body is still not responding" (Smith, 1992, p. 111).

Have you seen the bumper sticker "Life is hard. And then you die"? Cynical, perhaps, but we do not have to live long before we realize that as much as we would like for everything to be fair, it is not going to happen. Knowing this intellectually, however, does not necessarily reduce the disruptive effect of the imbalance.

Isolation

How many times have you thought, "No one knows what I'm going through!"? A sense of isolation or aloneness seems to accompany suffering. C. S. Lewis (1961) states, "You can't really share someone else's weakness, or fear or pain" (p. 13). Vanauken (1977), in writing about the death of his young wife, reveals that it was not only suffering his loss but having to go through the experience *without* her that made it so difficult: "Along with the emptiness . . . I kept wanting to *tell* her about it. We always told each other—that was what sharing was—and now this huge thing was happening to me, and I couldn't tell her" (p. 181).

The sense of aloneness reported by seriously ill clients is related in part to their actual physical separation from loved ones during treatments, hospitalizations, or clinic visits. But it also stems from their feeling that there is no one who is really "in their world." Having someone physically present does not necessarily remove the sense of aloneness:

> When I lay here it's lonely—very, very lonely. Because [my daughter] can't just sit here and talk to me all the time. She's got wash to do, fold and all that stuff. And then the kids to worry about. . . . The worst thing I've found about this whole disease is the loneliness. . . . Because your family can be with you and if they don't come and sit down and talk to you about different things, you're lonely. It's the loneliness that makes you sad inside. . . . It's like everybody's afraid of you or something. They're afraid that maybe they're gonna catch what you got or something. (Smith, 1992)

KnowledgeCheck 8-2

Identify at least four factors that disrupt health.

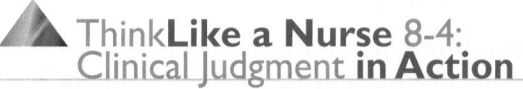

ThinkLike a Nurse 8-4:
Clinical Judgment in Action

- What impact do disruptions have on your life?
- How could you apply the information about disruptions to the health of a community? To the health of a nation?

WHY DO PEOPLE EXPERIENCE ILLNESS DIFFERENTLY?

Why is it that people vary greatly in terms of their response to life situations? Why do some people react to seemingly insurmountable problems with calmness and grace, whereas others fall apart over seemingly "small" disruptions? The human experience is too complex and interactive to fit into neat little categories or derive a score for predicting how a person will respond to a given situation. There are several factors, however, that may influence an individual's responses to illness. We focus now on four such factors, beginning with the stages of illness behavior.

Stages of Illness Behavior

How people react to an illness depends in part on their illness stage. Suchman (1972) identified five stages of illness behaviors that people move through as they cope with disruptions to health, as discussed in the following sections.

Experiencing Symptoms Symptoms are a signal that illness has begun. If the symptoms are recognizable, such as a runny nose, sneezing, and a cough, you may identify the problem as a common cold and turn to previously used remedies. Common problems rarely progress beyond this stage. However, if the symptoms are unusual, severe, or overwhelming, you may progress to the next stage.

Sick Role Behavior When you have identified yourself as ill, you assume the sick role, which relieves you of normal duties, such as work, school, or tasks at home. In Western biomedical culture, the prevailing view is that sick persons are not responsible for their illnesses and that a curative process outside the person is needed to restore wellness. We believe that the sick person has the duty to try to get well, to seek healthcare, and to cooperate with the care providers (Cockerham, 2017). The severity of the symptoms and anticipated length of illness determine whether you will progress further along the stages of illness.

Seeking Professional Care To reach this stage, you must determine that you are ill and that professional care is required to treat the illness. Persons who seek professional care are asking for validation of their illness, explanations for their symptoms, appropriate treatment, and information about the anticipated length of illness. Healthcare professionals often bypass this stage, relying on themselves to identify and treat the problem. This is not always the best course of action because it is difficult to be objective when examining yourself.

Dependence on Others When you accept the diagnosis and treatment of the healthcare provider, you typically also accept the need to depend on others. The severity of the illness and the type of treatment determine the extent of dependence. This may be limited to listening to the provider's instructions, filling the prescription, and following directions given in the office. However, illness that requires hospitalization is often associated with dependence on nursing staff and hospital personnel for activities of daily living, medications, and treatments. Some people easily make the transition to dependence; others remain as independent as possible even in the face of severe illness. Personal characteristics and values play a large role in determining how each of us will respond to the challenges of being dependent.

Recovery The final stage of illness is called **recovery.** The person gradually resumes independence and returns to normal roles and functioning. In minor illness, this is usually a return to the status quo. Severe illnesses may require a redefinition of optimal function. The greater the change in health status, the more difficult this transition will be. Learning to manage a chronic illness is the equivalent of a cure in an acute illness (Parsons, 1975). Both represent the recovery stage.

The Nature of the Illness

The nature of the illness (e.g., whether the illness is chronic or acute) affects the way persons react to disruptions and respond to illness.

Acute Illness An **acute illness** occurs suddenly and lasts for a limited amount of time. Acute illnesses, such as a cold, flu, or viral infection, may be minor and require no formal healthcare. Some acute illnesses, such as strep throat, may require a visit to a healthcare provider for treatment or even hospitalization or surgery, as in cholecystitis (gallbladder inflammation secondary to gallstone formation) or pyelonephritis (infection of the kidney). Although hospitalization and surgery can be quite traumatic, in each case the person is expected to recover. In acute illness, a person may experience the disruptions of pain, competing demands, and the unknown. However, an end is in sight. Relief is expected.

Chronic Illness In contrast, **chronic illness** lasts for a long period of time, usually 6 months or more, often for a lifetime. Chronic illness requires the person to make life changes. These changes might be regular visits to the clinic or hospital, daily medications, or lifestyle modifications such as a low-fat diet or smoking cessation. Common chronic illnesses include AIDS, diabetes mellitus, rheumatoid arthritis, and hypertension. Because of the lengthy period of illness, people with chronic disease often experience periods of remission or exacerbation.

- A **remission** occurs when symptoms are minimal to none.
- An **exacerbation** ("flare-up") occurs when symptoms intensify.

Clients with chronic illness often complain about the unrelenting nature of their health problems. A person with chronic illness may experience virtually all of the disruptions identified earlier. Box 8-2 identifies some interesting facts about chronic conditions.

Hardiness

Why does one client who drinks, smokes, overeats, and avoids exercise live into his 90s, yet another client who "follows all the rules" dies of a sudden heart attack at age 39? Our bodies do not react to the same stressors in the same way. One factor that may contribute to this difference is the person's hardiness.

BOX 8-2 ■ Facts About Chronic Conditions

- More than 117 million Americans live with chronic conditions.
- Chronic conditions account for about 70% of all deaths in the United States.
- About 80% of older adults have at least one chronic condition; 50% have at least two.
- Approximately 6% of adults older than age 65 have a diagnosable depressive illness.
- The top-three risks for functional decline are cognitive impairment, depression, and disease burden.
- The largest declines in functional abilities are associated with these physical conditions: arthritis of the hip or knee, sciatica, and chronic pulmonary diseases.
- Arthritis affects 1 in 4 U.S. adults; for more than 40% of those, arthritis limits their activities.
- More than 42% of the adult population and 19% of children and adolescents were obese in the period 2017–2018.
- In a large sample of Medicare beneficiaries, the following were the most frequent chronic physical conditions:

Hypertension (58%)	Depression (19%)
Hyperlipidemia (50%)	Alzheimer disease (4%)
Arthritis (35%)	Atrial fibrillation (8.8%)
Diabetes (28%)	Osteoporosis (7%)
Ischemic heart disease (28%)	Any cancer (other than skin cancer) (7%)
Chronic kidney disease (26%)	Emphysema, asthma, or chronic obstructive pulmonary disease (COPD) (12%)
Heart failure (14.5%)	

Sources: Centers for Disease Control and Prevention. (2021a). *Adult obesity facts.* http://www.cdc.gov/obesity/data/adult.html; Centers for Disease Control and Prevention. (2021b). *Child obesity facts.* http://www.cdc.gov/obesity/data/childhood.html; Centers for Medicare & Medicaid Services. (2022). *Chronic conditions data warehouse.* https://www.ccwdata.org/web/guest/medicare-charts/medicare-chronic-condition-charts; Centers for Disease Control and Prevention. (2022). *Chronic disease overview.* https://www.cdc.gov/chronicdisease/overview/index.htm; Ding, O. J., & Kennedy, G. J. (2021). Understanding vulnerability to late-life suicide. *Current Psychiatry Reports, 23*(9), 1–9.

Will to Live Hardiness has been described as developing a very strong positive force to live—and enjoying the ride (Fig. 8-5)! A man with heart problems said, "I guess everybody that's in the situation, who has to fight to live, and has learned the mental wizardry of it, you know, to make yourself want to live on. But if you want to, you develop this—this very, very strong positive force to make it go" (Smith, 1992, p. 131). Seigel (1986) reported a study by London researchers that revealed a 10-year survival rate of 75% "among cancer patients who reacted to the diagnosis with a 'fighting spirit,'" compared with a 22% survival rate "among those who

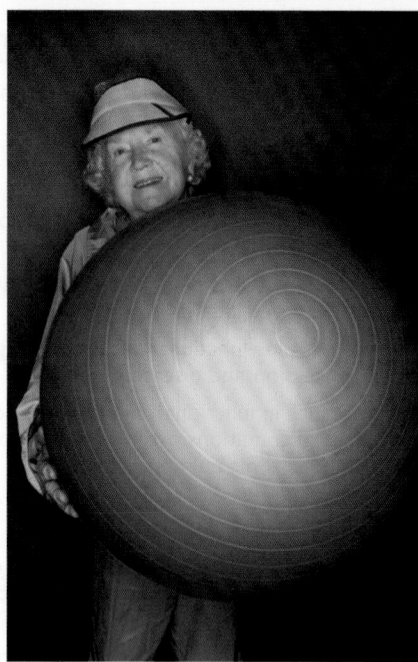

FIGURE 8-5 Hardiness has been described as developing a very strong positive force to live—and enjoying the fight!

responded with 'stoic acceptance' or feelings of helplessness or hopelessness" (p. 25).

Adapting to Change Another aspect of hardiness is the willingness to draw on resources within oneself or from others to break out of old patterns of living when life situations change. When disruption hits, some people don't have the cognitive, communicative, creative, and spiritual resources they need to make life changes, and they just give up. **Key Point:** *Hardy individuals are willing to seek out information and take initiative in dealing with life situations rather than sitting back and letting someone else control their lives.* Ironically, some people survive and thrive during times of adversity. Those who see themselves as hardy tend to approach changes with an "I can deal with this" attitude.

The Intensity, Duration, and Multiplicity of the Disruption

Everyone has limits. For healthcare providers, too many demands over too long a period of time can lead to *burnout*, a feeling of being overwhelmed and demoralized. For clients and their families, dealing with the cumulative effect of illness and other life disruptions can break down what might otherwise be excellent coping skills. After reaching a breaking point, their responses may not be typical of what they usually have demonstrated.

KnowledgeCheck 8-3

- Identify the factors that affect how a person responds to the disruptions of illness.
- Define *hardiness*.

Health Promotion Versus Health Protection

For the most part, the activities that promote health also protect health. Nevertheless, the ideas behind health promotion and health protection differ subtly but significantly. Murdaugh et al. (2018) explain that motivation is what distinguishes the two activities.

- Health promotion is motivated by the desire to increase well-being.
- Health protection is motivated by a desire to avoid illness.

For instance, the 40-year-old who begins an exercise program to improve strength and endurance is motivated by the benefits of health promotion. If they start exercising because their father died of a heart attack at age 50, they may be motivated by the need to protect their health.

Levels of Prevention

Leavell and Clark (1965) identified three levels of activities for health protection (illness prevention): primary, secondary, and tertiary. Interventions are classified according to their purpose in different stages of the disease process. This timing directs the types of interventions needed.

- Primary prevention activities are designed to prevent or slow the onset of disease. Examples include eating healthy foods, exercising, wearing sunscreen, obeying seat-belt laws, and keeping up with immunizations.
- Secondary prevention involves screening activities and education for detecting illnesses in the early stages. Examples are regular physical examinations, blood pressure and diabetes screenings, and tuberculosis skin tests.
- Tertiary prevention focuses on stopping the disease from progressing and returning the individual to the preillness phase. Rehabilitation is the main intervention during this level.

Patients and health providers move among these levels of prevention. For example, a patient hospitalized for a total hip replacement would receive the following:

- Tertiary prevention strategies focused on helping them recover from surgery, preventing complications of surgery, and later on, helping them regain their strength and learn to walk again.
- Secondary prevention strategies may have been used previously, for example, to screen for osteoporosis that leads to bone fragility and fractures.
- Primary prevention strategies help the patient after they return home, for example, limiting salt intake and eating a balanced diet that is low in fat and refined sugar.

Health-Promotion Models

A model illustrates a system or framework to help explain what you see in clinical practice. The most common frameworks used for designing health-promotion programs are described next.

Pender's Health Promotion Model

Pender's Health Promotion Model (HPM) (Fig. 8-6) identifies three groups of variables that affect health promotion: (1) individual characteristics and experiences, (2) behavior-specific cognitions and affect, and (3) behavioral outcome. The HPM is based on seven assumptions that reflect both nursing and behavioral science perspectives (Murdaugh et al., 2019).

The first two general assumptions concern the interpersonal environment:

1. Health professionals constitute a part of the interpersonal environment, which exerts influence on persons throughout their life span.
2. Self-initiated reconfiguration of person–environment interactive patterns is essential to behavior change.

The next five assumptions are characteristics of people, whom the theorist assumes:

3. Seek to create conditions of living through which they can express their unique human health potential.
4. Have the capacity for reflective self-awareness, including assessment of their own competencies.
5. Value growth in directions viewed as positive and attempt to achieve a personally acceptable balance between change and stability.
6. Seek to actively regulate their own behavior.
7. Interact with the environment in all their biopsychosocial complexity, progressively transforming the environment and being transformed over time.

Pender's model has been used extensively in several disciplines in research and professional practice focused on health promotion. As a nurse, you should find Pender's focus applicable to your work.

Wheel of Wellness

Several authors have likened the different facets of health to the spokes of a wheel (Hettler, 1984; Myers et al., 2000;

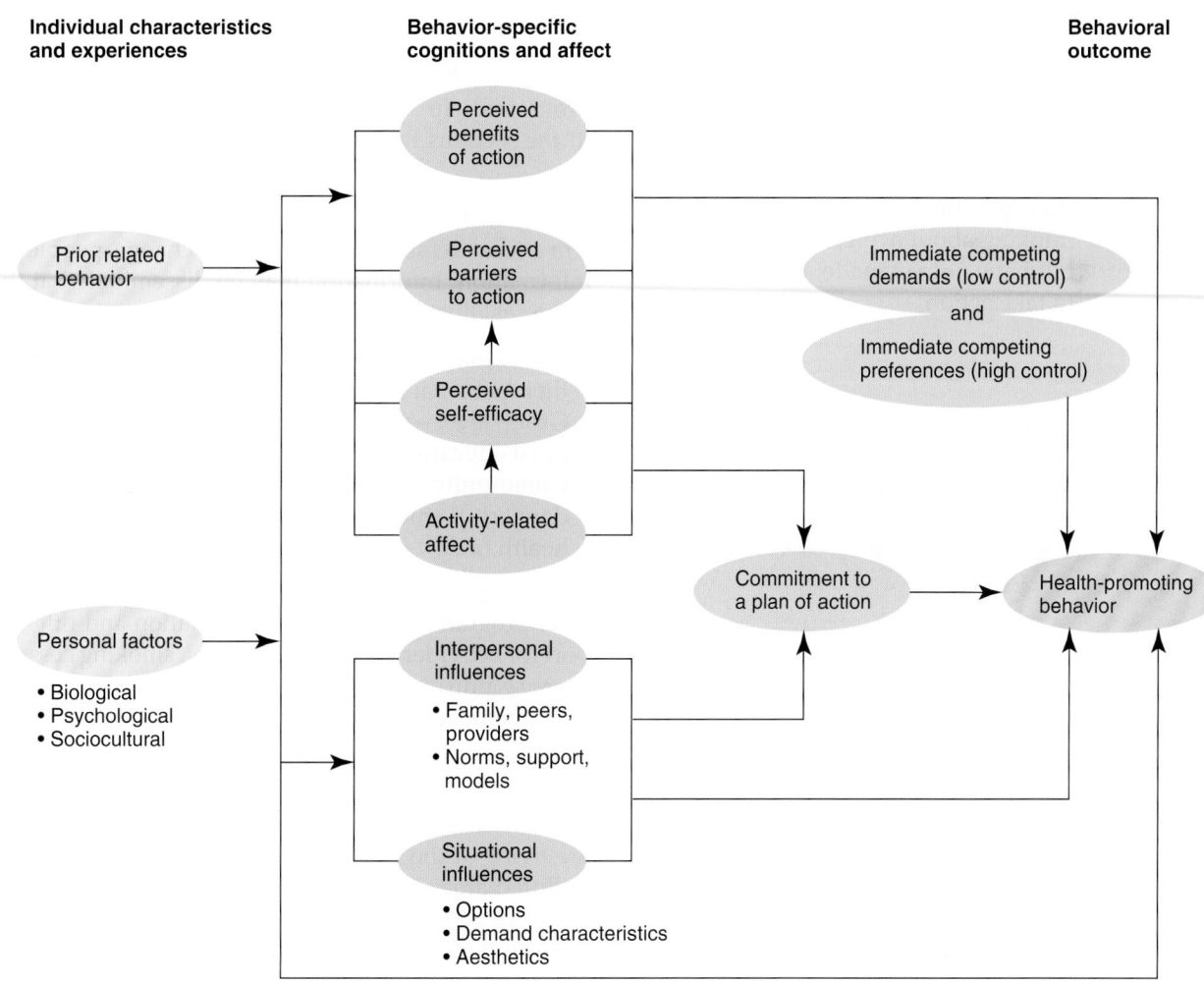

FIGURE 8-6 Pender's Health Promotion Model.

Witmer & Sweeney, 1992). If one of the spokes is weak, the whole wheel is weak. The "spokes" of the health wheel represent the dimensions of health: emotional, intellectual, physical, spiritual, social/family, and occupational (Fig. 8-7). The level of wellness progresses from the center to the outer part of the wheel. The center represents the least amount of wellness, and the outer part represents optimal wellness. If one area of an individual's life is not functioning at an optimal level, life will not be as fulfilling as it could be. As a nurse, you should assess each dimension for strengths and weaknesses.

Transtheoretical Model of Change

The Transtheoretical Model of Change (Prochaska & DiClemente, 1982) may serve to alter unhealthy behaviors. Health promotion and protection involve either changing the individual's response to the illness-producing stimuli or changing the environment so that the person will be less likely to encounter illness-producing stimuli. Either idea involves change. The Prochaska and DiClemente model identifies four stages of change: stages 2 through 5, in which change is occurring, and stages 1 and 6, which precede and follow the stages of change.

Stage 1	**Precontemplation**—Patients have no intention to change behavior in the foreseeable future because patients are unaware or underaware of their problems. They do not yet contemplate change.
Stage 2	**Contemplation**—Patients are seriously thinking about overcoming a problem but have not yet made a commitment to take action.
Stage 3	**Preparation**—Individuals are intending to take action in the next month and are reporting some small behavioral changes ("baby steps").
Stage 4	**Action**—The plan is implemented; this requires considerable **commitment** of time and energy.
Stage 5	**Maintenance**—Individuals are working to prevent relapse, and they grow increasingly more confident that the change can be sustained.
Stage 6	**Termination**—Persons who enter into the termination stage have changed the behavior and are not in danger of relapse.

Ideally, the stages would progress in this order. Realistically, a person may progress and regress in any of the stages. The change process in persons with some unhealthy habits (e.g., cigarette smoking, substance abuse, excessive eating) may best be described as a revolving door. An individual may exit at any point as the door goes around. If the exit occurs during or at the end of the maintenance period, the behavioral change is successful. If the exit occurs before the end of the maintenance period, relapse will occur, and the individual will return to the previous lifestyle.

Health Promotion Programs Health-promotion programs help a person advance toward optimal health. In the sections that follow, we discuss several program types.

Disseminating Information To recognize a problem and understand the options for change, people need information. Information may be disseminated at three levels, as illustrated in the following examples:

- Individual level—Teaching a client how to modify their personal dietary intake
- Group level—Classes offered at the local hospital, prenatal education programs, and worksite programs
- Community level—A billboard that presents the dangers of smoking, health blogs on the Internet, and health fairs

Changing Lifestyle and Behavior These are group-level programs that provide information and offer support for activities such as weight loss, smoking cessation, exercise, nutrition, and stress management. Some include a maintenance program to help sustain the change.

Protecting the Environment Environmental pollutants lead to health problems like respiratory diseases, heart disease, and some types of cancer. Individuals who are living at the poverty level are more likely to live in polluted areas and have unsafe drinking water. A main objective of *Healthy People 2030* is to promote healthier environments to improve health, including reducing exposure to harmful pollutants in air, water, soil, food, and materials in homes and workplaces.

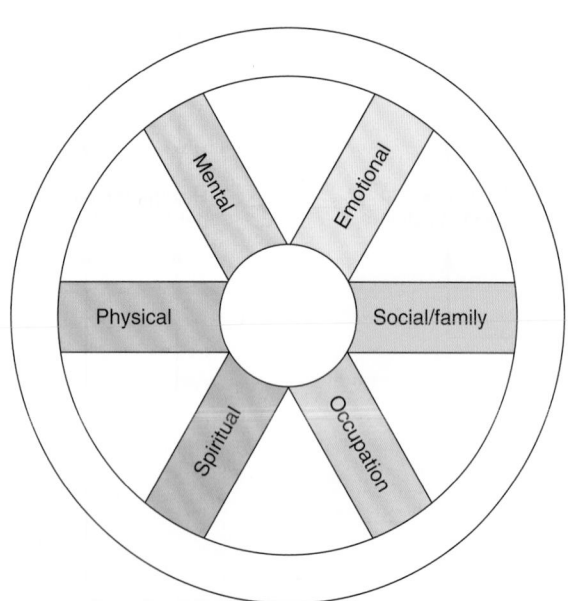

FIGURE 8-7 Wheel of wellness.

Assessing Wellness and Appraising Health Risk A wellness assessment tends to focus on the healthy behaviors. It supports positive change to improve health. A health risk appraisal identifies risky behaviors that promote disease. These tools are available on the Internet, in magazines, and at fitness centers.

KnowledgeCheck 8-4

- What are the six dimensions of health represented by the spokes on the wellness wheel?
- Identify the stages of change identified by Prochaska and DiClemente.
- Describe the four main types of health-promotion programs.

 ## ThinkLike a Nurse 8-5: Clinical Judgment in Action

J.T. drinks a vodka and tonic while eating lunch with coworkers. J.T. keeps a bottle of vodka in the office desk for use during the day. Later, J.T. stops at a local bar for a drink on the way home. At home, J.T. drinks a six-pack of beer while watching the game. What information do you need to determine which of Prochaska and DiClemente's stages of change J.T. is experiencing? How would you find this information?

Settings for Health-Promotion Programs The most common sites for health-promotion programs are health facilities, worksites, and schools.

- In healthcare settings, each interaction between patient and healthcare provider is an opportunity for health promotion. Unfortunately, most interactions focus on the disease process and compliance with treatments. You will need to make a conscious effort to help clients focus on behaviors that prevent illness and promote health.
- Nurses working in health clinics within large companies may be contracted to provide specific health-promotion programs, such as smoking cessation, stress management, weight reduction, and fitness training. Employers have found that health programs decrease work-related injuries and sick leave.
- Local school districts are another setting for health promotion. Health learning can begin at an early age, and nurses and teachers can regularly reinforce healthy behaviors and redirect unhealthy behaviors. Schools provide a setting that allows for continued exposure to information. Interventions may be directed at general health-promotion issues, such as physical activity, or they may focus on specific health risks, such as tobacco and alcohol use. School nurses work closely with teachers and parents to provide health-promotion services in the schools.

Health Promotion Throughout the Life Span

Health promotion is a lifelong process that begins at conception. Table 8-2 describes the focus of health-promotion programs at each developmental stage,

along with the types of screenings recommended for each age-group.

PracticalKnowledge knowing how

In the preceding section, you have learned how people experience health, wellness, and illness. In this section, we look at how this information can be applied to your nursing practice.

USING THE NURSING PROCESS TO PROMOTE HEALTH

Throughout this textbook, you will learn to use the nursing process to help clients deal with a variety of health problems. But how does the nursing process relate to the broader aspects of health, wellness, and illness described in this chapter? Overall, it involves helping clients—regardless of the stage of wellness—to look within themselves to develop creative ways to deal with the realities they are facing.

Murdaugh et al. (2019) summarized the health-promotion process as a series of nine steps that involve the client and the nurse. Notice that many steps of this process are similar to the nursing process:

1. Review and summarize data from assessment.
2. Reinforce the client's strengths and abilities.
3. Identify health goals and related behavioral change options.
4. Identify behavioral or health outcomes that will indicate that the plan has been successful from the client's perspective.
5. Develop a behavior-change plan based on the client's preferences, the stages of change, and "state-of-the-science" knowledge about effective interventions.
6. Reiterate the benefits of change and identify incentives for change from the client's perspective.
7. Address environmental and interpersonal facilitators and barriers to behavior change.
8. Determine a time frame for implementation.
9. Commit to behavior-change goals, and structure the support needed to accomplish them.

Patients may fail to comply with a proposed healthcare regimen if healthcare providers develop a plan of care that has no cultural or personal relevance for the patient (or family). Perhaps the plan does not consider the knowledge level of the patient or caregiver, or perhaps it is not feasible in terms of available support, time, energy, finances, or location. Patients may leave a hospital setting *against medical advice,* thereby endangering their chances of recovery. They may believe that the treatment offered to them will not help or that the illness is preferable to the proposed treatment. Noncompliance often occurs because the effort, inconvenience, or pain involved with a therapeutic plan of care is too much for them to handle.

Table 8-2 ➤ Health Promotion Throughout the Life Span

Conception to Birth

HEALTH PROMOTION FOCUS	HEALTH SCREENING
Education about pregnancy	Alpha-fetoprotein level
Abstinence from alcohol, cigarettes, and illicit drugs	Screening for gestational diabetes
Nutrition, including folic acid and iron requirements	Prenatal care
Exercise to maintain strength and muscle tone and control weight gain	Abuse
Parenting education	Additional screenings that may be offered:
	■ Ultrasound
	■ Amniocentesis
	■ Chorionic villus sampling

Infancy

HEALTH PROMOTION FOCUS	HEALTH SCREENING
Nutrition (breast vs. bottle)	Hearing evaluation
Introduction of solid foods	Screening for birth defects
Placing the infant on her back for sleep without a pillow to reduce the risk of sudden infant death syndrome (SIDS)	Blood work to rule out certain metabolic conditions
	Monthly examinations until at least 6 mo of age
Sensory stimulation	After age 6 mo, visits every 2 or 3 mo
Safety	Growth and development
Motor vehicle safety	Abuse
Oral health	

Toddler and Preschool

HEALTH-PROMOTION FOCUS	HEALTH SCREENING
Adequate supervision	Annual examinations
Safety, including storage of poisons	Growth and development
Toilet training	Cognitive skills
Motor vehicle safety	Abuse
Nutrition	Kindergarten readiness
Immunizations	
Oral health	
Sleep and rest	

School Age

HEALTH-PROMOTION FOCUS	HEALTH SCREENING
Nutrition	Annual examinations
Physical activity	Growth and development
Safety	Cognitive skills
Sexuality	Abuse
Stranger danger	
Oral health	

Table 8-2 ➤ Health Promotion Throughout the Life Span—cont'd

Adolescence

HEALTH-PROMOTION FOCUS	HEALTH SCREENING
Peer pressure	Growth and development
Motor vehicle safety	Sexually transmitted infection (STI) screening
Safety	Breast self-exam (BSE) (optional)
Self-esteem	Testicular self-exam (TSE) (optional)
Physical activity	Mental health
Suicide and depression	Stress
Firearm safety	Alcohol and drug use
Violence	Abuse
Sexuality	
Substance use and abuse	
Limiting sun exposure	
Update of immunizations	
Oral health	

Young Adult

HEALTH-PROMOTION FOCUS	HEALTH SCREENING
Physical activity	Comprehensive exam at least every 3 yr
Motor vehicle safety	Lifestyle
Safety	Pap smear
Violence	STI screening
Sexuality	BSE
Substance use and abuse	TSE
Limiting sun exposure	Mental health
Update immunizations	Stress
Oral health	Alcohol and drug use
	Abuse

Middle Adult

HEALTH-PROMOTION FOCUS	HEALTH SCREENING
Physical activity	Comprehensive exam at least every 3 yr to age 40, yearly after age 40
Safety	Blood pressure (BP) screening
Obesity	Lipid panel
Sexuality	Blood glucose
Lifestyle	Stress
Update of immunizations	Mammograms or thermography
Oral health	Digital rectal exam (DRE) for rectal polyps or prostate evaluation in men
Substance use and abuse	Prostate-specific antigen (PSA) for men
	Annual eye exam
	Sigmoidoscopy or colonoscopy
	Stool for occult blood with comprehensive exam
	Bone density
	Abuse

(Continued)

Table 8-2 ➤ Health Promotion Throughout the Life Span—cont'd	
Older Adult	
HEALTH PROMOTION	**HEALTH SCREENING**
Physical activity	Functional skills (activities of daily living [ADLs] and instrumental activities of daily living [IADLs])
Nutrition	Hearing
Safety	Falls risk
Obesity	Stress
Sexuality	Eye exam and glaucoma screen
Lifestyle	BP screening
Update of immunizations	Lipid panel
Oral health	Blood glucose
	Mammograms
	DRE for prostate evaluation in men
	PSA for men who have a life expectancy of at least 10 yr
	Stool for occult blood
	Bone density
	Follow-up sigmoidoscopy or colonoscopy
	Mental health
	Abuse

Remember that people probably do not refuse to carry out a plan of care simply out of stubbornness, hostility toward healthcare providers, or wanton disregard ♥ iCare for their own welfare. The challenge for nurses is to develop an individualized plan of care in collaboration with patients, based on mutual goals and respect.

ASSESSMENT/IDENTIFY CUES

In looking at an individual's overall wellness, it is easy to focus on the measurable aspects. Physical needs obviously are crucial, but competing issues, including social determinants of health, may be present and cause the client to view the therapeutic interventions as irrelevant or even disruptive.

Health-Promotion Assessment

A health-promotion assessment involves obtaining a health history, physical examination, fitness assessment, lifestyle and risk appraisal, life stress review, analysis of health beliefs, nutritional assessment, and screening activities.

History and Physical Examination

Assessment should begin with a thorough health history, review of body systems, and a physical examination.

- **Health History.** Ask the client about the family history of health disorders and cause of death of family members. Gather the history directly from the client. As always, provide privacy and comfort while conducting the history and examination.
- **Physical Examination.** The level of detail of the physical examination depends on the health history. At a minimum, the examination should include vital signs, weight, body mass index (BMI) or waist circumference, auscultation and palpation of the chest and abdomen, inspection of the skin, and palpation of peripheral pulses.
- **Laboratory Studies.** Recommended laboratory work depends on the history and examination findings. For most adult clients, a screening laboratory consists of a complete blood count, comprehensive metabolic panel, lipid panel, thyroid function panel, and urinalysis (American College of Sports Medicine [ACSM], 2017).
- **Disease-Specific Studies.** In clients with known cardiac or pulmonary disease, additional disease-specific studies may be performed (e.g., electrocardiogram [ECG], carotid ultrasound, or pulmonary function tests).

Physical Fitness Assessment

A physical fitness assessment includes the following:

- Cardiorespiratory fitness is reflected in the ability to perform large-muscle, moderate- to high-intensity exercise for prolonged periods of time (ACSM, 2017).

There are many different modes of testing, such as field tests (walking or running), treadmills, stationary bicycles, and step testing. Results depend on age and gender.

- *Muscular fitness* refers to both muscle strength and endurance. Muscle strength is a measure of the amount of weight a muscle (or group of muscles) can move at one time. *Muscle endurance* refers to the ability of a muscle to perform repeated movements.
- Flexibility is the ability to move a joint through its range of motion. The most common assessment is to evaluate low back and hip (trunk) flexion.

For information and guidelines for assessing physical fitness (cardiorespiratory, muscular, and flexibility),

 Go to **Chapter 8, Assessment Guidelines and Tools, Focused Assessment—Health Promotion: Physical Fitness Assessment**, in Volume 2.

Lifestyle and Risk Appraisal

Lifestyle refers to the manner in which a person conducts their life: physically, emotionally, spiritually, and mentally. Personal habits, recreation, and occupation are part of one's lifestyle. In the context of health and wellness, lifestyle includes all of the activities that promote optimal living, such as taking responsibility for one's health, physical activity, nutrition, interpersonal relations, spiritual growth, and stress management. You can gather this information by interview or by using a variety of questionnaires. A health risk appraisal (HRA) is a questionnaire that evaluates risk for disease based on current demographic data, lifestyle, and health behaviors. There are many HRA tools available; many are online. For one example of an HRA,

 Go to **Chapter 8, Assessment Guidelines and Tools, Focused Assessment: Lifestyle and Risk Assessment**, in Volume 2.

 Think**Like a Nurse** 8-6:
Clinical Judgment **in Action**

- Evaluate your own compliance with recommended health screenings for your age-group. What activities should you incorporate into your own health-promotion plan?
- Answer the questions in the Focused Assessment: Lifestyle and Risk Assessment. How did you score? What additional activities should be added to your health-promotion plan?

Life Stress Review

In 1976, Hans Selye proposed that stress triggers physiological responses that may, over time, induce illness.

Stressful Life-Change Events Likewise, Richard Rahe (1974) identified some stress-inducing life-change events and researched their possible effects on health. Rahe discovered that a high score on a life-change event

scale is associated with a greater likelihood of a negative health change—that is, the more stressful life-change events a person has, the more likely they are to experience a disruption in health. To see and use a life-change event scale,

 Go to the American Institute of Stress Web site at http://www.stress.org/holmes-rahe-stress-inventory/.

Alternatively, you might want to interview your patient to assess the following:

- The patient's belief in their ability to control the experience (e.g., an impending decision, an illness)
- How deeply the patient is involved in the activity that is producing stress (i.e., is it something they can change, or want to change?)
- Whether the patient is able to view such a change as a challenge to grow

Daily Stresses Other researchers have focused on daily stresses and their effects on actual health or on one's perception of health. Daily stresses involve travel to and from work, taking children to activities, daily chores, waiting in lines at shops, raising teenagers, and traffic jams. Researchers have found these stresses may gradually erode one's coping mechanisms, producing an inability to cope with daily events and an increased likelihood of illness.

Hardiness Research has also demonstrated that in the face of life events, some people develop hardiness rather than vulnerability (Abdollahi et al., 2016; Steptoe et al., 2015). Kobasa (1979) identified hardiness as a quality in which an individual experiences high levels of stress yet does not fall ill. There are three general characteristics of the hardy person:

- Control—belief in the ability to control the experience
- Commitment—feeling deeply involved in the activity producing stress
- Challenge—ability to view the change as a challenge to grow

If you need additional information on hardiness, review Chapter 9.

 Think**Like a Nurse** 8-7:
Clinical Judgment **in Action**

- Undoubtedly you are experiencing stress as a student in a nursing program. How would you rate your level of hardiness?
- What statements would demonstrate a hardy personality in each area (commitment, control, challenge)?

Health Beliefs

A health-promotion assessment would not be complete without investigating an individual's health beliefs. Health beliefs are embedded in one's culture and personal experiences. Culture influences beliefs and practices affecting wellness and disease prevention. For example, some people may use certain foods (e.g., garlic to prevent heart disease, orange juice to prevent a cold) or herbs to protect or restore health. Why do you think it is important for you to respect cultural and religious views while working with clients to adopt personal health goals?

Locus of Control It will be helpful to know whether health outcomes are a result of actions the person takes, actions of powerful others, or chance. The Multidimensional Health Locus of Control scale (MHLC) helps you obtain this information (Wallston et al., 1978). The MHLC measures the person's perception of the extent of control from each source. The person rates their level of agreement with statements such as "I am in control of my health," "No matter what I do, if I am going to get sick, I will get sick," and "Regarding my health, I can only do what my doctor tells me to do."

Identifying a patient's locus of control is of practical importance for several reasons:

- People who feel powerless about preventing illness are least likely to engage in health-promotion activities.
- People who respond to direction from respected authorities often prefer a health-promotion program that is supervised by a healthcare provider.
- Clients who feel in charge of their own health are the easiest to motivate toward positive change.

You can find a copy of the MHLC to print out and use with your patients if you

 Go to the University of Miami School of Nursing Web site at https://elcentro.sonhs.miami.edu/research/measures-library/mhlc/index.html

or do a Web search for "Multidimensional Health Locus of Control scale."

Nutritional Assessment

A nutritional assessment is a key component of an overall wellness assessment. Unhealthy eating habits occur across all ages, ethnicities, and socioeconomic classes. Assessment involves an evaluation of typical eating patterns correlated with physical examination findings and BMI. Body composition is important in identifying health risks. The usual methods for determining body fat composition clinically are by measuring height, weight, circumferences, and skinfolds (see Chapter 24 to review these).

The pattern of body fat distribution is an important predictor of health risks. People with fat stored around the trunk and abdominal area have a higher incidence of metabolic syndrome, hypertension, hyperlipidemia, heart disease, type 2 diabetes, and premature death than do those who have fat stored in the extremities (Ashwell & Gibson, 2016).

Health Screening Activities

Health screening activities are secondary prevention activities designed to diagnose specific diseases at an early stage so that treatment can begin before the disease can spread or become debilitating. Many of these screening activities are part of your usual care. For example, each time you check a client's blood pressure, you are performing a screen for hypertension. Table 8-2 identifies the typical health screening activities with each developmental stage. With regard to health screening guidelines, clinicians must take all of the following into consideration when they decide which screening tests to offer to their patients:

1. Different agencies and groups generate different guidelines for the type and frequency of screening. For example, the American Cancer Society has different Pap screening recommendations than the U.S. Preventive Services Task Force (USPSTF); the American Congress of Obstetricians and Gynecologists may have yet another recommendation.
2. Most evidence-based guidelines make use of cost–benefit analysis to arrive at their recommendations.
3. Various third-party payers have different policies regarding the type and frequency of screening for which they will reimburse.
4. Guidelines and recommendations change often.

Lipid Screening Activities
- Adults aged 20 years or older—Have a fasting lipid panel at least once every 5 years. If total cholesterol is 200 mg/dL or greater or high-density lipoprotein (HDL) is less than 40 mg/dL, frequent monitoring is required.
- Children aged 9 to 11 years—Universal screening is recommended, regardless of risk factors for cardiovascular disease (Bibbins-Domingo et al., 2016).
- Children aged 2 to 8 years—Screening is recommended if a parent, grandparent, aunt/uncle, or sibling has a history of myocardial infarction (MI), angina, cerebrovascular accident (CVA), coronary artery bypass graft (CABG)/stent/angioplasty, or hyperlipidemia (Bibbins-Domingo et al., 2016).

Dental Health Screening Clients should have regular dental checkups to detect early signs of oral health problems such as tooth decay, periodontitis (gum disease), and oral cancers.

Colon Cancer Screening For all persons at average risk for colorectal cancer, the American Cancer Society (2018) recommends starting regular screening at age 45. Screening can be a test that looks for signs of cancer in a person's stool (a stool-based test) or an examination that looks at the colon and rectum (a visual examination). If there is a strong family history of colorectal cancer or polyps, screening should begin at an earlier age and be conducted more frequently.

Breast Cancer Screening All female individuals should be familiar with how their breasts normally look and feel and report any changes to a healthcare provider right away. Although research does not show a clear benefit for physical breast examinations done by either a health professional or by patients for breast cancer screening (American Cancer Society, 2018; USPSTF, 2016), female individuals should be encouraged to discuss the risks and benefits of breast self-examination (BSE) and clinical breast examination with their healthcare provider. **Key Points:** *Beginning at age 45 years, individuals at average risk for breast cancer should have the choice to start annual breast cancer screening with mammograms (American Cancer Society, 2018; Kerlikowske et al., 2019).*

Cervical Cancer Screening A Papanicolaou (Pap) smear is used to detect cellular changes in the cervix.

- All female individuals should begin cervical cancer screening at age 21.
- Female individuals between the ages of 21 and 29 should have a Pap test every 3 years. They should not be tested for human papillomavirus (HPV) unless it is needed after an abnormal Pap test result.
- Female individuals between the ages of 30 and 65 should have both a Pap test and an HPV test every 5 years. This is the preferred approach, but it is also okay to have a Pap test alone every 3 years.
- Female individuals older than age 65 who have had regular screenings with normal results should not be screened for cervical cancer. Female individuals who have been diagnosed with cervical precancer should continue to be screened (American Cancer Society, 2018).

Testicular Cancer Screening In spite of the low prevalence of testicular cancer, male individuals should be aware that a lump in the testicle or a feeling of heaviness or swelling in the scrotum could be a sign of testicular cancer and should report these findings to their healthcare provider immediately (American Cancer Society, 2018).

Prostate Cancer Screening The USPSTF (2018) recommends against routine prostate-specific antigen (PSA)-based screening for prostate cancer but understands that some patients may request testing. PSA screening should be done only if it includes shared decision making that enables an informed choice by patients. However, healthcare professionals may consider offering the PSA and digital rectal examination (DRE) yearly to male individuals aged 50 years and older at risk for prostate cancer and with at least a 10-year life expectancy. If there are risk factors, testing should begin at age 40 to 45 years (American Cancer Society, 2018).

Skin Cancer Screening Screen during any health assessment or a specialized dermatological examination.

- A general survey of the skin using the ABCD criteria is a useful approach for assessing for skin malignancy: **A**symmetry, **B**order irregularity, **C**olor variability, **D**iameter greater than 6 mm.
- Rapidly changing lesions are also associated with an increased risk for cancer.

- Any suspicious lesions should be biopsied (Agency for Healthcare Research and Quality, 2014; National Cancer Institute, 2018, updated; Pignone & Bibbins-Domingo, 2017).

KnowledgeCheck 8-5

- Identify at least three common sites for health-promotion activities.
- What assessments are part of a health-promotion assessment?
- What role does stress play in health promotion?

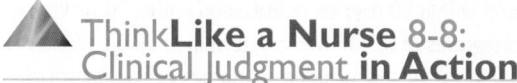

ThinkLike a Nurse 8-8: Clinical Judgment in Action

Your 55-year-old aunt tells you she hasn't had a physical examination in 20 years. She is a registered nurse. "I don't need one because I feel fine, and I can take care of myself." How would you respond?

NURSING DIAGNOSIS/ANALYZING CUES

A health-promotion diagnosis is a clinical judgment about an individual's, family's, group's, or community's motivation and desire to increase well-being and actualize health potential. Such motivation and desire are expressed by readiness to enhance specific health behaviors. The diagnosis can be used in any health state along the wellness–illness continuum. When the patient is unable to express their readiness, the nurse may make the health-promotion diagnosis and act on the patient's behalf (NANDA-I, 2018). NANDA-I health-promotion labels are preceded by the phrase "Readiness for Enhanced" and are now one-part statements with no etiology. Following are some examples of health-promotion diagnoses:

> Readiness for Enhanced Breastfeeding, Readiness for Enhanced Nutrition, and Readiness for Enhanced Self-Concept.

PLANNING/PRIORITIZING HYPOTHESIS/ GENERATING SOLUTIONS

NOC standardized outcomes related to health promotion vary depending on the focus area. For example, if the nursing diagnosis is Readiness for Enhanced Nutrition, an NOC outcome might be Nutritional Status. For examples of other NOC health-promotion outcomes, see the accompanying Standardized Language box.

Individualized goals and outcomes might include losing 20 pounds or exercising for 30 minutes five times per week. **Key Point:** *The nurse's role in health promotion is primarily to motivate clients and facilitate change. Clients are independently responsible for most of their health-promotion activities.* You may need to help them identify goals, but it is essential that the goals be the clients', not yours.

Healthy People 2030 **Goals** You may need aggregate wellness goals for groups as well as individualized goals. The following are four broad goals for the

Toward Evidence-Based Practice

Khalid, S. I., Maasarani, S., Shanker, R. M., Becerra, A. Z., Omotosho, P., & Torquati, A. (2022). Social determinants of health and their impact on rates of postoperative complications among patients undergoing vertical sleeve gastrectomy. *Surgery*, 171(2), 447–452.

This study compared the rate of complications after bariatric surgery in patients with social determinants of health (SDOH) to those without SDOH, specifically on the development of any complication within 60 days or readmission within 30 or 90 days. The five categories of SDOH were determined by the *Healthy People 2020* initiative and included economic, education, social, environmental, and healthcare. A total of 25,387 patients with morbid obesity underwent the surgical procedure during the study period; 9,044 had at least one SDOH, and the remaining 16,343 did not. The findings indicated that patients undergoing bariatric surgery who had at least one type of SDOH had a significantly longer length of stay and had increased rates of

complication (cardiac, wound complications, pneumonia, and/or urinary tract infection, for example). Additionally, the researchers found that patients with at least one type of SDOH were less likely to return for readmission.

1. You may think that postoperative complications would increase the likelihood of readmission; however, the study results demonstrate the opposite in patients with SDOH. From your knowledge about the social determinants of health, can you identify at least three reasons for this finding?

2. How is the SDOH economic instability (employment status, occupational environment, food insecurity, housing instability, or financial hardship) related to the findings in this study?

3. How might you contribute to improving outcomes for patients with SDOH?

U.S. population set by the *Healthy People 2030* initiative (*Healthy People*, n.d.):

- Attain high-quality, longer lives, free of preventable disease, disability, injury, and premature death.
- Achieve health equity, eliminate disparities, and improve the health of all groups.
- Create social and physical environments that promote good health for all.
- Promote quality of life, healthy development, and healthy behaviors in all life stages.

Interventions to achieve these goals are targeted at the health conditions and health behaviors shown in Box 8-3. Public health agencies at the local, state, and federal levels use these focus areas as a blueprint to design programs aimed at improving the health status of the community. To view those objectives,

 Go to the *Healthy People 2030* Web site at https://health.gov/healthypeople/objectives-and-data.

Whether standardized or individualized, expected outcomes for wellness diagnoses describe behaviors or responses that demonstrate health maintenance or achievement of an even higher level of health.

> Example: During the next year, Mr. Needham will continue to eat a balanced diet, with more emphasis on including whole grains and fiber.

By using the highest number (5) on the rating scale, you can use the NOC to write wellness outcomes.

> Example:
> Nursing diagnosis: Readiness for Enhanced Nutrition
> Expected outcome: Nutritional Status: (5) Not compromised

IMPLEMENTATION/TAKING ACTION

Community and public health nurses focus on the problems contributing to disease, such as poor housing conditions, sanitation, and nutrition; poverty; and substance abuse. The wellness focus in acute care is to educate patients about both health and disease.

Once the client identifies their goals, help them to identify the steps that they must take to reach the goals. Change occurs in stages. To create positive change, the client will need to understand the benefits of change, overcome the barriers to change, and make a commitment to follow through on the plan.

NIC does not have a special domain, or grouping, for wellness interventions. Instead, they are found throughout all areas of the taxonomy, particularly in the Behavioral, Safety, Family, Health System, and Community domains. Specific NIC nursing activities for health promotion include those in following subsections: Nutrition, Exercise, and Lifestyle Changes. The remainder of the chapter provides some strategies to promote their use.

Nutrition To guide people in making nutritional choices that promote health and prevent disease, the U.S. Department of Agriculture and the U.S. Department of Health and Human Services (USDHHS) revised the Dietary Guidelines for Americans (you will find these in Chapter 24) to include "MyPlate," a picture of a plate that is divided into four sections—fruits, vegetables, grains, and protein. My Plate is a quick, simple reminder to people to be more mindful of the foods they eat. The symbol is part of a healthy eating initiative that conveys seven key messages:

- Enjoy food but eat less.
- Avoid oversized portions.

BOX 8-3 ■ Topics Areas of *Healthy People 2030*

Health Conditions

1. Addiction
2. Arthritis, osteoporosis, and chronic back conditions
3. Cancer, blood disorders
4. Chronic kidney disease
5. Chronic pain
6. Dementias
7. Diabetes
8. Food safety
9. Healthcare-associated infections
10. Heart disease and stroke
11. Infectious disease
12. Oral conditions
13. Overweight and obesity
14. Pregnancy and childbirth
15. Respiratory diseases
16. Sensory or communication disorders
17. Sexually transmitted diseases

Health Behaviors

1. Child and adolescent development
2. Drug and alcohol use
3. Emergency preparedness
4. Family planning
5. Health communication
6. Injury prevention
7. Nutrition and healthy eating
8. Physical activity
9. Preventive care
10. Safe food handling
11. Sleep
12. Tobacco use
13. Vaccination
14. Violence prevention

Source: U.S. Department of Health and Human Services, Office of Disease Prevention & Health Promotion and Human Services. (n.d.). Healthy People 2030 *topics and objectives.* https://www.healthypeople.gov/2030/topics-objectives

- Make half of the plate fruits and vegetables.
- Drink water instead of sugary drinks.
- Switch to fat-free or low-fat (1%) milk.
- Compare sodium in foods.
- Make at least half your grains whole grains.

Exercise Regular physical activity each week, sustained for months and years, can produce long-term health benefits, including a lower risk for heart disease, stroke, type 2 diabetes, hypertension, high cholesterol, metabolic syndrome, certain types of cancer,

and depression. Regular physical activity also prevents weight gain; improves cardiorespiratory and muscular fitness; prevents falls by increasing muscle tone, strength, and balance, and promotes better memory and cognition in older adults (ACSM, 2017). Encourage physical fitness lifestyle habits in people of all ages and abilities. The most health benefits occur with at least 150 minutes (2 hours and 30 minutes) a week of moderate-intensity physical activity, such as brisk walking. Additional benefits occur with more physical activity. Children and teens should engage in at least 1 hour of age-appropriate physical activity daily. Activity should be vigorous in intensity and varied in type, not only to prevent boredom but also to promote muscle and bone strengthening as well as flexibility (Fig. 8-8).

For more information, do a Web search or,

 Go to the Presidential Youth Fitness Program Web site at https://pyfp.org/

Lifestyle Changes For healthy living, adults and teens must choose a lifestyle without smoking cigarettes or e-cigarettes (vaping) and recreational drugs and with little alcohol. Getting enough sleep and managing stress are also important. In general, adults need 6 to 9 hours of sleep a night. Children need more sleep (see Chapter 31). Inadequate sleep is linked to weight gain and obesity.

Role Modeling

A role model teaches by example, demonstrating the behaviors and/or attitudes to be learned. Models provide inspiration and strategies for health-promotion behavior.

> Example: A morbidly obese female joins an exercise group and wellness group led by a woman who has lost nearly 100 pounds. She admires the leader for her determination and selects her as a role model.

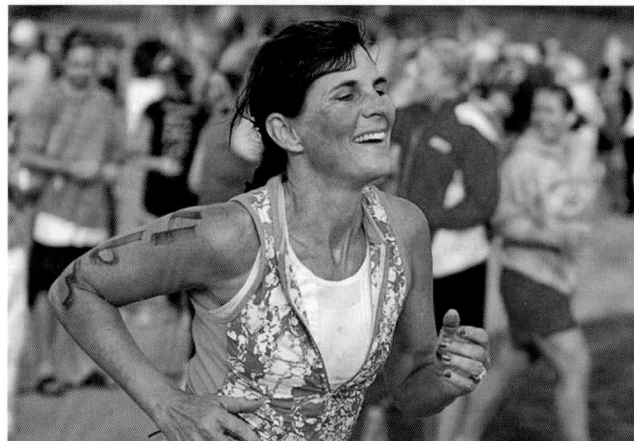

FIGURE 8-8 Vigorous-intensity exercise promotes muscle and bone strength and improves cardiovascular health.

It may be helpful for you to guide the client in choosing a role model and to keep the following in mind:

- Consider the client's age, culture, values, and preferred activities.
- The model should be someone with whom the client identifies.
- Ideally, the role model should be accessible to the client during the early stages of change.

    Example: During the next year, Mr. Needham will continue to eat a balanced diet. This allows for interacting and for exchanging information.

Nurses also serve as role models. Therefore, we should provide an example of healthy behaviors. It is difficult to advocate for healthy behavior if you do not follow the behavior that you recommend to clients. Imagine the trust a client loses when they find out that the nurse who tells him not to smoke cigarettes has a two-pack-per-day habit. To what extent do you model healthy behaviors?

Providing Counseling

Counseling is an interpersonal communication process that helps a client to identify problems and make changes. In the context of health promotion, counseling promotes personal growth and helps clients change their lifestyle. Counseling may be formal or informal, one to one or a small-group discussion, face to face or offered via phone or online. Each meeting with a client is a potential counseling session.

Individual Counseling

Face-to-face interaction may be helpful when clients are attempting a major lifestyle change. In an individual session, you can customize and map out the steps required to meet the client's goals.

- **Contracting.** Counseling may include writing a contract detailing the client's expected behaviors. Print out the contract and have the client sign it to reinforce their commitment. Suggest that the client post the plan in a location where they will see it often so that it serves as a frequent reminder.
- **Reinforcing.** During counseling sessions, remember to reinforce health-promoting behaviors that have already been established. For example, the client who uses e-cigarettes (vapes) may eat a balanced diet; reinforce the healthy habit to boost self-esteem. Stress to the client that you believe the client can succeed in making the desired behavior change.

Using Technology for Counseling

Many different forms of technology may be used as a primary counseling approach or as follow-up. Clients with hectic schedules may find it easier to arrange counseling using their cell phone (talking or texting) or computer than to schedule a face-to-face interaction. One recent study found that providers can offer resources, intervene earlier, and troubleshoot problems while patients are implementing behavior change more readily using

---

PICOT

Health Promotion

Situation: The student has noticed that many of his classmates have gained significant amounts of weight as the program has advanced. In addition, it seems as though there is always someone who is sick in class. Students are complaining about the cost of co-payments and over-the-counter medications. The student wonders whether there are practical ways to improve this situation at his school.

PICOT Components

P	Population/client	=	Young adult students
I	Intervention/indicator	=	Health-promotion information
C	Comparator/control	=	None
O	Outcome	=	Decreased risk of health problems
T	Time	=	None

Searchable Question

Do _____ (P) who receive/are exposed to _____ (I) demonstrate _____ (O) compared with _____ (C) during _____ (T)?

Example of Evidence: The World Health Organization defines health promotion as the process that enables people to improve their own health by improving control over the determinants of health. Health promotion is an important nursing activity. Healthcare spending in the United States exceeded $2 trillion in 2006. America's worsening health habits, particularly obesity, are contributing to this massive growth in spending. Cost-effective health-promotion measures include educating people about preventable health problems such as obesity, diabetes, hypertension, and other chronic diseases. Nursing educators will be at the forefront in evaluating nursing programs and teaching future nurses according to the needs of global health.

Practice Changes: The student talks to his professor about organizing a wellness group to share health-promotion ideas.

Source: Jadelhack, R. (2012). Health promotion in nursing and cost-effectiveness. *Journal of Cultural Diversity, 19,* 65–68.

technology than through traditional phone calls and office visits (Radovic et al., 2018).

- When using technology for counseling, set goals and map out the strategy for change just as you would in face-to-face counseling.
- Let the client know how and when you can be reached if questions arise.
- If you are using technology for follow-up counseling, it is best to schedule a time to speak. Having an appointment helps keep the client accountable to the expected behavior and helps to reinforce the information.

Providing Health Education

- Health education may focus on self-care strategies, caregiver concerns, or how to be an effective healthcare consumer.
  - Self-care programs typically cover nutrition, exercise, stress management, or disease prevention.
  - Caregiver education programs may teach caregivers how to perform nursing tasks or prevent injuries, or they may provide a list of community resources for respite care.
- Programs may consist of lectures, printed material, billboards, or posters. For example, the accompanying Self-Care box, Teaching Clients How to Prevent Upper Respiratory Infections, might be reproduced and posted in the lounge, restrooms, or locker areas of a worksite during the cold and flu season to decrease absenteeism.
- Nurses can teach clients how to be effective healthcare consumers, how to interact with healthcare providers, and how to maneuver through the healthcare system.
- For a review of patient education, see Chapter 16.

Providing and Facilitating Support for Lifestyle Change

Changing one's lifestyle is difficult, and most clients need support to do so. You can provide support during interactions and counseling sessions. You can also help the client to identify available resources within the community and from family, friends, and coworkers.

Group support exists for a variety of lifestyle changes. For example,

- WW®, Noom—for clients who want to lose weight.
- Alcoholics Anonymous—for clients who want to become and stay sober.

Group support provides the opportunity to meet people experiencing the same difficulties and perhaps find a role model. As a nurse, you should be familiar with the various programs available in your community and refer clients to them.

KnowledgeCheck 8-6

Identify four strategies to help a client engage in positive lifestyle changes.

Self-Care

Teaching Clients How to Prevent Upper Respiratory Infections

➤ **Maintain a healthy lifestyle.** That means get adequate sleep, ensure good nutrition, and engage in physical exercise. A balanced diet and physical fitness can boost your immune system to fight infection if it occurs.

➤ **Wash your hands often, and teach children to do so.** This helps prevent the spread of infection.

➤ **When using public restrooms, wash your hands.** Then turn off the faucet with a paper towel. Also use a paper towel to open the door as you leave the room.

➤ **Avoid touching your eyes, nose, and mouth** because doing so spreads any virus your hands have contacted (e.g., on doorknobs).

➤ **Avoid crowds when there is a cold or influenza epidemic.**

➤ **Throw away tissues as soon as you use them.**

➤ **When someone in the family has a cold,** keep bathrooms and the kitchen very clean, and do not drink from the same glass or use the same utensils.

➤ **When someone at home or at work has a cold,** wipe telephone receivers with soap and water or an antibacterial solution.

➤ **If children have a cold,** wash their toys and commonly used items well.

➤ **When choosing childcare, look for a clean environment;** ask what rules the facility or individual has about keeping the children clean (e.g., washing hands before snack time).

➤ **Don't smoke.** Cigarette smoke can irritate the respiratory tract, making you more susceptible to colds and illness.

➤ **Control stress.** People experiencing emotional stress tend to have weakened immunity to fight infection.

➤ **Consider taking echinacea or zinc lozenges,** although conclusive evidence of their effectiveness is not available at this time (Hemilä & Chalker, 2015). Consult your primary healthcare provider.

How Can I Honor Each Client's Unique Experience With Wellness, Health, and Illness?

As a nurse, you can be an instrument for wellness for clients and their families. Health promotion does not come automatically with your nursing license. Nor does it allow you the luxury of learning just one approach and applying it to every client. It means cultivating a holistic presence by listening and, in addition, by:

- Being maximally attentive
- Being aware of your own gifts and limitations of communication

- Being willing to learn from those in your care
- Recognizing and respecting others' ways of coping
- Enjoying others for who they are.

♥ **iCare** Patients may be impressed by your skill and knowledge and amazed by the healthcare technology used to diagnose and treat their illnesses. However, what they most often remember, perhaps throughout the rest of their lives, is that person who connected with them in a very special way. For example, a man who became quadriplegic after a car accident in his teens spoke of a senior nursing student who cared for him during his initial hospitalization. He said that after 26 years, he not only still remembered her but also still could sense the warmth of her caring presence.

During times of vulnerability, people seem acutely attuned to those who are helpful to them and also to those who slight them in hurtful ways, whether intentionally or not. What a challenge this creates for a nurse! In this section, we discuss steps you can take to prepare yourself for responding to your clients in ways that are meaningful to them.

Examine Life's Uncertainties

- **Wellness is a balancing act between living in the mostly known present and the mostly unknown future.** Encourage your clients to make active decisions that positively affect their future. You do not have control over a drunk driver who sails across the median and hits you head-on, but you do have control over getting the brakes on your car fixed or wearing your seat belt. Likewise, you do not know whether you will develop cancer or heart disease, but you can take responsibility for learning and practicing prevention and detection of problems.
- **Making health-promoting lifestyle choices is important, but it cannot protect us from risk.** Significant life experiences, such as getting married, having children, investing in friendships, venturing into business, and selecting a profession, all involve risk. Making a commitment to *anything* is a risk. Each person has a different "risk-comfort range." Some are willing to risk little and have fewer disappointments and less sparkling achievements. To others, security is not as important, and they are comfortable taking greater risks.
- **Life brings both joy and pain.** In *A Severe Mercy*, Sheldon Vanauken (1977) writes about finding and losing a great love. He reasons: "The joy would be worth the pain—if, indeed, they went together. If there were a choice . . . between, on the one hand, the heights and the depths and, on the other hand, some sort of safe, cautious middle way, he, for one, here and now chose the heights and the depths" (p. 9). He did, indeed, find a great love, and when he lost his wife at an early age, he was able to accept their time together as one of his life's greatest blessings.

- **As a nurse, you will face many uncertainties and dilemmas.** You will certainly face new experiences and challenges, situations you thought you would never have to deal with. You will observe pain, suffering, and death. You may never understand the apparent unfairness of it all. But often life brings new meaning when it takes a different direction from the one planned. For example, a couple formerly embittered over their third miscarriage found joy in adopting two children with disabilities.
- **You will also be privileged to witness many joys.** Some might even qualify as minor triumphs: a patient taking their first steps after major surgery, a pathology report that isn't as bad as feared, or even a peaceful death that brings closure to a grieving family. As you move from novice to expert, you may find that such witnessing causes you to stop questioning life's uncertainties and instead start treasuring them.

▲ Think**Like a Nurse** 8-9: Clinical Judgment **in Action**

- What uncertainties have you struggled with?
- What approaches have proved effective for you in dealing with uncertainties?

Envision Wellness for Your Clients and Yourself

Wherever there is a dream, there is someone there to tell you it can't be done, or at least not by you. There is something to be said, however, for "envisioning" wellness for your clients and yourself. Remember Evelyn (Meet Your Patient)? If her nurses had labeled her as debilitated and close to death, how would that have affected her? In contrast, their acceptance of her vision of herself as well and full of life supports her and aids her healing.

In the same way, think of how you view your own health. Is the life you envision for yourself characterized by zest and vigor? What are your family relationships like? What are your values? Does your work give meaning and purpose to your life? The wellness that you envision for yourself can be the blueprint for what you want to become. The skeptic in you might say, "What if I do everything that I know to do to maintain a healthy life and still have a heart attack at 45?"

As we have seen, life is full of uncertainties. That does not mean that you have to stop envisioning. Instead, use **flexible envisioning,** adjusting your goals and dreams to each new reality. Health does not mean always getting your first choice. Part of health is being able to dream a new dream, starting over if you need to but always envisioning that there is something worth striving for.

Establish Trust at Your First Patient Contact

When patients are admitted to a hospital or an ambulatory care facility, you will need to support them in their transition from wellness to illness, in dealing with the unknown, and in adjusting to a new environment. The relationship and trust you establish in your first contact with patients can go a long way toward relieving their anxiety and preserving the energy needed for healing. Take time to get to know your client. Try to set a tone of caring, respect, and understanding.

You can make the transition smoother for patients if you are prepared. The following activities should be incorporated into your nursing care:

- **Prepare the room.** A room that is prepared for the client conveys a message of acceptance. Room preparation depends on the type of unit or facility, the client's needs, and the anticipated treatment.

 Go to Chapter 8, **Clinical Insight 8-1: Preparing the Room for an Admission,** in Volume 2.

- **Greet the client.** Gather basic information ahead of time, such as name, diagnosis, and anticipated length of stay. Imagine how it might feel if you were a new patient and you heard the staff say, "Who's this? I didn't know we were getting an admission. How am I supposed to take care of this one, too?"
- **Introduce yourself to the client and family.** Explain who you are. Don't be afraid to tell a client that you are a nursing student. Many clients are aware that students have more time to spend with them.
- **Orient the client to the room and the unit.** Make sure the client knows how to use the bed, the call light, and any equipment that you expect them to use. Show the client the location of the restroom. If you will be measuring the client's intake and output, tell them so during your orientation. If the client is alert, they may be able to assist you with these measures. Remember that one of the disruptions associated with illness is anxiety about the unknown. If you tell your client what to expect, you help to minimize their anxiety.
- **Gather a health history.** In Chapter 3, you learned about assessment and recognizing cues. Chapter 19 provides a step-by-step approach to physical assessment. Be sure to include the client's expectations and concerns in your health history.
- **Establish a relationship with the client.** Take time to get to know your client. Try to set a tone of caring, respect, and understanding.

For detailed directions on how to admit a client to a hospital unit, including orienting the client to the room and gathering a health history, refer to the Highlights of Procedures box and also

 Go to Chapter 8, **Procedure 8-1: Admitting a Patient to a Nursing Unit,** in Volume 2.

Provide a Healing Presence

♥ **iCare** Part of what you do as a healing presence will never show up in a written care plan. However, your healing presence may be the most important aspect of care that you have to offer. A statement by a young woman undergoing chemotherapy illustrates the difference the healing presence of a nurse made:

> The nursing care I got was in response to the physical symptoms I showed. If I was not feeling good, they were sympathetic with me, you know. . . . But it was nothing further than that. There was no exploration of feelings or anything like that.
>
> Some of them were—seemed to be very caring. I remember [one nurse] . . . but she was just a really nice person. And I remember one time that I was throwing up dreadfully. . . . I rang for her and I said, "I'm sorry," and she was almost crying and she said, "No, I'm sorry you have to do this—you must feel awful." And she was just very empathetic with it, and I felt like, you know, I wasn't infringing upon her to make her empty my emesis basin or anything like that. (Smith, 1992, pp. 233–234)

Maintain Trust During Transitions

Just as you help patients transition into illness, your support is important in helping them transition to other units within the agency, other agencies, or home. As discussed in Chapter 3, planning for discharge begins with the admission assessment and continues until the patient is well enough to go home or is transferred to another unit or facility.

Handoffs and Transfers

Patients may transfer from one unit to another when their health status changes. For example:

- *A patient on a general nursing unit may be transferred to an intensive care unit* when they develop *sepsis* (a generalized, systemic infection that is often fatal).
- *Patients may transfer from the hospital to a long-term care facility or rehabilitation center* when they no longer require an acute care hospital or when their changed health status means that family members will not be able to care for them at home.
- *A patient residing in a long-term care facility may be transferred to a hospital* when they become acutely ill.

When the patient is transferred, they must adjust to a new environment, new routines, and new caregivers. This is yet another disruption for the patient and family. You can help by ensuring the transition is smooth and that there is continuity of care. Ensure the patient's comfort and safety, provide for teaching needs, and communicate with the agency or unit sending or receiving the patient. The process at time of transfer is similar. For detailed information on transfer reports (e.g., "SBAR"), see Chapter 17. Also refer to the accompanying Highlights of Procedures box and,

Go to **Procedure 8-2, Transferring a Patient to Another Unit in the Agency,** and **Procedure 8-3, Transferring a Patient to a Long-Term Care Facility,** in Volume 2.

Discharge From the Healthcare Facility

As much as patients usually look forward to being discharged, this, too, is a disruption. Patients are discharged when the outcomes of care are met. However, they are often dependent on family members for care and treatments they cannot manage alone. The inability to assume self-care can be stressful and anxiety producing. **Key Point:** *Successful discharge planning must begin at the first patient assessment, on admission to the facility.* The same conditions that require a formal discharge plan frequently also indicate the need for referrals for posthospital care in the community. Review Discharge Planning in Chapter 3, as needed.

Procedures for discharge vary among agencies. There may be a discharge planner or case manager to coordinate the transition to another agency or to home, but often you will need to manage the discharge. You can help by communicating and coordinating care and services and by teaching the patient and caregivers about the continuing care the patient needs. For more information, see the accompanying Highlights of Procedures box and,

 Go to **Procedure 8-4, Discharging a Patient From the Healthcare Facility; Forms, Discharge Assessment/ Instructions;** and **Patient Education Form,** in Volume 2.

KnowledgeCheck 8-7

Explain how you can promote patient trust during admissions, transfers, and discharges.

ThinkLike a Nurse 8-10: Clinical Judgment in Action

- How can you use the concepts of health when you are admitting a patient to a hospital setting? To a clinic? To an emergency department? To a rehabilitation or long-term care setting? In initiating home care?
- What questions can you ask or what observations can you make to help you gain information about individuals' health strategies, disruptions to health, and factors contributing to their responses to disruptions?
- How would you consider health concepts in planning for patients' discharge from healthcare settings?

Is a Healthy Life Attainable?

The concepts suggested in this chapter as ways to live a healthy life did not come from people who had easy lives. These themes were teased from literature, autobiographies, and interviews with people who were dealing with life situations that would be viewed as difficult from anyone's standpoint. However, in the midst of

---

Highlights of Procedures 8-1 Through 8-4

For steps to follow in all procedures, refer to the Universal Steps for All Procedures found on the inside back cover of Volume 2. Go to the full procedures in Volume 2 to practice and learn the skill. Use these Procedure Highlights later to help you review key steps.

Procedure 8-1 Admitting a Patient to a Nursing Unit

➤ Begin the admission: Introduce yourself, assist the patient into a hospital gown, weigh them, assist them into the bed.

➤ Validate patient identity.

➤ Obtain a translator, if needed.

➤ Complete the nursing assessment, including vital signs; validate the admission list of medications.

➤ Provide information: room, equipment, routines, Health Insurance Portability and Accountability Act (HIPAA), nurse call system, and advance directives.

➤ Answer any questions.

➤ Provide printed information.

➤ Complete nursing admission paperwork according to agency policy.

➤ Complete or ensure that admission orders have been completed.

➤ Inventory the patient's belongings; send home or lock up valuables.

➤ Finish the admission process.

  ➤ Ensure patient comfort (water, positioning, pain).

  ➤ Make one last safety check: call light, bed position, siderails.

  ➤ Ask: "Is there anything else I can do for you?"

Procedure 8-2 Transferring a Patient to Another Unit in the Agency

➤ Make a final, brief, focused assessment.

➤ Plan ahead the amount of help needed.

➤ Schedule the time of the transfer.

➤ Make appropriate notifications.

➤ Gather and label patient medications.

➤ Gather the patient's belongings, supplies, and treatment equipment.

➤ Bring the transfer vehicle to the bedside.

➤ Transfer the patient to the new room.

➤ Give oral handoff report and make final nursing notes entry.

Highlights of Procedures 8-1 Through 8-4

Procedure 8-3 Transferring a Patient to a Long-Term Care Facility

➤ Plan in advance: Notify the patient and family of the impending transfer.

➤ Prepare the patient's records; copy for the new facility if needed.

➤ Pack personal items and treatment supplies.

➤ Coordinate the transfer with the receiving facility and other hospital departments.

➤ Make the final assessment; document and sign.

➤ Move the patient to the transportation vehicle.

➤ Give an oral or telephone report to the receiving nurse; use standardized form if available.

➤ Notify the long-term care facility if the patient is colonized or infected with methicillin-resistant *Staphylococcus aureus* (MRSA) or other contagious microorganisms.

Procedure 8-4 Discharging a Patient From the Healthcare Facility

➤ Notify the patient and family well in advance of the discharge.

➤ A day or two before discharge:

Arrange for or confirm: transportation and services and equipment needed at home.

Make referrals.

Provide teaching about the patient's condition and medications.

Provide training in use of equipment.

Ask the caregiver to bring clothing for the patient to wear home.

➤ Day of discharge:

Make and document final assessments.

Confirm that the patient has house keys, heat is turned on, and food is available.

Make final notifications (community agencies, transportation).

Gather and pack the patient's personal items and treatment supplies.

Label and give take-home medications to the patient.

Give the patient prescriptions, instruction sheets, and appointment cards.

Review discharge instructions with the patient.

Answer questions.

Document the final nursing note and complete the discharge summary.

Accompany the patient out of the hospital.

Notify the admissions department of the discharge.

Ensure records are sent to the medical records department.

---

their circumstances, they were very much involved in *living*. Ripples or even waves of disruption or despair came into their lives, but through it all, they evolved an overriding sense of a life worth pursuing. This can be true for you as a nurse and also for those privileged to be under your care.

As a nurse, you offer your personal health and strength to your patients and their families every day. If you barely have enough physical, emotional, and spiritual strength to manage your own stressors, you will not have much available to offer others who are depleted. This is why it is so important for you to nurture yourself in all aspects of your life, to balance learning how to care for others with caring for yourself, to develop yourself as a healing presence in this world.

To explore learning resources for this chapter,

  Go to Davis Advantage **and find:**

Answers and Suggested Responses for all questions in this chapter

Concept Map

Knowledge Map

References and Bibliography

CHAPTER 9

Stress & Adaptation

Learning Outcomes

After completing this chapter, you should be able to:

➤ Define *stress*.

➤ Explain the difference between adaptive and maladaptive coping strategies.

➤ Explain the relationship between stressors, responses, and adaptation.

➤ Compare and contrast the stages of Selye's general adaptation syndrome (GAS) with the local adaptation syndrome (LAS), including both physical and psychological changes that occur.

➤ Describe physical changes occurring during the three stages of Selye's GAS.

➤ Discuss the inflammatory response: What triggers it, and what physiological changes occur?

➤ Explain how anxiety, fear, and anger relate to stress.

➤ Describe the specific psychological responses to stress, and discuss their relationships to the concept of stress.

➤ Provide examples and definitions of specific ego defense mechanisms.

➤ Briefly describe hypochondriasis, somatization, somatoform pain disorder, and malingering.

➤ Describe the physiological effects of prolonged stress and unsuccessful adaptation on the various body systems.

➤ Compare and contrast crisis and burnout.

➤ State three ways in which you could assess for each of the following: (1) stressors and risk factors, (2) coping methods and adaptation, (3) physiological responses to stress, (4) emotional and behavioral responses to stresses, (5) cognitive responses to stress, and (6) adequacy of support systems.

➤ Plan interventions or activities for preventing and managing stress.

Key Concepts

Adaptation

Coping

Stress

Related Concepts

See the Concept Map on Davis Advantage.

Example Client Conditions

Panic

Post-traumatic stress disorder (PTSD)

Meet Your Patients

Gloria and her husband, John, live in a residential community, from which John commutes to work in a nearby city. Gloria works as a certified public accountant from home. They have two teenage boys who need transportation to many extracurricular activities. Gloria and John teach Sunday school and are Eagle Scout leaders. Gloria's mother needs knee replacement surgery and cannot take care of Gloria's father, who has advanced Alzheimer disease. In addition to her own home responsibilities, Gloria must go to her parents' home to prepare meals and to provide care for them during the day. Gloria's sister sleeps in the parents' home during the night.

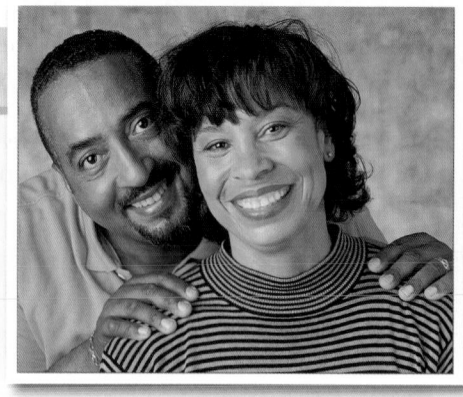

TheoreticalKnowledge
knowing why

Everyone experiences stress as a part of daily life, but we each perceive and respond to stress in our own unique way. Failure to adapt to stress has been linked to several physical and mental illnesses. You will encounter many stressful situations in your career, so you must develop healthful ways of responding and adapting.

ABOUT THE KEY CONCEPTS

The two overarching concepts for this chapter are **stress** and **adaptation.** To help you grasp those concepts, we present definitions and examples, as well as numerous subconcepts that relate to health and illness in various ways. Another important concept is **coping.** As a nurse, you need to understand stress and related concepts to help your clients cope effectively with anxiety and fear.

WHAT IS STRESS?

Stress is any disturbance in a person's normal balanced state. A **stressor** is a stimulus that the person perceives as a challenge or physical or emotional threat; it disturbs the person's sense of well-being by initiating a physical or emotional response. When stress occurs, it produces voluntary and involuntary **coping responses** aimed at reducing tension, pressure, or emotional strain. The changes that take place because of effective coping are called **adaptations.** We can also define *adaptation* as an ongoing effort to maintain external and internal equilibrium, or **homeostasis.**

Stress is not necessarily bad. It can keep you alert and motivate you to perform at a higher level. However, if you become too anxious, you may not be able to think clearly or focus on the task.

Types of Stressors

Stressors are commonly categorized in the following ways.

Distress/Eustress **Distress** threatens health; **eustress** (literally, "good stress") is protective. For example, a passionate kiss can produce as strong of a stress response as a slap in the face. Likewise, the Holmes–Rahe stress scale has similarly high scores for both marriage and divorce.

External/Internal Stressors may be **external** to the person, for example, the death of a family member, a hurricane, or even something as simple as excessive heat in a room. Stressors may also be **internal,** for example, diseases, anxiety, nervous anticipation of an event, or negative self-talk.

Developmental Stressors Developmental stressors can be predicted to occur at various stages of a person's life.

For example, most young adults face the stress of leaving home and beginning work as an independent adult, and many middle-aged adults may feel the demands of aging parents or even accepting their own physical changes. In a sense, developmental stressors may be easier to cope with because they are gradual and expected, and the person has time to prepare for them. For theoretical knowledge about developmental stages, refer to the theories of Erikson and Havighurst in Chapter 6.

See Box 9-1 for examples of developmental stressors.

Situational Stressors Situational stressors are temporary and typically unpredictable. For instance, you cannot anticipate or even control an automobile accident, a natural disaster, job conflict, or an illness. This type of stressor can occur at any life stage. There are also situational stressors that may also lead to a positive outcome, such as a wedding, job promotion, or family event.

Time Stressors Time stressors can lead to unsettled feelings or even fear or anxiety about the lack of opportunity to manage all the things that you have to do. Common examples of time stress include worrying about managing multiple demands or rushing to avoid being late for work or an appointment.

Anticipatory Stressors Anticipatory stressors are those that you experience concerning the future. Sometimes this stress can be focused on a specific event, such as an upcoming examination or clinical day. Anticipatory stress can also be undefined, such as a vague sense of concern about the future or a feeling that something will go wrong.

Physiological Stressors Physiological stressors affect body structure or function. You can categorize them as follows; a few examples are given for each category:

Chemical—environmental toxins, medications, tobacco
Physical or mechanical—trauma, cold, joint overuse
Nutritional—vitamin deficiency, high-fat diet
Biological—viruses, bacteria
Genetic—inborn errors of metabolism
Lifestyle—obesity, sedentary lifestyle

Psychosocial Stressors Psychosocial stressors are external stressors that arise from work, family dynamics, living situation, social relationships, financial strain, and other aspects of our daily lives. The Holmes–Rahe Social Readjustment Scale contains examples of psychosocial stressors.

KnowledgeCheck 9-1

Refer to the Meet Your Patients scenario at the beginning of the chapter.

- What are Gloria's stressors? Classify each of them as follows: (1) Are they physiological or psychosocial? (2) Are they developmental or situational?
- What are John's stressors?

BOX 9-1 ■ Stressors Throughout the Life Span

The following are common developmental stressors. Not everyone will experience these stressors.

Childhood

School-age children may also experience stressors at school or among peers; however, children's stressors occur primarily in the home:

- Absence of parental figures
- Failure of parents to meet needs for safety, security, love, and belonging
- Failure of parents to meet basic physiological needs for oxygen, food, elimination, rest, and cleanliness

Adolescence

- Exposure to an expanded environment and a wider circle of friends and acceptance by peers
- Rapid changes in body appearance
- Need for academic achievement, sports performance, or demonstration of other talents
- Peer pressure
- Maintaining self-esteem while searching for identity
- Decisions about the future in the areas of school, work, and relationships
- Conflicts between standards for behavior and the sex drive
- Decisions about alcohol and drugs

Young Adult

- Separation from family, starting college or a job
- Making the transition from youth to adult responsibilities
- Preparing for careers: graduation from college, learning a trade
- Establishing career goals and planning how to achieve success and career stability
- Financial stressors around relationships and providing a home for self or family

- Parenting children
- Conflicts between responsibilities for work and family or other relationships

Middle Age

- Concern with career achievement and continuing career challenges
- Continuation of child-rearing, marriage of the children, grandparenting
- Changes in appearance and health due to aging
- Dealing with numerous responsibilities (e.g., children, work, older parents, community activities)
- Empty-nest syndrome when the children leave home
- Being "sandwiched" between caring for aging parents as well as children or grandchildren
- "Midlife crisis"—time of transition when men and women may struggle with identity, goal attainment, and the concept of remaining time within the life span. Coping with aging in the middle-adult years may be characterized by a desire for change or excessively youthful behavior, dress, and attitude.

Older Adults

- Loss of family and friends due to illness or death, resulting in loneliness and isolation
- Changes in physical appearance and functional abilities, including mobility
- Major life changes (e.g., retirement, loss of life partner)
- Health issues with accompanying discomfort or pain
- The cost of healthcare
- Change in financial status
- Reduced level of independence
- Reduction in social status
- Alcohol abuse or dependence

Models of Stress

Some theorists (Lazarus & Folkman, 1984) conceptualize stress as a complex, dynamic, and reciprocal exchange between person and environment. Other theorists (Holmes & Rahe, 1967) view stress solely as a stimulus that causes psychological or physiological responses that in turn increase vulnerability to disease. Hans Selye (1974, 1976) found that physical, emotional, psychological, and spiritual stressors, or the anticipation of a stressor (as in anxiety), can initiate nonspecific physiological *responses*. Selye defined these responses as stress.

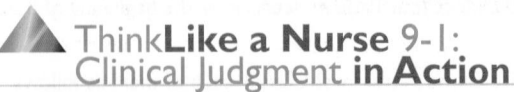

ThinkLike a Nurse 9-1:
Clinical Judgment in Action

- Make a list of your own stressors in the following areas: work, school, family, and living situation.
- What physiological stressors do you have?

HOW DO COPING AND ADAPTATION RELATE TO STRESS?

Coping strategies are the thoughts and behaviors a person uses to manage stressors. Coping strategies can be adaptive or maladaptive.

Adaptive (effective) coping involves making healthy choices that reduce the negative effects of stress (e.g., exercising to relieve tension; engaging in hobbies or sports; seeking support or advice). The difference between effective and ineffective coping may be in the extent to which a technique is used (for examples, see the Ego Defense Mechanisms section later in this chapter).

Maladaptive (ineffective) coping does not promote adaptation. Unhealthful coping choices include overeating, working too much, oversleeping, and substance abuse. Although a maladaptive behavior may temporarily relieve anxiety, this response may have other harmful effects. For example, a person who uses tobacco to relieve the tensions of a stressful work situation may experience an immediate decrease in anxiety but with long-term risks to health (e.g., cardiorespiratory disease).

Three Common Approaches to Coping

People use three approaches to cope with stress, at different times and in various combinations:

- **Altering the stressor.** In some situations, a person takes action to remove or change the stressor.
- **Adapting to the stressor.** It is not always possible to remove or change a stressor. Adaptation involves adjusting one's thoughts or behaviors related to the stressor. As Gloria (Meet Your Patients) gains experience as a caregiver, she may find more efficient, less stressful ways to care for her parents.
- **Avoiding the stressor.** Sometimes it is healthful to avoid a stressor. In other situations, avoidance may be maladaptive. For example, a woman who discovers a lump in her breast fears that she may have cancer. She copes with her anxiety by putting it out of her mind and avoids seeking medical care, perhaps making later treatment less effective.

The Outcome of Stress: Adaptation or Disease

Successful adaptation allows for normal growth and development and effective responses to changes and challenges in daily life. The outcome depends on the balance between the strength of the stressors and the effectiveness of the person's coping methods (Fig. 9-1). In the following equation, **E** is the event (stressor), **R** is the person's response (which is determined in part by past experiences, their perception of the stressor, and coping methods used), and **O** is the outcome:

Outcome:

E	+	R	=	O
stressful event		response (experience, perception, coping methods)		outcome (adaptation or disease)

Some events produce more stress than others. However, a person with good coping skills can usually adapt to a single stressful event, even a demanding one. But suppose several stressors occur in a short period of time. As with Gloria (Meet Your Patients), when there are many stressors or when stressors continue for a long period of time, adaptation is more likely to fail, with fatigue, despair, and depleted resources for coping.

Personal Factors Influence Adaptation

Why do some people succumb to overwhelming stress, whereas others adapt and thrive? Successful adaptation does not depend entirely on being able to alter or avoid stressors. Various personal factors also influence the outcome.

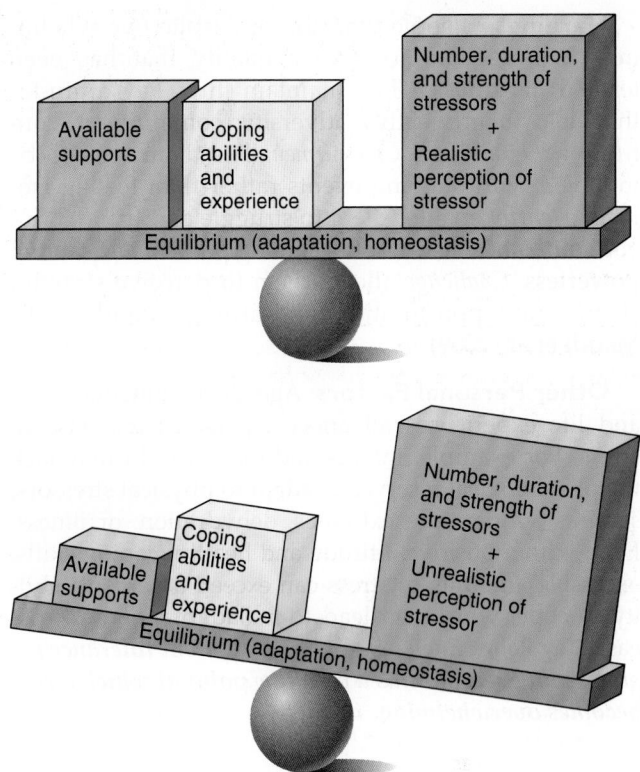

FIGURE 9-1 Adaptation occurs when a person has supports and coping abilities adequate to enable them to deal with the stressors. A realistic perception of the stressful event promotes adaptation, whereas an unrealistic perception makes adaptation more difficult.

Perception of the Stressor A person's perception may be realistic or exaggerated. Suppose two patients with similar coping skills and support systems both must have a mastectomy. One thinks, "Yes, I am losing a part of my body, but I am more than just my breasts. I am so grateful just to be alive." The other thinks, "I will be so ugly. I'll feel like less of a person after this." Which patient do you think is more likely to adapt successfully to this change in their body?

Overall Health Status Stressors may cause a healthy person to engage in constructive adaptive behaviors that improve health. For example, a person with high blood pressure may cope with this health stressor by modifying their diet and engaging in physical activity. However, if this same person is also coping with chronic pain and immobility, they may be too overwhelmed and exhausted to take action to lower blood pressure.

Support System Friends, family, faith-based groups, or people who share common interests often support each other in times of difficulty. A good support system can help a person adapt to stress and solve problems—for example, by providing emotional support, encouraging expression of feelings, and providing financial and other support. Talking to another caring person, whether it be a friend who is a good listener or a professional counselor, can help to release hormones that reduce stress.

Hardiness People who thrive despite overwhelming stressors tend to have a quality that has been termed **hardiness.** They maintain three key attitudes that help them weather adversity: commitment, control, and challenge. *Commitment* lets them seek to be involved with ongoing events rather than feeling isolated. *Control* enables them to struggle and try to influence outcomes instead of becoming passive and feeling powerless. *Challenge* allows them to perceive stressful changes as opportunities for learning (Maddi, 2002; Maddi et al., 2009).

Other Personal Factors Age, developmental level, and life experiences all affect a person's response to stress. For example, infants and the very old may lack the physiological reserves to adapt to physical stressors, such as temperature extremes, dehydration, or illness. Even with a positive attitude and healthy coping skills, excessive amounts of stress can exceed a person's ability to cope, which can lead to maladaptation and disease. **Key Point:** *Each person has a different tolerance for stress, but everyone has a breaking point at which stress becomes overwhelming.*

KnowledgeCheck 9-2

- True or False: The difference between adaptive and maladaptive coping is that maladaptive coping does not relieve stress.
- In addition to avoiding the stressor, what are two other approaches to coping?
- (Complete the sentence.) The outcome of stress (adaptation or disease) depends on the balance among the strength, number, and duration of the stressors and _____.

HOW DO PEOPLE RESPOND TO STRESSORS?

Although Selye's (1974, 1976) response-based model acknowledges physical, emotional, psychological, and spiritual *stressors*, his ideas about responses *(stress)* are primarily physiological. The body has various mechanisms for regulating its internal environment to maintain a balanced state, or homeostasis. Selye described the physiological responses to stress as either the general adaptation syndrome (GAS) or the local adaptation syndrome (LAS).

The General Adaptation Syndrome Includes Nonspecific, Systemic Responses

Would you be surprised to know that a near-miss automobile accident and kicking the winning field goal at a football game would both produce the same general body responses? Responses to stress involve the whole body, especially the autonomic nervous system and the endocrine system. The **general adaptation syndrome (GAS)** is Selye's name for the group of nonspecific responses that all people share in the face of stressors. The GAS has three stages: (1) the initial alarm stage, (2) resistance (adaptation), and (3) the final stage of either recovery or exhaustion (Fig. 9-2).

Alarm Stage—Fight or Flight

Has someone ever playfully grabbed you from behind and shouted, "Boo"? How did you feel? If you haven't had such an experience, think back to a time when something else startled you. Did your heart pound? Did you breathe fast? Was there a flutter in your stomach? Did your muscles tighten? What were your emotions? Did you want to run away, or were you "frozen"? That exercise in imagination should help you to understand the experience of the alarm stage. The alarm stage has two phases: shock and countershock.

- The **shock phase** begins when the cerebral cortex first perceives a stressor and sends out messages to activate the endocrine and sympathetic nervous systems. A surge of epinephrine (adrenaline) and various other hormones prepares the body for *fight* or *flight.* The shock phase usually lasts less than 24 hours, sometimes only a minute or two.
- In the **countershock phase,** changes produced in the shock phase are reversed, and the person becomes less able to deal with the immediate threat.

Various body systems produce responses when a stressor is perceived. See Figures 9-3, 9-4, and 9-5.

Endocrine System Responses In response to a perceived stressor, the following endocrine responses occur:

1. The *hypothalamus* releases corticotropin-releasing hormone (CRH).
2. *CRH,* together with messages from the cerebral cortex, directs the pituitary gland to release adrenocorticotropic hormone (ACTH) and antidiuretic hormone (ADH).
3. *ACTH* stimulates the adrenal cortex to produce and secrete glucocorticoids (especially cortisol) and mineralocorticoids (especially aldosterone).
   - *Cortisol,* in general, has a glucose-sparing effect. It increases the use of fats and proteins for energy and conserves glucose for use by the brain. Cortisol also has an anti-inflammatory effect. See Figure 9-3 for the effects of cortisol during the alarm reaction of the GAS.
   - *Aldosterone* promotes fluid retention by causing the kidneys to reabsorb more sodium. In that way, it helps to increase fluid volume and maintain or increase blood pressure.
4. *ADH* also promotes fluid retention by increasing the reabsorption of water by kidney tubules. See Figure 9-4 for the effects of aldosterone and ADH.
5. *Endorphins,* secreted by the hypothalamus and posterior pituitary, act like opiates to produce a sense of well-being and reduce pain.

General Adaptation Syndrome

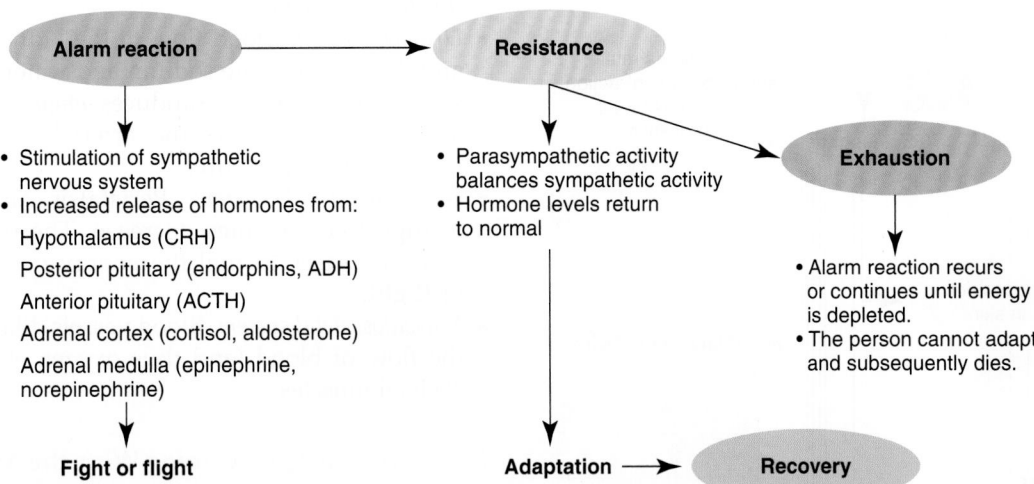

FIGURE 9-2 The stages of Selye's general adaptation syndrome (GAS) are (1) alarm (also called "fight or flight"); (2) resistance (or adaptation), in which the body enacts physical and psychological adaptive mechanisms to maintain homeostasis; and (3) either recovery or exhaustion (which usually ends in disease or death).

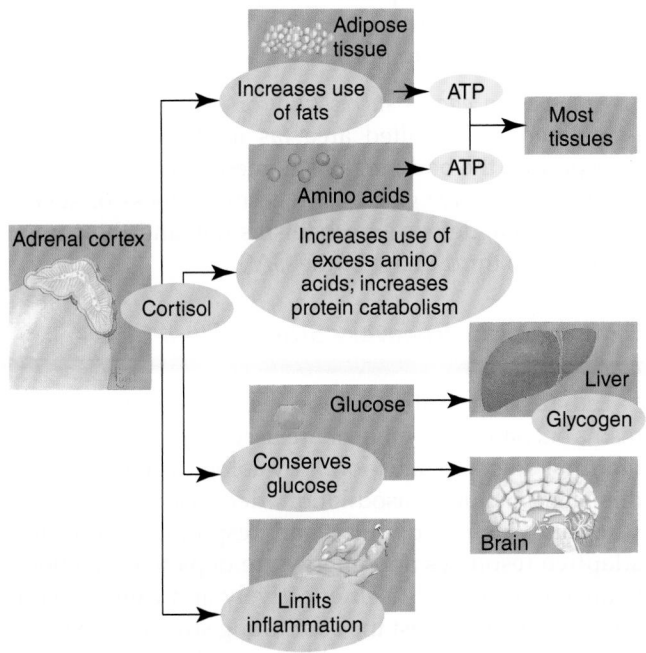

FIGURE 9-3 Functions of cortisol during the alarm stage of the general adaptation syndrome.

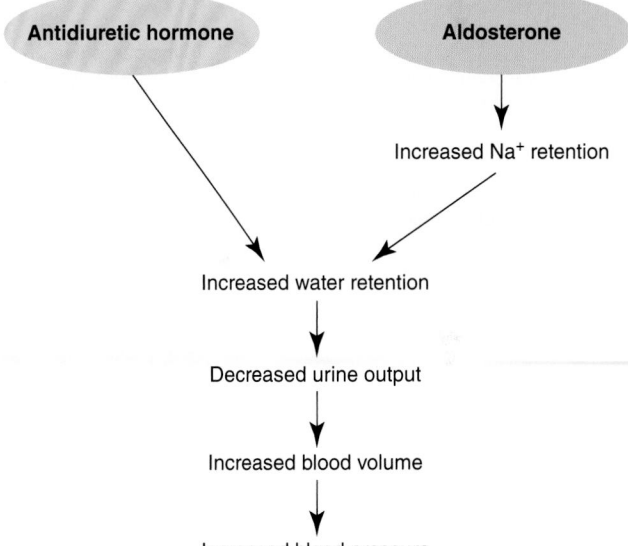

FIGURE 9-4 The release of antidiuretic hormone (from the posterior pituitary gland) and aldosterone (from the adrenal cortex) leads to sodium and water retention, increases blood volume, and increases blood pressure.

6. *Thyroid-stimulating hormone (TSH)* is secreted by the pituitary gland to increase the efficiency of cellular metabolism and fat conversion to energy for cell and muscle needs.

Sympathetic Nervous System Responses The cerebral cortex also sends messages via the hypothalamus to stimulate the sympathetic nervous system. The sympathetic nervous system then stimulates the adrenal glands to secrete adrenaline and norepinephrine,

which increase mental alertness. This allows the person to assess the situation and aids in a decision to stand and fight or run away in flight. Adrenaline also increases the ability of the muscles to contract and causes the pupils to dilate, producing greater visual fields. See Figure 9-5 for the effects of adrenaline during the alarm reaction of the GAS.

Other Body System Responses in the Alarm Stage The following are some body system responses

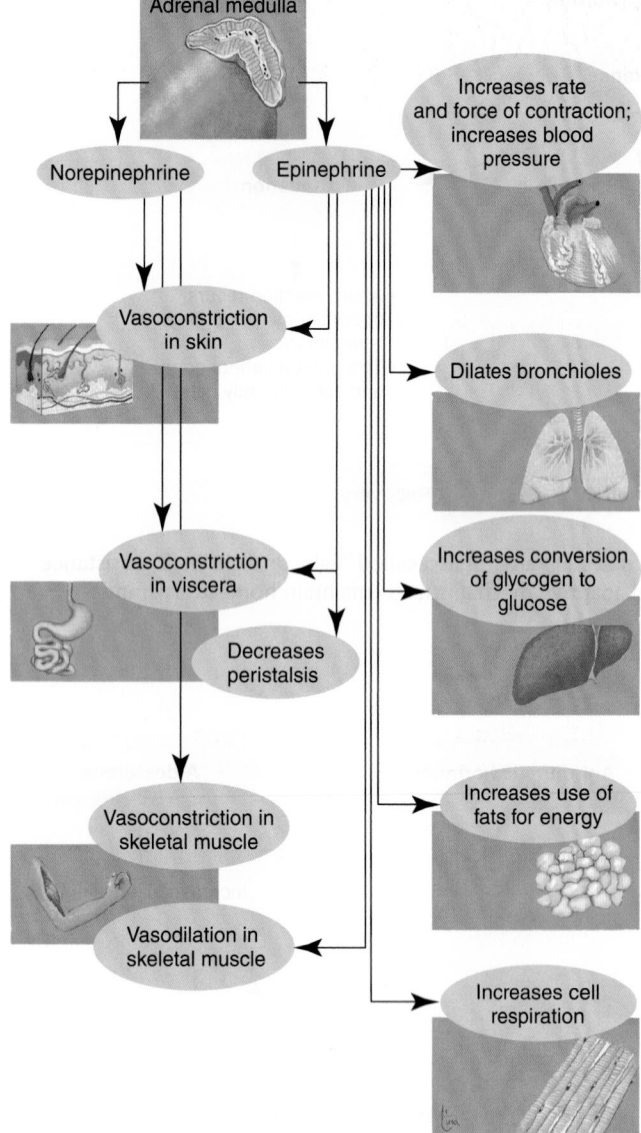

FIGURE 9-5 Functions of epinephrine and norepinephrine during the alarm stage of the general adaptation syndrome.

that occur in the alarm stage because of endocrine and sympathetic nervous system activity. Refer to Figures 9-2 through 9-5 to see how these changes are produced.

- *Cardiovascular system.* Heart rate and the force of heart contractions increase. Peripheral and visceral vaso-constriction increase blood flow to vital organs (e.g., brain, heart, lungs) and to muscles preparing for flight. Blood volume and blood pressure also increase, and the blood clots more readily.
- *Respiratory system.* The bronchioles dilate, thereby increasing the depth of respiration and tidal volume. This makes oxygen available for delivery to muscle, brain, and cardiac cells.
- *Metabolism.* The rate of energy expenditure increases. The liver converts more glycogen to glucose (*glycogenolysis*), making it available for fuel. Except in the brain, the body uses less glucose for energy. The use

of amino acids and the mobilization of fats for energy (*lipolysis*) increase.
- *Urinary system.* Blood flow to the kidneys decreases, and they retain more sodium and water. The kidneys secrete renin, which produces *angiotensin.* In turn, angiotensin constricts the arterioles and tends to increase blood pressure.
- *Gastrointestinal system.* Peristalsis and secretions of digestive enzymes decrease. The blood glucose level increases to fuel the energy needed for fight or flight.
- *Musculoskeletal system.* Blood vessels dilate, increasing the flow of blood (and thus oxygen and energy) to skeletal muscles.

Resistance Stage—Coping With the Stressor

During the second stage of the GAS, resistance (or adaptation), the body tries to cope, protect itself against the stressor, and maintain homeostasis. Stabilization involves the use of physiological and psychological coping mechanisms. Psychological defense mechanisms for coping are discussed in a subsequent section of this chapter. Physical adaptations help the heart rate, blood pressure, cardiac output, respiratory function, and hormone levels return to normal.

- *If the person adapts successfully* or if the stress can be confined to a limited area (as in the inflammatory response), the body regains homeostasis.
- *If the stress is too great* (as in serious illness or severe blood loss), defense mechanisms fail, and the person enters the third phase of the GAS.

Exhaustion or Recovery Stage—Final Effort to Adapt

Exhaustion If stress continues and adaptive mechanisms become ineffective or are used up, a person enters the final stage, exhaustion. Physiological responses in this stage include vasodilation, decreased blood pressure, and increased pulse and respirations. Physical adaptive resources and energy are depleted. The body is unable to defend itself effectively and cannot maintain resistance against the continuing stressors. Exhaustion usually ends in injury, illness, or death.

Recovery In contrast, if adaptation is successful, the final stage is **recovery;** for example, after a miscarriage, a couple participates in a support group and begins to focus more deeply on their relationship with each other. They are able gradually to resolve their grief.

KnowledgeCheck 9-3

- In general, what is the difference between the alarm stage and the resistance stage of the GAS?
- Name the gland that releases each of the following hormones in response to stress, and name each hormone's function: CRH, ADH, ACTH, aldosterone, cortisol, epinephrine, and norepinephrine.

- In the alarm stage of the GAS, what are the effects of the sympathetic nervous system on each of the following: heart, brain, glycogen stores, and skeletal muscle?
- What is the effect of Selye's resistance stage on the cardiovascular and respiratory systems? On hormone levels?

The Local Adaptation Syndrome Involves Specific Local Responses

Whereas the GAS is a whole-body response to a stressor, the LAS is a localized body response; that is, it involves only a specific body part, tissue, or organ. It is a short-term attempt to restore homeostasis. The two most common LAS responses you will deal with as a nurse are the reflex pain response and the inflammatory response. Others include blood clotting and pupil constriction in response to light.

Reflex Pain Response

When you perceive a painful stimulus, especially in one of your limbs, you immediately and unconsciously withdraw from the source of pain. If you've ever accidentally touched a hot stove, you certainly did not stop to ponder, "Hmmm, I think I will withdraw my hand"— you pulled your hand away before you could even think about it. This is a protective reflex, an involuntary, predictable response. Pain receptors send sensory impulses to the spinal cord, where they synapse with the spinal motor neurons. The motor impulses travel back to the site of stimulation, causing the flexor muscles in the limb to contract. This is a local, rather than a whole-body, response.

Inflammatory Response

The inflammatory response is a local reaction to cell injury, either by pathogens or by physical, chemical, or other agents (Box 9-2). **Key Point: *Regardless of the injuring agent (stressor), its mechanisms are the same, and they produce the classic symptoms of inflammation: pain, heat, swelling, redness, and loss of function.*** The inflammatory process includes a vascular response, a cellular response, the formation of exudate, and healing.

Vascular Response Immediately after injury, blood vessels at the site constrict (narrow) to control bleeding. The following also occur:

- *Response:* The injured cells release histamine.
    Effect: Local vessels dilate, increasing blood flow to the area **(hyperemia).**
- *Response:* The dying cells release kinin.
    Effect: Capillaries become more permeable, allowing fluid to move from capillaries into tissue spaces. This results in tissue **edema** (swelling).
- *Response:* **Leukocytes** (white blood cells) move into the area.
    Effect: Localized blood flow again decreases to keep white blood cells in the area to fight infection.

BOX 9-2 ■ Agents Causing Inflammatory Responses

The following agents stimulate the inflammatory response by causing cell injury:

- Autoimmune disorders
- Antigen–antibody responses
- Body substances (e.g., digestive enzymes leaking into the abdomen; accumulation of uric acid crystals in joints)
- Chemical injury (e.g., acid or alkali burns)
- Ischemia
- Neoplastic growth (i.e., cancer)
- Pathogens (e.g., bacteria, viruses)
- Physical agents:
    - Heat or cold
    - Radiation
    - Electrothermal injury
    - Mechanical trauma (e.g., abrasion, contusion, laceration, puncture, incision, fractures, sprains)

Cellular Response Specialized white blood cells **(phagocytes)** migrate to the site of injury and engulf bacteria, other foreign material, and damaged cells and destroy them. Sometimes they form a "wall" around an invading pathogen. The accumulation of dead white blood cells, digested bacteria, and other cell debris in the presence of infection is called *pus.*

Exudate Formation The fluid and white blood cells that move from the circulation to the site of injury are called **exudate.** The nature and quantity of exudate depend on the severity of injury and the tissues involved. For example, a surgical incision may ooze serosanguineous (clear or pinkish) exudate for a day or two.

Healing Healing is the replacement of tissue by regeneration or repair.

- **Regeneration** is the replacement of the damaged cells with identical or similar cells. However, not all cells can regenerate (e.g., some central nervous system neurons and cardiac muscle cells cannot regenerate).
- **Repair** occurs when scar tissue replaces the original tissue. Most injuries heal by repair. You will find a thorough discussion of wound healing in Chapter 32.

The inflammatory response is adaptive in that it protects the body from infection and promotes healing. However, chronic inflammation, as in arthritis, is itself a stressor.

Key Point: *Do not confuse inflammation with infection.* Inflammation is a mechanism for eliminating invading pathogens; therefore, you always see inflammation when there is infection. However, inflammation is stimulated by trauma as well as by pathogens (e.g., swelling of a sprained ankle); thus, it can occur when there is no infection.

KnowledgeCheck 9-4

- What are four characteristics of the LAS?
- Name two LAS responses.
- What are the classic symptoms of the inflammatory process?

Psychological Responses to Stress Include Feelings, Thoughts, and Behaviors

Health professionals understand most human health disorders to be *biopsychosocial.* This means that we respond and adapt to stress physically, cognitively, emotionally, behaviorally, and even spiritually, and our responses include feelings, thoughts, and behaviors (Box 9-3).

Just as the body responds physiologically to stress, psychological defense mechanisms are also triggered to diminish inner tension, protect against anxiety, and assist with coping and adaptation. Common defense mechanisms for dealing with stress described by Sigmund Freud and, later, Anna Freud include avoidance, compensation, conversion, denial, displacement, intellectualization, projection, rationalization, reaction formation, regression, repression and suppression, regression, and sublimation (Table 9-1). **Key Point:** *Although defense mechanisms are often thought of as negative reactions, they help to temporarily ease stress and protect self-esteem during critical times, allowing people to focus on what is necessary to overcome the stressor.*

Stress responses may be fleeting, as in a flash of anger that is gone in seconds, or chronic, as in the avoidance of relationships by an adult whose needs for love and security were not met as a child. As with physical responses, psychological responses can be adaptive or dysfunctional. Consider this example case:

> Both Laslow and Harvey have suffered heart attacks. Both feel anxious. To relieve anxiety, Laslow uses problem-solving measures. He educates himself about healthy nutrition, physical activity, and lifestyle changes that he must make to recover and prevent complications. Harvey uses denial as a method for coping, saying, "I feel fine. Even if I deny myself burgers, beer, and cigarettes, I could still get hit by a truck and die tomorrow." Although both may experience some relief from anxiety, which approach do you think is more adaptive in the long term?

Common emotional responses to stress include the concepts of anxiety, fear, anger, and depression.

Anxiety

Anxiety is "an emotion characterized by feelings of tension, worried thoughts, and physical changes like increased blood pressure" (American Psychological

---

BOX 9-3 ■ Psychological Responses to Stressors

Cognitive Responses

Difficulty concentrating

Poor judgment

Decrease in accuracy (e.g., in counting money)

Forgetfulness

Decreased problem-solving ability

Decreased attention to detail

Difficulty learning

Narrowing of focus

Preoccupation, daydreaming

Emotional Responses

Adjustment disorders

Anger

Anxiety

Depression

Fear

Feelings of inadequacy

Low self-esteem

Irritability

Lack of motivation

Lethargy

Behavioral Responses

Academic difficulties

Aggressiveness

Crying, emotional outbursts

Dependence

Nightmares

Poor job performance

Substance use and abuse

Altered sleep

Change in eating habits

Decrease in quality of job performance

Preoccupation and distraction

Illnesses

Increased absenteeism from work or school

Increased number of accidents

Strained family or social relationships

Avoidance of social situations or relationships

Rebellion, acting out

Association [APA], 2000). It is a response not to a threat but to the *anticipation* of threat—to imagining it. A person with anxiety worries; feels nervous, uneasy, and fearful; may be tearful; and may avoid certain situations out of worry. However, the person cannot always identify specifically what they are afraid of. A person

Table 9-1 ➤ Psychological Defense Mechanisms

DEFENSE MECHANISM	EXAMPLES	EXAMPLES AND CONSEQUENCES OF OVERUSE
Avoidance—Unconsciously staying away from events or situations that might open feelings of aggression or anxiety.	"I can't go to the class reunion tonight. I'm too tired; I have to sleep."	The person becomes socially isolated because of the tension they feel when around other people.
Compensation—Making up for a perceived inadequacy by developing or emphasizing some other desirable trait.	A small boy who wants to be on the football team instead becomes a great singer.	Use of drugs or alcohol to gain courage to enter a social situation.
Conversion—Emotional conflict is changed into physical symptoms that have no physical basis. The symptoms often disappear after the threat is over.	Feeling back pain when it is difficult to continue carrying the pressures of life; developing nausea that causes the person to miss a major examination.	Laryngitis, inability to speak on the anniversary of father's death. Continued anxiety can lead to actual physical disorders, such as gastric ulcers.
Denial—Transforming reality by refusing to acknowledge thoughts, feeling, desires, or impulses. This is unconscious; the person is *not* consciously lying. Denial is usually the first defense learned.	A student refuses to acknowledge that they are barely passing anatomy, does not withdraw from the class, and is now failing a nursing course. A person with alcohol dependence states, "I can quit anytime I want to."	Overuse can lead to repression and dissociative disorders (e.g., dual personalities, selective amnesia).
Displacement—"Kick the dog." Transferring emotions, ideas, or wishes from one original object or situation to a substitute inappropriate person or object that is perceived to be less powerful or threatening.	Husband loses his job, goes home, and yells at his wife. (This mechanism is rarely adaptive.)	In extreme situations, this mechanism leads to verbal and physical abuse.
Dissociation—Painful events are separated or dissociated from the conscious mind.	A person who was sexually abused as a child describes the events as though they happened to a sibling.	May result in a dissociative disorder, such as multiple personality disorder.
Identification—A person takes on the ideas, personality, or characteristics of another person, especially someone whom the person fears or respects.	Children play cowboy, police, firefighter, or mommy.	Assumes mannerisms, wears clothing, and arranges hair and physical appearance to match those of the other person.
Intellectualization—Cognitive reasoning is used to block or avoid feelings about a painful incident.	When her husband dies, the wife relieves her pain by thinking, "It's better this way; he was in so much pain." A person says "I think" rather than "I feel."	"My husband loves me, but he doesn't like it when another man talks to me; that's why he loses his temper and releases his anger physically by hitting me."
Minimization—Not acknowledging or accepting the significance of one's own behavior, making it less important.	"It doesn't matter how much I drink. I never drive when I'm drinking."	Person engages in unhealthy or antisocial behavior; there is no motivation to change behavior.
Projection—Blaming others. Attributing one's own personality traits, mistakes, emotions, motives, and thoughts to another; "finger pointing."	"The clinical instructor makes me nervous, so I cannot do well." "I forgot to bake cookies because you did not tell me that cookies were due at school today."	Person cannot see their own responsibility for a situation, so they cannot make adaptive behaviors. Person criticizes habits in others that are the same as one's own bad habits.

(Continued)

Table 9-1 ➤ Psychological Defense Mechanisms—cont'd

DEFENSE MECHANISM	EXAMPLES	EXAMPLES AND CONSEQUENCES OF OVERUSE
Rationalization—Use of a logical-sounding excuse to cover up or justify true ideas, actions, or feelings. An attempt to preserve self-respect or approval or to conceal a motive for some action by giving a socially acceptable reason. Similar to intellectualization but uses faulty logic.	"It was God's will that this happened to me." "If I didn't have to work, I would be a better wife."	This mechanism can lead to self-deception.
Reaction formation—Similar to compensation, except the person develops the opposite trait. The person is aware of their feelings but acts in ways opposite to what they are really feeling.	"It's okay that you forgot my birthday" (when it really is not okay).	Overuse can cause failure to resolve internal conflicts.
Regression—Using behavior appropriate in an earlier stage of development to overcome feeling of insecurity in a present situation.	Cooks and eats a comfort food (e.g., hot fudge sundae). A divorced 60-year-old dresses and acts like a teenager.	Can interfere with perception of reality.
Repression—Unconscious "burying" or "forgetting" of painful thoughts, feelings, memories, ideas; pushing them from a conscious to an unconscious level. It is a step deeper than denial.	Having no memory of sexual abuse by sibling or father. An adolescent forgets to put out the trash because being "bossed" makes him angry, but he feels guilty if he consciously chooses not to do it.	Flashbacks, post-traumatic stress disorder, and amnesia.
Restitution (undoing)—Making amends for a behavior one thinks is unacceptable to reduce guilt.	Giving a treat to a child who has been punished for wrongdoing.	May send double messages. Relieves the person of the responsibility for honesty about the situation.
Sublimation—Unacceptable drives, traits, or behaviors (often sexual or aggressive) are unconsciously diverted to socially accepted traits.	Anger is expressed by aggression when playing sports. A person who chooses not to have children runs a daycare center.	The "acceptable" behavior might reinforce the negative tendencies, and the person may still show signs of the undesirable trait or behavior. For example, a person indulges in child pornography to obtain sexual gratification.

Source: Adapted from Gorman, L. M., & Anwar, R. (Eds.). (2019). Neeb's fundamentals of mental health nursing (5th ed.). F.A. Davis.

---

with anxiety usually has recurring, intrusive concerns (American Psychological Association, 2000).

- *Mild to moderate anxiety*—may be adaptive because it motivates and mobilizes the person to action.
- *Severe anxiety*—consumes energy and interferes with the person's ability to focus on and respond to what is really happening.
- *Panic*—sudden surge of overwhelming fear or impending doom that comes without warning or obvious reason; more intense than the feeling of being "stressed out" that most people experience. See Example Client Condition: Panic.

See Chapter 10 for more information on theoretical knowledge of anxiety and fear, including levels of anxiety.

Fear

Fear is an emotion or feeling of apprehension (dread) from an identified danger, threat, or pain. The danger may be real or imagined. Anxiety and fear produce similar responses. However, some experts differentiate them as follows:

- Fear is related to a precipitating event; anxiety is related to a future (or anticipated) event.

EXAMPLE CLIENT CONDITION: Panic

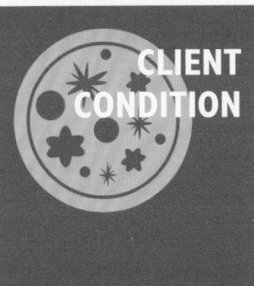
CLIENT CONDITION

General Definition
- Level of fear is out of proportion to the actual situation; often completely unrelated
- Persistent worry about having another episode
- Peak intensity typically in 10 minutes or less

Causes and Triggers
- First episodes occur out of the blue, without an obvious trigger.
- May be associated with major life transitions or stressful situations.

At Risk
- Occurs in 1 out of every 75; usually appears during the teens or early adulthood (APA, 2008). All ethnic groups are vulnerable to panic disorder. Women are twice as likely as men to have a panic disorder.
- Tend to run in families.
- May be associated with major life transitions or stressful situations.

RECOGNIZING COMPLICATIONS

- Can often lead to a phobia when repeatedly avoiding situations like the one when the attack occurred.
- Are more prone to alcohol and drug abuse.
- Have a greater risk of attempting suicide.
- Spend less time on satisfying activities.
- Tend to be financially dependent on others.
- Are afraid of driving more than a few miles from home.

- Over time, prolonged stress response can lead to high blood pressure, heart attack, stroke, migraines, high blood sugar, compromised immune system, irritable bowel syndrome, ulcers, weight gain, and reduced testosterone.

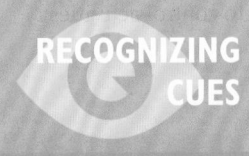
RECOGNIZING CUES

Assess for These Symptoms:

Physical
- Racing heartbeat, palpitations
- Feeling of not getting enough air
- Dizziness, lightheadedness, nausea
- Trembling, sweating, shaking
- Choking, chest pains
- Hot flashes, sudden chills
- Tingling in fingers or toes
- Reduced appetite
- Difficulty sleeping

Cognition and Emotion
- Feeling "crazy" and out of control
- *Depersonalization* (sensation of being detached from body)
- *Derealization* (feeling detached from your surroundings)
- Agitation, irritability, difficulty concentrating
- Fear of "going crazy," fear of dying

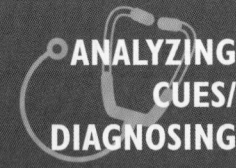
ANALYZING CUES/ DIAGNOSING

Nursing Diagnosis (NANDA-I)
Stress Overload

Other Nursing Diagnoses
Anxiety, Social isolation, Impaired social interaction, Low self-esteem, Ineffective coping

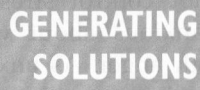
GENERATING SOLUTIONS

NOC Outcomes (Goals)
Mood Equilibrium, Personal Resiliency, Personal Well-Being

Individualized Outcome Statements
- Expects symptoms to improve gradually, not immediately
- Is active in trying to reduce stress and cope with panic

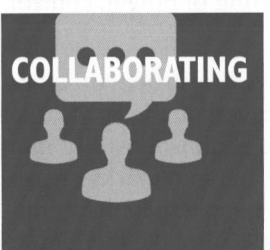
COLLABORATING

- Counseling or psychotherapy by a mental health professional who specializes in panic or anxiety disorders
- Cognitive–behavioral therapy (CBT)
- Cognitive restructuring—replace panic feelings with more realistic, positive thoughts
- Guided imagery
- Interoceptive exposure—go through the symptoms of an attack in a controlled setting

- Relaxation techniques
- Journaling; art therapy and other creative techniques
- Medication—selective serotonin reuptake inhibitors (SSRIs), selective norepinephrine reuptake inhibitors (SNRIs), antidepressants, anxiolytics, beta blockers

(continued)

EXAMPLE CLIENT CONDITION: Panic—cont'd

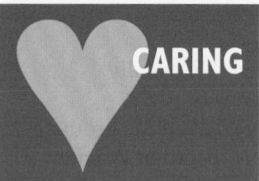

CARING

- Reassure that people with panic disorder can lead normal lives with treatment.
- Listen without interrupting or conveying judgment.
- Encourage a support group.

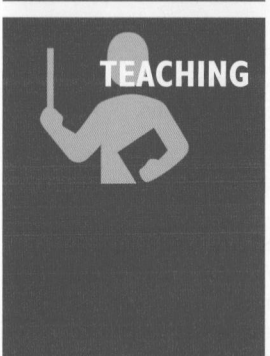

TEACHING

Many people are greatly helped by simply understanding exactly what panic disorder is and how many others suffer from it.

Help People To:

- Remind patient that fighting against the experience engages the "fear of fear" cycle that can make you feel even worse (Hofmann et al., n.d.).
- Teach patient that if panic symptoms creep up, they should label the experience and say, "I will be okay. This will pass in time." Accepting the experience, rather than

fighting against it, will likely help panic symptoms abate more quickly (Hofmann et al., n.d.).
- Break down a fearful situation into small, manageable steps.
- Approach situations that have been associated with a previous panic episode, rather than avoiding them.
- Slow breathing; cope with an attack.
- Limit caffeine; get adequate sleep; eat a healthy diet; and exercise regularly, especially aerobic exercise.

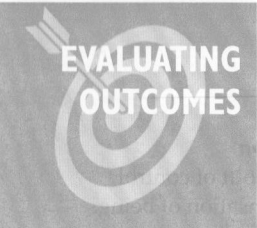

EVALUATING OUTCOMES

Assess for the following indicators of improvement:

- Exhibits responses that fit situations
- Verbalizes positive outlook
- Demonstrates ability to control activities
- Performs usual roles

- The source of fear is easily identifiable; the source of anxiety may not be specific.
- Fear can result from either a physical or a psychological event. Anxiety results from psychological conflict rather than physical threat.

 ThinkLike a Nurse 9-2:
Clinical Judgment in Action

Read the following two scenarios. In which situation are you most likely to feel fear rather than anxiety? Explain your reasoning.

1. You are a student assigned to a 6-hour day in the clinical area. Each time you have a clinical day coming up, you feel anticipation and look forward to working in the clinical area. However, you do not know what to expect. You think: "What will my patients be like? How will the day go? Do I know enough to handle it? Do I need to practice any procedures?" It is hard to answer these questions until you are on the unit and see your patients.
2. Given the same situation, suppose that when you begin your clinical day, your clinical instructor tells you that they will be in the agency, asking questions, supervising, evaluating your performance, and perhaps from your perspective, making your life miserable.

Anger and Depression

Anger is a strong, uncomfortable feeling of animosity, hostility, indignation, or displeasure.

- **Anger can be a healthy release of tension** when expressed appropriately and clearly. When the conflict is in the open, those involved have an opportunity to cope with it and resolve the issue at hand.
- **Anger is often a first protective response against anxiety.** A person who cannot control stressors may become apprehensive (anxious about what may happen) and respond with anger. As anxiety increases and the person recognizes fear, they feel more threatened and may resort to bullying behavior to increase the personal feeling of power, control, and self-esteem.

Hostility is anger that involves destructive behaviors (e.g., physical, emotional, or verbal abuse). Not all anger is expressed by aggressive actions; hostility may be more subtle, such as sarcastic, harsh remarks or passive-aggressive behaviors. Some people hide their emotions and suppress hurtful remarks or make them more socially acceptable through humor.

Depression may result from chronic stress. Parts of the brain are activated with stress, including the amygdala, which plays a critical role in emotional processing. Long-term stress induces a release of hormones, particularly cortisol (causes stress-related symptoms), as well as depletion of serotonin (acts as a mood stabilizer) (Tafet & Nemeroff, 2016). ✛ It is normal to feel down in response to stress, loss, or a traumatic event, but long-term depression is deeper than sadness and is a reason for concern. See Chapter 10 for more information about anxiety and depression.

KnowledgeCheck 9-5

- In addition to ego defense mechanisms, name four common emotional responses to stress.
- Explain how mild to moderate anxiety can be adaptive.
- True or False: One difference between anxiety and fear is that the danger in anxiety may be anticipated, whereas in fear, the danger is real.
- What are ego defense mechanisms?

Spiritual Responses to Stress

Many people trust in a higher power or faith-based community for support when coping with stress. Some search for a greater meaning for an illness, crisis, or other stressor. Others may view stressful situations as a test, a punishment, or a challenge.

Spiritual responses vary among individuals, as do all human responses. Examples include the following:

- Depending on a higher power or religious community for support when coping with stress
- Searching for a larger meaning in the illness or other stressor
- Viewing stress as a test, a punishment, or a challenge

Spiritual responses vary in different stages of stress.

- Alarm stage—A common first response is to pray or ask for help (e.g., for healing, coping).
- Adaptation stage—Prayer, meditation, and religious affiliation can also help during the second stage (adaptation).
- Exhaustion or recovery—Spiritual resources may become exhausted, creating spiritual distress, leaving the person feeling abandoned, helpless, and hopeless.

WHAT PROBLEMS OCCUR WHEN ADAPTATION FAILS?

Living with continual stress strains adaptive mechanisms and can lead to exhaustion and disease—which in turn can lead to more stress. Once established, this type of feedback loop is difficult to break. When adaptation fails, three types of disorders that can develop are stress-induced organic responses, somatoform disorders, and psychological disorders.

Stress-Induced Chronic Responses

As a result of repeated central nervous system stimulation and elevation of hormones, such as cortisol, chronic stress brings about physiological changes in various body systems. People who use maladaptive coping strategies (e.g., overeating, substance abuse) create additional stress on the body, further contributing to disease (Table 9-2).

Somatoform Disorders

Somatoform disorders are unexplained physical responses to stress and anxiety. The physical symptoms have no known organic cause. They are believed to result from unconscious denial, repression, and displacement of anxiety. The physical symptoms allow the person to avoid a situation that, if confronted, would provoke extreme anxiety.

The following are examples of somatoform disorders:

- **Hypochondriasis.** The person is preoccupied with the idea that they are or will become seriously ill. The person is abnormally concerned with their health and interprets their real or imagined symptoms unrealistically, fearing that they will get worse or become incurable. **Key Point:** *The person is not "faking it"; anxiety about their health may trigger the physical sensations.*
- **Somatization.** Anxiety and emotional turmoil are expressed in physical symptoms, loss of physical function, pain that changes location often, and depression. **Key Point:** *The patient is unable to control the symptoms and behaviors, and complaints are vague or exaggerated.* Movement disorders, weakness, dizziness, and fainting are common expressions of somatoform disorders, sometimes referred to as *anxiety neurosis.*
- **Pain disorder.** Emotional pain can manifest physically. Pain is the focus of the person's life. The physical cause is either disproportionate to the pain level the patient reports or cannot be found at all. The pain does not change location.
- **Malingering.** Malingering is different from the other disorders because it is a *conscious* effort to use the patient's symptoms to escape unpleasant situations or gain something (e.g., calling in sick because the person does not want to go to work).

KnowledgeCheck 9-6

- Name and describe three stress-induced organic or systemic responses to stress.
- Name and describe at least three somatoform disorders.

Stress-Induced Psychological Responses

Even if defense mechanisms are effective initially, with long-term stress, exhaustion develops, and the mechanisms begin to fail. The person may then try maladaptive ways to cope. As work and personal relationships deteriorate, the person loses self-esteem. Prolonged stress can eventually result in crisis and burnout, which we discuss

Table 9-2 ➤ Organic Responses Related to Failure of Adaptation

BODY SYSTEM	PHYSIOLOGICAL RESPONSE
Cardiovascular system	■ *Decreased cardiac output, oxygen depletion, and fatigue*—Continued secretion of epinephrine may cause angina (chest pain), myocardial infarction (heart attack), cardiomegaly (enlarged heart), and congestive heart failure, all of which lead to decreased cardiac output. As cardiac output decreases, less oxygen circulates to meet cellular metabolic demands, and the body becomes fatigued. Stress has been directly linked to stroke (Richardson et al., 2012). ■ *Vasoconstriction causes hypertension*—Prolonged secretion of epinephrine and renin results in vasoconstriction, causing hypertension (high blood pressure). ■ *Electrolyte imbalance and edema*—ADH, aldosterone, ACTH, and cortisol create electrolyte imbalance and retention of sodium and water, thus promoting peripheral edema.
Endocrine system	■ *Diabetes*—Consistent high levels of blood glucose and insulin can cause diabetes. ■ *Hyper- or hypothyroidism*—These metabolic disorders can result when persistent demands for thyroid hormone production cause a rebound failure of the gland. ■ *Prenatal effects*—Prenatal stress can increase the risk for preterm birth, low birth weight, and developmental delays and metabolic diseases later in life.
Immune system	■ *Autoimmune illness*—Stress reduces the ability of the body's immune cells to differentiate between self and non-self. Thus, the immune cells begin to attack body tissues, producing autoimmune illness (e.g., rheumatoid arthritis, allergies, fibromyalgia). ■ *Suppression of immunity*—Stress can weaken the immune system, leading to infection and illness. Indirectly, it is also linked to cancer (Ohio State University, 2013). Stress hormones can alter the behavior of neutrophils (type of white blood cells), potentially reducing protection against recurring cancer (American Cancer Society, 2021).
Gastrointestinal system	■ *Bowel inflammation and other disorders*—Stress can cause the bowel to react with constipation or diarrhea, gastroesophageal reflux, colitis, or irritable bowel syndrome. ■ *Gastric hyperacidity*—Continued secretion of hydrochloric acid produces gastric hyperacidity and erosion of the gastrointestinal tract, including the stomach, especially in the presence of *Helicobacter pylori*.
Musculoskeletal system	■ *Muscle tension and pain*—Constant readiness for fight or flight produces muscle tension and pain in various body sites. ■ *Tension headache and temporomandibular joint pain*—These can result from prolonged muscle tension in the head, neck, and spine.
Respiratory system	■ *Increased respiratory rate*—Epinephrine and circulating hormones dilate the bronchial tubes and increase the rate of respiration. ■ *Hyperventilation*—This can produce symptoms of alkalosis, including dizziness, tingling hands and feet, and anxiety. ■ *Exacerbation of existing asthma, hay fever, and allergies*—All of these can be provoked by distress in the respiratory system. In addition, stress aggravates chronic bronchitis and emphysema (Quick et al., 2006).

ACTH = adrenocorticotropic hormone; ADH = antidiuretic hormone; PTSD = post-traumatic stress disorder.

next (also see Fig. 9-6). More severe responses include mental and emotional illnesses, such as anxiety disorders, clinical depression, and post-traumatic stress disorder (PTSD). Anxiety and depression are discussed in Chapter 10.

Crisis

A crisis exists when (1) an event in a person's life drastically changes the person's routine, and they perceive it as a threat to self, and (2) the person's usual coping methods are ineffective, resulting in high levels of anxiety and an inability to function adequately. Such events are usually sudden and unexpected (e.g., serious illness or death of a loved one, serious financial losses, a motor vehicle accident, domestic violence, natural disasters) (Fig. 9-6).

Each person has a different tolerance for stress; an event that creates a crisis for one may be just a minor nuisance for another. Nevertheless, most experts agree

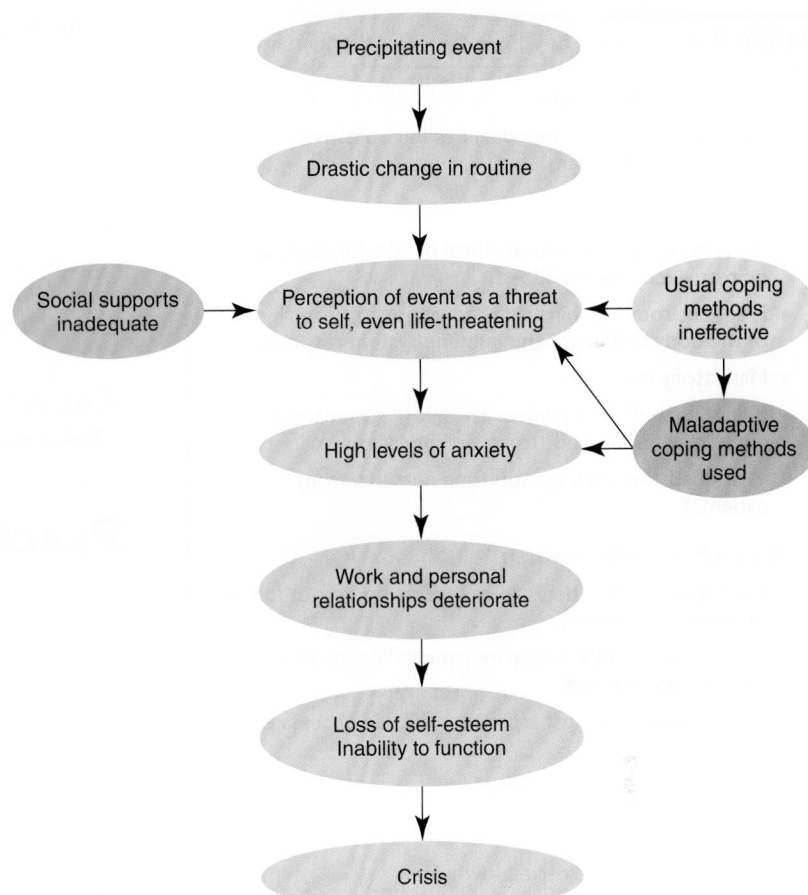

FIGURE 9-6 How a crisis develops.

that people experiencing a crisis go through phases (Gorman & Anwar, 2019; Stuart, 2013).

1. *Precrisis.* In response to the event or anxiety, the person uses their usual coping strategies, has no symptoms, denies feeling stress, and may even report a sense of well-being.
2. *Impact.* If the usual strategies are not effective, anxiety and confusion increase. The person may have trouble organizing their personal life and may feel the stress but minimize its severity.
3. *Crisis.* The person experiences more anxiety and tries new ways of coping, such as withdrawal, rationalization, and projection (refer to Table 9-1). The person recognizes the problem but denies that it is out of control.
4. *Adaptive.* The person redefines the threat and perceives the crisis in a realistic way. Rational thinking and positive problem-solving help the person to regain some self-esteem and begin socializing again. Adaptation is more likely if the person can use effective coping strategies and if situational supports are available.
5. *Postcrisis.* After a crisis, a person may have developed better ways of coping with stress, or the person may be critical, hostile, and depressed and use maladaptive strategies (e.g., overeating or engaging in substance abuse) to deal with what has happened.
Key Point: *People in crisis are at risk for physical and emotional harm, so intervention is essential (see Crisis Intervention in Volume 2).*

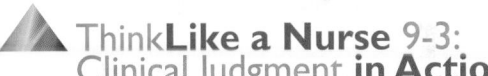

ThinkLike a **Nurse** 9-3:
Clinical Judgment **in Action**

Suppose you are the charge nurse on a 30-bed surgical unit. In addition, you must assume care of three more patients because another nurse called in sick. It is a normal, busy day with seven postoperative patients and eight discharges. In addition, a patient went into cardiac arrhythmia and was transferred to the coronary care unit. Because the nurse who called in sick was supposed to work an 8-hour shift and no replacement has been found, you are told you must stay and work 4 hours of overtime. You had plans to have dinner with your spouse this evening because it is your anniversary. Now you will surely not be home before 8:00 p.m., and you will be exhausted.

- What would be the stressors for you in this situation?
- What thoughts and feelings would you have?
- What physical responses would you probably notice?
- What are some psychological responses that you would use to help you adapt and cope with this day?
- How would you probably react if the same thing were to happen on the following day?

Burnout

Burnout involves more than working long hours and managing exceedingly demanding job responsibilities (Box 9-4). This type of stress occurs when coping

BOX 9-4 ■ Stressors That Can Lead to Burnout

Relationship Stressors

- Dealing with difficult personalities (e.g., patients, supervisors, physicians)

Staffing Stressors

- Working long shifts with minimal breaks for food, water, or rest; excessive workload
- Frequent rotating shifts that upset the circadian rhythm of the body and lower the immune system response
- Mandatory overtime
- Being "floated" to an unfamiliar unit (e.g., a maternity nurse may be "floated" to an orthopedic unit)
- Workload: low staffing ratio (one nurse to many patients)

Nurse–Patient Stressors

- Frustration with patients (e.g., those who do not follow therapeutic routines)
- Need to constantly anticipate patients' needs and cope with the unexpected
- Feeling helpless against a patient's disease process or lack of healing
- Dealing with death and dying

Employer Issues

- Lack of rewards; perceived low wage
- Few opportunities for growth or advancement
- Lack of support from administration, providers, colleagues
- Lack of participation in decision making
- Inability to delegate responsibilities
- Conflicting demands on time or unclear role expectations (APA, 2018)
- Organizational philosophy that conflicts with personal philosophy

is depleted, and the individual has a perception of not being in control of the work or personal situation. Burnout manifests as exhaustion; a sense of dread about work; and feelings of anger, irritability, and cynicism.

Excessive demands, lack of respect, or little support from an employer or coworkers can serve as a trigger for burnout. In response, the nurse experiences anger or frustration, feels overwhelmed and helpless, or suffers low self-esteem and depression. Some nurses experience grief, moral distress, and guilt when the situation prevents them from performing as well as they believe they should. As a result, a nurse may develop a physical illness or a negative attitude, or the nurse may use maladaptive coping techniques, such as smoking or substance abuse.

Compassion fatigue is a form of burnout that is not uncommon in the helping professions, such as nursing, and among others who are exposed to human suffering. Over time, those with compassion fatigue become

numb, feeling less able to display empathy for those in need.

Example Client Condition: Post-Traumatic Stress Disorder

Post-traumatic stress disorder (PTSD) is a severe form of anxiety that occurs after exposure to extreme psychological or violent trauma or to physical or emotional abuse. For nursing care, see the accompanying Example Client Condition for PTSD.

KnowledgeCheck 9-7

Define *crisis, burnout, panic,* and *PTSD.*

PracticalKnowledge
knowing how

In the remainder of this chapter, you will learn about planning and implementing care for patients experiencing stress. You will also have opportunities to practice clinical reasoning and critical thinking.

ASSESSMENT/RECOGNIZING CUES

People experiencing stress may not think clearly or communicate effectively; therefore, you will need to demonstrate empathy, develop rapport, and relieve their immediate anxiety as much as possible before beginning an assessment. Focus the patient by asking concise, direct questions and then proceeding to open-ended questions that will provide you with as much information as possible (see Chapter 15 for information on questioning techniques).

Assess Stressors, Risk Factors, and Coping and Adaptation

Data about the patient's stressors and risk factors should help you to:

- Determine whether the patient has a realistic or an exaggerated perception of the stressors.
- Identify factors that increase the risk for future stress.
- Identify interventions to reduce current stress and provide anticipatory guidance to prevent future stress.

You might begin gathering these data by having the patient complete a stress inventory. Then follow up with observations, such as those in the Focused Assessment box, Assessing for Stress: Questions to Ask.

Assess Responses to Stress

Stress responses are holistic; therefore, you will need to assess physiological, emotional, behavioral, and cognitive indicators of stress. **Key Point:** *Be aware that if coping is effective, clinical signs and symptoms of stress may not be evident.*

EXAMPLE CLIENT CONDITION 9-2: Post-Traumatic Stress Disorder (PTSD)

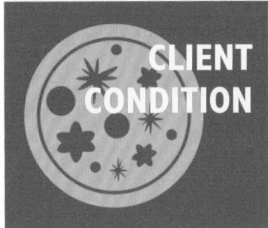

CLIENT CONDITION

General Definition

Prolonged anxiety after exposure to extreme psychological event or to physical or emotional abuse; feelings of harm and helplessness during a traumatic event. People with PTSD experience stress, anxiety, or fear even when there is no longer a direct threat or danger.

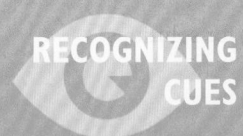

RECOGNIZING CUES

Assess for These Symptoms:

Physical
Increased blood pressure and heart rate, rapid breathing, muscle tension, nausea, diarrhea, dizziness. See Box 9-5.

Cognition and Mood
Can begin or worsen after the traumatic event but are not due to injury or substance use; may feel detached from friends or family
- Trouble remembering key features of the traumatic event
- Negative thoughts
- Distorted feelings (guilt or blame)
- Loss of interest in enjoyable activities
- Chemical abuse or dependence
- Difficulty forming new relationships

Reexperiencing
Words, objects, places, or situations that are reminders of the event can trigger nightmares, fear, and flashbacks (reliving the trauma), including physical symptoms like racing heart or sweating.

Avoidance
Reminders of the event may be the trigger to:
- Stay away from places, events, or objects that are reminders of the traumatic experience
- Feel emotionally numb
- Feel strong guilt, depression, or worry
- Lose interest in once enjoyable activities
- Have difficulty remembering the event

Reactivity
Usually constant instead of being triggered by a reminder of the event
- Easily startled
- Agitation, irritability
- Difficulty sleeping
- Angry outbursts for no apparent reason
- Excessive emotions
- Problems feeling or showing affection to others
- Difficulty concentrating

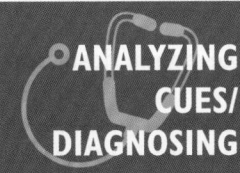

ANALYZING CUES/ DIAGNOSING

Nursing Diagnosis (NANDA-I)

Stress Overload

Post-trauma stress syndrome: Sustained maladaptive response to a traumatic, overwhelming event

Other Nursing Diagnoses

Anxiety, Social isolation, Impaired social interaction, Low self-esteem

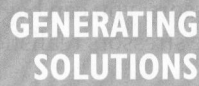

GENERATING SOLUTIONS

NOC Outcomes (Goals)

Mood Equilibrium, Personal Resiliency, Personal Well-Being

Individualized Outcome Statements

- Breaks up large tasks into small ones; sets priorities
- Spends time with other people; confides in a trusted friend or relative

- Expects symptoms to improve gradually, not immediately
- Is active in trying to reduce stress

(continued)

EXAMPLE CLIENT CONDITION 9-2: Post-Traumatic Stress Disorder (PTSD)—cont'd

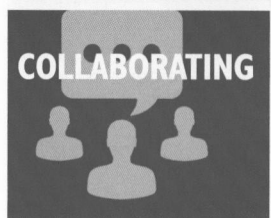

COLLABORATING

- Counseling or psychotherapy
- Exposure therapy
- Family therapy
- Group therapy
- Cognitive–behavioral therapy

- Eye movement desensitization and reprocessing
- Medications (antidepressants)
- Stress management

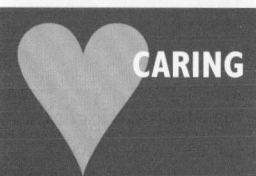

CARING

- Encourage the client to seek out comforting situations, places, and people.
- Listen to the client without interrupting, conveying judgment, or pushing for solutions.

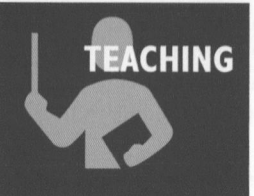

TEACHING

Help people to:

- Identify and deal with guilt, shame, and other feelings about the event.
- Change how they react to their PTSD symptoms (e.g., therapy helps people face reminders of the trauma).

Teach:

- Effects of trauma
- Relaxation and anger-control skills
- Tips for better sleep, diet, and exercise habits

EVALUATING OUTCOMES

Assess for the Following Indicators of Improvement:

- Exhibits affect that fits situation
- Verbalizes positive outlook
- Removes self from abusive relationships
- Expresses satisfaction with social relationships

- Demonstrates ability to control activities
- Performs usual roles

- **Assessing Physiological Responses** Because the GAS is nonspecific, you must obtain data from all body systems (for physical examination techniques, see Chapter 19).

  Vital signs—Elevations in pulse, respiration, and blood pressure will indicate whether the fight-or-flight response is present.

  General survey, or overview, of the patient—Note hygiene, grooming, facial expression, body language, posture, nonverbal expression, and ability to make eye contact.

  Box 9-5 summarizes physiological responses that indicate stress.

- **Assessing Emotional and Behavioral Responses** Assess for the emotional and behavioral responses to stress that are described in Box 9-3 and in the Focused Assessment box. The client may or may not be aware that the feelings or behaviors are related to stress, so be sure to:

  Observe nonverbal behaviors and body language for cues to mood and affect.

  Check client records for evidence about destructive behaviors (e.g., drug abuse).

- **Assessing Cognitive Responses** You can assess the client's cognitive functioning as you assess other functional areas. See Box 9-3 to review examples of cognitive responses. When you ask the client to describe and rate the intensity of the stressors, you can begin to assess whether they perceive the stressors realistically or in an exaggerated way.

Assess Support Systems

Determine the supports available and their ability to assist the client—that is, do the significant others have the sensitivity and skills to be supportive?

- Significant others are important to the success of a client's coping strategies.
- Support persons may be affected by the same stressors or by the client's responses to them.

 See the Focused Assessment box Assessing for Stress: Questions to Ask in Volume 2.

BOX 9-5 ■ Physical Responses to Stressors

- Dilated pupils
- Muscle tension
- Stiff neck
- Headaches
- Skin pallor
- Skin lesions (e.g., eczema, hives)
- Diaphoresis, sweaty palms
- Dry mouth
- Nausea
- Weight or appetite changes
- Increased blood glucose
- Increased heart rate
- Cardiac dysrhythmias
- Hyperventilation
- Chest pain
- Water retention
- Increased urinary frequency or decreased urinary output
- Diarrhea, constipation, abdominal pain, bowel incontinence
- Loss of sexual desire or ability
- Frequent colds and infections
- Low energy

examples of NANDA-I diagnoses (NANDA International, 2022) individualized with etiologies specific to a patient:

Physical	**Risk for Constipation** r/t decreased peristalsis secondary to stress
Behavioral	***Ineffective Health Management*** r/t use of denial as an ego defense mechanism to relieve anxiety
Cognitive	***Impaired Memory*** (short term) r/t overwhelming number and severity of stressors
Emotional	***Anxiety*** r/t uncertainty about the future and ineffectiveness of usual coping mechanisms
Interpersonal	***Impaired Parenting*** r/t maladaptive use of alcohol to cope with recent stress of divorce
Spiritual	***Hopelessness*** r/t perceived lack of support and ability to change the present situation

You may also wish to refer to the most recent NANDA-I *Nursing Diagnoses: Definitions and Classification* or to other nursing diagnosis handbooks.

It is important to identify the etiology of the diagnosis so that you can choose interventions to remove or modify the stressor. For example, if you believe a patient's diarrhea is being caused by stress, you intervene by modifying the stressor, helping the patient to perceive the stressor differently, and so on. If instead, the patient's diarrhea is caused by a gastrointestinal virus, your interventions would not be helpful.

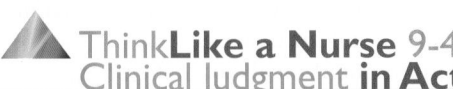

ThinkLike a Nurse 9-4: Clinical Judgment in Action

Review the scenario of Gloria and John (Meet Your Patients). How much does it really tell you about the clients' situation?

- Which aspect of stress do you have the most information about: their stressors, their coping methods and adaptation, their responses to stress, or their support systems?
- What facts do you have about either Gloria's or John's physiological responses to their multiple stressors? What can you infer their responses might be?
- What facts do you have about the clients' emotional and behavioral responses to their stressors?
- What information do you have about how well they are adapting to stress?
- What data do you have about their support systems? What information do you need?

■ NURSING DIAGNOSIS/ANALYZING CUES

Stress is nonspecific, so there is almost no limit to the number of nursing diagnoses that could be stress induced. Your theoretical knowledge of the holistic nature of stress should lead you to identify diagnoses in the physical, behavioral, cognitive, emotional, interpersonal, and spiritual domains. The following are some

KnowledgeCheck 9-8

- How might you identify and assess Gloria and John's stressors (Meet Your Patients)?
- List three questions you could ask to find out how Gloria is coping and adapting to stress.
- List three questions you could ask to assess Gloria's physiological responses to stress. What observations might you also make?
- List three questions you could ask to assess Gloria's emotional and behavioral responses to stress.
- How might you determine whether stress is affecting Gloria's cognitive functioning?
- You know Gloria's sister is providing some support. How could you find out more about the extent of Gloria and John's support system?

■ PLANNING /PRIORITIZING HYPOTHESES AND GENERATING SOLUTIONS

Nursing Outcomes Classification (NOC) standardized outcomes are outcomes that, if achieved, demonstrate resolution of the problem stated by the nursing diagnosis. For example, if you make a diagnosis of *anxiety* related to the client's perception that they will not be able to fulfill family responsibilities, you might use the NOC outcome Anxiety Self-Control (Moorhead et al., 2018). For a list and definitions of NOC outcomes to use for stress diagnoses, refer to the most recent edition of the NOC. Or you might choose to use a nursing diagnosis handbook with a current listing of accepted diagnoses.

Individualized goal or outcome statements are also specific to each nursing diagnosis. Broad, general goals for clients experiencing stress are to (1) reduce the strength and duration of the stressor, (2) relieve or remove responses to stress, and (3) use effective coping mechanisms. Examples of specific outcome statements you might use include the following:

- Reports (or physical examination reveals) reduction in physical symptoms of stress.
- Demonstrates less physical tension in facial expression and other muscle groups.
- Verbalizes increased feelings of control in the stressful situation.
- Uses problem-solving and anxiety-reducing techniques.
- Demonstrates relaxation and stress-reducing strategies.

Nursing Interventions Classification (NIC) standardized interventions for stress may be linked to both the problem and the etiology of the nursing diagnosis. Using the preceding example of Anxiety related to the client's perception that he will not be able to fulfill family responsibilities, some interventions may focus on supporting the client's ability to fulfill family roles; others may focus on general techniques for relieving anxiety (e.g., Anxiety Reduction, Calming Technique) (Butcher et al., 2019). For a list and definitions of NIC interventions to use for stress diagnoses, refer to the most recent edition of the NIC or a nursing diagnosis handbook.

Specific nursing activities should be individualized based on the patient's needs and the etiologies of the nursing diagnoses. Always consider the patient's ability and motivation to comply with the plan of care. See iCare 9-1.

IMPLEMENTATION/TAKING ACTION

Most stress-relieving interventions work by one or more of the following means:

- **Removing stressors** or modifying them
- **Supporting coping abilities** (e.g., changing the person's perception of the stressor)

♥ **iCare 9-1**

Will the Patient Comply?

- Is the patient willing to use complementary or alternative care measures? How open are they to deviating from traditional biomedical therapies?
- Is the patient willing to follow therapeutic suggestions?
- Collaborate with patients to determine what therapies will fit most comfortably into their lifestyle. Those are the interventions that will be most effective.

- **Treating responses** to stress (e.g., symptoms such as fatigue or diarrhea)

As you read through the following interventions, see whether you can identify which of the preceding means provides a rationale for the actions.

Health-Promotion Activities

People cannot always control the occurrence of a stressful event, and there are no high-tech treatments for coping with stress. However, a healthy lifestyle can prevent some stressors and improve the individual's ability to cope with others.

Nutrition Nutrition is important for maintaining physical homeostasis and resisting stress. For example, adequate nutrition boosts the immune system; proteins are needed for tissue building and healing. A healthy diet can reduce cortisol and adrenaline; these stress hormones take a toll on the body over time and can lead to illness. In addition, overweight and malnutrition are stressors that may lead to illness. Advise clients to do the following to achieve good nutrition:

- Maintain a normal body weight.
- Limit fat intake (especially animal fat) to no more than 30% of daily calories.
- Consume complex carbohydrates with fiber and a high nutrient composition—these *prompt the brain to produce more serotonin.*
- Limit the intake of sugar and salt—these lead to a spike and drop in serotonin.
- Eat more fish and poultry and less red meat *to reduce cholesterol and the risk of heart* disease.
- Eat smaller, more frequent meals *to aid digestion.*
- Eat citrus fruits—these strengthen the immune system and help to reduce levels of cortisol after a stressful trigger.
- Eat more green leafy vegetables, especially spinach—these are high in magnesium and beneficial for improving muscle and nerve function, regulating blood pressure, and supporting the immune system.
- Consume no more than one or two alcoholic beverages per day.

See Chapter 24 if you need detailed information about healthful nutrition.

Exercise Exercise promotes physical and emotional homeostasis. To achieve any health benefits, engage in exercise of moderate to vigorous intensity for at least 150 to 300 minutes per week (U.S. Department of Health and Human Services, 2018). Additional health benefits occur with more activity.

During exercise, the brain releases **endogenous opioids** (e.g., endorphins), which create a feeling of well-being. Exercise provides the following benefits:

- Improves muscle tone and helps to control weight
- Improves the functioning of the heart and lungs

- Reduces the risk of cardiovascular disease
- Promotes relaxation and reduces tension

Advise clients with obesity or chronic illness or who have always been sedentary to consult a primary caregiver before beginning a new exercise program. To promote adherence to the exercise routine, suggest that the client identify a variety of physical activities that they enjoy (e.g., swimming, bicycling, walking) and schedule regular sessions with one or more exercise "buddies," if possible.

See Chapter 29 for more specific physical activities to manage stress.

Sleep and Rest Sleep and rest restore energy levels, allow the body to repair itself, and promote mental relaxation. Most people need 7 or 8 hours of sleep a day; however, the amount of sleep varies among individuals. Stress, pain, and illness may interfere with the ability to sleep, so some clients may need help identifying and implementing techniques for relaxing and going to sleep (see Chapter 31 for more information on sleep, as needed).

Leisure Activities Compared with exercise, which not everyone enjoys, leisure activities are any activities that provide joy and satisfaction. They may involve physical activity, or they may be sedentary activities, such as reading, painting, or watching television. Leisure activities are a form of rest and, as such, are restorative.

Time Management People who manage their time efficiently and organize their life routines are likely to feel more in control and, therefore, less stressed. If clients feel overwhelmed, you can help them to prioritize tasks and make "to-do" lists. Assist them in learning to do the following:

- Delegate responsibilities and set boundaries on time.
- *Learn to say no.* Prompt clients to ask themselves:
  How much can I realistically do?
  What is essential to do?
  What would be nice to do?

If you would like more information on time management, see Chapter 40.

Avoiding Maladaptive Behaviors Some people use maladaptive behaviors as a response to stress. For others, the behaviors themselves become stressors. Advise clients to avoid unhealthful behaviors, such as the overuse of caffeine, alcohol, tobacco, recreational or prescription drugs, and even food. Counseling may be beneficial for those experiencing impaired social interactions (e.g., withdrawal and isolation, aggressiveness), sexual dysfunction (e.g., reduced libido, pain during sexual activity, painful periods, erectile dysfunction), poor sleep patterns (e.g., difficulty falling asleep or staying asleep, sleeping too much), stress eating (e.g., compulsive eating, anorexia, bulimia, restrictive eating), and risk-taking behaviors.

KnowledgeCheck 9-9

Name and discuss at least four aspects of a healthful lifestyle that can help prevent or relieve stress.

Relieving Anxiety

Because anxiety is a common response to illness, medical tests, and treatments, you will use anxiety-relief interventions every day of your professional life. For example, when

Toward Evidence-Based Practice

Pinho, L., Correia, T., Sampaio, F., Sequeira, C., Teixeira, L., Lopes, M., & Fonsecaab, C. (2021, April). The use of mental health promotion strategies by nurses to reduce anxiety, stress, and depression during the COVID-19 outbreak: A prospective cohort study. *Environmental Research, 195,* 110828. https://doi.org/10.1016/j.envres.2021.110828

Health professionals at the front line in providing care to patients during a pandemic are exposed to mental health issues, disease, and death in patients, as well as an array of other work-related stressors (work overload, lack of support, poor working conditions, intimidation, for example). To combat the profound effect of workplace stress, strategies to reduce nurses' stress and symptoms of anxiety and depression during the COVID-19 outbreak include physical activity, relaxation activity, recreational activity, healthy diet, adequate water intake, breaks between work shifts, maintenance of remote social contacts, and verbalization of feelings/emotions.

Kumar, S., Lee, K. N., Pinkerton, E., Wroblewski, K. E., Lengyel, E., & Tobin, M. (2021, October 14). Resilience: A mediator of the negative effects of pandemic-related stress on women's mental health in the USA. *Archives of Women's Mental Health, 25,* 137–146. https://doi.org/10.1007/s00737-021-01184-7

Resilience is the ability to resist illness, adapt positively, and function healthfully in the face of ongoing stress. In a sample of 3,200 women in the United States, those who demonstrated high resilience using a self-rated questionnaire experienced less anxiety and depression than those who demonstrated less ability to bounce back from stress. Strategies shown to enhance resilience, such as cognitive–behavioral therapy, mindfulness practices, and addressing socioeconomic factors, may help improve mental health outcomes.

Continued

Toward Evidence-Based Practice—cont'd

Lease, S. J., Ingram, C. L., & Brown, E. L. (2019). Stress and health outcomes: Do meaningful work and physical activity help? *Journal of Career Development, 46*(3), 251–264. https://doi.org/10.1177/0894845317741370

Researchers studied the impact of meaningful work and physical activity on perceived stress and health outcomes. Among 229 employed adults, those who perceived stress showed more risky lifestyle behaviors (i.e., poor diet, tobacco use, and alcohol use) and depressive symptoms. The negative effects of stress were reduced when adults rated their work as meaningful.

1. The negative effects of stress and burnout on the mental and physical health of nurses working during COVID-19 outbreaks are widely known. The study by Pinho and colleagues examined the effectiveness of strategies for mental health promotion in reducing nurses' perceived level of stress, anxiety, and depression. What other activities might nurses also use to aid in coping?

2. Resilience is the ability to recover quickly from difficulties. What strategies might nurses on the front line use to increase resilience during times of stress?

3. The negative effects of stress and burnout on mental and physical health are widely known. The study by Lease et al. examined the effect that perceived stress can have on behaviors. What other maladaptive outcomes might occur in people experiencing high levels of stress or chronic stress?

---

you tell patients what to expect before you perform a procedure or ask them to take deep breaths during a painful treatment, you lessen anxiety. If you have developed a therapeutic, trusting relationship, your very presence will help to ease the patient's anxiety. You will find specific interventions for anxiety in Chapter 8, and many of the interventions in the following sections provide anxiety relief as well. Also see the Holistic Healing box, Using CAM for Stress Reduction.

Anger Management

Anger is a common response to stress. However, clients usually do not openly say, "I am angry." They may not even recognize that they are angry. Instead, they engage in hostile behaviors (e.g., becoming hypercritical, verbally abusive, or demanding). You may have heard stories from nurses about the client who is "on the call light constantly." A sharp response from the nurse blocks communication and may escalate the person's anger. For tips on managing anger, refer to Violence, in Chapter 21; and Clinical Insight 9-1, Dealing with Angry Patients.

 Go to Chapter 9, Clinical Insight 9-1: Dealing with Angry Patients, in Volume 2

Stress-Management Techniques

Most stress-management techniques focus on discharging tension or simplifying one's life to modify stressors or control stress responses. **Relaxation,** a state of reduced physical and mental arousal, is an important intervention because it reverses some stress responses. By elongating muscle fibers, relaxation reduces neural impulses sent to the brain and decreases the activity of the brain and other body systems. In a relaxed state, blood pressure, heart rate, respiratory rate, and oxygen consumption decrease, whereas peripheral skin temperature and brain alpha-wave activity increase.

The techniques in this section are complementary and alternative medicine (CAM) therapies, and some require special training and licensing or credentialing. Many are discussed in detail in other chapters.

Physical Activity Not only an aid for coping with stress, physical activity can also prevent complications related to stress. Physical exertion releases tension held in muscles, improves muscle tone and posture, expresses emotions, and stimulates the secretion of endorphins, thus creating a feeling of well-being and relaxation.

Relaxation Techniques Relaxation techniques involve teaching the patient to relax individual muscle groups.

- **Progressive relaxation** in a quiet meditative state, which involves relaxing and contracting muscle groups, is much less traumatic and damaging to fragile joints and muscles than active exercise. Therefore, it may be used even by people who are not in good health.
- **Passive relaxation** occurs when the person relaxes the muscle groups without first contracting them.

Meditation Managing stress through meditation involves heightening one's attention or awareness. Regular meditation facilitates harmony among mind, body, and spirit, thereby reducing anxiety and giving the person a sense of control. **Mindfulness** is a type of meditation involving focus on the present moment. Mindfulness interventions can enhance health, wellness, and performance by reducing anxiety and psychological burnout (Hilton et al., 2019). **Yoga** is a form of meditation that involves strengthening and stretching muscles, improving balance, releasing stress, and improving psychological well-being (Mathad et al., 2017).

Visualization or Imagery Visualization (imagery) is a technique using the imagination to create a mental picture of something pleasant. This may be used to

Using Complementary & Alternative Modalities (CAM) for Stress Reduction

Holistic Healing

Exercise

Ma, W.-F., Wu, P.-L., Su, C.-H., & Yang, T.-C. (2017). The effects of an exercise program on anxiety levels and metabolic function in patients with anxiety disorders. *Biological Research for Nursing, 19*(3), 258–268. https://doi.org/10.1177/1099800416672581

This study examined the effectiveness of exercise in reducing stress in patients with anxiety. Participants using the exercise program had significant improvements in body mass index and high-density lipoprotein cholesterol levels with a level of moderate exercise compared with similarly matched patients who did not exercise.

Mindfulness Training

Rush, S. E., & Sharma, M. (2017). Mindfulness-based stress reduction as a stress management intervention for cancer care: A systematic review. *Journal of Evidence-Based Integrative Medicine, 22*(2), 347–359. https://doi.org/10.1177/2156587216661467

In a review of 13 studies, researchers found that patients with cancer who used mindfulness techniques that combined mindfulness meditation and yoga managed stress more effectively than before the technique. Mindfulness training may be an effective approach for stress reduction as part of cancer care.

Yoga

Vadiraga, H. S., Rao, R. M., Nagarathna, R., Nagendra, H. R., Patil, S., Diwakar, R. B., Shashidhara, H. P., Gopinath, K. S., & Ajaikumar, B. S. (2017). Effects of yoga in managing fatigue in breast cancer patients: A randomized controlled trial. *Indian Journal of Palliative Care, 23*(3), 247–252. https://doi.org/10.4103/IJPC.IJPC_95_17

Reduced cortisol levels in saliva suggest that yoga reduces fatigue in patients with advanced breast cancer.

Tai Chi

Tsai, P.-F., Kitch, S., Chang, J. Y., James, G. A., Dubbert, P., Roca, J. V., & Powers, C. H. (2017, March). Tai chi for post-traumatic stress disorder and chronic musculoskeletal pain: A pilot study. *Journal of Holistic Nursing, 36*(2), 147–158.

https://doi.org/10.1177/0898010117697617

Tai Chi may reduce pain and improve emotion, memory, and physical function in patients with post-traumatic stress disorder musculoskeletal pain.

relieve anxiety and complement the effects of relaxation techniques.

Biofeedback Biofeedback techniques use electronic instruments to measure bodily functions, such as brain activity, blood pressure, muscle tension, heart rate, skin temperature, and sweat gland activity. The immediate feedback helps the person become aware of and learn how to voluntarily control certain physiological responses, such as those produced by stress (DeWitt et al., 2019). Biofeedback practitioners require special training, and most are credentialed in biofeedback.

Acupuncture Acupuncture involves the insertion of a needle into "meridian points" to regulate the flow of energy or life force throughout the body. It can modify pain perception and restore normal physiological functions (e.g., decrease the heart rate). If you want more information, see Chapter 28.

Chiropractic Adjustment Chiropractic adjustment involves manual realignment of the vertebrae. The theory is that misalignment of the vertebrae leads to pain, loss of function, and illness. Realignment is performed to free energy, release muscle tension, and improve body function and health. Chiropractors undergo special education and training before they are qualified to perform adjustments.

Touch Therapies Therapies such as healing touch, Reiki, qigong, and therapeutic touch are types of energy therapies used to repattern the patient's energy fields. Healing energy is channeled through a practitioner's hands to improve well-being, reduce stress, improve mood, increase concentration, enhance productivity, manage pain, and accelerate healing (Kramer, 2018; Micozzi, 2019). Further studies are needed for use in children and conditions other than pain.

Massage Through manipulation of the soft tissues, massage relaxes muscles and releases body tension. This improves circulation and allows energy and blood to flow through muscles and soft tissues more readily. See Chapter 31 for more information.

Reflexology Reflexology is the application of pressure to specific points on the feet, hands, or ears. It is based on the premise that there are zones and reflexes in different parts of the body that correspond with certain organs or glands of the body. The goal is to relieve blockage, promote the flow of energy, and reduce tension—thus, reflexology may be helpful in treating stress-related illnesses (Micozzi, 2019).

Herbal Supplements Ashwagandha, also known as *Indian ginseng* or *Indian winter cherry*, has long been used in Ayurvedic medicine to reduce anxiety, pain, and inflammation. This herbal remedy works by normalizing cortisol levels, thus reducing the stress response and the symptoms that go along with it.

Other Activities The following are simpler activities you can recommend to most clients to aid in relaxation and stress reduction:

- **Humor.** Laughter releases endorphins and relieves feelings of stress (Fig. 9-7). It enhances respiration

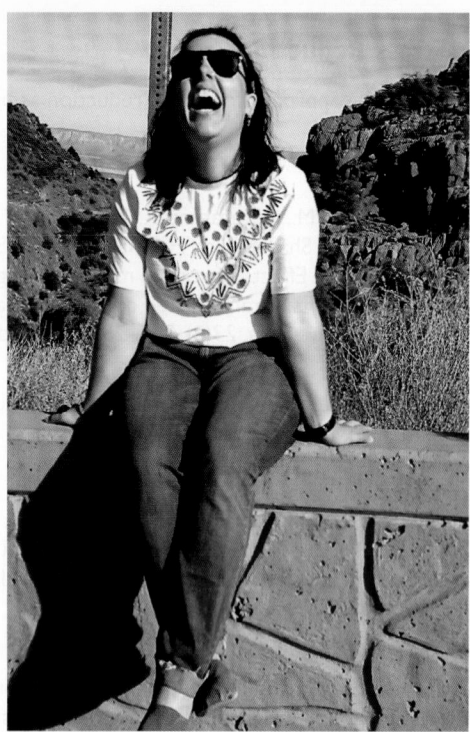

FIGURE 9-7 Laughter releases endorphins and helps to relieve stress.

and circulation, oxygenates the blood, suppresses the activation of stress-related hormones in the brain, and activates the immune system (Bennett et al., 2014; Cousins, 1979, 2005; du Pré, 1998; Tremayne, 2014). Some medical centers have begun implementing in-house humor programs for older adults as an intervention to reduce stress and preserve cognitive function. *Note: Humor is often useful in reducing anxiety in older adults* (Mallya et al., 2019). See iCare 9-2.

- **Music therapy.** Listening to relaxing music reduces the stress response. A study comparing the physiological and psychological effects of stress found that those exposed to relaxing music produced lower levels of cortisol and salivary alpha-amylase (endocrine markers produced with exposure to stress)

compared with rest alone or listening to soothing water. Music listening led to a lower perceived stress level and reduced anxiety, as well as quicker recovery after a stressful experience (Thoma et al., 2013; Umbrello et al., 2019).

- **Art activities.** Painting, working with clay, and engaging in other art activities can help to express emotions and release endorphins.
- **Dance and sports.** Like other forms of physical activity, dance and sports release physical tension and emotions. Steady-state exercises, such as running or swimming at a consistent pace, offer stress relief in a meditative manner through sustained deep breathing and movement. Physical activity can also enhance self-esteem and help people feel better through the simple act of accomplishing a personal goal.
- **Journal writing.** Journal writing helps the person to reflect on experiences and express emotions. The venting of emotion that can occur in journal writing often provides insights into the causes of stress and ways to modify stressors.

Changing Perception of Stressors or Self

Recall that altering one's perception is one way to improve adaptation to stress.

- **Cognitive restructuring** may be helpful for clients who have an unrealistic perception of the stressor and can imagine only negative outcomes. With this technique, you help clients to recognize their negative focus and restructure their thinking in more positive and realistic ways. For example, your patient is diagnosed with type 2 diabetes and can only think of losing his leg. You identify his negative thinking and encourage him to follow guidelines for controlling blood sugar, increasing physical activity, and adhering to a healthy American Diabetes Association (ADA) diet as the best way to avoid complications.
- **Identifying positive aspects of self and coping abilities** promotes self-esteem and helps clients to recognize and use the resources they have for coping with their stressors.
- **Self-affirmation** improves problem-solving under stress (Cresswell et al., 2013).
- **Positive self-talk** is another method for increasing self-esteem. Each time you hear negative self-talk, stop the client and ask them to rephrase the statement so that it is positive.

Identifying and Using Support Systems

You can facilitate successful adaptation by helping clients to identify and contact people and groups who offer various supports (e.g., listening, encouragement, advice, problem-solving, help with household tasks, financial support). Be aware of the groups available in your community (e.g., WW®, Alcoholics Anonymous, Reach for Recovery). You may need to teach socialization

---

♥ iCare 9-2

Using Humor

When using humor, the caring nurse considers the following:

- The nurse must be sensitive to patients' unique personalities, ethnic background, and other personal traits.
- Humor might not be appropriate when the patient is experiencing pain, is extremely ill, needs quiet time or privacy, needs to cry, or is stressed.
- When in doubt about whether to use humor or not, remember that there is no substitute for compassion, care, and touch.

skills to clients who are socially isolated so that they can begin to build a support system.

Reducing the Stress of Hospitalization

Illness and hospitalization are stressful for patients and their families. In addition to being sick, patients find themselves in unfamiliar surroundings, with little privacy and a certain loss of control.

- *Promote patient-centered care* in the healthcare agency as much as you can.
- *Involve patients and families actively in their care.* This helps them adapt to the stressors of hospitalization.
- *Teach patients what to expect* from hospitalization; give them a few tips to help plan ways to minimize the stress they experience (see the Self-Care box, Teaching Clients How to Reduce the Stress of Hospitalization).

Providing Spiritual Support

♥ iCare In addition to helping clients obtain spiritual support from church groups and clergy, you can help to strengthen the client spiritually. You may consider the following:

- Pray for or with clients, if they desire and if you are comfortable doing so. Prayer can help reduce their feelings of powerlessness and loneliness.
- Help clients to define their values and set boundaries that honor themselves and uphold their values.
- Teach clients to silently recite affirming phrases (e.g., on inhalation, say, "I am free"; exhale and say, "Stress, leave me"). The client may prefer to use relevant spiritual passages.

For other ways to provide spiritual support, see Chapter 13.

Crisis Intervention

As an entry-level nurse in acute and ambulatory care settings, you are more likely to see patients in the first three phases of crisis and not be present for the adaptive and postcrisis stages. Crisis centers often rely on telephone counseling (hotlines). If telephone counseling is not adequate, or if observations of the home environment are needed, home visits may be necessary. See Clinical Insight 9-2 for a description of how to intervene at an entry level of practice when a patient is in crisis.

 Go to Chapter 9, Clinical Insight 9-2: Crisis Intervention Guidelines, in Volume 2.

KnowledgeCheck 9-10

- Describe at least five specific interventions for dealing with an angry client.
- What is cognitive restructuring?
- What is the purpose of positive self-talk?
- List the seven steps of crisis intervention.
- Why is relaxation an important stress intervention?

Self-Care

Teaching Clients How to Reduce the Stress of Hospitalization

Share the following tips with clients, preferably before hospitalization.

What to Bring

➤ Make a list of necessities and pack carefully before you leave home. For example, bring your own soap, toothpaste, lotion, pajamas, and slippers or your favorite tea bags and sweetener. Having familiar things can make your stay more pleasant for you.

➤ Bring clothing that is washable, loose, and comfortable.

➤ If you will feel well enough, bring your computer, reading material, crossword puzzles, or whatever you like to do that can help prevent boredom and depression. You might want to bring a few family photos for your nightstand.

➤ Before your appointment, jot down a few notes of what you want to remember to ask when your healthcare provider comes into the room.

➤ Do *not* bring jewelry, cash, credit cards, or other valuables.

Family and Friends

➤ Do not allow family or friends to visit if they are ill.

➤ Ask family or friends to stay at the bedside, particularly when the healthcare provider is "making rounds." They can advocate when you feel too ill to ask for what you need.

➤ Family or friends can also help you interpret and remember the information and instructions that you will receive. There may be 30 care providers in your room each day, and when you do not feel well, it is hard to keep track of everything.

➤ Keep a bottle of hand sanitizer by your bed or insist visitors, including family members and care providers, use a hand-hygiene product at the door when entering the room, just as you do.

Caregivers

➤ Know the name of your primary nurse (or nurses) on each shift; ask as many questions as you need to.

➤ Even though some things seem to not make sense (e.g., taking your temperature at 3 a.m.), there is likely a medical reason for it. Try to be as patient and cheerful as possible.

Stress Management in the Workplace

Workplace stress is common, particularly in the helping professions, such as healthcare.

Caring for others can drain your physical, social, and mental energy. However, when you remain drained over a long period of time, your ability to care for others may be affected. Certain factors about the job can lead to feelings of stress, such as:

- Excessive workload, short staffing
- Few opportunities for growth or advancement

- Work that isn't engaging or challenging
- Lack of social support
- Not having enough control over job-related decisions
- Conflicting demands or unclear performance expectations
- Salary below expectations

You will need to pay attention to your feelings, your body, and your personal responses to stress.

- Do you notice that you are eating more than usual or have lost your appetite?
- Are you feeling edgy or impatient with family or coworkers, or are you not sleeping well?
- Do you feel tired or often have headaches or gastrointestinal distress?
- Are the muscles in your face and shoulders tense?
- Do you often take work home with you?
- Are you unable to stop thinking about work, even when you are at home?
- Do concerns about finances or personal situations consume your thinking and create a sense of doom?

If you answered yes to many of those questions, you probably need to start managing your stress. When stressors arise in the workplace, the following actions are especially important:

- *Set realistic expectations of yourself and others.* Do not be overcritical; most people, including you, are doing the best they can.
- *Ask for help.* Seeking the support of trusted friends and family does not indicate failure or incompetence. Your employer may offer stress-management support through an employee-assistance program. When overwhelmed by work stress, you may want to talk to a counseling professional who can help you manage stress and practice healthy coping behavior.
- *Strengthen relationships in the workplace and at home.* Having someone to connect with on the job can help you get through stressful situations. One way to relieve pressure is to offer support to colleagues who need help with tasks or with their feelings. This adds to the overall morale on a unit and improves the efficiency of performing many tasks.
- *Be proactive* about the things you can change and accept the things that you cannot change. Get involved in constructive efforts to change a particular stressor. If you cannot effect the changes, and if you cannot accept things as they are, you may need to think about removing yourself from the situation. Complaining and negative talk add to your own stress and that of others.
- *Join and support professional organizations* that address workplace issues (e.g., the National Student Nurses Association and the American Nurses Association).
- *Set boundaries.* In a fast-paced healthcare environment, which may be understaffed and undersupplied,

there are times to set healthy boundaries about working more shifts, taking more patients, or adding to your workload with more and more tasks and responsibilities. Saying no may be the best thing you can do for yourself to prevent burnout, and it also safeguards the safety of your patients.

- *Strive for balance* in these seven key areas: family; financial responsibilities; health; social contributions; career, vocation, or education; and spirituality or faith. Focus on the most important items and tasks; remember, work affects life, but your life also affects your work.
- *Take time to recharge.* When possible, be sure to use paid time off (PTO) and not let it go to waste. Rest and recovery are important for fending off work-related stress. 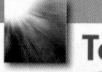 Whether you work the day or the night shift, getting restorative sleep helps you stay alert and keeps you from making careless errors on the job.

Making Referrals

This chapter has presented many assessments and interventions for reducing stress. Remember, though, that you are not yet an expert nurse, and no one, not even an experienced nurse, is an expert in all areas. It is important not to "get in over your head" and attempt to intervene beyond your abilities with clients who are showing maladaptive coping. You can help by recognizing your limitations and by referring the client to qualified professionals (e.g., a spiritual leader, a counselor, a social worker, a practitioner of complementary therapies, a physician, a psychologist, or a psychiatrist).

 ThinkLike a Nurse 9-5:
Clinical Judgment in Action

Saranyu is a registered nurse seeking employment at a local nursing home. She left her previous employer because of stress and frustration with agency policies, for which the bottom line was financial gain rather than quality patient care. What can Saranyu do to help ensure that she will not experience the same problem in the new agency?

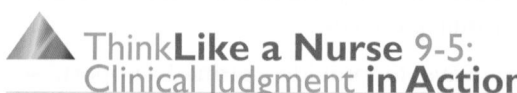

To explore learning resources for this chapter,

Go to Davis Advantage and find:

Answers and Suggested Responses for all questions in this chapter

Concept Map

Knowledge Map

References and Bibliography

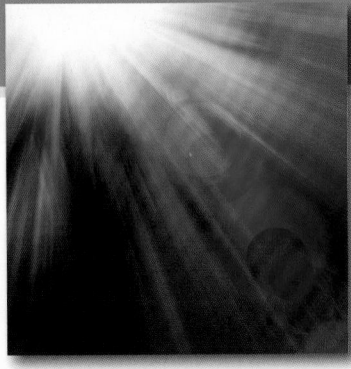

CHAPTER 10

Psychosocial Health & Illness

Learning Outcomes

After completing this chapter, you should be able to:

➤ Explain the relationship of psychosocial factors to overall health and development.

➤ Identify the factors that influence the development and stability of self-concept.

➤ List the four interrelated components of self-concept.

➤ Develop a nursing care plan for patients exhibiting disturbances in self-concept and self-esteem.

➤ Identify nursing diagnoses, prioritize hypotheses, generate solutions, and take action specific to body image disturbance.

➤ Describe interventions for preventing depersonalization.

➤ List the psychological and physiological effects of anxiety.

➤ Recognize the levels and symptoms of anxiety that are severe enough to merit referral to a mental health professional.

➤ Devise a nursing care plan for the nursing diagnosis of Anxiety.

➤ Differentiate between mild depression and that which should be referred to a mental health professional.

➤ Assess older adults for cues of depression.

➤ Prioritize hypothesis, generate solutions, and take action for patients who are depressed.

➤ Prioritize hypothesis, generate solutions, and take action for patients with a diagnosis of Risk for Suicide.

Key Concepts

Anxiety

Depression

Psychosocial health

Self-concept

Related Concepts

See the Concept Map on Davis Advantage.

Example Client Condition

Anxiety

Depression

Self-Concept Disturbance and Low Self-Esteem

Meet Your Patient

You are caring for a 16-year-old patient named Karli who is suffering from fractures to both arms and several ribs, as well as extensive first- and second-degree burns to 30% of her body, after a motor vehicle accident. Karli was driving her parents' car home from her part-time job when she lost control of the car and crashed into a wall. The car exploded in flames. A passerby quickly reported the accident, and fast action by the emergency response team saved Karli's life.

Karli is suffering from a moderate amount of shock and pain. She alternates among outbursts of anger, self-directed sarcasm, and despondence. She tells you that she cannot understand how the accident happened, that one moment she was adjusting the car radio, and the next moment she awoke in the hospital. Then suddenly, she explodes: "It's not fair! I just took my eyes off the road for a second; that's all!" She bursts into

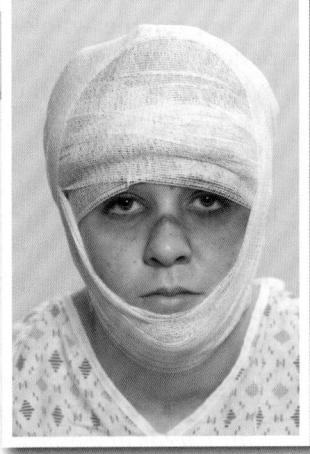

tears. Picking at her bandages, she sobs, "No one will ever love me the way I'm going to look. My life is over. I hate myself!" You take her hand. "I used to be pretty," she says, "but now I'll look like a freak! What did I do to deserve this? I know plenty of kids who drive drunk or high all the time. I wasn't doing anything wrong! Why did this happen to me?"

Before reading on, jot down a list of the multiple physical, psychological, and social issues that you would need to consider in developing a comprehensive care plan for Karli. You can revisit your list throughout this chapter to compare your answers.

ThinkLike a Nurse 10-1:
Clinical Judgment **in Action**

Review Chapter 6 as needed.

- What theoretical knowledge about Karli's developmental stage will assist you in determining nursing diagnoses, interventions, and outcomes?
- Considering that Karli will need a significant amount of assistance for activities of daily living (ADLs) because of her fractures and burns, how might you use the time to develop your therapeutic relationship?

ABOUT THE KEY CONCEPTS

This chapter introduces you to the key concepts of **psychosocial health, self-concept, anxiety,** and **depression.** As you study the related topics and terms in the chapter, you will gain a more complete understanding of the four key concepts. All of these will help you organize the content in your memory.

PSYCHOSOCIAL HEALTH

This chapter is designed to help you provide basic psychosocial care for patients in general practice settings. **Key Point:** *Remember, the physical body is only one dimension of a person. What patients are thinking and feeling is equally important to their healing process.*

Theoretical Knowledge knowing **why**

The interactions of the mind and body are continuous and complex. One of the strengths of nursing is that we can go beyond a *biomedical* (disease-oriented) focus to care for the whole person. Nurses recognize that patient responses to illness are influenced not only by the physical pathology but also by the person's psychosocial health and its relationship to their overall wellness.

The term *psychosocial* encompasses both psychological and social factors: a person's psychological state interacts with their social development and position within society to contribute to their overall—or biopsychosocial—well-being (Fig. 10-1). Figure 10-2 illustrates the interlocking psychosocial influences on health and personal development.

Key Point: *Any human dimension may dominate health needs at a given time.* For example, a patient suffering from a severe flare-up of psoriasis (a skin disease characterized by red, scaly patches) may require *physiological interventions* during the acute stage. They may not be ready to deal with body image issues *(psychological dimension)* until their skin lesions are better. Remember, though, that your patients' psychosocial needs are just as important as, for example, their dietary requirements or their level of pain.

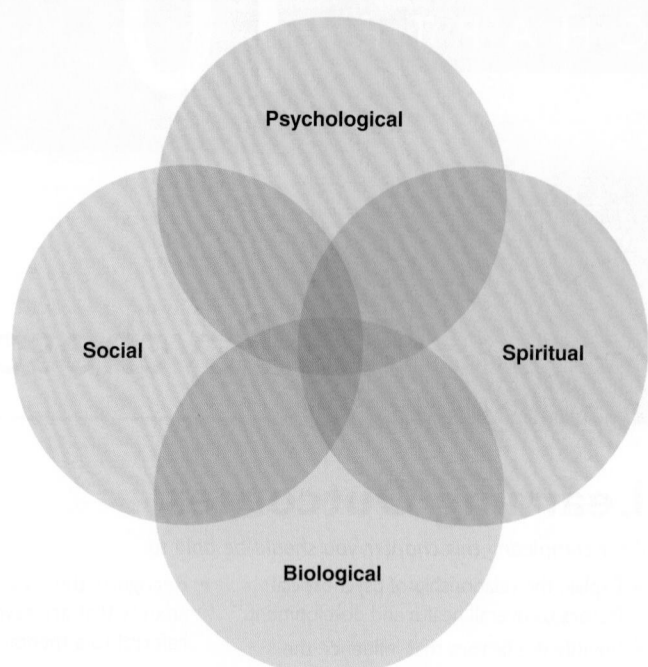

FIGURE 10-1 In the biopsychosocial view of health, biological, psychological, social, and spiritual factors interact to contribute to health.

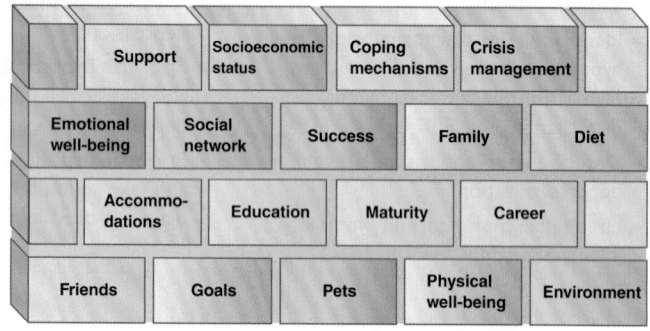

FIGURE 10-2 Interlocking psychosocial influences.

What Is Psychosocial Theory?

You can think of **psychosocial theory** as a method of understanding people as a combination of psychological and social events.

- **Erickson.** Of the many theories of psychosocial development, the works of the German psychologist Erik Erikson (1902–1994) are foremost. Using Erikson's theory, you can assess for successful completion of developmental tasks. Refer to Chapter 6 for more information about Erikson's theory.
- **Maslow.** Psychologist Abraham Maslow's theory of self-actualization and self-transcendence is another psychological theory that is relevant for healthcare providers (see Chapter 6). Maslow (1968) developed a widely accepted hierarchy of human needs and motivations, in which essential needs (e.g., air, water, and food) must be met before higher needs (e.g., learning, creating, understanding, and self-fulfillment).

Recall that, in order from most basic to highest need, Maslow's hierarchy includes physiological, safety and security, love and belonging, self-esteem, and self-actualization needs.

KnowledgeCheck 10-1

- Why is psychosocial theory relevant to healthcare?
- What does the term *biopsychosocial* mean?
- Explain the implication of Maslow's hierarchy of human needs for working with a homeless man with gangrene.

What Is Self-Concept?

Self-concept is one's overall view of oneself. It is your complete and unique answer to the question, "Who do you think you are?" (e.g., "I am a student"; "I am successful and competent"). **Key Point:** *Self-concept forms out of a person's evaluation of their physical appearance, sexual performance, intellectual abilities, success in the workplace, friendship and approval from others, problem-solving and coping abilities, unique talents, and so on. A person with a healthy self-concept has a mostly positive perception of these evaluations of self.*

- **Self-concept influences social functioning:**
  Example: Karli's self-concept is that she "looks like a freak." If this self-concept continues, she may withdraw from social interaction, and it will be difficult to form new relationships (social functioning).
- **Self-concept is influenced by social functioning:**
  Example: If others—for example, prospective employers—are not accepting of her injuries, she may have difficulty finding a place in society. This would reinforce her poor self-concept.

The "Dynamic Self" The self forms and changes in response to our environment. Margaret Mead (1934) states that we discover who we are through a life-long process of differentiating from and comparing ourselves to others. As we experience life events, we continually reconstruct and develop our understanding of who we are. Dickstein (1977) called this idea the **dynamic self,** meaning that who we are (the self) is subject to change through social and environmental influence. But if our concept of self is changeable, what factors cause it to change? Can it be harmed? If so, how? How does it first develop? These questions are explored next.

How Is Self-Concept Formed?

Humans are not born with a concept of self; rather, it develops during infancy and childhood as the child interacts with family members, peers, and others. The broad steps of self-concept formation are as follows:

Infant—Learning that the physical self is different from the environment: "Me; not me."
Child—Internalizing others' attitudes about the self, primarily parents and peers: "Who do *they* say that I am?"

Child and adult—Internalizing standards of society: "How do I compare to others?"
Adult—Self-actualization and self-adjustment: "This *is* who I am and who I will continue to be."

Change occurs gradually, and the steps overlap. Also, the age at which the stages occur varies widely among individuals.

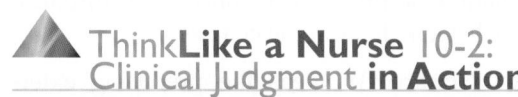

ThinkLike a Nurse 10-2: Clinical Judgment in Action

- Explain how each of Maslow's five basic needs is related to psychosocial development; that is, how might each of the needs affect psychosocial health if met or not met?
- To what extent do social relationships help or hinder a person in meeting each need?

What Factors Affect a Person's Self-Concept?

Some factors affecting a person's self-concept cannot be changed, for example, gender and developmental level. Others, such as socioeconomic status and family relationships, can be changed to a degree but are not fully under the person's control—and certainly not during childhood, when the self-concept is forming. Understanding that such factors are not within a patient's control may help you provide more sensitive, compassionate care to patients experiencing impaired self-concept.

Gender Certain aspects of self-concept differ by gender. Some of the differences appear to be related to the role expectations of boys and girls rather than any actual difference in ability. For example,

- Girls typically rate teamwork and cooperation as important to their sense of self, whereas most boys place a higher value on individual achievement.
- Physical appearance seems more important to girls throughout life.

As role expectations and career choices for both men and women expand, these gender-based differences in self-concept may fade.

Developmental Level As we mature, our self-concept becomes more inner-guided. That is, others (e.g., friends, the media) have less influence on our ideas about who we are. We become less likely to view our failures and shortcomings as evidence of worthlessness and more likely to see them as challenges common to all humans.

Family and Peer Relationships The family strongly influences a child's developing self-concept. As an infant's sense of self-permanence develops and becomes stable, categories of self begin to emerge. These include notions of gender, values, and a sense of having a distinct "place" among family members (Feiring & Taska, 1996). Social identity is first fostered by interactions between infants and their parents and broadens in toddlerhood through relationships with immediate and extended family members. For older children, peers become more important than family in this respect.

Illness and Hospitalization Illness, and especially hospitalization, can have a depersonalizing effect that alters the self-concept. The ill person may feel that they have become an object to be examined, poked, prodded, and discussed. (See Preventing Depersonalization in the Example Client Condition: Self-Concept Disturbance and Low Self-Esteem, later in the chapter.)

Locus of Control Whereas the preceding external influences contribute to the *formation* of our self-concept, internal influences help us to *moderate* it. For example, biochemical brain processes influence perceptual acuity, interpretation abilities, and level of insight and judgment.

- **Internal Locus of Control.** People who allow their inner "voice" to influence their self-concept have what is called an **internal locus of control.** Such people feel they can exert control over their lives. They take appropriate responsibility for their life experiences and for their responses to them. This enables them to interpret unexpected adverse events (e.g., injuries and illnesses) in a more positive light.
- **External Locus of Control.** In contrast, people who have an **external locus of control** attribute control of their situation to external factors, including other people, institutions, and God. They may feel they lack the ability to change what happens to them.

KnowledgeCheck 10-2
- When does self-concept become stable?
- What factors have been determined to have an impact on our self-concept?

What Are the Components of Self-Concept?

Self-concept embraces four interrelated components: body image, role performance, personal identity, and self-esteem.

Body Image
How often do you hear someone say something like the following?

"Look at those muscles. They look good!"
"Look at them pigging out. They need that candy like I need a hole in my head."

You probably grew up overhearing similar statements. Such preoccupations with food, weight, and appearance have led to prejudice against people who do not have perfect bodies. Therefore, it is not surprising that people engage in unhealthy behaviors in order to match social ideals or that patients like Karli have difficulty coping with disfiguring accidents or with surgeries such as limb amputation and mastectomy.

Body image is your mental image of your physical self, including physical appearance and physical functioning. Both cognitive understanding and sensory input influence body image. Our cognitive understanding is in turn influenced by family, social, ethnic, and cultural norms; education; and exposure to alternative values. The American media portray the ideal male as young, tall, and muscular; nevertheless, many men who do not meet that ideal maintain a positive body image because their cognitive understanding indicates they are in good health, are attractive to their partners, and so on.

Ideal, Perceived, and Actual Body Image People may not see their own bodies as objectively as others see them. Some psychological disorders interfere with the ability to interpret sensory data objectively.

Example: People with the eating disorder anorexia nervosa see themselves as fat even when their mirror reflects (and other people see) a normal or even an underweight body.

The closer the match between a person's ideal body image and sensory input about their body (perceived body image), the more positive the person's body image is likely to be.

Appearance and Function A physical disability, such as blindness, deafness, or paraplegia, can interfere with the development of a positive body image. Children born with a physical disability are at risk for poor self-concept and depression, perhaps related to the person's perception that they have low social value. In contrast, an attractive appearance and superior functioning, whether in a career, sports, or academics, make it easier to develop a positive body image. Keep in mind, though, that cognitive understanding (e.g., of one's success) can increase self-concept, regardless of a person's appearance or achievement.

Gradual Versus Sudden Body Changes Gradual changes in physical appearance occur naturally throughout life as the body matures and grows old. Most people adapt to such changes relatively easily, especially because their friends and colleagues are aging, too. In contrast, when changes in appearance or functioning occur abruptly (e.g., after an acute illness or an accident, as happened to Karli in the Meet Your Patient scenario), they are much more difficult to accept. Denial, anger, self-hatred, and despair are a few of the many reactions that can follow such an abrupt change in body image.

Influence of Body Image on Health Body image influences health and health behaviors. According to the Centers for Disease Control and Prevention (CDC, 2018), positive body image has been associated with a lower risk of illness and injury, better immune response, quicker recovery, and increased longevity.

Role Performance

Before you began your nursing program, what were your expectations? What activities did you imagine yourself engaged in, and what behaviors did you think would be expected of you? Together, these expectations make up your conception of the *role* of a nursing student. In addition to being a student, you probably play several roles, such as parent, sibling, friend, breadwinner, caregiver, volunteer, and so on. These are your **role expectations.**

Role performance can be defined as the actions a person takes and the behaviors they demonstrate in fulfilling a role. Instead of expectations, role performance is the reality.

- **Role strain.** If you expected that you would sail through your nursing program and instead, you find yourself so overwhelmed that you have begun to skip classes lately, then you are experiencing role strain, a mismatch between role expectations and role performance.
- **Interpersonal role conflict.** In addition, your ideas about how to perform the nursing student role may be very different from those of your instructors. When that type of mismatch occurs, you are experiencing an interpersonal role conflict.
- **Interrole conflict.** Imagine if you are a single parent and your child's sudden illness causes you to miss a week of classes and clinicals. When two roles make competing demands on an individual, interrole conflict occurs.

Personal Identity

Your **personal identity** is your view of yourself as a unique human being, different and separate from all others. Identity develops over time, beginning in childhood, when you identified with your parents. Unlike body image, which is expected to change over time, personal identity is relatively constant and consistent.

- **Cultural identity is culturally determined and learned through socialization.**
  - *People with a strong sense of personal identity* are less likely to compare themselves to others or to be unduly influenced by them. They tend to appreciate the unique perspective and contributions of others, yet they value their own perspectives and contributions.
  - *People with a weak sense of personal identity,* in contrast, have difficulty distinguishing their boundaries from those of others. They may interpret events in the environment personally or interpret their personal experiences as belonging to everyone.
    - *Example:* When the hospital's air-conditioning system fails, a patient with a weak personal identity may insist that it is a punishment for their complaint that the room was too cold.

- **Patients may experience an impaired sense of identity when they are challenged by a serious or chronic illness** (e.g., cancer, AIDS, or rheumatoid arthritis). They then place too many limitations on their activities or interpret the responses of others in light of their illness. For instance, a person with osteoporosis (loss of bone density) might say, "I can't go birdwatching anymore because I might trip and fall."

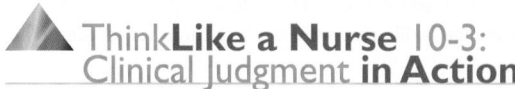 ThinkLike a Nurse 10-3: Clinical Judgment in Action

Think about Karli in the Meet Your Patient scenario. If you asked Karli to list 10 labels to identify herself, what do you think they would be? You may not have enough information to come up with 10, but think of as many as you can.

Self-Esteem

Self-esteem is, in the simplest terms, how well a person likes themselves. It is the difference between the "ideal self" and "actual self," that is, between "what I think I ought (or want) to be" and "what I really am." The area of overlap in Figure 10-3 illustrates the extent of self-esteem. The more overlap there is, the higher the self-esteem.

When we succeed beyond our ambitions, we experience a high sense of self-esteem, but when we aim for an ideal self beyond our capabilities, we risk a loss of self-esteem. Even mild illnesses and minor setbacks can cause some people to question their self-worth. It is not difficult to imagine how a sudden, disfiguring accident such as Karli's might provoke a crisis in self-esteem because Karli's ideal self is currently out of her reach. This is especially true if the problem is interpreted as one incident in a continuing pattern—for example, a couple hoping to become parents who experience a third pregnancy loss.

As another example, if you find that you are more successful as a nursing student than you expected to be when you enrolled in your nursing program, that is a boost to your self-esteem. If, however, your expectations

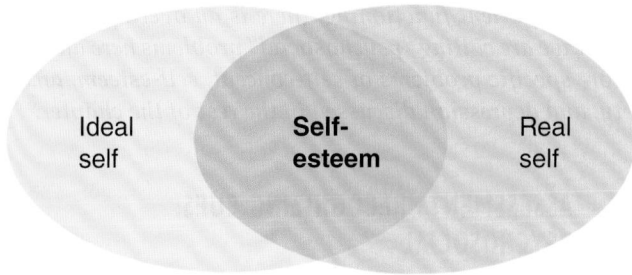

Ideal self: expectations and aspirations; "what I ought to be," "what I wish I were"

Real self: current skills, attributes, and successes; "what I really am"

FIGURE 10-3 Self-esteem is determined by the relationship between an individual's ideal self and real self.

of being a skillful nurse outweigh your current abilities, then lower self-esteem is likely.

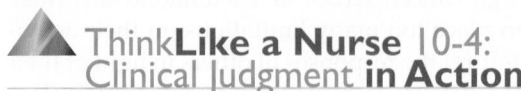

ThinkLike a Nurse 10-4: Clinical Judgment in Action

What if a person does not have any aspirations for success but is content to meet each day as a learner, vitalized by their daily discoveries? How do you think a high score on an examination would affect their self-esteem? How do you think a poor score on a clinical skills test would affect their self-esteem?

KnowledgeCheck 10-3

- What four components contribute to an individual's self-concept?
- What is self-esteem?

PracticalKnowledge
knowing how

Practical knowledge in this chapter consists of planning, implementing, and evaluating care to promote clients' mental health and provide support when they experience mental health problems. **Key Point:** *Remember, the physical body is only one dimension of a person. What patients are thinking and feeling may be equally important to their healing process.*

Communication and interpersonal skills are especially important in caring for patients' psychosocial needs (see Chapter 15). Physical illness may be particularly stressful when it occurs in combination with psychosocial issues. For example, think of Karli (Meet Your Patient). Might her condition have been less complicated if (1) she had no disfiguring injuries or (2) she were an older adult at a developmental stage when appearance is generally less crucial?

Nursing Care to Promote Psychosocial Health

As a nurse, you should be prepared to recognize and care for patients with psychosocial problems in all practice settings. **Key Point:** *Psychosocial problems involve nearly all areas of patient functioning; there is an overlap between what we are calling "psychosocial" problems here and the more specific problems of self-concept, self-esteem, anxiety, and depression discussed in the rest of the chapter.*

ASSESSMENTS/RECOGNIZING CUES: PSYCHOSOCIAL

No matter what the patient's medical diagnosis, you need to perform accurate and ongoing psychosocial assessments to develop holistic nursing diagnoses and interventions. Most admission assessment forms have questions to screen psychosocial status. If any of the answers indicate

the risk for a problem, you may need to conduct a more comprehensive special needs (or system-specific) assessment. For an example of a psychosocial assessment tool specific to Self-Esteem (self-esteem is one aspect of psychosocial health),

Go to Chapter 10. **Clinical Insight 10-2: Performing a Self-Esteem Inventory**, in Volume 2.

A comprehensive psychosocial assessment should include the following categories:

- Biological details
- Recent life changes or stressors (both positive and negative)
- Lifestyle and relationships with the wider social environment
- History of psychiatric disorders
- Functional abilities (behavioral performance)
- Self-efficacy (the belief that you can influence your own behaviors and outcomes)
- Family relationships
- Social resources and network
- Usual coping mechanisms
- Interpersonal communication
- Understanding of current illness
- Major issues raised by current illness
- Health priorities
- Spirituality (see the HOPE assessment tool in Chapter 13)
- Personality style. That is, personality traits that may affect care or compliance, such as a tendency to be dependent, hostile, dramatic, or critical (Gorman & Anwar, 2019).

Psychosocial information is personal and sometimes sensitive. To encourage patients to share this information, you will need to use your developing communication skills (see Chapters 3 and 15). For example:

- Be aware of your own biases and discomforts that could influence your assessment.
- Use active listening through eye contact and verbal response. Be sensitive, though; eye contact is uncomfortable for some people.
- Proceed from general details ("How do you get along with your parents?") to the specific ("Does your mother ever hit you?").
- Use an open and positive voice tone, facial expression, and body language (e.g., avoid frowning, criticizing, or expressing shock).
- Keep the focus on the patient.
- Be respectful and sensitive to cultural and gender-specific details.
- Use open-ended questions (questions that cannot be answered with a yes or no).
- Follow the patient's cues by using reflection and restating.
- Be flexible and use humor as appropriate.
- Provide empathetic feedback and touch as appropriate.

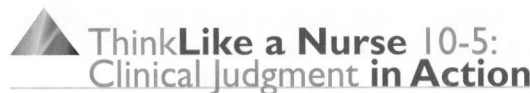

ThinkLike a Nurse 10-5: Clinical Judgment in Action

Psychologically, Karli is worried about the unfairness of her situation and is probably struggling with body image issues. In addition, what do you think her *social* concerns might be?

NURSING DIAGNOSIS/ANALYZING CUES: PSYCHOSOCIAL

What we are calling *psychosocial diagnoses* overlap with those used in the rest of the chapter for the more specific problems of self-concept, anxiety, and depression. That is, you may use some of these psychosocial diagnoses for clients who have problems involving self-concept, anxiety, and depression.

It would be impossible to list every possible psychosocial diagnosis; the following are but a few.

- *Family Coping Impairment.* Usual support (comfort and assistance) from a significant other is either insufficient, withdrawn, disabled, or maladaptive, causing a significant health challenge.
- *Parental Role Conflict.* A parent struggles with role confusion and/or conflict and parental position and responsibilities.
- *Impaired Individual Coping.* The patient fails to comprehend and effectively judge stressors, perceives incorrect or dangerous life choices as normal, is unable to identify strengths, and is unable to use available resources.
- *Post-Trauma Syndrome.* "[The person experiences a] sustained … maladaptive response to a traumatic overwhelming event" (Herdman & Kamitsuru, 2018, p. 316).
- 🍀 *Risk for Loneliness.* The person is separated from persons, culture, objects, or environments to which a person may have ongoing attachments.
- 🍀 *Social Isolation.* The person experiences aloneness (lack of interaction with others) that has a negative impact on their health.

Psychosocial issues can be a problem, a symptom of a problem, or the etiology of a problem. You must determine what is cause and what is effect, although this can be hard to unravel at times. What you identify significantly affects your choice of goals and nursing activities (Table 10-1).

PLANNING/PRIORITIZING HYPOTHESES AND GENERATING SOLUTIONS PSYCHOSOCIAL

Individualized goal/outcome statements will depend on the nursing diagnoses used, client input, and realistic expectations of what the client can achieve and agrees to. For example:

- For *Compromised or Disabled Family Coping,* examples of goal statements include "Involves family members

in decision making" and "Expresses feelings and emotions freely."
- For *Impaired Social Interaction,* goal statements may call for the client to develop the skills of "engagement, assertiveness, compromise, confrontation, and consideration."

The Psychosocial Health domain of the NOC taxonomy includes approximately 40 *NOC standardized outcomes* to describe psychological well-being, psychosocial adaptation, self-control, and social interaction. The following are a few examples:

> Abusive Behavior Self-Restraint
> Coping
> Child Adaptation to Hospitalization
> Psychosocial Adjustment: Life Change
> Role Performance
> Social Interaction Skills

Other NOC domains also include useful psychosocial outcomes. The following are only a few examples (Moorhead et al., 2018):

> Family Coping
> Family Functioning
> Family Participation in Professional Care
> Family Resiliency

PLANNING PSYCHOSOCIAL IMPLEMENTATION/ TAKING ACTION

Psychosocial nursing interventions and activities will be determined by the nursing diagnoses you identify, especially by the etiologies. In general, the purposes of the interventions in nursing activities are to provide conflict mediation, enhance socialization, or strengthen the family.

NIC standardized interventions for psychosocial diagnoses are found primarily in the Behavioral and Family domains of the NIC system. The following are some examples from the Behavioral domain:

> Anger Control Assistance
> Anxiety Reduction
> Coping Enhancement
> Decision-Making Support
> Socialization Enhancement

The following are examples of interventions from the Family domain:

> Family Involvement Promotion
> Family Support
> Family Therapy
> Parenting Promotion (Butcher et al., 2018)

Specific, individualized nursing activities used to help patients maintain a sense of personhood are discussed in the Example Client Condition: Self-Concept Disturbance and Low Self-Esteem.

Table 10-1 ➤ Implications of Identifying a Psychosocial Issue as Problem, Etiology, or Symptom

	AS PROBLEM	AS ETIOLOGY	AS SYMPTOM
Nursing Diagnosis	**Interrupted Family Functioning** r/t tumult from parental divorce	Delayed Development r/t lack of stimulation **secondary to Interrupted Family Functioning** (parental divorce)	Ineffective Individual Coping (Mother) r/t poor judgment and impaired reality perception, **as manifested by Interrupted Family Functioning** and risk-taking behaviors
Sample Goals (based on problem)	*NOC Outcome* Family Functioning	*NOC Outcome* Child Development: 4 years	*NOC Outcomes* Coping, Decision Making, Role Performance, Social Support, Impulse Control
	Goals Members perform expected family roles. Family cares for dependent members.	*Goals* Child demonstrates age-appropriate motor activities. Child uses four- and five-word sentences.	*Goals* Identifies coping strategies that have been effective in the past. Discusses the implications of decision alternatives with family.
Sample Interventions and Activities (based on etiology)	*NIC Interventions* Family Integrity Promotion Family Process Maintenance Normalization Promotion	*NIC Interventions* Developmental Enhancement: Child Parent Education Health Screening	*NIC Interventions* Coping Enhancement Decision-Making Support Impulse Control Training Family Involvement Promotion Support Group Support System Enhancement
	Specific Activities Promote parental involvement in healthcare. Assist the family with skills of and education for conflict resolution, coping, and problem-solving. Link the individual and family to the appropriate support and education services.	*Specific Activities* Establish time for one-on-one care. Provide for creative play (e.g., clay, blocks, painting). Teach parents appropriate stimulation. Teach parents about developmental milestones and expected behaviors. Assess changes in family processes.	*Specific Activities* Identify and discuss alternative behaviors. Encourage delaying decision making when under stress. Help the mother solve problems constructively. Assist her to evaluate her own behavior. Identify and discuss past successful coping behaviors that she has used.

Nursing Care for Example Client Condition: Self-Concept Disturbance and Low Self-Esteem

For assessment/recognizing cues, nursing diagnosis/analyzing cues, and planning/prioritizing hypothesis and generating solutions, as well as more nursing actions, see the Example Client Condition: Self-Concept Disturbance and Low Self-Esteem.

■ ASSESSMENT/RECOGNIZING CUES: SELF-CONCEPT AND SELF-ESTEEM

For an all-purpose assessment of self-concept you might use for screening in any setting,

Go to Chapter 10, **Clinical Insight 10-1: Assessing Self-Concept,** in Volume 2.

To assess self-esteem,

 Go to Chapter 10, **Clinical Insight 10-2: Performing a Self-Esteem Inventory,** in Volume 2.

▇ NURSING DIAGNOSIS/ANALYZING CUES: SELF-CONCEPT AND SELF-ESTEEM

Self-concept issues, like psychosocial issues, can be a problem, a symptom of a problem, or the etiology of a problem. It is important for you to determine what is cause and what is effect, although this may not always be clear. As you can see in Table 10-1, your analysis significantly affects your choice of goals and nursing activities. For diagnoses that may be useful for patients with either low overall self-concept or difficulties in specific domains of self-concept (e.g., self-esteem), see the Example Client Condition: Self-Concept Disturbance and Low Self-Esteem.

 ## Think**Like a Nurse** 10-6: Clinical Judgment **in Action**

In the Meet Your Patient scenario, Karli perceives herself as unlovable because of "looking this way." You should not assume that you know exactly what Karli means by this. Also from the scenario: "Picking at her bandages, she sobs, 'No one will ever love me the way I'm going to look. My life is over. I hate myself!' You take her hand. 'I used to be pretty,' she says, 'but now I'll look like a freak!'"

- Which of her words do you need to clarify with her?
- What might you say to her to get her to provide more information about the psychosocial meaning of her statement?

EXAMPLE PROBLEM: Self-Concept Disturbance and Low Self-Esteem

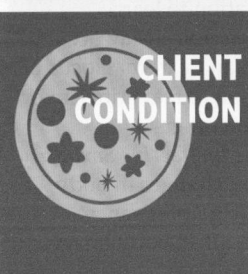
CLIENT CONDITION

Avoid Confusing Low Self-Concept With Clinical Emotional and/or Behavioral Psychiatric Diagnoses

There is no recognized diagnosis describing self-concept disorder in the American Psychiatric Association's *DSM-5* (2019). Self-concept (particularly self-esteem) plays a secondary role in a number of disorders but is not a primary disorder itself.

Basic Definitions

Self-Concept
One's overall view of self
The answer to "Who am I?"

Self-Esteem
The difference between ideal self and real self
An important component of self-concept

Defining Characteristics of the Problem

The person tends to:
- Avoid eye contact
- Have a stooped posture
- Move slowly
- Have poor grooming

Verbal behaviors include:
- Speaking hesitantly
- Being overly critical of others and of self
- Not accepting positive comments about self (e.g., "Oh, anybody could have done it")
- Apologizing frequently
- Feelings of powerlessness

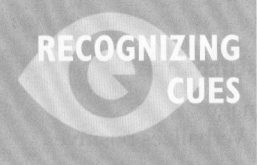
RECOGNIZING CUES

Key Point: *If you suspect serious problems with self-concept, document the patient's responses in your nursing notes and refer the patient for appropriate psychological testing.*

Self-Concept

- To screen for problems, assess body image, role performance, personal identity, and self-esteem.
- For specific details,

 Go to Chapter 10, **Clinical Insight 10-1: Assessing Self-Concept,** in Volume 2.

Self-Esteem

To assess for the self-esteem dimension of self-concept, look for these symptoms:
Avoids eye contact
Speaks hesitantly

Stooped posture
Overly critical
Moves slowly
- Observe for behaviors and comments associated with low self-esteem:
  Does not accept positive comments
  Poor grooming
  Apologizes frequently
  Overcritical of others and self (e.g., "I never do anything right")
  Verbalizes feelings of powerlessness (e.g., "Whatever you say is fine with me"; "It doesn't matter what I do; it won't change anything)
- For specific details,

 Go to **Chapter 10, Clinical Insight 10-2: Performing a Self-Esteem Inventory,** in Volume 2.

(continued)

EXAMPLE PROBLEM: Self-Concept Disturbance and Low Self-Esteem—cont'd

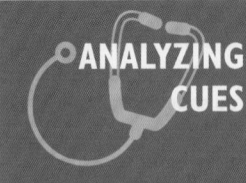

ANALYZING CUES

Analysis

When analyzing data for self-concept problems, avoid seeking simplistic cause-and-effect relationships. Determine whether the self-concept or self-esteem issue is the central problem or the etiology of another diagnosis.

Avoid confusing low self-concept with clinical, emotional, and/or behavioral psychiatric diagnoses.

Diagnoses as a Problem (Examples)

- **Chronic Low Self-Esteem**
  Definition: Ongoing, long-standing overall self-dissatisfaction and negative self-appraisal (i.e., wide differences between "ideal" and "actual" or "perceived" self). *Etiology example: Depression*
  - **Situational Low Self-Esteem.** *Definition:* Develops negative perception of self-worth and self-worth in response to a specific situation (e.g., loss or change) and wide differences between "ideal" or "actual" and "perceived" self. *Etiology example: Failure to adapt to change in functioning*
  - **Personal Identity Disturbance.** *Definition:* Incorrect assessment of self-identity, inability to integrate perception of self, and inability to distinguish self and nonself. *Etiology example: Mental illness*
  - **Body Image Disturbance.** *Definition:* Has a confused image of physical self (e.g., physical appearance) or negatively evaluates body or an aspect of it. *Etiology example:* Eating disorder, gender conflict, disfigurement

Diagnoses as an Etiology: Use as an etiology when Self-Concept or Body Image precedes and plays a central role in a condition such as depression.

Examples:
- *Impaired Individual Coping*—Use when a patient experiences difficulties in adapting perception and evaluation of self after changes in health status (e.g., loss of a limb).
- *Complicated Grieving*—May develop in anticipation of or after body changes (e.g., hysterectomy) or loss of a key role (e.g., resulting from death of a spouse).

Other Examples:
- *Deficient Knowledge*—Low self-esteem diminishes the motivation to learn.
- *Impaired Social Interaction*—May occur when low self-esteem and external locus of control cause the person to fear criticism or lack of acceptance from others.
- *Sexual Dysfunction* or *Ineffective Sexuality Pattern*—For example, changes in body structure or function (e.g., pregnancy, disease, arthritis) may affect body image.

PLANNING/ PRIORITIZING HYPOTHESES/ GENERATING SOLUTIONS

Examples:

For Chronic Low Self-Esteem

NOC Outcome: Quality of Life
Individualized Outcome: Expresses pleasure in participating in activities; is able to cue self to replace negative with positive self-talk

For Body Image Disturbance

NOC Outcome: Body Image
Individualized Outcome: Verbalizes positive aspects of body

EXAMPLE PROBLEM: Self-Concept Disturbance and Low Self-Esteem—cont'd

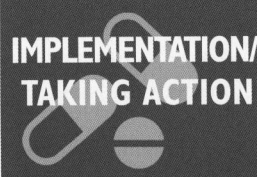

IMPLEMENTATION/ TAKING ACTION

Identify Patient Strengths

Help the client identify strengths and past achievements by pointing out areas of strength that you observe, such as the following:

- *Emotional strengths* include the ability to express emotions, to "feel" for others.
- *Relationship strengths* include being sensitive to others' needs and being a good listener.
- *Spiritual strengths* include faith in God and participation in church activities.

Evaluate the client's sense of humor, which can also be a strength; be sure the client considers special aptitudes, such as cooking, arts and crafts, sports, work, and education.

Promote Positive Body Image

When a negative body image is contributing to self-concept and self-esteem issues, refer to the discussion, Promoting Positive Body Image.

♥ iCare Prevent Depersonalization

You can help patients maintain a sense of personhood by using a caring approach:

- Introduce yourself if the patient does not know you.
- Address the patient by their preferred name each time you enter the room; always speak respectfully.
- Listen actively when the patient speaks.
- Do not talk *about* the patient to others in the room (e.g., do not say, "He seems better today, don't you think?"); speak *to* the patient.
- Use eye contact and touch; keep in mind that people vary in their desire to be touched.
- Always offer an explanation before beginning a procedure, and warn the patient before you touch them ("I'm going to touch your leg now").
- Move, turn, and position the patient gently.
- Provide privacy when performing procedures or discussing something personal or sensitive.

Other Interventions Specific to Self-Esteem:

- Establish a therapeutic nursing relationship emphasizing trust, consistency, honest communication, and unconditional positive regard.
- Encourage the client to be as independent as possible (e.g., by performing self-care).
- Monitor for and discourage self-criticism and negative self-talk.
- Teach client to substitute positive self-talk for negative self-talk. For example, the client says, "I know my blood sugar is high, but I still ate way too much again today." You might remind the client that they have been following their exercise program religiously.
- Be supportive and accepting, but do not invade the client's personal space.
- Help the client develop realistic goals.
- Encourage the client to take part in activities that offer opportunities for success.
- Role-model communication skills that will help improve interpersonal relationships. Provide opportunities for practice.
- Refer to self-help and support groups as needed.
- When possible, ask the client's advice (e.g., "How do you usually do this dressing change?")
- Point out good health practices and healthy aspects of the client's body function.

(continued)

EXAMPLE PROBLEM: Self-Concept Disturbance and Low Self-Esteem—cont'd

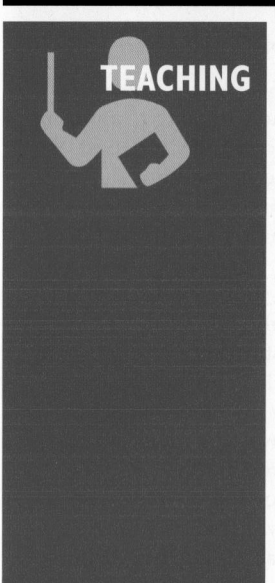

TEACHING

Promoting Self-Esteem in Children

Demonstrate love and acceptance by doing the following:

- Spending some one-on-one time with the child as often as possible: reading, playing, or just being together
- Being free with touches: a hug, a pat on the back
- Refraining from frequent negative criticism
- Providing nearly total acceptance of the child

Provide security by:

- Having clearly defined limits and consequences for breaking rules
- Being firm and consistent in applying the rules
- Being sure the rules are reasonable
- Allowing some latitude for individual actions within defined limits
- Treating the child with respect

- Establishing routines, such as bedtime activity, homework before play, dressing for school
- Clearly defining every family member's role

Promote competence by:

- Setting realistic expectations about behaviors
- Assigning a few chores that are within the child's capability (e.g., picking up toys, making the bed)
- Role-modeling values, such as respect for others, honesty, and responsibility
- Providing positive feedback
- Helping the child accomplish goals
- Providing a stimulating and responsive environment
- Providing support in meeting challenges

DSM-5 = Diagnostic and Statistical Manual of Mental Disorders, 5th edition.

PLANNING /PRIORITIZING HYPOTHESES AND GENERATING SOLUTIONS: SELF-CONCEPT AND SELF-ESTEEM

You will choose outcomes based on the client's specific nursing diagnosis. For examples, refer to Example Client Condition: Self-Concept Disturbance and Low Self-Esteem.

When self-concept is the etiology of other problems (e.g., Sexual Dysfunction related to negative body image), choose outcomes based on the problem label (e.g., Sexual Functioning). At least one outcome, if achieved, must demonstrate that the Sexual Dysfunction has been alleviated.

IMPLEMENTATION/TAKING ACTION: SELF-CONCEPT AND SELF-ESTEEM

Common *NIC standardized interventions* for self-concept and self-esteem diagnoses are found in the Example Client Condition for self-concept and self-esteem.

Specific, individualized nursing activities for patients with self-esteem and self-concept problems are discussed in the following sections.

Promoting Self-Esteem and Self-Concept

Although the foundation for self-esteem is laid in childhood and affected by many sociocultural variables, your nursing approach can help preserve and enhance a patient's self-esteem. For suggestions on promoting a patient's self-esteem, see the Example Client Condition: Self-Concept Disturbance and Low Self-Esteem.

Promoting Positive Body Image

A negative body image can contribute to broader self-concept and self-esteem issues, as well as to anxiety and depression. Therefore, some of the following body image interventions may also be useful for self-concept and self-esteem issues, as well as for anxiety and depression. You can help parents promote a positive body image in their children, and you can help patients develop a different attitude toward their bodies.

- Examine your own attitudes about what constitutes a healthy body, and pay attention to the messages you convey to others.
- Encourage patients to discuss body changes resulting from their illness, surgery, or trauma.
- Provide the opportunity to interact with people who have had similar body changes.

Teach clients the following and provide feedback as needed.

- **Healthy Does Not Mean Perfect.** Understand that healthy bodies come in a wide range of shapes and sizes. Social media may portray an ideal body that is unrealistic and unhealthy for most people. If they make you feel bad by comparison, don't look at them!

- **Focus on Activity and Healthy Eating.** Encourage clients to be active and focus on healthy eating rather than starving and depriving themselves to lose weight.
- **Don't Make Negative Comments About Your Body.** Be conscious of negative comments you make. Try not to talk negatively about body weight, size, or deformity; be kind to yourself. Ask a support person to point out when you are being unrealistically critical of your body.
- **Keep a List.** Keep a list of things you like about your body and refer to it when you are feeling down.
- **Accept Compliments.** Practice accepting positive comments about your appearance. Ask a support person to coach your responses as needed (e.g., say, "Thank you" after a compliment).
- **Challenge Critical Comments.** Practice challenging critical comments from others about your appearance.
- **Surround Yourself With Positive People.** Surround yourself with positive people who support the changes you are trying to make in your image of your body. Avoid people who are critical.
- **Use a Counter.** Buy a counter and click it each time you make a deliberate effort to accept positive feedback about your body or engage in positive body behaviors.

To see a Care Plan and Care Map for Disturbed Body Image,

 Go to Davis Advantage Resources, Chapter 10, **Care Plan and Care Map.**

 Think**Like a Nurse** 10-7: Clinical Judgment **in Action**

Refer to Karli in Meet Your Patient. Look at these five labels for self-concept problems: Chronic Low Self-Esteem Disturbance, Situational Self-Esteem Disturbance, Personal Identity Disturbance, Impaired Role Performance, Body Image Disturbance. Which one most clearly applies to Karli? Explain your thinking.

Facilitating Role Enhancement

Sometimes the difficulty with self-concept centers on an inability to fulfill one's usual or desired role. Specific actions to enhance role satisfaction include the following, some of which may also be useful for anxiety and depression:

- Help the client distinguish between ideal and actual role performance.
  - Help the person to identify their past, present, and future roles. For older adults, encourage reminiscence.
- Discuss boundaries, expectations, and management as defined by lifestyle and family networks.
- Facilitate communication between client and significant other regarding the sharing of role responsibilities to accommodate the role changes of the ill person.

- Help the client describe realistic roles and expectations tailored to specific health changes.
- Compare realistic roles with previous and less functional roles.
- Provide education about the difference between previous roles and current roles.
- Provide a learning environment that focuses on positive and supportive change.
- Help the client identify and role-play behaviors needed in new roles.

Knowledge Check 10-4

Without looking back at the preceding material, see whether you can:

- List three interventions for preserving self-worth and preventing depersonalization.
- List three interventions for promoting self-esteem.
- List three interventions for fostering positive body image.
- List three interventions for promoting role enhancement.

EXAMPLE CLIENT CONDITION: ANXIETY

I wake up in the middle of the night with a knot in my stomach and thinking about work. I go over and over my day and worry about my decisions and what I should have done instead. I replay the meetings in my head and think, "I know what that person said, but what did she mean by that?" I wonder whether I can handle the responsibility. My neck and shoulders are so tense that I get headaches. But when I try to relax and watch TV, I can feel my heart racing, and I feel shaky. I can't concentrate well enough to read.

Theoretical Knowledge knowing **why**

Anxiety is a common emotional response to stressors. Most anxious patients, even those with diagnosed obsessive–compulsive disorder or panic attacks, are not admitted to the hospital just for their anxiety. You will encounter them more often in community settings or when they are hospitalized for other illnesses.

Levels of Anxiety

Anxiety ranges from normal to abnormal, depending on its **intensity** and **duration**—how much anxiety is present and how long it has been present. Peplau (1963) described the four levels of anxiety found in Table 10-2.

Coping With Anxiety

People cope with anxiety in various ways.
  Mild anxiety:

- Exercising
- Talking with others
- Engaging in pleasurable activities

Table 10-2 ➤ Levels of Anxiety

DEFINITION OR DESCRIPTION	SYMPTOMS
Mild Anxiety	
Normal anxiety in response to the events of day-to-day living ▪ Heightens perception ▪ Sharpens the senses ▪ Enhances learning ▪ Enables the person to function at their optimal level	▪ If symptoms are present, they may include muscle tension, restlessness, irritability, and a sense of unease. ▪ The person usually does not experience distress.
Moderate Anxiety	
▪ As anxiety increases, the perceptual field narrows. ▪ The person begins to focus on self and the need to relieve their discomfort.	▪ Less alert to environmental events ▪ Distracts easily ▪ Shorter attention span ▪ May need help with problem-solving but can attend to their needs with direction ▪ Physical symptoms may include: 　Increased heart and respiratory rates 　Increased perspiration 　Gastric discomfort 　Increased muscle tension ▪ Rapid, loud, and higher-pitched speech
Severe Anxiety	
▪ Perceptual field is very narrow: The person can focus on only one particular detail or may shift focus to many extraneous details. ▪ Focus is totally on self and the need to relieve the anxiety	▪ Concentration and attention span are severely limited, so the person has difficulty completing simple tasks. ▪ Anxiety prevents problem-solving and learning. ▪ Feelings: May report dread, confusion, and other unpleasant emotions ▪ Physical symptoms: May include headaches, palpitations, tachycardia, insomnia, dizziness, nausea, trembling, hyperventilation, urinary frequency, and diarrhea
Panic Anxiety	
The person: ▪ Becomes unreasonable and irrational ▪ Is unable to focus on even one detail in the environment ▪ May misperceive environmental cues ▪ May lose contact with reality (e.g., hallucinations or delusions)	▪ May react wildly (e.g., shouting, screaming, running about, clinging to something) or withdraw completely ▪ Cannot function or communicate effectively (e.g., may speak incoherently or be unable to speak) ▪ May feel terror and impending doom, believe they have a life-threatening illness, or think that they are "going crazy" ▪ Physical symptoms include dilated pupils, labored breathing, severe trembling, sleeplessness, palpitations, diaphoresis, pallor, and muscular incoordination (Townsend, 2018).

▪ Deep-breathing
▪ Relaxation programs

Less adaptive behaviors include excessive sleeping, eating, smoking, crying, pacing, fidgeting, substance use, laughing, cursing, nail biting, or finger tapping.

Severe anxiety:
When anxiety is more severe, the person attempts to counteract the anxiety in some way.

Defense Mechanisms Each person develops unique patterns of coping with anxiety, called **defense**

mechanisms. Defense mechanisms are used consciously or unconsciously to relieve the anxiety, for example:

- **Denial**—refusing to acknowledge the existence of a real situation or associated feelings
- **Displacement**—transferring feelings from one target to another that seems less threatening (e.g., kicking the dog when you are angry at your boss)

See Chapter 9 for further discussion of defense mechanisms.

- When overused, defense mechanisms can be maladaptive and lead to psychological disorders such as phobias, obsessive–compulsive disorders, and dissociative disorders (e.g., amnesia). See Chapter 9 for further discussion of defense mechanisms.
- Excessive or unrelieved anxiety may contribute to
  - Psychosis—loss of ability to differentiate self from nonself
  - Impaired reality testing—knowing what is real and what exists only in one's mind
- Examples of psychotic responses to anxiety include schizophrenia and delusional disorders. *NOTE:* These

disorders are beyond the scope of this book. If you need more information, refer to a mental health text.

PracticalKnowledge
knowing **how**

Nursing Care for Example Client Condition: Anxiety

In general practice, the focus of nursing care for clients with anxiety is (1) to differentiate between mild anxiety and that which is severe enough to require referral to a mental health professional and (2) to provide interventions to relieve anxiety. You will find more theoretical knowledge, as well as nursing care, in the accompanying Example Client Condition: Anxiety.

KnowledgeCheck 10-5

- What is anxiety?
- When is anxiety a normal response to life?
- Identify at least three healthcare scenarios that might trigger anxiety in patients.

EXAMPLE CLIENT CONDITION: Anxiety

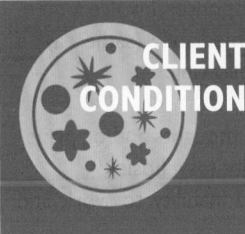
CLIENT CONDITION

Definition of Anxiety

- Anxiety is a common emotional response to a stressor.
- Fear and anxiety produce similar responses. However, you can differentiate them as follows:

  Fear: *Response:* Cognitive
  Threat: Known; physical or psychological
  Event: Present

  Anxiety *Response:* Emotional; psychological conflict
  Threat: Known or unknown; psychological conflicts
  Event: Anticipated, not existing yet

Key Point: *Anxiety is so common that mild anxiety is considered normal and even necessary for our survival.*

Defining Characteristics (Signs, Symptoms)

Behavioral—poor eye contact, restlessness, crying, trembling, rapid speech
Cognitive—confusion, difficulty concentrating, forgetfulness
Objective data—sweating, rapid pulse and respirations, dilated pupils
Subjective data—shortness of breath, nausea, insomnia, worry

Etiologies (Examples)

- Patients encounter anxiety-producing situations in healthcare settings because of threats to their basic needs (Stuart, 2012).
- Chronic anxiety has been associated with physical problems, such as the risk of heart attack.

Levels of Anxiety

Key Point: *Anxiety ranges from normal to abnormal, depending on its intensity and duration— "how much and how long." Each level requires different nursing actions.*

Normal anxiety level:
- Essential reaction to a real danger or threat to physical or psychological integrity
- Enables us to survive and, when the threat is no longer present, to move on

Abnormal anxiety level:
- Out of proportion to the situation
- Lasts long after the threat is over, perhaps causing the person to alter their lifestyle

(continued)

EXAMPLE CLIENT CONDITION: Anxiety—cont'd

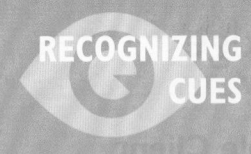

RECOGNIZING CUES

- Consider a comprehensive physical assessment to rule out underlying disease or disorders (e.g., hormone imbalance).
- Identify the presence, level, and source of anxiety. Each level requires different nursing actions.
- Determine whether the anxiety is normal and adaptive or whether it is severe enough to require nursing interventions, consultation, or referral to a mental health professional.

For a checklist to help you distinguish normal and severe anxiety,

 Go to Chapter 10, Focused Assessment: Anxiety Assessment Guide **in Volume 2.**

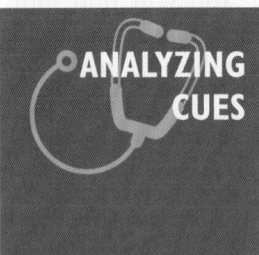

ANALYZING CUES

- **Anxiety**—Feeling of distress or apprehension whose source is unknown; the threat is psychological in nature.
- **Death Anxiety**—Apprehension, worry, or fear surrounding thoughts of dying

- **Decisional Conflict**—Struggle related to determining a course of action
- **Fear**—Feeling of dread or distress whose cause can be identified, often from a physical threat
- **Ineffective Denial**—Unsuccessful attempt to reduce anxiety by refusal to accept facts, feelings, or thoughts

PLANNING/ PRIORITIZING HYPOTHESIS/ GENERATING SOLUTIONS

For Anxiety

NIC Examples
Anxiety Reduction (priority intervention)
Anger Control Assistance
Anticipatory Guidance
Calming Technique
Coping Enhancement
Emotional Support

Individualized Nursing Activities
- Recognize that the client is anxious.
- Help the client identify the source of their anxiety.
- Deal with the symptoms of the client's anxiety.
- Provide a calm and safe environment to help the patient stay focused.
- Establish a relationship of trust, caring, and unconditional positive regard.
- Be present; stay with the client to help allay fears, create trust, and promote safety.
- Use clear and factual knowledge tailored to the individual's circumstances.
- Explain and, if necessary, explore details of all healthcare procedures.
- Advise regular physical exercise unless contraindicated by a physical condition.
- Help identify triggers and situations that create anxiety.
- Administer and monitor antianxiety medication prn.
- Assist with relaxation methods.

Severe Anxiety

NIC Examples
Same as for Anxiety

Individualized Activities

■ ✚ If you suspect severe or disabling anxiety, document the patient's responses. Involve a mental health professional immediately (same day) if you discover any of the following:
■ Suicidal thoughts
■ Assaultive or homicidal thoughts and/or plans
■ Loss of touch with reality (psychosis)
■ Significant or prolonged inability to work and care for self or family

Death Anxiety

NIC Examples
Emotional Support (priority)
Anxiety Reduction
Coping Enhancement
Decision-Making Support
Dying Care
Hope Instillation
Pain Management
Presence
Religious Ritual Enhancement
Spiritual Support

Individualized Activities
- Stay physically close to the fearful patient.
- Obtain spiritual support for the patient and family.
- Honor specific patient/family requests for care.

EXAMPLE CLIENT CONDITION: Anxiety—cont'd

GENERATING SOLUTIONS	Individualized Goal/Outcome Statements	NOC Examples
	For Anxiety	**For Anxiety**
	• Plans coping strategies for anxious situations	Anxiety Self-Control
	• Uses relaxation techniques as required	Anxiety Level
	• Reports absence of physical and psychological manifestations of anxiety	Concentration Coping
	For Death Anxiety	**For Death Anxiety**
	• Reports feeling less fearful	Acceptance: Health Status
	• Discusses funeral arrangements with family	Anxiety Self-Control Comfortable Death
	For Decisional Conflict	**For Decisional Conflict**
	• Identifies relevant information about the decision and its consequences	Decision Making Information Processing
	• Recognizes how various alternatives conflict with others' desires	
	For Fear	**For Fear**
	• Uses effective coping strategies	Fear Level
	• Maintains social relationships and control over life	Coping
	For Ineffective Denial	**For Ineffective Denial**
	• Verbalizes understanding of the complications that may occur if the disease is not treated	Acceptance: Health Status Fear Self-Control Symptom Control
	• Follows prescribed regimen for treatments and medications	

KnowledgeCheck 10-6

- List five nursing diagnoses you could use to describe a problem of anxiety.
- List four cues that would alert you that anxiety is severe enough to merit referral to a mental health professional.

EXAMPLE CLIENT CONDITION: DEPRESSION

Others imply that they know what it is like to be depressed because they have gone through a divorce, lost a job or broken up with someone. But these experiences carry with them feelings. Depression, instead, is flat, hollow, and unendurable.

—Kay Redfield Jamison (1997, p. 218), An Unquiet Mind

TheoreticalKnowledge
knowing why

Depression occurs in all age-groups, even in very young children. It affects about 5% of the adult population in the United States and is one of the top-three risks for functional decline. See Table 10-3 for common truths and myths about depression.

Table 10-3 ➤ Depression: Truths and Myths

TRUE	FALSE
Depressive disorders are more common among women than men (2:1).	"Getting on with life" will cure depression.
Spiritual distress is associated with depression.	Everyone likes to talk about how they feel.
Depression can be defined as a maladaptive emotional response.	Medication is the answer to depression.
Low-socioeconomic circumstances and social isolation correlate with depression.	Once depression has been cured, it does not return.

Key Point: *As a nurse generalist, your independent role is not to diagnose and treat mental illnesses. Rather, it is to assess and document the patient's behavioral state as it relates to their medical–surgical condition.* A depressed patient, for example, may not have the energy or motivation to recall or follow a medical regimen or keep appointments with health-care providers.

Unlike the feeling of true sadness, such as might accompany a divorce, death, or other loss, the depressed mood is typically marked by a sense of emptiness. This contributes to the depressed person's tendency to withdraw from social contacts and also explains the characteristically flat affect (Fig. 10-4).

Practical Knowledge
knowing how

Of course, you will not be conducting psychotherapy in your general practice. However, you *will* care for patients who are taking antidepressant medications and who have situational or even clinical depression. There is much you can do to make their care more effective.

Nursing Care for Example Client Condition: Depression

You will find more theoretical knowledge, as well as nursing care, in the accompanying Example Client Condition: Depression. See also Figure 10-5 and Box 10-1.

Assessment/Recognizing Cues and Taking Action for Older Adults: Depression, Delirium, or Dementia?

Cognitive disorders, such as delirium and dementia, are sometimes confused with depression because they share some symptoms. You can find more information about dementia in Chapter 7. Depression has been described previously.

Assessments/Recognizing Cues and Taking Action: Delirium Delirium, also called *acute confusion,*

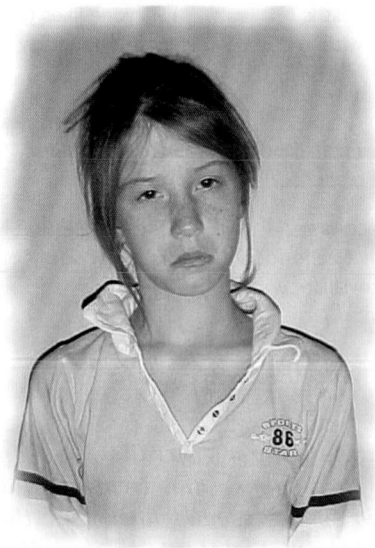

FIGURE 10-4 Depressed affect.

is an acute and potentially reversible disturbance of consciousness and cognition in response to underlying medical or mental illnesses, drug toxicity, and various other causes.

- Delirium is an important consideration in quality of care and patient safety; an estimated 30% of cases are preventable (Unal et al., 2022).
- Many aspects of nursing care—such as medication administration; evaluation of complications; and recognizing cues related to dehydration, nutrition, and sleep—are factors that can be modified to prevent the development of delirium.
- For patients with delirium, the nursing care focus is to keep the patient safe and identify and alleviate the source of the delirium.
- See the iCare Box 10-1, Relieving Anxiety for Patients with Confusion.

Assessment/Recognizing Cues: Dementia Dementia is an irreversible decline in mental abilities. The American Psychological Association (APA; 2019) defines dementia as one of the **neurocognitive disorders (NCDs),** a group of disorders in which the primary clinical deficit is in cognitive function. Dementia can occur at any age but is more common in older adults.

- NCDs are acquired rather than developmental.
- NCDs may be associated with Alzheimer disease, vascular disease, Parkinson disease, traumatic brain injury, HIV infection, or substance-/medication-induced NCD.
- Dementia affects about 10% of adults aged 65 years and older.
- Prevalence increases with age: the rate is about 33% in those older than age 85.

For a comparison of the symptoms of depression and dementia,

 Go to Chapter 10, **Focused Assessment: Differentiating Depression and Dementia,** in Volume 2.

Taking Action: Dementia The Progressively Lowered Stress Threshold (PLST) (Fletcher, 2012) provides a conceptual framework for the nursing care of patients with dementia:

- Monitor the effectiveness and side effects of medications given specifically to improve cognitive function or delay cognitive decline.
- Provide appropriate cognitive-enhancement techniques and social engagement.
- Ensure adequate rest, sleep, fluid, nutrition, elimination, pain control, and comfort measures.
- Avoid the use of physical and pharmacological restraints.
- Maximize functional capacity: maintain mobility and encourage independence as long as possible.
- Address behavioral issues: identify environmental triggers, medical conditions, or caregiver–patient conflict that may be causing the behavior.

EXAMPLE CLIENT CONDITION: Depression

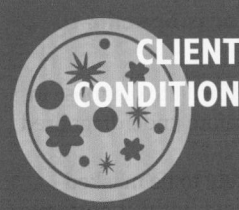

Definition

Depression

Commonly used to describe a feeling of sadness or "the blues." In healthcare, refers to a specific condition with characteristic symptoms and often devastating consequences if left untreated (Steptoe, 2007).

Criteria Established by the American Psychiatric Association (APA) for Major Depressive Disorder:

- Depressed mood most of the day nearly every day for at least 2 weeks, typically accompanied by markedly diminished interest or pleasure in activities previously enjoyed
- Insomnia or hypersomnia
- Loss of energy
- Feelings of worthlessness
- Diminished ability to concentrate
- Feelings of emptiness
- Recurrent thoughts of death (APA, 2019)

Facts & Figures

Depression occurs in all age-groups and is a leading cause of disability in the United States for those aged 15 to 44 years:
- Effects 16.1 million American adults.
- Median age at onset is 32.5 years
- More prevalent in women than in men
- Suicide is the second leading cause of death in 15- to 29-year-olds (World Health Organization, 2018).
  See Table 9-3 for common truths and myths about depression.

What Causes Depression?

Depression theories fall into the following four groupings:
- *Physiological theories* relate depression to biochemical imbalances stemming from hormonal, neurological, or genetic factors.
- *Psychodynamic theories* relate depression to loss, abandonment, and emotional detachment and to diurnal and seasonal mood variations.
- *Cognitive theory* relates depression to negative thinking.
- *Social/environmental theories* relate depression to poor family relationships, difficult interpersonal relationships, and socioeconomic and political factors.

Depression in Older and Middle Adults

- Depressive symptoms are an important indicator of general well-being and mental health among older adults.
- People who report many depressive symptoms often experience higher rates of physical illness, greater functional disability, and higher healthcare resource utilization.
- Although older adults were the demographic group with the highest suicide rates for decades, suicide rates for middle-aged adults (aged 24 to 62) have increased to comparable levels.
- In 2018, 13% of women aged 65 and over reported depressive symptoms compared with 9% of men (Federal Interagency Forum on Aging-Related Statistics, 2020).

Suicide

- Suicide can occur:
  - In patients on psychiatric units
  - In patients you care for on a medical–surgical unit or in their homes.
- Illnesses such as advanced cancer and AIDS are often accompanied by uncontrolled pain and delirium and are associated with higher suicide rates.
- People who are clinically depressed cannot just "snap out of it." If untreated, the symptoms may continue for weeks or even years.

(continued)

EXAMPLE CLIENT CONDITION: Depression—cont'd

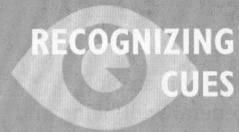
RECOGNIZING CUES

Assess for Risk Factors

Key Point: *If risk factors are present, perform focused assessment to determine whether depression is present.*

Risk Factors

Family history of depression, hormonal or nutritional imbalance; inability to externalize anger; low self-esteem: negative thinking: learned helplessness and hopelessness: prior failure of coping mechanisms; traumatic loss; catastrophic stressors (e.g., unemployment, disability, poor health, bereavement); chronic disease; female sex; sleep disturbance

Risk Factors Specific to Older Adults:
Disability, new illness, poor health status, prior depression, poor self-perceived health, sleep disturbance, bereavement, female gender (Cole & Dendukuri, 2014)

Assess for Signs and Symptoms (APA Criteria)

- Feelings (affect)
- Cognition (thoughts)
- Behaviors
- Lifestyle effects
- Physiological effects

Signs & Symptoms Specific to Older Adults

- Depression is difficult to diagnose in older adults and is therefore underdiagnosed and undertreated.
- Depression is more likely to be masked rather than exhibited by typical symptoms such as sadness.
- Symptoms are often physical or expressed as personality changes such as irritability.
- Some of the physical symptoms of depression (e.g., fatigue, anorexia, constipation, and psychomotor retardation) can be confused with physical illness, medication interactions, substance abuse, or "signs of old age."
- **Key Point:** *Depression may occur along with, or be mistaken for, dementia and delirium. In older adults, all three conditions may include the symptoms of confusion, distractibility, and memory loss.*

 Assess Suicide Risk

Be direct: "Have you thought about harming yourself? If so, what do you plan to do?"

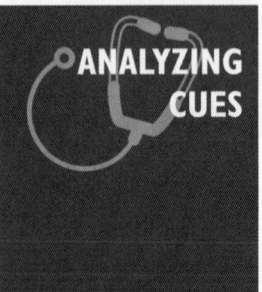
ANALYZING CUES

Depression is a psychiatric diagnosis, so you will not make that diagnosis. You should, however, describe associated problems that are amenable to nursing intervention. The following three diagnoses from Saba (2017) may be useful in describing the feelings and moods of patients who are depressed.

Primary Diagnoses

Hopelessness
Powerlessness
Suicide Risk—This must always be considered when a patient is depressed, especially when there is a history of prior attempts or the person verbalizes a desire to die or intent to kill themselves.

Associated Physical and Behavioral Diagnoses

Activity Alteration
Inadequate Health Management
Constipation
Obesity
Overweight
Limited Social Interaction
Inadequate Hygiene and Grooming
Difficulty Sleeping
Risk for Obesity
Inability to Perform Activities of Daily Living (Bathing, Feeding, Dressing, Toileting)

EXAMPLE CLIENT CONDITION: Depression—cont'd

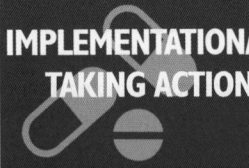

PLANNING/ PRIORITIZING HYPOTHESIS/ GENERATING SOLUTIONS

NOC Outcomes

- Depression Level
- Impulse Self-Control
- Suicide Self-Restraint
- Mood Equilibrium

Individualized Outcomes

- Participates in healthcare decisions to extent possible
- Sets realistic goals for self
- Expresses positive belief in self, others, and meaning of life

IMPLEMENTATION/ TAKING ACTION

General Interventions for Depression

Establishing a nurse–patient bond requires an empathetic approach involving warmth, acceptance, and understanding (unconditional positive regard) even in the face of an unresponsive, even angry, patient.

- Promote activity. Small-group activities help build self-esteem.
- Promote and teach good nutrition and hydration.
- Use therapeutic communication.
- Assess use of, and provide information about, complementary and alternative medicine for depression.

■ Continue to monitor for suicide risk. Be direct: "Have you thought about harming yourself?

- Institute measures to build self-esteem.
- Provide information on support groups.

Team Communication

If you identify signs of depression, be certain to communicate that to other members of the staff and to the primary care provider.

Medications

- Closely supervise patients being treated with antidepressants because severe side effects are possible.

■ When a patient is admitted to a hospital, there is a risk that self-administered medications may be overlooked. Missed doses of an antidepressant combined with a physical illness may cause depression symptoms to worsen.

 Nursing Interventions for Older Adults

Key Point: *Remember that (1) depression is not a normal part of aging, and (2) it is important to identify depression and not mistake it for dementia or "signs of old age."*

➤ Go to Focused Assessment: Differentiating Depression and Dementia, in this chapter

- **Medications.** Because metabolism changes with aging, the risk of adverse medication effects is high for older adults.
- **Reminiscence.** Encourage the patient to talk about significant experiences that have occurred during their life.

Key Point: *Keep in mind that depression is a significant predictor of suicide in older adults.*

- Rates of suicide for both men and women reach their highest peaks in the 85-and-older age-group.
- Depression alone cannot adequately explain late-life suicidal behavior, given that only a minority of depressed elders will actually attempt suicide.
- Other known risk factors for late-life suicide—such as loss of a significant other, disability, and prior suicide attempt—have limited explanatory power as well (Cheung et al., 2015).

Also see Box 10-1 and the accompanying CAM Box, Complementary and Alternative Modalities (CAM) used for Depression.

(continued)

EXAMPLE CLIENT CONDITION: Depression—cont'd

SUICIDE PREVENTION INTERVENTIONS

Suicide Prevention Interventions

Key Point: *Your most important nursing intervention is assessment. Be alert for risk factors and warning signs that may indicate the possibility of suicide (see Box 10-1).*

Key Point: *Remember that about 80% of those who attempt suicide give some prior verbal or indirect cues.*

- Evaluate the patient's medications (certain antihypertensive agents, steroids, cancer chemotherapeutic agents, and amphotericin-B can cause depression).
- If risk factors are present, put them prominently on the care plan and report them to other caregivers.
- Do not avoid the patient because you fear saying the wrong thing. Talking about suicide does not increase the risk.
- Be aware of your personal feelings and anxieties regarding suicide.
- If the patient mentions suicide specifically, be direct. Ask whether they are having thoughts of harming themselves.

- If they answer yes, do not leave them. Have someone contact the primary care provider so that a psychiatric consult can be ordered, and possibly transfer the patient to a psychiatric unit if physically stable.
- Ask whether the patient has a plan for suicide and, if so, what it is.

- ▪ Remove items that might be used for self-harm, for example, razor blades and other sharp objects, shoelaces, belts, intravenous tubing, telephone cords, pills, and glasses. Search the room and the bathroom.
- ▪ Make sure the windows cannot be opened.
- ▪ Follow agency policy for continuous monitoring, moving to a room close to the nurses' station, and so on (Gorman & Anwar, 2014; Maybury, 2008).

- **Key Point:** *Never attempt to work with a suicidal patient by yourself. Involve other members of the team immediately.*

COLLABORATING

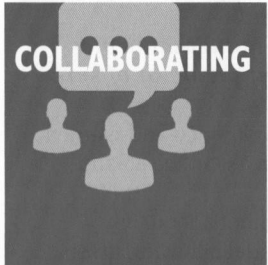

When Should I Refer the Patient to a Mental Health Specialist?

Figure 10-5 illustrates the continuum of mild to severe depression, incorporating aspects of mood, behavior, thoughts, and physical symptoms.

 The presence of any of the following should alert you to document the patient's responses in your nursing notes and make a referral to a mental health specialist:

- ▪ Personal or family history of recurrent depression or bipolar disorder
- ▪ Personal history of recurrence of depression within 1 year after stopping effective treatment

- ▪ Episode of major depression before age 20
- ▪ Severe, sudden, or life-threatening depressive episode (i.e., suicide attempt); if you believe there is a risk for suicide, make the referral immediately (Box 10-1)

Also,

▶ Go to Chapter 10, Clinical Insight 10-3: **Identifying Depressed Patients Who Should Be Referred for Evaluation,** in Volume 2.

EVALUATION

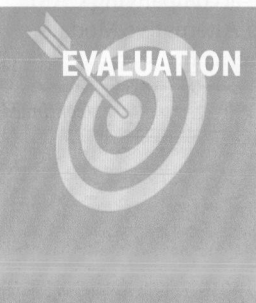

For Depressed Mood:

Reports feeling less sadness and depression
Interacts willingly and appropriately with others

For Powerlessness:

Participates in healthcare decisions to the extent possible
Sets realistic goals for self

For Hopelessness:

Expresses positive belief in self, others, and meaning of life
Demonstrates interest in life/activity

For Risk for Suicide:

Verbalizes any suicidal ideas to staff
Trusts staff enough to disclose any specific plans for suicide

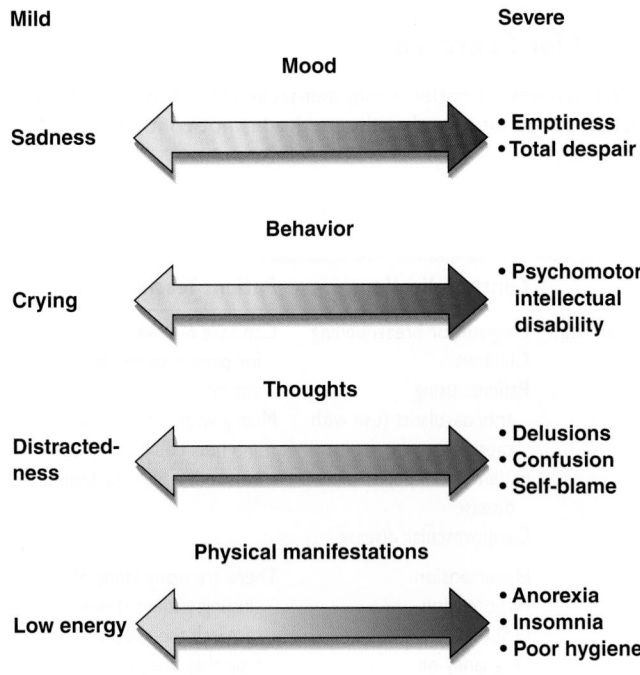

Mild   Severe

Mood

Sadness ←——————————→ • Emptiness
                                        • Total despair

Behavior

Crying ←——————————→ • Psychomotor
                                          intellectual
                                          disability

Thoughts

Distracted-ness ←——————————→ • Delusions
                                              • Confusion
                                              • Self-blame

Physical manifestations

Low energy ←——————————→ • Anorexia
                                            • Insomnia
                                            • Poor hygiene

FIGURE 10-5 Depression assessment continuum incorporating mood, behavior, thoughts, and physical state.

- Ensure a therapeutic and safe environment.
- Encourage and support advance-care planning: explain the trajectory of progressive dementia, treatment options, and advance directives.
- Provide caregiver education and support.
- Integrate community resources into the plan of care to meet patient and caregiver needs.

SUBSTANCE ABUSE AND MENTAL ILLNESS

Substance abuse is a major concern in the United States. It contributes to family crises, public health issues, and criminal justice concerns. Many people who regularly abuse drugs are also diagnosed with mental disorders. Mental illness and substance use disorders are among the leading causes of disability in the United States (Substance Abuse and Mental Health Services Administration [SAMHSA], 2022).

- *Persons diagnosed with mood or anxiety disorders,* antisocial personality, or conduct disorders are more likely to suffer from drug abuse or dependence as well (National Institute on Drug Abuse, 2020).
- *Similarly, persons diagnosed with drug disorder*s are roughly twice as likely to suffer from mood and anxiety disorders.

By far, the most common issue connecting mental illness and substance abuse is patients' use of alcohol and drugs in an attempt to relieve the mental health symptoms that they find disruptive or uncomfortable. Some examples include the following:

- A depressed patient who uses marijuana to numb the painful feelings
- A depressed patient with low energy and lack of motivation who abuses Adderall, cocaine, or crystal meth to increase the drive to get things done

Treatment for Substance Abuse Treatment helps reduce the powerful effects of drugs on the body and brain, thereby helping people improve their physical

---

BOX 10-1 ■ Cues Indicating a Possible Risk for Suicide

Risk Factors

- Alcohol or substance abuse
- Family history of mental disorders or substance abuse
- Family history of suicide
- Firearms in the home
- Family violence, including physical or sexual abuse
- A significant medical illness, such as cancer or chronic pain
- Compulsive gambling
- Recent losses: physical, financial, personal
- Age, gender, sex, race (older or young adult, unmarried white male, living alone)
- Recent discharge from an inpatient psychiatry unit

✚ **Warning Signs**

Patients with risk factors who exhibit any of the following warning signs clearly raise a red flag and merit immediate referral:

- Withdrawal from social contact
- Desire to be left alone

- Preoccupation with death and dying or violence
- Risky or self-destructive behavior, such as drug use or unsafe driving
- Changes in routine sleeping patterns
- Changes in eating habits
- Giving away belongings or getting affairs in order
- Personality changes, such as becoming very outgoing after being shy
- Saying goodbye to people as if they won't be seen again
- Talking about suicide (e.g., "I'm going to kill myself," "I wish I were dead," or "I wish I hadn't been born")

Source: Maybury, B. C. (2008, March 10). *Suicide prevention: Every nurse's responsibility.* Nurse.com. https://www.nurse.com/blog/2008/03/10/suicide-prevention-every-nurses-responsibility/

Complementary and Alternative Modalities (CAM) Used for Depression

Many people use herbal therapies to relieve symptoms of anxiety and depression. Patients may self-treat with herbal remedies, or CAM practitioners may prescribe them. You should assess for CAM use to be sure that the method is not contraindicated and that the patient has informed the primary care provider about its use.

DEPRESSION

CAM	Active Ingredients	Side Effects	Contraindications	Patient Teaching
Ginkgo biloba	Ginkgetin, ginkgolic acid, ascorbic acid, flavonols, sterols	Nausea, vomiting, diarrhea (usually mild) Headache	Pregnant or breastfeeding Children Patients using anticoagulants (use with caution) Patients with peptic ulcer disease Cardiovascular disease	Can take 6–8 weeks for patient to feel any better. Mixing with some fruits and nuts could produce poison ivy–like reaction.
Ginseng	Ginsenosides, beta-elemene, sterols, flavonoids, peptides, vitamins B$_1$, B$_2$, B$_{12}$, nicotinic acid, fats, minerals, enzymes	(Many) Nausea Vomiting Diarrhea Chest pain Headache Nosebleeds Palpitations Nervousness Insomnia	Hypertension Hypotension Diabetes Pregnancy or breastfeeding Patients with active bleeding Anticoagulants Antiplatelet medications	There are many kinds of ginseng; patient should research the specific type they are using. Discourage use by patients who are anticoagulated or who have hypertension or diabetes.
St. John's wort	Tannin, naphthodianthrones, flavonoids, bioflavonoids, phloroglucinols	Dry mouth Constipation Gastrointestinal upset Sleep disturbances Restlessness Photosensitivity Interferes with digoxin and indinavir	Pregnancy or lactation Children Use of monoamine oxidase inhibitors, selective serotonin reuptake inhibitors, alcohol, or over-the-counter cold and flu medications	Teach contraindications and side effects. Patients who are depressed should not take this herb without medical supervision.
S-Adenosyl methionine (SAMe)	Amino acid and adenosine triphosphate, which are produced naturally in the body and are now being reproduced artificially as well	Few side effects Gastric upset Hypomania (in patients with bipolar disorder) Anxiety (in patients with depression) Headache		Patients with bipolar disorder should not use this supplement unless under direct supervision of their physician. Use enteric-coated forms to decrease gastric irritation.

Source: Adapted from Beaubrun, G., & Gray, G. E. (2014). A review of herbal medicines for psychiatric disorders. Psychiatric Services, 51(9), http://ps.psychiatryonline.org/doi/10.1176/appi.ps.51.9.1130; Gorman, L. M., & Anwar, R. (2019). Neeb's fundamentals of mental health nursing (5th ed.). F.A. Davis.

♥ iCare 10-1

Relieving Anxiety for Patients With Confusion

People with dementia are often anxious and fearful. Find ways to reassure and help the person feel more comfortable as you converse, such as the following:
- Gently hold or pat the patient's hand.
- Realize that the person is probably distressed and is doing the best they can.
- Be affectionate, reassuring, and calm, even when things make no sense.
- Respond to the person's feelings instead of the content of their words. For example, if a person is constantly searching

for their partner, don't say, "Your partner is not here." Rather, say, "You must miss your partner," or "Tell me about your partner."
- If the person has difficulty finding the right word, supply it for them unless doing so upsets them. This helps control frustration.
- If you do not understand what the patient is trying to say, ask them to point to it or describe it (e.g., "What does a *zishmer* look like?").
- Consider using alternative therapy, such as music therapy, that may be soothing to the patient.

▼ Toward Evidence-Based Practice

Geipel, J., Koenig, J., Hillecke, T. K., & Resch, F. (2022). **Short-term music therapy treatment for adolescents with depression–a pilot study. The Arts in Psychotherapy, 77,** 101874.

Nine adolescents with mildly to moderate depression received twelve 50-minute sessions of music therapy in an outpatient setting as an adjunct to psychotherapy and/or medical treatment. Sessions were carried out by a trained music therapist. Pre-, post-, and follow-up surveys were used to examine acceptance, feasibility, and outcome measures. Short-term results demonstrated that participants experienced decreased depression severity, increased health-related quality of life, and more adaptive emotional coping strategies at postassessment. However, these effects were not shown to be sustained at the follow-up assessment.

Wibowo, W. D. A., Wijaya, S., & Amelia, N. (2021). **The effect of laughter therapy for depression level among geriatric patients at Pangesti Lawang Nursing Home. International Journal of Nursing and Health Services, 4(5),** 515–521.

A quasi-experimental research study was performed to determine whether laughter and classical music therapy positively affect mental health, particularly depression in elderly persons living in a nursing home. Thirty-two participants were divided into the experimental group ($n = 16$) and the control group ($n = 16$). All participants completed the Geriatric Depression Scale (GDS) before beginning the intervention and again after the intervention. The experimental group participated

in laughter therapy for 30 minutes, 2 times a week, for 2 weeks. The control group was given classical music therapy for the same duration as the laughter therapy. Results showed a difference in GDS score before and after the participants were given laughter therapy and classical music therapy. Both interventions had the same effect on decreasing the GDS score for the participants. There was no significant difference in GDS score between laughter therapy and classical music therapy, indicating that both interventions are effective.

İçel, S., & Başoğul, C. (2021). **Effects of progressive muscle relaxation training with music therapy on sleep and anger of patients at community mental health center. Complementary Therapies in Clinical Practice, 43,** 101338.

This study to determine the effects of progressive muscle relaxation training and music therapy on anger level and sleep quality included 66 patients diagnosed with a chronic psychiatric condition ($n = 32$ in the control group; $n = 34$ in the intervention group). In addition to their routine mental healthcare, the intervention group participated in progressive muscle relaxation training with music therapy for two sessions per week for 3 months. No intervention was implemented in the control-group patients except for their routine mental healthcare program. The results indicated that relaxation training and music therapy are effective strategies to increase sleep quality, reduce the level of trait anger, and help control anger in patients with chronic psychiatric conditions.

1. To help you with your analysis for the following questions, complete this table.

	STUDY A	STUDY B	STUDY C
Intervention			
Type of patient			
Result/conclusion			

2. Which of the studies tested an intervention?

3. Which of the interventions was most successful in improving well-being? Explain your thinking.

4. What is the value of the study findings (all three studies) for nurses or patients?

health and everyday functioning and regain control of their lives.

Depending on the substance(s) involved, treatment may include medications, behavioral treatments, or a combination.

Physicians, substance abuse counselors, and other health professionals play an important role in determining the right treatment for an individual.

Medications are available to treat addiction to opiates, nicotine, and alcohol, but none has yet been approved for treating addiction to marijuana, stimulants, or depressants. However, behavioral therapy can be helpful in these cases.

Nursing care for patients with addiction diagnoses is complex and requires special training. A major role for the nurse is to help the patient understand and adapt to the various medications. To find out more about substance abuse, see Chapter 6, particularly the Example Client Condition: Substance Abuse.

KnowledgeCheck 10-7

- What distinguishes clinical depression from feelings of sadness?
- How might a child manifest depression?
- Why is the nurse–patient (therapeutic) relationship important when caring for depressed individuals?

To explore learning resources for this chapter,

Go to Davis Advantage and find:

Answers and Suggested Responses for all questions in this chapter
Concept Map
Knowledge Map
References and Bibliography

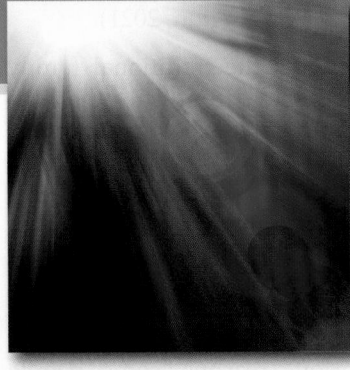

CHAPTER 11

Promoting Family Health

Learning Outcomes

After completing this chapter, you should be able to:

➤ Distinguish among different family structures.

➤ Describe approaches to working with various types of families to provide optimal care to both well and ill clients.

➤ Explain how family theories provide a framework for understanding family functioning.

➤ Identify family risk factors across five different stages.

➤ Discuss ways in which economic factors influence nursing practice, family care, and access to services.

➤ Discuss the effects of chronic and life-threatening illness on families.

➤ Identify populations most at risk for homelessness.

➤ Demonstrate an understanding of family violence.

➤ Conduct a family assessment.

➤ Identify common health beliefs and communication patterns in families.

➤ Identify appropriate nursing interventions when a family member is ill.

➤ Review how risk factors such as illness and death, substance abuse, violence, mental health disorders, financial hardship, unemployment, and other issues can change a family's structure, communication, and coping strategies.

➤ Discuss the sandwich generation and assessment and intervention strategies for caregiver burnout.

Key Concepts

Family
Family nursing

Related Concepts

See the Concept Map on Davis Advantage

Example Client Condition

Caregiver Role Strain

Meet Your Patient

Nicole is a 15-year-old high school student who is hospitalized with a broken right leg and shoulder injuries received in a motor vehicle accident. Two of the five passengers died in the car accident, including the driver (who was intoxicated). Nicole lives with her father, Jerrod; her stepmother, Audra; and her half siblings, Johnathon, age 5, and Sabrina, age 11. After Jerrod lost his job 2 weeks ago, they moved in with his mother, LeTanya Henderson, a 63-year-old single woman. LeTanya works two jobs to pay the mortgage on her 1,000-square-foot, two-bedroom, one-bathroom single-family home. She rents the detached casita to short-term renters to help cover the additional household expenses and her car payment.

The family has been adjusting to the new living arrangements. LeTanya has insulin-dependent diabetes and follows

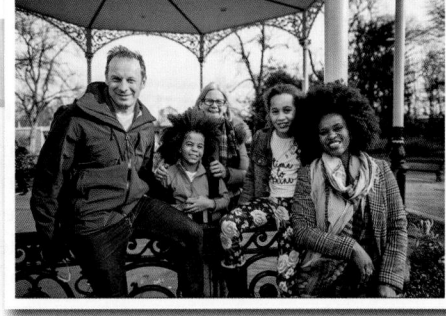

a strict diet and exercise regimen. Audra is a stay-at-home mom who home schools the 11- and 5-year-olds. The couple is expecting their third child in 3 months. Audra is currently on restricted activity due to pregnancy-related complications. Jerrod is taking on many of the household tasks and is concerned about how he will care for Nicole and Audra.

Theoretical Knowledge
knowing why

ABOUT THE KEY CONCEPTS

This chapter is about contemporary families and how they differ from those of the past. As you study the chapter, you will begin to see how **family, family nursing,** and other related concepts apply to the Hendersons (Meet Your Patient). The key concepts are the basis of the theoretical knowledge to which you will apply the nursing process and develop your clinical judgment. Integration of these concepts into your nursing care will help you meet the challenges of family health as a full-spectrum nurse.

WHAT IS A FAMILY?

Families come in many forms, with varied living arrangements and emotional connections. The concept of family can be defined from various perspectives: structure, function, or transition (Thompson et al., 2015).

- **Structure** (e.g., biological, legal): A **family** is formally defined as two or more people related by birth, marriage, or adoption residing in the same household (U.S. Census Bureau, 2021a). However, adult children living apart from their parents continue to be part of a family unit.
- **Function** (e.g., caretaking, financial, social support): A **family** is two or more individuals who provide physical, emotional, economic, or spiritual support to each other (Thompson, et al., 2017). They may or may not be related by blood but maintain involvement in each other's lives.
- **Transition** (e.g., cultural, tribal, rituals): A **family** is blended together through relationships, shared meaning, communications, rituals, and/or ideological unity.

Changes in Family Structures

We continue to see significant changes in the living arrangements of families, and the concept and purposes of family have become broader since the mid-20th century. Factors influencing changing views on the concept and purpose of family include the following:

- Increasing cultural diversity and cultural influences
- Less reliance on social traditions
- Wider acceptance of differing lifestyles
- Socioeconomic factors
- Absence of one or both parents
- Aging population (aging families) and improvements in their health and financial status
- Older average age at first marriage
- Changing residential preferences

Traditional Families Traditionally, people have thought of a family as consisting of a husband, wife, and their children. Although living with two parents is still the dominant living arrangement for children, a decline has occurred from 60 million (85%) in 1968 to 51.3 million (70%) in 2020 (Hemez & Washington, 2021).

Dual-Earner Families Like the traditional family structure, a similar shift occurred from only the husband in the labor force to both parents being employed. In 2016, 61% of households had dual family income (Bureau of Labor Statistics, 2019), compared to 64.4 % in 2019 and 59.8% in 2020 (Bureau of Labor Statistics, 2021). The decrease in 2020 coincided with COVID-19, which caused high unemployment rates and a shift to at-home learning for children.

Single Adults For various reasons, some people prefer to live alone. The number of adults living alone increased from 33 million (14%) in 2011 to 37 million (15%) in early 2021 (U.S. Census Bureau, 2021c). A large percentage of single adults prefer not to have children for various reasons (e.g., finances, global issues, medical concerns) (Brown, 2021). They usually have strong relationships with family, friends, or significant others who fulfill many of the familial roles.

Single Parent Families Single-parent families result from divorce, from the death of a partner, or when partners choose not to marry or live together. Aside from living with both parents, living with a mother only is the second-most-common living arrangement for children. The number doubled from 7.6 million (11%) in 1968 to 15.2 (21%) in 2020. Although it is less common, the number of children living with a father only quadrupled over the same period from 0.8 million (1%) to 3.3 million (4.5%) (Hemez & Washington, 2021).

Married Adults Without Children The percentage of childless married adults has remained consistent over 60 years. In 1960, 31% of married adults did not have children compared to 28% in 2000 and 30% in 2020 (VanOrman & Jacobsen, 2020).

Grandparent Families Grandparent households are a significant resource for single women with children and for families during economic distress. When parents are unable or unwilling to assume the parenting role, grandparents may raise their grandchildren to prevent foster care or other alternate placement. In 2020, an estimated 2.7 million grandparents were raising their grandchildren (Turner, 2022).

Military Families Members of the armed services must balance their military obligations with their family commitments. Military families are challenged with their active duty or reservist family member being separated from the family unit for extended periods of time to fulfill deployment assignments. The military has adopted a broad definition of "family" and offers support and resources to ensure the well-being of the deployed member's family and redeployment activities to facilitate a successful reintegration when the service member returns home.

Blended and Stepfamilies A **blended family** is established when single parents marry and either or both have children from a previous relationship. The nonbiological partner becomes the stepparent, and a stepfamily is created. Children will have more than two parental figures (biological and step) and may have step- or half siblings. Commonly, biological parents who are not living together in the child's home alternate the responsibilities for childcare.

Extended Families It is not unusual for extended family members (e.g., grandparents, aunts, uncles, cousins) to be considered immediate family and live within a single dwelling or in close proximity. Close friends may also be considered immediate family.

Sandwich Families The growing number of older adults has created **sandwich families** in which middle-aged adults who still have children at home must care for and share their household with aging parents. Although competent in the caregiver role, they experience stress and anxiety associated with financial burdens, feeling personally overwhelmed and emotionally conflicted, depression, guilt, and isolation (Hoyt, 2021; Kim et al., 2021).

♥ **iCare** You should carefully assess caregivers' needs and align them with available resources to provide the caregiver with respite care.

Multigenerational/Intergenerational Families Households that contain three or more generations of parents and their families or grandparents and grandchildren increased by 271% from 2011 to 2021 (Generations United, 2022). A common arrangement consists of a grandparent, adult child, and grandchildren. An estimated 66.7 million adults are living in a multigenerational household. In the Meet Your Patient scenario, what benefits would you infer from this living arrangement? What disadvantages would you infer?

LGBTQ+ Families Lesbian, gay, bisexual, transgender, or queer (LGBTQ+) families can be married, unmarried, cohabiting, divorced, separated, or single (Family Equality Council, 2021).

Other Family Structures In addition to families bound by marriage and bloodlines, other family types exist, such as unmarried individuals who may reside in a common household or individuals or couples who are foster parents to children. Although not biologically related, they assume a parenting role in the child's life and share experiences that create an emotional attachment; thus, they are very much a family.

- **Cohabiting adults** may choose to live together and not marry or live together as a "trial run" prior to marriage. Among the age-groups of 18 to 24 years, a greater share of women (24%) lived with an unmarried partner compared to men (7%). The percentage share was the same for both men and women between the ages of 25 to 34 years (U.S. Census Bureau, 2021b).

- **Foster families** provide care to children when the parents are unable to assume the parental role for various reasons. Over 407,000 children were in foster care in 2020. The majority of these children were cared for by nonrelatives (45%) compared to relatives (34%) (Children's Bureau, 2021).

♥ **iCare** You should show acceptance of and compassion toward the various family structures, functions, and relationships that you encounter throughout your nursing career. Focus on the significance of the family members in your patient's life. Reich (2020) notes that family relationships are unique and long lasting. The "family comprises relationships that are more intimate, emotionally powerful, and enduring than other connections" (p. 1). They do not have to be blood relatives to provide the emotional, social, spiritual, and other types of support that are characteristic of family relationships.

Approaches to Family Nursing

Family nursing refers to nursing care that is holistically directed toward the whole family as well as toward individual members (Fig. 11-1). Knowing the family unit is affected by acute or chronic illness, hospitalization, or healthcare interventions, the nurse best cares for the family by involving them in client care decisions.

The Henderson family demonstrates why nursing is directed toward the entire family to promote wellness and maximal function. If you focus only on Nicole, the

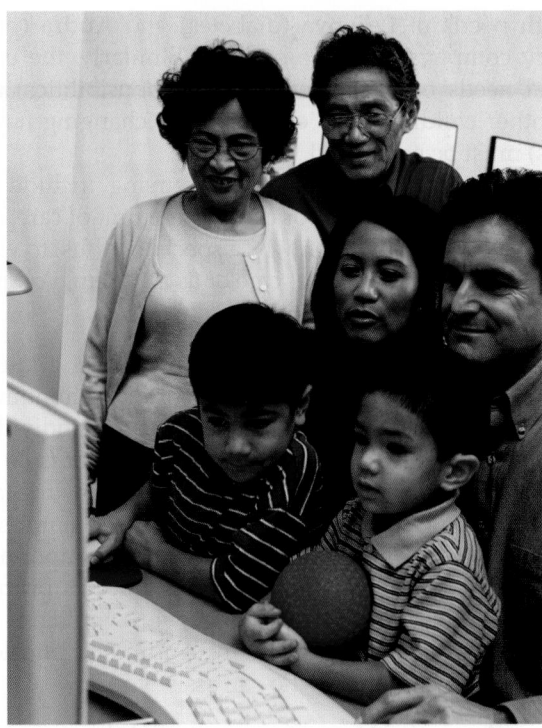

FIGURE 11-1 Family nursing refers to nursing care that is holistically directed toward the whole family as well as toward individual members.

Toward Evidence-Based Practice

Lee, H., Ryan, L. H., Ofstedal, M. B., & Smith, J. (2020). Multi-generational households during childhood and trajectories of cognitive functioning among U.S. older adults. *The Journals of Gerontology: Series B, 76*(6), 1161–1172. https://doi.org/10.1093/geronb/gbaa165

Researchers examined the impact of family structure during childhood on cognitive functioning in later life. The results revealed that older adults raised in multigenerational households (single parent with grandparents, two parents with grandparents) had higher levels of cognitive functioning. Childhood family structure was not associated with the rate of cognitive decline. Factors associated with a slower rate of cognitive decline included higher levels of education and income.

Tzoumakis, S., Burton, M., Carr, V., Dean, K., Laurens, K., & Green, M. (2019). *The intergenerational transmission of criminal offending behaviours*. Report to the Criminology Research Council, Grant CRG 19/14-15. Criminology Research Council. https://eprints.qut.edu.au/127298/

Researchers examined the relationships between the parents' criminal behaviors and the developmental outcomes of their children in early childhood (5 years) and conduct problems in middle childhood (11 years). Children with special needs were excluded from the study. Although intergenerational families can have positive impacts on children, those whose parents, especially the mother, engage in criminal behaviors were found to have a high risk for developmental and conduct disorders. These families will require early intervention programs and support to minimize this trend.

Jessee, V., & Adamsons, K. (2018). Father involvement and father-child relationship quality: An intergenerational perspective. *Parenting: Science and Practice, 18*(1), 28–44. https://doi.org/10.1080/15295192.2018.1405700

Researchers examined the transmission of father–child relationships across generations. The findings revealed positive relationships between the father's relationship with his paternal grandfather, his involvement with his own child at age 1 year, and the child's report of father–child relationship quality at 9 years of age. Fathers who were older, had higher household incomes, were more educated, and had more involvement with their child at age 1 showed better relationships with their child at age 9. Fathers engaged in emotional bonding activities that were reenacted in the next generation.

1. How can intergenerational influences affect children?

2. As a nurse, what cues would you assess in an intergenerational family?

3. Why do you think multigenerational households with grandparents had a positive effect on cognition in later life?

---

health needs of LeTanya (diabetes) and Audra (pregnancy complications) are omitted. Similarly, the emotional needs of Jerrod (caregiver responsibilities) and the other children (new environment, changing family roles) must be addressed.

Three perspectives on family nursing include the family as (1) the context for care, (2) the unit of care, and (3) a system. Family nursing is a specialty; thus, to work with the family as a unit of care or as a system, you may need additional preparation.

Family as the Context for Care As a graduate nurse, you should be prepared to work, at a minimum, with the family as the context for care of an individual person. **Key Point:** *Your focus in this approach is on the ill individual.* From this perspective, you view the family as either a resource or a stressor to your client. Using this knowledge, you would recognize the importance of Jerrod (Meet Your Patient), who is Audra's primary source of support. Before discharge, you would ask Jerrod, "Will you be able to care for Audra and Nicole at home? Are there others who can assist you?"

Family as the Unit of Care A slightly more complex approach views the family as the unit of care. You must assess and provide care to each member because wellness is critical to promoting family health. **Key**

Point: *Family health is viewed as the sum of all individual members; however, you might direct interventions to individual family members rather than the family as a whole.* For example, to use our earlier example, you might inquire about LeTanya's blood glucose or Jerrod's stress level and coping strategies to determine if interventions are needed to promote family health.

Family as a System Key Point: *In this approach, you focus on the family as a whole and as an interactional system.* Using this perspective, you direct your assessment and intervention to communications and interactions between family members. The systems approach sees the family as embedded in and interacting with a larger community. For example, you might ask, "How has your family adapted to the move and the new schools?"

KnowledgeCheck 11-1

- Name at least three types of family structures.
- What are two topics that the nurse can discuss with the family as a unit?

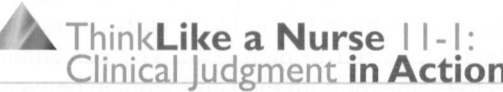

ThinkLike a Nurse 11-1: Clinical Judgment in Action

- How can you promote family cohesion for a family whose members live great distances from each other?

♥ iCare 11-1

The Family

- "The family" will be slightly different for every client you encounter.
- As a nurse, you must possess and exhibit a cultural awareness and competency for a broader definition of family as our society continues to change.
- Remember that what defines "the family" is very different for each person. There is no longer a traditional view of who and what constitutes a family.
- Ask the following: *"Can you introduce me to your family?"* Asking this avoids assumptions and allows the client to tell you about their family structure.

WHAT THEORIES ARE USEFUL FOR FAMILY CARE?

Several theories have been proposed to help us understand family functioning. Four such theories are general systems theory, structural–functional theories, family interactional theory, and developmental theory.

General Systems Theory

General systems theory (see Chapter 4) focuses on interactions between systems and the changes that result from these interactions.

- **Open system.** The family is considered an open system because the members function as individuals, are interdependent, and operate as a family unit (a whole, in systems language). Interactions can occur between members of the family or between multiple families.
- **Balance.** Healthy families strive to maintain a balance between external stress and internal relationships.
- **Interaction.** Changes in the behaviors or attitudes of an individual member affect the family unit, and changes in family structure and functioning affect individual members. Think of a system as a mobile; if one piece is moved, that movement sets the whole mobile in motion.
- **Suprasystems.** Broader systems that surround the family unit (e.g., the community, the city, the state, the healthcare system) are referred to as *suprasystems.*
- **Subsystems.** Smaller components that fit within the family system (e.g., the parent, the marital couple) are subsystems. Each subsystem has a particular function. For example, one family member might be viewed as the decision maker, another as the peacekeeper, and another as the disciplinarian for the children.

Structural–Functional Theories

Structural–functional family theories are based on the developmental theories of Freud, Erikson, and Havighurst (see Chapter 4) and include the concepts of family roles and interactions. The structural–functional

approach includes the following assumptions (Parsons & Bales, 1955):

- A family is a social system with functional requirements.
- A family is a small group possessing certain features common to small groups.
- The family accomplishes functions that serve both the individual and society.
- Individuals act according to internalized norms that are learned through socialization.

Key Point: *Although they view the family as a social system, structural–functional theories, unlike systems theory, focus on outcome rather than process.* You would use this theory to assess how well the family functions internally (among family members) and externally (with outside systems). Examples of family functions include socialization of children; meeting the physical, financial, and emotional needs of family members; caring for older members; and being productive members of society.

Family Interactional Theory

Family interactional theory views the family as a unit of interacting personalities (Hill & Hansen, 1960). **Key Point:** *The major emphasis is on family roles. This approach to understanding families de-emphasizes the influence of the external world on what occurs within the family.* Nurses working from an interactional perspective focus family healthcare on the interaction and communication between family members, their roles and power, family coping, and relationships with other people outside the direct family unit.

Developmental Theories

Key Point: *Developmental theories focus on the stage of family development.* Theorists typically identify eight stages in the family life cycle according to the ages of the children and parents: beginning family, childbearing family, family with preschool children, family with school-age children, family with teenagers and young adults, family launching young adults, postparental family, and aging family. Each stage is associated with developmental tasks the family needs to achieve. Most family development theories do not identify stages and tasks for families who remain childless throughout their lives. To learn about the developmental tasks associated with family stages, including those for families without children,

 Go to Chapter 11, Assessment Guidelines and Tools, Family Developmental Tasks, in Volume 2.

Generally, the stages follow one another in a linear progression; however, some families may be in more than one stage at a time or may revert to previous stages. This overlap or reversion is most common in families that have children spaced far apart, in blended families, and in stepfamilies. See Chapter 4 for developmental theories applicable to individual family members.

KnowledgeCheck 11-2

- Which type of theory focuses on interactions among families, family members, and groups in the environment?
- What is the name of the theory that views families as a social system with a focus on outcomes?
- What are some examples of family functions as defined by structural–functional theories?

ThinkLike a Nurse 11-2: Clinical Judgment in Action

- Using systems theory, you could view LeTanya, her son, her daughter-in-law, and her grandchildren as a system. Refer to the section on family structures—how would you categorize this family structurally?
- Using family interactional theory, what is the focus of the nurse for the Henderson family?
- Considering Jerrod and Audra, at what developmental stages are their "family"?

WHAT ARE SOME FAMILY HEALTH RISK FACTORS?

Many health risk factors are the same for families as for individuals, and they are similar across age-groups and family types. Basically, destructive behaviors remain destructive behaviors, regardless of who is performing them.

For specific topics related to families, also see Chapters 6 and 7 covering the life span, Chapter 9 on stress and adaptation, Chapter 15 on communication, and Chapter 16 on teaching clients.

Childless and Childbearing Couples

Adapting to new roles within the home creates stress for newly married couples; couples who are trying to become pregnant; and new parents who are inexperienced in the challenges and responsibilities of raising a healthy, happy, and safe child (Fig. 11-2). The use of maladaptive coping mechanisms can lead to health problems and deterioration in relationships. For example, for someone who uses alcohol to deal with stress:

- The individual is at risk for addiction, self-injury, and liver disease.
- The family can also suffer the harmful effects of neglect and family violence, as well as health risks related to pregnancy (e.g., miscarriage, congenital malformations, and genetic defects in the child).

Families With Young Children

Common parenting concerns center on the child's safety, development, socialization, education, discipline, nutrition, sleeping, and toileting.

- **Childcare.** Finding safe, nurturing, and affordable childcare can be a major source of family stress for parents working outside the home.

PICOT

Alcohol Treatment and Family Support

Situation: The nurse is meeting with a family before the discharge of the husband/father from alcohol treatment. The teenage daughter asks the nurse whether her father will ever drink again.

PICOT Components:

P—Population/client	=	Alcoholic adults
I—Intervention/indicator	=	Family support
C—Comparator/control	=	No family support
O—Outcome	=	Decreased risk of relapse
T—Time	=	Over time

Application of a Searchable Question:
Do _____ (P) who receive/are exposed to _____(I) demonstrate _____ (O) compared with _____ (C) during _____ (T)?

Example of Evidence: Alcohol abuse is a common social, family, and individual health problem. Research indicates that clients are less likely to relapse if they have spent more time in treatment and subsequent time in an abstinence-related group; home; if they engage in a structured intervention before detoxification, followed by aftercare; and they have sources of social support. In addition, approaches that

integrate family members into the treatment facilitate long-term recovery. Client support had a positive effect on sustained sobriety and motivation to change and was positively correlated with overall well-being and decreased stress and anxiety.

Practice Change: The nurse made certain to assess family relationships and sources of support for actual and future clients.

Source: Kouimtsidis, C., et al. (2016). Structured intervention to prepare dependent drinkers to achieve abstinence: results from a cohort evaluation for 6 months detoxification. *Journal of Substance Use, 21*(3), 331-34. https://doi.org/10.3109/14659891.2015.1029020; Matsuda, Y., Sharma, E., Charge, K.-J., & Smith, A. (2019). Predictors of parenting self-agency among mothers receiving substance abuse or mental health treatment. *International Journal of Mental Health Nursing, 28*(5), 1132–1141. https://doi.org/10.1111/inm.12624; McCrady, B., & Flanagan, J. (2021). The role of the family in alcohol use disorder recovery for adults. *Alcohol Research Current Reviews, 41*(1). https://doi.org/10.35946/arcr.v41.1.06; Moon, T., Mathias, C. W., Mullen, J., Karns-Wright, T. E., Hill-Kapturczak, N., Roache, J. D., & Dougherty, D. M. (2018). The role of social support in motivating reductions in alcohol use: A test of three models of social support in alcohol-impaired drivers. *Alcoholism: Clinical & Experimental Research, 3*(1), 123–134. https://doi.org/10.1111/acer.13911

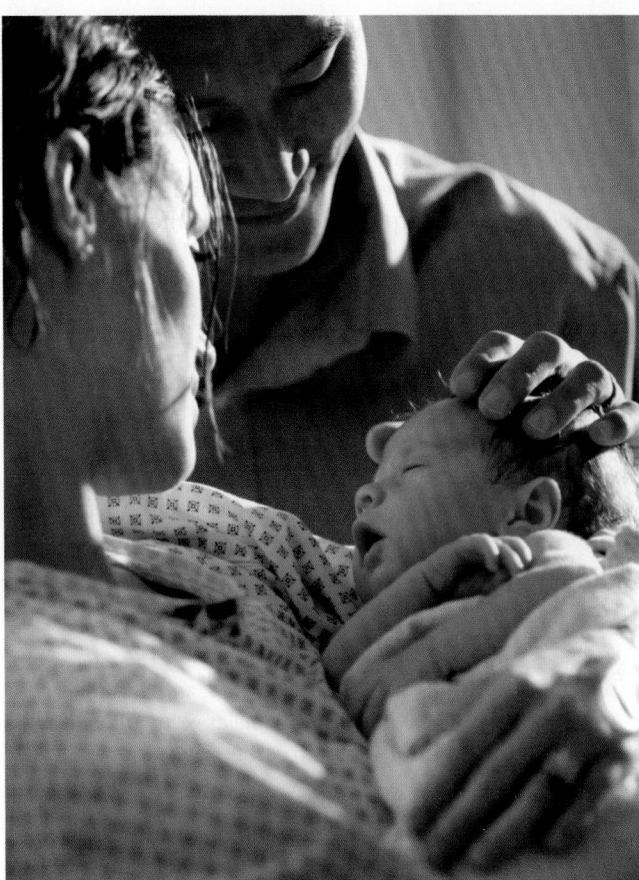

FIGURE 11-2 Newly married couples, couples who are trying to become pregnant, and new parents are vulnerable to stress as they adapt to new roles.

- **Marital relationship.** In addition, the demands of work and child-rearing mean less time is available to nurture the couple's relationship, leaving them at increased risk for marital discord.
- **Contagious diseases.** Injuries and illness create risks to family health. For example, children attending schools are exposed to contagious diseases that can spread to other family members. ✚ To reduce the risk for serious infectious diseases (e.g., measles, polio, or hepatitis B), parents need to adhere to the recommended childhood immunization schedule. You should teach the importance of vaccinations and provide accurate information to counter myths regarding vaccines.
- **Vaccinations.** Trend data show the importance of vaccinations for preventable diseases. In 2019, the number of measles cases among mostly unvaccinated individuals reached 1,281, which was the greatest number since 1992. This number decreased to 13 in 2020, with a slight increase to 49 cases in 2021 (Centers for Disease Control and Prevention [CDC], 2022). Parents who refuse immunizations for their children cite personal reasons, religious reasons, and concerns regarding the safety and effectiveness of vaccines (CDC, 2019a). In addition, a lack of insurance and lower income and education levels are associated with delayed, partial, or unvaccinated status (Ellithorpe, 2022).

- **Disability or chronic illness.** For families who live with a chronic illness (e.g., asthma, type 1 diabetes) or a developmental or learning disability (e.g., autism), the stress related to compromised health, falling behind in school, numerous medical appointments, and financial burdens can become overwhelming.

Families With Adolescents

Families with adolescents are often concerned about teen risk-taking behaviors.

- **Social Pressure and Risk Tolerance.** The formula "risk taking = curiosity + challenge + excitement + denial + reward" describes adolescent decision making in known and unknown situations (Hartley & Somerville, 2015; Pickhardt, 2014). Adolescents may participate in risky behaviors to impress others, to feel cool or important, or to experience a feeling of power. Research supports that the social reward of being accepted by their peers outweighs the known negative outcomes of risk-taking behaviors (Blakemore, 2018; Smith et al., 2014). You can educate parents about maintaining positive communications with their adolescent that include discussions of the hidden risks and costs of risky behaviors.
- **Specific Categories of Risk Behaviors.** Researchers used the CDC's risk domains to identify three categories of adolescent risk behaviors (Kwong et al., 2018):
  - Overt risk taking (e.g., smoking, alcohol, risky sexual behaviors, fighting, bullying, acting on dares)
  - Screen-time syndrome (e.g., combination of prolonged use of video games and watching TV with nonhealthy snacks, such as chips and high-sugar drinks)
  - Aversion to a healthy lifestyle (e.g., avoidance of healthy foods, low participation in moderate to vigorous exercise)

These categories can be used to develop specific preventive approaches to teach adolescents about healthy choices and lifestyles.

- **"Sandwich" Families.** Adolescents may also live in households with aging parents or grandparents, known as "sandwich" families (Fig. 11-3). Parents may become "sandwiched" between the needs of the adolescents and the needs of their aging parents. Adolescents reported more respect for caregivers, strengthened parent bonds, and limitations on family activities (Burke, 2017; Intriago, 2021).

Families With Young Adults

Young adults commonly move out of the parental home as their school years end, and many take on full-time jobs for the first time. The newly found autonomy and independence are exhilarating for some and anxiety-provoking for others. The boundary between adolescence and adulthood is blurred by societal forces (e.g., a contracting economy, changing labor force expectations, and

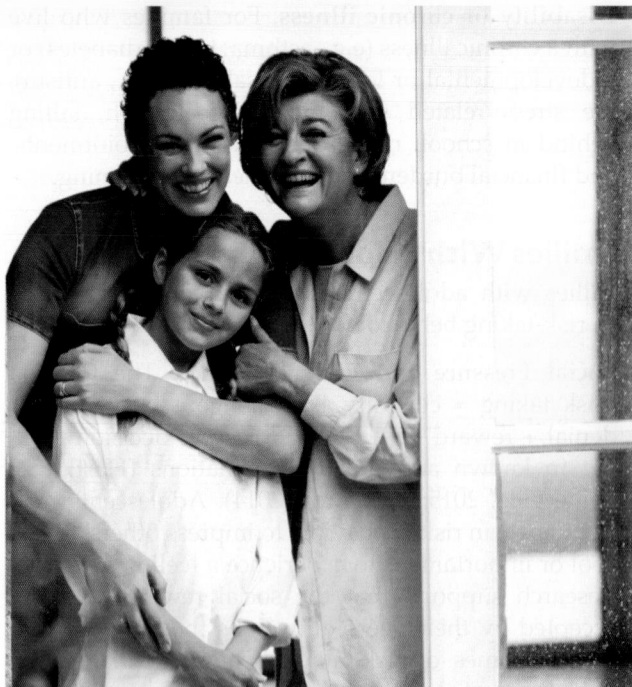

FIGURE 11-3 In families with adolescents or young adults, the parents may become "sandwiched" between the needs of the growing adolescents and the needs of their own parents.

expanding opportunities for women). Some confront such problems as tight finances, inability to find meaningful work, nontherapeutic personal relationships, or other life challenges.

"Return to the Nest" Financial strain might necessitate a young adult, alone or with a newly formed family, to move back with their parent(s) until they can "get back on their feet." Although returning to the home of origin can represent a new opportunity for family attachment, the presence of young adults in the household commonly changes the family dynamics. Role strain and poor communication are common. Roles within the family will evolve, and families will need to find healthy ways to adapt.

Families With Middle-Aged Adults

The middle years are a time of examining life goals and coping with aging and the empty nest. This can be not only a satisfying time but also a time of self-doubt. Keep in mind that the health of the middle-aged person also affects family health.

- **This can be a satisfying time** of role fulfillment, career success, financial security, and social comfort. Without the time demands of bringing up children, adults have more time available to pursue other personal interests or career paths. The quality of the spousal relationship might take on a new importance. The middle-aged adult may experience a new sense of freedom and need for self-exploration and personal growth.

- **The middle years can also be a time of self-doubt** triggered by the changes caused by aging, menopause, an empty nest, care or death of parents, heightened career demands, or change in relationships, all of which can create emotional strain.
- **Some people suffer a midlife crisis,** which is a period of intense questioning about the meaning of and their direction in life and what brings personal fulfillment. Adults battling a midlife crisis might display signs of depression, anxiety, or rebellion against the status quo.
- **The effects of long-standing unhealthy behaviors** often become apparent in middle adulthood. For example, people who have used tobacco for many years may begin to notice an increase in cough and chest congestion, or those who consume high-fat diets may develop high blood pressure or elevated cholesterol levels.

Families With Older Adults

Falls and Trauma Falls and trauma are a common health risk for families with older adults. For more information about this, see Chapters 7 and 21.

Social Isolation and Loneliness Social isolation and loneliness are common in older adults because of the loss of relationships that occurs with aging. Older adults have an increased risk for depression. Families should maintain frequent contact and communications to offset feelings of isolation and loneliness. Friends can also be a significant source of support (Fig. 11-4).

- *Family dynamics change* as the older person copes with the death of a spouse, sibling, friends, or other loved ones.
- *Loss and grief* can deeply affect an older person's quality of life, clarity of thinking, and physical and emotional well-being.
- *Retirement* can bring the simpler life that many people desire. However, retired individuals must deal

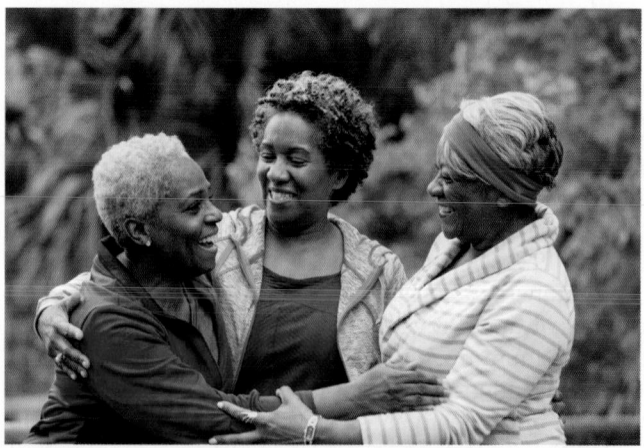

FIGURE 11-4 Friends play an important role in the support system of older people.

with the loss of daily contact with colleagues in the workplace; some experience a reduced sense of responsibility or purpose.

■ *Functional losses* may cause the person to limit physical activity, volunteer work, church attendance, and other social activities.

Nutrition and Hydration As a person ages, nutrition becomes more difficult to maintain. The following are situations that may compromise the nutrition of older adults:

■ Forgetting to eat (especially those who live alone)
■ Inadequate or unreliable transportation to shop for food
■ Lack of money to buy food
■ Physical changes that alter taste (e.g., reduced sensitivity in the taste buds and less saliva for taste and swallowing)
■ Loss of appetite
■ Poorly fitting dentures or absence of teeth

For more information about nutrition, see Chapter 24.

Memory and Problem-Solving Changes in cognitive function can occur with aging. Forgetfulness and confusion can pose risks to safety for older adults, particularly for those living alone or with other aging adults whose mental status is compromised. When older adults lose their ability to reason, they are vulnerable to physical harm. The demands of keeping the aging adult safe can lead to caregiver role strain and family stress.

ThinkLike a Nurse 11-3: Clinical Judgment in Action

■ What developmental stage is your family in? How do you know?
■ What basic attitudes, values, or beliefs influenced you in your childhood family?
■ How were decisions made in your childhood family? Were people's feelings and individuals' needs considered?
■ Can you remember good times and laughter that bonded you together as a family? In your present family life, how often do you laugh together?
■ In the Meet Your Patient scenario, what developmental stages do you see in the Henderson family?

WHAT ARE SOME CHALLENGES TO FAMILY HEALTH?

We have already mentioned the effects of some demographic changes, such as an aging population, on families. This section examines other regional and national trends that affect families.

Poverty and Unemployment

Poverty and unemployment involve interrelated social and economic factors.

Inadequate or No Health Insurance When families do not have adequate health insurance, they (1) do not seek preventive medical care or (2) use the emergency room for their medical needs. The Affordable Care Act (ACA), passed in 2010, provided healthcare coverage for people who cannot obtain private or employment-funded insurance. During the history-taking portion of your interaction with the client, you need to ask about insurance coverage. You can contact a case manager or social worker for clients with no or inadequate coverage.

Teenage Pregnancy The birth rate among teens aged 15 to 19 in the United States continues to decline and reached a record low in 2018 (Livingston & Thomas, 2019), with a continued decline from 17.4 per 1,000 female individuals in 2018 to 16.7 in 2019 (CDC, 2021). This is a positive trend for several reasons:

■ Many teens delay getting prenatal care, which can increase the risk that infants have health problems at birth.
■ Teen mothers are more likely to have greater health disparities and high unemployment rates.
■ Only a small percentage of teen mothers (10%) receive a 2-year or 4-year degree.
■ Children of teen mothers have higher involvement in the juvenile justice system (Youth.gov, n.d.).

Overall Economic Climate When the economy takes a downturn, families may struggle to provide for basic needs such as food, shelter, and healthcare.

■ *Single-parent and low-income families are hardest hit.* However, families in all socioeconomic levels can experience difficulties in an economic downturn. Most people living at or below the federal poverty level are minimum-wage or seasonal job workers. Jobs labeled nonessential may be eliminated in a sluggish economy. As a result, fewer workers are paying taxes in such an economy, so government programs supporting families in need may be underfunded. Although some families find creative solutions to economic difficulties (e.g., combining households), many experience extreme hardships.
■ *Middle-income families are also affected by corporate downsizing or stock market fluctuations.* Even families who were prospering may not have sufficient funds to cover a period of unemployment or economic recession. They may find it impossible to keep up with credit-card debt, home mortgages, car payments, insurance premiums, and perhaps school or other loans.

KnowledgeCheck 11-3

■ Which socioeconomic group of families is hardest hit during poor economic periods?
■ How are middle-income families affected by poor economic times?
■ What concerns are associated with teenage pregnancies?

Infectious Diseases

Family health may be affected by infections caused by a variety of pathogens. For in-depth information about preventing infections, refer to Chapter 20.

New or Drug-Resistant Pathogens Any number of new or resistant pathogens, such as severe acute respiratory syndrome (SARS), methicillin-resistant *Staphylococcus aureus* (MRSA), and influenza strains, can cause illness. For example, influenza viruses can cause severe illness in young children, pregnant women, people aged 65 years and older, and those with certain chronic diseases.

HIV Infection An HIV diagnosis can have a significant impact on the family. In addition to the physical and financial stressors, individuals who infect others may bear a tremendous burden of guilt. Some families keep the diagnosis a secret, whereas other families support each other and manage the illness as best they can.

- About 13% of the 1.18 million people in the United States living with HIV are unaware of their infected status (CDC, 2021a).
- Individuals at high risk include injection drug users and those who have unprotected sexual relationships with multiple partners.

✚ Early education and treatment are essential. Advances in treating HIV infection and preventing its spread have been made through public and client education, vaccination, antiviral therapy, the use of condoms with lubricants, and other antimicrobial treatments for HIV-related complications. Pregnant women who seek early prenatal care can minimize mother-to-child transmission of HIV (CDC, 2019b). The nurse should emphasize the use of proper protective precautions to minimize the spread of the disease.

"Old" (Comeback) Diseases Even old diseases once thought to be eradicated can threaten family health. In recent years, diseases once controlled by immunizations are making a comeback (e.g., measles, pertussis [whooping cough], polio, mumps, and smallpox). Many families either refuse or fail to comply with immunization schedules. As a result, a reduction occurs in **herd immunity,** which is a group's protection from disease that occurs because a large proportion of the group is immune. Parents should understand that childhood immunizations save lives and prevent diseases.

KnowledgeCheck 11-4
- What demographic groups are at highest risk of contracting HIV?
- Name two previously eradicated diseases that have become a threat again.

Chronic Illness and Disability

Chronic illness and disability of family members in the home profoundly change the way the family functions.

- **Caregiving.** Family members' roles evolve over time, especially that of the caregiver, who often must assist

with activities of daily living, such as getting around the home; feeding, bathing, dressing, and toileting; and getting in and out of a chair or bed.
- **Financial strain.** Disability may mean an inability to work or generate family income, creating financial strain or economic difficulties.
- **Mental strain**. Long-term illness and disability cause mental, emotional, or physical limitations that affect family communication patterns.
- **Relationships**. Because of caregiver strain and issues related to dependency, relationships within the family may be difficult.
- **Abuse**. Long-term care of a family member may increase the risk for abuse and neglect, including maltreatment of frail, elderly family members.

The Americans with Disabilities Act (ADA) Amendments Act of 2008 defines one component of **disability** as a physical or mental impairment that substantially interferes with a person's ability to engage in major life activities (U.S. Equal Opportunity Commission, 2008). Individuals have a disability if they meet criteria involving limitations in mobility/ambulation, hearing, vision, learning, cognitive, self-care, or independent living, to name a few. Mobility limitation is the most common type of disability, followed by cognitive disorders (e.g., problems with concentration, memory, decision making) and independent living (CDC, 2020).

Disabilities and other mobility limitations can lead to poor health outcomes in older adults because of the limited ability to access needed resources, such as fresh food and medical care. To achieve better long-term health outcomes, it is essential that nurses collaborate with social work/case management to ensure that older adults have the resources needed to remain independent as long as possible.

Homelessness

Homelessness is a growing problem for individuals and families in many U.S. cities. Many people who experience homelessness sleep on the streets, whereas others live temporarily with relatives or in mission shelters. Homelessness is far more complex than merely a lack of housing. Several factors are involved, such as financial crises, socially dysfunctional relationships, unemployment, lack of job skills, substance abuse, healthcare expenses, or the inability or lack of desire to live within the socially accepted norms of society. In the United States, severe economic difficulties and homelessness often result from mental illness, disability, or other factors (e.g., recession, loss of a job).

Social Isolation Families experiencing homelessness are often socially isolated. Many children in homeless situations do not attend school, and those who do tend to perform poorly. Families may not seek care for significant health problems because they may not know how to access the healthcare system or apply for healthcare services and fear they cannot afford care. Homelessness threatens family relationships and emotional and physical health. You should focus on helping the family meet the basic needs of food and shelter, which, according to Maslow's hierarchy of needs theory (see Chapter 6), must be met before the family can grow.

Groups at High Risk The homeless population is diverse. More men than women experience homelessness. Individuals represent a higher percentage (70%) of homelessness than people living in families with children (30%). The number of unsheltered homeless individuals has risen almost 30% over the last 5 years and affects "people of every race, ethnicity, gender, and most age groups" except children (National Alliance to End Homelessness [NAEH], 2021). Recessions and other economic barriers (e.g., high rent prices) increase the likelihood of individuals and families experiencing homelessness (Fig. 11-5).

♥ iCare Ending homelessness should continue to be a priority goal. Remain nonjudgmental and show compassion for your homeless clients. Advocate to ensure their needs are met by connecting them with the appropriate individuals (e.g., social worker, case manager) who can help them obtain needed resources.

Violence and Neglect Within Families

Intimate partner (domestic) violence—including physical abuse, psychological abuse, stalking, and sexual abuse—occurs among all racial, social, and economic groups.

- Approximately 1 in 4 women and 1 in 10 men have experienced sexual violence, stalking, and/or physical violence.
- More than 43 million women and 38 million men have been victims of psychological aggression, which is verbal and nonverbal communication designed to inflict mental or emotional harm or to exert control over the other person (CDC, 2021b).

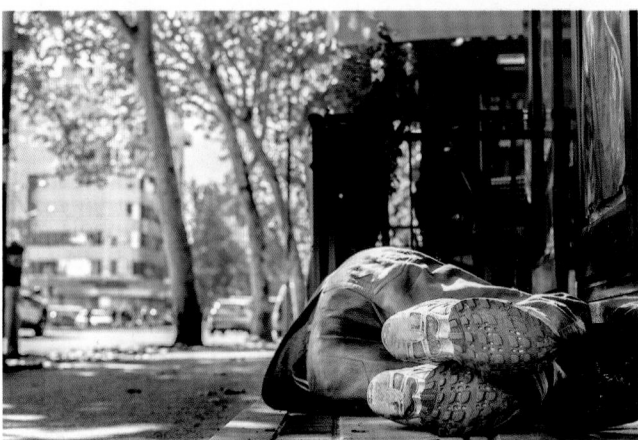

FIGURE 11-5 Unsheltered homelessness is a societal problem.

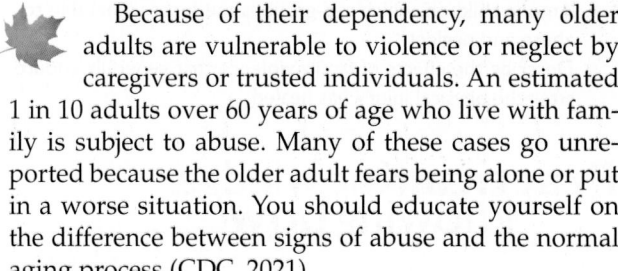

Because of their dependency, many older adults are vulnerable to violence or neglect by caregivers or trusted individuals. An estimated 1 in 10 adults over 60 years of age who live with family is subject to abuse. Many of these cases go unreported because the older adult fears being alone or put in a worse situation. You should educate yourself on the difference between signs of abuse and the normal aging process (CDC, 2021).

Victimization of Children Because of their dependency, small size, and inability to defend themselves, children are especially vulnerable to abuse (sexual, emotional, and physical) and neglect. This is usually at the hands of someone in a custodial role (e.g., parent, caregiver, teacher) (CDC, 2021).

- The number of children who have experienced some form of abuse and neglect is estimated at 1 in 7; however, many cases go unreported.
- Children in low-socioeconomic-status environments are at a higher risk for abuse and neglect.
- A reported 1,840 children died from abuse and neglect in 2019.
- Children in the age range from birth to 2 years are the most vulnerable to maltreatment (Children's Bureau, 2022).

Long-Term Effects Any type of violence is likely to have long-lasting effects on the victims and on the family.

- **Loss of Family Integrity**—Disintegration of family relationships and structure may occur (e.g., sending the children to foster care, escaping to a domestic violence shelter, living with others).
- **Health issues**—Effects of domestic violence include physical injury from the assault itself as well as chronic health problems that emerge as a complication of traumatic injury. Health problems may also result from the ongoing stress of violence or neglect:
  - *Families experiencing domestic violence* have more unintended pregnancies, miscarriages, abortions, and low-birth-weight babies.
  - *Victims' families have a higher incidence of* sexually transmitted infections (STIs) and higher rates of depression, post-traumatic stress syndrome, substance abuse, and suicide.
  - *Often there are long-term effects involving emotional injury,* marred self-esteem, or poor-quality relationships, even though the emotional and physical pain may stop when the victim leaves the family environment.
  - *Victims of family violence learn patterns of ineffective coping* that can be repeated in successive generations.

KnowledgeCheck 11-5
- Name two causes of homelessness.
- Name two groups of individuals who are vulnerable to homelessness.
- Name two types of violence.

- Among children, which age-group is the most vulnerable to abuse and neglect?
- Describe the effects of family violence that generally endure after the physical injury has healed.

PracticalKnowledge
knowing **how**

A holistic view of family health integrates the biological, social, cultural, and spiritual aspects of life and refers to individual members as well as the whole family. Nurses play a vital role in promoting family wellness across the life span. When working with families, you will encourage them to take responsibility for their own family health. Your interactions with families can empower them to practice healing and health-maintenance behaviors.

▮ ASSESSMENT

Family health assessment is similar to that for individuals. Gather all essential assessment information about each family member. Ensuring family privacy is essential to obtain an accurate and comprehensive family health assessment. (See Chapter 19 for additional information on physical assessment.) In addition to the individual's data, assess the health of the family unit. In general, a family assessment should include the following:

- Relevant medical data, social and family history for individuals within the family
- Family composition
- Family genogram showing health issues
- Family history and developmental stage
- Description of the home environment and surroundings
- Family structure, including communication patterns and power and role structures
- Family functions
- Health beliefs, values, and behaviors
- Family strengths
- Family stressors and coping
- Abuse and violence within the family.

To see an abuse assessment,

 Go to Chapter 6, **Procedure 6-1: Assessing for Abuse,** in Volume 2.

For a more complete description of the context of a family assessment,

 Go to Chapter 14, **Clinical Insights 11-1: Conducting a Family Assessment,** and the assessment tool, **Focused Assessment: Family Developmental Tasks,** in Volume 2.

The following sections discuss in more detail the assessment of family health history, family health beliefs, communication patterns, coping processes, and caregiver role strain.

Assessing the Family's Genetic History

The family history can provide clues about a person's health and susceptibility to disease. Genetic linkages have been discovered for common complex diseases, such as breast cancer, Alzheimer disease, diabetes, macular degeneration, seizures, inflammatory bowel disease, lupus, and heart disease, to name a few.

What Is Genomics? The study of human genes and their function, including the interactions among other genes and the environment is referred to as *genomics*. Simply said, it is about the interplay between a person's genetic makeup and food and environmental factors (e.g., lifestyle, stress).

How Can Genomics Be Useful? Genomics can be used to personalize a client's plan of care by:

- Identifying individuals at risk for certain conditions to provide more effective preventive care
- More accurately detecting illness, even before symptoms appear
- Tailoring healthcare to the individual while reducing a trial-and-error approach
- Evaluating a person's response to the care, considering multiple factors

Genomics helps us to understand how people respond differently to particular drugs and medical treatments. For example, whereas one client with a genetic predisposition for high cholesterol can reduce that risk through a change in diet and active exercise regimen, another may require cholesterol-reducing drugs.

How Is a Genogram Constructed? When assessing the family history, you can use a pictorial tool called a **genogram** to display the relationship of family members with pertinent health-related information (Fig. 11-6). This type of family tree can provide a quick and useful context in which to evaluate an individual's health risks.

To construct a genogram, you will use a three-generation (or more) diagram that shows the following for each family member:

- Causes of death
- Important health problems
- Genetically linked diseases
- Environmental (e.g., toxin) issues
- Mental health issues (e.g., depression, alcohol abuse, suicide)
- Occupational diseases (e.g., asbestos)
- Infections (e.g., MRSA)
- Obesity

When developing a genogram, use symbols and abbreviations to denote family members, and include a key for interpretation (Box 11-1).

Assessing the Family's Health Beliefs

Health beliefs can vary widely among families and among individuals within families, especially those of different generations. Generations may pass these

Family History by Genogram

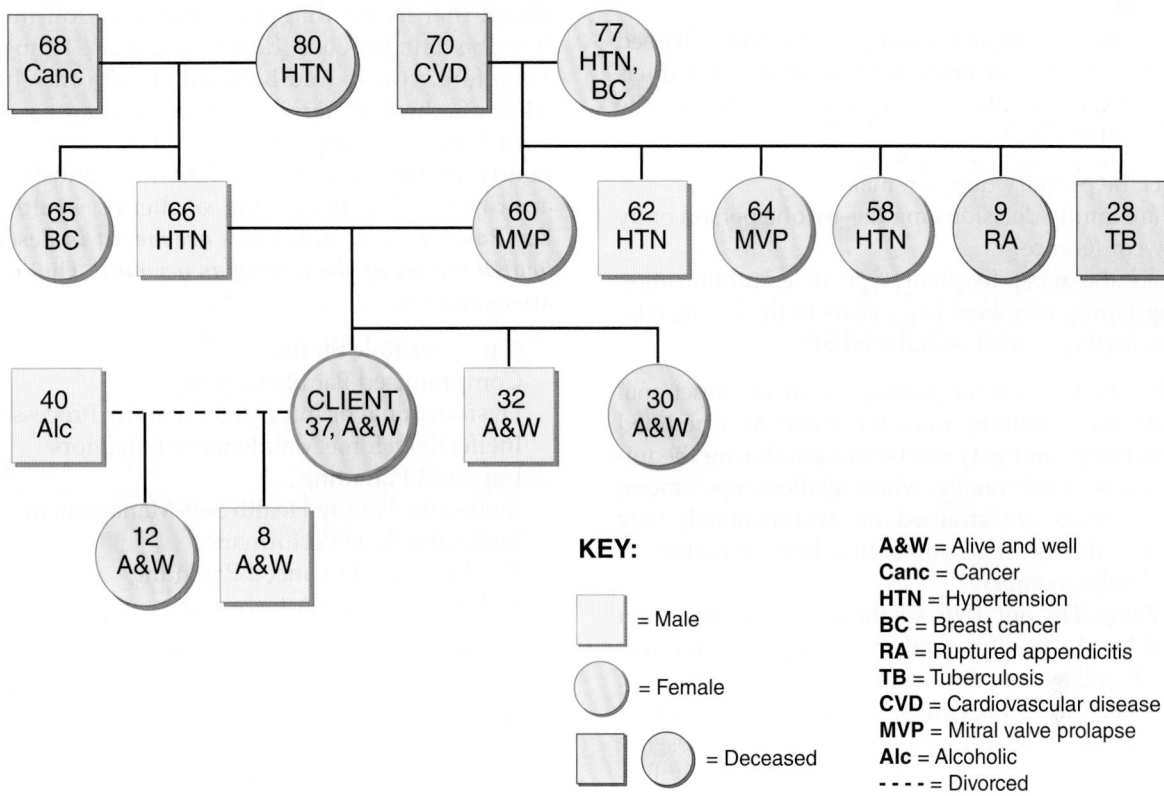

KEY:

☐ = Male

◯ = Female

☐ ◯ = Deceased

A&W = Alive and well
Canc = Cancer
HTN = Hypertension
BC = Breast cancer
RA = Ruptured appendicitis
TB = Tuberculosis
CVD = Cardiovascular disease
MVP = Mitral valve prolapse
Alc = Alcoholic
- - - - = Divorced

FIGURE 11-6 Family history by genogram.

BOX 11-1 ■ Family History by Listing Family Members

The following history is for a 37-year-old female client.

Client: Age 37, alive and well

Spouse: Age 40, divorced, alcoholism

Daughter: Age 12, alive and well

Son: Age 8, alive and well

Brother: Age 32, alive and well

Sister: Age 30, alive and well

Father: Age 66, hypertension (HTN)

Mother: Age 60, mitral valve prolapse (MVP)

Paternal aunt: Age 65, breast cancer

Maternal uncle: Age 62, HTN

Maternal uncle: Deceased age 28, tuberculosis (TB)

Maternal aunt: Age 64, MVP

Maternal aunt: Age 58, HTN

Maternal aunt: Deceased age 9, ruptured appendix

Paternal grandfather: Deceased age 68, cancer

Paternal grandmother: Age 80, HTN

Maternal grandmother: Age 77, HTN, breast cancer

Maternal grandfather: Deceased age 70, cardiovascular disease (CVD)

beliefs to future generations. Common health beliefs are expressed in such adages as "An apple a day keeps the doctor away," and "Feed a cold, starve a fever." Some families have an intense mistrust of medical care and hospitals and may seek treatment only when absolutely necessary (e.g., when the pain becomes unbearable).

The family's beliefs may influence individual decision making, even when a member shares only a few of the family's beliefs. Suppose a family is caring for a member who is older, frail, confused, and immobile. Imagine that one family member believes quality-of-life issues are more important than length of life. Yet another family member strongly disagrees with this belief and supports the right of the older adult to receive whatever care is needed for any length of time. In a situation like this, the family is at risk for interpersonal conflict, impaired communication, and caregiver strain. If you would like more information on health beliefs, see Chapter 8.

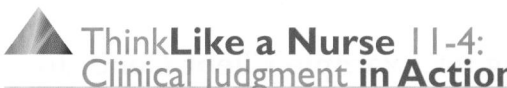

Think**Like a Nurse** 11-4:
Clinical Judgment **in Action**

- As a nurse, how can you promote overall wellness in a family with different needs and priorities?
- What changes in family function would you want to ask the Henderson family (Meet Your Patient) about?

Assessing the Family's Communication Patterns

To assess family communication patterns, you will need to interview the family and carefully observe the interactions between family members. Try to uncover the following information:

- Who is the primary decision maker?
- How are family decisions made—by one person or by family conference?
- What is the most frequent type of communication among family members (e.g., visits to the home, telephone, texting, e-mail, social media)?

Family members who participate in dysfunctional communication patterns may not come to scheduled family meetings and may not be present during the initial interview. Additionally, when relationships among family members are strained or dysfunctional, they may distort the information about a home situation or another family member.

Key Point: *Do not rely solely on the information provided by the family members during the interview process.* Families usually want to "put on the best face" for healthcare providers, so they may be careful to give socially desirable responses. Carefully observe the words people use and other cues, such as body language, direct eye contact, and other nonverbal expressions, particularly among family members.

Assessing the Family's Coping Processes

The physiological manifestations of stress (e.g., anxiety, increased pulse rate) may decrease the effectiveness of interventions and negatively affect a client's health. Similarly, family members who are not coping effectively may cause the client to become tense or anxious or have problems sleeping. Assessing family coping is a first step to helping them develop more effective coping patterns.

Observe for physical indications of stress, anxiety, or loss of sleep in the ill person and for relationships and communication patterns among family members. As a nurse, you can assess whether family members are irritable and speak harshly or curtly to one another. Pay attention to who is visiting. Family members who are not coping well may avoid coming to visit the client, so this may be an indicator of who is coping and who is not.

KnowledgeCheck 11-6

- Why is it important for you to ask about family health beliefs?
- What factors may impede a family's ability to cope with an individual's illness?
- What is the significance of a genogram?

Assessing for Example Client Condition: Caregiver Role Strain

To learn about this Caregiver Role Strain and relevant nursing care, see the Example Client Condition: Caregiver Role Strain.

ANALYSIS/NURSING DIAGNOSIS NP

Recall that in the diagnostic process, you must analyze the data for cues (data that deviate from norms). Therefore, you should be familiar with the characteristics of a healthy family so that you can use them as your basis for comparison (Box 11-2). For individual family members, any NANDA-I diagnosis may be appropriate for describing a client's health status. Key Point: *Family diagnoses are meant to describe the health status of the family as a whole.* The following are examples:

Caregiver Role Strain
Compromised Family Coping
Dysfunctional or Interrupted Family Processes
Ineffective Home Maintenance Behaviors
Impaired Parenting
Ineffective Family Health Self-Management
Ineffective Role Performance
Readiness for Enhanced Parenting
Risk for Impaired Attachment

For more NANDA-I standardized diagnoses, along with definitions and defining characteristics, refer to the most recent NANDA-I *Nursing Diagnoses Definitions and Classification* or to a nursing diagnosis handbook published by different authors. You may wish to visit the NANDA-I Web site at **www.nanda.org.**

PLANNING OUTCOMES AND EVALUATION

NOC outcomes specifically for families as units are found in the four NOC domains of Family Caregiver Performance, Family Member Health Status, Family Well-Being, and Parenting (Moorhead et al., 2018). Outcomes from other domains may apply as well, depending on the nursing diagnoses and hypotheses you have made.

Individualized goals/outcome statements you might write for a family include the following examples, which represent some of the traits of healthy families in Box 11-2. The family:

Teaches respect for others within and outside the family.
Observes rituals and traditions (e.g., celebrates birthdays).
Respects the privacy of each member.
Communicates effectively and openly.

Remember that the outcomes and solutions you develop for the care plan serve as the criteria for evaluating your client's responses to nursing interventions.

PLANNING INTERVENTIONS/IMPLEMENTATION

NIC interventions for families as units are found in the NIC domain of Family Integrity Promotion, which includes the classes for the Childbearing Family. Interventions from other domains may apply as well,

EXAMPLE CLIENT CONDITION: Caregiver Role Strain

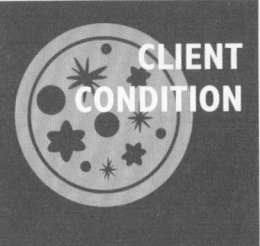

CLIENT CONDITION

Conflicts between caregiving and other responsibilities can produce tremendous family stress, and family caregiver experiences difficulties performing adequately in his role.

Causes and Triggers

The physical, emotional, and time demands involved in caring for family members who are chronically ill, disabled, or frail. Alternatively, you might describe the problem more specifically for a particular client, for example, as Caregiver Burden or Caregiver Role Stress.

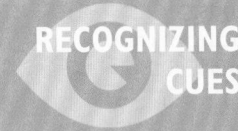

CONTRIBUTING FACTORS

Physical

- Physical, emotional, and time demands involved in caring for family members who are chronically ill, disabled, or frail
- Client physical care demands (complex treatments, frailty)

Emotional

- Poor communication
- Financial issues
- Conflicts between caregiving and other responsibilities
- Conflicts among family members

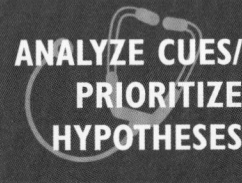

RECOGNIZING CUES

Recognize Caregiver Risk Factors & Symptoms

- Causes of role strain (see contributing factors)
- Dysfunctional communication, such as abusive language and aggression
- Apathy, withdrawal
- Emotional distress
- Caregiver depression, withdrawal, isolation, aggression, abusive communications

Recognize Family Functioning

- Conflicts
- Avoidance
- Attachment
- Demanding
- Criticism of healthcare personnel or family

Recognize Client Factors

- Physical injuries
- Withdrawal, isolation
- Neglect
- Depression
- Changes in daily routines, appetite, sleep patterns
- Support systems

ANALYZE CUES/ PRIORITIZE HYPOTHESES

Caregiver Role Strain

Definition: Difficulty in fulfilling care responsibilities, expectations, and/or behaviors for family or significant others (Herdman & Kamitsuru, 2018)

Defining Characteristics

Grouped into four main categories: caregiving activities, caregiver health status (physiological, emotional, and socioeconomic), caregiver–care receiver relationship, and family processes.

GENERATE SOLUTIONS

NOC Outcomes

- Caregiver Emotional Health
- Caregiver–Client Relationship
- Caregiver Well-Being

Individualized Outcome Statements

- Caregiver relief and respite
- Referral to family support groups

- Caregiver Physical Health
- Caregiver Performance: Direct Care
- Caregiver Performance: Indirect Care
- Treatment for depression
- Symptomatic relief to client and caregiver

(continued)

EXAMPLE CLIENT CONDITION: Caregiver Role Strain—cont'd

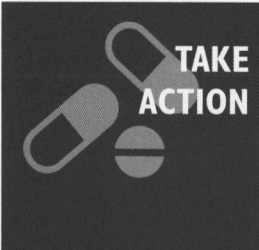

TAKE ACTION

NIC Interventions

- Caregiver Support, Coping Enhancement
- Caregiver Support, Respite Care
- Teaching: Disease Process (also Prescribed Diet, Prescribed Medication)
- Decision-Making Support, Health-System Guidance
- Energy Management
- Nutrition Management

Individualized Interventions

- Promote family cohesion during crisis (illness, hospitalization).
- Protect the client; assess for removal from environment.

Individualized Interventions (cont'd)

- Identify support systems to ensure caregiver support.
- Refer for anger-control assistance.
- Promote positive communications.
- Promote family wellness.
- Promote expression of feelings and open communication of fears, anxiety, and concerns.
- Praise positive relationships
- Praise/maintain family strengths
- Support family in problem-solving/decision making.
- Provide symptomatic treatment to client.
- Promote adequate self-care (e.g., nutrition, sleep, exercise).

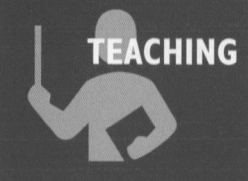

TEACHING

- Teach respect for others within and outside the family.
- Teach caregiver skills and techniques for effective coping.
- Teach how to address conflict.

- Teach health-promotion behaviors.
- Teach relaxation methods.
- Teaching proper balancing of care responsibilities with work.

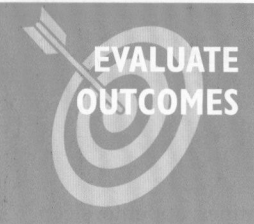

EVALUATE OUTCOMES

The caregiver will:
Demonstrate caregiver emotional health.
Exhibit competence in direct and indirect caregiver performance.

Develop a therapeutic caregiver–care receiver relationship
Ensure caregiver well-being and physical health.

BOX 11-2 ■ Characteristics of a Healthy Family

A healthy family requires more than merely the absence of family dysfunction or disease in an individual member. The following are characteristics of a healthy family:

- State of family well-being
- Sense of belonging and connectedness
- Clear boundaries between family members, where the responsibilities of adults are clear and separate from the responsibilities of growing children
- Sense of trust and respect
- Honesty and freedom of expression, including different opinions or viewpoints
- Spending time together, sharing rituals and traditions
- Relaxed body language, physical touch, and frequent eye contact
- Flexibility: adaptability and ability to deal with stress, openness to change

- Commitment: working together to maintain the family
- Spiritual well-being
- Respect for privacy of individual members
- Balance of giving and receiving
- Positive, effective communication
- Accountability, including acceptance when mistakes are made
- Appreciation and affection for each other
- Responding to the needs and interests of all members
- Health-promoting lifestyle of individual members
- Open discussions on disagreements and the ability to make compromises without ill feelings toward the other person.

depending on the nursing diagnosis you have made. The following are some examples:

> Caregiver Support
> Genetic Counseling
> Home Maintenance Assistance
> Respite Care
> Risk Identification.

Individualized nursing actions you might use with families include the following examples (Butcher et al., 2018); other interventions are described in succeeding sections:

- Establish trusting relationships with family members.
- Collaborate with family in problem-solving and decision making.
- Refer the family to support groups or other families dealing with similar problems.
- Refer for family therapy, as indicated.
- Monitor current family relationships.
- Assist family with conflict resolution.
- Encourage family to maintain positive relationships.
- Counsel family members on additional effective coping skills for their own use.
- Tell family members it is safe and acceptable to use typical expressions of affection when in a hospital setting.
- Encourage family members to verbalize their concerns, fears, and perceptions.

Promoting Family Wellness

Encourage families to value health promotion and incorporate it into their lifestyles. This will also affect the health of individual members. Health-promotion behaviors are typically learned within the family, so you can promote family wellness by addressing both individual and family needs. It is important to identify both the strengths (see Box 11-2) and basic weaknesses of the family to adequately meet healthcare needs.

Involving the family in each phase of the nursing process promotes positive health outcomes and helps establish trust between you and the family. Wellness interventions may include contracting, health teaching, anticipatory guidance, and promoting family cohesion during a crisis (e.g., hospitalization of a family member). For specific health-promotion activities, see Chapter 8.

Interventions When a Family Member Is Ill

When a family member is ill or hospitalized, other family members experience a range of emotions—especially when the illness is severe or of sudden onset. Family members may display signs of stress in a variety of ways, such as arguing with each other or with healthcare providers, being critical of the care that is provided, or frequently asking for information to be repeated or for status updates. These are normal reactions; do not take them personally.

The client and family need to understand the medical diagnosis, the plan of care, and the recovery process. In addition, the nurse often provides extensive discharge

---

> **BOX 11-3 ■** Interventions to Help the Family Cope With Hospitalization
>
> - Provide written materials explaining the client's diagnosis or condition.
> - Actively involve the family in team meetings.
> - Promptly follow up with family concerns or questions.
> - Encourage the family to go home and rest.
> - Encourage the family to call for updates when they cannot be present. Be sure to provide them with the code numbers or words.
> - Suggest ideas for stress-reducing activities (e.g., walking, meditating).
> - Inform the family about the on-site availability of a clergy member or chapel.
> - Encourage the family to participate in care activities as appropriate.
> - Keep the family informed of the client's progress.
> - Help the family to identify sources of stress and develop strategies to work through and dissolve the root cause.
> - Provide anticipatory guidance regarding outcomes and expectations for discharge.

instructions to the client and family before they leave the hospital. To help family members manage stress when a family member is ill, see Box 11-3.

Interventions for Example Client Condition: Caregiver Role Strain

For nursing interventions specific to Caregiver Role Strain, see Example Client Condition: Caregiver Role Strain.

 EVALUATION

Refer to the Example Client Condition for evaluation of outcomes and interventions specific to Caregiver Role Strain.

 To explore learning resources for this chapter,

 Go to Davis Advantage and find:

Answers and Suggested Responses for all questions in this chapter
Concept Map
Knowledge Map
References and Bibliography

CHAPTER 12

Caring in Multicultural Healthcare Environments

Learning Outcomes

After completing this chapter, you should be able to:

➤ Differentiate between diversity and multiculturalism.

➤ Explain why cultural competence is important for nurses.

➤ Explain what is meant by *culture* and *acculturation*.

➤ Discuss concepts pertaining to cultural diversity in nursing.

➤ Identify vulnerable populations in the United States.

➤ Define and give an example of culture universals and of culture specifics.

➤ Differentiate between cultural archetypes and cultural stereotypes.

➤ Describe the culture of the U.S. healthcare system, including professional subcultures.

➤ Describe the phenomena of culture, including how they can affect the

nursing care needs of clients and families.

➤ Discuss the differing views of culturally diverse clients, including biomedical, holistic, and alternative health systems, such as folk medicine.

➤ Explain guidelines for performing a transcultural assessment, including a cultural assessment model.

➤ Recognize the cultural implications inherent in nursing diagnoses.

➤ Describe nursing strategies that promote delivery of culturally competent care to clients and their families.

➤ Identify techniques for communicating with clients when there is a language barrier.

Key Concepts

Cultural competence

Culture

Related Concepts

See the Concept Map on Davis Advantage.

Meet Your Patients

Your clinical assignment is to spend the day in a walk-in clinic with a primary care provider. Your assignment while there is to greet the clients and help them complete a health history form. These are the clients you see that day:

▪ Romano Salvatore points to his head and moans. When you ask him what is wrong, he makes a gesture to convey to you that he does not understand what you are saying and replies in Italian.

▪ Rosanna is a frantic young mother, carrying her 4-year-old son, José, who is crying and coughing. Rosanna informs you that José complains of a sore throat and has a fever. She tells you she has been to her *curandero*, but José is not getting any better. You notice that José

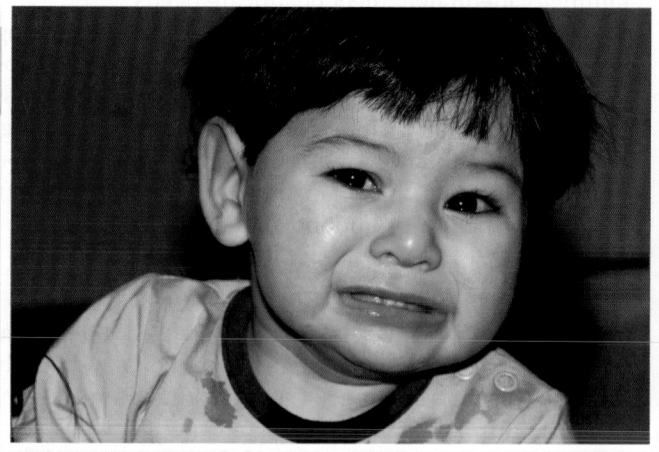

is wearing a heavy coat and knit hat although it is quite warm outside. When you ask Rosanna about the child's clothing, she says that José is cold.

Meet Your Patient (continued)

- Lee Chan, an older Chinese American man, is accompanied by eight family members. Because the waiting area is small, everyone except his daughter Kim is asked to wait outside. Mr. Chan is quiet and does not make eye contact with you. His daughter explains that

her father has stomach cancer and is in a lot of pain because of disharmony. When you ask him to rate his pain, he just shakes his head and looks away. Would you wonder what "disharmony" means in this situation?

TheoreticalKnowledge
knowing why

Try to answer the following questions about the patients you have just met. You may not have the theoretical knowledge to answer them all—you will acquire that in this chapter—but do your best based on the background you now have.

ThinkLike a Nurse 12-1:
Clinical Judgment in Action

- Think about Romano Salvatore.
  If you could speak Italian, what would you ask him?
- Think about Rosanna and her child.
  One question that might spring immediately to your mind is, "What is a *curandero*?" How would you find out this information?
  Why do you think that the child is dressed more warmly than you would expect for the weather?
- Think about Mr. Chan and his family.
  How would you feel about so many of his family members coming with Mr. Chan to the clinic?
  Why do you think he is not looking at or speaking to you?
  How could you communicate with Mr. Chan? Would you assume that he does not speak your language? Explain your reasoning.

ABOUT THE KEY CONCEPTS

The overarching concepts for this chapter are **culture** and **cultural competence.** These and the concepts of *diversity, multiculturalism, assimilation,* and *culture universals* are important for nurses to understand and apply to the care of clients.

WHY LEARN ABOUT CULTURE?

You will care for clients from various cultures and likely work on a multicultural healthcare team (see Fig. 12-1). Having cultural knowledge can help you to provide culturally competent care.

Diversity and Multiculturalism Are Related Concepts Diversity and multiculturalism are related but different concepts. Diversity looks at the differences among people in society, based on numerous factors, such as race, gender, religion, socioeconomic status, sexual orientation, religion, culture, and so on. In contrast,

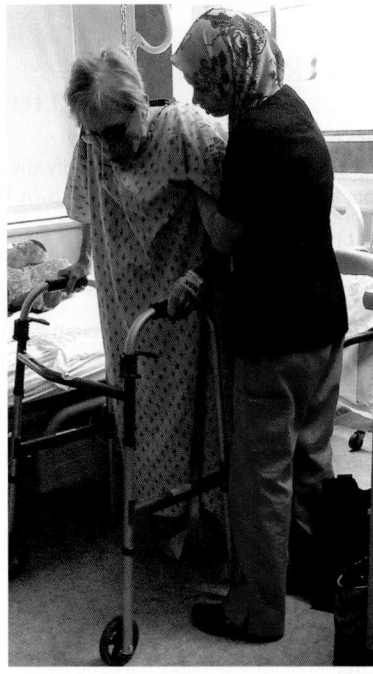

FIGURE 12-1 Nurses work with patients from many cultures.

multiculturalism accommodates diversity and incorporates inclusion. At its best, multiculturalism promotes the acceptance of and respect for individual differences. It requires one to become aware of both advantages and challenges encountered by various groups (Plaut et al., 2018). This awareness and knowledge is essential for all nurses because they need to provide care to all patients.

The Population Is Diverse The United States is a multicultural society. We continue to see a trend of increasing immigration from other nations. In 2021, 43.9% of U.S. foreign nationals who obtained lawful permanent resident status in the United States were from Mexico, China, India, the Philippines, Cuba, and the Dominican Republic (Gibson, 2021). Of the 11,411 refugees admitted into the United States in fiscal year 2021, 75.2% were from Congo, Syria, Afghanistan, Ukraine, and Myanmar (Rush, 2021). By 2030, U.S. population growth will be attributed to net international migration (1.1 million) compared with natural population increases (1 million). By 2060, net international migration (1.1 million) will be the significant driver of U.S. population compared with natural increases (500,000) (Vespa et al., 2020).

Demographically, the fastest-growing racial or ethnic group is made up of individuals who identify as two or more races, followed by individuals of Asian and Hispanic descent (Vespa et al., 2020). Additionally, data show that by 2060, the non-Hispanic White population is expected to decrease to 179 million people, a drop of 20 million from 2016. The United States is expected to become a minority nation by 2045 or earlier, meaning no single population group will have a majority share of the total population (see Box 12-1) (Frey, 2018, 2020; Vespa et al., 2020).

ThinkLike a Nurse 12-2: Clinical Judgment in Action

- With what cultural groups do you identify?
- In the neighborhood where you live, identify the cultural or ethnic groups that are different from your own. How many are there?
- In the school you are now attending, how many different cultural or ethnic groups are represented? What are they?

Health Disparities Exist Among Racial and Ethnic Groups A *Healthy People 2030* overarching goal is to eliminate disparities, achieve health equity, and attain health literacy to improve the health and well-being of all people in the United States (*Healthy People 2030*, n.d.).

- **Health Status.** One general disparity is that some minority racial groups experience higher rates of illness and death and, in general, poorer health status compared with the non-Hispanic White population. For example:
  - Compared with rates for the White population, infant mortality rates are significantly higher for the Black, Native Hawaiian/Pacific Islander, and American Indian/Alaska Native populations (Ely & Driscoll, 2021).
  - Black (of non-Hispanic origin), Hispanic, and American Indian/Alaska Native adults have a higher prevalence of asthma (Centers for Disease Control and Prevention [CDC], 2022a).
  - Black Americans are eight times more likely to have an HIV/AIDS diagnosis than are Whites, and their rate of diagnosis is more than twice that of Latino men (Kaiser Family Foundation, 2020).

However, non-Hispanic White individuals experienced a slightly higher rate of death from heart disease (21.3%) compared with individuals who are Native Hawaiian/Other Pacific Islanders (20.8%) and individuals who are Black (non-Hispanic) (20.7%).

- **Quality of care.** The overall quality of healthcare improved in the United States, including person-centered care, patient safety, care coordination, effective treatment, and healthful living. However, disparities still exist for individuals experiencing economic instability, individuals who are uninsured, and among racial and ethnic groups (Agency for Healthcare Research and Quality [AHRQ], 2022).
- **Access to care.** From 2002 to 2018, the percentage of people under 65 years covered by health insurance and who had a usual provider of care increased. In line with this, personal spending on health insurance and healthcare services decreased. However, access to dental and oral healthcare services did not show a substantial improvement, especially for low-income and rural populations (AHRQ, 2022).

Nursing Is Challenged to Provide Culturally Competent Care As you know, nurses care for patients from many different races and cultures. Nursing care that is appropriate for the dominant cultural group may be ineffective and inappropriate for people who have a different cultural heritage. In the United States, the healthcare culture reflects the dominant European American culture. The majority of nurses in the healthcare sector are White (81%) and are not representative of the racial makeup of the general population, with only 19% of registered

---

BOX 12-1 ■ Population Projections per Racial Group, 2016–2060

Group	2016 Population (in millions)	2030 Population (in millions)	2060 Projections (in millions)
Non-Hispanic Whites	198.0	198.0	179.1
Hispanic	57.5	74.8	111.2
Black/African American	43.0	49.0	60.7
Asian	18.3	24.4	36.8
American Indian and Alaska Natives	4.1	4.7	5.6
Native Hawaiian and other Pacific Islander	771 (thousand)	913 (thousand)	1.1

Source: Vespa, J., Armstrong, D. M., & Medina, L. (2020). *Demographic turning points for the United States: Population projections for 2020 to 2060.* Current Population Report P25-1144. U.S. Census Bureau.

nurses (RNs) identifying themselves as minorities (Smiley et al., 2021). **Key Point:** *It is impossible to know about every culture, but it is important to learn about those you will encounter most often.* An understanding of culture, ethnicity, and race will help you in providing direct care, teaching, supervising, and modeling culturally competent care to other care providers.

KnowledgeCheck 12-1

- What do recent demographic trends in the United States indicate?
- Why should nurses know about the culture, ethnicity, and race of clients?

WHAT IS MEANT BY CULTURE?

Culture is a complex and dynamic concept that includes the social norms, behaviors, and beliefs of groups of people. Culture is dynamic because individuals' attitudes, values, customs, and so on change over time as they interact with other groups, expand their knowledge, and learn new ways of being. Although people have a desire to honor tradition, they also want to be interconnected with the world. The following are some other definitions of culture:

- *Spector* (2017) explained culture in a unique way by asserting that we should view it by picturing the entire luggage each of us carries around on our lifetime journey. According to Spector, the luggage can be beliefs, habits, practices, likes and dislikes, and so on that we can learn from our families and can transmit to our children.
- *Leininger and McFarland* (2002) view culture as "the learned, shared, and transmitted knowledge of values, beliefs, and lifeways of a particular group that are generally transmitted intergenerationally and influence thinking, decisions, and actions in patterned or in certain ways" (p. 47).
- The *Office of Minority Health* (2013) defines culture as "the integrated pattern of thoughts, communications, actions, customs, beliefs, values, and institutions associated, wholly or partially, with racial, ethnic, or linguistic groups, as well as with religious, spiritual, biological, geographic, or sociological characteristics" (p. 10).

Characteristics of Culture

In understanding more about the meaning of *culture* and *cultural*, recall the following characteristics:

- **Cultural beliefs provide identity and a sense of belonging** if they continue to satisfy its members and do not conflict with the dominant culture.
- **Cultures consist of common beliefs and practices.** Most members of a culture share the same beliefs, traditions, customs, and practices, as long as they continue to be adaptive and satisfy the members' needs.

Culture can influence everything its members think and do.

- **Culture is both** *universal* **(everyone has it) and** *dynamic* **(it changes).** Cultural customs, beliefs, and practices are not static. They change over time and at different rates as members adapt and respond to their environment and external influences.
- **Culture exists at many levels.** Culture exists in both the material (art, writings, dress, or artifacts) and the nonmaterial (customs, traditions, language, beliefs, and practices). See Figure 12-2.
- **Cultural values, beliefs, and traditions are passed down from generation to generation.** Learning occurs through life experiences shared with other members of the culture, either formally (e.g., in schools) or informally (e.g., in families). Some generations totally adopt the values, beliefs, and traditions of their elders, some partially accept them, and others reject them.
- **Cultural assumptions and habits can be unconscious.** Thus, they may be difficult for members of the culture to explain to others or to identify as different from another culture.
- **Culture is diverse** and demonstrates the variety that exists among groups and among members of a particular group.

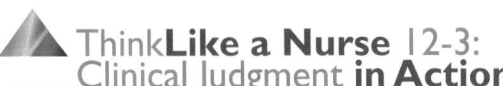

ThinkLike a Nurse 12-3: Clinical Judgment in Action

Figure 12-2 depicts an example of ways in which members of particular cultural groups express their cultural uniqueness in dance. Can you think of other ways that people express their culture?

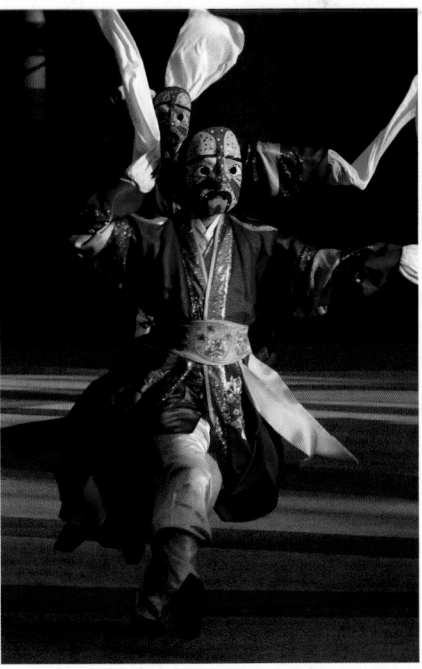

FIGURE 12-2 Traditional lunar New Year dancer in South Korea.

Ethnicity, Race, and Religion

You may hear the terms *culture, ethnicity,* and *race* used interchangeably, but in fact, they have separate, specific meanings. Distinctions between culture, ethnicity, race, and religion might seem confusing, but think of it this way: You are a member of:

- The subculture of nursing
- An ethnic group (e.g., Portuguese Americans from the Azores)
- A racial group (e.g., White)
- A religion (e.g., Roman Catholicism)

Each of those groups has its own set of beliefs and values, so your culture is a blend of all of them.

Ethnicity

Examples of ethnic groups include French Canadians, Hmong, and Latinos.

- **Ethnicity is similar to** *culture* in that it refers to groups whose members share a common social and cultural heritage that is passed down from generation to generation.
- **Ethnicity is also similar to** *subculture*, in that the members of an **ethnic group** have some characteristics in common (e.g., race, ancestry, physical characteristics, geographic region, lifestyle, religion) that are not shared or understood by others.
- **Ethnicity may include race, but it is not the same as race.** To demonstrate, the U.S. Census Bureau (2020) has separate categories for race and ethnicity. The question related to ethnicity inquire as to whether the respondent is of Hispanic, Latino, or Spanish origin, with choices of:
  - (1) No, not of Hispanic, Latino, or Spanish origin
  - (2) Yes, Mexican American or Chicano
  - (3) Yes, Puerto Rican
  - (4) Yes, Cuban
  - (5) Yes, another Hispanic, Latino, or Spanish origin, with a box to identify.
  - **Hispanic** Americans are people who originally came from any Spanish-speaking country (e.g., Mexico, Spain).
  - **Latino/Latinx,** strictly speaking, refers only to people from Central or South America.
  - **Spanish** implies origin in Spain.

Key Point: *You can reference your patient's ethnicity (e.g., Mexican American, Puerto Rican, Cuban, Colombian American) rather than using the term* **Hispanic, Latino/Latinx,** *or* **Spanish.**

Race

Race is often used to identify someone by similar phenotypic traits, such as skin color, blood type, or bone structure. However, you cannot tell race from a person's appearance or skin color. The terms *race* and *ethnicity* overlap somewhat because race can be a characteristic of a specific ethnic group. The U.S. Census Bureau (2020) asks people to choose the race with which they identify and divides the population into the following list of racial categories:

- White
- Black or African American
- American Indian or Alaskan Native
- Asian Indian
- Chinese
- Filipino
- Japanese
- Korean
- Vietnamese
- Other Asian
- Native Hawaiian
- Chamorro
- Samoan
- Other Pacific Islanders

People of Hispanic, Latino, or Spanish origin may be of any race because the U.S. Census Bureau includes Hispanic/Latino/Spanish as an ethnicity rather than a race category.

♥ **iCare Race as a Social Construct** You cannot determine a person's race by their appearance. As a culturally sensitive nurse, ask people what race they identify with and what name they prefer to use for it. For more information on race as a social construct,

 Go to the article "Race Is a Social Construct, Scientists Argue," at http://www.scientificamerican.com/article/race-is-a-social-construct-scientists-argue/

Key Point: *We tend to group and categorize data to make them meaningful and useful, but we must be careful to avoid using these categories as the basis for interacting with people or providing care. When you need to designate a name for a racial or ethnic group, be as specific as possible (e.g., "Syrian American" instead of "White").*

Religion

Religion may be confused with ethnicity because people within an ethnic group may share the same religion. For example, individuals who consider themselves part of the Jewish culture are often also part of the Jewish faith community. **Religion** refers to an ordered system of beliefs regarding the cause, nature, and purpose of the universe, especially the beliefs related to the worship of a God or gods (Andrews et al., 2020). In many cultures, religion is a high priority (Figure 12-3).

Concepts Related to Culture

The term *bicultural* describes a person who identifies with two cultures and integrates some of the values and lifestyles of each into their life. A child whose father is Jewish and whose mother is an Italian Catholic may

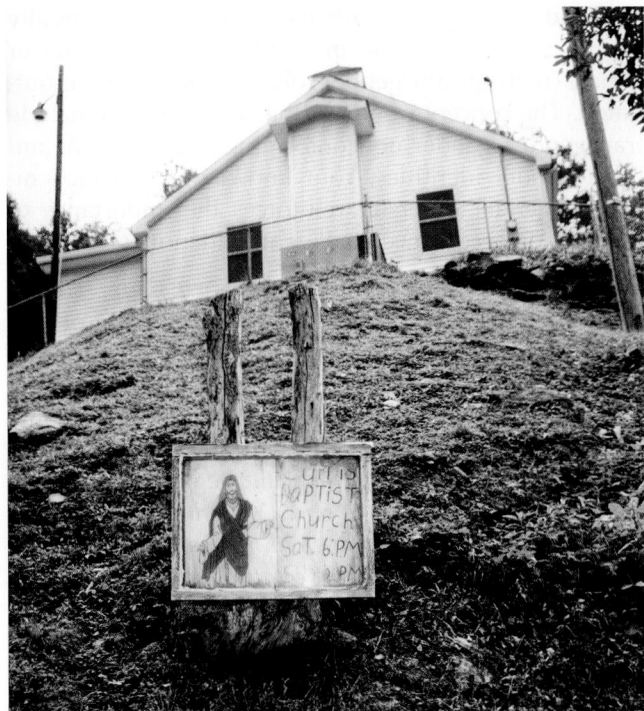

FIGURE 12-3 Even in this tiny community of rural Appalachia, people have built a place for worship.

choose to follow Jewish tradition while still holding some of the values and beliefs of their Italian heritage. A bicultural person may experience divided loyalties or enjoy the best of both cultures.

Multicultural refers to many cultures and is used to describe groups rather than individuals. Many regions of the United States are multicultural, meaning that the region is populated by individuals from many different cultural groups. The same can be said about workplace environments.

Think of a hospital: caregivers may be members of various ethnic, racial, and religious groups, and the nurses, providers, physical therapists, and students each make up a different subculture. A hospital is thus a multicultural setting.

Socialization, Acculturation, and Assimilation

Socialization Socialization is the process of learning to become a member of a society or a group. A person becomes socialized by learning social rules and roles; by learning behaviors, norms, values; and by being exposed to the perceptions of others in the same group or role. Your education program is socializing you into the role of a professional nurse. Families, schools, churches, peer groups, and the media are agents of socialization and foster their members' identification with the culture.

Acculturation Acculturation is a learning process through which **immigrants** (new members of a group or country) assume the characteristics of that culture. The best way to understand acculturation is that it is a concurrent process of cultural and psychological change occurring when individuals or groups from one culture are placed into contact with another culture and acquire some of those new elements (Frazer et al., 2017). A person who is acculturated accepts both their own and the new culture, adopting elements of each. Acculturation is the outgrowth of the underrepresented group's need to survive and flourish in the new culture. It may take several years, perhaps three generations, for an immigrant group to become acculturated.

Assimilation Assimilation occurs when the new members gradually learn and take on the essential values, beliefs, and behaviors of the dominant culture. Assimilation is complete when the newcomer is fully merged into the dominant cultural group. A person becomes assimilated by, for example, learning to speak the dominant language; marrying a member from the new (host) culture; and establishing close, personal relationships with members of the new group. For example, if you emigrated from your home in the United States to Mexico, you would take with you your own language and food preferences. But over time, you might gradually begin to eat more of the local foods and learn to speak the native tongue, Spanish.

Dominant Cultures, Subcultures, and Underrepresented (Minority) Groups

Ethnocentrism is the tendency to think that your own group (cultural, professional, ethnic, or social) is superior to others and to view behaviors and beliefs that differ greatly from your own as somehow wrong, strange, or unenlightened. The tendency to ethnocentrism exists in all groups, not just in the dominant culture.

Dominant Culture The dominant culture is the group that has the most authority or power to control values and reward or punish behaviors. It is usually, but not always, the largest group. The dominant group may assume their ways are the norm and that everyone else is culturally different. What do you think is the current dominant culture of the United States? If you said White or European American, you would be only partially correct. The ancestors of most White Americans emigrated from Europe, and many were Protestant or part of other Christian religions. Thus, the dominant culture in the United States and Canada is considered White Anglo-Saxon Christian of European descent. The dominant or common culture changes over time (Johansson et al., 2017).

Subcultures Subcultures are groups within a larger culture or social system that have some characteristics that are different from those of the dominant culture (e.g., values, behaviors, ancestry, ways of living, abilities [e.g., deaf]). People in subcultures have had different experiences from those in the dominant group because of factors common to the group (e.g., social class, residence, gender, sexual orientation, ethnic background)

(Oyserman, 2017). You may be able to recognize subcultures by their speech patterns, hearing deficits, dress, gestures, eating habits, lifestyles, or other factors (e.g., providers, nurses, women, older adults, persons with disabilities, rural Midwesterners). However, you should not make assumptions about a patient's behavior based on their subculture.

Key Point: *Subculture diversity in healthcare settings can be a powerful determinant of collaborative work and can lead to cultural reform that can strengthen outcomes (Mannion, 2018).*

Underrepresented (Minority) Groups Underrepresented, or minority, groups are also made up of individuals who share race, religion, or ethnic heritage. They usually have fewer members than the majority group but are no less important to U.S. society. Depending on the type of group, members may or may not share beliefs, practices, or physical characteristics. The term *minority* can also be used to refer to a group of people who receive different and inequitable treatment from others in society. You should consider that this use of the term may be offensive to some because it suggests inferiority and marginalization.

KnowledgeCheck 12-2

- Define *culture*.
- Give an example of each: ethnic group, race, religion.
- How does culture provide identity for an individual?
- Give an example of *acculturation*.

Vulnerable Populations as Subcultures **Vulnerable populations** are groups that are more likely to develop health problems and experience poorer outcomes because of limited access to care, high-risk behaviors, and/or multiple and cumulative stressors (e.g., people experiencing homelessness, economic instability, or mental illness; people with physical disabilities; the very young; and older adults). Some ethnic and racial minority groups are also vulnerable. For example, among American Indian and Native Alaskan populations, there is a high prevalence of type 2 diabetes in those under 20 years of age (Poudel et al., 2018). **Key Point:** *Vulnerable populations are subcultures of all of the major cultural groups.*

People of various socioeconomic classes are found in all ethnic groups. In fact, the subculture of poverty can be found throughout the world. When caring for patients from vulnerable populations, it is important to focus on their strengths and resources, not exclusively on their difficulties and risks.

The framework of the public health initiative *Healthy People 2030* addresses the care of vulnerable populations. One of its overarching goals is to achieve health equity, eliminate disparities, and attain health literacy to improve the health and well-being of all groups. One plan to meet this goal is to "facilitate the development and availability of affordable means of health promotion, disease prevention, and treatment" (*Healthy People 2030,* n.d.).

Gender as a Subculture Society is continually evolving, and the view of gender as either male or female (with specific gender roles and behaviors) is outdated. The concept of gender has expanded to include transgender, gender nonconforming, gender-fluid, and other gender identities. Your knowledge and recognition of gender diversity reinforces the importance of respect and acceptance of all gender identities.

 Old Age as a Subculture Older adults, especially the very old, can be thought of as a vulnerable population in some respects. For example, they are more susceptible to illness and may encounter barriers in access to care. In addition, some older individuals experience varying types of abuse (e.g., physical, sexual, financial, neglect, psychological) (CDC, 2021). **Key Point:** *You should assess for elder abuse in all cultures and not assume that indicators of abuse are a result of a cultural practice.* The violence can be perpetuated by the caregiver, family member, or someone else they trust.

HOW DO CULTURAL VALUES, BELIEFS, AND PRACTICES AFFECT HEALTH?

Values help to shape health-related beliefs and practices. Do you know what values are? Think for a minute about what you "value" in your own life. You may name, for example, learning, family, independence, faith, and cleanliness. Or you may have said something entirely different. Simply put:

- A **personal value** is a principle or standard that has meaning or worth to an individual (e.g., cleanliness).
- A **belief,** in contrast, is something one accepts as true (e.g., "I believe that germs cause disease").
- A **practice** is a set of behaviors that one follows (e.g., "I always wash my hands before preparing food").

Do you now see how values, beliefs, and practices are related?

- Cultural values, beliefs, and practices are the principles, standards, ideas, and behaviors that members of a cultural group share. Some values of the dominant U.S. culture include cleanliness, youth, beauty, success, and independence.
- You should not assume a client shares your values, beliefs, and practices—nor those of the dominant culture.
- **Key Point:** *Remember, also, that individuals within an ethnocultural group vary widely and that learning commonalities is no substitute for careful assessment of each person.*

What Are Culture Universals and Specifics?

- **Culture universals** are the values, beliefs, and practices that people from *all* cultures share. Leininger and McFarland (2002) call these *culture commonalities.*

- **Culture specifics** (*culture diversities* in Leininger's theory) are those values, beliefs, and practices that are special or unique to a culture.

For example, all cultures celebrate the birth of a new baby in some way (a culture universal), but different cultures celebrate birth *rites* in different ways (a culture specific). Similarly, people from all cultures practice marriage rites in rituals that are culture specific (Figure 12-4).

Archetype or Stereotype?

At this point in your efforts to be culturally sensitive, you might be thinking, "My friends are Chinese American, and their wedding was the same as my own wedding with my Italian family"; or "I know plenty of people with Greek heritage who don't put amulets on their babies." Of course, you are correct. However, acknowledging that there are commonalities within a group is not the same as saying that *all* people in the group have those characteristics. You now understand the difference between an archetype and a stereotype.

- A **cultural archetype** is a symbol for remembering some of the culture specifics and is usually not negative. For example, you might think Mexican Americans are more likely to have brown skin or European Americans as having blue eyes—these are not negatives.
- A **cultural stereotype** is an unsubstantiated belief that all people of a certain racial or ethnic group are alike in many respects. Stereotypes are often, but not always, negative. They are, however, assumptions that should

not factor into an objective assessment or evaluation of any patient.

Remember, there is probably more variation among people *within* an ethnic or cultural group than there is *between* the groups, and that variation stems from socioeconomic differences or regional origin as much as from race or ethnicity. **Key Point:** *The guiding principle for your practice is that each person must be seen as unique—they may be a member of an ethnic group, influenced by their heritage but are not defined by it.*

How Do Culture Specifics Affect Health?

Culture specifics affect our health beliefs and behaviors. Thus, knowledge of the culture specifics of groups in your community will help explain why clients from different cultures have different expectations of healthcare. Ultimately, it will help you to provide culturally competent care. The following are six culture specifics that influence health, as described by Giger (2016).

Communication

Communication is an exchange of information, ideas, and feelings. It includes verbal and nonverbal language (i.e., spoken language, gestures, eye contact, and even silences). Think how difficult it would be if you became ill in a country where you did not speak the language. How would you tell the caregivers your symptoms or understand the treatment plan? Language differences present one of the most difficult obstacles to providing care. Even when you and the client speak the same language, culture influences how feelings and thoughts are expressed and which verbal and nonverbal expressions are appropriate to use. See Chapter 15 for communication strategies.

Space

Space refers to a person's personal space, or the boundaries that determine how close another person can be to another person. A person's comfort level is related to space. If you are invading someone's personal space, a common reaction is for the person to move away from you. A similar concept, **territoriality,** means the geographic space a person views as owned or claimed, such as an area or room (Spector, 2017). When an individual's personal space is protected, they feel secure and safe, less anxious, and in control.

Within all cultural groups, personal space varies depending on the relationship between the people speaking: intimates versus acquaintances, people of a different position within the social hierarchy, or other variables.

Time Orientation

Time orientation varies among people of different cultures. Individuals can be past, present, or future oriented. Differences in time orientation can be important as you plan nursing interventions. For example, clients

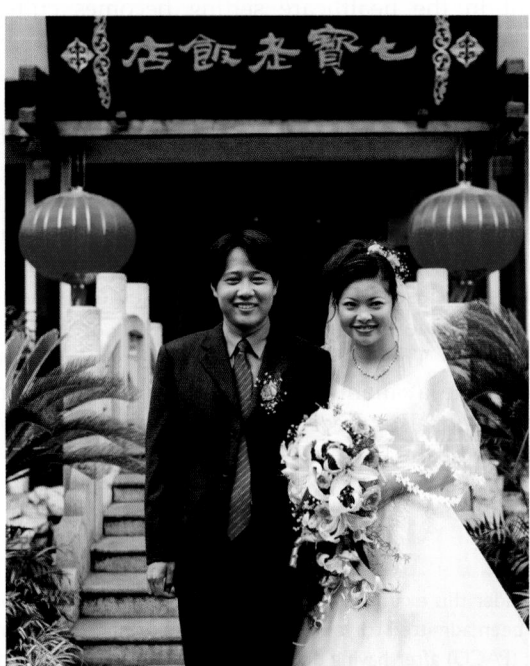

FIGURE 12-4 People of all cultures practice marriage rituals.

who are past oriented may show up late (or not at all) for follow-up appointments; therefore, they may respond better if you provide a written or telephone reminder of their appointment. In contrast, clients who are future oriented may be more focused on illness prevention; thus, they may be more receptive to teaching on health promotion.

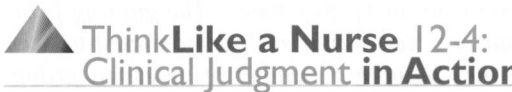

ThinkLike a Nurse 12-4: Clinical Judgment in Action

- Suppose you say to a client, "You will need to exercise and follow a low-calorie diet to lose weight and control your diabetes." What kind of time orientation would make it easier for a client to follow your directions?
- Suppose a client says, "I know I need to lose weight, but I work so much, and the children take so much time. I just don't have time to shop and cook for the right foods or to exercise." What time orientation does this illustrate?

Social Organization

Social organization includes the family unit (e.g., nuclear, single parent, or extended family) and the wider organizations (e.g., community, religious, ethnic) with which the individual or family identifies (Spector, 2017).

- **A close social organization can be found in all cultures; however, the specifics vary**. For example, in some cultures, men are likely to be the dominant family members. But in other cultures, families are matriarchal—that is, the decision makers and family leaders are women.
- **The social organization of your clients' cultures can provide clues about how they will act during life events**, such as birth, death, illness, and mourning. For example, a client who does not trust large institutions or government agencies is likely to use home remedies and delay seeing a conventional medical provider, even though insurance pays for their healthcare.
- **Kinship and social ties also determine who receives healthcare, and in what priority**. In the United States, for example, someone of high status (e.g., a celebrity or political figure) is likely to receive better care than a person who is economically disadvantaged and socially unknown in the community. In some cultures, men receive care before women and children.

Environmental Control

Environmental control refers to a person's perception of their ability to plan activities to control nature or direct environmental factors (Spector, 2017). A person's beliefs and practices toward health and illness are directly related to this concept. For example, if a person does not believe they have control over their health outcomes, they may not seek medical care, take their medications, or exercise. Some patients may not view circumstances as something to be "controlled"; therefore, they tend to accept pain stoically and not demand relief. Think about why Mr. Chan (Meet Your Patients) just shook his head and looked away when asked to rate his pain.

Biological Variations

Biological variations include ways in which people are different genetically and physiologically. They include body build and structure, skin color, vital signs, enzymatic and genetic variations, and drug metabolism (Spector, 2017). Biological variations create susceptibility to certain diseases and injuries and explain differences in responses to treatment. For example, Black patients statistically have poorer responses to certain categories of antihypertensive drugs compared with White patients on similar medications (Clemmer et al., 2020). Consequently, clinical trials (drug studies) now recommend incorporating biological variations. For more information about biological variations,

 Go to **Chapter 12, Clinical Insight 12-1: Assessing for Biological Variations,** in Volume 2.

Other Culture Specifics

Other aspects of life may also be culture specific. Religion/philosophy and education vary among subcultures in the United States, whereas technology, politics/law, and the economy exert broader effects that can be seen among different countries but less so among subcultures within a country.

- **Religion and Philosophy.** A person's religion may determine what healthcare treatments will be accepted. For example, some religions (e.g., Jehovah's Witnesses) do not accept blood transfusions.
- **Education.** Education influences perceptions of wellness and illness and the knowledge of options that are available for healthcare. These, in turn, affect the person's expectations for care.
- **Technology.** The availability of supplies and equipment in the healthcare setting becomes culturally expected. For example, nurses in most of the United States assume they will have bed linens, water, electricity, prescribed medications, and diagnostic machines. In many parts of the world, however, these items are not available.
- **Politics and the Law.** Governmental policies (e.g., Medicare, Medicaid) affect healthcare by determining eligibility, allocation of funds, reimbursement for providers, and acceptable standards. Review Chapter 1 for an overview of governmental healthcare programs.
- **Economy.** The condition of the economy directly affects the availability of funds for publicly funded services. It also affects the individual's ability to pay for healthcare.

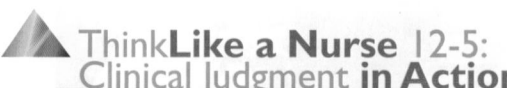

ThinkLike a Nurse 12-5: Clinical Judgment in Action

Consider this example: Mrs. Myers, a Japanese American woman, has been admitted to your care from the postanesthesia care unit (PACU) after having undergone a major surgical procedure. She refuses pain medicine, although she appears to be in pain.

As the hours pass, Mrs. Myers continues to refuse the pain medication, so eventually the nurses stop asking.

- Do you assume that she is experiencing no pain?
- Are you or the other nurses stereotyping her for her cultural response to pain?
- What would you do?

KnowledgeCheck 12-3

- Explain the difference between an archetype and a stereotype.
- Identify at least six culture specifics affecting health.
- How could you use this information about culture specifics to provide better care to your clients?

WHAT IS THE "CULTURE OF HEALTHCARE"?

The conventional and indigenous healthcare systems can exist side by side in any culture (Leininger & McFarland, 2002; McFarland & Wehbe-Alamah, 2018). Each has its own culture.

The Conventional Healthcare System The conventional healthcare system is run by healthcare providers who have been formally educated and trained in a structured environment for particular roles and responsibilities. In the United States, conventional healthcare is dominated by a biomedical healthcare system that combines Western biomedical beliefs with traditional North American values of self-reliance, individualism, and aggressive action. Table 12-1 summarizes the norms of this system, also called *Western* or *allopathic medicine.*

The conventional healthcare system also includes practitioners formally trained in alternative healthcare, such as diet therapy, mind–body control methods, therapeutic touch, acupressure, reflexology, naturopathy, kinesiology, and chiropractic.

The Indigenous Healthcare System The indigenous healthcare system consists of *folk medicine* and *traditional healing methods,* which may also include

♥ iCare 12-1

Caring in Multicultural Healthcare Environments

Farik, an 84-year-old Middle Eastern Muslim man who does not speak English, has come to the intensive care unit (ICU) for multisystem failure. He arrives with multiple family members, all in a highly emotional state. His brother explains to the nurse that it is expected that the male members of his family collectively make decisions, in accordance with Muslim tradition. They may elicit guidance from an Imam, an experienced Muslim leader, regarding medical treatment decisions. The nurse's priority focus is Farik's immediate physical needs. However, it is equally important that the nurse demonstrates caring by being respectful and sensitive to Muslim norms and practices and, specifically, Farik's family's preferences. This is essential to providing appropriate, culturally sensitive, competent, and holistic care.

Table 12-1 ➤ Summary of Cultural Norms of the U.S. Healthcare System

NORM	EXAMPLES
Beliefs and Values	Standardized definitions of *health* and *illness*
	Significance of technology
	Reliance on the biomedical system
	Desire to conquer disease
	Defines health as absence or minimization of disease
Practices	Maintaining health and preventing disease through such practices as immunizations and avoidance of stress
	Annual physical examinations and diagnostic tests
Habits	Hand washing
	Use of jargon (e.g., "take your vitals")
	Use of problem-solving methods
	Documentation
Likes	Punctuality
	Neatness and organization
	Compliance (e.g., with medical "orders")
Dislikes	Tardiness
	Disorganization
	Messiness, lack of cleanliness
Customs	Use of procedures (e.g., circumcision, last rites) surrounding birth and death
	Professional respect and observance of hierarchy found in autocratic and bureaucratic systems
	Adherence to a set of ethical standards and codes of conduct
Rituals	Annual physical examination
	The surgical procedure

Sources: Adapted from Giger, J. (2016). *Transcultural nursing: Assessment and intervention* (7th ed.). Elsevier; Leppa, C. (2005). Transcultural communication within the health care subculture. In C. Munoz & J. Luckmann (Eds.), *Transcultural communication in health care* (2nd ed., pp. 74–83). Thomson Delmar Learning; Ladha, T., Zubairi, M., Hunter, A., Audcent, T., & Johnstone, J. (2018). Cross-cultural communication: Tools for working with families and children. *Paediatrics & Child Health, 23*(1), 66–69. https://doi.org/10.1093/pch/pxx126; Spector, R. (2017). *Cultural diversity in health and illness* (9th ed.). Pearson Education.

over-the-counter (OTC) and self-treatment remedies. Different groups have different folk practices, but all cultural groups probably use the conventional healthcare system to at least some degree.

Conflicts may occur when the conventional provider does not understand the beliefs and practices of the indigenous healthcare systems and its traditional healers. The view that a practice is not important because it is not grounded in scientific biomedical knowledge creates distrust between the client and provider and benefits no one.

Evidence shows that indigenous-led health partnerships that integrate traditional indigenous knowledge with some biomedical practices provide an inclusive approach that incorporates physical, emotional, spiritual, and psychosocial aspects of healthcare (Allen et al., 2020). This holistic approach to care improves health outcomes.

Key Point: *As a nurse, you should become aware of and understand a variety of health beliefs and practices so that you can better meet the needs of your clients.*

What Are Health and Illness Beliefs?

Generally speaking, people follow one of the following health belief systems (Andrews et al., 2020).

- The **scientific/biomedical health system** is one with which you are already familiar.
- In the **magico-religious system,** belief in supernatural (mystical) forces dominates. One example is Voodoo, which is practiced by people of various cultures.
- The **holistic belief system** focuses more on the need for harmony and balance of the body with nature. The concept of **holism** emphasizes the relationships among all living things. It considers the body working together with an individual's spirituality, emotions, culture, relationships, environments, and other aspects of life.

 ThinkLike a Nurse 12-6: Clinical Judgment in Action

- What do you do to keep yourself healthy?
- What do you do to treat minor illnesses when you do not want to see a healthcare provider?

What Are Health and Illness Practices?

In addition to knowing their values and beliefs, you need to know health practices of people in various cultural groups to maintain wellness. Think about the patients in the Meet Your Patients scenarios. As you consider the following questions, keep in mind that cultural health practices can be efficacious (helpful), neutral (neither helpful nor harmful), or dysfunctional (harmful) (Giger, 2016):

- Would you support or discourage Mr. Chan's daughter's request for a Chinese spiritual leader to come to

Mr. Chan's room and perform a ceremony to restore his harmony?
- Would you support Rosanna's dressing her child in a heavy coat and knit hat although it is quite warm outside?
- Do you think the ceremony or dress is harmful or helpful in each case?

You should encourage practices that could be helpful and discourage those that are harmful.

KnowledgeCheck 12-4

- What are magico-religious belief systems?
- As a nurse, in which of the following cultural health practices would you support your client: efficacious, neutral, dysfunctional, uncertain? Why?
- Refer to the Meet Your Patients feature. Identify an efficacious practice.

 ThinkLike a Nurse 12-7: Clinical Judgment in Action

- What aspects of the indigenous and conventional systems have you used for yourself or your family? Give examples.

Nursing and Other Professional Subcultures

The biomedical healthcare system in the United States is a culture with its own set of norms. That culture can be further divided into subcultures, such as those of providers, nurses, or therapists. Nursing is the largest subculture within the overall healthcare culture. Leininger (1978) defines the **culture of nursing** as the learned and transmitted lifeways, values, symbols, patterns, and normative practices of members of the nursing profession that are not the same as those of the mainstream culture. The beliefs and values of the nursing subculture have been formed in part by the U.S. society at large, which historically has been dominated by White, Anglo-Saxon, Protestant beliefs.

Nursing Values In addition to beliefs and values of the broader healthcare system (see Table 12-1), nurses tend to value:

- Nursing autonomy
- Caring
- Use of the systematic critical thinking processes
- Objective reporting and description of pain; an unemotional response

Key Point: *In this book, we add "using knowledge and experiences to develop the competencies of critical thinking and clinical judgment" to the list of nursing values.* Although these values may not be consistently rewarded in practice, we believe the nurse's knowledge, thinking, and decision making are essential to the safety and well-being of patients.

The Need to Examine Your Values As you become more socialized into the nursing culture, you should continue to examine professional values to see how strongly you identify with them and how they affect your work with patients. For example, suppose you value silent suffering in response to pain. If your client in the very early stages of labor is screaming and crying, even though the contractions are very mild on palpation, you might be tempted to view them as a whiner. Be careful not to lose your ability to understand health and illness from the patient's point of view.

Example Scenario Review the case of Rosanna and José (Meet Your Patients). After a positive strep test, the primary care provider prescribes an antibiotic for José's fever and sore throat. You observe that Rosanna does not seem to be happy with the medicine, so you stress to her that it is important for her to give the medication immediately to make José better. On her way out of the clinic, Rosanna throws the prescription in the trash. Why do you think she threw away the prescription? Some people believe that illness is caused by the body's imbalance of "hot" and "cold" (not related to temperature). The scenario doesn't tell you for sure, but it could be that Rosanna did not believe the medication would help her son, so she decided not to spend money on it. This problem could have been prevented if you or the primary care provider had assessed Rosanna's health beliefs and practices and discussed with her the treatment options for José. For example, if she considered his ear infection to be "hot," then the provider might have been able to explain that the prescribed medication would get rid of the heat and pain that José is experiencing from the infection.

Key Point: *This is an example of what can happen when healthcare providers are so rigidly grounded in the beliefs of the professional healthcare culture that they fail to recognize and understand the health beliefs and practices of their clients. Such rigidity is a barrier to culturally competent care.*

KnowledgeCheck 12-5

What are the norms of the healthcare system in the United States?

Alternative Healing Systems

You need to know how healers from various cultures cure and care for members of their group. All cultures think of their healthcare system and beliefs as "traditional." We use *alternative* in this chapter to refer to beliefs and practices that are not of the Western, North American, biomedical, or conventional healthcare system (previously discussed). You have already learned about different *healthcare beliefs and practices* that clients may have (e.g., biomedical or scientific, holistic, magico-religious). The following section focuses on the types of *healing systems* that you may find in all cultures throughout the world.

Folk Medicine

Defined as the beliefs and practices that the members of a cultural group follow when they are ill, folk medicine includes both self-treatment and the use of folk healers (Andrews et al., 2020). When you feel as if you're getting a cold or the flu, what do you do? If you said that you take vitamin C or eat chicken soup, then you are practicing folk medicine. You most likely do what your mother or some other relative did for you in similar situations. Knowledge of these treatments is passed down from generation to generation through oral, and sometimes written, tradition.

- *Folk medicine* often involves natural medicines (e.g., herbs, plants, minerals, animal substances).
- *Magico-religious folk medicine* involves the use of charms, holy words, rituals, and holy actions to prevent and treat illnesses (Spector, 2017).

Why People See Folk Healers Why would someone want to see a folk healer rather than a professional healthcare provider? People may seek out folk healers because the healers speak their native language, share their values and beliefs, charge less money, are readily available, and visit the sick at home—or simply because people perceive that the professional healing system cannot meet their needs.

Many folk healing traditions are guided not only by cultural practices but also by religious beliefs and rituals. Religious rituals are often associated with births (e.g., circumcision) and deaths (e.g., who is allowed to wash the body and prepare it for burial). **Key Point:** *Although there is a strong association between culture and religious beliefs, you should never assume that because your patient is a member of a certain culture, they will also be of a certain religion. You should always ask as a part of your cultural assessment.*

Holistic Healthcare

Holistic and biomedical approaches consider health and disease from different perspectives. Consider the case of a person with bacterial pneumonia. **Western** or **conventional biomedical treatment** would use antibiotics to kill the bacteria, an antipyretic to suppress fever and discomfort, an expectorant to liquefy secretions, increased fluids, and rest. Treatment is successful when the pathology (i.e., infection) and symptoms (e.g., fever) are gone. Western medicine is often referred to as **allopathy,** a term used to indicate medical practice that treats disease with remedies that counteract the effects of the disease. In contrast, holistic approaches would include other treatments, such as herbal teas, warm-air inhalants, a focus on diet and rest, and other simple things.

Holistic healthcare is often used interchangeably with *complementary healthcare* and *alternative healthcare,* but the terms do not have the same meaning. Refer to the Holistic Healing box, Complementary and Alternative Medicine.

Complementary and Alternative Medicine

Complementary and Alternative Medicine (CAM)

➤ **Complementary medicine** is the use of rigorously tested therapies to complement those of conventional (i.e., biomedical) medicine.

Examples include chiropractic care, biofeedback, and the use of certain supplements.

➤ **Alternative medicine,** in contrast, is used instead of conventional medical care. CAM encompasses a range of philosophies, approaches, and therapies that the conventional healthcare system does not commonly use, accept, understand, study, or make available.

Examples include iridology, aromatherapy, and magnet therapy.

Some CAMs are derived from the ancient and indigenous healthcare systems of people of other countries.

➤ **Ayurveda** is a system that covers all aspects of health and wellness. Ayurveda's core belief is that a sense of harmony with nature and our inner being produces health. Ayurveda attributes health to balance between three forces, or energies, called **dosha:** (1) creation *(kapha)*, (2) preservation *(pitta)*, and (3) destruction *(vata)*. Humans have a physical and psychological constitution made up of those three forces. Imbalance between these forces leads to illness and disease.

The ideal *dosha* is *vata–kapha–pitta* in equal proportions. Imbalances may be caused by age; lifestyle; diet; too much

or too little physical exertion; the seasons; or inadequate protection from weather, chemicals, or germs. Ayurveda interventions include exercise, breathing, meditation, visualization, aromatherapy, therapeutic massage, and herbs to treat illness and maintain health.

➤ **Traditional Chinese medicine (TCM)** practitioners consider that each person has their own energies and elements. Energies focus on the balance of *yin* and *yang* energies (complementary but opposing life forces). The five elements are earth, water, wood, fire, and air/metal. Each element is associated with specific characteristics, such as color, smell, flavor, sound, and so on.

If these balances are disturbed, ill health will result. Interventions include lifestyle modifications, herbal remedies, massage, and/or acupuncture.

Integrative healthcare refers to coordinated care that encompasses all treatments and health practices a patient uses. To provide integrative care, a practitioner must know about the interactive effects of conventional and CAM treatments and be able to coordinate all the care modalities. The practitioner must establish trust so that the patient will disclose CAM use and must communicate with other health providers for referral and coordination of care. Integrative healthcare is holistic because it considers all aspects of the patient's care.

KnowledgeCheck 12-6

- What are some common folk medicine practices?
- What is integrative healthcare?
- Why might members of some cultural groups seek out the local folk healer rather than the conventional healthcare provider?

WHAT IS CULTURALLY COMPETENT CARE?

The terms *cultural awareness, cultural sensitivity,* and *cultural competence* are often used interchangeably; however, they are not the same.

- **Cultural awareness** refers to an appreciation of the external signs of diversity.
- **Cultural sensitivity** is an awareness or knowledge of the uniqueness of other cultures. It is a set of competencies that help one recognize and understand similarities and differences among people of other cultures.
- **Cultural competence** is the ability to effectively incorporate culture into the provision of care, to show respect, accept differences, and empower decision making. You cannot achieve cultural competence overnight because it is a developmental process.

As you gain more knowledge and awareness of the needs of individuals from various ethnocultural groups,

you will move forward on the journey toward cultural competence. The following are descriptions of culturally competent nursing practice.

American Nurses Association

The American Nurses Association (ANA) publication *Nursing: Scope and Standards of Practice* (2015) devotes an entire standard to promoting cultural competency. Standard 8 highlights that RNs should practice in a manner that is congruent with cultural diversity and inclusion to ensure culturally congruent practice. Among other competencies, the nurse should:

- Demonstrate respect, equity, and empathy when dealing with a culturally diverse and vulnerable population.
- Understand one's own beliefs, values, and heritage while undertaking activities to understand other individuals' cultural preferences, along with application of that understanding.
- Identify acculturation and the effects of discrimination and oppression.

Safe, Effective Nursing Care

Several of the safe effective nursing care (SENC) competencies ensure culturally competent care. For example, the client-centered care competency recognizes that nurses provide care that shows respect for client values, religious beliefs, needs, and preferences. Understanding cultural needs and preferences ensures the implementation of interventions to promote client comfort and safety. To review SENC competencies, see the SENC box, What Is Safe, Effective Nursing Care? in Chapter 1.

Leininger

Although Madeline Leininger does not use the term *cultural competence,* her theory fits with that concept. The goal of her theory is to guide research that will assist nurses in providing *culturally congruent care* using her three modes of nursing care actions and decisions (to be explained later in the chapter).

♥ **iCare** Nurses can achieve this goal by:
- Discovering cultural care and caring beliefs, values, and practices
- Analyzing the similarities and differences of these beliefs among the different cultures

WHAT ARE SOME BARRIERS TO CULTURALLY COMPETENT CARE?

Your ability to provide culturally competent care may be hampered by various prejudices, biases, and language barriers. Self-knowledge and critical thinking are essential in helping you identify and manage them. You should avoid the following barriers in your practice:

- **Bias.** A lack of impartiality, one-sidedness; can be positive or negative.
- **Ethnocentrism.** The tendency of people to believe their own beliefs and values are right and that those of other cultures are wrong (or unusual). This can cause your patient to feel that you disapprove of or don't understand or respect their culture.
- **Cultural stereotype.** The unsubstantiated belief that all people of a certain racial or ethnic group are alike in certain respects. A stereotype may be positive or negative.
  - **Prejudice.** Negative attitudes toward other people based on faulty and rigid stereotypes about race, gender, sexual orientation, status, and so on.
  - **Discrimination.** The behavioral manifestations of a prejudice (e.g., refusing to provide services or opportunities to certain racial or ethnic groups). Members of underrepresented groups still experience discrimination in education housing, banking, and the job market.

Racism

Racism results in racial inequity. Kendi (2019) defines racism as "a marriage of racist policies and racist ideas that produces and normalizes racial inequities" (pp. 17–18). Similarly, institutional racism is described as "the existence of systematic policies or laws and practices that provide differential access to goods, services and opportunities of society by race" (Morgan et al., 2020).

The overall impact of racism, at any level, is inequalities in healthcare that result in negative health outcomes and conditions for people of color. The COVID-19 pandemic has shown how racism and institutional racism can have significant negative health consequences for people of color (e.g., the Latinx and Black American populations) (Gross et al., 2020). Due to systemic social

---

Safe, Effective Nursing Care

How Cultural Competency Improves Patient Outcomes

Chapter Key Concepts: Cultural Competency

SENC Competency: Goal-Directed Client-Centered Care

Full-Spectrum Model: The full-spectrum nursing model concept that is most pertinent is "doing": *Show respect for client values, religious beliefs, needs, and preferences.*

Background. Every client is entitled to healthcare that is respectful of their cultural beliefs and practices. The SENC competency of providing goal-directed, client-centered care protects and promotes the dignity of the client. Culturally competent healthcare empowers the client and facilitates participation in healthcare decisions. Culturally skilled providers incorporate trust, respect, and therapeutic communication in their relationships with patients (Robinson, 2019). The provider was able to establish a good interpersonal relationship with the patient, which is the foundation for mutual goal setting. Cultural competency promotes better nurse–patient and patient–provider communications and relationships (Brown et al., 2016; Robinson, 2019). This contributes to a cultural partnership and sensitivity, which results in the following:

➤ Both nurse and patient better understand the disease process and treatment management.
➤ The patient is more likely to adhere to the treatment protocols.
➤ Patient outcomes are improved.

Think about it:

What is the relationship between cultural competence and healthcare disparities?

How can cultural competence by healthcare providers affect patient outcomes?

Source: Brown, O., Ham-Baloyi, W., Rooyen, D., & Marais, L. C. (2016). Culturally competent patient–provider communication in the management of cancer: An integrative literature review. *Global Health Action, 9*(1), Article 33208. http://doi.org/10.3402/gha.v9.33208; Robinson, J. (2019). *Cultural competency can improve healthcare for all.* https://www.physicianspractice.com/view/cultural-competency-can-improve-healthcare-all

issues, people of color are more likely to have comorbidities, lack health insurance, and lack access to healthcare. Thus, people of Hispanic or Latin origin and non-Hispanic African Americans were 2.8 times more likely to die of COVID-19 than their non-Hispanic, White counterparts (CDC, 2020).

Nurses have an essential role in recognizing and addressing the adverse impacts of racism. You can ensure all patients are treated fairly and with respect and dignity. In addition, you can use strong advocacy skills to facilitate equitable treatment and remove barriers to care or delays in care. Finally, to fulfill your professional obligations, you must confront your internal biases; speak up when you observe racism, discrimination, or injustices against vulnerable patients or your colleagues; and advocate for your patient to reduce health disparities.

Language Barriers

More than 60 million people in the United States speak a language other than English at home (Ziegler & Camarota, 2019). Language barriers, including dialects, regionalisms (words or pronunciations particular to a specific region), street talk, and jargon, will obviously affect your ability to communicate with clients. Recall Mr. Salvatore in the Meet Your Patients scenario. Suppose he has a condition requiring immediate surgery, and you need his consent even though he and his family do not speak English. You will need a certified interpreter. If Mr. Salvatore uses a different dialect or slang, the interpreter may have difficulty understanding him. In that case, you should review the policies of your healthcare facility to obtain additional resources. If there were no other immediate options for translation help, you would have to temporarily resort to nonverbal language and pictures to communicate.

Key Point: *If a consent issue is involved, the hospital must ensure adequate resources to comply with informed consent requirements.*

Street Talk, Slang, and Jargon Words or expressions used by a subculture are called *jargon*. Street talk, slang, and jargon can be as challenging as another language. Their meanings change, and not everyone has the same interpretation of a word or a phrase. For example:

- The word *bad* can mean "bad" or "good" depending on the context.
- Texting can be another form of jargon—not everyone understands the abbreviations used in texting.

Healthcare Jargon In healthcare, we often use jargon: peculiar terminology and abbreviations that our clients do not understand. For example, many patients may not understand the question, "Have you voided today?" Even worse, patients may hesitate to ask for clarification because they do not want to admit their lack of understanding of your words.

Other Barriers

- *Lack of knowledge* about the cultural and ethnic values, beliefs, and behaviors of people within their community is not unusual among healthcare providers. It can cause them to misinterpret a client's behaviors.
- *Emotional responses,* such as fear and distrust (both yours and the client's), can arise when members of different cultural groups meet.
- *Self-knowledge* is essential in removing barriers and helps you to communicate effectively with your clients.

WHAT IS CULTURAL HUMILITY?

As an emerging trend, some professionals advocate the concept of *cultural humility* to overcome some of the limitations of cultural competence as an endpoint. The focus of cultural humility is the following:

- Self-reflection to examine one's biases, assumptions, and beliefs
- Lifelong learning to hear and comprehend what each client is saying and to learn from them
- Incorporating patient beliefs and practices into the plan of care, when appropriate
- Ensuring sufficient resources that align with services needed

In essence, cultural humility is an orientation to care that is patient centered and continuously evolving (Lekas et al., 2020).

KnowledgeCheck 12-7
- Define *cultural competence.*
- How do the barriers of ethnocentrism and language impede nursing care of multicultural populations?

PracticalKnowledge
knowing **how**

Each phase of the nursing process presents an opportunity to provide culturally sensitive, congruent, and competent care. You must establish rapport before beginning data collection.

ASSESSMENT/RECOGNIZING CUES

Various regulating bodies (e.g., The Joint Commission and the Office of Minority Health) require healthcare organizations to integrate cultural data into a patient's health records. Cultural assessment consists of an interview and a physical assessment. When you perform a cultural assessment, you should gather data directly from your client, but if this is not possible, you may ask for help from a friend or family member of the client. **Key Point:** *Because of privacy concerns and legal guidelines, you should not rely on a family member to serve as an interpreter.*

Toward Evidence-Based Practice

Byrne, D. (2020). Evaluating cultural competence in undergraduate nursing students using standardized patients. *Teaching and Learning in Nursing, 15*(1), 57–60. https://doi.org/10.1016/j.teln.2019.08.010

The researcher examined the differences in cultural competence between students who received lecture plus simulation using standardized patients and those who received only the lecture. Posttest results revealed no significant differences between the two groups and that both groups improved from cultural awareness to the cultural competence range. However, the lecture-plus-simulation group experienced less anxiety in interacting with culturally diverse patients as the simulation progressed.

Knecht, J., Fontana, J., Fischer, B., Tetrault, J., & Spitz, K. (2019). An investigation of the development of cultural competence in baccalaureate nursing students: A mixed-methods study. *Journal of Cultural Diversity, 26*(3), 89–95.

Researchers compared the impact on cultural competence of students who had traditional clinical placements with those who provided care to the underserved population in ethnically diverse environments, followed by guided reflection. The results revealed that students who participated in the diverse-setting group had higher cultural competence scores than those in the traditional group. Other essential qualitative themes in the diverse groups were enlightenment (eye-opening), nursing role competence, and connections. Students indicated that a book could not capture their experiences. The immersion experience in the community enhanced the students' connection with people in various neighborhoods.

Kaihlanen, A., Hetapakka, L., & Heponiemi, R. (2019). Increasing cultural awareness: Qualitative study of nurses' perceptions about cultural competence training. *Biomedical Central Nursing, 18*(38), Article 38. https://doi.org/10.1186/s12912-019-0363-x

Researchers examined the perceptions of nurses after a 4-week cultural competence course designed to focus awareness of cultural features using a variety of learning activities (e.g., lectures, discussions, Web-based learning tasks). The participants explored the basis for and pitfalls of cross-cultural communications and used the information presented to develop new perspectives on their own communication patterns and to explore the justifications for certain workplace practices. Participants indicated the training was valuable and provided them with needed insights, and they appreciated that the educator was a nonhealthcare provider. For example, they expressed an awareness of how their own "cultural cage" guided their behavior and the interpretation of the behavior of others. With this awareness, participants felt more encouraged to encounter culturally diverse patients. In addition, participants developed increased respect for equality in care and the need to remain respectful and nonjudgmental. Self-awareness of cultural features provided a foundation for culturally appropriate communications and care.

Instructions: Some nurses have expressed concerns that their nursing curricula did not prepare them to address the cultural needs of diverse patients. They requested for themselves and asked that nursing students receive more education on cultural care. Answer the following questions:

1. Which studies or results support the belief that education and learning activities on culture will improve cultural competence?

2. What is the importance of encounters with clients from various cultures in acquiring cultural competency?

3. Which study provides the best evidence for ensuring that nurses receive training on cultural competence?

The Health History

Some information you obtain from a patient's health history may be sensitive or personal. Ask open-ended questions when beginning a cultural assessment to encourage patients to talk about themselves. In addition, you must convey empathy, show respect, establish trust, listen actively, and provide appropriate feedback.

■ Always ask clients about their use of alternative medicine and folk remedies so that any effects on traditional biomedical medications and treatments can be evaluated. Some remedies may interfere with traditional treatments; others can be dangerous. Many people use folk remedies, but they may be reluctant to tell you because they fear ridicule or disapproval.

You will not need to perform an in-depth cultural assessment on every client, but you will need to recognize situations in which this is needed. For a list of questions to help you gather essential information for a cultural assessment,

 Go to **Chapter 12, Assessment Guidelines and Tools, Focused Assessment: Obtaining Minimal Cultural Information**, in Volume 2.

Physical Assessment

Physical assessment may reveal biocultural variations. To assess and evaluate clients accurately, you need to know the normal physiological variations among healthy members of selected populations (e.g., body proportions, vital signs, general appearance, skin, musculoskeletal system, and illness).

■ **Assessing the Skin.** Knowledge of biocultural variations is essential in assessing for pallor, cyanosis, jaundice, erythema, rashes, and petechiae in clients with dark skin. You must be observant and detailed in your assessment. For helpful suggestions and for more information about assessing the skin, see Chapter 32, and

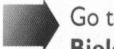 Go to **Chapter 12, Clinical Insight 12-1:Understanding Biological Variations,** in Volume 2.

- **Assessing for Pain Key Point:** *Culture influences the patient's responses to pain. Because pain and comfort are subjective, you need to quantify them as objectively as possible by using a pain measurement scale. It is essential to investigate the meaning of pain to each patient and their view of acceptable ways to express or cope with pain.*

Cultural Assessment Models and Tools

Some agencies have special tools for in-depth cultural assessments. If yours does not, you can structure your assessments using any culture model. For example, you may want to search the Internet for the following models:

- Transcultural Nursing Assessment Guide (Andrews et al., 2020)
- Leininger's Sunrise Model Depicting the Theory of Cultural Care, Diversity, and Universality
- Transcultural Assessment Model (Giger & Davidhizar, 2008)
- Spector's Heritage Assessment Tool. Unlike the preceding tools, which assess culture specifics, Spector's tool assesses heritage *consistency:* the degree to which a person's lifestyle reflects their traditional culture (country of origin, race, or ethnic group). This assessment tool also reveals the degree to which the client still identifies with their cultural origins.

For another example of a focused cultural assessment,

 Go to **Chapter 12, Assessment Guidelines and Tools, Focused Assessment Cultural Assessment Using the Transcultural Model,** in Volume 2.

NURSING DIAGNOSIS/ANALYZING CUES

There are Clinical Care Classification (CCC) diagnoses that specifically address culture. However, cultural factors can be the etiology of various problems. Any of the diagnostic labels can be used for patients of any culture, provided that the defining characteristics are present. Some possible examples include the following (CCC, n.d.):

- **Nutrition Alteration: Body Nutrition Deficit** might apply to a patient who is hospitalized and cannot obtain foods prepared in the traditional way of their ethnic group.
- **Parenting Alteration** could occur if the patient's traditional methods of discipline are not acceptable or appropriate in the dominant culture.

- **Powerlessness** might occur when the patient is unable to make healthcare personnel understand the importance of their cultural rituals or healthcare practices.
- **Verbal Impairment** is sometimes used for patients who do not speak or understand the nurse's language.
- **Health Maintenance Alteration** might be used for clients and/or caregivers who do not follow a health-promoting or therapeutic plan. For example, the plan may be inconsistent with the patient's beliefs.
  - Example: Suppose that a 60-year-old woman who works as a hotel housekeeper is repeatedly admitted to your hospital for uncontrolled hypertension. You diagnose Health Maintenance Alteration because she does not take her prescribed medication. But do you know that the cost of the antihypertensive medication does not fit into her budget? Or perhaps she believes that herbs, diet, and other practices will decrease her blood pressure.

Using your understanding of cultural norms or differences, you should know that nonadherence or problems managing health needs are defining characteristics of *Health Maintenance Alteration.* This requires you to examine the cultural impact of care.

Key Point: *The preceding example illustrates the concern that standardized nursing diagnoses are not always culturally sensitive and therefore may not apply accurately to patients who are not from the dominant culture. Nursing diagnoses should describe responses that patients see as problematic.* A nurse and patient who are from different cultures may not have the same perceptions of health and illness, which can lead to misdiagnosis. The nurse may either diagnose a problem that doesn't exist for the patient or diagnose a real problem but fail to describe it accurately (Wilkinson, 2012).

The following are a few examples of standardized nursing diagnoses that could be interpreted differently by people from different cultures. Undoubtedly there are others.

Acute Pain	Anxiety
Decisional Conflict	Coping Impairment
Health Maintenance	Role Performance
Alteration	Alteration
Socialization Alteration	Noncompliance
Powerlessness	

You should use all labels carefully and validate nursing diagnoses with the patient to be sure that the statement describes their health status as they see it.

PLANNING/PRIORITIZING HYPOTHESES AND GENERATING SOLUTIONS

The outcomes you choose, whether standardized or individualized, depend on the nursing diagnoses you have identified. If the diagnoses are culturally sensitive, the outcomes should be as well. However, you must involve the patient to be certain. For example, suppose you and a dying patient agree that their diagnosis is Acute Pain.

Nevertheless, your goals will be different if you want the patient to be free from pain, whereas they want to stay alert enough to interact with their family, even if it means enduring some pain. When your cultures differ, it is even more important to validate the goals with the patient. Some individualized goal/outcome statements associated with cultural differences might include the following:

- Agrees to take prescribed analgesic (pain medication) before bedtime and after family leaves for the evening.
- Talks to their spiritual adviser about conflicts between the treatment plan and their religious beliefs.
- Freely shares information about folk practices and OTC medications with the provider.

IMPLEMENTATION/TAKING ACTION

To plan culturally appropriate care, you should become familiar with the cultural groups that are dominant in your area and that you will encounter in your nursing practice.

Nursing Interventions Classification (NIC) standardized interventions related to culture and the provision of culturally competent care include the following examples:

Mutual Goal Setting (for Ineffective Health Management)
Self-Responsibility Facilitation (for Decision-making, Readiness for Enhanced)
Culture Brokerage (for Comfort, Impaired)

Culture Brokerage is defined as "the deliberate use of culturally competent strategies to bridge or mediate between the patient's culture and the biomedical health-care system" (Butcher et al., 2018, p. 126).

Individualized nursing activities and focused assessments are important for all patients. However, patients from different cultural and ethnic groups may have unique needs that require culturally competent care.

Nursing Strategies for Providing Culturally Competent Care

You will need information about clients' cultural values, beliefs, and practices to identify and implement the interventions that will support these practices (Wilkinson, 2012). For example:

- When you are teaching about a specific treatment regimen prescribed by the provider, you should find out whether it conflicts with the patient's folk beliefs or alternative treatments. If so, suggest modifications.
- Remember to identify educational methods that are most appropriate for your client's needs (e.g., translated materials and/or diagrams) and to make community referrals as necessary.
- When caring for patients from vulnerable populations, it is important that you focus on their strengths and resources, not exclusively on their difficulties and risks.

How Should I Respond to a Client's Cultural Health Practices?

Theorists describe different situations in which nursing decisions and actions are needed regarding a client's cultural health practices. A practice may be helpful, harmful, or neutral, or the effects may be unknown (Giger, 2016; Leininger, 1991; McFarland & Wehbe-Alamah, 2018). See Table 12-2.

Negotiation The client's perspective may differ from yours about the effects of a particular practice. Negotiation acknowledges that gap. **Key Point:** *You must negotiate when folk or traditional practices might be harmful to the client.*

Example: The nurse negotiates with the client to continue seeing the *curandero* but also to come to the clinic every 6 weeks to have their blood pressure checked. If the client refuses all nursing or biomedical interventions, the avenue is still open to continue monitoring the client to identify changes in their health status. If a health crisis occurs, it may be possible to renegotiate the care.

Repatterning/Restructuring Repatterning or restructuring occurs when you attempt to change your actions or the client's lifestyle (Leininger, 1991; McFarland & Wehbe-Alamah, 2018). While still respecting their cultural values and beliefs, you would support and encourage the client to significantly modify their behaviors and to adopt new, different, and beneficial health behaviors.

Example 1: Change in nurse's actions. When the client refuses to take the prescribed pain medication, the nurse uses massage, distraction, and other nonpharmacological techniques to help relieve their pain.
Example 2: Modification of the client's behaviors. A client refuses to see a biomedical provider for their family's needs. However, when the folk healer is unsuccessful in treating their child's illness and the child becomes critically ill, the nurse convinces the client to bring the child to the emergency department.

How Do I Communicate With Clients Who Speak a Different Language?

Communicating with clients who do not speak your language can be especially challenging. The Internet and computer software allow patients to type information in their native language and translate it into English as a way to communicate with providers. However, the best way to provide culturally competent care to such clients

Table 12-2 ➤ Possible Effects of a Patient's Cultural Health Practices

THE EFFECTS ARE:	EXAMPLE	NURSING APPROACH
Efficacious (Helpful)	Family or friends bring ethnic foods that are appropriate for the client's prescribed diet.	Encourage practices that will likely improve client health and help preserve cultural values related to health.
Neutral (Neither Helpful Nor Harmful)	Some people associate good health with eating properly and fasting to cure disease. Some may treat illness with prayers or simple foods.	There should be no harm in allowing a patient to continue a neutral health practice. You would not want to interfere with these neutral practices.
Uncertain (Unknown by You)	A client drinks a daily smoothie that consists of certain herbs and spices, such as ginger, cinnamon, and basil, for "good health."	You can neither encourage nor discourage these practices until you obtain more information about them. Do this as soon as possible.
Dysfunctional (Harmful)	A client may refuse to give prescribed medication to their child.	Discourage folk practices that may cause harm. In such instances, you should support and enable the client to adapt to biomedical therapies (repatterning/restructuring) or negotiate with the client to achieve satisfying outcomes.

is to use a professional medical interpreter or translator. Each must meet predetermined standards to participate in translation services.

- **Interpreters** are specially trained to provide the meaning behind the words. They serve as a cultural brokers by conveying the client's responses to questions and by providing general information about the client's culture.
- **Translators** just restate the words from one language to another. You should review your facility's policies and procedures for translation resources. The Joint Commission views communication as an essential aspect of patient care (The Joint Commission, 2014). For guidelines when using an interpreter and for when an interpreter is not available,

 Go to **Chapter 12, Clinical Insights 12-2: Communicating with Clients Who Speak a Different Language,** in Volume 2.

Culturally and Linguistically Appropriate Services (Clas) Standards

CLAS standards promote culturally and linguistically appropriate services to ensure that care is respectful of and responsive to the person's cultural and linguistic needs. **Key Point: *Healthcare facilities must provide language assistance services by, in order of preference, bilingual staff, face-to-face interpretation by trained persons, or telephone interpreters. Healthcare interpreters should be used to obtain informed consent and to assist the patient to understand the treatment plan***

(Office of Minority Health, 2021). For a complete listing of the National CLAS standards,

 Go to the Office of Minority Health website at https://thinkculturalhealth.hhs.gov/clas/standards

Developing Strategies

There are several strategies for you to consider and many resources to help you develop strategies specific to various cultural groups (Box 12-2). Consider the following as you move forward on your journey toward cultural competence:

Reflect and Know Yourself

- Understand your own cultural values and practices and appreciate how they may differ from those held by people of other cultures.
- Recognize your own biases about people and groups and consider how they may affect the care you provide.
- Learn from your mistakes and don't make them again.

Keep Learning

- Learn as much as you can about the cultural groups in your community and work area.
- Study nursing theories and principles pertaining to culture.
- Take advantage of every opportunity to interact with persons from different cultural groups.

BOX 12-2 ■ Being Considerate of Cultural Specifics

Consider Verbal and Nonverbal Communication.

- Know, or find out, whether touch (e.g., a handshake) is expected or prohibited.
- Know, or find out, whether eye contact is expected or avoided. Avoiding eye contact, for some, is a sign of respect.
- Ask the client how they wish to be addressed.
- Know, or find out, the ways people welcome each other.

Consider the Person's Need for Personal Space.

- Know the person's cultural and religious customs regarding touching and contact.
- Know the usual comfortable distance for conversing in the client's culture.

Consider Body Language.

- Gestures that are acceptable in one culture may be taboo in another. Know what is acceptable to the client.
- Be aware that smiling does not universally indicate friendliness.

Consider Time Orientation.

- Tell clients when you are coming and be on time.
- Avoid surprise visits.
- Share your own expectations about time.

- Ask clients what they expect regarding time, appointments, and so on.
- Be sure you know the times for and meanings of the client's religious and ethnic holidays.

Consider Social Organization.

- Know which person in the family is the leader or decision maker.
- Know what dates are important and whether gifts are expected or not.
- Know how special events, such as births and funerals, are celebrated; whether certain colors have meaning; and what the expected rituals are.

Consider the Person's Perspective on Environmental Control.

- Find out what the client's health traditions and practices are.
- Know whether the person believes they have any ability to "change things."
- Know the general influence of the culture on perception and tolerance of pain.
- Know what foods are forbidden, what foods may or may not be eaten together, and which utensils are used and in what manner.

Accommodate and Negotiate

- Make an effort to incorporate beliefs and practices from various cultures into your nursing care and teaching materials.
- Encourage helpful or neutral cultural practices and discourage those that are dysfunctional (harmful).
- Suggest alternatives to harmful practices.
- Accommodate cultural dietary practices when possible. For inpatients, some dietary departments can make special foods, and you can encourage families to bring food from home. In all situations, help patients and families adapt cultural foods to therapeutic diets.

Collaborate

- Work with the folk medicine practitioner in the interest of the client.
- Advocate for all of your clients, but especially for those not from the dominant culture.
- Consider the cultural role of the family member who makes the primary decisions. To ignore this person is to doom your interventions to failure.

Respect

- Consider each client as a unique individual, influenced but not defined by their culture.
- Respect your clients regardless of cultural background, and never force, pressure, manipulate, or

coerce them to participate in care that conflicts with their values and beliefs.

This is by no means an exhaustive list. Most likely, you can think of other strategies. It may help you to "take a trip to BALI":

Be aware of your own cultural heritage.
Appreciate that the client is unique: influenced but not defined by her culture.
Learn about the client's cultural group.
Incorporate the client's cultural values/behaviors into the care plan.

KnowledgeCheck 12-9

- List five factors to consider to help you develop strategies to become more culturally competent.
- What does the acronym "BALI" stand for?

How Can I Become Culturally Competent?

Of course, you can't become culturally competent just by reading. Recall that people acquire cultural competence gradually, progressing through stages.

Theoretical knowledge can increase your awareness and appreciation of cultural differences, but you can achieve cultural competence only if you are motivated and, even then, only by interacting with people from different cultures (Galanti, 2018). Carballeira (1997) sums up this process with the LIVE and LEARN model for culturally competent family services:

Like		Listen
Inquire		Evaluate
Visit	and	Acknowledge
Experience		Recommend
		Negotiate

Key Point: *If there were only one intervention you could use to improve your cultural competence, it should be to routinely ask patients what matters most to them in their illness and treatment.* No matter how busy you are, you can find time to do that. You can then use that information to incorporate cultural needs into the client plan of care.

Think**Like a Nurse** 12-8:
Clinical Judgment **in Action**

What kind of knowledge do you need to become culturally competent (theoretical, practical, self, ethical)? Explain your answer. (Refer to Chapter 2 to review types of knowledge, if necessary.)

To explore learning resources for this chapter,

Go to Davis Advantage and find:

Answers and Suggested Responses for all questions in this chapter
Concept Map
Knowledge Map
References and Bibliography

CHAPTER 13

Spirituality

Learning Outcomes

After completing this chapter, you should be able to:

➤ Describe the differences and similarities between religion and spirituality.

➤ Discuss what is meant by *spirituality*.

➤ Understand the implications for nursing care based on the religious beliefs or practices of patients.

➤ Identify five barriers to spiritual care.

➤ Perform a spiritual assessment.

➤ Recognize the differences between spiritual care diagnoses and those that

may serve as etiologies of other nursing diagnoses.

➤ Plan nursing interventions based on the data obtained in a spiritual assessment.

➤ Examine your own level of comfort in terms of performing spiritual interventions.

➤ Describe collaborative efforts to ensure the spiritual care of clients.

Key Concepts

Spirituality

Religion

Spiritual care

Related Concepts

See the Concept Map on Davis Advantage

Meet Your Patient

Charles Johnson is a 75-year-old divorced man with newly diagnosed lung cancer. He is unsure whether he wants to have the chemotherapy his provider recommends to try to increase his life span.

Mr. Johnson was brought up in the Christian church, but he has fallen away from practicing his faith over the years. He began smoking at age 15 and has been a heavy drinker all of his adult life. As a young man, he distanced himself from church. He explains: "Church folks are all a bunch of hypocrites, if you ask me. I choose not to be a part of any of that." Nevertheless, he says that he tries to be kind to and tolerant of others. "I've messed up my life, so I figure I don't have any business telling other people how to live. I guess I just figure that how a person lives is between him and God."

Mr. Johnson has one surviving relative, a sister, who is concerned about him. His sister is a devout Jehovah's Witness, and she has tried several times to talk to Mr. Johnson about the importance of Jehovah in her life. She continually leaves religious pamphlets and materials in his mailbox to encourage him to think about religion again.

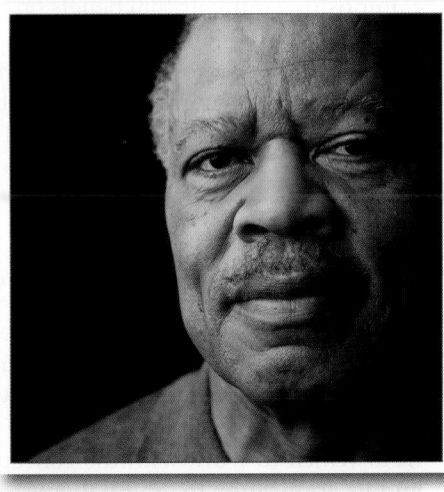

Mr. Johnson's wife divorced him 20 years ago because of his drinking behaviors, and he has alienated his two middle-aged children, so he rarely sees his grandchildren. He lives alone, is retired, and is having financial difficulties. He has one avid hobby: he loves to go out in a boat and fish all day with his buddy, Jim.

■ Mr. Johnson clearly has some physical and psychosocial difficulties. Can you identify them?

■ Assess Mr. Johnson's support system. Whom can he rely on for help?

■ How might you help Mr. Johnson to add some spiritual supports to his available resources?

This chapter presents a holistic interpretation of spirituality—one that views spirituality as a component of every person's life. It also encourages you to consider how spirituality can be incorporated into nursing care to improve your clients' health and wellness. As you read through the content and answer some of the questions posed for Mr. Johnson, consider your own feelings about spirituality.

TheoreticalKnowledge knowing why

Spirituality in nursing has multiple layers. The following layers of competing concerns must be properly balanced to minimize your confusion, frustration, and avoidance of spiritual care:

- **Spirituality of the Nurse.** Each nurse's spirituality (or feelings about spirituality) serves as part of the guiding framework for their practice.
- **Spirituality of the Patient and Family.** Spirituality will be understood in different ways by your patients and their families. Their spirituality may be deeply ingrained or totally separate from formal religion.
- **Effects of Nursing Education.** The emphasis placed on spiritual care differs among the various nursing programs; however, it is important to remember to treat each patient as a unique individual and avoid imposing your spiritual beliefs on the patients.
- **Demands of Nursing Practice.** Time constraints imposed by day-to-day patient care can have a negative impact on your ability to meet patients' spiritual needs. A therapeutic nurse–patient relationship is the foundation for meeting your patients' spiritual needs (Keenan & Kirwan, 2018).

ABOUT THE KEY CONCEPTS

As you study this chapter, try to relate what you are reading to the key concepts of **spirituality** and **religion,** and try to understand how those two concepts relate to each other. This will provide you with a foundation from which to work with the concept of **spiritual care** and its application to your patients.

HISTORY OF SPIRITUALITY IN NURSING

History shows that religiosity and spirituality were important components of medical care. People prayed to the gods or God for healing and as an adjunct for primitive medical procedures. Religious communities throughout the world combined the healing arts with religious care. They viewed caring for the sick as an expression of the values of hospitality, charity, and the vital tenant of loving one's neighbor.

Through the ages, nurses and other caregivers have demonstrated deep concern for the spiritual as well as the physical and psychological needs of those who are sick and infirm. Historical nursing leaders like Florence Nightingale and Rufaidah Al-Asalmiya established the role of spirituality as a key component of nursing care. They viewed spirituality as fundamental to healing and instilled this value in their nurses, nursing students, and professional standards of practice (Lovering, 2012; Yesilcinar et al., 2018).

Modern nursing (and the broader health community) has reclaimed the spiritual dimension as a vital part of its identity and recognized its power to influence health.

Key Point: *Today, spiritual care cannot be the "overlooked" area of nursing practice. It is an essential element in global nursing care. Professional standards of care make clear that meeting patients' spiritual needs is essential to provide holistic nursing care.* The Joint Commission (2018a, 2018b) has established standards for spiritual care. In addition, the American Nurses Association (ANA) *Code of Ethics for Nurses* (2015) instructs that nurses must incorporate factors such as culture and religious and spiritual beliefs into the plan of care for clients.

WHAT ARE RELIGION AND SPIRITUALITY?

Spirituality and religion are related, yet they are two distinct and different concepts (Smith-Trueau, 2019; Paul Victor & Treschuk, 2020). One way to distinguish religion from spirituality is to think of spirituality as a journey and religion as a map or transport vehicle, as shown in Table 13-1. For example, atheists and agnostics have no religious foundation, but they may have spiritual needs (Sinclair & Rosielle, 2020).

What Is Religion?

Religion is a set of beliefs, practices, and codes of conduct associated with a structure (e.g., church, mosque, synagogue) or organized group that integrates beliefs and values into a way of living (Smith-Trudeau, 2019). It is similar to a map to get to a certain location—it tells you what to believe and identifies what values are essential. The map itself may be in the form of a religious tradition (e.g., Christianity) or denomination (e.g., Baptist), which provides an identity and a "lens" for reading the world. The rituals, symbols, sacraments, and holy writings associated with religions serve as bases of authority and provide diverse ways to go beyond the physical and access the divine (e.g., God) (Fig. 13-1). Regardless of their differences, many of the world religions have the following in common:

- **Theology**—that is, discussions and theories related to the divine's relation to the world
- Sacred writings that are regarded as authoritative and/or reveal the nature of the divine
- Notion of created order and purpose
- Definition of *human being* that includes important life events

The Impact of Nurse Self-Awareness on Client Spiritual Care

Chapter Key Concepts: Spirituality; Goal-Directed, Client-Centered Care; Nurse Self-Awareness

Competencies: Provide goal-directed, client-centered care; show respect for client values, religious beliefs, needs, and preferences. (Thinking, Doing, Caring)

Background: Goal-directed, client-centered care includes addressing physical, psychosocial, and spiritual needs. Spirituality is not always linked with religion. Rather, it is what the individual professes it to be (Fowler, 2017a; Ubaidi, 2017). The SENC competency of goal-directed, client-centered care recognizes that the nurse must respect and incorporate the client's values, religious/spiritual beliefs, needs, and preferences into the plan of care. This implies holistic care.

> Establishing mutual goals with the client promotes holistic assessment and ensures the inclusion of this vital aspect of client care.

> To provide holistic care, the nurse must understand the meaning of spirituality and have spiritual self-awareness.

Such self-awareness contributes to the ability to relate meaningfully to clients and to support their spiritual needs (Smith-Trudeau, 2019).

Think about it:

> Describe nursing interventions that would meet the spiritual needs of the client.

> How does providing goal-directed, client-centered care attend to the spiritual needs of the client?

> Discuss how spiritual self-awareness by the nurse might influence the spiritual care provided for the client.

Sources: Smith-Trudeau, P. (2019). Spirituality: A very misunderstood work. *Vermont Nurse Connection.* https://d3ms3kxrsap50t.cloudfront.net/uploads/publication/pdf/1810/Vermont_4_19.pdf; Fowler, J. (2017a). Spiritual care part 1: The importance of spiritual care. *British Journal of Nursing,* 26(8), 478; Ubaidi, B. (2017). Integration of spiritual needs into patient care. *Journal of Family Medicine and Disease Prevention,* 3(2). https://doi.org/10.23937/2469-5793/1510056.

Table 13-1 ➤ Comparison of Religion and Spirituality

RELIGION (THE MAP)	SPIRITUALITY (THE JOURNEY)
A "roadmap" that defines: Beliefs Values Code(s) of conduct and ethics	One's journey through life; a personal quest to define meaning, fulfillment, and satisfaction in life; a will to live; a belief in self; an exploration of who you are
A tradition or system of worship that provides: Rituals Answers Norms Connection with God	A dynamic relationship with that which transcends; a capacity to know and be known (a sense of openness, expectation); connectedness with self, others, nature, and a higher power (Fowler, 2017a); the source of inspiration, hope, and fulfillment (Hrabe, et al., 2019)
The roadmap and tradition define: What is to be believed How beliefs affect life Self-image and identity	A lifelong process of growth (which may involve joy and/or struggle); a constant process of taking in "truth" and then adding individual insight to arrive at a way of perceiving and acting in the world
Issues: Faith, belief, trust, the nature of good and evil, the meaning of suffering, judgment, enlightenment	Issues: Faith, hope, love

- Notion of sin (primarily in Western religions), origin of evil, and the nature of suffering
- Conception of either salvation (in Judeo-Christian religions), enlightenment (in Eastern religions), or atonement
- **Eschatology,** or doctrines about the human soul and its relation to death, judgment, and eternal life (primarily a Western concept)

- Explanation of the nature of reality, the higher self or soul, the relationship between humans and the divine, and the purpose of human existence.

What Is Spirituality?

Spirituality is the day-to-day, moment-by-moment journey in life and living. Like a journey, spirituality involves personal subjective experiences that take place

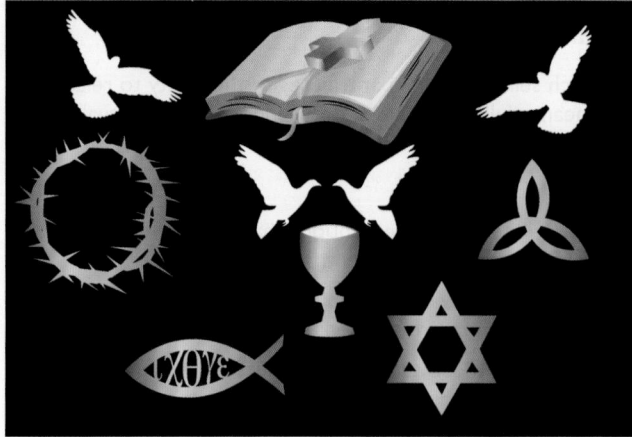

FIGURE 13-1 Associated with religion are various symbols and holy writings. For example, the Bible, cross, crown of thorns, trinity symbol, doves, chalice, and fish are all associated with Christianity, whereas the Star of David is associated with Judaism.

over time. It encompasses hope, purpose, meaning, connections/relationships, appreciations, and understanding. Many life events that prompt spiritual growth are fulfilling and joyful, but growth can also result from painful situations that cause internal upheaval, struggle, and challenge. To effectively provide spiritual care to clients, you must have insight into your own beliefs and thoughts about spirituality (Hawthorne & Gordon, 2020).

It is critical for you to recognize and respect the different ways that clients understand religion and spirituality. **Key Point:** *Most people are comfortable with their beliefs (or lack thereof); your primary goal is to support their healing, not convert them to a different view.* You must also be able to recognize when a client may be experiencing spiritual distress and recognize that this is a time to show compassion and caring (Smith-Trudeau, 2019). You may also need to collaborate with professionals who have more specialized training. These aspects of spiritual care are discussed later in this chapter.

KnowledgeCheck 13-1

- Regardless of their differences, what do many world religions have in common?
- Which can be compared with a journey: religion or spirituality?
- True or false: Both religion and spirituality allow a person various ways to access the divine.
- What is Mr. Johnson's religion (Meet Your Patient)?
- What is his sister's religion?

 ThinkLike a Nurse 13-1:
Clinical Judgment in Action

- What do you know, or what can you speculate, about Mr. Johnson's (Meet Your Patient) spirituality?

What Are the Core Issues of Spirituality?

By now you know that spirituality has many dimensions. In the New Testament of the Bible, the Apostle Paul identified "three things that last": faith, hope, and love. We limit discussion here to these three core issues (Aspen Reference Group, 2002). These virtues are expressed in or provide the foundational practice of various religions (Smith-Trudeau, 2019; Stavresky,1999):

- Islam—reading of the Qur'an, daily prayer, meditation, fasting.
- Buddhism—journey toward possession of spiritual power; overcoming the illusion of self.
- Hinduism—Dharma guides to use the inner life of spiritual truth toward discovery of truth.
- Judaism—originates with Jewish ethnic identity; establishes a relationship and eternal covenant with God; reading of the Torah.
- Christianity—reading of the Holy Bible; belief in the power of prayer; adherence to the Ten Commandments.

Faith

Faith is a global framework of beliefs, the strength of which guides and grounds many people, helps many make sense of the world, and empowers people to confront challenges (Canada et al., 2016; Paul Victor & Treschuk, 2020).

- Faith allows us to trust, to maintain an optimistic perspective on life events, and to find purpose in life.
- Like spirituality, faith represents a set of beliefs developed over time.
- People who experience the *joys of faith* exhibit a sense of self, as well as insights into their gifts and talents (Feder, 2021; Navales, 2021; Wanderlust, n.d.).
- *Faith struggles* are common among people who experience illness and significant loss. People experiencing faith struggles might feel anger, guilt, self-judgment, and worthlessness.

C. S. Lewis, a devout Christian, reveals that after the death of his wife, his grief caused him to doubt whether God exists at all, or if so, whether He is perhaps a "Cosmic Sadist" (1961, p. 35) who deliberately tortures us. Finally, Lewis came to understand that such shattering experiences are "one of the marks of His presence" (Lewis, 1961, p. 76).

Hope

Hope is an expectation of positive outcomes that is consistent with a desired future goal (Hong et al., 2015; Jensen, 2022). It reinforces the motivation to engage in goal-seeking behaviors.

- Hope includes the basic human need to achieve, create, and shape something of our lives that will endure.
- Hope is rooted in purpose—who am I, what is my purpose, and why have I been created?

- Hope is a major factor in how a person copes with a debilitating or terminal illness. People may cling to hope and endure aggressive noncurative treatments (Blackler, 2017), or they may lose hope and give up.

After suffering a near-fatal spinal cord injury, actor Christopher Reeve struggled with hope, yet he wrote in an essay, "Hope … is different from optimism or wishful thinking. When we have hope, we discover powers within ourselves we may have never known—the power to make sacrifices, to endure, to heal, and to love. Once we choose hope, everything is possible" (Reeve, 2002, p. 176).

Love

Love is often considered the core of one's strength, the basis for caring relationships (Hemberg et al., 2017), and one's greatest spiritual need (Blevins, 2021; Christman & Mueller, 2017). In combination, love, faith, and hope create one's perspective of health (Hemberg et al., 2017).

- Some view love as a trade: We extend our love because we hope to have it returned in some way or to simply experience the emotional satisfaction of loving others.
- Even when our love is shared, we must inevitably face separation at our death or the death of our loved ones.
- Love and health are interconnected; thus, illness and sudden injury commonly prompt "struggles with love." For example, clients with debilitating illnesses who require increasing levels of care may see themselves as a burden to their loved ones.
- Unconditional love can be demonstrated through kindness, patience, endurance, and truthfulness. The love and support of family and caregivers is invaluable in helping to restore a client's inner integrity and self-worth and strengthen the desire for health. They help patients to overcome negative states (e.g., loneliness, despair), increase healing, and promote better-quality outcomes (Hemberg et al., 2017).

Reeve stated that the most powerful words his wife spoke to him in the first days after his injury, "the words that saved my life," were "You're still you. And I love you" (Reeve, 1998, p. 32).

Cures, Miracles, and Spiritual Healing

A **miracle** is anything that allows for the presence of the transcendent (e.g., God, a higher being, a divine presence). Miracles may be spiritual phenomena, mysterious, and difficult to define or explain.

- **Key Point:** *We typically think of miracles as events that break with the natural order of things; however, miracles may proceed according to natural law.*
  Example: After the death of her client, a provider described the client's long-resisted acceptance of his impending death as the miracle, which prevented fruitless interventions and unnecessary suffering (La Madrid, 2012).

- **One aspect of miracle events is that they far exceed our expectations.** Although *medical miracle* refers to an unexpected recovery that is contrary to the prognosis (Gallegos, 2022), miracles do not always involve physical cures.
  Example: An older woman, bitter for decades over the death of her young daughter, "feels" her daughter's presence and dies in peace.
- **Miracles can be viewed as perfectly ordinary events or explained as the act of a "deity"** (McGrew, 2019). For example, a blind person suddenly can see, with no treatment or explanation.

Clients May Request a Prayer for Cure The client or family may request a prayer for a cure when your expertise tells you that all curative measures have been exhausted.

- **You should not say that a cure is impossible;** however, you should avoid giving the client and family false hope.
- **It may be possible for you to reframe the situation for them.** Perhaps healing does not necessarily have to imply the elimination of suffering or of the disease. Instead, there may be various forms of healing. A transformation in a client's thinking or feeling or in acknowledging beliefs can be seen as a miracle.

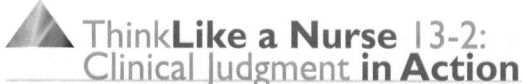

ThinkLike a Nurse 13-2: Clinical Judgment in Action

What are your beliefs about miracles? How would you respond to a patient who asks if you believe a miracle can occur to heal them?

How Might Spiritual Beliefs Affect Health?

Religion and spirituality are two separate and distinct constructs: religion usually encompasses formal rituals, beliefs in higher beings or higher meaning, and personal level of importance, whereas spirituality measures one's sense of spiritual well-being, connectedness, emotional well-being (e.g., peace, comfort), and stability. However, current research tends to address both concepts and their influence on health because they are tightly connected (Dombo, 2022).

> *Example:* Sharma et al. (2017) found that higher levels of religion and spirituality were associated with posttraumatic growth, purpose in life, and decreased risks for major depressive disorder and alcohol use disorders among U.S. military veterans.

Key Point: *A large body of literature suggests that religion and spirituality have a positive influence on health outcomes but does not yet answer the how or why.*

KnowledgeCheck 13-2

- What is the difference between faith, hope, and love?

ThinkLike a Nurse 13-3:
Clinical Judgment in Action

- How might religion negatively influence health?
- Has there been a pivotal moment in your life, a moment of crisis or despair, that eventually provided an opportunity for spiritual growth?

MAJOR RELIGIONS: WHAT SHOULD I KNOW?

Learning about other religions requires you to be open and nonjudgmental. When you care for a client from a known religious background, you need to think about how the person's beliefs affect their ideas of health, healing, hospitalization, and the experience of dying. To help you make these connections, the following brief descriptions of several of the world's major religious traditions provide you with several different worldviews. They will also provide you with insight into areas to ask about when you conduct a religious assessment. To learn about the influence of various religions on end-of-life care, see Chapter 14.

- **Key Point:** *The more you know about the differences and similarities among the world's major religions, the more you will be able to offer comprehensive and compassionate care to clients.*

- **Key Point:** *There may be various beliefs and practices within any religious group, so always validate with your client to avoid stereotyping.*

Judaism

Judaism is one of the Western world's oldest religions and the foundation on which Christianity and Islam were built. The Jewish law is set down in the collective writings of the Torah. Judaism is based on the worship of one God (monotheism), obeying the Ten Commandments, and practicing charity and tolerance toward others. The degree to which Jewish people celebrate rituals and holy days depends on whether they identify with Orthodox, Liberal, Conservative, or Reconstructionist beliefs (Amore et al., 2019).

- *The Sabbath.* Jews celebrate the Sabbath from sunset on Friday to sunset Saturday evening. For Orthodox Jews, work is prohibited on the Sabbath. This includes writing, traveling, and switching on lights and appliances.
- *Holidays.* During Passover (in March or April), some Jewish clients may require special foods, dinnerware, and utensils. The Day of Atonement, or Yom Kippur (in September or October), is the holiest day of the

Toward Evidence-Based Practice

Cannon, E., Bauer, R., Finch, M., Wallen, H., & Shaw, A. (2019). **Prayer circles and the perception of work environment.** *MEDSURG Nursing, 28*(5), 311–316.

The healthcare team asked the chaplain to pray with them after the death of a patient for whom they were unable to achieve adequate pain control. They continued to invite the chaplain to pray with them for 1 to 2 minutes each morning. This study examined the perception of the group prayer among clinical and nonclinical healthcare workers. Three major themes emerged from the results: (1) prayer provided a more positive tone to start the day (created unity, elevated moods, improved attitudes); (2) better attitudes and moods were reflected in the care provided to patients (greater empathy, better rapport); and (3) prayer helped some, but not all, participants feel comfortable praying and discussing spirituality with patients.

Phillips, G., MacKusick, C., & Whichello, R. (2018). **Workplace incivility in nursing: A literature review through the lens of ethics and spirituality.** *Journal of Christian Nursing, 35*(1), E7–E12. https://doi.org/10.1097/CNJ.0000000000000467

Researchers examined the effects of spirituality on workplace incivility. The literature synthesis revealed a consistent theme of improved job satisfaction and organizational commitment. Findings showed that workers with greater spirituality did not experience the low self-esteem associated with bullying. Results also revealed that spirituality and religion positively influenced

job performance, productivity, and behaviors. In addition, feeling valued and supported enhanced spirituality.

Simmons, A., Rivers, F., Gordon, S., & Yoder, L. (2018). **The role of spirituality among military en route care nurses: Source of strength or moral injury?** *Critical Care Nurse, 38*(2), 61–67. https://doi-org.su.idm.oclc.org/10.4037/ccn2018674

En route care nurses provide care to seriously ill or injured military members during air, ground, or sea transport to medical treatment facilities that can provide higher levels of care. Researchers investigated the effect of spirituality among these nurses who see the most devastating injuries of war. The results revealed a common theme that the nurses' spirituality helped them to stay mentally fit and deal with the stressors of deployment. Some nurses indicated that their spirituality was the greatest contributor to their suffering. The type of patients and the things they saw created significant internal turmoil and resulted in moral injury.

1. Which study supports group prayer in the work environment, and what were the benefits?

2. Suppose you are a chief nurse administrator and have been asked to support chaplain-led group prayer at the beginning of each shift for healthcare team members who desire to participate. Explain how the findings from each of the studies would be useful in supporting your decision.

Jewish calendar. It is a special day of fasting (abstaining from food), but fasting is not required if it would be a danger to the client. A Jewish client may wish to keep that day to pray and rest. For Orthodox clients, you might offer approved alternatives to oral medication (e.g., injections or suppositories).

- *Dietary Practices.* Conservative Jews observe strict dietary laws: only kosher foods are accepted. Kosher foods have strict guidelines for animal slaughter and food preparation. These foods do not contain pork, certain types of seafood, or combinations of dairy and meat (Fowler, 2017f). Meals are also double-packaged if kosher foods are heated in nonkosher heating units (Rich, 2022). If possible, consult a rabbi or dietitian who is knowledgeable about Jewish dietary laws for assistance in planning dietary and activity modifications.
- *Clothing Practices.* Orthodox Jewish women often prefer to have their bodies and limbs covered. They may also prefer to keep their hair covered with a scarf and may often wear a wig. Orthodox men are likely to keep their heads covered with a hat or skullcap *(kappel)*.
- *Medical and Reproductive Practices.* Some Orthodox Jewish sects forbid contraception unless the woman's health is at risk. Nearly all Jewish boys are circumcised, usually 8 days after birth. Orthodox Judaism usually forbids organ transplants, but opinions vary, and decisions may rest with the rabbinic authority.

Both Reconstructionist and Reform Judaism incorporate current societal values. Reconstructionists view Judaism not as a religion with rituals mandated by God but as a spiritual path with unity and connections developed among persons (My Jewish Learning, 2022; Rich, 2022). Likewise, followers of Reform Judaism adhere to the traditional tenets but practice inclusion, such as the acceptance of women as rabbis (ReformJudaism, 2022).

Christianity

Christianity is a major world religion. Christians worship Jesus Christ and believe that his death atoned for their sins by granting them forgiveness from God, which allows for eternal life. Their sacred text, the Bible, includes the Judaic Old Testament and the New Testament relating to the life of Christ. Rituals and practices vary among the Christian denominations, but the following are some similarities:

- *Baptism.* Many Christians practice baptism, which is a sign of moral cleansing and correlates to being born again. The baptism of an infant, also known as *christening,* indicates that the child will be raised with Christian values and influences. When infants or children are very ill, parents may request baptism.
- *Dietary Practices.* Christians usually have no special dietary requirements, although some choose to abstain from eating meat on Fridays and/or during Lent, and some abstain from alcohol. Others may fast for personal reasons.
- *Health and Reproductive Practices.* Most Christians do not object to blood transfusion or organ transplantation. Perspectives vary on using artificial birth control methods; however, natural family planning methods (e.g., rhythm) are widely accepted.

Christianity has many denominations, including Roman Catholicism, Orthodoxy, Protestant denominations (e.g., Lutheran, Baptist, United Methodist), and others (e.g., Jehovah's Witnesses, Mormons, Christian Scientists). Table 13-2 identifies specific factors a nurse may need to address for patients of selected denominations.

Islam

Islam was the third monotheistic religion to emerge, after Judaism and Christianity (Fowler, 2017d). The word *Islam* means "submission." A Muslim follower is one who submits to Allah (God). Muhammad is the founder of Islam and a respected prophet. The sacred book of authority in Islam, the Holy Qu'ran, is the result of messages from the angel Gabriel sent from God to the prophet Muhammad. It contains one common message of many faiths: there is a Supreme Being whose sovereignty is acknowledged in worship and whose teaching and commandments must be obeyed.

As related to healthcare and practice, followers of the Muslim faith have diverse views. The most common are listed here, but you should always ask your patients about their beliefs and preferences.

- *Blood Transfusion/Transplants.* There is no specific religious rule prohibiting blood transfusion or organ transplantation.
- *Dietary Practices.* Muslims do not eat pork. Other meat must be *halal* meat, which is killed in a special manner stated in Islamic law. Fruits, vegetables, fish, and eggs are allowed, but not if they are cooked near pork or nonhalal meat.
- *Holidays.* During the month of Ramadan, Muslims fast between sunrise and sunset; however, those who are sick are not expected to fast. Essential drugs and medicines are allowed at all hours during Ramadan.
- *Hygiene Practices.* Muslims always wash their hands before eating, and it is customary to eat with the right hand (unless prevented by injury). The left hand is considered unclean (Attum et al., 2022). Clients usually prefer to wash in free-flowing water, so if a shower is not available, provide a pitcher to use in the bath (Attum et al., 2022).
- *Modesty.* Women usually prefer to be treated by female staff. Some women may refuse vaginal examination by a male nurse or provider.
- *Reproductive Practices.* After the birth of a baby, many Muslims may whisper prayers in the newborn's ear so that the first thing heard are words of prayer. Orthodox Muslims do not approve of contraception;

Table 13-2 ➤ Nursing Considerations for Specific Religions

RELIGION	PRACTICES/BELIEFS	KEY IMPLICATIONS FOR NURSES
Jehovah's Witness	Many clients who identify as Jehovah's Witnesses would accept death rather than accept blood or blood products, which can be a serious medical concern (Fowler, 2017e; Jehovah Witness, 2022).	■ Remain nonjudgmental. ■ Accept the client and/or family's decision. ■ Provide emotional support.
Roman Catholicism	In Roman Catholicism, the sacraments are a means to obtain grace. There are different types of sacraments and religious rituals.	■ Ask the patient if they would like you to call a priest. ■ Inquire as to any other special needs or desires.
Christian Science	Christian Scientists can choose the healthcare that meets their needs and that of their families (Christian Scientist, 2022). Therefore, you may encounter varying practices, based on your clients' degree of adherence to Christian Scientist beliefs and practices.	■ It is imperative to do an individualized assessment to determine how to best incorporate their spiritual values into the plan of care.
Mormonism	The Church of Jesus Christ of Latter-Day Saints (LDS) is commonly called the Mormon Church. Mormons believe in Jesus and one God and adhere to the sacred writings of the Holy Bible and the Book of Mormon.	■ Ask if there is someone they would like called. Mormons look to their church leaders and family for support and comfort. ■ Remove sacred undergarments before surgery or in emergency situations and treat with respect or give to family members (Andrews et al., 2020).
Seventh-day Adventism	Members of the Seventh-day Adventist Church observe Saturday as the Sabbath, a day of rest and worship, with no secular work or unnecessary business. Members believe that a healthy mind and body are essential elements of faith and worship and that both spiritual health and physical health are enhanced by good nutrition.	■ Inquire as to dietary preferences. ■ Ask patients about choices to keep the Sabbath day holy if hospitalized on a Saturday.

however, individuals vary widely in their practices. Abortion is frowned on but may be tolerated for medical reasons (Mohammed, 2022).

Hinduism

Hinduism, viewed as the oldest major religion, does not embrace a single body of beliefs and practices or the existence of a single deity. Hindus may worship several or even hundreds of gods and goddesses, including elements in the natural world, such as rivers, fire, and so forth. Sacred Hindu texts include the *Vedas,* the *Bhagavad Gita* (Song of the Blessed One), and the *Ramayana,* the story of the life of the god Rama.

■ *Dietary Practices.* Most Hindus are lactovegetarians, consuming milk but no eggs. Many will not eat beef and avoid bovine-derived medication because of the reincarnation of certain gods (Fowler, 2017c). Fasting, which may mean eating only "pure" foods, such as fruit or yogurt, is common during major festivals but is not expected of the sick.

■ *Hygiene Practices.* Many Hindu patients prefer to wash in free-flowing water (e.g., a shower instead of a tub). If a shower is not available, provide a jug of water for the person to use in the bath.

■ *Lifestyle and Health Practices.* Hindus practice ayurvedic medicine, which encompasses all aspects of life, including diet, sleep, elimination, and hygiene. Some believe in the medicinal properties of "hot" and "cold" foods (does not refer to temperature or spicy qualities). There is no religious objection to contraception, blood transfusion, or organ donation. The use of alcohol or tobacco may be accepted.

■ *Modesty and Respect.* Modesty is encouraged, and women usually prefer to be treated by female medical staff. Some Hindus may consider touching a person's feet or head a sign of disrespect.

■ *Religious Beliefs.* The core concepts of Hinduism are karma, dharma, and reincarnation (Fowler, 2017c). Karma teaches that every action has or causes an effect. A person who does not fulfill their destiny or given purpose in life (dharma) will have bad karma.

After death, persons begin a new life in a different body or spiritual form (reincarnation).

- *Religious Symbols.* Some Hindus wear a "sacred thread" around the body or wrist. Do not remove or cut this thread without permission from the client or next of kin. Jewelry often has a religious significance.

Buddhism

To followers, the Buddha, or the "Awakened One," is revered not as a god but as an example of a way of life (Fig. 13-2). Siddhartha Gautama was born into a royal family in 624 BCE in a part of northern India that is now in Nepal, gained enlightenment at age 35, and then began to teach others how to attain liberation from suffering for themselves and others.

One of the Buddha's core teachings is that suffering can be ended by following the eightfold path: right understanding, right intention, right speech, right action, right livelihood, right effort, right mindfulness, and right contemplation (Knierim, n.d.). **Nirvana,** similar to the Christian concept of heaven, can be attained only through an absence of desire, the achievement of perfection, and the lack of a unique identity. Buddhism is about finding spirituality within oneself. Like Hindus, Buddhists believe in karma and reincarnation.

- *Dietary Practices.* Food is an essential component of maintaining spiritual focus, meditation, and interactions with others. Many Buddhists follow a vegetarian diet; in some cases, the diet may include both milk and eggs. Fasting customs vary by tradition (Fowler, 2017b).

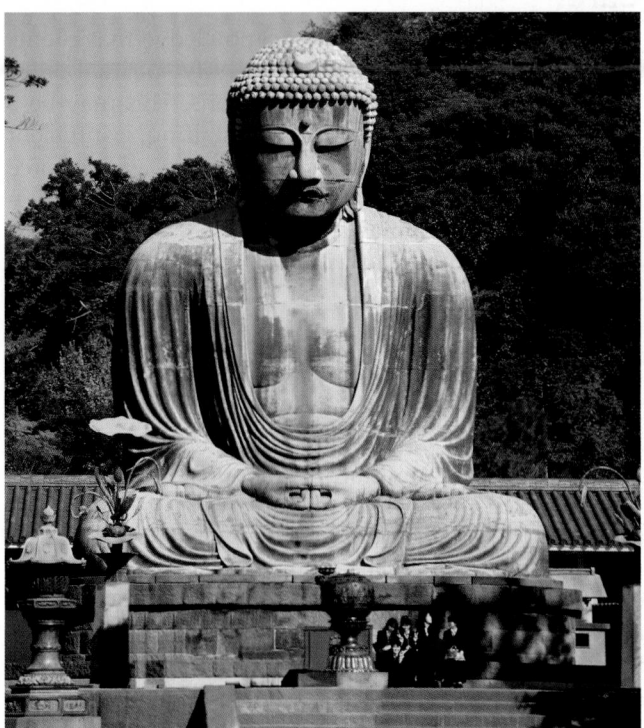

FIGURE 13-2 The Buddha is revered as an example of a way of life.

- *Reproductive Practices.* Buddhists accept contraception but typically condemn abortion and active euthanasia.
- *Transfusions and Transplants.* They will usually accept blood transfusion and organ transplantation.

Native American Religions

There are more than 570 federally recognized Native American nations or tribes in the United States (National Congress of American Indians [NCAI], 2020). Although each group has its own traditions and cultural heritage, some general beliefs underlie the more specific tribal ideas. To most Native American groups, Earth is considered to be a living organism, the body of a higher individual, and humankind has an intimate relationship with this organism through nature. Thus, rather than having a designated sacred place to worship, Native American traditions place value on the land, mountains, rivers, and meadows (NCAI, 2019; Kleinsmith, 2022).

- *Communication.* Note-taking by the professional is forbidden in some Native American cultures. Ask the patient if they are comfortable with you taking notes during the interview. Explain that it is okay if they are not. This may mean that when you take a history or perform an examination, you must rely on your memory and record findings later.
- *Health Practices.* Most Native American traditions consider health as a state of harmony with nature. Whenever disharmony exists, disease or illness can occur. Patients may want to engage a traditional Native American healer to restore this harmony (Fig. 13-3).

Atheism

Atheists do not believe in Gods or supernatural deities. Rather than receiving directives on living from external sources, atheists have their own personal moral code that is derived from their value systems, beliefs, and life experiences. They can be spiritual and even religious, but they often focus on the humanistic, secular perspectives (Lipka, 2019).

Even though many atheists do not participate in structured religion, they may have a desire to discuss their fears or other concerns with others in a nonsecular way. A nurse recalls a patient's comment that he regretted putting "Atheist" on his admission paperwork because he would have welcomed the presence of a chaplain to discuss where he was spiritually (Mais, 2010).

Key Point: *This comment does not imply that all atheists would react in the same way as this one. It does, however, reinforce the importance of a thorough assessment of each client's needs instead of relying on categories and labels.*

KnowledgeCheck 13-3

- Which major religion requires halal meat in the diet?
- Which denomination or religion does not believe in blood transfusions?
- True or false: Atheists are not religious or spiritual.

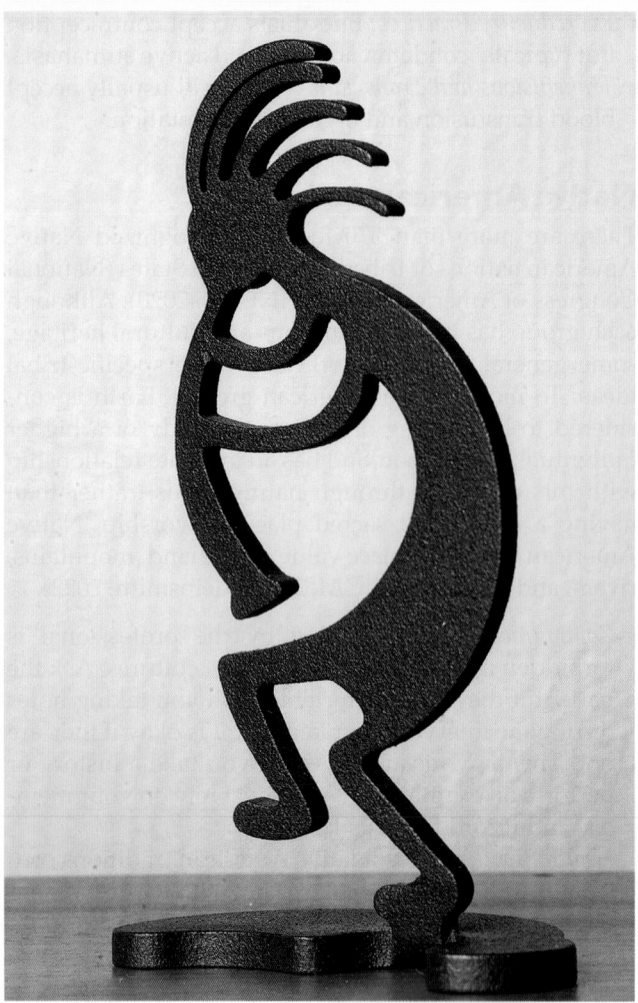

FIGURE 13-3 Kokopelli, the humpbacked flute player, has been a sacred figure to Native Americans of the Southwest for thousands of years.

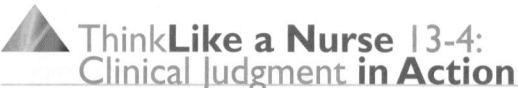

ThinkLike a Nurse 13-4:
Clinical Judgment in Action

What are some ways that world religions might influence nursing care?

Self-Knowledge: what every nurse should know

As you have seen, your clients' spiritual and religious backgrounds may be diverse and may involve ways of thinking and doing that seem strange to you or that you do not fully understand. Before trying to understand their experience, you must give considerable thought to your own religious or spiritual journey to avoid implicit or explicit bias. Attaining self-knowledge is an important aspect of becoming a full-spectrum nurse. This section will help you in your reflections.

What Are Your Personal Biases?

We always carry our own perspectives with us. We tend to view the world through lenses we acquired in childhood, adolescence, and early adulthood. In addition, religious education often teaches that certain religious beliefs and practices are superior to all others. When you view your own experience as the norm or as the preferred way of organizing the world, you tend to limit the range of care you provide to the client who believes differently.

- **Key Point:** *Spiritual care demands nonjudgmental attitudes and an open manner of thinking that invites rather than excludes.*
- **Key Point:** *If you are aware of your biases, it will be easier to avoid abuses of spiritual care.*

ThinkLike a Nurse 13-5:
Clinical Judgment in Action

Consider the following examples. For each person, what moral/spiritual judgments should the nurse avoid?

- A nurse is caring for a postoperative patient who is also HIV positive.
- A patient has come to the clinic to be treated for gonorrhea (a sexually transmitted infection). They convey having at least six sexual partners this year.
- A man comes to the emergency department (ED) at least once a month to ask for morphine to treat his back pain. He is known to abuse drugs and to visit other EDs for the same purpose.

What Are Some Barriers to Spiritual Care?

Although most nurses would acknowledge that clients have a spiritual dimension, few identify spiritual problems or provide spiritual interventions. This may be a result of economic constraints, poor staffing, insufficient time, lack of privacy, and high-tech care, which force nurses to focus only on physical needs to the exclusion of spiritual health. It may also be caused by inconsistencies in the meaning of "spirituality" (Britt & Acton, 2021; Smith-Trudeau, 2019).

Lack of General Awareness of Spirituality

A greater awareness of spirituality in general will help you tune into the spiritual needs of clients and improve your comfort in communicating about spiritual matters. Technological advances and other factors (e.g., workloads, institutional demands) in the healthcare environment have shifted the focus from "being with" the client to "doing for" the client (Maphosa, 2017; Ordons et al., 2020). This creates a mutual spiritual disconnect because the "spirit" component of caring for the whole client (mind–body–spirit) is neglected, which in turn diminishes the nurse's attunement to the client's spiritual dimension. The result is missed opportunities to show caring, compassion, sensitivity, and empathy.

Lack of Awareness of Your Own Spiritual Belief System

To feel comfortable making spiritual interventions, you will need more than just theoretical knowledge. You will also need introspection and an awareness of your own spiritual journey. Nurses who are aware of their own spirituality are better able to incorporate spiritual care into their practice (Hrabe et al., 2019; Trudeau-Smith, 2019). You can take steps to enhance your spiritual growth, take care of and nurture your own spiritual needs, gain a broader view of spirituality, and increase sensitivity to the spiritual needs of others. You must:

1. Understand the differences among religion, spirituality, spiritual care, and spiritual wellness.
2. Develop an awareness of your own spirituality and how it is applied (or not) in meeting the client's spiritual needs.
3. Understand the connection between meeting the client's spiritual needs and nurturing your spiritual dimension.
4. Open yourself by being totally present with the client, including being an active listener. Allow the client to share their feelings and emotions without reserve, and reflect in your attitude and demeanor that you care and have the time to listen.
5. Develop your critical and reflective thinking abilities. Explore through reflection and discussions with others. Write your own epitaph: one or two lines summing up how you would like to be remembered.
6. Reflect on your thoughts and feelings about the care you provided at the end of each shift. Identify your spiritual work.
7. Reflect on your thoughts, feelings, and personal experience with grief, loss, and end-of-life issues. For example, what is the first death you can remember? What were your feelings at the time? How do you usually cope with loss? What actions by others comforted you? Imagine you have only a few weeks to live; think how you would feel.

Differences in Spirituality Between Nurse and Patient

When a client's spiritual beliefs are very different from your own, you must be careful not to impose your beliefs on the client or discount the importance of their beliefs and rituals. For example, if a client has a serious or terminal illness, the client and their family might be offended if their nurse inquires whether they are "saved" Christians. By remaining focused on the client's need to talk about meaning, salvation, or other issues, you provide full-spectrum spiritual care. In the Meet Your Patient scenario, do you think Mr. Johnson feels supported by his sister?

When the client's views or beliefs are similar to yours, take care not to make false assumptions about their spiritual needs. Although you share some commonalities, this does not mean you will have the same perspectives or needs in all areas of spirituality or religion.

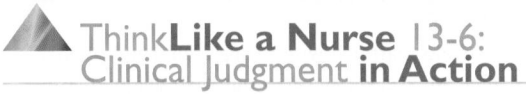

ThinkLike a Nurse 13-6: Clinical Judgment in Action

- How does your religion or spirituality differ from Mr. Johnson's (Meet Your Patient)?
- How is it similar?
- Can you think of problems these differences and similarities could cause you in caring for him?

Fear That Your Knowledge Base Is Insufficient

Nurses sometimes avoid giving spiritual care because they feel they lack knowledge of spirituality or of the client's religion. This is a realistic concern. In several studies, nurses were found to be unsure of what constituted spiritual problems and spiritual interventions (Ordons et al., 2020; Ross et al., 2022). In some cases, they did not identify the spiritual dimension of care, or they took religious aspects into account but did not place them into a broader spiritual perspective. Your ability to incorporate spiritual care into practice will increase with experience.

Fear of Where Spiritual Discussions May Lead

Many nurses fear that inquiring into the spiritual domain might cause harm to the client. For example, what if a client asks, "Do you think active euthanasia is morally wrong? Would it jeopardize my salvation?" Here are some fears that may arise:

- You may not feel prepared to answer the questions.
- You might have an answer based on your personal religious beliefs but fear the client may think you are imposing your beliefs on them.
- You might wonder whether communicating your own beliefs (e.g., if you favor active euthanasia) might jeopardize the client's spiritual life if your ideas turn out to be "wrong."

Key Point: *The following are some ideas that may help counter your fears:*
- *The fact that the patient is addressing this concern with you indicates that you are open to the spiritual domain of care.*
- *The patient's questions about euthanasia could lead to discussions about their fears of pain, dependence, being a burden on family members, and dying alone.*
- *You should realize that being open to the spiritual realm and assessing the patient's need for spiritual intervention does not mean that you must be a chaplain or have the extraordinary ability to deal with all spiritual or religious questions or requests. You can collaborate with a chaplain, who is more prepared to deal with specific religious issues.*

KnowledgeCheck 13-4

- What qualities can you demonstrate that may help you improve the quality of spiritual care you provide?
- What common barriers to spiritual interventions do nurses encounter?
- True or false: No matter how nonjudgmental and open we may think we are, we all carry our own unique biases and prejudices that have the potential to affect patient care.

 ## ThinkLike a Nurse 13-7: Clinical Judgment in Action

- What are possible errors made by nurses in relation to spiritual care?
- What are some ways that you can develop a greater awareness of the "spirit within the self"?
- Discuss ways that nurses and clients can nurture their own spiritual needs.

PracticalKnowledge
knowing how

Most hospital admission forms include a place to record the client's religious preferences. Unfortunately, some nurses believe that by completing such forms, they have addressed the patient's spiritual needs. However, armed with your basic theoretical knowledge of spirituality and your growing spiritual self-knowledge, you should be able to provide a level of support that extends beyond paperwork to compassion and caring. The good news is that spiritual care has never been more welcomed by patients. You now know the importance of and can provide care to meet your patient's spiritual needs. The Practical Knowledge section will provide a more detailed understanding of your role in spiritual care.

To see a care plan and care map for a client with Spiritual Distress,

 Go to Davis Advantage, **Resources, Chapter 13, Nursing Care Plan: Spiritual Distress,** and **Care Map: Spiritual Distress**.

▌ RECOGNIZING CUES

People of the same religion often vary greatly in the degree to which they follow religious practices. It is not enough to "fill in the religion blank" on an assessment form. You should always do a careful assessment of your client's religion and associated needs, practices, and desires. Keep in mind that this may be a sensitive area for some clients.

Key Point: *It may be difficult to obtain meaningful information on the initial admission assessment due to time constraints in completing the paperwork, collaboration with the healthcare team, and the stresses involved in getting the client introduced to the healthcare setting.* Obtain the essential data of the client's church preference, name of clergy, whom to call in case of emergency, dietary requirements/restrictions, and any religious implications for medical care (e.g., refusal of blood transfusions). As you interact further with the client and family, trust will develop, and you will be able to obtain more sensitive, complex, and meaningful spiritual/religious information.

Key Point: *Timing is essential in conducting a spiritual assessment. Use the discussion about the reason for hospitalization to assess the client's coping processes. Ask, "How are you handling this spiritually?" or "How does this affect your faith or spiritual foundation?"*

Sources of Spiritual Data

You can acquire information about a patient's spirituality from a variety of sources other than interviews:

- *Patient's Environment.* Observe the client's environment for hints about their spirituality (e.g., pictures of family, the presence of sacred texts or reading materials, articles used in worship [a crucifix, rosary beads, statues], or copies of church bulletins).
- *Patient's Questions.* The patient may ask questions that are indicative of spiritual comfort, longing, or distress. For example, the patient may ask whether church attendance provides you with a sense of comfort and meaning.
- *Patient's Behaviors, Moods, and Feelings.* Emotional behaviors give a clear and certain indication that the patient is struggling with issues that have spiritual overtones (Gilbertson et al., 2022). These warrant further assessment and nursing intervention. For example, a patient may ask you if you have ever felt really guilty about something you did as a child.
- *Nonverbal Communication.* Body language may indicate hope or distress. For example, you may observe a patient praying. Or when asking about spirituality, you may see the patient roll their eyes, shake their head, and tense their muscles.

Spiritual Assessment Tools

Some healthcare agencies have focused spiritual assessment tools tailored to their particular setting. Others may use externally developed tools, including those discussed next.

HOPE The HOPE questions (Gowri & Hight, 2001) are an easy-to-use screening method. HOPE is a mnemonic, as follows:

H—sources of Hope
O—Organized religion
P—Personal spirituality/Practices
E—Effects on medical care and end-of-life issues

The HOPE model is recognized as the most comprehensive assessment tool in palliative care (Blaber et al., 2015) and useful for older adults (Wiltjer, 2019) because it:

- Explores in greater detail the relationship between the client's spirituality and healthcare needs
- Assesses those areas that are essential to the client's spiritual well-being
- Facilitates the development of individualized plans for ongoing spiritual care (Blaber et al., 2015; Wiltjer, 2019)

 JAREL The JAREL spiritual well-being scale was developed by nurses and is especially intended for use with clients 65 years and older. Cutting across religious and atheistic belief systems, the 21-question tool assesses three key dimensions: (1) faith/belief, (2) life/self-responsibility, and (3) life satisfaction/self-actualization (Hungelmann et al., 1996; Lu et al., 2019).

SPIRIT The comprehensive spiritual assessment tool developed by Maugans (1996) and Highfield (2000) involves obtaining information on six key areas designated by the acronym SPIRIT:

S—Spiritual/religious belief system
P—Personal spirituality
I—Integration within a spiritual community
R—Ritualized practices and restrictions
I—Implications for medical care
T—Terminal events planning

To see a copy of a spiritual assessment based on the SPIRIT model, and for questions to use for the HOPE approach,

 Go to **Chapter 13, Assessment Guidelines and Tools, Focused Assessment: The HOPE Approach to Spiritual Assessment: Examples of Questions** and **Focused Assessment: S-P-I-R-T Assessment**, in Volume 2.

KnowledgeCheck 13-5

What are the six areas for spiritual assessment summarized in the SPIRIT tool?

ThinkLike a Nurse 13-8: Clinical Judgment in Action

Complete the SPIRIT assessment (in Volume 2) on yourself. Discuss it with your classmates.

▰▰ ANALYZE CUES/PRIORITIZE HYPOTHESES

When analyzing spiritual assessment data, you must consider the person's developmental stage. People progress through stages of spiritual development in much the same way as they develop physically and cognitively. Spiritual behaviors that seem problematic in one stage may not be so in an earlier stage. To review developmental stages, refer to Chapters 6 and 7.

Spirituality and Religiosity Diagnoses

Box 13-1 contains diagnostic labels that specifically deal with religion and spirituality. The following are examples of full diagnostic statements for spiritual problems:

- *Spiritual Distress* related to overwhelming anxiety associated with the need to have a surgical procedure that is not accepted by her religion.
- *Impaired Religiosity* related to altered ability to exercise reliance on beliefs or practice rituals associated with religious faith.
- *Risk for Spiritual Distress* related to the potential for altered ability to integrate or find meaning in life through connectedness within self that may compromise health or health decisions.

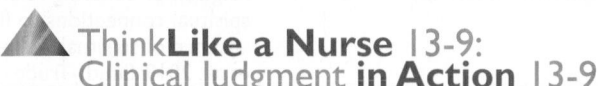 ThinkLike a Nurse 13-9: Clinical Judgment in Action 13-9

Which of these nursing diagnoses would you use for Mr. Johnson (Meet Your Patient): Spiritual Distress, Risk for Spiritual Distress, or Impaired Religiosity? Why? See Box 13-1 as needed.

Spirituality as Etiology

It is sometimes difficult to determine the problem from the etiology. Does the patient experience Spiritual Distress because of pain and hopelessness? Or did the patient first lose faith in their religious teachings, which led to hopelessness and anxiety? Either way, spiritual support is needed.

Several diagnoses relate to spirituality as the problem, etiology, or symptom. Examples include Noncompliance/Nonadherence to Treatment; Hopelessness; and Powerlessness. The following are examples of diagnostic statements with spiritual etiologies:

Decisional Conflict related to confusion about the religious implications of the decision to forgo heroic treatment measures

Nonadherence to treatment regimen related to the patient's belief that the illness is "God's will" and that healing will occur (without treatment) for the same reason.

KnowledgeCheck 13-6

Consider the following statement: A nursing diagnosis that reflects either an actual or a potential problem may reflect religious and/or spiritual dimensions of the human condition.

- Is this statement true?
- Would it be true for a *physical* diagnosis (e.g., Disturbed Sleep Pattern)? Explain your thinking.

▰▰ GENERATE SOLUTIONS

The outcomes you establish in the planning stage of the nursing process serve as the criteria for your evaluation of the patient's progress and the success of the nursing interventions.

BOX 13-1 ■ Spirituality Diagnoses, Examples

Moral Distress	The psychological disequilibrium and negative feeling state experienced when a person makes a moral decision but does not follow through by performing the behavior indicated by that decision. Usually this is because there are various constraints on that behavior (Wilkinson, 1987/88).
Impaired Religiosity*	Difficulty in exercising, or impaired ability to exercise, reliance on beliefs or to participate in rituals of a faith tradition (e.g., go to church, take communion) (Herdman et al., 2021).
Risk for Impaired Religiosity*	Occurs when risk factors are present but symptoms are not. Risk factors may be categorized as developmental, environmental, physical, psychological, sociocultural, or spiritual. Examples include life transitions, lack of transportation, pain, depression, social isolation, and suffering.
Risk for Spiritual Distress*	"Susceptible to a state of suffering related to the impaired ability to integrate meaning and purpose in life through connection with self, others, and the world, and/or a power greater than oneself, which may compromise health" (Herdman et al., 2021, p. 462). For example, may question religious rituals, such as prayer ("God has forgotten about me") or may seek spiritual guidance or help (Smith-Trudeau, 2019)
Spiritual Distress	Anguish or suffering related to an inability to make interpersonal, intrapersonal, and/or spiritual connections to find meaning and purpose in life (Herdman et al., 2021, p. 462). The absence of spiritual wellness and the therapeutic quest for purpose and meaning (Hrabe et al., 2019; Smith-Trudeau, 2019).
	Defining characteristics (signs and symptoms) include the following:
	■ *Connections to self:* Expressing a lack of love, courage, acceptance, or peace; a lack of meaning and purpose in life; feelings of anger or guilt
	■ *Connections with others:* Refusing to see religious leaders; refusing to interact with family or friends; feeling disconnected from support system; expressing feelings of alienation
	■ *Connections with art, music, literature, nature:* Decreased or no interest in nature, music, writing, art; no interest in spiritual reading
	■ *Connections with power greater than self:* Inability or refusal to pray or to participate in religious activities; feeling abandoned by their chosen deity; expressions of anger toward deity; sudden changes in spiritual practices (increased or decreased)
Spiritual Pain	A deep nonphysical pain in one's soul/being that occurs when a person experiences a combination of awareness of death, loss of relationships, loss of self, loss of purpose, and loss of control (Schultz et al., 2017). However, this combination of negative experiences can be balanced by having a life-affirming and transcending purpose and an internal sense of control (Fig. 13-4). The presence and quality of Spiritual Pain is determined by the degree to which the person is experiencing each symptom and by the relationship of the components to each other (Millspaugh, 2005).

Sources: Adapted from Millspaugh, C. (2005). Assessment and response to spiritual pain: Part II. *Journal of Palliative Medicine, 8*(5): 1110–1117; Herdman, H., Kamitsuru, D., & Lopes, C. (Eds.). (2021). *Nursing diagnoses: Definitions & classification, 2021–2023* (12th ed.). Thieme; Schultz, M., Meged-Book, T., Mashiach, T., & Bar-Sela, M. (2017). Distinguishing between spiritual distress, general distress, spiritual well-being, and spiritual pain among cancer patients during oncology treatment. *Journal of Pain & Symptom Management, 54*(1), 66–73. https://doi.org.su.idm.oclc.org/10.1016/j.jpainsymman.2017.03.018; Smith-Trudeau, P. (2019). Spirituality: A very misunderstood work. *Vermont Nurse Connection.* https://d3ms3kxrsap50t.cloudfront.net/uploads/publication/pdf/1810/Vermont_4_19.pdf; Wilkinson, J. (1987/1988). Moral distress in nursing practice: experience and effect. *Nursing Forum, 23*(1), 12–29.

*In order to make safe and effective judgments using NANDA-I nursing diagnoses, it is essential that nurses refer to the definitions and defining characteristics of the diagnoses listed in this work.

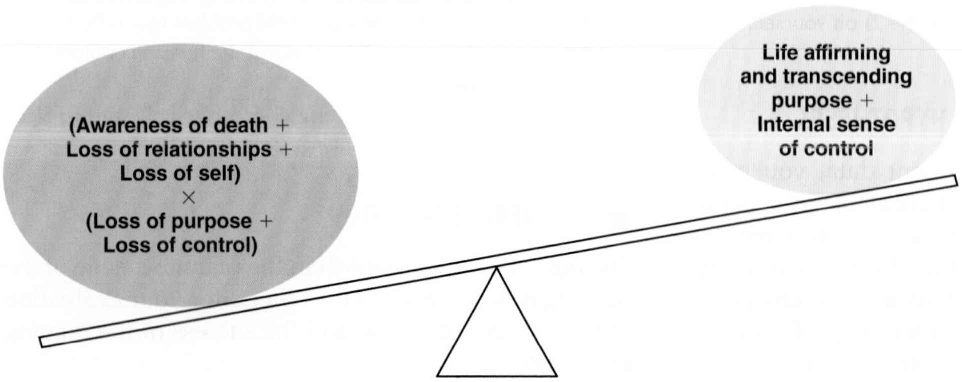

(Awareness of death + Loss of relationships + Loss of self)
×
(Loss of purpose + Loss of control)

Life affirming and transcending purpose + Internal sense of control

FIGURE 13-4 Components of spiritual pain.

Nursing Outcomes Classification (NOC) standardized outcomes associated with spirituality diagnoses include, but are not limited to, the following: Anxiety Level, Comfortable Death, Dignified Life Closure, Hope, Loneliness Severity, Personal Resiliency, Personal Well-Being, Quality of Life, Spiritual Health, and Will to Live (Moorhead et al., 2018).

Individualized goals/outcome statements you might write for spiritual diagnoses include the following:

- For Risk for Spiritual Distress—Exhibits no signs or symptoms of spiritual distress (e.g., finds meaning in life, expresses hope and faith, follows usual religious practices).
- For Spiritual Distress—Returns to previous state of spiritual well-being and comfort (e.g., expresses a sense of peace, asks to see religious adviser).
- For Impaired Religiosity—Experiences the desire and ability to participate in the rituals of a particular faith.

▰ GENERATE SOLUTIONS/TAKE ACTION

Spiritual interventions are those used to treat and prevent spiritual problems related to the patient's illness. You will direct some nursing activities toward resolving the problem, others toward removing the etiology, and still others toward relieving symptoms. You will, of course, base your nursing activities on the patient's symptoms and the problem etiologies. However, there are some nursing interventions that are useful for all, or most, spiritual problems.

A few Nursing Interventions Classification (NIC) standardized interventions to promote spirituality are discussed in this section. The evidence base for these is specific to older adults (Jackson et al., 2016; Toivonen et al., 2015); however, they can be useful for other age-groups, as well.

When you are performing interventions of a spiritual nature, remember the following:

- **Key Point: *You absolutely must follow the patient's lead and be caring and respectful without inserting your own beliefs into the conversation.***
- **Choose your language carefully**—words similar to *saved, repentance,* and *born again,* which may be a part of everyday conversation for people who follow religion, may cause some patients to feel pressured or uncomfortable. Try to mirror, and not go beyond, the patient's religious terminology.

It requires knowledge, skill, and practice to provide religious support without imposing your own beliefs. The safest course of action is to offer to contact a chaplain for the patient. However, patients cannot always— or may not always want to—wait for a chaplain.

Active Listening (NIC)

The Active Listening intervention allows the nurse to establish a trusting relationship and to hear, understand, and interpret what the client is saying. Listening actively involves four NIC interventions and one non-standardized activity.

Presence (NIC) Presence means to be with patient and family in meaningful ways. It requires:

- Your actual presence at the bedside
- Being open to the issues and concerns of the patient
- Allowing the patient to lead discussions rather than setting the agenda or controlling the conversation
- Sincere communication
- Being fully available to the client
- Listening to the patient's stories about their illness

Touch (NIC) Caring touch, such as hand holding or touching an arm or shoulder, facilitates communication. It conveys concern, comfort, and acceptance, especially during stressful experiences. At least one study has shown touch to improve life satisfaction and faith. Some people prefer not to be touched, so carefully observe the patient's responses.

Exploring Meaning (Non-NIC) *Meaning* refers to a clear understanding of the illness or loss (e.g., loss of independence). It also refers to the concepts of finding meaning and purpose in life or a sense of personal worthiness. You can facilitate the patient's search for meaning by asking probing questions, providing explanations, and reframing maladaptive interpretations of life events.

Reminiscence Therapy (NIC) Reminiscence is the recalling and sharing of past life events with another person. It promotes meaning-making through rethinking and clarifying previous experiences. As the patient reminisces, they may make spiritual links by expressing personal beliefs that helped them live through difficult life events. This intervention is more effective within a long-term relationship.

Spiritual Support (NIC)

NIC defines Spiritual Support as "assisting the patient to feel balance and connection with a greater power" (Butcher et al., 2018, p. 353). Effective Spiritual Support is based on a focused spiritual assessment, including the person's belief system. It may include assisting with forgiveness, encouraging hope, praying, and reading scriptures or other texts the patient requests.

Forgiveness Facilitation (NIC) Forgiveness is the act of pardoning or being pardoned for an offense, debt, or obligation. Letting go of the resentment felt for another promotes constructive changes in a person's life; a sense of renewal; and reconciliation with God, church, and one's inner being. To provide this intervention, you must first assess the patient's needs for reconciliation with self, others, and God. If, like Mr. Johnson (Meet Your Patient), the person has lost contact with family members because of disagreements, you could collaborate with the social worker and chaplain about ways to facilitate a meeting if that is what the patient desires.

Forgiveness is considered one aspect of love. People have a spiritual need to forgive others, to be forgiven, and to forgive themselves (Cao et al., 2021; Harvard Health, 2021; Long et al., 2020).

- When a person cannot forgive others, it separates them from others and may interfere with the ability to move forward.
- When a person cannot forgive themselves, they may feel the pain of shame, guilt, and anger.
- The person may be hurting because they want forgiveness from someone they have wronged or from a higher power.
- Many people interpret their illness as punishment for sins.

You can help the person achieve spiritual peace by listening when the person expresses self-doubt or guilt, providing guidance, praying with the patient if they request it, or offering to contact their chosen spiritual leader if intensive spiritual support is needed.

Hope Inspiration (NIC) **Hope** is a subjective state of confidence in the possibility of a better future. It includes a positive orientation, faith, and will to live. **Hopelessness** is a state in which the person perceives limited or no alternatives or personal choices. To intervene effectively, it is important to know the source of the person's hope and the factors underlying the feelings of hopelessness. As a nurse, you can encourage spiritual growth, which is thought to facilitate hope, and you can refer your patient to a support group to help in stress reduction, coping, and hope.

Prayer (Non-NIC) Prayer is an integral component of almost every religion. Research shows that clients who received intercessory prayer had an improved quality of life (Struve et al., 2015). The purpose of prayer may be for health or simply to transform illness into a positive experience (Reimer-Kirkham et al., 2018). So, it is quite possible that a patient or a family member may ask you to pray for them or with them. It is important to distinguish between *praying with* and *praying for*.

- If the patient asks you to pray *with* them, determine whether the patient simply wants you to be present while they or another person leads the prayer. You should ask whether they want you to begin the prayer or whether they want to begin the prayer.
- If a patient asks you to pray *for* them, assess what it is that the patient wants you to pray for. Often the patient is merely asking you to pray for them on your own time, as frequently as your schedule allows.

Regardless of the situation, if you feel comfortable doing so, then you should enter the experience of prayer with confidence; after all, the patient or family member has asked you to be present because they feel at ease with you and trust in your abilities. However, if you feel at all uncomfortable about offering prayer, then you should state those feelings and offer to find someone who is comfortable with prayer. For example, you might say either of the following to the patient or family:

- "Thank you for asking me to pray with you; there is another nurse on the floor who is better at this than I am. May I have your permission to seek that person out for you?"
- "I am confident that the chaplain can help you in many ways with your request. May I make a referral to the chaplain for you?"

Prayer consists of those ways that we respond to and interact with the divine, whether by words, thoughts, or actions (e.g., the painting in Fig. 13-5). People tend to think of prayer in its narrowest sense as being requests for something (intercession), and this is an important and useful type of prayer. If you wish to pray with clients, understanding the different types of prayer may help. For various types of prayers,

 Go to **Clinical Insight 13-1: Types of Prayers** in Volume 2.

The following is an excerpt from an aunt's e-mail to a distribution group of her family and friends. It movingly demonstrates a belief in the powerful nature of prayer and is an example of how people rely on intercessory prayer during illness.

Example: I would really appreciate your prayers … for my nephew … who is newly diagnosed with Hodgkin's lymphoma. We go to the clinic at 10 a.m. to get his labs and then [to] the Children's Hospital to start his chemotherapy. … He is very sad and scared. His chest symptoms have increased … [and] we know the mass is still growing. Please pray … for wisdom and communication with the doctors and nurses. Pray all who come in contact with my nephew give peace, comfort, and soothing touch. Pray the side effects … are minimal. More than anything, … pray the chemo targets every cancerous cell … and specifically for greater than 70% shrinkage. [Pray also for] no more … fever, night

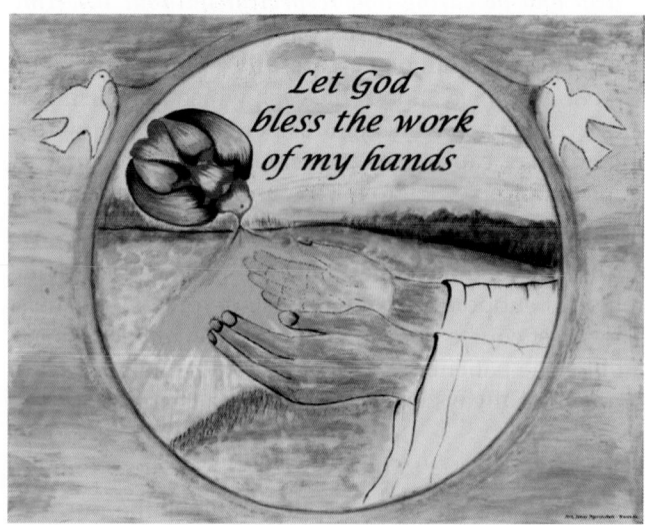

FIGURE 13-5 This painting may be an expression of prayer.

Holistic Healing

Intercessory Prayer

Many people pray when they are ill, and prayer seems to have positive effects. But what about the effects of *intercessory prayer*—the prayers of people for *others* who are ill? How useful is intercessory prayer? The following studies support the use of intercessory prayer as a complementary and alternative medicine (CAM):

➤ **Abu et al. (2019)**—In a study of 1,039 patients with acute cardiac syndrome, in which 88% were aware of intercessory prayers, results showed a clinically meaningful increase in their generic physical health–related quality-of-life score between 1 and 6 months after hospitalization compared with those who were unaware. In addition, patients receiving intercessory prayer had clinically meaningful improvements in their physical limitations.

➤ **Simao et al. (2016)**—Researchers found that prayer helped patients cope with illness and crisis, decreased anxiety and depression, and promoted better physical functioning. Recognizing prayer as a nonpharmacological intervention, they recommended its incorporation into clinical practice.

➤ **Struve et al. (2015)**—Researchers studied the effect of intercessory prayer on disruptive behaviors in six clients with late-stage dementia over a 12-week period. The results showed a reduction in disruptive behaviors in 27 categories per week. The use of antipsychotic medication was reduced or discontinued in four clients. The researchers concluded that intercessory prayer improved the clients' quality of life by reducing their disruptive behaviors.

sweats, weight loss, [and] chest pain. God truly can work miracles in times of trial and we are trusting fully in Him at this great time of need. (D. Wojcik, personal communication, March 1, 2013)

Prayer has a variety of purposes, expressions, and meanings to patients and their families, as well as to nurses. Prayer may provide for periods of intimacy with God, reveal the presence and love of God, and serve as a powerful source of comfort and hope.

 Go to **Clinical Insight 13-2: Praying With Patients,** in Volume 2.

Other Nursing Activities

Spiritual care in nursing often involves working with people who have come face to face with a significant life event that calls forth a new sense of meaning and purpose. Specific nursing activities, to be individualized to each client's needs, are discussed in the following list:

■ Make referrals when needed. Priests, ministers, rabbis, and other spiritual advisers are all resources for you and the client. There are times when you should refer a client to others with more knowledge and experience in religion and spirituality. For example, a client may be experiencing Spiritual Distress because they believe they need forgiveness for a past act, or a client may refuse medical treatment because they think their church would not approve.

■ For hospitalized and hospice clients, you can usually ask the chaplain's office to refer the client and family to clergy or religious counselors in the community.

■ For nonhospitalized clients, access an electronic or paper directory for local places of worship.

■ Encourage expression of feelings. The best way to do this is simply to ask the client how they are feeling or what they think about a particular situation.

■ Help the client identify feelings of guilt. You might ask the following after a client has voiced a concern: "How do you feel about that?" or "You seem to feel sad about saying/doing that."

■ Help significant others understand the client's feelings and needs. Encourage family members to talk with the client or simply to have a seat at the bedside. Periods of silence often lead to the most therapeutic of discussions.

■ Maximize the client's comfort. This is one of the most important spiritual activities a nurse can perform. A client cannot think about spiritual issues when plagued with physical pain or discomfort.

■ Listen to the patient's stories. These tell the life history surrounding the person's illness and spiritual comfort or distress.

■ Assess the client's needs for reconciliation. This may include reconciliation with self, others, and the divine. If the client has lost contact with family members because of disagreements related to past events, you could collaborate with the social worker and chaplain about ways to facilitate a meeting.

■ Explore with the client the possible meanings of *healing, miracle,* and *cure.*

■ Collaborate with the dietary department. Provide foods compatible with the person's religious needs. Encourage family members to bring foods from home, as appropriate.

■ Respect the client's dress (and other) requirements as determined by their religion. This may include religious icons, jewelry, or special clothes.

■ Do not make assumptions about the client's and family's beliefs. When a client dies, for example, making a seemingly harmless statement such as "They've gone to a better place" assumes the family believes in an afterlife. If they ask, you can briefly share your beliefs, but reflect their questions back to them (e.g., "Tell me what *you* think happens after death").

KnowledgeCheck 13-7

■ What is prayer?
■ What are ways you can support a client's prayer needs?
■ When a client asks you to pray for them, what might be your most effective first response?

♥ iCare 13-1

Older adults have identified their spiritual needs in healthcare settings as understanding their spiritual practices; relationship with God or other deity; hope, meaning, and purpose of life; and interpersonal connections and therapeutic professional staff interactions (Palmer et al., 2018).

Taking those needs into account, what are some concrete things you might do to demonstrate caring with older adult patients?

♥ iCare 13-2

Spirituality

- Spirituality means different things to different people.
- Spirituality has a great impact on a person's well-being and outlook on healthcare situations.
- A caring nurse is respectful and open to different religious beliefs, recognizing that spirituality is an accumulation of life experiences and is very personal in nature.
- Exhibiting empathy and a nonjudgmental attitude can be supportive and helpful.
- Often, you will not need to say anything. Simply listening and "being present" in the moment is beneficial.

ThinkLike a Nurse 13-10: Clinical Judgment in Action

A patient dying of lung cancer asks you to pray with him early one morning. You agree and ask him what he would like you to pray for. He responds: "That I may be cured of my cancer and go back home." He is on oxygen therapy, has pain medications given as prescribed, and is in a room by himself. You validate his information in the electronic health record (EHR) and note that he is a Christian. Construct a prayer that might be meaningful and helpful.

Return to the scenario for Charles Johnson (Meet Your Patient). See whether you can answer the three questions more completely now after reading this chapter.

Summary

In summary, the more you know about yourself, the more effectively you care for others. To work effectively with a diverse population, you must first obtain a great degree of self-knowledge. Try the following:

- Be open to the many possibilities for diverse thinking.
- Welcome challenging experiences that allow for personal growth.
- Take time to think about how your actions and biases might affect the care of others. As you know, communication and therapeutic relationships are important in supporting spirituality.

To explore learning resources for this chapter,

Go to Davis Advantage and find:

Answers and Suggested Responses for all questions in this chapter

Concept Map

Knowledge Map

References and Bibliography

CHAPTER 14

Experiencing Loss

Learning Outcomes

After completing this chapter, you should be able to:

➤ Name and describe at least four types of loss.

➤ Identify the stages of grief as described by major theorists.

➤ Compare and contrast four types of grief.

➤ List and discuss at least five factors that affect grieving.

➤ Define *death* according to the Uniform Determination of Death Act.

➤ Give a definition of *higher-brain death.*

➤ Create a timeline of the dying process, indicating the physiological signs and symptoms common to each stage.

➤ List and describe the models and theories of grief and bereavement.

➤ Define *end-of-life care, hospice care,* and *palliative care.*

➤ Identify the legal and ethical issues involved in death and dying.

➤ Apply the nursing process in the care of dying patients and their families.

➤ Describe the responsibilities of the nurse regarding postmortem care.

➤ Identify nursing interventions to help clients who are grieving.

Key Concepts

Death and dying

End-of-life care

Grief

Loss

Related Concepts

See the Concept Map on Davis Advantage.

Meet Your Patient

Thomas Manning is a 47-year-old man who is in the oncology unit with end-stage cancer of the pancreas. He is married and has three children, ages 18, 15, and 13 years. His oldest daughter has been away at college for only 6 months. Mr. Manning's father died 3 months ago from complications of alcoholism, and his mother has been withdrawn and grieving. His wife, Mary, tells you that Thomas "just wants to die" and does not want anyone trying to revive him or "push on his chest" if he dies. Mary is distressed and wants him to "keep fighting."

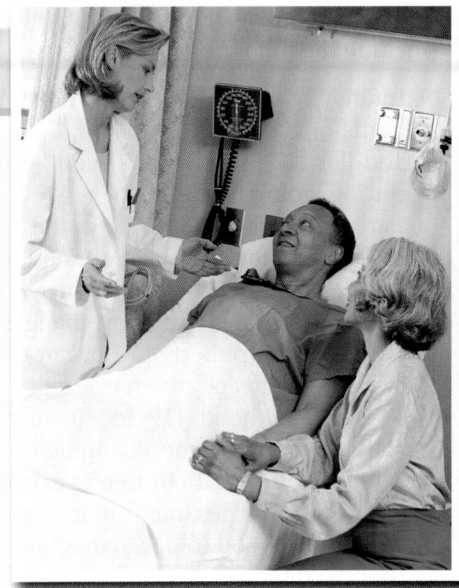

Theoretical Knowledge
knowing why

Throughout your nursing career, you will care for patients coping with loss—of youth, beauty, previous health, functioning, or quality of life. Many of your patients, like Thomas Manning, will be confronting their own approaching death, whereas family members will be facing the loss of their loved one. You can use your theoretical and practical knowledge to help these people cope with their losses and grieve in a way that is healing, even transformative. As a foundation, you must understand your own feelings and attitudes about loss, grief, and dying and have the competencies to intervene with skill and compassion.

ABOUT THE KEY CONCEPTS

To provide care for patients experiencing loss, you will need to understand the key concepts of **loss, grief, death and dying,** and **end-of-life care.** Related concepts, such as stages of death, depression, and grief education, will expand the way you think about the key concepts.

WHAT IS LOSS?

Do you associate *loss* with death? Many people think of losing a loved one through death. Loss is a daily occurrence. **Loss** can be defined as the undesired change or removal of a valued object, person, or situation. It begins at birth when we lose the warmth and security of the womb and ends with the ultimate loss, the death of self. Examples of losses at each stage of development include the following:

- Infancy (1 month to 1 year)—weaning from breast or bottle
- Toddler (12 months to 3 years)—loss of the familiar setting, going to preschool
- Early childhood (3 to 6 years)—going to full-day school, moving, and losing friends
- Middle childhood (6 years to puberty)—loss of the familiar, dealing with body changes
- Adolescence (puberty to 18 years)—loss of childhood, expectation to act grown up
- Young adulthood (19 to 40 years)—loss of single status/parents' home, changing relationships
- Middle adulthood (40 to 65 years)—children leaving home, job changes, medical issues
- Older adulthood (older than 65 years)—loss of health, friends; retirement

Categories of Loss

Loss can be categorized in the following ways.

Actual Versus Perceived Loss

- **Actual loss** includes the death of a loved one (or relationship), theft, deterioration, destruction, and natural

disaster. The loss can be identified by others, not just by the person experiencing it (e.g., hair loss during chemotherapy).
- **Perceived loss** is internal; it is identified only by the person experiencing it (e.g., a person who is now in middle adulthood may feel that they have lost their youth.).

Physical Loss Versus Psychological Loss

- **Physical loss** includes (1) injuries (e.g., when a limb is amputated), (2) removal of an organ (e.g., hysterectomy), and (3) loss of function (e.g., loss of mobility).
- **Psychological losses** challenge our belief system. Also known as *perceived losses,* they are commonly seen in the areas of sexuality, control, fairness, meaning, and trust.
- **Some losses may be mixed.** For example, after the removal of a prostate gland, a man may feel both the physical and psychological loss of sexuality.

External Versus Internal Loss

- **External losses** are actual losses of objects that are important to the person because of their cost or sentimental value (e.g., jewelry, a home). These losses can be brought about by theft, destruction, or disasters such as floods and fire.
- **Internal loss** is another term for perceived or psychological loss.

Loss of Aspects of Self These losses include physical losses such as the loss of body organs, limbs, and body functions and/or body disfigurement. Psychological and perceived losses in this category include aspects of one's personality, developmental change (as in the aging process), loss of hopes and dreams, and loss of faith.

Environmental Loss This loss involves a change in the familiar, even if the change is perceived as positive. Examples include moving to a new home, getting a new job, and going to college. These losses can be perceived or actual.

Loss of Significant Relationships This includes, but is not limited to, actual loss of spouses, siblings, family members, or significant others through death, divorce, or separation (e.g., military deployment).

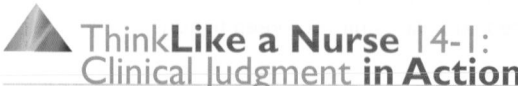

Think Like a Nurse 14-1:
Clinical Judgment in Action

- Which kinds of loss do you think Thomas Manning (Meet Your Patient) is experiencing?
- Why is it important to recognize loss?

WHAT IS GRIEF?

Whenever there is a significant loss, there is grieving. **Key Point:** *Although grieving requires energy and can interfere with health and delay healing, it is positive and essential to psychological healing after a loss.*

Consider the following losses and the different reactions of the patients involved:

Both Mr. Epse's and Mr. Maldona's spouses died 2 months ago. Mr. Epse's wife died after a 3-year battle with cancer. He and the family were at her bedside. Mr. Maldona's wife died of COVID-19 after being hospitalized for 2 days. He could not be at her bedside. Which spouse do you think will grieve the loss more? Why? Discuss this situation with a classmate. Do you both have the same opinion about this?

It is really impossible to decide who would feel "more" grief because the meaning of the circumstances surrounding each situation and the significance of the relationship may be different for each spouse. Both men are most likely grieving. **Key Point: *The intensity of the grief depends on the meaning the person attaches to the loss.***

The length and history of the relationship are most likely different for each spouse. One spouse had the opportunity to share the illness with his wife, whereas the other spouse experienced a fairly sudden loss. One person may feel as if he lost his companion, friend, confidant, soulmate, and source of stability, whereas another may simply feel as if he lost himself. **Key Point: *The grief response and the intensity of the grief will depend on the meaning the person attaches to the loss.*** This is true for everyone who experiences grief.

- **Grief** is the physical, psychological, and spiritual responses to a loss.
- **Mourning** consists of actions associated with grief (e.g., crying, wearing black clothing). These processes are normal and natural responses to a loss.
- **Bereavement** is the period of mourning and adjustment after a loss.
- **Key Point: *Although each person may express grief differently, some aspects of grief are shared by almost everyone.***

KnowledgeCheck 14-1

What types of losses commonly occur in our lives?

Theoretical Foundations of Grief

Traditional models of grief present the process as occurring in stages, cautioning that there is no single, correct way to grieve and that people do not move neatly from one stage or step of grief to the next. Rather, grieving is a fluid, ongoing process. Some theorists are moving away from stage models of grieving and toward the idea of grieving as a process of reconstructing meaning; that is, the meaning of and emotions surrounding the loss are constantly changing for the bereaved. See Table 14-1.

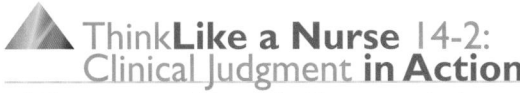

ThinkLike a Nurse 14-2: Clinical Judgment in Action

What are some of the similarities you see in the models/theories described in Table 14-1?

Factors Affecting Grief

To begin thinking about factors affecting grieving, consider the next exercise.

ThinkLike a Nurse 14-3: Clinical Judgment in Action

Mr. Klein is an 86-year-old man whose wife died of heart disease 2 months ago. He has two adult children, both of whom visit him regularly. He also has a very supportive pastor, Mr. Owens, who meets him in the park to share stories. Mr. Owens is 30 years old and has been raising his 5-year-old daughter alone after the sudden death of his wife 6 months ago in an automobile accident. His parents and siblings live out of state. Each man misses his wife very much.

- What factors do you think play a role in each man's grief?
- Who do you think will "get over it" faster?
- What are some issues that may make each man's grief uniquely difficult?

No two people ever grieve in the same manner because many factors play a role in the grieving process. They include the following:

- **Significance of the loss.** The meaning the person has attached to the person or object lost will be different for each person. The greater the attachment, the more difficult the grief will be.
- **Support system.** People with strong emotional and psychosocial support typically have less complicated grief.
- **Unresolved conflict.** Prolonged or dysfunctional (complicated) grief can occur with unresolved conflict. A conflict (e.g., an argument) left unresolved may cause prolonged grief.
- **Circumstances of the loss.** The manner and circumstances of the death can leave the bereaved feeling guilty, responsible, or unprepared. Violent deaths (e.g., homicide, suicide, accident) can result in prolonged or dysfunctional (complicated) grief.
- **Previous or multiple losses.** A person who has sustained several losses in a short period of time may experience dysfunctional (or complicated) grief. In the hospital, you will frequently care for patients with multiple losses; for example, a patient who has had a stroke with paralysis has lost their mobility, independence, and familiar surroundings when moved to a skilled care facility.
- **Spiritual/cultural beliefs and practices.** Spirituality and religious beliefs can help or hinder the grieving process. One person might believe the deceased is in a place of contentment and happiness, where all suffering is over. Another may believe that the deceased person will be reborn into another form. Yet another may believe that death is final, and there is no afterlife. Most cultures engage in rituals (e.g., funerals) that allow the bereaved to openly express their grief and pain (Fig. 14-1), whereas others may limit expressions of grief to private settings.
- **Timeliness of the death.** The death of a child or a young person is almost universally more difficult to accept than the death of an older person. In addition to the loss of the person, there is a sense of unfairness

Table 14-1 ➤ Theories and Models of Grief

STAGES	DESCRIPTION
George Engel (1961)—Three Stages of Grief	
Uncomplicated grief is universal, has a clear onset and a predictable course (with modifications), and does not require treatment.	
Shock and Disbelief	Initial phase. The sufferer denies the loss in an attempt to protect against the shock of reality.
Developing Awareness of the Loss	■ Painful feelings of sadness, guilt, shame, helplessness, hopelessness, loss, and emptiness ■ Loss of interest in usual activities; impaired work performance ■ Loss of appetite, sleep disturbances, physical symptoms of pain or other discomfort
Restitution and Recovery	■ Final phase; prolonged and gradual ■ Carries on the work of mourning and overcomes the trauma of the loss ■ A state of health and well-being is reestablished.
John Bowlby (1982)—Phases of Grief	
This attachment theory describes the reaction to strong emotional bonds that have been developed. The individual must work through each process to avoid complicated grief. Grief is a mature way of dealing with loss of attachment.	
Shock and Numbness	■ Initial stage ■ Disorientation ■ Feelings of helplessness
Yearning and Searching	■ The grieving person yearns to be reconnected with the deceased and searches for connections.
Disorganization and Despair	■ Permanence of the loss is now real ■ Feelings of pain ■ Emotions of grief to the fullest ■ Feels there is no hope of reconnection
Reorganization	■ Adjusting to life without the deceased (or lost object) ■ Developing new coping skills
Theresa Rando (1984, 1986, 1991, 1993, 2000)	
Rando identified the three Processes of Grieving described next. In addition, she identified six tasks (6Rs) associated with grieving: (1) recognizing the loss, (2) reacting to the separation, (3) recollecting memories of the deceased, (4) relinquishing the old attachment, (5) readjusting to the new environment, and (6) reinvesting self.	
Avoidance	■ Shock, disbelief, denial, anger, bargaining
Confrontation	■ Begins to face the loss ■ A very emotional and upsetting time when grief is felt most acutely
Accommodation	■ Begins to live with the loss ■ Feels better ■ Resumes some routine activities

Table 14-1 ➤ Theories and Models of Grief—cont'd

STAGES	DESCRIPTION
William Worden (2002)—Four Tasks of Grieving	
Accepting the Reality of the Loss	***Realizing that the loved one (or object) is gone*** ■ In the hours and days after a significant loss, the grieving person typically feels numb and unable to accept the fact of the loss. ■ Numbness is thought to be a helpful form of denial, which allows the person to "take in" only what the psyche is capable of handling. ■ The task of realizing the loved one or object is gone may take several days or, in the case of a sudden death, weeks.
Working Through the Pain and Grief	***Feelings and emotions that surface are intense and can change rapidly.*** ■ Feels "out of control" ■ May say they feel as if they are "going crazy" ■ Usually the longest phase for two reasons: 　• Because none of us likes to be in pain, we become expert at finding ways not to feel it. We overeat, overmedicate, overwork, and drink to excess to avoid feeling the pain, and we thereby prolong the process of grief. 　• Caring people do not like to see their loved ones in pain, so they make attempts to remove the pain (e.g., by distraction) rather than letting the person experience it. Like avoidance, this well-meaning behavior also prolongs the process.
Adjusting to the Environment in Which the Deceased Is Missing	***Adjusting to the environment without the deceased*** ■ This may mean performing activities and tasks, such as going for walks or shopping, that were once shared by themselves. ■ It may include taking on roles and responsibilities that the deceased previously held. ■ Such experiences can be extremely sad, frustrating, and challenging or very rewarding. ■ Once the person has established the new pattern, they typically feel satisfaction and increased self-esteem.
Emotionally Relocating the Deceased and Moving on With Life	***Investing emotional energy.*** ■ Initially all energy is focused on the deceased: thinking about the person, talking about them, reliving memories, and so on. It is nearly impossible to think of anything else. ■ Concentration is difficult, so the grieving person finds it hard to engage in activities such as reading. ■ When the person's energy begins to flow toward others or to different or former interests (e.g., working, socializing), the healing process is in progress.
Elisabeth Kübler-Ross (1969)—Five Stages of Grieving	
Individuals may not experience every stage or go through the stages in a linear order. In addition, individuals may experience two or more stages simultaneously.	
Denial	■ "Not me"; "This cannot be happening"; "I don't believe it" ■ The person is usually in a state of shock. ■ Denial is not necessarily negative; it gives the person a chance to prepare psychologically for accepting the news.

(Continued)

Table 14-1 ➤ Theories and Models of Grief—cont'd

STAGES	DESCRIPTION
Anger	■ "Why me?"; "Why is this happening?" ■ Anger can be obvious or subtle. ■ Anger is the person's response to the feeling that the situation is unfair. ■ The person may take their anger out on people who are "safe" (e.g., family, spouse) or from whom there will be no reprisals (e.g., nurses, provider).
Bargaining	■ "If only I can live until …"; "Yes, but …" Usually this takes the form of a bargain with God or a higher power, in which the person asks to live to see a birth, graduation, wedding, and so forth.
Depression	■ A withdrawn sadness, not to be confused with clinical depression. This is a response to the current loss as well as to any accumulated and/or future losses.
Acceptance	■ Not necessarily *wanting* death (or the loss) but coming to terms with it and ceasing to fight it. The person may seem almost devoid of feelings.

Margaret Stroebe and Henk Schut (1999)—Dual-Process Model

Mourning is cyclical. People oscillate between two dimensions in bereavement.

Loss-Oriented Response	■ Focuses on grief work ■ Concentrates on appraising and processing the loss; searches for meaning ■ Experiencing pain
Restoration-Oriented Response	■ Focuses on dealing with the consequences of the loss ■ Establishes new routines and takes on new roles (paying bills, doing laundry) ■ Reorients to the world without the deceased person

Dennis Klass, Phyllis R. Silverman, and Steven L. Nickman (1996)—Continuing Bond Model

Bereavement, or grief, is never fully resolved.

■ The focus should not be on individuals obtaining closure but instead on finding new ways to relate to the deceased.

■ The griever maintains a continuing bond with the deceased.

Negotiate and Renegotiate	■ The meaning of the loss is negotiated and renegotiated over time. ■ However, the emphasis is not on achieving closure or forgetting. ■ The emphasis is on establishing therapeutic expressions of continuing bonds to adapt to the loss (e.g., memorabilia, pictures).

Robert Neimeyer (1999)—Meaning-Making Model of Grief/Bereavement

Grieving is a process of meaning reconstruction. The best predictor of a positive adaptation to loss is the ability to find meaning in the loss. The unsuccessful struggle to find meaning can result in complicated forms of grief.

Sources: Bowlby, J. (1982). *Attachment and loss* (Vols. 1–3). Basic Books; Colvin, C. & Ceide, M. (2021). Review of grief therapies for older adults. *Current Geriatrics Reports, 10,* 116–123. https://doi.org/10.1007/s13670-021-00362-w; Engel, G. L. (1961). Is grief a disease? A challenge for medical research. *Psychosomatic Medicine,* 23(1), 18–22; Kübler-Ross, E. (1969). *On death and dying.* Macmillan; Neimeyer, R. (1999). Narrative strategies in grieving therapy. *Journal of Constructivist Psychology,* 12(1), 65–68; Rando, T. (1984). *Grief, dying and death: Clinical interventions for caregivers.* Research Press; Smit, C. (2015). Theories and models of grief: Applications to professional practice. *Whitireia Nursing and Health Journal,* 22(1), 33–37; Stroebe, M., & Schut, H. (1999). The dual process model of coping with bereavement: Rationale and description. *Death Studies,* 23(3), 197–224; Stroebe, M., & Schut, H. (2010). The dual process model of coping: A decade on. *Omega: Journal of Death and Dying,* 61(4), 273–289; Worden, J. W. (2002). *Grief counseling and grief therapy: A handbook for the mental health practitioner* (3rd ed.). Springer.

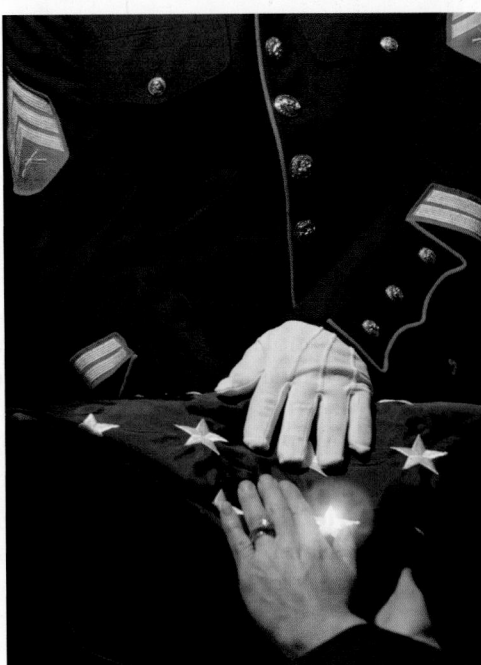

FIGURE 14-1 Rituals are used to facilitate grieving.

because of the loss of *potential*—of what the child might have become or achieved.

Developmental Stages and Grief

Based on Erik Erikson's stages of psychological growth, we all must achieve certain psychological milestones during a lifetime. Grief can affect the healthy development of life stages, and in turn, the person's stage of development can affect the grieving process. Refer to Chapter 6, Life Span: Infancy Through Middle Adulthood, if you need to review Erikson's theory.

Childhood Because cognitive development is not yet complete, preschool children believe that death is temporary and reversible, as with cartoon characters that "die" and then "come to life" again.

- During early childhood, children begin to understand that death is permanent, but they believe that it will never happen to them or anyone they know.
- Young children believe they are the cause of what happens around them. This is known as *magical thinking*. Such thinking may cause them to feel guilt when someone close to them dies.
- Other responses include regressing to a previous developmental stage: "acting like a baby," demanding food and attention, becoming incontinent, and talking "baby talk."

During the weeks after a death, a child may feel immediate grief, may or may not display sadness, or may continue to believe the person is still alive. These are normal reactions.

Adolescence The bereavement and emotions felt by adolescents, along with confusion regarding their

identity and role, can create major uncertainty. The adolescent is struggling to learn who they are as a person as they break away from parental control. The loss of a parent during this time may create a sense of guilt and unfinished business.

At the same time, the bereaved teen also faces psychological, physiological, social, and academic pressures. Although teens may look mature, they often lack emotional maturity but are often expected to be "grown up" and support a surviving parent or younger siblings. When they feel this responsibility, they do not have the opportunity, or the permission, to mourn and may turn to those outside of the family to discuss their feelings.

Research shows that bereaved youths who have lost a parent or sibling experience a wide range of unhealthy symptoms and behaviors (e.g., anxiety, depression, delinquency, aggression, suicidal ideation or attempts, post-traumatic stress disorders) (Shulla & Toomey, 2018; Slomski, 2021). Adult caregivers must be alert to these behaviors and take appropriate interventions to meet the bereavement and safety needs of children and adolescents.

Adulthood Adults are cognitively able to understand the nature of death and have usually experienced other types of loss. Over time, they perceive loss as a normal part of living. How they respond to loss depends on factors, such as the person's self-esteem and the availability of support.

Older Adulthood A special difficulty for older adults is the cumulative effects of the many losses that they experience. Most deaths occur among older adults, so they are likely to lose friends and siblings in rapid succession, in addition to physical and functional losses and the loss of independence. However, the loss of a child can create significant and sometimes irreparable mental and physical outcomes, accelerated disabilities, and loss of the ability to function independently. To minimize these negative outcomes, caregivers should use listening skills and metaphors and promote storytelling (Alftberg et al., 2018; Gerber et al., 2022). In addition, professional counseling can help older adults deal with the devastating emotional impact of losses and guide them as they begin the process of preparatory grief in anticipation of their own death (Colvin & Ceide, 2021; Meichsner et al., 2020).

KnowledgeCheck 14-2
- What are the main tasks of the grieving process?
- What factors affect the grieving process?

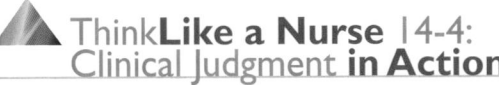
ThinkLike a Nurse 14-4: Clinical Judgment in Action
Refer to Thomas Manning and his wife (Meet Your Patient). Apply each of the factors affecting grief to Thomas and to Mary (they may be different for each spouse). If the scenario does not provide enough information for you to comment, say so and then describe how you would obtain the data you need.

Types of Grief

Grief can be categorized in several ways, most of which have to do with timing and intensity.

Uncomplicated Grief (Normal/Functional Grief) This is the natural response to the loss of a person or object. The bereaved person may experience a range of feelings, behaviors, and thoughts related to the loss. Emotions are initially intense but gradually diminish over time (several months to several years). The recognition and meaning of the loss will always be present, but the intensity of the responses will lessen.

Dysfunctional (Complicated Grief) Also known as *prolonged acute grief*, this is characterized by intensity of emotion and length of time. The person's responses are maladaptive, dysfunctional, unusually prolonged, or overwhelming (Iglewicz et al., 2020). For example, the bereaved may become severely depressed, violent, or suicidal; a "workaholic"; socially isolated; or demonstrate addictive behavior. After several years, the person may still be experiencing as much pain and disruption as in the first months after the loss. Chronic grief, masked grief, and delayed grief are all examples of dysfunctional (complicated) grief:

- **Chronic grief** begins as normal grief but continues long term, with little resolution of feelings and an inability to rejoin normal life.
- **Masked grief** occurs when the person is grieving but expressing the grief through other types of behavior. For example, a person whose spouse has died may begin drinking heavily, or a couple who have lost a child may start to argue more intensely with each other. They may not recognize this change in behavior as part of their grief response.
- **Delayed grief** is grief that is put off until a later time (e.g., "I'll think about it later; right now, I'm busy trying to keep a roof over our heads and care for my children").

The following scenario is an example of complicated grief. In each of these instances, the bereaved person lacks coping mechanisms and/or the familial or communal support that is helpful in overcoming grief.

John and Cyndi Kieryls had been married for 15 years. This is a second marriage for both. Cyndi's older brother, Craig, and his daughter, Lyllie, live with them. They moved into a new neighborhood 4 years ago, and the family has been very active in local events. Cyndi has fibromyalgia, and John has type 2 diabetes. After returning home from a fishing trip, John found Cyndi deceased in the house. Craig and Lyllie were away on vacation. John was extremely upset and heartbroken.

The neighbors were very supportive of the Kieryls. They prepared meals for the first month after Cyndi's death. However, 15 months later, John still cries inconsolably every time he talks to anyone. He only wants to talk about his love for Cyndi and what a dark place the world has become. He refused his provider's referral to grief counseling, asserting that no one can understand what he is feeling. The neighbors have started to avoid him, and Craig and Lyllie moved back to their home state. John started to neglect his health and his environment. He is currently hospitalized with hyperglycemia and dehydration.

Complicated grief can have social, physical, emotional, and financial consequences.

Disenfranchised Grief This is experienced in connection with a loss that is not socially supported or acknowledged by the usual rites or ceremonies. Some examples include the unplanned termination of a child's foster placement or a mistress whose lover dies (Albuquerque, 2021; Lockton et al., 2020). In each of these instances, the bereaved person lacks the familial or communal support that is helpful in grieving.

Anticipatory Grief This type of grief is experienced before a loss occurs. Think back to Mr. Epse, whose wife died after a 3-year battle with cancer. He most likely grieved as he watched the vibrant woman he once knew change before his eyes and as he anticipated her death. Family members experience anticipatory grief as they watch a loved one with Alzheimer disease lose mental capacity and realize that the person they once knew is becoming progressively removed from them. Potential negative outcomes of anticipatory grief are that the survivor may detach from a dying person too early in the dying process, leaving the dying person without emotional support, or it may prolong the grief of the survivor.

ThinkLike a Nurse 14-5: Clinical Judgment in Action

Thomas Manning (Meet Your Patient) had a strained relationship with his father for most of his life. His father was an alcoholic and constantly fought with his mother while Thomas was growing up. A few months ago, his father was hospitalized for the third time for complications of alcoholism. Thomas visited and confronted his father regarding his drinking and the problems and pain it had caused him and the family. The confrontation ended in an argument. That night, Thomas' father slipped into a coma. He died a few days later, without recovering consciousness.

- What issues does Thomas have to deal with?
- Why might this be a dysfunctional (complicated) grief process?

DEATH AND DYING

In mainstream North American culture, death is not seen as a natural part of life but rather as something to avoid at all costs. Death is associated with the loss of physical control and function, independence, relationships, and possibilities. Death is the ultimate loss.

How Is Death Defined?

The definitions of death have evolved with considerations of technology.

- **Higher-brain death.** Historically, some practitioners used the term **higher-brain death,** which defined

EXAMPLE CLIENT CONDITION: Complicated Grief

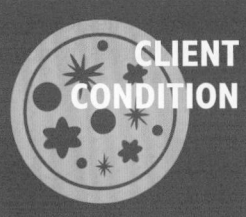
CLIENT CONDITION

Problem:

Complicated (Dysfunctional) Grief Also known as *prolonged acute grief*, this is characterized by intensity of emotion and length of time. The person's responses are maladaptive, dysfunctional, unusually prolonged, or overwhelming (Iglewicz et al., 2020). For example, the bereaved may become severely depressed, violent, or suicidal; may become highly socially isolated; or may demonstrate addictive behavior. After several years, the person may still be experiencing as much pain and disruption as in the first months after the loss. Chronic grief, masked grief, and delayed grief are all examples of dysfunctional (complicated) grief:

- **Chronic grief** extends beyond the normal grief period and negatively affects the ability to rejoin normal life.
- **Masked grief** occurs when the person is grieving but expressing the grief through other types of behavior. For example, a person whose spouse has died may begin drinking heavily or a couple who lost a child may start to argue more intensely with each other. They may not recognize this change in behavior as part of their grief response.
- **Delayed grief** is grief that is put off until a later time (e.g., "I'll think about it later; right now, I'm busy trying to keep a roof over our heads and care for my children").

In each of these instances, the bereaved person lacks coping mechanisms and/or the familial or communal support that is helpful in overcoming grief.

Incidence

After a loss, most people will experience intense grief that decreases over time. However, a small percentage (7%–10%) will experience prolonged grief disorder, characterized by continued high levels of grief symptoms (Szuhany et al., 2021).

Contributing Factors

- The factors that contribute to prolonged grief disorders are varied and not well defined.
- Literature reviews identify several factors, including, but not limited to, sudden unexpected loss, sense of blame, lack of coping skills, inability to process the loss, avoidance behaviors, inadequate social support, and preexisting mood disorders.

Consequences

- Individuals suffering from prolonged grief disorders are not focused on the future.
- They are feeling an intense amount of emotional pain.
- This can lead to depression, suicidal ideations; suicide attempts; lack of engagement in life activities; and health problems, often due to neglect of preventive and maintenance interventions.

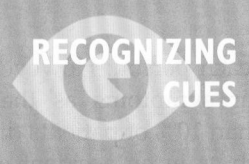
RECOGNIZING CUES

- Use a compassionate, accepting, nonjudgmental approach.
- Assess for history of mental health disorders.
- Assess for suicidal ideations.
- Assess history of previous losses.

- Assess for alteration in daily activities (eating, sleeping, hygiene, engagement, etc.).
- Assess for physiological functioning (vital signs, weight loss/gain, hydration status).
- Assess support network and resources (e.g., church, family, friends).

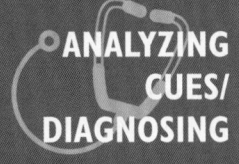
ANALYZING CUES/ DIAGNOSING

- Ineffective coping strategies related to difficulty adapting to loss of a spouse as evidenced by excessive crying, expressions of meaningless life.

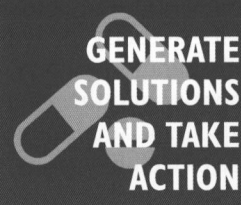
GENERATE SOLUTIONS AND TAKE ACTION

- Implement actions to promote physiological well-being.
- Collaborate with the interprofessional team to facilitate referral to appropriate resources.
- Determine the patients' support sources (e.g., family church, community).

- Discuss with patient the benefits of bereavement counseling and support groups.
- Explore previous losses and coping strategies.
- Provide emotional support.
- Encourage patient to identify activities they find meaningful and enjoyable.

(continued)

EXAMPLE CLIENT CONDITION: Complicated Grief—cont'd

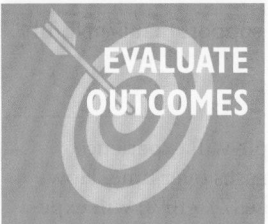

EVALUATE OUTCOMES

The patient will:
- Have a sense of peace, well-being, and acceptance of their loss.

- Demonstrate effective coping strategies.
- Demonstrate less emotional distress, which continues to resolve over time.

death as the irreversible cessation of all "higher"-brain functions (e.g., cognitive functioning, consciousness, memory, reasoning). By this definition, a functioning brainstem could maintain both respiratory and cardiac activity, although the person does not make purposive responses to external stimuli, cephalic reflexes are absent, and the electroencephalogram shows no activity.

- In 1978, the **Uniform Law Commission** redefined death broadly as the "irreversible cessation of all functioning of the brain, including the brainstem" as determined by reasonable medical standards. This definition did not provide clear guidance to states.

- In 1981, the **Uniform Determination of Death Act** was adopted to further clarify (see Box 14-1) and expand the previous definition to include the "irreversible cessation of circulation and respiratory functions" based on acceptable medical standards. Providers use several methods to assess for functioning of the brainstem (e.g., pupils fixed and unresponsive to light, no corneal reflex, absence of vestibulo-ocular reflexes).

What Are Coma and Persistent Vegetative State?

A **coma** is a prolonged, deep state of unconsciousness lasting days or even years. The patient cannot be aroused and may or may not have decreased brainstem

reflexes. The degree of damage to the higher-brain area or cortex determines whether the coma is reversible or irreversible.

The loss of higher cerebral functions can result in a **persistent vegetative state (PVS)**, in which the person does not purposefully respond to stimuli, is unaware of the environment, and has no cognition or affective mental functions. Thus, the person cannot speak or obey commands. Patients in a PVS may look somewhat normal and may occasionally grimace, cry, or laugh. They continue to have a sleep–wake cycle, may have some spontaneous movements, and may open their eyes in response to external stimuli. The family may believe that the patient is responding to the environment and thus not want to give up hope for recovery. The grieving process can be continuous, delayed, or prolonged.

What Are the Stages of Dying?

To help dying patients and their families understand the dying process, your theoretical knowledge base must include information on both physiological and psychological processes.

Physiological Stages of Dying

The dying process is unique to each person. However, people experience many similar symptoms as they approach the end of life. Fewer than 10% of patients die suddenly and unexpectedly, such as in an accident or massive heart attack. Ninety percent die after a long illness, progressively deteriorating until entering an active dying phase at the end (Emanuel et al., 2015; Knight & von Gunten, n.d.). The following timeline describes the physiological responses of that group (Burgess, 2020; DerSarkissian, 2020; Emanuel et al., 2015; Lee et al., 2019).

One to Three Months Before Death The dying person begins to withdraw from the world and people. Sleep increases; it becomes difficult for the body to digest food, especially meat; and appetite and food intake decrease. Liquids are preferred. Anorexia and the resulting ketosis may be protective because they can diminish pain and increase the person's sense of well-being.

One to Two Weeks Before Death A host of physical changes indicates the body is beginning to lose its ability to maintain itself. Cardiovascular deterioration

---

BOX 14-1 ■ Uniform Determination of Death Act

1. **[Determination of Death]** An individual who has sustained either (1) irreversible cessation of circulatory and respiratory functions or (2) irreversible cessation of all functions of the entire brain, including the brainstem, is dead. A determination of death must be made in accordance with accepted medical standards.

2. **[Uniformity of Construction and Application]** This Act shall be applied and construed to effectuate its general purpose to make uniform the law with respect to the subject of this Act among states enacting it.

Source: President's Commission for the Study of Ethical Problems in Medicine and Biomedical and Behavioral Research. (1981). *Defining death: A report on the medical, legal, and ethical issues in the determination of death* (p. 73). Government Printing Office.

brings reduced blood pressure, changes in pulse and skin color (e.g., a yellowish pallor), and extreme pallor of the extremities. Temperature fluctuates, and perspiration increases. Respiratory rate may increase or decrease. During sleep, the dying person may experience brief periods of apnea. Congestion may cause a rattling sound and/or a nonproductive cough.

Days to Hours Before Death Often a surge of energy brings mental clarity and a desire to eat and talk with family members. However, as death approaches, patients tend to become dehydrated and have difficulty swallowing, which results in decreased blood volume. The tissues of the tongue and soft palate sag, and the gag reflex declines, so secretions accumulate in the oropharynx and/or bronchi. Often the mucous membranes become dry and tacky, and the lips become cracked. Dehydration during the last hours of dying is thought not to cause distress and perhaps to stimulate endorphin release (DerSarkissian, 2020; Emanuel et al., 2015).

- **Respirations**—Breathing may be shallow, rapid, or irregular; periods of apnea may lengthen to 10 to 30 seconds before breathing resumes.
  - Congestion causes a "death rattle" that can be quite loud.
  - **Cheyne-Stokes respirations** may occur. This is a cyclic pattern consisting of a 10- to 60-second period of apnea and then a gradual increase in the depth and rate of respirations. Respirations gradually become slow and shallow, and then the cycle begins again with apnea.
- **Peripheral circulation** decreases, and the person perspires and feels "clammy."
  - Blood pressure decreases; pulse may be hard to detect.
  - Extremities become cool and mottled; the underside of the body may be much darker.
  - Decreased circulation also results in reduced kidney function and decreased urinary output.
- **Elimination**—As peristalsis slows, the patient may retain feces. Urine output decreases, and the urine often becomes more concentrated and foul-smelling. Sphincters relax, and bowel and bladder incontinence can occur.
- **Muscles** throughout the body relax, causing the face to "droop."
- **Vision** blurs; the eyes may be open or partially open but unseeing. Instead, the patient may see things that are not visible to others.
- **Cognition**—In the final hours of life, many patients become restless and agitated. This response may be caused by medications, liver failure, cerebral hypoxia, renal failure, stool impaction, distended bladder, increased pain, or unresolved emotional or spiritual issues. Near the time of death, some people unexpectedly become more coherent and energized for a time. Others become less communicative, quiet, and withdrawn (DerSarkissian, 2020; Emanuel et al., 2015). Fatigue is common.

Moments Before Death The dying person does not respond to touch or sound and cannot be awakened. Typically, there is a short series of long-spaced breaths before breathing ceases entirely and the heart stops beating.

Psychological Stages of Dying

Perhaps the best-known author on the psychology of dying is Dr. Elisabeth Kübler-Ross (1969). She felt that if people understood what dying patients are experiencing, they would be more competent in caring for them. She found that people tend to experience one or more of five psychological stages during the period from the terminal diagnosis to the actual death (Table 14-1). When you study the Kübler-Ross stages, it is important to understand that a dying person:

- May not go through every stage.
- May not go through the stages in a linear fashion but rather in random order.
- Does not necessarily complete one stage and move on to the next.
- May experience two or three stages simultaneously.

Key Point: *Remember that it is not the nurse's responsibility to move people to the next stage so that dying patients accept death. It is our responsibility to accept and support people "where they are" and help them to verbalize their feelings. We need to understand patients, not change them.*

What Is End-of-Life Care?

When, precisely, is the end of life? There is no set, agreed-upon definition or set of criteria. A recent set of guidelines provides a working definition that includes the following three situations:

- The patient has a fatal condition.
- Death is likely with the next exacerbation of disease.
- The patient acknowledges the seriousness of the situation.

The goal is to ensure that end-of-life care is delivered with compassion, sensitivity, and competency. Some of these competencies include the following (Ferrell et al., 2018):

- Making a holistic assessment of patients and families (i.e., physical, psychological, social, and spiritual)
- Acknowledging diversity in patients' beliefs and customs
- Promoting the provision of comfort care to the patient by addressing symptoms (e.g., pain, dyspnea, constipation, anxiety, fatigue, nausea, vomiting, altered cognition)
- Evaluating the impact of traditional, complementary, and technological therapies on patient, families, and established outcomes
- Incorporating essential communication strategies that meet spiritual and cultural needs

- Applying legal and ethical principles to end-of-life care
- Demonstrating respect for the patients' views and wishes during end-of-life care
- Assessing patient, family, colleagues, and one's own success in coping with suffering, grief, loss, and bereavement at the end of life
- Recognizing one's own attitudes, feelings, values, and expectations about death and dying
- Providing quality postmortem care

End-of-life care includes palliative care and hospice care, which are similar in that both may involve caring for dying patients, and neither focuses on cure. Some people use the terms interchangeably; however, there are subtle differences.

Palliative Care

Palliative care is actually aggressively planned comfort care. It addresses end-of-life care concerns that include supporting families and caregivers, promoting continuity of care, ensuring respect for persons, addressing emotional and spiritual concerns, managing symptoms (e.g., pain, dyspnea, depression), and ensuring informed decision making.

When patients reach a stage in their illness in which cure is no longer possible, or when they refuse further treatment, they may be eligible to receive "comfort care"—meaning that no further efforts will be made to stop the disease process or prevent the patient from dying. However, the patient will receive treatment to minimize unpleasant symptoms (e.g., nausea, pain). Although the correct interpretation of the term *comfort care* is, "Nothing more *can* be done to cure your loved one," family members may interpret it as "Nothing more *will* be done." In this situation, the term *palliative care,* which refers to care provided by a holistic team of professionals, may be more acceptable. Palliative care can occur in a variety of settings (e.g., at home, assisted living facilities, acute care facilities, long-term care facilities). Providers should understand and educate patients and families on end-of-life care and be comfortable with providing care (Emanuel et al., 2015; National Institute on Aging, 2021; Schroeder & Lorenz, 2018).

A patient does not necessarily have to be "actively dying" to receive palliative care. It is also provided over a long period of time for those who have slowly progressive diseases. The overall goal of palliative care is increased patient/family satisfaction, improved symptom control, and cost savings for hospitals (Schroeder & Lorenz, 2018).

Hospice Care

The first modern-day hospice was founded in 1968 by Dame Cicely Sanders in a London hospital.

- **Hospice care focuses on holistic care of patients who are dying or debilitated and not expected to improve.** Unlike palliative care, for a patient to be eligible for hospice insurance benefits, a provider must certify that the patient is likely to die within 6 months.
- **Hospice care is based on two key premises:**
  - The quality of life is as important as the length of life.
  - Those who are terminally ill should be allowed to face death with dignity and while surrounded by the comfort of their homes and families.
- **The purposes of admitting a patient to hospice are to:**
  - Provide a family with some respite for a period of time
  - Stabilize a patient who requires symptom management
  - Care for a patient who is in the end stage of a disease (e.g., cancer) and needs a level of expert care that family members cannot provide at home
- **An interprofessional team plans holistic care with the patient and family.**
  - Family members are encouraged to be active in the team to the extent they are able.
  - Nursing support is available 24 hours a day, and families are taught what to expect as the disease progresses. As the patient nears death, hospice workers remain as long as necessary.
  - After the patient dies, there is follow-up bereavement care for the families.

Legal and Ethical Considerations at End of Life

The technology of life support makes it possible to prolong bodily functions almost indefinitely, leaving patients and families struggling with decisions about prolonging life. More clients depend on nurses for education regarding patient rights and end-of-life care choices. Each situation is unique, and you should be able to explore with clients the various options available. See Chapter 5, Ethics & Values, and Chapter 39, Legal Accountability, more information about the ethical and legal aspects of each of the following topics.

Advance Directives

An **advance directive** is a group of instructions (written or oral) stating a person's wishes regarding their healthcare if they are incapacitated or unable to make

---

♥ iCare 14-1

Rebecca

Rebecca is a 30-year-old woman who has end-stage colon cancer; she has been hospitalized for 21 days. You have gotten to know her very well, and she shares with you that she always loved walking on the beach and feeling the sun on her face. After lunch, you inform Rebecca there is another important test that has been prescribed. You have obtained administrative approval and surprise Rebecca by taking her outside for a little while and allowing her to feel the warmth of the sun on her face and get a breath of fresh air.

End-of-Life Care

➤ **Dingley et al. (2021)** found that a synthesis of the research literature demonstrated overall support for complementary therapies on physical symptom management (e.g., fatigue, dyspnea, nausea, vomiting, appetite) and psychosocial and spiritual support (e.g., mood, inner peace, quality of life, agitation). However, flaws in research methodologies limited the significance of the studies related to consistency in findings and sustainment of positive findings.

➤ **Candy et al. (2020)** found that the evidence was inconclusive on the effectiveness of massage and aromatherapy in reducing anxiety and pain and improving quality of life. There was low-quality evidence that reflexology reduced pain.

➤ **Zeng et al. (2018)** found that common complementary and alternative medicine (CAM) methods (e.g., acupressure, breathing, hypnotherapy, meditation, reflexology, Reiki) provided only short-term benefits in the improvement of various symptoms (e.g., fatigue, anxiety, pain, dyspnea, nausea, vomiting) in patients receiving hospice and palliative care.

that decision. An ordinary power of attorney does not give another person the right to make healthcare decisions for the patient; only a durable power of attorney for healthcare decisions can do that.

The **Patient Self-Determination Act (PSDA),** passed by Congress in 1990, requires that all healthcare providers who receive Medicare funds (e.g., hospitals, home care agencies, hospices, nursing homes) must (1) educate staff and patients, (2) provide patients with information on their rights to accept or refuse treatment, and (3) provide an opportunity for all patients to complete an advance directive. Hospital providers and staff must comply with the wishes of the patient regarding end-of-life decisions (Centers for Medicare & Medicaid Services [CMS], 2020). The laws in each state vary regarding advance directives. It is important for you to understand the federal and state laws and the policies of your institution. Two types of advance directives serve different purposes:

- A **living will** is a document that provides specific instructions about the kinds of healthcare the person would wish (e.g., pain medications) or would wish *not* to have (e.g., ventilator support) in particular situations.
- A **durable power of attorney (DPOA)** for healthcare, or **healthcare proxy,** identifies another person to make decisions for the individual regarding healthcare choices when an individual is unable to do so based on circumstances (e.g., irreversible coma, dementia). The individual should provide specific instructions about their desires regarding hydration, feeding tubes,

medication, resuscitation, and mechanical ventilation. Because this is a legal document, it should be properly prepared (executed) and can be changed or canceled at any time by the patient. Nurses should document whether the patient has an advance directive in the medical records.

Key Point: *Some people fear that once an advance directive is signed, no further care will be provided. Explain to families and patients that this is not true; instead, the directive is intended to make sure they will get the level of care they desire.* Remind patients that they should formulate advance directives while they are healthy. Such explanations are independent nursing activities, for which you are responsible. To download a copy of your state's advance directives,

 Go to **https://www.caringinfo.org/planning/advance-directives/by-state/**

Respecting Patient and Family Needs

Chapter Key Concepts: Loss, grief, dying, end-of-life care

Competency: Goal-Directed Client-Centered Care (Thinking, Doing, Caring)

Situation: Karen Litvak is a 64-year-old woman who has lived her entire life with her mother. Her 86-year-old mother is hospitalized with pneumonia. Karen spends each day at her side. "I don't know how to help her," Karen says to the nurse. "She always took care of me." When her mother stopped breathing, a code was called, and doctors, nurses, and therapists ran into the room and began aggressive resuscitation (CPR). Karen stood out of the way but did not leave the room. The chaplain asked her to come out into the hallway with him, but she refused. The chaplain continued to urge her until she said forcefully, "No, I want to stay." Karen looked to the nurses, who nodded yes, she could stay.

The CPR efforts were not successful. The nurses asked Karen whether she would like to come closer while they washed her mother's body. Karen talked about her mother as the nurses wiped her mother's face and hands, put a clean hospital gown on her, and folded a clean sheet up to her waist. Karen thanked the nurses and turned to go. The nurses asked her where she would go and whether she had anyone to stay with her. She said she had a sister and would stay with her for a while.

Think about it: Client-centered care means showing respect for the client's values, religious beliefs, needs, and preferences.

➤ Should the nurses have allowed Karen to stay during CPR? Why or why not?

➤ How did the nurses show respect for Karen?

Prescriptions for DNR/DNAR

A **do-not-resuscitate (DNR) prescription** is written by a provider and means do *not* resuscitate the patient (or DNAR—do not attempt resuscitation) in the event of cardiac or respiratory failure. You may also see the previously widely used acronym "No CPR" (no cardiopulmonary resuscitation). Some people may advocate for the acronym **AND** (allow natural death) as a more positive term in end-of-life situations. However, evidence did not support the continued use of the AND acronym because although it is viewed as positive, its use contributed to confusion about the multiple concepts related to the do-not-resuscitate focus. The most recent guidance from the American Nurses Association (ANA) is the acronym DNR (ANA Ethics Advisory Board, 2020). **Key Point:** *You must know the terminology used by your healthcare organization and pay careful attention to agency policies and advance directives so that you are prepared if the patient suffers a cardiopulmonary arrest.* An important responsibility of the nurse is to ensure that information is provided in a clear and helpful manner to promote the patient's understanding.

In many healthcare environments, when patients experience a cardiopulmonary arrest, resuscitation (CPR) is performed almost automatically in the absence of advance directives indicating otherwise. Given certain situations (e.g., intense patient suffering with little chance of survival), this practice may cause you to experience moral distress. The ANA recommends that you should seek support and guidance to promote your well-being (ANA Ethics Advisory Board, 2020).

You should carefully explain to patients and families what CPR involves and their available options. For example, the provider cannot write a DNR prescription without their permission, and they have the right to refuse CPR. Nurses have a duty to communicate with patients and the interprofessional team regarding the patient's wishes regarding end-of-life care and to clarify the treatment plan. Do-not-resuscitate language must be clearly documented, reviewed, and updated to reflect changes in the patient's condition. Avoid language that is subject to interpretation or confusing (e.g., chemical code only—give drugs but no chest compression or respiratory assistance; slow code—do not immediately start CPR; do nothing). **Key Point:** *Providers must clearly specify any limitations to a full code ("limited code"), and the prescription should align with agency policy.*

Interventions such as family meetings and interprofessional collaboration with the palliative care team improve decisions about end-of-life care (Brent et al., 2018). See Box 14-2 for the additional recommendations by the ANA on the nurse's role in end-of-life decisions.

Medical Aid in Dying (MAiD) The ANA acknowledges that nurses have a role in MAiD in those states in which it is legal (ANA, 2019). MAiD permits a competent adult with a terminal illness to self-administer oral or enteral medications that may hasten death. Nurses must respect the patient's right to self-determination

in end-of-life decisions and remain nonjudgmental and supportive while evaluating their own value system related to this issue. **Key Point:** *In keeping with the Code of Ethics, nurses are ethically prohibited from administering MAiD medications but must be knowledgeable of the arguments for and against MAiD and of their own personal value systems.*

BOX 14-2 ■ Highlights of American Nurses Association Recommendations Concerning Do-Not-Resuscitate (DNR) Prescriptions

- The nurse should assist patients and decision makers in making informed choices regarding end-of-life desires. The information provided can include clinical factors that incorporate risks of resuscitation, benefits, burdens, patient wishes, and so on.
- The competent patient's choices have the highest priority when there is conflict, which is consistent with autonomy and the right to self-determination.
- When the patient is not competent, give the highest priority to advance directives or the surrogate decision makers.
- DNR orders should be discussed explicitly with the patient and significant others, preferably before a life-threatening illness.
- DNR orders must be documented, reviewed, and updated, especially for patients in surgery.
- Nurses should provide quality patient care regardless of DNR status.
- DNR does *not* mean "discontinue care" or substandard care. Nurses must ensure that the quality of care is not compromised.
- Nurses should be aware of and have an active role in developing DNR policies in the institutions where they work; they should participate in interdisciplinary mechanisms for resolving disputes among patients, families, and healthcare practitioners concerning DNR orders.
- Nurses have a responsibility to use evidenced-based guidelines in performing resuscitation to avoid harm to the patient and breach of professional integrity, such as participation in "slow codes" or "partial codes."
- Nurses have a duty to educate patients and families about technologies and termination-of-treatment decisions and to encourage them to think about end-of-life preferences and make their wishes known in advance.
- Nurses have a duty to communicate relevant information and to advocate for a patient's end-of-life preferences to be honored.

Source: Adapted from American Nurses Association (ANA). (2012). *Revised position statement: Nursing care and do not resuscitate (DNR) and allow natural death (AND) decisions.* https://www.nursingworld.org/~4ad4a8/globalassets/docs/ana/nursing-care-and-do-not-resuscitate-dnr-and-allow-natural-death-decisions.pdf; ANA Ethics Advisory Board (2021). ANA Position statement: Nursing care and do-not-resuscitate (DNR) decisions. *The Online Journal of Issues in Nursing (OJIN),* 26(1). https://doi.org/10.3912/OJIN.Vol26No01PoSCol02

Palliative Sedation Some advocate the use of continuous sedation until death as an alternative to assisted suicide. The Hospice and Palliative Nurses Association (HPNA) promotes **palliative sedation** as the controlled and monitored use of sedatives and nonopioid medications to induce unconsciousness to relieve suffering from refractory and unendurable symptoms (HPNA, 2016). The goal is to manage intractable symptoms, which distinguishes it from aiding in death.

Assisted Suicide

Assisted suicide means making available that which is needed for the patient to end their own life (e.g., pharmacological agents or weapons). The patient is physically capable of ending their own life, has expressed the intention to do so, and has turned to the healthcare provider merely to supply the means. Although physician-assisted suicide is legal in some states, the ANA opposes assisted suicide because it is not consistent with the commitments of the nursing profession and violates public trust (ANA, 2019).

Euthanasia

The term **euthanasia** comes from the Greek word *euthanatos*, which means "good death." It refers to the deliberate ending of the life of someone suffering from a terminal or incurable illness. The ANA opposes euthanasia for the same reasons given for assisted suicide—both violate core commitments of the profession and public trust (ANA, 2019); thus, nurses cannot participate in euthanasia scenarios.

Active euthanasia occurs as a result of a direct action (e.g., giving an overdose of medication). It can be *voluntary* (patient consents), *involuntary* (patient refuses), or *nonvoluntary* (patient is unable to consent, or someone else makes the decision and the patient is unaware of it). Unlike assisted suicide, in which the person assisting makes available the means for the person to take their own life, in euthanasia, the assistant also serves as the direct agent of death (e.g., administers the medication).

Passive euthanasia occurs as a result of a *lack* of action (e.g., withholding medications or food necessary to sustain life). Honoring the refusal of treatments is not generally considered passive euthanasia and can be ethically and legally permissible. For more information about the ethical and legal issues surrounding euthanasia, see Chapter 5, Ethics & Values, and Chapter 39, Legal Accountability.

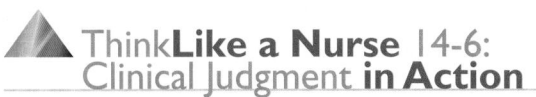

ThinkLike a Nurse 14-6: Clinical Judgment in Action

What are your feelings about medical aid in dying, assisted suicide, palliative sedation, and euthanasia? Focus on your feelings, not on principles, explanations, and rationales.

Autopsy

An autopsy is a medical examination of the body to determine the cause of death. Autopsies also provide relevant data about disease processes and causes. The pathologist performs a detailed internal and external evaluation of the body, removes body organs, and extracts sample tissues for further examination. The organs are then replaced in the body, and the body cavities are closed with sutures. An autopsy requires signed permission from the next of kin, except in cases in which autopsy is required by law (e.g., suspicious or unwitnessed deaths).

Organ Donation

The Uniform Anatomical Gift Act (UAGA) provides guidance on tissue, eye, and organ donation (National Conference of Commissioners on Uniform State Laws, 2009). The act was amended to add language that would prevent others from overriding an individual's prior decision regarding organ donation. However, there remain ethical concerns that the UAGA might result in donors being maintained on life support against their family's wishes.

Key Point: *A conflict between a potential organ donor's advance directives and measures to ensure the viability of the donor's organs (e.g., life support) must be resolved as soon as possible by one of the following, in this order: (1) the donor (if able), (2) the surrogate decision maker, or (3) another person as authorized under state law. Until resolution, maintaining the suitability of the organs has the highest priority. You should advocate that your patient's advance directives are clear on end-of-life care and organ donation.*

The UAGA has been adopted in most states. In general, the UAGA states the following:

- As a rule, general donors must be at least 18 years of age or an emancipated minor.
- Next of kin can donate organs when a person dies unless an objection is known.
- Relatives cannot revoke a person's donation, even after death.
- The person making the gift can amend or revoke it at any time.

Many states issue identification cards or allow driver's licenses to be amended to identify a person as an organ donor. However, even though donor cards are legal in all states, to minimize litigation and unwanted media, many institutions will obtain family consent (Organ Donation and Transplant Alliance, 2017). Therefore, if a patient is planning to donate organs or tissues, be sure that they discuss these wishes with family members. If death is imminent, a healthcare team member (provider or nurse) should ask whether the patient has agreed to be an organ donor, has a donor card, or is registered with the state's donor database. In many institutions, a transplant coordinator contacts the family and makes the request for organ and tissue donation.

KnowledgeCheck 14-3

- What are advance directives?
- What is the ANA's position on assisted suicide?

PracticalKnowledge
knowing how

 ASSESSMENT

When a patient is dying or has experienced a loss, you must carefully assess the patient and significant others for the common physical, emotional, behavioral, and cognitive grief reactions. For a list of these, along with guidelines to follow when assessing dying and grieving patients,

> Go to **Chapter 14, Assessment Guidelines and Tools**, in Volume 2.

You should also assess the knowledge base, history of loss, coping patterns and abilities, meaning of the loss or illness, support systems, and cultural and spiritual needs. For dying patients, assess the following:

- Determine whether there are burial or cremation plans or other such tasks (e.g., calling family members) when the client and family are ready to discuss these topics.
- Determine whether the dying client has advance directives (e.g., living will, DPOA for healthcare) and organ donation documents.

Is It Grief or Depression?

When you are performing a focused assessment for grief or loss, you will need to distinguish between grief and depression. Sadness and depression are an integral part of grief, with several common symptoms (e.g., sadness, insomnia, poor appetite, and weight loss). However, lasting depression may be a sign that the stress of grieving has triggered a major depressive episode (Clark et al., 2021). Grief tends to come and go—it can be triggered, for example, by a holiday or other reminder. For help in differentiating between grief and depression,

> Go to **Chapter 14, Assessment Guideline and Tools, Assessing Grief and Loss**, in Volume 2.

KnowledgeCheck 14-4

What assessments should you make for your terminally ill patient and their family?

 ANALYSIS/DIAGNOSIS

When you are analyzing patient data, keep in mind that most grief is normal, not complicated or dysfunctional. You must determine whether loss and grieving are the problem or the etiology because the etiology will influence your interventions. Also note that the same diagnoses can be used in the context of death, dying, grief, or loss.

Loss and Grieving as Problem Various nursing diagnoses may be appropriate for a person who is dying or grieving. The most obvious ones are Grieving, Anticipatory Grieving, and Dysfunctional Grieving (HCA, n.d.) and Complicated Grieving (Herdman et al. 2021).

Key Point: *Do not use a Dysfunctional or Complicated Grieving diagnosis for every person who is grieving a loss.* Dysfunctional and Complicated Grieving describe disabling pain and grief, characterized by long-term grieving (perhaps years), functional impairment, and/or intense emotions. The person may deny or have difficulty expressing feelings of loss or may experience physical symptoms because of suppressing feelings.

Loss and Grieving as Etiology Loss, grief, and dying are an etiology when they create problems in other areas of patient or family function. The following are examples of such nursing diagnoses:

- Anxiety related to inability to cope with the loss or related to unknown outcome of situation
- Fear or anxiety related to impending death
- Decisional Conflict related to end-of-life treatment measures (e.g., knowledge that the treatment may lengthen life but decrease the quality of life)
- Fatigue related to demands of caring for a dying loved one
- Spiritual Distress related to loss of trust in a loving God (HCA, n.d.)

Several other diagnoses may be related to coping or feelings associated with the loss, such as Coping Impairment, Denial, and Hopelessness. This list is not exhaustive, so carefully synthesize your assessment data to formulate an accurate diagnosis.

⚠ ThinkLike a Nurse 14-7:
Clinical Judgment in Action

Refer to the scenario for Thomas Manning and his wife in the Meet Your Patient scenario and the preceding Think Like a Nurse: Clinical Judgment in Action exercises 14-1, 14-4, and 14-5. Also refer to a nursing diagnosis handbook, the Clinical Classification System (https://careclassification.org/framework/), and manuals for Nursing Interventions Classification (NIC) and Nursing Outcomes Classification (NOC), as needed.

- Does Thomas Manning (Meet Your Patient) have any symptoms of Grieving?
- How do you think that outcomes and interventions will differ for Grieving and Dysfunctional (Complicated) Grieving?

■ **PLANNING OUTCOMES/EVALUATION**

Encourage the patient and family to play an active role in planning care. Involving family members helps facilitate their acceptance of the diagnosis and may put the patient more at ease. Questions such as the following will help to elicit the patient's goals for the end of life (Medline Plus, 2020; National Academies of Sciences, 2015; O'Brien et al., 2019):

- What do you want to accomplish or do?
- What are the things you wish you could still do?

- What are your fears or things that cause you anxiety?
- Whom would you like to see?
- What would make you more medically comfortable?
- What is an acceptable pain level for you on a scale from 0 to 10?
- Where do you want to spend the rest of your life? Where are you most comfortable?
- If spiritual peace is important to you, what would help you achieve it?

Outcomes are determined by the diagnostic label you use. Outcomes established for patients allow you to evaluate the success of your interventions.

Individualized goals/outcome statements you might write for a grieving or dying person include the following examples. The patient and/or family will:

- Communicate openly among themselves and health-care providers (e.g., express fear, concerns, pain).
- Obtain satisfactory pain relief and symptom management.
- Exercise control in the management of care to the extent possible.

As always, you will use the goals set in the planning stage as criteria for evaluating the patient's or family's health status.

KnowledgeCheck 14-5

- List three nursing diagnosis labels you might consider when dying or grieving is the primary problem.
- List three nursing diagnosis labels that might occur as a result of dying or grieving.

▨ PLANNING INTERVENTIONS/IMPLEMENTATION

Specific nursing activities for death, dying, and bereavement are determined by the nursing diagnosis, especially by the etiology. A compassionate approach is essential but may be challenging. Watching patients struggle with pain, loss, grief, and death may stir our own deepest doubts and fears, and we may reject the challenge to respond from the heart. Employers usually reward nurses for what they *do* rather than who they *are* as people, so it is easy to rationalize that we have other tasks to accomplish that may be equally important. When we do that, we ignore the real gift we have to offer the suffering patient: our willingness to "walk the walk" with them, if even for a short time. **Key Point: *Your ability to help someone who is grieving or dying is largely determined by your attitude. Full-spectrum nurses combine their psychomotor and thinking skills with compassion in ministering to those who are suffering.***

Some important nursing interventions involved in the care of the dying person are discussed in the following sections. Also see the following Example Client Condition and Care Map for Grieving.

Therapeutic Communication

Therapeutic communication is critical to building a trusting relationship with the dying or **grieving** patient and their significant others. It is most important to listen to the dying patient and to be alert for and respond to nonverbal cues. Encourage patients and family members to express their feelings, and reassure them that their feelings are normal and not "wrong." In discussions about DNR or withholding or withdrawing treatments, it is important to find out why the patient is seeking that option: Do they wish to avoid suffering, or do they fear being a burden to loved ones?

Providers and nurses should always work to improve their communication skills because they are essential for achieving better outcomes at the end of life (O'Brien et al., 2019; Pfeifer & Head, 2018). See Box 14-3 for some barriers to end-of-life communication. For tips on communicating with people who are dying or bereaved,

 Go to **Chapter 14, Clinical Insight 14-1: Communicating With People Who Are Grieving**, in Volume 2.

If you need more information on communication and therapeutic relationships, refer to Chapter 15.

Facilitating Grief Work

Regardless of the source of grief (e.g., a loss of health, an impending death), you can help patients and families express their feelings, recall memories, and find meaning in their lives.

Expressing Feelings

It is the family, not just an individual patient, who grieves a death or loss. Grief is a normal process, and people must communicate their feelings to effectively deal with it (Fig. 14-2). Sometimes people hold in their feelings, which interferes with their grief resolution. You may need to facilitate the process, using your therapeutic communication skills to help them feel comfortable (refer to Chapter 15 as needed). The following are several ways to facilitate the expression of feelings:

- Encourage questions, and respond to them within a reasonable time.
- Sit beside the head of the bed; do not appear rushed.
- When you observe the patient or family member expressing feelings, either verbally or nonverbally, encourage them to continue.
- Expect and accept a wide range of feelings, including anger, fear, and loneliness.
- Ask, "How would you like me to help?" or "What do you need?"
- Be sure that everyone on the healthcare team understands and follows the care plan.

♥ iCare 14-2

Loss, Grief, and Dying

Dealing with loss, grief, and dying is very difficult. As caregivers, we can display "caring" to patients, friends, and families by merely being present. Some people need space, whereas others may need acknowledgment and comfort.

When a death occurs, it is important to acknowledge the loss of life. Consider the patient's culture and beliefs to determine how this is done. A moment of silence and/or spiritual reflection can exhibit "caring" to acknowledge the sacredness that a life has been lost for friends and family members as well as caregivers.

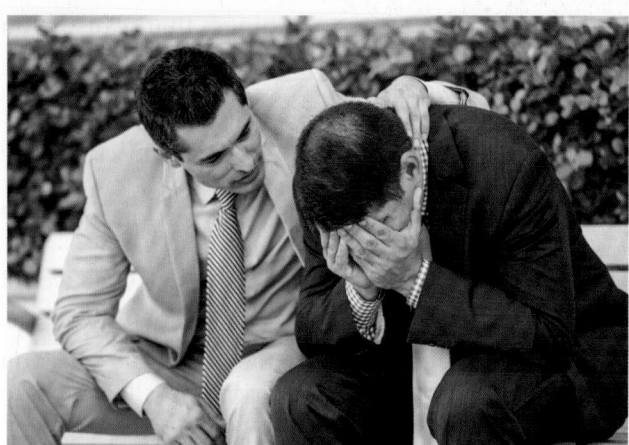

FIGURE 14-2 Family openly expressing grief.

BOX 14-3 ■ Barriers to End-of-Life Communication

- Fear of one's own mortality
- Unresolved personal grief issues (e.g., the loss of one's own parent)
- Lack of experience with death and dying
- Fear of expressing emotion (e.g., crying)
- Fear of not knowing the answer to a question
- Fear of destroying hope or causing harm to the patient
- Not knowing whether to give an honest (and possibly unwelcome) answer to a question
- Not understanding the family's culture
- Keeping physical distance (e.g., standing away from the person or avoiding eye contact)
- Insensitivity: interrupting communication, patronizing, giving false reassurance

Sources: Anderson, R., Bloch, S., Armstrong, M., Stone, P. C., & Low, J. T. S. (2019). Communication between healthcare professionals and relatives of patients approaching the end-of-life: A systematic review of qualitative evidence. *Palliative Medicine*, 33(8), 926–941. https://doi.org/10.1177/0269216319852007; Pfeifer, M., & Head, H. (2018). Which critical communication skills are essential for interdisciplinary end-of-life discussion? *AMA Journal of Ethics*, 20(8), E724–731. https://doi.org/10.1001/amajethics.2018.724; Saretta, M., Doñate-Martínez, A., & Alhambra-Borrás, T. (2022). Barriers and facilitators for an effective palliative care communication with older people: A systematic review. *Patient Education and Counseling*, 105(8), 2671–2682. https://doi.org/10.1016/j.pec.2022.04.003; Sinuff, T., Dodek, P., You, J. J., Barwich, D., Tayler, C., Downar, J., Hartwick, M., Frank, C., Stelfox, H. T., & Heyland, D. K. (2015). Improving end-of-life communication and decision making: The development of a conceptual framework and quality indicators. *Journal of Pain and Symptom Management*, 49(6), 1070–1080. http://dx.doi.org/10.1016/j.jpainsymman.2014.12.007

- Ask yourself what you would do if this were your family member.
- Do not compare another person's loss with your own experience. Avoid comments such as "I know how you feel." Instead, say, "Tell me how you feel."

Recalling Memories

Grieving patients and family members may need to recall memories, both good and difficult. One way to encourage recall is to go through photos with them and ask questions about the people in the pictures. Also look for objects of sentiment (e.g., a family heirloom) in the environment and ask the dying or bereaved person to share their significance.

Finding Meaning

Another way to support grief work is to help the patient or family find meaning in their lives or in their past. Facilitating life review is one technique to help the patient and/or family recognize the unique contributions this person has made to family, friends, and society. You can begin by asking about the various aspects of the patient's life (e.g., "What were some of his favorite hobbies/activities?"), commenting on pictures in the room, or picking up on verbal cues that are expressed.

Bibliotherapy

Bibliotherapy is a counseling technique used when grief therapy is indicated. It uses guided reading of self-help literature or fiction to increase client awareness and understanding and promote healing. Poems, novels, and essays can help produce new insights, either as the client retells the story or is guided to discuss their feelings and thoughts about the characters in the story (Monroy-Fraustro et al., 2021; Suvilehto et al., 2019).

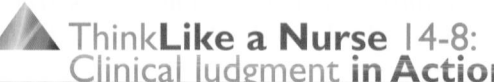

ThinkLike a Nurse 14-8: Clinical Judgment in Action

- You walk into the room and find Mrs. Manning (Meet Your Patient) sitting in a chair and softly weeping while Mr. Manning sleeps. What would you say to her?
- Mr. Manning waves his hand in the air and says to you, "I'm not taking any more of those damn pills." What response would you make to him?

- A young woman approaches you in the hall and says, "I want to visit Mom and stay with her, but I just can't stand to see her like that. I feel guilty for wanting to leave." What would be your therapeutic response?

Helping Families of Dying Patients

When a patient is dying, it is important to view the family as your unit of care. If the patient is unresponsive, you may find yourself spending most of your care time with the family, providing education, support, and a listening ear. Observing their loved one dying can leave family members feeling confused, angry, helpless, and even devastated. Sensitive, compassionate nursing care is always essential, especially during this time. You can use the interventions in the preceding sections as you help family members to understand that what they see may be very different from what the patient is experiencing. For more specific interventions for helping families of dying patients,

 Go to **Chapter 14, Clinical Insight 14-2: Helping Families of Dying Patients,** in Volume 2.

KnowledgeCheck 14-6

- Describe four ways to facilitate the grief work of a grieving or dying person.
- List two specific interventions, in addition to facilitating grief work, for helping grieving families.

Caring for the Dying Person

To effectively care for terminally ill patients, you must meet their physiological, psychological, social, sexual, and spiritual needs. Most hospitals and hospice facilities have an interprofessional team (e.g., provider, nurse, social worker, nutritionist, allied health therapists, clergy) to provide holistic care to dying patients and their families.

Meeting Physiological Needs

Active dying usually occurs over a period of 10 to 14 days (although it can take as little as 24 hours). In the "final hours," the last 4 to 48 hours of life, most patients need skilled care around the clock as body systems fail. Physiological needs during this time include mobility, oxygenation, safety, nutrition, fluids, elimination, personal hygiene, and control of pain and symptoms (nausea, vomiting).

 A top priority for older adults is comfort at the end of life. Older adults have unique palliative care needs (Santivasi et al., 2020). Research shows that fewer than 10% of the very old experience unconsciousness during the final stage of dying; thus, attention to the most common symptoms of pain and distress must be addressed. This is especially true with older adults who have cognitive-impairment conditions. There was a strong positive association between end-of-life comfort and dying in a long-term care facility (Fleming et al., 2017).

For specific interventions and guidelines to use when caring for a dying patient,

 Go to **Chapter 14, Clinical Insight 14-3: Caring for the Dying Person: Meeting Physiological Needs,** in Volume 2.

Meeting Psychological Needs

When a patient is terminally ill, the primary provider is usually responsible for deciding what and how much to tell the person. Ideally, everyone involved with the patient should have input into this decision, and you should know exactly what they and the family have been told. Most patients want to know their prognosis as soon as possible so that they can put personal affairs in order, share their feelings with family members, and come to terms with their life and death. The ethical concept of autonomy guides that providers should not withhold information from the patient. The provider and members of the interprofessional team must consider cultural beliefs and practices in meeting patients' psychological needs. Also, many patients realize that they are dying without being told. For specific interventions to help meet the psychological needs of dying patients,

 Go to **Chapter 14, Clinical Insight 14-4: Caring for the Dying Person: Meeting Psychological Needs,** in Volume 2.

KnowledgeCheck 14-7

- Describe six nursing interventions to use in meeting the physiological needs of a dying person.
- Describe six nursing interventions to use in meeting the psychological needs of a dying person.
- What should be the focus of your interventions when the patient is very near death?

Addressing Spiritual Needs

When a person is terminally ill, their spirituality may become very important as they search for meaning in the illness and suffering. The person may be looking for forgiveness and/or acceptance or be reaching out to feel connected. Ways to address this need include (but are not limited to) empathetic listening, contacting pastoral care or clergy if the patient asks for this service, special rituals, praying with the patient, music, meditation, or special readings.

Information about specific religious practices may help you provide appropriate interventions at the end of life. For example, Orthodox Jewish religious doctrine says that after the death of an Orthodox Jewish patient, you should handle the body as little as possible if you are not Jewish. Remember, though, that there are wide

Toward Evidence-Based Practice

Davidson, J., Bojorquez, G., Upvall, M., Stokes, F., Bosek, M. S. D., Turner, M., & Lee, Y.-S. (2022). Nurses' values and perspectives on medical aid in dying: A survey of nurses in the United States. *Journal of Hospice and Palliative Nursing, 24*(1), 5–14. https://doi.org/10.1097/NJH.0000000000000820

Nurses were surveyed to gain insight into their values and perspectives on the issue of medical aid in dying (MAiD). Results from 2,043 data sets revealed that many nurses would not hesitate to provide care to patients concerning MAiD (86%). However, the percentage decreased to 67% for those who would provide care during the final act. In their professional context, 57% of nurses supported MAiD, whereas only 49% would personally support it. Nurses who identified as religious were less supportive than nurses who identified as spiritual. Respondents identified a need for more information and guidance on their role in MAiD.

Davidson, J., Stokes, L., Bosek, M. S. D., Turner, M., Bojorquez, G., Lee, Y. S., & Upvall, M. (2022). Nurses' values on medical aid in dying: A qualitative analysis. *Nursing Ethics, 29*(3), 636–650. https://doi.org/10.1177/09697330211051029

Researchers analyzed comments from 1,213 nurses related to MAiD. Results centered around four major themes:

1. Autonomy With Judgment: Some nurses would focus on and respect patients' autonomy. They viewed MAiD as a component of their professional role as a nurse.

2. Honoring With Limitations: Some nurses identified specific concerns that would affect their decisions, such as legal liability, personal ethical boundaries, negative stigma of being viewed as a facilitator of death, and not having to administer the medication.

3. Not Until …: Nurses felt that more information was needed to make an informed decision regarding their participation in MAiD. In addition, nurses questioned the impact on individuals with physical disabilities who were unable to self-administer the medication.

4. Adamantly Against: Nurses who were adamantly against MAiD cite several reasons, such as personal values, religious beliefs, and the view that it is the same as suicide or murder.

Researchers concluded that nurses need more information on the legislative specifics of MAiD and how they translate into actual nursing practice. Nurses should assist in developing policies and standards related to MAiD.

---

1. Based on these research results, what is the importance of including topics such as MAiD in nursing curricula for students and in-services for nurses?

2. What strategies could promote more involvement among nursing students and nurses in policy planning related to MAiD?

---

individual differences and that you must assess each patient and family to determine how closely they adhere to the rituals of their religion. Review Chapters 12 and 13, as needed.

Addressing Cultural Needs

Cultural values can influence a person's openness to discussions regarding death and end-of-life healthcare preferences. End-of-life concerns important to most people include comfort; open, accurate, honest communications; ensuring needs are met; support, hope, and optimism; mutual forgiveness; honoring spiritual beliefs; and saying goodbye (American Psychological Association [APA], 2019; Fleming et al., 2017).

There is some overlap between religious and cultural practices. For example, most cultural groups engage in some type of religious ceremony that helps the bereaved begin the grieving process (Fig. 14-3). Nevertheless, some death rituals and expressions of grief may be culture based but not necessarily involve religion. For example, some cultures may emphasize keeping emotions more subdued and limiting expressions of grief to private settings, whereas others gauge the value of the deceased by the amount of crying that occurs.

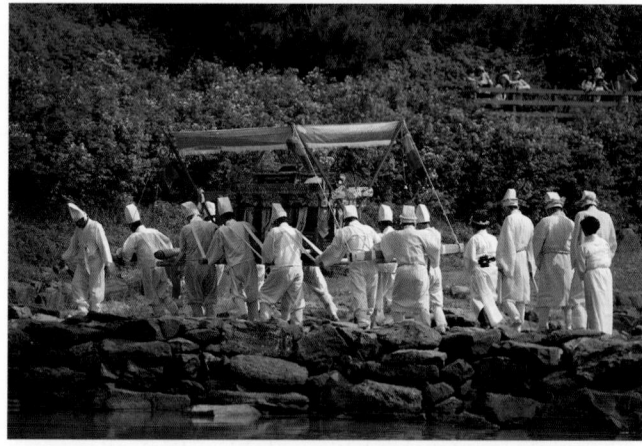

FIGURE 14-3 After death, rituals, such as funerals, are viewed as respect for the deceased and help friends and family bring closure.

To provide culturally sensitive care at the end of life, you will need some patient-specific information about relevant cultural practices surrounding death. **Key Point:** *As with spiritual care, remember that you cannot assume that a person follows the practices of their cultural group; you must assess to be sure.* For general cultural information, see Chapter 12.

ThinkLike a Nurse 14-9: Clinical Judgment **in Action**

Reflect on this reading by Theresa Rando in *The Gift of Presence:*

It is one of the most difficult things in the world to do to sit and listen while another's heart is breaking with grief, to hold the hand of a dying patient who cries silently while staring into space. The gift of presence, the gift of being with those in pain, is the only gift we can give. It is the sole armor patients have against the anguish. The very most we can do for dying patients is to make it better, with our presence and concern, than it would be if we were not there. . . .We cannot "do" anything that can get rid of the psychic pain of impending loss and death. (Rando, 1984, p. 272)

Close your eyes and visualize yourself sitting quietly beside a dying patient and holding their hand. Visualize the patient crying silently. Can you still your mind and remain silent, or do you feel you must say something to make the patient feel better?

Providing Postmortem Care

Postmortem care includes care of the patient's body after death and fulfilling any legal obligations, such as arranging transportation to the morgue or funeral home and determining the disposition of the patient's belongings. You will follow agency policies and respect cultural and spiritual preferences, along with giving the care that is commonly provided. In most states, the provider must pronounce death; in some areas, however, a coroner or a nurse may also perform this task. Changes in the body after death include the following:

- **Rigor mortis** (the stiffening of the body after death) is caused by contraction of the muscles from a lack of adenosine triphosphate (ATP). It occurs about 2 to 4 hours after death. Rigor mortis begins in the involuntary muscles (e.g., the heart). It appears next in the head, neck, and trunk, and finally in the extremities. It disappears about 96 hours after death.
- **Algor mortis** occurs when the blood stops circulating. The body temperature drops about 1.88°F (1°C) per hour until it reaches room temperature.
- **Livor mortis** occurs when the dependent parts of the body appear bluish and mottled. That happens when the blood stops circulating and the red blood cells break down, releasing hemoglobin.

♥ **iCare** If the family wishes to be alone with the body, straighten the bedcovers, remove all tubes (unless contraindicated), and make the patient look as natural as possible. Give family members whatever time they need before you prepare the body. Ideally, you will have already established a relationship with the family and will have begun to facilitate their grieving during the patient's dying period. And you will have prepared them as the death becomes imminent.

For specific guidelines for care of the body and other immediate postmortem interventions to support family members,

Go to **Chapter 14, Clinical Insight 14-5: Providing Postmortem Care**, in Volume 2.

KnowledgeCheck 14-8

- Why is it important to position the body with a pillow under the head and shoulders soon after death?
- Why is it important to close the eyes and mouth of the deceased and position the body within at least 2 to 4 hours after death?

Providing Grief Education

At some point after the immediate postmortem period, reteach the stages of grief and point out that it may take months or even years to resolve. Explain that grief may become more intense on the anniversary of the death (or other loss) and on significant dates (e.g., birthdays).

Recall that once the bereaved person accepts that the loss is real, their feelings may be so intense that they may wonder whether they are losing their sanity. The grieving person may be fatigued from not sleeping, may be disoriented or unable to concentrate, and may have numerous other symptoms. Reassure the person that such responses are expected and that there is no single right way to grieve (APA, 2020). Also assure the person that although the grief process takes time, the symptoms will not last forever.

Helping Children Deal With Loss

Some families may need information about helping children deal with grief, especially when there is a death in the family. You may need to explain that children perceive death differently from adults and the importance of addressing death and grief with children. See the accompanying Self-Care box, Helping Children Deal With Loss, for teaching surviving relatives how to help children deal with grief.

Taking Care of Yourself

When caring for dying patients, you will confront your own feelings of mortality. It is important to understand your own attitudes, fears, and beliefs concerning death, so think about these before you encounter dying patients. This will enable you to deal with patients and their families in a healthier way. In addition, suppressing feelings associated with the death of patients can take a heavy toll on you emotionally.

When you become involved with dying persons and their families at such an intimate time in their lives, you become connected to them. There is nothing wrong with this emotional involvement; it helps you to be effective in your work. But just as you care for these families, you also need to care for yourself during these times.

- **Recognize that feelings of grief and loss are normal,** so do not be afraid to confront grief. If you deny your

Self-Care

Helping Children Deal With Loss

Teach surviving relatives the following:

➤ If a child is frightened about attending a funeral, do not force them to go. It is important, however, to include the child in some service or observance, such as lighting a candle, saying a prayer, or visiting the gravesite, at a later time.

➤ Spend as much time as possible with the child, making it clear that the child has permission to show feelings openly or freely.

➤ Let the child know that it is okay to want attachment items (e.g., picture, jewelry, special object).

➤ Be prepared for intermittent expressions of sadness and anger from the child over a long period of time.

➤ Be prepared for the possibility of regression to earlier developmental stages (e.g., talking "baby talk").

➤ Assure the child that they were in no way responsible for the death.

Warning signs that may indicate the need for professional help, especially if they are prolonged, include an extended period in which the child loses interest in daily activities and events, inability to sleep, loss of appetite, fear of being alone, extended regression, repeated statements about wanting to join the dead person, withdrawal from friends, refusal to attend school, or a drop in academic performance.

Special Considerations Related to COVID-19

➤ Children may be extremely fearful they will lose the remaining parent to COVID-19.

➤ The child may feel guilty or depressed, believing they brought home the virus.

➤ The death of a parent is exacerbated by the isolation, depression, anxiety, and other adverse mental health concerns caused by imposed barriers to socialization.

➤ Children with preexisting mental health issues are at a greater risk for maladaptive grieving.

➤ Educate parents to consult a provider if the child exhibits major behavioral changes (e.g., risky behaviors, suicidal ideation/attempts, depression). Healthcare providers, like the remaining parent and family, are major sources of support.

➤ Emphasize that the child needs a trusted support source to openly discuss their feelings. In addition, the child may benefit from a bereavement group.

Source: Adapted from Slomski A. (2021). Thousands of US youths cope with the trauma of losing parents to COVID-19. *Journal of the American Medical Association, 326*(21), 2117–2119. https://doi.org/10.1001/jama.2021.20846

feelings and focus on caring for others, you will begin to wear down physically and emotionally.

■ **Talk with other colleagues about your feelings.** Nurses are known for being able to take care of everyone but themselves. Do not be afraid to ask for what you need. Also recognize that your coworkers may need support. Form a nurses' support group that meets regularly to talk about the feelings of grief or loss and to remember those who have died. If you need or want a facilitator, pastoral care workers and social workers may be available for these services.

■ **When away from work, do some nice things for yourself** on a regular basis (e.g., facial, quiet bubble bath, massage, a sports event). Set aside a special relaxation spot in your home; decorate it with items that help you focus on peaceful thoughts (e.g., candles, pictures, religious objects).

■ **If you wish, it is appropriate to attend calling hours and/or funeral services** when one of your patients dies to help diffuse some of your feelings of loss. Also, it is meaningful to family members to know that you took the time to remember them and their loved one.

Interventions for Example Client Condition: Complicated Grief

For nursing interventions specific to Complicated Grief, see Example Client Condition: Complicated Grief.

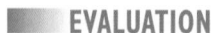 **EVALUATION**

Refer to the Example Client Condition for evaluation of outcomes and interventions specific to Complicated Grief.

 To explore learning resources for this chapter,

 Go to Davis Advantage and find:

Answers and Suggested Responses for all questions in this chapter

Concept Map

Knowledge Map

References and Bibliography

Care Map

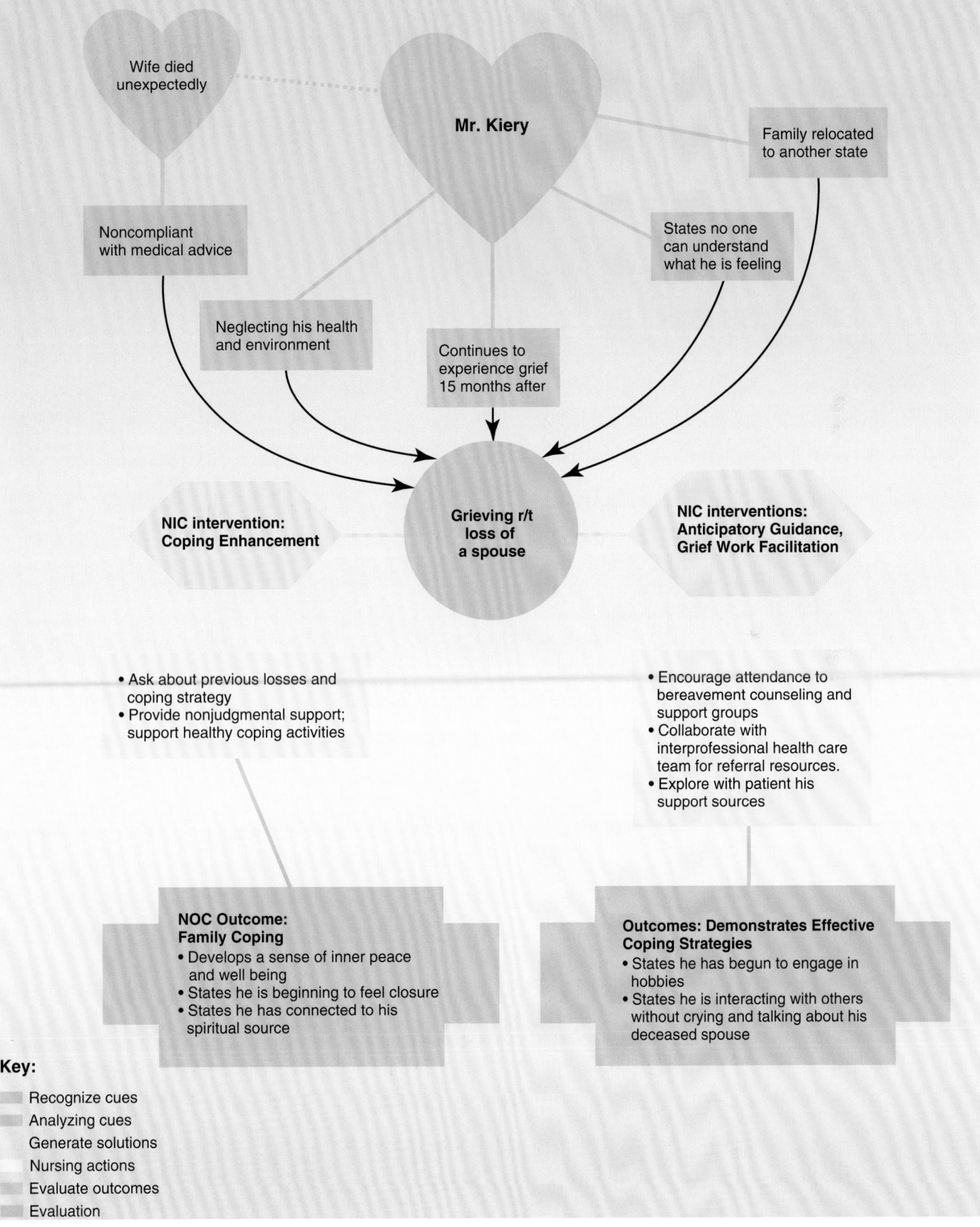

Wife died unexpectedly

Mr. Kiery

Family relocated to another state

Noncompliant with medical advice

States no one can understand what he is feeling

Neglecting his health and environment

Continues to experience grief 15 months after

NIC intervention:
Coping Enhancement

Grieving r/t loss of a spouse

NIC interventions:
Anticipatory Guidance, Grief Work Facilitation

• Ask about previous losses and coping strategy
• Provide nonjudgmental support; support healthy coping activities

• Encourage attendance to bereavement counseling and support groups
• Collaborate with interprofessional health care team for referral resources.
• Explore with patient his support sources

**NOC Outcome:
Family Coping**
• Develops a sense of inner peace and well being
• States he is beginning to feel closure
• States he has connected to his spiritual source

Outcomes: Demonstrates Effective Coping Strategies
• States he has begun to engage in hobbies
• States he is interacting with others without crying and talking about his deceased spouse

Key:
Recognize cues
Analyzing cues
Generate solutions
Nursing actions
Evaluate outcomes
Evaluation

UNIT **3**

Essential Nursing Interventions

CHAPTER  15

Communicating & Therapeutic Relationships

Learning Outcomes

After completing this chapter, you should be able to:

➤ Discuss the three basic levels of communication.

➤ Describe the process of communication between sender and receiver; include all five elements.

➤ List the characteristics of verbal and nonverbal communication.

➤ Analyze factors that influence the communication process.

➤ Describe some characteristics of collaborative professional communication.

➤ Explain how relationships and roles influence communication.

➤ Describe the role of communication in each of the four phases of the therapeutic relationship.

➤ Compare and contrast techniques that enhance communication with those that hinder communication.

➤ Communicate with clients with impaired hearing, speech, or cognition.

➤ Communicate with clients whose culture, language, or gender identification is different from yours.

➤ Plan nursing care for a client experiencing impaired communication.

Key Concepts

Communication
Communication techniques
Therapeutic relationships

Related Concepts

See the Concept Map on Davis Advantage.

Meet Your Patient

You have been assigned to care for John Barker, a 76-year-old man admitted to the hospital with bleeding in the lower gastrointestinal tract. When you enter the room to introduce yourself, his wife is at the bedside. They are holding hands, and both have clearly been crying. You begin by saying, "Good afternoon, Mr. Barker. I am a nursing student from the university. I've been assigned to care for you tomorrow." Mr. Barker swallows hard and says, "I don't think you'll be able to do anything for me!" His wife says, "Don't take it personally. It's not a good time right now. Please just leave us alone."

You leave the room, unsure how to respond. At the unit station when you review the chart, the charge nurse says, "Oh my! You've been assigned to him? I hope you've got a lot of experience." As you read the electronic health record, you realize that Mr. Barker was just informed that he has advanced-stage colon cancer.

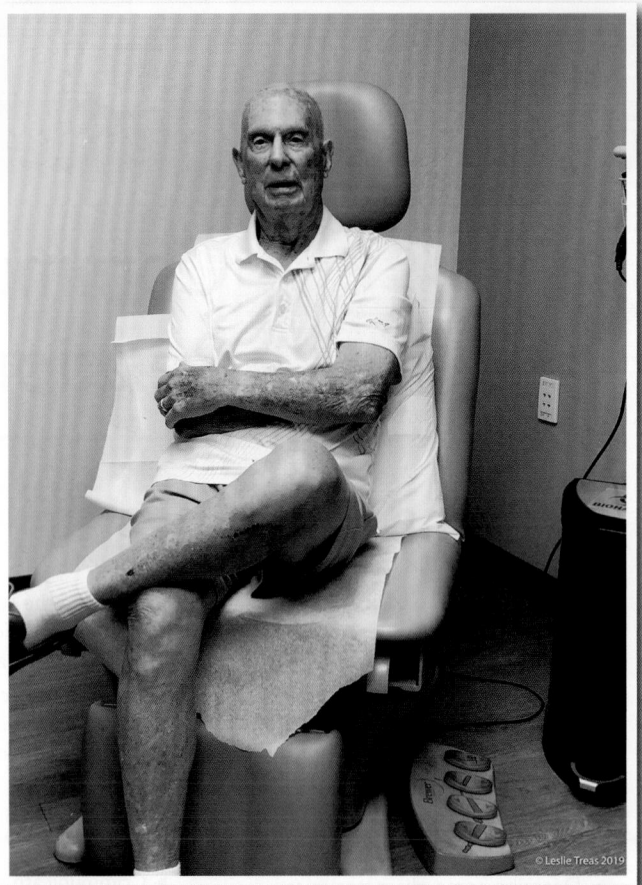
© Leslie Treas 2019

TheoreticalKnowledge
knowing why

As a resource to you while you are learning what it means to care for patients in difficult situations such as Mr. Barker's, you might look to the following professional and regulatory agencies that stress the importance of good communication:

- The Joint Commission:
  National Patient Safety Goal 2, effective 2020. This aims to improve patient safety by improving communication among caregivers.
  The Joint Commission *Speak Up Campaign.* The goal of this safety program is to help patients and their advocates become active in their care (Box 15-1). Topics covered include safe surgery, pain management, medication safety, and discrimination reduction. Patients have the right to:
  Receive care that is free from discrimination and have a language interpreter, if necessary
  Receive effective, understandable information
  Make decisions about their healthcare and even refuse care
  Be treated with courtesy and know the names of their caregivers
  Receive copies of tests and medical records (The Joint Commission, n.d., 2019).

- The **National Academy of Medicine (NAM) (formerly the Institute of Medicine [IOM])** values patient-centered care by communicating in a way that respects patients' differences, values, preferences, and expressed needs. The NAM focuses on providing

---

BOX 15-1 ■ Teaching Patients to Speak Up

The Joint Commission Speak Up program helps to prevent healthcare errors by helping patients and advocates to be actively involved in their care.

- Ask a trusted family member or friend to be your advocate to listen to your providers and ask questions on your behalf.

- Learn about your health conditions and your plan for care. Participate in your healthcare decisions.

- Pay attention to the care you are receiving and make sure you are receiving the right treatments and medication.

- Speak up if you have questions or if there is something you don't understand.

- Obtain healthcare from reputable providers and facilities.

Source: The Joint Commission. (2019). *SpeakUP: Know your rights.* https://www.jointcommission.org/-/media/tjc/documents/resources/speak-up/speak-ups/for-your-rights/speak-up-for-your-rights-85-x-11_.pdf patient education to foster informed decisions, promote involvement in care, and enhance health maintenance and healing.

- The **National League for Nursing (NLN)** promotes excellence in nursing practice with the core values of caring, integrity, diversity, and excellence. Open, clear, and respectful communication is the foundation for nurses providing quality care that contributes to patient well-being.

ABOUT THE KEY CONCEPTS

In this chapter, you learn how **communication techniques** link to the concept of **communication** and how both help you to form **therapeutic relationships** with patients, families, and members of the healthcare team.

WHAT IS COMMUNICATION?

Communication is a dynamic, reciprocal process of sending and receiving messages using words, sounds, expressions, body movements, written symbols, and behaviors. Communication is more than the act of talking and listening.

Communication Occurs on Many Levels

Communication is not just an exchange of words between two individuals. It occurs in inner dialogue, between people, and among groups.

Intrapersonal Communication Conscious internal dialogue, sometimes known as *self-talk,* describes *intrapersonal communication.* For example, if you discover your patient is pale, diaphoretic (perspiring profusely), and moaning, you may ask yourself, "What's happened? This patient appears to be in a lot of pain."

- *Constructive affirmation,* or *positive self-talk* (e.g., "This will work! I can do it"), promotes success in a task.
- *Negative self-talk* (e.g., "I can't do this, it's too difficult") may adversely affect a person's ability to complete a task.

Interpersonal Communication Communication that occurs between two or more people is interpersonal. Nurses use interpersonal communication to gather information during assessment, to teach about health issues, to explain care, and to provide comfort and support. In addition, professional nurses communicate with other nurses and healthcare team members to provide comprehensive care for clients. To appropriately delegate activities, they must also communicate effectively with unlicensed assistive personnel (UAP).

Group Communication *Group communication* occurs when you engage in an exchange of ideas with two or more individuals at the same time. Examples of small-group communication include staff meetings, committee meetings, educational groups, self-help groups, and family teaching sessions. Working with groups requires effective communication skills and a basic understanding of group processes—discussed later in the chapter.

Public Speaking Nurses make presentations to groups to educate people about health issues, to lobby for health legislation, and to address colleagues at professional conferences.

KnowledgeCheck 15-1

- What is the purpose of communication?
- Describe the three levels of communication.
- What level of communication was used in the Meet Your Patient scenario?

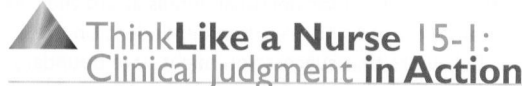 ThinkLike a Nurse 15-1: Clinical Judgment in Action

Evaluate your own skills with the three levels of communication.

Communication Involves Content

The **content** of communication is the actual subject matter, words, gestures, and substance of the message. It is the message that everyone can hear or see. For example, suppose your client said, "I slept through lunch." The content of that statement is open to interpretation. It does not tell you whether they think this is a good thing because they needed rest or a bad thing because they are so exhausted. As you can see, the words are just a part of the communication. You must also consider the process.

Communication Is a Process

Process refers to the act of sending, receiving, interpreting, and reacting to a message. Figure 15-1 illustrates the relationship among the following five elements of the communication process.

- The **sender** (source or encoder) uses verbal and nonverbal methods to deliver a message (content) to another person.
- **Encoding** refers to the process of selecting the words, gestures, tone of voice, signs, and symbols used to transmit the message. For example, as a beginning nursing student, you might feel anxious about caring for Mr. Barker (Meet Your Patient). To communicate your concerns to your instructor, you might say directly, "It makes me nervous to be assigned to him." Or you might avoid eye contact and tell your instructor, "I'm going to need some help today." Both styles communicate your anxiety, but they are expressed differently.
- The **message** is the verbal and nonverbal information the sender communicates. It might be the content of a conversation, a speech, a gesture, a note, and so forth. Effective messages are complete, clear, concise, organized, timely, and expressed in a manner that the receiver can understand. **Key Point: *The message must***

Safe, Effective Nursing Care

Limits and Boundaries of Therapeutic Relationships

Chapter key concept: Therapeutic Relationships

Competency: Provide goal-directed, client-centered care (Thinking, Doing)

What are boundaries? Boundaries define personal space and allow people to communicate comfortably. This box illustrates the effects of boundaries on the competency of Patient-Centered Care and the key concept of therapeutic relationships. Therapeutic (professional) relationships have stricter boundaries than personal relationships: questions and comments made to friends may be inappropriate between colleagues or with clients. Moreover, boundaries between patients and care providers are not equal and are not always clear. Patients are asked for personal details about their lives, are physically exposed, and are often dependent on the care provider. Behaviors that suggest you might have boundary issues include the following:

➤ Thinking about or socializing with the patient while away from work

➤ Disclosing personal information

➤ Engaging in physical contact, flirting, or discussing sexual attraction, including by texting or online messaging

Think about it: How do those factors make patients vulnerable? What knowledge and skills do you need to develop trust-based therapeutic relationships with patients and families? What can you do to help them maintain their dignity?

Actions: In developing professional and therapeutic boundaries, try to achieve the "zone of helpfulness." That is, find a balance between underinvolvement on one end and overinvolvement on the other (National Council of State Boards of Nursing [NCSBN], 2018). The NCSBN calls for nurses to:

➤ Show respect for human dignity.

➤ Avoid personal gratification at the patient's expense.

➤ Never interfere in the patient's personal relationships.

➤ Promote patient autonomy and self-determination.

➤ Understand that the nurse–patient relationship is based on trust.

Nurses have a moral duty to protect patients from inappropriate relationships. Patient-centered care is only possible when boundaries are respected and patients and their families feel safe.

Source: National Council of State Boards of Nursing (2018, August). *A nurse's guide to professional boundaries.* https://www.ncsbn.org/ProfessionalBoundaries_Complete.pdf

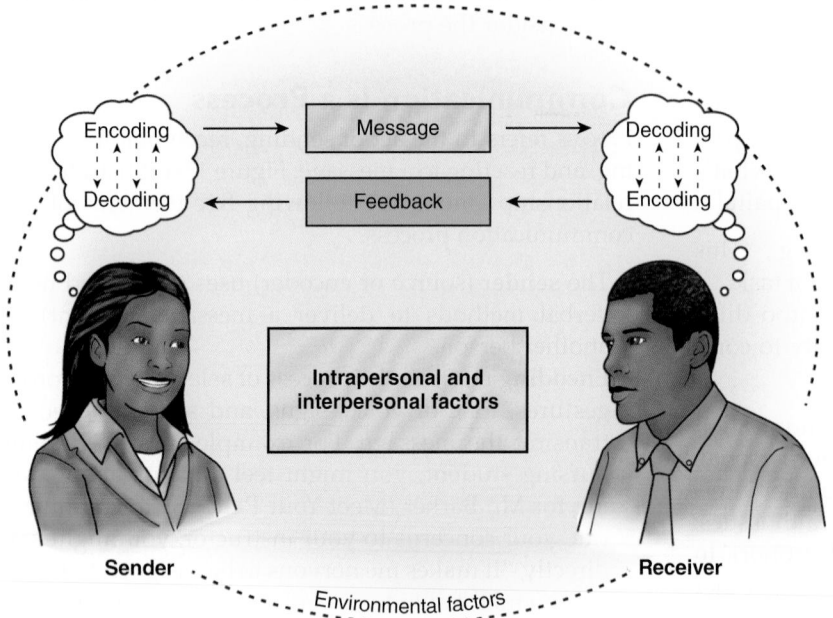

FIGURE 15-1 Communication: A sender encodes and transmits a message to a receiver, who decodes it and transmits feedback.

be appropriate for the situation and for the developmental level of the person receiving the message.
■ The **channel** is the method by which the message is conveyed. Face-to-face communication is a commonly used channel. Nurses may use touch as a nonverbal way to communicate caring and concern. Other channels include written pamphlets, audiovisual aids, recordings, telephone and text messages, and the Internet. When choosing the best channel for communicating, consider the type of message, its purpose, and the size of the audience.
■ The **receiver** is the observer, listener, and interpreter of the message. The receiver interprets **(decodes)** by relating the message to past experiences to determine

the sender's meaning. The receiver uses visual, auditory, and tactile senses to decode the message. If the sender's intended meaning matches what the receiver thinks it means, then the message was effective. Messages are sometimes misinterpreted, especially when the receiver is not physically or emotionally ready to receive the message.

For example, if you approach your instructor to discuss your concerns about your patient when they were assisting with an emergency, they might be unable to receive your message.

- **Feedback** may be verbal, nonverbal, or both. Once the receiver has received and interpreted the message, they may be stimulated to respond by providing feedback to the sender. Feedback validates that the receiver received the message and understood it as the sender intended.

KnowledgeCheck 15-2

Using the Meet Your Patient scenario, identify at least one sender, one message, one receiver, one channel, and one example of feedback.

Verbal Communication

Verbal communication is the use of spoken and written words to send a message. It is influenced by educational background, culture, language, age, gender identification, and past experiences. Verbal communication is generally a conscious act in which the sender chooses the most effective words to communicate a message. The goal of a verbal message is for the receiver to understand both your words and your intended meaning. The following factors affect how a message is received.

Vocabulary

Healthcare workers have a vocabulary of technical terms and jargon. However, patients may be unfamiliar with the language of healthcare and find its use intimidating or, at best, unclear. Consider the following example, in which a nurse says:

You need to be NPO after 2400. I'll be in to prep the op site at 0800. You'll need to void before your premed. Then we'll transfer you to a gurney and take you to the holding area.

Do you think most patients would understand this message? Do *you* understand all the words? Consider how much better it would be if the nurse had said the following:

You will not be able to eat or drink anything after midnight. I'll come in about 8 in the morning to clean your hip and get it ready for your surgery. You'll need to empty your bladder before I give you some medicine to relax you. Then, we'll put you on a cart and take you to the surgical area.

Key Point: *Use medical terms only when you are certain that the listener will understand them. Otherwise, using plain language is more effective.*

Denotative and Connotative Meaning

Denotation is the literal (dictionary) meaning of a word. **Connotation** is the implied or emotional meaning of the word. Consider the following examples:

A mother says to her infant, "Don't cry, baby."
A 40-year-old man says to his spouse, "Would you rub my back, baby?"
A 10-year-old boy says to another boy, "You're a baby!"

The denotative meaning of *baby* is a very young child who is less than a year old. However, the connotative meaning is different in each example. In the first example, the connotative meaning is the same as the denotative meaning. The nurse might interpret the second example as a sexist remark, whereas in the last example, the 10-year-old boy undoubtedly meant *baby* as an insult. As you can see, words are often value laden or biased. **Key Point: *Use terms that provide clear, objective data and are not open for misinterpretation.***

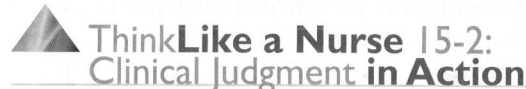

ThinkLike a Nurse 15-2: Clinical Judgment in Action

Think of two other examples in which the connotative meaning of a word may be different from its denotative meaning.

Pacing

The pace and rhythm of the delivery can alter the receiver's interpretation of the message. The pace must be slow enough for the receiver to interpret one thought before the sender moves on to the next thought but must also be fast enough to maintain the listener's interest. When a lecturer talks too slowly, does your mind wander?

Intonation

"Tone of voice," or **intonation,** reflects the feeling behind the words. We listen for:

- *Pitch* (high or low)
- *Cadence* (rising and falling of the pitch)
- *Volume* (soft or loud)

For example, experiment with different ways you might say, "Your test results are in."

Pitch, cadence, and volume can reinforce or contradict the message while conveying various emotions. People tend to tune out when someone speaks in a **monotone** (does not vary the pitch, cadence, and volume). Before presenting lengthy information, whether to an individual or to a group, try different ways to speak to ensure that the listener remains engaged with your topic.

In an electronic message (e.g., text, e-mail), the receiver does not have the benefit of intonation or body language. This may lead to miscommunication. People sometimes insert *emojis, emoticons* (symbols such as "smiley faces"), or animations or use uppercase text to provide cues to the emotional tone of a message.

Clarity and Brevity

A conversation that is clear and brief holds the interest of all parties and effectively conveys the intended messages.

- **Clarity** requires (1) that you select words that convey your intended meaning and (2) that you make sure your spoken words and the nonverbal language send the same message.
- **Brevity** can be achieved by using the fewest words possible.

Timing

Timing is crucial. Before starting a conversation, assess your client. A person who is unable to concentrate (e.g., pain, hunger, distraction) will not receive the message as you intended it. Similarly, a client attempting to cope with stressors (e.g., limited finances, an upcoming surgery) may be too distracted to listen effectively. Consider the following principles:

- *Timing:* **Consider the presence of others.** If you ask a client about a personal issue in the presence of others, you may receive a different response than if you ask the question privately. In contrast, if you are instructing a client about a recommended diet, be sure that the person who does the shopping and cooking is also present.
- *Timing:* **Interaction must allow ample time for response.** A rapid flow of questions or one-sided conversations inhibits interaction.

Relevance

Key Point: *Communication is effective when those involved find the discussion to be important.* When teaching your client about their medication, begin by reminding them of the purpose of the discussion: "Let's talk about how you can take this medication to get the best control of your pain."

Credibility

Patients judge the **credibility** (or believability) of the message by the trustworthiness of the sender. Your credibility depends on a pattern of honest, factual, and timely responses to patient concerns, as well as congruence between your verbal and nonverbal communication.

- **Always be open and honest with patients.** When you unintentionally offer unrealistic reassurance, the patient may feel that you are not being honest and genuine. This ends up impairing trust between the patient and nurse.
- **Give information only if you are certain of the facts.** A response such as, "I don't know, but I will find out for you," is far better than an incorrect answer, guess, or opinion.
- **Keep your promises.** Doing what you say you are going to do builds trust and cooperation with your

patient. This is especially important in healthcare because patients often feel stressed, vulnerable, and emotional (Bladh & Van Leewen, 2017). Timely responses are respectful and help to build a therapeutic relationship.

- **If a situation makes you uncomfortable, it is better to acknowledge your discomfort than to risk a loss of credibility.** For instance, you may feel uncomfortable talking to Mr. Barker (Meet Your Patient) about his recent diagnosis. You may be tempted to say, "Maybe the test results are wrong," or "Everything is going to be okay."
  - If your discomfort is because you need more information or facts, a more honest approach would be to acknowledge that your patient's diagnosis is a serious matter. You might then say, "You must have many questions. I will explain as much as I can, and we can ask your provider to talk to you, too, if you like."
  - If you are uncomfortable addressing Mr. Barker's fears and feelings, you might say, "It might help you to talk to someone about your concerns. Would you like for me to arrange for a more experienced counselor or hospital chaplain to come visit you when you're ready?"
  - To be credible, your body language must be consistent with your spoken words.

Humor

Laughter can create physiological changes that contribute to well-being and provide an emotional release in a tense situation, thus positively influencing the patient's attitude and healing. Patients may also express serious concerns and deal with emotional issues through humor (Schöpf et al., 2017). Humor is highly subjective and personal, and it is influenced by cultural norms. **Key Point:** *Use humor cautiously, and never direct humor at the client, disease process, or treatment team. Misused humor is inappropriate, offensive, and unprofessional.*

Nonverbal Communication

Because nonverbal communication emerges from feelings on a more unconscious level, your patient's body language, including posture, gesture, movement, facial expression, and eye gaze, can tell you how they are coping with what they are hearing and how they are processing the information.

♥ **iCare** Your body language is equally important. When speaking to your patient who is sitting or lying in bed, it is helpful to sit on the side of the bed or to be at eye level, rather than speaking from an elevated, standing position. This can put your patient at ease and help form a genuine connection. Eye contact and face-to-face interactions are certainly important; however, genuine empathy and warmth are the most powerful in making a connection with your patient and fostering good communication (McCabe, 2004; Newell & Jordan, 2015).

Facial Expression Movement of the face and especially the eyes are the most obvious forms of nonverbal communication. Facial expressions communicate joy, anger, sadness, concern, interest, skepticism, apathy, or fear. Raised eyebrows, staring, squinting, or darting eyes all convey meaning. A mismatch between your verbal message and facial expression may be confusing or cause the client to doubt your credibility (Fig. 15-2).

The interpretation of facial expressions is culturally dependent. For example, downcast eyes may indicate a wide variety of messages, including shyness, sadness, poor self-esteem, desire to avoid the conversation, respect, powerlessness, or submissive behavior. Direct eye contact may indicate an interest in the conversation and a willingness to communicate; however, it may make some patients uncomfortable. You must determine the best way to communicate with each individual client.

Posture and Gait Body position, gait, and posture offer clues to a person's attitudes, emotions, physical well-being, and self-concept. When you see someone with an erect posture, head held high, and a quick gait, what do you think? In Western culture, these are nonverbal indicators of health and self-assuredness. In contrast, a slow, shuffling gait may signify someone who is ill, is depressed, or has poor self-esteem.

Personal Appearance First impressions matter, and poor first impressions are hard to change. Professional appearance sets the stage for the initial connection between nurse and patient and shouldn't be overlooked. A professional appearance with clean, appropriate attire conveys competence, confidence, attention to detail, and a valuing of cleanliness (Blahd & Van Leewen, 2017).

Personal appearance provides clues to a person's feelings, socioeconomic status, culture, and religion. A certain style of dress or religious jewelry, piercings, or tattoos may not represent the patient's actual cultural or religious beliefs. **Key Point: *Have you thought about what your own personal appearance conveys to your patients and colleagues?***

Gestures Hand and body gestures emphasize and clarify the spoken word.

- Gestures are good indicators of the feeling tone behind the words. Imagine that your patient says, "I'm okay." What might it mean if they accompany their statement with raised arms? What might it mean if, instead, they lower their head to their hands?
- Gestures vary among individuals, so use them with caution. Suppose someone makes a V with the second and third fingers of the hand. To some people, this is a peace sign; to others, it could be a victory sign, the number two, or have no meaning to it at all.
- Gestures can help you communicate with individuals with impaired verbal communication.

♥ iCare Touch Touch can convey affection, caring, concern, and encouragement (Fig. 15-3). Avoid using touch when dealing with someone who is angry or emotionally unstable because the touch may be misinterpreted (e.g., as a sign of aggression or sexual intention). Although touch can be highly effective, use it with sensitivity and appropriateness to the situation, environment, culture, and receptivity of the patient.

For examples of therapeutic nonverbal behaviors and how patients may interpret them, see Box 15-2.

KnowledgeCheck 15-3
- Identify the components of verbal and nonverbal communication.
- What action should you take when there is a discrepancy between the client's spoken word and nonverbal body language?

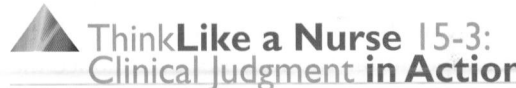
ThinkLike a Nurse 15-3: Clinical Judgment in Action
- Observe an interaction between family members or your fellow students. Look for congruence between verbal and nonverbal communication. Strategize what you would say

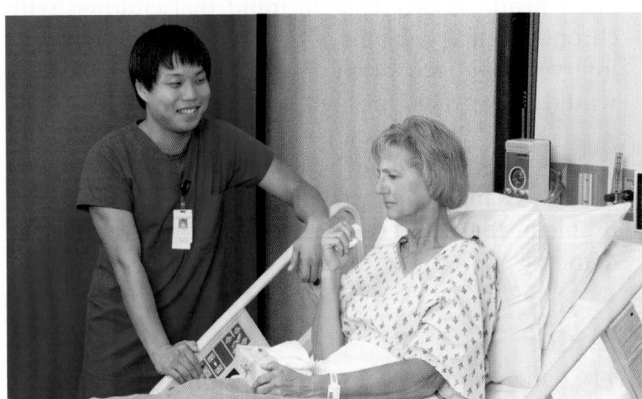
FIGURE 15-2 The nurse's facial expression is not appropriate because the patient appears to be in distress.

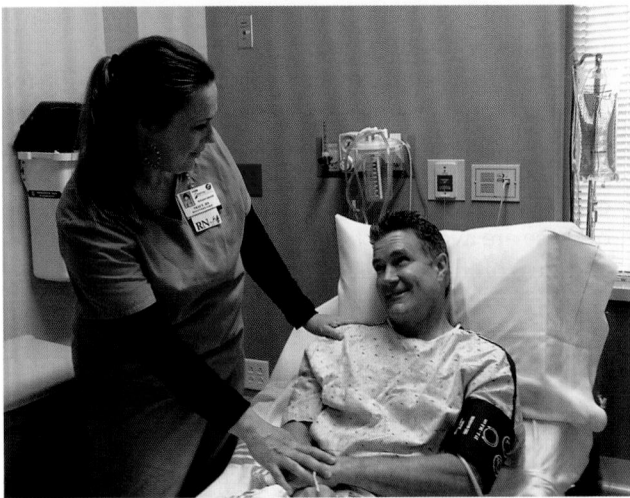
FIGURE 15-3 The nurse conveys genuine caring using touch.

BOX 15-2 ■ Enhancing Communication Through Nonverbal Behaviors

Nonverbal Behaviors	Interpretation
Direct eye contact	Demonstrates interest and attention. Consider the client's cultural heritage when determining how much eye contact is appropriate.
Leaning forward	Shows interest in the conversation.
Personal space	A distance of 18 inches to 4 feet allows most clients to feel comfortable during the interaction. Adjust the distance within that range based on the client's preference.
Concerned facial expression	Lends credibility, if congruent with conversation.
Professional appearance	Gives people an impression of how you may act in your role as a healthcare provider.
Sitting down to talk	Communicates willingness to listen and a sense of not wanting to rush the interaction with the client.
Touch	Conveys caring and concern when used appropriately.
Context	Consider the situation and make sure your body language, tone, gesture, and other nonverbal signals are appropriate and comfortable for the situation.

to validate the intended meaning when the two modes of communication are not in agreement.

■ Recall the brief interaction with the charge nurse in the Meet Your Patient scenario. What might you say or do in response?

WHAT FACTORS AFFECT COMMUNICATION?

The following sections discuss the major factors other than verbal and nonverbal language that affect communication.

Environment

Communication is most successful in an environment that is quiet, private, free of unpleasant smells, and at a comfortable temperature. You may not even notice the noise and distractions in the healthcare setting, but you need to be sensitive to how the environment is affecting your client. Background noise is distracting, interferes with hearing, and can create confusion. Being around others who are in pain or distress creates anxiety and fear; lack of privacy may cause embarrassment. Those feelings may keep your patient from sharing personal information or understanding your message.

♥ iCare To discuss private matters, find a location for conversation that will allow patients and their families to hear important information, freely ask questions, and express emotion. Consider using the hospital chapel, a conference room, or a private room. If none of these are available, be sure to close privacy curtains and turn off the television or other distractions.

Life Span Variations

Physical and cognitive development, language skills, level of education, and maturity influence communication. Therefore, you will need to modify your strategies to communicate effectively, respectfully, and compassionately with patients at all developmental stages. For detailed information on each developmental stage, see Chapters 6 and 7.

■ **Infants** require attachment to a parent or caregiver, nurturing, social interaction, and physical stimulation, such as soothing talk and gentle touch, to achieve normal neurological development.

■ **Young toddlers** with limited language skills communicate nonverbally. Your response may combine verbal and nonverbal communication. For example, if a hospitalized 1-year-old cries out for their mother, you might cuddle the child with their favorite toy and reassure them by saying, "Mama will be back very soon."

■ **Older toddlers and preschoolers** have more verbal ability. Although they may prefer to have a parent present, they are likely to talk with you and answer questions.

■ **School-age children** are usually comfortable interacting verbally. Pay attention to their vocabulary as they speak and match it as closely as possible, using words and phrasing that the child will understand.

■ By the time children reach **adolescence,** most can process abstract concepts. As a result, they are usually able to understand disease processes, treatments, and other health issues. Bear in mind that children with chronic health problems, who have required frequent interventions, are often more knowledgeable than would be expected for their age.

■ **Older adults** are often affected by sensory alterations, such as hearing loss or vision changes, or any of a variety of healthcare problems that affect cognition and expression, such as dementia.

Gender

Every patient or family interaction is unique; there is no "one-size-fits-all" approach even with respect to gender. People have different life experiences that reflect gender identity, gender expression, and sexual orientation. **Key Point:** *Patterns of communication are person specific, not necessarily gender specific.*

♥ **iCare** To create a caring and gender-affirming environment for all individuals:

- Use inclusive, gender-neutral language. For example, when working with a patient who was born male but identifies as transgender or nonbinary, refer to the patient's testicular health rather than men's health.
- Ask patients about their preferred gender pronouns and use them consistently.
- Listen to and reflect patients' language when describing their own sexual identity and how they refer to their relationships or partner.
- Reflect on your own personal biases, preconceptions, and areas for growth.

Regardless of gender, be aware that patients and nurses may express or interpret the same message differently. For example, a patient might state, "I feel so lousy today." One nurse may interpret this comment as a desire to talk, whereas another nurse may discuss pain control.

Personal Space

People vary in the amount of physical space they prefer when communicating. The distance they maintain is influenced by the relationship of the individuals, the nature of the conversation, personal preference, the setting, and culture (Fig. 15-4). Also see Chapter 12 for cultural preferences for personal space. Hall (1992) describes four distinct distances for communication: intimate, personal, social, and public.

Intimate Distance People engaging in personal conversation are typically about 18 inches apart, although it depends on their individual preferences. Within this distance, people can easily interpret facial expressions, maintain eye contact, hear each other speaking at a low volume, and even sense each other's smell and body heat.

♥ **iCare** It is also at this distance that body contact occurs. As a nurse, you invade a client's personal space to perform assessments and procedures, or even while using touch to offer support. This may make some clients uncomfortable. Before providing nursing interventions in the client's intimate distance, discuss what you are about to do. It is best to ask the client's permission, even for gentle touch, if you have the slightest doubt about their receptivity. If the touch is not optional, say, "I'm going to touch you now because [whatever the reason]."

Personal Distance Personal distance is typically from 18 inches up to 4 feet. Interactions with clients and healthcare team members will commonly occur in this range.

♥ **iCare** This distance facilitates sharing of feelings or personal thoughts and is appropriate when communicating caring or concern.

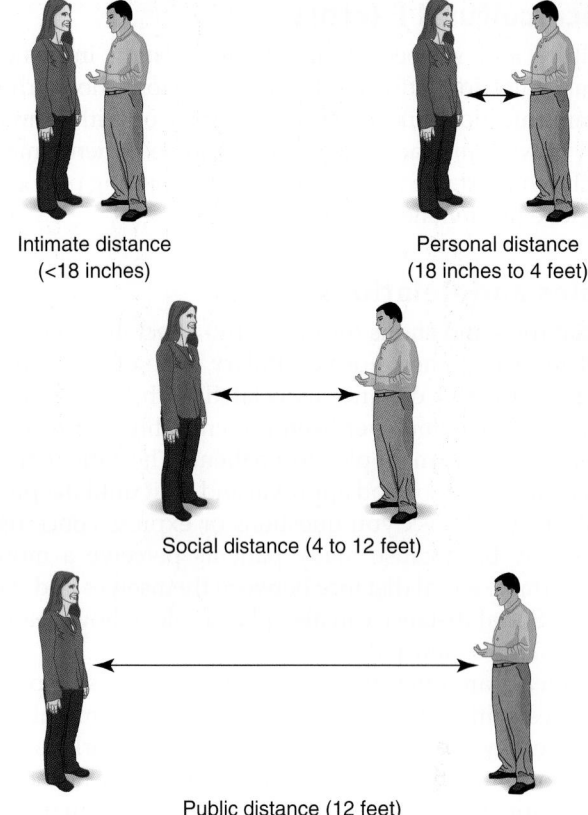

Intimate distance (<18 inches)

Personal distance (18 inches to 4 feet)

Social distance (4 to 12 feet)

Public distance (12 feet)

FIGURE 15-4 The distance that individuals engaged in communication maintain between one another is influenced by their relationship, the nature of the conversation, the setting, and cultural background(s).

Social Distance Social distance is generally between 4 and 12 feet. This is common for formal interactions or when communicating with a group. At this distance, individuals are not within range to be physically touched. The volume of the spoken words may be loud enough for others to overhear, so people share personal feelings and thoughts less often at this distance. For example, if you stand at the client's bedside and ask how they are feeling, you will likely receive a more personal response than if you were to ask the same question while standing at the door.

Public Distance Public distance is beyond 12 feet. This distance requires loud and clear enunciation for communication. This distance is characterized by a lack of individuality and a greater focus on the group or community, as in a lecture.

Territoriality

♥ **iCare Territoriality** refers to the space and things that an individual identifies as their own. In a hospital setting, many patients consider the hospital room and their personal belongings to be their territory. Patients may be uncomfortable if you change, rearrange, or interfere with this personal space. To establish trust, you must request permission to handle, move, or discard any personal item, even if hospital property.

Sociocultural Factors

Culture and socioeconomic status strongly influence communication, affecting facial expressions, nonverbal communication, and even the selection of with whom and how to interact. For example, some patients may not be comfortable with a male nurse providing perineal hygiene to a female patient.

Roles and Relationships

Social roles and status (or hierarchy) affect the sender's and receiver's choice of vocabulary, tone of voice, use of gestures, and distance associated with the communication. Have you ever been present while a provider explained a treatment plan to a patient? The patient may ask no questions or nod approval and wait until the provider leaves to ask you questions or express concerns. This may be because many patients perceive a more comfortable social distance between themselves and the nurse. Social distance can also play a role in how health professionals view patients.

Patients are often unclear about the nurse's responsibilities within the healthcare team. Some might be confused by the fact that many healthcare workers, all of whom may be wearing "scrub apparel," call themselves nurses even though they are not legally qualified to use the title. If you are working with UAPs, medical assistants, or other team members, be sure to clarify their roles with the patient so that they can communicate their questions and concerns to the appropriate healthcare provider. Some agencies are assigning colors for various workers' scrubs (e.g., blue for physicians, purple for nurses) to help patients to identify healthcare workers.

KnowledgeCheck 15-4

- What are the major factors that affect communication?
- At what distance(s) do most nurse–client interactions occur?

WHAT IS COLLABORATIVE PROFESSIONAL COMMUNICATION?

Communication is essential to collaborative practice among nurses, physicians, and health professionals from other disciplines. You might recognize collaborative professional communication by the following characteristics:

- Uses an assertive style
- Makes use of standard communication tools

Communication Styles

Teamwork and communication in the workplace are vital not only for safe and effective patient care but also for work satisfaction and the emotional health of caregivers. Understanding communication styles can help you manage and improve your own approach for effectively communicating with coworkers, patients, and their families.

Passive

Those who adopt a passive approach avoid conflict and allow others to take the lead. Passive communicators may exhibit timid posture or negative body language; they tend to be submissive, indecisive, apologetic, or whining. For example, "Whatever you want. I'll just wait for you to decide what you're going to do." Not taking phone calls or ignoring texts are other examples of a passive approach.

Passive Aggressive

This style of communication avoids direct confrontation but subtly achieves goals through manipulation. Passive-aggressive communicators may appear cooperative or passive on the surface, yet they typically undermine the efforts of others. As a result, passive-aggressive communicators often become alienated from others. Facial expressions and body language do not match with how the person feels.

Incivility and Bullying Passive-aggressive behavior in the workplace can take the form of incivility and bullying. Not only can this type of behavior foster errors and poor patient outcomes (ANA, 2021; The Joint Commission, 2010), but it can also lead to physical and emotional issues among coworkers, such as anxiety, depression, absenteeism, substance abuse, sleep disorders, and in some cases, suicide (Danza, 2018). Passive-aggressive actions may include the denial of support to a coworker, a refusal to communicate, excluding someone from the conversation, withholding information, rudeness, staring, glaring, sighing, eye rolling, or making faces (Kinser, 2018). **Key Point:** *Nurses experiencing bullying in the workplace need to report behaviors to a nurse manager or supervisor; or, if there is no resolution, refer the issue to the agency's human resources department.*

Aggressive

The goal is to win and be in control. Aggressive communicators try to dominate others using intimidation and humiliation. They often blame or criticize others, events, or situations. They are poor listeners, tend to be impulsive, and have a low tolerance for frustration. Intimidating posture and overbearing voice tone are common. "My way is the correct way. You don't know what you're talking about," typifies an aggressive approach.

Workplace violence. The Joint Commission (2021, p. 1) defines workplace violence as "an act or threat occurring at the workplace that can include any of the following: verbal, nonverbal, written, or physical aggression; threatening, intimidating, harassing, or humiliating words or actions; bullying; sabotage; sexual harassment; physical assaults; or other behaviors of concern involving staff, licensed practitioners, patients, or visitors." Of those reporting workplace violence, patients are overwhelmingly most often inflicting physical harm or verbal abuse on nurses. Among those experiencing emotional abuse, managers/administrations, followed by patients, most commonly are the offenders. However, underreporting of workplace violence incidents is believed to be a major problem (The Joint Commission, 2021).

Assertive

Assertive communication is the expression of a wide range of positive and negative thoughts and feelings in a style that is direct, open, honest, spontaneous, responsible, and nonjudgmental. When using this style of communication, you take responsibility for your own thoughts and actions without blaming others, encourage feedback, and enable yourself to find mutually satisfying solutions to conflict by confronting people constructively.

How Do I Communicate Assertively?

Caring for patients relies on the healthcare team working together and communicating effectively. Teamwork and effective communication also contribute to job satisfaction, professional engagement, and growth. Mutual support and awareness of signs of stress and overload are key. Techniques for communicating assertively and professionally include the following:

- **Maintain professional composure.**
  - Maintain eye contact, as culturally appropriate.
  - Speak clear language to accurately convey your intention.
  - Project a clear tone of voice in a respectful manner.
  - Communicate self-confidently.
  - Convey a can-do attitude.
  - Refrain from sarcasm.
  - Do not invite negative responses.
- **Use *I* statements.** An *I* statement should include the elements of behavior (or facts), feeling, and effect (on you) (American Heart Association, 2021). For example, instead of saying, "Why haven't you ordered Ms. Sadiq's pain medications yet?" you might say, "I contacted you this morning about Ms. Sadiq's lack of pain relief, but I don't see a change in her analgesic order. I am concerned about her discomfort and the effect it may have on her willingness to ambulate."
- **Focus on the issue, not the participants.** For example, "I think this approach might be the best, but I'd like to hear your thoughts."
- **Use effective nonverbal language.** Your body and verbal language should be congruent. Eye contact demonstrates interest and shows sincerity. Posture also communicates your attention and interest in the dialogue.
- **Invite positive responses.** For example, say, "I would really appreciate it if you could help me weigh Mr. Kudari on the bed scale," rather than, "Would you want to help me weigh him?"
- **Learn to accept criticism without becoming anxious or defensive.** Acknowledge that you might not have had experience with a particular patient situation or might not have the required depth of knowledge in an area. Suppose Ms. Nobu's prescriber says, "Are you playing pharmacist today?" You might respond, "It's true—I am not an expert on analgesics. However, Ms. Nobu needs pain relief, and I need your help prescribing pain medication."
- **Strive for a workable compromise,** but not if it affects patient well-being or your feelings of self-respect. Suppose an administrator comes to a patient's room while you are inserting a nasogastric tube and says, "I need to see you right now. Come to the desk immediately." An example of a workable compromise would be to say, "I understand that you need to talk to me right away, but I need to finish what I am doing. What about meeting you at the nurses' station as soon as I finish, in about 10 minutes?"
- **Assertiveness is a learned skill.** Role-playing with a colleague can build your confidence and improve your approach to communicating with patients, especially when conveying bad news or other difficult information (Laranjeira et al., 2021).

How Do I Communicate Safely?

 Effective communication and teamwork are essential for the delivery of high-quality, safe patient care. To avoid communication failures that can lead to unanticipated adverse events in patients, nurses must speak up when they have concerns and take the necessary steps to communicate assertively and collaboratively with the healthcare team (The Joint Commission, n.d.).

For additional guidelines from professional organizations about collaborative communication for patient safety,

Go to Clinical Insight 15-1, Collaborative Professional Communication, in Volume 2.

- **Question care decisions openly and honestly.** To advocate for clients, you must question care decisions that do not seem right to you and assertively discuss errors or poor clinical judgment with coworkers. Avoid beginning your statements with timid or self-effacing statements that fail to take credit for your contributions (e.g., "You may disagree with this …"). For example, a nurse at handover might say to the nurse who has been caring for a critically ill patient, "I want to be sure that I have everything right and that I am clear about what is most important for this patient."
- **Use "critical (CUS) language."** Use your CUS words: **concerned, uncomfortable, and safety,** as in, "I'm concerned, I'm uncomfortable, this is unsafe, or I'm scared" (Agency for Healthcare Research and Quality, 2020; Leonard et al., 2004). Some organizations identify a code phrase for themselves, for example,

"I need clarity." In this situation, the receiver of the request must stop and listen attentively while the sender asserts the issues that need to be clarified (Amer, 2013; The Joint Commission, 2010).

- **Practice closed-loop communication.** In closed-loop communication, both the sender and receiver confirm that the information is correctly communicated and understood. The following is an example of how this method reduces error:

The resuscitation team arrives for an adult patient in cardiac arrest. The physician orders 1.0 mg of epinephrine 1:10,000 dilution to be given IV bolus. The nurse repeats aloud to the team before administering the drug: "1.0 mg of epinephrine, 1:10,000 dilution, IV bolus." The physician repeats: "That is correct. 1.0 mg epinephrine, 1:10,000 dilution, IV bolus."

This method reduces the risk of errors caused by miscommunication, assumptions, or misinterpretation. Read-back measures also verify information and are especially useful for preventing medication errors.

- **Use checklists.** Lists are a simple, clear, and effective way to communicate necessary information and interventions for patient care and safety, thus preventing care that might be missed or delayed (Robson, 2016).
- **Add debriefs at the end of the shift.** Another way to ensure communication is to gather at the end of a shift for a short meeting to discuss what went well and what could be improved. Consider this time to be a "teachable moment" (Robson, 2016).

Using Standardized Communication Tools

Nurses are taught to be more descriptive of clinical situations and patient responses, whereas physicians learn to be concise and precise. Standardized communication tools are effective in overcoming differences in nurse–physician communication styles and conveying key information clearly and concisely. Structured communication tools ensure accuracy and create an environment in which individuals can express concerns. This facilitates the exchange of information for healthcare professionals involved in the patient's care.

A well-known and highly effective method for team communication and collaboration is the **SBARQ** model. The acronym represents **S**ituation, **B**ackground, **A**ssessment, **R**ecommendation, and **Q**uestion. For further explanation of this model,

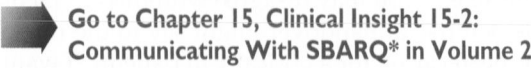
Go to Chapter 15, Clinical Insight 15-2: Communicating With SBARQ* in Volume 2.

For more information about giving a verbal report, also see Chapter 17.

Using the Patient Rounds Approach

Patient rounding is an example of collaborative communication in which the healthcare team gathers at the patient care area to discuss goals for care and/or changes in the plan of care and to respond to the questions of the patient, family, and healthcare staff. Meeting for rounds allows the nurse to provide input that leads to improved interprofessional working relationships and professional satisfaction.

A **handoff report** is the process of communicating patient information to another healthcare provider, commonly at the end of a shift or when transferring the patient's care to a provider in another unit or facility or at home.

WHAT IS THE ROLE OF COMMUNICATION IN THERAPEUTIC RELATIONSHIPS?

♥ **iCare** Caring is integral to a therapeutic nurse–patient relationship, which, according to Benner (1984), is a core value of nursing practice. She uses the terms *connectedness* and *involvement* to describe nursing. In demanding environments, nurses multitask and function with many competing priorities. Because of this, they run the risk of conveying a rushed, noncaring attitude to patients. This can be frustrating to patients and exhausting for nurses.

- A **therapeutic relationship** focuses on improving the health of the client, whether an individual or community.
- Therapeutic communication is essential for providing high-quality nursing care. It increases patient satisfaction, decreases patient anxiety, and improves patient cooperation and compliance with treatment. It is used to establish the therapeutic relationship, provide and obtain healthcare information, and express interest in and concern for the client and family.

Communication Is Essential to All Phases of the Therapeutic Relationship

The therapeutic relationship consists of four phases. As you read about each phase, notice the fundamental role of client-focused communication.

Preinteraction Phase The preinteraction phase occurs before you meet the client. You lay the groundwork for communication by gathering information about the client, but you do not communicate directly with the client. As a student, you initiate this phase as you prepare for clinical shifts. The client also experiences a preinteraction phase, which begins when they identify the need for healthcare.

Orientation Phase The goal of the orientation phase is to establish rapport and trust using verbal and nonverbal communication. This phase begins when you meet the client and introduce yourself and your role in the relationship. When rapport is established, clients are more likely to express their concerns openly and seek emotional support. Because the clients may not be immediately ready to communicate, it is important to be sensitive to mood, experience, and overall physical and psychological state. Try to understand the cause of your client's behavior, comments, and attitudes, and respond with patience and wisdom. Orientation ends when the relationship has been defined.

Working Phase Most therapeutic communication occurs in the **working phase,** the active part of the relationship. During this phase, the nurse communicates caring, the patient expresses thoughts and feelings, mutual respect is maintained, and honest verbal and nonverbal expression occurs. Key communication goals are to assist the client to clarify feelings and concerns. A professional relationship is courteous, trustworthy, and confidential and is accomplished by active listening.

Termination Phase The conclusion of the relationship marks the **termination phase,** whether at the end of the nurse's shift or on the client's discharge from the unit, facility, or service. Reviewing and summarizing help to bring the relationship to a comfortable closure. If communication has been effective, the termination phase prepares the nurse and client for future interactions. Unsuccessful communication may affect the client's health outcomes or understanding of their disease process, as well as affect the nurse's job satisfaction.

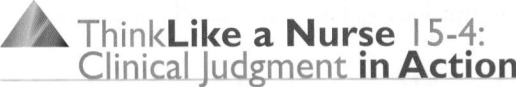

ThinkLike a Nurse 15-4: Clinical Judgment in Action

Recall the scenario of Mr. Barker (Meet Your Patient).

- What phase of the therapeutic relationship is illustrated in the scenario?
- How might the interaction between you and Mr. Barker change if it occurred in a different phase of the therapeutic relationship?
- What could you have done differently?

Therapeutic Communication Has Five Key Characteristics

The therapeutic relationship requires *therapeutic use of self:* conscious use of your knowledge and skills to effect change in the patient. This requires practice so that you will be able to recognize boundaries and focus on the patient rather than on your own feelings and experiences.

Five qualities characterize communication in the therapeutic relationship: empathy, respect, genuineness, concreteness, and confrontation. Later in the chapter, you will learn specific strategies for enhancing communication, as well as barriers to therapeutic communication. Look for these techniques and barriers in any conversation you analyze.

♥ **iCare Empathy** The desire to understand and be sensitive to the feelings, beliefs, and situation of another person is called **empathy.** It requires you to adapt your style, tone, vocabulary, and behavior to create the best approach for each client situation. It is

relatively easy to have empathy for people who are like you and who are likable. It is more difficult to connect with people you see as difficult or different. To empathize with a client, you must look beyond outward appearance or behavior and put yourself, mentally and emotionally, in the client's place. The empathy with which you care for your patients, deliver difficult news, or guide them through complex decisions can have an enormous impact on patients' and family members' experience and adaptation to illness.

♥ **iCare Respect** In the therapeutic relationship, you communicate respect by valuing the client and being flexible to meet the client's needs. You show respect when you introduce yourself to your clients and ask for their preferred way to be addressed. Making even minor adjustments in patient care, such as delaying breakfast for an hour to allow the client to sleep, communicates that you respect the client's wishes. When a relationship is grounded in respect, both parties maintain power and self-esteem. Be appreciative. A word of gratitude and recognition also goes a long way in building collegial relationships and promoting cooperation (American Heart Association, 2021).

♥ **iCare Genuineness** When interviewing clients, we expect them to respond truthfully. Similarly, clients have a right to truthful responses from healthcare providers.

- **Genuineness requires honesty.** If you are unable to answer a client's question, do not offer guesses. Make a response such as, "I don't know, but I'll find out and let you know."
- **Genuineness also involves a willingness to self-evaluate.** How well did I communicate? Did I handle that situation appropriately and respectfully? How could I improve my communication?

Concreteness In a therapeutic relationship, you must offer understandable responses to a client's questions and concerns. To do so requires you to express what you mean in concrete, specific terms. The message must be constructed and delivered in a manner that is suitable for the client.

Confrontation If your client is unable to express thoughts clearly, ask them directly to say it another way or clarify the point further. Similarly, you must be willing to be challenged if you are unclear.

Communication Is Important in Group Helping Relationships

Nurses frequently communicate with groups, for example, when interacting with a family, a community, or a committee. Groups can enhance problem-solving and creativity, generate understanding and support, enhance morale, and provide affiliation. However, *groupthink,* a pattern of communication in which consensus overrides creativity in problem-solving, can emerge, particularly in cohesive groups or those with an unbalanced power structure.

In small groups, all members have an opportunity to communicate their opinions. In larger groups, patterns of communication form; some members voice their opinion regularly, whereas others are often quiet. When only a few members participate in discussion, it is essential to examine nonverbal behavior to determine whether the nonspeaking members are understanding the discussion.

Task Groups Task groups are formed to address a task or fulfill a need. Typically, members are chosen based on their ability to complete the activity. Other times, members are selected for reasons of convenience, such as availability, interest, or agenda, rather than for the skills needed to accomplish the goal of the group. Short-term groups disband once the task is completed (e.g., a task force to address holiday scheduling or a panel to critique response to a disaster drill). Because the group members' time together is limited, the focus of communication is on the task at hand. Therefore, time to develop rapport or relationships is limited.

Ongoing Groups Ongoing groups address recurrent issues. Committees are a form of an ongoing task group. Ongoing committees in healthcare organizations include quality improvement, infection control, and discharge planning. Members have designated roles within the group (e.g., presenter, recorder, timekeeper). A leader or chairperson is usually appointed or elected.

Self-Help Groups Self-help groups are voluntary organizations composed of individuals with a common need, experience, or concern.

- They are typically peer-led groups. Members decide on shared goals and tasks, and they share responsibilities. Members are encouraged to share experiences and seek support from other members of the group. Communications are to be open and honest to promote self-healing and contribute to positive group experiences.
- Self-help groups most often have face-to-face meetings, but they may also participate in online formats.
- Nurses or experts in the field may be consulted to offer guidance or education to the group.
- Self-help groups are open. People attend when they feel the need for support. Generally, there are no registration or attendance requirements. Sometimes, depending on its purpose, people attend for a specific period, depending on their needs.
- There is generally no or little cost to attend. Groups may ask for donations to cover the cost of refreshments, publicity, rental of meeting space, copying of materials, and so on; no one profits financially.

Therapy Groups Therapy groups are organized to help individual members cope with challenging personal issues or stressful life events, such as divorce, death of a spouse, or new motherhood. Therapy groups may also address ways to improve relationships and improve communication. Also called *self-awareness* or *growth groups*, they may be ongoing or have a designated length of operation.

Work-Related Social Support Groups These support groups help members of a profession cope with the stress associated with their work. The helping professions can be emotionally draining. Members have an opportunity to share concerns and offer mutual support through facilitated formal meetings or informal drop-in events. To be successful, a group must have characteristics that allow the group to function and achieve its goals (Box 15-3).

KnowledgeCheck 15-5

- Identify and describe the phases of the therapeutic relationship.
- What are the five characteristics of therapeutic communication?
- Describe the difference between a task group and a self-help group.
- Compare and contrast the role of a therapy group with that of a work-related support group.

ThinkLike a Nurse 15-5: Clinical Judgment in Action

Review the local newspaper, the hospital social media group, the Internet, and the school intranet. Identify at least three group helping experiences available. How might you learn more about these organizations? How would you determine whether they are resources that you might make available to your patients?

PracticalKnowledge knowing how

Therapeutic communication is used throughout the nursing process. In the next few sections, we explore communication problems as well as therapeutic interventions.

 ASSESSMENT/RECONGIZING CUES

Assessment is essential to effective communication. You should assess for factors that alter a client's ability to receive, process, or transmit information, such as

---

BOX 15-3 ■ Characteristics of a Successful Group

A successful group includes the following:
- Clearly defined purpose
- Shared set of guidelines under which the group functions
- Sense of shared responsibility
- Shared leadership
- Mutual trust
- Comfort among members
- Climate that is cohesive but does not stifle individuality
- Members who are willing to share feelings, concerns, or beliefs
- Flexibility to change what is not working

developmental delays, physical and cognitive impairment, substance abuse, and so forth.

For further information, refer to guidelines for a focused assessment of patient communication,

 Go to Chapter 15, Assessment Guidelines and Tools, Focused Assessment: Communication, in Volume 2.

NURSING DIAGNOSIS/ANALYZING CUES

Communication can be the problem or the etiology of a nursing diagnosis. The following NANDA-I diagnosis labels describe communication problems. Note that communication problems may involve the inability to receive, interpret, or express spoken, written, and nonverbal messages.

- **Readiness for Enhanced Communication** is recommended by NANDA-I when the client expresses a willingness to enhance communication that is already effective.
- **Impaired Oral Communication** is an appropriate diagnosis if the client has (1) expressive aphasia or a physiological problem, such as dyspnea, stuttering, or laryngeal cancer, that impairs the ability to speak or (2) receptive aphasia or sensory deficits that impair the ability to receive messages.
- **Impaired Communication** is the preferred diagnosis if the client is unfamiliar with the dominant language or has some other difficulty in receiving and sending messages.

Etiologies of Communication Diagnoses

Your assessment data will help you determine whether communication impairment is the primary problem or whether it is a result of other health problems. Some nursing diagnoses may cause or contribute to communication problems, for example:

- Acute or chronic confusion may cause difficulty in expressing or receiving verbal and nonverbal messages. Confusion may be related to physical (e.g., stroke, head trauma) or mental health issues (e.g., dementia), a side effect of medications, or sleep deprivation.
- Mental health problems can also lead to communication problems, for example:
  - Anxiety impairs the ability to deliver and receive messages.
  - Chronic or Situational Low Self-Esteem often results in limited interaction with others.

Communication as Etiology of Other Nursing Diagnoses

Impaired Verbal Communication may be the etiology of other nursing diagnoses, for example:

- Anxiety r/t inability to communicate needs
- Impaired Social Interaction r/t inability to carry on conversation

- Chronic Low Self-Esteem r/t fear of conversing with others secondary to stuttering

PLANNING/PRIORITIZING HYPOTHESES AND GENERATING SOLUTIONS

Individualized client outcomes and goals depend on the nursing diagnosis you identify. For example, for Impaired Verbal Communication, you might write the following desired outcomes for a client:

- Uses alternative methods of communication (e.g., writing, picture board, gestures) effectively.
- Demonstrates minimal frustration with communication difficulties.
- Communicates effectively using a translator or interpreter.
- Interprets messages accurately, as evidenced by appropriate verbal or nonverbal feedback.

IMPLEMENTATION/TAKING ACTION NP

Specific nursing activities for communication problems depend on the etiology of the problem and on the goals selected. The focus of nursing interventions is to facilitate communication and resolve or reduce the factors interfering with it.

NIC standardized interventions for Impaired Verbal Communication are Active listening, Assertiveness Training, Communication Enhancement (Hearing or Visual Deficit), Presence, and Touch.

Enhancing Therapeutic Communication

The following sections contain techniques and activities you can implement immediately to improve your communication with patients and others.

Addressing the Patient

♥ **iCare** In the orientation phase of the relationship, ask your patients how they would prefer to be addressed. For patients who are unable to respond, ask family members how you might best address them. This conveys respect, which is essential to a therapeutic relationship.

Active Listening

People often think of listening as a passive activity. If you have ever been in a one-sided conversation, you know that listening can be passive. In contrast, an active listener uses all senses to focus on the sender's message and allows the sender the opportunity to complete comments without interruption (Fig. 15-5).

Failure to listen to your client will result in missed messages or misinterpretation. Consider the following example:

Patient: I guess I'm going to have surgery tomorrow.
Nurse: [Checking the IV fluids and hanging a medication.] Uh-huh.

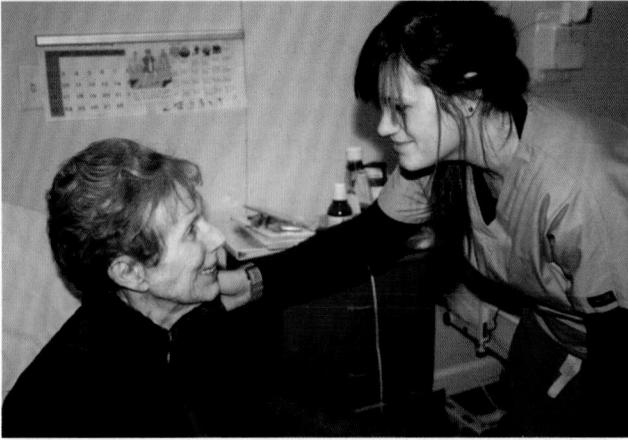

FIGURE 15-5 Active listening using full attention, direct eye contact, and caring touch.

> *Patient:* The surgeon says I'll be in intensive care for a few days.
>
> *Nurse:* [*Looking at the drainage in the urine collection bag.*] Okay. Your urine looks good.
>
> *Patient:* I guess this is a pretty risky surgery.
>
> *Nurse:* [*Recording on the flow sheet.*] Yep.

How do you think the patient must feel in this situation? The patient is clearly expressing concern about their upcoming surgery and seems to want to talk about it with the nurse. However, the nurse is busy with a variety of tasks and is not paying attention to the conversation. Undoubtedly, the patient will continue to feel anxious. In fact, their unsuccessful attempts to communicate may even increase their anxiety. If the nurse were listening, this would be an excellent opportunity to discuss the patient's concerns, provide preoperative teaching, and help the patient ease their anxiety.

Establishing Trust

Honesty and disclosure cannot exist without trust. That is why mutual trust is an essential component of professional and therapeutic communication. As trust grows, the client can more easily relay information and share feelings. To establish trust, always greet the client by name and preferred pronoun, listen actively, respond honestly to the client's concerns, and provide competent and consistent care.

Being Assertive

An assertive person can express themselves effectively and directly communicate their point of view while still respecting the viewpoints and beliefs of others. Because assertive communication is based on mutual respect and the confidence to confront difficult issues, the therapeutic relationship is a safe place for clients to convey their needs and concerns without feeling judged.

♥ **iCare 15-1**

Caring Using Active Listening

Active listening behaviors convey caring, signal a willingness to listen, and provide a comfortable environment for the client to share their concerns. To listen actively:

- Keep your attention in the moment and on the patient. Do not multitask.
- Do not look at your smartphone or watch; never text while the patient is talking.
- Do not interrupt the patient.
- Pay attention to verbal and nonverbal communication and look for congruence.
- If a message is unclear, seek clarification through the use of probing questions or reflective comments, such as, "Tell me more," or "When you say … what do you mean?"
- Face your client, lean in, and make eye contact.
- Focus the conversation on issues of importance to the client (see Fig. 15-5).
- Using a mobile device during a conversation distracts you from active listening. If you must take notes, use audio recording or take notes using only key words to stimulate your memory at another time.
- Do not casually talk with coworkers while the patient is waiting.

Restating, Clarifying, and Validating Messages

These three techniques help to identify client concerns and focus communication. They are especially helpful if the client is unclear or vague about a message.

- **Restating** means using your own words to summarize the message you received from the client. This demonstrates concern, active listening, and understanding of what the patient has said. The following is an example:
  - *Client:* I'm so worried about my diabetes. I have young kids. I want to see them grow up. I know too many diabetics who have died young.
  - *Nurse:* Diabetes is a serious disease. I understand your worry about its effects on you. That's why we want to focus on becoming well controlled so that you can avoid complications.
- **Clarifying** messages helps ensure that you have accurately interpreted the information. For instance, you might state, "I'm not sure what you mean when you say you're so worried about your diabetes." Or "When you say you're worried, what do you mean?"
- **Validate** the message by asking the client whether you are making a correct interpretation: "When you say you're worried about your diabetes, do you mean you are afraid you will die soon?"

Interpreting Body Language and Sharing Observations

Be attentive to what the patient says and how they say it. Note the tone of voice, rate of speech, distance, eye movement, facial expressions, and gestures. If the spoken and the nonverbal messages are inconsistent, you can share your observations by describing the patient's body language or tone of voice. For example, you might say, "I know you said you feel well, but your voice and hands are trembling. How can I help you?" Or more simply, "You're frowning. Has something upset you?"

Exploring Issues

Ask open-ended questions to obtain a clear understanding of an issue and follow your client's thoughts. Probing comments, such as "Tell me more," encourage your client to share information.

Using Silence

Learn to be comfortable with silence, especially when your client is emotionally upset. When you remain attentive, silence demonstrates acceptance and allows the client to organize their thoughts and thus provide further information.

Summarizing the Conversation

At the end of the conversation, summarize what you have heard. For example, you might say, "Today we talked about diet, exercise, and medications for high blood pressure. Your assignment now is to review the handouts and start taking your medication every morning. I'll see you in 2 weeks at your follow-up visit." Summarizing demonstrates active listening and allows the client to clarify misunderstandings.

Using Process Recordings

A strategy commonly used to improve therapeutic communication skills is called **process recording.** In process recording, ideally, two people converse while a third records the conversation. Documentation of the conversation is objective and not influenced by memory.

- **Audio recording** captures the words and intonation of the conversation, but it must be supplemented by notes describing the nonverbal communication.
- **Video recording** allows participants to examine both verbal and nonverbal communication.

Afterward, the participants analyze the interaction. As you examine an interaction, evaluate how well you showed empathy, respect, and genuineness. Identify techniques you used to enhance the communication (e.g., active listening, restating, reflective listening). Be alert for barriers to therapeutic communication.

Barriers to Therapeutic Communication

As you learn to communicate therapeutically, you may find yourself thinking, doing, or saying things that seem to shut down your conversation. If so, acknowledge your error and return to therapeutic patterns. The following sections describe the most common barriers to therapeutic communication.

Asking Too Many Questions

Asking questions at the appropriate time is important. However, asking too many questions, especially closed questions (requiring only a yes or no answer), can make clients feel that they are being interrogated. It may also suggest insensitivity or a lack of respect for the client's issues, as in the following dialogue:

Patient:	I feel lousy today.
Nurse:	Didn't you sleep well?
Patient:	No, hardly at all.
Nurse:	Did you take anything to help you sleep?
Patient:	No.
Nurse:	Do you think you should have taken something?
Patient:	I guess.
Nurse:	Why didn't you tell the night nurse you needed something?
Patient:	I don't know.

As you can see, this approach controls the range and nature of client responses. In contrast, open-ended questions stimulate conversation and exploration. Consider the preceding conversation in comparison with the following conversation:

Patient:	I feel lousy today.
Nurse:	Lousy? Tell me more.
Patient:	Well, my back and neck hurt, and I hardly slept at all. I thought it would go away, but I just lay in bed last night worrying.
Nurse:	What kind of things are you worrying about?
Patient:	I'm worried about …

Notice that the nurse's open-ended questions encouraged the patient to discuss their concerns.

Fire-Hosing Information

Sometimes a healthcare provider might meet with a patient or family and deliver an overwhelming amount of information in a short time. Those involved might understand what the provider said but afterward remember only a portion of it. Or they might feel stunned, confused, intimidated, or helpless. It is better to engage your patient in a dialogue in which you give important information and prompt your patient to share their own concerns and questions. You can then ask them about their understanding of what has been shared and clarify when needed.

Asking Why

Sometimes we need to learn why a patient acted or responded as they did. However, directly asking for reasons suggests criticism to some people. If you ask, "Why did you stop taking your medication?" the patient may become defensive and stop talking. A subtle approach is more comfortable for the patient. You might ask, "What concerns do you have about your medication?" or "Tell me more about your experience with the medication."

Both approaches will help you obtain more information about the client's concerns without suggesting criticism.

Changing the Subject Inappropriately

Try not to abruptly change the topic of discussion because you will seem uninterested. This often occurs when the nurse is intent on one issue and the patient is focused on another, or if the topic is difficult to discuss (e.g., abnormal test results, poor prognosis).

Notice when a person changes the subject, as in the following example:

Nurse:	Your wife is very sick. Do you think she will get better?
Patient's spouse:	It's tough, I know. Her condition reminds me of a movie I saw last night. She even looks like the lead actress.

Your relationship with your patient's partner and the facts of the situation determine whether you would redirect this conversation back to the original subject or allow the digression. You may choose to give the partner more time to be comfortable with you before approaching this topic again.

Failing to Probe

Failing to ask relevant questions can convey a lack of caring. It can also result in incomplete assessment and affect the quality of your care. When assessing, you should explore issues in detail. Review the following conversations:

Patient:	I'm having a lot of discomfort in my back.
Nurse:	How much does it hurt?
Patient:	Quite a bit. I had trouble sleeping last night.
Nurse:	I'll get you something for pain.

Compare that conversation with the next example, in which the nurse gathers additional data:

Patient:	I'm having a lot of discomfort in my back.
Nurse:	Tell me about the discomfort.
Patient:	It hurts a lot. I had trouble sleeping last night.
Nurse:	When did you first notice this pain?
Patient:	It started in the middle of the night.
Nurse:	What does it feel like?
Patient:	I feel sore. I'd like to turn over to my side, but I can't because of this heavy cast.
Nurse:	Let me help you turn. *[Assists patient to turn and uses pillows to hold the patient on her side.]*
Patient:	Oh, that feels better!
Nurse:	I'm glad you're feeling better. Would you like something for pain as well?
Patient:	I think I'm okay now.

In the second example, the nurse followed her original question with additional probing questions. A few additional questions helped clarify what the patient needed and led to immediate comfort.

Expressing Approval or Disapproval

Nurses need to be sensitive about expressing both approval and disapproval to a patient. Although it may seem supportive, expressing approval can inhibit further sharing—it puts you in the position of being the judge of what is "right." This often prompts the patient to continue to seek approval. The patient thinks, "I'd better be careful; she may not approve of the next thing I was going to tell her. She expects me to be this way." Instead, consider offering recommendations and allowing the patient to choose. Read the following exchange:

Patient:	I've decided I'm going to have the surgery.
Nurse:	That's great. I think you made the right choice.

Compare that conversation with the following example:

Patient:	I've decided I'm going to have the surgery.
Nurse:	Tell me about your decision.
Patient:	Well, my shoulder has been bothering me for several months now. I know I said I wanted to put off surgery, but I think I'll have a faster recovery if I just get the surgery done now.
Nurse:	Your choices are to do a trial of physical therapy and anti-inflammatory medications, to try a steroid injection, or to have surgery.
Patient:	Right. But there's a good chance I'll still need surgery even if I try the therapy or medication. The only thing that will actually fix the problem is surgery. The others don't guarantee improvement.

Can you see how the conversation changes if the nurse does not express approval? By encouraging the patient to discuss the choices, the nurse empowers the patient to make their own healthcare decisions.

Offering Advice

Avoid statements such as "If I were you …" or "You should …" These statements impose your opinion on your clients. In effect, your statements function as approval if they agree with the client's thoughts or disapproval if they do not. As with other forms of approval or disapproval, the conversation halts. If the client asks, "What should I do?" help clarify the options and provide the client with information about the choices. Giving the client your solution deprives the client of the opportunity to participate as a partner in the decision-making process.

Providing False Reassurance

- **Providing realistic reassurance helps to ease concern, offers comfort, and communicates empathy.** Therefore, it is an appropriate and therapeutic action—if the reassurance is warranted.

> Example: *A patient presents to the emergency department (ED) for treatment of an acute episode of asthma. Because anxiety can trigger asthma, it is certainly therapeutic to reassure the patient that they will be cared for promptly and effectively.*

■ **False reassurance is a barrier to therapeutic communication.** When patients or family members ask for information or tell you that they are worried, it is easy to reassure them that everything will be fine. However, such responses are uninformed and inaccurate and may feel dismissive and disingenuous, even condescending.

> Example: *You are a nurse working at the triage station in the local ED. Your role is to evaluate the condition and prioritize the care of all clients presenting for treatment. An ambulance arrives with a man experiencing severe chest pain. He is ashen and short of breath. He tells you his pain is "crushing." Suspecting a heart attack, you immediately move him to the critical care bay of the ED and request urgent evaluation. Several minutes later, his wife arrives. She anxiously asks you, "How is my husband?" How would you respond?*

It may feel natural to offer a response such as, "Don't worry; everything will be all right." But do you really know that will be the case? A better approach is to provide accurate information: "I had him immediately taken in for treatment. I'll get you in to see him as soon as I can. Please have a seat, and I'll check on him." This comment is accurate and calming and avoids misleading the person.

Stereotyping

As discussed in Chapter 12, racial, cultural, religious, age-related, or gender stereotypes distort assessment and prevent you from recognizing the patient's uniqueness. Examples of statements reflecting a stereotype include the following: "He's old; he won't remember anything you tell him," and "Men are always the biggest wimps about pain." Such comments block communication and escalate tension.

Stereotypes and generalizations may be blatant or subtle. Obvious examples, such as the preceding ones, are easily recognized and may create an intense reaction. Others are harder to identify but may be equally disruptive to care, for example:

■ Believing a patient will be calm and know what to expect because they had previous hospitalizations for the same diagnosis, had previous surgeries or other procedures, or was given information about the condition
■ Assuming patients will understand their plan for healthcare because of educational level or work experience (e.g., expecting that a physician who has suffered a heart attack needs little or no explanation of care)

■ Expecting all patients with the same surgery or diagnosis to experience similar responses

Using Patronizing Language

Patronizing language communicates superiority or disapproval. Statements such as, "You ought to know …" are patronizing and offensive to the client. Condescending approaches, such as, "You should have used the call button before you got up; you're lucky you didn't hurt yourself," do not communicate respect for the client.

Elderspeak, another form of patronizing behavior, describes ways that healthcare workers may unintentionally show disrespect to elderly patients by speaking to them in a high-pitched, louder, slower, repetitive, childlike voice and calling patients "sweetie," "dearie," or "mama." Staff may also alter pronouns, saying, for example, "Are we ready for our bath?" Although the intent is to communicate caring, many patients are offended because it sounds as though you are speaking to a child. Research indicates that mentally competent nursing home residents are irritated by elderspeak and that people with moderate dementia or Alzheimer disease become more agitated and resistant to care if they are addressed in this manner (Williams et al., 2009).

Other barriers to therapeutic communication include:

■ Excessive nurse workload and nursing shortage
■ Language differences between the nurse and patient
■ Environment unconducive to patient privacy
■ Patients' and nurses' emotional fluctuations, moods, and personality (Arkorful et al., 2021).

KnowledgeCheck 15-6
Identify at least five barriers to communication.

Enhancing Communication With Clients From Other Cultures

The way you address your patient will vary according to culture. In the United States and many other countries, people use a formal salutation (Mr., Mrs., Ms., Dr.). The given name (personal name) precedes the surname. Other countries, such as Korea and China, go by surname, followed by first name. Be sensitive to the practices of your patients and ask their preference.

For patient- and family-centered communication and respect for cultural care, healthcare facilities should provide qualified interpreter services for patients with limited English proficiency (LEP) (The Joint Commission, 2010, 2018).

■ Many health facilities offer on-site and phone-accessed interpreter or video remote interpreter (VRI) services.
■ Internet-based and mobile technologies with applications are commonly available for translating English into various other languages. You may try learning a

Toward Evidence-Based Practice

Arkorful, V. E., Hammond, A., Basiru, I., Boateng, J., Doku, F., Pokuaah, S., Kwadwo Agyei, E., Asamoah Baoteng, J., & Kweku Lugu, B. (2021). A cross-sectional qualitative study of barriers to effective therapeutic communication among nurses and patients, *International Journal of Public Administration, 44*(6), 500–512. https://doi.org/10.1080/01900692.2020.1729797

The most prevalent patient-related communication barriers noted in this study included individual sociodemographic factors, relationship between nurse and patient, and language differences. Nurse-related barriers had more to do with excessive workload, human resource challenges, inadequate knowledge, and difficulty dealing with patients' emotional fluctuations. Environmental-related barriers, such as noise, lack of privacy, and room arrangement, had a negative impact on communication.

Crawford, T., Candlin, S., & Rogers, P. (2017). New perspectives on understanding cultural diversity in nurse-patient communication. *Collegian Journal: The Australian Journal of Nursing Practice, Scholarship & Research, 24*(1), 63–69. https://doi.org/10.1016/j.colegn.2015.09.001

Differences in language and culture among patients and caregivers pose a significant risk for misunderstanding and miscommunication that may affect health outcomes and patient safety. Researchers found that pronunciation, word stress, intonation, and speech delivery were the factors that most often contributed to misunderstandings of the spoken language. Other problems with communication were attributed to poor grammar and limited vocabulary.

Howe, C. J., Walker, D., & Watts, J. (2017, October). Use of recommended communication techniques for diabetes educators. *HLRP: Health Literacy Research and Practice, 1*(4), e145–e152. https://doi.org/10.3928/24748307-20170810-01

In a study involving 522 diabetes educators, researchers examined the 14 techniques they used to communicate with their patients. The most common approach was using plain language with three to five main points. To ensure patients' understanding of information, educators frequently used the teach-back method for improving self-care and diabetes control.

1. After participating in an educational activity to improve your communication skills, suppose you are the nurse providing care for a patient with diabetes.

    a. What nonverbal cues might you use to convey caring?

    b. What nonverbal behaviors communicate a noncaring attitude or poor listening?

    c. What verbal skills might you use to establish a therapeutic relationship with the client?

    d. What nonverbal behaviors interfere with the therapeutic relationship between the nurse and the client?

2. Suppose you are a graduate nurse working in the intensive care unit of a large teaching hospital. You are providing care to the following four patients. What are some ways you would establish a therapeutic relationship and communicate caring to these patients and their families? List at least three strategies for each patient.

    a. A 65-year-old man 3 hours postop after repair of an abdominal aortic aneurysm. Your patient is intubated and breathing with the assistance of a mechanical ventilator. He is fully alert and responsive after surgery.

    b. An 88-year-old frail woman with delirium receiving a blood transfusion for a lower gastrointestinal bleed.

    c. A 3-year-old child with acute epiglottitis whose parents are not in the unit.

    d. A pregnant woman from Somalia with limited English language and literacy skills who is in the active phase of labor.

3. What pitfalls in communicating would you avoid in caring for your patients with language barriers?

few key words in your patients' primary language to communicate basic care and understand their basic needs. For a list of a few useful Spanish terms and for guidelines for communicating with clients who speak Spanish,

Go to Chapter 15, Clinical Insight 15-3: Communicating With Clients From Another Culture, in Volume 2.

Use bi- or multilingual healthcare workers or family members as interpreters only if there are no other options. It may be culturally unacceptable to have family members ask personal questions. As a result, messages may be altered, or questions may remain unasked. Additionally, patients' privacy may be violated by having personal contacts serve as interpreters.

See Chapter 12 for additional information on the use of interpreters.

Enhancing Communication With Clients Who Have Impaired Speech

Use the following guidelines to help you communicate with clients who have speech or language impairments:

- Nonverbal communication is the key to communication with clients with impaired speech.
- Ask the client to use hand gestures and a picture board, as appropriate.
- Solicit family assistance in understanding the client's speech.
- Provide a comfortable environment for the client to practice speaking.

- Be positive and patient.
- Although the client may have difficulty speaking, you should continue to speak and explain all procedures.
- A referral to a speech pathologist may be necessary (The Joint Commission, 2010).

Enhancing Communication With Clients Who Have Impaired Cognition or Reduced Level of Consciousness

Communicating with cognitively impaired clients can be difficult, time consuming, and frustrating for even the most experienced nurse. This might be a patient with acute illness or neurological injury, congenital abnormality, sensory or language deficits, or dementia. In the hospital setting, impairments are heightened because of illness, changed routines and environment, and medication. As a result, the patient may be unable to understand explanations, follow directions, ask for help, or report symptoms (Zembrzuski, 2013).

♥ **iCare 15-2**

Communicating With Caring Presence

Lisa is admitting Ana, a 30-year-old female. Ana is visiting from Brazil and speaks only Portuguese. While shopping, she experienced severe right-lower-quadrant abdominal pain and was rushed to the hospital by ambulance. She is alone and scared. Although medical interpreters have been provided, none of her family or friends has arrived yet. Lisa, recognizing Ana's fear, takes the time to sit with her, reassuring her through nonverbal communication such as smiling, making eye contact, and gently touching her shoulder. She sits quietly, holding her hand. Her presence seems to reassure Ana, who stops crying and remains calm until her friends arrive.

For guidelines to help you communicate with clients with impaired cognition or consciousness, see Box 15-4.

BOX 15-4 ■ Communicating With Patients Who Have Impaired Cognition or Consciousness

Clients Who Are Cognitively or Developmentally Impaired or With Dementia

Always try to communicate.	Make every effort to communicate, even if you think that the client cannot understand you.
Do not use the in-room intercom to speak with the patient.	A voice sounding from the intercom on the bedside call system might frighten the patient and cause confusion, delirium, or other cognitive impairments. It is better to talk face to face.
Don't rush the client.	Be patient and provide adequate time to allow the client to communicate. The client needs time to respond to your questions or commands.
Reduce environmental distractions.	Extraneous noises, lights, and even smells can compete for attention when talking with or providing instructions to the patient. For example, you might turn off the TV or close the door if you want to reduce distractions.
Approach the patient directly.	To avoid frightening the patient, approach the patient from the front, make eye contact, address the person by name, smile, and speak in a calm and friendly voice.
Talk first and touch second.	Touching a patient before establishing basic trust might frighten the confused or cognitively impaired patient.
Do not argue or insist the patient agree with you.	The patient with altered perception or cognition might not have the capacity to understand or accept reality. Pushing them to agree with you can create anxiety or hostility.
Use multiple communication modalities.	Provide verbal and written discharge instructions. Review the instructions several times with the client before discharge. Include family members in the teaching.
Provide reminders.	Use memory aids, schedules, and reminder notices to reinforce information.
Orient the client.	Verbally orient to time, person, and place, and provide visual orientation materials, such as a calendar or schedule.
Stimulate memory.	If the client loses their place in the conversation, stimulate memory by repeating their last expressed thought (e.g., "We were talking about your back pain. Tell me more about your back pain.").
Use short, simple sentences, but avoid elderspeak.	Use short sentences containing a single thought (e.g., "Are you hungry?"). Avoid complex statements (e.g., "You look hungry. Would you like a sandwich or a milkshake, or can you hold off until dinner?").
Ask yes or no questions.	Ask direct questions that require only a yes or no answer (e.g., "Are you hungry?").
Limit choices.	Limit choices to avoid confusing or frustrating the patient.
Be concrete and specific.	Do not use vague comments to indicate that you are listening. The client may be unable to interpret comments such as, "I see." Instead, repeat the client's words and directly state your response (e.g., "You are cold. I will bring you a blanket").

(Continued)

BOX 15-4 ■ Communicating With Patients Who Have Impaired Cognition or Consciousness—cont'd

Avoid slang and jargon.	The client may not understand and may become anxious.
Use gestures.	Model desired behaviors. You might say, "Brush your teeth now," and then pantomime brushing your teeth.
Don't assume.	Bear in mind that the client cannot behave differently and that they may be confused about reality. When the person is talking about superficial, routine matters, they may seem more competent than they are.

Patients Who Have Expressive Difficulties

- If you are sure of the word the person is trying to say, repeat it. Do not guess, though.
- Pay close attention to nonverbal communication.
- Assess for and anticipate unmet needs, such as hunger, thirst, and pain.
- Respond to the emotion, not the words.

Patients Who Are Unconscious

- Touch and speak to unconscious or sedated patients; inform them of the care you are providing. Although the patient may not be able to respond, they may be able to hear your comments. The patient may also benefit physiologically when hearing your voice or that of their loved ones.
- Consult with previous caregivers or the family to determine what the patient responds to.
- Begin each interaction by identifying yourself and calling the patient by name.
- Speak calmly and slowly, even if the patient does not seem to be alert and oriented.
- Explain all healthcare procedures as you are doing them.
- Provide soothing music and periods of rest.

Patients Who Have Suffered a Stroke

- Remember that many stroke survivors may have trouble communicating their thoughts. They also commonly experience emotional ups and downs and frustration. Do not take these moods personally.
- Use simple language and allow time for the person to respond.
- Yes or no questions also work well when someone has expressive aphasia after a stroke.
- Paraphrase to be sure you understand what your patient is saying.
- When a patient has aphasia, speak slowly, not louder. Be careful not to use a patronizing tone.
- **Augmentative and alternative communication** (AAC) is a tablet, laptop, or voice-generating device that helps someone with a speech or language impairment to communicate. AAC includes all forms of communication other than speech to express thoughts, needs, wants, and ideas, such as communication boards and electronic devices.
- Be a good listener and allow time for the patient to express their thoughts.

Practice Resources

Sources: Alzheimer's Society (2019); American Heart Association (2021); American Speech-Language-Hearing Association (n.d.); Cleveland Clinic (2019); National Institute of Health, National Institute on Deafness and Other Communication Disorders (2019); Zembrzuski (2013, revised).

To explore learning resources for this chapter,

    Go to Davis Advantage and find:

Answers and Suggested Responses for all questions in this chapter

Concept Map

Knowledge Map

References and Bibliography

CHAPTER 16

Patient Education

Learning Outcomes

After completing this chapter, you should be able to:

➤ Present three factors contributing to the expanding role of teaching in professional nursing.

➤ Describe the concepts of teaching and learning.

➤ Name, define, and give one example of each of Bloom's three updated domains of learning.

➤ Describe the six levels of cognitive thinking in the modified (Krathwohl) Bloom's classification.

➤ Discuss factors that can affect learning.

➤ List at least six barriers to teaching and learning.

➤ Describe some strategies for motivating learners.

➤ Develop strategies for working with clients of various cultures or with learning differences.

➤ Perform learning assessments.

➤ Develop teaching plans for clients.

➤ List four methods for evaluating the outcomes of teaching and learning.

➤ Document teaching content, methods, and patient responses to learning.

Key Concepts

Health literacy

Learning

Learning environment

Teaching

Related Concepts

See the Concept Map on Davis Advantage.

Meet Your Patient

Heather, a 20-year-old mother, and her 4-year-old, Jade, come to the clinic for a well-child checkup. During the visit, you notice that Jade speaks only in one- or two-word phrases. The mother's tone is impatient. "Stop using that baby talk." Heather says, "All her friends are taller and talking more. She was even small when she was born, so I suppose it's my fault."

Your assessment shows the child is below the fifth percentile for height and weight. You assess for teaching needs and provide anticipatory guidance to the mother. How would you begin to address Heather's learning needs without reinforcing her feelings of self-blame? What health teaching could you provide that might help resolve this problem?

Your teaching plan should include safety measures, immunizations, and nutrition for a 4-year-old, as well as

expected growth and development. How can you evaluate whether the teaching has been effective and enhance the mother's retention of this new information?

By the time you finish working through this chapter, you should be able to answer these questions and provide teaching to meet the unique needs of other patients you encounter.

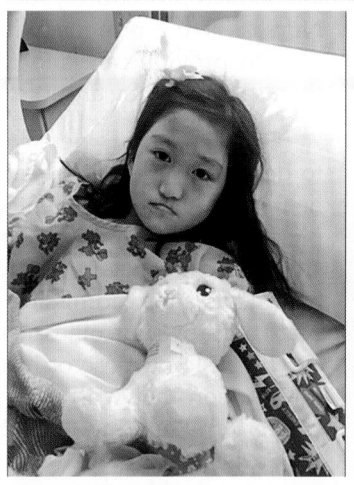

ABOUT THE KEY CONCEPTS

This chapter covers concepts that underlie how people take in and offer information within the healthcare setting. A firm grasp of **teaching, learning, health literacy,** and the **learning environment** will allow you to call to mind the information that you will need in your professional role when teaching patients in a variety of settings.

TheoreticalKnowledge
knowing **why**

Nurses have been teaching patients since Florence Nightingale taught about the value of good nutrition, fresh air, exercise, and personal hygiene (Nightingale, 1860/1992). Since that time, teaching has become progressively more important, due in part to the following factors.

Patients Participate in Healthcare Decisions Primary care providers expect patients to share the responsibility for their own health. Patients and families require accurate, clear, and complete information so that they can make *informed* decisions. You can help patients find answers to their questions, identify reliable resources, and develop self-care and health-promotion behaviors.

Hospital Stays Are Brief A great deal of complex care is provided in patients' homes and the community. Patients are often discharged home while still requiring medication, wound care, stoma or tube feedings, and skilled procedures, such as urinary catheterization. Nurses have a responsibility to teach family members how to provide care and to teach patients to care for themselves as they are able.

Healthcare Is Expensive Patient education can help to decrease the overall cost of healthcare. It does so by helping to increase patient understanding of and compliance with medical and nursing regimens, which can shorten hospital stays, reduce the frequency of medical treatments and readmission (Bastable, 2019; Peter et al., 2015), improve outcomes, and prevent complications.

The basic purpose of health education is to provide information that will empower clients and families to (1) perform self-care and (2) make informed decisions about their healthcare options. Like other interventions, you can use education to promote wellness; prevent or limit illness; restore health; adapt to changes in body function; and facilitate coping with stress, illness, and loss.

WHO ARE THE LEARNERS?

As a nurse, your learners are clients, families, and others who care for the client. You will often provide informal, one-to-one teaching while performing other nursing actions. For example, as you give a medication, you will teach about both therapeutic and adverse effects. Or you may do more formal teaching to groups of people in a variety of healthcare settings.

As a nurse, you will also be responsible for teaching the healthcare workers whom you supervise. For example, you may instruct unlicensed assistive personnel (UAP) how to perform various patient care tasks or even when you observe an error in technique. Or you may help a newly hired nurse learn how to use new equipment on the unit.

Nurses in practice are also involved in the clinical instruction of nursing students, new graduates, and other members of the healthcare team. Most of this teaching may be informal, although you might also present specific topics at unit meetings and conferences. For example, you might teach the nurses on your shift how to reduce falls for high-risk patients on your unit or how to ensure back safety when performing patient care.

WHAT ARE MY TEACHING RESPONSIBILITIES?

Nurses are responsible for educating patients on preventing and managing health conditions and promoting their own health. The benefits of patient education include the following:

- Empowers patients to take control of their own healthcare (Yeh et al., 2018)
- Improves patient adherence to prescribed healthcare (Oldenmenger et al., 2018)
- Reduces health complications and hospital readmission (Peter et al., 2015)
- Promotes safety with medication usage (Waszak et al., 2018)
- Improves patient satisfaction
- Increases (nursing) role satisfaction

The American Nurses Association (ANA) The ANA's *Code of Ethics for Nurses With Interpretive Statements* (2015) holds that nurses are responsible for promoting and protecting the health, safety, and rights of patients. Patient teaching is essential in fulfilling that responsibility.

In *Nursing: Scope and Standards of Practice*, Standard 12 states, "The registered nurse seeks knowledge and competence that reflects current nursing practice and promotes futuristic thinking" (ANA, 2022, p. 76). Registered nurses' teaching activities include the following:

- Providing health teaching that addresses topics such as healthy lifestyles, risk-reducing behaviors, developmental needs, activities of daily living, and preventive self-care
- Using health-promotion and health-teaching methods appropriate to the situation and the healthcare consumer's values, beliefs, health practices, developmental level, learning needs, health literacy, readiness and ability to learn, language preference, spirituality, culture, and socioeconomic status

- Seeking opportunities for feedback and evaluation of the effectiveness of the strategies used
- Using information technologies to communicate health-promotion and disease-prevention information to the healthcare consumer in a variety of settings
- Providing healthcare consumers with information about intended effects and potential adverse effects of proposed therapies

The Joint Commission Standards require educators in healthcare organizations to provide education based on patients' assessed needs and to consider the literacy, motivation to learn, developmental and physical limitations, barriers to communication, culture, and religious beliefs of every patient (The Joint Commission, 2010).

American Hospital Association's (2003) Patient Care Partnership Previously called the Patient's Bill of Rights, the Patient Care Partnership describes in plain language the right of consumers to receive accurate and easily understood information about health plans, healthcare professionals, and healthcare facilities. If patients speak a language other than English, have a physical or mental impairment, or simply do not understand something, they have the right to receive help so that they can make informed healthcare decisions.

WHAT ARE SOME BASIC LEARNING CONCEPTS AND PRINCIPLES?

The educational process consists of both teaching and learning. **Teaching** is an interactive process that involves planning and implementing instructional activities to meet intended learner outcomes or providing activities that allow the learner to learn (Bastable, 2019). Nurses must have effective communication skills to:

- Adequately convey information
- Assess verbal and nonverbal feedback
- Accommodate various learning styles

In patient education, nurses can use teaching, counseling, and behavioral modification together to achieve effective client learning.

Key Point: *Learning is a change in behavior, knowledge, skills, or attitudes.* Information alone will not change behaviors. Change occurs because of motivation to learn and with planned or spontaneously occurring situations, events, or exposures. The "five rights" in Box 16-1 describe how some basic principles of learning help with planning patient education.

Learning Theories

Social learning theory explains the characteristics of the learner. *Self-efficacy* is an important concept in social learning theory. It refers to a person's perceived ability to bring about a desired result.

- **Behavioral learning theory** is characterized by explicit identification of information to be taught and

BOX 16-1 ■ Five Rights of Teaching

When you are making a teaching plan, you can use this list to ensure that you consider each of the five "rights" of teaching.

Right Time
- Is the client ready, free of pain and anxiety, and motivated?
- Have you and the client developed a trusting relationship?
- Have you set aside sufficient time for the teaching session?

Right Context
- Is the environment quiet, free of distractions, and private?
- Is the environment soothing or stimulating, depending on the desired effect?

Right Goal
- Is the client actively involved in planning the learning objectives?
- Are you and your client both committed to reaching mutually set goals of learning that achieve the desired behavioral changes?
- Are family or friends included in planning so that they can help follow through on behavioral changes?
- Are the learning objectives realistic and valued by the client; do they reflect the client's lifestyle?

Right Content
- Is the content appropriate for the client's needs?
- Is it new information or reinforcement of information that has already been provided?
- Is the content presented at the client's level?
- Does the content relate to the client's life experiences, or is it otherwise relevant to the client?

Right Method
- Do the teaching strategies fit the learning style of the client?
- Do the strategies fit the client's learning ability?
- Are the teaching strategies varied?

immediate reward for correct responses. It has roots in psychology and the belief that the environment influences behavior and, in fact, is the essential factor in determining human action. Pavlov (1927), Skinner (1953), and Bandura (1971) are behavioral theorists.
- **Cognitive theory** sees learning as a complex cognitive (mental) activity. Learning is an intellectual or thinking process in which the learner structures and processes information. Cognitive theory also recognizes the importance of developmental stage and social, emotional, and affective influences on learning. Bloom (1956) is one of the major cognitive theorists.
- **Humanism** focuses equally on the learner's affective (emotional), cognitive (intellectual), and attitudinal

qualities. It emphasizes the learner's active participation and responsibility in the learning process. Learning is thought of as self-motivated, self-initiated, and self-evaluated, and its purpose is self-development and achievement of the learner's full potential.

KnowledgeCheck 16-1

- Identify at least three reasons nurses have a responsibility to teach clients.
- Define *teaching*.
- Define *learning*.

Learning Occurs in Three Domains

People learn in three ways, or *domains:* cognitive, psychomotor, and affective (Bloom & Krathwohl, 1956). You should include each of these domains, involving thinking, doing, and caring/feeling, when writing objectives and planning teaching and evaluation strategies.

Table 16-1 provides examples of client learning in each of the domains.

Krathwohl (2002) adapted Bloom's model describing learning using a more outcomes-based approach: remember, understand, apply, analyze, evaluate, and create (Fig. 16-1).

Cognitive Learning

Cognitive skills are the mental activities for processing incoming information. **Key Point:** *Learning is not about how many facts you can recall but rather how meaningful the information is and how effectively you can use it when needed.* After capturing your patients' attention and getting them to perceive the need to learn the information you are trying to teach, your goal is then to expand their learning beyond simple *remembering* and *understanding*. You will promote their thinking to a higher level that involves *applying, evaluating,* and *creating* ways to meet their own healthcare needs.

Table 16-1 ➤ Bloom's Domains of Learning	
DOMAIN AND LEVELS OF BEHAVIOR	**EXAMPLES OF CLIENT BEHAVIORS**
Cognitive (thinking) Includes memorization, recall, comprehension, and the ability to analyze, synthesize, apply, and evaluate ideas.	Reports the names and doses of the three medications they are taking. Explains the expected effect of the medication they have been prescribed. Designs a planned schedule for dressing changes for a wound on their leg. Describes how to distinguish between normal inflammation and signs of infection in a wound. Recognizes the need for behavioral changes to decrease the chance of recurrence of infection.
Psychomotor (skills) Includes sensory awareness of cues involved in learning, as well as imitation and performance of skills and the creation of new skills.	Identifies that they need to read directions before starting a project. Brings personal equipment to a teaching session. Follows the instructor who is demonstrating diapering of a newborn, imitating their movements. Diapers a newborn after observing a demonstration. Independently changes the complex dressing; the wound heals with no signs of infection. Creates a new approach to giving their daily injections.
Affective (feelings) Includes receiving and responding to new ideas, demonstrating commitment to or preference for new ideas, and integrating new ideas into a value system.	Makes eye contact with the nurse as they explain the admission process. Asks questions about what to expect during a procedure they will undergo. A parent of a child who has just been admitted to the hospital expresses commitment to staying with their child after the nurse explains the impact of hospitalization. A client who has overcome drug addiction chooses to present their story to high school groups.

Source: Adapted from Bloom, B. S., & Krathwohl, D. R. (1956). Taxonomy of educational objectives: The classification of educational goals. In *Handbook I: Cognitive domain.* Longmans, Green; Bloom, B. S., Mesia, B. B., & Krathwohl, D. R. (1964). *Taxonomy of educational objectives: Vol. 1. The affective domain. Vol. 2. The cognitive domain.* David McKay.

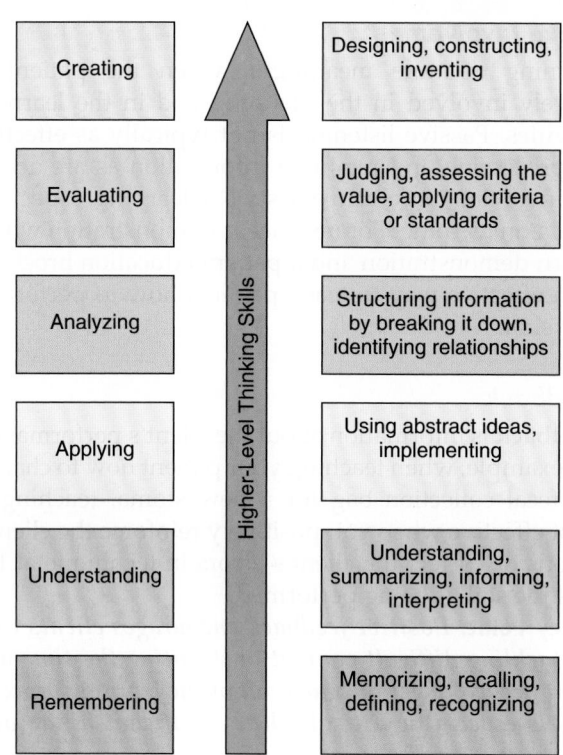

FIGURE 16-1 Bloom's revised taxonomy for higher-order thinking skills.

Psychomotor Learning

Psychomotor learning involves performing skills that require both mental and physical activity. It requires the learner to value learning the skill (the affective domain) as well as understand and implement the skill (the cognitive domain). Strategies and tools used to teach patients and caregivers the skills they need for their own healthcare may include demonstration and return demonstration, simulation models, streaming video, journaling and self-reflection, and the use of electronic applications, especially those containing interactive functions.

Affective Learning

Affective learning involves changes in feelings, beliefs, attitudes, and values. It is considered the "feeling domain." Strategies and tools for promoting learning that motivate patients and caregivers to want to adopt the knowledge and skills may include role modeling, support groups, storytelling, discussion, role-playing, mentoring, one-to-one counseling and discussion, interactive applications, video, photographs and illustrations, and some text-based materials.

KnowledgeCheck 16-2

- What are the three domains of learning?
- What strategies and tools are used to promote learning within each of the three domains of learning?
- Give an example of each of the domains of learning.

▲ ThinkLike a Nurse 16-1: Clinical Judgment in Action

By now, you have probably already learned how to assess a patient's blood pressure (BP).

- Think about how you were taught to perform that *skill*. What would have been the best way for *you* to learn to take a BP reading? To read a book and look at the photos closely? To watch an online video? To have someone tell you how to do it? To have someone demonstrate the skill? Perform the BP measurement yourself? Some other way?
- Now think about the *principles* involved with BP (e.g., normal ranges, the physiological regulation of the BP). What, for you, would have been the best way to learn the principles? Read a book? Listen to a lecture or podcast? Watch a video? Physically obtain a BP reading for a patient? Work a case involving BP? Some other way?
- From your answers to the two preceding questions, what (if anything) can you conclude about different domains of learning and the kinds of activities to use in teaching and learning in each domain?

Many Factors Affect Patient Learning

Learning is complex. Many factors can either enhance or interfere.

Motivation

Motivation is desire from within. Little learning can occur without it. Motivation is greatest when clients:

- Recognize the need for learning
- Believe it is possible to improve their health
- Are interested in the information they are being given

Think about classes you have taken. Have you worked harder in some than in others? What motivated you? Was it because you were intrigued by the information, wanted to earn a good grade, respected the instructor, or had other incentives?

Motivation may be based on physical, emotional, and social needs; the need for task mastery or success; and health beliefs. In your client teaching, try to apply the following principles for motivating learners:

- **Convey your interest in and respect** for your clients to help motivate them to be engaged and successful in the learning experience.
- **Create a warm, friendly, and nonjudgmental environment.** This can enhance social needs motivation, as can your enthusiasm.
- **Help the client to identify a practical need.** For example, Heather (Meet Your Patient) may not be aware that her child is at risk for injury from home hazards. Helping her to understand the normal behavior of a 4-year-old may motivate her to childproof her home.
- **Use rewards and incentives.** The need for achievement and competence is related to task mastery and self-efficacy. When a person succeeds at a task, they are usually motivated to continue learning.

- **Help the client to realize that health and safety really matter.** For example, Heather may understand that a 4-year-old likes to explore and may recognize there are safety hazards in the home; however, she will not be motivated to learn safety measures if her attitude is that "it is no big deal."

Readiness

Readiness is the demonstration of behaviors that indicate the client is both *motivated* and *able* to learn *at a specific time*. You must consider readiness in your planning. For instance, a client may not be "ready" for teaching right before scheduled diagnostic tests or treatments because anxiety makes it difficult to concentrate.

Physical Condition Physical factors (e.g., pain, strength, coordination, energy, senses, mobility) and attention contribute to a patient's readiness to learn—for example:

- Pain interferes with the ability to concentrate on the teaching.
- The patient needs adequate strength, coordination, energy, and mobility to demonstrate psychomotor learning.
- Patients with impaired hearing or vision require adaptations in your teaching and evaluation strategies.

Emotions Severe anxiety, stress, or emotional pain interferes with the ability to learn (Rajala et al., 2018). In addition, the learning itself, and the idea that behaviors must be changed, can create anxiety. However, a mild level of anxiety can enhance learning by providing motivation. For example, a patient newly diagnosed with diabetes may not be experiencing physical complications related to the disease, so they may not be interested in learning about diabetes. You may be able to motivate them (i.e., create some anxiety) by pointing out the potential and serious complications (e.g., blindness, kidney damage) of uncontrolled diabetes. But do so carefully so that the client does not interpret your words as a threat, excessive negativity, or preaching.

Timing

You must present information at a time when the client is open to learning. Timing is therefore everything.

- **People retain information better when they have an opportunity to use it soon after it is presented.** For example, one nursing student reads about insulin; another reads the same information and administers different types of insulin to several patients. At the test 2 weeks later, the second student will have an advantage at test time.
- **For some concepts, the client might need more time to absorb and apply information,** especially when complex thinking is required.

Active Involvement

Learning is more meaningful when the patient is actively involved in the planning and in the learning activities. Passive listening is not typically as effective for processing and retaining information as are activities involving more than one style of learning, especially hands-on learning. For instance, a demonstration with a return demonstration and a patient education brochure is an effective way to teach patients how to perform a new skill.

Feedback

Feedback is information about the client's performance. For example, when teaching your patient how to change the fecal collection bag for a new stoma, teaching is most effective when you positively reinforce the client's actions or correct the client's errors in technique at the time the skill is being performed.

Key Point: *Positive feedback encourages clients who are tackling difficult content or devoting the time and effort needed to get the most out of the learning process. This is especially critical when significant behavioral changes are required.*

When teaching or coaching, you may sometimes need to suggest alternatives or point out errors. Do so in a positive way when you can. Be careful not to seem judgmental when clients are learning a new skill or are giving home care. Fear of failure or judgment can be a barrier to learning at what could be the client's most teachable moment.

Repetition

The patient is more likely to retain information and incorporate it into their life if the content is repeated. For example, patients often forget what medication is prescribed for certain conditions. Repeating the name of the drug can help patients remember it. This is especially true for learning psychomotor skills. Do you remember the first time you counted a radial pulse? Even that simple skill may have been difficult at first. By now it is probably very easy for you.

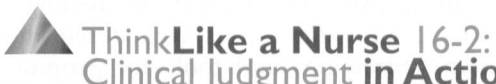

ThinkLike a Nurse 16-2: Clinical Judgment in Action

Use examples from your own experience if you can. Do not use examples you have read in the preceding sections.

- Give an example to illustrate the importance of *relevance* in learning.
- Give an example to illustrate the importance of *repetition* in learning.
- Give an example to illustrate the importance of *timing* in learning.

Learning Environment

For most people, an ideal learning environment is private, quiet, physically and psychologically comfortable, and free from distractions. If a separate space

Safe, Effective Nursing Care

Teaching Clients Through Collaborative Partnership

Chapter Key Concepts: Teaching, Learning

Competency: Provide goal-directed, client-centered care; collaborate with the interprofessional healthcare team

Background

To meet the learning needs of patients with chronic illnesses or multiple comorbidities, the nurse must empower the patient by:

➤ Engaging the patient in the entire teaching/learning process

➤ Establishing a partnership with the patient as the core member of the healthcare team

➤ Using health education to help the patient to make informed health decisions (Russo et al., 2019).

Empowering the patient as a full partner in care potentially improves health outcomes (Karazivan et al., 2015; Russo et al., 2019). The goal of effective patient teaching is to increase patient knowledge, thereby facilitating patient decision making regarding health issues.

Think About It

➤ Using a patient-centered, collaborative approach, what should be your first step in teaching effectively?

➤ Discuss how you would engage the patient in the teaching/learning process.

➤ Discuss how patient partnership and empowerment have the potential to change health behaviors.

➤ Describe how you would arrive at the desired outcomes for a teaching/learning session.

Sources: Karazivan, P., Dumez, V., Flora, L., Pomey, M.-P., Del Grande, C., Ghadiri, D. P., Fernandez, N., Jouet, E., Las Vergnas, O., & Lebel, P. (2015, April). The patient-as-partner approach in health care: A conceptual framework for a necessary transition. *Academic Medicine, 90*(4), 437–441. https://doi.org/10.1097/ACM.0000000000000603; McAlnearney, A. S., Fareed, N., Gaughan, A., MacEwan, S. R., Volney, J., & Sieck, C. J. (2019, January). Empowering patients during hospitalization: Perspectives on inpatient portal use. *Applied Clinical Informatics, 10*(1), 103–112. https://doi.org/10.1055/s-0039-1677722; Russo, G., Tartaglione, A., & Cavacece, Y. (2019). Empowering patients to co-create a sustainable healthcare value. *Sustainability, 11*(5), 1315. https://doi.org/10.3390/su11051315

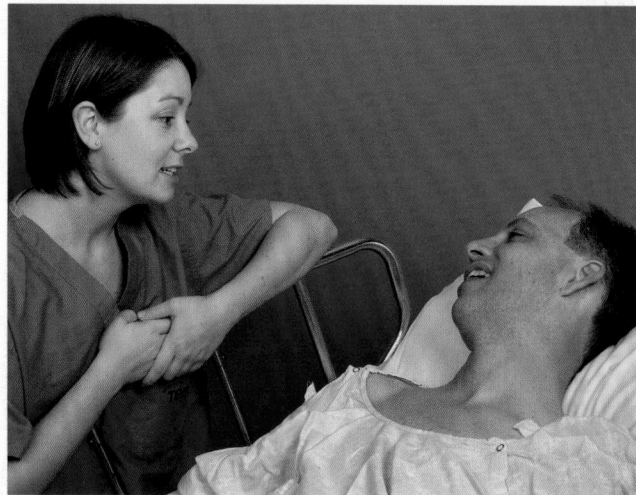

FIGURE 16-2 Sit or stand close to the patient so that you can talk privately.

try to use inspirational or motivational accessories (e.g., photographs, video).

Scheduling the Session

Plan for uninterrupted time to allow you to adequately assess and understand the patient. The teaching time does not need to be long, just uninterrupted (e.g., by procedures, physical therapy). Based on the patient's condition (e.g., activity intolerance, attention span, fatigue, pain), shorter teaching sessions may be best for comprehension and retention. Finding a suitable time to teach can be a challenge, but a moment can be a teaching session, as shown in Box 16-2.

Amount and Complexity of Content

The more complex or detailed the content is, the more difficult it is for most people to learn and retain, as you probably know from your own learning experiences.

is not available, you can at least try to find a quiet corner, pull the bed curtain shut, close the door, or sit close to the patient so that you can talk softly (Fig. 16-2). Make the best of what you have to work with. However, some clients are best motivated and engaged when teaching occurs in a group.

When you are planning a teaching session, provide good lighting and comfortable seating that are conducive for conversations. Have your teaching materials at hand to avoid unnecessary interruptions in the teaching session. If you have an area that is set aside for teaching,

---

BOX 16-2 ■ Teachable Moments

A student nurse walks into her patient's room. This week in class, she has been learning patient education. Her instructor has informed the students that they expect students to incorporate teaching into each clinical day. But the student ponders, "I am way too busy to find time to teach. What am I going to do?" Later in the day, she asks the nurse who is coassigned to her client for suggestions. The nurse asks, "Did you take the patient's blood pressure (BP)?" When the student answers that she did, the nurse says, "Did you explain why you were doing that and what the BP readings mean?" Again, the student says, "Yes." The nurse asks, "When you gave your patient their medications, did you explain why you were giving each one?" The student says, "Yes, and the side effects, too." A light goes on! The student begins to understand that almost every patient contact presents an opportunity for teaching, even when the contact is brief.

For example, which of these situations would you expect to be more challenging?

- Teaching parents about the need for isolation precautions for their preterm infant who has just been diagnosed with an immune disorder.
- Teaching parents how to diaper their preterm infant.

The greater the change, the greater will be the challenge for both nurse and patient. For example, which of these clients would you expect to experience a more demanding learning challenge?

- A client rehabilitating after a stroke who has to relearn using eating utensils, swallowing, and other basic tasks for daily hygiene and self-care
- A client who must learn only a daily schedule for taking medications

Communication

Communication is central to the teaching and learning process in which nurses and clients exchange information, perceptions, and feelings. Recognize cues to verbal and nonverbal feedback that the client gives; they can tell you whether the client is attentive and focusing on the learning activities. For more information about communication, see Chapter 15.

Special Populations

For clients who have special needs (e.g., those with learning disabilities, attention deficit-hyperactivity disorder [ADHD], mental illness, affective or communication disorders, developmental delay, or brain injury), you must plan carefully to ensure that you maximize learning by adapting teaching strategies to the patient's special learning needs. Consider a variety of approaches—one size does not fit all. For example, you may need to do one or more of the following:

- Plan brief, frequent learning sessions.
- Consider the client's strengths and opportunities for learning rather than limitations.
- Pay special attention to minimizing distracting stimuli in the environment.
- Present information slowly.
- Use repetition.
- Understand and be satisfied with slower progress.

If you are not familiar with the patient's condition, you must acquire theoretical knowledge of it. Include a family member, caregiver, or other significant person in the teaching to reinforce the learning and act as a safety net for implementing the information.

Developmental Stage

An understanding of intellectual development will help you to gear your teaching strategies and content to the level of the client. When teaching psychomotor skills, you will need to assess the person's fine and gross motor development. For example, after a stroke, a patient may not have adequate fine motor skills to complete a task. If you would like to review an extensive discussion of intellectual development, including Piaget's theory (1966), refer to Chapter 6.

ThinkLike a Nurse 16-3: Clinical Judgment in Action

A client who has a brain injury needs to learn how to administer insulin. Another client who must learn to change a wound dressing has ADHD.

- How do you think these clients' health status might affect the following:
  - Their motivation to learn?
  - Their ability to be actively involved in the learning?

What approaches or changes might you need to make in the following:

- The learning environment?
- The timing of the teaching session?
- The use of repetition?
- Your communication?
- The amount and complexity of content presented in a session?
- Your use of feedback?
- The amount of nurse support?

STAGES OF COGNITIVE DEVELOPMENT

Piaget identified three stages of cognitive development that are especially important in client teaching in the cognitive domain:

- **Preoperational stage** (2 to 7 years old), in which the child begins to acquire language skills and find meaning through the use of symbols and pictures.
- **Stage of concrete operations** (7 to 11 years old), in which the child learns best by manipulating concrete, tangible objects and can classify objects in two or more ways (e.g., identify a shape as a triangle and also as green). Logical thinking begins, and the child can understand the relationship between numbers and the idea of reversibility. The child also can begin to recognize and adapt to the perspective of others. Before reaching the stage of formal operations, clients learn best from examples instead of definitions, and they understand concrete terms rather than abstract terms.
- **Formal operational stage** (age 11 years or older), in which the person can use abstract thinking and deductive reasoning. The person can relate general concepts to specific situations, consider alternatives, begin to establish values, and try to find meaning in life. Not everyone reaches this stage, including some adults.

Teaching Older Adults

When teaching older adults, consider the many factors that can adversely affect the teaching.

- **Allow extra time** for teaching, and stop occasionally for rest periods as needed.
- **Assess for hearing and vision deficits,** and adapt your style according to any restrictions, such as

using large print or visual aids; speak slowly and repeat information as necessary.

- **Refer to Table 16-2 for some learning principles** that apply to older adults, as well as tips for effectively teaching older adults.

Teaching Children

When you work with children, use strategies to gain trust, reduce their anxiety, promote cooperation, and enhance their emotional readiness to learn. For instance, for a child who needs surgery:

- Encourage caregivers to schedule a tour of the hospital at least 1 week before the admission date and introduce the child to staff members and other patients of the same age (if possible).
- Teach the child to practice breathing exercises or other aspects of tests or treatments that they will be involved in.
- With the parents' permission, provide the child with ice cream or some other type of food, game, or material "reward."
- Give the child a coloring book to take home, or suggest using a mobile application about what surgery might be like.

For children in the preoperational stage, simplify the information and use pictures or video and concrete

Table 16-2 ➤ Incorporating Principles of Adult Learning Into the Teaching of Older Adults	
CHARACTERISTICS OF ADULT AND OLDER ADULT LEARNERS	**TIPS FOR TEACHING ADULTS**
Attitudes **Adults are independent and self-directed.**	■ Help them to identify their own learning needs.
Adults must recognize the need to learn before they become willing to learn.	■ Explain why the information or new skill is important. Be sure to include materials with practical tips and realistic goals for learning.
Some adults may be uneasy about the learning process because of (1) fear of failure anxiety, (2) past unsatisfactory experiences with educational processes, (3) having received their formal education many years ago, or (4) feeling that "being taught" is for children.	■ Present content in a nonthreatening environment where there is no risk of judgment or embarrassment in front of peers. Privacy is often necessary. ■ Offer feedback simply to improve important skills. ■ Consider that the intent of patient education is to improve clinical outcomes. Privacy is often necessary. ■ Respect clients for what they already know.
Adults are more motivated to learn if they can use the information or skills immediately.	■ Plan the teaching session close to the time the patient will need the information or need to perform a new skill.
Adults prefer to be partners in the learning process—to have some control over what they learn and how they learn it.	■ Encourage clients to tell you first what they intend to gain from the educational session. ■ Plan the goals of your session in advance and allow the client to customize them.
Some adults are resistant to the need to learn new information. They may feel, "I've been just fine all these years without needing to know that; why should I learn it now?" Or they may believe that they are "too old to learn." These may be defenses to avoid failure or to resist change.	■ Work with the client to establish the "need to know" at the onset of the program. ■ Involve the client in defining what they intend to gain from the educational session. ■ Reassure the client about the importance of the information. ■ Encourage the client to tackle a little at a time.
Older adults tend to be socially less connected and might perceive bias, ageism, or isolation.	■ As for any individual, you must honor cultural backgrounds, local customs and practices, and personal preferences.
Experience **Adults have previous life experiences that can enhance learning.**	■ Assess what they already know. Then build teaching based on what they need to know. ■ Relate new content to clients' past experiences and knowledge; have them use their experiences to solve problems.

(Continued)

Table 16-2 ➤ Incorporating Principles of Adult Learning Into the Teaching of Older Adults—cont'd

CHARACTERISTICS OF ADULT AND OLDER ADULT LEARNERS	TIPS FOR TEACHING ADULTS
Messages are best received when they are part of a real-life experience.	■ Model the message you are conveying to your audience: "Walk the walk" and not just "talk the talk."
Learning Environment **Many adult learners do well when a hands-on approach is used.** Older adults learn best by practicing a new skill or rehearsing new information to learn it.	■ Offer active participation and opportunities for interaction with the instructor and other clients. ■ Demonstrations and practical tips are useful for adult clients, particularly older adults.
Many older adult learners need to review new information away from the initial learning environment to retain it. The information might not sink in until later.	■ Use take-home materials, such as colorful posters, table tents, tip sheets, and patient-friendly brochures, to reinforce information.
Older adult learners can be distracted and annoyed by cellular phones and other electronic devices.	■ Request that phones, radios, or other electronic devices be turned off for the educational session. Silence your own phone as well.
Most older adults were raised during a time when technology was not as prevalent as it is today. Learning occurred primarily through the reading, discussion, and retelling of stories.	■ Use informal teaching sessions that include storytelling. Keep your stories short. ■ Convey your genuine interest in your clients before sharing personal stories. ■ To elicit stories, you must be a patient and empathetic listener. ■ Allow more time for older adults, especially those with chronic illness, to tell their own stories. ■ Tie the patient's past experiences to the lesson. ■ Ask open-ended questions and be willing to wait for the answers.
Older people may bring family members or other caregivers to the teaching session to help interpret or remember the information presented. Sometimes the extra people in the room can be noisy and distracting to the patient's learning situation.	■ If others in the room are distracting, it may be helpful to ask them to minimize their conversations or, in some circumstances, to leave the room for a time.
Older adults usually learn better when they are not overwhelmed with multiple needs, topics, or skills at one time.	■ Introduce only a few topics at a time. Usually, tackling one to three new topics or skills is enough. ■ Identify the information that is most important for your client to walk away with. Define those topics and cover them well. ■ Remember, slow and steady wins the race, especially when it comes to learning information that is essential to the patient's health.
Sensory and Physical **Changes in visual, distance, depth, acuity, and light perception occur with aging,** diminishing the ability to take in information. Older adults experience increased sensitivity to glare and reduced color perception. Processing of sensory information is slower in the later decades of life.	■ Avoid colors such as blue, green, and lavender because they are difficult for older adults to differentiate. ■ Remove physical barriers that could compromise the field of vision (e.g., projector position, tables). ■ Choose fonts that are bold, black, and a minimum size of 18 points. Fancy lettering is harder to decipher. ■ A nonglare background without a stylized pattern is easier to see and process than are complex designs. ■ For those who cannot read or who have severe visual impairment, consider recording instructional material.

Table 16-2 ➤ Incorporating Principles of Adult Learning Into the Teaching of Older Adults—cont'd	
CHARACTERISTICS OF ADULT AND OLDER ADULT LEARNERS	**TIPS FOR TEACHING ADULTS**
Older adults may have experienced changes in hearing. Older adults may have reduced: ▪ Hearing acuity ▪ Perception for various tones ▪ Filtration of extraneous noise	▪ Speak slowly, using a normal tone of voice. ▪ If you must speak more loudly than normal, be careful not to sound condescending, as though speaking to a child. Clients should not perceive annoyance in your tone. ▪ Many adults with hearing impairment do some lip-reading, although they may be unaware of it. You can facilitate lip-reading by not distorting your facial features with exaggerated pronunciation. ▪ Provide a quiet setting and decrease background noise. Close the door or windows if outside noise interferes.
Some older adults learn better when they have a source of supplemental information or support to help them compensate for the short-term memory loss that may occur with aging.	▪ Reinforce your teaching with follow-up opportunities and connections to the community for information and support in grasping new information or acquiring a new skill.
Older adult learners can be particularly affected by fatigue, illness, medication, pain, stress, and other personal factors.	▪ Plan the teaching session for a time when the patient is well rested, as pain-free as possible, and comfortable.

examples. Instead of giving a detailed rationale for taking medication, tell the child that the medicine will make them feel better, use pictures of a child drinking from a medicine cup, or give the child a calendar to mark each time a dose is taken.

Cultural Factors

"Learning and culture are inseparable" (Wlodkowki & Ginsberg, 2017, p. ix). Awareness of norms, values, communication, social structure, time orientation, and cultural identification is important in planning patient teaching. If the client is not fluent in the prevailing language, you may need to use an interpreter or a translator application.

♥ **iCare** Nurses care by being culturally sensitive. This involves respect for clients' identity and needs, regardless of who they are, where they are from, how they speak, how old they are, their religious and spiritual practices, whether they have disabilities or learning differences, their financial status, how much they weigh, how socially popular they are, or any other aspect that can lead to unfair treatment.

Box 16-3 highlights key concepts of teaching with a culturally competent approach.

Health Literacy

Health literacy is a central focus in the *Healthy People 2030* initiative. The definition of health literacy was updated to: "Personal health literacy is the degree to which individuals have the ability to find, understand, and use information and services to inform health-related decisions and actions for themselves and others (USDHHS, & ODPHP,

n.d.)". It does not refer simply to a person's ability to read and write but rather to how a person can effectively:

▪ Find information and services to meet health needs for self and others.
▪ Communicate health needs to others.
▪ Understand and apply information and services to meet health needs.

Health illiteracy exists when the person is unable to apply language skills to understand information about their healthcare. This occurs, for example, when the language spoken is not the patient's preferred language or when the format through which the information is communicated is not suited to the patient. Learning gaps can occur in the following examples:

▪ The patient has a hearing impairment, and discharge teaching is done verbally, so the client fails to understand the words.
▪ A healthcare provider uses medical terminology, jargon, and acronyms that are unfamiliar or misinterpreted by the patient, thus resulting in an unintended message or a lack of meaningful information.
▪ A patient is diagnosed with a serious illness and is fearful, making it difficult to process the information.
▪ Limited health literacy is more common among the medically underserved community, minority populations, and older adults.

Patients with low health literacy are not as likely to understand the connection between risky behavior and health. They encounter problems such as difficulty taking medications as prescribed; difficulty managing complex or chronic health problems; and higher rates

BOX 16-3 ■ Culturally Competent Teaching

Assessments

- Inquire about or observe interactions between family members so that you can identify the decision maker and how decisions are made.
- Assess for preferences that may conflict with the information you plan to present.
- Observe verbal and nonverbal communication patterns.
- Assess whether the family is past, present, or future oriented.
- Determine whether the patient and/or family prefers a same-sex or same-gender nurse to teach the client about personal topics, such as birth control and sexually transmitted infections. Different patients vary in their ideas about what is appropriate for discussion between different sexes or genders.
- Determine whether the client's values and wishes are in congruence or conflict with those of the family.

Self-Knowledge

- Admit unfamiliarity with the patient's culture or preferences, but express willingness to learn.
- Find sources of information that can help you learn about the patient's culture and preferred healthcare practices.

♥ iCare Caring

- Respect, accept, and validate the client's beliefs.
- Find ways to incorporate the client's current healthcare practices and beliefs into the plan of care, unless there is potential for harm.

Interventions

- Include the patient's cultural practices and preferences in the plan of care.
- Speak slowly and clearly; avoid slurring syllables.
- Do not use slang expressions or unfamiliar jargon, acronyms, and medical terminology.
- Use short sentences and concrete rather than abstract words. Present only one idea in each sentence.
- Use pictures and other visual aids to help communicate your meaning, as needed.
- Provide teaching materials in the client's preferred language. If you cannot read it, have it translated so that you can judge its appropriateness.
- Avoid using humor; jokes often do not translate well because of connotations and culture-specific context.

Feedback

- Obtain feedback carefully. Do not assume that a client who smiles, nods, and says "yes" really understands what you are teaching. The client may be embarrassed to ask questions or may feel that it will embarrass you.
- Encourage the client to ask questions; stop often to evaluate client understanding.

---

of emergency department (ED) visits, hospitalization, rehospitalization, and death.

Promoting Health Literacy To enhance understanding between you and your patients, refer to the following tips for promoting health literacy:

- **For those with limited English proficiency, provide information in the patient's primary language,** use online or software translation tools, or seek an interpreter to translate.
- **Speak using everyday words and plain-language sentences.** Explain technical terms when using them for the first time. Avoid jargon and unfamiliar acronyms.
- **Ask questions that involve "how" and "what"** rather than "yes" and "no."
- **Provide a take-home summary** of the main points they need to remember. Having something to refer to later can be useful for reinforcing important information.
- **Assist patients in completing forms** and/or health histories as needed.
- **Provide an opportunity for clients to ask questions.**
- **For children, use age-appropriate** printed books, apps, coloring books, and electronic applications.

See Patient Teaching box, Creating Patient Teaching Materials.

Barriers to Teaching and Learning

As you gain teaching experience, you will begin to recognize the factors we have just discussed (e.g., timing, the environment) and to manipulate those that can be changed to enhance teaching and learning. The following are the most common barriers for the nurse and the patient and those encountered when using technology-based learning.

Barriers for the Nurse

The following are barriers to effective teaching:

- **Competing demands** on the nurse's time (e.g., to prepare for teaching)
- **Conflicting schedules** between the nurse's available time for teaching and the client's available time to learn
- **Ineffective coordination** between the nurse's clinical demands and the client's best opportunity to learn
- **Lack of space and privacy,** which can interfere with effective patient education

Toward Evidence-Based Practice

Mobile applications (apps) are commonly used for patient and caregiver health education as well as for healthcare provider education.

Gabrielli, S., Dianti, M., Maimone, R., Betta, M., Filippi, L., Ghezzi, M., & Forti, S. (2017). Design of a mobile app for nutrition education (TreC-LifeStyle) and formative evaluation with families of overweight children. *JMIR mHealth and uHealth, 5*(4), e48. http://doi.org/10.2196/mhealth.7080

The mobile application used in this study (TreC-LifeStyle) offers information for a healthy diet and physical activity. It allows for customized interventions matched to the specific needs of each child. The app also uses food monitoring, feedback, reward, and virtual coaching to support weight loss. Combined with wearable technology that tracks children's physical activity (steps), mobile technology supports health education for children's weight management in primary care.

Oudkerk Pool, M. D., Hooglugt, J-L. Q., Schijven, M. P., Mulder, B. J. M., Bouma, B. J., de Winter, R. J., Pinto, Y., & Winter, M. M. (2021, February). Review of digitalized patient education in cardiology: A future ahead? *Cardiology, 146,* 263–271. https://doi.org/10.1159/000512778

In a review of digital patient education literature, researchers found that online text and video resources contributed to patient empowerment and shared decision making in healthcare. Key elements of effective digital education include clear, structured, comprehensible information.

Scott, K. M., Nerminathan, A., Alexander, S., Phelps, M., & Harrison, A. (2017, January). Using mobile devices for learning in clinical settings: A mixed-methods study of medical student, physician and patient perspectives. *British Journal of Educational Technology, 48*(1), 176–190. https://www.doi.org/10.1111/bjet.12352

Mobile technology is commonly used for healthcare professionals' education in the clinical setting. In this study, physicians and medical students used mobile devices to conveniently access health information. Some users had difficulty because of Internet access. Another downside to using mobile devices at the patient's bedside was distraction when communicating with the patient. However, researchers concluded that the benefits outweigh the risks because healthcare providers need to access and verify health information.

1. In the first article discussing mobile technology for patient education and compliance, why do you think a weight-management application with education, feedback, virtual coaching, and wearable technology was found to be more effective for patient teaching than traditional methods?

2. Have you used a mobile application for your own health education? Was it beneficial to you for learning new information or reinforcing information you received during your own healthcare visit? Why or why not?

3. What are some of the limitations of mobile technology for patient education?

4. What is the responsibility of the nurse when suggesting specific mobile apps to patients and caregivers?

5. As the use of mobile devices becomes increasingly more common in the clinical setting, what is needed to keep healthcare providers' focus on direct patient interaction in the clinical setting?

- **Teaching not seen as a priority** by the nurse or the organization
- **No third-party reimbursement** for teaching
- **Frustration** with the amount of documentation needed

Barriers for the Learner (Patient)
The following are barriers to learning effectively:

- Illness, fatigue, other physical conditions
- Anxiety, personal stress
- Low literacy, low health literacy
- Environment not conducive to learning
- Lack of time to learn
- Overwhelming amount of behavioral change needed
- Overwhelming complexity of the condition or treatment
- Lack of support and ongoing positive reinforcement

- Lack of motivation, willingness to take responsibility
- Language barrier
- Teaching not suited to learning preferences and style
- Provider use of jargon and technical terms
- Does not perceive need for the information taught

Barriers to Technology-Based Learning
Although technology is an asset to learning, it may also create some barriers. Some of the barriers are the same as in the classroom; others are unique, including the following:

- Reduced or lack of social interaction
- Poor learner motivation
- Diverse learning styles
- Time issues

- Technical problems (software or devices)
- Access to the Internet, for some clients

KnowledgeCheck 16-3

- List and define six factors that affect the learning process.
- What is one strategy you could use to motivate a client who seems uninterested in learning?
- What are some aspects of the environment that can enhance or interfere with learning?
- What two strategies might you use with a client functioning with low cognitive ability?

 ThinkLike a Nurse 16-4:
Clinical Judgment in Action

- List some actions you can take to avoid each of the teaching barriers.
- Give an example of each of the barriers to patient education. Take the example of stress of illness: A patient is frightened after having a heart attack, worried about the cost of the medical treatment, and worried about not being able to go to work, so they cannot concentrate on the material being presented to them.

Note: These questions may be difficult, depending on your knowledge and experience. Work with others to answer the questions, as necessary.

PracticalKnowledge
knowing how

The teaching process parallels the nursing process. You will assess learning needs and readiness, make educational diagnoses, write learning objectives, plan and implement teaching strategies, and evaluate client learning.

ASSESSMENT/RECOGNIZING CUES

A learning assessment will help you to determine the right format for teaching your clients, the content to cover, the learning goals, and the teaching strategies. Your initial assessment consists of general information about the amount of time and resources available for your teaching. For example, with Heather (Meet Your Patient), assess the following:

- **Learning needs.** Heather needs to learn about the normal growth and development, age-appropriate behaviors, and nutritional needs of 4-year-olds. She will need safety and health instructions for the next year because her child may not return for another checkup until age 5 years.
- **Client's knowledge level.** You need to identify Heather's understanding of her child's development so far, as well as her expectations of her preschool-age child. Also find out what Heather knows about nutrition and language development for 4-year-olds.
- **Health beliefs and practices.** Determine Heather's (and Jade's) healthcare practices as well as trust in the healthcare system. For example, what kinds of meals does she offer Jade?

- **Physical readiness.** Some interruptions are likely because 4-year-olds have short attention spans. Will Heather be too distracted to listen to the information presented? You may need to provide appropriate play materials for Jade so that she will require less attention from Heather.
- **Emotional readiness.** Emotional maturity is a factor in Heather's readiness to learn. She has expressed concern that her child is so small; you could begin the teaching based on Heather's interest in Jade's progress and health. However, Heather's responses to the care provider during the visit may not have been well thought-out if her child is restless or if she has limited time for the visit.
- **Ability to learn.** During the interview, you can begin to assess Heather's ability to learn, based on her responses to questions. Also ask about her educational level.
- **Literacy level.** You might ask Heather to read a short paragraph related to the topic you are teaching. Then ask questions to determine how well she understood the information.
- **Neurosensory factors.** You can assess Heather's vision, hearing, and manual dexterity as you observe her interactions with her child. Also observe her response to visual and auditory clues that you and the child give. Watching her manipulate a pen, pencil, or toy could provide data about manual dexterity.
- **Learning styles.** Ask Heather how she learns best. Understanding that she probably does not have extensive blocks of time or focused attention to read or listen, you might give her single-page handouts, videos, or pamphlets instead of books or more detailed booklets.

You will recognize cues in your initial comprehensive assessment of the client. You will recognize cues in your initial comprehensive assessment of the client. For guidelines and questions to ask when conducting a learning assessment.

 Go to Chapter 16, Assessment Guidelines and Tools, Focused Assessment Box: Learning Assessment Guidelines, in Volume 2.

NURSING DIAGNOSIS/ANALYZING CUES

Deficient Knowledge is the most frequently used (and often misused) nursing diagnosis for a client teaching plan. It may be either a problem or the etiology of a diagnosis.

Deficient Knowledge as the Primary Problem

Key Point: *You should use Deficient Knowledge only if you believe that the lack of knowledge is the primary problem. Use it to describe conditions in which the patient needs new, additional, or extensive knowledge.*

To generate a nursing diagnosis for a specific client condition, first identify the specific area where the client lacks knowledge. Then relate it to the cause for the knowledge deficit and add the client cues that indicate the need for nursing action, which is to provide client teaching, for example, *Deficient Knowledge (diabetic foot care) related to lack of prior experience, as manifested by anxiety and many questions about foot care.*

Incorrect Uses of Deficient Knowledge

Key Point: *Always look beyond the knowledge deficit to see what problematic responses it produces.*

- **Beware of routine or misdiagnosing the client's need for health information.** It is easy to see that a client lacks information, label it as a Deficient Knowledge problem, and try to solve the problem by giving information—but information may not be what the patient needs at all.
- **Do not use Deficient Knowledge routinely as a problem label for all patients** (Jarrell et al., 2011). There are information needs associated with almost every client condition. However, you cannot assume a particular client needs to be taught that information. For example, a person with a foot ulcer secondary to long-standing diabetes may already know more than you do about foot care. **Key Point:** *For most nursing diagnoses, you can write a nursing order to provide the informal teaching needed instead of formulating a Deficient Knowledge diagnosis.*
- **Do not use Deficient Knowledge for problems involving the client's** *ability to learn.* To accurately describe such situations, use non–NANDA-I diagnoses such as the following:
  - Impaired Ability to Learn r/t fear and anxiety
  - Impaired Ability to Learn r/t delayed cognitive development
  - Lack of Motivation to Learn r/t feelings of powerlessness

Deficient Knowledge as the Etiology

Deficient Knowledge is usually most effective as the etiology of other nursing diagnoses, such as the following:

- Ineffective Health Maintenance related to (r/t) Deficient Knowledge of immunizations
- Risk for Impaired Parenting r/t Deficient Knowledge of child's developmental need for stimulation
- Ineffective Family Health Management r/t Deficient Knowledge of the procedure for drawing up and injecting insulin

▰ PLANNING/ PRIORITIZING HYPOTHESES AND GENERATING SOLUTIONS

Before making a teaching plan, determine what clients want to accomplish by making a **learning contract.** This is a statement of understanding between nurse and client about how to achieve mutually set goals. A contract increases commitment by the client to reach those goals. It usually describes:

- The responsibilities of both nurse and client
- The time frame for the teaching
- Content to be included
- Expectations of all participants

Teaching goals are broad in scope and describe what is expected as the outcome of the teaching and learning process. They should address all three domains of learning. In contrast, **learning objectives** are single, specific behaviors that must be completed to accomplish the goal. They are short term and ideally are accomplished in one or two sessions.

Similar to patient outcomes in the nursing process, learning objectives/goals should include:

- Action verb
- Activity that can be measured or observed
- Circumstances of the learner's performance
- How learning will be measured

Consider, for example:

Goal: Demonstrate ability to perform newborn care in 3 days.

Learning Objectives: (1) Changes infant's diaper, making sure that umbilical cord remains outside the diaper. (2) Demonstrates bathing while maintaining newborn's axillary temperature of greater than 98.5°F (36.9°C).

See Table 16-3 for examples of active verbs for each domain of learning.

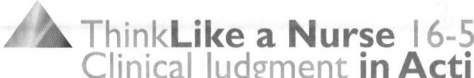

ThinkLike a Nurse 16-5: Clinical Judgment in Action

A client has just been diagnosed with diabetes mellitus. They must monitor and record their blood glucose three times a day. The two of you establish as a goal that they will be able to perform glucose testing independently within 1 week. What objectives would you need to write to achieve this goal?

▰ PLANNING INTERVENTIONS/IMPLEMENTATION

In Chapter 3, you learned about creating a nursing care plan. For clients and families with special learning needs, you will create individualized teaching plans. The teaching plan is often a part of the client's complete nursing care plan.

Creating Teaching Plans

When planning teaching, first and foremost, you will organize content that addresses your client's needs. Creating a conducive environment that is free of distractions is important for learners and is necessary for learning to occur.

Table 16-3 ➤ Examples of Active Verbs for Domains of Learning		
COGNITIVE DOMAIN	AFFECTIVE DOMAIN	PSYCHOMOTOR DOMAIN
Compare	Cry	Apply
Define	Choose	Arrange
Describe	Defend	Assemble
Differentiate	Discuss	Change
Explain	Display	Construct
Give examples	Express	Create
Identify	Initiate	Demonstrate
List	Justify	Inject (e.g., medication)
Name	Relate	Manipulate
Plan	Revise	Move
State	Select	Organize
Summarize	Share	Start
	Smile	Work

Let us apply these aspects of a teaching plan, using Heather (Meet Your Patient) as an example. You have recognized the client's need for anticipatory guidance regarding safety for her 4-year-old. Your nursing diagnosis is Deficient Knowledge (safety for a 4-year-old) related to the mother's inexperience.

Teaching Strategies A teaching strategy is the method used to present content. For Heather, this might include one-to-one instruction and printed information. You must always use plain language. The Joint Commission recommends "teach-back" and "show-back" techniques to assess and ensure patient understanding (Agency for Healthcare Research and Quality, 2020; The Wellness Network, 2016;). You may use drawings, models, technology, or devices to demonstrate your teaching message (Fig. 16-3). Always encourage your patients to ask questions to avoid misunderstanding.

Content The content of your teaching includes the information your client must understand to reach the desired goal. It can include facts, skills, or emotions. For Heather (Meet Your Patient), the content of your informal teaching might include the following:

- *Poison control and prevention*—Curiosity and lack of ability to understand danger put the preschooler at greater risk.
- *Accident prevention*—This would include the need for car seats, increased supervision when exploring, and the use of a helmet when the child rides a bicycle.
- *Risk of choking*—Foods that are hard to swallow or chunky (e.g., hot dogs) are a concern for a 4-year-old.

Patient Teaching

General Tips for Effective Patient Teaching Sessions

Create a Conducive Learning Environment.

➤ **Provide private space to talk** with your patient and other designated family members. Be sure the setting allows for privacy and is free of distractions and interruptions.

➤ **Provide health education when the patient is in the best state of mind to concentrate** on what you are saying. For example, you will want to be sure the patient has pain under control but is not drowsy from pain relievers. Anxiety, depression, and fatigue also interfere with learning.

➤ **Help your patient decide who should be involved in the teaching session.** On the one hand, caregivers assisting in the care after discharge would benefit from the learning process. On the other hand, some patients may not want others to be present because of modesty or cultural practices.

Plan and Communicate Information According to Your Patient's Needs.

➤ **Be considerate of cultural, religious, or other preferences** that might influence the way your patient receives information.

➤ **Learning differences or cognitive impairment can also hamper learning.** Adjust the learning style and level of complexity accordingly. Likewise, modify the teaching approach for patients with visual or hearing deficits. Consider limited English proficiency, mental health, and emotional stress when communicating with patients.

➤ **Find out what your patient needs to know before making a teaching plan.** Involve them in the learning process. This not only improves your patient's motivation to learn but also helps your patient to get more out of the education.

➤ **Be sure you provide the vital information needed for home care.** Because time, staffing, and resources are limited in the healthcare setting, decide what is most important and set that as priority teaching.

- *Need for immunizations and physical checkup*—These are important and should be scheduled during the next year.

Scheduling and Sequencing These terms refer to both the information and the timing of the teaching session.

- **Sequencing**—*how you organize the information.* This refers to the order in which you present the content. As a rule, you should begin with simple and nonthreatening topics and then present complex and difficult ones. To enhance the client's understanding, limit the information you present to two or three important points at a time.

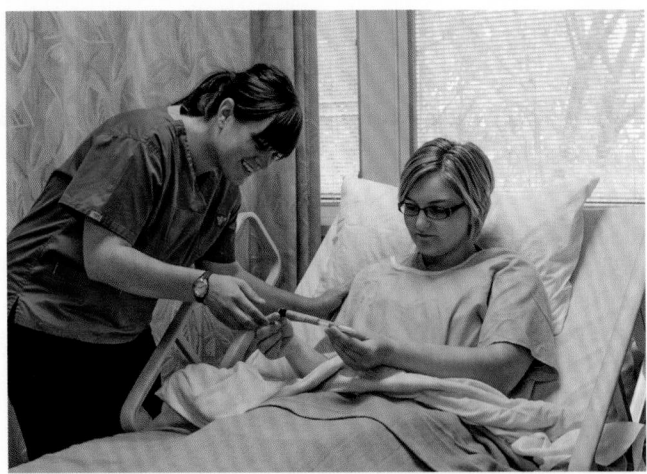

FIGURE 16-3 The nurse uses demonstration and return demonstration to teach a patient how to give herself an insulin injection.

- **Timing**—*when the teaching session(s) are to be scheduled.* This should be based on the client's and nurse's needs. When extensive content is involved, it is best to schedule a teaching session in advance; the nurse and client are then committed and prepared for the session. Meeting for short periods of time can be most effective if teaching is succinct and organized.

In the example at the beginning of this chapter, you could teach Heather about poison control and accident prevention in the lobby while she and her preschooler are waiting for the child to be examined. During the child's examination, you could review immunizations and the need for an annual checkup. At the end of the examination, when discussing the child's nutrition, you might include a discussion of foods that are a choking hazard, such as hot dogs.

Instructional Materials You will use instructional materials to introduce information and reinforce learning. You might give Heather printed handouts with the contact number for the Poison Control Center hotline or a link to an online video demonstrating how to properly install a child car seat. To involve the child, you might include a coloring book and stickers about one of the topics or a mobile tablet with a gaming app that teaches a child about taking medication.

Selecting Specific Teaching Strategies

Before selecting one of the many teaching strategies, consider the client's needs and learning style and the advantages and disadvantages of each method. For a comparison of the advantages and disadvantages of each of the following teaching formats discussed, see Table 16-4.

The nurse may reinforce material taught by various methods by asking, "What questions do you have?" However, when asking, "Do you understand?" some patients are likely to answer "yes" out of embarrassment or a need to cooperate. **Key Point: *A patient's lack of questions does***

not necessarily mean that they understand what has been taught; it could in fact mean the opposite.

Printed Materials Printed materials may be available in the form of fact sheets, discharge instructions, printed pamphlets, or detailed booklets. See Patient Teaching box, Creating Patient Teaching Materials for tips for creating teaching material for patients and caregivers that is easily understood.

Digital Sources of Information Clients obtain extensive information through applications (apps) for smartphones, tablets, and computers, as well as authority source, scientific, and credible Web sites (e.g., Centers for Disease Control and Prevention [CDC]). Clients connect with others and share a common interest through blogs, chats, threaded discussions, and social media special-interest groups. They exchange information, express opinions, offer support, promote interests and activities, and network for personal or professional reasons.

Mobile technology offers convenient access to a variety of learning tools. For example, smartphone and tablet apps include customizable medication reminders, reward systems for healthy behaviors, and educational components. Health-tracking devices and apps offer data regarding activity, diet, and other healthy lifestyle behavior, which can be the basis for a customized health teaching plan.

Demonstration and Return Demonstration In this method, the nurse explains and demonstrates a skill or task. The patient or caregiver then shows comprehension by returning the demonstration. Return demonstrations should occur close to the initial teaching of the skill. Mannequins can be useful for teaching certain skills, such as cardiopulmonary resuscitation (CPR) (Fig. 16-4).

Lecture Patients may attend a seminar or other presentation of health information. Presenters can engage clients with an attention-getting opening and support teaching points with stories, quotes, images, analogies or metaphors, and humor. Lectures can be enhanced by including discussion and question-and-answer periods for clarifying content and by using audiovisuals such as specialized applications, computer-projected slides, streaming video, flip charts, posters, brochures, and models.

Group Meetings and Support Groups Participants discuss topics, share personal experiences and feelings, learn coping strategies from others in the group, and receive firsthand information about diseases or treatments. The discussion leader acts as a facilitator to achieve objectives shared with the group at the beginning of the session. Effective group discussion requires:

- An atmosphere of trust that encourages everyone to participate
- Openness to new ideas and information
- Confidentiality of the content expressed

One-to-One Instruction The most common approach for patient education is direct sharing of information between the nurse and patient. It offers

Text continued on page 417

Teaching Plan

Client Data

Emily O'Connor is the advanced practice nurse in charge of the student health center on campus at State University. A research project revealed that 60% of students surveyed on campus reported that they spent 300 minutes per week on moderate-intensity exercise, which was consistent with a study examining compliance with the *Physical Activity Guidelines for Americans.* However, the researchers found 62% adherence by self-report but only 10% when measured via accelerometer. Thus, Emily decided to teach students and interested campus staff members about the importance of physical activity for physical and emotional well-being. To reinforce the content, Emily developed colorful brochures with photos and charts to make the information more visually appealing and an interactive teaching session to capture clients' attention. She also provided food so that people would have additional motivation to attend.

Nursing Diagnosis

Potential Deficient Knowledge (health behaviors) about physical activity as evidenced by campus-wide survey results showing that less than two-thirds of students comply with the U.S. Department of Health and Human Services recommendations for physical activity.

NOC Outcome

Knowledge: Health Behavior (1805)

NIC Intervention

Teaching: Group (5604)

Teaching Environment

1. Provide an environment conducive to learning that is free of noise, confusion, and distractions. Promote comfort by making personal introductions and offering refreshments during break time.

   Rationale: When adult clients are in an environment in which they feel comfortable, they are less distracted and more able to learn. Participants' physical and emotional comfort are important for creating a positive atmosphere for adult learning. The environment influences a client's interest level and actual motivation to acquire new knowledge (Heik, 2018).

Overall Strategy/Approach

1. Focus on patient problems.
2. Relate content to life experience.
3. Explain how the education will solve a problem.
4. Involve clients in the educational process.
5. Use a variety of methodologies.

   Rationale: Utilizes principles of adult learning. Using a variety of methodologies is important because different people learn in different ways.

Instructional Materials

1. Printed materials (brochures, fact sheets)

   Rationale: Print materials at an appropriate reading level (the National Institutes of Health recommend fifth to eighth grade) for the target audience to allow participants to review information when it is convenient for them (Agency for Healthcare Research and Quality, 2020; Choudhry et al., 2015; Leonard, 2017; National Institutes of Health, 2018). In a study looking at the effectiveness of five types of media (print materials, online PDF, audio files, audio with text Web page, and streaming video demonstration) for improving patients' learning, the findings showed that although participants preferred multimedia presentations, patients retained information from the supplementary materials regardless of the form the content was presented in (Wilson et al., 2012).

2. Streaming video, wearable technologies, or other interactive applications.

   Rationale: In a study investigating the effectiveness of video for teaching patients how to perform cardiopulmonary resuscitation (CPR), the findings indicated that patients who used audiovisual aids reported video as better than text for presenting health information (Chowdhury et al., 2018).

Teaching Plan (continued)

Nursing Diagnosis (continued)

3. Animation, storytelling, and other interactive multimedia (animation, narration, and text) programming

Rationale: To improve patient safety by reducing alarm fatigue in healthcare staff, researchers found that using animation and storytelling combined with an efficient and engaging multimedia training program was effective in motivating staff to change clinical behavior (Alexander & Baker, 2017).

Learning Objective	Schedule/ Sequence	Content	Teaching Strategy
By the end of the first educational session, participants will be able to explain why physical activity is important.	April 1–8	1. Determine date, time, and content of class to be held.	Advertise the educational session by using posters on campus, the campus newspaper, newsletters, social networking sites, and text and e-mail blasts.
	April 9 6:30–7:00 p.m.	2. Social hour. Healthy snacks and beverages. Get acquainted.	
	7:00–7:30 p.m.	3. Identify barriers to engaging in at least 300 minutes of moderate-intensity physical activity or 150 minutes of vigorous-intensity physical activity per week.	Lecture with PowerPoint slides, including photos
	7:30–7:50 p.m.	4. Describe how physical activity helps to promote health, prevent illness, control weight, and enhance overall quality of life.	Projected information (e.g., PowerPoint, YouTube)
	7:50–8:00 p.m.	5. Provide thorough instruction on proper technique for exercises to build strength, improve balance, and increase flexibility.	Video demonstration of various types of exercises with playback of class participants' technique
	8:00–9:00 p.m.	6. Promote awareness and track activity recorded in fitness logs in follow-up contact with participants.	Questions and answers
		7. Provide access to group fitness classes at the local community center.	Hand out printed passes or URL for downloading them from the community center's Web site, if available.

Rationale: Content is based on the Health Belief Model, designed by the U.S. Public Health Service. It identifies four key factors that promote health-seeking behavior (adapted for this setting): (1) person perceives they are at risk for disease (low activity level), (2) person perceives that poor fitness is harmful and has serious consequences, (3) person believes the suggested intervention (300 min/week of physical activity) will improve health, and (4) person believes treatment (physical activity) effectiveness is worth overcoming barriers (Hochbaum, 1958).

(continued)

Teaching Plan (continued)

Evaluation

Eighteen women and 20 men attended the session. When Emily began the educational session, the participants were seated in chairs facing the front of the room, where the screen was set up for a YouTube video presentation. She distributed the printed handout materials and provided a short introduction. Before she began teaching, two women began talking about their battle with obesity and difficulty getting out to exercise. Three women shared stories about friends and family members who had suffered poor health and immobility. One had a question about sports-related injuries. During this discussion, the participants turned their chairs to face each other and talked among themselves.

Emily realized that learning takes place when participants share stories with facilitation by the group leader. Teaching does not have to be led exclusively by the facilitator. Even though she had a teaching plan, she was flexible enough to modify the plan to meet participants' needs. She turned off the PowerPoint, turned on the lights, and instead of lecturing or showing videos from the Centers for Disease Control and Prevention (CDC) Web site, she shared information by answering questions and guiding the discussion.

During this process, Emily realized she had made assumptions about the participants' goals for this educational program and their educational needs. She learned that the women who attended came to the program with an understanding of the benefits of exercise and the consequences of low levels of physical activity; they knew that exercise is important for health and fitness. They wanted to talk about their obstacles, concerns, and questions; they wanted to separate myths from facts; and they wanted to learn proper techniques and how they could maintain motivation to perform at least 300 minutes per week of moderate-intensity physical activity.

After the session, Emily realized that she needed to revise her plan and offer a second session in a week or two. Her assumption that a lack of knowledge was responsible for the low number of people adhering to the *Physical Activity Guidelines for Americans* was not confirmed through discussion with the participants. She developed the following new goals for the second session:

1. By the end of the educational intervention, participants will:
   a. State that questions pertaining to weekly physical fitness have been addressed.
   b. Identify the factors that act as a barrier to engaging in physical activity.
   c. Share strategies for overcoming barriers to engaging in physical activity.
   d. Suggest at least five ways to perform at least 300 minutes of moderate-intensity physical activity per week.
   e. List steps to follow if an injury occurs while engaging in physical activity.
2. At the 1-year follow-up visit, participants will report that they increased physical activity by 60 minutes per week during the past 12 months.

References

Alexander and Baker (2017); Choudhry et al. (2015); U.S. Department of Health and Human Services, National Institutes of Health (2018, updated); Wilson et al. (2012); Wlodkowski and Ginsberg (2017).

Table 16-4 ➤ Formats for Patient Teaching: Advantages and Disadvantages

Lecture

BENEFITS	LIMITATIONS
■ Efficient and cost-effective way to impart information, especially to large groups. ■ Useful for conveying basic concepts and information that serve as the foundation for higher-level, critical thinking later. ■ Presenter can use media-rich formats within the lecture to reach clients with auditory and visual learning styles. ■ Lectures can be recorded for future use.	■ Does not allow for individualization of teaching. ■ Passive-learning technique; usually not suited for optimal retention of information. ■ May not be geared to the level of the client. ■ Less effective for teaching in the psychomotor or affective domains. ■ Can lead to oversaturation if too much information is presented in too short a time. ■ Boredom is common. ■ Not a good strategy for promoting critical thinking. ■ Little opportunity for assessing client comprehension.

Group Discussion

BENEFITS	LIMITATIONS
■ A learner-centered and effective method for teaching in the affective and cognitive domains. ■ Many students enjoy a learning environment with opportunities for interaction with peers. ■ Social involvement can enhance content.	■ Less effective with large groups. ■ The nurse must be comfortable with less structure and with unpredictable client responses. ■ Managing group discussion requires that the instructor have good leadership skills. ■ Not well suited for teaching in the psychomotor domain. ■ Quality of group work can be negatively affected by "groupthink," a force that stifles creativity when individuals succumb to the subtle pressure of agreeing with the group even though affirmation does not reflect the client's individual opinion. ■ Brainstorming fails when participants are distracted or fail to contribute ideas because of fears of rejection or ridicule by peers. Some might even hold back with brainstorming when anticipating the ideas to be unpopular with the instructor. ■ Individuals who dominate can be equally problematic when crowding out less confident participants. ■ Those who are disruptive or intentionally sabotage the activity can interfere with successful group discussion.

Demonstration and Return Demonstration

BENEFITS	LIMITATIONS
■ Is most effective in teaching psychomotor skills (e.g., use of equipment, self-injection, dressing changes). ■ Can be used in small groups if enough equipment is available. ■ When the task or skill is performed correctly, return demonstration can increase self-confidence. ■ Allows for targeted questions and answers and discussion of practical matters, rather than theory.	■ Does not work well with large groups or for those who do not learn best by observing others. ■ May not be well suited for participants who learn at different rates; some might need repeated demonstration or slow enactment of steps, whereas others do not. ■ Time consuming and labor intensive. ■ Involves preparation time to set up equipment. ■ Space must be suitable for the demonstration format. ■ Demonstrator must have specialized expertise if technical skills are involved.

(Continued)

Table 16-4 ➤ Formats for Patient Teaching: Advantages and Disadvantages—cont'd

One-to-One Instruction and Mentoring

BENEFITS	LIMITATIONS
■ Gives the nurse the opportunity to establish a relationship with a client, convey interest in their learning needs, and tailor the teaching to the client's needs as the session proceeds.	■ Can be labor intensive and reaches the fewest numbers of clients.
■ Mentoring allows reluctant clients to ask questions more readily.	■ May overwhelm clients if a large quantity of information is given in a short period of time and therefore may not promote retention.
■ Enables the nurse to provide frequent feedback so that information can be repeated and clarified as needed.	■ Tends to isolate the client from peers who may share the same learning needs and who could provide support.
■ Can be a subtle but powerful method to increase motivation and ability to perform a desired behavior.	■ Can be hampered by personality conflicts.
■ Useful for teaching in all three domains: affective, psychomotor, and cognitive.	■ Relies heavily on the instructor, preceptor, or nurse being a good role model and having effective teaching skills.

Printed Materials

BENEFITS	LIMITATIONS
■ Allows for standardized information to be presented to each client but with some room for individualization.	■ Assumes literacy, proficiency in the dominant language, motivation to read the content, organization to keep track of materials, and visual acuity to decipher the print.
■ Hard-copy documents are a good way to reinforce information, demonstration and return demonstration, or one-to-one instruction.	■ Most general materials should be written at a sixth-grade reading level with words that most people understand (Choudhry et al., 2015).
■ Handouts allow the nurse to cover just the main ideas while using the time more efficiently for face-to-face instruction.	
■ Printed materials are portable, so people can read the information when most convenient.	

Online Sources of Information and Mobile Technologies

BENEFITS	LIMITATIONS
■ The Internet makes a vast amount of health-related information readily available. This makes it possible for consumers to participate in self-care and make informed decisions.	■ The nurse has little control over the quality of information that clients access via the Internet.
■ Patients feel empowered when they have access to relevant and understandable information.	■ Before recommending Web sites to a patient, you need to read them yourself to be sure the information is accurate and the format and reading level are best suited to your patient.
■ Patients often cope better and experience less uncertainty when health information is available.	■ See Chapter 37 for information about evaluating materials you obtain from a Web site.
■ The use of audiovisual materials engages both sight and hearing and can accommodate large groups.	■ Audiovisual hardware and software can be expensive and must be replaced, upgraded, or updated.

Patient Teaching

Creating Patient Teaching Materials

➤ **Organize information** so that the most important material stands out and is repeated for emphasis and clarity. Keep it short and concise.

➤ **Use everyday words and plain-language sentences.** Avoid jargon, abbreviations, or acronyms that are not familiar to clients. Simple sentences are best.

➤ **Include specific step-by-step actions** you want clients to take.

➤ **Use headings, bullets, and easy-to-read font.** Lists are easier for patients to read and help them retain information.

➤ **Use many drawings and photographs** to emphasize the information.

➤ **Phrase directions positively** to reinforce what you want patients to remember (e.g., say "do" rather than "don't" or "never").

➤ **Use active verbs** (e.g., "Take the pill" rather than "The pill should be taken").

➤ **Personalize the information** by using "you" as if you are teaching in person.

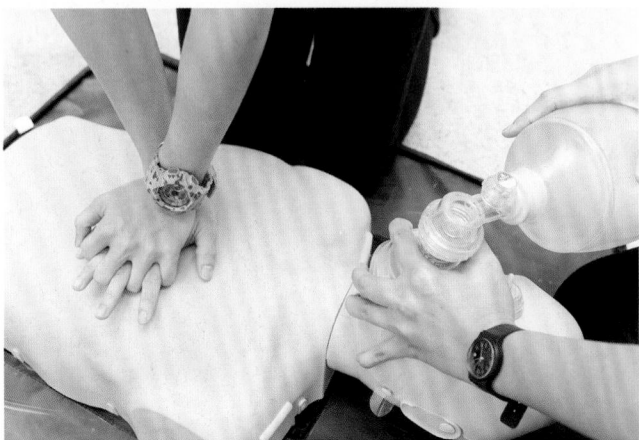

FIGURE 16-4 Mannequins can offer realism and relevance to an educational experience.

an opportunity for patients and caregivers to ask questions as the nurse is providing instruction. The nurse can directly observe and offer feedback on the client's performance.

Role-Modeling In role-modeling, the nurse teaches by example, demonstrating the behaviors and attitudes that clients should adopt. For children, role-modeling using a puppet, stuffed animal, or a child's own doll can be helpful in reducing anxiety and enhancing the child's learning. For instance, you can suggest that the child be "the nurse" and "feel Miss Bunny's pulse," or have a puppet "suggest" to a child, "When I get a shot, I say, 'Ouch!' real loud, and then it's all over!"

KnowledgeCheck 16-4

- True or False: When a patient has a learning disability, you should use a non–NANDA-I diagnosis (e.g., impaired ability to learn) to describe the problem.
- True or False: Learning objectives are short term and, ideally, should be accomplished in one or two teaching sessions.
- List and state the advantages and disadvantages of at least six teaching strategies.

EVALUATION OF LEARNING

Evaluation of the effectiveness of the teaching plan is essential to improving the quality of instruction.

- Were your teaching objectives realistic and in line with the client's and caregivers' goals for health information?
- Did you accurately recognize client and caregiver cues for readiness to learn?
- Were your teaching methods, the timing of the teaching, content, amount of information, and quality of teaching materials suited to the client's and caregiver's needs?

The client is your best source for feedback. Be sure to ask whether the materials and methods were helpful or uninteresting and offer other comments. The following methods are commonly used to evaluate client learning:

- **Oral questions/interviews/questionnaires/checklists** allow clients to evaluate their own progress. You may obtain additional information by talking with the client about whether your teaching was effective; however, you may obtain more honest responses by using an anonymous online survey after the delivery of healthcare services.
- **Direct observations of client performance** are descriptive notes that you make of the client's performance. They will help you in providing feedback, either to reinforce accurate learning or to correct misinformation.
- **Client's reports and client records** of performance and results. You can evaluate the data and give feedback. Provide criteria and clear expectations to help the client document.
- **Tests and written exercises** can be used in a formal learning setting to measure retention and progress toward meeting content objectives (e.g., CPR training). This method requires the client to have adequate literacy skills.

Key Point: *Clients will not remember everything you teach them.* Repetition, reinforcement, and practice are necessary for retention, and so is information that is made memorable.

Documentation of Patient Education

As is true for all nursing actions, it is important to document the responses of the client and caregivers to teaching. Documentation also is evidence that teaching was done and communicates the information to other health professionals. Write objective statements about what was taught and the client skills and behaviors that demonstrate learning. For informal teaching that occurs during other care activities, you may simply record in the nursing notes or use agency-provided documentation forms.

To explore learning resources for this chapter,

Go to Davis Advantage and find:

Answers and Suggested Responses for all questions in this chapter

Concept Map

Knowledge Map

References and Bibliography

CHAPTER 17

Interprofessional Partnerships: Documenting & Reporting

Learning Outcomes

After completing this chapter you should be able to:

➤ Explain the purposes of documentation.
➤ Compare and contrast electronic and written documentation.
➤ Identify a variety of documentation formats and their purposes.
➤ Follow documentation guidelines for accurate recording of the health status of patients, nursing interventions,

and patient outcomes in written and electronic formats.
➤ Identify approved abbreviations to use in documenting in clinical environments.
➤ Discuss the key elements of giving a verbal patient report.
➤ Explain the process for verifying or questioning a medical prescription.

Key Concepts

Documentation
Oral reporting

Related Concepts

See the Concept Map on Davis Advantage.

Meet Your Patient

Steven Stellanski is a 16-year-old male who has just been released from the postanesthesia care unit (PACU) after an emergency appendectomy. You are assigned to his care on your unit. Steven is groggy but moaning in pain. "Help me, help me," he whispers. He is holding his abdomen and grimacing. The PACU nurse tells you that Steven has Down syndrome and functions at an elementary school–age level.

Steven's vital signs are as follows: tympanic membrane temperature, 37.7°C (99.9°F); pulse, 104 beats/min; respirations, 24 breaths/min; and blood pressure, 104/68 mm Hg. An IV bag of lactated Ringer's solution is infusing at 125 mL/hr. The dressing on Steven's right lower abdomen is dry and intact. An indwelling catheter is draining pale-yellow urine.

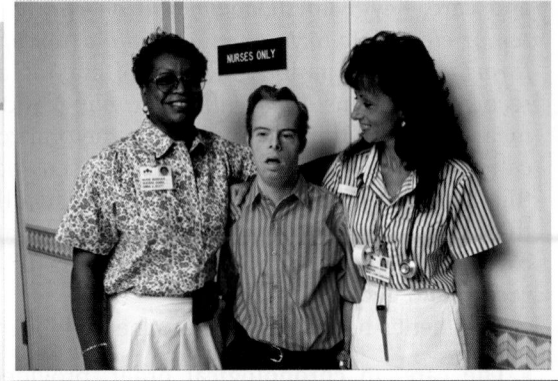

The provider has prescribed a patient-controlled analgesia (PCA) pump that will deliver morphine sulfate at 1 mg every 15 minutes, up to 4 mg per hour. Steven is to remain NPO (nothing by mouth) for now. His postoperative dressing is to be changed tomorrow morning, and the nurses are to institute progressive ambulation as tolerated.

Theoretical Knowledge
knowing why

When you imagine yourself working as a nurse, what do you think of? Most people picture themselves at the bedside working with patients. When you look at ads for nursing jobs, they often show a nurse performing interventions (e.g., hanging an IV bag, listening to heart sounds). The ads rarely show the nurse documenting or verbally reporting care. Yet healthcare professionals rely on these two methods of communication to coordinate patient care. In this chapter, we discuss paper, electronic, and oral communication.

ABOUT THE KEY CONCEPTS

Documentation and **oral reporting** are the two broad concepts linked to all other concepts in this chapter. As you read, think: "What does this have to do with documentation?" and "How does this relate to oral reporting?"

DOCUMENTATION

Documentation is the act of recording patient status and care. **Key Point: *Documentation can be in written or electronic form or in a combination of the two forms.*** Documentation is the act of making a written record. The terms *documenting, recording,* and *charting* mean the same thing. **Reporting** is the oral communication about a patient's status and is discussed later in this chapter. Similarly, the concept of a **health record** that contains documentation, prescriptions, and other care information replaced the concepts of **medical record** and **chart.**

A patient's health record permanently documents:

- **The care, in chronological order,** provided by all healthcare providers
- **The patient's responses to interventions** and treatments
- Important facts about a patient's health history, including past and present illnesses, examinations, tests, treatments, and outcomes

As a nurse, you are responsible for managing and implementing the interprofessional plan of care. That responsibility includes documenting the care provided and the progress made toward achieving patient goals. Research shows that most electronic health record (EHR) systems increase the nurses' documentation time; however, nursing researchers and EHR software manufacturers are making great efforts to streamline the documentation process to decrease the time burden associated with its use (Moore et al., 2020; Studwick et al., 2022).

How Do Healthcare Providers Use Documentation?

Clear, complete, concise, comprehensive, and correct documentation in a client health record serves the following purposes:

Communication Members of the interprofessional team use the health record to communicate about the client's status and care. For example, if it is not possible to speak directly to the respiratory therapist on your shift, you can at least review the progress notes. This documentation communicates essential information that enables healthcare professionals to plan and evaluate treatment and monitor health status over time.

Continuity of Care Communication promotes continuity of care. For example, if you are concerned that the client is at high risk for infection, you can include a nursing diagnosis of Infection on the written or electronic plan of care. You would then initiate nursing prescriptions for other nurses to regularly observe for and document signs of infection.

Quality Improvement To improve overall quality of care, healthcare agencies must identify ways to decrease length of stay, control costs, and identify knowledge and practice gaps that can be addressed through in-services and continuing education. In an internal review, they

- Perform **manual medical records audits** (directed reviews) of written documentation.
- Run reports to analyze large amounts of data in EHR systems.

External accrediting agencies, such as The Joint Commission, review written and electronic records to ensure delivery of quality care and public safety.

Planning and Evaluation of Client Outcomes Documentation enables providers, nurses, and other healthcare professionals to plan and evaluate treatment and monitor health status over time.

Legal Record The health record will be scrutinized by legal experts if a dispute about a client's care arises. In court, the health record is legal evidence of the care given to a client and is used to judge whether the interventions were timely and appropriate. Expert reviewers look for documentation of the client's baseline status, changes in status, interpretation of the changes, interventions implemented, and the client's responses to those interventions.

Professional Standards of Care The American Nurses Association (ANA) recognizes the importance of documentation, which is contained in many of its standards. To review the specific standards that include documentation, review the ANA's publication *Scope and Standards of Practice* (2021) on the ANA's Website (https://www.nursingworld.org).

Reimbursement and Utilization Review Insurance companies, government and third-party payers, budget managers, and organization billing staff use client health records to determine the cost of care. They also use the health record for **utilization review** to determinate whether the medical treatments and interventions were necessary and appropriate.

✚ **Education and Research** As a student, you are well aware that the health record provides a snapshot of what is going on with the client, enabling you to research unfamiliar diagnoses, prescriptions, and treatments before beginning direct care. This helps you to deliver safe care.

The health record is also used to gather data for clinical research. The increasing use of EHRs enables rapid analysis of large numbers of health records. The use of large samples of health records and clinical data sets is an essential step toward better understanding the cause and progression of disease, treatment methods, and outcomes across varied populations and diseases.

Why Are Standardized Nursing Languages Important?

- **Make nursing visible.** As healthcare costs escalated, it became necessary to demonstrate the value of nursing—that is, to describe what nurses do and the outcomes that result. Standardized nursing terminology makes nursing care and its effect on patient outcomes more visible in patient records.
- **Support nursing research.** Documentation systems that use ANA-recognized terminology (e.g., Clinical Care Classification [CCC], NANDA-I, Nursing Interventions Classification [NIC], Nursing Outcomes Classification [NOC]) allow researchers to retrieve nursing data for aggregation and analysis and establish standards for the delivery of evidence-based nursing care. Such standards help close the gap between what research shows to be the best nursing practices and the interventions nurses use in practice.
- **Provide standardized terminology for use in EHR systems.** Computers require standardized information that can be converted to numerical codes.

Several standardized language models have been created and are used in nursing documentation, such as CCC and NANDA-I (for nursing diagnoses), NIC (for interventions), and NOC (for patient outcomes). To review how to use standardized nursing language in your own practice, see the standardized language sections in Chapter 3.

How Are Health Records Systems Organized?

A **health records system** is the overall process by which to create, store, and retrieve client records in an organization. Each healthcare agency determines the health record system and standardized language that it will use. Some agencies develop their own standardized terminology for their EHRs. Nursing leaders in each organization usually determine the documentation forms that nurses will use within the records system.

Source-Oriented Record Systems

Patients in hospitals and long-term care facilities commonly use **source-oriented records.** Members of each discipline record their findings in a separate section of the medical record. A typical source-oriented record includes the following sections:

- **Admission data**—demographic information, insurance data, contact information
- **Advance directive**—information on client's wishes for end-of-life care
- **History and physical**—a detailed summary of the current health problem; past medical, surgical, and social history; medications taken; allergies; review of systems and physical examination data
- **Provider's prescriptions**—plan of care that includes medications, treatments, and activities
- **Progress notes**—chronological documentation by healthcare team members, including client examinations, problem identification, and response to therapy
- **Diagnostic studies**—reports detailing the findings of tests that have been performed, such as x-ray examination, ultrasound, or pulmonary function tests
- **Laboratory data**—results from diagnostic tests, such as complete blood count (CBC)
- **Nurses' notes**—documentation of client care and response to treatment recorded by nurses (usually chronological)
- **Graphic data**—numerical data collected over time and displayed visually to allow for analysis of trends. Examples include intake and output (I&O) records; vital sign flowsheets; rating scales; and checklists of client activity, dietary intake, and activities of daily living (ADLs).
- **Rehabilitation and therapy notes**—chronological documentation by therapists (e.g., physical, occupational, respiratory) about assessments, treatment plan, and client response to therapy.
- **Discharge planning**—includes data from utilization review, case managers, or discharge planners on anticipated client needs after discharge

Advantages You can easily find the care provided by each discipline and laboratory and diagnostic test results.

Disadvantages A drawback of this system is that data may be fragmented and scattered throughout the client's record. That means that you need to review all sections of the medical records to track treatments and client outcomes associated with a particular problem. For example, suppose a client with congestive heart failure is retaining fluids, causing her to be short of breath on exertion. To find the interventions implemented for this problem, you would need to look in the following sections:

1. Prescriptions from primary care providers (PCPs) to see the drugs (e.g., cardiac or diuretics) prescribed to treat fluid retention
2. Respiratory therapist's notes for the client's response to breathing treatments
3. Nursing notes to determine assessments, care provided, and outcomes (e.g., head of the bed elevated to facilitate breathing)
4. Graphic section to evaluate urinary output in response to the medication

Problem-Oriented Record (POR) Systems

Problem-oriented records (PORs) are organized around the client's problems. There are no separate sections for each discipline. The POR consists of four parts: database, problem list, plan of care, and progress notes.

- The **database** consists of various components, such as demographic data, the history and physical, nursing assessment data, and family and social history. As the client's condition changes, the database is updated to reflect their status.
- The **problem list** is a concise listing of actual and resolved problems identified from the database. If a problem changes or is redefined, the problem list is updated to reflect the change. See Figure 17-1 for an example of a problem list.

Problem number	Date entered	Date resolved	Client problem
1	mm/dd/yyyy	mm/dd/yyyy	Abdominal pain (unknown etiology) Redefined mm/dd/yyyy
1A	mm/dd/yyyy		Appendicitis resulting in emergency appendectomy
1B	mm/dd/yyyy		Acute pain r/t abdominal incision 2 appendectomy
2	mm/dd/yyyy		Down syndrome — functions at school-age level
3	mm/dd/yyyy		Risk for constipation r/t opioid use for pain control and h/o appendicitis

FIGURE 17-1 A problem list for Steven Stellanski (Meet Your Patient). Note that Problem 1 has been redefined now that the cause of Steven's pain has been determined. Note also that the list contains both medical and nursing diagnoses.

- The **plan of care** includes the PCP's prescriptions and the nursing care plan to address the identified problems. Other disciplines may also contribute to the plan.
- **Progress notes** are organized according to the problem list. Each discipline records on shared notes. The documentation is labeled according to problem number.

Advantages A problem list allows for input from all disciplines, making it easy to monitor the client's progress and enhance collaboration.

Disadvantages To work well, the POR system requires a cooperative spirit among healthcare providers as well as diligence in maintaining a current database and problem list.

Charting by Exception

Charting by exception (CBE) is a system of charting in which you only document significant findings or exceptions to standards and norms of care. To use the CBE effectively, you must know and adhere to professional, legal, and organizational guidelines for nursing assessments and interventions.

You document on preprinted flowsheets that contain normal findings for the facility. **Key Point: *CBE assumes that the patient has responded normally to all standards, unless a separate entry is made (an exception).*** Each flowsheet has entries for expected aspects of care and thus can vary by specialty areas or diagnosis.

Advantages CBE reduces the amount of time spent on documentation of routine care, provides a record that is easily read and understood, and clearly highlights variations from the expected plan of care. EHRs can standardize common processes and list abnormal findings from the menu bar. These abnormal findings are often displayed in the patient summary or the opening page to a patient record (Park et al., 2022).

Disadvantages The main problem associated with CBE is omission of pertinent information. Critics of CBE believe it:

- Requires nurses to be overly familiar with the organization's documentation standards and policies
- Makes it difficult to capture the skilled judgment of nurses
- Reduces care to such rote repetitions that the nurse may forget to document an exception to the established standards

- ✚ CBE can lead to errors because nurses may conclude that care has been completed when in fact, it was not done. This system requires you to carefully assess and validate the care provided.

Here is an example of what part of a CBE flowsheet for Steven Stellanski (Meet Your Patient) might look like. Notice in the first section that the day-shift nurse merely initials that they have made an assessment or taken one of the listed actions at each of the designated times:

DATE: 00/00/0000				
Hour	0800	0900	1000	1100
ACTIVITY				
Bedrest		LP		
Ambulate	LP*			
Sleeping				
BRP				
HOB elevated	LP	LP		

	DAY	EVENING	NIGHT	
Neurological		√		
Cardiovascular		√		
Pulmonary		√		
Gastrointestinal		*		Vomited 3x1, 100 mL clear yellow fluid at 0730. Given Promethazine 7 mg IV with relief.

Key: √ = normal findings, * = significant finding.

Notice also that the second table (with the check marks) is a summary for the day shift. This is where the nurse describes and discusses any of the significant findings noted at the individual assessment times.

Electronic Health Record (EHR) Systems

The EHR consists of records entered into the computer. EHRs typically combine source-oriented and problem-oriented record styles, although the source-oriented system is most common. For example, a client's EHR often contains prescriptions, clinical documentation, laboratory results, and other test and procedure results, as well as a problem and diagnosis list, the integrated plan of care (IPOC) of the various providers (e.g., physicians, advanced practice nurses, therapists, case managers), and their documented progress notes.

A section of an electronic form for recording I&O in source-oriented format is shown in Figure 17-2. As you can see, the I&O screen records numerical data. It also allows the nurse to add brief narrative comments in each field. Figure 17-3 is an electronic IPOC in problem-oriented format. The IPOC can be updated at the times specified by the organization, and I&O data can be entered at any time. Both exist within the same electronic records system.

Advantages

- **Enhanced communication and collaboration.** Improved communication among healthcare providers.
- Allow for computerized provider entry prescriptions
- **Improved access to information**
  - Multiple healthcare providers can access the same information at the same time.
  - Authorized persons can access information remotely (e.g., from a client's home).
  - EHRs integrate client information between multiple departments so that new information is immediately available to users in all areas. For example, when the laboratory enters a critical result, such as a clotting time, you have immediate access.
- **Time savings**
  - Retrieves stored information quickly and easily
  - Creates reports quickly because of the computer's ability to aggregate data (e.g., a 24-hour graph of the client's vital signs)
  - Reduces repetition and duplication
- **Improved quality of care**
  - The system can use protocols to automatically enter prescriptions based on the client's condition. For example, some EHR systems will automatically enter a prescription to observe and document the risk of falls when a client's "fall score" exceeds a certain level.
  - Embedded protocols enhance caregiver knowledge and the ability to follow clinical practice guidelines. For example, the nurse can activate an immediate link to the tables of information needed to decide how much insulin to give based on the client's blood glucose results.
  - Minimizes medical errors through programmed alerts that are automatically displayed when a provider takes an action that could be harmful (e.g., prescribes a drug to which a client is allergic).
  - Analyzes data at the time of collection, making immediate nursing decision making possible.
  - Facilitates EHR evidence-based practice by analyzing thousands of records across populations and geographic locations to support nursing decisions and guide professional and organization quality improvement.
- **Information is private and safe.**
  - Information is permanently stored with minimal risk of loss.

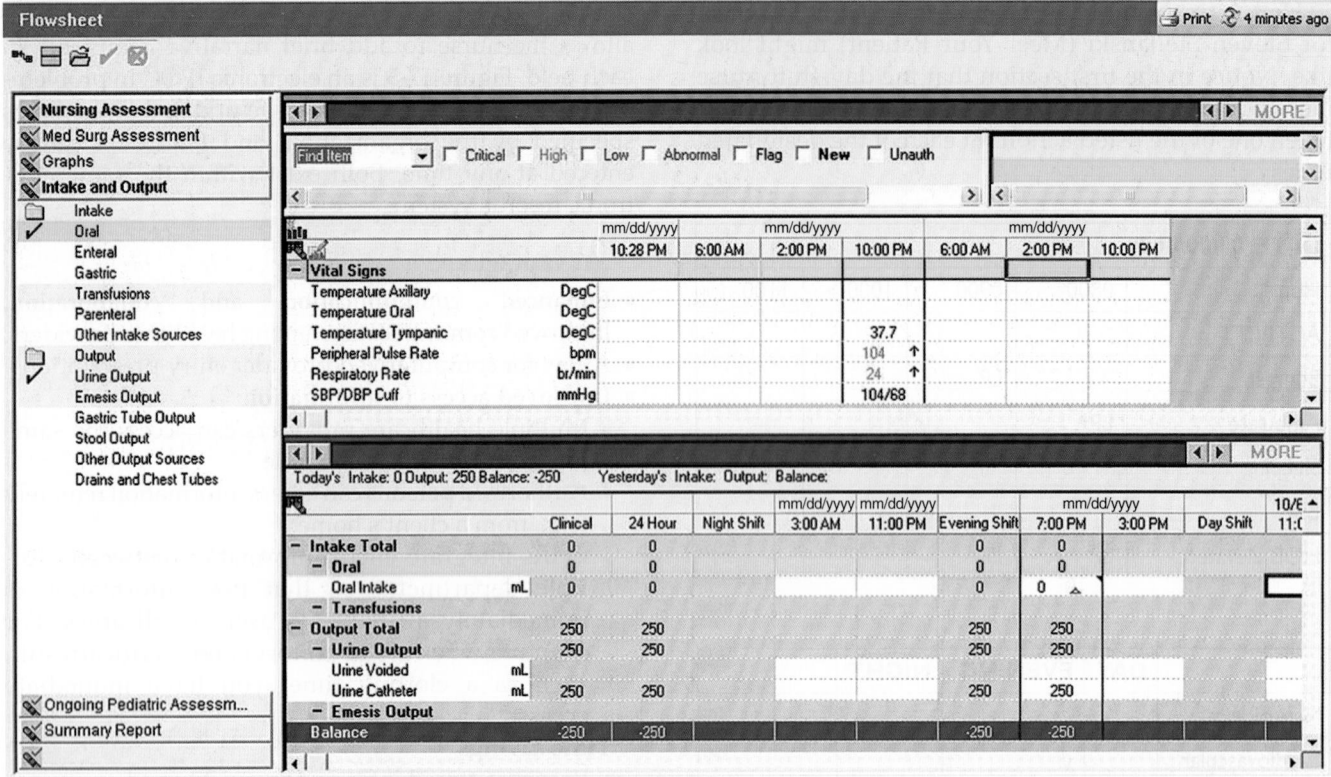

FIGURE 17-2 An electronic intake and output (I&O) entry form.

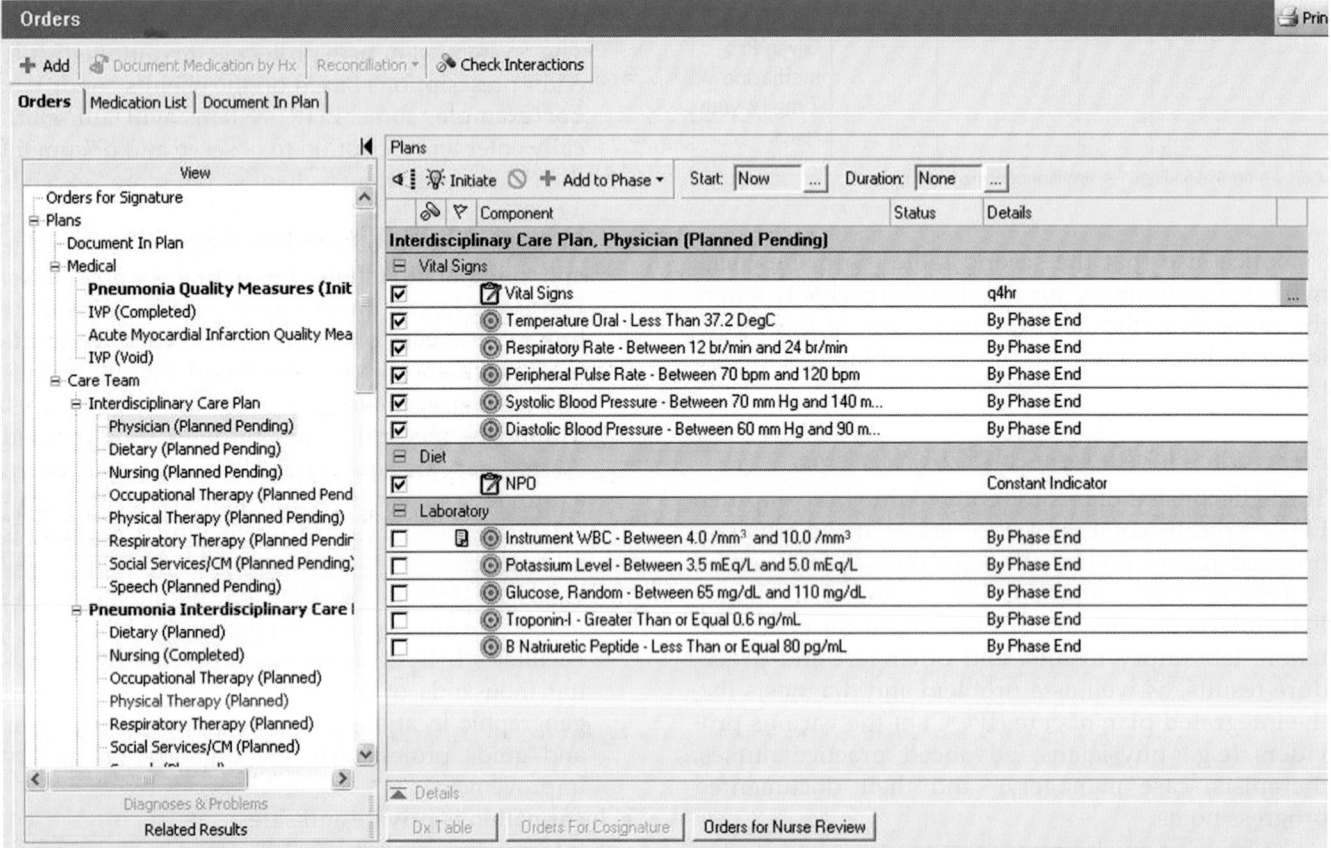

FIGURE 17-3 A portion of an electronic integrated plan of care (IPOC) form.

- Confidentiality of client information is enhanced by restricting access, tracking everyone who accesses the healthcare record, and requiring proper security clearances and unique passwords.
- Front-view screen protectors prevent others from looking at your computer screen.

Disadvantages of Electronic Health Records

- **Expense:** Electronic documentation systems are expensive.
- **Downtime:** Downtime processes must be in place for times when parts of the EHR are not available (e.g., because of power outages and system upgrades).
- **Difficulties associated with change:**
  - Learning to use some documentation systems can be challenging and time consuming.
  - Some EHRs are not user-friendly (e.g., difficult to access information needed to make care decisions).
  - Some systems do not control redundancy well, requiring the client to provide repetitive information.
- **Lack of integration:** Some EHRs are not integrated across the different departments or systems, which decreases the sharing of information.
- EHRs can be a safety concern due to interoperability, lack of federal regulations, ineffective designs, fraudulent inputting, user errors, mix-ups in patient profiles, and other factors (Pfeifer, 2020; Schulte & Fry, 2019).

Paper Records

You will probably not work in facilities that still use paper records. However, they may be used as a backup for outages of electronic systems. For a summary of the advantages and disadvantages of paper records, see Box 17-1.

KnowledgeCheck 17-1

- Identify the purposes of the client health record.
- What are the key differences in the organization of source-oriented records, problem-oriented records, electronic documentation systems, and charting-by-exception systems?
- What are three advantages of EHRs?
- What are three advantages of paper health records?

Documentation and Clinical Judgment

The goal of all nursing documentation is a clear, concise, and complete representation of the client's healthcare experience that is easily accessible and understood by all members of the healthcare team. Effective documentation allows you to help clients make sound health decisions by trending cues, hypotheses, and evaluation of outcomes.

The quantitative drop-down boxes and checklists in EHRs may not adequately reflect the nursing process nor capture the work of nurses (Stein et al., 2019). Current EHR systems may not utilize terminology, such as Recognize or Analyze Cues from the Clinical Judgment

---

BOX 17-1 ■ Advantages and Disadvantages of a Paper Health Record

Advantages

- Care providers are comfortable with it because it is familiar. There is little "learning curve."
- Paper records do not require large databases and secure networks to function.
- There is no downtime for system changes, weather, and so on.
- It is relatively inexpensive to create new forms and update old ones.

Disadvantages

Access may be delayed. Only one care provider can access the record at a time; the provider must be in the same location as the record.

Retrieving information may be slow.

- Healthcare providers may need to search through multiple pages to find needed information.
- Specific documentation is difficult to retrieve when needed, especially when files are archived in another part of the building.

Documentation is time consuming.

- Documentation may take more time because writing by hand is slower than computer entry.

- Documentation is often redundant and repetitive.
- Paper records require a manual audit of many charts to create reports and collect client data. This is time and resource intensive.

There is a relatively high risk for patient care error.

- Narrative documents are hard to read if the handwriting is illegible or messy. This means nurses have to take time from patient care to contact providers to clarify handwritten prescriptions.
- Papers can be lost from the records or damaged, leading to duplicate assessments or medication errors.
- Paper records are often inconsistent in how the same patient information is documented, even within the same organization. Standardized terminology often is not used.

Storage of paper records is expensive.

Confidentiality is difficult to protect. There is no way to know who may have access to the paper health record without proper authorization.

Model discussed in Chapter 2. However, you should strive to incorporate the nursing process and clinical judgment in your documentation.

Assessment/Recognize Cues: Document cues that may indicate actual or potential client problems. At an initial assessment, document comprehensive data about all client systems.

Nursing Diagnosis/Analyzing Cues: After analyzing cues/assessment data, document your hypotheses about the client's response to actual or potential health conditions or needs.

Planning/Prioritizing Hypotheses and Generating Solutions: Document measurable and achievable short-term and long-term solutions, with goals directed at preventing, minimizing, or resolving identified client problems or issues.

Implementation/Taking Action: After putting the plan of care into effect, document the specific actions taken based on the solutions generated that align with the hypothesis (diagnosis).

Evaluation: Document client responses to nursing care; document whether the plan of care was effective in preventing, minimizing, or resolving the identified problems; and then modify the plan as needed.

What Are Some Common Formats for Nursing Progress Notes?

Nursing documentation can take many forms, including computerized electronic documents, audio or video files, e-mails, faxes, scanned paper documents, electronically stored photographs, x-ray findings, and other images. The choice of format used in your organization will determine your nursing documentation system. In all formats, you must learn to use abbreviations appropriately.

Use of Abbreviations

Recall the case of Steven Stellanski (Meet Your Patient). Following is a brief admission note using a narrative documentation format. Underline any words or entries that you do not understand:

00/00/0000 1600 Pt received on unit from PACU. VSS. TM temp 37.7°C (99.9°F), P 104, and BP 104/68. LOC unstable. Arouses when name called but quickly drifts off to sleep. PERRLA. Moaning, grimacing, holding abd, whispers "Help me. Help me." LR at 125 mL/hr infusing in R forearm. IV site patent. Urinary catheter in place, draining pale yellow urine. Abd dsg dry & intact. Morphine sulfate PCA prescribed. Will initiate. ———————————— *Ron Allen, RN*

You can see from this entry that nurses use many abbreviations in their documentation. Every healthcare institution has a list of approved abbreviations that may be used in documentation. Be sure to consult your organization's list before you document. For a list of commonly used abbreviations in healthcare and another list of abbreviations that pertain to medication administration,

 Go to **Chapter 17, Abbreviations Commonly Used in Healthcare,** in Volume 2.

 Also go to **Chapter 23, Common Medication-Related Abbreviations,** in Volume 2.

The Joint Commission (2018) "do not use" list directs medical personnel in healthcare organizations to write out certain words rather than using the abbreviations (see Table 17-1).

Narrative Format

Narrative format is used with written source-oriented and problem-oriented charts. The **narrative chart entry**

Table 17-1 ➤ Joint Commission "Do Not Use" List	
DO NOT USE THIS ABBREVIATION	**WRITE OUT THE WORD OR DOSE**
U or u	Unit
IU	International Unit
Q.D., QD, q.d., qd	Daily
Q.O.D., QOD, q.o.d., qod	every other day
MS, MSO4, and MgSO4	either morphine sulfate or magnesium sulfate
The trailing zero for medications (X.0 mg)	X mg (e.g., 10 mg)
Lack of leading zero (.X mg)	0.X mg (e.g., 0.1 mg)

Other Recommendations

In consideration of furthering The Joint Commission's Patient Safety Goals, some institutions require the following to minimize common errors that occur in healthcare organizations:

- Write out "greater than" or "less than"—rather than using the symbols > or <.
- Write drug names in full—rather than using abbreviations.
- Use metric units—instead of apothecary units.
- Write "at" or "each"—rather than using the @ symbol.
- Write "mL" or "milliliters"—in place of the "cc" abbreviation.
- Write "mcg" or "micrograms"—instead of the "µg" abbreviation.

tells the story of the client's experience in the order that it happens.

- It provides information on the details of the client's care—status, activities, nursing interventions, psychosocial context, and response to treatment.
- It tracks the client's changing health status and progress toward goals.
- It is especially useful when attempting to construct a timeline of events, such as a cardiac arrest or other emergency situations.
- A disadvantage is that the lack of standardization can result in lengthy notes, making it difficult to retrieve relevant data in a timely manner.
- A concern is that with the focus on EHR, clinicians may not read narrative notes, despite their value as an important communication tool, due to their length and variations in format (Payne et al., 2021).

Problem–Intervention–Evaluation (PIE)

The **Problem–Intervention–Evaluation (PIE) system** organizes information according to the client's problems. It requires keeping a daily assessment record and progress notes. PIE eliminates the need for a separate care plan and provides a nursing-focused rather than medical-focused record.

> *Problem:* Use data from your original assessment to identify appropriate nursing diagnoses.
> *Intervention:* Document the nursing actions you take for each nursing diagnosis.
> *Evaluation:* Document the client's response to interventions and treatments.

Problems are identified from the admission assessment. Subsequent entries begin with identification of the problem number. This type of documentation establishes an ongoing care plan. A PIE charting entry for Steven Stellanski (Meet Your Patient) might look like this:

00/00/0000   1630
P: 1B
I: Pt $\bar{c}$ 1 mg doses up to 4 mg morphine/hr. Groggy yet c/o pain. Has not triggered PCA independently. Rates pain as 8 on scale of 1–10. PCA use reviewed with pt. Demonstrated use $\bar{c}$ 1st dose at 1615.
E: Still moaning & grimacing. Has not initiated another dose via PCA. Reinforced teaching with 2nd dose given. May need continuous infusion if unable to use to control pain. ─────────────────── Ron Allen, RN

This style of documentation tends to focus only on the listed problems and not on the client as a whole. However, the primary disadvantage of PIE charting is that it does not document the planning portion of the nursing process. There is no seamless flow of client data/cues, nursing hypotheses (diagnosis), and actions/interventions, such as that seen in a patient's plan of care.

SOAP/SOAPIE/SOAP(IER)

The **SOAP format** is often used to write nursing and other progress notes. It can be used in source-oriented, problem-oriented, and electronic health records. The following list explains the acronyms SOAP, SOAPIE, and SOAP(IER).

- *Subjective data*—What the client or family members tell you about the client's signs and symptoms and the reason for seeking healthcare. Typically, this is documented by quoting the actual words said.
- *Objective data*—Factual, measurable clinical findings, such as vital signs, test results, and quality of breath sounds. Refer to Chapter 3 to review subjective and objective data.
- *Assessment*—Conclusions drawn from the subjective and objective data, usually client problems or nursing diagnoses. **Key Point: *SOAP terminology is different from nursing process terminology. In the nursing process chapter, we referred to conclusions about data as inferences or problems and stated that assessment does not include conclusions about data. When using SOAP, you should document your conclusions or hypothesis about the data under "A."***
- *Plan:* Short-term and long-term goals and strategies that will be used to relieve the client's problems.
- *Interventions:* Actions of the healthcare team performed to achieve expected outcomes.
- *Evaluation:* An analysis of the effectiveness of interventions.
- *Revision:* Changes made to the original care plan.

Components of a POR Recall that a POR is organized according to specific client problems and has five components: database, problem list, initial plan, progress notes, and a discharge summary. You will refer to and use the following four parts when documenting in SOAP format:

- **Problem List.** A numbered list of the client's current problems in chronological order is compiled so that you can refer to the number when entering your notes.
- **Initial Plan.** This includes expected outcomes and plans for further care interventions and teaching. There is only one initial plan, so you must update and change the plan in subsequent progress notes.
- **Progress Notes.** This is where you record the SOAP(IER) information. As a rule, you enter a note for each current problem every 24 hours or when the client's condition changes.
- **Discharge Summary.** At discharge, each problem on the list is addressed and a notation made about its status. Unresolved problems, with plans for each, are included when communicating with the client, other facilities, and home health agencies.

Following is an example of SOAP progress notes using the admission data of Steven Stellanski (Meet

Your Patient). In the previous section, these same data were used to create a narrative note. Notice that the data are similar; however, the narrative note is organized by data source. Steven's SOAP(IER) charting entry related to his postoperative nausea and pain could look like this:

00/00/0000	1630	#1 – Nausea related to anesthesia_____ S – Pt states, "I feel sick to my stomach. Help me." O – Vomited 100 mL clear, light-yellow fluid. _____ A – Nauseated secondary to anesthesia. P – Monitor nausea and give antiemetic as needed. _____ I – Administered Promethazine 7 mg IV at 1640.
	1700	E—States he feels less sick to his stomach. Ron Allen, RN_____
00/00/0000	1600	#1B – Acute pain related to abdominal incision 2° appendectomy _____ S – States, "Help me, help me." Moaning and grimacing. _____ O – Moaning and grimacing; holding abd. Drsg dry & intact. BP 104/68, P 104, R24, and TM temp 99.9°F. PERRLA. _____ A – Postoperative pain P – Give analgesic as needed. _____ I – Morphine PCA initiated at 1615. Instructed on its use. 1st dose (1 mg) administered as demonstration. _____
	1715	E – Still moaning & grimacing even after 2nd dose given as additional demo. Still has not initiated additional PCA dose.———— Ron Allen, RN _____
	1730	R – Still no pain relief; still has not used PCA independently. Discussed w/ Dr. Jadu. Continuous infusion begun at 2 mg/hr. Will supplement up to 4 mg/hr prn. _____ Ron Allen, RN _____

Disadvantages This type of documentation can be inefficient and ineffective.

- You may find the same interventions and responses repeated in more than one section for patients with overlapping problems.

- You may also find that nurses write a complete narrative rather than a single problem entry because the SOAP format does not clearly document changes over time (Podder et al., 2020)

Some believe that rearranging the order to APSO is more beneficial because it provides essential information at the beginning of the note, streamlines communication, and maintains the relevant relations between the S/O and A/P relationships (Podder et al., 2020).

Focus Charting

The term *focus* is used to encourage you to view the client's status from a positive rather than a problem-oriented perspective. **Focus Charting** uses assessment data to evaluate client care concerns, problems, or strengths. It also identifies necessary revisions to the care plan as you record each entry. The focus is often:

- **A nursing diagnosis** (e.g., Breathing Pattern Impairment)
- **A sign or symptom** (e.g., shortness of breath)
- **Client behavior** (e.g., inability to follow inhaler instructions)
- **A special need** (e.g., non–English-speaking)
- **An acute change in condition** (e.g., sudden appearance of chest pain)
- **A significant event** (e.g., surgery).

Focus Charting works well in acute care settings, in areas with the same care, and where procedures are repeated frequently.

In Focus Charting, the first column contains the time and date, the second column identifies the focus or problem addressed in the note, and the third column contains charting in a DAR format. DAR is an acronym for *data, action,* and *response.*

- **Data.** Subjective and objective data (e.g., laboratory and diagnostic test results) that support the focus. This section reflects the assessment phase of the nursing process.
- **Action.** Describe interventions performed, such as medication administration or nurse–provider communications. This section reflects the planning and implementation phases of the nursing process.
- **Response.** The client's response to your interventions. This section reflects the evaluation phase of the nursing process.

Advantages Focus Charting is attractive because it addresses the client's concerns holistically.

Disadvantages The absence of a common problem list may lead to inconsistent labeling of the focus of notes, thus causing difficulty in tracking client progress. The following is an example of a Focus note.

00/00/0000 1700	Focus: developmental delay	**D:** 16 y.o. rec'd on unit at 1600 from PACU; postappendectomy. Has Down syndrome. Morphine PCA initiated. Pt unable to use PCA to control pain. Continuous infusion at 2 mg/hr begun at 1730. PERRLA. Alert, drifting in & out of sleep. PACU RN reports pt functions at elementary school–age level. **A:** Will discuss pt status w/ parents and adjust plan of care accordingly. ———— —— *Ron Allen, RN*
1730		**R:** Met w/ parents, who report that pt has significant developmental delays and needs supervision w/ all ADLs. Pt comfortable on 2 mg/hr infusion of Morphine. Use of PCA for supplementary pain control reviewed with parents. Parents demonstrated understanding. Stated they will assist pt w/ PCA when meds are needed. ———— —— *Ron Allen, RN*

DATE/TIME	00/00/0000 0900	00/00/0000 1330
Neurological Alert and oriented to time, place, and person. PERRLA. Symmetry of strength in extremities. No difficulty with coordination. Behavior appropriate to situation. Sensation intact without numbness or paresthesia.	√	√
Orient client		
Refer to neurological flowsheet		
Pain No report of pain. If present, include pain scale intensity choice by patient (0–10) with location, description, duration, radiation, precipitating and alleviating factors.	Abdominal incision pain – score 10	√
Location	RLQ	
Description	Dull, constant	
Relief measures	Percocet 1 tablet PO (by mouth)	
Pain relief: Y = yes / N = no	Y	
Cardiovascular Apical pulse 60 to 100. S_1 and S_2 present. Regular rhythm. Peripheral pulses (radial, pedal) present bilaterally. No edema or calf tenderness. Extremities pink, warm, moveable within patient's ROM.		
IV Solution and Rate	Lactated Ringer's at 125 mL/hr	Lactated Ringer's at 125 mL/hr

FACT System

Noted for its individual elements, the **FACT documentation model** incorporates many charting-by-exception (CBE) principles and disadvantages. It includes four key elements:

Flowsheets individualized to specific services
Assessment features standardized with baseline parameters
Concise, integrated progress notes and flowsheets documenting the client's condition and responses
Timely entries documented when care is given

FACT documentation includes only exceptions to the norm or significant information about the client. It eliminates the need to document normal findings. The disadvantages of the FACT system are the same as for CBE. The following is a FACT example for Steven Stellanski (Meet Your Patient).

Electronic Entry

The Health Information Technology for Economic and Clinical Health (HITECH) Act has been instrumental in the movement to electronic health records. Electronic clinical information systems streamline documentation processes, make them more accurate and efficient, and reduce the risk of human error. This frees you to do the expert work that only nurses can do. Electronic documentation requires changes in how you document your work.

- EHRs change documentation formats from paper to electronic.
- Documentation occurs at the bedside, instead of at the nurse's station.
- Decision-making processes change from gradual to immediate.

As a nurse, you will almost certainly need to have computer skills (Fig. 17-4). You will play a crucial role in the development and evaluation of EHR systems that are effective and efficient for nurses. You may even participate directly in the design–implementation–redesign cycle of the EHR system in your organization.

Electronic documentation forms and flowsheets (such as Fig. 17-2) include the information that your organization has decided is important to document. Reminders to document specific kinds of information (e.g., late medications; overdue nursing interventions) display automatically to help ensure your documentation is accurate. The extensive use of clearly named data-entry fields, drop-down menus, check boxes, and specially created templates allows you to enter your nursing documentation quickly and efficiently, usually with minimal keyboard typing.

Depending on the EHR system used and the associated documentation form, progress notes may be entered electronically in prebuilt note formats. In some electronic systems, you may still need to write progress notes on lined paper, in narrative, SOAP, PIE, Focus, or FACT formats. Using electronic documentation systems can be challenging, and it may take a few days to know where to correctly document your nursing care and feel confident that you have not overlooked anything. EHR software is user-friendly. Many organizations have printed information, classes, and Web-based tutorials that provide information about electronic documentation. Take advantage of opportunities to build your knowledge when they arise.

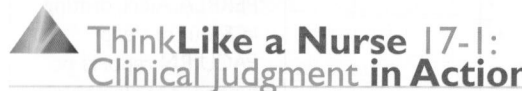
KnowledgeCheck 17-2

- Summarize the characteristics of each of the different kinds of nursing documentation formats (narrative, PIE, SOAP, Focus, CBE and FACT, and electronic entry).

ThinkLike a Nurse 17-1: Clinical Judgment in Action

Compare the documentation examples (narrative, PIE, SOAP, Focus, CBE and FACT, and electronic documentation). If you have had experience with documenting in the clinical setting, apply this experience as well. With which documentation format do you feel most comfortable? Why?

What Forms Do Nurses Use to Document Nursing Care?

Documentation forms vary by purpose, institution, and unit. However, regardless of the system or forms used, nursing documentation reflects a systematic problem-solving approach, such as the nursing process that incorporates critical thinking and clinical reasoning. **Key Point: *You document assessments/recognizing cues, diagnoses/analyzing cues, planning/prioritizing hypothesis and generating solutions, implementation/taking action (what you actually did), and evaluation of client responses.*** This section discusses the forms that are commonly used in addition to the nursing progress notes discussed in the preceding sections.

Nursing Admission Data Forms

You will use admission forms in all settings—for example, in ambulatory clinics, long-term care facilities, and hospitals. The nursing admission form may be separate or a combined interdisciplinary form that is completed at the time the client enters the healthcare system. Accurate and timely completion of this form is essential because baseline assessment data:

- **Establishes a benchmark** to monitor changes in the client's status.
- **Provides information** about the client's support system and helps forecast future needs.
- **Contains critical information** (e.g., presenting illness or reason for admission, vital signs, allergy information, current medications, ADL status, physical assessment data, and discharge planning information). The form completed by Stanley Williams (in Volume 2) at his first clinic visit is an example of an ambulatory care admission form. To see Mr. Williams' completed form,

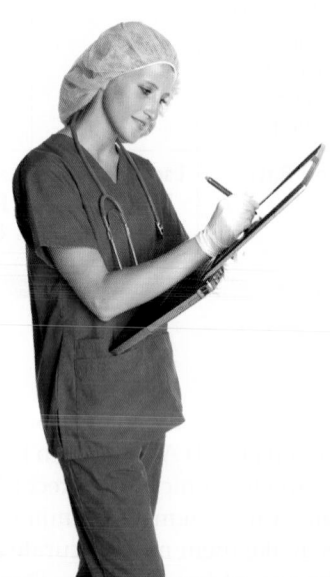
FIGURE 17-4 Many healthcare institutions are adopting computerized patient records.

 Go to **Meet the Williams Family** at the beginning of Volume 2.

For an example of an electronic admission form,

 Go to **Documentation Forms, Adult Admission History Electronic Screen**, in Volume 2.

Discharge Summary

Discharge data are obtained with the admission assessment but are often recorded on a separate form. **Key Point:** *A general principle in nursing is that discharge planning begins on admission. Therefore, discharge needs should be evaluated when the patient first enters a healthcare facility, especially in acute care facilities.* Ask yourself what this patient would need if they were to go home in the next few days. For example, would they need help with food preparation? With their medicines? With their hygiene?

A **discharge summary** can be started any time after admission and revised throughout the hospitalization in the electronic medical record. In contrast, it is the last entry made in the paper record. A summary is completed when the patient is transferred within the same organization or to another facility or discharged to home. The discharge summary may be an interprofessional document, or each discipline may write a separate summary. The forms are different in each organization, but they contain similar data. For an example of an electronic discharge planning form,

 Go to **Chapter 7, Forms, Discharge Assessment/ Instructions**, in Volume 2. Also refer to **Chapter 7, Procedure 7-4: Discharging a Patient from the Healthcare Facility**, in Volume 2.

Also see Chapter 8 for more information about discharge planning.

As you can see in Figure 17-5, there is a drop-down menu to locate the Nursing Discharge Note. It is important to clearly document the patient's condition on discharge because the discharge summary serves as baseline data for the healthcare professionals who will provide follow-up care.

Flowsheets and Graphic Records

Flowsheets and graphic records are used to do the following:

- **Document assessments and care that are performed frequently, on a recurring schedule, or as a part of unit routines** (e.g., I&O, weight, hygiene measures, ADLs, and medications).
- **Perform and document care activities.** How often you do so depends on your client's condition and the unit policy. In the first hour after surgery, for example, you would probably document vital signs every 15 minutes, then every 30 minutes for 1 hour, and then every 4 hours.
- **Allow you to see patterns of change in client status.** For instance, you may view a steady increase in the line representing a client's blood pressure compared with their pain score on an electronically generated graph. On a paper form, you may scan across a row to see that your client has not had a bowel movement for several days.

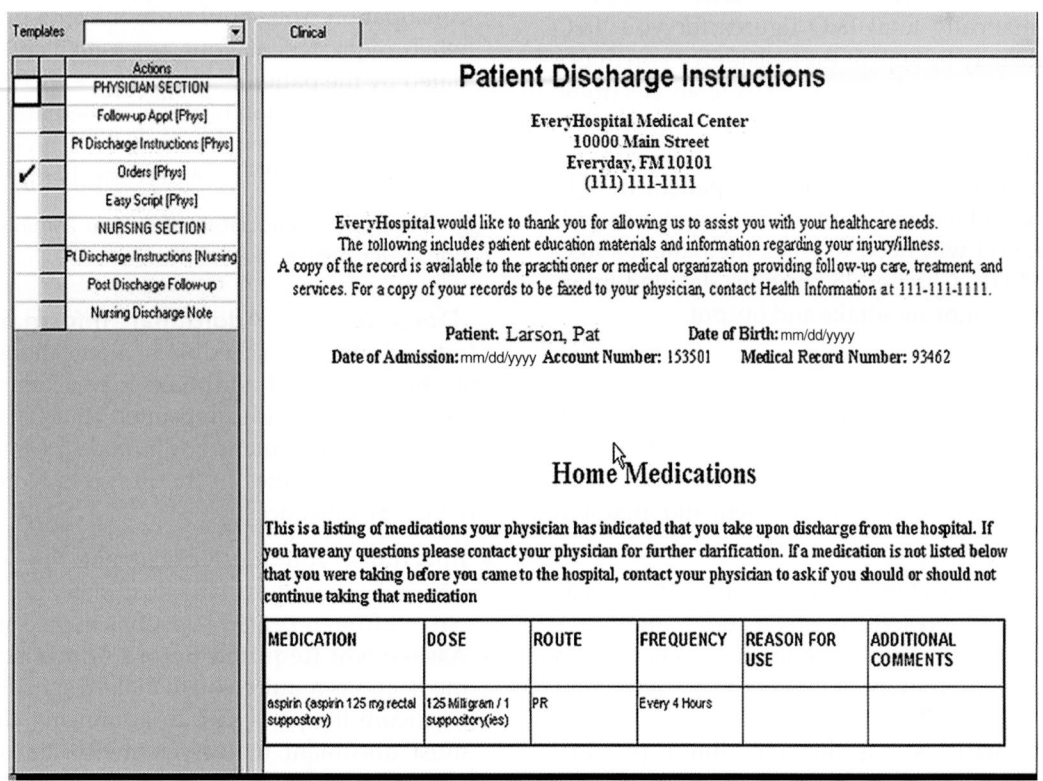

FIGURE 17-5 A portion of an electronic discharge planning form.

For an example of a paper graphic flowsheet, see Figure 3-1. For an electronic flowsheet for I&O, see Figure 17-2.

Checklists

Assessments and care may also be documented on paper and electronic checklists. Common normal and abnormal findings are usually organized according to body systems. Figure 17-6 is an example of a paper checklist.

- **Using a paper form,** the nurse checks the box that reflects the current assessment findings. Some checklists include nursing actions, such as wound care, treatments, or IV fluid administration. Essentially these forms are used to promote comprehensive documentation. Client care activities, responses, and exceptions (deviations) are documented in the narrative note section of the paper form.
- **Using an electronic field-based checklist,** the nurse enters values or text in the appropriate fields and saves the documentation. Electronic flowsheets contain information similar to paper checklists, but they also include a greater range of potential documentation areas that can be opened as needed (e.g., treatments, IV fluid administration, and other parameters).

Intake and Output Records

You will enter data about the patient's fluid balance on a separate I&O form or flowsheet. Electronic systems have flowsheet sections or I&O forms to enter I&O and save it into the patient's EHR (see Fig. 17-2). I&O is totaled by shift and by 24-hour periods. Paper forms must be totaled manually, whereas electronic systems usually automatically total I&O figures for you. I&O paper graphics may be kept at the bedside, or you might input the I&O totals at the bedside using an electronic device (e.g., tablet). For a paper record, see Figure 3-1.

If your patient or a family member can assist with measuring the patient's I&O, teach the patient how to track their own intake and output on the paper record. Nevertheless, you will need to enter the patient's I&O data into the EHR. Chapter 25 provides detailed information about monitoring intake and output.

Medication Administration Records

Medication administration records (MARs) contain information about the medications prescribed for the client. The information and format vary by setting, with significant differences between outpatient and inpatient facilities.

- **Inpatient facilities.** Inpatient medication records contain a list of prescribed medications and track their administration and usage for the agency. For a comparison of the content of inpatient and outpatient MARs, see Table 17-2.
- **Outpatient facilities** (e.g., include clinics, primary care offices, and treatment facilities). Because patients do not stay at the facility, usually the MAR primarily contains information about how the patient is to use the medications prescribed. Patients retain responsibility for administering their own medications, either independently or with the help of family or caregivers.

Some electronic MARs allow providers to look up detailed information about the medication, including indications, contraindications, expected and adverse effects, and safe dosage ranges based on routes of administration. Figure 17-7 shows a portion of an electronic medication record. See Figure 23-7 for a paper MAR.

Terminology for Medication Administration Times You will document medications according to the times they are given: scheduled, unscheduled, continuous, prn, STAT, and so on.

- **Scheduled medications** are medications that are to be given on a regularly scheduled basis.
- **Unscheduled medications** are medications that are given on call at the appropriate time. An example of an unscheduled medication is a preoperative medication to be administered immediately before the patient goes to the surgical holding area.
- **Continuous infusions** are IV fluids that are running consistently unless stopped to administer an incompatible medication or a blood transfusion.
- The letters **prn** mean "as needed." Medications administered prn are given only when the patient meets certain conditions that were established in the medication prescription. Typically, medications are prescribed prn for relief of pain, fever, nausea, and constipation. You should administer a prn medication when requested or your assessment of need is validated by the patient.
- A **STAT** medication is given immediately, only once.
- A **single-prescribed** medication is given once at the designated time, but not necessarily immediately.

✛ Document immediately after you administer the medication, never before.

Documenting Additional Information About Medications For scheduled medications, you may only have to initial and make a checkmark in the column with times with preprinted times at the top. You will need to document additional information on the MAR and sometimes in the Progress Notes in the following circumstances:

- **Injections.** You must document the type and the site of the injection. This documentation protects the patient from repeated injections in the same location.
- **Assessment Required Before Administration.** Some medications require you to make a specific assessment to ensure that it is safe to administer the drug. You must document that assessment data on the MAR, along with the time of administration and other

DATE ____ / ____ / ____

PHYSICAL ASSESSMENT - SHIFT _____

NEURO

LOC	ORIENTATION	SPEECH
❑ ALERT	❑ X3 ❑ FOR AGE	❑ APPROPRIATE
❑ SEDATED	❑ PERSON	❑ APHASIA
❑ LETHARGIC	❑ PLACE	❑ SLURRED
❑ UNRESPONSIVE	❑ TIME	❑ RAMBLING

SENSATION	FONTANELS	
❑ INTACT	❑ FLAT	❑ NA
❑ NUMBNESS	❑ SUNKEN	
❑ TINGLING	❑ BULGING	

CARDIOVASCULAR

RHYTHM	PULSE	EDEMA	CAP. REFILL
❑ REGULAR	❑ STRONG	❑ ABSENT	❑ < 3 SEC.
❑ IRREGULAR	❑ WEAK	❑ _____	❑ > 3 SEC.
❑ MURMUR	❑		

MONITOR RHYTHM

RESPIRATORY

EFFORT		BREATH	
		LU LL SOUNDS RU RL	
❑ NORMAL	❑ DYSPNEA	❑ ❑ CLEAR ❑ ❑	
❑ LABORED	❑ COUGH	❑ ❑ CRACKLES ❑ ❑	
❑ NASAL FLARING	❑ SPUTUM	❑ ❑ RHONCHI ❑ ❑	
❑ RETRACTIONS	❑ CRYING	❑ ❑ WHEEZING ❑ ❑	
❑ IRREGULAR		❑ ❑ DIMINISHED ❑ ❑	
		❑ ❑ ABSENT ❑ ❑	

GASTROINTESTINAL

ABDOMEN		
❑ FLAT	❑ FIRM	❑ NAUSEA
❑ ROUNDED	❑ TENDER	❑ VOMITING
❑ DISTENDED	❑ NON-TENDER	
❑ SOFT		
❑ GIRTH_____ CM		

BOWEL SOUNDS	STOOL	
❑ ACTIVE	❑ REGULAR	LAST BM
❑ ABSENT	❑ CONSTIPATED	
❑ HYPER	❑ DIARRHEA	_____
❑ HYPO	❑ INCONTINENT	

SUCTION
❑ INTERMITTANT   ❑ CONSTANT   ❑ CLAMPED
❑ FEEDING TUBE   ❑ PATENT
❑ NG   ❑ PLACEMENT ✔
DRNG COLOR:

GU

URINE	❑ CATHETER
❑ CLEAR, YELLOW / AMBER ❑ QS	❑ PAIN
❑ OTHER _____	❑ FREQUENT
	❑ RETENTION ❑ INCONTINENT

MUSCULOSKELETAL

MOBILITY	MUSCLE TONE	ROM
❑ NORMAL	❑ GOOD	❑ FULL
❑ ASSIST X _____	❑ OTHER	❑ LIMITED
❑ AMBULATORY		
❑ BED REST		
❑ OTHER	❑ P.T. CONSULT	

SKIN

CONDITION	TURGOR	MUCOUS MEM
❑ WARM, DRY INTACT	❑ ADEQUATE	❑ MOIST
❑ BREAKDOWN	❑ DECREASED	❑ DRY

COLOR ❑ NORMAL
❑ PALE ❑ CYANOTIC ❑ FLUSHED ❑ _____

WOUND/INCISION/DRESSING

LOCATION/CONDITION/DRAINAGE	HEALING NO S/S INFECTION
_____	❑
_____	❑
_____	❑

TUBES/DRAINS

LOCATION/CONDITION/DRAINAGE	GRAVITY	SUCTION
_____	❑	❑
_____	❑	❑
_____	❑	❑

IV'S

IV SITE / CONDITION	PATENT, NO REDNESS OR SWELLING	PUMP
_____	❑	❑
_____	❑	❑
_____	❑	❑

NURSING ASSESSMENT   PATIENT NAME

PAIN
❑ ABSENT   PAIN SCALE _____
❑ PRESENT   LOCATION _____
❑ CONTROLLED

PSYCHOSOCIAL

EYE CONTACT ❑ YES ❑ NO
❑ APPROPRIATE   ❑ RESTLESS   ❑ COMBATIVE
❑ FLAT AFFECT   ❑ AGITATED   ❑ BELLIGERENT
❑ UNCOOPERATIVE ❑ CRYING   ❑ ODOR
❑ ANXIOUS   ❑ SUBSTANCE USE

DISCHARGE

DISCHARGE PLAN
❑ NA   ❑ ONGOING   ❑ COMPLETED
❑ D.P. CONSULT   ❑ O.T CONSULT   ❑ H.H. CONSULT

EQUIPMENT

❑ BED ALARM	❑ CARDIAC MONITOR
❑ CPM	❑ FEEDING PUMP
❑ IV PUMP X_____	❑ K - PAD
❑ OXIMETER	❑ PCA PUMP
❑ PASSPORT	❑ POLAR ICE
❑ SUCTION	❑ TELEMETRY
❑ _____	❑ _____
❑ _____	❑ _____

SIGN

SIGNATURE X_____ TIME_____
REASSESSED BY X_____ TIME_____

OBSERVATION / INTERVENTION / EVALUATION
(TIME & INITIAL ENTRIES)

PHYSICAL ASSESSMENT - SHIFT _____

NEURO

LOC	ORIENTATION	SPEECH
❑ ALERT	❑ X3 ❑ FOR AGE	❑ APPROPRIATE
❑ SEDATED	❑ PERSON	❑ APHASIA
❑ LETHARGIC	❑ PLACE	❑ SLURRED
❑ UNRESPONSIVE	❑ TIME	❑ RAMBLING

SENSATION	FONTANELS	
❑ INTACT	❑ FLAT	❑ NA
❑ NUMBNESS	❑ SUNKEN	
❑ TINGLING	❑ BULGING	

CARDIOVASCULAR

RHYTHM	PULSE	EDEMA	CAP. REFILL
❑ REGULAR	❑ STRONG	❑ ABSENT	❑ < 3 SEC.
❑ IRREGULAR	❑ WEAK	❑ _____	❑ > 3 SEC.
❑ MURMUR	❑		

MONITOR RHYTHM

RESPIRATORY

EFFORT		BREATH	
		LU LL SOUNDS RU RL	
❑ NORMAL	❑ DYSPNEA	❑ ❑ CLEAR ❑ ❑	
❑ LABORED	❑ COUGH	❑ ❑ CRACKLES ❑ ❑	
❑ NASAL FLARING	❑ SPUTUM	❑ ❑ RHONCHI ❑ ❑	
❑ RETRACTIONS	❑ CRYING	❑ ❑ WHEEZING ❑ ❑	
❑ IRREGULAR		❑ ❑ DIMINISHED ❑ ❑	
		❑ ❑ ABSENT ❑ ❑	

GASTROINTESTINAL

ABDOMEN		
❑ FLAT	❑ FIRM	❑ NAUSEA
❑ ROUNDED	❑ TENDER	❑ VOMITING
❑ DISTENDED	❑ NON-TENDER	
❑ SOFT		
❑ GIRTH_____ CM		

BOWEL SOUNDS	STOOL	
❑ ACTIVE	❑ REGULAR	LAST BM
❑ ABSENT	❑ CONSTIPATED	
❑ HYPER	❑ DIARRHEA	
❑ HYPO	❑ INCONTINENT	

SUCTION
❑ INTERMITTANT   ❑ CONSTANT   ❑ CLAMPED
❑ FEEDING TUBE   ❑ PATENT
❑ NG   ❑ PLACEMENT
DRNG COLOR:

GU

URINE	❑ CATHETER
❑ CLEAR, YELLOW / AMBER ❑ QS	❑ PAIN
❑ OTHER _____	❑ FREQUENT
	❑ RETENTION ❑ INCONTINENT

MUSCULOSKELETAL

MOBILITY	MUSCLE TONE	ROM
❑ NORMAL	❑ GOOD	❑ FULL
❑ ASSIST X _____	❑ OTHER	❑ LIMITED
❑ AMBULATORY		
❑ BED REST		
❑ OTHER	❑ P.T. CONSULT	

SKIN

CONDITION	TURGOR	MUCOUS MEM
❑ WARM, DRY INTACT	❑ ADEQUATE	❑ MOIST
❑ BREAKDOWN	❑ DECREASED	❑ DRY

COLOR ❑ NORMAL
❑ PALE ❑ CYANOTIC ❑ FLUSHED ❑ _____

WOUND/INCISION/DRESSING

LOCATION/CONDITION/DRAINAGE	HEALING NO S/S INFECTION
_____	❑
_____	❑
_____	❑

TUBES/DRAINS

LOCATION/CONDITION/DRAINAGE	GRAVITY	SUCTION
_____	❑	❑
_____	❑	❑
_____	❑	❑

IV'S

IV SITE / CONDITION	PATENT, NO REDNESS OR SWELLING	PUMP
_____	❑	❑
_____	❑	❑
_____	❑	❑

FIGURE 17-6 A portion of a nursing assessment checklist.

Table 17-2 ➤ Comparison of Content of MARs for Inpatient and Outpatient Facilities

INPATIENT MARS	OUTPATIENT MARS
▪ Drug name	▪ Drug name
▪ Dosage	▪ Dosage
▪ Route of administration	▪ Route of administration
▪ Frequency	▪ Number of pills, patches, and so on to be dispensed at each prescription refill
▪ Duration	▪ Number of refills prescribed
▪ Scheduled times of administration	▪ Directions for using the medication, including frequency and duration
▪ Documentation of medication administration	▪ Historical information about prescriptions, pharmacies used, and refills authorized
▪ Signatures (written or electronic) of nurses administering medication	

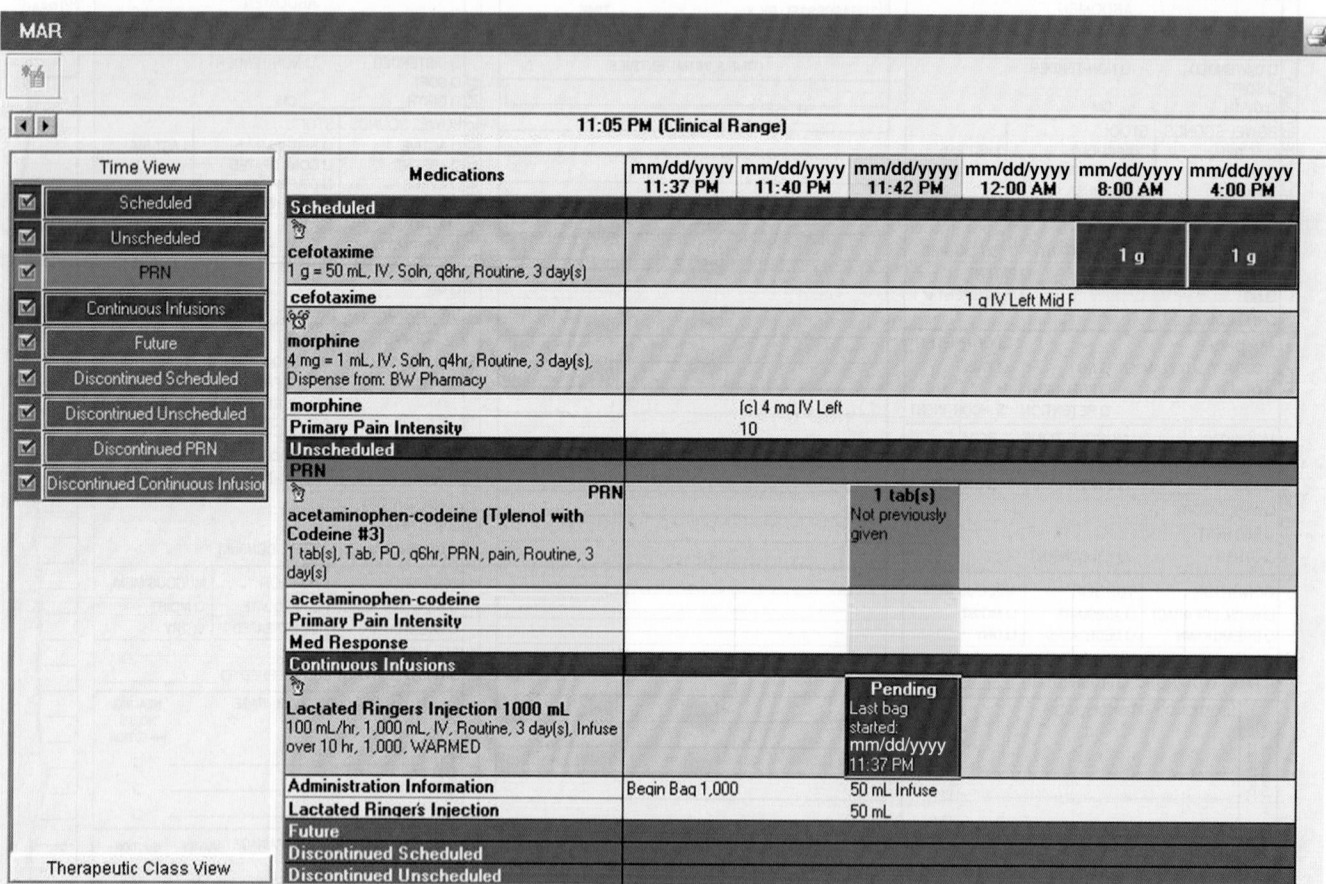

FIGURE 17-7 A portion of an electronic medication administration record.

required information (see Chapter 23). For example, you should not administer digoxin (a cardiac medication) if the apical heart rate is below 60 beats/min, so you must auscultate the rate before giving the drug. Blood pressure, insulin, and anticoagulant medications also require assessments before administration.

▪ 🕂 **Drug Allergies.** Drug allergies are always noted on the MAR. This makes them easily visible for caregivers who are prescribing or administering medication. If the patient has an allergic

reaction to a medicine, you must report this to the provider and document the response on the MAR and in the nurses' notes.

▪ **STAT, prn, Unscheduled, and Single-Order Medications.** Enter on the MAR the time the medication is given. Make a narrative note of your assessment findings and the patient's response to the medication in the appropriate location on the MAR. In an EHR, some documented data, such as the pain score before administration of an analgesic, may automatically migrate from other documentation sources to become visible on the MAR.

- **Dosage range prescriptions.** You may occasionally see a prn prescription that provides a range of medication to be given based on your assessment of the patient. For example, "Titrate morphine 2–3 mg IV every 1–2 hours to achieve pain control."
  ✚ In the electronic MAR system, medication range prescriptions (e.g., 1 to 2 mg) are difficult to prescribe, so The Joint Commission and most agency protocols no longer allow dosage range prescriptions.

- **Patient Refusal.** If the patient refuses a medication, note the refusal on the MAR. Your organization's policy will determine how this is documented. On paper, you might draw a circle around the scheduled time of administration. When documenting electronically, you can click on an option offered in the MAR, such as Not Given, and then select *Patient Refused* from a drop-down field listing multiple reasons why a medication was not administered.

- **Omitted Medication or Delayed Administration.** It may be necessary to withhold a medication or delay its administration if the patient is not available or is experiencing health changes that require immediate interventions. On the paper MAR, you may find a boxed section at the bottom with a code to indicate why the medication was withheld or given at a different time. Circle the scheduled time and fill in the symbol. You will also have to document the omission or delay in your nurses'

notes. However, in the electronic MAR, it is often possible to reschedule administration times for a single dose or permanently going forward. Many systems will require you to enter the reason and the action taken.

Patient Care Summary

Electronic patient care summaries typically pull patient data from multiple areas of the health record (medical and nursing diagnoses, prescriptions, treatments, results). Figure 17-8 is an example of an electronic patient care summary screen.

In an electronic summary, each patient has a separate screen. All authorized members of the care team can access the electronic care summary at the same time, even if they are away from the patient or outside the organization in a remote location, depending on the institution's permission for access. The electronic care summary is usually not a permanent part of the patient's health record.

Integrated Plan of Care

Integrated plans of care (IPOCs) are a combined documentation and care plan form. An IPOC maps out, day by day, patient goals, outcomes, interventions, and treatments for a specific diagnosis or condition from admission to discharge. Major aspects of the treatment plan (e.g., laboratory and diagnostic testing, medications, standardized interventions, therapies) are included in the pathway. IPOCs help administrators predict length

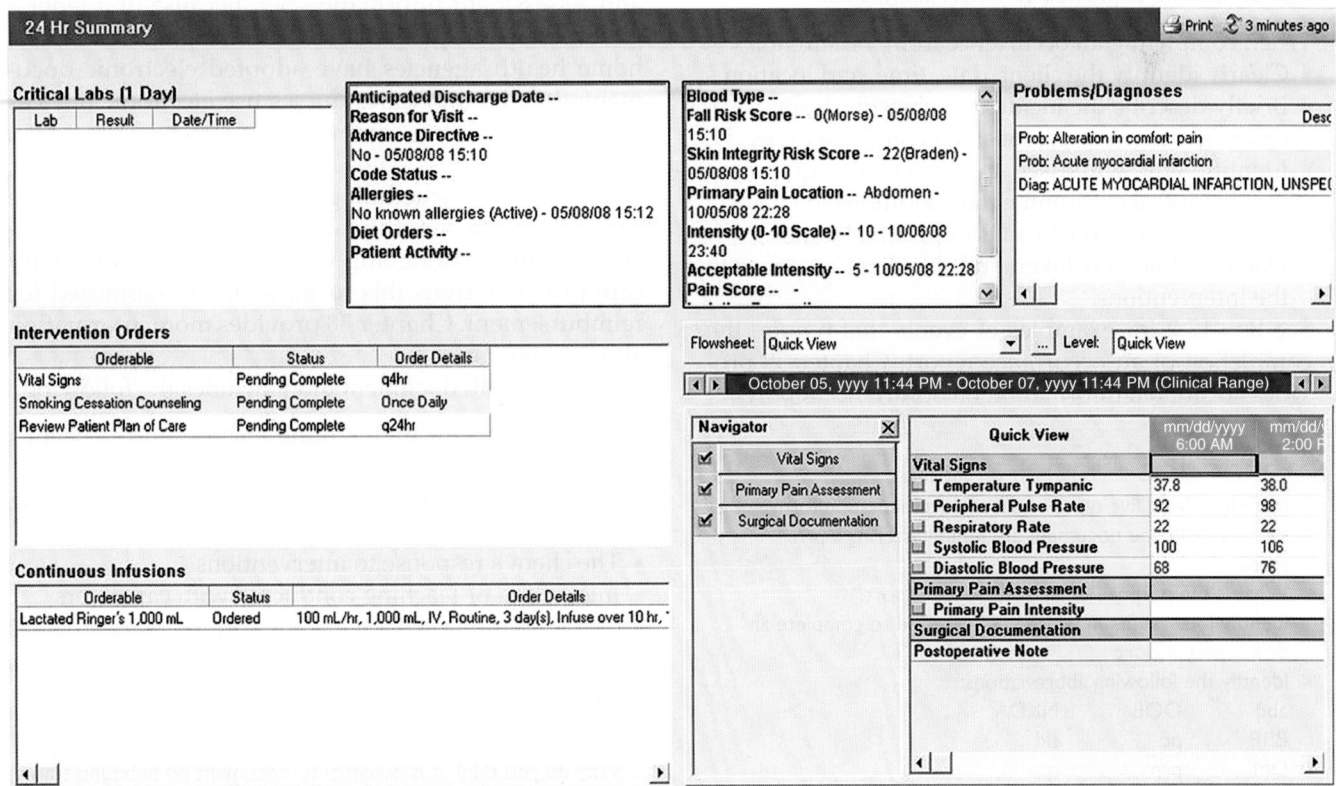

FIGURE 17-8 A portion of an electronic patient care summary screen.

of stay and monitor costs of care and can assist with staffing. They also eliminate duplicate documentation, increase team effort, and enhance the nurse's teaching about what the patient can expect during the hospital stay. Figure 17-3 is an example of an electronic IPOC.

Multiple patient diagnoses can be captured easily in an electronic IPOC. However, in special situations, you may need to individualize the paper IPOC by commenting on special issues in the space provided for narrative comments (e.g., developmental delay with our patient Steven Stellanski).

Occurrence Reports

An **occurrence report,** or *incident report,* is a formal record of an unusual occurrence or accident. It is an organizational report used to analyze the event, identify areas for quality improvement, and formulate strategies to prevent future occurrences.

- The overall goal is to create safer processes and procedures for clients and staff.
- **Key Point:** *An occurrence report is not part of the client's health record and thus should never be referenced in the nurses' notes or in other sections of the health record.*
- The paper report is sent to risk management, according to agency protocol, whereas the electronic form is completed on the organization's secure internal network.
- ✚ You should report all errors, even if there was no adverse impact on the patient. This is important from a safety standpoint for improving your institution's quality of care and from a legal perspective to provide defensible information.
- When completing an occurrence form, be sure to:
  - Clearly identify the client, date, time, and location.
  - Briefly describe the incident in objective terms.
  - Quote the client or persons involved if possible.
  - Identify any witnesses to the event, equipment involved, and environmental conditions.
  - Avoid drawing conclusions or placing blame.
  - Document actions taken and the client response to the interventions.
- See Box 17-2 for examples of events that require the completion of an occurrence report. Chapter 39 provides additional information on occurrence reports.

KnowledgeCheck 17-3

- Identify at least five types of paper documentation forms.
- What should you document after administering a prn medication?
- What is the purpose of an occurrence report?
- Identify four events in which you will need to complete an occurrence report.
- Identify the following abbreviations:

abd	OOB	NKDA
BRP	pc	tid
DM	prn	q
fx	STI	LUQ

BOX 17-2 ■ Events Requiring an Occurrence Report

- Patient fall or other injury
- Medication error
- Incorrect implementation of a prescribed treatment
- Needlestick injury or other injury to staff
- Loss of patient belongings
- Injury of a visitor
- Unsafe staffing situation
- Lack of availability of essential patient care supplies
- Inadequate response to emergency situation

What Is Unique About Documentation in Home Healthcare?

Although you will perform many of the same assessments and interventions in home care that you do in other areas of healthcare, the documentation is unique. The Centers for Medicare & Medicaid Services (CMS) guidelines govern home healthcare documentation. Among the requirements for care are the following:

- Certification of homebound status
- A plan of care
- Ongoing assessment of the need for skilled care

The most commonly used paper home health documentation form is known as OASIS—the Outcome and Assessment Information Set. Because of a federal government emphasis on electronic health records, home health agencies have adopted electronic documentation. Home health nurses use electronic devices (e.g., tablets, laptop computers) to retrieve client data, document progress notes in the home, order supplies, and coordinate scheduling of follow-up visits. Home care requires a monthly summary describing the client's status and ongoing needs. The client's primary care provider signs this form, which is submitted for reimbursement. Chapter 38 provides more information about home care.

Home health documentation includes the following:

- Your assessment highlighting changes in the client's condition
- Interventions performed (e.g., wound care, dressing changes, teaching)
- The client's response to interventions
- Interaction or teaching conducted with caregivers
- Communications with the client's primary care provider

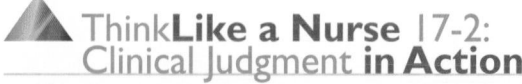

ThinkLike a Nurse 17-2: Clinical Judgment in Action

Why do you think it is essential to document homebound status and the ongoing need for skilled care?

What Is Unique About Documentation in Long-Term Care?

Documentation requirements for long-term care depend on the level of care the client requires.

- All clients in long-term care facilities must have a comprehensive assessment at admission.
- Federal law further requires that a resident be evaluated using the Minimum Data Set (MDS) for Resident Assessment and Care Screening within 14 days of admission.
- The MDS must be updated at specified intervals and with any significant change in client condition.

For an example of an MDS Basic Tracking form,

Go to the **CMS** Web site at http://www.cms.gov/, and do a search for Minimum Data Set (MDS).

 Legal requirements to protect older adults mandate that you report changes in a client's condition to the primary care provider as well as the client's family. You must document your communications on the appropriate forms. If you are caring for a client receiving Medicare-reimbursed services (e.g., IV therapy, wound care, or rehabilitation services), documentation is required with each shift. In addition, a nurse must record a weekly summary that includes the following:

- A summary of the client's condition
- An evaluation of the client's ability to perform ADLs
- The client's level of consciousness and mood
- Hydration and nutrition status
- Response to medications
- Any treatments provided
- Safety measures (e.g., bed rails, bed alarm, wander guard)

Long-term care facilities also provide intermediate-care services for clients who need assistance with medications, nutrition, and ADLs. These clients require a nursing care summary every 2 weeks.

KnowledgeCheck 17-4

How do home care and long-term care documentation differ from hospital-based documentation?

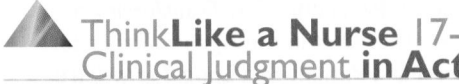 ThinkLike a Nurse 17-3: Clinical Judgment in Action

Why do long-term care clients require less frequent documentation than clients in acute care settings?

ORAL REPORTING

The purpose of giving an oral report is to maintain continuity of care, engage in professional communications, build team relationships, and collaborate to improve client care. The quality of the report you give and receive influences how you and others plan the shift work. Restrict your oral reports to client-focused discussion and limit unimportant details and social conversation. The patient care summary provides a foundation for the oral report.

How Do I Give a Handoff Report?

The purpose of a **handoff report** (sometimes called a *change-of-shift report* or *handover report*) is to promote continuity in care. The nurse is alerted to the client's status, recent status changes, planned activities, diagnostic tests, or concerns that require follow-up. A handoff report may be given at the bedside or in a conference room, using paper notes or an EHR device.

As a student nurse, you will receive reports either from the offgoing nurse or from the oncoming shift nurse assigned to the client. Report any changes to the nurse assigned to the client during your shift, and always give a report before leaving the unit.

- **A bedside report,** sometimes known as "walking rounds," allows you to observe important aspects of care, such as appearance, IV pumps, and wounds. With a bedside report, the outgoing nurse can introduce you to the patient. If the patient is alert, give them the opportunity to participate in the report and ask questions. Although this type of report is time consuming, it encourages continuity of care, team collaboration, and client/family communications. **Key Point:** *Ensure that the patient's privacy rights are protected when using bedside reports.*
- **A face-to-face oral report** may involve only the outgoing and oncoming nurse or may include the entire oncoming shift. When given in a conference room, an oral report does not let you directly observe the client, but it is time efficient and still allows interaction between nurses.
- **An audio-recorded report** is a convenient but sometimes time-consuming way to transmit information. The outgoing nurse audio-records a report on their clients. This method does not allow you to ask questions about the client; occasionally the audio quality is poor, and the report is not clear. However, an advantage of this method is that the outgoing nurse continues to provide client care while the incoming nurse receives report. To minimize communication errors, the outgoing and incoming nurses should speak directly to each other to update information or answer any questions about the clients.

Standardized Report Formats

Inadequate communications during handoffs can contribute to adverse client events. One study found that communication failures were the most common attributable causes of sentinel events and a major contributing factor in 70% of adverse events (Guttman et al., 2021). Sentinel events are those events that result in death or severe harm to a patient. **Key Point:** *No matter where or how the handoff report is given, nurses should use a consistent, structured (standardized) process that contains critical key* *items, which has been shown to significantly reduce client care errors (The Joint Commission, 2017).*

- The **IPASS** format is a multifaceted approach that promotes sustained improvements over time. The acronym stands for **I**llness severity, **P**atient summary, **A**ction list, **S**ituation awareness and contingency plans, and **S**ynthesis by receiver (The Joint Commission, 2017).
- The **PACE** format is one example of a standardized approach developed specifically to organize patient data in handoffs. The acronym stands for **P**atient/Problem, **A**ssessment/Actions, **C**ontinuing/Changes, and **E**valuation (Schroeder, 2006).
- The **SBAR** (**S**ituation–**B**ackground–**A**ssessment–**R**ecommendation) is an easy-to-remember, concrete acronym useful for framing any conversation. Because nurses and providers communicate in very different ways, SBAR is useful for interprofessional communication, especially critical situations requiring a clinician's immediate attention and action. SBAR allows for an easy and focused way to set expectations for how and what will be communicated between team members. The SBAR technique can be adapted for handoff reports. The iSBAR acronym can be used when calling a healthcare provider and includes identification of the person answering the phone and identification of the patient.

For additional information about communicating with IPASS, SBAR, and PACE.

 Go to **Chapter 17, Clinical Insight 17-1: Giving Oral Reports**, in Volume 2.

KnowledgeCheck 17-5

- What data should be included in a handoff report?
- What are the types of handoff reports?

What Is a Transfer Report?

Transfer reports are given when a patient is transferred from unit to unit or from facility to facility. If the patient is being transported to another unit in the same facility, you will need to transport their paper medical records unless the receiving unit can electronically access the records. Detailed information about the patient's health history can be communicated between healthcare professionals or transmitted before transfer. You should review your facility's policy about what can be copied or electronically transmitted during client transfers.

 Research shows that older adults are vulnerable to errors in care when transitioning from one healthcare facility to another. Medication errors were dominant, resulting in increased hospital readmissions, injuries, or death. Medication Reconciliation and Medication Review (MBAR) should be completed either electronically or in writing to ensure a safe transition (Beuscart, 2021).

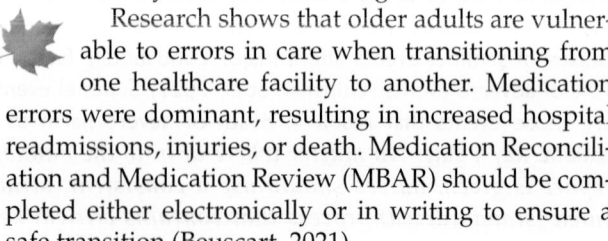

Safe, Effective Nursing Care

Ensuring Safe, Effective Handoff Reports

Chapter Key Concepts: Documentation, Oral reporting

Competencies: Provide Safe, Quality Client Care; Embrace/Incorporate Technological Advances

Thinking: Consider the number of client handoffs per day among nurses and other providers. Factors that contribute to miscommunication and breakdowns in client care during handoff reports include a lack of a standardized protocol or form, a lack of experience, and a lack of dedicated time for reporting.

Caring: A primary role of the nurse is to ensure safe, quality client care. Caring influences the way you think and act and motivates the nurse to be attentive to safety. Because they care, nurses perform interventions to prevent harm to clients (e.g., report critical laboratory values, follow principles of documentation).

Doing: Collaborate with others in your facility to suggest the following strategies for improving quality of care, teamwork, and patient safety:

- Standardize the information (e.g., SBAR) to be conveyed.
- Include "if . . . , then . . ." statements for current problems (e.g., *if* the glucose level is still elevated, *then* call the provider for insulin prescriptions).
- Develop an electronic form or other tool to reinforce and clarify the transfer of knowledge and responsibility.
- Conduct training sessions to lessen the chance of reporting errors.

What strategies can you adopt to promote an effective handoff report?

Sources: Cloete, L. (2015). Reducing medication errors in nursing practice. *Nursing Standard, 29*(20), 50–59; Ernst, K., McComb, S., & Ley, C. (2017). Nurse-to-nurse shift handoffs on medical-surgical units: A process within the flow of nursing care. *Journal of Clinical Nursing, 27*(5–6), e1179–e1201. https://doi.org/10.1111/jocn.14254; The Joint Commission. (2017). Inadequate hand-off communication. *Sentinel Alert Event, 58.* https://www.jointcommission.org/resources/sentinel-event/sentinel-event-alert-newsletters/sentinel-event-alert-58-inadequate-hand-off-communication/

For a review of transfers and discharges,

 Go to **Chapter 7, Procedure 7-2: Transferring a Patient to Another Unit in the Agency, Procedure 7-3: Transferring a Patient to a Long-Term Care Facility, and Procedure 7-4: Discharging a Patient from the Healthcare Facility**, in Volume 2.

How Do I Receive and Document Verbal and Telephone Prescriptions?

Although computerized order entry systems have decreased the use of verbal and telephone orders, licensed nurses may, on occasion, have to accept these types of orders. Because of the increased risk of hearing or writing the prescription incorrectly, nurses must strictly follow The Joint Commission's longstanding guidance that requires the person receiving a prescription (order) or test result to "read back" the information to validate its accuracy before taking any action (The Joint Commission, 2007). SBAR-R is a revised version that adds the read-back component to promote compliance and minimize errors and failures in communication between the nurse and provider.

Telephone Prescriptions

Telephone prescriptions can lead to error because of differences in pronunciation, dialect, or accent; background noise; poor reception; and unfamiliar terminology. Taking a telephone prescription is strongly discouraged, but may be acceptable in the following situations:

- When there has been a sudden change in your client's condition and the provider is not in the hospital or cannot transmit prescriptions electronically.
- In a life-threatening emergency—but you must apply the "document and read-back" safeguard.

Computerized provider order entry, fax machines, and e-mail have reduced the need for telephone prescriptions; however, their use may never disappear entirely. For guidelines to use when taking telephone prescriptions,

 Go to **Chapter 17, Clinical Insight 17-2: Receiving Telephone and Verbal Prescription**, in Volume 2.

Verbal Prescriptions

Verbal prescriptions are spoken directions for patient care given to you in person, usually during an emergency. **Key Point:** *Providers should never use verbal communication as a routine method of giving prescriptions.* For guidelines to promote safety in the receipt of verbal prescriptions,

 Go to **Chapter 17, Clinical Insight 17-2: Receiving Telephone and Verbal Prescriptions**, in Volume 2.

KnowledgeCheck 17-6

- What important factors should you document when receiving a telephone prescription?
- What is the purpose of a verbal prescription? When should it be used?

How Do I Question a Prescription?

If you feel uncertain about a prescription, you must question it. As a student, you will first want to discuss your concerns with your clinical instructor or the patient's nurse. If you have concerns, do not remain quiet—act on them.

- **Follow organization policy** for clarifying prescriptions.
- **If a prescription is written illegibly on paper or is entered into the EHR with certain details or**

components missing, contact the provider directly for clarification. Generally, you should contact the provider who wrote the prescription.

- **If, after contact, the provider leaves the prescription as is and you still don't feel comfortable** with it or believe there is an error, you may refuse to implement it. Also:
  - Inform the chain of command at your organization about your refusal.
  - Usually, you will speak with the charge nurse, who may then contact the nurse manager or nursing supervisor.
  - The nature of the prescription will determine how this situation is handled.
  - If you do refuse to follow a prescription, you must document your refusal and the actions you took to clarify the prescription.

As a new nurse, you may feel uncomfortable about questioning a prescription. Even experienced nurses sometimes feel uneasy with this challenge. If you are uncertain how to proceed, you can discuss your concerns with your colleagues, the charge nurse, or the supervisor before contacting the provider. Your efforts to clarify the prescription help to protect your patient.

Key Point: *If you believe a prescription is inappropriate or unsafe, you are legally and ethically required to question the prescription.*

PracticalKnowledge
knowing **how**

To document care effectively, you need to be familiar with the forms and requirements of your institution. Document routine nursing actions (e.g., skin care) on the designated paper or electronic flowsheets or forms, and record your assessments, interventions, and patient responses to care in the format approved by your organization. It is important to document accurately, completely, and consistently so that the patient's progress can be tracked and appropriate care given.

♥ **iCare** Remember that the client's health record is permanent and that information contained in the record is confidential. As a student, you are granted access to a client's medical record for educational purposes. You have a duty to keep the information private and confidential. The Health Insurance Portability and Accountability Act (HIPAA) regulations govern access, storage, transfer, and discussion of client information. For more information about privacy, confidentiality, and HIPAA, refer to Chapters 5 and 39.

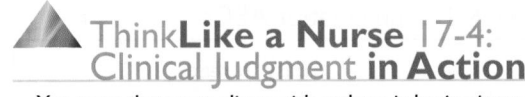 Think**Like a Nurse** 17-4:
Clinical Judgment **in Action**

You note that your client with asthma is having increasing difficulty breathing. You call the provider, who gives you a telephone prescription for an asthma medication and then hangs up. When you enter the verbal prescription electronically, you discover your pharmacy does not carry this nonformulary medication.

- Was this an acceptable reason to take a verbal prescription?
- The provider gets irritated when you call back and says, "I prescribed what I wanted." How would you handle this situation?
- You entered the prescription electronically after the provider hung up. How could this situation have been avoided?

GUIDELINES FOR DOCUMENTING CARE

Key Point: *Your documentation should convey the care that you provided to the patient during your shift.* Thus, if you read your documentation 3 years later, as happens in malpractice lawsuits, it should attest that the care you provided to the patient adhered to minimum standards of nursing practice.

- For a brief set of documentation tips, see Box 17-3.
- For detailed guidelines for documentation,

 Go to **Chapter 17, Clinical Insight 17-3: Guidelines for Documentation** and **Clinical Insight 17-4: Guidelines for Paper Health Records**, in Volume 2.

- For guidelines for documenting using paper health records, see Clinical Insight 17-4.

Guidelines for Electronic Health Records

Well-designed nursing documentation forms and systems help you organize your work, manage your care plans, track client diagnoses and outcomes, and support decision making by healthcare providers.

How Can I Document Efficiently and Effectively?

To ensure your documentation in the EHR is most efficient and effective, keep the following in mind:

- **You must have basic computer and software skills** to document effectively in the EHR.
- **If you are uneasy or more stressed using unfamiliar software or computers,** it may take you longer to make the transition to documenting in the EHR.
- **Help keep client rooms clutter-free** so that you have a place to use a portable computer in the room to document care.

What Is Unique About Entering the Data?

- **Before Documenting.** Before opening the documentation forms, you must ensure that the client's name,

identification number, and any other unique health record identifiers are correct.

- **Saving Documentation.** If your EHR allows you to save partially completed documentation before signing it, plan to complete the documentation and sign it as quickly as possible. In some EHR systems, saved documentation cannot be seen by others until it is signed.
- **Checklists.** Electronic forms and flowsheets are often built in a format similar to a checklist. This can make it more difficult to capture detailed client changes and findings.
- **Errors.** If you make an error (e.g., make entries in the wrong patient record or enter and sign the wrong information), you can correct it. The entry can never be completely deleted; however, the corrected information will be visible to anyone viewing the patient record.

What Happens If the Computer Doesn't Work?

EHR systems can have periodic downtimes due to scheduled maintenance or network or interface problems. Client care does not stop, so you need to know the procedures to follow when the EHR is offline and inaccessible. Follow organization policies regarding the amount of time the EHR needs to be "down" before you begin documenting on paper forms.

How Do I Maintain Confidentiality and Data Security?

Although the specific risks to and safeguards of confidentiality differ in detail between paper and electronic records, confidentiality is equally important in both. The following safeguards are specific to EHRs:

- **Ensure confidentiality and privacy.** Close the screen, lock the computer, or permanently log off the system when moving away from an open EHR. Most computer stations will automatically log off after a specified period of inactivity. This helps keep unauthorized viewers from having access to client information.
- **Use privacy filters.** Some computer screens are equipped with privacy filters to prevent unauthorized viewers from seeing the information.
- **Create a secure password.** Do not use something obvious, such as your birth date, Social Security number, or family members' names. Instead, you might choose a password that is at least eight characters long and includes at least one capital letter (if the system is case sensitive), one number, and (if allowed by the system) one symbol. The system you are using will determine the specifications.
- **Change your password at regular intervals.** Do this even if your organization does not require it. Some systems will lock you out of the system if your password is not changed as required.
- **Do not share your personal username or password with anyone.** You are responsible for the data entered using your electronic identity. If someone else enters data or accesses records under your identity, you may be held responsible if the client initiates legal action.

BOX 17-3 ■ Documentation ABCs	
Accurate	**E**asy to read
Bias-free	**F**actual
Complete	**G**rammatical
Detailed	**H**armless (legally)

- **Do not leave client data displayed on the screen where others can see it.**
- **Do not leave the computer unattended after you have logged on.** This allows others access to confidential data and to document under your name.
- **Do not leave a portable device (e.g., a laptop or PDA) unattended in a public location,** such as on a countertop in the nurses' station. This increases the possibility of theft or unauthorized access to secured client information.
- **Never access client health records that you have no professional reason to view.** This is a severe breach of client privacy rules. Know your state and federal laws and the consequences for privacy violations.
- **Become familiar with your organization's policies** regarding network and client health record information security and confidentiality.

KnowledgeCheck 17-7

Refer to **Clinical Insight 17-3: Guidelines for Documentation** and **Clinical Insight 17-4: Guidelines for**

Paper Health Records, in Volume 2, to help you answer the following questions:

- What aspects of care should be documented?
- When should care be documented?
- How is documentation on paper different from documentation in an EHR or on an electronic digital form?

 ## ThinkLike a Nurse 17-5: Clinical Judgment in Action

You are caring for two patients on a medical-surgical unit. One of your patients is short of breath and complaining of chest pain. Your other client is recovering from abdominal surgery. Currently, the patient is alert, stable, and pain-free. After stabilizing your first patient, you realize you are 45 minutes late in administering a medication to the abdominal surgery patient. You are not sure how to proceed.

- What theoretical knowledge do you need?
- You give the medicine as soon as you can (60 minutes late). How and where should you document the medication administered?
- If you had been aware that you were going to be late with the medication, what could you have done to be sure it was given on time?

Toward Evidence-Based Practice

Davison, K., Queen, R., Lau, F., & Antonio, M. (2021). Culturally competent gender, sex, and sexual orientation information practices and electronic health records: Rapid review. *JMIR Medical Informatics, 9*(2). https://doi.org/10.2196/25467

Nurses have a responsibility to improve diversity, equity, and inclusion efforts in their healthcare facility not only to support their employer's initiatives but also to better serve patients and their families. Outdated gender, sex, and sexual orientation information practices in electronic health records, in patient care, and elsewhere can lead to health inequities for sexual and gender minorities (SGMs). Researchers found a lack of inclusive and gender-affirming language in some clinical documentation. They also noted that the use of inclusive and gender-affirming language during clinical interactions led to quality and therapeutic relationships between providers and SGM patients that supported their psychological safety.

Nes, A., Steindal, S. A., Hamilton Larsen, S., Camilla Heer, H., Lærum-Onsager, E., & Roth Gjevjon, E. (2021). Technological literacy in nursing education: A scoping review. *Journal of Professional Nursing, 37*(2), 320–334. https://doi.org/10.1016/j.profnurs.2021.01.008

Technology continues to evolve in all aspects of healthcare, from patient monitoring devices to electronic patient records. Technological literacy is a fundamental skill that is essential to nursing practice. Researchers investigated informatics in nursing curricula. Findings revealed that the acquisition, measurement, and maintenance of technological literacy is lacking in most nursing education curricula. Integrating nursing informatics competencies into nursing education could improve the knowledge and skills students need to enable them to provide

safe, effective patient care and ensure nursing students have an active role in technology development and implementation.

Badowski, D., Horsley, T. L., Rossler, K. L., Mariani, B., & Gonzalez, L. (2018). Electronic charting during simulation. *Computers, Informatics, Nursing, 36* (9), 430-437. https://doi.org/10.1097/CIN.0000000000000457

Information literacy (informatics, computer technology) is a core competency for nursing students. However, students may have limited access to electronic health records (EHRs) in clinical practicum. Researchers investigated how nursing programs incorporated EHRs in nursing curricula. Findings revealed that 56% of the 146 participants used EHRs in simulation-based learning experiences (SBLEs). Integration occurred primarily in the skills (89%) and simulation labs (92%). Participants who did not incorporate EHRs into the curricula cited costs and budgetary constraints as inhibiting factors. Most of the participants (54.6%) were satisfied with the time students spent using EHRs for SBLEs, whereas 45.6% were dissatisfied for various reasons (e.g., faculty resistance, technology bugs, use difficulties). Only 35% of participants indicated their graduates were adequately prepared to use EHRs, 9% indicated unprepared, and the majority (55.8%) did not include this question on graduate surveys. Researchers concluded that nursing programs should identify innovative ways to integrate EHRs into nursing curricula.

1. How can nurses help to ensure health equity for sexual and gender minorities? Why is this important?

2. Why is technological literacy important in nursing practice?

3. Based on these three studies, what is the role of clinical practice and education in helping students acquire essential nursing competencies?

Can I Delegate Documentation in the Medical Records?

In some facilities, each member of the team is responsible for documenting care provided to the client. Nursing assistants or other unlicensed assistive personnel (UAP) often document ADLs, activity, and I&O on graphic records. You are responsible for documenting the nursing care you provide. Never document the actions of others as though you performed them. If an action is crucial to a chain of events, you may document that action on paper or in the EHR, clearly referring to the person who did the action. For example, "Became dizzy; assisted to chair by Nora Roverdale, UAP."

KnowledgeCheck 17-8

- Can documentation in the patient records be delegated?
- You are a student nurse on a medical-surgical unit. You review your client's record and notice that the provider entered prescriptions that do not appear to be appropriate for your client. The provider is still in the area. How would you handle this situation?

To explore learning resources for this chapter,

Go to Davis Advantage and find:

Answers and Suggested Responses for all questions in this chapter

Concept Map

Knowledge Map

References and Bibliography

CHAPTER 18

Measuring Vital Signs

Learning Outcomes

After completing this chapter, you should be able to:

➤ Describe the physiological processes involved in regulating body temperature, pulse, respirations, and blood pressure.

➤ Convert between the Fahrenheit and centigrade temperature scales.

➤ Discuss expected normal vital signs findings for various age-groups.

➤ Recognize patient vital signs readings that should be referred to the primary care provider.

➤ Define *arterial oxygen saturation, hypoxia, hyperventilation,* and *hypoventilation.*

➤ Define *hypotension, hypertension, essential hypertension,* and *secondary hypertension.*

➤ Select the correct site and equipment for measuring the temperature, pulse, respiration, and blood pressure of patients in various age-groups.

➤ Demonstrate correct technique and procedures for measuring temperature, pulse, respiration, and blood pressure.

➤ Explain the importance of several measurements to interpret a patient's blood pressure.

➤ State at least one nursing diagnosis to describe a problem for each of the vital signs: temperature, pulse, respirations, and blood pressure.

➤ Describe nursing interventions for the patient (1) with temperature alterations, (2) with impaired respiratory status, (3) diagnosed with high blood pressure (hypertension), and (4) with alterations in pulse parameters.

➤ Identify important tips to teach your patients in managing their hypertension.

Key Concepts

Oxygenation (respirations)
Perfusion (pulse, blood pressure)
Thermoregulation
Vital signs

Related Concepts

See the Concept Map on Davis Advantage.

Example Client Conditions

Hyperthermia/Heatstroke
Hypothermia
Hypertension
Hypotension

Meet Your Patients

Your instructor has scheduled a clinical day at a local community health fair for students to answer health-related questions, administer flu vaccines, check blood sugar levels, and take vital signs: temperature, pulse, respirations, and blood pressure (BP). You have been asked to check vital signs.

Jason. The first person who arrives at the booth is Rosemary, a young mother, with Jason, her 2-year-old son. She tells you he has been eating poorly and is very irritable. The child's skin is warm and dry, and he is flushed. Rosemary explains that she does not have a thermometer, and she would like you to take her son's temperature. Jason's axillary temperature is 101.8°F (38.8°C).

Now it is time to think like a nurse! What could this temperature reading mean? What, if any, additional data

should you collect? How will you explain your findings to Rosemary? What action would you advise Rosemary to take? You may not yet have all the theoretical knowledge you need to answer these questions, but try to do so anyway, based on your present knowledge and your life experiences.

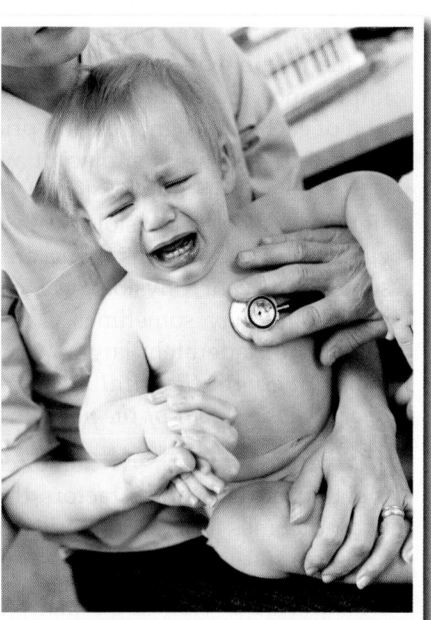

(Continued)

443

666

Meet Your Patients (continued)

Ms. Sharma. The next person to arrive at the booth is Ms. Sharma, an active 80-year-old woman who works part-time in a local literacy program and walks 3 miles four times per week. Ms. Sharma notes that she has "lost a little pep. I don't feel sick, but I'm tired lately." Her pulse is difficult to feel. The rhythm is irregular, and the strength of the pulse is uneven—some beats are strong, whereas others are weak. What might this finding mean? What questions do you have for Ms. Sharma? What, if any, additional data should you collect? How will you explain your findings to Ms. Sharma? What action would you advise her to take?

Mr. Jackson. As Mr. Jackson sits down next to you, you notice he is short of breath. His respiratory rate is 28 breaths/min, and he appears to be struggling to breathe. What do you think this respiratory rate means? What should be your next action? What would you say to Mr. Jackson?

Lucas. The next patient to arrive is Lucas, a 35-year-old accountant who works for a firm in a nearby office building. Lucas tells you he has been under a lot of stress and is worried about his BP. You measure his BP as 150/98 mm Hg. Is this an acceptable BP? What does this reading mean? What should you discuss with Lucas? What advice should you offer?

You will gain the theoretical knowledge you need to answer the preceding questions as you work through this chapter and learn more about vital signs.

ABOUT THE KEY CONCEPTS

The key concepts of **thermoregulation, perfusion,** and **oxygenation** pertain to specific **vital signs** you will learn about in this chapter (temperature, pulse, respirations, and BP). A grasp of these underlying concepts will help you understand and remember the rationale for what you do when measuring and interpreting vital signs.

WHAT ARE VITAL SIGNS?

The concept of **vital signs (VS)** suggests assessment of vital or critical physiological functions. Variations in temperature, pulse, respirations, or BP are indicators of a person's state of health and function of the body systems. These four assessments are among the most frequent you will make as a nurse. Because of their importance, accurate measurements and documentation of each vital sign are a top priority.

Do not become complacent when a patient's vital signs are within normal limits. Although stable vital signs may *indicate* physiological well-being, they do not *guarantee* it. Vital signs alone are limited in detecting some important physiological changes. For example, vital signs may sometimes remain stable even when there is a moderately large amount of blood loss. **Key Point:** *Evaluate the vital signs in the context of your overall assessment of the patient.*

Other Vital Signs Some experts have recommended adding other factors that affect patient care and outcomes to the four traditional measures of physiological status:

- *Pain.* This is viewed by many as the fifth vital sign (Pozza et al., 2021; Rosenberg, 2018). See Chapter 28. Some argue that viewing pain as a fifth vital sign has not improved the problem of undertreated pain and has contributed to opioid addiction. They recommend a more interprofessional, multidimensional approach to promoting patients' comfort (Levy et al., 2018; Scher et al., 2019)
- *Oxygen saturation.* Pulse oximetry provides important information on arterial blood oxygen concentration.
- *Smoking status* is important to assess based on the impact of smoking on body functions and thus vital signs.
- *Emotional distress.* This can have an impact on overall physiological functioning.

Rather than being overly concerned about whether these parameters should be referred to as vital signs, we recommend that nurses include them in all their ongoing assessments of patients.

♥ iCare 18-1

Measuring Vital Signs

Measuring vital signs seems pretty straightforward. How can you incorporate caring into this technical task?

Simple Solution: Approach every patient unhurriedly. Introduce yourself, make eye contact, and explain what you will be doing before you touch the person. Ensure your voice is low, calm, and kind. "*Hello, Mr. Smith. My name is Annie Gates. I'm a student nurse. I need to take your vital signs, which includes taking your blood pressure and measuring your temperature, pulse, and breathing rate. Is it okay with you that I perform these tasks?*"

Introducing yourself and explaining your actions show respect for the person's autonomy. In addition, you are informing and educating the patient about the plan of care and allowing them an opportunity to consent or refuse. A warm and kind voice conveys caring.

When Should I Measure a Patient's Vital Signs?

In the Meet Your Patients scenario, patients asked you to take their vital signs. However, in many clinical settings, vital signs are measured and documented in the following commonly occurring circumstances:

- On admission to the hospital
- For inpatients, at the beginning of a shift
- At a visit to the healthcare provider's office or clinic
- Before, during, and after surgery or certain procedures
- To monitor the effects of certain medications or activities
- Whenever the patient's condition changes

The ideal frequency for assessing vital signs depends on the patient's condition and the events taking place (Ghosh et al., 2018; Sapra et al., 2022). Agency policies also determine the frequency for monitoring and recording vital signs. The following list contains commonly used frequencies:

- In the hospital: once every 4 to 8 hours
- In the home health setting: at each visit
- In the clinic: at each visit
- In skilled nursing facilities: weekly to monthly

✚ You must always obtain an initial set of vital signs to establish the patient's baseline. When a patient's vital signs vary from their baseline, you should assess and document them more frequently to determine a trend in the degree and severity of the variation. As a beginning practitioner, you should validate your clinical assessments with a more experienced nurse and determine how often to reassess.

Key Point: *A baseline is important for evaluating a change in the patient's physiological status. Such a change may be caused by a disease state, the effect of therapies, or changes in physical activity or environment.*

Many healthcare facilities are using smart beds that contain under-the-mattress sensors for contact-free, continuous monitoring of patients' respiratory and heart rates. When the rates deviate from the preset parameters, alerts notify the nurse. Continuous monitoring facilitates early detection of clinical deterioration. ✚ Even with smart beds, the nurse must continue to assess the patient's BP and temperature. You can decide, based on cues, whether vital signs need to be monitored more frequently than prescribed by the primary care provider.

Table 18-1 shows average or normal findings for adults, but it is important to remember that each person has his or her own baseline for "normal." If a patient's vital signs vary from established norms, compare the finding with that person's baseline.

How Do I Document Vital Signs?

Most agencies have special flowsheets for documenting vital signs. If the vital signs are not within normal limits, you will also document them in the nurses' notes, along

Table 18-1 ➤ Vital Signs: Average Normal Findings for Adults	
Mean Adult Temperature	
Oral	36.7°C–37°C (98°F–98.6°F)*
Rectal	37.2°C–37.6°C (99°F–99.6°F)*
Pulse	
Normal range	60–100 beats/min
Average	80 beats/min
Respirations	
Normal range	12–20 breaths/min
Blood Pressure	
Normal range	<120 mm Hg systolic and <80 mm Hg diastolic
Elevated	120–129 mm Hg systolic and <80 mm Hg diastolic
Hypertension stage 1	130–139 mm Hg systolic or 80–89 mm Hg diastolic
Hypertension stage 2	≥140 mm Hg systolic or ≥90 mm Hg diastolic
Hypertensive crisis	>180 mm Hg systolic and/or >120 mm Hg diastolic

*This is revised downward from the traditional norms to reflect more recent research (Geneva et al., 2019; Mackowiak et al., 1992; Sapra et al., 2022; Sund-Levander et al., 2002; Whelton et al., 2018).
- The systematic review reported the following mean normal temperatures: oral, 36.3°C (97.3°F); rectal, 36.9°C (98.3°F).
- The traditional Wunderlich (1871) average normal temperature is 37.0°C (98.6°F) to 37.5°C (99.5°F), depending on measurement site.

with any associated symptoms (e.g., cyanosis [blue-gray skin] with abnormal respirations). Nurses are required to take appropriate actions based on their assessment findings cues; therefore, you must also document your interventions (e.g., elevating the head of the bed when the patient has shortness of breath) in the electronic health record.

BODY TEMPERATURE

Body temperature is the degree of heat maintained by the body. It is the difference between heat produced by the body and heat lost to the environment.

TheoreticalKnowledge
knowing why

You must understand the concept of *thermoregulation* to assess and support regulation of body temperature at a professional level. You will learn the normal temperature range, how heat is produced by and lost from the body, and factors that influence body temperature.

What Is Thermoregulation?

Thermoregulation is the process of maintaining a stable internal body temperature. To keep the body temperature constant, the body must balance heat production and heat loss. This balance is controlled by the hypothalamus, located between the cerebral hemispheres of the brain. Similar to a thermostat, the hypothalamus recognizes and responds to even small changes in body temperature that are sent to it by sensory receptors in the skin.

Core Temperature This is the temperature deep within the body, such as in the viscera and liver. The hypothalamus regulates body temperature. The pulmonary artery catheter measures the temperature of the blood and is the most accurate indicator of core body temperature. It is not routinely used in clinical practice because it requires an invasive procedure.

- **Key Point:** *Rectal measurements are used to represent core temperatures, whereas oral and axillary measurements reflect surface temperatures.*
- An adult's normal internal (core) temperature ranges from about 36.1°C to 38.2°C (97°F to 100.8°F).
- Core temperature is typically 0.6°C to 1.2°C (1°F to 2°F) higher than surface (skin) temperature.

What Is a Normal Temperature?

No single number can be considered "normal" because body temperature varies among individuals because of differences in metabolism. Furthermore, each person's temperature fluctuates with age, exercise, and environmental conditions. However, the body does function optimally within a narrow temperature range.

"Average" Normal Temperature There is little definitive evidence about what, exactly, is a normal temperature. You may see different values in the many sources you read. We can at least conclude that the traditional belief of 37°C (98.6°F) for an average normal reading is too high, based on available research (Protsiv, 2020).

- Older research found a mean normal adult oral temperature of 36.3°C (97.3°F) (Sund-Levander et al., 2002). (See Table 18-1.)
- Research results found a mean body temperature of 36.6°C (97.9°F), with a range of 35.3°C to 37.7°C (95.5°F to 99.8°F). It also found that older adults have lower body temperatures and noted variations in temperature based on sex (Obermeyer et al., 2017).

Body temperature can be evaluated based on individual norms and variability (Marui et al., 2017; Sapra, 2022; Sund-Levander et al., 2004). Table 18-2 shows age-related variations for all vital signs, including temperature.

Slight Variations in Temperature Variations of temperature above or below normal, if temporary, usually are not significant. Greater variations indicate a disturbance of function in some system or region of the body (Fig. 18-1). However, the degree of temperature elevation does not always indicate the seriousness of the underlying disease or condition. For example, some acute, even fatal, infections may cause only a mild temperature elevation. **Key Point:** *A continuous elevation,*

Table 18-2 ➤ Comparison of Normal Vital Signs for Various Ages*

AGE	TEMPERATURE AVERAGE, °C (°F)	PULSE RANGE (beats per min)	RESPIRATIONS RANGE (breaths per min)	BLOOD PRESSURE AVERAGE (mm Hg)
Newborn	36.8 (98.2)** axillary	130 (80–180)	30–60	80/40
1–3 years	37.7 (99.9)** rectal	110 (80–150)	20–40	98/64
6–8 years	37.0 (98.6)** oral	95 (75–115)	20–25	102/56
10 years	37.0 (98.6)** oral	90 (70–100)	17–22	110/58
Teen	37.0 (98.6)** oral	80 (55–105)	15–20	110/70
Adult	36.7 (98) oral	80 (60–100)	12–20	<120/80
Adult older than 70 years	35 to 36.0 (95 to 96.8) oral	80 (60–100)	12–20	120/80, up to 160/95

*NOTE: Pulse and respirations are shown as ranges, not averages. This means that you might see either the low or high extreme for a short period of time without alarm. Ranges and averages should be used as guides, not absolutes.

Example 1: A normal newborn's respiratory rate may be as much as 60 when crying or 30 when at rest.

Example 2: An older adult being treated for hypertension may regularly have a blood pressure reading of up to 160/95. Although this is not desirable or "normal," it may be normal for that patient but should be managed by a provider.

To interpret vital signs, you must know the patient's baseline and the activity at the time of the measurement.

** We speculate that based on recent literature for adult temperatures, these may all be slightly high (Protsiv, 2020).

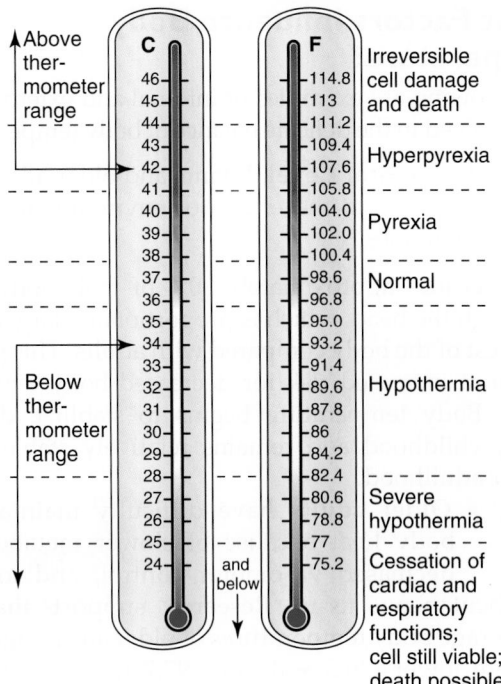

FIGURE 18-1 Ranges of normal and altered body temperatures.

even if slight, is cause for concern and indicates a need for further evaluation.

What Is the Response to Variations in Temperature?

The neurological feedback mechanism in the hypothalamus senses internal temperature changes and initiates compensatory mechanisms to maintain a stable environment.

Decreasing the Body Temperature When heat sensors in the hypothalamus are stimulated, they send out impulses to reduce the body temperature.

- This activates compensatory mechanisms, such as peripheral vasodilation, sweating, and inhibition of heat production.
- **Vasodilation** (increase in the diameter of the blood vessels) diverts core-warmed blood to the body surface, where heat can be transferred to the surrounding environment.

Increasing the Body Temperature When sensors in the hypothalamus detect cold, they send out impulses to increase heat production and reduce heat loss.

- To produce heat, the body responds by shivering and releasing epinephrine, which increases metabolism.
- To reduce heat loss, the blood vessels constrict. **Vasoconstriction** (narrowing of the blood vessels) conserves heat by shunting blood away from the periphery (where heat is lost) to the core of the body, where the blood is warmed.

- **Piloerection** (hairs standing on end) also occurs, but it is not an important heat-conserving mechanism in humans.

Behavioral Control of Temperature People also engage in behaviors to maintain a comfortable body temperature. In response to feeling cold, you turn up the thermostat, put on more clothing, or move to a warmer place. When you feel too warm, you turn on an air conditioner, remove some clothing, or take a cool shower.

How Is Heat Produced in the Body?

The body produces heat through the interaction of three factors: metabolism, the movement of skeletal muscles, and nonshivering thermogenesis.

Metabolism Metabolism is the sum of all physical and chemical processes and changes that take place in the body. Metabolism uses energy and generates heat. The **basal metabolic rate (BMR)** is the amount of energy required to maintain the body at rest. Body size, lean muscle mass, and numerous hormones influence BMR. For example:

- **Hyperthyroidism** (an increase in the thyroid hormone **thyroxine**) increases the BMR. Patients with hyperthyroidism often complain of feeling warm even when in a cool environment.
- **Hypothyroidism** (a decrease in the thyroid hormone **thyroxine**) decreases the BMR, and less heat is produced. Your patient may complain of feeling cold in a warm environment.

The hormones epinephrine and norepinephrine also increase BMR and heat production.

Skeletal Muscle Movement Skeletal muscles are used in all body movements. Muscles need fuel to function.

- The breakdown (catabolism) of fats and carbohydrates in muscle produces energy and heat. It requires very little muscle activity to sit and read this text, but if you were to go for a run, you would use more skeletal muscles. After your run, your body temperature would be higher, perhaps as high as 38.3°C to 40°C (101°F to 104°F).
- In contrast, if you were to go outside without a coat when the temperature was 1.6°C (35°F), your hypothalamus would sense a drop in body temperature, and you would begin to shiver to produce heat. This mechanism is so efficient that body heat production can rise to about four times the normal rate in just a few minutes.

Nonshivering Thermogenesis Nonshivering thermogenesis is the metabolism of brown fat to produce heat. It is used by infants because they cannot produce heat through shivering like adults and children. This mechanism disappears in the first few months after birth.

How Is Heat Exchanged Between the Body and the Environment?

Heat moves from an area of higher temperature to an area of lower temperature; that is, cool air and objects "pick up" heat from warmer ones. The mechanisms that affect the exchange of heat between the body and the environment are radiation, convection, evaporation, and conduction (Fig. 18-2). **Radiation** is the loss of heat through electromagnetic waves emitting from surfaces that are warmer than the surrounding air.

- If the uncovered skin is warmer than the air, the body loses heat through the skin. This is why a cool room warms when it is filled with many people.
- If the skin is cooler than the air, a person can acquire heat by turning on a heat lamp or being in the sunlight.

Radiation accounts for almost 50% of body heat loss.

Convection is the transfer of heat through currents of air or water. Nurses use this principle to intentionally raise or lower a patient's body temperature.

- Immersion in a warm bath can raise body temperature for a hypothermic patient.
- The currents of cool air produced by a fan can reduce a fever in a hyperthermic patient.

Evaporation occurs when water is converted to vapor and lost from the skin (as perspiration) or the mucous membranes (through the breath). Evaporation causes cooling.

- Water loss by evaporation is called **insensible loss.**
- Evaporation is affected by the moisture in the environment **(humidity).** In areas with high humidity, less moisture evaporates from the skin, and less cooling occurs.

Conduction is the process whereby heat is transferred from a warm to a cool surface by direct contact. For example, you should not put patients on uncovered cool surfaces such as metal radiology tables or weighing scales. It could cause a drop in the patient's temperature. Together, the processes of convection and conduction account for approximately 15% to 20% of all heat loss to the environment.

What Factors Influence Body Temperature?

The following are examples of internal and external factors involved in the delicate balance of body temperature.

Developmental Level Infants and older adults are most susceptible to the effects of environmental temperature extremes.

- **Infants** lose approximately 30% of their body heat through the head, which is proportionally larger than the rest of the body compared with adults. This places them at increased risk for decreased body temperature. Body temperature begins to stabilize during early childhood and remains relatively stable until older adulthood.

   ■ **Older adults** have difficulty maintaining body heat because of slower metabolism, decreased vasomotor control, and loss of subcutaneous tissue. Research supports that the average body temperatures of older adults age ≥ 60 were lower (36.5 ± 0.48°C; 97.7 to 98.56°F) than those of adults < age 60 (36.69 ± 0.34°C; 98.04 to 98.65°F) (Geneva et al., 2019). **Key Point: *You should ask your older patients their usual temperature range to establish a baseline temperature and be alert for changes. Some research findings have identified the average normal temperature for older adults as about 35°C to 36°C (95°F to 96.8°F).***

Environment The environment strongly influences body temperature. For example:

- Warm room temperatures, high humidity, or hot baths can increase body temperature.
- Very high external temperatures can significantly increase internal temperatures, causing heatstroke.
- Cold environments, especially with strong air currents, can lower body temperatures and, in severe cases, lead to hypothermia.

Sex The female body temperature varies (as much as 1°F [0.6°C]) due to the menstrual cycle and pregnancy.

- Body temperature is lower when progesterone levels are low and increases as progesterone levels increase.

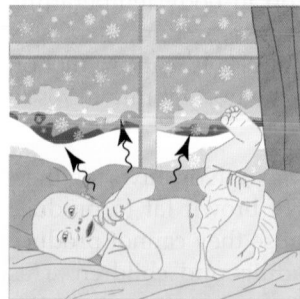 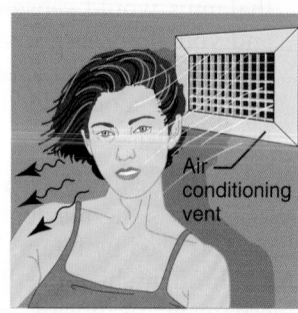 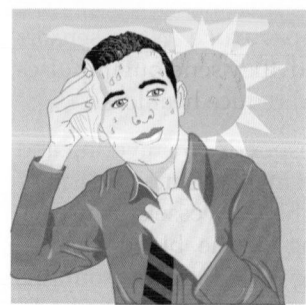 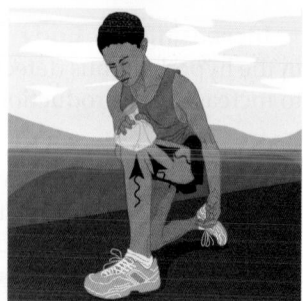

FIGURE 18-2 Mechanisms of heat exchange with the environment: radiation, convection, evaporation, and conduction.

- Hormonal fluctuations during menopause, when menstruation stops, often cause temperature fluctuations commonly known as *hot flashes,* which can produce episodes of intense body heat and sweating.

Exercise The increase in metabolism from hard work or strenuous exercise can increase body core temperature to 38.3°C (101°F) or higher depending on environmental conditions. The sweat that is produced during exercise evaporates and helps to cool the body.

Emotions and Stress Emotional stress, excitement, anxiety, and nervousness stimulate the sympathetic nervous system, causing the production of epinephrine and norepinephrine. These trigger an increase in the metabolic rate, which in turn increases body temperature.

Circadian Rhythm The body has an internal physiological 24-hour cycle called the *circadian rhythm.* Certain physiological processes (e.g., changes in temperature and BP) occur every 24 hours. Temperature can fluctuate 0.6°C to 1.2°C (1°F to 2°F) and is usually lowest in the early-morning hours and highest in late afternoon or early evening. You need to take several readings at different times of the day.

ThinkLike a Nurse 18-1: Clinical Judgment in Action

- You notice the following temperature readings in your patient's electronic health record:
  0400: 97.4°F
  0800: 97.9°F
  1200: 98.4°F
  1600: 99.6°F
  2000: 100.9°F
- When you assess the patient's temperature at midnight, it is 38.4°C (101.2°F). What do you notice about the pattern of the temperature readings?
- What is important in this scenario?
- As a nursing student, what should you do?

KnowledgeCheck 18-1

- Which age-groups are most susceptible to thermoregulation problems, and why?
- List five factors that affect body temperature.
- What are the compensatory mechanisms for decreasing body temperature?
- What are the compensatory mechanisms for increasing body temperature?

What Is a Fever (Pyrexia)?

- **Fever, or pyrexia,** is an oral temperature higher than 37.8°C (100°F) or a rectal temperature of 38.3°C (101°F) in an adult. A person with a fever is said to be **febrile;** one without fever is **afebrile.**

 - **Baseline effects**—Because older adults have a lower-than-average baseline, they may experience fever at a temperature lower than the traditional definition given previously.

- A **moderate fever** is the body's natural defense against infection (up to 39.5°C [103°F]), and although uncomfortable, it does not pose a threat to most patients. A fever is beneficial because it enhances the immune response. Specifically, it
1. Kills or inhibits the growth of many microorganisms
2. Enhances phagocytosis
3. Causes the breakdown of lysosomes and self-destruction of virally infected cells
4. Causes the release of interferon, a substance that protects cells from viral infection

- **Key Point:** *Older adults may be unable to reach the fever temperature range necessary to develop a strong inflammatory response to infectious diseases (Geneva et al., 2019).*
- **Key Point: Hyperpyrexia,** *a fever above 41.0°C (105.8°F), is dangerous and requires intervention to prevent damage to body cells, especially in the brain, leading to confusion, delirium, seizures, or coma.* In addition, vascular collapse may follow, producing cerebral edema, shock, and death. Death usually results if body temperature becomes higher than 43°C to 44°C (109°F to 112°F) (McCance & Huether, 2019).

Some patients who are sensitive to slight temperature elevations (e.g., those with epilepsy) may experience these detrimental effects at temperatures lower than 41.0° (105.8°F).

What Causes a Fever? Fever occurs when, in response to **pyrogens** (fever-producing substances), the body's thermostat resets at a higher temperature. The following occur:

- **Pyrogens**—When bacteria or other foreign substances invade the body, they stimulate **phagocytes** (specialized white blood cells), which ingest the invaders and secrete pyrogens (e.g., interleukin-1).
- **Hypothalamus and set point**—Pyrogens induce the secretion of **prostaglandins** (substances that reset the hypothalamic thermostat at a higher temperature). The reset value is called the **set point.**
  - The body's heat-regulating mechanisms then act to bring the core temperature up to this new setting.
  - When the stressor is removed, the set point resets at normal.

Fever Occurs in Three Phases

1. **Initial phase (febrile episode or onset):** The period during which body temperature is rising but has not yet reached the new set point. The onset of fever may be sudden or gradual, depending on the condition causing it. The person usually feels chilly and generally uncomfortable and may shiver.
2. **Second phase (course):** The period during which body temperature reaches its maximum (set point) and remains fairly constant at the new higher level. The person is flushed and feels warm and dry during this phase, which may last from a few days to a few weeks.

3. **Third phase (defervescence or crisis):** The period during which the temperature returns to normal. The person feels warm and appears flushed in response to vasodilation. Diaphoresis occurs, which assists with heat loss by evaporation. This phase is commonly referred to as the fever's "breaking."

Four Ways to Describe a Fever

- **Intermittent fever:** Temperature alternates regularly between periods of fever and periods of normal or below-normal temperature without pharmacological intervention, or the temperature returns to normal at least once every 24 hours.
- **Remittent fever:** Fluctuations in temperature (greater than 2°C [3.6°F]), all above normal, during a 24-hour period.
- **Constant (sustained) fever:** Temperature may fluctuate slightly (less than 0.55°C [1°F]) but is always above normal.
- **Relapsing (or recurrent) fever:** Short periods of fever alternating with periods of normal temperatures, each lasting 1 to 2 days.

Example Client Condition: Hyperthermia/Heatstroke

Hyperthermia, like hyperpyrexia (fever), is a body temperature above normal. **Key Point:** *However, in hyperthermia, the elevated body temperature is higher than the set point.* The hypothalamic regulation of body temperature is overwhelmed and does not reset the set point as it does in fever. Hyperthermia occurs because the body cannot promote heat loss fast enough to balance heat production or high environmental temperatures.

Example Client Condition: Hypothermia

Hypothermia is an abnormally low core temperature, usually less than 35°C (95°F) (Peiris et al., 2018). However, you must know the person's usual normal range of temperature because some people, especially older adults, have a normal temperature of less than 35°C (95°F). See the accompanying Example Client Condition: Hypothermia.

PracticalKnowledge
knowing **how**

Now that you understand the concept of thermoregulation, you are ready to gain the practical knowledge of how to assess and support a patient's body temperature.

ASSESSMENT/RECOGNIZE CUES

In our daily routines, we commonly assess temperature by touch. For example, you can use simple touch to detect fever; however, you cannot differentiate degrees of fever. Because vital signs are used as indicators of a patient's health status, it is essential to have an accurate measure. To see the sequence of steps to take when measuring a patient's temperature, see the Highlights of Procedures box; for the full procedure,

 Go to **Chapter 18, Procedure 18-1: Assessing Body Temperature**, in Volume 2.

Temperature Measurement Scales: Fahrenheit and Centigrade

Two scales are used for recording temperature: Fahrenheit and centigrade (or Celsius), a metric scale. Most people in the United States are familiar with the

---

EXAMPLE CLIENT CONDITION: Hyperthermia/Heatstroke

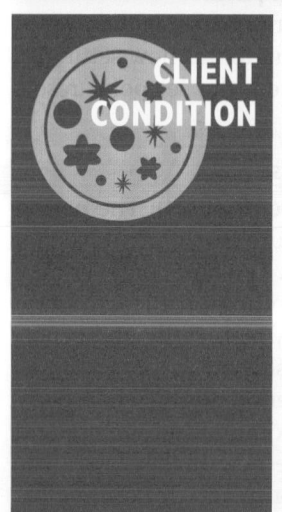

Definitions

NOTE: Based on variations in normal body temperatures, you should not rely solely on temperature reading as the distinguishing factor between heatstroke and heat exhaustion. Conduct a thorough assessment.

Hyperthermia

- Body temperature above normal and higher than the set point
- Body temperature dangerously high (39.4°C–41.1°C or 103°F–106°F, or higher)

Heat Exhaustion

May occur with a core temperature of 37°C (98.6°F) to 39.4°C (103°F). For symptoms, see Assessment section.

Heat Stroke

Occurs when the body's temperature regulation fails, usually when the hyperthermia progresses to a temperature above 39.4°C (103°F). Temperatures of 41.1°C (106°F) and higher may be reached.

Complications

Untreated heatstroke can cause damage to the heart, brain, kidneys, and other vital organs, resulting in permanent disability and even death.

EXAMPLE CLIENT CONDITION: **Hypothermia**

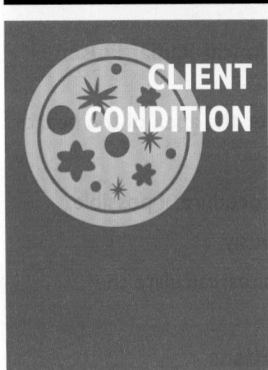

CLIENT CONDITION

Definition:
- Abnormally low core body temperature of <35°C (<95°F)
- As the body temperature drops, metabolic processes slow. The prolonged exposure to cold is no longer correctible by shivering and may prove fatal.
- Environmental exposure to extreme cold
- Surgery
- Medically induced hypothermia (to reduce the need for oxygen in tissues)

Hypothermia causes vasoconstriction, coagulation in the microcirculation, tissue ischemia (lack of oxygen), and poor organ perfusion that can lead to failure of vital organs (e.g., heart, kidneys, brain).
- Metabolic or nervous system dysfunction
- Drug intoxication

Fahrenheit scale; however, some healthcare agencies use centigrade.

- Electronic and tympanic membrane thermometers can usually measure temperature in either scale; often, all you need to do is to flip a switch.
- Some types of thermometers only provide one scale (Fig. 18-3 shows both scales), so you may need to convert a reading from one scale to the other.
  - You may have a conversion app on your cell phone, or you can find a conversion tool on the Internet.
- If you need to convert scales and do not have access to a conversion chart, you can use a mathematical formula.

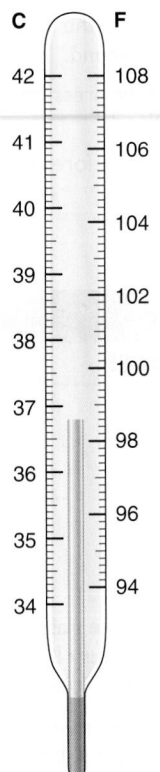

FIGURE 18-3 Some thermometers are available with degree markings in Fahrenheit or centigrade. *Left,* Centigrade scale. *Right,* Fahrenheit scale.

Key Point: *To convert from Fahrenheit to centigrade, subtract 32 from the Fahrenheit temperature and multiply by 5/9.*
Example: A patient has a temperature of 102°F. What is the temperature measured in centigrade?

$$(102 - 32) \times \tfrac{5}{9} = (70 \times 5) \div 9 = 39°C$$

Key Point: *To convert a centigrade reading to Fahrenheit, multiply the centigrade temperature by 9/5, and add 32.* As a cross-check, we can verify the preceding example:
Example: A patient has a temperature of 39°C.

$$(39 \times \tfrac{9}{5}) + 32 = (351 \div 5) + 32 = 102°F$$

What Equipment Do I Need?

Nurses measure temperature with various kinds of thermometers. Each type has advantages and disadvantages (Table 18-3), so you need to think critically about the type of thermometer best suited for each patient situation.

Glass Thermometers Historically, the thermometer was a glass mercury-filled tube marked in degrees Fahrenheit or centigrade and read visually. Because of dangers associated with broken glass and exposure to mercury, healthcare facilities have complied with the U.S. Environmental Protection Agency and the American Hospital Association advice against the use of equipment containing mercury (Environmental Protection Agency [EPA], 2018). Electronic digital thermometers or glass or plastic thermometers containing other liquids, such as alcohol or gallium–indium–tin (Galinstan), have replaced those containing mercury.

Electronic Thermometers Electronic thermometers are rechargeable units consisting of an electronic probe attached to a portable unit by a thin wire. A beep sounds when the peak temperature is reached. The probe is covered with disposable plastic sheaths to prevent transmission of infection. You must discard the sheath after each use. **Key Point: *Most units have a red probe for rectal temperatures and blue probe for oral. Use the correct probe for each site.***

Highlights of Procedures

For steps to follow in *all* procedures, refer to the Universal Steps for All Procedures found on the inside back cover of Volume 2. Go to the full procedures in Volume 2 to practice and learn the procedure steps. Use these procedure highlights later to help you review key points.

Procedure 18-1: Assessing Body Temperature

➤ Clean thermometer before and after use if it is not disposable.

➤ Select the appropriate site and thermometer type.

➤ Turn on or otherwise ready the thermometer.

➤ Insert the thermometer in its sheath, or use a thermometer designated only for the patient.

➤ Insert and leave an electronic thermometer in place until it beeps; for other thermometers, use the recommended times.

➤ Cleanse and store in recharging base (store glass thermometers safely to prevent breakage).

➤ For an oral temperature, obtain a reading 20 to 30 minutes after the patient consumes hot or cold food or fluids or smokes.

➤ Hold a rectal thermometer securely in place, and never leave it unattended.

Procedure 18-2: Assessing Peripheral Pulses

➤ Make sure the client is resting while you assess the pulse.

➤ Count for 15 or 30 seconds if the pulse is regular; count for 60 seconds if it is irregular.

➤ Note pulse rate, rhythm, and quality.

➤ Compare pulses bilaterally.

Procedure 18-3: Assessing the Apical Pulse

➤ Position the patient supine or sitting.

➤ Palpate and place the stethoscope at the fifth intercostal space at the midclavicular line.

➤ Count for 60 seconds.

➤ Note pulse rate, rhythm, and quality and the S_1 and S_2 heart sounds.

Procedure 18-4: Assessing for an Apical-Radial Pulse Deficit

➤ Palpate and place stethoscope over the apex of the heart.

➤ Palpate the radial pulse.

➤ Have two nurses carry out the procedure, if possible.

➤ Count for 60 seconds, simultaneously.

➤ Compare the pulse rate at both sites; calculate the difference.

Procedure 18-5: Assessing Respirations

➤ Count unobtrusively (e.g., while palpating the radial pulse).

➤ Count for 30 seconds if respirations are regular; count for 60 seconds if they are irregular.

➤ Observe the rate, rhythm, and depth of respirations.

Procedure 18-6: Measuring Blood Pressure

➤ If possible, place the patient in a sitting position, with the feet on the floor and the legs uncrossed.

➤ Measure blood pressure after the patient has been inactive for 5 minutes.

➤ Support the patient's arm at the level of the heart.

➤ Use a cuff of the appropriate size.

➤ Wrap the cuff snugly.

➤ Inflate the cuff while palpating the artery. Inflate to 30 mm Hg above the point at which you can no longer feel the artery pulsating.

➤ Place the stethoscope on the artery, and release pressure at 2 to 3 mm Hg per second.

➤ Record systolic/diastolic pressures (first and last sounds heard—e.g., 110/80).

➤ Wait at least 2 minutes before remeasuring.

Table 18-3 ➤ Advantages and Disadvantages of Various Thermometers

ADVANTAGES	DISADVANTAGES
Glass Thermometer	

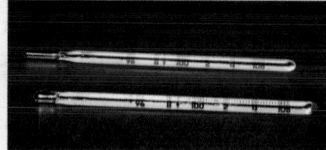

■ Flexibility of use: Can be used for measuring oral, rectal, or axillary temperature	■ ✚ Do not use glass thermometers containing mercury. If you find one, recommend that it be replaced immediately.
■ Inexpensive initial cost	
■ Accuracy, as indicated by several studies	■ Easily broken, so there is ongoing cost of replacement and risk for injury
■ Easily disinfected	■ Slow: It takes 3–8 min to obtain an accurate reading, depending on the site.
	■ Difficult for some people to read accurately

Table 18-3 ➤ Advantages and Disadvantages of Various Thermometers—cont'd

ADVANTAGES	DISADVANTAGES

Electronic Thermometer

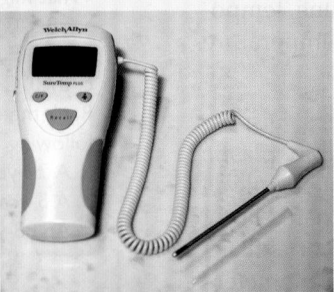

ADVANTAGES	DISADVANTAGES
■ Flexibility of use: Can be used for measuring oral, rectal, or axillary temperature ■ Ease of use ■ Rapid measurement: It takes 2–60 sec to obtain reading, depending on the unit.	■ Expensive initial cost ■ Requires regular inspection and maintenance to ensure accuracy ■ Data are conflicting regarding their accuracy compared with other types of thermometers. ■ Need to be kept charged

Electronic With Infrared Sensor

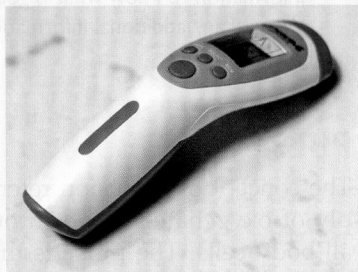 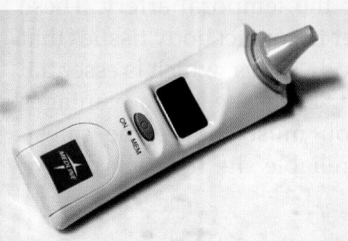

ADVANTAGES	DISADVANTAGES
■ Ease of use ■ Rapid measurement: It takes 2–5 sec to measure the temperature. ■ May be the most cost-effective method because of time and labor savings from their rapid reading capabilities ■ Low rate of operator error	■ Expensive initial cost ■ Less accurate than electronic or glass/plastic thermometers when used for tympanic membrane temperatures, as some studies indicate ■ Requires regular inspection and maintenance to ensure accuracy ■ Batteries require recharging.

Disposable Chemical Thermometer

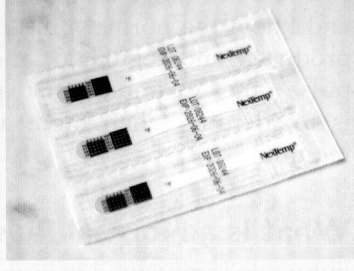 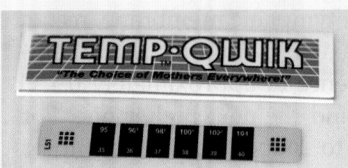

ADVANTAGES	DISADVANTAGES
■ Ease of use; requires no special training ■ Equally as accurate as the electronic thermometer ■ Less expensive than purchasing supplies for and maintaining an electronic thermometer ■ Because it is disposable, it may prevent spread of infection among patients. ■ Recommended for measuring axillary temperature among pediatric patients over the age of 2 years.	■ Less accurate/reliable than glass or plastic thermometers ■ The skin must be dry. ■ Indicates only body surface temperature; does not reflect core temperature ■ Guidelines presently recommend only for pediatric patients

Electronic Infrared Thermometers Electronic infrared thermometers are rechargeable units. They contain a sensor that detects heat in the form of infrared energy given off by the body. The thermometer does not touch the actual sites (e.g., tympanic membrane, temporal artery). A beep sounds when the peak temperature is reached.

Disposable Chemical Thermometers Disposable chemical thermometers consist of a thin plastic strip, patch, or tape that contains a matrix of chemicals designed to produce color changes at a designated body temperature. Most are used once for an oral or axillary reading and then discarded. Disposable thermometers are useful in the home and for patients in protective isolation. When using this method, abnormal temperatures should be validated with a more reliable thermometer (Brassey & Heneghan, 2020).

What Sites Should I Use?

You must choose the safest, most accurate, and most reliable site for each patient. The sites for intermittent measurement are the mouth, rectum, axillae, tympanic membrane, and skin over the temporal artery. These sites allow the thermometer to contact body tissues that are well supplied with blood vessels, which is essential for accurate measurement. Each site has advantages and disadvantages, so you must choose the safest, most accurate, and most reliable site for each patient (Table 18-4).

Sites for Core Temperature Sites in the pulmonary artery, esophagus, and bladder accurately measure core temperature. These sites are used in surgery and intensive care, but they are invasive, expensive, and impractical for most clinical environments. Measurements from these sites require the use of specially designed thermometers and practitioners with advanced training. **Key Point:** *Pulmonary artery temperature is considered the gold standard with which other sites are compared.*

Temperature Variations at Different Sites Although research on site differences is conflicting, generally, from lowest to highest readings, the sites are thought to be axillary, oral, tympanic membrane, rectal, and temporal artery. For axillary, oral, and rectal temperatures, there is a difference of approximately 0.4°C (0.8°F) between each site and the next higher one. For convenience, nurses tend to round the fraction up to 0.5°C (1°F). For example, an axillary temperature of 36.7°C (98.06°F) is similar to an oral reading of 37.3°C (99.1°F) or a rectal reading of 37.8°C (100.1°F).

✚ Use this only to help you understand your patient's data. You cannot reliably convert temperatures mathematically between sites. When you measure a temperature, record the value you obtain and the site used.

◤ ThinkLike a Nurse 18-2: Clinical Judgment in Action

- Convert the following temperatures and analyze the readings. What might they mean?
  a. 38.5°C _____ °F
  b. 96.5°F _____ °C
  c. 37.0°C _____ °F
- Rank the expected early-evening temperatures of the following individuals from lowest to highest:
  a. A 22-year-old college athlete
  b. A 5-year-old kindergarten student
  c. An 88-year-old nursing home resident

◤ ThinkLike a Nurse 18-3: Clinical Judgment in Action

Recall the patients in the Meet Your Patients scenario. Two-year-old Jason's axillary temperature was 38.8°C (101.8°F), and his skin was warm, dry, and flushed. His mother told you that he had been eating poorly and was very irritable.

- What changes in behavior alert you that something is wrong?
- Do you have enough theoretical knowledge or patient information to know what is going on?
- What, if any, additional information about the patient situation do you need?

PULSE

The concept of perfusion refers to the continuous supply of oxygenated blood through the blood vessels to all body cells. The **pulse** is the rhythmic expansion of an artery produced when a bolus of oxygenated blood is forced into it by contraction of the heart. How do you think the pulse affects perfusion? How might perfusion affect the pulse?

TheoreticalKnowledge knowing why

To assess and support regulation of a patient's pulse, you will need to understand the concept of perfusion and know the normal pulse range, how the pulse is produced and regulated, and factors that influence pulse rate. An important reason to assess the pulse is to identify when more advanced monitoring is required.

What Is a Normal Pulse Rate?

Pulse rate is measured in beats per minute. The normal range for healthy young and middle-aged adults is 60 to 100 beats/min, with an average rate of 70 to 80 beats/min (see Table 18-1).

When the heart rate is of concern, you will most likely use a cardiac monitor to determine not only the rate but also the rhythm and intensity of the pulse.

Table 18-4 ➤ Disadvantages and Contraindications of Various Sites for Measuring Temperature

ADVANTAGES	DISADVANTAGES	CONTRAINDICATIONS
Temporal Artery—Passing the probe of an infrared thermometer over the front of the forehead to the temporal area.		
<ul><li>**Most accurate** representation of core temperature</li><li>**Fast.** Most scanners provide a reading in about 3 sec.</li><li>**No discomfort** is associated with the procedure.</li><li>**Safe.** Can be used even for those who cannot follow instructions (e.g., infants).</li><li>**Less prone to error** than tympanic thermometer</li></ul>	<ul><li>Requires special scanning thermometer</li><li>Any covering (hat, hair, etc.) prevents heat from dissipating and causes the reading to be falsely high. This is also true for the side of the head lying on a pillow.</li></ul>	Wounds on or near the forehead; may be affected by diaphoresis (sweating), exercise, and environmental temperatures (Robertson & Hill, 2019)
Rectal—Inserting the thermometer into the rectal cavity		
<ul><li>Accurately represents core (internal) body temperature. Seen as the "gold standard" for routine measurement of body temperature (Sapra et al., 2022).</li><li>Use for patients who are unable to follow directions for oral temperature monitoring or in situations in which accuracy is crucial</li></ul>	<ul><li>Most patients find this method objectionable or embarrassing.</li><li>✥ Not recommended as the first choice of site because of the risk for injury to the rectal mucosa, especially in infants</li><li>Requires special positioning of the patient</li><li>Presence of stool may cause inaccurate reading and present a hygienic concern.</li><li>May be frightening for young children and embarrassing to older children</li></ul>	<ul><li>✥ Patients who may be injured by the method (e.g., patients who have a rectal disease, severe diarrhea, or rectal surgery)</li><li>Patients with cardiac surgery and some heart conditions; this method can stimulate the vagus nerve and slow the heart rate.</li><li>Patients with hemorrhoids</li><li>Immunosuppressed patients or those with clotting disorders</li></ul>
Oral—Thermometer placed under the tongue (sublingual)		
<ul><li>Simple, convenient</li><li>Comfortable for most patients</li><li>Safe for adults and children who are old enough to follow simple directions</li></ul>	<ul><li>✥ Glass thermometers can break if bitten.</li><li>Slow; requires up to 8 min to ensure an accurate reading (if glass thermometer used)</li><li>Patient must keep their mouth closed for several minutes (glass thermometers).</li><li>Eating, drinking (e.g., ice water, hot tea), and smoking in the 30 minutes before measurement affect the accuracy of the reading.</li><li>Bradypnea may create false temperature elevations.</li><li>Tachypnea is associated with lowered readings because it increases evaporative cooling of the oral cavity.</li></ul>	<ul><li>✥ Patients who cannot cooperate with the instructions or who might be injured (e.g., infants and small children; patients who have had oral surgery, breathe through the mouth, have chills, or are confused or unconscious)</li></ul>

(Continued)

Table 18-4 ➤ Disadvantages and Contraindications of Various Sites for Measuring Temperature—cont'd

ADVANTAGES	DISADVANTAGES	CONTRAINDICATIONS
Axillary—Placed under the armpits		
▪ Safe ▪ Easy to use; accessible ▪ Can be used for children and for uncooperative or unconscious patients ▪ Recommended over rectal site for routine measurements	▪ Not reflective of core temperature. At the onset of fever, peripheral vasoconstriction is intense, so the skin is cooler. ▪ Considered one of the least accurate sites ▪ Diaphoresis (sweating) can cause the reading to be lower. ▪ Thermometer may need to be left in place for a long time (8 minutes if glass is used).	▪ Patients who are perspiring heavily ▪ Does not accurately diagnose fever. If fever is suspected, confirm with measurement from another route.
Tympanic Membrane—Thermometer is inserted into the ear canal		
▪ Fast (2–5 sec) ▪ Easy to use ▪ Can be used for children over age 6 months (Massaro & Schmitt, 2018) and for uncooperative or unconscious patients	▪ Requires a special thermometer, a relatively expensive initial purchase ▪ More variable than oral and rectal sites ▪ Must be carefully positioned to ensure accuracy; prone to caregiver measurement errors ▪ Presence of cerumen (earwax) may affect accuracy. ▪ Significant differences have been found between readings in left and right ear of same patient. ▪ Risk of injury to tympanic membrane if not positioned carefully to avoid touching it ▪ May be uncomfortable for the patient ▪ Research is mixed on the accuracy and reliability of tympanic membrane instruments. ▪ Hearing aids must be removed.	▪ ✚ Patients who have had recent ear surgery ▪ Contraindicated in the presence of ear infection
Skin—Disposable; placed against the skin (e.g., on the forehead)		
▪ Safe, convenient ▪ Easy to use for nonprofessionals ▪ Can be used when other sites are contraindicated ▪ Inexpensive (Chemical paper or tape is used.)	▪ Forehead skin temperature is generally 1°C–2°C (2°F–4°F) less than core temperature; if marked deviations in skin temperatures are detected, the readings must be confirmed via a more reliable route.	▪ Should not be used when accurate, reliable readings are required (e.g., in the presence of hypothermia or heatstroke) ▪ Skin temperatures may be accurate and reliable when obtained with an infrared skin thermometer (Chen et al., 2020).

How Does the Body Produce and Regulate the Pulse?

The pulse wave begins when the left heart ventricle contracts and ends when it relaxes. Each contraction forces blood into the already-filled aorta, increasing pressure within the arterial system. The intermittent pressure and expansion of the arteries cause the blood to move along in a wavelike motion toward the capillaries. You can palpate a light tap at the peak of the wave, when the artery expands. The trough (low point) of a pulse wave occurs when the artery contracts to push the blood along its way.

- The **peak** of the wave corresponds to **systole,** or the contraction of the heart.
- The **trough** corresponds to **diastole,** or the resting phase of the heart.
- **Stroke volume** is the quantity of blood forced out by each contraction of the left ventricle. You will not usually know your patient's actual stroke volume, although it averages 70 mL in most healthy adults. If stroke volume decreases (as in a large blood loss, or *hemorrhage*), the body tries to maintain the same cardiac output by increasing the pulse rate.
- **Cardiac output** is the total quantity of blood pumped per minute. It is expressed in liters per minute and calculated as follows:

$$\text{Cardiac output} = \text{stroke volume} \times \text{pulse (heart) rate}$$

For a person with a pulse of 80 beats/min and an average stroke volume (70 mL), the cardiac output would be about 5,600 mL (or 5.6 L) per minute.
- **The autonomic nervous system** regulates the heart rate. Sympathetic stimulation increases the heart rate (and thus the cardiac output), whereas parasympathetic stimulation decreases it. For more information on the autonomic nervous system, see Chapter 34.

What Factors Influence the Pulse Rate?

In a healthy adult, the peripheral pulse rate is the same as the heart rate. Therefore, taking the pulse is a quick and simple way to assess the condition of the heart, blood vessels, and circulation. The pulse varies in response to:

- Changes in the volume of blood pumped through the heart
- Variations in heart rate
- Changes in the elasticity of the arterial walls
- Any condition that interferes with heart function.
- Impaired functioning of the nervous system. The heart and blood vessels are regulated by the nervous system, so conditions that interfere with the normal functioning of the nervous system also affect the pulse.

Other factors that may cause variations in pulse rate, rhythm, or quality include the following:

- **Developmental level.** Newborns have a rapid pulse rate. The rate stabilizes in childhood and gradually slows through old age. The resting heart rate may not significantly change with age; however, variability changes. It may take longer for the pulse rate to increase with stress and exercise and also to decrease afterward (Medline Plus, 2020). Thus, you should not rely solely on changes in the pulse rate of older adults to detect their response to external stressors.
- **Sex.** Adult female individuals have a slightly higher pulse rate than do adult male individuals.
- **Exercise.** Muscle activity normally increases the pulse rate. After exercise, a well-conditioned heart returns to a normal rate more quickly. People who are well conditioned have lower heart rates, both before and during exercise, than those who are less conditioned.
- **Food intake.** Ingestion of a meal causes a slight increase in pulse rate for several hours.
- **Stress.** Stress triggers the fight-or-flight sympathetic nervous system response, which increases both pulse rate and strength of the heart contractions (stroke volume).
- **Fever.** The pulse rate tends to increase about 10 beats/min for each degree Fahrenheit of temperature elevation. The reasons are that (1) the metabolic rate increases, and (2) peripheral vasodilation occurs in response to the fever, causing a decrease in BP. The body then causes the heart to beat faster to compensate for the decreased BP.
- **Disease.** Diseases, such as heart disease, hyperthyroidism, respiratory diseases, and infections, are generally associated with increased pulse rates. Hypothyroidism is associated with decreased pulse rates.
- **Blood loss.** A small blood loss is generally well tolerated and produces only a temporary increase in pulse rate. Theoretically, a large blood loss stimulates the sympathetic nervous system, bringing about an increase in pulse rate to compensate for the decreased blood volume. However, research suggests that vital signs are limited in their ability to detect large blood losses; thus, a stable pulse and BP are unreliable measures of the amount of loss.
- **Position changes.** Standing and sitting positions generally cause a temporary increase in pulse rate as a result of blood pooling in the veins of the feet and legs. This causes decreased blood return to the heart, decreasing BP, and subsequently, an increase in heart rate.
- **Medications.** Stimulant drugs (e.g., epinephrine) increase pulse rate. Cardiotonics (e.g., digitalis), opioids (e.g., narcotic analgesics), and sedative drugs decrease pulse rate.

Toward Evidence-Based Practice

Geneva, I., Cuzzo, B., Fazili, T., & Javaid, W. (2019). Normal body temperature: A systematic review. *Open Forum Infectious Diseases, 6*(4), ofz032. https://doi.org/10.1093/ofid/ofz032.

Evidence-based practice from research evolves over time. In the largest meta-analysis to date, the researchers' findings questioned the normothermia baseline axillary temperature range of 37.0°C to 38°C (98.6°F to 100.4°F) established by Wunderlich in 1868 and the current published overall mean body temperature of 36.8°C (98.2°F). Their analysis established a lower overall mean of 36.59°C (97.86°F). Further, per measurement site, the average temperatures were calculated as follows: axillary, 35.97°C (96.75°F); oral, 36.57°C (97.8°F); urine, 36.61°C (97.9°F); tympanic, 36.64°C (97.95°F); and rectal, 37.04°C (98.67°F). Researchers attributed the differences between rectal and urine temperatures, both core body temperatures, to the noninvasive processes used in previous research to measure urine temperatures. The findings supported the lower body temperature in healthy older adults but found that sex differences in body temperature were not clinically significant. The researchers concluded that body temperature is influenced by several variables, most importantly the patient's age and the site of measurement.

Takayama, A., Takeshima, T., Nakashima, Y., Yoshidomi, T., Nagamine, T., & Kotani, K. (2019). A comparison of methods to count breathing frequency. *Respiratory Care, 64*(5), 555–563.

Changes in or abnormal respiratory rates are one of the first indicators of deterioration in patients' clinical condition. Numerous researchers have found that it is the vital sign most neglected by healthcare providers. In addition, numerous methods are used to assess respirations. Researchers examined the reliability of two quick assessment methods: (1) 15-s quadruple—count for 15 seconds and multiply by 4, and (2) breathing time—count the time needed for a single breath and divide by 60, with the standard method 1-minute breath count—counting respirations for 1 full minute (60 seconds). Results revealed that the 15-s quadruple method overestimated breathing frequency. The breathing time method (the duration between the beginning of inspiration and the beginning of the next inspiration) had better agreement with the 1-minute breath count.

---

1. How can research findings affect clinical practice?

2. What are important considerations when evaluating a patient's temperature?

3. Why do you think the breathing time measurement method would more closely align with the 1-minute breath count?

Practical Knowledge
knowing **how**

Now that you understand some of the concepts and factors that produce the pulse, you are ready to learn the practical knowledge to assess and support this aspect of physical functioning.

ASSESSMENT/RECOGNIZING CUES

Assess the pulse by **palpation** (feeling) or **auscultation** (listening with a stethoscope). To palpate the pulse, select the pulse site and lightly compress the patient's artery against the underlying bone with your index and middle finger. When a patient's pulse is difficult to palpate, you may need to use a Doppler device, which has an ultrasound transducer that transmits the pulse sounds to an audio unit. For a summary of the steps for assessing a patient's peripheral pulse, see the Highlights of Procedures box. For the full procedure,

Go to **Chapter 18, Procedure 18-2: Assessing Peripheral Pulses**, in Volume 2.

What Equipment Do I Need?

To count the pulse, you need a watch or clock with a second hand or digital display. To auscultate the pulse, you will use a stethoscope. The stethoscope does not magnify sounds, but rather, blocks out noise so that you can hear the heartbeat and other faint sounds.

- A **stethoscope** consists of a sound-transmitting device (bell and diaphragm) attached to earpieces by rubber tubing and hollow metal tubes (Fig. 18-4).
    Bell—Use to hear low-frequency sounds (e.g., certain heart sounds)
    Diaphragm—Use to assess high-frequency sounds (e.g., lung sounds)
- **Stethoscopes can be either single lumen or double lumen.** A single-lumen stethoscope has one tube connected to the chest piece. A double-lumen stethoscope has two tubes attached to the chest piece. Double-lumen stethoscopes are more sensitive than single-lumen instruments.
- **Most stethoscopes come with soft earpieces** that help seal your ear canal to block room noise from interfering with the sound.

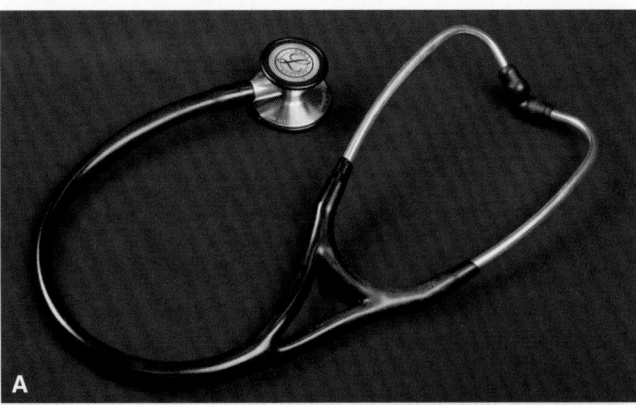

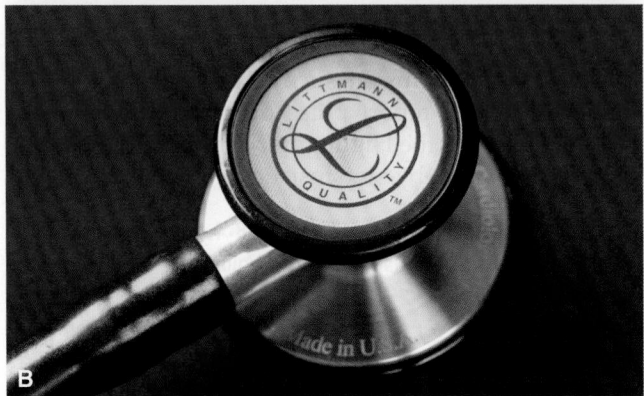

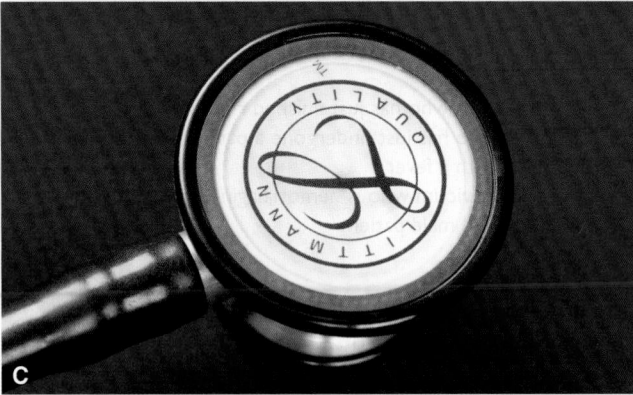

FIGURE 18-4 (A) A stethoscope. (B) The bell, for low-frequency sounds. (C) The diaphragm, for high-frequency sounds.

■ **Stethoscopes have varying lengths of tubing.** Short tubing requires you to be close to the patient and bend more, but the sound may be a bit better than with longer tubing, which is more likely to rub against the body or clothing. Some stethoscopes are made to work effectively through clothing. Unless you have that type, place the instrument directly on the skin.

■ **Digital stethoscopes** are also available to provide sound clarity in noisy environments, for obese patients, and for care providers who have a hearing impairment.

■ ✦ **To prevent injury,** do not wear a stethoscope around your neck.

■ **To prevent cross-contamination,** always clean your stethoscope before and after using it to examine a patient.

Use a 70% isopropyl alcohol, sodium hypochlorite, or benzalkonium chloride wipe. Alcohol pads are highly recommended because in addition to cleaning, they do not damage the rubber components (Littman/3M, 2022). To inhibit recontamination of stethoscope membranes, some researchers also recommend using chlorhexidine (Alvarez et al., 2016; Napolitani et al., 2020).

What Sites Should I Use?

Nurses assess the pulse at the apex of the heart (**apical pulse**) or at a place where an artery can be pressed by the fingers against a bone (**peripheral pulses**). Peripheral sites are shown in Figure 18-5.

The choice of pulse site depends on the reason for assessing the pulse and/or the accessibility of a site. You would, for example, use the:

■ *Radial artery* for routine assessment of vital signs. This is the most used site because it is easily found and readily accessible.
■ *Brachial artery* when performing cardiopulmonary resuscitation (CPR) of infants
■ *Carotid artery* during CPR of adults and for assessing circulation to the brain

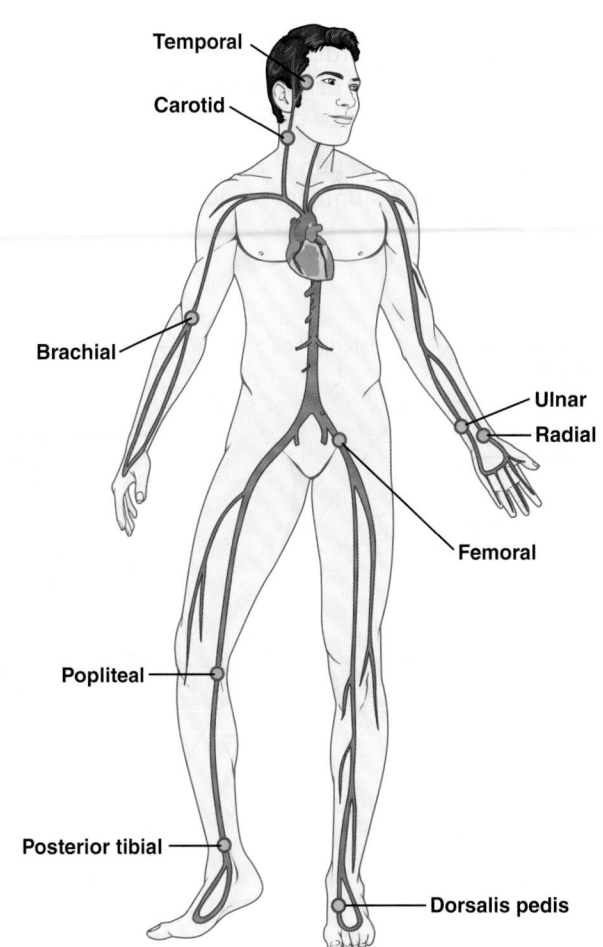

FIGURE 18-5 Sites commonly used for assessing a pulse.

- *Temporal artery* when assessing circulation to the head or when other sites are not easily accessible
- *Dorsalis pedis* (also called *pedal pulse*) and *posterior tibial arteries* for assessing peripheral circulation to the feet and legs
- *Femoral artery* to determine circulation to the legs and for children
- *Popliteal artery* for assessing circulation to the lower leg

ThinkLike a Nurse 18-4: Clinical Judgment in Action

- If you obtain a very slow radial pulse, how might you check to be sure your count is accurate?
- What kind of nursing knowledge does this require (i.e., theoretical, practical, self, or ethical)?

When Should I Take an Apical Pulse? Key Point: *The apical pulse reading is the most accurate of the pulses.* In a healthy person, the apical and peripheral pulses should be about the same rate. However, in some cardiovascular diseases, they can differ. If the heartbeat is weak, for example, some beats may be too weak to feel in a peripheral site. In this case, you would obtain a lower count for the radial than for the apical pulse. Use the apical site when:

- The radial pulse is weak or irregular.
- The rate is less than 60 beats/min or greater than 100 beats/min.
- The patient is taking cardiac medications (e.g., digitalis).
- The patient is an infant or is a child up to age 3 (because peripheral pulses may be difficult to palpate).

For children, the location is different, depending on age (Fig. 18-6). For a summary of steps for assessing an

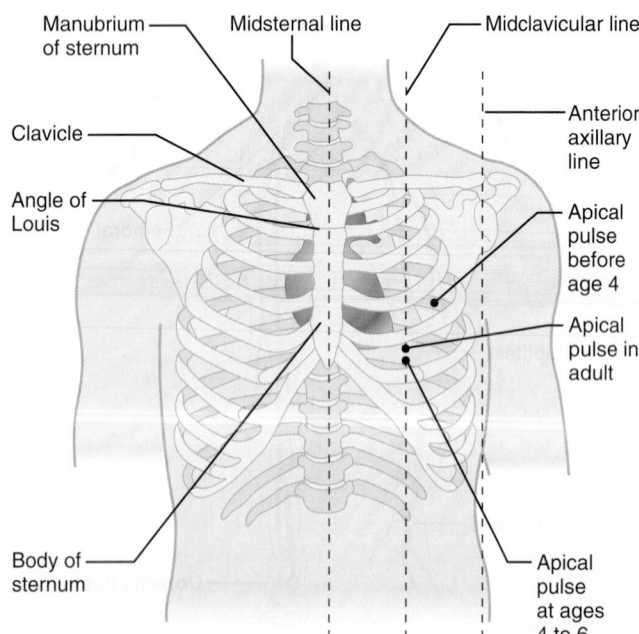

FIGURE 18-6 Location of apical pulse for adults and children.

Labels in figure: Manubrium of sternum — Midsternal line — Midclavicular line — Anterior axillary line — Clavicle — Angle of Louis — Apical pulse before age 4 — Apical pulse in adult — Body of sternum — Apical pulse at ages 4 to 6

apical pulse, see the Highlights of Procedures box. For step-by-step instructions,

 Go to **Chapter 18, Procedure 18-3: Assessing the Apical Pulse,** in Volume 2.

When Should I Take an Apical-Radial Pulse? You will sometimes need to obtain a radial and apical pulse reading at the same time to assess for heart function or the presence of heart irregularities. A difference between the two counts **(pulse deficit)** indicates that not all apex beats are being transmitted or felt at the radial artery. As you are listening at the apical site, you will hear a beat without feeling a pulse at the radial artery. You may detect a pulse deficit in conditions that interfere with peripheral perfusion, such as atrial fibrillation. You should promptly report pulse deficits to the primary care provider. See the Highlights of Procedures box for a summary; for step-by-step instructions,

 Go to **Chapter 18, Procedure 18-4: Assessing for an Apical-Radial Pulse Deficit,** in Volume 2.

KnowledgeCheck 18-2

For each of the following, would you expect the pulse rate to be greater or less than the normal adult rate of 80 beats/min?

- A healthy, professional tennis player
- A newborn infant
- An adolescent who has just finished running track
- A patient who has just undergone a painful procedure
- A patient with a fever
- An accident victim who is hemorrhaging
- A 90-year-old male patient

What Data Should I Collect?

You will need data about three characteristics of the patient's pulse: rate, rhythm, and quality.

Pulse Rate

To assess the pulse **rate,** count the number of beats per minute while palpating or auscultating. Begin the count with a beat that is counted as zero (Centers for Disease Control and Prevention [CDC], 2022); however, because of discrepancies in the literature, follow your agency's policy.

- **For normal, healthy adults,** you can determine the rate of a regular heart rhythm by counting the pulse for 15 seconds and multiplying the result by 4 or 30 seconds and then multiplying by 2.
- **If the pulse is irregular or slow,** always count for 1 full minute.

Table 18-1 identifies average pulse rates for adults, and Table 18-2 provides pulse rates for other age-groups.

- **Bradycardia** (*brady* = slow, *cardia* = heart)—Rates below 60 beats/min
- **Tachycardia** (*tachy* = rapid, *cardia* = heart)—Rates over 100 beats/min

Pulse Rhythm

The intervals between heartbeats establish a pattern known as the **rhythm.** Normally, the heart beats at regular intervals, much like a metronome. When the intervals between beats vary enough to be noticeable, the rhythm is abnormal (**dysrhythmia**). Abnormal rhythms may be (a) single beats that occur too early or too late or (b) a group of irregular beats that form a pattern. When assessing an irregular pulse, it is important to determine whether the beat is *regularly irregular* (an irregular rhythm that forms a pattern) or *irregularly irregular* (an unpredictable rhythm). To make this distinction, you must count the rate for a full minute. An irregular heart rhythm can be very serious and may require additional assessment by **electrocardiogram (ECG),** a procedure that traces the electrical pattern of the heart.

Pulse Quality

The quality of the pulse is assessed by determining the pulse volume and bilateral (both sides) equality of pulses.

Pulse Volume This refers to the amount of force produced by the blood pulsing through the arteries. Normally, the pulse volume for each beat is the same.

- The following terminology refers to the characteristics of the pulse volume; the numbers are assigned on a scale of 0 to 3.

0—Absent: Pulse cannot be felt.
1—Weak or thready: Pulse is barely felt and can be easily obliterated by pressing with the fingers.
2—Normal quality: Pulse is easily palpated, not weak or bounding.
3—Bounding or full: Pulse is easily felt with little pressure; not easily obliterated.

Bilateral Equality Bilateral equality is useful in determining whether the blood flow to a body part is adequate.

- Assess bilateral equality by comparing the pulses on both sides of the body for equal volume. For example, if you are concerned about the circulation to the left hand, assess both the right and left radial arteries to determine whether the volume is the same.
  - **If the pulses feel the same,** they are said to be *equal in strength bilaterally.*
  - **If one pulse is stronger than the other,** then the pulses are *unequal bilaterally.* You would record, "Radial pulses unequal in strength bilaterally; weaker in left arm." You may also document the equality by using a pulse volume scale. For example, you might record, "Radial pulses unequal in strength bilaterally; Right 2, Left 1."

Absent or Weak Pulse If a peripheral pulse is absent or weak, it may be because the circulation is compromised in that extremity. Assess for pallor or cyanosis to confirm this.

- **Cyanosis** is a bluish or grayish discoloration of the skin resulting from deficient oxygen in the blood.

- **Pallor** refers to the paleness of skin in one area compared with another part of the body. For example, when circulation to the lower extremities is compromised, the feet often appear pale in comparison with the trunk or arms, and the feet may feel cool to the touch. In addition, the dorsalis pedis and/or posterior tibial pulses may be weak or absent.

NURSING DIAGNOSIS/ANALYZING CUES

Pulse changes are symptoms, not problems. Therefore, nursing diagnoses are useful for describing the condition that is *causing* the pulse changes.

- **Tissue Perfusion Alteration (Peripheral)** can be used when a pulse is absent or weak and cool, pale skin is present.
- **Skin Integrity Impairment Risk** and **Risk for Impaired Tissue Integrity** may be used as secondary diagnoses when Ineffective Tissue Perfusion is present. If tissue is not adequately perfused, tissue ischemia and *necrosis* (death of tissue) may occur.
- **Fluid Volume Deficient** may cause the pulse to be weak and thready.
- **Fluid Volume Excess** may cause the pulse to be bounding and full.
- **Cardiac Output Alteration.** A decrease may cause tachycardia, bradycardia, or changes in pulse volume.

NOTE: *By itself, a change in pulse (e.g., weak and thready) is not adequate to support the preceding diagnoses. Other symptoms must also be present (e.g., fatigue, delayed capillary refill).*

PLANNING/PRIORITIZING HYPOTHESES AND GENERATION SOLUTIONS

Nursing Outcomes Classification (NOC) standardized outcomes include the following:

- Vital Signs Status is the only outcome that directly pertains to assessing the pulse.
- Other outcomes depend on the nursing diagnosis causing the pulse changes. For example, Ineffective Peripheral Tissue Perfusion can be monitored with the NOC label of Circulation Status.

Some *individualized goal/outcome statements* you might write for pulse status follow:

- Apical pulse 60 to 80 beats/min when at rest.
- Pedal pulses 80 to 100 beats/min, 2 (on a scale of 0 to 3), and equal bilaterally.

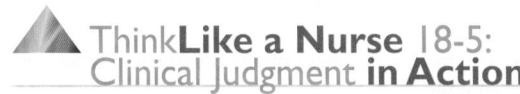

ThinkLike a Nurse 18-5:
Clinical Judgment **in Action**

Did you notice that the pulse rates in the preceding two goals are not the same as the full normal range shown in Table 18-1? What do you think might be a reason for this?

IMPLEMENTATION/TAKING ACTION

Nursing Interventions Classification (NIC) standardized interventions include the following examples:

- Dysrhythmia Management, which applies to monitoring an abnormal pulse
- Vital Signs Monitoring, which may be used for general evaluation of patients who do not have an identified problem with the pulse.

Specific nursing activities and focused assessments for a patient with a dysrhythmia depend on the cause of the problem and on specific prescriptions from the provider. For example, a patient with a pulse rate of 50 beats/min is usually considered to have bradycardia. However, such a slow resting heart rate would be perfectly normal for a well-trained athlete. Some dysrhythmias are *benign;* that is, they are not dangerous to the patient and require no interventions.

Nursing strategies that address dysrhythmias, regardless of cause, include the following:

- **Closely monitor the patient's vital signs**. A reduced heart rate may alter BP and tissue perfusion. The extent of intervention depends on the effect of the dysrhythmia on the patient's other vital signs.
- **Monitor the patient's activity tolerance**. Degree of activity, orientation, and level of fatigue while the dysrhythmia is present are indicators of the patient's ability to tolerate the dysrhythmia. Monitor vital signs before, during, and after activity.
- **Collect and assess laboratory data as prescribed**. Cardiac function depends on normal electrolyte balance, particularly potassium, calcium, and magnesium levels. If a patient is receiving medications that affect cardiac rhythm, serum levels of these medications must be checked periodically.
- **Help determine the cause of the dysrhythmia.** Determine when the patient experiences the dysrhythmia. Are there precipitating or alleviating factors?
- **Administer antidysrhythmic medications.** These are prescribed to control the heart rhythm.
- ♥ **iCare** ▪ **Provide emotional support.** The patient experiencing a dysrhythmia may be frightened by the experience. Explain all procedures to the patient and maintain a calm presence. Family members may also be frightened. Be sure to include them in your explanations and teaching.

▲ ThinkLike a Nurse 18-6: Clinical Judgment in Action

- Which of the following findings should be referred to the primary healthcare provider so that an ECG can be prescribed? Why?
  Patient A, who has a radial pulse of 100 beats/min, regular, and equal bilaterally
  Patient B, who has a regular apical pulse of 100 beats/min
  Patient C, who has a very irregular apical pulse of 78 beats/min

- Recall the patients in the Meet Your Patients scenario. Ms. Sharma is an active 80-year-old woman who works part-time and exercises four times per week. She is complaining of feeling tired. You find that her pulse is irregular and uneven.
  What other patient data do you need to know? How would you go about getting this additional information?
  What actions should you consider taking while meeting with Ms. Sharma?
  What theoretical knowledge (rationale) supports your beliefs and actions?

RESPIRATION

Respiration is the exchange of oxygen and carbon dioxide in the body. The process of respiration has two aspects: mechanical and chemical.

- **Mechanical.** The mechanical aspects of respirations involve the active movement of air into and out of the respiratory system. This is known as **pulmonary ventilation** or, more commonly, *breathing.*
- **Chemical.** The chemical aspects of respiration include the following:
  External respiration—The exchange of oxygen and carbon dioxide between the alveoli and the pulmonary blood supply.
  Gas transport—The transport of these gases throughout the body.
  Internal respiration—The exchange of these gases between the capillaries and body tissue cells.

This chapter focuses on the mechanical aspects of respiration. Chapters 33 and 34 explore gas exchange and transport throughout the body.

TheoreticalKnowledge knowing why

To assess and support patients' respirations, you will need to know the normal range of respiratory rates, how respiration is regulated, the mechanics of breathing, and factors that affect respiration.

What Is a Normal Respiratory Rate?

Respiratory rate normally varies with age, exertion, emotions, and other factors. Normal adult respirations are identified in Table 18-1, and normal respiratory rates at other developmental stages are shown in Table 18-2.

How Does the Body Regulate Respiration?

Special respiratory centers in the medulla oblongata and pons of the brain, along with nerve fibers of the autonomic nervous system, regulate breathing in response to minute changes in the concentrations of oxygen (O_2) and carbon dioxide (CO_2) in the arterial blood.

Key Point: *The primary stimulus for breathing is the level of CO₂ tension in the blood.*

- **Central chemoreceptors,** located in the respiratory centers, are sensitive to CO_2 and hydrogen ion (pH) concentrations. Minor increases in either stimulate respirations.
- **Peripheral chemoreceptors** are located in the carotid and aortic bodies. The partial pressure of oxygen in arterial blood (Pao₂) is normally between 80 and 100. When the Pao₂ falls below normal, peripheral chemoreceptors stimulate respirations.

Usually, breathing is an involuntary action that requires little effort. However, it is possible to exert conscious control over respiration (e.g., a young child holding their breath during a temper tantrum; a person holding their breath when swimming).

What Are the Mechanics of Breathing?

Pulmonary ventilation depends on changes in the capacity of the chest cavity (Fig. 18-7).

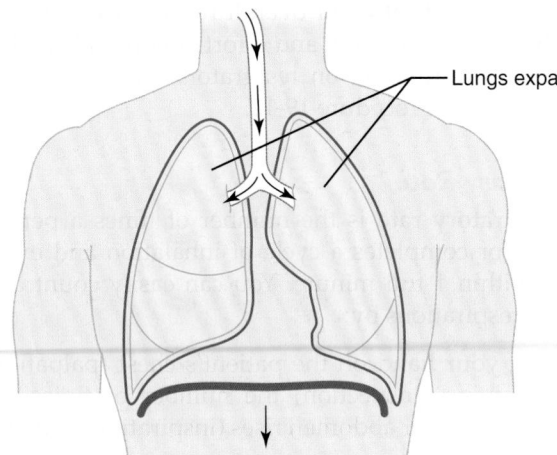

A During inspiration (diaphragm contracting)

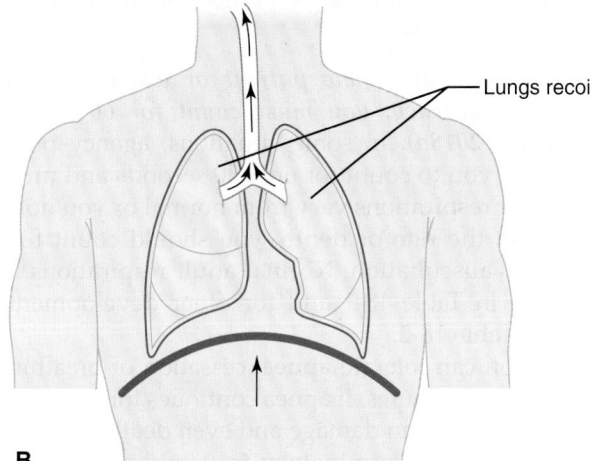

B
During expiration (diaphragm relaxing)

FIGURE 18-7 Changes in thoracic cavity during inspiration and expiration. (A) During inspiration. (B) During expiration.

Inspiration In response to impulses sent from the respiratory center along the phrenic nerve, the thoracic muscles and the diaphragm contract. The ribs move upward from midline ½ to 1 inch (1.2 to 2.5 cm), the diaphragm moves downward and out about 0.4 inch (1 cm), and the abdominal organs move downward and forward, expanding the thorax in all directions. As expansion causes airway pressure to decrease below atmospheric pressure, air moves into and expands the lungs. This stage of respiration (drawing air into the lungs) is termed **inspiration.**

Expiration When the diaphragm and thoracic muscles relax, the chest cavity decreases in size, and the lungs recoil, forcing air from the lungs until the pressure within the lungs again reaches atmospheric pressure. This stage, which involves the expulsion of air from the lungs, is called **expiration.** Expiration is passive and normally takes 2 to 3 seconds, compared with 1 to 1.5 seconds for inspiration. During normal breathing, the chest wall and abdomen gently rise and fall.

KnowledgeCheck 18-3

- Which two gases are exchanged through respiration?
- Which respiratory process involves the movement of air into and out of the lungs?
- What is external respiration?
- What is the primary stimulus for breathing?
- What mechanical forces allow the lungs to expand?

What Factors Influence Respiration?

Key Point: *A change in respiratory rate/altered breathing frequency is an early indication of clinical deterioration in patients. Therefore, you must conduct further assessments to formulate hypotheses about contributing factors.*

To interpret the meaning of your patients' respiratory data, you need to be aware of factors that influence breathing.

- **Developmental level.** A newborn's respiratory rate usually ranges from 40 to 60 breaths/min. However, some references give an upper limit of 90 breaths/min so long as it is for a short period of time (transient tachypnea). The rate gradually decreases until it reaches the normal adult rate of 12 to 20 breaths per minute. The respiratory rate decreases slightly in older adults.

  Respirations, often thought of as the forgotten vital sign (Nicolò et al., 2020; Sapra, 2022), provide essential information on your patient. In older adults, respiratory rates greater than 28 beats/min are considered tachypneic (Charilaos & Bhardwaj, 2019). You should conduct a more assessment of older adults to identify other cues of adverse events.

- **Exercise.** Muscular activity causes a temporary increase in respiratory rate and depth to increase oxygen availability to the tissues and rid the body of excess carbon dioxide.

- **Pain**. Acute pain causes an increase in respiratory rate but a decrease in depth.
- **Stress**. Psychological stress, such as anxiety or fear, may markedly influence respiration due to sympathetic stimulation. The most common change is an increase in rate.
- **Smoking**. Chronic smoking increases the resting respiratory rate because of changes in airway compliance (elasticity).
- **Fever**. When heart rate increases because of fever, the respiratory rate also increases. For every 1°F (0.6°C) the temperature rises, the respiratory rate may increase up to 4 breaths/min.
- **Hemoglobin**. Respiratory rate and depth increase as a result of anemia (reduced hemoglobin), sickle cell anemia (abnormally shaped red blood cells), and high altitudes. When hemoglobin is decreased or abnormal, the rate and depth of respirations, as well as the heart rate, may increase to maintain adequate tissue oxygenation. High altitudes inhibit the binding of oxygen to hemoglobin and trigger similar compensatory efforts.
- **Disease**. The rate of breathing may be increased or decreased by various diseases. For example, brainstem injuries and increased intracranial pressure may interfere with the respiratory center, inhibiting respirations or altering respiratory rhythm.
- **Medications**. Central nervous system depressants, such as morphine or general anesthetics, cause slower, deeper respirations. Caffeine and atropine can cause shallow, fast breathing.
- **Position**. Standing up maximizes respiratory depth; lying flat reduces respiratory depth. Slumping (sitting with shoulders forward and the back curved in a C shape) prevents chest expansion, which impedes breathing.

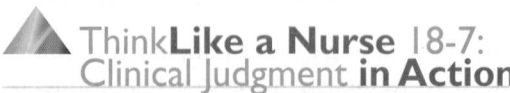

ThinkLike a Nurse 18-7:
Clinical Judgment in Action

Consider the following patient situations. What effect would they have on respirations?

- A patient with four fractured ribs
- A patient who is 9 months pregnant
- A young child excited at their birthday party
- An adult who has consumed alcoholic beverages

PracticalKnowledge
knowing **how**

Although you may assess the adequacy of external and internal respiration in various ways, it is pulmonary ventilation (breathing) that you assess as a vital sign. Accurate assessment of respirations depends on your ability to recognize normal breathing, abnormal breathing, and factors that affect breathing. This chapter discusses only assessment of respirations and analysis/diagnosis. For outcomes and interventions for respiratory problems, see Chapter 33.

ASSESSMENT

Because people can control their breathing rate, it is best to count respirations when the patient is unaware of what you are doing. One way to do this is to palpate and count the radial pulse and then count the respirations before removing your fingers from the patient's wrist. For a summary of the procedure, see the Highlights of Procedures box. For the entire sequence of steps,

Go to **Chapter 18, Procedure 18-5: Assessing Respirations**, in Volume 2.

What Equipment Do I Need?
- For measuring respiratory rate—a watch with a second hand or digital display
- For auscultating respirations—a stethoscope
- Many electronic thermometers have counter displays and signals that indicate 15-, 30-, and 60-second time intervals for counting respirations.

What Data Should I Obtain?

In addition to measuring the respiratory rate, you will also observe indicators of overall respiratory function, including depth, rhythm, and effort, among others. For additional information on respiratory assessment, see Chapter 19 and Procedure 19-12.

Respiratory Rate

The **respiratory rate** is the number of times a person breathes (or completes a cycle of inhalation and exhalation) within 1 full minute. You can easily count and observe respirations by:

- Placing your hand on the patient's chest (palpation) or observing (inspection) the number of times the patient's chest or abdomen rises (inspiration) and falls (expiration)
- Placing your stethoscope on the patient's chest (auscultation) and counting the number of inhalation and exhalation cycles.

Key Point: *For a new patient or when you need to ensure accuracy, you must count for 60 seconds (Wheatley, 2018a).* In some situations, agency policy may allow you to count for only 30 seconds and multiply by 2. If respirations vary from normal or you notice changes in the rate or depth, you should count for 1 minute by auscultation. Normal adult respirations are identified in Table 18-1 and for other developmental stages in Table 18-2.

A person can tolerate **apnea**, cessation of breathing, for only a few minutes. If apnea continues for more than 4 to 6 minutes, brain damage and even death can occur. See Table 18-5 for terminology to describe respiratory rhythms.

Key Point: *Respiratory rate is a measure of the patient's general condition, but rate alone is not a good*

Table 18-5 ➤ Respiratory Rates and Rhythm

TYPE	DESCRIPTION	ILLUSTRATION
Eupnea	Normal respirations, with equal rate and depth, 12–20 breaths/min	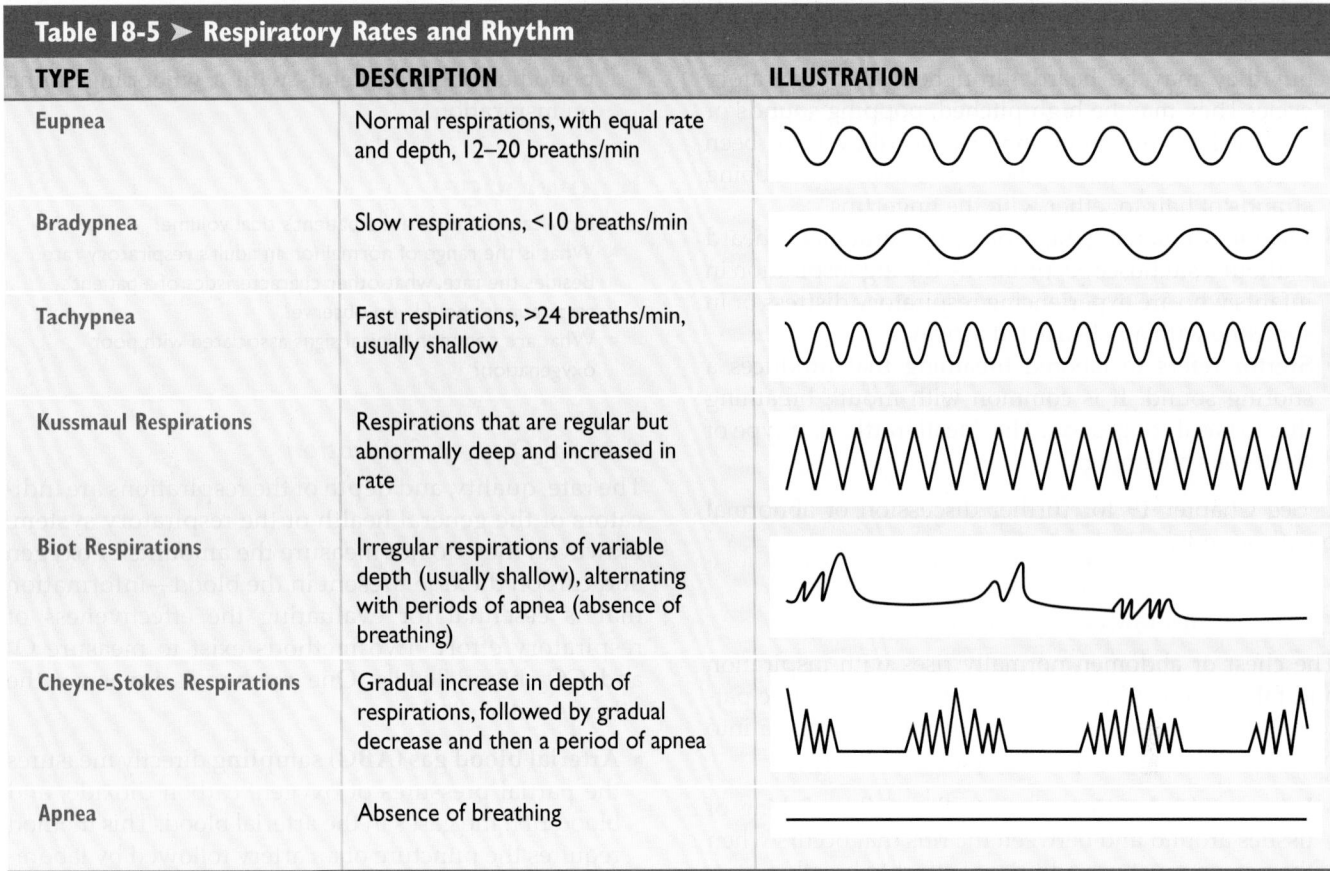
Bradypnea	Slow respirations, <10 breaths/min	
Tachypnea	Fast respirations, >24 breaths/min, usually shallow	
Kussmaul Respirations	Respirations that are regular but abnormally deep and increased in rate	
Biot Respirations	Irregular respirations of variable depth (usually shallow), alternating with periods of apnea (absence of breathing)	
Cheyne-Stokes Respirations	Gradual increase in depth of respirations, followed by gradual decrease and then a period of apnea	
Apnea	Absence of breathing	

indicator of the adequacy of respiration. You must also assess other characteristics of the respirations.

Respiratory Depth

Tidal volume is the amount of air taken in on inspiration—about 300 to 500 mL for a healthy adult. Specialized equipment is required to measure tidal volume. However, you can estimate the adequacy of tidal volume by observing the depth of a patient's respirations. This is a subjective evaluation of how much or how little the chest or abdomen rises during breathing. Respiratory depth is described as:

- **Deep**—Taking in a very large volume of air and fully expanding one's chest or abdomen)
- **Shallow**—When the chest barely rises and is difficult to observe
- **Normal**—Falling between shallow and deep

Respiratory Rhythm

Rhythm is assessed simply as *regular* or *irregular*. Generally, the period between each respiratory cycle is the same, and there is a regular breathing pattern (see "Eupnea" in Table 18-5). Infant breathing rhythms are more likely to be irregular than adult rhythms. An abnormal breathing pattern may indicate other healthcare problems and deserves further assessment. Two abnormal breathing patterns, Cheyne–Stokes and Biot breathing, are discussed in Chapter 33.

Respiratory Effort

Respiratory effort refers to the degree of work required to breathe. Normal breathing is effortless. When diseases such as asthma or pneumonia are present, the person must work harder to breathe.

- **Dyspnea** is increased effort with breathing or labored breathing.
- **Orthopnea** is difficulty or inability to breathe when in a horizontal position. You will observe this in some patients with respiratory or cardiac conditions.

♥ **iCare** Breathing difficulties are uncomfortable for the patient and frequently produce fear, anxiety, and fatigue. Remain with the patient, initiate actions to improve breathing (e.g., positioning, respiratory treatment), and speak to the patient in a low and calming voice.

Breath Sounds

You will use a stethoscope to listen for breath sounds. Normal respirations are quiet. Abnormal (adventitious) sounds include the following:

- **Wheezes** are high-pitched, continuous musical sounds, usually heard on expiration. They are caused by narrowing of the airways. Wheezes can often be heard without a stethoscope.
- **Rhonchi** are low-pitched, continuous gurgling sounds caused by secretions in the large airways. They often clear with coughing.

- **Crackles** are caused by fluid in the alveoli. They are discontinuous sounds usually heard on inspiration, but they may be heard throughout the respiratory cycle. They may be high-pitched, popping sounds or low-pitched, bubbling sounds, and they have been described as similar to the sound made by rubbing strands of hair together with the fingertips.
- **Stridor** is a piercing, high-pitched sound that is heard without a stethoscope, primarily during inspiration in infants who are experiencing respiratory distress or in someone with an obstructed airway.
- **Stertor** refers to labored breathing that produces a snoring sound. It is common with mouth breathing due to nasal congestion. The "death rattle" is a type of stertorous breathing.

See Chapter 19 for further discussion of abnormal breath sounds.

Chest and Abdomen Movement

The chest or abdomen normally rises with inspiration and falls with expiration in a gentle and rhythmic pattern. When a person is having difficulty moving air into or out of the lungs, respiratory patterns change.

- **Intercostal retraction** refers to the visible sinking of tissues around and between the ribs that occurs when the person must use additional effort to breathe.
- **Substernal retraction** exists when tissues are drawn in beneath the sternum (breastbone).
- **Suprasternal retraction** exists when tissues are drawn in above the clavicle (shoulder girdle).

Associated Clinical Signs

When you assess respiration, it is important to assess for clinical signs of oxygenation.

- **Hypoxia**—Signs of **hypoxia** (inadequate cellular oxygenation) include pallor or cyanosis, restlessness, apprehension, confusion, dizziness, fatigue, decreased level of consciousness, tachycardia, tachypnea, and changes in BP.
  - When evaluating cyanosis, the tongue and oral mucosa are the best indicators of hypoxia.
  - Cyanosis of the nails, lips, and skin may be caused by hypoxia but may also be related to cold or reduced circulation in that area.
  - Chronic hypoxia causes **clubbing** (loss of the nail angle) of the fingers.
- **Cough**—A **cough** is a forceful or violent expulsion of air during expiration. Coughs may be symptoms of allergic reactions, lung disease, respiratory infection, or heart conditions.
  - Coughs may be *constant* (occurring frequently and consistently) or *intermittent* (occurring occasionally).
  - The cough is **productive** if secretions are expectorated (coughed up). The cough is **nonproductive** or **dry** if no secretions are produced.

- A **hacking cough** is a series of dry coughs that occur together, whereas a **whooping cough** is a sudden, periodic cough that ends with a whooping sound on inspiration.

KnowledgeCheck 18-4

- How can you estimate a patient's tidal volume?
- What is the range of normal for an adult's respiratory rate?
- Besides the rate, what other characteristics of a patient's respirations should you observe?
- What are common clinical signs associated with poor oxygenation?

Arterial Oxygen Saturation

The rate, quality, and depth of the respirations are indicators of the general health of the respiratory system. However, they do not measure the amounts of oxygen and carbon dioxide present in the blood—information that is essential for evaluating the effectiveness of respiratory effort. Two methods exist to measure O_2 and CO_2 blood levels. One method is invasive; the other is not.

- **Arterial blood gas (ABG) sampling** directly measures the partial pressures of oxygen, carbon dioxide, and blood pH, the gases in the arterial blood. This method requires the puncture of an artery followed by laboratory testing of the sample. It provides comprehensive data, but it is invasive, painful, time consuming, and relatively expensive. If you need more information about this diagnostic test, consult a medical–surgical nursing or laboratory tests text.
- **Pulse oximetry** is a noninvasive method of monitoring oxygenation with a device that measures **oxygen saturation** (an indication of the oxygen being carried by hemoglobin in the arterial blood). The oximeter emits light, and a photosensor placed on the patient's finger or earlobe measures the light passing through the site and calculates a pulse saturation (SpO_2) that is a good estimate of arterial oxygen saturation. The only risk in pulse oximetry is that clinicians may become too dependent on it or trust erroneous readings. Do not neglect the other aspects of a holistic respiratory assessment. In many situations, oxygen saturation is monitored routinely along with the other vital signs. To learn how to apply a pulse oximeter,

 Go to **Chapter 33, Procedure 33-2: Monitoring Pulse Oximetry**, in Volume 2.

ThinkLike a Nurse 18-8: Clinical Judgment in Action

- Mrs. Dowell has smoked two packs of cigarettes per day for 45 years. She has recently been diagnosed with pneumonia—an infection of the lungs. What vital signs assessments would be important for Mrs. Dowell, and why?
- Recall the patients in the Meet Your Patients scenario. Mr. Jackson is short of breath and struggling to breathe. His

respiratory rate is 28 breaths/min. What else do you need to know about the patient situation? What is important and what is not important in this scenario?

NURSING DIAGNOSIS/ANALYZING CUES

As noted earlier, *hypoxia* refers to inadequate cellular oxygenation. It results from decreased oxygen intake, decreased ability of tissues to remove oxygen from the blood, impaired ventilation or perfusion, impaired gas exchange between the blood and alveoli, or inadequate levels of hemoglobin. The following are two common alterations in respiration:

- **Hyperventilation** occurs when rapid and deep breathing results in excess loss of CO_2 **(hypocapnia).** A patient who is hyperventilating may complain of feeling lightheaded and tingly. Causes of hyperventilation include anxiety, infection, shock, hypoxia, drugs (e.g., aspirin, amphetamines), diabetes mellitus, and acid–base imbalance.
- **Hypoventilation** occurs when the rate and depth of respirations are decreased, and CO_2 is retained or alveolar ventilation is compromised. Hypoventilation may be related to chronic obstructive pulmonary disease, general anesthesia, impending respiratory failure, or other conditions that result in decreased respirations.

Two nursing diagnoses commonly used to describe various respiratory problems are Impaired Gas Exchange and Ineffective Breathing Patterns. For a more complete list, see Chapter 33.

BLOOD PRESSURE

BP is the pressure of the blood as it is forced against arterial walls during cardiac contraction.

- **Systolic pressure** is the peak pressure exerted against arterial walls as the ventricles contract and eject blood.
- **Diastolic pressure** is the minimum pressure exerted against arterial walls, between cardiac contractions when the heart is at rest.

Adequate BP is essential for healthy tissue perfusion and is an important indicator of overall cardiovascular health. BP is measured in millimeters of mercury (mm Hg) and is recorded as systolic pressure over diastolic pressure (e.g., 110/74 mm Hg).

Pulse Pressure Pulse pressure is the difference between the systolic and diastolic pressures. For a BP of 120/80 mm Hg, the pulse pressure is 40 mm Hg. It is an indication of the volume output of the left ventricle. Generally, the pulse pressure should be no greater than one-third of the systolic pressure, as in the example of a BP of 120/80 mm Hg, with a pulse pressure of 40 (⅓ × 120 = 40). Pulse pressure provides an indicator of heart health. A high pulse pressure may be a predictor of heart attacks or atherosclerosis, whereas a low pulse pressure can indicate poor heart functioning (Mankad, 2022).

KnowledgeCheck 18-5
- For a patient whose BP is 150/80 mm Hg, what is the pulse pressure?
- Is that normal? If so, explain. If not, what should the pulse pressure be?

TheoreticalKnowledge
knowing **why**

To assess and support patients' BP, you will need to understand how the concepts of systolic and diastolic BP contribute to **tissue perfusion**.

1. Contraction of the heart (systolic pressure) forces a bolus of oxygenated blood into the arterial circulation to provide a continuous supply of oxygen to all body cells *(perfusion)*.
2. The heart then rests and refills with blood (diastolic pressure), which is pumped out to the tissues.
3. Any factor that interferes with this cycle can cause impaired tissue perfusion.

You will also need to know that an expert panel has classified a normal BP and the stages of hypertension (Whelton et al., 2018).

How Are Blood Pressure Readings Categorized?

The 2017 guidelines on the prevention, detection, evaluation, and treatment of high BP classify a "normal" BP as a systolic BP of <120 and a diastolic BP of <80. Table 18-6 identifies the classification of adult BP and the corresponding treatment.

How Does the Body Regulate Blood Pressure?

BP regulation is a highly complex process. It is influenced by three factors: cardiac function, peripheral vascular resistance, and blood volume. The body constantly regulates and adjusts arterial pressure to supply blood to body tissues via perfusion of the capillary beds. For an in-depth discussion, see Chapter 34.

Cardiac Function

Recall that **cardiac output** is the volume of blood pumped by the heart per minute, and it reflects the functioning of the heart. An increase in cardiac output causes an increase in BP; a decrease in cardiac output causes a decrease in BP (if all other factors remain the same). A change in either stroke volume or heart rate alters cardiac output.

Increased Stroke Volume Conditions that increase cardiac output by increasing stroke volume include the following:

- Increased blood volume (e.g., as occurs during pregnancy)

Table 18-6 ➤ Classification of Adult Blood Pressure (BP)*

CATEGORY	SYSTOLIC (mm Hg)		DIASTOLIC (mm Hg)	FOLLOW-UP
Normal	<120	and	<80	Encourage lifestyle modification if there are risk factors. Recheck in 1–2 years or sooner if there are risk factors.
Elevated	120–129	and	≤80	Encourage lifestyle changes. Recheck in 3–6 months of nonpharmacologic therapy.
Stage I Hypertension	130–139	or	80–89	**Low atherosclerotic cardiovascular disease (ASCVD):** Encourage lifestyle changes. Recheck in 3–6 months of nonpharmacologic therapy. **High ASCVD:** Manage with both nonpharmacologic and antihypertensive drug therapy with repeat BP in 1 month.
Stage II Hypertension	≥140	or	≥90	Evaluation by a primary care provider within 1 month of diagnosis; treat with nonpharmacologic therapy and two different classes of antihypertensive drugs. Recheck BP in 1 month.
Hypertensive Crisis	>180	and/or	>120	Consult your provider immediately.

Note: If systolic BP and diastolic BP fall within two categories, classify based on the higher category.
Source: Data from Whelton, P., Carey, R. M., Aronow, W. S., Casey, D. E. Jr, Collins, K. J., Dennison Himmelfarb, C., DePalma, S. M., Gidding, S., Jamerson, K.A., Jones, D.W., MacLaughlin, E. J., Muntner, P., Ovbiagele, B., Smith, S. C. Jr, Spencer, C. C., Stafford, R. S., Taler, S. J., Thomas, R. J., Williams, K.A. Sr, ... Wright, J.T. (2017). 2017 ACC/AHA/AAPA/ABC/ACPM/AGS/APhA/ASH/ASPC/NMA/PCNA guideline for the prevention, detection, evaluation, and management of high blood pressure in adults: A report of the American College of Cardiology/American Heart Association Task Force on Clinical Practice Guidelines. Hypertension, 71(6), e13–e115. https://doi.org/10.1161/HYP.0000000000000065; Whelton, P., Carey, R. M., Aronow, W. S., Casey, D. E. Jr, Collins, K. J., Dennison Himmelfarb, C., DePalma, S. M., Gidding, S., Jamerson, K.A., Jones, D.W., MacLaughlin, E. J., Muntner, P., Ovbiagele, B., Smith, S. C. Jr Spencer, C. C., Stafford, R. S., Taler, S. J., Thomas, R. J., Williams, K.A. Sr, ... Wright, J.T. (2018). 2017 ACC/AHA/AAPA/ABC/ACPM/AGS/APhA/ASH/ASPC/NMA/PCNA guideline for the prevention, detection, evaluation, and management of high blood pressure in adults. Journal of the American College of Cardiology, 71(19), e127–e248. https://doi.org/10.1016/j.jacc.2017.11.006

- More forceful contraction of the ventricles (e.g., as occurs during exercise)

Decreased Stroke Volume Conditions that decrease cardiac output by decreasing stroke volume include the following:

- Dehydration
- Active bleeding
- Damage to the heart (as seen after myocardial infarction, or heart attack)
- A very rapid heart rate (up to a point). Although an increase in heart rate increases cardiac output, a very rapid heart rate limits the time allotted for the ventricles to fill, resulting in decreased stroke volume and, ultimately, decreased cardiac output.

Peripheral Resistance

Peripheral resistance refers to arterial and capillary resistance to blood flow as a result of friction between blood and the vessel walls. Increased peripheral resistance creates a temporary increase in BP. The amount of friction or resistance depends on blood viscosity, arterial size, and arterial compliance. The walls of the veins are thin and very distensible, so they have little influence on peripheral resistance and BP.

- **Blood Viscosity** (thickness). Blood viscosity influences the ease with which blood flows through the vessels. Viscosity is determined by the **hematocrit** (the percentage of red blood cells in plasma).
  - **High hematocrit**—elevates BP. (Any disorder that increases hematocrit [e.g., dehydration] increases blood viscosity and, therefore, BP.)
  - **Low hematocrit**—may reduce BP. (A low hematocrit, as seen in anemia, lowers viscosity and may reduce BP.)
- **Arterial Size.** The sympathetic nervous system controls vasoconstriction and vasodilation. The smaller the radius of a blood vessel, the more resistance it offers to blood flow.
  - Constricted arteries prevent the free flow of blood and, subsequently, increase BP.
  - Dilated arteries allow unrestricted flow of blood, thereby reducing BP.

■ **Arterial Compliance** (elasticity). Arteries with good elasticity can distend and recoil easily and adequately. When age- or disease-related changes in arterial structure cause a loss of elasticity, peripheral resistance, and possibly BP, increase. **Arteriosclerosis** (hardening of the arteries) is a common contributor to increased BP in middle-aged and older adults.

Blood Volume

The normal volume of blood in the body is about 5 L (5,000 mL). A significant loss of blood, as occurs with hemorrhage, reduces vascular volume, and BP falls. When vascular volume is increased above the norm, as occurs with renal (kidney) failure and fluid retention, BP increases.

What Factors Influence Blood Pressure?

Key Point: *BP normally changes from minute to minute with changes in activity or changes in body position. Therefore, you must establish BP patterns rather than relying on individual BP readings when determining whether a patient's BP is normal or abnormal.* This is even more important for older adults because their BP tends to fluctuate even more. The following are some factors that affect the BP:

■ **Developmental Stage.** The BP of an average newborn varies widely, with a systolic BP of about 60 to 90 mm Hg and a diastolic BP of 20 to 60 mm Hg (Batton, 2020; University of Iowa Children's Hospital, 2022). It increases gradually throughout childhood. A child's or adolescent's BP depends on body size; therefore, a smaller child or adolescent has a lower BP than does a larger child or adolescent. Both systolic and diastolic BP continue to increase with age as a result of decreased arterial compliance and changes in the left ventricular wall. These changes resulting from the normal aging process can lead to cardiovascular instability (Sapra et al., 2022).

■ **Sex.** The average BP for male individuals is slightly higher than that for female individuals of comparable age. After menopause, BP tends to increase in female individuals, possibly due to a decrease in estrogen.

■ **Family History.** A family history of hypertension markedly increases the likelihood of an individual's developing hypertension.

■ **Lifestyle.** Increased sodium consumption, smoking, and consumption of three or more alcoholic drinks per day have been shown to elevate BP. Caffeine may raise BP for a short while after ingestion, but it has no long-term effect on the BP.

■ **Exercise.** Physical fitness has been shown to reduce BP in many individuals. However, muscular exertion temporarily increases BP as a result of increased heart rate and cardiac output. You should therefore wait about 30 minutes before you assess the BP of someone who has been physically active.

■ **Body Position.** BP is higher when a person is standing than when they are sitting or lying down. Readings are higher if taken with the patient's arm below heart level or if the arm is unsupported at the patient's side. Seated readings are higher if the patient's feet are dangling rather than resting on the floor or if the legs are crossed.

■ **Stress.** Fear, worry, excitement, and other stressors cause BP to rise sharply because of sympathetic nervous system stimulation (fight-or-flight response). For example, "white-coat hypertension" occurs when a patient's BP is elevated in the provider's office or clinic—a situation in which they are likely to experience stress—but not at other times. However, if BP is consistently elevated with stress, treatment may be indicated.

■ **Pain.** Pain often causes an increase in BP. However, severe or prolonged pain can significantly decrease BP.

■ **Race.** Individuals who are Black have a higher rate of hypertension and a higher incidence of complications and hypertension-related deaths than other demographic groups (Whelton et al., 2018)

■ **Obesity.** As a rule, obesity increases BP due to (1) the additional vascular supply required to perfuse the large body mass and (2) the resultant increase in peripheral resistance.

■ **Diurnal Variations.** Generally, BP varies according to the person's daily schedules and routines. BP is lower while the person is sleeping and upon wakening, rises during the day, and drops again toward bedtime.

■ **Medications.** Many medications alter BP. This effect may be intended, as with antihypertensive medications, or unintended, such as the drop in BP that often results when a patient receives pain medication. ✚ Many over-the-counter preparations, herbal products, and illicit drugs can affect BP. Teach your patient to consult with a pharmacist to identify the effect these products can have when taken with regularly prescribed medications.

■ **Diseases.** BP may be affected by diseases that affect the circulatory system or any of the major organs of the body (e.g., the kidneys).

■ **Genetic Variations/Genes.** Research has shown a link between genetic factors and hypertension (CDC, 2020).

▲ ThinkLike a Nurse 18-9: Clinical Judgment in Action

■ Evaluate the following adult blood pressures. Are they high, low, or normal?
  116/90 mm Hg
  80/50 mm Hg
  184/102 mm Hg
  140/90 mm Hg
  40/0 mm Hg
■ What theoretical knowledge did you use to evaluate the blood pressures?

PracticalKnowledge
knowing **how**

Now that you understand the concept of perfusion and how BP is maintained and regulated, you are ready to gain practical knowledge of how to assess and support this aspect of physical functioning.

■ ASSESSMENT/RECOGNIZING CUES

BP may be assessed directly or indirectly.

Direct Method In the *direct method,* a catheter is threaded into an artery under sterile conditions and attached to tubing that is connected to an electronic monitoring system. The pressure is constantly displayed as a waveform on the monitor screen. This method of measuring BP is very accurate and is mostly used in critical care and surgery because of the risk of sudden arterial blood loss.

Indirect Method Usually, you will measure BP via the *indirect,* or *noninvasive method.* This provides an accurate estimate of arterial BP that can be performed in any setting. For a summary of a procedure for noninvasive BP monitoring, see the Highlights of Procedures box. For the complete procedure

 Go to **Chapter 18, Procedure 18-6: Measuring Blood Pressure,** in Volume 2.

What Equipment Do I Need?

You will need a stethoscope, a BP cuff and sphygmomanometer, or an electronic BP monitor to assess BP. Electronic monitoring is gradually replacing the stethoscope and sphygmomanometer in patient care settings. However, a common stethoscope and sphygmomanometer are sufficient to hear most patients' BPs. When BP is weak, ultrasonic stethoscopes are useful for magnifying sound waves occurring during systole.

The stethoscope can have a bell and a diaphragm or simply a diaphragm. The bell is better for transmitting lower-frequency sounds, compared with higher-frequency sounds transmitted by the diaphragm (Meyer, 2022). Most people use the diaphragm because it is easily placed and because some stethoscopes do not have a bell (see Fig. 18-4). The key to clarity of sound is to use a high-quality stethoscope with short tubing.

Sphygmomanometers A **sphygmomanometer** consists of a vinyl or cloth cuff, a pressure bulb with a regulating valve, and a manometer (Fig. 18-8). BP cuffs contain an inflatable rubber bladder. The cuff is attached to a gauge or manometer and a valved pressure bulb that inflates the bladder (Fig. 18-9). Cuffs can be placed on either the upper arm or midthigh and are supplied in various sizes.

Aneroid manometers are the type of sphygmomanometers commonly used in practice. They have dials that register BP by pointers attached to a spring.

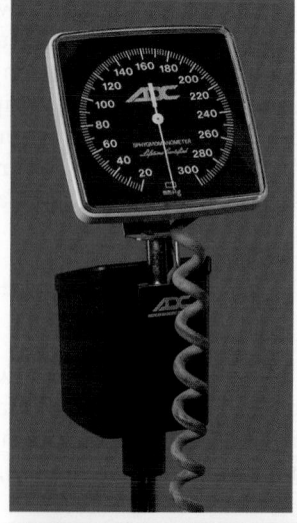

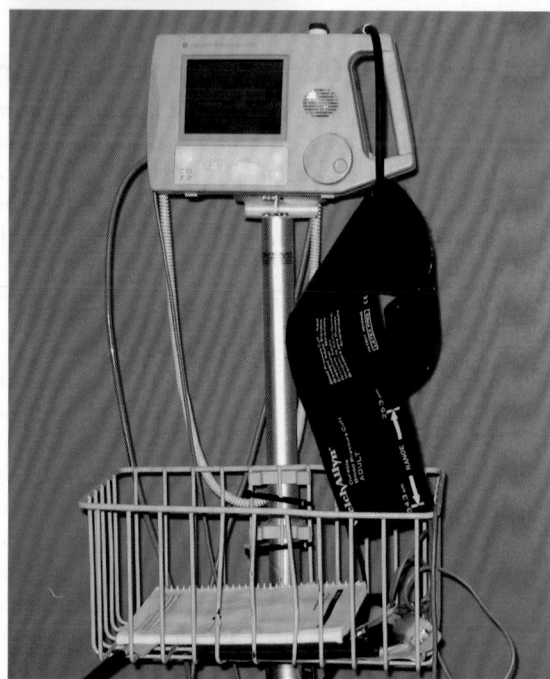

FIGURE 18-8 Types of manometers. *Top left,* Aneroid. *Bottom,* Electronic.

Mercury manometers have been eliminated in most healthcare agencies.

Electronic Blood Pressure Monitors Electronic BP monitors use either microphones to sense sounds or sensors that detect pressure waves as blood flows through arteries (Fig. 18-8, bottom). They can be set to monitor and record BP at timed intervals and do not require the use of a stethoscope. They measure systolic, diastolic, and mean arterial pressures. Electronic monitors are useful when you must monitor BP frequently (e.g., during surgery, in critical care units). To ensure accuracy, you should auscultate a baseline BP before initiating automatic monitoring. Electronic monitors may be less accurate than those with an aneroid monitor, or they may malfunction.

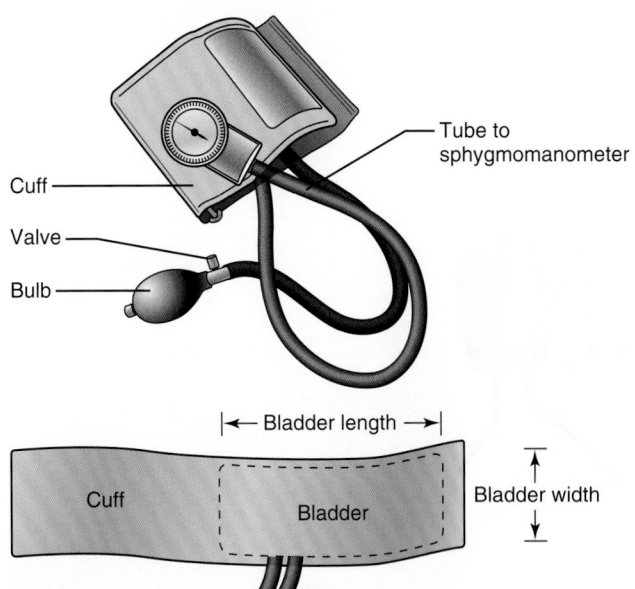

FIGURE 18-9 (A) Parts of the blood pressure cuff. (B) Placement of bladder within the cuff.

Numerous types of electronic BP monitors can be purchased for patient home use. Teach patients to know their baseline and seek follow-up care when readings are not within their normal range. See the accompanying Home Care box, Teaching Your Patient Self-Monitoring of Blood Pressure, for further topics to teach patients about using electronic BP monitors.

What Cuff Size Should I Use?

The *width* of the bladder of a properly fitting cuff will cover approximately two-thirds of the *length* of the upper arm (or other extremity) for an adult and the entire upper arm for a child (Fig. 18-10) (Mattoo, 2018; McEvoy, 2019). Alternatively, you can check that (1) the *cuff width* is 40% of the arm circumference, and (2) the *length* of the bladder encircles 80% of the arm in adults (Mishra et al., 2017).

Using a cuff or bladder of the incorrect size can result in a measurement error of as much as 30 mm Hg. If the cuff is too narrow, your reading will be too high; if it is too wide, the reading will be too low. Although cuffs are

Home Care

Teaching Your Patient Self-Monitoring of Blood Pressure (BP)

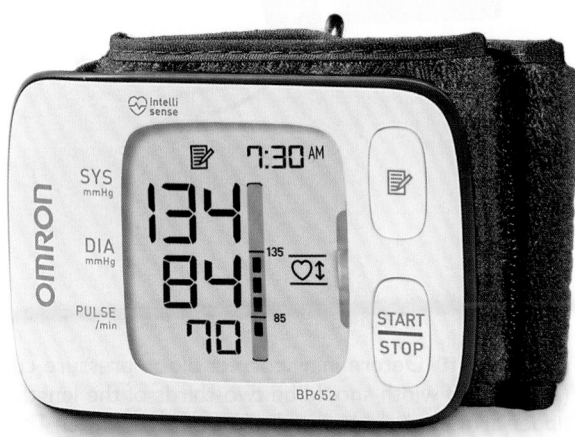

➤ With a portable home device, the patient simply pushes a button, and the cuff inflates and deflates automatically. The device provides an electronic digital readout of the BP. Because these devices are sensitive, arm movement or improper cuff placement can cause inaccurate readings.

➤ Some grocery stores, fitness clubs, and other public places have stationary automatic BP devices for public use. The machine gives a visual display of the BP reading. The accuracy of these machines varies.

Benefits of Self-Monitoring

➤ May detect high BP in those who have not previously had a problem (screening)

➤ Allows for observation of the BP *pattern* over time, rather than a one-time office reading. The results can be analyzed to distinguish "white-coat hypertension" from actual hypertension.

➤ For patients with hypertension, self-monitoring increases participation in treatment and may improve compliance with treatment.

Disadvantages of Self-Monitoring

➤ Possible incorrect use of the BP device

➤ May cause needless anxiety over a single elevated reading

➤ Patients with hypertension may make adjustments to their medications based on the BP readings without consulting their care provider.

Nursing Implications

➤ Teach proper use of the self-measurement devices.

➤ Periodically evaluate the patient's technique.

➤ Teach the meaning of BP readings and the need to look for patterns from multiple readings, not just a single reading.

➤ Explain the need for calibration of the home-monitoring device according to the manufacturer's instructions or at least twice a year. Note any differences in readings after calibration.

➤ Have the patient bring the home-monitoring device to clinical visits so that readings can be compared with simultaneously recorded auscultatory readings.

➤ Teach the patient to establish a baseline range with their healthcare provider and to have abnormally high or low readings (occurring on more than one occasion) rechecked by the provider.

➤ Advise the patient to keep a written record of BP readings, including the date and time for each, and bring it to each clinic or office visit.

Using Evidence to Support Clinical Practice

Chapter Key Concept: **Perfusion (blood pressure)**

Competency: **Validate and Incorporate Evidence-Based Research Into Practice**

Background: It is essential to measure blood pressure accurately for appropriate treatment and management (Munter et al., 2019; Park et al., 2022). Accuracy and reliability of blood pressure measurement are improved with proper patient position, arm position, and timing. Research shows a correlation between increased readings and timing of the measurement, positioning of the patient (standing versus sitting in a chair versus lying on an examining table), and positioning of the arm at the level of the heart (Jahangir, 2018; Mayo Clinic Staff, 2018; Munter et al., 2109; Whelton et al., 2018).

Scenario: A 70-year-old obese patient with a history of hypertension and peripheral vascular disease is seen in the ambulatory care setting. You are assessing their vital signs to provide data for medication management. Before taking the patient's blood pressure, you obtain an aneroid sphygmomanometer and then request the patient sit in a chair for 5 minutes, after which you ask them to extend one arm while supporting the arm at the level of the heart. Another nurse states, "You don't need to do all that."

Think about it:

➤ What factors could influence the accuracy of the blood pressure assessment in this patient?

➤ What evidence will you give the other nurse for your actions, and how will you locate best evidence to support your response?

➤ What other actions should you institute to maintain accuracy in blood pressure measurement?

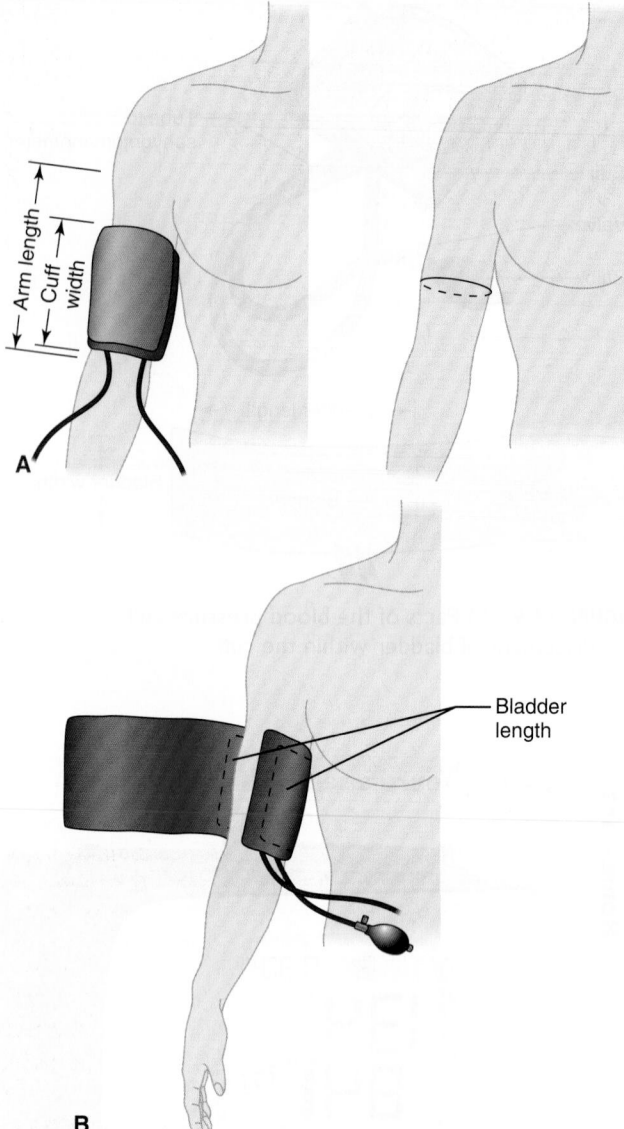

FIGURE 18-10 Determining correct blood pressure cuff size. (A) The cuff width should be two-thirds of the length of the upper arm or should encircle 40% of the arm. (B) The length of the bladder should encircle 80% of the upper arm.

manufactured in various sizes, in practice, you will probably have access to only two or three different adult sizes. If you must use a cuff of the improper size, (1) it is better to use one that is too large than one that is too small, and (2) be sure to document the cuff size along with the BP reading. Refer to Figure 18-10 and Table 18-7 for information about cuff sizes in centimeters. In addition,

 Go to **Chapter 18, Clinical Insight 18-1: Choosing a Blood Pressure Cuff Size**, in Volume 2.

Which Site Should I Use?

You usually use the *brachial artery* for assessing BP. However, the condition of the patient's arm, as well as other factors, can interfere with accurate BP measurement.

▪ Avoid assessing BP in an arm that has an IV access device, renal dialysis fistula, skin graft, extensive trauma, a cast, or a dressing.

▪ Do not use the arm that is paralyzed or on the same side as previous breast or shoulder surgery.

▪ Alternative sites that you can use are the forearm, thigh, or calf. However, systolic pressure may be 20 to 30 mm Hg higher in the lower extremities than in the arms, but diastolic pressures are similar. Also, forearm and upper arm readings may not be interchangeable.

▪ Always document the site used.

Auscultating Blood Pressure

BP can be measured indirectly by auscultation or palpation. The preferred, and most used, method is auscultation; however, palpation is useful in certain situations. When auscultating BP, place your stethoscope over an artery:

1. **Inflate the cuff**. As you *inflate* the cuff, the artery is occluded as the pressure of the cuff exceeds the

Table 18-7 ➤ Blood Pressure Cuffs: Acceptable Bladder Sizes

CUFF TYPE	NEWBORN	INFANT	CHILD	SMALL ADULT	ADULT	LARGE ADULT	ADULT THIGH
Arm circumference at midpoint (cm)*	<6	6–15	16–21	22–26	27–34	35–44	45–52
Bladder width (cm)	3	5	8	12	16	16	16
Bladder length (cm)	6	15	21	22	30	36	42

Sources: Perloff, D., Grim, C., Flack, J., Hill, M., McDonald, M., & Morgenstern, B. Z. (1993). Human blood pressure determination by sphygmomanometry. *Circulation,* *88,* 2460–2470; Pickering, T., Hall, J. E., Appel, L. J., Falkner, B. E., Graves, J., Hill, M. N., Jones, D. W., Kurtz, T., Sheps, S. G., & Roccella, E. J. (2005). Recommendations for blood pressure measurement in humans and experimental animals: Part 1: Blood pressure measurement in humans: A statement for professionals from the subcommittee of Professional and Public Education of the American Heart Association Council on High Blood Pressure Research. *Hypertension, 45*(1), 142–161; Whelton, P., Carey, R. M., Aronow, W. S., Casey, D. E. Jr, Collins, K. J., Dennison Himmelfarb, C., DePalma, S. M., Gidding, S., Jamerson, K. A., Jones, D. W., MacLaughlin, E. J., Muntner, P., Ovbiagele, B., Smith, S. C. Jr, Spencer, C. C., Stafford, R. S., Taler, S. J., Thomas, R. J., Williams, K. A. Sr, ... Wright, J. T. (2018). 2017 ACC/AHA/AAPA/ABC/ACPM/AGS/APhA/ASH/ASPC/NMA/PCNA guideline for the prevention, detection, evaluation, and management of high blood pressure in adults. *Journal of the American College of Cardiology, 71*(19), e127–e248. https://doi.org/10.1016/j.jacc.2017.11.006.
*Arm circumference is half the distance (midpoint) from the acromion to the olecranon process. If correct size not available, use next larger (rather than smaller) size.

pressure in the artery. At that point, blood flow through the artery is halted, and no sound can be heard.

2. **Deflate the cuff slowly**. Blood begins to flow rapidly through the partially open artery, producing turbulence that you will hear through the stethoscope as a tapping sound.

The sounds you listen for when you assess BP are called **Korotkoff sounds.** These sounds, described by Russian neurologist Nicolai Korotkoff in 1906, are used to describe the sounds of blood pulsating through arteries (Fig. 18-11) (Meyer, 2022).

- **First sound—Systolic.** The first sound you hear as you deflate the cuff is the *systolic pressure.* It is a tapping sound that corresponds to a palpable pulse.
- **Second sound—Turbulence.** This sound is soft and swishing. It becomes longer and occasionally disappears. When the artery is no longer compressed, blood flows freely, and no sound is heard.

- **Third sound—Rhythmic Tapping.** The third sound begins midway through the BP and is a sharp, loud rhythmic tapping sound.
- **Fourth sound—Muffled.** The fourth sound is softer, faded, and muffled.
- **Fifth sound—Diastolic.** The last sound is the diastolic BP. It corresponds with the absence of sound (silence).

You will not always be able to identify each of the five sounds. In some patients, the sounds are distinct, but in others, you will note little difference between beginning and ending sounds.

Palpating Blood Pressure

When the BP is difficult to hear (e.g., in patients with shock) you can use palpation alone. You can usually palpate only the systolic BP because diastolic pressure is difficult to feel. To learn this technique,

 Go to **Chapter 18, Procedure 18-6: Palpating the Blood Pressure, Variation D,** in Volume 2.

Using Palpation With Auscultation

Using palpation with auscultation helps ensure the accuracy of your readings when measuring BP. To learn how to perform this method,

 Go to **Chapter 18, Procedure 18-6: Measuring Blood Pressure,** in Volume 2.

For tips that will help ensure the validity of your BP measurements,

 Go to **Chapter 18, Clinical Insight 18-2: Taking an Accurate Blood Pressure,** in Volume 2.

Calculating Proper Inflation Pressure The first time you measure a patient's BP, you do not know what the systolic BP is or how high to inflate the cuff. Should

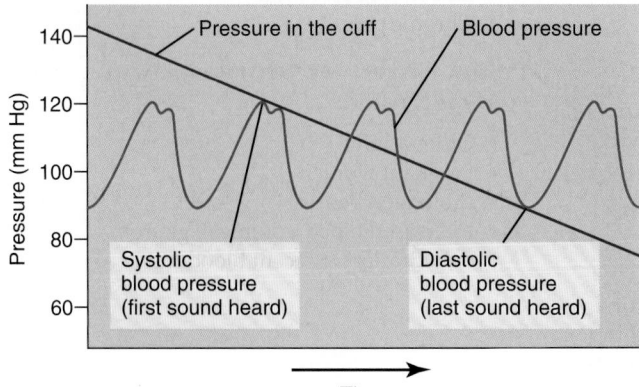

FIGURE 18-11 Relationship of blood pressure to changes in cuff pressure and the first and fifth Korotkoff sounds (blood pressure 120/80).

you pump the cuff to 200 mm Hg just to be sure you don't miss the first sound? The answer is *no*.

- *If you overinflate* the cuff (e.g., inflate to 200 mm Hg), the patient will feel discomfort.
- *If you underinflate* it (e.g., stop inflating at 110 mm Hg), you may miss the first sound and obtain an incorrect reading.

You can use palpation with auscultation to estimate the systolic BP. This helps ensure that you inflate the cuff to the proper level to obtain an accurate reading. To learn how to perform this method, see Procedure 18-6, Measuring Blood Pressure.

Recognizing an Auscultatory Gap If the patient has hypertension, as you auscultate the BP during deflation of the cuff, you may note the loss of sounds for as much as 30 mm Hg, followed by the return of sound. This loss and later return of sound is referred to as an **auscultatory gap**. Palpating first and then auscultating (as described in the preceding paragraph and Procedure 18-6) ensures that you will not miss the isolated first sound. Failure to recognize an auscultatory gap can result in a serious misreading of the systolic BP, namely, a falsely low systolic value and/or a falsely high diastolic value. You should record the range of pressures in which the gap occurs (e.g., BP left arm, sitting, 170/90 with an auscultatory gap from 170 to 140).

KnowledgeCheck 18-6
- Which of the Korotkoff sounds would you record as the systolic pressure?
- Which of the Korotkoff sounds would you record as the diastolic pressure?

- A nurse is auscultating a BP. They hear the first sound at 170 mm Hg. The sound disappears immediately. At 150 mm Hg, the sound appears again and continues until there is silence at 80 mm Hg. The pressures were taken in the right arm with the patient supine.
  How should the nurse record these pressures?
  How do you explain what happened?

NURSING DIAGNOSIS/ANALYZING CUES
- Hypotension and hypertension are medical diagnoses or, more commonly, symptoms rather than nursing diagnoses. However, they may be the etiology of nursing diagnoses—for example, Risk for Falls related to orthostatic (postural) hypotension or Fear of Falling related to fainting 2¼ orthostatic (postural) hypotension.
- You may use the diagnosis Blood Pressure Alterations when the patient experiences or is susceptible to changes in or modification of the systolic or diastolic pressures (HCA Healthcare, n.d.).

Example Client Condition: Hypotension
Hypotension is diagnosed when the systolic BP is 90 mm Hg or lower, or when the diastolic BP is 60 mm Hg or lower (National Institutes of Health, 2022). For more information about hypotension and for goals and interventions, see the Example Client Condition: Hypotension.

Example Client Condition: Hypertension
A transient elevation in BP is a normal response to physiological or psychological stress (e.g., after exercise). To confirm a diagnosis of hypertension, use an

EXAMPLE CLIENT CONDITION: Hypotension

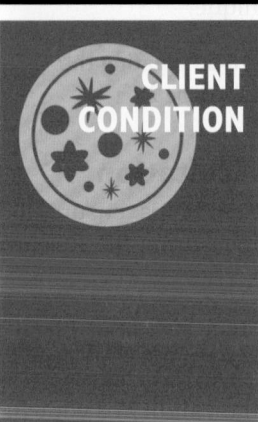
CLIENT CONDITION

Definitions

Hypotension (low blood pressure [BP]) occurs with either of the following:
- Systolic BP of 90 mm Hg or lower
- Diastolic BP of 60 mm Hg or lower (National Institutes of Health, 2022)
- It is usually not a problem unless the decrease from baseline BP causes dizziness, fatigue, concentration problems, activity intolerance, or shortness of breath.

  - Very low BP (hypovolemic shock) is a medical emergency.

Orthostatic (Postural) Hypotension— Sudden drop of ≥10 mm Hg diastolic or a drop in systolic BP of ≥20 mm Hg within 2–5 minutes of moving from a lying or sitting position to a standing position (Ringer & Lappin, 2022), causing dizziness and/or fainting

Risk Factors for Hypotension
- Low hematocrit
- Medical conditions (e.g., hypothyroidism, diabetes, heart failure)
- Chronic pain

Risk Factors for Orthostatic Hypotension:
- Older adults
- Pregnant women
- Prolonged bedrest
- Decreased blood volume (e.g., from dehydration or recent blood loss)

average based on two or more readings obtained on two or more occasions. See Table 18-6 for parameters of elevated BP, Stage 1 hypertension, and Stage 2 hypertension. For more information about hypertension, and for nursing diagnoses, goals, and interventions, see the Example Client Condition for Hypertension.

▮ PLANNING/PRIORITIZING HYPOTHESES AND GENERATING SOLUTIONS

Because hypotension and hypertension are collaborative problems, you may need goals for overall BP monitoring, but more likely, you will use goals for problems related to hypotension and hypertension (e.g., risk for falls). For a diagnosis of risk for falls, a goal might be, "Patient will experience no falls this week."

▮ IMPLEMENTATION/TAKING ACTION

NIC standardized interventions and *individualized interventions* are both used for planning patient care. Refer to the Example Client Conditions: Hypotension and Hypertension. Also see Holistic Healing box: Alternative Therapies for Lowering Blood Pressure. For tips on teaching patients about hypertension,

 Go to **Clinical Insight 18-3: Teaching Your Client About Hypertension**, in Volume 2.

KnowledgeCheck 18-7

- Which type of hypertension does each patient have, if any?
  Patient A: 150/80 on two separate occasions
  Patient B: 180/100 on one occasion
  Patient C: 138/88 on two occasions

EXAMPLE CLIENT CONDITION: Hypertension

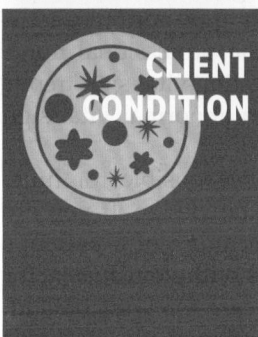
CLIENT CONDITION

Definitions

See Table 18-6.
- *Elevated:* Systolic blood pressure (BP) of 120 to 129 mm Hg and diastolic BP of <80 mm Hg
- *Hypertension Stage 1:* Systolic BP 130–139 mm Hg or diastolic BP 80–89 mm Hg
- *Hypertension Stage 2:* Systolic BP 140 mm Hg or greater or diastolic BP 90 mm Hg or greater

  Key Point: *To confirm a diagnosis of hypertension, use an average based on ≥2 readings obtained on ≥2 occasions to estimate the individual's level of BP. A combination of office/clinic and self-monitoring of BP measurements is recommended to confirm a diagnosis and to obtain correct medication dosage* (Whelton et al., 2018).

Risk Factors

Modifiable: Smoking/second-hand smoke, overweight, obesity, sedentary lifestyle, unhealthy diet, high cholesterol levels, stress, heavy alcohol consumption
Nonmodifiable: Family history, increased age, race, chronic kidney disease

Complications

Hypertension increases the stress on the heart and blood vessels. If untreated, it may lead to heart attack, heart failure, peripheral vascular disease, kidney damage, or stroke (National Heart, Lung, and Blood Institute, 2019).

Alternative Therapies for Lowering Blood Pressure

Holistic Healing

According to an American Heart Association's Scientific Statement, some alternative methods—particularly aerobic exercise and resistance training—can be considered adjunctive to the medical therapies of diet and medication to reduce blood pressure. Biofeedback techniques (isometric handgrip exercise and device-guided slow breathing) are likely to reduce blood pressure by a small amount, but the evidence is not as strong. Research suggests that the following, as adjunctive treatments, may help to reduce blood pressure in people with hypertension: meditation, yoga, relaxation therapy, stress-reduction techniques, and acupuncture. The National Center for Complementary and Integrative Health (2021) reinforces that complementary

approaches should be used as components of a lifestyle-change program with approval by the primary care provider.

Source: Brook, R., Appel, L. J., Rubenfire, M., Ogedegbe, G., Bisognano, J. D., Elliott, W. J., Fuchs, F. D., Hughes, J. W., Lackland, D. T., Staffileno, B. A., Townsend, R. R., Rajagopalan, S., American Heart Association Professional Education Committee of the Council for High Blood Pressure Research, Council on Cardiovascular and Stroke Nursing, Council on Epidemiology and Prevention, and Council on Nutrition, Physical Activity. (2013). AHA Scientific Statement. Beyond medications and diet: Alternative approaches to lowering blood pressure. *Hypertension, 61*(6), 1360–1383; National Center for Complementary and Integrative Health (2021). *Complementary health approaches for hypertension.* https://www.nccih.nih.gov/health/providers/digest/complementary-health-approaches-for-hypertension

■ Which of the following patient(s) has/have *primary* hypertension?
  Patient A, who is obese and has a high sodium intake
  Patient B, who is in renal failure
  Patient C, who has hypertension induced by pregnancy
  Patient D, who has a family history of hypertension

ThinkLike a Nurse 18-10: Clinical Judgment in Action

Recall the patients in the Meet Your Patients scenario. Lucas is 35 years old. He has been under a lot of stress. His BP is 150/98 mm Hg.

■ To evaluate his BP, what else do you need to know about Lucas' situation (the context)?
■ What possible actions should you consider while meeting with Lucas?
■ What is the theoretical knowledge (rationale) to support your decisions?

PUTTING IT ALL TOGETHER

In the hospital setting, you will usually take a complete set of vital signs on patients at regular intervals. In ambulatory care settings, this may vary according to the patient's chief complaint. Regardless of clinical setting, you will need to use clinical judgment about which vital signs to measure and how often to measure them.

Evaluating Vital Signs

You should evaluate the patient's vital signs based on known norms and on their particular trends. When you note a deviation in the vital sign, evaluate it in the context of their medication, diagnosis, procedures, environment, activity, and other factors to understand the theoretical basis for the change. You must put all the vital signs and other clinical signs together to determine the best course of action.

Example A: A high fever can cause BP to drop precipitously. Suppose this patient's temperature is 103.5°F (39.7°C). In that case, in addition to the drop in BP, you should also anticipate a rise in pulse and respiratory rate. What should you do? Your action depends on the patient's condition and the context. What else is going on in the situation? If medication for the fever has been prescribed for the patient, you would administer the medication and evaluate the vital signs again at frequent intervals. If the vital signs do not improve, you would then notify the primary care provider.

Example B: Now change the context slightly. Add to your preceding data that the patient has

undergone a surgical procedure and is not taking any antibiotics. Now what should you do? If your answer is to notify the primary care provider, you are correct. Always evaluate all the vital signs as a unit.

Key Point: *A sudden change in the patient's condition requires a thorough assessment. You must report your findings to the primary care provider.*

Delegating Vital Signs

In many healthcare settings, vital signs are commonly obtained by unlicensed assistive personnel (UAP). When working with complex or critical patients, you should carefully consider whether to delegate vital signs to a UAP. The significance of the vital sign results must be analyzed in relation to other clinical and environmental cues (assessment data).

■ **If you are the registered nurse (RN)** working in a team nursing model, you are responsible for reviewing and interpreting the findings of all UAPs. This includes evaluating their technique and the accuracy of their measurements. The professional nurse is *always* responsible for interpreting vital sign trends and making decisions based on abnormal vital sign findings.
■ **As a student nurse,** you are responsible for functioning within your scope of knowledge. If you are unsure how to interpret the meaning of a patient's vital signs, discuss the findings with your instructor and/or the nurse assigned to care for your patient. Even though you are participating in the patient's care, the assigned nurse maintains responsibility for patient oversight.

To explore learning resources for this chapter,

➤ **Go to Davis Advantage and find:**

Answers and Suggested Responses for all questions in this chapter

Concept Map

Knowledge Map

References and Bibliography

CHAPTER 19

Health Assessment

Learning Outcomes

After completing this chapter, you should be able to:

- Identify the purposes and components of a physical examination.
- Discuss the differences among a comprehensive, focused, and ongoing physical examination.
- Describe how to prepare for a physical examination.
- Demonstrate the skills used in physical examination.
- Explain adaptations that may be required when you examine clients of various ages and abilities.
- Identify the components of the general survey.
- Conduct a full physical examination of a client.
- Discuss the expected findings of a physical examination.
- Document the findings of a physical examination.
- Perform a brief bedside physical examination.

Key Concepts

Health assessment
Nursing assessment
Physical examination

Related Concepts

See the Concept Map on Davis Advantage.

Meet Your Patient

Stanley Williams is scheduled for a comprehensive physical examination at the family health center at 1400 today. As you recall, he has previously been seen and evaluated by Assad Johnson, RN, FNP. Mr. Williams has medical diagnoses of hypertension, degenerative joint disease, obesity, and heavy tobacco use. During his earlier visit, Assad instructed Mr. Williams about a low-salt, low-fat diet and advised him to lose weight and quit smoking. Assad also ordered laboratory work to establish a baseline for wellness and detect abnormalities that might indicate illness.

At today's visit, Assad will perform a comprehensive physical examination of Mr. Williams and review his laboratory results. You can review the results of Mr. Williams' laboratory work in the accompanying image. After Stanley's appointment, Nadine Williams will also have a comprehensive examination.

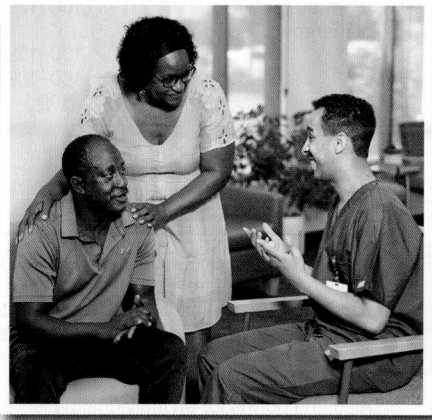

Laboratory Data for Stanley Williams

Name: Stanley Williams **Age:** 56
Acct#: K00205412   Family Medicine Center, A. Johnson

Test	Result	Reference Range*
CBC/Differential		
WBC	5.6 x 10³/mm³	5–10 x 10³/mm³
Hemoglobin	14.8 g/dL	M: 14–18 g/dL F: 12–16 g/dL
Hematocrit	45.1%	M: 42–52% F: 37–47%
RBC count	5.1 million/mm³	M: 4.7–5.14 million/mm³ F: 4.2–4.87 million/mm³
MCV	84 mm³	85–95 mm³
MCH	29 pg	28–32 pg
MCHC	34%	33–35%
Neutrophils	57%	59%
Lymphocytes	30%	34%
Monocytes	5%	4%
Eosinophils	2.5%	2.7%
Basophils	0.7%	0.5%
Platelet count	197,000/mm³	150,000–400,000/mm³

Test	Result	Reference Range*
Comprehensive Metabolic Panel		
Sodium	138 mEq/L	135–145 mEq/L
Potassium	4.3 mEq/L	3.5–5.0 mEq/L
Chloride	101 mEq/L	97–107 mEq/L
Carbon dioxide	27 mEq/L	23–29 mEq/L
BUN	16 mg/dL	10–31 mg/dL
Creatinine	0.8 mg/dL	M: 0.6–1.2 mg/dL F: 0.5–1.1 mg/dL
Glucose	156 mg/dL	75–110 mg/dL
Albumin	4.0 g/dL	19–60 years: 3.2–4.8 g/dL
Total protein	7.2 g/dL	6.8–8.0 g/dL
ALT (alanine aminotransferase, also called SGPT)	18 units/L	M: 10–40 units/L F: 7–35 units/L
ALP (alkaline phosphatase)	43 units/L	M: 35–142 units/L F: 25–125 units/L
AST (aspartate amino transpeptidase, also called SGOT)	26 units/L	M: 19–48 units/L F: 9–36 units/L
Bilirubin, total	0.7 mg/dL	0.3–1.2 mg/dL
Calcium	8.5 mg/dL	8.2–10.2 mg/dL

Test	Result	Reference Range*	
Lipid Panel**			
Total cholesterol	201 mg/dL	<200 200–239 >240	-Desirable -Borderline high -High
LDL cholesterol (Primary target of therapy)	140 mg/dL	<100 mg/dL 100–129 mg/dL 130–159 160–189 >190	-Optimal -Near optimal/above optimal -Borderline high -High -Very high
HDL cholesterol	34 mg/dL	<40	-Low
Triglycerides	196 mg/dL		

**To interpret lipid panel results, follow the most recent guidelines of the National Cholesterol Education Program (NCEP) Expert Panel on Detection, Evaluation, and Blood Cholesterol in Adults available at www.nhlbi.nih.gov/guidelines/cholesterol/atglance.pdf. The reference range figures in this table will undoubtedly be revised (and lowered) by NCEP in the near future.

Also, the norms for an individual patient's lipid panel depend on the calculation of risk factors. Stanley is hypertensive, is obese, and has an elevated blood sugar. His norms reflect high risk for coronary heart disease; they would be about <160 for total cholesterol, <100 for triglycerides, <100 for LDL, and >45 for HDL.

Test	Result	Reference Range*
Urinalysis		
Appearance	Clear	Clear
Color	Amber	Light yellow to amber
Odor	Aromatic	None–aromatic
pH	6.0	5.0–9.0
Specific gravity	1.012	1.001–1.035
Leukocyte esterase	Negative	Negative
Nitrites	Negative	Negative
Ketones	Negative	Negative
Protein	5 mg/dL	<20 mg/dL
Crystals	None	In acid urine: uric acid, calcium oxalate, amorphous urates In alkaline urine: triple phosphate, calcium phosphate, ammonium biurate, calcium carbonate, amorphous phosphates
Casts	None	None, except rare hyaline
Glucose	Negative	Negative
WBC	1/hpf	<5/hpf
RBC	1/hpf	<5/hpf
PSA (prostate-specific antigen)	2.8 ng/mL	<4 ng/mL
Fecal occult blood screen		
Sample #1 — negative Sample #2 — negative Sample #3 — negative		

*For most studies, each laboratory establishes its own reference range.

TheoreticalKnowledge
knowing why

In this chapter, theoretical knowledge consists mostly of information about the key concepts. You will see how an understanding of the key concepts will prepare you and the client for the examination and help you to modify your assessments for different age-groups.

ABOUT THE KEY CONCEPTS

A **health assessment** is a comprehensive assessment of the physical, mental, spiritual, socioeconomic, and cultural status of an individual, group, or community. **Nursing assessments** focus on the client's functional abilities and physical responses to illness and other stressors. In contrast, medical assessments focus on disease and pathology. As a nurse practitioner, Assad Johnson combines the nursing and medical approaches. A **physical examination** consists of the techniques used in a health or nursing assessment to gather objective data about the body.

PHYSICAL EXAMINATION

A complete health assessment includes both a nursing history and a physical examination. In addition to physical examination, you will also ask questions to obtain subjective data about each body system or area. This may be done in a separate nursing interview or as you perform the physical examination. Both the interview and the examination require tact and sensitivity.

Purposes of a Physical Examination

A physical examination is performed for any of several reasons:

- **To obtain baseline data.** Data about the patient's physical status and functional abilities serve as a baseline for comparison as the patient's health status changes.
- **To identify nursing diagnoses, collaborative problems, and wellness diagnoses**. Problem statements form the basis for the plan of care and help you to address the patient's nursing care needs.
- **To monitor the status of a previously identified problem**. For example, Mr. Williams has already begun treatment for hypertension. Today's examination will be linked to the laboratory results to further explore the status of his hypertension.
- **To screen for health problems**. Regular checkups can help to identify health problems at early stages. Because Mr. Williams has an enlarged prostate, a prostate-specific antigen (PSA) test was done to screen for prostate cancer.

To assess for access to healthcare resources. Ask your client about the following factors to find out if they have access to appropriate health resources (*Healthy People 2030*, 2020):

- Coverage: Ability to pay for healthcare resources and entry into the healthcare system. Uninsured people are less likely to access medical care and more likely to have poor health outcomes.
- Services: Having access to healthcare is associated with clients receiving recommended screening and prevention services.
- Timeliness: Ability to access healthcare when the need is recognized.
- Workforce: Access to capable, qualified, culturally competent providers.

Types of Physical Examinations

The type of physical examination you perform will depend on the client's health status, the nature of the client encounter, and the setting.

- **Comprehensive physical examination** (also called *physical assessment*) includes a health history interview and a complete head-to-toe examination of every body system. For example, you would perform a comprehensive physical examination at an outpatient appointment for an annual physical, a client's admission to an inpatient setting, and at the initial home health visit.
- A **focused physical assessment** (or examination) pertains to a particular topic, body part, or functional ability rather than overall health status, and it adds to the database created by the comprehensive assessment. For example, in an emergency situation, your assessment will be rapid and focused on the presenting problem.
- A **system-specific assessment** is a focused assessment limited to one body system (e.g., the lungs, the peripheral circulation). The following are examples of focused and system-specific physical assessments, respectively:
  - Assessing bowel sounds when a client has abdominal pain
  - Listening to breath sounds, counting respirations, and obtaining pulse oximetry readings to assess a patient's respiratory status
- **Ongoing assessment** is performed as needed, after the initial database is completed, and ideally, at every interaction with the patient. For example, on a medical–surgical unit, each nurse who provides care to a client conducts a brief ongoing assessment to determine changes in the client's status.

For more details on the types of assessment, see Chapter 3. To learn how to perform a brief bedside assessment,

Go to **Chapter 19, Procedure 19-20: Brief Bedside Assessment,** in Volume 2.

Preparing to Perform a Physical Examination?

Develop a systematic approach and follow the same order each time you perform a physical examination. This will help you recall the steps and include all the important data.

- A **head-to-toe approach** starts at the head and neck and progresses down the body, examining the feet last.
- A **body systems approach** examines each system in a predetermined order (e.g., musculoskeletal, cardiovascular, neurological).

Whatever the approach, prepare yourself, the environment, and the client before you begin.

Prepare Yourself

- **Preparing for a physical examination requires theoretical knowledge of**:
  - Anatomy and physiology
  - Examination equipment and techniques
  - Therapeutic communication
  - Documentation
- **Self-knowledge is also important:**
  - How comfortable are you when performing an examination?
  - What skills do you need to review or practice?
  - Will you need assistance to perform some aspects of the examination?
  - Will you need help documenting your findings?
  - Honestly evaluate your strengths as well as areas that need improvement.
  - Be sure to seek help from your instructor, an experienced nurse, fellow students, or other healthcare providers as needed.
- **Before approaching the patient, familiarize yourself with their situation.**
  - What are the patient's main health concerns?
  - What is the purpose of your examination? For instance, if you are doing a focused assessment of a patient's wound, you will need to learn about the wound being examined.
  - Is there a dressing over the wound? What supplies will you need to remove and replace the dressing?
  - Has the patient required pain medication before examinations in the past?
- **Finally, unless this is an initial assessment, review the nursing plan of care** and keep it in mind as you examine the patient. Reviewing previous findings helps you work efficiently and to formulate any questions you might want to ask the patient. Furthermore, your assessment data may lead to modification or updating of the care plan.

Prepare the Environment

- **Privacy. Key Point:** *Physical examination requires you to observe and touch the client's body, so privacy is essential.*
  - You will need a room with curtains or a door to shield the client from view.
  - For additional privacy, drape your client and uncover only the area you are examining. Consider cultural differences, but don't assume everyone from a particular culture has the same values or sensitivities. That goes for age and gender, too.
  - For convenience, you may use bed linens and/or a gown to drape. Disposable paper drapes are also available.
- **Noise.** Because you will need to hear the patient and listen to a variety of sounds during the examination, turn off the television, radio, or other media.
- **Lighting.** You will need good lighting to observe subtle changes in skin and body contours.
- **Temperature.** Adjust the temperature of the room according to patient comfort.
- **Equipment.** Determine the instruments and equipment you will need. Take everything you need so that you will not have to leave the client to obtain supplies. To see commonly used equipment,

 Go to the box **Equipment Needed for Physical Examination** in Procedure 19-1 in Volume 2.

Prepare the Client

In most clinical settings, you must examine a client often to evaluate changes in status, and timing will be decided by the client's condition rather than by convenience. However, when possible, select a time when the client is comfortable and receptive to the examination. Avoid conducting the examination when the client is in pain or is hungry, tired, anxious, or unwilling to cooperate in the assessment.

♥ **iCare** Take the time to establish rapport with the client; this will help the client relax and cooperate fully in the assessment.

- Introduce yourself, ask the client how they wish to be addressed, and explain what you will be doing.
- Ask the client to void before the examination; this promotes relaxation and also makes it easier to palpate the abdomen.
- Always alert the client before touching them. For example, before you start to palpate the neck for lymph nodes, say, "I'm going to feel your neck now."
- Proper positioning during the examination also promotes comfort (see the following section).
- Pay attention to the pace of your examination, being careful not to prolong it and tire the client.

Key Point: *Consider developmental and cultural differences. For example, some clients may wish to have a family member present during an examination; some may require a same-sex clinician. If you and the client do not speak the same language, arrange to have an interpreter present.*

Be prepared to ask culturally sensitive questions as a way to reduce anxiety and stress for patients and family members. Performing a health assessment requires close contact with the patient and requires you to be prepared by asking appropriate questions. After explaining what is usual in Western medicine (drapes, closed doors, and knocking before entering), ask the patient:

- Is there anything I should know about your privacy or modesty concerns before I conduct an examination?
- In your culture, how would a healthcare provider show respect for a female/male patient during the examination?

KnowledgeCheck 19-1

- What are the purposes of a physical examination?
- Describe how you would prepare for a physical examination.

ThinkLike a Nurse 19-1:
Clinical Judgment in Action

- The nurse conducts a physical examination for Stanley and Nadine Williams (see Meet Your Patient) at an outpatient clinic. Discuss the differences between their planned experience and a focused physical examination of a hospital inpatient.
- Identify a plan to practice and improve your assessment skills.

Positioning the Client for a Physical Examination

The client will need to assume a variety of positions during a comprehensive physical examination. As you place your client in positions that allow you to best observe the body system you are examining, be alert to special needs that call for you to modify the position. If your patient is unable to move without assistance, use available devices to position the patient and maintain body alignment. Pillows are the most common devices used to assist with positioning, provide support, and elevate body parts (see Chapter 29 if you need more information). You will need a variety of sizes to position patients who are unable to assist with positioning. If pillows are not available, you can use folded blankets or towels. Foam wedge pillows are useful for elevating the upper body when an adjustable bed is not available and for abducting the hips. Table 19-1 illustrates and describes the major positions you will need to use.

KnowledgeCheck 19-2

Identify the best position for examining the lungs, heart, pulses, and abdomen.

Physical Examination Techniques

You will use the physical examination techniques in the following order, with one exception: inspection, palpation, percussion, auscultation, and sometimes olfaction. *Exception:* When performing an abdominal assessment, perform auscultation before percussion and palpation to avoid disturbing the abdominal sounds.

Inspection **Inspection** is the use of sight to gather data. You begin to use inspection the moment you meet the client and continue as you observe the person's gait, personal hygiene, affect, and behavior during the general survey. You will also use inspection as you evaluate each body system.

- Adequate lighting and proper positioning aid inspection.
- The otoscope, ophthalmoscope, and penlight also enhance your inspection abilities.

Safe, Effective Nursing Care

Health Assessment and Cultural Adaptation

Related Concepts: Developmental Stages

SENC Competencies: Goal-directed, client-centered care (Thinking, Doing, Caring)

Background: When performing a health assessment, adaptation for the developmental age of the client is a widely accepted nursing practice. It is also important to adapt for the client's culture. In order to engage diverse clients and respond to their preferences and values, culturally competent communication must be an integral component when initiating the health assessment (Kwame et al., 2021; Shahzad et al., 2021). The Thinking, Doing, Caring dimensions of goal-directed, client-centered care promotes the same principle. Four areas that demonstrate cultural adaptation in the health assessment are eliciting client preferences regarding the following: (1) comfort with touch, (2) comfort with exposure (modesty), (3) need for personal space, (4) and need for the presence of a support person.

Scenario: A client who speaks Portuguese requires an interpreter while hospitalized. You are assigned to complete the initial health assessment.

Think about it: The following items are for your own reflection or discussion with peers.

1. The nurse directs questions and makes eye contact with which of the following when obtaining the history: the interpreter or the client? Discuss how your response supports cultural adaptation.

2. Formulate questions for the nursing history to elicit client preferences regarding comfort with touch, comfort with exposure, personal space, and the presence of a support person.

Source: Kwame, A., & Petrucka, P. M. (2021). A literature-based study of patient-centered care and communication in nurse-patient interactions: barriers, facilitators, and the way forward. *BMC Nursing, 20*(1), 1–10; Shahzad, S., Ali, N., Younas, A., & Tayaben, J. L. (2021). Challenges and approaches to transcultural care: An integrative review of nurses' and nursing students' experiences. *Journal of Professional Nursing, 37*(6), 1119–1131.

Table 19-1 ➤ Positioning the Client

 Note: *Clients with disabilities, clients who are weak, and clients who have poor balance may require assistance to safely attain or maintain various positions.*

POSITION AND DESCRIPTION	COMMENTS
Standing	
Upright posture with both feet flat on the floor	Use to examine the musculoskeletal and neurological systems and to assess gait and cerebellar function.
	If the client uses an assistive device, allow the client to use it during your assessment.
	Clients with physical disabilities, clients who are weak, and clients who have poor balance may not be able to assume this position.
Sitting	
Sitting upright at side of bed or examination table 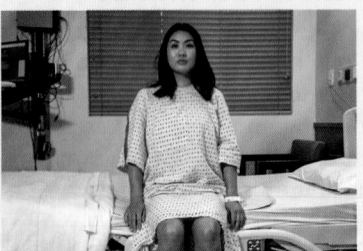	Use to assess vital signs, head and neck, chest, cardiovascular system, and breasts.
	If your client has a physical disability or is weak, they may need assistance to maintain this position. If the client uses a wheelchair, they may feel more comfortable remaining in the wheelchair during this part of the assessment.
Supine	
(Including Fowler's and semi-Fowler's positions) Lying flat on the back with arms and legs fully extended 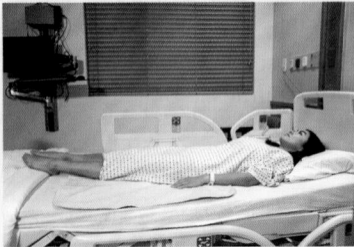	Use to assess the abdomen, breasts, extremities, and pulses. If your client becomes short of breath, raise the head of the bed (HOB).
	■ In **Fowler's position,** the head is elevated 60°.
	■ In **semi-Fowler's position,** the head is elevated only 30°–45°.
Dorsal Recumbent	
Supine with knees flexed 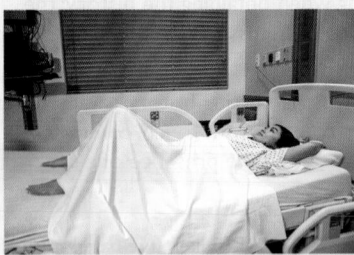	Use for abdominal assessment if your client has abdominal or pelvic pain. Flexing the knees promotes relaxation of the abdominal muscles.

Table 19-1 ➤ Positioning the Client—cont'd

POSITION AND DESCRIPTION	COMMENTS
Lithotomy	
Dorsal recumbent position at end of table with feet in stirrups, legs flexed, and widely open 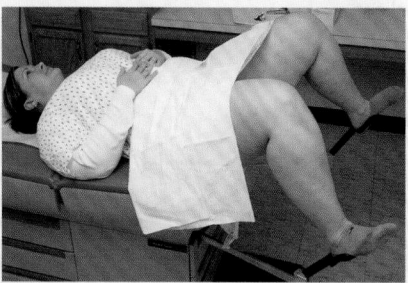	Use for a female pelvic examination; provides maximum exposure of genitals. Older patients or patients with physical disabilities may need support to assume and maintain this position. The patient's legs are exposed here to illustrate position.
Sims'	
Flexion of the hip and knees in a side-lying position 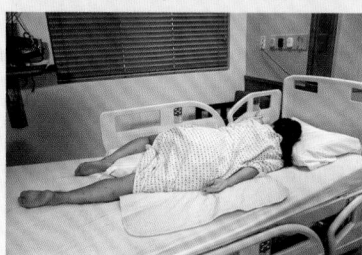	Use to examine the rectal area. Use for a female pelvic examination if the patient is unable to assume the lithotomy position. Do *not* use if the client has had total hip replacement.
Prone	
Lying on stomach (A small pillow under the abdomen makes this position more comfortable.) 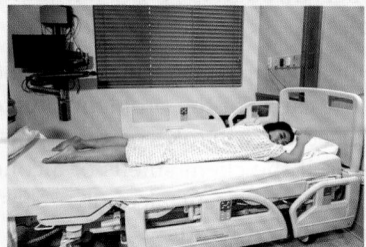	Use to examine the musculoskeletal system, especially hip extension; may also be used to examine the back and buttocks. May be difficult to assume by clients with physical disabilities or respiratory problems.
Lateral Recumbent	
Lying on the side in a straight line 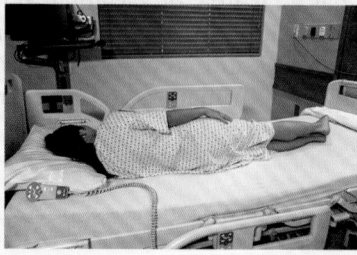	Left lateral recumbent is used to evaluate heart murmur or during a thorough cardiovascular assessment. This position brings the heart closer to the chest wall. If the client cannot assume this position, listen to the heart with the client seated and bending forward.

(Continued)

Table 19-1 ➤ Positioning the Client—cont'd

POSITION AND DESCRIPTION	COMMENTS
Knee–Chest	
On hands and knees with head down and buttocks elevated 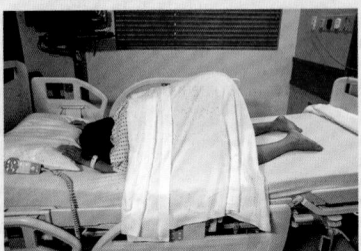	Provides good visualization for examining the rectal area. However, it is not used often because it is embarrassing and uncomfortable for the client.

Palpation Palpation is the use of touch to gather data. Use palpation to assess temperature; skin texture; moisture; anatomical landmarks; and such abnormalities as edema, masses, or areas of tenderness. As you begin and move through the assessment of each body system, always inform the client that you are about to touch them. Use a gentle approach and be certain your hands are warm. Begin with light pressure to detect surface characteristics. Then move to deep palpation to assess the underlying structures. Examine last any areas of discomfort or sensitivity. Following is a list of the most common palpation techniques, using different parts of the hand.

- *Fingertips:* Use for fine tactile discrimination, including assessment of skin texture, swelling, and specific locations of pulsations and masses.
- *Dorsum of hand:* Use for temperature determination.
- *Palmar surface of hand:* Use for locating general area of pulsations.
- *Grasping with fingers and thumb:* Use to detect the position, shape, and consistency of a mass.

Percussion Percussion is tapping your fingers on the skin using short strokes. Tapping (percussing) produces vibrations, and the resulting sound allows you to determine the location, size, and density of underlying structures. Percussion is especially useful when assessing the abdomen and lungs. A quiet environment allows you to perceive the subtle differences in percussion notes.

Percussion takes practice. To learn more about percussion, including direct and indirect percussion and terminology for the notes you may hear,

 Go to **Chapter 19, Clinical Insight 19-1: Performing Percussion,** in Volume 2.

Auscultation is the use of hearing to gather data.

- **Direct auscultation** is listening without using an instrument. If you have heard wheezing or chest congestion without the use of a stethoscope, you have already performed direct auscultation.
- **Indirect auscultation** is listening with the help of a stethoscope.
- To improve your skill in indirect auscultation,

 Go to **Chapter 19, Clinical Insight 19-2: Performing Auscultation,** in Volume 2.

Olfaction is the use of the sense of smell to gather data. Some clinicians may not consider **olfaction** a formal assessment skill; however, you will certainly use this skill in the clinical setting. Olfaction adds information to the data you collect through the other techniques. Consider these examples:

- If a client is slurring their words, you will want to look for data that reveal the cause of the problem. Slurred speech might be caused by a stroke or by sedative medications. However, if the client smells of alcohol, you would first investigate recent alcohol use as a probable cause for the slurred words.
- If an older client smells of urine, you would want to assess for problems with leakage of urine or inability to perform self-care.
- If the client's breath has a "fruity" or "acetone" odor, you would suspect ketoacidosis, which may accompany diabetes. You would know to assess the urine for ketones and contact the primary care provider if necessary.

KnowledgeCheck 19-3

- Identify five physical assessment skills.
- In what order are these skills performed?

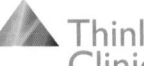 Think**Like a Nurse** 19-2: Clinical Judgment **in Action**

Think about olfaction as an assessment technique. Give two or three additional examples of data you might collect through the use of smell.

Modifications for Different Age-Groups

The basic techniques of physical examination remain the same for everyone. However, your approach will vary according to the developmental stage of your patient. As a rule, encourage parents of infants and children to be present for the examination.

Infants Use the assessment as an opportunity to teach the parent about normal growth and development. Infants usually feel most secure if a parent holds them during the examination, either against the chest or, for older infants who can sit without support, on the parent's lap. Otherwise, position an infant on a padded examination table. ✥ If there are siderails, raise them to prevent falling. Do not leave the infant's side or turn your back on the infant.

Toddlers The following list includes some tips for examining toddlers:

- **Include parents.** Toddlers are interested in exploring the environment, but they also like to stay close to a parent, often in the parent's lap.
- **Perform invasive procedures last.** Toddlers may be fearful of invasive procedures, such as examination of the oral cavity or inner ear. If they are upset, it will be more difficult to examine other body areas.
- **Give the child choices.** Most toddlers enjoy making choices, so this will promote cooperation. For example, you might provide a choice by saying, "Should I listen to your chest first, or should we see how much you weigh?"
- **Allow the child to show you his developmental skills.** If the child needs assistance to remove clothing, have the parent help, and observe how the parent and child interact.
- **Use praise freely.** Praise the toddler for their abilities and cooperation. This sets the stage for positive feelings about healthcare.

Preschoolers Preschool children are developing initiative and, as a result, usually cooperate with an examination. However, children of this age have fantasies and fears that may arise during the examination. For example, they may object to a noninvasive procedure because they believe it will cause pain or injury, or they may refuse to step on the scale because to them, it resembles a monster.

- **Combat fears** by demonstrating the procedure on a doll or having the parent step on the scale before you approach the child.
- **Allow the preschool child to sit in a parent's lap if they wish.** By age 5, most children will be comfortable enough to lie on the examination table if a parent is present.
- **Let the child help with the examination.** For example, have the child hold equipment or remember their height and weight.
- **Give reassurance** as you go through the examination—for example, "Your lungs sound very healthy."
- **Always compliment the child on cooperating.**

School-Age Children The school-age child has a rapidly expanding vocabulary and usually seeks the approval of parents, teachers, and healthcare providers.

- **Develop rapport** by asking the child about their favorite school or play activities.
- **Support independence.** Allow the child to undress and get up and down from the examination table independently.
- **Demonstrate your equipment** and let the child touch it before you use it. This makes the equipment seem less threatening.
- **Allow time for teaching.** The school-age child will be interested in how their body works, so use this opportunity for teaching.

Adolescents The adolescent is often self-conscious and introspective and may wish to be examined without parents or siblings present, at least during the more personal aspects of the examination. Offer the adolescent this choice.

- **Provide privacy.** Adolescents often worry about the "normalcy" of their changing bodies and appreciate respect for their privacy.
- **Be certain to discuss the normal physiological changes** that accompany puberty. If you need to review those changes, see the section on adolescence in Chapter 6.
- **Be aware that adolescent behavior may be strongly influenced by peer values.**
- **Emphasize lifestyle habits that promote wellness,** including a healthful diet; adequate rest and exercise; and avoidance of tobacco, alcohol, and other drugs.
- **Discuss sexually transmitted infections and cancer,** particularly testicular cancer and human papillomavirus.
- **Prepare the adolescent, if necessary, for a pelvic examination and breast examination,** which usually begin in the teen years. Be familiar with cultural norms that may require a modification in standard care. For example, some cultures/religions do not allow procedures that will tear the hymen if a female patient has not yet had sexual intercourse. Additionally, some cultures may require certain accommodations for younger patients. If you are not familiar with specific cultural practices, be sure to ask.
- **Screen for depression and suicide risk.** Suicide is the third-leading cause of death among adolescents (see Chapter 10 for a review of depression and suicide).

Young and Middle Adults Most young and middle adults are able to cooperate during a physical examination and do not require a modified approach. Modifications may be required if the client has an acute or chronic illness or cannot understand or follow instructions. ⚇ Adults with disabilities often face significant barriers when seeking to access healthcare (e.g., lack of knowledge, anxiety about the examination process and dependency on others, environmental or physical limitations, and inadequate knowledge of health-care professionals about their disability). These barriers affect the health of and health outcomes for adults with disabilities (Kilic et al. 2019).

According to the Centers for Disease Control and Prevention (CDC, 2022), adults with disabilities

- are three times more likely to have heart disease, stroke, diabetes, or cancer than adults without disabilities;
- are more likely than adults without disabilities to be current smokers; and
- are less likely than adults without disabilities to have received a mammogram (if needed) during the past 2 years.

Older Adults Allow extra time to interview and examine older adults. Many older adults are adjusting to changes in physical abilities and health. As part of a comprehensive examination:

- **Assess the client's support** system and ability to perform activities of daily living. Observe your client's energy level during the physical examination and provide rest periods if needed.
- **Limit position changes.** If the client tires easily, arrange the examination sequence to limit position changes.
- **Difficulty assuming positions.** Be aware that stiff muscles and arthritic joints may make it impossible for the client to assume certain positions.
- **Adapt your techniques** when examining older adults with impaired vision or hearing. Obtain feedback to be sure the patient is seeing and hearing you adequately.

The acronym SPICES will help you to remember common problems of the elderly that require nursing intervention (Fulmer, 1991, 2007) and to focus your assessment as you perform a comprehensive physical examination:

S—Sleep disorders
P—Problems with eating or feeding
I—Incontinence
C—Confusion
E—Evidence of falls
S—Skin breakdown

Modifications for Clients With Disabilities (Differently Abled)

Health assessment in clients with cognitive, sensory, or mobility impairments can be challenging but is important to perform. Consider modifying your routine and scheduling a realistic health assessment appointment length, utilizing portable accessible medical equipment, learning safe transfer techniques, and maintaining respectful etiquette when working with patients who present with adaptive resources like a wheelchair, service animal, personal care assistant, or sign language interpreter.

Ask patients with disabilities if they need help before providing assistance and, if they do, how to best help. People with mobility disabilities are not all the same; many use mobility devices of different types, sizes, and weights; transfer in different ways; and have varying levels of physical ability. Make sure to ask questions. Understanding what assistance, if any, is needed and how to provide it will allow you to provide safe and accessible healthcare for people with disabilities.

KnowledgeCheck 19-4

What examination modifications, based on developmental stage, should you consider for the following clients (Meet Your Patient)?
- Stanley Williams
- Stanley's 3-year-old granddaughter, Kayla Robinson
- Stanley's elderly mother, Charlene Williams

PracticalKnowledge
knowing **how**

The remainder of the chapter discusses each of the components of a comprehensive physical examination. The Highlights of Procedures box near the end of this chapter summarizes the entire comprehensive physical assessment, including a summary of the general survey. For a step-by-step approach to performing each assessment,

 Go to **Chapter 19, Procedures,** in Volume 2.

To understand your patient's overall health status, you will need to be aware of the various diagnostic tests associated with each of the systems you assess. Refer to the agencies' laboratory "norms" and to diagnostic studies handbooks, as needed, to interpret the tests.

THE GENERAL SURVEY

The **general survey** is your overall impression of the client. It begins at first contact and continues throughout the examination. **Key Point: *Be sure to consider cultural background because this may influence your findings and interpretations.***

When you discover a deviation from the expected results in the general survey, you will explore it further during the focused assessment of that body system. For example, if on meeting the patient you notice a drooping eyelid **(ptosis)** on one side of the face, you will keep that in mind as you perform the neurological assessment. Ptosis may be caused by a stroke or neurological injury.

Once you have completed your general survey of the client, you can begin to focus on each body system. Whether you are doing a complete or focused physical examination, remember that all body systems are interrelated. A problem in one system may affect or be affected by other systems. The following are aspects of the general survey. For a step-by-step approach, see the Highlights of Procedures box near the end of this chapter, and

Go to **Chapter 19, Procedure 19-1: Performing the General Survey,** in Volume 2.

Personal Identity Identifying personal information early in the examination is important to establish trust and to make the patient more comfortable. The nurse should collect information about the patient's gender, preferred pronouns/name, and sexual orientation, as well as racial identity and cultural identity. You should discuss this information before the examination to determine whether any accommodations need to be made in the standard procedures.

Appearance and Behavior Refer to Volume 2, Procedure 19-1: Performing the General Survey, steps 1, 2, and 3, for details about assessing appearance and behavior.

Body Type and Posture Posture is also a cue about overall health status. Focused assessments in the remainder of the examination will help to reveal the exact meaning of such cues.

Speech As you speak with the client and ask health-related questions, look for clues offered by his speech.

- **Inappropriate or illogical responses** may be associated with psychiatric disorders.
- **Difficulty speaking or changes in voice quality** may indicate a neurological problem.
- **Rapid speech** may be a sign of anxiety, hyperactivity, or the use of stimulants.
- **Hoarseness** could indicate inflammation in the throat from infection, overuse, a foreign body, or perhaps a tumor or other obstructive material.
- **Slow speech** may be due to depression, sedation from medications, or neurological disorders.
- **Vocabulary and sentence structure** provide information about the client's educational level and comfort with the language.
- **Language barriers** occur when two people do not understand one another and there is a breakdown in communication. Language barriers can come from physical language disabilities, which include stuttering, articulation disorder, and hearing loss, or when healthcare providers and patients do not share a common language. Patients experiencing language barriers are more likely to miss medical appointments and have more difficulty arranging appointments because of the language barrier. As a result, they experience poorer health outcomes.

Mental State Mental state includes level of consciousness and capacity to interact. If the client has an altered mental status, ask a family member about the onset of the change. Keep in mind that many medications, especially in older adults, may contribute to confusion or other changes in mental status.

Dress, Grooming, and Hygiene A client's ability to dress and perform personal hygiene is affected by physical and emotional well-being. Many challenges and barriers to good hygiene exist, including the lack of access to clean water. You should document your observations and determine whether the client has access to the resources needed to perform personal hygiene. Avoid making judgments about the patient; instead, use your observations to investigate for healthcare disparities and to provide teaching and resources for the client.

Vital Signs You should assess vital signs as a part of the general survey and with subsequent assessments. Analyze for trends. See Chapter 18 for a complete discussion of vital signs, if needed.

Height and Weight Height and weight provide valuable information about your client's growth and development, nutritional status, and overall general health while informing risk for various diseases such as diabetes and heart disease (Fig. 19-1). These data are important for proper dosing of medication. When possible, the client should wear minimal clothing (gown) and no shoes. Because children have frequent changes in growth, their measurements are documented on growth charts for easy monitoring and comparison to age- and sex-related standards.

Body mass index (BMI) evaluates the relationship between height and weight. You can calculate the BMI for adults using a BMI calculator or table. For a BMI table,

Go to Chapter 19, **Procedure 19-1: Performing the General Survey,** in Volume 2.

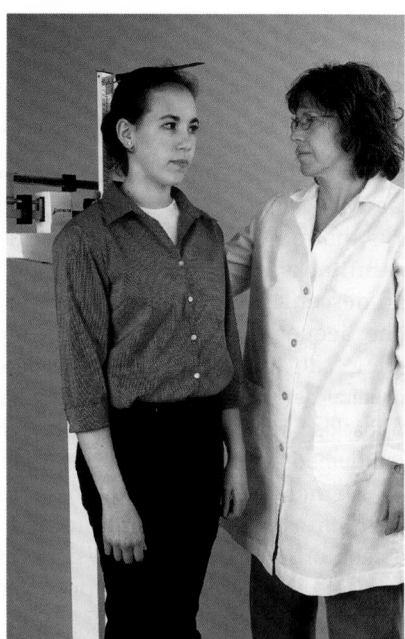

FIGURE 19-1 For adults, measure height with the client's back to the platform scale.

Key Point: *Because the proportion of fat to muscle affects BMI calculation, the BMI is not useful for the following:*

- *Athletes (who have a larger proportion of muscle)*
- *Pregnant and lactating women (who have a larger blood and tissue volume)*
- *Growing children*
- *Frail and sedentary older adults*

THE INTEGUMENTARY SYSTEM

The integumentary system consists of the skin, hair, and nails. In a comprehensive examination, you assess this system briefly in the general survey and then in greater detail as you move to examine other areas of the body. This allows the client to remain draped as long as possible. For step-by-step instructions,

 Go to **Chapter 19, Procedure 19-2: Assessing the Skin,** in Volume 2.

The Skin

To perform a skin assessment, observe skin color, lesions, and other characteristics. Also notice unusual odors. For a summary of procedure steps, see the Highlights of Procedures box near the end of this chapter.

- An unpleasant body odor may be a sign of poor hygiene, the presence of a wound, or underlying disease.
- Excessive sweating may be related to activity (e.g., if the client has just finished exercising), thyroid problems, or overactive sweat glands.
- An odor of urine or stool may indicate a nursing diagnosis of Self-Care Deficit or Bowel or Urinary Incontinence.

Skin Color

Skin color varies according to age and race. Variations seen in neonates and infants include the following:

- Congenital dermal melanocytosis (previously known as *Mongolian spots*) are benign, blue-black birthmarks that occur most commonly on the lower back and buttocks of children of African, Hispanic, and Asian descent. They are the result of pigmented cells in the deeper areas of skin. Most fade by age 2, but they can persist until early adolescence. Congenital dermal melanocytosis must be differentiated from marking resulting from abuse, especially due to the location (lumbosacral region) and color (bluish).
- **Capillary hemangiomas,** sometimes known as "stork bites," are small, irregular, pink-red areas that are often seen around the face and nape of the neck in newborns. They typically disappear in infancy, although they can persist until age 5.
- **Café-au-lait spots** are light-brown birthmarks that can occur anywhere on the body. The name of these

birthmarks is French for "coffee with milk" because of their light-brown color. Most often, café-au-lait spots are not associated with medical problems, although they can sometimes signal a genetic disorder.

Gua sha, or coining, translates to "scraping or bruising." It is an important part of medicine in various cultures, including those in Southeastern Asia. Skin, lubricated with an oil, is scraped with a ceramic spoon, worn coin, or metal cap. The elongated bruises resulting from this procedure are considered signs of balance, stimulated blood flow, and the restoration of health. Cupping, another type of ancient therapy, consists of circular suction cups made of glass, bamboo, or earthenware being applied to dry skin. The suction causes a bruise or hematoma. Wet cupping involves small skin incisions made in the suction area. Patient care should always be culturally sensitive, so be sure to ask if you see something you are not familiar with. Skin markings may be misconstrued for maltreatment or abuse.

Table 19-2 discusses the significance of other skin color variations that may be seen in clients of any age. To view illustrations of color changes,

 Go to **Chapter 19, Procedure 19-2, Assessing the Skin,** in Volume 2.

Skin Characteristics

Similar to skin color, the tone, temperature, texture, and turgor of the skin offer cues about the client's health status. Although it is not technically a skin characteristic, you should also check for edema while you are assessing the skin.

Skin Tone   Observe the color of the patient's skin and compare your findings to what is expected for their skin tone. Note changes such as pallor (paleness), cyanosis (blueness), jaundice (yellowness), or erythema (redness).

Skin Temperature   The skin should feel warm, but keep in mind that the temperature should be consistent with the room temperature and the patient's activity level.

Skin Moisture   Excessive moisture may result from hyperthermia, thyroid hyperactivity, anxiety, or **hyperhidrosis** (excessive sweating). Dry skin may result from dehydration, chronic renal failure, hypothyroidism, excessive exposure, or overzealous hygiene.

Skin Texture   The following factors affect skin texture:

- **Exposure.** Exposed areas tend to be drier and coarser in texture, as do the elbows and knees.
- **Age.** The skin of infants and young children is very smooth because of the lack of exposure to the environment.
- **Hyperthyroidism and other endocrine disorders.** These may cause the skin to become coarse, thick, and dry.

Table 19-2 ➤ Common Skin Color Variations

COLOR VARIATION AND DESCRIPTION	SIGNIFICANCE
Pallor	
In clients with light skin: extreme paleness; skin appears white; loss of pink or yellow tones. In clients with dark skin: a loss of red tones	May be related to poor circulation or a low hemoglobin level (anemia). The best sites to assess for pallor include the oral mucous membranes, conjunctiva, nailbeds, palms, and soles of feet.
Cyanosis	
A blue-gray coloration of the skin, often described as ashen	If seen in the lips, tongue, mucous membranes, and facial features, it is known as *central cyanosis* and is associated with hypoxia. **Acrocyanosis,** bluish discoloration of palms and soles in the first few hours to days of life, is normal in newborns. Cold causes the lips to turn blue, but the tongue is not affected. Cyanosis may also be seen in the extremities, especially the hands and feet, after exposure to extreme cold.
Jaundice	
A yellow-orange cast to the skin	Often associated with liver disorders The best sites to assess for jaundice include the sclera, mucous membranes, hard palate of the mouth, palms, and soles of the feet. Jaundice in the newborn is a normal finding in the first few weeks of life unless there is blood incompatibility or a congenital disorder.
Flushing	
A widespread, diffuse area of redness	Generalized redness of the face and body may occur as a result of fever, excessive room temperature, sunburn, polycythemia (an abnormal increase in red blood cells), vigorous exercise, or certain skin conditions (e.g., rosacea).
Erythema	
A reddened area	Associated with rashes, skin infections, prolonged pressure on the skin, or application of heat or cold
Ecchymosis	
Bruised (blue-green-yellow) area	May be seen anywhere on the body The color will vary based on the age of the injury. May indicate physical abuse, internal bleeding, side effect of medication, or bleeding disorder To review assessing for abuse, refer to the **Example Problem: Abuse, Neglect, and Violence**, in Chapter 6 in Volume 1. Also, ➤ Go to **Chapter 6, Procedure 6-1, Assessing for Abuse**, in Volume 2.
Petechiae	
Tiny pinpoint red or reddish-purple spots	Visible in the skin due to extravasation (leakage from vessels) of blood into the skin May be associated with a variety of disorders and medications
Mottling	
Bluish marbling	Occurs in clients with light skin, especially when cold In newborns, mottling indicates overstimulation of the autonomic nervous system.

■ **Impaired circulation.** Peripheral arterial insufficiency is associated with smooth, thin, shiny skin with little to no hair. In contrast, venous insufficiency leads to thick, rough skin that is often hyperpigmented.

Skin Turgor This refers to the elasticity of the skin, which provides data about hydration status. **Edema,** which is an excessive amount of fluid in the tissues, is an abnormal finding. It is common in clients with congestive heart failure, kidney disease, peripheral vascular disease, or low albumin levels. A client with edema may tell you their skin feels "tight" or say, "My shoes don't fit anymore." Swollen tissue may feel tender to the touch. Edema is not actually a condition of the skin, but it is convenient to assess for it while assessing the skin. For a grading system to describe edema,

 Go to **Chapter 19, Procedure 19-2, Assessing the Skin,** in Volume 2.

Skin Lesions

Any **lesion,** variation in pigment, or break in continuous tissue requires assessment. When you observe a lesion, evaluate it for size, shape, pattern, color, distribution, texture, surface relationship, exudate, tenderness, pain, or itching.

Key Point: *Evaluate all skin lesions for the possibility of malignancy, especially those located in a site exposed to chronic rubbing or other trauma.* You can remember the warning signs of malignant lesions by thinking of the letters ABCDE: (**A**symmetry, **B**order irregularity, **C**olor variation, **D**iameter greater than 0.5 cm, **E**levation above the skin surface).

Normal Lesions Lesions considered to be normal variations and not harmful include:

■ **Milia.** White raised areas on the nose, chin, and forehead of newborns. These lesions, which resemble "whiteheads," are due to retention of sebum in the maturing sebaceous glands. They disappear during infancy.
■ **Nevi (moles), freckles, birthmarks.**
■ **Skin tags.** Tiny tags or buds of skin, usually around skin creases, in middle and older adults.
■ **Striae.** Silver-to-pink "stretch marks" in pregnant women, women who have had children, and anyone who has experienced significant weight fluctuations.

Abnormal Lesions Abnormal lesions are classified as primary or secondary.

■ **Primary skin lesions.** Develop as a result of disease or irritation. The pustules of acne are an example.
■ **Secondary skin lesions.** Develop from primary lesions as a result of continued illness, exposure, injury, or infection, such as the crusts that form from ruptured pustules.

To help you categorize and describe lesions, and to view abnormal lesions associated with particular conditions (e.g., cellulitis),

 Go to the table **Describing Skin Lesions** and **Step 7** in **Chapter 19, Procedure 19-2: Assessing the Skin**, in Volume 2.

KnowledgeCheck 19-5
■ What aspects of the skin should you assess?
■ What assessments should you perform if you find a lesion?
■ What warning signs lead you to suspect a malignant lesion?

The Hair

When assessing the hair, inspect and palpate for color, texture, and distribution and the condition of the scalp. The hair should be clean and free of debris. A client who does not properly groom their hair may need help with other self-care tasks.

■ **Color.** There is a wide range of naturally occurring hair color. Age-related graying of the hair varies among individuals according to their genetic background.
■ **Texture.** Normal hair texture varies from fine to coarse.
■ **Distribution.** Generally, the hair is evenly distributed on the scalp, and fine body hair is present over the body. Men often have more hair on the face, chest, and back. Alterations in hair distribution may be signs of disease if the distribution is abnormal for the patient.
■ **Alopecia.** Hair loss along the temples and in the center of the scalp is considered a normal balding pattern in men and is largely genetically based.
  ■ Diffuse alopecia can be caused by chemotherapy for the treatment of cancer, by nutritional deficiencies, or by endocrine disorders.
  ■ Thinning hair can also occur in the perimenopausal period when hormone levels are fluctuating or may indicate an endocrine disorder.
  ■ Patchy hair loss may be caused by fungal infections of the scalp, hair pulling, constant wearing of caps, or **alopecia areata,** a benign autoimmune disorder.
■ **Hirsutism.** This excess facial or trunk hair may be due to endocrine disorders or steroid use.
■ **Scalp.** Normally the scalp is smooth, firm, symmetrical, nontender, and without lesions.
■ **Pediculosis.** The hair should be free of debris and **pediculosis** (head lice infestation). Head lice are tiny, very mobile, and difficult to see. You may find it easier to see the eggs, or **nits,** that are deposited on the hair shaft close to the scalp.

For a step-by-step description of assessing the hair, see the Highlights of Procedures box near the end of this chapter, and

 Go to **Chapter 19, Procedure 19-3: Assessing the Hair,** in Volume 2.

The Nails

Variations in color, shape, or texture may indicate health problems. For a summary of nail assessment, see the Highlights of Procedures box near the end of this chapter. For illustrations of nail variations and a step-by-step description of nail assessment,

 Go to **Chapter 19, Procedure 19-4: Assessing the Nails,** in Volume 2.

Nail Color Pink nails with rapid capillary refill indicate circulation to the extremities. Other color abnormalities that you may encounter include the following:

- **Half-and-half nails,** in which a distal band of reddish-pink covers 20% to 60% of the nail. These occur in clients with low albumin levels or renal disease.
- **Mees' lines,** which are transverse white lines in the nailbed. They are seen in clients who have experienced severe illnesses or nutritional deficiencies.
- **Splinter hemorrhages,** which are small hemorrhages under the nailbed. They are associated with bacterial endocarditis or trauma.

Nail Shape A change in nail shape may indicate underlying disease. Clubbing, in which the nail plate angle is 180° or more, is associated with long-term hypoxic states, such as occur with chronic lung disease (see Procedure 19-4 in Volume 2).

Nail Texture Nails and surrounding epidermis are normally smooth. Chronic nail-picking results in callus formation around the nail. Occasionally, the surrounding skin becomes inflamed. This condition, known as **paronychia,** is painful and may require drainage if infection is present.

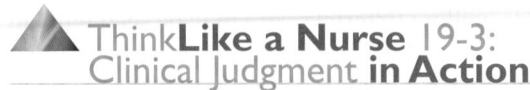

ThinkLike a Nurse 19-3: Clinical Judgment in Action

You are caring for a female client who has no hair on the head. How might you determine the cause of the hair loss? What other assessments should you perform?

THE HEAD

Assessment of the head is often referred to by the acronym HEENT: **H**ead, **E**yes, **E**ars, **N**ose, and **T**hroat. You will use all the assessment techniques—inspection, palpation, percussion, and auscultation—in the HEENT examination.

The Skull and Face

Taking individual variation into account, on inspection, the skull should be rounded and the face symmetrical in appearance and movement. Head size is familial.

- A large head in an adolescent or adult may be associated with **acromegaly,** a disorder associated with excess growth hormone.

- **Microcephaly,** an abnormally small head size in infants, is caused by a variety of genetic and environmental factors.
- **Asymmetry** may be the result of trauma, surgery, neuromuscular disorder, paralysis, or congenital deformity.
- In infants, **abnormal shape or flattening of the skull** may result from trauma during a vaginal birth or placing the baby in the same position for several hours every day.
- In infants and children, a head that is growing disproportionally faster than the body may be a sign of **hydrocephalus** (an accumulation of excessive cerebrospinal fluid).
- **Facial appearance** that is inconsistent with gender, age, or racial/ethnic group may indicate an inherited or chronic disorder, such as Graves disease, hypothyroidism with myxedema, or Cushing syndrome.

The Highlights of Procedures box near the end of this chapter summarizes the assessment of the face. For the entire procedure,

 Go to **Chapter 19, Procedure 19-5: Assessing the Head and Face,** in Volume 2.

The Eyes

In examining the eyes, you will inspect and palpate the external eye structures, assess vision, and examine the internal eye structures. The Highlights of Procedures box near the end of this chapter summarizes the eye examination. For step-by-step instructions,

 Go to **Chapter 19, Procedure 19-6: Assessing the Eyes,** in Volume 2.

For convenience, you may wish to perform some cranial nerve testing along with the eye examination (e.g., corneal reflex, pupillary reaction, accommodation, and extraocular movements). For instructions on performing a cranial nerve examination,

 Go to **Chapter 19, Procedure 19-16: Assessing the Sensory-Neurological System,** in Volume 2.

Visual Acuity

Visual acuity is a measure of the eye's ability to detect the details of an image. When testing visual acuity, you will assess distant, near, peripheral, and color vision, usually with a Snellen chart. Nurses commonly perform screening tests of visual acuity. Other testing is performed by nurses in advanced or specialty practice or by an optometrist or ophthalmologist as needed. To test visual acuity, see Procedure 19-6 in Volume 2.

Distance Vision **Normal vision** is clear vision at 20 feet (20/20) in the right eye, left eye, and both eyes.

Myopia Diminished distant vision, **myopia,** is associated with a smaller fraction. For example, 20/100

vision means that to see text a person with normal vision can read at 100 feet, the client has to stand just 20 feet from the Snellen chart.

Near Vision A client with normal near vision will be able to read the newsprint from a distance of 35.5 cm (14 in.) without hesitation with either eye and with both eyes.

Color Vision **Color vision** is the ability to detect color. Color blindness may be genetically inherited (usually seen in males), or it may result from macular degeneration or other diseases that affect the cones of the eye. Use the color bars at the base of the Snellen chart to test color vision. **Ishihara cards** are specialized cards that enable thorough testing for color blindness. They contain embedded figures within a field of color (see Procedure 19-6 in Volume 2).

Visual Field Visual field is the area the eye is able to observe. It is related to peripheral vision and extraocular muscle (EOM) function. Visual field abnormalities may be caused by problems with cranial nerves (CNs) III, IV, and VI or with the retina. Poorly controlled diabetes, cataracts, macular degeneration, and advanced glaucoma are other disorders that limit the visual field.

- **Peripheral vision** describes the boundaries of the visual field while the eye is in a fixed position. The common phrase "I see you out of the corner of my eye" refers to peripheral vision.
- **EOMs** control the movement of the eye and eyelids and allow you to track movement. Three CNs innervate the EOM: CN III (oculomotor), CN IV (trochlear), and CN VI (abducens). CN III also works together with CN II (optic) to control the pupillary reaction to light. Figure 19-2 illustrates the eye positions affected by the EOM and the corresponding cranial nerves.

External Structures of the Eye

To review the structure of the external eye, see Figure 19-3. There should be no pallor, dryness, or edema.

Eyelids and Lashes The following are common abnormal findings on the eyelids:

- A **pterygium** is a growth or thickening of conjunctiva from the inner canthus toward the iris.

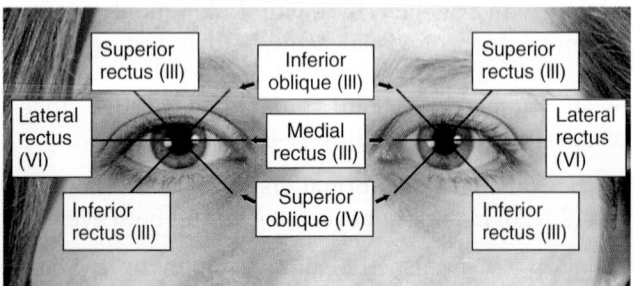

FIGURE 19-2 Cranial nerves and the extraocular muscles.

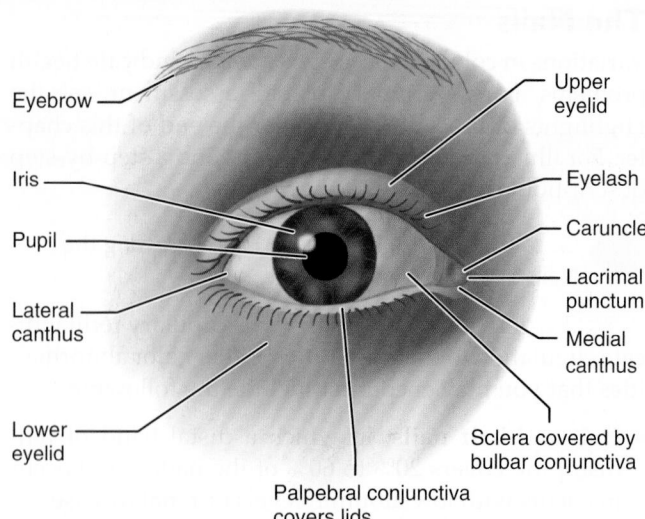

FIGURE 19-3 The external eye and eyelid.

- **Ectropion**, an everted eyelid, is commonly seen in older adults secondary to loss of skin tone. It can lead to excessive dryness of the eyes.
- **Entropion,** an inverted eyelid, can lead to corneal damage.
- **Ptosis,** or drooping of the lid, may be seen in clients who have experienced a stroke (cerebrovascular accident [CVA]) or Bell's palsy (paralysis of the facial nerve). To see ptosis and other abnormalities,

Go to **Chapter 19, Procedure 19-5: Assessing the Head and Face** and **Procedure 19-6: Assessing the Eyes,** in Volume 2.

Sclera and Conjunctiva Associated disorders may include infection, allergies, injuries, and liver disorders. For example, yellow **(icteric)** sclera may be seen with an elevated bilirubin. Blood visible in the sclera is known as a **subconjunctival hemorrhage** and may be related to trauma or hypertension.

Lens and Cornea The lens and the **cornea,** or outermost layer of the eyeball, are transparent, smooth, and moist. Roughness or irregularity of the cornea is seen with trauma or a corneal abrasion.

Pupils The **pupils** should be uniform in color, equal in size, and round. They should **accommodate** equally; that is, the pupils constrict, and the eyes converge (cross) as a person attempts to focus on an object moving toward them. This is typically charted as PERRLA: **P**upils **E**qual, **R**ound, **R**eactive to **L**ight and **A**ccommodation. The following are common pupillary abnormalities:

- **Sluggish accommodation** may be caused by anticholinergic drugs or advanced age.
- **Failure of one or both pupils to accommodate** may reflect a CN III problem or **exophthalmos** (associated with hyperthyroidism).
- **Congenital cataracts,** although rare, may be seen in infants and are checked during an eye examination

using the "red reflex." Congenital cataracts cause "lazy eye" or amblyopia and can lead to other eye problems, such as nystagmus, strabismus, and an inability to fix a gaze upon objects.

- **Cloudy pupils,** a finding related to cataracts, are commonly seen in older adults.

- **Mydriasis** (enlarged pupils) may be seen with glaucoma, an increase in intraocular pressure.
- **Many medications** affect pupil size (e.g., **mydriatics** are used to dilate the pupil to allow better visualization of the internal eye during examination).
- **Miosis** (constricted pupils) often results from medications to treat glaucoma.
- **Anisocoria** (unequal pupils) may be seen with central nervous system disorders such as stroke, head trauma, or cranial nerve injuries. In some individuals, anisocoria may be normal.

Internal Structures of the Eye

Use an ophthalmoscope to visualize the internal structures of the eye (the optic disc, physiological cup, retinal vessels, retinal background, and macula). This is an advanced assessment technique; however, advanced practice nurses and registered nurses on specialty units do perform it with training. This technique provides information about certain diseases that affect the eye, such as hypertension and diabetes.

KnowledgeCheck 19-6

- What are the major components of an eye assessment?
- Identify the cranial nerves involved with eye movement and function.

The Ears and Hearing

The ears are involved in both hearing and equilibrium.

- The **external ear** collects and conveys sound waves to the middle ear. It protects the middle ear from environmental factors such as humidity and temperature and prevents entry of foreign matter.
- The **middle ear** contains the tympanic membrane and cavity, the eustachian tube, and the **ossicles** (the small bones of the middle ear: the malleus, incus, and stapes). The middle ear conducts sound waves to the inner ear.
- The **inner ear** is responsible for hearing and equilibrium. Figure 19-4 illustrates the structures of the ear.

For procedure steps and guidelines for using the otoscope and tuning fork, as well as for other aspects of ear examination, see the Highlights of Procedures box near the end of this chapter and

Go to **Chapter 19, Procedure 19-7: Assessing the Ears and Hearing,** in Volume 2.

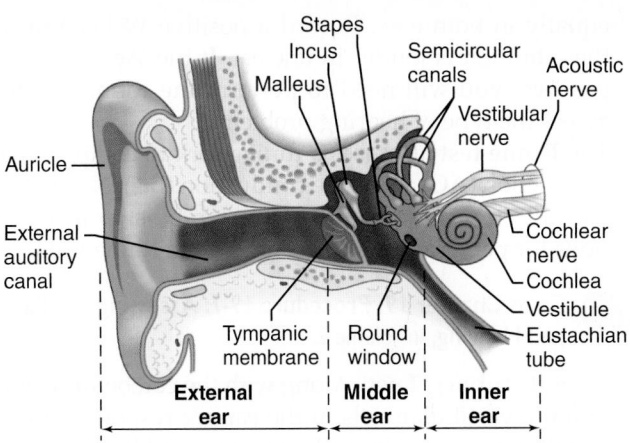

FIGURE 19-4 Cross section of the ear.

Examining the External and Middle Ear

- **On inspection,** the ears should be of equal size and similar appearance. Normally, the pinna is level with the corner of the eye and within a 10° angle of vertical position (shown in Procedure 19-7 in Volume 2).
- **On palpation,** the external structures of the ear are smooth, nontender, pliable, and without nodules. A painful auricle or tragus may be associated with **otitis externa** (an outer ear infection), whereas tenderness behind the ear is seen with **otitis media** (a middle ear infection).

Otoscopic Examination As you begin the otoscopic examination, you may notice that the external auditory canal contains **cerumen** (wax), which protects the middle ear from excessive drying. However, it should not completely obstruct the ear canal. Cerumen may be black, dark red, yellowish, or brown in color and waxy, flaky, soft, or hard, with no odor; all are normal variations. Be careful as you manipulate the otoscope because the inner two-thirds of the canal can be tender with the pressure and manipulation of the otoscope head.

Normally, the **tympanic membrane (TM)** is pearly gray, shiny, and translucent. The structures of the middle ear should be visible through the membrane. Changes in its appearance arise from abnormalities such as otitis media (infection or inflammation of the ear), which causes a red, bulging TM, and the presence of pressure equalization tubes in young clients with chronic ear infections.

Assessing Hearing

To assess hearing, you will need a quiet room and a tuning fork. Gross hearing ability includes the ability to hear both high- and low-pitched tones.

The Weber and Rinne Tests Hearing involves the transmission of sound vibrations and the generation of nerve impulses along CN VIII.

- The **Weber test** assesses both aspects. When you place a vibrating tuning fork on the center of the client's head, they should be able to sense the vibration equally in both ears. Record a positive Weber test if the vibration is louder in one ear. If the Weber test is positive, you will need to perform the Rinne test to assess the type of hearing problem.

- The **Rinne test** also uses a tuning fork to compare air conduction (AC) and bone conduction (BC). Normally AC is twice as long as BC. For step-by-step instructions for performing the Weber and the Rinne tests,

 Go to **Chapter 19, Procedure 19-7: Assessing the Ears and Hearing,** in Volume 2.

The Romberg Test   Along with the cerebellum and midbrain, vestibular cells in the ear are responsible for maintaining equilibrium. To assess equilibrium, perform the Romberg test. You may prefer to perform the Romberg test with examination of the neurological system instead of with the ears.

KnowledgeCheck 19-7
Your client has a negative Weber test. What further testing is required?

 ## ThinkLike a Nurse 19-4: Clinical Judgment in Action
What type of symptoms would you expect a client to be experiencing if they had a positive Romberg test?

The Nose
The nose and sinuses (Fig. 19-5) are the organs of smell and are part of the respiratory system. Vaporized molecules sniffed into the upper nasal cavities trigger receptors that generate impulses along the olfactory nerve (CN I) that travel to olfactory centers in the temporal lobes.

See the Highlights of Procedures box near the end of this chapter for a summary of the examination steps. For the complete procedure, along with expected findings,

 Go to **Chapter 19, Procedure 19-8: Assessing the Nose and Sinuses,** in Volume 2.

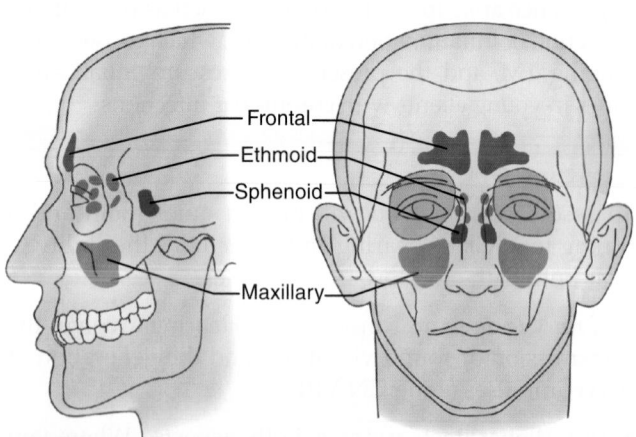

FIGURE 19-5 Paranasal sinuses: frontal, ethmoid, sphenoid, and maxillary.

The Mouth and Oropharynx
The structures of the mouth include the lips, tongue, teeth, **gingiva** (gums), uvula, hard and soft palate, and salivary glands and ducts (Fig. 19-6). On external inspection, the mouth and lips should be symmetrical and without lesions, swelling, or drooping. For an illustration of abnormal conditions and instructions for examining the mouth and oropharynx,

 Go to **Chapter 19, Procedure 19-9: Assessing the Mouth and Oropharynx,** in Volume 2.

Also see the Highlights of Procedures box near the end of this chapter.

- The **lips, buccal mucosa, and gingiva.** The lips, **buccal mucosa** (mucous membrane of the cheeks), and gums should be smooth, moist, and pink in color. Increased pigmentation (e.g., bluish or dark patches) occurs in clients with dark skin. When inspecting the mouth, be sure to ask your client about the use of tobacco, either smoked or chewed. Both forms are associated with an increased risk for oral cancer.
- The **teeth.** Tooth decay and periodontal (gum) disease are common. Poor oral hygiene is a major contributing factor to both. As you examine the mouth and teeth, talk to the patient about oral care and ask about access to dental care. Reasons for delaying or not getting dental care include high costs, lack of insurance or access to services, and fear and anxiety (*Healthy People 2030*, 2020). Recommend tooth brushing after each meal, daily flossing, and dental checkups every 6 months. See Chapter 22 for a more complete discussion of oral hygiene and prevention of periodontal disease.
- The **tongue and oropharynx.** When inspecting the mouth, carefully examine the oropharynx and all aspects of the tongue: dorsal, ventral, and lateral. For illustrations of abnormalities,

 Go to Chapter 19, **Procedure 19-9: Assessing the Mouth and Oropharynx,** in Volume 2.

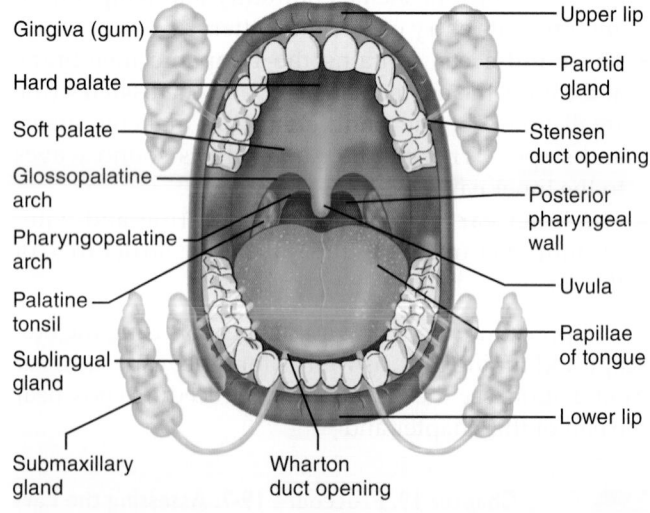

FIGURE 19-6 Structures of the mouth.

THE NECK

The neck has components of the musculoskeletal, neurological, vascular, respiratory, endocrine, and lymphatic systems. The sternocleidomastoid and trapezius muscles form the landmarks of the neck, known as the **anterior and posterior triangles.** The symmetrical neck muscles center and coordinate movement of the head.

The trachea, thyroid gland, anterior cervical nodes, and carotid arteries are positioned in the anterior triangle; the posterior cervical nodes are in the posterior triangle. You will palpate the tracheal rings and the cricoid and thyroid cartilage in the midline of the anterior neck.

For a summary of assessment steps, see the Highlights of Procedures box near the end of this chapter. For the complete procedure and for illustrations of structures of the neck,

 Go to **Chapter 19, Procedure 19-10: Assessing the Neck,** in Volume 2.

The Cervical Lymph Nodes The cervical lymph nodes occur in three chains. The lymph nodes are generally not palpable, although occasionally nodes can be felt, especially in young children. Normal nodes are small in size (less than 1 cm), mobile, soft, and nontender.

The Thyroid Gland Normally, the thyroid is smooth, firm, nontender, and often nonpalpable. However, thyroid abnormalities are common. An enlarged thyroid may be associated with either hypothyroidism or hyperthyroidism. Thyroid masses may be malignant or benign.

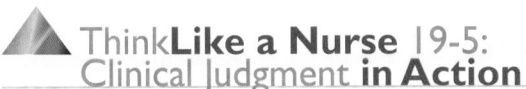
ThinkLike a Nurse 19-5:
Clinical Judgment in Action

A client complains of sore throat, fever, chills, and runny nose. What assessments should you perform?

THE BREASTS AND AXILLAE

The breasts consist of glandular, adipose, and connective tissue; smooth muscle; and nerves (Fig. 19-7). The functions of the female breast are sexual stimulation and milk production for nourishing offspring. Female breast size and shape vary, and commonly one breast is slightly larger than the other. At puberty, the ovaries produce estrogen and progesterone, which stimulate the development of the breasts. The menstrual cycle, pregnancy, and breastfeeding also enlarge breast tissue. Although breasts are thought of as female organs, male individuals also have breasts. However, because of limited estrogen and progesterone levels, male breasts develop only minimally. In the United States, fewer than 1% of all breast cancers occur in men.

Breast tissue and lymph drainage for the breast extend up into the axilla. The majority of breast tumors are found in the tail of Spence, in the axilla. A breast

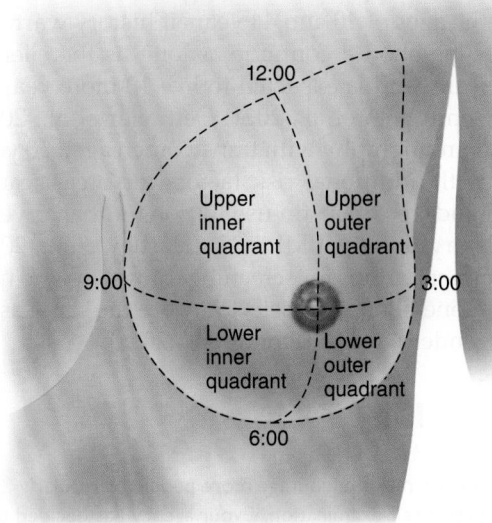

FIGURE 19-7 Breast tissue extends up into the axilla.

examination therefore always includes an examination of the axillae. Clients may have breast reconstruction after breast removal as a result of cancer or breast augmentation for cosmetic reasons. Following breast reconstruction or augmentation, clients should not omit breast examination, and it is performed in exactly the same way as for natural breasts.

Clinical Breast Examination You should perform a breast examination for the client if they cannot do it themselves, and you should demonstrate the procedure as part of client teaching for self-care. Clinical breast examinations are not recommended for average-risk individuals at any age (American Cancer Society, 2022).

Breast Self-Examination Key Point: *Researchers agree that patients who perform a breast self-examination (BSE) should be trained in proper technique in order to avoid falsely negative findings (American Congress of Obstetricians and Gynecologists, 2014, reaffirmed 2021; Phipps et al., 2019).* Men and women should be familiar with how their breast tissue normally looks and feels so that they can be aware of any changes.

For a summary of breast examination, see the Procedure Highlights box at the end of this chapter. For a step-by-step guide to examining the breasts and axillae,

 Go to **Chapter 19, Procedure 19-11: Assessing the Breasts and Axillae,** in Volume 2.

Mammography and Thermography The American Cancer Society (2022) recommends that individuals with average risk of breast cancer undergo regular screening mammography or breast thermography starting at age 45 years. Individuals aged 45 to 54 years should be screened annually; individuals 55 years and older should transition to biennial screening or have the opportunity to continue screening annually. Clients should have the opportunity to begin annual screening between the ages of 40 and 44 years if history warrants, and screening should continue as long as the client is in good health and is expected to live 10 more years or longer (Monticciolo et al., 2021; Oeffinger et al., 2015). Discuss mammography with transwomen aged 50 years or older with additional risk factors for breast cancer (estrogen and/or progestin use for longer than 5 years, family history, and/or BMI > 35) (Hartley et al., 2018). The recommendations for screening transmen who have not undergone bilateral mastectomy are the same as for nontransgender women (Stone et al., 2018).

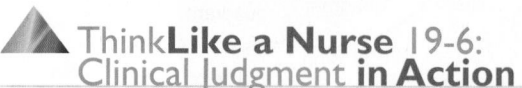

ThinkLike a Nurse 19-6: Clinical Judgment in Action

What strategies might encourage more people to regularly perform breast self-examination, if your agency has decided to promote that measure?

THE CHEST AND LUNGS

The chest, or thorax, is the bony cage that protects the heart, lungs, and great vessels. The ribs, sternum, and vertebrae form the chest. **Key Point:** *Be systematic in your assessment: Always assess the areas of the chest and lungs in the same order.* To learn how to assess the chest and lungs,

 Go to **Chapter 19, Procedure 19-12, Assessing the Chest and Lungs**, in Volume 2.

For a summary, see the Highlights of Procedures box near the end of this chapter.

Chest Landmarks

Before beginning the thoracic examination, review the following important landmarks that will help you visualize the underlying structures and perform an accurate assessment:

- **Anterior chest**—Identify positions vertically on the anterior chest in relation to the ribs. For example, the space between the fifth and sixth ribs is known as the fifth intercostal space (5th ICS). You can easily palpate the ribs and count the spaces if you remember that the 1st rib is tucked up next to the clavicle (Fig. 19-8A).
- **Anterior chest**—Use a series of imaginary vertical lines (Fig. 19-8B) with the rib spaces to further aid in identifying locations on the anterior chest. For instance, the apex of the heart is usually located in the fifth intercostal space at the left midclavicular line (5th ICS MCL).
- **Posterior chest**—Identify positions vertically in relation to the vertebrae (Fig. 19-9B). The prominent vertebra at the base of the neck is the seventh cervical vertebra (C7). The next one down is T1 (first thoracic). Counting down to about T9 should be adequate.
- **Lateral and posterior chest**—Use imaginary lines on the lateral and posterior chest as well. Figure 19-9,

parts A and C, illustrates the location of these lines. Notice that the anterior axillary line can be used to locate sounds on both the anterior and lateral chest.

Chest Shape and Size

The chest diameter expands up to 3 inches (7.6 cm) with deep inspiration. The anteroposterior diameter of the chest is about half the size of the lateral diameter (written as AP: Lateral = 1:2).

 Musculoskeletal changes associated with aging result in a gradual increase in the anteroposterior diameter. This change is also seen, regardless of age, in clients who have chronic obstructive pulmonary disease (COPD), a disorder associated with long-term smoking. Figure 19-10 illustrates normal and "barrel" chest shapes.

Osteoporosis, a common disorder associated with aging, is associated with increased porosity of the vertebrae. As a result, vertebrae may compress or collapse, shortening the length of the spine and pushing the ribs forward and downward.

Breath Sounds

Listen to breath sounds in a quiet room by auscultating one full respiratory cycle at each site. Directly apply the stethoscope to the client's skin. Compare breath sounds bilaterally. Three types of normal breath sounds are heard (Fig. 19-11).

- **Normal sounds.** Three types of normal breath sounds are heard: bronchial, bronchovesicular, and vesicular.
- **Abnormal sounds.** Breath sounds that differ from those three are abnormal (adventitious), for example, wheezing or sounds that are difficult to hear.

For more information about the respiratory system, see Chapter 33. For a table describing normal and abnormal breath sounds and the procedure for performing a respiratory assessment, see the Highlights of Procedures Box and

 Go to **Chapter 19, Procedure 19-12: Assessing the Chest and Lungs**, in Volume 2.

KnowledgeCheck 19-8

- List and describe the location of the horizontal and vertical landmarks of the anterior chest.
- List and describe the location of the horizontal and vertical landmarks of the posterior chest.
- List and describe the location of the vertical landmarks of the lateral chest.

THE CARDIOVASCULAR SYSTEM

The cardiovascular system consists of the heart and the blood vessels. The heart is a muscle that pumps blood throughout the body. In a healthy adult, it is about the size of a clenched fist. The blood vessels, which make

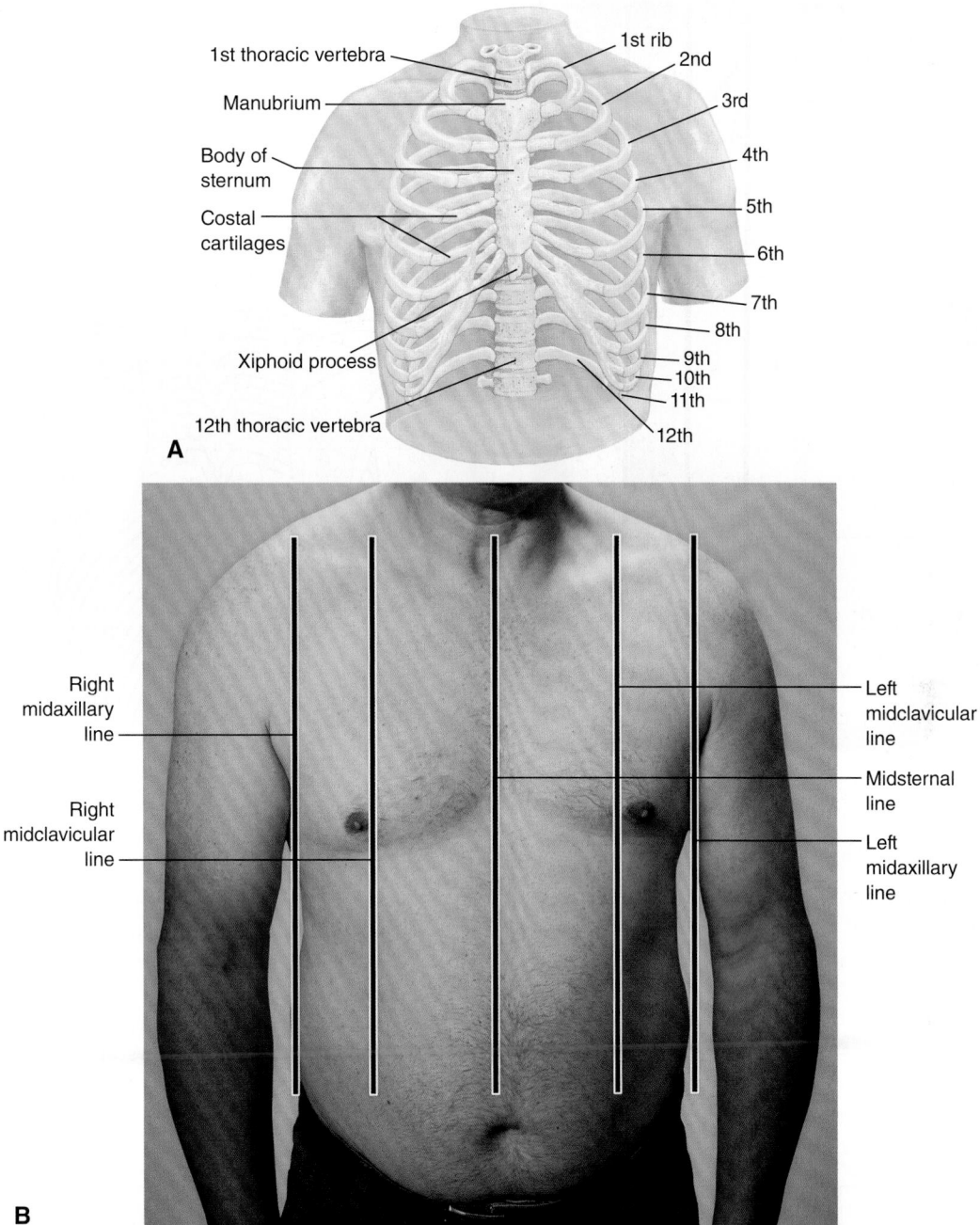

FIGURE 19-8 *A,* The anterior thoracic cage and the bony landmarks. *B,* A series of imaginary vertical lines is used to describe locations on the chest.

up the vascular system, have two main networks: the pulmonary circulation and the systemic circulation. See Chapter 34 if you need to review the anatomy of the cardiovascular system.

- **Pulmonary circulation.** Oxygen-depleted blood circulates from the heart into the lungs, where it is oxygenated, then back to the heart. This system is known as the **pulmonary circulation.**
- **Systemic circulation.** The left ventricle pumps blood into the **systemic circulation** via the arterial system.
- **Capillaries.** The arteries subdivide many times, becoming smaller and smaller until they separate,

in the tissues and organs, into **capillaries.** It is at the capillary level that oxygen is delivered to the tissues.
- **The venous system** collects the oxygen-depleted blood and returns it to the right atrium of the heart to begin the circuit again.
- **The coronary circulation,** which circulates blood through the heart itself, is a part of the systemic circulation.

For further discussion on pulmonary circulation and oxygenation, see Chapter 34. The Highlights of Procedures box at the end of this chapter summarizes

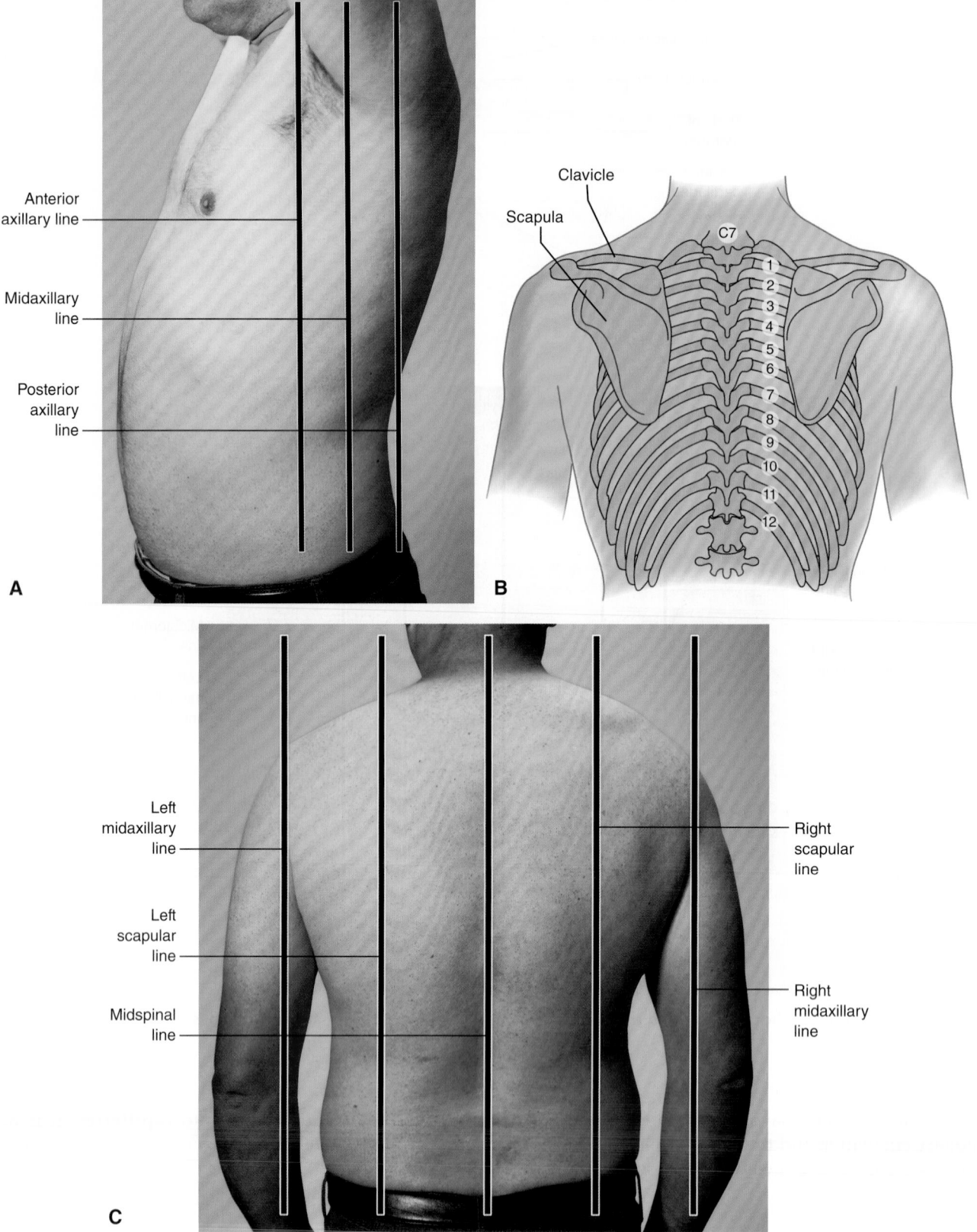

FIGURE 19-9 *A*, Lateral chest landmarks. *B*, The vertebrae are the landmarks on the posterior chest. *C*, Landmark lines on the posterior chest.

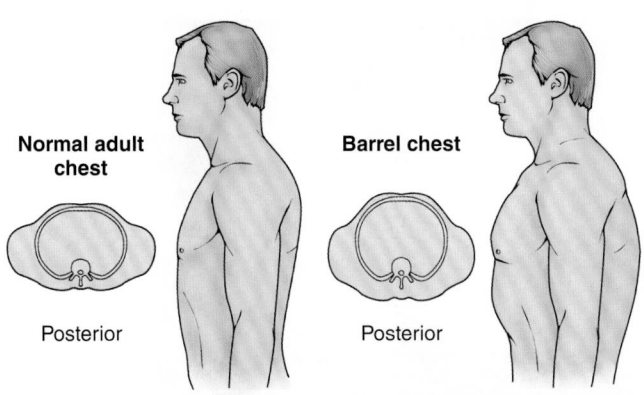

Normal adult chest

Barrel chest

Posterior

Posterior

FIGURE 19-10 The normal anteroposterior to lateral ratio is 1:2. The lateral aspect of the chest increases dramatically with COPD, leading to a barrel-chest appearance.

assessment of the heart and vascular system. For a complete step-by-step procedure,

 Go to **Chapter 19, Procedure 19-13: Assessing the Heart and Vascular System,** in Volume 2.

The Heart

The heart is positioned at an angle on the left side of the chest in the third, fourth, and fifth ICSs. To facilitate auscultation of specific heart sounds,

perform the cardiac assessment with the client in three positions: sitting, supine, and left lateral recumbent. Clients with chronic heart or lung problems may have little cardiac reserve, so minimize position changes to conserve your client's energy.

♥ **iCare** To help minimize your client's anxiety, explain that it always takes time to examine the heart and circulatory system.

The Cardiac Cycle

During a cardiac cycle, the atria and ventricles alternately contract and relax to fill and empty; while the atria are contracting (emptying), the ventricles are relaxing (filling), and vice versa.

- **Systole** refers to the contraction, or emptying, of the ventricles.
- **Diastole** refers to the relaxation, or filling, phase of the ventricles.

Inspecting and Palpating the Heart

Begin your assessment of the heart with the client sitting.

- *Observe the **precordium**,* the area of the chest over the heart, for visible pulsations. A small pulsation at the 5th ICS MCL, also known as the **point of maximal impulse (PMI),** is normal.

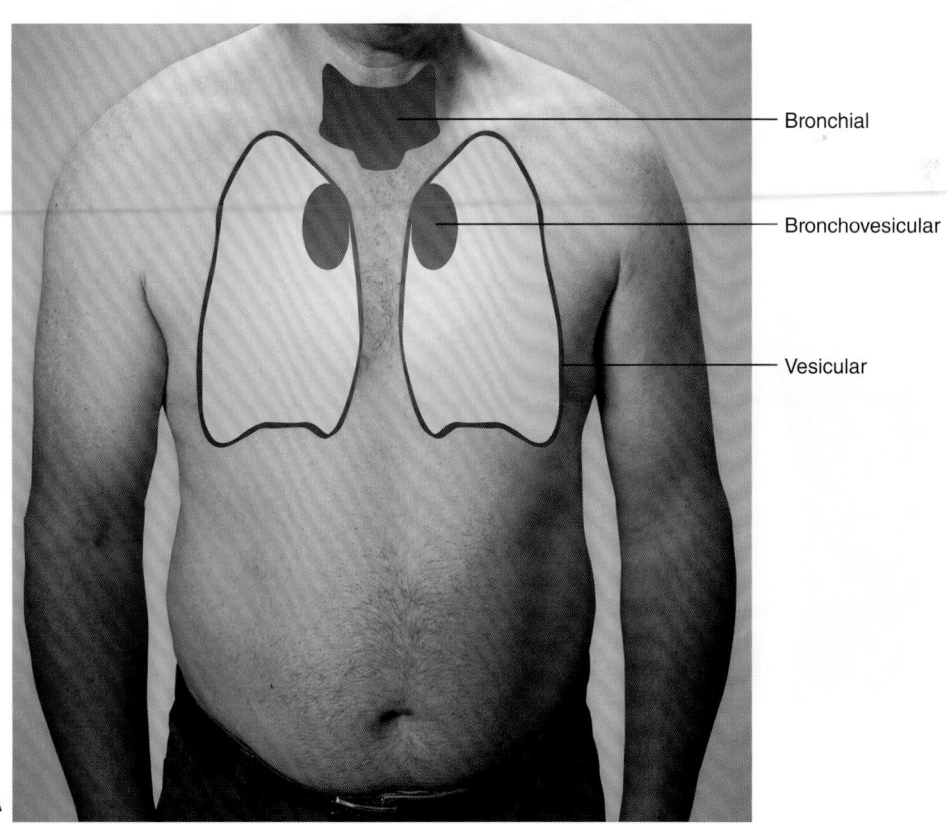

Bronchial

Bronchovesicular

Vesicular

A

FIGURE 19-11 Normal breath sounds. A, Anterior.

Continued

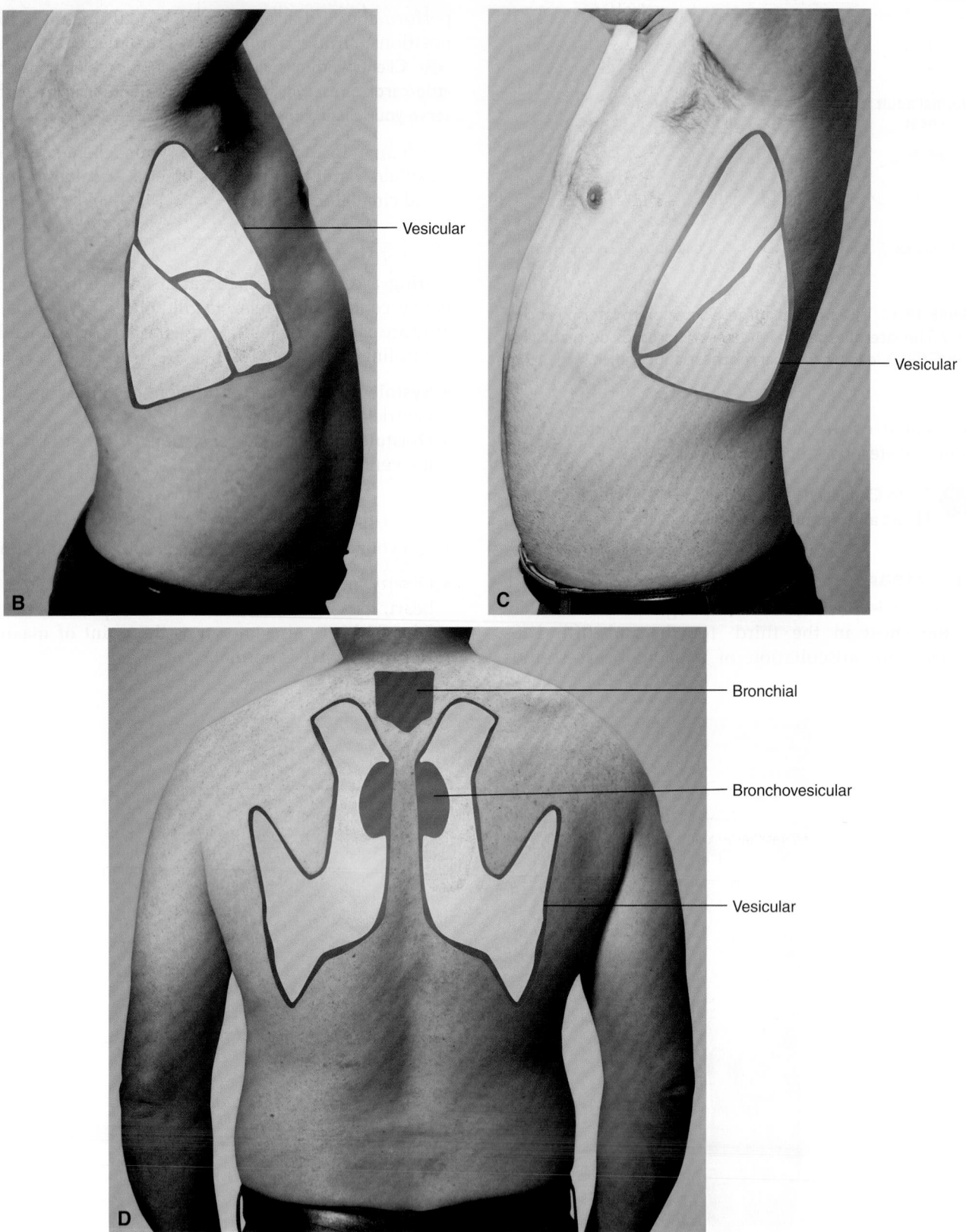

FIGURE 19-11—cont'd *B,* Right lateral. *C,* Left lateral. *D,* Posterior.

■ *Also palpate for vibrations.* A **thrill** is a vibration or pulsation palpated in any area except the PMI. A thrill is associated with abnormal blood flow and usually has an accompanying **murmur** (additional heart sound).

Auscultating the Heart

Auscultate to establish cardiac rate and rhythm and to identify normal and abnormal heart sounds. A quiet room is essential.

■ **The four sites located over the heart valves are the preferred listening areas.** However, you can hear heart sounds from any location on the anterior chest wall. Table 19-3 and Figure 19-12 describe

Table 19-3 ➤ Locations for Assessing the Heart

STRUCTURE TITLE	VALVE ASSESSED	LOCATION
Base Right	Aortic valve	2nd ICS right sternal border
Base Left	Pulmonic valve	2nd ICS left sternal border
Left Lateral	Tricuspid valve	4th ICS left sternal border
Apex	Mitral valve	5th ICS MCL

ICS, Intercostal space; *MCL*, midclavicular line.

BASE

— Base right (aortic)
— Base left (pulmonic)
— Erb point
— Left sternal border (tricuspid)
— Apex (mitral), PMI

APEX

FIGURE 19-12 Cardiac auscultation sites.

these locations. To learn more about auscultating the precordium,

 Go to **Chapter 19, Procedure 19-13: Assessing the Heart and Vascular System,** in Volume 2.

■ **Auscultate in an orderly fashion.** Start at the aortic area, and move gradually through each landmark. The following is a mnemonic you may use to recall the order of the heart sound landmarks:

Aunt	Aortic
Polly	Pulmonic
Takes	Tricuspid
Meds	Mitral

Heart Sounds Listen carefully at each site to each component of the heart sounds. For more information about abnormal heart sounds,

 Go to **Chapter 19, Procedure 19-13: Assessing the Heart and Vascular System, step 8,** in Volume 2.

■ **First heart sound.** S_1 (or "lub") results from the closure of the valves between the atria and ventricles. "Lub" is a dull, low-pitched sound, loudest over the mitral and tricuspid areas. S_1 marks the beginning of systole.

■ **Second heart sound.** S_2 (or "dub") corresponds to closure of the semilunar valves (between the ventricles and the great arteries exiting the heart). "Dub" is higher in pitch and shorter than the S_1 "lub." The S_2 is loudest at the aortic and pulmonic areas. S_2 marks the beginning of diastole. Normally, the mitral and tricuspid valves and the aortic and pulmonic valves close within a fraction of a second from each other. This near-simultaneous closure results in a singular S_1 and S_2 sound. However, a split sound may occur, at either S_1 or S_2, if there is a delay in closure of one of the valves.

■ **Third heart sound.** A third heart sound (S_3), heard immediately after S_2, has a gallop cadence that follows the rhythm of the word "KenTUCKy." It is best heard at the apical site with the client lying on his left side.

■ **Fourth heart sound.** A fourth heart sound (S_4), heard immediately before S_1, has a rhythm that follows the word "FLOrida." S_4 is best heard at the apical site, using the bell of the stethoscope, with the client lying on their left side.

■ **Murmurs** are additional sounds produced by turbulent flow through the heart. Some murmurs are "innocent," but others represent pathology, such as an alteration in valve structure. Identifying and classifying a murmur are advanced skills that require practice. To learn more about assessing murmurs,

Go to **Chapter 19, Procedure 19-13: Assessing the Heart and Vascular System,** in Volume 2.

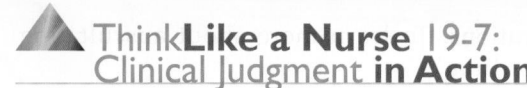

ThinkLike a Nurse 19-7: Clinical Judgment in Action

What findings would you anticipate when assessing Mr. Williams' (Meet Your Patient) thorax?

The Vascular System

The vascular system is a network of arteries and veins that transport oxygen, carbon dioxide, and nutrients to the cells of the body.

- **Arteries carry blood away from the heart.**
  - The *pulmonary arteries* carry oxygen-depleted blood from the right ventricle to the lungs.
  - The *systemic arteries* carry oxygenated blood from the left ventricle to the body periphery.
- **Veins carry blood toward the heart**.
  - The *pulmonary veins* transport oxygenated blood from the lungs to the left atrium.
  - The *systemic veins* return oxygen-depleted blood from the periphery to the right atrium of the heart.

The Central Vessels

The carotid arteries and internal jugular veins run alongside the sternocleidomastoid muscle on both sides of the neck. These central vessels provide circulation to the brain. For illustrations,

 Go to **Chapter 19, Procedure 19-13: Assessing the Heart and Vascular System,** in Volume 2

The Carotid Arteries Because the carotid arteries are large and close to the heart, you can easily feel a pulse over the carotid artery, even when it is difficult to palpate a peripheral pulse.

- ✚ Never palpate both carotid arteries at the same time because bilateral pressure may impair cerebral blood flow.
- As a general rule, avoid palpating the carotids except during cardiopulmonary resuscitation or when it is necessary to assess them for a specific reason (such as in a comprehensive physical examination or when an underlying pathology makes it necessary to establish that circulation to the head is adequate).

- Turbulent blood flow through the carotid artery produces a whooshing sound known as a **bruit.** Bruits are common among older adults.

The Jugular Veins return blood from the brain to the superior vena cava. The best position for assessment of jugular venous distention (JVD) is semi-Fowler's (30° to 45° angle).

- The *external jugular veins* are superficial; the *internal jugular veins* are deep.
- Normally, the jugular veins are flat when the client is in an upright position and distend when the client lies flat.
- JVD is seen when the right side of the heart is congested because of inadequate pump function.

The Peripheral Vessels

The peripheral vessels supply blood to all the body cells. The **arteries** are a high-pressure system with several palpable pulse sites. The **veins** are a low-pressure system with valves to prevent backflow caused by gravity. The veins return blood to the heart via the continuing pressure from the arterial system and the pumping action of the adjacent skeletal muscles. You will assess the peripheral vascular system by:

- *Measuring the blood pressure* (see Chapter 18). Usually you will measure the blood pressure at the start of the examination as part of the general survey.
- *Palpating the peripheral pulses* (see Chapter 18). In a healthy individual, pulses will be regular, strong, and equal bilaterally. Weak, absent, or asymmetrical pulses may indicate partial or complete occlusion of the artery. Other signs of arterial occlusion include pain, pallor, cool temperature, paresthesia, or paralysis.
- *Inspecting and performing tests for adequate perfusion.* The data you obtain when inspecting and palpating the integumentary system provide some information about peripheral tissue perfusion. Recall that when an area is not adequately oxygenated, the skin may be pale, cyanotic, cool, and shiny; hair growth may be sparse compared with other areas; and there may be clubbing of the nails. Inadequate tissue oxygenation may be a result of chronic pulmonary problems; however, it can also result from impaired central or peripheral circulation.

For more information on assessment of peripheral vessels,

 Go to **Chapter 19, Procedure 19-13: Assessing the Heart and Vascular System,** in Volume 2.

KnowledgeCheck 19-9

Identify the precautions to take when evaluating the carotid arteries.

THE ABDOMEN

The method most commonly used to identify the location of assessment findings is the four-quadrant method, which divides the abdomen into four sections by "drawing" a line vertically from the xiphoid process to the symphysis pubis and a horizontal line at the level of the umbilicus (Fig. 19-13).

- To promote comfort, ask the client to empty their bladder before the examination.
- **Key Point: *When examining the abdomen, inspect and auscultate first, before percussing and palpating. Percussion and palpation stimulate the bowel and may alter bowel sounds; therefore, the examination sequence differs from that for other body systems.***

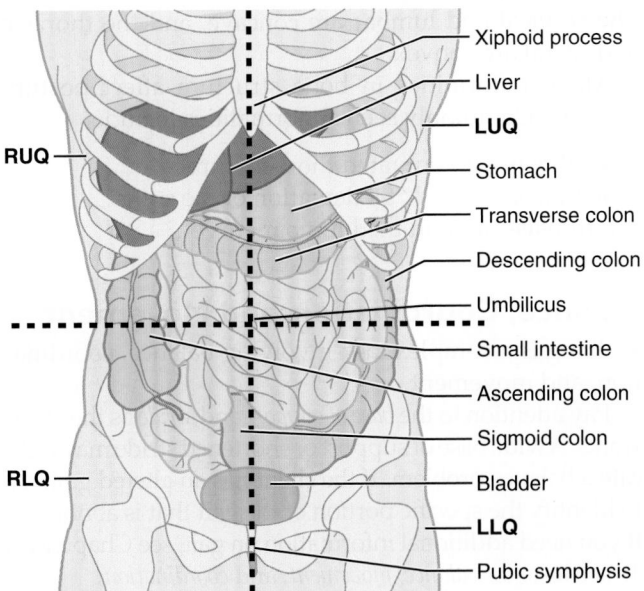

FIGURE 19-13 The four abdominal quadrants.

Xiphoid process
Liver
LUQ
RUQ
Stomach
Transverse colon
Descending colon
Umbilicus
Small intestine
Ascending colon
Sigmoid colon
RLQ
Bladder
LLQ
Pubic symphysis

 iCare ▪ If the client has a painful area, examine that area last to minimize discomfort during the rest of the examination.

Inspecting the Abdomen The skin over the abdomen is usually paler than that over other parts of the body. In clients with abdominal distention, the skin will appear taut. Distention may be normal, as with pregnancy, or it may be due to gas or fluid retention or bowel obstruction. Note the position, contour, and color of the umbilicus. Swelling or bulging near the umbilicus may indicate an **umbilical hernia.** Umbilical hernia is fairly common in infants due to delayed closure around a small muscle around the umbilicus (belly button). In adults, being overweight or having multiple pregnancies may increase the risk of developing an umbilical hernia. For an illustration of an umbilical hernia,

 Go to **Chapter 19, Procedure 19-14: Assessing the Abdomen,** in Volume 2.

See Figure 19-14 for typical variations in abdominal shape.

Auscultating the Abdomen Proceed in an organized manner, listening in several areas in all four quadrants. Use the same pattern for every examination so that it becomes routine.

▪ **First, auscultate bowel sounds.** Bowel sounds are high-pitched, irregular gurgles or clicks lasting 1 to several seconds and occurring every 5 to 15 seconds (or 5 to 30 times per minute) in the average adult. For information on abnormal bowel sounds,

 Go to **Chapter 19, Procedure 19-14: Assessing the Abdomen,** in Volume 2.

▪ **Next, auscultate the major arteries.** Major arterial vessels lie in the abdomen below the intestines. Listen over the aorta and the renal, iliac, and femoral arteries for the presence of bruits.

Percussing the Abdomen Use indirect percussion to assess for fluid, air, organs, or masses. Some practitioners include percussion of the kidney with the abdominal examination.

Palpating the Abdomen Begin with light palpation to put the patient at ease. Palpate for tenderness and guarding in all four quadrants. Palpation of the liver and spleen is an advanced technique not usually performed by staff nurses, except perhaps in some specialty areas.

The Highlights of Procedures box at the end of this chapter summarizes abdominal assessment. For the complete procedure,

Go to **Chapter 19, Procedure 19-14: Assessing the Abdomen,** in Volume 2.

KnowledgeCheck 19-10

▪ What strategies can you use to make the client more comfortable during an abdominal assessment?
▪ Identify the sequence of assessment for the abdominal examination.

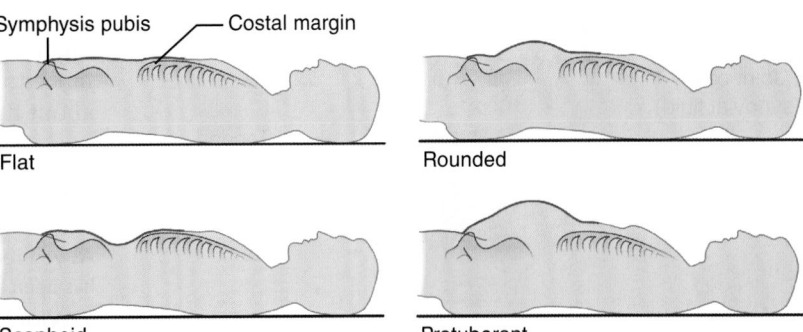

FIGURE 19-14 Normal variations in abdominal contour.

Symphysis pubis — Costal margin

Flat

Rounded

Scaphoid

Protuberant

THE MUSCULOSKELETAL SYSTEM

The musculoskeletal system consists of bones, muscles, and joints. Bone is complex, living tissue that responds to nutrition, stress, and illness.

- **The bones** include
  - *Long bones,* such as the humerus and tibia;
  - *Flat bones,* such as the sternum and ribs; and
  - *Irregular bones,* such as the vertebrae and pelvis.
  - **Tendons, ligaments, and cartilage** serve as connecting structures.
  - **Bursae,** small disc-shaped, fluid-filled sacs, act as cushions to reduce friction between the joint and the tendons that cross over the joint (Fig. 19-15).

The musculoskeletal system provides shape and support to the body, allows movement, protects internal organs, produces red blood cells in the bone marrow, and stores calcium and phosphorus. Assessment of the musculoskeletal system includes evaluation of the client's posture, gait, bone structure, muscle function, and joint mobility. The procedure is summarized in the Highlights of Procedures box at the end of this chapter. For step-by-step instructions,

 Go to **Chapter 19, Procedure 19-15: Assessing the Musculoskeletal System,** in Volume 2.

Body Shape and Symmetry

To assess bone structure, examine body shape and symmetry. The client should be able to stand upright with the neck and head midline. There are four normal curvatures of the spine (see Procedure 19-15 in Volume 2).

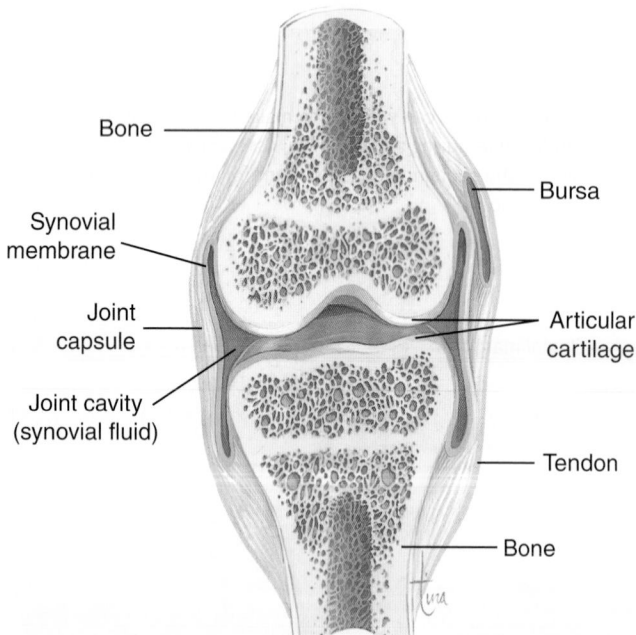

FIGURE 19-15 Many synovial joints have bursae that act as cushions against friction.

The cervical and lumbar are concave, and the thoracic and sacral are convex.

Major deformities in bone structure affect posture and gait. Commonly seen abnormalities include:

- **Kyphosis**—accentuated thoracic curve
- **Scoliosis**—lateral "S" deviation of the spine
- **Lordosis**—accentuated lumbar curve

Balance, Coordination, and Movement

Walking is a complex task involving balance, coordination, and movement.

Pay attention to the *base of support* and *stride* as the client walks. A wide base of support or shortened stride may indicate a balance problem. If the client has an altered gait, try to identify the specific portion of the gait that is abnormal. If you need additional information on gait, see Chapter 29. To see tests for *balance, movement,* and *coordination,*

 Go to **Chapter 19, Procedure 19-15: Assessing the Musculoskeletal System,** in Volume 2.

♥ **iCare** As you perform each assessment, pay attention to the client's stability and level of comfort. Do not attempt movements that may produce pain or cause the client to fall. For example, recall that Stanley Williams (Meet Your Patient) has bilateral knee pain. Before asking him to perform deep knee bends or hop in place, you would want to assess his pain and its triggers.

Joint Mobility and Muscle Function

Joints should move freely, without pain or crepitus (clicking or grating sounds).

- **Color changes** in a joint indicate inflammation or infection. If you see erythema or swelling, investigate further by feeling for warmth.
- **Joint deformity** requires investigation. Determine any effect the deformity has on function.
- To **assess function,** test range of motion (ROM) and muscle strength.
  - **Active ROM** requires the client to move the joint through its full ROM.
  - **Passive ROM** is used when the client is unable to exercise each joint independently. Instead, you support the body and move each joint through its ROM.
- **Assess muscle strength** along with movement by asking the patient to perform ROM while you apply resistance to the part being moved. For more information about the musculoskeletal system, see Chapter 29.

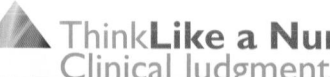 Think**Like a Nurse** 19-8:
Clinical Judgment **in Action**

As you recall, Mr. Williams (Meet Your Patient) is overweight and has been having pain in both of his knees.

- What history questions would you ask him to assess his knee pain?
- What would you do to examine his knees?

THE NEUROLOGICAL SYSTEM

The neurological system controls or affects the function of all body systems and allows interaction with the external world. Its work is carried out through the transmission of chemical and electrical signals between the brain and the rest of the body. The basic functions of the nervous system are cognition, emotion, memory, sensation and perception, and regulation of homeostasis.

A comprehensive neurological assessment takes hours to complete and is usually reserved for clients with symptoms of neurological problems. As a staff nurse in general practice, you usually perform only portions of a neurological examination. In the next few sections, we look at the components of a focused neurological examination. For a summary, see the Highlights of Procedures box at the end of this chapter. For the complete procedure

 Go to **Chapter 19, Procedure 19-16: Assessing the Sensory-Neurological System,** in Volume 2.

Developmental Considerations

When interpreting a neurological examination, consider the following developmental changes and modifications.

Infants Reflexes present at birth include rooting, sucking, palmar grasp, tonic neck reflex (fencing), and Moro. These reflexes disappear during infancy. With neurological injury, as may occur with stroke or trauma, these reflexes may return, indicating severe neurological problems (see Chapter 6).

Young Children Because language skills and motor development are age-dependent, the Denver Developmental Screening Test (Denver II, 1990) is used as a neurological screen for young children. The Denver II examines motor, language, and coordination skills. It requires specialized training to administer and evaluate. For toddlers and older children, you can usually perform a comprehensive neurological examination with age-appropriate modifications. For example, when testing for smell, use materials that a young child knows, such as bananas or apples.

With advanced age, changes commonly observed are slower reaction time, a decreased ability for rapid problem-solving, and slower voluntary movement. The number of functioning neurons decreases. However, intelligence, memory, and discrimination do not change with normal aging.

Neurological deficits in older adults are usually the result of adverse effects of medications or medication interactions, nutritional deficits, dehydration, cardiovascular changes that alter cerebral blood flow, diabetes, degenerative neurological conditions (e.g., Parkinson disease or Alzheimer disease), alcohol or drug use, depression, or abuse.

Cerebral Function

Cerebral function refers to the client's intellectual and behavioral functioning. It includes level of consciousness (LOC), orientation, mental status and cognitive function, and communication.

Level of Consciousness

LOC includes arousal and orientation.

Arousal Arousal may range from alert to deeply comatose. Arousal is classified based on the type of stimuli (auditory, tactile, or painful) required to produce a response from the client. An alert client responds to *auditory stimuli* (e.g., verbal communication or noise). **Key Point:** *Remember, if your client does not speak the same language as you do, they may not respond to questions or instructions.*

Orientation *Orientation* refers to the client's awareness of time, place, and person.

- **Orientation to time** includes awareness of the year, date, and time of day. Hospitalized patients are subjected to lights and noise around the clock, are roused in the middle of the night for medications or time-sensitive treatments, and are given anesthesia and pain medications that alter their sense of awareness, so they easily become disoriented to time.
- **Orientation to place** involves awareness of surroundings. The patient should know that they are, for example, in the hospital and not in church. Patients who have been moved (e.g., from the emergency department to a ward bed) may not recall their room number but are easily reoriented.
- **Orientation to person** involves recognition of familiar persons and self-identity. The client should be able to state their name or identify people in photographs at the bedside. Because a client may meet many health professionals during a hospitalization, they may not be able to recall your name unless you have had repeated encounters.

Mental Status and Cognitive Function

Mental status and cognitive function include behavior, appearance, response to stimuli, speech, memory, communication, and judgment. By this point in the examination, you would have already interviewed the client and talked with them while performing the examination, so you would have a good deal of information about their mental status and cognitive function. You would have already assessed posture, gait, motor movements, dress, and hygiene through the general survey and the musculoskeletal examination, and you would be aware of the client's mood based on the tone of voice, actions, and statements.

Many clinicians choose to screen for mental status and cognitive function by working questions into the interaction with the client as they assess other body systems. This type of informal assessment is not only more natural for the client, but it is also more accurate. If you choose this method, observe for clarity of thought, appropriate content, concentration, memory, and ability to perform abstract reasoning.

Documenting Cerebral Function

Glasgow Coma Scale (GCS) Document LOC by describing the client's response or using the GCS to grade eye, motor, and verbal responses. The GCS evaluates eye opening, motor responses, and verbal responses. Its limitations are that it relies heavily on vision and verbal interaction, and it does not evaluate brainstem reflexes.

Full Outline of UnResponsiveness (FOUR) A systematic review of evidence suggests that best practice should include the use of the GCS plus other evaluation of brainstem reflexes, eye examination, vital signs, and respiratory assessment. The **FOUR** provides additional information beyond that of the GCS. To see and use both scales,

 Go to **Chapter 19, Procedure 19-16: Assessing the Sensory-Neurological System**, in Volume 2.

Documenting Responses If you are not using the GCS, use the following terms to describe arousal:

- **Alert**—Follows commands in a timely fashion.
- **Lethargic**—Appears drowsy; easily drifts off to sleep.
- **Stuporous**—Requires vigorous stimulation before responding.

- **Comatose**—Does not respond to verbal or painful stimuli.

Although these terms are widely used, a thorough description is preferable. Look at the following two chart entries:

Example 1: Pt. lethargic.
Example 2: Pt. responds to repeated tactile and verbal stimulation. Quickly drifts off to sleep if stimulation is discontinued.

As you can see, the second charting entry provides significantly more information than the first.

Cranial Nerve Function

CN assessment is a key component of the neurological examination. The cranial nerves control a variety of sensory and motor functions (Table 19-4 and Fig. 19-16).

Reflex Function

A reflex produces a rapid, involuntary response that occurs at the level of the spinal cord. Because the brain is not involved, muscle response is instantaneous. Intact sensory and motor systems are required for a normal reflex response.

- **Deep tendon reflexes (DTRs)** are automatic responses that do not require conscious thought from the brain.

Table 19-4 ➤ Cranial Nerves

CRANIAL NERVE NUMBER AND NAME	TYPE OF NERVE	FUNCTION OF NERVE
I. Olfactory	Sensory	Smell
II. Optic	Sensory	Visual acuity, visual fields, and ocular fundi
III. Oculomotor	Motor	EOM, pupil constriction
IV. Trochlear	Motor	EOM
V. Trigeminal: 3 branches	Sensory and motor	Corneal reflex; scalp, teeth, and facial sensation; and jaw movement
VI. Abducens	Motor	EOM
VII. Facial	Motor and sensory	Facial movement, sense of taste
VIII. Auditory	Sensory	Hearing and equilibrium
IX. Glossopharyngeal	Motor and sensory	Swallowing, gag response, tongue movement, taste, secretion of saliva
X. Vagus	Motor and sensory	Sensation of pharynx and larynx; motor activity of swallowing and vocal cords; sensory in cardiac, respiratory, and blood pressure reflexes; peristalsis; digestive secretions
XI. Spinal accessory	Motor	Head movement and shoulder elevation; motor to larynx (speaking)
XII. Hypoglossal	Motor	Tongue movement

EOM, **Extraocular muscle.**

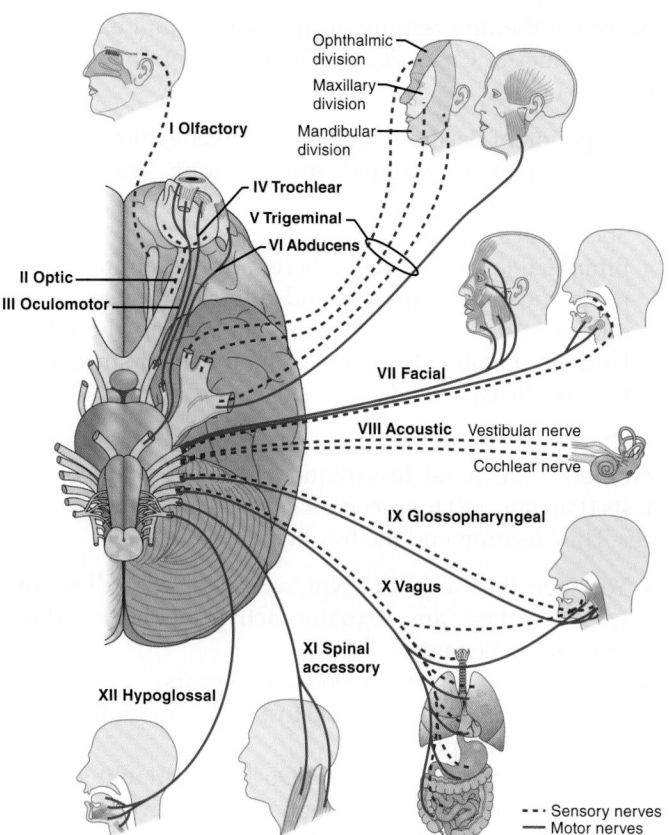

FIGURE 19-16 Origin of cranial nerves.

Motor and Cerebellar Function

The neurological system coordinates the function of the skeleton and muscles. Motor pathways transmit information between the brain and muscles, and the muscles control movement of the skeleton. The cerebellum helps coordinate muscle movement, regulate muscle tone, and maintain posture and equilibrium. The cerebellum is also largely responsible for **proprioception,** or body positioning. Disorders of motor and cerebellar function result in pain or problems with movement, gait, or posture. Thus, when you assess the musculoskeletal system, you also assess the motor functions of the neurological system.

KnowledgeCheck 19-11

- Identify and describe the components assessed in the neurological examination.
- What approach to assessment should you take in the following scenarios?
  Your client has no neurological problems, but you are performing a comprehensive examination.
  Your client is hospitalized for a documented cerebrovascular accident.
  Your client has been admitted with an acute head injury, and the extent of neurological injury is unknown.

THE GENITOURINARY SYSTEM

In most practice settings, nurses assess only the patient's external genitalia and inguinal lymph nodes. Nurse practitioners and physicians perform comprehensive examinations of the reproductive and urinary systems, as do nurses working in specialty areas. However, even as a novice nurse, you may assist with examinations or just be present as a witness or to provide emotional support to the client. Transgender patients should undergo assessments and screenings for all organs present, regardless of transition status. Established guidelines for cisgender individuals should be applied to transgender patients (Sterling et al., 2020).

♥ iCare The genitourinary system includes both the reproductive system and the urinary system. Because assessment focuses on elimination and sexual and reproductive function, it might be embarrassing or uncomfortable for many people. A competent, professional approach is needed. Your confidence and ease with these topics will help the client to feel more relaxed.

The Male Genitourinary System

A complete examination includes assessment of the external genitalia, evaluation for hernias, and a rectal examination for prostate screening. The penis and scrotum are examined by inspection and palpation. You will assess some of the urinary system organs when examining the back (kidneys, ureters) and the abdomen (bladder); the prostate gland is palpated during the examination of the rectum and anus (discussed later in

Each DTR corresponds to a certain level of the cord and is graded on a scale from 0 to 4+.
- **Superficial reflexes** are elicited by swiftly and lightly stroking a body part (e.g., with the reflex hammer). Superficial reflexes are graded as positive or negative.

For an overview of steps for assessing reflexes, see the Highlights of Procedures box near the end of this chapter. To see illustrations and the DTR scale,

 Go to **Chapter 19, Procedure 19-16: Assessing the Sensory-Neurological System,** in Volume 2.

Sensory Function

To assess sensory function, ask the client to keep their eyes closed as you apply various stimuli. Ask the client to indicate when they feel a sensation. Vary your location and approach so that you test sensation, not pattern recognition. If you notice an area of altered sensation, systematically assess the area to define the border of the change. Usually, you will limit your testing to the upper and lower extremities and the trunk. If the client has known or suspected deficits, you should test at numerous other sites. For techniques for assessing reflexes and sensory function, see the Highlights of Procedures box, and

 Go to **Chapter 19, Procedure 19-16: Assessing the Sensory-Neurological System,** in Volume 2.

this chapter). For steps to follow in examining the male genitourinary system, see the summary in the Highlights of Procedures box at the end of this chapter, and

 Go to **Chapter 19, Procedure 19-17: Assessing the Male Genitourinary System,** in Volume 2.

When examining the patient's penis, be aware that they may or may not have been **circumcised** (excision of the foreskin of the penis). Because clear scientific evidence is scarce, the American Academy of Pediatrics (AAP) no longer recommends newborn male **circumcision** as a routine practice (Pokarowski et al., 2022). Instead, the AAP recommends that parents be provided with factually correct, nonbiased information on male circumcision so that they can make an informed decision. For some, circumcision is tied to religious and cultural beliefs (e.g., among Jewish and Muslim populations) or is a matter of family tradition or personal hygiene. For others, however, circumcision seems unnecessary or disfiguring and is not performed.

A **hernia** is a protrusion of the intestine (or other organ) through the wall that contains it. An **inguinal hernia** may be a small protrusion with minimal symptoms, or it may cause pain and distention as a loop of bowel extends into the scrotum. In male individuals, this is most likely to be a protrusion of the intestine, either through the abdominal wall **(direct hernia)** or into the inguinal canal and possibly into the scrotum **(indirect hernia).**

KnowledgeCheck 19-12

- What assessment techniques are used when examining the male genitourinary system? Refer to Procedure 19-17 to answer this question.
- What is the most common hernia occurring in male individuals?

The Female Genitourinary System

You may be called upon to assist with a comprehensive examination. For a procedure for inspecting external female genitalia and palpating inguinal lymph nodes, see the Highlights of Procedures box at the end of this chapter, and

 Go to **Chapter 19, Procedure 19-18: Assessing the Female Genitourinary System,** in Volume 2.

External Examination

For adolescents and young patients who are not sexually active, an external genitourinary examination includes an inspection of the amount and distribution of pubic hair, the skin of the pubic area, and the external genitalia, along with palpation of the inguinal lymph nodes.

Internal Examination

Patients who are sexually active; who have abnormal findings on external examination; who have abdominal, pelvic, or genitourinary complaints; or who are on

hormone therapy require an internal genital examination (Ahuja & Cron, 2021). The examination includes the following:

- Palpation of Bartholin glands and Skene ducts
- Assessment of vaginal muscle tone and pelvic musculature
- Speculum examination
- Bimanual examination, wherein the examiner palpates the cervix, uterus, and adnexal tissues using one or two fingers within the vagina and the other hand on the outside to help bring the inner structures toward the two hands.

Pap Smear Recent changes to major guidelines recommend, in general, less frequent routine Papanicolaou tests (Pap smears) to screen for cervical and uterine cancer. They recommend the following:

- Younger than age 21: Not screened, regardless of whether they are sexually active or have other risk-taking behaviors.
- Ages 21 through 29: Screen every 3 years.
- Ages 30 to 65: Screen every 3 to 5 years (and follow the advice of their provider).

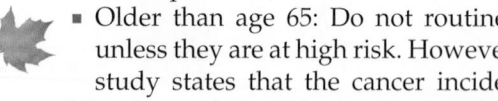
- Older than age 65: Do not routinely screen unless they are at high risk. However, a recent study states that the cancer incidence rates used for the guidelines do not account for the high prevalence of hysterectomy in the United States. This has the largest impact on older Black women. The authors recommend that the risk and screening guidelines be reconsidered (Beavis et al., 2017)

- Most transmen retain their cervixes and need comprehensive genitourinary healthcare, including cervical cancer screening, following the recommendations for cisgender women. 🍀 In general, transmen are screened less frequently for cervical cancer and are less likely to be up to date on their Pap tests compared with cisgender women. Healthcare providers play a key role in minimizing emotional discomfort before, during, and after a pelvic examination; decreasing physical discomfort during the examination; and adapting techniques to account for testosterone-induced anatomic changes (Potter et al., 2016).
- Those with certain vulnerabilities (e.g., weakened immune system, HIV positive) should have a Pap test every year (Agency for Healthcare Research and Quality [AHRQ], 2019; American Cancer Society, n.d.-b)

Key Point: *National screening guidelines vary, and they change frequently.*

Additional cultures or screens may be done if there is unusual discharge or risk of sexually transmitted infection. A **speculum examination** is performed to collect specimens and assess the cervix. To learn about assisting with a speculum examination,

 Go to **Chapter 19, Clinical Insight 19-3: Assisting with a Speculum Examination,** in Volume 2.

KnowledgeCheck 19-13

What are the responsibilities of the nurse during an internal examination of the female genitourinary system?

The Anus, Rectum, and Prostate

Examining the rectum and anus is the last aspect of a comprehensive examination. For the female client, this examination is usually performed at the end of a bimanual pelvic examination while the client is still in the lithotomy position. Usually, a male client assumes the Sims' position, and you perform the examination after completing your examination of the genitals. For a summary of this procedure, see the Highlights of Procedures box at the end of this chapter. For a step-by-step procedure,

 Go to **Chapter 19, Procedure 19-19: Assessing the Anus and Rectum,** in Volume 2.

Inspect the anus and rectum for skin condition and hemorrhoids and palpate for muscle tone, masses, and tenderness. Skin irritation and erythema are common in clients who have diarrhea and infants and toddlers who wear diapers. **Hemorrhoids** (dilated, usually painful, anal vessels) may be seen in clients with a history of constipation. Many people develop hemorrhoids with pregnancy and childbirth.

A comprehensive examination for a man should include a digital rectal examination to assess for prostate enlargement. An enlarged prostate may indicate benign enlargement of the prostate, which is common in male clients older than age 50, or it may indicate prostatitis. A hard nodule or multiple nodules may indicate prostate cancer.

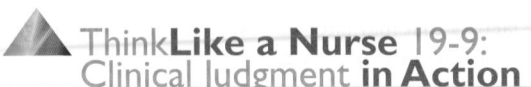 ThinkLike a Nurse 19-9:
Clinical Judgment in Action

How will examination of the rectum and anus differ for Stanley and Nadine Williams (Meet Your Patient)?

DOCUMENTING PHYSICAL EXAMINATION FINDINGS (STANLEY WILLIAMS)

Assad Johnson has completed his physical examination of Stanley Williams (Meet Your Patient). What follows is his charting entry. Recall that Assad is an advanced practice nurse and has performed a comprehensive physical examination. Therefore, this examination and charting entry are more extensive than what would be expected of a staff nurse. Keep in mind that you should use only abbreviations on your clinical agency's approved list.

General Survey A 56-year-old overweight man presents to the clinic for a physical examination in no apparent distress. Pt. appears stated age; is dressed in gray pants and black sweater, appropriate for climate;

hair short and brushed; exposed skin appears clean and dry; and alert and oriented to time, place, and person. Speech is clear; response and affect appropriate. Moves all extremities well; gait steady and balanced. Smells of cigarettes.

Height	5 ft 7 in.
Weight	202 lb (92 kg)
BP	166/100
Pulse	88 beats/min
RR	19 breaths/min
Temp	98.5°F (36.9°C), oral
BMI	32

Integumentary Skin even in color, warm & dry, good turgor, no suspicious lesions. Well-healed scar in right inguinal area. Hair clean, coarse, evenly distributed. Some graying. Nails pink, brisk capillary refill, no clubbing.

Head & Neck Normocephalic, erect, midline. Scalp mobile, no lesions, tenderness, or masses. Facial features symmetrical. Thyroid gland symmetrical and not enlarged; cervical lymph nodes not palpable or tender.

Eyes Snellen = right eye 20/100, left eye 20/100, both eyes 20/100. Color vision intact. Difficulty noted with near vision. Visual fields normal by confrontation. Extraocular movements intact. PERRLA at 3 mm by direct and consensual. Eyes clear and bright, + blink, no lid lag or abnormalities. Anterior chamber clear. Cornea & iris intact. Sclera white, conjunctiva clear. Lacrimal glands and ducts nontender. + red reflex bilateral, discs flat with sharp margins, vessels intact, retina & macula even in color.

Ears, Nose, & Throat Skin intact, no masses, lesions, or discharge. Position WNL. External ears nontender to palpation. + whisper test. Weber—no lateralization. External canals clear without redness, swelling, lesions, or discharge. Tympanic membranes intact, light reflex and bony landmarks visible; frontal and maxillary sinuses nontender. Nares patent, able to distinguish familiar odors, mucosa pink, no discharge, septum intact with no deviation.

Mouth Lips, oral mucosa, gingivae pink with no lesions. All teeth present and in good repair. Pharynx pink, tonsils absent, palate intact. Symmetrical rise of the uvula, + gag and swallow reflex. Tongue smooth, pink, symmetrical, mobile, without lesions, taste intact (correctly identified sweet, salty, and sour).

Respiratory Respirations 19 breaths/min and unlabored. Trachea midline, AP less than transverse chest diameter. Chest expansion symmetrical. No tenderness, scars, masses, or lesions. Diaphragmatic excursion 5 cm. Lungs clear to auscultation.

Cardiovascular PMI @ MCL at 5th ICS, P 85, regular, no murmurs, gallops, or thrills present; pulses +2, no bruits or thrills, no varicosities; jugular venous pulsation 2 cm at 45°. Carotids without bruits.

Breasts Symmetrical. No masses, lymphadenopathy, or discharge.

Abdomen Abdomen soft, rounded, no masses or pulsations. Surgical scar R inguinal area. + bowel sounds, + tympany throughout.

Musculoskeletal Normal spinal curvature. Joints and muscles symmetrical, no deformity. + Bilateral knee pain (right more than left). Full ROM in upper and lower extremities, + 5 muscle strength, moderate crepitus right knee.

Neurological Awake, alert, and oriented to time, place, and person. CN I–XII intact. Gait steady and coordinated; negative Romberg; unable to do deep knee bends due to pain. Point-point localization, superficial and deep sensation intact, + 2 deep tendon reflexes.

Genitourinary Circumcised male; penis nontender, no masses, urethral meatus midline, no discharge; testicles descended bilaterally, nontender, inguinal and femoral canals free of masses, prostate small, smooth, mobile, nontender. Rectal wall smooth, no masses, stool hemoccult negative.

Highlights of Procedures 19-1 through 19-20

For steps to follow in *all* procedures, refer to the Universal Steps for All Procedures found on the inside back cover of Volume 2. Go to the full procedures in Volume 2 to practice and learn the skill. Use these procedure highlights later to help you review key steps.

Note: Throughout the assessment, compare findings on both sides of the body.

Procedure 19-1: Performing the General Survey

➤ Identify any signs of distress.

➤ Observe the patient's apparent age, sex, race, facial expression, body size and type, posture, movements, speech, grooming, dress, hygiene, mental state, and affect.

➤ Measure vital signs.

➤ Measure height and weight, and calculate body mass index (BMI).

➤ Consider the client's cultural/ethnic background, sex, gender, and developmental stage.

➤ Review history data that may influence general survey findings, including usual state of health, current health problem, allergies, and unexplained changes in weight.

 ➤ Perform functional and SPICES assessments for older adults.

➤ Note verbal and nonverbal responses throughout examination.

Procedure 19-2: Assessing the Skin

➤ Techniques: Inspection, palpation, and olfaction

➤ Assess both exposed and unexposed areas.

➤ Inspect skin color; note any unusual odors.

➤ Inspect and palpate any lesions. Describe their size, shape, color, distribution, texture, surface relationship, and exudate.

➤ Evaluate the lesions for possible malignancy, remembering the mnemonic ABCDE.

➤ Use dorsal aspect of your hand to palpate skin temperature.

➤ Check skin turgor.

➤ Palpate skin for texture, moisture, and hydration.

➤ Review history that may influence skin findings.

Procedure 19-3: Assessing the Hair

➤ Techniques: Inspection and palpation

➤ Assess scalp hair and body hair.

➤ Inspect hair for color, quantity, distribution, condition of scalp, and presence of lesions or pediculosis.

➤ Palpate the texture of the hair.

➤ Palpate the scalp for mobility and tenderness.

Procedure 19-4: Assessing the Nails

➤ Techniques: Inspection and palpation

➤ Inspect the nails for color, condition, and shape.

➤ Palpate the texture of the nails.

➤ Assess capillary refill.

➤ Assess factors that may alter nail assessment findings (e.g., a cold environment may slow capillary refill).

➤ Examine nails on both hands and feet.

➤ You may defer examination of the toenails until you assess peripheral circulation.

Procedure 19-5: Assessing the Head and Face

➤ Techniques: Inspection, palpation

➤ Inspect the head for size, shape, symmetry, and position.

➤ Compare side to side throughout the examination.

➤ Inspect the face for expression and symmetry.

➤ Palpate the head for masses, tenderness, and scalp mobility.

➤ Palpate the face for symmetry, tenderness, muscle tone, and temporomandibular joint (TMJ) function.

Highlights of Procedures 19-1 through 19-20

Procedure 19-6: Assessing the Eyes

➤ Techniques: Inspection and palpation

➤ Assess distance vision using a Snellen chart.

➤ Test near vision by measuring the client's ability to read newsprint at a distance of 14 inches (35.5 cm).

➤ Test color vision by using color plates or the color bars on the Snellen chart.

➤ Assess peripheral vision by determining when an object comes into sight.

➤ Assess extraocular muscles (EOMs) by examining the corneal light reflex, observing the six cardinal gaze positions, and performing the cover/uncover test.

➤ Inspect the external eye structures.

➤ Test the corneal reflex with a cotton wisp, if appropriate.

➤ Check pupil reaction for direct and consensual response.

➤ Assess accommodation by having the patient focus on an approaching object.

➤ Palpate the external eye structures.

➤ Assess internal structures via ophthalmoscopy.

Procedure 19-7: Assessing the Ears and Hearing

➤ Techniques: Inspection and palpation

➤ Inspect the external ear for placement, size, shape, symmetry, and the condition of the skin.

➤ Palpate the external structures of the ear for skin condition and tenderness.

➤ Inspect the tympanic membrane and bony landmarks.

➤ Assess gross hearing with the whisper and watch-tick tests.

➤ Perform the Weber test to assess hearing loss.

➤ Perform the Rinne test to identify whether hearing loss is conductive or sensorineural.

➤ Perform Romberg test (may also be done with neurological examination).

Procedure 19-8: Assessing the Nose and Sinuses

➤ Techniques: Inspection and palpation

➤ Inspect the external and internal structures of the nose.

➤ Insert the speculum about 1 cm, and then open it as much as possible.

➤ Transilluminate and palpate the sinuses.

➤ Palpate the external structures of the nose.

Procedure 19-9: Assessing the Mouth and Oropharynx

➤ Techniques: Inspection and palpation

➤ Inspect the lips, oral mucosa, gums, teeth, and bite.

➤ Inspect the tongue and frenulum; inspect under the tongue.

➤ Inspect the hard/soft palate, tonsils, and uvula.

➤ Palpate the lips and tongue for tenderness and muscle tone.

➤ Test the gag reflex by touching the back of the soft palate with a tongue blade.

Procedure 19-10: Assessing the Neck

➤ Techniques: Inspection and palpation (auscultation as needed)

➤ Inspect the neck. Note symmetry, range of motion (ROM), and skin condition.

➤ Palpate the cervical lymph nodes. Note the size, shape, symmetry, consistency, mobility, tenderness, and temperature of any palpable nodes.

➤ Palpate the thyroid. If it is enlarged or if there is a mass, auscultate.

Procedure 19-11: Assessing the Breasts and Axillae

➤ Techniques: Inspection and palpation

➤ Inspect the breasts and axillae for skin condition, size, shape, symmetry, and color.

➤ Inspect the nipples for discharge. Culture any discharge, if present.

✚ If you notice an open lesion or nipple discharge, wear procedure gloves to palpate the breasts.

➤ Palpate the breasts using the vertical strip method, pie wedge method, or concentric circles method.

➤ Palpate the nipples, areolae, axillae, and clavicular lymph nodes.

Procedure 19-12: Assessing the Chest and Lungs

➤ Techniques: Inspection, palpation, percussion, auscultation

➤ Assess respirations by counting the rate and observing the rhythm, depth, and symmetry of chest movement.

➤ Inspect the chest for anteroposterior-to-lateral ratio, costal angle, spinal deformity, respiratory effort, and skin condition.

➤ Palpate the trachea.

➤ Palpate the chest for tenderness, masses, or crepitus; chest excursion; and tactile fremitus.

➤ Percuss the chest; percuss diaphragmatic excursion.

➤ Auscultate breath sounds.

Procedure 19-13: Assessing the Heart and Vascular System

➤ Techniques: Inspection, palpation, auscultation

➤ If possible, work from your patient's right side.

➤ Inspect the neck for pulsations.

Continued

➤ Measure jugular venous pressure (JVP).

➤ Inspect the precordium for pulsations.

➤ Palpate the carotid arteries.

➤ Palpate the precordium for pulsations, lifts, heaves, or thrills.

➤ Auscultate the carotid arteries with the bell of the stethoscope.

➤ Auscultate the jugular veins with the bell of the stethoscope.

➤ Auscultate the precordium at the apex, left lower sternal border, base left, and base right.

➤ Use the bell and then the diaphragm of the stethoscope.

➤ Palpate the peripheral pulses. Any abnormalities require further evaluation.

➤ Perform manual compression test to evaluate venous system.

Procedure 19-14: Assessing the Abdomen

➤ Techniques: Inspection, auscultation, percussion, palpation (in that order)

➤ Have the client void before the examination.

➤ Position the client supine with the knees slightly flexed.

➤ Inspect the abdomen.

➤ Auscultate the abdomen for bowel sounds and bruits.

➤ Use indirect percussion to assess at multiple sites in all four quadrants.

➤ Using your fist or blunt percussion, percuss the costovertebral angle bilaterally to assess for kidney tenderness.

➤ Lightly palpate throughout the abdomen by pressing down 1 to 2 cm in a rotating motion. Identify surface characteristics, tenderness, muscle resistance, and turgor.

➤ Use deep palpation to palpate organs and masses.

Procedure 19-15: Assessing the Musculoskeletal System

➤ Techniques: Inspection and palpation

➤ Compare bilaterally during the assessment.

➤ Assess posture, body alignment, and symmetry.

➤ Assess the spinal curvature.

➤ Examine the gait by assessing the base of support, stride, and phases of the gait.

➤ Assess balance through tandem walking, heel-and-toe walking, deep knee bends, hopping, and the Romberg test.

➤ Assess coordination by testing finger–thumb opposition, rhythmic movements of lower and upper extremities, and rapid alternating movements.

➤ Test the accuracy of movements by having the client touch their finger to their nose with their eyes closed.

➤ Measure limb length and circumference.

➤ Inspect muscle and joint symmetry.

➤ Perform range of motion of all joints.

➤ Assess muscle strength by having the client perform ROM against resistance.

Procedure 19-16: Assessing the Sensory-Neurological System

➤ Assess behavior.

➤ Determine level of arousal.

➤ Determine level of orientation.

➤ Assess memory.

➤ Assess mathematical and calculation skills.

➤ Assess general knowledge.

➤ Evaluate thought processes.

➤ Assess abstract thinking.

➤ Assess judgment.

➤ Assess communication ability.

➤ Test cranial nerves.

➤ Test superficial sensations; begin with most peripheral part of the limb.

➤ Test deep sensations: vibratory and kinesthetic.

➤ Test kinesthetic sensation (position sense).

➤ Test discriminatory sensations: stereognosis, graphesthesia, two-point discrimination, point localization, and sensory extinction.

➤ Test deep tendon reflexes: biceps, triceps, brachioradialis, patellar, and Achilles.

➤ Test superficial reflexes.

➤ Assess for dementia in institutionalized older adults.

Procedure 19-17: Assessing the Male Genitourinary System

➤ Techniques: Inspection and palpation

➤ Inspect the external genitalia, including color, discharge, and the pattern of hair distribution.

➤ Palpate penis, scrotum, testes, and epididymis for lumps, masses, hernias, or enlarged lymph nodes.

Procedure 19-18: Assessing the Female Genitourinary System

➤ Techniques: Inspection and palpation

➤ Inspect the external genitalia, including hair distribution; skin, mucosa; urethral meatus; and vaginal introitus, color, discharge, and lesions.

➤ Inspect the clitoris, urethral meatus, and vaginal introitus. Observe for color, size, and presence of discharge or lesions.

➤ Palpate Bartholin, urethral, and Skene glands.

Highlights of Procedures 19-1 through 19-20

➤ Assess vaginal and pelvic muscle tone.

➤ Palpate inguinal and femoral are for hernias.

➤ Palpate lymph nodes.

Procedure 19-19: Assessing the Anus and Rectum

➤ Inspect the external anal area, sphincter tone, and stool for occult blood.

➤ Palpate the anus and rectum for muscle tone and masses.

➤ For women, assessment of the anus and rectum is usually performed at the end of the internal pelvic examination; for men, it is done after the genitourinary examination.

Procedure 19-20: Brief Bedside Assessment

➤ Modify the procedure to fit the patient's health status.

➤ Observe the environment and the patient's general appearance.

➤ Measure vital signs, pain status, and pulse oximetry.

➤ Use a systematic (e.g., head-to-toe) approach.

➤ Assess the integument (hair, nails, and skin).

➤ Assess the head and neck (ears, eyes, lips, tongue and oropharynx, carotids).

➤ Assess the heart (auscultate heart sounds).

➤ Assess the back with patient sitting (including breath sounds).

➤ Assess the anterior chest (heart and lungs).

➤ Assess the abdomen with patient supine.

➤ Assess urinary status.

➤ Assess upper extremities, including edema and capillary refill.

➤ Assess lower extremities, including edema and capillary refill.

➤ Assess for spinal deformities with patient standing.

➤ Assess balance, coordination, ROM, and gait.

➤ Check Babinski and Homan reflexes.

To explore learning resources for this chapter,

Go to Davis Advantage and find:

Answers and Suggested Responses for all questions in this chapter

Concept Map

Knowledge Map

References and Bibliography

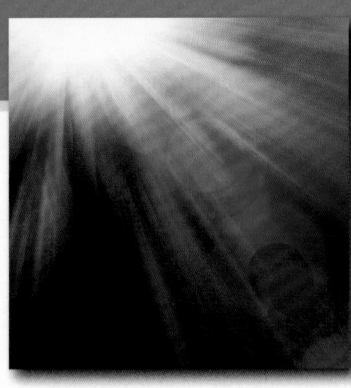

CHAPTER 20

Promoting Asepsis & Preventing Infection

Learning Outcomes

After completing this chapter, you should be able to:

➤ Discuss the six links in the chain of infection.

➤ Describe the stages of a typical infectious process.

➤ Describe four processes involved in primary, secondary, and tertiary defense.

➤ Identify activities that promote immune function.

➤ Discuss the factors that place an individual at increased risk for infection.

➤ Explain why it is important to be aware of emerging infectious diseases.

➤ Explain why multidrug-resistant pathogens are of special concern in healthcare.

➤ Use standard precautions to prevent transmission of infection through blood and body fluids.

➤ Describe additional precautions that must be taken when there is concern about contact, droplet, or airborne disease transmission.

➤ Compare and contrast methods of preventing infection by breaking the chain of infection.

➤ Implement measures to prevent healthcare-related infections.

➤ Use medical asepsis and sterile technique when appropriate.

➤ Discuss infection prevention and control measures in the home and community.

➤ Discuss the nurse's role in recognizing, preventing, and helping to contain the spread of a biological epidemic.

Key Concepts

Body defenses

Infection

Infection prevention and control

Medical asepsis

Surgical asepsis

Related Concepts

See the Concept Map on Davis Advantage.

Example Client Conditions

Multidrug-Resistant Organism (MDRO) Infections

Meet Your Nursing Role Model

Jarek Shvets works as a nurse on a busy labor and delivery unit in a major medical center. One night at the dinner table, his 7-year-old daughter, Stephanie, asks, "Daddy, what was the most important thing you did at work today?" Jarek considers his reply. Finally, he answers, "I washed my hands—a lot." Jarek says that he also assisted in the birth of five infants, resuscitated one of the infants who was struggling for breath, and identified several problems that prevented complications for mothers in labor. "Daddy, I don't understand why washing your hands was so important," Stephanie protested. "Look at all the *really* important things you did today!"

As you read this chapter, think back to Jarek's discussion with his daughter. Perhaps you will someday say the same thing to your child or anyone who asks about your day.

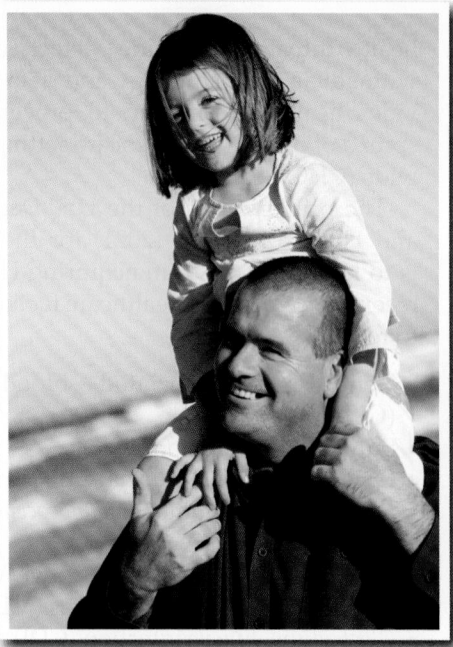

Theoretical Knowledge
knowing why

In the theoretical knowledge section, you will learn how infections occur and about measures to prevent them. We will discuss healthcare-associated infections and related professional standards and guidelines.

ABOUT THE KEY CONCEPTS

Infection is the invasion of and multiplication in the body by a pathogen (a microorganism capable of causing disease). A grasp of the broad concept of **infection** will enable you to promote biological safety for your clients, using **infection prevention and control** activities. Those activities include **medical and surgical asepsis** and interventions to support patients' body defenses.

WHY MUST NURSES KNOW ABOUT INFECTION PROCESSES?

The goals of infection prevention and control discussed in this section are to:

- Protect patients from infections.
- Meet professional standards and guidelines.
- Protect yourself and others from diseases.
- Reduce the severity of illness and complications resulting from infection.

Healthcare-Associated Infections

The term **healthcare-associated infections (HAIs)** refers to infections associated with healthcare given in any setting. The term **nosocomial infection** refers more specifically to hospital-acquired infections. HAIs aggravate existing illness and lengthen hospital stay and recovery time.

- HAIs are the leading complication of hospital care and one of the 10 leading causes of death in the United States (Agency for Healthcare Research and Quality [AHRQ], 2018).
- Approximately 1 in 31 hospitalized patients has at least one HAI (Centers for Disease Control and Prevention [CDC], 2018).
- *Clostridium difficile* is one of the most common and most serious infections. Those who take antibiotics, especially older adults, are at greatest risk for acquiring *C. difficile* (CDC, 2019b).

The following are some reasons for the high incidence of healthcare-related infections:

- In hospitals and other facilities, patients encounter many care providers, facility staff, and others who can transmit pathogens to them.
- Ill patients are vulnerable to infection because of their lowered resistance. Likewise, they are a source of infection for others.
- Inpatients undergo many invasive procedures (e.g., injections), which can be a source for microbes to invade the body.

Professional Standards and Guidelines

Various government, professional, and accrediting organizations have created quality-control guidelines for healthcare agencies and professionals. The following are important examples.

The Centers for Disease Control and Prevention. The CDC, an agency of the U.S. Department of Health and Human Services, responds to new and emerging health threats worldwide, detects and tracks disease with advanced technology and data analytics, and provides health information to prevent and control the spread of disease in healthcare settings and community-wide (CDC, 2022).

The primary goal of the U.S. Department of Health and Human Services (2021) for the healthcare setting is to keep patients from acquiring HAIs while they are receiving care in any healthcare facility. Specific aims are to reduce:

- Central line–associated bloodstream infection (CLABSI)
- Surgical site infection (SSI)
- Catheter-associated urinary tract infection (CAUTI)
- Methicillin-resistant *Staphylococcus aureus* infection (MRSA)
- Ventilator-associated pneumonia (VAP)
- Multidrug-resistant organisms (MDROs)
- *Clostridium difficile* infection (CDI) and hospitalization

Agency for Healthcare Research and Quality The AHRQ is an agency within the U.S. Department of Health and Human Services. The agency's mission is to provide scientific evidence to make healthcare safer and make health information, tools, and resources available for both healthcare providers and consumers.

The Joint Commission The Joint Commission (TJC) is a quality oversight agency. Its standards for performance include extensive criteria describing what healthcare organizations must do to minimize the risks of infection. In addition, Goal 7 of the TJC National Patient Safety Goals for 2022 is to reduce the risk of HAIs. The Infection Control Initiatives include strategies for healthcare providers to prevent infection in inpatient and community-based settings. Goals focus on improving hand cleaning and using evidence-based guidelines to prevent infections that are difficult to treat, blood infections from central lines, infections after surgery, and illnesses caused by catheters in the urinary tract (TJC, 2021).

Quality and Safety Education for Nurses Quality and Safety Education for Nurses (QSEN) is a group of educators that addresses the challenge of preparing nurses with the knowledge, skills, and attitudes necessary to improve the quality and safety of their places of work (Cronenwett et al., 2007).

American Nurses Association Standard 5 of the American Nurses Association (ANA) *Nursing: Scope & Standards of Practice* (ANA, 2015) applies to infection prevention and control:

- Partners with the healthcare consumer to implement the plan in a safe and timely manner.
- Implements the plan in a timely manner in accordance with the patient safety goals. (ANA, 2015, p. 61)

Limiting the Spread of Infectious Diseases

Cooperative efforts among many disciplines and organizations worldwide are required to limit the spread of infectious diseases. The World Health Organization (WHO) is committed to reducing healthcare-associated complications, preventing SSIs, combating MDROs, preventing sepsis and catheter-associated bloodstream infections, preventing CAUTIs, and improving response to and recovery from infection (WHO, 2009). The CDC tracks critical global infection rates and provides health information and resources for limiting the spread of infection. TJC (2012) requires hospitals to have an emergency management plan for responding to large numbers of infectious patients who might need to be treated as a result of an epidemic or pandemic event.

HOW DOES INFECTION OCCUR?

Imagine that your clinical instructor alerts you to an outbreak of an infectious disease in the hospital where you have your assignment. So far, 14 patients have become infected, and one has died. Would that prompt you to learn how infection is spread and why certain bacteria seem to affect some people more than others?

Infections Develop in Response to a Chain of Factors

Infections spread through a **chain of infection.** It is made up of the six links described in the following subsections, all of which must be present for the infection to be transmitted from one individual to another (Fig. 20-1). Later in the chapter, we discuss how to interrupt the chain to limit the spread of infection.

Infectious Agent

Some microorganisms are harmful. Others live on or in the human body without causing harm (e.g., the *Staphylococcus* bacteria growing on human skin). Other microorganisms are beneficial or even essential for human health and well-being. They are referred to as **normal flora.**

Normal Flora Normal flora live in the intestine and aid in digestion; synthesize vitamin K; and release vitamin B_{12}, thiamine, biotin, niacin, and riboflavin (Rowland et al., 2018; Hill, 1997). In addition, they limit the growth of harmful bacteria by competing with them for available nutrients. There are two types of normal flora: transient and resident.

- **Transient flora** are normal microbes that you acquire by coming in contact with objects or another person (e.g., when you touch a soiled dressing). Hand washing can remove these.
- **Resident flora** are permanent inhabitants of the skin and cannot usually be removed with routine hand

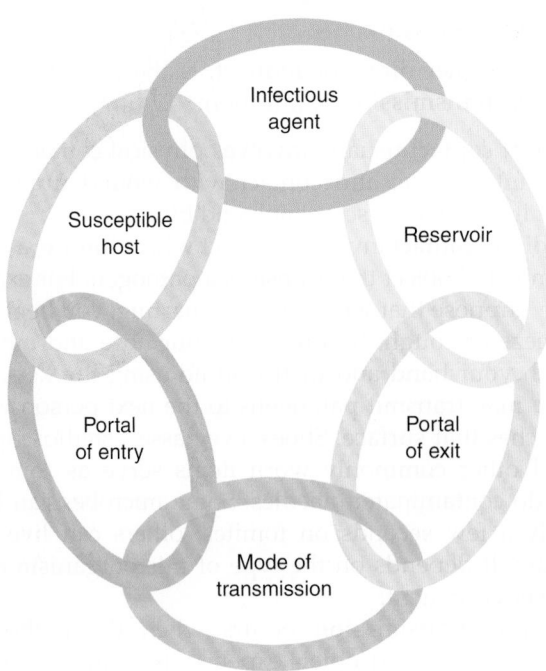

FIGURE 20-1 All of the six links in the chain of infection must be present for infection to be transmitted from one person to another.

washing. They live and multiply harmlessly deep in skin layers.

Pathogens are microorganisms that are capable of causing disease.

- **The largest groups of pathogens** are bacteria, viruses, and fungi (which include yeasts and molds).
- **Less common pathogens** are protozoa, helminths (commonly called worms), and **prions,** which are infectious protein particles that cause certain neurological diseases.
- **Normal flora may become pathogenic** when a patient is especially vulnerable to disease or if they enter regions of the body they do not normally inhabit (*Escherichia coli,* harmless in the bowel, cause infection when they multiply in the urinary tract).

Once a pathogen enters a host, four factors determine whether the person develops infection:

- **Virulence of the organism** (its power to cause disease)
- **Host environment**—ability of the organism to thrive in it
- **Number of organisms** (the greater the number, the more likely they are to cause disease)
- **Host defenses**—ability to prevent infection

Reservoir

A **reservoir** is a source of infection: a place where pathogens survive and multiply. Some reservoirs are:

- **Living organisms**. **Key Point:** *Most pathogens flourish in a warm, moist, dark environment. This is why the human body is the most common reservoir*

for pathogens. Animals and insects can act as living reservoirs. Some people, called **carriers,** can defend themselves from active disease but harbor the pathogenic organisms within their bodies. They may have no symptoms, yet they serve as reservoirs and can pass the disease to others.

- **Nonliving reservoirs.** These include soil, water, food, and environmental surfaces (e.g., contaminated water, garbage, fecal matter, exudate on wound dressings). In healthcare facilities, many surfaces act as reservoirs (e.g., sinks, toilets, bed rails, bed linens) because of their proximity to patients, visitors, and healthcare providers carrying pathogens on their skin, clothing, and equipment.

Characteristics of Environments Supportive to Microbes Most pathogens need the following to survive:

- **Nutrients.** To live and thrive in humans, microbes must be able to use the body's precise balance of nutrients, electrolytes, pH, and temperature. Bacteria can rapidly multiply in food left at room temperature. For example, the bacteria *Salmonella enteritidis,* which causes salmonellosis ("food poisoning"), can contaminate raw and undercooked meat and eggs.
- **Moisture.** Pathogens require hydration for survival and often prefer the moist environment of wounds, the genitourinary tract, the throat, and the airways. However, the spores formed by some bacteria allow them to live without water (e.g., the *Bacillus* and *Clostridium* species, both of which cause foodborne disease).
- **Temperature.** For most pathogens, the ideal temperature for survival is 95°F (35°C). Environments that are either too hot or too cold for a particular species will slow its growth or even kill the population of organisms. In part, the microbes that are pathogenic to humans are so because they thrive at about the same temperature as the human body. Thus, a fever in response to infection can inhibit and even kill invading pathogens.
- **Oxygen.** Many bacteria and most protozoa and fungi are **aerobic.** That is, they must have oxygen to live and grow (e.g., *Candida albicans* [yeast]). **Anaerobic organisms** do not require oxygen for growth and may even be killed in its presence. One example is *Clostridium tetani,* which causes tetanus when a spore enters the body through an open wound.
- **pH and Electrolytes.** To live in humans, pathogens need the body's precise balance of moisture, sugars, pH (acidity), and electrolytes. Most prefer a pH range of 5 to 8. Therefore, they cannot survive in the highly acidic environment of the stomach. When patients take antacids, stomach pH increases and lessens this natural bodily defense. The organisms multiply and can then cause infection in other systems, such as the lungs or gut.
- **Light.** Microbes grow best in dark environments (e.g., inside the body, deep in wounds, and under

dressings). Ultraviolet light is sometimes used to remove pathogens such as *Staphylococcus, Salmonella,* and viruses from surgical instruments and other objects. It is also used to disinfect drinking water.

KnowledgeCheck 20-1

- What is a pathogen?
- What is the role of normal flora?
- Identify at least five reservoirs of infection.

Portal of Exit

A contained reservoir is only a potential source of infection. For infection to spread, a pathogen must exit the reservoir. In the case of human or animal reservoirs, the most frequent **portal of exit** is through body fluids.

- **Expelling foreign materials.** The body's natural response to foreign materials, including pathogens, is to try to expel them. If you have a pathogen in the respiratory system, you cough and sneeze. If it is in the gastrointestinal system, they exit when you vomit or experience diarrhea.
- **Nonintact skin.** Wounds, bites, and abrasions provide an exit for body fluid. Blood, serous fluid, and pus seeping from a wound help transport pathogens away from the broken skin. In healthcare-related infections, puncture sites, drainage tubes, feeding tubes, and intravenous lines serve as exit routes for pathogens.

Mode of Transmission

Contact, either direct or indirect, is the most frequent **mode of transmission** of infection.

- **Direct contact** usually involves physical contact, sexual intercourse, and contact with wound drainage, but it can involve scratching and biting.
- **Indirect contact** involves contact with a **fomite,** a contaminated object that transfers a pathogen. For example, suppose that while you are charting, you begin to sneeze or cough. If you cover your nose and mouth with your hand and then resume using the keypad, you may transmit pathogens to the next person who touches that surface. Shoes, eyeglasses, stethoscopes, and other commonly worn items serve as fomites, as do contaminated needles. Some microbes can live only a few seconds on fomites; others can live for years. It depends on the type of microorganism and the environment.
- **Droplet transmission** occurs when the pathogen travels in water droplets expelled as an infected person exhales, coughs, sneezes, or talks, in addition to during suctioning and oral care. The droplet can then be inhaled or enter the eye of a susceptible person. Although droplets can travel only a few feet, within that distance, they may readily contaminate fomites that then transmit the organism by contact.
- **Airborne transmission** occurs when microorganisms float considerable distances on air currents to infect large numbers of people. Sweeping a floor or shaking out contaminated bed linens can stir up airborne

---

PICOT

Situation: The handoff report has been concluded in an intensive care unit (ICU). The unit manager alerted the staff that there has been an increase in enterococci-related urinary tract infections (UTIs) on the unit, and the infection control team will be following several of the unit's patients. The primary nurse is preparing to bathe a client in the ICU and notices that the basin is wet from the previous bath. Knowing that the patient is more vulnerable to infection and that bacteria need a damp environment to grow, the nurse considers the bath basin as a possible reservoir for enterococci. What question might the nurse ask to guide the search for evidence?

PICOT Components

P	Population/client	=	ICU patients
I	Intervention/indicator	=	Dry bath basin
C	Comparator/control	=	Wet bath basin
O	Outcome	=	Enterococci urinary tract infection
T	Time	=	During ICU stay

Searchable Question: How do _____ (P) who receive/are exposed to _____ (I) develop _____ (O) compared with _____ (C) during _____ (T)?

Example of Evidence: Hospital-associated infections (HAIs) are linked to a high number of patient illnesses and deaths every year. Musuuza et al. (2016) examined the benefit of using chlorhexidine gluconate (CHG) for bathing hospitalized patients in both ICU and non-ICU settings on the occurrence of HAIs. They examined the findings of 26 studies involving 861,546 patient days over 12 years. The researchers found that bathing patients with CHG significantly reduced the incidence of HAIs. This may be a result of reduced microbial colonization of the patient's skin and the hands of healthcare workers.

Practice Change: As a result of the findings in the literature, the nurse resolved to use disposable bath kits with chlorhexidine antimicrobial cleanser and to encourage colleagues to do the same. The nurse also suggested to the unit manager to establish a hospital protocol to require disposable bath kits with 4% CHg wash for patient bed baths.

Source: Musuuza, J. S., Guru, P. K., O'Horo, J. C., Bongiorno, C. M., Korobkin, M. A., Gangnon, R. E., & Safdar, N. (2019). The impact of chlorhexidine bathing on hospital-acquired bloodstream infections: A systematic review and meta-analysis. *BMC Infectious Diseases, 19:* Article 416. https://doi.org/10.1186/s12879-019-4002-7

microorganisms into the air. Common airborne patho-gens are the agents of measles and tuberculosis, in addition to many fungal infections.

- A **vector** is an organism that carries a pathogen to a susceptible host. The mosquito is a common vector for diseases, including malaria, yellow fever, and the Zika and West Nile viruses. Ticks, fleas, mites, and some animals can also be vectors for other infections (e.g., Lyme disease).

Portal of Entry

Pathogens can enter the body through various **portals of entry.** Normal body openings, such as the conjunc-tiva of the eye, the nares (nostrils), mouth, urethra, vagina, and anus, are potential portals of entry, as are abnormal openings, such as cuts, scrapes, and surgical incisions. Vectors, such as mosquitoes, create portals of entry when they bite through the skin. In healthcare settings, common portals of entry include wounds, surgical sites, and insertion sites for tubes, lines, or needles.

Susceptible Host

A **susceptible** (or compromised) **host** is a person who is at risk for infection because of inadequate defenses against the invading pathogen. Among the factors that can increase susceptibility are:

Age (very young, very old)
Compromised immune system (immune suppres-sion for organ transplantation or treatment of cancer)
Immune deficiency conditions (e.g., HIV, leukemia, malnutrition, lupus)

KnowledgeCheck 20-2

- Identify the six links in the chain of infection.
- What kinds of microbes favor the human body as a reservoir of infection?

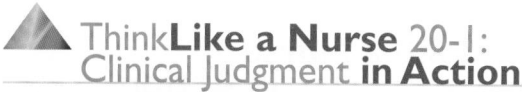

ThinkLike a Nurse 20-1: Clinical Judgment in Action

You are working as a nurse on a medical-surgical unit. What roles might you play in the chain of infection?

Infections Can Be Classified by Location and Duration

An infection is classified according to its location in the body, whether it is the patient's first infection, where it was acquired, and how long it lasts.

Local or Systemic

- **Local infections** are those that cause harm in a limited region of the body, such as the upper respiratory tract, skin, urethra, or a single bone or joint.

- **Systemic infections** occur when pathogens invade the blood or lymph and spread throughout the body.
  - **Bacteremia** is the clinical presence of bacteria in the blood.
  - **Septicemia** is a symptomatic systemic infection spread via the blood.

Primary or Secondary

- **A primary infection** is the first infection that occurs in a patient.
- **A secondary infection** is one that follows a primary infection, especially in immunocompromised patients.
  Example: A frail client infected with pneumonia may develop herpes zoster (shingles, a viral infection related to past infection with varicella) related to the stress of illness.

Exogenous or Endogenous

Healthcare providers need to determine the source of pathogens in a patient who becomes infected while they are in the facility.

- In **exogenous healthcare-related infections,** the patho-gen is acquired from the healthcare environment.
- In **endogenous healthcare-related infections,** the pathogen arises from the patient's normal flora when some form of treatment (e.g., chemotherapy or antibi-otics) causes the normally harmless microbe to multi-ply and cause infection.
  Example: A yeast infection may develop in a client receiving antibiotics after surgery.

Acute, Chronic, or Latent

- **Acute infections** have a rapid onset but last only a short time (e.g., the common cold, urinary tract infection).
- **Chronic infections** (e.g., a wound abscess, hepatitis) develop slowly and last for weeks, months, or even years. Some chronic infections, such as relapsing fever, recur after periods of remission.
- **Latent infections** cause no symptoms for long periods of time, even decades. Tuberculosis and HIV are examples.

Infections Follow Predictable Stages

Many infections follow a fairly predictable course, although the precise duration and intensity of symp-toms in each stage vary from one individual to another:

- **Incubation.** Infection begins in the stage between suc-cessful invasion of the pathogen into the body and the first appearance of symptoms. In this stage, the per-son does not suspect that they have been infected but may be capable of infecting others. This stage may last only a day, as with the influenza virus, or as long as several months or even years, as with tuberculosis.
- **Prodrome.** The prodromal stage is characterized by the first appearance of vague symptoms. For example, a person infected with a cold virus may experience a

mild throat irritation. Not all infections have a prodromal stage.

- **Illness.** The patient becomes ill when the signs and symptoms of the disease appear. If the patient's immune defenses and healthcare treatments (if any) are ineffective, this stage can end in death.
- **Decline.** When the patient's immune defenses, along with any medical therapies, successfully reduce the number of pathogenic microbes, the signs and symptoms of the infection begin to fade.
- **Convalescence.** Healing begins as the remaining number of microorganisms approaches zero. Convalescence may require only a day or two or, for severe infections, as long as a year or more.

Why Should Nurses Be Aware of Emerging Pathogens and Diseases?

Continental and intercontinental travel allow for many ways of spreading emerging diseases. Infected travelers serve as reservoirs for pathogens. The closed spaces and recirculated air systems in airplanes provide an ideal environment for the transmission of airborne pathogens and for both direct and indirect contact contamination between passengers. Air travel also enables a person to infect many people headed for widespread locations, sometimes before the reservoir person shows symptoms of the disease.

- An **endemic** condition occurs at a stable, predictable rate within a particular environment, region, or population. In some areas of Africa, malaria is an example of an endemic disease.
- An **outbreak** is when there is a sudden increase in the number of people with a condition that is greater than expected. Outbreaks are limited to relatively small areas (e.g., cholera after the 2010 Haiti earthquake).
- An **epidemic** is an outbreak of a disease that spreads over a large geographic region or in a defined population group (e.g., elderly, healthcare workers). The Zika virus, which started in Brazil and spread to the Caribbean, is an example of an epidemic.
- A **pandemic** is an exceptionally widespread epidemic—that is, one that affects a large number of people in an entire country or worldwide. Examples of pandemics are SARS-CoV-2 (also known as *COVID-19* or *coronavirus*), H1N1 influenza 2009 (commonly known as *swine flu*), and bubonic plague in the 14th century.

Emerging Infectious Diseases Although there are various definitions, you can think of emerging infectious diseases as:

- **Newly identified diseases** caused either by an unrecognized microorganism (e.g., the virus causing AIDS, unknown before 1980; SARS-CoV-2, not previously identified before 2019]) or by a known organism causing a new response (e.g., enterovirus D68, *Streptococcus* infection triggering toxic shock syndrome).

- **Diseases occurring in new geographic areas** (e.g., Ebola virus originating in western Africa; SARS-CoV-2, first identified in Wuhan, China) or settings (e.g., *C. difficile* was primarily an HAI and now occurs in the community).
- **Microorganisms in animals or insects that extend their host range to begin infecting humans** (e.g., avian influenza, or "bird flu"; H1N1 virus from swine; or Zika virus, which is carried by mosquitos and can cause birth defects when acquired during pregnancy).
- **Microbes that evolve to become more virulent** (e.g., a strain of *E. coli,* which now causes severe illness).
- **Known diseases that dramatically increase in incidence as a result of failed or poor compliance with public health measures** that are meant to control outbreaks, such as immunization (e.g., mumps and pertussis, also known as *whooping cough*) and water treatment (cholera).
- **Many viruses show a high mutation rate and can rapidly yield new strains.** For example, the influenza virus is difficult to eradicate and immunize against because of its adaptability.
- **Organisms that are deliberately altered for bioterrorism** (e.g., the contamination of mail with *Bacillus anthracis* [anthrax]).
- **Most emerging pathogens are viruses.** The WHO has prioritized the following emerging pathogens for which few or no medical countermeasures exist: SARS-CoV-2 virus, Ebola virus, Zika virus, severe acute respiratory syndrome (SARS), Middle Eastern respiratory syndrome (MERS), Crimean Congo hemorrhagic fever.
- Some viruses are exceedingly contagious (measles), whereas others are less so.

Multidrug-Resistant Organisms

Antibiotic resistance is one of the most significant challenges in treating patients with severe infectious diseases. To learn about MDROs, see the accompanying Example Problem: Multidrug-Resistant Organism (MDRO) Infections.

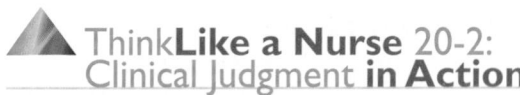

ThinkLike a Nurse 20-2: Clinical Judgment in Action

- Why are emerging infections of special concern in healthcare?
- Why are MDROs of special concern in healthcare?

WHAT ARE THE BODY'S DEFENSES AGAINST INFECTION?

The human body has three "lines of defense" against infectious disease:

- Certain anatomical features limit the entry of pathogens.
- Protective biochemical processes fight pathogens that do enter.
- The presence of pathogens activates immune responses against specific, recognized invaders.

The first two (primary and secondary) lines of defense are nonspecific; that is, they have no means of adapting their response to each specific invader. Instead, they act in precisely the same way against any and all intruders, from a simple cold virus to deadly fungal spores.

Primary Defense

The "soldiers" in the first line of defense are the structural barriers of the human body. **Primary defense** prevents organisms from entering the body.

- **Normal flora of the body.** Any treatment that disturbs the balance between the normal flora and other microorganisms can increase the client's risk of developing disease. For example, when broad-spectrum antibiotics are used to treat infection, they may eliminate normal flora in addition to those causing the infection. This allows other kinds of pathogens to multiply, producing a **superinfection** or another opportunistic infection.
- **Skin.** Intact, healthy skin prevents the entry of many pathogens. The normal flora of the skin keep a healthy balance by limiting the multiplication of other organisms that come in contact with the skin.
- **Respiratory tract.** The nares, trachea, and bronchi are covered with mucous membranes that trap pathogens, which are then expelled. The nose contains hairs that filter the upper airway, and the nasal passages, sinuses, trachea, and larger bronchi are lined with cilia, tiny hairlike cells that sweep microorganisms upward from the lower airways. Coughing and sneezing forcefully expel organisms from the respiratory tract.
- **Eyes.** The lacrimal glands produce tears that contain lysozyme, an antimicrobial enzyme. Tears help the body to wash infective organisms from the eyes.
- **Mouth.** The mouth normally has a large number of pathogenic microorganisms, but saliva, similar to tears, contains lysozyme and helps continually wash microbes from the teeth and gums. The rich blood supply of the mouth swiftly transports defensive blood cells, and the normal flora of the mouth compete with invading organisms for nutrition, thus keeping the microorganisms in check.
- **Gastrointestinal tract.** Many pathogens that reach the stomach are destroyed in its **acidic** environment. Those that successfully enter the small intestine face the antimicrobial action of bile. In addition to normal peristalsis, diarrhea and vomiting eliminate pathogens that invade the gastrointestinal tract. Moreover, normal flora in the intestine secrete antibacterial substances.
- **Genitourinary tract and the anus.** The epithelial cells lining the urethra and anus secrete mucus, which adheres to pathogens to promote their excretion through urine and stool. Urine is highly acidic and contains lysozyme. Mucous membranes lining the vagina also help keep pathogens from establishing colonies there. In addition, the high acidity and normal flora of the vagina keep pathogens in balance.

Secondary Defense

Pathogens that dodge the primary defense and enter the body begin to release wastes and secretions and cause the breakdown of cells and tissues. The presence of such chemicals activates a set of **secondary defenses.**

- **Phagocytosis** is the process by which phagocytes (specialized white blood cells [WBCs]) engulf and destroy pathogens directly. Phagocytes can also signal to other WBCs to aid in eliminating microorganisms that cause disease. They can also kill pathogens by releasing enzymes that lead to their destruction. Table 20-1 summarizes the types of WBCs and their roles in defending against infection.
- **Complement cascade** is a process by which a set of blood proteins, called *complement,* triggers the release of chemicals that attack the cell membranes of pathogens, causing them to rupture. Complement also signals basophils (WBCs) to release histamine, which prompts inflammation.
- **Inflammation** is a process that begins when histamine and other chemicals are released, either from damaged cells or from basophils being activated by complement. With inflammation, blood vessels dilate and become more permeable, which increases the flow of phagocytes, antimicrobial chemicals, oxygen, and nutrients to the affected area. **Key Point:** *The classic signs and symptoms of inflammation are localized warmth and erythema (redness), which develop as blood flow is increased.* In addition, fluid leaking from the more permeable blood vessels accumulates in the surrounding tissue, causing edema that in turn prompts pain.
- **Fever** is a rise in core body temperature that increases metabolism, inhibits the multiplication of pathogens, and triggers specific immune responses (discussed shortly). Believing that low-grade fevers are a necessary natural defense mechanism, most clinicians do not treat a fever unless it is greater than 102°F (38.9°C).

Tertiary Defense

Immunity against an infection is achieved through the presence of antibodies that neutralize or destroy toxins or disease-producing organisms.

- **Active immunity** occurs when the body makes its own antibodies or T lymphocytes (also called *T cells*) to protect the body against a pathogen.
- **Passive immunity** can also be achieved when an individual receives antibodies that come from someone else rather than producing them through their own immune system, such as through immunizations or breastfeeding (Box 20-1).
- **Specific immunity** is the process through which the immune cells "learn" to recognize and destroy

Table 20-1 ➤ Types and Functions of White Blood Cells (WBCs)

TYPE	FUNCTION
Granular	
Basophils: 0.5%–1% of total WBCs	Release histamine and heparin granules as part of the inflammatory response
	Percentage normal during infections
Eosinophils: 1%–3% of total WBCs	Have a role in allergic reactions and control inflammation; have limited role in phagocytosis
	Percentage increases in parasitic infections
	Not commonly found
Neutrophils: 55%–70% of total WBCs	Break down pathogens by releasing enzymes
	Although short-lived, neutrophils can be aggressive and can kill some healthy cells.
	The collection of dead neutrophils is called *pus*.
Agranular	
Lymphocytes: 20%–35% of total WBCs	T cells—responsible for cell-mediated immunity; recognize, attack, and destroy antigens
	B cells—responsible for humoral immunity; produce immunoglobulins to attack and destroy antigens
	Percentage of total lymphocytes increases in viral infection and chronic bacterial infection; it decreases in sepsis.
Monocytes: 3%–8% of total WBCs	Able to phagocytize directly and to differentiate into macrophages, which help clean up damaged or injured tissue
	Percentage increases in tuberculosis, protozoal infections, and rickettsia infections.

Note: Laboratory values alone are not adequate for diagnosing infection. The presence of clinical signs (e.g., fever, pain, swelling) must be assessed.

BOX 20-1 ■ Four Types of Immunity

Natural Active Immunity. After a person becomes ill with an infection, the body produces its own antibodies to fight the disease-causing organism and protect it from infection in the future (e.g., influenza).

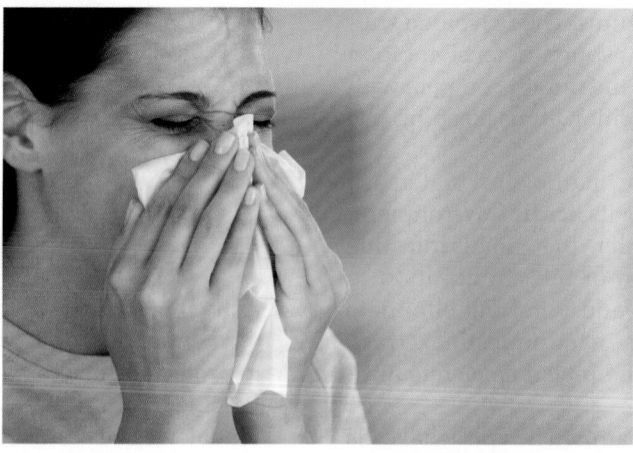

BOX 20-1 ■ Four Types of Immunity—cont'd

Artificial Active Immunity. An immune response occurs when the body is exposed to weakened or dead pathogens in a vaccine. The body then makes T cells or antibodies that keep it from actually developing the illness (e.g., tetanus, measles). This type of immunity offers long-lasting or even lifetime protection.

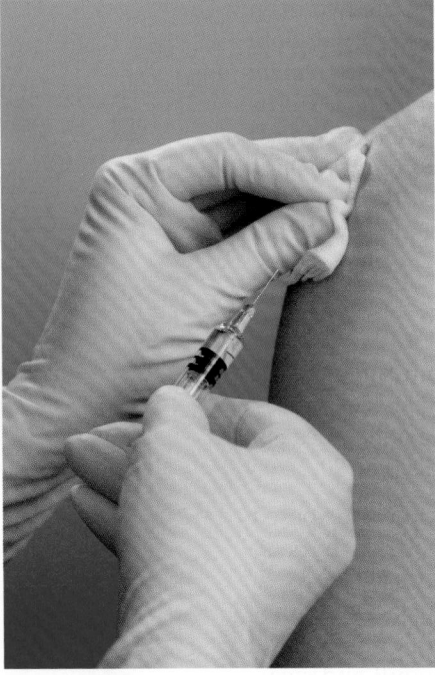

Natural Passive Immunity. Immunity results when natural antibodies are passed from one body to another, such as from mother to baby through the placenta or through breastfeeding.

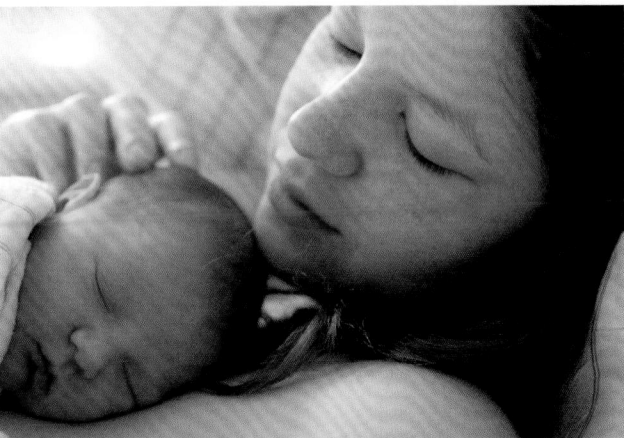

Artificial Passive Immunity. Protection from infection is achieved when a person receives serum from another person or animal that has already produced antibodies against the pathogen (e.g., serum for treatment of rabies or botulism).

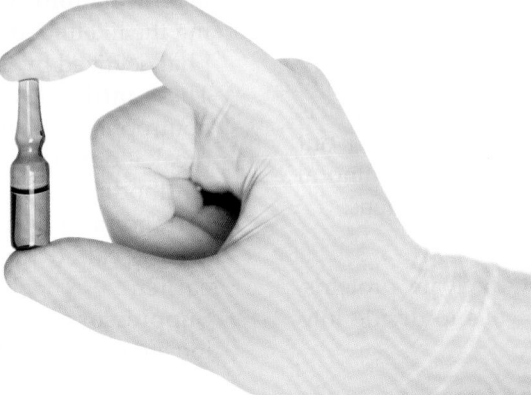

BOX 20-1 ■ Four Types of Immunity—cont'd

pathogens they have encountered before. This is why people who recover from an infectious disease like measles never get the disease again, even if they are repeatedly exposed to the virus. The cells involved in specific immunity are the **lymphocytes,** WBCs produced from stem cells in the red bone marrow. There are two main types of lymphocytes: T cells and B cells. **Key Point:** *Both B cells and T cells form in the bone marrow. B cells remain in the bone marrow until they are fully mature. T cells go to the thymus to mature. Both are activated against pathogens within the lymphatic system (lymph nodes, spleen, tonsils) to protect and preserve health and prevent infection.* The receptors on the surface of these two types of lymphocytes allow them to recognize invaders.

Cellular Immunity

The **cellular (cell-mediated) immune response** acts directly to destroy infection-causing pathogens (i.e., viruses, fungi, protozoans, cancers) without using antibodies but rather by activating phagocytes and T cells (Fig. 20-2).

1. The immune process starts when the body is exposed to a particular **pathogen.** Infecting microbes in the body invade cells and signal for more microbes to take over.
2. **Antigens** are proteins on the outer surface of pathogens that evoke an immune response.
3. Along come WBC **phagocytes** that engulf and swallow the pathogen.
4. After the pathogen is destroyed, the phagocyte now displays pieces of itself on the antigens of the destroyed pathogen. This is known as an **antigen-presenting cell** (APC).
5. Now **memory T cells** bind to the APC to fight similar pathogens in the future. With subsequent infections, memory T cells increase the speed and intensity of the T-cell response to recognize similar intruders.
6. Nearby **helper T cells** come in and fight against the infecting agent by activating T cells and alerting B cells to get involved.
7. **Active T cells** multiply to fight the infection by releasing proteins and enzymes to destroy the pathogen. These are called **cytotoxic (killer) T cells.**
8. **Suppressor T cells** stop the immune response when the infection has been contained (also see Fig. 20-3).

Humoral Immunity

The humoral immune response (or antibody-mediated response) protects the body by circulating antibodies to fight against pathogens. The body's defense system acts by producing specialized WBCs (leukocytes) to seek out and destroy invaders (Fig. 20-3). This is how a humoral immune response works to fight against pathogens:

- A person is exposed to a **pathogen.**
- **Helper cells** in the bone marrow activate proteins, called **interleukins,** that cause B cells to divide into **memory cells** and **active B cells.**

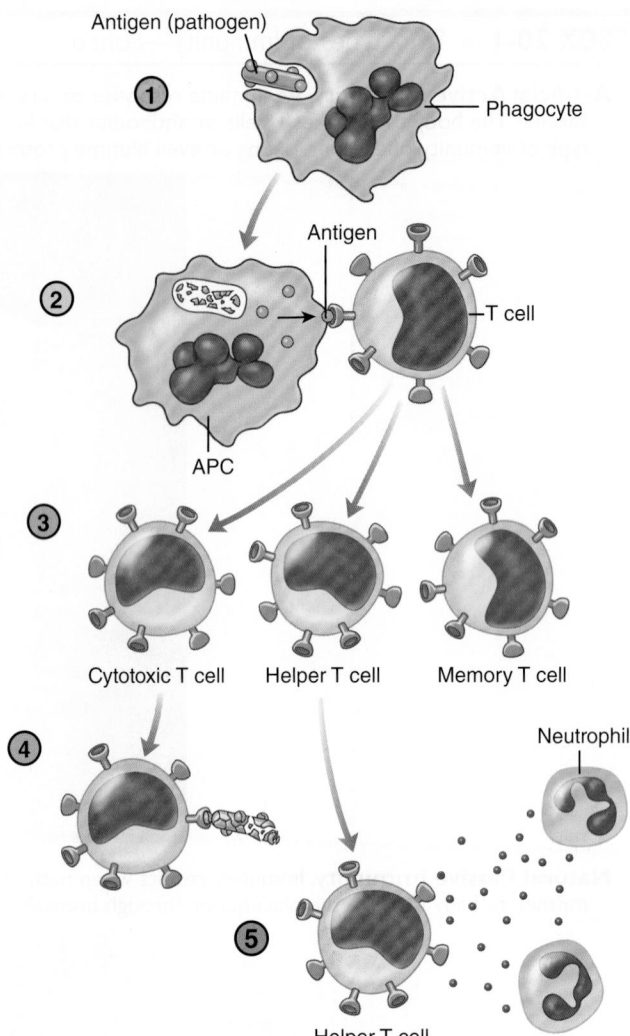

FIGURE 20-2 The cell-mediated immune response causes white blood cells to attach to antigens.

- **Active B cells** produce Y-shaped **antibodies** that bind to the pathogen's attachment site **(antigen)** and interfere with its ability to infect other cells (Box 20-2). This process, called **neutralization,** does not destroy pathogens; it just makes them ineffective.
- Antibodies also cause pathogens to clump together **(agglutination),** reducing their activity and increasing the likelihood that the clump will be detected and phagocytized by leukocytes.
- These **antibodies** signal leukocytes (macrophages and neutrophils) to come in and engulf the pathogen and break it down.
- Antibodies also fight infection by triggering **inflammatory chemicals** to destroy the pathogen. This is called the **complement cascade,** described earlier.
- **Suppressor cells** stop the immune response when the infection is contained.

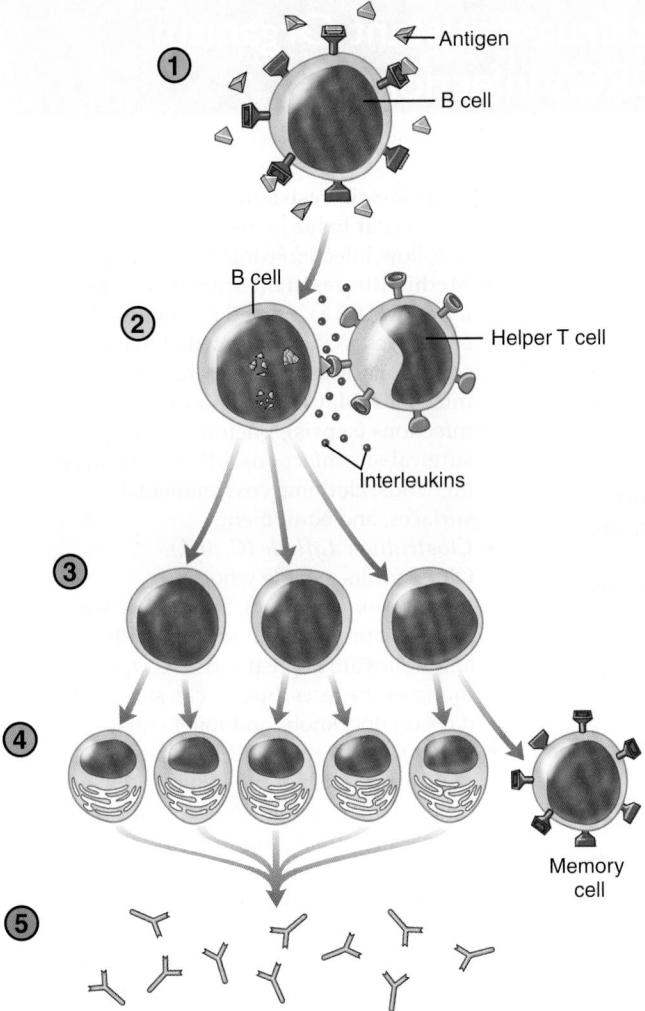

FIGURE 20-3 The humoral immune response produces antibodies to destroy antigens.

KnowledgeCheck 20-3

- Identify and describe the purpose of the body's three major lines of defense against infection.
- If a patient's laboratory work reveals that immunoglobulin M (IgM), but not immunoglobulin G (IgG), is present in the blood, what could you conclude about this infection?

WHAT FACTORS INCREASE HOST SUSCEPTIBILITY?

Anything that weakens the body's defense system makes a person more susceptible to infection. In addition, any factors that increase the person's exposure to pathogens, such as working at a day care facility or being a nurse, increase the risk for infection.

Developmental Stage Young children are vulnerable because their immune systems are immature and they have had limited exposure to pathogens. Children frequently begin to have more infections when they start having contact with people outside their family (e.g., when they attend day care or start school). Acquiring active immunity is a part of the developmental process.

Older adults are also susceptible hosts because the immune response declines with aging. Skin, a primary defense, becomes less elastic and more prone to breakdown with aging. Older adults also tend to be less active, tend to have other underlying illnesses, and their nutrition may be inadequate.

Breaks in the First Line of Defense A break in the skin, whether caused by a surgical procedure, injury, skin breakdown, an insect bite, or insertion of an IV device, creates a portal of entry for infectious microorganisms.

Illness or Injury A coexisting infection, illness, or injury limits the physical resources available to combat a new pathogen.

Tobacco Use
- Smoking is a major risk factor for pulmonary infections because it interferes with normal respiratory functioning, including the ability to move the chest, cough, sneeze, and have full air exchange.
- Chemicals in tobacco immobilize cilia; thus, secretions pool in the lower airways, creating a favorable environment for bacteria to live and replicate.
- Smoking and vaping adversely affect the immune system by compromising the antibacterial function of leukocytes. As a result, chronic exposure to secondhand smoke increases the risk for respiratory infection, ear and sinus infection, meningitis, and postsurgical and nosocomial infections (Bagaitkar et al., 2008).

Substance Abuse
- **Alcohol** curbs hunger. As a result, many chronic alcohol users do not consume an adequate diet, leading to vitamin, mineral, and protein deficiency. Over time,

BOX 20-2 ■ Immunoglobulin (Ig) Classes

- **IgM** is the first antibody to appear when an antigen (e.g., pathogen) is encountered. It is also involved in agglutination with incompatible blood types.
- **IgG** is the most common immunoglobulin in the body. It takes at least 10 days for IgG to be produced in response to an initial infection. IgG is the only immunoglobulin that can cross the placenta to provide temporary immunity to the fetus/infant.
- **IgE** is the immunoglobulin primarily responsible for the allergic response.
- **IgA** is found in mucous membranes in the intestines, respiratory and urinary tracts, saliva, tears, and breast milk. IgA provides additional immune protection by secreting around the body openings.
- **IgD** forms on the surface of B cells and traps the potential pathogen to prevent it from replicating and causing disease.

EXAMPLE CLIENT CONDITION: Multidrug-Resistant Organism (MDRO) Infections

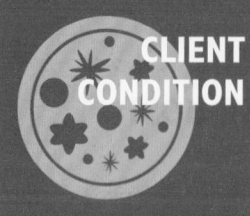
CLIENT CONDITION

Definition of MDROs

Microbes that have mutated to develop resistance to one or more classes of antimicrobial drugs; associated with serious illness, increased hospitalization, higher death rates

Background

During the past several decades, the prevalence of MDROs in U.S. hospitals and medical centers has increased steadily.

Importance/Implications

- Antibiotic resistance is one of the most significant challenges in treating patients with severe infectious diseases.
- Options for treating MDRO infections are limited.
- MDROs are associated with serious illness, increased mortality, and increased hospital lengths of stay and costs.

Transmission

(1) One person to another via the hands of healthcare personnel and visitors; (2) bed linens, bed rails, medical equipment, personal items, and other contaminated inanimate objects.

Types

- **Vancomycin-resistant enterococci (VRE).** Most occur in hospitals. Spread by failure to follow infection control measures.
- **Methicillin-resistant *Staphylococcus aureus* (MRSA).** Spread by skin-to-skin contact, especially in crowded living conditions. Most are skin and soft tissue infections. May cause bloodstream infections **(sepsis)**, pneumonia, and surgical-site infections. MRSA can survive on hands, clothing, environmental surfaces, and equipment.
- ***Clostridium difficile (C. diff.).*** Older adults, people who are immunocompromised, and people who have had prolonged treatment with antibiotics are at greater risk. *C. diff.* are found in the feces. Spores can survive for days on doorknobs and toilet seats.
- **Other significant MDROs** include multidrug-resistant tuberculosis (MDR-TB), penicillin-resistant *Streptococcus pneumoniae*, multidrug-resistant *E. coli*, and *Klebsiella pneumoniae*.
- **Antibiotic-resistant superbug.** Mutant strains that are resistant to conventional antibiotic therapy (e.g., a strain of drug-resistant *E. coli* that can pass its resistance to other species of bacteria).

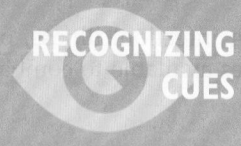
RECOGNIZING CUES

Assess risk factors, symptoms, and diagnostic test results.

Risk Factors

- Previous exposure to antibiotics
- Impaired body defense (e.g., caused by underlying disease or immune deficiency)
- Severe illness
- Invasive procedures and devices
- Repeated hospitalization, especially intensive care units (ICUs)
- Advanced age

Symptoms

- Wounds that are slow or fail to heal with antibiotics
- Observe for symptoms of infections: fever, swelling, redness, excessive warmth, pain, or drainage.
- Diarrhea, abdominal cramping

Diagnostic Tests Results

- Cultures and sensitivities of wound and skin, blood, sputum, urine, cerebral spinal fluid (CSF)
- Complete blood count (CBC) with differential
- Some institutions require screening cultures at admission or on specialty units (ICU).

EXAMPLE CLIENT CONDITION: Multidrug-Resistant Organism (MDRO) Infections—cont'd

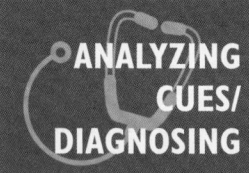

ANALYZING CUES/ DIAGNOSING

Infection Risk (MDRO) r/t open skin lesions and long-term antibiotic use

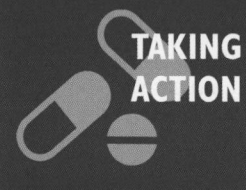

GENERATING SOLUTIONS

Patient Goals

- No signs of localized infection (e.g., fever, inflammation)
- Verbalizes improved comfort
- Effective coping behaviors while isolated

Nurse Goals

- Practices MDRO prevention measures
- Recognizes the signs of MDRO infection

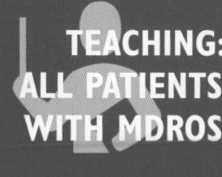

TAKING ACTION

Care of All Patients With MDROs

- Adhere strictly to guidelines for hand hygiene, glove use, and isolation precautions for all patient contact until cultures are negative.
- Observe standard precautions for all patients.
- Ensure patient areas are cleaned well and often.
- Disinfect high-touch surfaces (bed rails, door handles, sink). For *C. diff.*, use a bleach-containing disinfectant.
- Use private rooms as needed.

- Wear gowns and gloves for all contact with patient and contaminated items.
- Dedicate noncritical equipment (stethoscope, thermometer) for use with individuals with MDRO infection.
- Use masks and eye protection, especially when splashes are possible.
- Assign patient to single room if available. If not, place with a patient with the same MDRO.
- Special measures to prevent lower respiratory infections in intubated patients

TEACHING: ALL PATIENTS WITH MDROS

For All Patients with MDROs

Teach patient and caregiver:

- Ways to limit further spread of infection to close contacts, including meticulous hand hygiene and standard precautions. See the box Holistic Health: Preventive Actions Limiting Spread of Infection.
- Difference between bacterial and viral infection
- Importance of avoiding overuse of antibiotics

- Those unable to keep infected wounds covered and practice strict hand washing should be excluded from activities involving close contact with others (e.g., day care, contact sports).

NOTE: To teach about preventing all types of infections, which would include MDROs, see the box Home Care: Preventing Infection in the Home and Community in this chapter.

(continued)

EXAMPLE CLIENT CONDITION: Multidrug-Resistant Organism (MDRO) Infections—cont'd

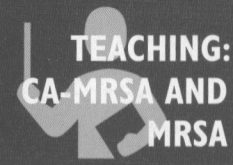

TEACHING: CA-MRSA AND MRSA

For Clients Who Are Infected With Community-Acquired MRSA

Teach patient and caregiver:

Medications
- Take antibiotics as prescribed and take *all* the doses.
- Contact your provider if the infection doesn't improve after a few days of antibiotic use.
- Do not use antibiotics prescribed for someone else or give your drugs to others.
- Follow your provider's recommendations for flu and pneumonia vaccinations. This will decrease your use of antibiotics.

Personal Hygiene

- **Key Point: *Be sure providers clean their hands before touching you.***
- Wash your hands often with soap and water. Wash for 20 seconds.
- Use 60% alcohol-based hand sanitizer if soap and water are not available or hands are not visibly soiled.
- Avoid sharing personal items (e.g., towels, makeup, combs, clothing).

Other Measures

- Watch for signs of infection (e.g., drainage or inflammation of a wound); contact your provider at once.
- Cough and sneeze into your elbow and wash your hands after using a tissue.

For Clients Who Are Infected With MRSA

Teach patient and caregiver:
- Keep all wounds clean and covered with bandages.
- When changing a dressing:
  Don't touch the wound with your bare hands. Wear gloves.
  Immediately discard the soiled dressing and gloves in a plastic bag where no one else can touch them.
  Wash your hands after removing the gloves.
- Don't touch other people's wounds or dressings.
- Avoid close-contact activities until your skin infection is healed, unless you can ensure that your sore will not come in contact with another person.
- Shower daily, using antibacterial soap if your healthcare provider advises it.
- Wash your clothing, towels, and bedding separately from other family members' items. Use warm or hot water and bleach, if possible. Use warm or hot setting on the dryer.
- Wash workout clothes after each use.

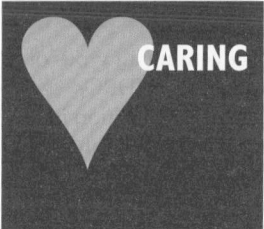

CARING

♥ **iCare** • Be sensitive to patients' emotional needs because many feel shamed by the odor of wound infection. Others may become angry or depressed during extended isolation.

- Provide measures to relieve boredom (isolation reduces sensory input).
- Patients may be socially isolated because other people fear they will be infected.
- Encourage visitors to spread out visits and be mindful of patient's feelings of loneliness.

---

excessive alcohol use is toxic to the liver and to the cells lining the intestinal mucosa of the esophagus and gut, which can lead to inflammation, infection, and injury.
- **Inhaled substances** affect the respiratory cilia in a manner similar to tobacco.
- **Any substances that affect orientation and energy** level will diminish food intake, activity, rest, and hygiene—factors that support host defenses.
- **Injecting substances** leads to breaks in skin integrity, further increasing the risk of infection.

Multiple Sexual Partners The more sexual partners a person has, the greater the risk of acquiring sexually transmitted infections and cervical cancer. Microbes are transmitted via semen, vaginal secretions, or blood that is present during sexual intercourse.

Environmental Factors Increased exposure to pathogens and pollutants in the environment irritate the respiratory airways and lead to infection. Breaks in the skin increase the risk for local or systemic infection. Exposure to pathogens can also occur in the work setting (e.g., teacher, healthcare worker) and in living situations (e.g., skilled nursing care, parents with children in preschool) and can increase the risk for infection.

Chronic Disease Poor circulation prevents antibodies and T cells from reaching the pathogens and damages tissue, making it easier for pathogens to enter and thrive.

- **Diseases that impair peripheral circulation,** such as uncontrolled hypertension (high blood pressure) and diabetes mellitus, make the patient prone to infection in the extremities. Poor circulation prevents antibodies and T cells from reaching the pathogens and damages tissue, making it easier for pathogens to enter.
- **Leukemia,** a form of cancer of the blood, increases the production of abnormal WBCs, but these cells are ineffective in combating infection.
- **Immunodeficiency and HIV exposure.** Because HIV infects T cells, a patient with AIDS has a reduced ability to fight off secondary infections.

Medications Some medications are given for the purpose of reducing the immune response. For example, patients receiving organ or tissue transplants usually are given medications to prevent organ rejection. Drugs used to treat allergies, arthritis, lupus, and irritable bowel syndrome (IBS) also reduce the immune response. For most patients, though, decreased immunity is an unwanted side effect of treatment.

- Even common medications, such as NSAIDs (e.g., ibuprofen), lessen the immune response.
- As a side effect, some medications, such as chemotherapeutic agents, impair the production of WBCs or cause the cells produced to be abnormal.
- Antibiotics can also increase the risk for infection. For example, an antibiotic given for a respiratory infection may cause a vaginal yeast infection because it destroys colonies of normal vaginal flora, allowing the harmful microbes to thrive. Such **superinfections** (opportunistic growth of harmful transient pathogens that are normally kept in check) can be challenging to treat.

Poor Nutrition A diet with low-quality foods can lead to a weakened immune system. A high-fat diet can disrupt the healthy balance of normal bacteria in the gut, whereas a diet high in fruits, vegetables, nuts, and seeds containing beta-carotene and vitamins A, B, C, and E, along with other nutrients, helps the body fight off infection. Plant-based foods and lean meats, poultry, and fish contribute to healthy body weight, which can also strengthen the immune response.

Lack of Physical Activity A sedentary lifestyle contributes to the risk of various health issues, including reduced immunity. Physical activity promotes circulation that delivers WBCs and other immune-boosting complexes, such as T cells, phagocytes, and antibodies, to the site of infection. Outdoor activity can even bolster T-cell activity to aid in immune protection.

Poor Sleep Sleep is restorative; not getting enough sleep can compromise the effectiveness of the immune system. During sleep, the body produces antibodies and cytokines to help stave off infection.

Stress and Grief Emotional state contributes to the body's state of well-being. Prolonged stress, anxiety, depression, and grief can depress the immune system's effectiveness in fighting infection, such as the flu, herpes, shingles, and other viruses.

Nursing and Medical Procedures Several procedures are associated with an increased risk of infection. For example, urinary catheterization may injure the fragile urethral mucosa, provide a direct pathway for pathogens into the bladder, and prevent the normal flushing of the urethra. An IV line may also serve as a portal of entry for pathogens to enter a patient's body.

KnowledgeCheck 20-4

- What factors increase a client's risk for infection?

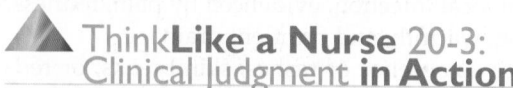

ThinkLike a Nurse 20-3: Clinical Judgment in Action

- Consider your current lifestyle. How would you evaluate your ability to support your body's defenses?

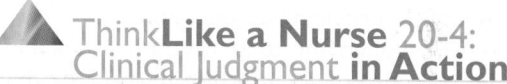

ThinkLike a Nurse 20-4: Clinical Judgment in Action

Recall the scenario of Jarek Shvets, the labor and delivery nurse, and his daughter (Meet Your Nursing Role Model). Why did Jarek say that hand washing was the most important thing he did at work that day? Explain your answer by referring to all the links in the chain of infection.

PracticalKnowledge
knowing how

As a nurse, you will have direct contact with patients who are infected with a variety of pathogens or who are at increased risk for infection. The remainder of this chapter provides practical information for preventing infection in your clients and for caring for clients with infection.

ASSESSMENT/RECOGNIZING CUES

Some elements of the nursing history and physical assessment focus specifically on the risk factors for and symptoms of infection.

Nursing History

To elicit information related to infection, ask the client about the following:

- Any exposure to pathogens in the environment, including work site, recent or international travel, contact with people who are ill, and unprotected sexual behavior
- Any unusual foods or products ingested
- Health status (e.g., diabetes, immunodeficiency, autoimmune disorder); injury history

- Medications, over-the-counter preparations, herbal products, and any substances currently in use
- Current level of stress
- Immunization history
- Symptoms of illness

Physical Assessment

The following observations focus specifically on infection:

- **General appearance.** Does the patient seem fatigued? Are they diaphoretic (perspiring profusely)? Are they wrapped in blankets or complaining of feeling chilled? Does the patient appear well nourished? Are the mucous membranes dry?
- **Skin.** Examine the skin thoroughly for:
  - Normal elasticity (turgor)
  - Signs of local infection, evidenced by pain, redness, swelling, warmth, and purulent drainage
  - Presence or absence of rashes, skin breaks, or reddened areas
  - *Note:* Patients with poor peripheral circulation often have skin discoloration rather than signs of inflammation when experiencing an infection.
- **Lymph nodes.** Swollen and tender lymph nodes may indicate the presence of an infection in the area that drains into the nodes.
- **Temperature and pulse.** Elevated temperature and pulse rate are classic signs of an infection.

The presence of one infection does not eliminate the risk for an additional infection. For example, a patient being treated with IV medications for a wound infection is at risk for infection at the IV site, as well as for a superinfection or an infection related to insufficient immunizations. Each specific test should be evaluated based on the patient's condition, age, and coexisting conditions.

 See **Chapter 20, Diagnostic Testing, Common Tests for Evaluating the Presence of or Risk for Infection**, in Volume 2.

NURSING DIAGNOSIS/ANALYZING CUES

Only one NANDA-I diagnosis directly pertains to infection: Risk for Infection.

Risk for Infection Virtually any patient in a healthcare setting is at Risk for Infection as a result of exposure to pathogens in the environment. **Key Point:** *Use this diagnosis only for patients who are at higher-than-usual risk (e.g., those with poor nutritional status) and who need nursing interventions to help prevent infection. Do not use it for the generic assessments you do routinely for all patients (e.g., assessing temperature, routine examination of surgical incision).* Examples of appropriate use of this diagnosis include the following:

- **Risk for Infection** (NANDA-I) r/t altered immune response secondary to corticosteroid therapy

- **Infection Risk** (Clinical Care Classification [CCC], 2012) r/t impaired skin integrity and poor nutritional status
- **Risk for Surgical Site Infection** (NANDA-I) r/t low WBC count and undernutrition

For a care plan and care map for Risk for Infection,

 Go to Davis Advantage, Resources, **Chapter 20, Care Plan** and **Care Map.**

Actual Infection Once an infection develops, it is not precisely a nursing problem; it is managed collaboratively with the healthcare team. Infection is confirmed by medical diagnosis and diagnostic tests.

- **NANDA-I** does not have a diagnostic label for actual infection.
- **CCC** uses the diagnosis **Infection** (CCC, 2012).
- **Collaborative Problem.** This text and some nurses prefer to state an actual infection as a collaborative problem, allowing for a focus on the complications of infection, as in the following examples:
  - Potential Complications of Urinary Tract Infection: Sepsis
  - Potential Complications of Communicable Disease (e.g., tuberculosis): Social Isolation

Infection as an Etiology Patients with infection may have other actual nursing diagnoses as a result of their infected status. For example:

Social Isolation r/t communicable disease (e.g., tuberculosis [TB])

Decreased Diversional Activity r/t inability to leave room secondary to protective isolation

PLANNING/PRIORITIZING HYPOTHESES AND GENERATING SOLUTIONS

Nursing Outcomes Classification (NOC) standardized outcomes for a diagnosis of Risk for Infection include:

Community Risk Control	Infection Severity
Communicable Disease	Risk Control: STDs
Immune Status	Wound Healing: Primary Intention
Immunization Behavior	Wound Healing: Secondary Intention

Individualized goals/outcome statements depend on the specific nursing diagnosis and etiology. For example, for an undernourished woman, if the nursing diagnosis is Risk for Infection r/t intravenous puncture site, an appropriate goal would be:

Patient will show no signs of localized infection at the infusion site, as evidenced by the absence of swelling, redness, excessive warmth, pain, or drainage.

You will evaluate the nursing care plan by examining the extent to which such goals have been met.

IMPLEMENTATION/TAKING ACTION

When caring for a patient at risk for infection, nursing activities are aimed at breaking the chain of infection at every possible link. Some common reasons patients are diagnosed with Risk for Infection are exposure to pathogens, compromise of normal defense mechanisms, increased physiological stress, or inadequate immune response. Provide the following broad interventions to direct care to those issues:

- Use aseptic technique to reduce exposure to pathogens.
- Maintain skin integrity and support natural defenses against infection.
- Reduce stress.
- Promote immune function through collaborative care, healthy diet and activity, sleep, and lifestyle.
- Provide supportive measures to decrease the length of time that invasive devices (e.g., IV lines, urinary catheters) are needed.

Nursing Interventions Classification (NIC) standardized interventions for patients with infections include:

Communicable Disease Management
Immunization/Vaccination Management
Incision Site Care
Infection Control
Surveillance
Teaching: Safe Sex
Wound Care

Specific nursing activities will be based on the unique situation of the client, described in the etiology of the diagnostic statement. The following are examples of activities:

- **For clients who have had surgery and general anesthesia** or who are at risk for pneumonia, promote coughing and deep breathing on a regular basis.
- **For clients being mechanically ventilated,** provide special oral care designed to prevent VAP. (See the accompanying Promoting Safe, Effective Nursing Care box for an example.)
  - For older adults, especially those who are frail or in a debilitated state and those living in a group residence, encourage immunizations that can help them to acquire immunity for some communicable diseases, such as influenza.
- **Healthcare workers** can also benefit from immunizations to protect them from HAIs.
- **Community health nurses** can limit disease transmission through surveillance of the community, tracking of disease patterns, and initiation of prompt treatment.
- **For clients who have breaks in the skin or surgical incisions,** assess regularly for infection, and follow appropriate medical or surgical asepsis guidelines.
- **For all clients at risk for infection,** provide care that is based on the principles of medical asepsis.

Teaching Infection Prevention in the Home and Community

Clients and caregivers are usually at less risk for infection in their homes than they are in the hospital because:

- They share the same potential pathogens and antibodies.
- There is limited exposure to others with illness.

Nevertheless, to protect their own health and the health of others, clients need to understand basic principles of medical asepsis, personal hygiene, and infection control. You should also teach them to recognize the signs and symptoms of infection and, for those who have an infection, help them to understand that particular organism and disease process. See the box Home Care: Preventing Infection in the Home and Community and the Example Client Condition: Multidrug-Resistant Organism (MDRO) Infections.

Promoting Wellness to Support Host Defense

Lifestyle factors that strengthen host defense and help break the chain of infection are healthful nutrition, good hydration, adequate hygiene, rest and exercise, stress reduction, and immunizations.

Nutrition Monitor and support client nutrition, including protein, vitamins, minerals, and water. An acute infection depletes the body's nutritional stores. Nutrients are required to replace lost stores, maintain production of WBCs, and repair damaged tissues. Common bodily defenses against infection involve increased mucus secretions and fever, which increases the metabolic rate. These defenses also increase water loss. Chapter 24 further discusses the importance of adequate nutrition.

Hygiene Encourage frequent hand washing and regular showering or bathing to decrease the bacterial count on the skin. However, be aware that overzealous sanitation diminishes the skin's natural oils and may lead to cracking of the skin. Chapter 22 focuses on the importance of hygiene for health. Also, see the box Home Care: Preventing Infection in the Home and Community.

For the immunocompromised or bed-bound hospitalized patient, provide daily bedside baths (or more often upon patient request) using filtered tap water, disposable basins, and prepackaged bathing products. Nurses should use disposable basins and cloths with 2% chlorhexidine gluconate (CHG) to reduce colonization of specific bacteria and infections with MDROs (American Association of Critical-Care Nurses, 2013; Cassir et al., 2015; Huang et al., 2016; Musuuza et al., 2019; Petlin et al., 2014; Power et al., 2012). Apply emollients after bathing to prevent dry skin.

Rest and Sleep Advise patients that 6 to 9 hours per night is considered fully restorative for most people. However, sleep needs and patterns vary. Rest and sleep conserve energy needed for healing.

Home Care

Preventing Infection in the Home and Community

➤ Use antiseptic and antibacterial wipes or sprays to disinfect the home environment, or make up diluted bleach mixture to wipe down frequently touched surfaces. This may be stored for a month in an opaque container. ✚ NEVER mix a bleach solution with other household cleaners.

➤ Procedures performed using sterile technique in the hospital (e.g., urinary catheterization) are often performed by clean procedure in the home.

➤ Healthcare workers can carry pathogens into the home; they must use good hand hygiene to avoid infecting clients.

➤ If clients or family members are capable and willing to perform the required treatment, provide the necessary teaching.

➤ Assess for signs of infection: fever, chills, and fatigue; lymph gland enlargement; delayed healing of wounds, drainage; skin that is warm to the touch, reddened, and tender.

➤ Teach clients and family members the signs and symptoms of infection and when to report these findings to their primary care provider.

➤ Advise those planning international travel to get their vaccinations before departing, especially for travel to Africa, South-Central Asia, or Central America, where they may contract COVID-19, malaria, dengue, rickettsiosis, hepatitis, and Zika virus.

Teaching Basic Infection Prevention Measures in the Home

➤ Always wash hands before, during, and after preparing food and before eating; before putting the hands near the face; after toileting or after changing diapers; after blowing the nose, coughing, or sneezing or before or after being around someone who's sick; before and after treating any wound; after touching an animal, pet food, or pet waste; and after contact with trash or contaminated items.

➤ Keep the home environment clean.

➤ Prepare and store food safely. Growth of pathogens in foods can be prevented by:

Cooking at high temperatures and storing in a cool place

Using highly concentrated solutes (e.g., salting meat and preserving fruit jellies, jams, and preserves)

➤ Do not share personal care items (e.g., towels, washcloths, toothbrushes, combs).

➤ Washing dishware and eating utensils in a dishwasher with hot water and detergents is sufficient decontamination.

Avoiding Infection Outside the Home

➤ Wash hands with soap and water for a full 20 seconds; do not touch surfaces in a public bathroom.

➤ Carry and use antibacterial hand gel as needed while in public places.

➤ Wash hands upon returning home.

➤ Ask healthcare providers to wash their hands before touching you if they have not done so.

Sources: Centers for Disease Control and Prevention. (2019, April 29, updated 2022, March 14, March 21). *Handwashing: Clean hands saves lives.* https://www.cdc.gov/handwashing/when-how-handwashing.html; Centers for Disease Control and Prevention. (2021, August 26). *Healthy habits to help prevent flu.* https://www.cdc.gov/flu/prevent/actions-prevent-flu.htm

---

Safe, Effective Nursing Care

Preventing Ventilator-Associated Pneumonia (VAP)

Key Concepts: Infection Prevention and Control

Competencies: Provide safe, quality client care; collaborate with the interprofessional healthcare team

You and your colleagues can help improve the quality of patient care. Think about the following project and consider what Thinking, Doing, and Caring skills are required for its success.

Scenario: Nurses and physicians at the Mercy Medical Center wanted to reduce the rate of VAP in the intensive care unit.

1. **They collected data** to establish the current VAP rate of 12.6 cases per 1,000 ventilator days.

2. **Then they developed and implemented an intervention.** Nurses provided oral care with cetylpyridinium chloride using a suction toothbrush every 4 hours. After that, they cleaned the patient's mouth with a hydrogen peroxide–treated suction swab, performed deep oropharyngeal suctioning, and applied mouth moisturizer.

3. **The result.** Incidence of VAP declined 72%, and after changing the tooth cleanser to chlorhexidine gluconate, VAP declined by 90% (Hutchins et al., 2009).

Other researchers interested in preventing VAP reviewed 28 clinical trials in the scientific literature. They found that chlorhexidine rinses, gels, and swabs also lower the risk for HAIs for patients receiving mechanical ventilation (El-Rabbany et al., 2015).

Think About It.

Reflect on the following and discuss the questions with your peers:

➤ What information did nurses and team members need before changing the care of patients on ventilators?

➤ How does the intervention improve patient comfort?

➤ How significant do you think the team's work was? How will their efforts affect patients?

➤ What do you think the team should measure to determine whether the intervention worked?

Exercise and Activity Emphasize that exercise is just as important as rest and sleep. Too little activity causes circulation to slow and the lungs to supply less oxygen. Excessive exercise leads to fatigue and joint injury. Chapters 29 and 31 provide in-depth discussion of rest, sleep, activity, and exercise.

Stress Reduction Inform clients of the need to reduce stress. Laughing increases immune responses, improves oxygenation, and promotes body movement. In contrast, physical or mental stress decreases the body's immune defense. Studies demonstrate a correlation between stress and disease (Cousins, 1979; Franco et al., 2003). See Chapter 9 if you want additional details about stress.

Immunizations Encourage clients to follow recommendations for immunizations (e.g., via vaccination) to protect against several common infectious diseases (e.g., COVID-19, measles, mumps, pertussis, polio, pneumonia, influenza, smallpox, and shingles). Unfortunately, some pathogens, such as the common cold virus, mutate too rapidly for an immunization to be developed. **Key Point: *For most diseases, at least 85% of the population must be immunized in order to protect the entire population from the disease.*** Refer to the CDC for recommended vaccination schedules for infants, children, adolescents, and adults; during pregnancy, and prior to international travel.

KnowledgeCheck 20-5

What actions improve the host's ability to prevent infection?

PRACTICING MEDICAL ASEPSIS

Asepsis is a term that refers to the absence of contamination by disease-causing microorganisms. **Medical asepsis** ("clean technique") refers to procedures that decrease the potential for the spread of infection. You likely already practice medical asepsis in other settings without realizing it. For example, at home, you wash your hands before and after handling food. In the healthcare setting, medical asepsis includes hand hygiene, environmental cleanliness, standard precautions, and protective isolation.

Infection prevention and the patient's safety depend on nurses' ability to rigorously and consistently follow the principles of asepsis. When you are hurrying, you may be tempted to take shortcuts or forget to follow a guideline. **Key Point: *Cutting corners can put your patient, and possibly yourself, at risk for a serious infection.***

Maintaining Clean Hands

Key Point: *Hand hygiene is the single most important activity for preventing and controlling infection.*

The WHO (2011) chose the reduction of HAIs as the first "global patient safety challenge," with the theme "clean care is safer care." Hand hygiene is the cornerstone

strategy because it is simple, standardized, low cost, and based on solid scientific evidence.

Although you may think you already know how to wash your hands, decisions about the type of hand hygiene to use, how long to wash, when to wash, and so on are based on the amount of contact you have with patients or contaminated objects, as well as the patient's infection status and susceptibility to infection. Hand washing involves five key factors: time, water, soap, friction, and drying.

- **Time.** In a nonsurgical setting, wash the hands vigorously for at least 15 seconds for a soap-and-water wash, longer if hands are visibly soiled. Wash for 20 to 30 seconds when using an alcohol-based hand rub. In a surgical setting, wash for 2 to 6 minutes, depending on the soap or other product used.
- **Water.** Use warm water and rinse off soap completely.
- **Soap.** Use agency-approved soap. The CDC (2002) recommends using a 60% alcohol-based solution (rubs, sprays, gels) for routine hand cleansing and plain or antimicrobial soap and water when hands are visibly dirty (Boyce & Pittet, 2002). Iodine compounds are also effective, but they are usually too irritating for regular hand hygiene.

If there is a potential for contact with bacterial spores (e.g., when caring for a client with a *C. difficile* infection), you must wash your hands with soap and water; alcohol-based solutions are not effective against spores.

- **Friction.** Rub all surfaces of the hands and wrists vigorously, including the backs of the hands and between the fingers. Remove jewelry and clean areas underneath. Clean thoroughly underneath the fingernails using a brush or nail pick.
- **Drying.** Use single-use towels or hand dryers to remove all moisture after washing the hands. If using antimicrobial hand gels, apply and rub hands until dry.

For more specific details, guidelines, and step-by-step instructions for hand hygiene,

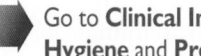
Go to **Clinical Insight 20-1: Guidelines for Hand Hygiene** and **Procedure 20-1: Hand Hygiene** in Volume 2.

Key Point: *Failure to perform standards of care constitutes medical negligence and can result in harm to the patient.* In addition, Medicare does not reimburse for patient complications arising from certain HAIs, many of which result from poor hand washing. Despite the importance of clean hands, research demonstrates that clinical staff members do not consistently observe hand hygiene guidelines (Pittet et al., 2017). You can help improve clinical practice by serving as a role model for good hand hygiene.

Maintaining a Clean Environment

A clean environment includes the surfaces in a patient's room, as well as supplies, equipment, and other objects brought into the room. The floor, soiled dressings and

About Protecting Patients From the Spread of Infection

Care enough to:
- Be knowledgeable about your organization's policy and procedures.
- Spend the time for thorough hand washing and strict aseptic technique when needed.
- Never use shortcuts when it comes to hand hygiene and asepsis.
- Remind others about diligent hand hygiene and the use of personal protective equipment and sterile techniques.
- Be bold and call people out on breaks in aseptic technique when violations occur.
- Caring is being an advocate for infection prevention.

tissues, sinks, commodes, and bedpans are examples of contaminated items. An object becomes contaminated or unclean if it contacts a contaminated surface—or if you suspect, for whatever reason, that it may contain pathogens. Agency policies determine whether a reusable item is cleaned, disinfected, or sterilized, based on how the item is used.

Cleaning

Cleaning is the removal of visible soil (organic and inorganic) from objects and surfaces. In healthcare agencies, it is usually accomplished manually or mechanically using water with detergents or enzymatic products formulated to inhibit microbial growth. A goal of medical asepsis is to keep all public and patient care areas within the facility clean and free from dust, debris, and contamination. Any spilled liquids, dirty surfaces, or potentially contaminated areas should be cleaned immediately. Items must be cleaned thoroughly before they can be disinfected or sterilized.

Disinfecting

Disinfection removes pathogens on inanimate objects by physical or chemical means, including steam, gas, chemicals, and ultraviolet light.

Levels of Disinfection Chemical germicides can achieve three levels of disinfection:

1. **High-level disinfection** kills all organisms except high levels of bacterial spores.
2. **Intermediate-level disinfection** kills bacteria, mycobacteria, and most viruses.
3. **Low-level disinfection** kills some viruses and bacteria.

Semi- and Noncritical Items Disinfection is used for semicritical and noncritical items:

- **Semicritical items** are those that contact mucous membranes or nonintact skin. They must be free of all

microorganisms except bacterial spores, so they must at least be disinfected and sometimes sterilized.
- *Examples:* Reusable devices, such as flexible endoscopes and respiratory therapy and anesthesia equipment.
- **Noncritical items** are supplies and equipment that come in contact with intact skin but not mucous membranes. They do not carry a high risk of infection transmission, and they can be decontaminated where they are used.
  - *Examples:* Bedpans, stethoscopes, and blood pressure cuffs
  - *Examples of noncritical environmental surfaces:* Floors, food utensils, bed linens, and bed rails.

Sterilizing

Sterilization is the elimination of all microorganisms (except prions) in or on an object. The most common sterilizing methods used in hospitals are (1) autoclaving with moist heat, also called *immediate use steam sterilization;* (2) gas or vapor (e.g., ethylene oxide gas at low heat); (3) dry heat; (4) ozone; (5) liquid chemicals (e.g., peracetic acid); and (6) low-temperature hydrogen peroxide gas (Association of periOperative Registered Nurses [AORN], 2018).

Key Point: Sterilization is used when the absolute purity of an object or surface is critical.

- **Critical items** are ones that pose a high risk for infection if they are contaminated with any microorganism—that is, those that enter the vascular system or sterile tissue or those items through which blood flows.
  - *Examples:* IV catheters, needles for injections, urinary catheters, surgical instruments, some wound dressings, and chest tubes

As a nurse, you must be familiar with the agency's policies and procedures for cleaning, handling, and transporting items to be disinfected and sterilized and for working collaboratively with other departments (e.g., Environmental Services) to keep the patient care area as clean and free of clutter as possible.

For more specific information about maintaining a clean environment in institutional and home care,

 Go to **Clinical Insight 20-2: Providing a Clean Patient Environment** in Volume 2.

CDC Guidelines for Preventing Transmission of Pathogens

In addition to hand washing and maintaining a clean environment, you should follow other precautions to protect yourself and your patients. CDC guidelines provide for two tiers of protection (Siegel et al., 2022):

- **Standard precautions,** the first tier of protection, apply to the care of all patients. You must assume that every patient is potentially colonized or infected with an organism that could be passed to others in the healthcare setting.

- **Transmission-based precautions,** the second tier of protection, are for patients with known or suspected infection or colonization with pathogens. Recall from the discussion on the chain of infection that pathogens may be transmitted by contact, droplet, or air. Each mode of transmission requires a different approach to prevent infection.

♥ **iCare** For all transmission-based precautions, institute measures to counteract the negative effects of isolation on patients (i.e., anxiety, depression, perceptions of stigma, reduced contact with staff, and increases in preventable adverse events).

Table 20-2 provides a summary comparison of standard and transmission-based precautions.

For detailed guidelines to aid you in following both types of precautions, see **Clinical Insight 20-3: Following CDC Standard Precautions,** and **Clinical Insight 20-4: Following Transmission-Based Precautions** in Volume 2.

Personal Protective Equipment The CDC recommends the use of personal protective equipment (PPE) for healthcare workers, and the U.S. Occupational Safety and Health Administration requires employers to provide PPE for healthcare workers (e.g., gloves, gowns, face masks, and eye protection [Fig. 20-4]) (U.S. Department of Labor, n.d.-b). This equipment is to be used in standard precautions and transmission-based precautions. To learn how to don and remove PPE,

Go to **Procedure 20-2: Donning Personal Protective Equipment (PPE)** and **Procedure 20-3: Removing Personal Protective Equipment (PPE)** in Volume 2.

KnowledgeCheck 20-6

Under what circumstances are standard precautions used?

Protective Environment in Special Situations The CDC recommends a protective environment (isolation) for the special class of stem cell transplant patients who are neutropenic (and therefore immunocompromised) secondary to chemotherapy. You may, in

Table 20-2 ➤ Comparison of Centers for Disease Control and Prevention (CDC) Standard and Transmission-Based Precautions	
STANDARD PRECAUTIONS	**TRANSMISSION-BASED PRECAUTIONS**
Tier I Precautions Use with all clients, in all settings, regardless of suspected or confirmed presence of infection	Tier 2 Precautions Use for patients known or suspected to be infected or colonized with infectious agents
Principle: All blood, body fluids, secretions, excretions except sweat, nonintact skin, and mucous membranes may contain pathogens.	*Principle:* Routes of transmission for some microorganisms are not completely interrupted using standard precautions alone. Used *in addition to* standard precautions.
Include: Hand hygiene; use of gloves, gown, mask, eye protection, or face shield (depending on expected exposure); and safe injection practices	
Note: Standard precautions do not completely protect against microorganisms spread by contact, droplets, or through the air.	
New Elements of Standard Precautions *Added for protection of patients* more than of healthcare personnel: Respiratory hygiene and cough etiquette, safe injection practices, wearing a mask when performing special lumbar puncture procedures	Three Categories of Precautions *Contact Precautions*—For organisms spread by direct contact with the patient or their environment. This is the most common form of transmission. *Droplet Precautions*—For pathogens spread through close respiratory or mucous membrane contact with respiratory secretions (e.g., sneezing, coughing, talking); pathogens that do not remain infectious over long distances. *Airborne Precautions*—For pathogens that are small and remain infectious over long distances when suspended in the air and are easily transmitted through air currents (e.g., fanning linens, ventilating systems)

Source: Siegel, J. D., Rhinehart, E., Jackson, M., Chiarello, L., & Healthcare Infection Control Practices Advisory Committee. (2022). *2007 guideline for isolation precautions: Preventing transmission of infectious agents in the healthcare setting.* https://www.cdc.gov/infectioncontrol/pdf/guidelines/isolation-guidelines-H.pdf

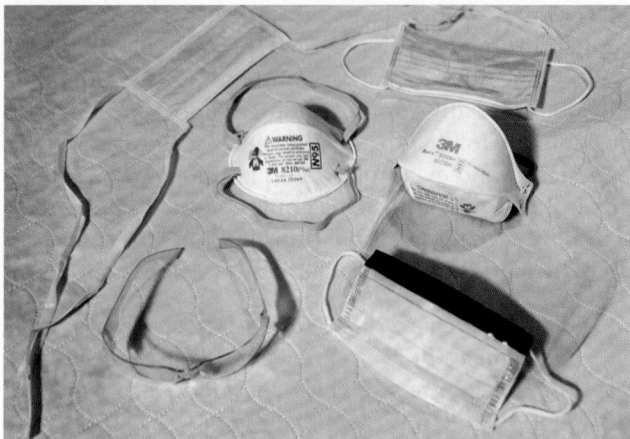

FIGURE 20-4 Several types of face masks and eye shields are available.

some facilities, encounter protective isolation for other types of patients as well. However, in most instances, standard and transmission-based precautions are adequate protection for those patients.

- **Follow standard precautions** meticulously, including hand hygiene before and after patient contact.
- **Follow transmission-based precautions** as indicated by a suspected or proven infection.

When providing care to patients who are immunosuppressed (e.g., receiving chemotherapy), keep in mind:

- Only healthy caregivers should provide care. Do not provide care if you have an upper respiratory infection or were exposed to someone with an infection.
- Healthcare workers caring for patients in protective isolation should not also be providing care for other patients with active infections.
- Restrict visitors who have viral or other contagious illnesses.

Patients with compromised immunity are more likely to become infected by pathogens harbored in their own bodies than from pathogens transmitted by other people (Siegel et al., 2022). Therefore, except for the special situations described, standard and transmission-based precautions should protect even unusually vulnerable patients from organisms brought in by healthcare workers and visitors.

Control of Potentially Contaminated Equipment and Supplies

Whenever possible, use disposable equipment in an isolation room. Nondisposable equipment and supplies require special handling.

- **Protective Isolation.** If a client is in protective isolation, be sure that equipment has been disinfected before it is taken into the room. Take linens and dishes directly to the protective isolation room, and hand them to someone wearing the required protective clothing.

- **Transmission-Based Isolation.** If the client is in transmission-based isolation, disinfect the equipment upon removal from the room. When removing linens or nondisposable items from a room with contact, droplet, or airborne isolation, place them in special biohazard bags.

Disposing of Used Isolation Supplies Place contaminated disposable, nonsharp equipment and materials containing body fluids in biohazard bags. This process requires two healthcare workers.

- The worker inside the room wears protective clothing and handles only contaminated items.
- The second worker stands at the door and holds the isolation bag open.
- The first worker places solid, nonsharp solids or liquids up to 25 mL inside the bag without touching the outside of the bag. If the bag contains linens, the isolation bag is closed and placed in a laundry hamper.
- Securely close an isolation disposal bag and place it in a special isolation trash container.
- Special disposal methods are used to prevent these objects from going into a landfill, where they could become a reservoir of infection.

Sharps Disposal Always place disposable needles, syringes, and other sharp items, such as broken glass, in special disposable sharps containers immediately after their use. Never recap a contaminated needle. Refer to Chapters 21 and 23 for further information on preventing needlestick injuries.

Laboratory Specimens Laboratory specimens contain blood and body fluids and are always considered contaminated. Label the specimen container in a clean area before taking it to the patient. Have the specimen collected by a healthcare worker who is wearing appropriate protective clothing. Once the specimen is collected, place it in a special transport bag. Do not allow the outside of the bag to touch any contaminated item, including your gloves.

KnowledgeCheck 20-7
- If you needed to disinfect a sink in a client's home, what would you use?
- List at least three actions clients can take to help avoid infection when they are out in the community.

PRACTICING SURGICAL ASEPSIS
Sterile means "without life" and therefore no infectious organisms. Inanimate objects, such as surgical equipment, gauze dressings, or wound irrigation fluid, may be sterilized. However, it is impossible to rid the human body of all microorganisms, either in or on it.

Surgical asepsis, or **sterile technique,** requires the creation of a sterile environment and the use of sterile equipment. It differs from medical asepsis in that it is more complex, and it is not required for use with all

♥ iCare 20-2

About Supporting the Psychological Needs of Patients in Isolation

Keep in mind that it is the disease that is being isolated, *not* the person who has the disease. Patients in isolation continue to have a need for human contact. In fact, isolation may produce anxiety and increase the desire for human contact. Search for ways to reassure and maintain contact with the patient in protective isolation.

- Use touch as much as possible (when wearing required protective equipment).
- Set aside time to ask about how the client is coping with isolation.
- If the patient is in droplet isolation, remember that the transmission area is 6 feet from the patient. You can go to the door of the room and speak to the patient without a mask.
- Reassure the patient that precautions are temporary.
- Explain that the precautions and the personal protective equipment protect you and the patient, as well as family members and other patients.

patients. Sterilization can be accomplished through the use of special gases or high heat. Surgical equipment and implanted devices are examples of materials that must be sterilized.

To create a sterile area, housekeeping personnel perform extensive cleaning using special solutions and procedures. All health personnel working in the area must wear appropriate surgical attire and perform a surgical hand scrub.

Levels of Asepsis Use modified sterile technique for many bedside procedures that have traditionally used sterile technique (e.g., tracheostomy care, wound care).

- **Sterile technique** is the use of sterile gloves and sterile supplies (e.g., drapes, wound dressings, instruments, water).
- **Modified sterile technique** is the use of nonsterile procedure gloves with sterile supplies.
- **Clean technique** is the use of clean hands or nonsterile gloves and clean, rather than sterile, supplies (e.g., tap water).

Performing a Surgical Scrub

A **surgical scrub** is a modification of the hand-washing procedure described earlier (see Table 20-3 for a comparison). It traditionally involves an extended scrub of the hands using a sponge, nail cleaner, and a bactericidal scrubbing agent. Another method uses a brushless scrub, using a bactericidal scrubbing agent. All methods require a prewash before the surgical scrub.

 Go to **Procedure 20-4: Surgical Hand Washing: Traditional Method** and **Procedure 20-5: Surgical Hand Washing: Brushless System** in Volume 2.

Table 20-3 ➤ Different Types of Hand Hygiene

METHODS	AGENT	PURPOSE	AREA	DURATION (MINIMUM)
Routine hand wash	Water and nonantimicrobial soap (i.e., plain soap)	Remove soil and transient microorganisms	All surfaces of the hands and fingers	15 seconds
Antiseptic hand wash	Water and antimicrobial soap (e.g., chlorhexidine, iodine, and iodophors)	Remove or destroy transient microorganisms and reduce resident flora (persistent activity)	All surfaces of the hands and fingers	15 seconds
Antiseptic handrub	Alcohol-based handrub	Remove or destroy transient microorganisms and reduce resident flora (persistent activity)	All surfaces of the hands and fingers	Until the hands are dry
Surgical antisepsis	1. Water and antimicrobial soap (e.g., chlorhexidine, iodine, and iodophors) 2. Water and nonantimicrobial soap (i.e., plain soap) followed by long-acting, alcohol-based surgical hand scrub product	Remove or destroy transient microorganisms and reduce resident flora (persistent activity)	Hands and forearms	1. 2–6 minutes 2. Follow manufacturer instructions for surgical hand scrub product with persistent activity

Source: Centers for Disease Control and Prevention. (2019). *Hand hygiene in healthcare settings.* https://www.cdc.gov/handhygiene/

Donning Surgical Attire

Burn units; labor and birth units; and some surgical wards, intensive care units, nurseries, and oncology wards require surgical attire for patient caregiving. In each of these units, nurses care for clients who are at increased risk for infection or are undergoing an invasive procedure that places them at higher risk. The goal on all of these units is to protect the patient from infections transmitted by healthcare workers.

Clean Surgical Attire Staff members working in these areas don *clean* surgical attire, or scrub suits, when they arrive on the unit. These scrub suits should not be worn outside the unit. If you must transport a patient to another area or leave the unit to gather supplies, wear a covering over the scrub suit. Remove the covering on your return to the unit. Additional precautions include a disposable hat to cover the head, shoe coverings, and face masks.

Sterile Surgical Attire Personnel in the surgical setting or involved in certain invasive procedures must dress in *sterile* surgical attire. As a beginning student, your role will initially be limited to observation, but later you will need to prepare for your clinical experience in the surgical setting.

First, you will change into scrub apparel, apply shoe coverings, and put on a disposable hat, then wash your hands and apply a face mask. If there is a potential for spray of fluids, wear a face mask with eye shield. Be sure to adjust the mask so that it is comfortable to breathe through. Then perform the surgical scrub. If a surgical gown is required, put it on after the hand scrub.

- **Closed Gloving.** If you are applying full surgical attire, you will need to apply gloves using a closed method, after you have put on your gown. Once you don sterile gloves, you may touch only sterile items. For complete instructions,

 Go to **Procedure 20-6: Sterile Gloves and Gown (Closed Method)** in Volume 2.

- **Open Gloving.** You will often wear sterile gloves for procedures that do not require full surgical attire. For this, you will use the open method of gloving. For complete instructions for open-method sterile gloving,

 Go to **Procedure 20-7: Sterile Gloves (Open Method)** in Volume 2.

Using Sterile Technique in Nursing Care

Healthcare providers use sterile technique to perform a variety of procedures. Some of the procedures require full surgical PPE; others do not. Examples of procedures that use both sterile technique and principles of medical asepsis are administering an injection, starting an IV line, and performing a sterile dressing change. To clarify, when administering an injection, you prepare the patient, cleanse the injection site, and remove the needle cap using standard precautions. You do not don sterile gloves, but for the rest of the procedure, you observe sterile technique by taking care not to touch or otherwise contaminate the exposed needle. **Key Point:** *Keep in mind that sterile touches sterile, and unsterile touches unsterile.*

Preparing and Maintaining Sterile Fields There are some variations in how you might set up sterile fields. Sometimes it is as simple as opening a package of supplies wrapped in a sterile disposable cover. At other times, you may work with a larger reusable or disposable sterile drape (wrapped in an outer wrapping). To learn a procedure for maintaining a sterile field, as well as adding supplies and sterile liquids to it,

 Go to **Procedure 20-8A: Setting Up a Sterile Field** in Volume 2.

Adding Supplies to a Sterile Field Some supplies (e.g., urinary catheter kits) are packaged in a wrapper that can form a sterile field. The outside of these packages is considered clean, and the inside is sterile. Consider a 1-inch margin around the drape unsterile, even if it remains on a horizontal surface. You must open these packages in a way that does not contaminate the inside of the wrapping.

✚ Be cautious when adding supplies to the sterile field. If any object falls only partly on the field, it is no longer sterile. Never assume an item is sterile. If there is any doubt about its sterility, consider it contaminated. For detailed instructions on how to add supplies to a sterile field,

 Go to **Procedure 20-8B: Adding Supplies to a Sterile Field** in Volume 2.

Adding Sterile Solutions to a Sterile Field Add sterile liquids to a sterile field by gently pouring them into a container on the field. Some sterile drapes contain an impermeable membrane between layers that serves as a barrier to moisture and prevents wicking. With this type of drape, you may pour sterile liquid directly on gauze pads on the field. Pour only an amount of liquid that is sufficient to make the gauze pads damp; otherwise, excess fluid may run off the field, causing the field to become contaminated. A wet field is not sterile because it does not provide a barrier to microorganisms on the unsterile surface under the drape. See Box 20-3 about common breaks in sterility. For step-by-step instructions on how to add sterile solutions to a sterile field,

 Go to **Procedure 20-8C: Adding Sterile Solutions to a Sterile Field** in Volume 2.

KnowledgeCheck 20-8

- When will you need to don sterile gloves using the closed method?
- True or false: Some procedures require both standard precautions and sterile technique.
- What part or parts of a sterile field are considered to be unsterile?

For steps to follow in *all* procedures, refer to the Universal Steps for All Procedures found on the inside back cover of Volume 2. Go to the full procedures in Volume 2 to practice and learn the procedure steps. Use these procedure highlights later to help you review key points.

Procedure 23-1: Hand Hygiene

If using alcohol-based handrubs:

1. Use alcohol-based handrubs when hands are not soiled.
2. Cover all surfaces of fingers and hands.
3. Rub together 20–30 seconds, until dry.

Procedure 23-2: Donning Personal Protective Equipment (PPE)

➤ Before exposure, don appropriate PPE according to standard precautions or transmission guidelines.

➤ Wear an N-95 respirator mask for airborne isolation.

➤ Wear a surgical mask for droplet isolation.

Procedure 23-3: Removing Personal Protective Equipment (PPE)

➤ Remove PPE at doorway before leaving patient room, or in an anteroom.

➤ Avoid contaminating self, others, or environment when removing equipment.

➤ Considered contaminated: front areas, sleeves, head cover, mask, and gloves of the PPE.

➤ Considered clean: the inside of the gown, gloves, and head cover; the ties on the mask; and ties in the back of the gown.

➤ Always remove gloves first when removing PPE, unless gown ties in front.

Procedure 23-4: Surgical Hand Washing: Traditional Method

➤ Don surgical shoe covers, cap, and face mask before the scrub.

➤ Use warm water.

➤ Perform a prewash using soap and water.

➤ Clean under your fingernails under running water.

➤ Wet the scrub sponge; apply a generous amount of antimicrobial soap.

➤ Using a circular motion, scrub all surfaces of nails, hands, and forearms at least 10 times or for the length of time specified by agency policy.

➤ Rinse hands and arms by keeping your fingertips higher than your elbow.

➤ Grasp a sterile towel and back away from the sterile field.

➤ Thoroughly dry your hands before donning sterile gloves.

Procedure 23-5: Surgical Hand Washing: Brushless System

➤ Don surgical shoe covers, cap, and face mask before the scrub.

➤ Use warm water.

➤ Perform a prewash using soap and water.

➤ Clean under your nails under running water.

➤ Apply a generous amount of antimicrobial soap.

➤ Using a circular motion, scrub all surfaces of nails, hands, and forearms at least 10 times or for the length of time specified by agency policy.

➤ Rinse hands and arms by keeping your fingertips higher than your elbow.

➤ Grasp a sterile towel and back away from the sterile field.

➤ Thoroughly dry your hands before donning sterile gloves.

Procedure 23-6: Sterile Gown and Gloves (Closed Method)

➤ Put on shoe covers, hair covers, and mask before scrub.

➤ Perform surgical scrub.

➤ Grasp the gown at the neckline; slide your arms into the sleeves without extending your hands through the cuffs.

➤ Have a coworker pull the shoulders of the gown up and tie behind the neck.

➤ Don gloves using the closed method by keeping your hands always covered, first with the gown cuffs and then with the sterile gloves.

➤ Secure the waist tie on your gown by handing it to a coworker and turning to receive it.

➤ Keep your hands within your field of vision at all times.

➤ Do not turn your back to a sterile field.

Procedure 23-7: Sterile Gloves (Open Method)

➤ Remove all jewelry, including rings and watches.

➤ Place the glove package on a clean, dry surface.

➤ Open the inner package so that the cuffs are closest to you.

➤ Apply the glove of your dominant hand first by touching only the inside of the glove (the folded-over cuff) with your nondominant hand.

➤ Apply the second glove by touching only the outer part of the glove with your already-gloved hand; keep your sterile thumb well away from your bare skin.

➤ Do not touch the gloves to any unsterile items.

Procedure 23-8: Sterile Fields

➤ Prepare the sterile field as close as possible to the time of use.

➤ Do not cover the sterile field once established.

➤ Do not turn away from the sterile field.

➤ Inspect for package integrity, inclusion of sterile indicator, and/or expiration date. Do not use outdated items.

➤ Clear a space and prepare the patient before setting up the sterile field.

➤ Establish the sterile field with a sterile drape or sterile package wrapper.

➤ Add items to the sterile field by gently dropping them onto the sterile field.

➤ Pour sterile solutions into a sterile bowl or receptacle without touching the bowl or splashing onto the sterile field.

➤ Don sterile gloves and perform the procedure.

BOX 20-3 ■ Avoiding Common Breaks in Sterility

To avoid common breaks in sterility:

- Never reach across a sterile field.
- Make sure your clothing or laboratory coat never touches any part of the sterile field.
- Keep your fingernails short and clean. Avoid nail polish, acrylics, and artificial nails.
- Avoid wearing jewelry that dangles or can fall into the sterile field.
- Keep long hair pulled back or covered by a head covering designed for sterility.
- Change your gown or reinforce with additional sterile drapes if it is soaked through.
- Avoid splashing any kind of solution onto the sterile field.
- Keep doors closed so that turbulent airflow does not contaminate a sterile area with airborne microbes.
- Make sure you are opening equipment packaged with labels indicating it has been sterilized properly.
- Clean wounds and prep sterile sites from clean to dirty.
- When witnessing someone else contaminate a sterile field or object, identify the break and cover the area with sterile drapes or replace with a new sterile setup, gown, or gloves.

Source: Adapted from Simko, L. (2012). Breaking sterility: Procedural violations in healthcare. *Nursing, 42*(8), 22–26.

INFECTION CONTROL AND PREVENTION FOR HEALTHCARE WORKERS

It is critical that you learn how to protect yourself from infections. You not only want to avoid personal illness but also avoid becoming a reservoir for infection. Nurses and other patient care workers are at great risk of acquiring infections because they come in contact with a large number and variety of pathogens. Skin contact, mucous membrane contact, and puncture wounds often serve as portals of entry.

As a nurse, you need to monitor other healthcare workers, patients, and visitors for adherence to infection control measures. As a patient advocate and promoter of health and safety, you have a responsibility to protect patients, coworkers, families, and yourself from potential hazardous exposure, as well as from microorganisms brought into the unit.

What Role Does the Infection Preventionist Nurse Play?

The task of the infection prevention nurse is to minimize the number of infections in the healthcare facility. Infection preventionists must keep current with information about pathogens, antibiotic resistance, and infection control. The infection prevention nurse also functions as an epidemiologist, tracking down the source of HAIs and strengthening measures to prevent their recurrence. Finally, all members of the infection prevention team enforce compliance with federal, state, and local regulations in addition to hospital protocols related to infection control and prevention.

What Should I Do If I Am Exposed to Bloodborne Pathogens?

Exposure to blood, body secretions, or body tissues containing blood or secretions requires immediate action. See Box 20-4 for complete instructions. The first step is to minimize the exposure by washing the area thoroughly. Then notify the appropriate people, complete an injury report, and seek medical attention.

- Anyone exposed to bloodborne pathogens should have baseline laboratory work done to check for hepatitis and HIV. If the patient source is known, the infection preventionist will arrange to have the patient tested.
- Subsequent testing and possible preventive treatment are based on the type of exposure and what is known about the source and the injured person.
- To limit risks from the exposure, the infection prevention team will provide counseling and recommendations as soon as possible after the event.
- Chapters 21 and 23 present information on preventing needlestick injuries.

BOX 20-4 ■ If You Are Exposed to Blood or Other Body Fluids

If you are stuck by a needle or other sharp or get blood or other potentially infectious materials in your eyes, nose, mouth, or on broken skin:

1. Immediately flush the exposed area with water and clean any wound with soap and water or a skin disinfectant if available.
2. Report the exposure immediately to the supervisor in the agency. If you are a student, also report immediately to your instructor.
3. Seek immediate medical attention. Consent to testing and follow-up treatment as advised.
4. Complete an incident or injury report.
5. Attend counseling sessions provided by the agency.

Source: U.S. Department of Labor. (n.d.-b). *Healthcare wide hazards: Bloodborne pathogens.* https://www.osha.gov/SLTC/etools/hospital/hazards/bbp/bbp.html

How Can I Minimize the Effects of Bioterrorism and Epidemics?

Bioterrorism is the intentional release, or threatened release, of disease-producing organisms or substances for the purpose of causing death, illness, harm, economic damage, or fear. Six diseases with recognized bioterrorism potential are anthrax, botulism, pneumonic plague, smallpox, viral hemorrhagic fevers, and tularemia.

Recognize an Outbreak Should a biological event occur, either as a result of bioterrorism or a naturally occurring epidemic, a key factor in minimizing its effects is the ability to quickly recognize unusual disease patterns and detect the presence of infectious diseases. Some electronic health record systems include specific pattern-identification programs. However, there is no substitute for direct clinical observation skills and judgment.

Key Point: *Nurses need to assess not only the individual patient's condition but also clusters of symptoms.* Hospital, emergency department, and clinic nurses are in key positions to recognize outbreaks because they see patients from multiple primary care providers. Nurses must keep the following questions in mind:

- Am I seeing an unexpected number of infectious diseases or diseases possibly caused by infectious organisms?
- Am I noticing similar cases that are not responding to medical treatment?
- Are healthcare workers and others who come in contact with infectious patients becoming ill?

Notify the Safety Officer After identifying a suspicious pattern, you should notify the institution's interventionist or safety officer as soon as possible. Appropriate cultures will be needed to determine infection. If cultures are positive, federal and state health departments should be notified. If the infectious organism is unknown, samples must be preserved for future analysis.

Institute Appropriate Level of Standard Precautions **Key Point:** *In the event of an epidemic or pandemic, the essential principles of hand hygiene and standard precautions will be the core of your measures for infection prevention and control.*

- Patients with similar symptoms should be cared for by a minimum number of healthcare providers, and those providers must use appropriate isolation precautions.
- If the etiology and transmission route of the causative organism are unknown, standard, contact, and airborne precautions should be implemented as needed.
- The U.S. Department of Labor (n.d.-b) defines types of PPE and situations for use.

Prepare Clients for a Pandemic Disease Outbreak Teach clients that preparing for pandemic diseases is similar to other general kinds of emergency preparedness, including risk assessment, everyday preventive actions (see the box Holistic Health: Preventive Actions Limiting Spread of Infection), and limitations on activity and travel.

Preventive Actions Limiting Spread of Infection

The best way to prevent illness is to avoid exposure to the virus.

- **Stay at home when sick,** especially during the contagious phase of illness. If you have symptoms, wear a face mask when you are near other people and before you enter a healthcare setting.
- **Avoid close contact** and **practice social distancing** when potentially exposed to a contagious illness. This means keeping at least 6 feet away from others.
- **Socializing outdoors** provides extra space for safe physical distancing and fresh air flow for avoiding airborne illnesses. You are also less likely to encounter high-contact surfaces when meeting outside.
- **Gather in groups of 10 or fewer** and **avoid discretionary travel** to reduce exposure to others. Most viruses are spread from person to person between people who are in close contact (within 6 feet) or through airborne droplets when an infected person sneezes or coughs.

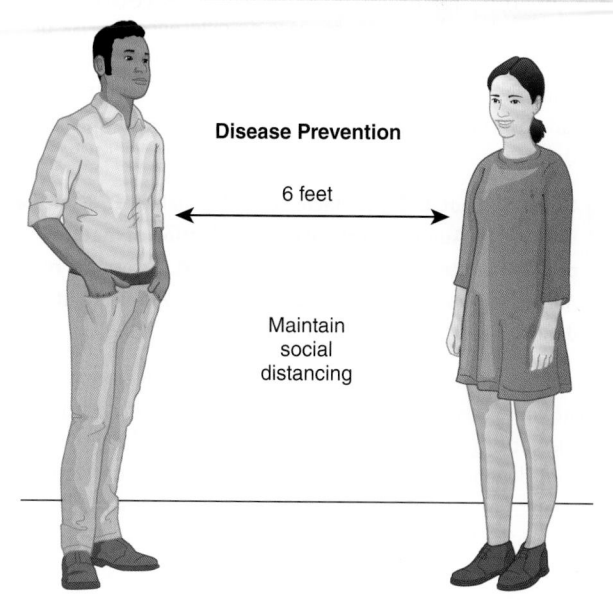

Disease Prevention

6 feet

Maintain social distancing

Continued

Preventive Actions Limiting Spread of Infection

➤ **Clean hands.** Thorough hand washing with soap and running water for 20 seconds is the best way to prevent the spread of infection. Scrub palms, in between fingers, knuckles, nailbeds, and wrists. If water is not available, use an alcohol-based hand sanitizer (at least 60% alcohol) (CDC, 2022).

➤ **Cover mouth and nose.** Sneeze or cough into a clean tissue or bent elbow. Discard tissues in the trash.

➤ **Avoid touching eyes, nose, and mouth.** *Germs thrive in moist environments such as these.* Avoid handshakes and other direct contact if exposed to a virus.

➤ **Clean and disinfect frequently touched surfaces.** Carry sanitizing wipes with you to wipe surfaces down with alcohol-based product, or use a diluted bleach solution or soap and warm water.

➤ **Practice good health habits.** Get plenty of sleep. Eat nutritious food. Drink plenty of water. Be physically active. Manage stress.

Source: Centers for Disease Control and Prevention. (2021, August 26). *Healthy habits to help prevent flu.* https://www.cdc.gov/flu/prevent/actions-prevent-flu.htm; Centers for Disease Control and Prevention. (2022, March 14). *Handwashing: Clean hands save lives: When and how to wash your hands.* https://www.cdc.gov/handwashing/when-how-handwashing.html

Toward Evidence-Based Practice

Wills, B. W., Smith, W. R., Arguello, A. M., McGwin, G., Ghanem, E. S., & Ponce, B. A. (2020). Association of surgical jacket and bouffant use with surgical site infection risk. *JAMA Surgery,* 155(4):323–328. https://doi.org/10.1001/jamasurg.2019.6044

Researchers gathered evidence to determine whether mandated surgical jackets and bouffant head covers in the surgical suite lessen the risk of postsurgical complications. In a study involving 34,042 surgical patient contacts over a 22-month time span, there were no differences in risk of surgical site infection, mortality, postoperative sepsis, or wound dehiscence between groups who wore the mandated head covering and surgical jackets compared with those who did not.

Goyal, S., Khot, S. C., Ramachandran, V., Shah, K. P., & Musher, D. M. (2019, August). Bacterial contamination of medical provider white coats and surgical scrubs: A systematic review. *American Journal of Infection Control,* 46(8), 994–1001. https://doi.org/10.1016/j.ajic.2019.01.012

Common findings among 22 scientific studies demonstrated that white coats and scrubs are colonized with multidrug-resistant organisms (MRDOs). Contamination of attire varies depending on laundering practices (frequency, water temperature, use of dryer). White coats are laundered less often than scrubs. Scrubs made with antimicrobial materials may reduce contamination.

Kanamori, H., Rutala, W. A., & Weber, D. J. (2017, October 15). The role of patient care items as a fomite in healthcare-associated outbreaks and infection prevention. *Clinical Infectious Disease,* 65(8), 1412–1419. https://doi.org/10.1093/cid/cix462

Researchers examined multiple hospital-acquired infection (HAI) outbreaks related to contaminated patient care items, including infection with MDROs. Most fomite-related HAIs resulted from inappropriate disinfection practices, especially involving medical equipment.

Jencson, A. L., Cadnum, J. L., Piedrahita, C., & Donskey, K. J. (2017, November 13). Hospital sinks are a potential nosocomial source of *Candida* infections. *Clinical Infectious Diseases,* 65(11), 1954–1955. https://doi.org/10.1093/cid/cix629

Contaminated sinks have been implicated in the transmission of MDROs, particularly from moist sites such as sink drains and countertops from splattered water. Researchers found frequent *Candida* species contamination of sinks in multiple hospitals.

Chapman, L., Hargett, L., Anderson, T., Galluzzo, J., Zimand, P. (2021). Chlorhexidine gluconate bathing program to reduce health care-associated infections in both critically ill and non-critically ill patients. *Critical Care Nurse,* 41(5), e1-e8. https://doi.org/10.4037/ccn2021340

Toward Evidence-Based Practice—cont'd

Consistent bathing of patients in the medical-surgical intensive care unit with 4% chlorhexidine gluconate (CHG) solution was associated with a 52% reduced risk of HAIs, specifically MDROs, vancomycin-resistant enterococci, *Clostridium difficile,* and methicillin-resistant *Staphylococcus aureus.*

> Makhini, S., Umscheid, C.A., Soo, J., Bartlett, A., Landon, E., & Marrs, R. (2021). Hand hygiene compliance rate during the COVID-19 epidemic. *JAMA Internal Medicine, 181*(7), 1006–1008. https://doi.org/10.1001/jamainternmed.2021.1429

In a study of 1159 patients hospitalized during the COVID-19 pandemic over a 1-year period, compliance with hand hygiene increased at the beginning of the pandemic as a result of (1) fear and increased awareness of the importance of hand hygiene associated with transmission of infection, (2) fewer room entries and exits by the staff, (3) fewer visitors, (4) remote rounding by the healthcare team, (5) clustering patient care activities, and perhaps (6) improved touchless hand-hygiene dispensers. However, high compliance was not sustained over time, even with automated monitoring of hand-hygiene practices.

1. From these studies, what can you conclude about the transmission of HAIs?

2. What measures do these studies suggest for reducing microbial colonization that could lead to the spread of HAIs? What else could nurses do to further lessen the risk of spreading microbes in the clinical setting?

3. Why might nurses fail to clean hands before and after contact with potentially contaminated items or direct patient care?

4. What strategies can you think of to improve healthcare worker compliance with hand hygiene in your hospital setting? Think creatively.

SUMMARY

After studying this chapter, you should be armed with the basic knowledge you need to protect yourself and your clients from infection. However, knowledge is not enough. **Key Point:** *Healthcare professionals too often fail to comply with guidelines for infection prevention, even the seemingly simple measures such as hand hygiene and standard precautions.* Although healthcare workers must wash their hands, patients do not necessarily feel comfortable asking them to do so (Musu et al., 2017). Your role as a nurse is to integrate the best current evidence with your clinical expertise and, through your own individual performance, minimize harm to patients and others. This includes using technology and standardized practices that support patient safety and quality care.

To explore learning resources for this chapter,

Go to Davis Advantage and find:

Answers and Suggested Responses for all questions in this chapter
Concept Map
Knowledge Map
References and Bibliography

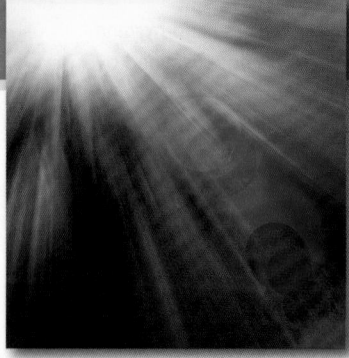

CHAPTER 21

Promoting Safety

Learning Outcomes

After completing this chapter, you should be able to:

➤ List the three leading causes of accidental death in the United States.

➤ Discuss developmental and individual factors that create safety risks.

➤ Identify at least five safety hazards in the home environment and interventions to prevent injury from them.

➤ Discuss the steps to follow when you suspect that a client has ingested a poisonous substance.

➤ Describe the choking rescue maneuver, and identify instances when it is appropriate to use it.

➤ Describe the four main physical hazards that are found in the community and interventions to prevent injury from them.

➤ Describe and give examples of hazards that we encounter in the healthcare agency.

➤ Identify four interventions to prevent falls in the healthcare agency.

➤ Discuss the appropriate use of siderails in the healthcare agency.

➤ Properly apply restraints, and discuss measures to prevent injury in clients who are restrained.

➤ Discuss at least one data-collection instrument that is used to assess the client who is at risk for falls.

➤ Plan and implement nursing care to promote safety and prevent injury in clients who are at risk for falls.

Key Concepts

Safety

Patient safety

Related Concepts

See the Concept Map on Davis Advantage.

Example Problem

Falls

Meet Your Patient

- **Alvin Lin.** Alvin Lin is a 79-year-old man who was just transferred from a long-term care facility to your medical unit. His admitting diagnosis is dehydration and pneumonia. The night nurse reported that he had rested well during the night and was alert and oriented. When you enter his room, he is confused and does not know where he is. He becomes combative and tries to get out of bed. How should you respond to the situation?

- **Teresa.** Suppose you are a nurse making a home visit to Teresa, who lives in a rural area. Teresa is 20 years old and has a 2-year-old daughter. She is also responsible for caring for her elderly grandmother, who is recovering

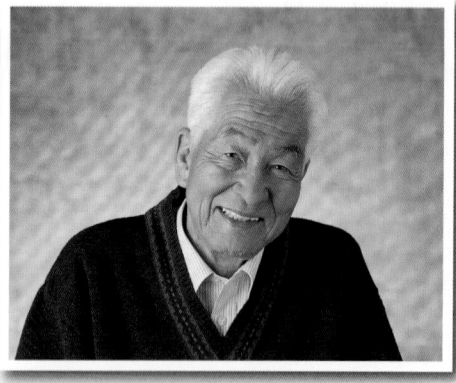

from a hip fracture. Teresa says that it is getting more difficult to keep up with her toddler, who is "into everything," and to care for the needs of her grandmother. Her grandmother has a fear of falling and is reluctant to do anything for herself.

Theoretical Knowledge
knowing why

This chapter will increase your ability to recognize safety hazards in the home, community, and healthcare facility and to plan interventions that promote safety for clients of all ages, such as the two in the Meet Your Patients scenario. Many accidental injuries can be prevented by being aware of hazards and taking reasonable precautions.

ABOUT THE KEY CONCEPTS

Safety is a basic human need, second only to survival needs such as oxygen, nutrition, and fluids. As a nurse, the concept of safety is fundamental to providing safe, effective, high-quality care to your clients. Nurses contribute to **patient safety,** in any setting, by coordinating and integrating the multiple aspects of quality into their nursing care, as well as the care delivered by others in the setting. You must also be concerned with your own safety and the safety of other care providers. Many accidental injuries can be prevented by being aware of hazards and taking reasonable precautions.

IMPORTANCE OF SAFETY

According to the Centers for Disease Control and Prevention (CDC, 2022a), accidents, or unintentional injuries, are the third leading cause of death in the United States. An estimated 173,000 people die each year as a result of accidents. Expressed another way, one person dies from an accident every 5 minutes. Poisoning is now listed as the number-one cause of unintentional death, followed by motor vehicle accidents, falls, accidental hanging/strangulation/suffocation, and drowning (see Table 21-1). Of course, the death rate is not the only noteworthy number in the CDC report: millions of people received injuries that disabled them beyond the day of injury.

Many healthcare organizations are campaigning for safer patient care in an effort to reduce the cost of healthcare and the burden of suffering. The following are examples:

- **The Joint Commission**, the accrediting body for healthcare facilities, each year publishes its *National Patient Safety Goals.* For example, the 2022 goals include improving the accuracy of patient identification, improving the effectiveness of communication among caregivers, reducing the harm associated with clinical alarm systems, reducing the risk of healthcare-associated infections, and implementing evidence-based practices for preventing surgical site infections. For a link to the 2022 *National Patient Safety Goals,*

 Go to the website of the Joint Commission at https://www.jointcommission.org/standards_information/npsgs.aspx

Table 21-1 ➤ Leading Causes of Unintentional Deaths in the United States	
MECHANISM OF INJURY	**TOTAL ANNUAL DEATHS, ALL AGE-GROUPS**
Poisoning and exposure to noxious substances	65,773
Falls	39,443
Motor vehicles	39,107
Accidental hanging/strangulation/suffocation	7,076
Drowning	3,692

Source: Xu, J. Q., Murphy, S. L., Kochanek, K. D., & Arias, E. (2021). Deaths: Final data for 2019. *National Vital Statistics Reports, 70*(8).

- The **Institute of Medicine's (IOM,** 1999) report *To Err Is Human: Building a Safer Health System* brought public attention to patient safety. It stated that it is simply not acceptable for patients to be harmed by the same healthcare system that is supposed to offer healing and comfort. The report identified five critical principles to ensure safe healthcare systems:

   Provide leadership.
   Recognize human limits in process design.
   Promote effective team functioning.
   Anticipate the unexpected.
   Create a learning environment. (IOM, 1999)

   To learn what is meant by a "culture of safety" in the healthcare setting, read the accompanying Safe, Effective Nursing Care (SEND) box.

- **American Nurses Association (ANA).** The ANA advocates for healthcare reforms, with the priority being access to high-quality healthcare for all persons. With the passage of the Patient Protection and Affordable Care Act (PPACA), the ANA is committed to educating the public about how changes to the system affect patients' lives and the nursing profession (ANA, 2018). The ANA's main aim is to support patient safety.

- The **Quality and Safety Education for Nurses (QSEN Institute),** a task force to improve nursing education, identified and described six competencies that all nursing students should have by graduation. Safety is one of those competencies (Cronenwett et al., 2007; Cronenwett et al., 2009).

- **Medicare** is a federal agency that has identified "**never events,**" or hospital-acquired conditions (HACs): costly errors that cause serious injury or death and that are mostly preventable (e.g., falls, injury from restraints). Medicare will no longer pay institutions for the care required to treat the effects of such errors (Centers for Medicare & Medicaid Services [CMS], 2006, modified 2020).

Creating a Culture of Safety

Chapter Key Concept: Safety (Thinking, Doing, Caring)

Competency: Collaborate with the interprofessional healthcare team; provide safe, quality client care

Background: In the recent past, patient safety was more or less taken for granted. It was assumed that all dedicated practitioners would perform correct actions and that people who made mistakes were "bad apples" and would be fired. Mistakes were hushed up. Certainly, the patient or family was never told an error had occurred. This culture of secrecy and blame still exists in some settings.

In the past 20 years, advisory bodies have reported the cost to society and the huge impact of medical mistakes on patients and their families. The National Academy of Medicine (NAM), previously called the Institute of Medicine (IOM), has called for (a) healthcare organizations to work to dismantle the culture of secrecy and blame and create a culture of safety and (b) that nurses be leaders in these efforts.

Safe, Effective Nursing Care (SENC) activities were created specifically to help prepare nurses for these roles. SENC describes the skills you need to become part of the new culture of safety. Baseline knowledge and skills you will need to acquire include:

➤ Thinking in terms of systems.

➤ Understanding how systems create a mistake-prone environment.

➤ Understanding the types of errors that occur in your facility

Key Point: *People make the mistakes. Systems set the stage for them.*

Think about it: It is equally important to determine what systems need to be in place to build the culture of safety. Some critical system features include the following, along with questions for your reflection or discussion:

➤ All levels of leadership make safety a visible priority and take actions that promote safety. *Why is leadership important in changing culture?*

➤ All staff members providing care are formally encouraged to communicate their concerns to the team. *Why do you think nurses or junior doctors might not communicate concerns?*

➤ All information needed to appropriately manage the patient across shifts, units, and facilities or after other handoffs is available at all times. *What types of errors can occur during handoffs?*

➤ Facility adopts a nonpunitive response to error and uses strategies such as root-cause analysis to identify system issues. *What effect might a punitive culture have on error reporting?*

➤ Facility recognizes both individual and system causes of error but emphasizes a systems approach to error reduction. *Describe one system that can break down and make errors more likely.*

➤ Each person providing care acknowledges their own potential for error and values their own role in preventing errors. *What can you do to help prevent errors?*

Sources: Institute of Medicine (IOM, 2001, 2011).

WHAT FACTORS AFFECT SAFETY?

To promote client safety, you will need theoretical knowledge about developmental stages and individual risk factors that affect clients' ability to avoid accidental injury. This chapter discusses specific risk factors and describes hazards in three environments: the home, the community, and the healthcare agency.

Developmental Factors

The type and incidence of accidents vary among age-groups. You will find interventions for all age-groups integrated into the topics throughout this chapter. The descriptions given for each age-group are characteristics common to most people in that group. However, individuals progress through developmental stages at their own pace, so there will always be some people who do not fit the group description closely. For supplemental discussion of safety needs during different developmental stages, review Chapters 6 and 7.

Infant/Toddler Infants and toddlers are completely dependent on others for their care. They are able to walk and manipulate objects before they have the judgment to recognize dangers. Infants and toddlers are curious and tend to explore the environment by putting objects in their mouths. This is why the incidence of choking is highest between 6 months and 3 years of age. As mobility continues to improve, toddlers gain more freedom, and their curiosity leads them to explore cupboards, stairs, open windows, swimming pools, and other hazards (CDC, 2012; Sleet, 2018).

■ Drowning is the leading cause of death for children ages 1 to 4, followed by motor vehicle accidents (Xu et al., 2021).
■ Falls, choking, sudden infant death syndrome (SIDS), and ingesting poisons are other critical safety concerns.

Preschooler After age 3 years, children are a little less prone to falls because their gross and fine motor skills, coordination, and balance have improved. However, as they begin to play outside more often (e.g., playgrounds, pools, front yards, and so on), there are additional safety concerns.

■ *Accidental deaths*—Motor vehicle injuries are a major cause, along with drowning, fires, and poisoning.

- *Nonfatal injuries*—Falls are the primary cause of nonfatal injuries.

Although preschoolers become more aware of dangers and limitations, adult supervision is essential.

School-Age Child School-age children have developed more refined muscle coordination and control and improved decision-making skills. However, because they become more involved in activities outside the home, bone and muscle injuries are common. Injuries are often related to sports, skateboarding, bicycle riding, and playground injuries. Most school-age children are less fearful than are toddlers, and they are often ready to try any new skill with or without practice or training. Exposure to the wider school and neighborhood environment also increases the safety risks for children from people outside the home (e.g., abduction).

- *Accidental deaths*—Motor vehicles continue to be the leading cause in this age-group.
- *Nonfatal injuries*—Falls are the leading cause of nonfatal injuries.

Adolescent Peak physical, sensory, and psychomotor abilities give teenagers a feeling of strength and confidence, yet they lack the wisdom and judgment of adults. This, along with feelings of being indestructible, makes them more likely to participate in risk-taking behavior and, in turn, more prone to injury.

- *Accidental death*—Motor vehicle accidents are the leading cause of death, followed by suicide.
- *Accidental injuries*—Sports and recreational injuries, including diving and drowning incidents, are also common, especially when drinking and drug use are involved.

Adult Workplace injury may be a significant concern. Other injuries to adults are related to lifestyle (e.g., excessive drug or alcohol use), stress, carelessness, abuse, and decline in strength and stamina.

- *Accidental death*—Unintentional poisoning, followed by intentional self-harm (suicide), causes more deaths than motor vehicle accidents (Xu et al., 2021).

- *Accidental injuries*—For many, work and family responsibilities leave little time for regular physical activity, increasing the risk of musculoskeletal injury in the so-called weekend athlete.

Older Adult Although many older adults have intact senses and continue to enjoy life as they age, physiological changes do occur (e.g., reduced muscle strength and joint mobility; slowing of reflexes; decreased ability to respond to multiple stimuli; and sensory losses, particularly hearing and vision). These changes increase the older adult's risk for falls, burns, car accidents, and other injury.

- *Accidental death*—Falls are the most common cause of accidental death for adults age 65 and older (Xu et al., 2021).

Individual Risk Factors

In addition to developmental stage, individual factors also influence a person's risk for unintentional injury. These include lifestyle, cognitive awareness, sensoriperceptual status, ability to communicate, mobility status, physical and emotional health, and awareness of safety measures. Table 21-2 summarizes individual risk factors.

KnowledgeCheck 21-1

- What are some important developmental considerations when providing a safe environment for a preschool child?
- What is the main cause of injuries during the adolescent period?
- What are some ways that the aging process makes the older adult more prone to injury?
- Based on your theoretical knowledge and the scant patient data you have, why do you think Teresa's toddler (Meet Your Patients) is at risk for accidents? What about Teresa's grandmother?

SAFETY HAZARDS IN THE HOME

What safety issues in the home environment would you need to assess with regard to Teresa's toddler and grandmother (see Meet Your Patients)? The overview

Table 21-2 ➤ Individual Risk Factors for Injury

RISK FACTORS	BEHAVIOR MANIFESTATION
Lifestyle	Smoking, alcohol abuse, risk-taking behaviors
Cognitive awareness	Confusion due to stress and loss of short-term memory
Sensory and perceptual status	Loss of senses (e.g., vision, hearing, pain) that provide first line of defense
Impaired communication	Language barriers and hearing and speech impairment related to disease processes
Impaired mobility	Impaired strength, with accompanying problems in mobility, balance, and endurance
Physical and emotional well-being	Reduced physical stamina and depression, with feelings of loss of control and helplessness
Safety awareness	Reduced cognitive awareness (e.g., of older adult) and immature development of the child

of home safety hazards in this section should help you answer this question.

Except for motor vehicle accidents, most fatal accidents occur in the home. The leading causes of death in the home are poisonings, falls, fires and burns, and choking. For children, maternal mental health problems and having older siblings are associated with less safe homes (Zonfrillo et al., 2018).

Poisoning

Poisoning death rates have more than quadrupled in the past 20 years. Although young children are frequent victims, the increase has been mainly among adults. In many cases, the person does not die but becomes ill or suffers other effects. Poisoning exposure accounts for more than 2 million emergency department visits per year in the United States (CDC, 2022).

- **Young children** are poisoned most often by improper storage of household chemicals, medicines and vitamins, and cosmetics (see Box 21-1).

  The use of lead in paint has been banned since 1978, but lead-based paint can still be found in older homes and toys produced in some foreign countries. Some soil (which young children often put in their mouths) contains high levels of lead. 🌼 In the United States, poor, urban, and immigrant populations are at higher risk for lead exposure than other groups.
- **Older children and adolescents** may attempt suicide by overdosing with medicines or be poisoned accidentally when experimenting with recreational or prescription drugs.
- **Adults** experience poisoning as a result of illegal drug use or misuse or abuse of prescription drugs, especially narcotic medications, tranquilizers, and antidepressants.

BOX 21-1 ■ Poisonous Agents Commonly Ingested by Children

- Household cleansers, including oven cleaner, drain cleaner, toilet bowl cleaner, and furniture polish
- Medicines, including cough and cold preparations, vitamins, pain medications, antidepressants, anticonvulsants, and iron tablets, which may look like candies to children
- Indoor houseplants, including poinsettia, *Dieffenbachia*, *Philodendron*, and many others
- Cosmetics, hair relaxer, nail products, mouthwash
- Kerosene, gasoline, lighter fluid, paint thinner, lamp oil, antifreeze, windshield washer fluid, lighter fluid, and other chemicals
- Alcoholic beverages
- Wild plants and mushrooms
- Pesticides, rodent poisons

- **Death from prescription analgesics and prescription opioids** has reached epidemic levels in the past decade, greater than deaths from heroin and cocaine combined. A big part of the problem is nonmedical use—using pain medications without a prescription or using them just for the high they cause. In 2018, an estimated 10.3 million people aged 12 years or older misused opioids in the past year (Substance Abuse and Mental Health Services Administration [SAMHSA], 2022).
- **Treatment choice** depends on the poison ingested. For most poisonings, the most effective intervention is professional administration of activated charcoal orally or via gastric tube. However, charcoal is not effective for ethanol, alkali, iron, boric acid, lithium, methanol, or cyanide. Depending on the situation, other options for medical treatment include gastric lavage, dialysis, administration of antidotes (i.e., Narcan), and forced diuresis.

Carbon Monoxide Exposure

Carbon monoxide (CO) is a colorless, tasteless, odorless toxic gas. Exposure can cause headaches, weakness, nausea, and vomiting; prolonged exposure leads to seizures, dysrhythmias, unconsciousness, brain damage, and death. Each year in the United States, CO poisoning causes approximately 350 unintentional deaths (CDC, 2017a).

- Most CO exposures occur at home.
- Most CO exposures involve females, children under the age of 17 years, and adults aged 18 to 44 years.
- CO poisoning accounts for a majority of deaths at the scene of fires and is also a relatively common cause of death by suicide.
- Many CO deaths occur during cold weather among older adults and the poor who seek nonconventional heat sources (e.g., gas ranges and ovens) to stay warm.

Scalds and Burns

The following are common causes of scalds and burns:

- **Scald injuries** (e.g., from hot water, steam, or grease) are the most common cause of burns in children younger than age 3. Scalding burns (especially on both feet or both hands) and cigarette burns in children and vulnerable older adults should always prompt you to assess for abuse (see Procedure 6-1).
- **Warming food or formula in the microwave** may cause the food to become hotter than intended, leading to burns in infants and young children.
- **Sunburn** can cause a first- or second-degree burn.
- **Contact burns** may occur from contact with metal surfaces and vinyl seats when cars are parked in the sun. 🌼 The risk of contact burns in all age-groups is greater in the presence of such heating devices as kerosene heaters, wood-burning stoves, and home sauna heating elements. People may use these as heat

sources when they cannot afford the cost of traditional furnace fuels.

- **Chemical agents**, such as acid, alkali, or other organic compounds, can also cause localized burns.

Fires

Home fires are a major cause of death and injury. Older adults and children younger than age 5 years have the greatest risk of fire death. Most *fatal home fires* occur while people are asleep, and most fire-related deaths occur from smoke inhalation. The following are common causes of fire in the home:

- **Smoking** (e.g., cigarettes) is the leading cause of fatal home fires.
- **Heating equipment** is equally responsible during the winter.
- **Home oxygen administration equipment**—In 75% of home fires involving oxygen, smoking materials are the ignition source.
- **Other causes of fire include** unsupervised children playing with matches, improper use of candles, and faulty wiring.

Example Problem: Falls

Falls are the third leading cause of injury-related deaths—and the leading cause for older adults. More than half of all falls occur in the home, and about 80% of home falls involve people aged 65 years and older. The rate triples for adults older than 75 years (Clemson et al., 2019). See the Example Problem: Falls, later in the chapter, for more information.

Firearm Injuries

Gun ownership is a controversial issue, so keep that in mind when you address patients. Some people keep guns in the home for protection and/or recreation (e.g., hunting, target shooting). However, guns are a source of unintentional injury and death.

- Household access to firearms has been implicated as a risk factor for youth suicide and domestic homicide, as well as unintentional injury (Knopov et al., 2019; Monuteaux et al., 2019).
- Gun safety and security are especially important when there are children in the home or someone who abuses substances.
- Because of the frequency and severity of unintentional firearm injuries involving children, the American Academy of Pediatrics and other groups have mounted efforts to educate parents about firearm safety.

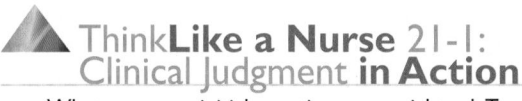

ThinkLike a Nurse 21-1: Clinical Judgment in Action

- What are some initial questions you might ask Teresa (Meet Your Patients) regarding her home environment?

- What are some basic interventions you might suggest to Teresa to help childproof the home?

To answer this question, you will need to recall information about:

Safety hazards encountered in the home

Developmental and lifestyle factors that affect safety

Specific nursing activities that can be used to prevent accidents or injuries related to the environmental hazards (e.g., firearms)

Suffocation/Asphyxiation

Suffocation by smothering is the leading cause of death for infants younger than 1 year. Suffocation may also be caused by drowning, choking on a foreign object, or inhaling gas or smoke.

- **Infants**—Suffocation of infants is often related to bed or crib hazards, such as excess bedding or pillows, or toys hung from long ribbons inside the infant's crib. Infants can become entangled in cords from window blinds or in the ribbon or string used to hang a pacifier around an infant's neck.
- **Ages 1 to 18 years**—Drowning is an important cause of accidental death in children 1 to 18 years old. **Key Point:** *Children up to age 4 are especially at risk for drowning.*
- **Nonfatal incidents**—Food items (e.g., hot dogs, raw vegetables, popcorn, hard candies, nuts, and grapes) are responsible for most nonfatal choking incidents.
- **Fatal** incidents—Nonfood items (e.g., latex balloons and plastic bags) cause the majority of suffocation deaths in young children.

KnowledgeCheck 21-2

- What are the most common poisonous agents ingested by children?
- Name one source of carbon monoxide (CO) poisoning.

Take-Home Toxins

Take-home toxins are hazardous substances transported from the workplace to the home. The National Institute for Occupational Safety and Health (NIOSH) reports that pathogenic microorganisms, asbestos, lead, mercury, arsenic, pesticides, caustic farm products, and dozens of other agents cause significant morbidity and mortality in workers' homes (NIOSH, 1997, updated June 2014). These toxins are most likely transported to workers' homes on the workers themselves, on their clothing, or on objects brought from the workplace. In the home, contamination occurs via any of three sources:

- Direct skin-to-skin contact or direct contact with contaminated clothing
- Arthropod vectors, such as ticks
- On dust particles that are inhaled (e.g., anthrax spores, arsenic in mine and smelter dust)

SAFETY HAZARDS IN THE COMMUNITY

This section discusses four hazardous agents: motor vehicle accidents, pathogens, pollution, and electrical storms. These are a major contributor to illness, disability, and death worldwide.

Motor Vehicle Accidents

Motor vehicle accidents (MVAs) are the second leading cause of accidental death in the United States. Teens and young adults aged 16 to 24 years are more likely to be distracted by devices, resulting in more MVAs than for drivers in other age-groups (CDC, 2022b). Older drivers are at higher risk of being injured or killed in a car crash. Every day, on average, 500 people over age 65 are injured in an automobile accident.

Contributing Factors

- **Key Point:** *Failure to use seat belts and failure to use proper child car seats are the major contributing factors.*
- **Air-bag deployment** when young children are improperly placed in the front passenger seat also causes severe injuries and death.
- **Driver distraction** is driver inattention, thought to be mostly due to cell-phone use and texting, which are banned or curtailed in most states.
  - Distracted driving also includes activities such as eating, talking to other passengers, and adjusting the radio or climate controls.
  - In 2019, more than 3,000 people were killed and 424,000 were injured in crashes involving a distracted driver.
  - Also in 2019, 20% of those who died in MVAs involving a distracted driver were nonoccupants (pedestrians, bicyclists, and others) (CDC, 2022b).
- **Other contributing and risk factors** for MVAs and related injuries and deaths include speed, alcohol, and nonuse of motorcycle helmets.

Pathogens

A **pathogen** is any microorganism capable of causing an illness. Pathogens can enter the body through several sources in the environment: food, mosquitoes and other insects, rodents and other animals, and unclean water.

Food-Borne Pathogens

Food poisoning is a nonspecific term that describes illness caused by ingesting bacteria and other microorganisms, or their toxins, in food. Contributing factors include:

- Improper food storage and preparation (a major cause of food poisoning)
- Raw foods, for example, raw meat, poultry, eggs, shellfish, raw fruits and vegetables, and unpasteurized milk and fruit juice

- Poisonous chemicals in the environment that may contaminate foods (e.g., mercury, arsenic, zinc, and potassium chlorate)

Vector-Borne Pathogens

Vectors are organisms that transmit pathogenic bacteria, viruses, and protozoa from one host to another. The following are examples:

- **Mosquitoes.** The severity of the reaction to a mosquito bite depends on the degree of allergy to the mosquito's saliva. In addition to the discomfort caused by their bites, infected mosquitoes can transmit diseases, such as West Nile virus and malaria. They can also transmit parasites to domestic animals (e.g., dog heartworm, equine encephalitis).
- **Other Insects.** Other insects, such as roaches, fleas, sand flies, lice, and ticks (which are, technically, arachnids and not insects), can also transmit serious diseases and produce a wide variety of allergens. Allergic sensitivity to cockroaches, for example, is a predictive factor for asthma severity (Shamsollahi et al., 2019).
- **Animals.** Structural defects in a building (e.g., roofs and walls) can permit the entry of birds, rodents, and other small animals, and dead spaces in walls permit their circulation among apartments in multiunit dwellings. Rodents and other animals can also act as vectors and allergens. Examples include the following:
  Rabies can be spread through the bite of a rabid animal.
  Some fungal diseases can spread via the inhalation of bird droppings.
  Mouse proteins have been implicated in the occurrence of asthma.

Water-Borne Pathogens

Sanitation refers to measures to promote and establish favorable health conditions, especially those related to the community's water supply. People who live in substandard housing may not have safe drinking water, hot water for washing, or adequate methods of waste disposal. People in rural areas often depend on private wells, which may not be adequately maintained and tested for pathogens such as *Giardia lamblia, Cryptosporidium,* and *Escherichia coli.* These are primarily community health problems.

Pollution

Pollution is any harmful chemical or waste material discharged into the air, water, or soil. Examples of pollutants are gaseous fumes, asbestos, carbon monoxide, and cigarette smoke. Each year Americans generate 292 million tons of trash. Of this, approximately 69 million tons are recycled, and 25 million tons are composted (U.S. Environmental Protection Agency [EPA], 2020).

Air Pollution Air pollution occurs indoors as well as outside.

- **Outdoor air pollution** includes motor vehicle emissions; asbestos; toluene; metals, such as mercury and lead compounds; and emissions from sources such as factories and power plants.
- **Indoor pollutants** include radon; carbon monoxide; and allergens from dust mites, cockroaches, mold, rodents, and pets.

Passive exposure to tobacco smoke is associated with respiratory disease and cancer, and environmental air pollution is linked to cardiovascular disease and respiratory viral infection (Dai et al., 2017; U.S. Department of Health and Human Services, 2014).

Water Contamination Contamination in lakes, rivers, and streams ultimately affects both recreation and food production. Pollution occurs when inadequately treated or inappropriate quantities of human, industrial, or agricultural wastes are released into the water systems. If the pollution is severe enough, the water may become unsafe for human consumption.

Noise Substantial exposure to noise has been associated with a range of adverse health effects, including hearing loss, stress, elevated blood pressure, and loss of sleep. Noise is pervasive in our society, caused by, among other sources, road traffic, airplanes, garbage trucks, construction equipment, lawn mowers, and loud music. People who live or work near major roads, bus depots, airports, and trucking routes are at greater risk, as are those in certain work environments (e.g., railroad workers).

Soil Improper waste disposal and excessive use of pesticides can contaminate soil. Agricultural, industrial, and manufacturing processes create solid and toxic waste. Animal, radioactive, and medical wastes pose special problems. Household products (e.g., paints, cleaners, oils, batteries, and pesticides) contain corrosive or toxic ingredients that contaminate the environment when disposed of improperly.

Weather Hazards

More than 1,000 people die each year in the United States due to weather hazards. Heat-related deaths are the most common. The number of deaths due to lightning, tornadoes, and hurricanes has fallen steadily during the 21st century, and deaths related to floods have declined more recently, mostly because of advances in technology and warning systems (National Weather Service [NWS], 2021). For additional information about Weather Hazards,

 Go to the website of the National Hazard Statistics at http://www.nws.noaa.gov/om/hazstats.shtml

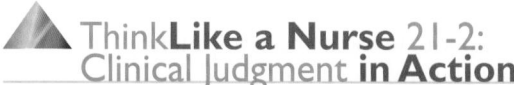

KnowledgeCheck 21-3

- What are the major causes of injuries from motor vehicle accidents (MVAs)?
- List at least three tips for preventing food poisoning.
- List three sources of noise pollution.

 ThinkLike a Nurse 21-2: Clinical Judgment **in Action**

Identify an environmental problem in your neighborhood. What are some possible solutions?

SAFETY HAZARDS IN THE HEALTHCARE FACILITY

According to Leap Frog Hospital Safety Grade (2022), more than 200,000 avoidable deaths occur in U.S. hospitals each year. Healthcare facilities embody several safety hazards for residents and workers. We have discussed the hazard of infection in Chapter 20. Box 21-2 lists The Joint Commission's *National Patient Safety Goals* for 2022, which should give you an idea of the types of accidents that occur in healthcare agencies. If you would like to see a full explanation of the patient safety goals,

 Go to the website of The Joint Commission at https://www.jointcommission.org/standards/national-patient-safety-goals/.

BOX 21-2 ■ The Joint Commission (TJC) 2022 *Patient Safety Goals*

For a full understanding of TJC *Patient Safety Goals,*

Go to http://www.jointcommission.org/

Goal 1. Identify patients correctly.

Goal 2. Improve staff communication.

Goal 3. Use medicines safely.

Goal 6. Use alarms safely.

Goal 7. Prevent infection.

Goal 15. Identify patient safety risks (specifically, suicide risk).

*UP 1. Prevent mistakes in surgery.

---

*Universal Protocol (UP 1), Prevent mistakes in surgery, is a preprocedure verification process to make sure that all documents, information, and equipment are available and that the correct procedure is performed on the correct person and site.

Source: Adapted from The Joint Commission. (2022a). *The Joint Commission: Accreditation program, Hospital.* 2022 *National patient safety goals.* https://www.jointcommission.org/standards_information/npsgs.aspx

Organizational factors contribute to errors and safety problems in healthcare, including the following:

- Poor design
- Maintenance failures
- Unworkable procedures
- Shortfalls in training
- Less-than-adequate tools and equipment
- Inadequate staffing
- Disruptive behavior and intimidation in the workplace
- Culture of disrespect among healthcare professionals

Healthcare Culture Healthcare has traditionally been a hierarchy, with the physician at the top. However, healthcare professionals, including nurses, have been taught to practice with autonomy. This combination of factors has helped create a culture that does not respond well to questions about possible problems with patient care, particularly from subordinates. It is clear that such a culture needs to be repaired, and many healthcare organizations are working to address disrespectful behavior, staff reluctance to speak up about risks and errors, and blatant disregard of expressed concerns.

Quality Nursing Care Key Point: *Because nurses are the healthcare professionals who spend the greatest amount of time with patients, research has documented what physicians, patients, and nurses themselves have long known: the quality of nursing care affects patient health and outcomes and sometimes can be a matter of life or death.* In providing quality care and patient safety, nurses are indispensable. Studies have shown that:

- Employing fewer nurses to provide care is associated with greater numbers of patient deaths (Aiken et al., 2001, Kutney-Lee & Aiken, 2015; Olds et al., 2017).
- Providing less nursing time to patients is associated with higher rates of infection, gastrointestinal bleeding, pneumonia, cardiac arrest, and death from these and other causes (Driscoll et al., 2018; Tvedt et al., 2017).

What Are Never Events?

Never events, also known as **Serious Reportable Events (SREs),** are healthcare-acquired complications that (1) can cause serious injury or death to a patient and (2) should never happen in a hospital. In addition, never events have the following characteristics. They are:

1. Clearly identifiable and measurable
2. Serious
3. Usually preventable

You can gain insight into healthcare facility hazards by examining the following list of serious reportable events (National Quality Forum, 2020). Be aware that this list may grow and change more over time.

- Foreign object (such as a sponge) left in patients after surgery
- Air embolism

- Administration of the wrong type of blood
- Severe pressure injuries
- Falls and trauma
- Infections associated with urinary catheters
- Infections associated with intravenous catheters
- Symptoms resulting from poorly controlled blood sugar levels
- Surgical site infections after certain elective procedures (e.g., certain orthopedic surgeries, bariatric surgery for obesity)
- Deep vein thrombosis or pulmonary embolism after total knee and total hip replacement procedures

The Institute for Healthcare Improvement (IHI, n.d.-b), an independent, not-for-profit organization, recently completed the 5 Million Lives Campaign as a follow-up to its 100,000 Lives Campaign. The IHI Campaign recommended healthcare changes to reduce morbidity and death in American healthcare. At least three of the 5 Million Lives goals supported the list of never events: prevent adverse drug events, prevent central line infections, and prevent surgical site infections. To read the entire list of recommendations and the results of the campaign,

 Go to the IHI website at http://www.ihi.org/engage/ initiatives/completed/5MillionLivesCampaign/Pages/ default.aspx

 Think**Like a Nurse** 21-3: Clinical Judgment **in Action**

Many never events can be reduced by good nursing care. By preventing complications and maximizing reimbursement, nurses can prove their value to an organization and make the case for better staffing. Over which of the never events do you think nurses have the most control? Explain your thinking.

Understanding Errors in Healthcare—Root Cause Analysis

Root-cause analysis (RCA) tries to solve problems by identifying and correcting the underlying cause(s) of events, as opposed to simply addressing their symptoms. The goal is to decrease the likelihood that the problem will recur. A root cause is typically a finding related not to individual error but to a process or system that has the potential for redesign to reduce risk. Therefore, a root-cause finding is usually used for the purpose of redesigning a process or system rather than preventing an individual error. RCA provides an organized structure for the analysis of errors and is designed to answer three basic questions:

1. What happened?
2. Why did it happen?
3. What can be done to prevent it from happening again?

The Joint Commission requires healthcare agencies to perform RCA for all unexpected occurrences involving death or serious physical or psychological injury, also known as **sentinel events.**

Toward Evidence-Based Practice

Inanloo, A., Mohammadi, N., & Haghani, H. (2017). The effect of shift reporting training using the SBAR tool on the performance of nurses working in intensive care units. *Journal of Client-Centered Nursing Care, 3*(1), 51–56.

This study investigated the effect of training nurses *(intervention)* in intensive care units on the use of the SBAR tool for shift-to-shift reporting. This observational study used a checklist based on the SBAR tool to record data. Researchers observed nurses' use of the SBAR tool before training and again after training. Findings indicated that shift-to-shift report performance significantly improved after the intervention.

Bonds, R. L. (2018). SBAR tool implementation to advance communication, teamwork, and the perception of patient safety culture. *Creative Nursing, 24*(2), 116–123.

An evidence-based project (EBP) was implemented using a standardized multidisciplinary situation, background, assessment, recommendation (SBAR) tool to improve communication, teamwork, and the perception of a patient safety culture among the surgical nurses, physicians, and

anesthesia providers. All participants received training on the SBAR tool, followed by a 7-week implementation period. Findings indicated that communication utilizing the SBAR method increased by 100%. Results of a survey to measure participants' perception of a patient safety culture revealed that the use of a standardized communication tool improved the overall perception of a patient safety culture and teamwork across disciplines.

1. Identify a recent interaction you have had in which communication was difficult. What issues specific to the healthcare setting may encourage communication difficulties?

2. Communication problems among healthcare personnel can jeopardize patient safety. SBAR, a structured communication technique, has been adapted from aviation and the military as a strategy for clear communication based on a statement of the situation, background, assessment, and recommendations related to a clinical issue. Based on the findings from each of the studies, identify specific ways that the use of SBAR can affect patient safety.

Culture of Safety

A positive nursing unit culture helps improve patient outcomes. Culture is a way of thinking, behaving, or working in a place or organization. **Key Point:** *In a culture of safety, nurses practice in an environment where all staff members work together to create a safe unit, disclose errors without fear, and address any safety concerns.* Key components of a culture of safety include the following (Helbling & Huwe, 2015; Lee et al., 2019):

- **Team empowerment.** Every individual has the opportunity to be heard, feel important, and be a valued team member for the contribution offered.
- **Communication.** Open and honest lines of communication are needed between the team members and from the team to other hospital units.
- **Transparency.** Team members are united in their efforts to eliminate rumors and operate with only the facts, contributing to mutual team goals.
- **Accountability.** Staff claim ownership for human error and are willing to disclose the error and help prevent similar errors

Also refer to the accompanying iCare box.

Equipment-Related Accidents

Equipment-related accidents usually occur when equipment malfunctions or as a result of improper use, for example, when suction devices and infusion pumps are not working properly, oxygen cylinders are transported

♥ iCare

Caring Is Creating a Culture of Safety

Safety is a basic need for all persons. Your commitment to safety is one way for you to show caring. As the person closest to and most constantly with the patient, you can facilitate a culture of safety by:

- Speaking up for safety. Use CUS words:
  - **C**—State your concern.
  - **U**—Say why you are uncomfortable.
  - **S**—State, "This is a safety issue"; explain how and why.
- Stopping the line (e.g., calling for a preprocedure "time out" when there is a concern)
- Escalating the safety issue when needed, communicating through the appropriate chain of command
- Being open and transparent with patients/families/colleagues
- Participating in *safety huddles* (quick conversations with a focus on safety)
- Opening all meetings with the topic of safety, allowing time for stories/concerns
- Using situation, background, assessment, recommendation (SBAR) communication
- Validating and verifying when unsure (have another nurse check)
- Ensuring *200% accountability* (calling other nurses or healthcare disciplines on handwashing or use of personal protective equipment)
- Reporting both actual and "near-miss" medication errors, policy deviations, treatment and outcome variations, and adverse events
- Participating in your organization's patient and caregiver safety committee

incorrectly, or wheelchairs and beds are not locked during transfer activities.

Alarm Safety

Missed alarms cause harm most commonly when (a) the medical device does not detect the alarm condition, (b) the alarm is not communicated to a medical practitioner, or (c) the alarm is communicated but not adequately addressed.

Thousands of alarms go off every day in hospitals. **Alarm fatigue** occurs when nurses become overwhelmed by the number of alarm signals and begin to ignore alarms, delay response to alarms, or even deactivate them. Missed alarms or delayed responses have resulted in sentinel events, including patient deaths. The Joint Commission named alarm desensitization a National Patient Safety Goal and requires that healthcare facilities provide:

- A comprehensive alarm-management program that includes input from nurses, other healthcare workers, and management
- Education for staff about the purpose and proper operation of the alarms systems for which they are responsible (The Joint Commission, 2022a).

Fires and Electrical Hazards

Fire in a healthcare agency is more often related to anesthesia or improperly grounded or malfunctioning electrical equipment than to smoking. Most healthcare agencies have policies for preventing electrical hazards. Nevertheless, patients and visitors do break the rules, so smoking cannot be discounted as a hazard.

When a fire occurs, an announcement is made over the communication system. Often, words such as "Code Red" or "Code Yellow" are used in an effort to prevent panic among patients and visitors. The announcement may ask visitors to leave the building.

Restraints

A **restraint** is a device or method used for the purpose of restricting a patient's freedom of movement or access to their body, with or without their permission. The most obvious form of restraint is the use of physical force by another person. A restraint may also be (1) a mechanical device, material, or equipment, such as a cloth vest or side-rails, or (2) a chemical restraint (e.g., sedatives and psychotropic medications) given to control disruptive behavior.

- Devices such as casts and traction are not considered restraints (Barber, 2017; CMS, 2008).
- **Physical holding of a patient is not always considered restraint.** Sometimes it is necessary to use devices or methods that involve the physical holding of a patient for routine physical examinations or tests.
- **Restraints are classified according to the reason for their use:** medical-surgical restraints or restraints

used for behavior management. Medicare has specific guidelines for each circumstance. Guidelines are more restrictive when restraints are used for behavior management.

Nurses traditionally restrained highly dependent older adults, patients with poor mobility, those with impaired cognitive status, and those they judged to be at risk for falls. However, it has been found that restraints make care more time consuming and do not reduce falls. Restraints are themselves a safety hazard and actually increase the likelihood of injury. A restrained person has a natural tendency to struggle and try to remove the restraint. As a result, the person can become entangled and suffer nerve damage, circulatory impairment, or even suffocation.

- **Potential Physical Effects.** Restraint-imposed immobility can cause pressure injuries and contractures, result in a loss of strength, and affect nearly every body part.
- **Potential Emotional Effects.** The person may suffer anger, fear, humiliation, and diminished self-esteem.

Restraint-Free Environments

Research indicates that less restraint use saves time and money and reduces patient injuries (Bauer & Weust, 2017; Chou et al., 2019).

The ANA, along with other healthcare organizations, has established evidence-based guidelines showing that a restraint-free environment is the standard of care. When the decision is made to avoid restraints, alternatives must be provided to keep the patient safe. **Key Point: *Restraints never resolve the underlying problem; addressing the reason behind the patient's behavior is key to calming the patient (Mitchell et al., 2018).***

To provide the safest possible care environment, The Joint Commission encourages healthcare facilities to do the following:

- Promote a commitment to reducing the use of restraints and seclusion among all direct-care staff.
- Educate caregivers before they take part in any restraint-related activity.
- Document restraint episodes specifically, in detail.
- Maintain one-on-one viewing of patients in restraint and seclusion.
- Include staff members when deciding whether to explore new technology that is considered a safe alternative to traditional restraint devices.
- Budget for an adequate number of qualified staff to attend to patients.

Restraint Is Sometimes Necessary

Organizational guidelines differ slightly, depending on whether restraints are used to support medical healing or for a behavioral health reason (e.g., when a patient is irrational and pulling out their IV lines). Use restraints only as a last resort. As much as possible, use technology (such as bed alarms) and better anticipation of patient needs instead of restraints.

➕ If you must use restraints, Medicare, The Joint Commission, and other regulators require both of the following:

- Restraints be medically prescribed.
- All less restrictive interventions are tried first.

Do Not Depend on Siderails

Based on the CMS standards, siderails can be viewed as a restraint.

- *A full-length siderail* is a restraint when it is used to prevent the patient from getting out of bed, regardless of whether the patient is able to do so safely.
- *A half- or quarter-length upper siderail* can be an aid to independence if it is used by the patient for the purpose of getting into and out of bed.
- *Split rails* are not considered restraints if a client requests them in order to feel more secure.

Remember that older or cognitively impaired adults may regard siderails as a barrier rather than as a reminder that they need assistance. **Key Point: *Several studies have shown that siderails may lead to serious falls and injuries. These findings have led healthcare providers to reevaluate the use of restraints and to recommend that siderails not be used routinely (Bleijlevens et al., 2016; Brugnolli et al., 2020).***

KnowledgeCheck 21-4
- What is a typical cause of fire in healthcare facilities?
- What measures should you take, and in what order, if a fire occurs in the hospital?

Mercury Exposure

Mercury is a heavy, odorless, silver-white liquid metal. **Key Point: *Mercury is toxic in both acute and chronic exposure.*** It can be inhaled, ingested, or absorbed through the skin. It accumulates in muscle tissue and can cause renal and neurological disorders, especially in fetuses and neonates. Because of its shiny color and ability to form beads or balls, mercury is appealing to curious children. See Table 21-3 for potential health effects.

Products that may contain mercury include thermometers, thermostats, batteries, fluorescent light bulbs, blood pressure devices, and electrical equipment and switches. Since 1998, the American Hospital Association (AHA) and the Environmental Protection Agency (EPA) launched a program to eliminate mercury-containing waste in the healthcare industry and prevent it from entering the environment via incinerators, landfills, and wastewater.

- **Thermometers and Sphygmomanometers.** Mercury thermometers are no longer being made in the United States. However, some people may still have them in their homes. Most, but not all, healthcare facilities have eliminated mercury thermometers and sphygmomanometers. Some hospitals conduct thermometer exchanges, providing free or low-cost nonmercury thermometers to anyone who brings in a mercury thermometer.
- **Mercury Spills.** Healthcare facilities must have policies and procedures for hazardous waste spills, as required by The Joint Commission, the EPA, and the Occupational Safety and Health Administration (OSHA). You are not likely to encounter mercury exposure in acute care and ambulatory agencies.

Table 21-3 ➤ Potential Health Effects of Mercury

PRIMARY ROUTE	POTENTIAL HEALTH EFFECTS
Acute Effects	
Toxicity	Symptoms of chills, nausea, malaise, chest tightness and pain, dyspnea, coughing, stomatitis, gingivitis, excess salivation, and diarrhea. High levels can cause severe respiratory irritation, digestive disturbances, and severe renal damage.
Inhalation	Respiratory damage, wakefulness, muscle weakness, anorexia, headache, ringing in the ears, chest pain, inflammation of the mouth, and pneumonitis
Eye	Irritation and corrosion
Skin	Irritation and allergic dermatitis
Ingestion	Intestinal obstruction
Chronic Effects	
Primarily central nervous system	Numbness or tingling of the hands, lips, and feet; behavior and personality changes
Other	Fatigue, weakness, anorexia, weight loss, and gastrointestinal disturbances

Biological Hazards

As a nurse, you will place a high priority on the biological safety of patients. Institutionalized patients are at especially high risk from infectious microorganisms, some of which are highly resistant to antibiotics. To learn about or review healthcare-related infections, asepsis, and infection control, refer to Chapter 20.

Hazards to Healthcare Workers

Nursing is an active profession, and workplace injuries are all too common. Common accidents include back injuries, needlestick injuries, radiation injury, and violence. Nurses sometimes hesitate to report that they have been injured because they fear being labeled a complainer or troublemaker or being denied opportunities for promotion and other consequences. However, OSHA (1) requires that employers show employees how to report a workplace injury and (2) prohibits discrimination against employees who make such reports.

 You should always report an injury. By doing so, you help (1) pinpoint trends and areas of need in safety and (2) ensure you will receive necessary treatment and follow-up.

Back Injury

Nursing personnel are consistently listed in the top 10 occupations for work-related musculoskeletal disorders (MSDs). Most often the MSD involves the shoulders and back (U.S. Bureau of Labor Statistics, 2019). Recent literature reveals that the frequency of back pain in nurses ranges between 62% and 87% (Clari et al., 2021; Gilchrist et al., 2021), likely because many nursing tasks require bending and twisting of the torso, activities that can cause injury when the nurse does not use correct body mechanics or equipment. Among the most stressful activities are transferring patients (e.g., from toilet to chair), weighing patients, lifting a patient in bed, repositioning patients in beds or chairs, and changing bed linens.

The ANA (2008) supports actions and policies that result in the elimination of manual patient handling. The ANA aims to:

- Create a culture of safety by requiring employers to develop a safe handling and moving program with policies, appropriate equipment, training, and accommodations for injured employees.
- Empower nurses to (1) actively participate in creating and implementing safe handling measures and (2) promptly report hazards, incidents, and injuries in a "blame-free" environment.

♥ iCare Safe patient handling procedures improve the quality of care for patients by enhancing safety, comfort, and dignity. The use of assistive equipment and devices can reduce the potential for patient injuries from falls, skin tears, and shoulder dislocations, to name a few.

Refer to Chapter 29 for information about body mechanics and how to safely lift and move patients. For more information about ANA's campaign to prevent musculoskeletal injuries,

Go to the ANA's **Safe Patient Handling Web site** at https://www.nursingworld.org/practice-policy/work-environment/health-safety/safe-patient-handling/

Needlestick Injury

Since the 1990s, the number of needlestick injuries has declined due to the increased of devices with safety mechanisms. As safer technologies have become available, injuries occurring from disposable syringes have decreased significantly. However, the number of injuries from sutures and scalpel blades, particularly among physicians and operating room staff, continues to be high. More than half of the injuries from disposable syringes affect nurses (CDC, 2019). In addition, a quarter of all injuries occur to the nonuser (e.g., UAP, housekeeping, laundry worker, etc.). **Key Point:** *It is important to remember that the use and activation of safety mechanisms and proper disposal are essential to protect not just the user of the device but also those who come into contact with that device.*

The federal Needlestick Safety and Prevention Act and OSHA standards require employers to maintain a log of sharps injuries and to purchase needleless systems and safer needle devices. Needlestick injury rates declined by more than 36% during the 3-year period after the passage of that law. Nevertheless, needlestick injuries and other sharps-related injuries continue to occur.

The risk of needlestick injury increases for nurses who:

- Work in stressful environments
- Work varying or long shifts (longer than 12 consecutive hours)
- Have a low skill level, based on education level or experience

Other risk factors include a lack of protective equipment, recapping needles, and working in an area that requires higher-than-average use of needles.

For suggestions about how you can prevent needlestick injuries,

 Go to Chapter 21, **Clinical Insight 21-2: Preventing Needlestick Injury,** in Volume 2.

Radiation Injury

Radiation is the process of emitting radiant energy in the form of waves or particles. Ionizing radiation is used in computerized tomography (CT) scans in diagnostic radiology, linear accelerators in radiotherapy, and positron emission tomography (PET) scans in nuclear medicine. Patients are deliberately exposed to radiation during diagnostic tests and certain medical treatments. Healthcare workers who care for these patients are unavoidably exposed to small doses of radiation.

Take precautions to avoid excessive radiation exposure for the patient and yourself during x-ray procedures. **Key Point:** *Follow the principles of time, distance, and shielding when caring for a patient who is being treated with an internal radioactive implant:*

- **Time:** Organize nursing care to limit the amount of time with the patient.
- **Distance:** Perform nursing care near the patient only if absolutely necessary.
- **Shielding:** Wear protective shielding (e.g., a lead apron) and wear a film badge if you deliver care that exposes you to radiation regularly. The film badge will indicate any radiation exposure.

Violence

The impact of violent acts on healthcare workers is widespread and includes injuries, higher-than-average staff turnover, increased requests for medical leaves, unusually high time-off and attendance issues, and stress-related illnesses (Liu et al., 2019). Hospital security may not be sufficient to protect you from injury if violence breaks out among patients, visitors, and/or staff. This is especially true in the following situations:

- **A crowded or chaotic environment**—For example, the emergency department (ED), which has 24-hour accessibility and may sometimes be crowded and chaotic.
- **Anxiety and anger**—Under the stress of an acute illness, patients and family members alike may become anxious and angry and act out in ways that are unpredictable and atypical. **Key Point:** *Violence typically begins with anxiety and escalates in stages through verbal aggression and then physical aggression. If you can relieve a patient's anxiety, you may be able to halt the progression to physical violence.*
- **Certain emotional and physical conditions** increase the risk for patient aggression (refer to Assessing the Risk for Violence in the following Practical Knowledge section).

The Joint Commission (2022b) recently established a new standard to address the prevention of workplace violence in hospitals. The requirements clarify that workplace violence is an organizational issue and that a systems approach is necessary to address workplace violence. The new standards require hospitals to establish a strong culture of safety and violence prevention. One goal is that there will be a change in the employee mindset that violence is "part of the job" to a view of workplace violence as an occupational hazard that can be managed and prevented.

KnowledgeCheck 21-5

- What measures can healthcare workers use to reduce exposure to radiation?
- What safety measures help reduce equipment-related injuries in the healthcare facility?
- As a nurse, what can you do to help prevent injuring your back?

PracticalKnowledge
knowing **how**

This section provides focused assessments, general interventions for addressing patient safety, and specific nursing interventions for safety hazards discussed in the preceding Theoretical Knowledge section.

■ ASSESSMENT/RECOGNIZING CUES

It is important to assess the client's immediate environment, developmental stage, and individual risk factors. The following will help you to perform focused assessments for fall risk, home safety, and risk for violence.

Assessing/Recognizing Cues for Example Client Condition: Falls

The use of a standardized fall-prevention tool has been shown to decrease fall rates (Coppedge et al., 2016). You will find more information about fall assessment and standardized tools in the Example Client Condition: Falls. Also,

 Go to Chapter 21, **Assessment Guidelines and Tools, Get Up and Go Test** and the **Times Up & Go Test,** in Volume 2.

The Morse Fall Scale This scale is a rapid and simple method for assessing a patient's likelihood of falling. Ideally, the scale should be calibrated specifically for each nursing unit so that fall-prevention strategies are targeted to those most at risk. Institutions implementing the Morse scale should train personnel in the proper use of the scale (Morse, 1997, 2008, 2009). To see the Morse Fall Scale,

 Go to the Network of Care Web site, at **www. networkofcare.org/library/Morse Fall Scale.pdf**

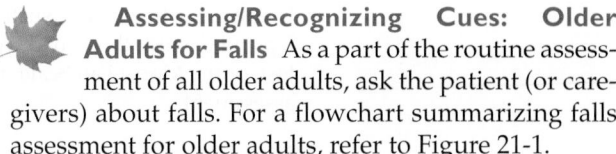 **Assessing/Recognizing Cues: Older Adults for Falls** As a part of the routine assessment of all older adults, ask the patient (or caregivers) about falls. For a flowchart summarizing falls assessment for older adults, refer to Figure 21-1.

- **Get Up and Go. Use if there is a history of falls.** If a patient or caregiver reports a single fall or risk factors, conduct the Get Up and Go test to identify whether the patient is presently at risk for falls or needs further evaluation.
- **Timed Up & Go. If the patient is seeking care because of a fall or if you observe any difficulty with ambulation,** refer the patient to a practitioner with advanced skills and experience for a Timed Up & Go test and a comprehensive fall evaluation. Primary care providers should perform a Timed Up & Go test annually for fall risk assessment for all patients over age 65 (American Academy of Neurology, n.d.-a., n.d.-b.; Grossman et al., 2018; Podsiadlo & Richardson, 1991).

EXAMPLE PROBLEM: Falls

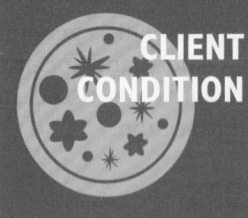

CLIENT CONDITION

Facts About Falls

- Third leading cause of injury-related deaths—the leading cause for older adults.
- Over 800,000 patients a year are hospitalized because of a fall injury.

Falls in the Home

- More than half of all falls occur in the home.
- Infants and older adults are especially at risk for injury from falls.
- About 80% of home falls involve people aged 65 years and older. The rate triples for adults older than 75 years.

Falls in the Healthcare Facility

- Most agencies have established procedures and safety features to prevent falls.
- Falls are the most common incident reported in hospitals and long-term care facilities,
- Falls occur in 1 of every 2,000 patient stays (Centers for Disease Control and Prevention [CDC], 2021e).
- Many cases involve falling from a bed.
- Falls occur more frequently on nights, weekends, and holidays.

Risk Factors

Key Point: *Clients usually have multiple risk factors.*
- History of falls
- Age >80 years
- Impaired vision
- Weakness/dizziness (e.g., from disease or therapy)
- Gait or balance problems
- Pain
- Hypotension
- Orthostatic hypotension
- Cognitive impairment
- Chronic conditions (e.g., arthritis)
- Medication side effects (e.g., drowsiness)
- Polypharmacy
- Home hazards
- Unfamiliar environment
- Alcohol use

Complications of Falls

Falls may cause serious injuries, disability, loss of independence, and even death.

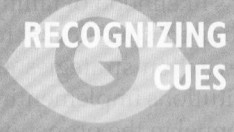

RECOGNIZING CUES

- Assess all inpatients for fall risk when they are admitted.
- Identify modifiable risk factors (different conditions require different nursing interventions.)
- For clients at risk for falls, repeat the risk assessment every 8 hours, and increase the frequency of monitoring.
- Identify medications that increase the risk for falling (e.g., opioid analgesics, sedatives, and antihypertensives).
- Use standardized tools, such as the Get Up and Go test, the Timed Up and Go test, or the Morse Fall Scale, for fall risk assessment.

Morse Fall Scale

The risk of falling varies greatly with different patient populations, different times of day, and different stages of the patient's illness.

Key Point: *Age alone is not a predictor of falls, but the items scored by the scale are more common in older adults (Morse, 2001).*

The Morse Fall Scale uses the following questions to assess a person's risk for falls:
1. Does the patient have a history of falling?
2. Does the person have more than one medical diagnosis?
3. Does the person use ambulatory aids, such as crutches or a walker?

 Assessing Older Adults for Falls

Ask older adults (or caregivers) about falls at least once a year. If there is a history of falls, use the Get Up and Go Test.

Get Up and Go Test

- Move from sitting to standing without using arms to help them rise.
- Walk several paces, turn, and return to the chair.
- Sit back in the chair without using arms for support.

If patient has difficulty or unsteadiness, require the following assessment:
- Sit.
- Stand without using arms for support.
- Close their eyes for a few seconds while standing in place.
- Walk a short distance and come to a complete stop.
- Sit in the chair without using arms for support.

Timed Up & Go

Refer to a practitioner with advanced skills and experience for a Timed Up & Go and a comprehensive fall evaluation if one of the following exists:
1. The patient is seeking care because of a fall.
2. You observe difficulty with ambulation.

EXAMPLE PROBLEM: Falls—cont'd

4. Does the person have an IV line or a saline lock?
5. Is the person's gait normal or stooped or otherwise impaired?
6. What is the person's mental status (e.g., disoriented, forgetful)?

The nurse then uses the tool to score, tally, and record those six variables on the patient's chart.

To see the Morse Fall Scale,

 Go to the Network of Care Web site at **www.networkofcare.org/library/Morse Fall Scale.pdf**

In this test, the patient is asked to get up and walk 8 feet in 8.5 seconds or less. To see the Timed Up & Go Test,

 Go to the CDC Website at **hepps://www. cdc.gov/steadi/pdf/TUG**

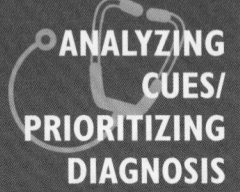
ANALYZING CUES/ PRIORITIZING DIAGNOSIS

Primary Diagnosis:

Fall Risk

Related Diagnoses:

Activities of Daily Living (ADLs) Alteration
Fear (of falling)
Injury Risk
Self-Care Deficit
(Clinical Care Classification System [CCC], n.d.)

Examples:

- Fall Risk r/t weakness and impaired vision
- Self-Care Deficit (Hygiene/Toileting) r/t fear of falling when ambulating

---

GENERATING SOLUTIONS

NOC Outcomes

- Balance
- Fall Prevention Behavior
- Personal Safety Behavior
- Safe Home Environment

Individualized Goal Statements

- Remains injury-free
- Maintains independence
- Home is free from falls hazards (e.g., throw rugs)

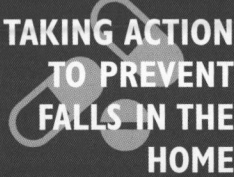
TAKING ACTION TO PREVENT FALLS IN THE HOME

Key Point: *Prevention is key!*
Fear of falling should not inhibit a person from living an active life.

- Teach clients measures for increasing the safety of their home environment.

Exercise Regularly

Provide gait training and advice on the safe use of assistive devices.

- Exercise at least 30 minutes every day. Amount of activity depends on age, physical condition, and intensity of the exercise. Any activity is better than none (see Chapter 29).
- Tai chi, yoga, exercise classes, and weight training help improve balance, coordination, flexibility, and strength.
- Learn to use assistive devices, such as walkers and canes safely. Be sure rubber tips are not worn.
- Keep the walking aid by the bed at night.

Childproof the Home

- Install window guards; never leave a window wide open.
- Use gates at the top and bottom of stairways for small children.
- Never leave a child alone on a changing table, even for a moment.
- Supervise young walkers to protect from falls.
- Remove chairs near counters or other areas where young children would be likely to climb. Push chairs all the way under dining tabletops.
- Teach children to pick up their toys.
- Be sure that children wear helmets and appropriate protective gear for bicycling, skateboarding, and other active sports.

(continued)

EXAMPLE PROBLEM: Falls—cont'd

Take Your Time

- You are more likely to fall when you are tired, sick, rushed, or emotionally upset.
- Walk and go up stairs carefully, without hurrying; be careful not to be distracted while walking.
- Do one thing at a time; complete it before going on to the next task.
- Get out of a bed or chair slowly and check your balance before standing or walking—especially if you are taking medications for high blood pressure and other conditions.

Lighten Loads—Brighten Paths

- Carry things in several small loads instead of one very large load so that you are able to see over them, especially on stairs.
- Use bags with handles instead of large boxes or laundry baskets to carry items.
- Make sure rooms are adequately lit, use dim light (e.g., a night light) at night, and turn on the lights before entering a room.
- Have your eyes checked at least once a year.
- Clean eyeglasses frequently.

Don't Trip Yourself Up

- Ensure that shoes fit properly; wear slippers with nonskid soles. Do not go barefoot.
- Avoid loose, trailing clothes. Keep hems of clothing at a length to prevent tripping.

- Older adults with leg or hip stiffness and pain may shuffle when walking; the use of a cane or walker may help.
- Use nonskid covers on tips of assistive devices, such as canes, walkers, and crutches. Replace when worn.
- Use a ladder or step stool; do not stand on the top step of a stepladder; never climb on a chair.

For Older Adults or Those With Limited Mobility

- Use beds that are low to the floor.
- Keep a cordless phone in each room and by the bedside to make it easier to call for help if needed.
- Ask your doctor or pharmacist to review your medicines—both prescription and over the counter—to reduce side effects and interactions (especially important for psychotropic medications).
- Get treatment for postural hypotension and cardiovascular disorders, including dysrhythmias.

Use Caution on Stairs

- Keep stairs well lit.
- Keep stairs free of clutter.
- Install sturdy handrails and slip-resistant floor coverings on staircases.
- Fasten stair coverings securely.
  - For older adults and those with vision problems, paint the top and bottom steps white or put white stripes on the front edges of steps.

Minimize Bathroom Hazards

- Use shower chairs and raised toilet seats.
- Install grab bars and use a nonskid mat in the shower and tub.
- Install handheld shower attachments to make it easier to sit while showering and minimize the need to move and turn.

Clear the Floor

- Tape or otherwise fasten phone and electrical equipment cords to the baseboard.
- Arrange furniture to provide wide walking areas.
- Keep clutter (e.g., toys, magazines, clothing) out of the walkways.
- Remove all scatter or throw rugs (or at least be sure they have nonskid padding under them).
- Wipe up all foods and fluids from the floor immediately.
- Apply an ice-melt product, salt, or sand to icy sidewalks, steps, and porches.

EXAMPLE PROBLEM: Falls—cont'd

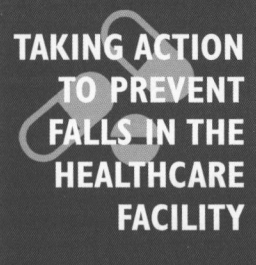

TAKING ACTION TO PREVENT FALLS IN THE HEALTHCARE FACILITY

Nursing Care in the Healthcare Facility

- Review medications, especially psychotropic medications. Modify as needed.
- Place call light within reach. Have patient demonstrate ability to call for the nurse.
- Orient patient to surroundings (e.g., bathroom, chairs); you may need to label items.
- Place disoriented patients in rooms near the nurses' station.

- Keep water, urinal, bedpan, and tissues within easy reach of patient.
- Provide a night-light.
- Keep floors dry and free of clutter.
- Teach fall-prevention strategies to patient and family.
- For patients at risk for falls, place a warning sticker on the chart or door.
- Use bed and chair monitoring devices for patients with altered levels of consciousness or orientation.

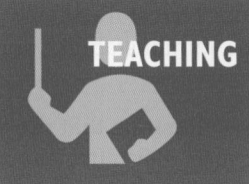

TEACHING

Home Care

Teach what to do if a fall occurs
- Don't panic.
- Stay still for a few minutes to get over the shock.

- If you think you are okay, slide over to a sturdy piece of furniture, assume a kneeling position, and push yourself up; then sit down until you recover.
- If you cannot move, try to cover yourself to keep warm until help arrives.

Sources: Adapted from Centers for Disease Control and Prevention. (2021e). National Center for Injury Prevention and Control. Important facts about falls. https://www.cdc.gov/homeandrecreationalsafety/falls/adultfalls.html; American Academy of Neurology. (n.d.-c). Get Up and Go Test. https://www.aan.com/Guidelines/Home/GetGuidelineContent/265; American Academy of Neurology (AAN). (n.d.-d). The Timed Up and Go Test. https://www.aan.com/Guidelines/Home/GetGuidelineContent/266; Avin, K. G., Hanke, T. A., Kirk-Sanchez, N., McDonough, C. M., Shubert, T. E., Hardage, J., Hartley, G., & Academy of Geriatric Physical Therapy of the American Physical Therapy Association. (2015). Management of falls in community-dwelling older adults: Clinical guidance statement from the Academy of Geriatric Physical Therapy of the American Physical Therapy Association. Physical Therapy, 95(6), 815–834; Centers for Disease Control and Prevention. (2017c). Take a stand on falls. http://www.cdc.gov/features/older-adult-falls/index.html; Clinical Care Classification System. (n.d.) Coding for nurses. https://careclassification.org/

Assessing/Recognizing Cues for Home Safety

Many accidents occur in the home (e.g., fire, poisoning). Everyone should take a few minutes to check for environmental safety hazards.

- A **home safety checklist** is a convenient way for clients to identify potential hazards. Many such lists are available; for example, conduct an Internet search for "home safety checklist."
- **The safety assessment scale (SAS)** is an objective way to evaluate the dangers incurred by people with memory and cognitive deficits who live alone at home. In addition to assessing for injury, this scale evaluates whether the person with cognitive impairment is capable of taking medications and performing other activities of daily living (ADLs) independently. To use the short version of the SAS to assess risk status and decide whether the person should have an in-depth evaluation,

 Go to **Assessment Guidelines and Tools, SAS Safety Assessment Scale**, in Volume 2.

Assessing/Recognizing Cues for the Risk for Violence

You can be prepared to intervene and perhaps even prevent violence if you recognize risk factors and early warning signs (Arnetz, 2022; Copeland & Henry, 2017).

1. **Assess for factors that increase the risk for aggression:**
   - Mental disorders, such as dementia, delirium, schizophrenia, and bipolar disorder
   - Being under the influence of alcohol or other drugs
   - Withdrawal from alcohol or other drugs
   - History of violence
   - Clinical conditions such as high fever, epilepsy, head trauma, and hypoglycemia
2. **Assess for anxiety:**
   - Agitation and restlessness
   - Pacing
   - Talking loudly, speaking rapidly
   - Gesturing wildly
   - Verbal aggression, such as threats, sarcasm, and swearing

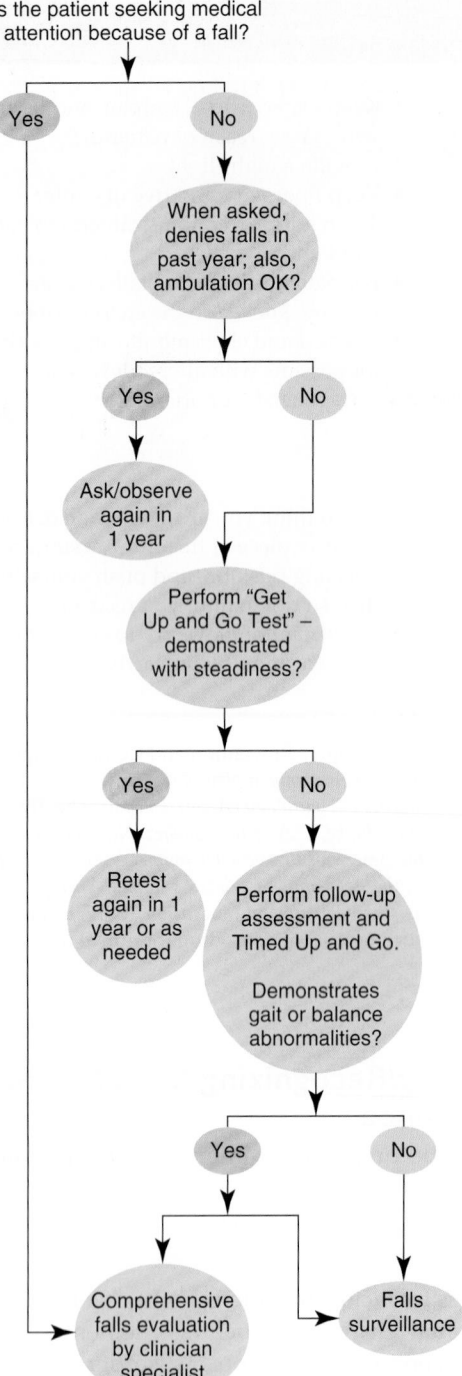

FIGURE 21-1 Falls assessment flowchart.

KnowledgeCheck 21-6

- Which assessment tool would you use for a slightly confused home care client to assess their ability to safely live alone and perform activities of daily living?
- List the six risk factors that are assessed on the Morse Fall Scale.
- How should you screen older adults to see if they need a comprehensive fall evaluation?

NURSING DIAGNOSIS/ANALYZING CUES

A few examples of Nursing Diagnosis labels (Clinical Care Classification System [CCC], n.d.) to use in describing safety problems are:

Hyperthermia	Injury Risk
Hypothermia	Poisoning Risk
Swallowing Impairment	Suffocation Risk
Falls Risk	Trauma Risk

Key Point: *Use the diagnosis Injury Risk only when the risk cannot be described by one of the more specific nursing diagnoses.*

Etiologies How would your interventions differ for each of the following two nursing diagnoses?

Fall Risk r/t poor vision secondary to cataracts
Fall Risk r/t to muscle weakness, joint instability, and poor sense of balance

The preceding nursing diagnoses illustrate that problem etiologies are important because they affect your choice of interventions. Etiologies may include environmental hazards as well as the developmental and individual risk factors discussed in the preceding sections. Keep in mind that you must state *specific* etiologies for each individual—not just general ones such as "environmental hazards." For example:

Correct: Fall Risk r/t cluttered home environment and joint instability
Incorrect: Fall Risk r/t environmental and physical factors

PLANNING/PRIORITIZING HYPOTHESIS AND GENERATING SOLUTIONS

The *NOC standardized outcomes* you use will depend on the nursing diagnosis. The following are some examples:

Community Disaster Response
Fall Prevention Behavior
Parenting Performance: Infant/Toddler Physical Safety
Personal Safety Behavior
Physical Injury Severity
Respiratory Status: Airway Patency
Safe Home Environment
Thermoregulation

Individualized goals/outcome statements you might write for a client's safety diagnoses include the following examples:

- The child will be free of injury.
- (Client) will experience no physical injury due to environmental hazards.
- Family members will describe their planned escape routes in case of fire.

IMPLEMENTATION/TAKING ACTION

NIC standardized interventions will be determined by the nursing diagnosis you use. A few examples of NIC interventions are:

Aspiration Precautions
Dementia Management
Emergency Care
Environmental
    Management:
    Worker Safety
Fall Prevention

First Aid
Home Maintenance
    Assistance
Sports-Injury
    Prevention: Youth
Surveillance

General Interventions Related to Safety

Specific nursing activities are designed to monitor and manipulate the physical environment to promote safety. The following are some general activities that provide an overview of your role in safe, effective nursing care (Thinking, Doing, Caring) in all types of settings and circumstances:

- Assess and continually monitor the safety needs of patients, based on their level of physical and cognitive function and past history of behavior.
- Provide client education to foster informed decisions and involvement in care and to facilitate postdischarge health.
- Evaluate and use techniques/processes to avoid medical/nursing errors in the delivery of client care.
- Remove hazards from the environment or modify the environment to minimize hazards and risk.
- Use technology to deliver safe, effective care.
- Establish mutual goals with clients, and teach clients about specific safety measures.
- If an accident or injury occurs in the healthcare setting, file an incident report according to agency policy. See Chapters 17 and 40 for more information on this topic.
- Urge patients to be active members of the healthcare team.

For more information to help patients participate in their care,

 The Joint Commission (TJC) website and watch **Speak Up: Know Your Rights** at http://www.jointcommission.org/multimedia/speak-up-know-your-rights/

Home Care Safety Interventions

In this section we discuss some specific interventions to address particular hazards in home care.

Prevent Poisoning in the Home

In all cases of suspected poisoning, call 911 or the local emergency number right away. Even if the person is having no

symptoms, call the Poison Control Center (PCC) as soon as possible. **The national PCC number is (800) 222-1222; they will connect you to a local PCC.**

Never induce vomiting when the ingested material is acidic or caustic to the esophagus.

- Although the American Academy of Pediatrics no longer recommends inducing emesis (e.g., with syrup of ipecac), some practitioners may still do so.
- The national PCC does not support the routine stocking of ipecac in households with young children.
- Ipecac should be given only on specific recommendation from a poison center or qualified medical personnel (Haijer et al., 2013).

For Children Nursing actions focus on teaching parents how to childproof the home and what to do if a child ingests a poisonous substance. All homes should be equipped to handle an emergency if poisoning occurs. Teach parents:

- To keep the telephone number for the nearest PCC easily accessible.
- If they suspect a child has ingested a poisonous substance, it is crucial to obtain help immediately so that there is less time for the substance to enter the child's system.

For Adults Unintentional poisoning can affect people of all ages and from all walks of life. However, middle-aged adults have the highest unintentional poisoning death rates. Advise clients of the following:

- Take only prescription medications prescribed by a healthcare professional.
- Never take larger or more frequent doses of medications to try to get faster or more powerful effects, particularly prescription pain medications.
- Never share or sell your prescription drugs.
- Be sure to follow the directions on the label when taking medications, and read all warning labels.

Advise families with older adults to prevent accidental overdose or misuse of prescribed medications by using a medication organizer for the days/times the pills are to be taken. The patient or family member may fill the organizer once a week.

For steps to prevent poisoning, see the box Home Care: Preventing Poisoning in the Home. For actions to take if poisoning occurs at home,

 Go to the Mayo Clinic website, **Poisoning First Aid,** at http://www.mayoclinic.org/first-aid/first-aid-poisoning/basics/art-20056657

Home Care

Preventing Poisoning in the Home

Young children will eat and drink almost anything. Most victims of accidental poisoning are children younger than the age of 5. Tips to prevent poisoning include the following:

Careful Words and Actions

➤ Never leave a small child unattended near household cleaning supplies or medicines, even for a moment. If you must answer the phone or doorbell, take the child with you. *Children act fast; it takes only a moment for them to swallow something.*

➤ Avoid taking medicines in front of children. *Children tend to imitate adults.*

➤ Never call medicines or vitamins "candy." Instead, use the correct name ("cough medicine," and so on).

Careful Storage

➤ Store medicines or household chemicals on high shelves or in locked cabinets and drawers. Never leave them on kitchen or bathroom counters.

➤ Store all household chemicals away from food.

➤ Keep medicines and household chemicals in their original containers. Leave the original labels on. Do NOT store chemicals in containers that normally hold food.

➤ Use child-resistant packaging for medicines and household chemicals. Close the container securely after each use.

➤ Do not assume your child is safe around substances in child-resistant containers. *Research has shown that many toddlers and preschoolers can open them.*

Careful Disposal

➤ Teach clients to take advantage of any community programs that take back unwanted medications for safe disposal (e.g., call the local trash service or a local pharmacy for options in your area).

➤ Teach clients how to safely dispose of outdated prescription medications:

  ➤ Crush the medication or add water to dissolve it.

➤ Mix the drugs with an undesirable substance such as kitty litter or used cooking grease *To make it less desirable for pets and children to eat.*

➤ Place the mixture in an empty can or resealable bag and put it in the trash.

➤ Remove all identifying information from prescription labels before throwing containers in the trash or recycling them.

➤ If disposal options are not available, medicines can be flushed down the sink or toilet when they are no longer needed (U.S. Food and Drug Administration, 2020). For a list of medicines recommended for disposal by flushing,

 Go to the FDA web site at https://www.fda.gov/drugs/safe-disposal-medicines/disposal-unused-medicines-what-you-should-know#Flush_List

Careful Environment Checks

➤ Verify that houseplants are nontoxic. Examples of toxic plants are rhododendron, philodendron, English ivy, holly, mistletoe, and lily of the valley.

➤ Find out whether any plants growing in your yard are poisonous, and if so, remove them.

➤ Teach children that they must never eat berries, wild mushrooms, or other edible-looking plants in yards, fields, and forests. *A wide variety of plants can cause illness and even death in young children.*

➤ Warn parents to keep children from chewing on windowsills and to carefully clean up flakes of paint. Advocate for clients who need to have lead-based paint replaced in their homes. *Lead-based paint can still be found in older homes, and some soil contains a high lead content. Young children often put dirt in their mouths and chew on furniture and windowsills, especially when they are teething.*

Prevent Carbon Monoxide Poisoning

Nursing interventions include teaching prevention measures, such as the following:

■ Buy, install, and maintain a home CO detector.
■ Ensure that gas or wood-burning appliances are adequately vented to the outside.
■ Repair rust holes or defects in vehicles that could allow exhaust fumes to enter the passenger compartment.
■ Do not use a kerosene heater, gas oven, or gas range to heat a house, even for a short time.
■ Never operate gasoline-powered engines, such as automobiles, generators, or lawn mowers, in confined spaces, such as garages or basements, or near open doors or windows.

■ Never burn charcoal inside a home, cabin, recreational vehicle, or tent—not even in a fireplace.

If CO intoxication is suspected, the person should be treated with 100% humidified oxygen. A simple blood test may be done to confirm CO levels in the blood.

Prevent Home Fires

Nursing interventions include teaching families how to prevent fires and measures to take should a fire occur. Stress the following:

■ **Have a warning system.** Have working smoke alarms and change the batteries every 6 months or more often. Keep a phone near the bed or chair for people who have limited mobility.

- **Have an escape plan.** Develop a home fire escape plan and practice it at least twice a year.
  - Keep a rope or other type of ladder for escape from rooms above ground level.
  - Have a fire extinguisher in the home, and know where it is located and how to use it.
  - Check fire extinguishers regularly, and replace them when they become outdated.
- **Have a preventive frame of mind.** When decorating holiday trees and the exterior of your home, always use fire-safe lights. Do not leave light sets hung on the outside of your home year after year. Always unplug holiday tree lights before leaving home, and remove the tree from the home when it becomes dry. Other cautions include:
  - Never leave burning candles unattended. Do not use candles near curtains or other flammable materials.
  - For charcoal grills, use only charcoal starter fluids designed for barbecue grills.
  - For gas grills, be sure that the hose connection is tight, and check hoses for leaks.
  - Store flammable materials (e.g., oil-soaked rags) in appropriate containers (e.g., metal container with a tight lid).
  - Do not smoke, especially in bed—and especially in a home where oxygen is in use.
  - Never use an open flame when oxygen is in use.
- **Promote electrical safety in the home.** Make sure electrical outlets have covers. Routinely inspect electrical appliances for damaged cords; replace frayed cords. Do not place electrical cords under carpets, and make sure cords do not hang off tables and countertops.
- **Know what to do if a fire occurs.** The actions you take to extinguish a small fire depend on the source of the fire. For example:
  - Never pour water on a grease fire.
  - Never discharge a fire extinguisher into a pan fire.
  - If there is an oven fire, turn off the heat and keep the door closed.
  - If there is a microwave fire, keep the door closed and unplug the microwave.

  Key Point: *If the house is on fire, follow your escape plan. Crawl or stay low to the floor as much as possible to avoid the smoke.*

Prevent Scalds and Burns in the Home

Fire is not the only cause of thermal injuries. Teach clients how to avoid scalds and burns from other causes:

- Turn pot handles toward the back of the stove so that children cannot tip them over.
- Never wear loose-fitting clothing when cooking.
- **Key Point:** *Avoid warming infant formula and food in the microwave. Many parents ignore this advice, so also tell them to always check the temperature of formula and food carefully before giving it to the child.*

- Remove lids or other coverings from microwaved food carefully.
- Do not smoke, use matches, or drink hot liquids while holding an infant.
- Do not leave burning cigarettes unattended.
- Always check bath water temperature for children and older adults, and set the water heater temperature low enough to prevent scalds.
- Place guardrails in front of radiators and fireplaces.
- Wear protective clothing and sunscreen when outside.

KnowledgeCheck 21-7

- Identify four safety measures that decrease the risk of scalds or burns in the child.
- What are some specific activities that reduce the possibility of fires in the home?

Prevent Firearm Injuries

Education is an essential intervention to prevent unintentional firearm injuries involving children. The American Academy of Pediatrics (2021) and other groups have mounted efforts to educate parents so that they will be able to make smart choices related to gun safety. You can help by teaching gun owners that it is important to store firearms unloaded and in a secure, locked container when not in use and to store ammunition in a different location from the firearm. Suggest that they participate in gun safety courses and know the following rules for safe gun handling (National Rifle Association Headquarters, n.d.-a.):

- Always keep the gun pointed in a safe direction so that even if it were to go off, it would not cause injury or damage.
- Never put your finger on the trigger until you are ready to shoot.
- Always keep the gun unloaded until ready to use it.
- Before cleaning a gun, make absolutely sure that it is unloaded. If you do not know how to open the gun and inspect the chamber(s), leave it alone and get help from someone who does.

Teaching Children Even if parents avoid having guns in their own home, it is possible that children will encounter them in other places. Urge parents to teach children safe behavior around firearms and to be sure children know what to do if they see a gun (e.g., at a friend's house or in school):

1. Stop.
2. Don't touch it.
3. Leave the area.
4. Tell an adult. (National Rifle Association Headquarters, n.d.-b.)

Prevent Suffocation

Clients should recognize and teach children the universal sign for choking: grasping the neck between the thumb and index finger or clutching the neck with both hands (Fig. 21-2). It is also important to teach

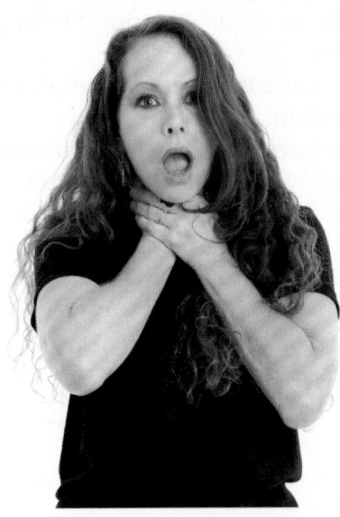

FIGURE 21-2 The universal sign for choking.

clients the following measures to prevent suffocation or asphyxiation:

- Inspect toys for small, removable parts.
- Do not attach pacifiers, rattles, or other infant toys to ribbons or strings.
- Do not use sweatshirts or jackets with necktie strings.
- Position mobiles well above the crib, and remove them once the baby begins to push up on hands and knees or by age 5 months, whichever comes first.
- Keep window blind cords out of the child's reach.
- Store plastic bags away from young children in a secure place.
- Ensure that the crib is designed to meet federal regulations: Crib slats must be less than $2\frac{3}{8}$ inches (6 cm) apart, and the mattress must fit snugly.
- When feeding children meat, cheese, or other firm foods, cut the food into very tiny pieces.
- Do not give a young child hard candy, chewing gum, nuts, popcorn, grapes, or marshmallows.
- Supervise children's balloon play, and dispose of burst balloons promptly.

Choking Rescue

Teach adults, and suggest they teach their children, the universal sign for choking (see Fig. 21-2). Also teach the basic first aid for choking, but explain that choking rescue is a skill that is best taught using supervised practice with a mannequin. Recommend that clients attend classes presented by organizations such as the Red Cross or the American Heart Association. **Key Point:** *The most important thing to remember when someone is choking is to have someone call 911 immediately.*

The Choking Rescue Maneuver This maneuver is an emergency procedure for removing a foreign object lodged in the airway. It lifts the diaphragm and forces enough air from the lungs to create an artificial cough. The cough should move and expel the obstruction from the airway. The **Heimlich maneuver** makes use of

abdominal thrusts only. The American Red Cross (2015) alternates five back blows with five abdominal thrusts until the blockage is dislodged. For more details about the choking rescue procedure,

 Go to Chapter 21, **Clinical Insight 21-1: Choking Rescue Maneuver,** in Volume 2.

- You can obtain a summary and illustration of the Heimlich at the U.S. National Library of Medicine, MedlinePlus, at this URL:

 https://medlineplus.gov/ency/imagepages/18152.htm

- There is also a YouTube video at:

 https://youtu.be/XOTbjDGZ7wg

Prevent Drowning

Drowning is a form of suffocation but is discussed separately here for convenience. Teach clients the following water safety measures:

- Supervise activity when the child is near any source of water.
- Children up to age 4 are especially at risk for drowning and should never be left unattended in or near a bathtub, hot tub, swimming pool, or other source of water. Even wading pools, toilets, and mop buckets hold enough water to drown a small child.
- Do not allow children to run around a pool or dive in shallow areas.
- If you have a pool, be sure it has a barrier (e.g., tall fence) to prevent children from gaining access.
- Insist that children use personal flotation devices (e.g., lifejackets, not float toys). This is controversial, however. Some authorities regard flotation devices as toys that provide false security; others say anything that reduces a child's fear of the water is positive because it is the fear reaction that leads to drowning.

Prevent Take-Home Toxins

Most preventive measures apply to the workplace. However, you can teach clients who are at risk to remove work clothing and to shower, preferably in an open-air shower, before leaving work. If facilities for showering are not available, patient advocacy may be appropriate. (To learn about advocacy, see Chapter 40.)

- If exposed workers have not showered at work, they should remove their clothing, then shower immediately upon entering the home.
- When handling contaminated clothes or objects, they should wear gloves to reduce the risk of skin transmission.
- Laundering may not be effective in removing certain toxins from clothes.

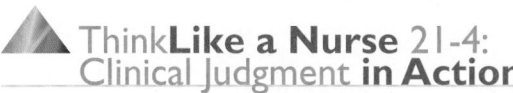

ThinkLike a Nurse 21-4: Clinical Judgment in Action

You are having dinner in a restaurant and notice that the guest at the table beside you seems to be choking.

- What is the universal sign for choking?
- What is the first action you should take?

KnowledgeCheck 21-8

- List two things a person who works around workplace toxins can do to prevent bringing them into the home.
- What specific safety measures would you discuss with a mother to prevent choking in her 9-month-old child?

Community Interventions: Teaching for Safety Self-Care

In addition to teaching home safety to clients, you should also teach to promote safety self-care related to particular hazards in the community and environment.

Motor Vehicle Safety

Anticipatory guidance and educational programs are important measures for improving motor vehicle safety for all age-groups. You may also wish to become politically active on the issue of motor vehicle safety. For instance, you might petition your city council for a

stop sign at a particularly dangerous intersection or a reduced speed limit on a highway.

Also teach clients the following measures for avoiding motor vehicle injuries:

- Be cautious when walking or bicycling on the roadway, and observe all laws.
- Do not drink alcohol or take unprescribed or recreational drugs and drive. Have a designated driver.
- Do not engage in distracting activities while driving (e.g., using cell phones, texting, changing the music, applying cosmetics).
- Observe the speed limits.
- Always wear seat belts while driving, and periodically check belts to ensure safe operation.
- Buckle children properly in age-appropriate safety seats in the back seat of the car. If in doubt about how to use safety seats, ask the local police department to check the installation of your child safety seat. See Table 21-4.

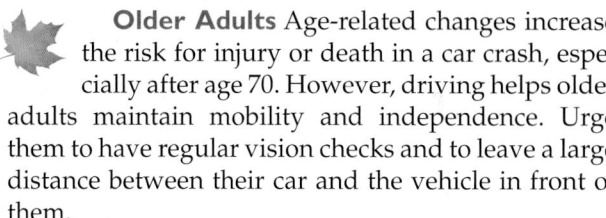 **Older Adults** Age-related changes increase the risk for injury or death in a car crash, especially after age 70. However, driving helps older adults maintain mobility and independence. Urge them to have regular vision checks and to leave a large distance between their car and the vehicle in front of them.

Table 21-4 ➤ Types of Car Safety Seats

AGE	TYPE OF SEAT	GUIDELINES
Infants younger than 1 year old	"Infant-only" (These are small and may have carrying handles or be part of a stroller system.)	Use rear-facing seats from birth to ages 2–4 years old or until they reach the upper weight or height limits specified by the seat manufacturer).

FIGURE 21-3 Infant car seat with infant in rear-facing position in the middle of the back seat.

(Continued)

Table 21-4 ➤ Types of Car Safety Seats—cont'd

AGE	TYPE OF SEAT	GUIDELINES
Toddlers and preschoolers	"Convertible" (can be used rear-facing, then converted to forward facing)	Rear-facing seats are safer for toddlers up to age 4 yr. It is best to ride rear-facing as long as possible (until they reach the height and weight maximum specified by the seat manufacturer).
School-age children	Booster seats	After outgrowing their car safety seat, children should stay in a booster seat until the car seat belts fit properly (usually at about 4 ft 9 in. tall and between 9 and 12 years old). Booster seats are safer than a seat belt alone.
Older children	Car lap and shoulder belts	Children can use a seat belt once it fits them properly. Seat belts fit properly when the lap belt lays across the upper thighs (not the stomach) and the shoulder belt lays across the chest (not the neck). Some experts recommend that anyone weighing <110 lb, regardless of age, ride in the back seat. Riding in the back seat is associated with a 40% reduction in the risk of fatal injury and up to a 46% reduction in cars with airbags.

Note: These are guidelines, not legal requirements. Some states may also have laws governing the types and use of car safety seats. You should be familiar with the laws in your area.

For in-depth information about child safety seats,

 Go to the **American Academy of Pediatrics Web site** at https://healthychildren.org/English/safety-prevention/on-the-go/Pages/Car-Safety-Seats-Information-for-Families.aspx

Sources: American Academy of Pediatrics (2021). *Car seats: Information for families.* https://healthychildren.org/English/safety-prevention/on-the-go/Pages/Car-Safety-Seats-Information-for-Families.aspx; Centers for Disease Control and Prevention. (2021b). *Child passenger safety.* http://www.cdc.gov/features/passengersafety/

Food Safety

Teach clients safe food handling and other preventive measures, such as the "4 Cs of food safety": **C**lean, **C**ook, **C**ombat cross-contamination, **C**hill. For further explanation of the 4 Cs, refer to the Self-Care box, Food Safety.

Fighting Vector-Borne Pathogens

The following are points you can use to teach clients about strategies to combat the vectors of mosquitoes, ticks, and rodents (CDC, 2021d; EPA, 2022a).

Mosquitoes Public strategies to control mosquitoes include spraying programs and digging ditches to promote drainage from stagnant areas. Individuals can help by taking the following actions:

- Remove sources of stagnant water.
  - Empty standing water in old tires, buckets, toys, or other outdoor containers.
  - Change water in birdbaths, fountains, wading pools, and potted plant trays at least once a week to destroy mosquito habitats.
  - Keep rain gutters unclogged.
  - Treat swimming pools with the proper chemicals, and keep the water circulating.
- **Kill or repel mosquitoes.**
  - Use "bug zappers" or citronella candles for evening outdoor activities.

Self-Care

Food Safety

Clean

➤ Wash hands and surfaces often. Always wash your hands with soap and water before handling or preparing food and before eating.

➤ Don't be a source of foodborne illness yourself:

➤ Avoid preparing food for others if you have a diarrheal illness.

➤ Avoid changing a baby's diaper while preparing food.

➤ Wash produce. Rinse fresh fruits and vegetables in running tap water to remove visible dirt.

➤ Remove and discard the outermost leaves of a head of lettuce or cabbage.

➤ Never use a cutting board, knife, or other object that was used to prepare meat, poultry, or fish for any other purpose until it has been thoroughly washed in hot, soapy water.

➤ Be careful not to contaminate foods while slicing them up on the cutting board. Bacteria grow well on the cut surface of fruits or vegetables.

➤ Wash hands with soap after handling reptiles, birds, or baby chicks and after contact with pet feces.

Cook

➤ Use a thermometer to measure the internal temperature of meat.

➤ Cook to temperatures sufficient to kill bacteria:

Ground beef to an internal temperature of 160°F (71°C).

Leftovers and casseroles, 165°F (74°C)

Beef, lamb, and veal, 145°F (63°C)

Pork and ground beef, 160°F (71°C)

Whole poultry and thighs, 180°F (82°C)

Poultry breasts, 170°F (77°C)

Ground chicken, 165°F (74°C)

Stuffed fish, 165°F (74°C)

Roast meats at an oven temperature of 300°F (149°C) or above.

➤ Cook eggs until the yolk is firm. Do not eat raw or partially cooked eggs.

➤ Hold hot food above 140°F (60°C) and for no more than 2 hours.

Combat Cross-Contamination (Separate)

➤ Avoid cross-contaminating goods by washing hands, utensils, and cutting boards after they have been in contact with raw meat or poultry and before they touch another food.

➤ Put cooked meat on a clean platter, rather than back on one that held the raw meat.

Chill

➤ Refrigerate leftovers within 4 hours. Bacteria multiply quickly at room temperature.

➤ Avoid leaving cut produce (e.g., fruits, vegetables) at room temperature for a prolonged time.

➤ Chill cooked foods rapidly in a shallow (2-inch-deep) container. Large volumes of food will cool more quickly if they are divided into several shallow containers for refrigeration.

➤ Do not buy partially thawed items. Be sure they are frozen solid.

➤ Use a cooler to transport foods when the temperature is above 80°F (27°C).

➤ Store deli meat for only 1 or 2 days.

➤ Use thermometers in the refrigerator and freezer.

Keep freezer temperature at 0°F (−18°C) or below.

Keep refrigerator temperature at 40°F (4°C) or below.

➤ Thaw foods in the refrigerator or under cold running water. Use the microwave to thaw foods only if you are going to continue cooking them at that time.

➤ Pack lunches in insulated containers. You can refrigerate or freeze sandwiches before packing to keep them cold.

Store

➤ Cover and date food.

➤ Store vegetables and fruit separately from uncooked meats.

➤ Do not store food in decorative containers unless they are labeled safe for food. Some types of crystal and pottery, for example, have high lead content.

➤ Store cleaning supplies away from food.

Report

Report suspected foodborne illnesses to your local health department. The local public health department is an important part of the food safety system. Often, calls from concerned citizens are how outbreaks are first detected.

Other

➤ Never eat any food that has an odor or that might be spoiled.

➤ Be aware that some imported folk remedies, such as *greta* (which is used by some Hispanic patients for colic), may be contaminated with lead.

➤ Observe sanitation reports before selecting eating establishments in the community.

Sources: Centers for Disease Control and Prevention. (2021c). *Food safety.* https://www.cdc.gov/foodsafety/; FoodSafety.gov. (2021). *Keep food safe.* http://www.foodsafety.gov/keep/index.html; U.S. Food and Drug Administration. (n.d.). *Food.* https://www.fda.gov/food

- Use EPA-registered mosquito repellents when necessary, and follow label directions carefully.
- All repellents and pesticides should have the name and amount of active ingredient on the label. **Key Point:** *No pesticide is 100% safe, so people must use them cautiously.*

- **Avoid mosquitoes if you can.**
  - Repair holes in window and door screens.
  - Replace outdoor lights with yellow "bug" lights. They will attract fewer mosquitoes but are not repellents.
  - If you go into areas with high mosquito populations (e.g., salt marshes, deep woods), wear head nets, long sleeves, and long pants.
  - If there is a mosquito-borne disease alert, stay indoors during the evening when mosquitoes are active.
- **Consult the experts.** Contact your local health department if you have questions about mosquitoes or about a spraying program.

Ticks   When walking in tick-infested areas:

- Use DEET-containing insect repellent. Reapply it every few hours (or according to the label). Formulations as high as 50% are recommended for adults and children over the age of 2 months. Use with caution for children. Wash off repellent at night before going to bed.
- When wearing sunscreen, apply sunscreen first and then repellent.
- Treat clothing with permethrin-containing or other insect repellents.
- Wear light-colored clothing. Ticks are attracted to dark colors; also, it is easier to see a tick on light-colored clothing.
- Wear long-sleeved shirts, tucked in. Pull socks up over pant legs.
- After walking in wooded areas, inspect your body, especially in the hair and skin folds. Use a mirror to view all parts of your body.
- Remove ticks right away. This can prevent some infections, such as Lyme disease or Rocky Mountain spotted fever. For instructions on how to remove attached ticks,

 Go to the CDC Web site at http://www.cdc.gov/ticks/removing_a_tick.html

Rodents and Other Animals   To control rodents, raccoons, and other small animals, remove as many food and water sources as possible. Advise clients to do the following:

- Cover food and clean up immediately after meals.
- Do not leave unwashed dishes on counters and in sinks.
- Keep garbage in closed containers that cannot be overturned.
- Repair holes and cracks in the exterior structure of the home, as well as in walls, closets, and attics; around sinks and cabinets; and so on.

- Use commercial traps or hire professional exterminators.
- Participate in neighborhood cleanup projects.

Keep in mind that rat and mice poisons and baits can be fatal and should not be used in areas accessible to children and pets.

Reducing Pollution

Teach families that they can help to reduce pollution from solid and hazardous wastes, as well as air and noise pollution of the environment. Refer to the following tips:

Air Pollution   To help reduce air pollution, pay attention to air-quality warnings, and restrict time spent in high-traffic areas. You might also participate in carpools or use public transportation whenever possible.

Noise Pollution   Two specific interventions you can teach clients to help prevent irreversible hearing loss are to:

- Avoid exposure to high noise levels.
- Wear protective devices (e.g., ear plugs) in environments with a high noise level.

Hazardous Waste   The following are tips for safe disposal:

- **Information.** Contact the local refuse-disposal company for instructions about the proper disposal of hazardous waste (e.g., paints, solvents, pesticides, cleaners, rechargeable batteries).
- **Products.** Use the least hazardous products available; use only the amount necessary for a project. Share leftover materials with neighbors.
- **Motor oil.** Never dump motor oil into storm drains. For old oil and tires, call your local waste-management company or a local quick-lube or tire dealer for recommendations regarding disposal.
- **Batteries.** Talk to an automotive dealer or repair service about recycling or trading in car and other batteries.

Solid Waste   Proper disposal and recycling of solid wastes helps to prevent pollution. Remember the 4 **R**s: **R**educe, **R**euse, **R**ecycle, and **R**espond

Reduce the amount of trash discarded (e.g., don't buy products that have unnecessary packaging).

Reuse containers, bags, and products; sell or donate instead of throwing items out.

Recycle by using and buying recyclable and recycled products; compost yard trimmings.

Respond by educating others, expressing preferences for less waste (e.g., to manufacturers, merchants).

Weather Hazard Safety Measures

Teach clients that if they are aware of what weather event is about to affect their area, they are more likely to survive it. Before severe weather strikes, suggest that clients:

1. **Develop a disaster plan** at home, work, school, and when outdoors. The American Red Cross offers planning tips and information on putting together a disaster supply kit at:

 the American Red Cross website at http://www.redcross.org/

2. **Identify a safe place to take shelter.** For information on how to build a safe room in your home or school,

 go to the Federal Emergency Management Agency Web site at https://www.fema.gov/emergency-managers/risk-management/safe-rooms

3. **Know the county/parish in which you live or visit** and in what part of that county you are located. The National Weather Service issues severe weather warnings on a county/parish basis or for a portion of a county/parish.

4. **Keep a highway map nearby** to follow storm movement from weather bulletins.

5. **Have a Weather Radio receiver unit with a warning alarm** tone and battery backup to receive warning bulletins.

6. **Check the weather forecast before leaving for extended periods outdoors.** Watch for signs of approaching storms.

7. **If severe weather threatens, check on people** who are older, very young, or physically or mentally disabled. Don't forget about pets and farm animals.

Implementation/Taking Action: Promoting Safety in the Healthcare Facility

The following interventions will help you to prevent common accidents in the healthcare setting.

Implementation/Taking Action for Example Client Condition: Falls

Key Point: *Perhaps the most important thing you can do to prevent falls is to identify those who are at risk for them.* Nursing actions to prevent falls are based on the cues identified at the initial assessment. For a summary of actions, review the Example Problem: Falls.

To see a care plan and care map for Fall Risk,

 Go to Davis Advantage, Resources, Chapter 21, **Care Plan** and **Care Map.**

Reducing Electrical Hazards

Electrical hazards are a major cause of fires in healthcare agencies. The following interventions help reduce electrical hazards:

- Before use, have all electrically powered equipment and accessory equipment evaluated by facilities management.

- The Joint Commission standards mandate that all employees participate in education and training programs for electrical safety.
- If an electrical safety hazard is suspected, clearly label the malfunctioning equipment and send it for inspection.
- Use three-pronged electrical plugs whenever possible.
- Observe for breaks or frays in electrical cords.

Preventing and Responding to Fires

You must know your agency's procedures for responding to a fire, including how to evacuate patients from the building. Remember: **R-A-C-E.**

- **Rescue the patient**—Remove the patient from immediate danger. Move patient(s) into the corridor, and close doors to the affected area.
- **Activate the alarm**—Report the location and kind of fire, and identify yourself. Activate the nearest alarm.
- **Confine the fire**—Close all doors and windows. Turn off all oxygen valves after coordinating with the charge nurse.
- **Extinguish the fire**—Use the proper extinguisher. Stay between the fire and the path to safety. Keep low.

Key Point: *If you discover a fire, your first instinct may be to contain or put out the fire. Fight that instinct. Your first action is to rescue the patient.* You should try to extinguish (the E step) the fire only after the R-A-C steps are completed and only if it is a small fire that is contained to one area, such as a trash can. If the fire gets out of control, leave the area immediately.

Extinguisher Classifications You should know where the extinguishers are located in your facility and know how to use them. Most agencies use multipurpose (Class ABC) extinguishers.

Class A—Wood, paper, rubber, textiles, plastics
Class B—Flammable liquids, gases, oils, solvents, paints, or greases
Class C—Live electrical wires or equipment
Class D—Combustible metals (e.g., potassium, magnesium, titanium)
Class K—Kitchen fires involving cooking oils and fats

Preventing the Need for Restraints

Key Point: *Restraints are a last resort. The current standard of care is restraint-free.* The following nursing interventions provide less restrictive alternatives to using restraints for patients who are confused or otherwise cognitively impaired.

Provide Consistency Keep the environment and the caregivers as consistent as possible. To help relieve anxiety, encourage family and friends to:

- Remain with the patient around the clock for a few days after admission
- Help with the patient's care
- Bring familiar objects from home

Review the Patient's Medications Determine whether they may affect mental status or balance.

Provide Relaxation and Relieve Anxiety Relieving anxiety helps to prevent wandering. You may wish to try some of the following measures:

- Orient patients and families to their surroundings; reorient as often as necessary.
- Provide consistency of caregivers and environment.
- Use therapeutic touch and relaxation techniques, such as massage.
- Use the least invasive and most comfortable method to deliver care. For example, use a toileting schedule or provide a bedpan instead of inserting a urinary catheter, or encourage and provide oral fluids to avoid inserting an IV for hydration.
- Discontinue treatments that cause discomfort or agitation as soon as possible. For example, some patients become agitated and pull at or try to escape sensations from indwelling catheters, intravenous catheters, and nasogastric tubes.

Provide Frequent Assessment and Surveillance Use one-to-one supervision as needed and encourage family members and friends to stay or to hire sitters for clients who need supervision. Place patients with cognitive deficits or patients who need supervision for other reasons near the nursing station. Check on them frequently. Assess all patients regularly for cognitive changes.

Find Ways to Communicate This is essential, even though it may be difficult to communicate with patients who have cognitive deficits. Assess the patient's communication abilities to determine whether they can let you know what they need and want. You will need to be especially alert for body language, such as gestures, nods, and eye contact, because these may be the patient's only way of communicating.

- Speak clearly, calmly, and slowly.
- Smile and face the patient.
- Ask the patient directly what they need, for example, "Do you need the bathroom?"
- Word questions so that the patient can answer with a yes or no.

Modify the Environment Some simple ways to prevent agitation and confusion are to:

- Reduce noise on the unit and provide adequate light.
- Use music therapy for a calming effect.
- Use wedge cushions and body props for patients sitting in chairs to help them maintain good posture in the chair. These help keep patients from slumping and falling out of the chair.
- Use low beds for patients who are likely to fall or wander.
- It may be best to remove bed rails in some situations.
- Keep doors to the unit locked if this is feasible and acceptable.

- In long-term care facilities, also lock outside doors. Have a staff member at main entrances and exits.

For types of alarms and specific instructions about using bed alarms,

 Go to **Procedure 21-1: Using Bed and Chair Monitoring Devices,** in Volume 2.

Anticipate Unmet Needs Patients often try to get out of bed because they have a need they cannot express. The best way to achieve restraint-free care is to individualize care to avoid the risky behavior. Look for the meaning of disruptive behaviors (e.g., the wandering patient may be thirsty or in pain). The following are examples of actions to anticipate patient needs:

- Plan an elimination routine based on the patient's history; patients often try to get out of bed because they need to go to the toilet.
- Provide pain relief and other comfort measures to decrease agitation.
- Provide diversional activities.

Key Point: *Sometimes restraints are necessary to ensure the immediate physical safety of the patient or others.* When that occurs, follow organization policies, and always use the least restrictive restraint that ensures safety.

For a summary of using restraints, see the Highlights of Procedures box. To learn in more detail about applying and using restraints,

 Go to **Procedure 21-2: Using Restraints,** and **Clinical Insight 21-3: What You Should Know About Using Restraints,** in Volume 2.

Responding to Mercury Spills

If a mercury spill is not properly cleaned, the mercury can remain in cracks and crevices for long periods of time and cause continuous exposure to mercury vapors. Large spills usually must be cleaned by a pollution control agency and can be very costly. It is especially difficult to remove mercury spills from carpets, so carpets usually have to be disposed of as hazardous waste. If you must clean mercury spills of 25 mL or less (e.g., from a broken glass thermometer), consult Box 21-3.

Keeping Equipment Safe

The following interventions help ensure safe use of equipment:

- Seek advice if you are unsure how to operate the equipment.
- Make sure medical equipment has been properly inspected.
- Be alert to signs that the equipment is not functioning properly.
- Make sure that rooms are not cluttered with equipment.

Highlights of Procedures 21-1 and 21-2

 For steps to follow in *all* procedures, refer to the Universal Steps for All Procedures found on the inside back cover of Volume 2. Go to the full procedures in Volume 2 to practice and learn the procedure steps. Use these procedure highlights later to help you review key points.

Procedure 21-1: Using a Bed Monitoring Device

➤ Select the correct type of alarm for your patient.

➤ Explain to the patient and family that the device alerts the staff when the patient tries to get out of the chair or bed.

➤ Apply or place the device; connect the control unit to the sensor pad.

➤ Connect the control unit to the nurse call system, if possible.

➤ Explain that the patient will need to call for assistance when wanting to get up.

➤ Disconnect or turn off the alarm before assisting the patient out of the bed or chair.

➤ Reactivate the alarm after assisting the patient back to the bed or chair.

➤ Understand that bed alarms do not prevent falls by themselves; they are used to improve the timeliness of staff response. Patients who are at risk for falls require increased observation and surveillance.

Procedure 21-2: Using Restraints

➤ Follow agency policy, state laws, and professional guidelines.

➤ Try alternative interventions, such as the following, first:

Bed/chair alarms

Patient sitters (nonprofessional staff hired to watch the patient)

➤ Use the least-invasive method among the various types of restraints:

Verbal restraints

Chemical restraints (e.g., antipsychotic or sedative medication)

Seclusion (safe containment to deescalate)

Physical restraints (4-point devices, tie-on, Velcro, leather)

➤ Use restraints only as a last resort to protect a patient and/or caregiver from injury, not for the convenience of the caregiver or as a punishment.

➤ Obtain the required consent form.

➤ Obtain a medical order before restraining, except in an emergency.

➤ Secure restraints in a way that allows for quick release.

➤ Ensure that restraints do not impair circulation or tissue integrity.

➤ Check restraints every 30 minutes.

➤ A prescriber must reassess and reorder the restraints every 24 hours.

➤ Release restraints and assess every 2 hours (more often for behavioral restraints).

BOX 21-3 ■ What to Do If There Is a Mercury Spill

✚ Do not touch mercury droplets. Mercury vaporizes; the toxic vapors can be inhaled or absorbed through the skin.

In the Healthcare Agency

✚ If you are not trained in the procedure, do not attempt to clean up a mercury spill. Notify the environmental services department.

- Keep people and animals away from the area.
- Clean the spill promptly.
- If you are trained, use a commercially made mercury spill kit. All healthcare facilities should have them. Spill kits should contain gloves, protective glasses, mercury-absorbing powder, special mercury sponges, and a disposal bag. Some kits have filtered vacuum equipment.
- Follow agency guidelines and instructions in the kit.
- Clean beads off skin, clothing, and disposable items. Place cleaning materials and disposable items in the disposal bag and seal. Follow agency policy for laundering clothing.
- On hard surfaces, use a flashlight to search for beads.
- Change clothing that has been contaminated.

- Wash well. Shower and wash your hair as soon as possible so that you do not unknowingly carry mercury home.
- Ventilate the area well to reduce the concentration of mercury vapors. Promote exhaust ventilation if possible.
- Complete an occurrence report.

In the Home and Community

- If you do not have a spill kit, wear rubber gloves and eye protection; use paper towels for cleanup and a plastic bag for disposal.
- Keep people and pets away from the area.
- Wipe beads off skin, clothing, and disposable items. Place disposable items in a plastic bag and seal with tape.
- On hard surfaces, use cardboard to scrape up the beads and pour them into a can or jar with a lid. Then wash the area.
- Shower or wash well.
- Keep the area well ventilated for several days.
- Do not use a broom or vacuum cleaner. These will just spread the mercury around and be contaminated by it.
- Do not flush mercury or cleaning materials down a toilet or drain.
- Do not wash and reuse contaminated materials.

- Follow agency policies regarding equipment brought from the patient's home (e.g., hair dryers, electric shavers, radios); usually these should be inspected for proper grounding and safe cords.

Reducing Alarm Fatigue

The American Association of Critical-Care Nurses (AACN, 2018) suggests the following nursing actions:

- Provide proper skin preparation for electrocardiogram (ECG) electrodes.
- Change ECG electrodes at least daily.
- Set alarm parameters and levels on ECG monitors to meet individual needs.
- Collaborate with the interprofessional team to customize delay and threshold settings on oxygen saturation via pulse oximetry (SpO_2) monitors.
- Provide education about devices with alarms.
- Establish interprofessional teams to address issues such as the development of policies and procedures related to alarms.
- Monitor only those patients with clinical indications for monitoring, as determined by the interprofessional team.

For more explanation about the AACN strategies to reduce alarm fatigue and improve patient safety:

 Go to the AACN Practice Alert: Alarm Management at https://www.aacn.org/clinical-resources/practice-alerts/managing-alarms-in-acute-care-across-the-life-span

Coping With Violence

Some agencies have a "public safety room." Patients who have been arrested and brought to the hospital for blood and urine testing or any hostile patient who has risk factors for violence should receive care in the public safety room. The following are other interventions for preventing and protecting yourself from violence (Ackley & Ladwig, 2019; Butcher et al., 2018; Doenges et al., 2019):

- Intervene to relieve anxiety. Anxiety often precedes violent behavior.
- Treat underlying medical conditions. For example, give medications or check blood glucose levels.
- Administer sedatives such as diazepam or lorazepam. There may be standing prescriptions for these.
- Use a calm, reassuring approach.
- Avoid using threatening, aggressive body language.
- Don't respond to anger with anger.
- Don't defend when the patient is verbally aggressive.
- Don't wear a stethoscope around your neck, dangling jewelry, or anything a patient might use to hurt you.
- If you know you will be receiving a patient who is angry or violent, remove objects from the room that could be used as a weapon.
- Don't go into a room alone with a patient who is angry or violent.

- Keep the room door open; do not let the patient get between you and the door.
- Remain at least an arm's length away from the patient who is angry or violent.
- Do not turn your back on a patient who is angry or violent.
- Do not touch the patient without permission, unless you intend to physically restrain them.
- Protect others in the environment. Follow the department's safety guidelines.
- As a last resort, use mechanical restraints if ordered and as necessary.
- **Key Point:** *Your priority must be your own safety and the safety of others in the area.*

Which Safety Interventions Can I Delegate?

As a nurse manager or a primary care nurse, you may need to delegate safety promotion interventions to UAP. For all delegation decisions, refer to the discussion and guidelines in Chapter 3.

- **Restraints.** One safety activity you might delegate is applying restraints. As in all delegation, you must first be sure that the UAP is competent to perform the skill. You may delegate the application of the restraints; however, you may *not* delegate the assessment of the patient's status or the evaluation of the patient's response to the restraints. You may assign the UAP to:
  - Remove and reapply restraints to provide skin care and allow for supervised movement.
  - Observe for skin excoriation under or around the restraint location and report it to you.
- **Other measures.** You should be sure UAPs are aware of and follow all safety measures and institutional procedures. For example, you can expect the UAP to remove clutter and spills in patient rooms, to provide patients with nonskid slippers, and to lock beds and wheelchairs.

 To explore learning resources for this chapter,

 Go to Davis Advantage **and find:**

Answers and Suggested Responses for all questions in this chapter

Concept Map

Knowledge Map

References and Bibliography

CHAPTER 22

Facilitating Hygiene

Learning Outcomes

After completing this chapter, you should be able to:

➤ Explain how personal hygiene relates to health and well-being.

➤ Identify factors influencing personal hygiene practices.

➤ Discuss delegation of hygiene activities to unlicensed assistive personnel (UAP).

➤ Discuss the nurse's role in determining a client's self-care ability.

➤ Identify nursing diagnoses related to self-care ability and hygiene practices.

➤ Describe assessments to make when providing hygiene care of the skin, feet, nails, mouth, hair, eyes, ears, and nose.

➤ Describe the following types of baths: complete, assist, partial, towel, bag, shower, tub, and therapeutic.

➤ Apply the nursing process to common hygiene-related problems of the skin, feet, nails, mouth, hair, eyes, ears, and nose.

➤ Demonstrate nursing skills to promote patient hygiene (such as bathing, foot care, and bed making).

➤ Demonstrate care of the eyes, ears, and teeth, including glasses, contacts, hearing aids, and dentures.

➤ Discuss the relationship between a patient's overall well-being and the immediate environment.

Key Concepts

Activities of daily living
Hygiene
Self-care ability

Related Concepts

See the Concept Map on Davis Advantage.

Example Problem

Hygiene Self-Care Deficit

Meet Your Patients

You and an unlicensed assistive personnel (UAP) are to assist the following patients with their hygiene.

■ Mrs. Rosha, a 76-year-old Asian woman of Indian heritage who was admitted yesterday after suffering a stroke that paralyzed her right side. She is now unable to speak clearly and becomes frustrated as she attempts to communicate her needs. Her daughter says Mrs. Rosha is a proud and tidy woman who has been living alone and caring for herself independently since her husband's death last year, even maintaining the yard and garden. She wears eyeglasses for reading and driving and has a hearing aid.

■ Mr. Fuller, a 68-year-old Orthodox Jewish man admitted last week after a massive heart attack. Although his eyes are open, he does not respond to external stimuli. Because of impaired swallowing, Mr. Fuller is unable to take food or fluid orally. A feeding tube was placed to ensure adequate nutrition and hydration. His oral mucous membranes and lips are dry and crusty. He is

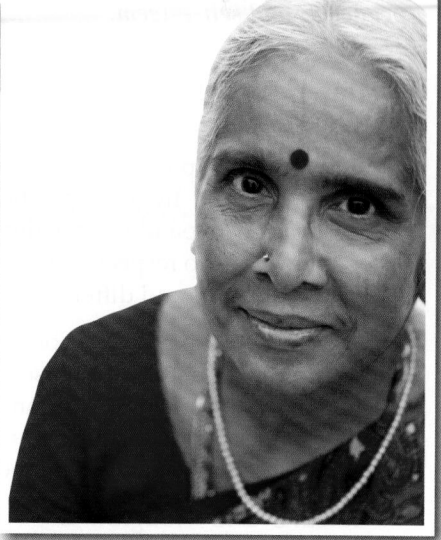

incontinent of urine and stool. Mr. Fuller's son, John, tells you that throughout his life, Mr. Fuller adhered to Orthodox Jewish law and requests that you respect this in his care.

Think about the following questions now, then again after you have read the chapter. What immediate concerns come to your mind about each of these patients? How will you ensure that their hygiene needs are met? Are there any safety issues? Which parts of their hygiene care can you delegate, if any?

Theoretical Knowledge
knowing why

This chapter provides the theoretical knowledge you need to answer the preceding questions, as well as others that will arise as you care for patients. It begins first with an explanation of the concepts of hygiene, activities of daily living (ADLs), and self-care.

ABOUT THE KEY CONCEPTS

Hygiene is the broadest of the key concepts because everything in the chapter is related to hygiene. However, **ADLs** and **self-care ability** must also be considered key concepts because every aspect of hygiene must include consideration of these two ideas. That is, you need to know the patient's ability to perform an ADL in order to know how to give appropriate hygiene care (e.g., can they wash their entire body or just their hands and face?).

HYGIENE AND SELF-CARE

Hygiene describes activities involved in maintaining personal cleanliness and grooming. **ADLs**, such as taking a bath or shower, washing hair, or brushing and flossing teeth, promote comfort, improve self-image, and decrease infection and disease. Healthy people perform their own personal hygiene; however, some patients need assistance because of illness or injury. **Key Point:** *As a nurse, you are responsible for providing the necessary assistance and, at the same time, encouraging as much self-care as possible to promote activity, independence, and self-esteem.*

What Factors Influence Hygiene Practices?

♥ **iCare** Every patient is unique, so as you would expect, personal hygiene practices vary greatly. To reflect caring, expand your understanding of the concept of hygiene to respect and accommodate each person's preferences and differences whenever possible.

Personal Preferences Some people prefer a shower, others a bath. One person may shower in the morning to wake up and feel clean for the day, whereas another bathes in the evening to relax before going to sleep. Choice of soaps and shampoos varies as well.

Culture and Religion or Spirituality Cultural and spiritual values and beliefs about hygiene form the foundation for our beliefs as adults. Many people consider daily bathing, use of deodorant, and brushing the teeth necessary to eliminate body odors, whereas other people may find a weekly bath sufficient. Religious or spiritual beliefs may also influence hygiene practices. For example, Orthodox Judaism prohibits

receiving personal care from a member of the opposite sex. You should always confirm your patient's personal preferences.

Economic Status or Living Environment Inadequate bathing facilities or lack of money for hygiene supplies (e.g., lack of access to running water or soap) can influence how often a person bathes. People living in poverty must focus on meeting basic needs for food and shelter before they can spend money and energy on hygiene.

Developmental Level

- **Infants and young children.** Parents and other caregivers perform hygiene care for infants and young children. Older children learn practices that become habits, such as brushing and flossing the teeth.
- **Preteens and teenagers.** As older children begin to perform their own hygiene, they are influenced by media and societal norms. For example, some preteens may avoid water and bathe only under parental duress, but teenagers, who are typically very self-conscious, may begin to take several showers a day. Many teenagers have oily skin and can tolerate frequent bathing.
- **Adults.** As we age, the oil-producing sebaceous glands become less active. Frequent bathing and the use of deodorant soap further dry the adult skin. Older adults may find it necessary to bathe only every 2 or 3 days, use less soap, and increase the use of skin moisturizers.

Knowledge and Cognitive Levels Not everyone has the knowledge needed to make appropriate decisions. Patient teaching is an important part of your hygiene care because even if they are ill at the moment, most people will eventually be responsible for their own personal hygiene. For example:

- Some people may not know the importance of flossing their teeth.
- Some female patients may not be aware of the importance of cleansing the perineum from front to back.

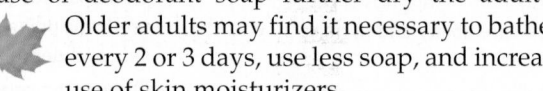

ThinkLike a Nurse 22-1: Clinical Judgment in Action

Think about Mrs. Rosha and Mr. Fuller (Meet Your Patients). After reviewing each of the factors presented, determine the following for each patient:

- Which factor(s) will have the most influence on the hygiene practices of this patient?
- Why do you think so?
- How will this factor affect the individual plan of care?

How Does Health Status Affect Self-Care Ability?

Both physiological and emotional factors can interfere with a person's ability or willingness to perform hygiene measures.

Pain Pain limits the person's ability and motivation to perform ADLs. The pain itself, limited mobility caused by the pain, and drowsiness from analgesics used to manage the pain may all contribute to a self-care deficit.

Limited Mobility Limited mobility (e.g., from joint and muscle problems, casts or traction, injury, weakness, fatigue, surgery, prescribed bedrest, or pain) makes it difficult to perform hygiene activities. For example:

- A patient may be unable to bend over to wash the lower legs and feet or cut the toenails or may be unable to raise the arms to wash and dry hair.
- A patient who is weak or "lightheaded" may be afraid of falling and be reluctant to move about. Such a person needs help, especially getting into the bathtub or shower.
- Obstacles, such as IV lines, oxygen tubing, nasogastric tubes, indwelling urinary catheters, or casts, may also interfere with the patient's ability to perform self-care.

Sensory Deficits Sensory deficits diminish a person's ability to perform hygiene measures safely and independently. Safety is a priority for patients with sensory deficits. Consider these examples:

- A patient with a visual deficit is admitted to the hospital. Because they are unfamiliar with the new surroundings, the patient is unable to gather the necessary supplies for grooming. You would need to provide direction, assistance, and understanding.
- A patient with hearing loss is taking an anticoagulant (a medication to delay blood clotting). You may need to provide explicit written instructions about the importance of using an electric razor instead of a preferred double-edged razor.

Cognitive Impairment Patients with conditions such as dementia, delirium, psychoses, stroke, Alzheimer disease, or traumatic brain injury may be unable to initiate their own grooming. The patient may be unable to determine the need for hygiene, much less know how to accomplish related tasks.

- *Example:* A patient with advanced Alzheimer disease may forget how to care for themselves and will need step-by-step direction. Because the person may also have difficulty interpreting stimuli in the environment, they may be fearful and resistant to hygiene measures performed by the nurse. Such cognitive deficits may require new or modified hygiene plans.

Emotional or Other Mental Health Disturbances A person with depression may neglect grooming and hygiene because of a profound lack of energy or motivation. Patients experiencing altered reality states, such as psychoses, delusions, or hallucinations, may:

- Dress inappropriately for the weather or the situation.
- Have poor hygiene practices.

- Be unable to make decisions about "what to do next" when bathing, dressing, and so on.

KnowledgeCheck 22-1

- What are the benefits of personal hygiene?
- Why should you respect and accommodate your patients' hygiene preferences?
- Identify two economic or living-environment factors that may influence how frequently a person bathes.
- Identify one example of a cognitive impairment that may make independent initiation of grooming impossible.
- Why may people experiencing depression neglect their grooming and hygiene?

PracticalKnowledge
knowing**how**

This section of the chapter will assist you in assessing for and promoting self-care abilities and planning care for patients with self-care deficits. **Key Point:** *Plan hygiene care around the patient's needs, not facility routines or staff convenience.* For guidelines for assessing, diagnosing, planning, and evaluating deficits in hygiene self-care, see the Example Client Condition: Hygiene Self-Care Deficit.

ASSESSMENT/RECOGNIZING CUES (SELF-CARE)

Assess your patient's functional status regularly. Focus on the patient's *ability* to perform hygiene measures and the need for assistance, not necessarily on the *quality* of these measures. To learn what to include in an assessment of functional ability, self-care, and hygiene,

 Go to the **Focused Assessment Box, Guidelines for Assessing Hygiene, Functional Assessment Abilities,** in Volume 2.

NURSING DIAGNOSIS/ANALYZING CUES (SELF-CARE)

The general concept of **self-neglect** occurs when the person is capable of performing self-care but fails to maintain socially accepted standards of health and well-being (which might include hygiene). The following are nursing diagnoses (Clinical Care Classification System [CCC], n.d.) specific to self-care abilities—except for the NANDA-I diagnosis Self-Neglect, which NANDA-I defines as follows: "A constellation of culturally framed behaviors involving one or more self-care activities in which there is a failure to maintain a socially accepted standard of health and well-being" (Herdman & Kamitsuru, 2021, p. 248)

Bathing/Hygiene Deficit
Dressing/Grooming Deficit
Feeding Deficit
Toileting Deficit
Self-Neglect

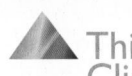

ThinkLike a Nurse 22-2: Clinical Judgment in Action

Answer the following questions for Mrs. Rosha (Meet Your Patients):

- What factor(s) may interfere with Mrs. Rosha's self-care ability?
- How can you ensure maximum independence with hygiene for her?
- How might you encourage her to strive toward optimal functioning?

PLANNING/PRIORITIZING HYPOTHESIS AND GENERATING SOLUTIONS (SELF-CARE)

NOC standardized outcomes for Self-Care Deficit diagnoses are determined by the specific diagnosis. Useful outcomes might be:

- *For patients who have more than one activity deficit*—Use Self-Care: Activities of Daily Living (ADLs).
- *For patients who have a single self-care deficit*, choose from these outcomes:
  Self-Care: Bathing
  Self-Care: Oral Hygiene
  Self-Care: Dressing
  Self-Care: Eating
  Self-Care: Toileting

When using NOC outcomes to write goals, rank the patient's abilities by using the NOC scale for self-care indicators: (1) dependent, does not participate; (2) requires assistive person and device; (3) requires assistive person; (4) independent with assistive device; and (5) completely independent. For example:

- Chooses clothing (5)
- Buttons clothing (4)

IMPLEMENTATION/TAKING ACTION (SELF-CARE)

For NIC standardized interventions for Self-Care Deficits, refer to the Example Client Condition: Hygiene Self-Care Deficit.

Individualized interventions depend on the extent of the client's Self-Care Deficit, as well as the etiology of the problem. Refer to the Example Client Condition, Hygiene Self-Care Deficit. The following are examples for Dressing/Grooming Deficit:

- Demonstrate the use of assistive devices (e.g., to help patient grasp and pull on socks).
- Use Velcro fasteners instead of buttons and zippers.

You will find a thorough discussion of specific hygiene-care interventions (e.g., care of the skin, oral hygiene) in the remainder of this chapter. For additional examples, see the bathing and hygiene plan of care and care map in this chapter.

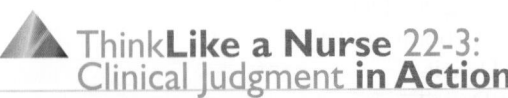

ThinkLike a Nurse 22-3: Clinical Judgment in Action

- Which of the preceding self-care diagnoses apply to Mrs. Rosha and Mr. Fuller (Meet Your Patients)?

- Explain the reasoning for your choices.
- For each patient, what are the related factors for his or her Self-Care Deficit?
- Write a self-care diagnostic statement for Mrs. Rosha and Mr. Fuller.

Types of Scheduled Hygiene Care

The following types of scheduled hygiene care are provided in most inpatient facilities (e.g., hospitals and long-term care settings).

- **Hourly rounds (comfort rounds or safety rounds),** which consist of seeing the patient every hour, on schedule, to offer help with self-care needs (e.g., pain relief, positioning, and toileting). Hourly rounding improves patient safety and greatly reduces call light use.
- **Early morning care** is provided soon after the patient awakens to prepare the patient for breakfast or other activities, such as diagnostic tests. As needed, assist with toileting, washing the face and hands, giving mouth care, and providing comfort measures.
- **Hygiene care (bathing)** can occur anytime during your shift. Ideally, you would find a time that is convenient for both you and the patient. Depending on the patient's self-care ability, assist with toileting, bathing, oral hygiene, skin care, hair care (including shaving if needed), dressing, and positioning or helping the patient transfer to a chair. Change or straighten bed linens, according to agency policy, and tidy the room.
- **H.S. (hour of sleep) care** is given before the patient goes to sleep. Offer the same care as given during the bath, adding a back massage to help the patient relax. Also, place the call light, water glass, urinal, or anything else the patient may need during the night within easy reach. Turn off lights and TV and close the door before leaving the room (according to patient needs and preferences). For a back massage procedure,

 Go to **Chapter 31, Procedure 31-1,** in Volume 2.

Delegating Hygiene Care

In some institutions, UAPs perform most of the hygiene care, but in others, registered nurses (RNs) are responsible for all patient hygiene with total patient care.

♥ iCare 22-1

Hygiene Routines

When performing hygiene care for your patient, ask how they would prefer their routine. This can be as simple as asking:

What part of your care are you able to participate in?
What soap do you prefer?
How would you like your hair styled?
What clothes do you like to wear?

These questions show caring, compassion, and respect for each patient.

If you are working with a UAP, you will need to carefully assess patients to ensure that it is safe to delegate their care. If the patient is unstable or the UAP is inexperienced or unfamiliar with the patient's limitations, you must assist or perform the care yourself. Read What Should I Know About Delegation and Supervision? in Chapter 3 for a review of making delegation decisions. Also see Figure 22-1.

Before assigning a UAP to assist with a bath, shower, or toileting, give instructions about the following:

- Patient's limitations and restrictions and the amount of assistance necessary
- Use of any assistive devices (e.g., cane, walker, or gait belt)
- Specific safety precautions to follow (e.g., use of gait belt or shower chair)
- Presence of obstacles (e.g., drainage tubes, catheters, IV tubing, or bandages) and how to maintain them during bathing or toileting
- Observations to make during the procedure and why the observations are important. Examples include the following:
    Skin condition; presence of lesions; areas of special concern over bony prominences and under abdominal folds and breasts
    Presence, appearance, and amount of urine or stool or the need to collect a specimen

Key Point: *Remember, as the professional nurse, you are responsible for determining the meaning of the data reported to you by the UAP.* Assisting with or supervising care (especially a bath) is an excellent opportunity for you to assess the patient's level of consciousness,

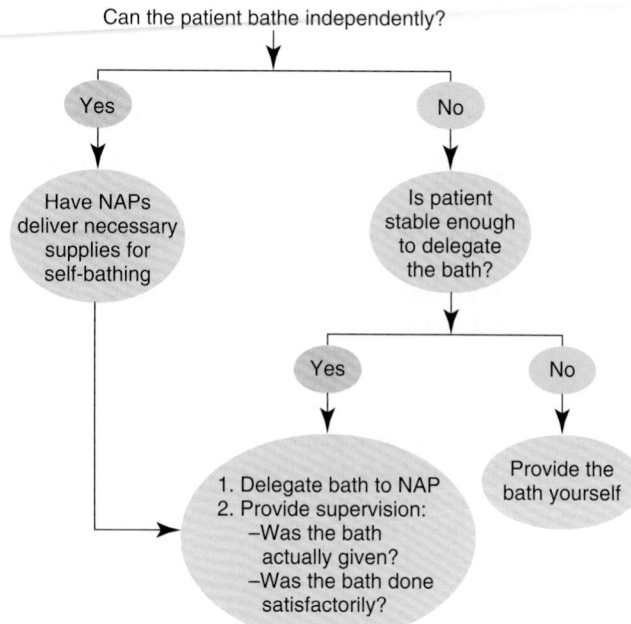

FIGURE 22-1 The registered nurse should assess the patient, delegate bathing as appropriate, and provide supervision.

short- and long-term memory, ability to follow instructions, range of motion (ROM), skin condition, activity tolerance, and overall self-care ability.

ThinkLike a Nurse 22-4: Clinical Judgment in Action

Think of Mrs. Rosha (Meet Your Patients). You have delegated her bathing and oral hygiene to a UAP.

- What information do you need to share with the UAP about this patient's needs, limitations, or preferences?
- What, if any, specific observations will you ask the UAP to make for Mrs. Rosha?
- What, if any, specific observations will *you* need to make for Mrs. Rosha?
- What action will you take if you determine that the patient's needs and preferences were not met by the UAP?

 Go To Davis Advantage, Resources, Chapter 22, Care Plan and Care Map: Bathing Self-Care Deficit

CARE OF THE SKIN

The preceding sections introduced you to the broad topic of hygiene, self-care, and activities of daily living. The rest of the chapter will deal with specific topics, such as care of the skin.

TheoreticalKnowledge knowing why

To assist patients with skin care, you must have theoretical knowledge about personal hygiene measures and the structure and function of the **integument** (skin).

Anatomy and Physiology of the Skin

The **integumentary system** consists of the skin, the subcutaneous layer directly under the skin, the hair, nails, and the sweat and sebaceous glands. The skin has two distinct layers, the epidermis and the dermis (see Fig. 32-1):

1. The **epidermis** (the thicker, outer layer) consists of stratified squamous epithelial tissue composed of keratinized (dead) cells, which are fused to make the skin waterproof.
    - The epidermis continually sheds (**desquamates**) and is completely replaced every 3 to 4 weeks.
    - The epidermis contains melanin, a pigment that provides protection against the ultraviolet rays of the sun and that, together with circulating blood, gives skin its color.
2. The **dermis** (the thinner, second layer) contains blood and lymphatic vessels, nerves, bases of hair follicles, and sebaceous and sweat glands.

Promoting Safe, Effective Nursing Care

Promoting Health and Safety Through Self-Care Management

Chapter Key Concept: Hygiene, Self-Care Ability (Thinking, Doing, Caring)

Competency: Provide goal-directed, client-centered care

Background. Promotion of health and safety requires patient engagement and patient–provider partnership. An active partnership establishes trust and encourages self-care management. **Key Point: *Hand hygiene is considered the most significant action in breaking the chain of infection.*** Best practice regarding hand hygiene has infrequently considered the role of the patient in the chain of infection (Caine et al., 2016; Nash, 2019). Salcido (2012) reported an increase in hand-hygiene compliance in healthcare workers (HCWs) when engaging patients and having them ask the HCW, "Did you wash/sanitize your hands?" (p. 342).

Scenario: The student is caring for a patient with a surgical incision. A nurse enters the room and begins to remove the dressing without initiating hand hygiene.

Think about it: Reflect on the following questions or discuss them with your peers.

1. In this situation, what are the implications for the student nurse in maintaining safe and effective care and prevention of infection?

2. Identify specific strategies to engage the patient in self-care management to reduce the risk of infection.

3. Debate the value of utilizing the patient-engagement strategy, "Did you wash/sanitize your hands?" as reported by Salcido (2012).

Resources: Caine, L. Z., Pinkham, A. M., & Noble, J. T. (2016). Be seen and heard being clean: A novel patient-centered approach to hand hygiene. *American Journal of Infection Control, 44*(7), e103–e106; Nash, J. (2019). Patient as observer: Practical steps to launching a hand hygiene quality assurance program in the medical imaging outpatient setting. *Journal of Medical Imaging and Radiation Sciences, 50*(3), S9; Salcido, R. (2012). Patient safety: It is in our hands. *Advances in Skin and Wound Care, 22*(8), 342.

EXAMPLE CLIENT CONDITION: Hygiene Self-Care Deficit

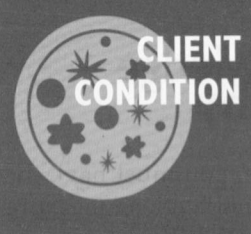
CLIENT CONDITION

Factors Affecting Self-Care

The ability to perform and engage in hygiene self-care is determined by many factors, including:

- Age
- Developmental stage
- Life experience
- Sociocultural orientation
- Health
- Available resources

Problem Definition

- **Self-care deficit** exists when a person is unable to perform consistent and effective self-care (e.g., when a person is unable to perform one or more activities of daily living [ADLs], such as bathing or toileting).
- **Hygiene self-care deficit** occurs when the person lacks the ability to bathe independently, including washing the whole body, combing hair, brushing teeth, doing skin care and nail care, and applying makeup.

Possible Adverse Effects of Hygiene Care

Although cleanliness can contribute to well-being, comfort, and health, it can also be stressful—for example, for critically ill patients, the frail elderly, and those with dementia. Adverse events include:

- Decreased oxygenation or ventilation
- Hypertension
- Hypotension
- Intracranial hypertension
- Cardiorespiratory arrest

Etiologies

- Pain
- Fatigue, activity intolerance, decreased strength or endurance (e.g., emphysema, pneumonia, heart failure)
- Impaired cognitive ability
- Impaired sensation or perception
- Limited mobility
- Emotional or mental health disturbances
- Environmental barriers (e.g., doorway too narrow to accommodate walker)
- Medication side effects (e.g., drowsiness)
- Substance abuse
- Lack of knowledge
- Lack of motivation

EXAMPLE CLIENT CONDITION: Hygiene Self-Care Deficit—cont'd

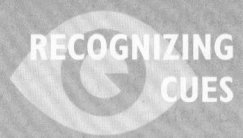

RECOGNIZING CUES

Assess Self-Care Ability

Use a standardized functional status rating to assign a score to each response.
- For the commonly used Katz ADL,

Go to the Clinical Nursing Web site at https://consultgeri.org/try-this/general-assessment/issue-2.pdf

- You can also create your own scale, such as the following:
  1. Completely independent; needs no assistance.
  2. Needs device or special equipment (e.g., walker, large-handle spoon).
  3. Requires help, supervision, or teaching from another person.
  4. Requires help from a person, as well as a device or special equipment.
  5. Totally dependent; does not participate in the activity.

Obtain a Health History

- Identify underlying illness, injury, or disease.
- Identify cognitive impairment.
- Identify cues for depression, psychoses, or delusions.
- Identify cues for other factors (see list of etiologies).
- Determine preferences and practices.
  To learn what to include in an assessment/identifying cues of self-care and hygiene,

Go to the **Focused Assessment** box, **Guidelines for Assessing Hygiene,** in Volume 2.

NURSING DIAGNOSIS/ ANALYZING CUES

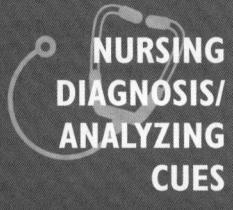

Hygiene Self-Care Deficits

NOTE: These nursing diagnoses focus on **hygiene** self-care deficits. For other self-care deficits, refer to the discussions in this chapter on care of the skin, feet, nails, oral cavity, hair, eyes, ears, and nose.
- **Self-care diagnoses related to hygiene** are Self-Care Deficit: Bathing, Dressing, Toileting, and Feeding and sometimes Activities of Daily Living (ADLs) Alteration (Saba, 2017).

Classify Functional Level in the diagnostic statement. Use one of the following:
- The scale in the earlier Assessment row
- Descriptive terms such as *mild, moderate, severe,* and *total*

Examples:
- **Diagnostic statement, using a scale:**
- Bathing/Hygiene Deficit (2) related to severe knee pain 2° degenerative joint disease
- **Diagnostic statement using descriptors:**
- Toileting Deficit (severe) related to Activity Intolerance 2° heart failure

PLANNING/ PRIORITIZING HYPOTHESIS AND GENERATING SOLUTIONS

NOC Outcomes

Self-Care: Activities of Daily Living (ADLs) is appropriate for all of the Self-Care Deficit diagnoses.
  Other NOC outcomes depend on the nursing diagnosis, for example:
- Ostomy Self-Care
- Self-Care: Bathing
- Self-Care: Oral Hygiene
- Self-Care: Dressing
- Self-Care: Toileting

Individualized Goal Statements (Examples)

- By May 4, will complete bath independently, except for back and feet, after nurse provides equipment and assists patient to the bathroom.
- Verbalizes satisfaction with body cleanliness and oral hygiene after hygiene care.
- Accepts assistance with ADLs or total care, as needed.

(continued)

EXAMPLE CLIENT CONDITION: Hygiene Self-Care Deficit—cont'd

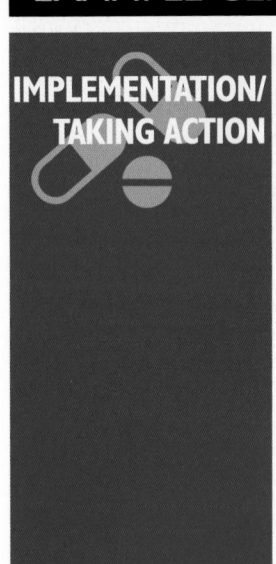

IMPLEMENTATION/ TAKING ACTION

NIC Interventions

- Bathing
- Bowel Management
- Ear Care
- Energy Management
- Environmental Management
- Foot Care
- Hair and Scalp Care
- Nail Care
- Oral Health Maintenance
- Perineal Care
- Self-Care Assistance: Bathing/Hygiene
- Self-Care Assistance: Dressing/Grooming
- Self-Care Assistance: Toileting
- Urinary Elimination Management

Individualized Interventions

- Offer pain medication before ADLs.
- Allow sufficient time for all ADLs to prevent fatigue and frustration.
- Modify care to meet individual needs.
- Evaluate patient responses continually as you work.
- Provide care in small segments, allowing the patient to rest after brushing teeth.
- Promote eventual self-care.

Special Circumstances

Critically ill patients need rest, so you will not push them to perform at their highest level of function.

    If the patient is able to perform self-care, allow them to rest while you perform part of the care—for example, washing the feet and legs.

Functions of the Skin

The skin has the following five main functions:

1. *Protection.* Intact skin is the body's first line of defense against bacteria and other microorganisms that can enter the body. Skin protects underlying tissues from thermal, chemical, and mechanical injury to underlying tissues. **Sebaceous glands** secrete an oily substance called **sebum**, which helps to waterproof and lubricate the skin and decrease bacterial growth.
2. *Sensation.* The skin contains sensory organs or receptors for heat, cold, pressure, touch, and pain.
3. *Regulation.* The skin helps maintain fluid and electrolyte balance by preventing the escape of excess water and electrolytes from the body. It helps to regulate body temperature by dilating and constricting blood vessels and activating or inactivating sweat glands. **Sweat glands,** concentrated in the axillae and external genitalia, excrete water in the form of perspiration; evaporation produces a cooling effect on the skin.
4. *Secretion/excretion.* The sweat glands secrete fatty acids and proteins and excrete nitrogenous wastes *(urea),* sodium chloride, and water in perspiration.
5. *Vitamin D formation.* The skin contains a form of cholesterol that is changed to vitamin D on exposure to ultraviolet light from the sun.

See Chapter 32 for more information about the structure and functions of the skin.

Common Skin Problems

You should be familiar with the following common skin problems and observe for them as you provide skin care:

- **Pruritus** (itching) may lead to scratching and breaks in the skin.

- **Dry skin** tends to crack, burn, or itch.
- **Maceration** is softening of the skin from prolonged moisture (e.g., urinary incontinence). It makes the epidermis more susceptible to injury.
- **Excoriation** is a loss of the superficial layers of the skin caused, for example, by scratching and by the digestive enzymes in feces.
- **Abrasion,** a rubbing away of the epidermal layer of the skin, especially over bony areas or prominences, is often caused by friction or shearing forces that occur when a patient moves or is moved in bed.
- **Pressure injuries** are lesions caused by tissue compression and inadequate perfusion. See Chapter 32.
- **Acne** is an inflammation of the sebaceous glands that is common among adolescents and young adults.
- **Burns** are a type of traumatic injury caused by thermal, electrical, chemical, or radioactive agents.

To see illustrations of most of these skin problems,

 Go to Chapter 19, **Procedure 19-2** in Volume 2.

Risk Factors

In addition to a person's hygiene practices, health status and developmental stage also affect skin condition.

Health Status Anything that interferes with the hydration, circulation, and nutrition of the skin creates a risk to skin integrity. As you read about each of the following risk factors, think whether it would be present for Mr. Fuller (Meet Your Patients):

- **Dampness.** Excessive perspiration (e.g., in fever) and incontinence of urine or bowel cause the skin to become damp. The skin breaks down more easily when it is damp, especially in the skinfolds. This is called **maceration**.

■ **Dehydration.** Fluid loss (e.g., from vomiting, diarrhea, or fever) and insufficient fluid intake can cause dehydration. This causes the skin to become dry and crack easily.

■ **Nutritional status.** Very thin or very obese people are at increased risk for skin irritation and injury. *Morbid obesity* can make it physically difficult for a person to reach all areas of the body and can lead to the development of odor and fungal conditions. Having a low body mass index (BMI) can cause dry, thin skin, which is at higher risk for skin breakdown or injury.

■ **Insufficient circulation.** Immobility, vascular disease, and overall inadequate nutritional status may compromise circulation. This predisposes the patient to local tissue death and ulceration when skin cells do not receive enough oxygen.

■ **Skin diseases.** Skin diseases such as impetigo (a bacterial infection of the skin) and *systemic diseases,* such as measles and chickenpox, cause lesions that create discomfort and require special hygiene care.

■ **Jaundice.** Certain diseases can cause a yellow discoloration brought about by accumulation of bile pigments in the skin. Jaundice causes the skin to be itchy and dry.

■ **Lifestyle and personal choices.** Some people damage their skin by exposure to ultraviolet rays (e.g., sunbathing, tanning beds). Some use sunscreen; some do not. As another example, many people have skin tattoos or piercings, creating the risk for systemic and local infection and scarring.

Developmental Stage

■ Infants have fragile, easily injured skin.

■ As a child matures, the skin becomes more resistant to injury and infection, but children need adults to provide or supervise the cleanliness of their skin.

■ In adolescence, the sebaceous glands enlarge, and secretions increase. The skin becomes oily and susceptible to acne.

 ■ With aging, the skin changes in numerous visible ways, increasing the older adult's risk for skin problems, such as ulcers and reduced ability to heal. Refer to Table 22-1 for a description of normal skin changes in older adults.

KnowledgeCheck 22-2

■ What are five functions of the skin?
■ How does the skin help regulate body temperature?
■ What changes take place in the skin as a person ages?

Table 22-1 ➤ Normal Skin Changes in Older Adults

STRUCTURE	CHANGE IN STRUCTURE AND ACTIVITY	CLINICAL EFFECTS
Epidermis	Thinner; decreased rate of cell turnover.	Skin appears pale and somewhat translucent; slower healing.
Subcutaneous tissues	Thinner and more fragile, less fat.	Decreased protection of bony prominences and thermoregulation.
Collagen and elastin fibers in the dermis	Weaken and become less elastic.	Skin becomes wrinkled.
Sebaceous and sweat glands	Activity decreases.	Skin becomes dry, scaly, and itchy. Temperature regulation in hot weather becomes more difficult.
Hormones (estrogen and progesterone)	Production decreases.	Contributes to drying and thinning of the skin.
Skin	Vascularity decreases.	Skin becomes cool and pale.
Hair follicles	Diminish in number and activity.	Hair becomes thin; grows more slowly.
Melanocytes (pigment cells)	Numbers decrease.	Hair turns gray or white; skin may become unevenly pigmented.
Nails	Thicken, become softer, growth rate diminishes.	Nails tear easily.
Skin growths	Become more common (e.g., warts, "liver spots," "age spots").	Most are caused by years of sun exposure; most are harmless (except for skin cancers, which are fairly common but not normal changes).

PracticalKnowledge
knowing how

ASSESSMENT/RECOGNIZING CUES (SKIN)

♥ **iCare** Patients may be sensitive about skin problems or poor hygiene practices, so as you interview and examine the patient, do so in a nonjudgmental, respectful manner. Protect the patient's privacy by closing the curtain and exposing only the area being bathed or examined. Be mindful of the room temperature, and try to reduce drafts to avoid chilling the patient.

For a thorough discussion of skin assessment, including how to describe and document your observations, see Chapter 19. Also,

 Go to **Chapter 22, Assessment Guidelines and Tools, Focused Assessment: Guidelines for Assessing Hygiene** (section entitled Skin), in Volume 2.

Subjective Data Ask the patient about their usual bathing and skin care practices and preferences, as well as the following:

- Past and current skin concerns, including their effects on the patient's life
- Prescription and over-the-counter (OTC) or herbal remedies used to treat any skin concerns
- Allergic skin reactions to food, medications, plants, skin care products, and so on
- History of diseases or other factors that are known to cause skin issues

Objective Data Inspect each area of the skin in an orderly, head-to-toe manner, noting overall cleanliness, condition, color, texture, turgor, hydration, and temperature. Observe for rashes, lumps, lesions, and cracking. Look for drainage from wounds or around tubes. Observe for the following changes in skin color:

- **Pallor** in a person with light skin may appear as pale skin without underlying pink tones. In a person with dark skin, observe for an ashen-gray or yellow color.
- **Erythema** is redness of the skin. It is related to vasodilation and inflammation. Erythema looks different in patients with dark skin, so you may discover it by palpating the skin for areas of increased warmth.
- **Jaundice,** a yellow discoloration of the skin, occurs in patients with impaired liver function. It is best seen in the sclerae of the eyes.
- **Cyanosis,** a bluish coloring of the skin, is caused by decreased peripheral circulation or decreased oxygenation of the blood. It may be related to cardiac, pulmonary, or peripheral vascular problems. You can best see cyanosis by examining the conjunctivae, tongue, buccal mucosa, and palms and soles for a dull, dark color.

KnowledgeCheck 22-3

- True or False: The professional nurse is responsible for making assessments.
- True or False: Assisting with the bath is an excellent time to assess the patient.
- To inspect for pallor in a person with dark skin, which areas would you assess for an ashen-gray or yellow color?
- What is the term that means "a bluish color of the skin"?
- Name two physiological causes of erythema.
- Where can you best see jaundice?

NURSING DIAGNOSIS/ANALYZING CUES (SKIN)

Impaired Skin Integrity as the Problem

When you wish to focus on prevention or treatment of the *skin condition,* use the following diagnostic labels (CCC, n.d.):

- **Skin Integrity Impairment Risk.** *Definition:* Increased chance of skin breakdown.
  Risk factors: The general conditions that affect the skin: dampness, dehydration, insufficient circulation, nutritional status (thin or obese), skin diseases, systemic diseases, and jaundice.
  Example: Skin Integrity Impairment Risk related to immobility secondary to casts and traction
- **Skin Integrity Impairment.** *Definition:* Diminished ability to maintain the integument (dermis and epidermis).
  Characteristics: interruption of body structures, breakdown of skin layers (dermis), crack or break of skin surface (epidermis).
  Example: Skin Integrity Impairment related to decreased peripheral circulation secondary to arteriosclerosis

Skin Integrity Impairment as the Etiology

Skin Integrity Impairment may be the etiology of other nursing diagnoses. Certain skin conditions place the patient at risk for infection by causing cracks or breaks in the skin. Others may contribute to discomfort and low self-esteem. The following are examples:

Infection Risk related to skin lacerations and abrasions
Situational Self-Esteem Disturbance related to appearance and self-consciousness about skin lesions secondary to severe eczema

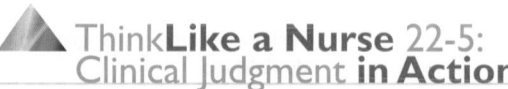 ThinkLike a Nurse 22-5:
Clinical Judgment in Action

- Why are Mrs. Rosha and Mr. Fuller (Meet Your Patients) at risk for Impaired Skin Integrity?
- What are the specific kinds of skin integrity conditions that pose an increased risk to both patients?

PLANNING/PRIORITIZING HYPOTHESIS AND GENERATING SOLUTIONS (SKIN)

NOC standardized outcomes for problems of the skin include the following:

Immobility Consequences: Physiological	Self-Care: Hygiene Self-Esteem
Tissue Integrity: Skin and Mucous Membranes	Wound Healing: Primary Intention Wound Healing: Secondary Intention

Individualized goals/outcome statements you might write for a patient with skin problems include the following:

- Skin will remain intact and free of secretions.
- Skin will remain free of lesions.
- Patient will follow regimen to improve skin dryness.

IMPLEMENTATION/TAKING ACTION (SKIN)

Examples of *NIC standardized interventions* for skin integrity and skin care include the following:

- For **Skin Integrity Impairment**—Bathing, Cutaneous Stimulation, Perineal Care, Pressure Management, Pressure Ulcer Care, Skin Surveillance, and Wound Care
- For **Skin Integrity Impairment Risk**—Add to the previous items: Bed Rest Care, Circulatory Precautions, Pressure Ulcer Prevention, and Positioning

Individualized nursing activities for patients with Skin Integrity Impairment include bathing and massage, which are presented in this section. If you delegate patient bathing to UAPs (Fig. 22-1), you must make certain that the patient actually gets a bath.

Bathing Bathing serves three purposes: health, social interaction, and pleasure or relaxation.

- Bathing removes perspiration and bacteria from the skin surface, helping to prevent body odor.
- The warmth from the bath solution and the friction of bathing dilate the blood vessels near the surface of the skin, increasing the circulation.
- Bathing stimulates depth of respirations and provides sensory input.
- Bathing can be a time to strengthen the nurse–patient relationship.
- Bathing promotes relaxation and comfort, enhances well-being, and improves self-image.

Back Massage Regardless of the type of bath used, when possible, end the bath with a back massage to provide relaxation and stimulate circulation. As with all procedures, be sure there are no contraindications to massage (e.g., fractured ribs, burns, recent heart surgery). To learn a procedure for giving a back massage,

Go to **Chapter 31, Procedure 31-1: Giving a Back Massage**, in Volume 2.

Choosing the Type of Bath to Meet Patient Needs

The type of bath you give depends on your nursing judgment; the patient's preference, self-care ability, and endurance; and the medical plan of care.

- **Assist bath**—The nurse helps the patient with areas that may be difficult to reach, such as the back, feet, and legs.
- **Complete bath**—The nurse washes the patient's entire body without assistance from the patient. For complete instructions,

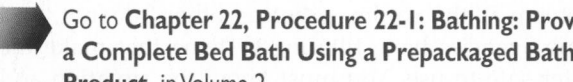

Go to **Chapter 22, Procedure 22-1: Bathing: Providing a Complete Bed Bath Using a Prepackaged Bathing Product**, in Volume 2.

- **Partial bath**—The nurse cleanses only the areas that may cause odor or discomfort, such as the axillae and perineum. If a complete bath would be stressful to the patient, you may choose to give a partial bath.

The following sections discuss other types of baths in detail.

Bed Baths and Modified Bed Baths

A **bed bath** is for patients who must remain in bed but who are able to bathe themselves. You will assist by placing the bath supplies on the bedside stand or overbed table. The following are four types of bed baths:

Prepackaged Bathing Products Recent evidence supports the now widespread use of **prepackaged bathing products** (Groven et al., 2017; Martin et al., 2017; Matsumoto et al., 2019; Veje et al., 2019). These are sets of commercially prepared and packaged, premoistened, disposable washcloths that are warmed before use. Recent guidelines recommend the use of prepackaged bathing products. Studies suggest the following benefits:

- Helps assure consistency of bathing technique among caregivers
- Prevents inconsistent applications of emollients (moisturizers)
- Decreases the skin damage due to rough washcloths
- ✚ Decreases the potential for colonization of the skin and the spread of microorganisms with the use of tap water and basins. This is especially true of products containing chlorhexidine (Huang et al., 2019; Matsumoto et al., 2019; Patel et al., 2019).

Bag Bath A bag bath uses 8 to 10 washcloths moistened with water (preferably sterile, filtered, or distilled) or a pH-balanced no-rinse soap. The washcloths are warmed, and each part of the patient's body is cleansed with a fresh cloth.

Basin and Water Bath This is a type of bed bath in which you use a disposable basin with water; washcloths; lotion; and a pH-balanced, no-rinse soap or a chlorhexidine-and-water solution. This may be done, for instance, if a patient prefers this type of bath to the prepackaged bathing products or if the patient is grossly soiled (i.e., large amounts of blood or feces). When you use a basin and water bath, you must be aware of the potential for healthcare-acquired infections (HAIs) related to (1) reusable basins and (2) the presence of bio-film in hospital waterlines and plumbing.

- **Bathwater.** Depending on the patient's condition, it may be safer to use distilled, sterile, or filtered water in place of tap water to prevent skin contamination with bacteria biofilm. Some agencies have a serious problem with biofilm, whereas others do not, and some agencies have filtering systems that make the water safe to use. You must know the situation and the policy in your institution. When using tap water, it is a good idea to bathe the patient with a solution of chlorhexidine and water to combat any bacteria that may be present (Lewis et al., 2019; Rutala & Weber, 2019). **Key Point:** *One size does not fit all! The more vulnerable the patient, the more caution you must exercise regarding basin and water bathing.*

For guidelines for bathing adults, see Box 22-1. **Key Point:** *Guidelines change frequently; be alert for practice changes.*

Shower

Most ambulatory patients prefer a shower. It is a time-saver and refreshing as well as cleansing. In a hospital or long-term care facility, some clients can manage a shower mostly on their own. For complete information,

 Go to **Chapter 22, Clinical Insight 22-1: Assisting With a Shower or Tub Bath,** in Volume 2.

Tub Bath

If a client is ambulatory but requires assistance with bathing (e.g., because of pain and stiffness in the hands and arms), you may prefer a tub bath (see Clinical Insight 22-1 in Volume 2). It will be easier for you to wash and rinse the patient, and you will not get as wet as when you help with a shower. Immersion in the water also helps to soak areas that are crusty, scaly, or soiled and relaxes stiff, sore muscles and joints. Overall, tub baths are thought to be of greater benefit than a bed bath.

The tub should have handrails and a nonskid surface to prevent falls. Some patients need assistance getting into and out of a tub. Some kneel or squat first and then sit in the tub. For completely dependent patients, there are specially designed tubs that reduce the effort necessary to lift patients into and out of the tub. You can also use a hydraulic lift and a regular tub.

Therapeutic Bath

The primary care provider may prescribe **therapeutic baths** for some patients. These baths are given for a

---

BOX 22-1 ■ Guidelines for Bathing the Adult Patient

Bathing Frequency

For patients who are unable to provide self-care, assist with or provide a bath:

- Daily or more frequently for comfort purposes (on patient request)
- To respond to diaphoresis
- To address a significant incontinence episode

Privacy and Timing of the Bath

Maintain patient privacy throughout the procedure.

Bath time should be determined based on:

- Patient preference
- Clinical stability
- Patient's physiological tolerance to activity
- Sleep pattern (uninterrupted sleep is essential to the healing process)

Bath Supplies and Products

Prepackaged bath products should be used in place of basin and tap water for regular bathing:

- Remove reusable basins from the environment to encourage the use of prepackaged bathing products.
- If using a basin, use sterile or distilled water in place of tap water, unless the hospital has a filtering system that prevents biofilm in the waterlines.
- No-rinse pH-balanced cleansers with emollients help to protect the barrier function of the skin and reduce the risk of dry skin.

Chlorhexidine gluconate (CHG) 2% prepackaged cloths are recommended to decrease the colonization of bacteria on the skin.

- Do not rinse; retain 2% CHG on the skin at all times.
- Do not use on mucous membranes (face or perineal area).

Source: Veje, P. L., & Larsen, P. (2014). The effectiveness of bed bathing practices on skin integrity and hospital-acquired infections among adult patients: A systematic review protocol. *The JBI Database of Systematic Reviews and Implementation Reports, 12*(2), 71–81.

---

specific purpose (e.g., to relax muscles, to remove scales and crust from the skin). Given that current research suggests that hospital water supplies may serve as a reservoir for pathogens and play a role in HAIs, the use of distilled, specially filtered, or sterile water would seem preferable if in accord with provider prescription and facility policy.

It is your responsibility to add the medically ordered substance, ensure appropriate temperature, and assist the patient into the tub. Use a disposable sitz tub if one is available. If not, clean the tub thoroughly at the end of the bath, preferably with a chlorhexidine-based product. Examples of therapeutic baths include the following:

- Oatmeal or coal tar baths are therapeutic baths used to treat specific skin conditions, such as psoriasis.
- A warm sitz bath is another type of therapeutic bath. It helps to cleanse the perineum and soothe inflammation of perineal, vaginal, or rectal tissues.

Perineal Care

The **perineum** (the area between the anus and vulva in a female, or the anus and scrotum in a male) is a dark, warm, moist area that supports bacterial growth. Perineal care promotes comfort and prevents odor, skin excoriation, and infection. You will usually give perineal care (including the external genitalia) along with a complete bed bath, but it may be needed at other times as well. Give perineal care more frequently if the patient is incontinent of urine or feces or has drainage from the area.

Whether you and the patient are of the same or different sex, perineal care may be embarrassing for you both. Perform care in a professional manner, and provide the patient with privacy (e.g., shut the door, pull bed curtains, drape properly). A matter-of-fact, sensitive approach puts most patients at ease. For complete information about providing perineal care,

 Go to **Chapter 22, Procedure 22-3: Providing Perineal Care,** in Volume 2.

KnowledgeCheck 22-4
- What causes body odor?
- What is the best intervention to rid the skin of body odor?
- What is the rationale for providing perineal care?
- How can you protect patient privacy during perineal care?

 ## ThinkLike a Nurse 22-6: Clinical Judgment in Action
- Which of your patients (Meet Your Patients) will require nurse-assisted perineal care? Explain your reasoning.
- Which patient, if you are a woman, is most likely to be embarrassed by perineal care? Explain your reasoning.
- If you need more theoretical knowledge to answer these questions, what is it? Where could you find the information?

Bathing Patients Who Have Dementia

Bathing should be a pleasant experience, not a stressful one. But patients who have dementia tend to become agitated when told it is time to bathe, and they often yell, scream, pinch, or hit their caregivers (Nygaard et al., 2022; Osuoha et al., 2021). The reason for the patients' agitation is usually that they experience pain, cold, fear, and loss of control. When you meet patient comfort needs (e.g., by adjusting the water temperature or taking special care when washing arthritic joints), the patient becomes less agitated, and aggressive behavior declines significantly.

You can significantly reduce aggressive behaviors by giving a bag bath instead (Konno et al., 2021). Despite the common myths about bathing, keep in mind that:

- The patient does not always need to have a daily tub bath or shower. It does not take a large amount of water (e.g., a shower) to get a person clean. Using prepackaged bathing products can help you finish the bath more quickly, possibly reducing the patient's agitation.
- The bath does not have to be performed at the same time every day, nor in the way "we have always done it here." You can educate families that showers and tub baths are not the only ways to get clean.
- It is not necessary to bathe a person who is resisting. You can adapt the approach, method, and time.
- Patients who are forced to bathe do not "just forget about it"; many stay upset and agitated for hours.

For more discussion of bathing myths and for instructions about providing a bath for a person with dementia, see iCare Box 22-2.

 ## ThinkLike a Nurse 22-7: Clinical Judgment in Action

Suppose you have been providing baths with prepackaged wipes to a patient who has mild dementia. One day a visiting family member says, "My father tells me he has not had a bath all week. What's going on here?" What would you do? How could you help to prevent this misunderstanding in the future?

♥ iCare 22-2

Caring Tips for Bathing a Patient With Dementia
- **Focus on the patient,** not the task; provide choices.
- **Distract** with food or by playing relaxing music.
- **Use a gentle type of showerhead** for rinsing. A strong spray may frighten the patient.
- **Be creative:** Try bathing one part of the body each day.
- **Bathe at a regular time,** preferably at the same time that the patient bathed at home.
- **Ensure continuity of care** so that the patient can build a relationship with the caregiver and be less fearful.
- **Provide privacy.** Patients with dementia do not necessarily lose their modesty and sense of privacy.
- **Avoid sensory overload:** Turn down lights, warm the room, play soft music, and speak calmly. People with dementia have difficulty processing information. Sensory overload may trigger aggression.
- **Foster independence.** Encourage the patient to wash their own face if able so that they may feel like an active participant.
- **Explain the procedure simply,** using short sentences.
- **Let the patient know before you touch or spray them** with any fluids. Sudden actions are often frightening.
- **Do not rush.** The patient will feel the tension and may become agitated.
- **Teach techniques to caregivers at home** (e.g., being flexible with time, using a bag bath).
- Also refer to the "What if …" section of Procedure 22-1.

Bathing Patients Who Have Morbid Obesity

Obesity is defined as a BMI of 30 or higher (about 20% to 40% above one's ideal weight). Severe, or **morbid,** obesity exists when the BMI is 40 or higher (or body weight is 50% more than ideal weight).

For a person with morbid obesity, a thorough skin assessment is essential, but it is difficult. Be sure to obtain adequate assistance to reposition the patient during the skin examination so that you do not miss any areas. Pay special attention to skinfolds. The following are preventive interventions for problems related to hygiene, moisture, pressure, shear and friction, and nutrition (Ewens et al., 2022).

Hygiene Clients with morbid obesity may find it physically difficult to reach all areas of the body. In addition, they may have limited mobility. An inability to maintain good hygiene may lead to odor and fungal infections.

- Ask how the patient handles skin care at home. Use the same adaptations, if possible.
- Provide a trapeze to assist the patient to lift and access areas that are difficult to reach.
- Provide a handheld shower and long-handled brushes.
- Experts vary on the use of soap. Certainly, the skin should be rinsed and dried well.

Moisture Skin in skinfolds stays damp because perspiration cannot evaporate.

Moisture contributes to the development of fungal and other skin infections.

- Use moisture barrier creams, particularly in skinfolds and the perineal area.
- Use fans, if permitted.
- Change linens often.
- Manage incontinence.
- If fungal infections occur, you may need a medical prescription for antifungal powders, sprays, cream, or ointment.

Pressure Pressure can be caused by limited mobility, skinfolds where skin rubs on skin, tight clothing, catheters, and so on.

- Reposition the patient frequently to redistribute the pressure of the skinfolds.
- Reposition catheters and tubes often; use tube holders to prevent rubbing.
- Separate the skinfolds with towels.

Shear and Friction The patient is at risk for friction and shearing injury from pulling skin across the linens when moving in the bed and chair.

- Provide a trapeze.
- Do not use sheepskins.
- Use a waterproof and breathable mattress cover.
- Keep linens wrinkle-free.

 The American Nurses Association's position is that you should use specialized lifts and other equipment to move patients safely and avoid injury to yourself (de Castro, 2004). If you must move the patient in an emergency situation, obtain sufficient help to avoid pulling the skin across the sheet or other surface.

Bathing Older Adults

Key Point: *For older adults, especially the bed-bound and frail elderly, the goals are to prevent drying and injury to the skin.* At the same time, you should promote comfort and encourage independence in ADLs. This requires proper skin care and bathing techniques.

- Bag baths adequately address the problems of skin dryness, itching, and irritation. They also improve skin integrity and may be less distressing to frail older adults (Archer et al., 2021).
- Use a no-rinse pH-balanced cleanser to further protect the barrier function of the skin.
- Other interventions include avoiding the use of soap, being sure to clean the skin immediately after soiling, and applying skin moisturizer.
- Also see What If . . . Your Patient Is an Older Adult, when you

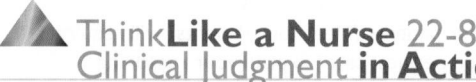 Go to **Chapter 22, Procedure 22-1: Bathing: Providing a Complete Bed Bath Using a Prepackaged Bathing Product,** in Volume 2.

KnowledgeCheck 22-5

- A nurse has bathed the entire body of a patient who is bedridden without assistance from the patient. What is the term for this bath?
- What are the advantages of a prepackaged bag bath?
- For which type of bath will you most likely have a medical prescription?

ThinkLike a Nurse 22-8: Clinical Judgment in Action

Which type of bath would be most appropriate for each of your patients (Meet Your Patients)? Provide rationales for your choices.

CARE OF THE FEET

Foot care is a necessary part of hygiene and essential at any age for tissue health, proper posture, and ambulation.

TheoreticalKnowledge knowing why

When providing foot care, you will need theoretical knowledge about the structure of the feet, life-span variations, and common foot problems. The feet provide support for the weight of the entire body and absorb a significant amount of shock during walking. Their structure is complex, consisting of 26 bones and many muscles, tendons, and ligaments.

 Foot problems tend to increase with aging. Because of diseases such as arteriosclerosis and peripheral vascular insufficiency, older adults often have decreased circulation to the lower extremities. This increases their risk for foot ulcers and infection. The incidence of diabetes is high among older adults, further increasing the risk for infection secondary to delayed healing. In addition, the skin becomes dry, predisposing it to cracking.

Common Foot Problems

Eight out of 10 Americans report having experienced a foot problem—nail problems and foot odor are the most common. Many foot problems are the result of improperly fitting shoes.

- A **corn** is a cone-shaped thickening of the epidermis caused by continuous pressure (e.g., from improperly fitting shoes) over bony prominences (e.g., toe joints).
- **Calluses** are usually found over bony prominences on the weight-bearing part of the foot: the heels, soles, or plantar surfaces of the feet. They are similar to corns but cover a wider area and are not painful.
- **Tinea pedis,** or athlete's foot, is a fungal infection of the skin, aggravated by moisture accumulation in unventilated shoes. Symptoms include itching and burning skin with blisters, scaling, and cracking, especially between the toes. Athlete's foot may be contracted by walking barefoot in public showers.
- An **ingrown toenail** grows inward into the soft tissues around it, and the tissue at the nail border becomes swollen, inflamed, and painful. It may result from improperly trimming the toenails and wearing poorly fitting shoes. The nail may need to be surgically removed.
- **Foot odor** is produced when microorganisms growing on the feet interact with perspiration. The warm, moist environment created by shoes encourages both perspiration and bacterial growth.
- **Plantar warts** are painful growths caused by a virus. They may occur on any part of the sole of the foot but often develop under pressure points, such as the heel or ball of the foot.
- **Pressure injuries** are lesions caused by unrelieved pressure that impairs the circulation; this usually occurs over a bony prominence. In patients who are immobile, the back of the heels, the ankles, and the great toes are common locations, but pressure injuries do, of course, occur over other bony prominences.
- A **bunion** (hallux valgus) is a progressive disorder that begins at the enlargement of the first metatarsal joint at the base of the great toe and then progresses to leaning of the big toe, gradually changing the angle

of the bones over time. A characteristic bump occurs slowly and continues to become increasingly prominent with aging. Tight-fitting shoes (particularly with high heels) are thought to be the cause of bunions in most patients. Genetics and some diseases, such as arthritis, also play a role. For optional illustrations and more information about bunions,

 Go to the American College of Foot and Ankle Surgeons Web site at https://www.acfas.org/.

PracticalKnowledge
knowing **how**

The nursing focus for foot care is on assessment, prevention, and early identification of problems.

ASSESSMENT/RECOGNIZING CUES (FEET)

This chapter describes routine observations that you can make when giving foot care. The color and temperature of the feet provide data about circulation and oxygenation. For example, cold, dusky, or pale feet may indicate impaired circulation or tissue perfusion secondary to peripheral vascular disease. For a thorough discussion of foot assessment, see Chapter 19, and

Go to **Chapter 22, Procedure 22-4, Pre-Procedure Assessments;** also see **Assessment Guidelines and Tools, Focused Assessment: Guidelines for Assessing Hygiene,** in Volume 2.

NURSING DIAGNOSIS/ANALYZING CUES (FEET)

The feet can be affected by congenital malformations, injuries, improper footwear, and medical conditions. The following are examples of using NANDA-International terminology (Herdman & Kamitsuru, 2021) to write nursing diagnoses related to the feet:

- Impaired Skin (or Tissue) Integrity (feet) related to mechanical pressure from wearing shoes that do not fit properly
- Risk for Impaired Skin Integrity (feet) related to (1) decreased sensation secondary to diabetes mellitus and (2) decreased circulation to the feet secondary to arteriosclerosis
- Impaired Walking related to foot pain secondary to arthritis

PLANNING/PRIORITIZING HYPOTHESES AND GENERATING SOLUTIONS (FEET)

NOC outcomes for foot care are the same as for other areas of the body, as they relate to circulation, infection, tissue integrity, and wound healing. Examples include:

Tissue Integrity: Skin and Mucous Membranes
Wound Healing: Primary (and Secondary) Intention

Individualized goals/outcome statements you might write for a patient with foot problems include the following:

- Avoids trimming calluses
- Wears shoes that fit properly
- Inspects feet regularly

◼ IMPLEMENTATION/TAKING ACTION (FEET)

Examples of *NIC standardized interventions* include:

Foot Care
Circulatory Care: Arterial Insufficiency
Circulatory Care: Venous insufficiency
Infection Protection
Self-Care Assistance
Skin Surveillance
Teaching: Individual; Wound Care

Individualized nursing activities related to care of the feet are those that prevent infection, odor, and trauma to the soft tissues of the feet. To learn how to administer foot care,

 Go to **Chapter 22, Procedure 22-4: Providing Foot Care,** in Volume 2.

Teaching Your Client About Foot Care

While performing foot care, use the opportunity to teach the patient self-care for the feet. This is especially important for clients who have diabetes. Include the information in the accompanying Self-Care Box in your patient teaching.

Diabetic Foot Care The following self-care measures are especially important for people who have diabetes or poor peripheral circulation. Those who have diabetes should have their feet checked regularly by a professional. People who have diabetes are at high risk for foot problems because they often have impaired circulation and delayed healing, as well as an increased risk for infection. Furthermore, if they have neuropathy, they may not experience pain with a foot injury, so treatment may be delayed. If untreated, a seemingly minor foot lesion can progress to gangrene and require amputation.

KnowledgeCheck 22-6

- What are some causes of ingrown toenails?
- What is the cause of foot odor?
- Why should you *not* apply lotion between the toes?

CARE OF THE NAILS

The nails are part of the integumentary system. Like the hair and skin, they are composed of epithelial tissue. Healthy nailbeds are usually clean, pink, smooth,

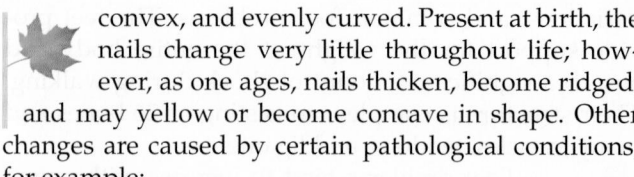 convex, and evenly curved. Present at birth, the nails change very little throughout life; however, as one ages, nails thicken, become ridged, and may yellow or become concave in shape. Other changes are caused by certain pathological conditions, for example:

- Trauma to the nail can lead to nail bruising or the nail falling out.
- Inadequate diet or metabolic changes can cause the nails to become brittle.
- Patients with diabetes mellitus are much more prone to infection.

◼ ASSESSMENT (NAILS)

Unclean or rough fingernails may scratch or abrade the skin and create a risk for infection. Other nail changes may reflect an underlying disease process. In addition, the area under the nail can harbor bacteria, which can be another source for transmitting microbes. When assessing the nails:

- *Obtain subjective data* about the patient's usual nail care practices, any history of nail problems, and their treatments.
- *To obtain objective data,* inspect the nails for shape, contour, and cleanliness, and observe whether they are neatly manicured and trimmed appropriately, straight across.

◼ NURSING DIAGNOSIS/ANALYZING CUES (NAILS)

The following are examples of nursing diagnoses related to nail care (CCC, n.d.):

- Risk for Impaired Tissue Integrity related to ingrown nails secondary to trimming too close to the cuticle
- Risk for Infection related to loss of skin integrity secondary to hangnails, cracked cuticles, or trauma from using sharp scissors or nail clippers

◼ PLANNING/PRIORITIZING HYPOTHESES AND GENERATING SOLUTIONS (NAILS)

There are no *NOC outcomes* that relate especially to nail care, but you can use outcomes that relate more generally to circulation, infection, tissue integrity, and wound healing, for example:

Knowledge: Health Behavior
Self-Care: Hygiene

Individualized goals/outcome statements you might write for a patient with problems related to the care of the nails may include the following:

- Demonstrates proper care of the nails
- Seeks care of a **podiatrist** (physician who specializes in foot care) for toenail care

Teaching Your Client About Foot Care

While performing foot care, use the opportunity to teach the patient self-care of the feet. This is especially important for people who have diabetes. Include the following in your teaching.

Daily Foot Inspection

➤ Inspect the feet daily, using a mirror to view all surfaces. Check between the toes for cracks or redness. Look for calluses, blisters, wounds and lesions, or dry areas.

➤ If you cannot check your own feet, have someone else do it.

Hygiene for Feet and Nails

➤ Wash, rinse, and dry the feet well.

➤ Avoid soaking the feet if you have diabetes or if there is decreased circulation to the feet.

➤ Apply a water-soluble lotion to feet, but do not use lotion between the toes because it may cause maceration.

➤ Use an antifungal powder, if necessary, for athlete's foot.

➤ Do not cut or file callused areas.

➤ Cut and file toenails straight across. Do not use a razor blade on the nails or feet.

Shoes and Stockings

➤ Wear cotton or wool socks, which absorb perspiration.

➤ Wear well-fitted, sturdy shoes with nonskid soles and arch support. Natural materials, such as canvas and leather, are best because they allow air to circulate and perspiration to evaporate. Shoes should allow 1/2 to 3/4 inch of toe room.

➤ Avoid open-toed shoes, sandals, high heels, and flip-flops. They do not protect the feet.

➤ Before putting on shoes, check for foreign objects; check that the inside of the shoe is smooth.

Protecting the Feet

➤ Avoid measures that impair circulation to the feet, such as wearing tight garters or knee stockings, or crossing the legs.

➤ Do not go barefoot, even when getting out of bed at night. Wear slippers.

➤ Do not put tape or over-the-counter corn medicines or pads or other medications (e.g., hydrogen peroxide) on the feet.

➤ Do not smoke. This further decreases circulation to the feet.

When to Seek Medical Attention

➤ Pain in the feet or legs. This may be a sign of loss of circulation, serious infection, or nerve damage (neuropathy).

➤ Wounds or ulcers on the feet, especially if they don't seem to be healing

➤ Cut to the feet or lower legs that extends deep into the skin and bleeds significantly

➤ Cuts or cracks in the feet

➤ Generalized redness or red streaks surrounding a wound or ulcer on the feet or lower legs. This might be a sign of infection of the tissue (cellulitis).

➤ Fever greater than 101°F (38.5°C).

➤ Confusion. This can be a sign that a wound infection has entered the bloodstream (septicemia). A change in mental status might indicate low blood sugar, which occurs with serious infection or if the patient has diabetes.

➤ Numbness or tingling, decreased sensation, cold skin temperature, corns, ingrown toenails, and for trimming very thick nails—especially if you have diabetes.

 IMPLEMENTATION/TAKING ACTION (NAILS)

Examples of *NOC standardized interventions* for nail care include Infection Protection, Nail Care, Self-Care Assistance, and Teaching.

Individualized nursing activities related to proper care of the nails include providing nail care for dependent patients. The procedure for care of the fingernails is the same as that for care of the toenails. For that procedure,

➤ Go to **Chapter 22, Procedure 22-4: Providing Foot Care,** in Volume 2.

Teaching Your Client About Nail Care Teach clients the following self-care measures:

- Inspect the nails daily.
- Trim nails with a nail clipper. (People with diabetes or circulatory problems should file only because cutting poses a risk for injury to the tissues.)
- File the nails straight across, rounding the corners slightly to prevent scratching. Do not cut deeply into the lateral corners because this may cause ingrown nails.
- Carefully remove hangnails using a cuticle clipper.
- Clean under the nails with an orangewood stick or other blunt instrument.
- Push back the cuticles gently.
- Use a moisturizing lotion to soften cuticles.
- Avoid biting nails.
- Consult a podiatrist for ingrown toenails or other nail problems.
- Recommend to patients with diabetes, circulatory insufficiency, or nail problems that they seek nail care from a podiatrist.

KnowledgeCheck 22-7

- True or False: Healthy nails are usually clean, smooth, and convexly curved.
- List at least three nail changes that occur with aging.
- List at least four things you should teach clients about self-care of their nails.

Oral Hygiene

To maintain the integrity of the mucous membranes, teeth, and gums and to prevent tooth loss and gum disease, it is important to have (1) routine dental checkups, (2) adequate nutrition, and (3) daily mouth care (oral hygiene). The following are benefits of mouth care:

- It removes food particles and secretions.
- A clean mouth helps to promote a better appetite.
- It reduces the incidence of healthcare-acquired pneumonia in older adults and critically ill patients in acute care settings.

Theoretical Knowledge
knowing **why**

Digestion of food begins in the mouth (oral cavity). The tongue and teeth begin digestion by breaking up food and mixing it with saliva. The structures of the mouth pertinent to oral hygiene include the tongue, **gingiva** (gums), and teeth.

- **Incisors** (front teeth) are for biting and tearing,
- **Molars** (in the back of the mouth) are used for chewing.
- **Wisdom teeth** are the very back molars on either side of the jaw bone.
- **Saliva**, produced by three pairs of salivary glands in the mouth, also acts as a mechanical cleaner of the mouth.

Developmental Variations

The first set of teeth (the **deciduous teeth**) erupts between 6 months and 2 years of age. By age 2, a child usually has 20 teeth (Fig. 22-2). Between the ages of 6 and 12 years, the deciduous teeth loosen, fall out, and are eventually replaced with 32 permanent teeth (Fig. 22-3).

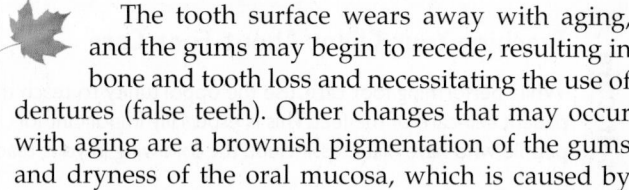

The tooth surface wears away with aging, and the gums may begin to recede, resulting in bone and tooth loss and necessitating the use of dentures (false teeth). Other changes that may occur with aging are a brownish pigmentation of the gums and dryness of the oral mucosa, which is caused by decreased saliva production.

Risk Factors for Oral Problems

Oral health is influenced by heredity, nutrition, and oral hygiene. Therefore, any condition that prevents good oral hygiene can lead to oral problems. Risk factors include the following:

- **History of periodontal disease**
- **Lack of money or insurance** for dental care
- **Pregnancy.** The gums may bleed easily and become puffy and tender during pregnancy because of increased estrogen, which increases the vascularity of the gingiva. Good hygiene is needed to prevent infection.
- **Poor nutrition or eating habits.** Adequate intake of calcium, phosphorus, and vitamin D is essential for healthy teeth and gums. Excessive intake of refined sugars leads to dental decay. One example of this is **baby-bottle tooth decay,** which occurs when parents put an infant or toddler to bed with a bottle or sippy cup of milk, fruit juice, or other sugary beverages. Carbohydrates in the fluid cause demineralization of the tooth enamel, leading to major decay of the upper and lower teeth.
- **Medications.** The anticonvulsant phenytoin (Dilantin) causes gingival hyperplasia (excessive growth of cells). Other medications cause dryness of the mouth (e.g., diuretics, medications used to treat cancer, numerous calcium channel blocker agents [especially nifedipine], and tranquilizers such as chlorpromazine [Thorazine] and diazepam [Valium]).

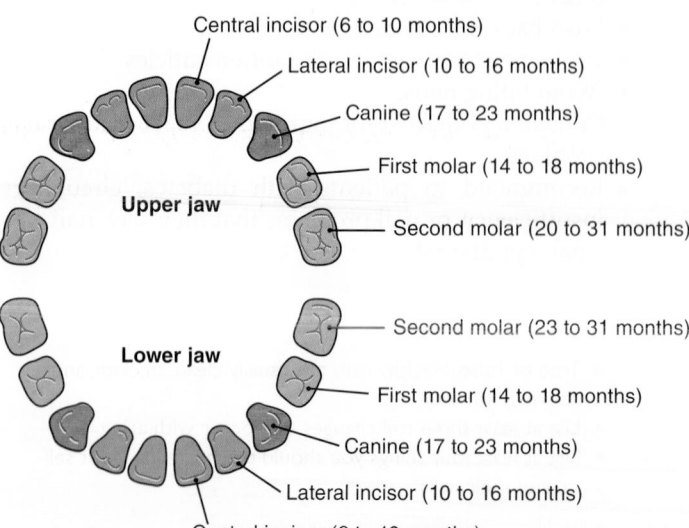

Central incisor (6 to 10 months)
Lateral incisor (10 to 16 months)
Canine (17 to 23 months)
First molar (14 to 18 months)
Upper jaw
Second molar (20 to 31 months)

Second molar (23 to 31 months)
Lower jaw
First molar (14 to 18 months)
Canine (17 to 23 months)
Lateral incisor (10 to 16 months)
Central incisor (6 to 10 months)

FIGURE 22-2 The 20 deciduous teeth.

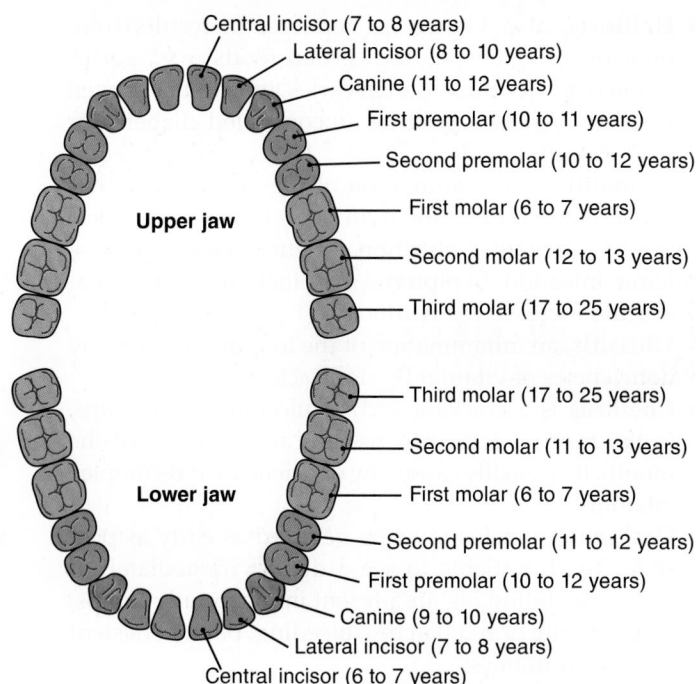

Central incisor (7 to 8 years)
Lateral incisor (8 to 10 years)
Canine (11 to 12 years)
First premolar (10 to 11 years)
Second premolar (10 to 12 years)
First molar (6 to 7 years)
Second molar (12 to 13 years)
Third molar (17 to 25 years)

Upper jaw

Third molar (17 to 25 years)
Second molar (11 to 13 years)
First molar (6 to 7 years)
Second premolar (11 to 12 years)
First premolar (10 to 12 years)
Canine (9 to 10 years)
Lateral incisor (7 to 8 years)
Central incisor (6 to 7 years)

Lower jaw

FIGURE 22-3 Most adults have 32 permanent teeth.

■ **Medical treatments** affecting the oral cavity include the following:

Jaw surgery, which requires scrupulous oral hygiene to prevent infection

Radiation treatments of the head and neck, which can damage teeth and jaw structure and permanently damage the salivary glands

Oxygen therapy, which dries the oral mucosa

■ **Any situation that causes dry mouth** predisposes to cracking of the mucosa, including cigarette smoking, excessive alcohol use, inadequate fluid intake (e.g., being NPO), dehydration, and mouth breathing.

■ **Compromised self-care abilities** may be caused by:

Decreased level of consciousness (e.g., a person who is comatose or heavily sedated), serious illness or injury, weakness, activity intolerance, or paralysis

Cognitive impairment (e.g., developmental delay, dementia)

Depression

Lack of knowledge or motivation to perform self-care

KnowledgeCheck 22-8

■ How do the teeth aid in digesting food?
■ How many deciduous teeth does a child usually have?
■ List at least three factors that cause dry mouth.
■ List at least two medications or medical treatments that can cause oral problems.
■ Name four situations that can compromise self-care ability for oral hygiene.

 ThinkLike a Nurse 22-9:
Clinical Judgment **in Action**

■ For which of your patients, Mrs. Rosha or Mr. Fuller, does the scenario provide *actual data* to indicate that the patient is at risk for oral problems? What are the data?

■ Why is the patient's nursing diagnosis Risk for Oral Mucous Membrane Impairment instead of Oral Mucous Membrane Impairment?

Common Problems of the Mouth

Dental **caries** (cavities) and periodontal disease are the two most frequent problems affecting the teeth. They are discussed here, along with other common mouth problems.

■ **Dental caries** are primarily caused by the failure to remove plaque.

■ **Plaque** is an invisible bacterial film that builds up on the teeth and eventually leads to the destruction of the tooth enamel. Untreated plaque can result in tooth loss. The plaque builds up with dead bacteria and forms hard deposits at the gumlines **(tartar).**

■ **Tartar** causes deterioration of the supporting structures that hold the teeth in the gums and also attacks the bone tissue, causing the teeth to become loose.

■ **Other factors** that contribute to the formation of cavities include excessive intake of refined sugars, a lack of brushing and flossing, and infrequent visits to the dentist.

■ **Periodontal disease (pyorrhea)** is the major cause of tooth loss in adults 35 years and older. It is an inflammation characterized by bleeding and receding gums and destruction of the surrounding bone structure. The patient experiences halitosis and complains of a bad taste in the mouth. When pyorrhea is advanced, the gums become infected, and the teeth loosen and may fall out or need to be removed.

■ **Gingivitis** is inflammation of the gum tissue surrounding the teeth. If untreated, it may progress to periodontal disease.

- **Halitosis,** also known as bad breath, results from poor oral hygiene, eating certain foods (e.g., garlic, onions), tobacco use, dental caries, infections, or even systemic diseases, such as uncontrolled diabetes or liver disease.
- **Stomatitis,** an inflammation of the oral mucosa, has numerous causes, including bacteria, mechanical trauma, irritants, nutritional deficiencies, and systemic infection. Symptoms may include pain, halitosis, and increased salivation.
- **Glossitis,** an inflammation of the tongue, is caused by deficiencies of vitamin B$_{12}$, folic acid, and iron.
- **Cheilosis** is a cracking and/or ulceration of the lips, in the form of reddened fissures at the angles of the mouth. It is usually caused by deficiencies in B-complex vitamins.
- **Oral malignancies** must be detected as early as possible. Teach patients to see a dentist immediately if any of the following are present in the mouth: lumps, ulcers, white or red patches, bleeding, pain, persistent sores, or numbness.

KnowledgeCheck 22-9

- Identify and define several causes of halitosis.
- What are the two most common problems affecting the teeth?
- What is the end result of severe periodontal disease?

PracticalKnowledge
knowing **how**

 You should assess the patient's oral cavity when performing or assisting with oral hygiene. This is particularly important for older adults because of the association between oral health and systemic disease.

ASSESSMENT/RECOGNIZING CUES (ORAL CAVITY)

You might begin your subjective assessment by asking the patient about their usual hygiene practices. You should also interview the patient or examine patient records for the risk factors for oral problems discussed in the preceding section. Ask about tobacco and alcohol use.

As part of your objective assessment during hygiene care, inspect the lips, oral mucosa, gums, and tongue. The mucosa and gums should be pink and moist, without lesions or bleeding. Look for loose, missing, or decaying teeth; tartar; and stomatitis; also note any unusual odors or halitosis. Check to be sure the tongue is normal in color and without lesions.

 The Kayser–Jones Brief Oral Health Status Examination (BOHSE) is used to assess the oral cavity of older adults. It was specifically designed for nursing home residents who have either normal or impaired cognitive functioning, and it can be used by a variety of nursing personnel. The tool

assigns a numerical rating to findings for the following: the lymph nodes, lips, tongue, tissue inside the mouth, gums, saliva, condition of natural teeth, condition of artificial teeth, pairs of teeth in chewing position, and oral cleanliness. To learn more about the BOHSE and see a copy of the tool, you can search the web, or

Go to the Clinical Nursing Web site and search for Kayser–Jones BOHSE at http://consultgeri.org/try-this/general-assessment/issue-18.pdf

To learn more about physical assessment of the oral cavity, refer to Chapter 19. Also,

Go to **Chapter 22, Assessment Guidelines and Tools, Guidelines for Assessing Hygiene,** in Volume 2.

NURSING DIAGNOSIS/ANALYZING CUES (ORAL CAVITY)

In addition to Self-Care Deficit, discussed in the first part of the chapter, the following are examples of nursing diagnoses that may be useful in describing problems of the mouth:

- Infection Risk related to mouth lesions
- Caries related to an inability to afford dental care
- Oral Mucous Membrane Impairment related to an inability to manage mouth care secondary to impaired mobility

Oral and dental problems can be the etiology of other nursing diagnoses, for example:

- Knowledge Deficit related to lack of interest in learning about oral hygiene
- Inadequate Nutrition related to lack of teeth for mastication
- Pain related to mouth lesions

PLANNING/PRIORITIZING HYPOTHESES AND GENERATING SOLUTIONS (ORAL CAVITY)

NOC standardized outcomes for oral problems include Oral Hygiene, Self-Care: Oral Hygiene, and Knowledge: Health Behavior.

Individualized goals/outcome statements you might write for mouth problems include the following:

- Oral mucous membranes will remain pink, moist, and intact.
- Demonstrates correct technique for brushing and flossing
- Makes preventive dental visits every 6 months

IMPLEMENTATION/TAKING ACTION (ORAL CAVITY)

For some clients, you may need only to provide the necessary supplies for mouth care. For others, you will need to assist or even completely provide care as often as necessary to keep the mouth clean and moist. Rinsing with mouthwash is not a substitute for a thorough cleaning of the teeth and mouth.

NIC standardized interventions for mouth care include Oral Health Maintenance, Self-Care Assistance, and Teaching: Individual.

Individualized nursing activities related to oral hygiene include (1) teaching for self-care (see the box Self-Care: Teaching Your Client About Oral Hygiene) and (2) assisting with and providing oral hygiene for dependent patients.

Teaching Your Client About Oral Hygiene

Teach the following self-care measures to promote oral health and prevent periodontal disease.

Preventing Caries and Periodontal Disease

- Eliminate high-sugar snacks between meals (ice cream, soft drinks, candy, gum, jams and jellies).
- Include cleansing, fibrous foods, such as raw fruits and vegetables, in the diet.
- Include an adequate intake of calcium; phosphorus; and vitamins A, C, and D.
- Have regular dental checkups every 6 months.
- Brush teeth with a soft brush and toothpaste after each meal and at bedtime (some dentists say twice a day). Bacteria do the most damage to the teeth in the first 24 hours after eating.
- Floss between the teeth daily to remove food debris and stimulate the blood flow to the gingiva.
- Use a fluoride toothpaste to strengthen tooth enamel.
- You can make your own cleanser by combining one part baking soda with two parts salt.
- Follow the dentist's recommendations for topical applications of fluoride.

Brushing and Flossing

The following are self-care measures. For a procedure to use for nurse-administered brushing and flossing,

 Go to **Chapter 22, Procedure 22-5: Brushing and Flossing the Teeth,** in Volume 2.

- Make sure the brush is small enough to reach all teeth. If it is too firm, it can injure enamel and gum tissue.
- Electric toothbrushes are effective; however, you should consult your dentist about using water-spray units because they can force debris into pockets of the gums.
- Brush at a 45° angle, from the gum to the tooth crown, using small circular or vibrating motions.
- When flossing: (1) Wrap one end of the floss around each of your middle fingers. (2) Hold about 1 to 2 inches of floss tightly between the fingers. (3) Insert floss between each tooth by gently moving it back and forth; do not force it. (4) Floss adjacent sides of each tooth to

the gum tissue but not into the gum because you may injure the tissue. (5) Use a fresh section of floss when it becomes soiled or frayed. (6) Rinse your mouth well when you are finished. A variety of convenient flossing devices are available as an alternative to this method (Fig. 22-4).

Oral Hygiene for Children

- Begin oral hygiene when the first tooth erupts. Use a washcloth, cotton ball, or gauze pad moistened with water.
- Do not put the child to bed with a bottle or sippy cup. Milk, juice, or any other liquid with sugar can lead to dental caries in the young child when the liquid sits on the teeth at night or for naps.
- Begin brushing the child's teeth with a soft toothbrush at about 18 months old. Start first using water only. Later, switch to a fluoride-containing toothpaste.
- Follow your dentist's instructions for giving a fluoride supplement.
- Schedule a visit to the dentist when all 20 deciduous teeth have erupted.
- See your dentist if you notice any problems, such as chipping, redness or swelling, caries, or misalignment.
- For school-age children, parents may need to supervise mouth care to be sure it is done adequately.

Denture Self-Care

- If you have dentures or other removable prostheses ("bridges"), wear them. If you do not, the gums are likely to shrink, and you will have further gum loss.
- Clean dentures and bridges at least once a day, preferably after each meal.
- Remove dentures from the mouth to clean them.
- Use regular toothpaste or special denture-cleaning compounds.
- Do not use hot water on dentures; it may damage them.

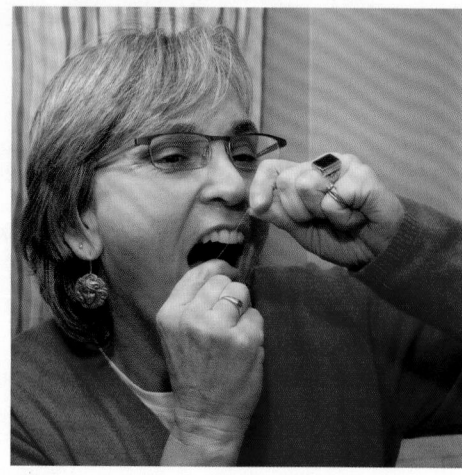

FIGURE 22-4. Flossing between the teeth is an essential part of oral hygiene.

- If the dentures have metal parts, do not soak them overnight in cleaning solutions.
- Store dentures in a denture cup, in distilled, sterile, or filtered water, to prevent drying. Do not wrap them in tissues because they may accidentally be thrown away.
- Clean dentures over a plastic pan or towel in the sink (Fig. 22-5). They are fragile and may break if dropped.

Assisting With Denture Care

A patient may have a complete set of removable dentures or just an upper or lower plate. A **bridge,** or partial plate, consists of one or more artificial teeth. A bridge may be permanently fastened to other teeth, or it may be removable. Artificial teeth are fitted to the individual and should not be used by anyone else. If the person leaves the prosthesis out of their mouth for long periods, the shape of the gums will change, and it will no longer fit properly. Poorly fitted or loose dentures can lead to chewing difficulties and even nutritional deficiencies.

 Research suggests that elderly persons should remove dentures at bedtime to prevent problems such as tongue and denture plaque and gum inflammation. In addition, elderly persons who wear dentures during sleep are more likely to develop pneumonia (Bartlett et al., 2018).

As a nurse, your role is to ensure cleanliness by teaching for self-care (as described previously) or to provide denture care for dependent clients. For further information,

Go to **Chapter 22, Procedure 22-6: Providing Denture Care,** in Volume 2.

Oral Care for Critically Ill Patients

Critically ill patients in acute care settings are at high risk for healthcare-associated pneumonia. This is especially true for those dependent on a ventilator. Ventilator-associated pneumonia (VAP) is the most common HAI

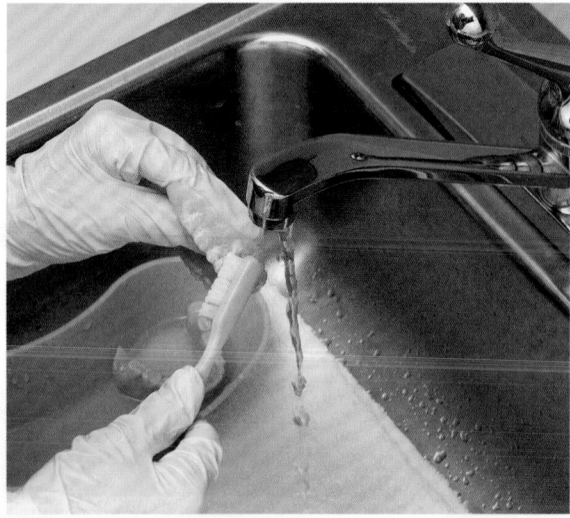

FIGURE 22-5 Dentures must be cleaned thoroughly as a part of daily oral hygiene.

in critically ill patients. A simple and inexpensive way to reduce the risk of pneumonia for critically ill patients is to keep their teeth clean, thus reducing the number of bacteria (American Association of Critical Care Nurses, 2010; Cooper, 2021; Reese et al., 2021). The regimen includes the following:

- Brush the teeth two to four times a day.
- Use a soft toothbrush.
- Moisturize oral mucosa and lips every 2 to 4 hours.
- Use chlorhexidine gluconate (0.12%) swabs for mechanically ventilated intensive care unit (ICU) patients.
- Use mouthwash inside the mouth twice a day for adult patients who are on a ventilator.

Oral Care for Unconscious Patients

Oral care for unconscious patients is particularly important because they often breathe through the mouth. If the patient is receiving oxygen per cannula or has a nasogastric or feeding tube inserted, the mucous membranes become even drier. To learn more about how to provide oral care for unconscious patients,

Go to **Chapter 22, Procedure 22-7: Providing Oral Care for an Unconscious Patient,** in Volume 2.

 An unconscious patient often responds to oral stimulation by biting down, so use a padded tongue blade instead of your fingers to hold the mouth open. Also use a padded tongue blade when providing oral care for a patient with seizures to avoid the patient biting you.

- Follow agency practices for the type and frequency of special mouth care. Some patients may need it every hour or two.
- You may use commercially packaged applicators or foam swabs to clean the mouth.
- **Do not use lemon-glycerine swabs** because they are drying to the mucosa and may cause changes in tooth enamel.
- **Do not use hydrogen peroxide** because it is irritating to oral mucosa and may alter the balance of normal flora of the mouth.

Oral Care for Patients Who Have Dementia

Poor oral health and dental pain affect general well-being and quality of life—specifically, they have effects on the ability to eat, type of diet, weight changes, speech, hydration, appearance, and social interactions. This is especially true for older adults who have dementia, who have a high level of oral diseases and dental problems. Dental disease and pain may be the source of some of the behavior problems in this population.

Because it is a challenge to provide oral hygiene for patients who have dementia, staff sometimes neglect care. Residents may be uncooperative: refusing care, refusing to open the mouth, biting the toothbrush, and

Toward Evidence-Based Practice

American Association of Critical-Care Nurses (AACN). (2017). *AACN practice alert. Oral care in the critically ill.* https://www.aacn.org/clinical-resources/practice-alerts/oral-care-for-acutely and-critically ill-patients

This evidence report reviewed references and graded the evidence for the conclusions the researchers drew. They used an alpha scale (Level A = strongest support, Level M = weakest [manufacturer's recommendations only]). The following are two AACN recommendations for oral care in the critically ill:

- Use oral chlorhexidine gluconate (0.12%) rinse twice a day in intubated patients to reduce the risk of ventilator-associated pneumonia (VAP), not routinely for all patients. (Level A)
- Brush teeth, gums, and tongue at least twice a day. (Level E)

Kes, D., Yildirim, T. A., Kuru, C., Pazarlioglu, F., Ciftci, T., & Ozdemir, M. (2021). Effect of 0.12% chlorhexidine use for oral care on ventilator-associated respiratory infections: A randomized controlled trial. *Journal of Trauma Nursing, 28*(4), 228–234.

Researchers explored the effects of a chlorhexidine rinse (CHX) compared with a sodium bicarbonate rinse in preventing VAP in hospitalized patients. Nurses provided oral care in patients in the CHX group three times a day using 0.12% CHX. Patients in the placebo group received oral care with sodium bicarbonate three

times a day by nurses. VAP significantly decreased in the 0.12% CHX group compared with the placebo group.

Ory, J., Raybaud, E., Chabanne, R., Cosserant, B., Faure, J. S., Guérin, R., et al.. (2017). Comparative study of 2 oral care protocols in intensive care units. *American Journal of Infection Control, 45*(3), 245–220.

Over 2,000 patients in five adult intensive care units (ICUs) were studied over two time periods. During period 1, caregivers used a foam stick with chlorhexidine for oral care, and during period 2, oral care included a foam stick with chlorhexidine and tooth brushing with aspiration. Results indicated that oral health was significantly better and VAP rates decreased significantly after the implementation of tooth brushing with aspiration (period 2). In addition, caregivers reported greater satisfaction with the quality of oral health conditions after implementing the period 2 protocol.

1. Suppose you are a critical care nurse using the AACN Practice Alert guidelines. For which of the two AACN recommendations would you most want to have further research evidence?

2. Which of the latter two studies described provides additional support for the AACN guideline? Explain your thinking.

3. How are the patients in the latter two studies alike or different from the patients for whom the AACN Practice Alert was designed?

---

so on. Research is needed to identify the best interventions (Delwel et al., 2018). Meanwhile, for experts' suggestions for ways to provide oral care to patients with dementia,

 Go to **Chapter 22, Procedure 22-5: Brushing and Flossing the Teeth (What if …? section),** in Volume 2.

KnowledgeCheck 22-10

How would you position Mr. Fuller (Meet Your Patients) to perform oral hygiene?

CARE OF THE HAIR

Hair is an accessory structure of the skin.

- **Vellus hair** is the short, fine hair present over much of the body.
- **Terminal hair,** which is coarser, darker, and longer, is found on the scalp, eyebrows, axillae, perineum, and legs.

The hair helps to maintain body temperature, serves as a receptor for tactile sensation, and influences a person's self-image. Sebaceous glands found at the base of the hair follicle secrete sebum, or oil, to lubricate hair and scalp. The condition of the hair is a measure of a person's overall health. See Chapter 19 for more

information about changes in hair that occur throughout the life span and as a result of illness.

ASSESSMENT (HAIR)

For the purposes of hygiene, you will need information about the patient's history of hair problems or current conditions needing treatment (e.g., pediculosis), diseases or therapy that affect the hair (e.g., chemotherapy), and factors influencing the patient's ability to manage their hair and scalp care (e.g., Physical Mobility Impairment). Ask the patient about special products used and about their preference for styling their hair. Inspect the condition and cleanliness of the hair, and inspect the scalp for dandruff, lesions, and so forth. For more complete information about assessing the hair, see Chapter 19. Also,

 Go to **Chapter 22, Assessment Guidelines and Tools, Focused Assessment: Guidelines for Assessing Hygiene,** in Volume 2.

NURSING DIAGNOSIS/ANALYZING CUES (HAIR)

Common problems associated with the hair and scalp include the following (also see Chapter 19):

- **Dandruff** is a condition in which there is excessive shedding of the epidermal layer of the scalp. Primary symptoms include itching and flaking of the scalp, which may be caused by a fungal infection.

- **Pediculosis** is an infestation of head lice. Although frequently associated with poor hygiene practices, it knows no socioeconomic boundaries. Head lice spread through the sharing of combs, brushes, hair ornaments, hats, and caps.
- **Alopecia,** or hair loss, can be very stressful and affect self-image. Abnormal hair loss, which may be gradual or sudden, can be caused by an autoimmune disorder, hormonal imbalance, thyroid disease, stress, fever, certain medications, or chemotherapy.

When the difficulty lies with self-care ability, you can use Self-Care Deficit: Dressing/Grooming, and Self-Care Deficit: Bathing/Hygiene. Examples of other nursing diagnoses that may apply include the following:

- Skin Integrity Impairment Risk related to secretions on the scalp
- Situational Self-Esteem Disturbance related to alopecia secondary to chemotherapy

KnowledgeCheck 22-11

- List at least four assessments you should make of a patient's hair.
- What is pediculosis?
- What is alopecia?

PLANNING/PRIORITIZING HYPOTHESES AND GENERATING SOLUTIONS (HAIR)

NOC standardized outcomes for problems of the hair and scalp include Self-Care: Activities of Daily Living (ADL); Tissue Integrity: Skin and Mucous Membranes; and Self-Esteem. As always, select outcomes based on the client's nursing diagnosis.

Individualized goals/outcome statements you might write for a patient with problems related to the hair include the following:

- Scalp and hair are clean.
- By 9/18, brushes own hair
- Hair and scalp are free from infestation, infection, irritation, or dryness.
- Verbalizes improved comfort and self-esteem

IMPLEMENTATION/TAKING ACTION (HAIR)

NIC standardized interventions specific to hair care are as follows: Hair and Scalp Care, Skin Surveillance, and Infection Prevention.

Individualized nursing activities related to the care of the hair include daily brushing and combing of the hair, shampooing, and for men, shaving and beard care.

Providing Hair Care

- Brush the hair daily to remove tangles, massage the scalp, stimulate the circulation, and distribute oil down the hair shaft.

- Use a stiff-bristled brush, but be sure the bristles are not sharp enough to injure the patient's scalp. Likewise, a comb with broken or uneven teeth or one that is too fine can break or snarl the hair or scrape the scalp.
- Comb tightly curled hair with a wide-toothed comb or pick.
- Encourage patients to brush and comb their own hair if they are able to do so.
- Encourage family members to assist with hair care as a way to involve them in the patient's care and reduce feelings of helplessness.
- Do not cut a patient's hair unless they consent to the haircut.

Shampooing the Hair Shampooing cleans the hair and scalp. It is soothing and relaxing to many patients. Hair can be shampooed while the person is in the shower, standing or sitting over a sink, or in bed. Protect the patient's eyes with a dry washcloth, and make sure the water temperature is appropriate for the patient. For patients who are unable to tolerate a standard shampoo procedure, you can use a dry shampoo as an alternative. However, it is not as effective as shampooing with water. Commercially prepared shampoo caps are available and have, in most institutions, replaced the dry shampoo method. For a summary of a procedure for shampooing the hair, see the Highlights of Procedures box. For complete steps,

 Go to **Chapter 22, Procedure 22-8: Shampooing the Hair**, in Volume 2.

Hair Care for Black Clients The hair of Black clients varies in texture from some other ethnicities—it may be long or short, straight or curly, thick or thin. Worn naturally, very curly hair can easily become entangled or matted, and it tends to be fragile and easily broken.

Shampoo and groom the hair according to the person's preference. In general, though, you should comb and brush the hair daily and apply a light oil to the scalp. Ask a family member to bring in the product the patient prefers to use. Do not apply chemical relaxers to a patient's hair. Only a licensed beautician should do this.

Beard and Mustache Care

Beards and mustaches tend to collect food particles. They should be washed daily during a bath or shower and combed and trimmed as necessary. Use agency-approved (e.g., filtered) water. Do not shave a patient's mustache or beard without permission to do so. For details on beard and mustache care, see the Highlights of Procedures box and

 Go to **Chapter 22, Procedure 22-9: Providing Beard and Mustache Care,** in Volume 2.

Shaving

Depending on the culture, shaving is an important part of grooming and helps patients feel better about their appearance. Many men shave their facial hair every day. Women may shave to remove axillary and leg hair. If the patient has a bleeding disorder or is taking anticoagulant medication, you should use an electric razor. For important points about shaving, see the Highlights of Procedures box. Also,

▶ Go to **Chapter 22, Procedure 22-10: Shaving a Patient,** in Volume 2.

Some dark-haired men have tightly curled facial hair, which curls back into the skin when shaved. An inflammatory reaction may occur, resulting in the formation of papules and pustules ("razor bumps"). If the man wishes to use a **depilatory** (hair-removing agent) instead of shaving, be sure to keep the chemical from contacting the patient's eyes, nose, mouth, and ears. Do not use a straight or safety razor to remove the depilatory because it will irritate the skin. Some men with this condition prefer to grow a beard, especially when they are ill and unable to care for themselves.

CARE OF THE EYES

Usually you will not need to provide special hygiene care for the eyes. The eyelids and lashes keep dust and debris from entering the eyes, and tears continually cleanse and lubricate them. When necessary, you may gently cleanse the eyes, from the inner to the outer canthus, with a moistened washcloth, with no soap. If there is drainage or crusting, use a different cloth for each eye to prevent cross-contamination.

ASSESSMENT/RECOGNIZING CUES (EYES)

When performing hygiene care, inspect the eyes for redness, lesions, swelling, crusting, excessive tearing, or discharge. Also check the color of the conjunctivae. You should also ask the patient or check patient records to see whether they wear glasses or contact lenses. If the patient wears glasses, ask when they use them (e.g., for reading, for driving), and ask how well they see without them. If the patient wears contact lenses, determine the following:

- The type of lens (hard, soft, long-wearing, disposable)
- How often they wear them (daily, occasionally) and for how long at a time
- Whether they are worn during sleep
- History of or current problems with lens usage (e.g., cleaning, removal)
- Usual practices for cleaning and storage
- History of or current problems with the eyes (e.g., redness, tearing, irritation, dryness, or "scratchy feeling")

These should be adequate data for hygiene care. However, it is not a complete eye assessment. For detailed information about assessing the eyes, see Chapter 19.

NURSING DIAGNOSIS/ANALYZING CUES (EYES)

Other than Bathing/Hygiene Self-Care Deficit, there is only one standardized nursing diagnosis specific to the eyes: Visual Alteration (CCC, n.d.). This label is of limited use for hygiene care. Other diagnoses you might use include the following:

- Risk for Infection related to improper hand washing and improper lens cleaning
- Risk for Injury (to eyes) related to wearing lenses longer than recommended

PLANNING/PRIORITIZING HYPOTHESIS AND GENERATING SOLUTIONS (EYES)

The only *NOC standardized outcome* specific to the eyes is Sensory Function: Vision. For hygiene care, you could use Self-Care: Bathing or Self-Care: Activities of Daily Living.

Individualized goals you might write for eye care include these examples:

- Demonstrates proper cleaning and storage of contact lenses
- Eyes appear clean and without redness or drainage.

IMPLEMENTATION/TAKING ACTION (EYES)

NIC standardized interventions specific for eye care include Eye Care and Self-Care Assistance: Bathing. However, for an Infection Risk or Injury Risk diagnosis, you could use Infection Protection, Self-Care Assistance, and Individual Teaching.

Individualized nursing activities related to the care of the eyes include providing eye care to unconscious clients, caring for eyeglasses and contact lenses, and caring for artificial eyes.

Eye Care for the Unconscious Patient

 Having lost the blink (corneal) reflex, comatose or critically ill patients need more frequent eye care (every 2 to 4 hours).

- Keep their eyes lubricated with saline or artificial tears to protect them from corneal abrasions and drying.
- You may also need to use a protective eye shield to keep the patient's eyes closed.
- Instill eye ointment or drops in the lower lids as ordered.

To review a procedure for administering eye medications,

▶ Go to **Chapter 23, Procedure 23-2: Administering Ophthalmic Medications,** in Volume 2.

Caring for Eyeglasses and Contact Lenses

Eyeglasses need to be cleaned at least once a day. Using warm water and a soft cloth, clean gently to prevent scratching of the lens. Ask the patient whether the lenses require a special cleaning solution; some patients bring their own. **Key Point:** *Label each patient's glasses, and store them in a safe place within the patient's reach, preferably in a glasses case in the drawer of the bedside table. They are expensive, so take care that they are not lost or damaged.*

Contact lenses, an alternative to glasses, are plastic discs worn on the cornea over the pupil. They float on the tears of the eye and stay in place because of surface tension. The cornea is nourished mainly by oxygen from the atmosphere and from tears, so in order to ensure an optimal supply of oxygen, contact lenses must be removed periodically. Wearing time varies from daily wear to up to around 30 days, depending on the type of lens. People usually care for their own contact lenses.

- **Users must be careful to keep contact lenses free of microorganisms** that could cause eye infections and to avoid eye irritation.

- **Lenses should be kept away from all water,** according to the CDC (n.d., updated 2021).
  Water can cause soft lenses to swell and stick to the eye, possibly scratching the cornea.
  Water is not germ-free, and serious eye infections can result.
  The CDC recommends contact lens removal before showering, swimming, or using a hot tub.
  Users should not store lenses in water.
  If water touches the lenses, the wearer should remove and discard them.

- **Teach cleaning and disinfecting measures to clients as needed** (see the box Self-Care: Teaching Your Clients About Cleaning and Storing Contact Lenses), and follow those measures when you must care for a client's lenses.
- **If you need to remove a patient's lenses during an emergency, follow universal precautions** and handle the lenses as you would any other valuable patient property.

- **Never use your fingernails to remove a lens** because you may scratch the eye or damage the lens.

For more detailed instructions,

 Go to **Chapter 22, Procedure 22-11: Removing and Caring for Contact Lenses,** in Volume 2.

Caring for Artificial Eyes

An artificial eye is made to look like a natural eye. It can be made of glass or plastic. Some artificial eyes are permanently implanted in the socket, but others must be removed daily for cleaning of the prosthesis and the eye socket. If the patient is not able to perform eye care, ask

Self-Care

Teaching Your Clients About Cleaning and Storing Contact Lenses

- ➤ Cleaning and disinfecting procedures and solutions vary among manufacturers. Depending on the type of lens, use saline solutions or special rinsing and soaking solutions.

- ➤ Use a special container for the lenses, with a cup labeled for the left and right lens. Some lenses are stored in a solution; others are stored dry. Follow the manufacturer's instructions.

- ➤ Always wash your hands before touching the eyes or the lenses.

- ➤ Be careful not to allow the lenses to come in contact with soaps, hair sprays, or cosmetics.

- ➤ Do not wear soft lenses while using eye drops or ointment (wait 1 hour after using drops and at least 4 hours for ointment).

- ➤ Be aware of the risk for eye irritation when in the presence of smoke or chemical vapors.

about and follow their usual routines when possible. For details about removing, cleaning, and replacing an artificial eye, see the Highlights of Procedures box and

 Go to **Chapter 22, Procedure 22-12: Caring for Artificial Eyes,** in Volume 2.

KnowledgeCheck 22-12

- True or False: Eyes should be cleansed from the outer to the inner canthus.
- How can a contact lens wearer help prevent eye infections?
- After you have cleaned a prosthetic eye, should you dry it before reinserting it or leave it wet?

CARE OF THE EARS

Healthy ears require minimal care. However, you will need to help patients who have limited self-care abilities and teach others about self-care. For example, **cerumen** (wax) impaction is a common cause of hearing loss, especially in older adults. People sometimes believe hearing loss is a normal part of aging and fail to seek treatment. Encourage them to see their primary care provider whenever hearing loss occurs.

- **Teach patients to avoid using rigid objects,** such as bobby pins or toothpicks, to clean their ears. Such instruments can traumatize the ear canal and may rupture the tympanic membrane (eardrum).
- **Likewise, never use cotton-tipped applicators;** they will push the cerumen farther into the ear, causing a blockage.

- **For dependent patients, assess for drainage, excess cerumen, and hearing loss during the bath.** Clean the auricle, and remove wax from the canal with the tip of the moistened washcloth or disposable wipe. If cleansing does not effectively remove excess cerumen buildup, obtain a prescription for cerumenolytic drops and water irrigation.

- **You can delegate ear cleaning and hearing aid care to the UAP** if you are sure that the UAP knows how to perform these tasks. Describe what you want the UAP to observe and report to you.

See Chapter 27 for information about ear irrigations.

Care of Hearing Aids A hearing aid is a battery-powered device that amplifies sound. Three types of hearing aids are shown in Figure 22-6. Also, some patients wear a hearing aid in the temple pieces of their eyeglasses. People with severe hearing loss may wear a body hearing aid that clips onto the clothing or a harness-type carrier that connects by a cord to the earpiece. Digital hearing aids are rapidly replacing the analog models.

Hearing aids are expensive and often essential to the patient, so handle and store them properly. They require regular cleaning and replacement of batteries. Even with good care, they usually need to be replaced every 5 to 10 years, and earmolds usually need adjustment more often than that. **Key Point:** *Never place a hearing aid in water.*

For guidelines to remove, clean, and replace a hearing aid, see the Highlights of Procedures Box, and

 Go to **Chapter 22, Procedure 22-13: Caring for Hearing Aids,** in Volume 2.

CARE OF THE NOSE

Usually the nose requires no special care. Have the patient remove excess secretions by gently blowing into a tissue with both nostrils open. Holding one nostril shut can force secretions into the eustachian tubes.

- **In debilitated or unconscious patients,** dried secretions can interfere with respiration. Remove secretions by gently inserting a moistened cotton-tipped applicator into the nostrils. Occasionally you may need to

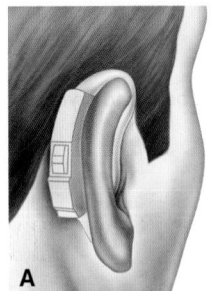 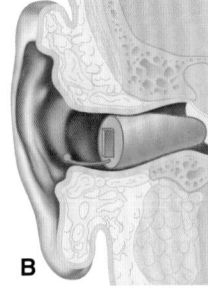 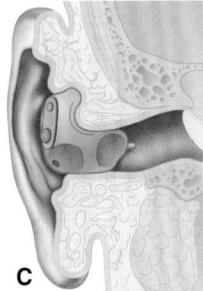

A   **B**   **C**

FIGURE 22-6 Hearing aids. *A,* The postaural (behind-the-ear) aid is the most widely used. A plastic tube connects it to an earmold. *B,* An in-the-canal aid is the least visible. *C,* The in-the-ear aid is made in one piece; all components are in the earmold.

instill saline into the nares and suction secretions to keep the airway patent.

- **If the patient has an NG tube,** the constant pressure on the skin may cause breakdown. Provide special skin care and a lubricant at the point where the tube touches the nares.

THE CLIENT'S ENVIRONMENT

♥ **iCare** A comfortable environment contributes to the client's well-being. It is your responsibility, as a nurse, to see that the bedside unit and surroundings are clean, safe, and comfortable.

ASSESSMENT/RECOGNIZING CUES (SCANNING THE ENVIRONMENT)

Each time you enter a patient's room, you should scan the environment to see whether you need to make adjustments to ensure patient safety and comfort:

- Is the room temperature comfortable?
- Are the siderails up, when indicated?
- Is the bed in a low position, and are the wheels locked?
- Are bed linens clean and free of wrinkles?
- Is the patient's call device within reach?
- Is the overbed table clean and uncluttered?
- Is there uncluttered walking space?
- Are there unpleasant odors?

Each time you leave the room, ask, "What else can I do for you?" This ensures that you have not overlooked anything.

IMPLEMENTATION/TAKING ACTION (THE ENVIRONMENT)

NIC standardized outcomes related to the patient's environment for hygiene are:

Environmental Management
Environmental Management: Comfort
Environmental Management: Safety

♥ **iCare** Adequate ventilation; proper room temperature; low noise level; and neat, clean surroundings are important to ensure the patient's comfort. A caring nurse provides for patient well-being by paying attention to environmental details.

Prevent and Eliminate Odors

Body secretions such as urine, feces, vomitus, or draining wounds cause odors in both inpatient facilities and the home. Odors can be offensive, and patients often feel embarrassed by them, so work quickly to free the environment of any sources of odors.

- Cleanliness is the best way to prevent odors.
- Provide good ventilation, if this is under your control. For example, open a window or use a fan.

For steps to follow in *all* procedures, refer to the inside back cover of Volume 2. Go to the full procedures in Volume 2 to practice and learn the procedure steps. Use these Procedure Highlights later to help you review key points.

Procedures 22-1 and 22-2: Bathing: Providing a Complete Bed Bath Using a Prepackaged Bathing Product, and Bathing: Using a Basin and Water

➤ Use prepackaged bathing products.

➤ Check the temperature of the packaged bath wipes after microwaving.

➤ Avoid chilling or tiring the patient.

➤ Bathe the patient following the principles of "head to toe" and "clean to dirty."

➤ For extremities, cleanse from distal to proximal.

➤ Use a new wipe for cleansing the perineum and whenever the wipe becomes soiled.

➤ Perform hand hygiene when moving from a contaminated body part to cleanse a clean body part.

➤ If performing a basin and water bath, use a disposable basin and distilled, filtered, or sterile water, according to agency requirements. Use a solution of chlorhexidine gluconate (CHG) and water to bathe the patient and clean the pan. Store the basin upside down.

➤ CHG 2% prepackaged cloths decrease the colonization of bacteria on the skin and should not be rinsed.

Procedure 22-3: Providing Perineal Care

➤ Provide privacy; keep the patient covered as much as possible.

➤ Place waterproof underpad to protect the bed linens.

➤ Use warmed prepackaged wipes.

➤ Perform perineal care following the principle of "clean to dirty" (front to back).

Procedure 22-4: Providing Foot Care

➤ Inspect the feet thoroughly for skin integrity, circulation, and edema.

➤ Clean the feet with warmed prepackaged wipes; clean the toenails, rinse, and dry well.

➤ Trim the nails straight across, unless contraindicated. Check institutional policy; many institutions do not allow nurses to trim nails.

➤ File the nails with an emery board.

➤ Lightly apply lotion, except between the toes.

➤ Ensure that footwear or bedding is not irritating to the feet.

Procedure 22-5: Brushing and Flossing the Teeth

➤ Assess the teeth, mucous membranes, and swallowing ability.

➤ Position the patient to prevent aspiration (sitting or side-lying position).

➤ Hold the brush at a 45° angle, and brush the patient's teeth (or assist).

➤ Floss and rinse, using sterile, filtered, or distilled water according to agency policy.

➤ If the patient is at risk for choking, suction secretions as needed.

Procedure 22-6: Providing Denture Care

➤ Refer to Procedure 22-6, Brushing and Flossing the Teeth.

➤ Remove (and replace) the top denture before the lower denture.

➤ Tilt dentures slightly when removing and replacing.

➤ Handle dentures carefully, and place a towel in the sink to avoid breaking the dentures if you drop them.

➤ Use cool, agency-approved water and a stiff-bristled brush.

Procedure 22-7: Providing Oral Care for an Unconscious Patient

➤ Assess the condition of the teeth (or dentures), gums, and mucous membranes.

➤ Assess for the gag reflex.

➤ Position the patient to prevent aspiration.

➤ Brush and floss the patient's teeth.

➤ Suction secretions as needed.

Procedure 22-8: Shampooing the Hair

➤ Determine the type of procedure needed. Assess the patient's ability to help and the condition of the hair and scalp.

➤ Identify hair-care products needed for the procedure.

➤ Wash the hair with no-rinse shampoo or no-rinse shampoo cap.

➤ If basin and water are used, protect the bed from getting wet.

➤ Protect the patient's eyes and ears from soap and water.

➤ Towel-dry the hair.

➤ Take care not to burn the patient with the hair dryer if one is used.

Procedure 22-9: Providing Beard and Mustache Care

➤ Assess the skin for redness, dry areas, or lesions.

➤ Trim the beard and mustache to the desired length with a comb and scissors or beard trimmer.

➤ Shampoo the beard and mustache.

➤ Apply conditioner, if desired.

➤ Towel-dry the beard and mustache, and comb and style as desired.

Procedure 22-10: Shaving a Patient

➤ Wear procedure gloves.

➤ Assess the skin for redness or dry areas.

➤ To soften the beard and moisten the skin:

➤ Apply a warm, damp towel to the face.

➤ Apply shaving cream or soap.

Highlights of Procedures 22-1 to 22-16

- To prevent skin irritation:
  - Hold the skin taut and shave the face and neck.
  - If using a safety razor, hold the blade at a 45° angle to the skin.
  - Apply aftershave product, if desired.

Procedure 22-11: Removing and Caring for Contact Lenses

- Instill one or two drops of wetting solution.
- Gently remove contact lenses; use your finger pads, not your fingernails.
- Clean and store contact lenses in sterile solution.
- Mark the containers "L" and "R" to identify the correct eye.

Procedure 22-12 Caring for Artificial Eyes

- Have the patient lie down.
- Remove the artificial eye: Raise the upper eyelid; with dominant hand, depress the lower lid and apply slight pressure below the eye (or use a small bulb syringe).
- Clean the eye: Clean the eye with saline; store in saline or distilled, sterile or filtered water (per agency policy); label the container.
- Clean the edge of the eye socket with a moistened cotton ball.
- Reinsert the eye: Be sure the prosthesis is wet. Hold it with your dominant hand. Spread the patient's eyelids apart with nondominant hand and guide prosthesis into the eye socket.

Procedure 22-13: Caring for Hearing Aids

- Keep hearing aids away from heat and moisture.
- Clean hearing aids with a damp cloth only.
- Avoid hairspray and other hair-care products.
- Turn off hearing aids when not in use.
- Replace dead batteries immediately.
- Store hearing aids in a case with the battery compartment open.
- Keep hearing aids and batteries away from children and pets.
- To clean a hearing aid: Turn it off, remove it from the ear, cleanse the outer ear and the hearing aid, check the battery, reinsert it, turn it on, and check the volume with the patient.

Procedure 22-14: Making an Unoccupied Bed

- Remove soiled linens without cross-contaminating other items in the room.
- Remake the bed with clean linens.
- Do not "shake" or "fan" linens.
- Work efficiently and safely.
- Ensure that there are no wrinkles in the bottom sheet or drawsheet.

Procedure 22-15: Making an Occupied Bed

- Maintain patient safety during the procedure.
- Assess the patient's ability to move and need for assistive equipment and patient-handling devices.
- Position the patient laterally near the far siderail, and roll soiled linens under the patient.
- Place clean linens on the side nearest you, and then tuck under the soiled linens.
- Roll the patient over the "hump," and position the patient on their other side, near you. Raise the near siderail.
- Move to the other side of the bed; pull soiled and clean linens through, and complete the linen change as in Procedure 22-14: Making an Unoccupied Bed.
- Place the bed in a low position, raise the siderails, and fasten the call light to the pillow.

- Empty and clean urinals, bedpans, or emesis basins promptly.
- Dispose of soiled dressings or other malodorous items in appropriate containers, and immediately remove them from the room.
- Unless contraindicated by the patient's illness, you can use a room deodorizer to help eliminate odors.
- Smoking is not allowed in patient rooms and in most institutions, in part because of the odor.

Control Room Temperature

Although preferences may vary, a room temperature between 68°F and 74°F (20°C and 23°C) is usually comfortable for most patients. Those who are very ill, very young, or very old may need a higher-than-normal room temperature. If there is no thermostat in the room, you may need to provide blankets, open a window, provide a fan, and so on to adjust the room temperature.

Limit Noise

People who are ill are often sensitive to various environmental noises, such as an ice machine, suction equipment, paging systems, loud talking, and laughter. Make it a priority to control noise. Keep unnecessary conversations to a minimum, and speak quietly. Some hospitals have instituted a "quiet hour" to promote better rest. Others have installed decibel meters to help nurses be mindful of noise escalation during activity in the nurses' station.

Standard Bedside Equipment

In a hospital, standard bedside equipment usually includes a bed, bedside stand (end table), overbed table, and one or two chairs. The wall unit may consist of a call light, oxygen, suction and electrical outlets, and light fixtures and switches. The patient's personal items are usually kept in the bedside stand. Therefore, you should request permission from the patient before opening the stand. Personal hygiene items, a bedpan, and a urinal may also be kept in the lower cabinet of this stand.

Hospital Beds Hospitalized patients spend a significant amount of time in bed. Hospital beds can be uncomfortable and may contribute to restlessness and poor sleep.

- Memory foam and moisture-control mattresses are available and provide more comfort. However, they are expensive and not used routinely.
- Hospital beds are generally standard in size and higher and narrower than a home bed. This allows you to reach the patient more easily and safely.
- Hospital beds are usually electronically controlled, so the patient and nurse can raise and lower the head and foot separately by the push of a button (see Fig. 22-7 for bed positions).

Safety Concerns for Beds To help prevent falls, a common cause of injury, be aware of and use bed safety features.

- ✚ **Bed height.** Patient safety is your priority, so although you should raise the entire bed to a working level that is comfortable for you, be sure to place the bed in the lowest position before leaving the bedside. Long-term care settings usually have low beds to make it easier for ambulatory patients to transfer into and out of bed. As a part of the admission procedure, you will teach patients how to use the bed controls.

- **Siderails.** Patients may use siderails when moving into and out of bed. Although siderails may help to prevent falls by patients with decreased consciousness, they are considered a passive restraint and may pose a risk to a patient with a cognitive impairment. See Chapter 21 for additional information about the safe use of siderails and other equipment.

- ✚ **Wheel locks.** To help prevent falls, always lock the wheels on a hospital bed when it is stationary, when you are helping the patient to a sitting position on the side of the bed, or when assisting with a transfer to a chair or stretcher. An unlocked bed could roll out from under an ambulatory patient or one you are assisting to get out of bed.

Mattresses and Linens Mattresses are usually firm and covered in a water-repellent material that resists staining and soiling and may be easily wiped down with a germicidal cleaner. Various special therapeutic mattresses are available to help reduce the effects of pressure over the bony prominences (e.g., sacrum, heels). See Chapter 32 for further discussion of special mattresses.

- **Mattress and Mattress Covers.** A mattress cover and/or pad promotes patient comfort and prevents soiling of the mattress. Mattress covers may lose their effectiveness over time, allowing moisture, blood, or bacteria to penetrate the mattress.
  - Regularly check each medical bed mattress cover. If you find any visible signs of damage or wear (e.g., cuts, tears, cracks, pinholes, snags, or stains), the cover should be immediately replaced to reduce the risk of infection.
  - Routinely remove the hospital bed mattress cover and inspect the mattress for wet spots, staining, or signs of damage or wear. Check all sides and the bottom of the mattress.
  - If a mattress is found to be damaged, worn, or visibly stained, it should be removed and discarded according to the healthcare facility's procedures and the manufacturer's instructions. (U.S. Food and Drug Administration, 2017).
- **Linens.** Sheets may be fitted or flat. Other linens include drawsheets, washable incontinence pads, pillowcases, blankets, bedspreads, and gowns. If a plastic

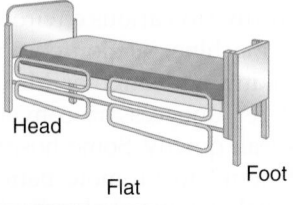

Head

Flat   Foot

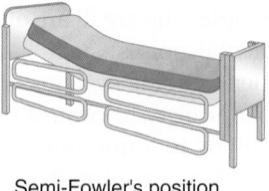

Semi-Fowler's position (30° angle)

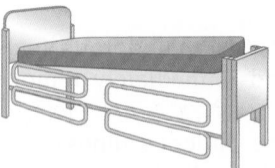

Trendelenburg's position

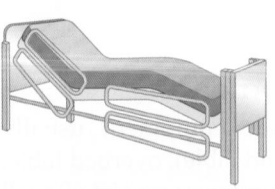

Fowler's position (45° angle)

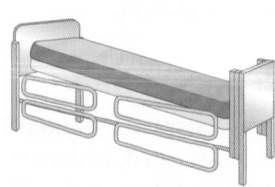

Reverse Trendelenburg's position

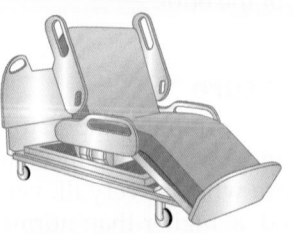

Sitting position (special wound-care beds; also adjust to standing position)

FIGURE 22-7 Hospital beds adjust to several positions.

surface lies directly under the sheet, you should place a cloth or other absorbent pad between the patient and the sheet. Because plastic mattress covers and pads do not allow moisture to escape, they contribute to skin maceration for patients who are incontinent or diaphoretic.

Bed Making   Clean, wrinkle-free bed linens help to promote comfort and a sense of well-being. In contrast, wrinkled and soiled linens can contribute to skin breakdown and pressure areas. Linens are generally changed daily after the bath and when soiled. If patients are up and about during the day, such as on a rehabilitation unit, beds are made daily, but bed linens may be changed weekly or only when soiled. If the patient is immobile or on bedrest, you or the UAP can make the bed while the patient occupies it. For more information about bed making, see the Highlights of Procedures Box, and

 Go to **Chapter 22, Procedure 22-14: Making an Unoccupied Bed** and **Procedure 22-14: Making an Occupied Bed,** in Volume 2.

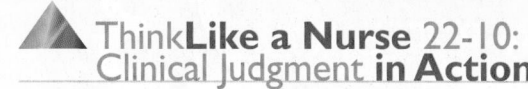 ThinkLike a Nurse 22-10: Clinical Judgment in Action

In the Meet Your Patients scenario, for which of your patients will you most surely need to make an occupied bed? Why?

 To explore learning resources for this chapter,

 Go to **Davis Advantage** and find:

Answers and Suggested Responses for all questions in this chapter

Concept Map

Knowledge Map

References and Bibliography

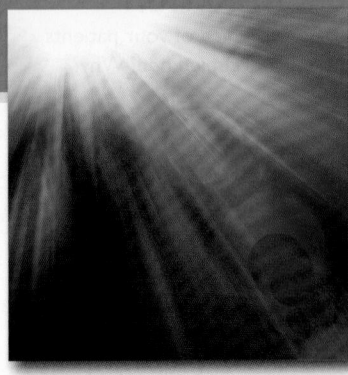

Administering Medications

Learning Outcomes

After completing this chapter, you should be able to:

➤ Name at least five sources of medication information.

➤ Distinguish among various nomenclature systems for naming and classifying drugs.

➤ Discuss the concepts and processes of pharmacokinetics, including drug absorption, distribution, metabolism, and excretion.

➤ Define *onset, peak,* and *duration* of drug action; *therapeutic level, peak level,* and *trough level;* and *biological half-life.*

➤ Compare and contrast primary, secondary, cumulative, and side effects and adverse, toxic, allergic, anaphylactic, and idiosyncratic reactions.

➤ Define *drug–drug interaction, antagonistic drug relationship, synergistic drug relationship, drug incompatibility,* and *medication contraindications.*

➤ Correctly calculate drug dosages, including (1) conversion among the metric, apothecary, and household measurement systems and (2) working with units and milliequivalents (mEq).

➤ List the types and methods for communicating medication prescriptions.

➤ Discuss the agencies and legislation that help to ensure drug quality and safety.

➤ Describe nursing assessment before, during, and after the administration of a drug.

➤ Plan care for clients with diagnoses of Risk for Injury and Ineffective Health Management related to medications.

➤ Administer medications using the "three checks" and "rights of medication."

➤ Describe appropriate steps to take when communicating a medication error.

➤ Demonstrate the correct procedure for administering medications by the oral, enteral, inhalant, and parenteral routes.

➤ Demonstrate the intramuscular injection procedure at the following sites: ventrogluteal, deltoid, and vastus lateralis.

➤ Explain the disadvantages of using the dorsogluteal site for intramuscular injections.

➤ List five steps to incorporate in your practice to ensure safe medication administration and prevent a medication error.

Key Concepts

Medication administration

Medication safety

Pharmacology

Related Concepts

See the Concept Map on Davis Advantage.

Meet Your Patients

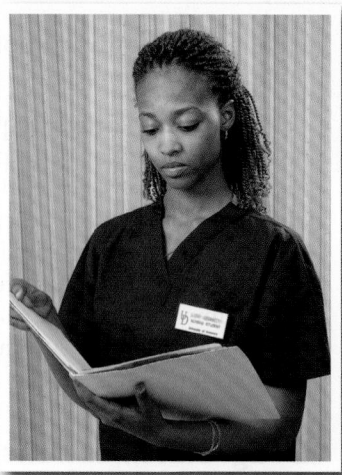

As a new nurse, you are scheduled to administer medications to five clients on the medical–surgical unit today for the first time. Your preceptor will be available as a resource. Your clients are:

- Margaret Marks, an 82-year-old woman who has a fractured hip and experiences periods of confusion
- Cary Pearson, a 70-year-old man with feeding and swallowing difficulties who receives his medications through a gastrostomy tube
- Cyndi Early, a 32-year-old woman with diabetes who is scheduled for surgery at 1000 today
- James Bigler, a 44-year-old man who had a repair of a compound fracture of the right arm and is receiving IV fluids and medications
- Rebecca Jones, an 84-year-old woman with compression fractures of two lumbar vertebrae resulting from a fall.

You have reviewed your assignment but are unsure of where to begin. Should you visit your clients first and perform an assessment? Should you first review the medical records? What should you do with the medication administration records (MARs)? There are so many questions running through your head, and you are a little nervous being on your own. Perhaps you could use the model of full-spectrum nursing (Chapter 2) to focus your thinking. In general, anytime you give a medication, you will need to incorporate the following:

1. *Theoretical Knowledge:* Find out about the actions and expected effects of the medications you are to give.
2. *Client Situation:* Assess the health status (e.g., disease process) of each client as it relates to their medications.
3. *Critical Thinking:* Why is the drug being given? Is there anything about the client's physiology that may alter their responses to the drug? Do you need to modify the administration procedure in any way?
4. *Practical Knowledge:* Be sure that you know the procedures for administering each medication safely.

By the time you complete this chapter, you will have the information you need to make those kinds of judgments. And remember that while you are a student, your instructor and the staff nurses will be there for support.

Theoretical Knowledge
knowing **why**

Pharmacology is the science of drug effects. It deals with all drugs used in society, legal and illegal, prescription and nonprescription. Because drugs can have both a therapeutic and a harmful effect, you should thoroughly understand the medications you administer.

ABOUT THE KEY CONCEPTS

The broadest concepts identified in this chapter are **medication administration** and **medication safety.** An understanding of the theoretical knowledge of **pharmacology** (another key concept) and practical knowledge about safe procedures will help you safely administer medications. As you learn other concepts (e.g., pharmacodynamics, pharmacokinetics), relate them to the three key concepts. This helps to organize information so that you can apply it to clinical situations.

HOW ARE DRUGS NAMED AND CLASSIFIED?

A **drug** is a chemical that interacts with a living organism and alters its activity. In healthcare, drugs are used in diagnosing, treating, or preventing a disease or other medical condition. The term *drug* is used interchangeably with *medication,* although some people mistakenly may think the term *drug* refers only to an illegal substance.

Drug Names

A drug may have multiple names. It is important for you to know the brand name and the generic name.

- The **chemical name** is the exact description of the drug's chemical composition and molecular structure. For example, *2-(p-isobutylphenyl) propionic acid* is the chemical name of the anti-inflammatory drug ibuprofen. The chemical name is rarely used in nursing practice.
- The **generic (nonproprietary) name** is assigned by the United States Adopted Name Council (USAN Council) when the developing manufacturer is ready to market the drug. This is usually similar to the chemical name, but in a simpler form.
- The **official name** is also the generic name that is listed in publications such as the *United States Pharmacopeia–National Formulary (USP-NF).* For example, *ibuprofen* is both a generic and an official name.
- The **brand (trade** or **proprietary) name** is what the drug is sold as in stores. The brand name is easily recognized because it begins with a capital letter and sometimes has a registration mark (®) at the upper right of the name. Different manufacturers of the same medication may give it different brand names.

For example, Advil, Nuprin, and Motrin are all brand names for ibuprofen.

Prescription drugs require a prescription from a healthcare provider (e.g., physician or advanced practice nurse) who is licensed by the state to prescribe or dispense drugs. **Nonprescription, or over-the-counter (OTC),** drugs may be purchased without a prescription and are assumed to be safe for the general population if consumers follow the manufacturer's directions. For example, ibuprofen 200 mg is sold over the counter, whereas ibuprofen 800 mg requires a prescription.

Drug Classifications

It is not realistic to know everything about every drug, so "looking it up" must become second nature. If you learn the common characteristics of a drug classification, then when you encounter a new drug, you will be able to associate it with its classification and make inferences about its basic characteristics.

- By usage—why the drug is used
- By body system—where the drug works
- By chemical or pharmacological class—what the drug is made of

A drug can be placed in more than one category in a classification system. Classified by usage, for example, ibuprofen (Motrin) can be an analgesic, anti-inflammatory, and an antipyretic agent. A drug can act on more than one body system, as well; in fact, most do. For example, diazepam (Valium) is used for its antianxiety effects, but it also decreases the activity of the intestinal system and other smooth muscles and can be used to treat seizures and muscle spasms.

KnowledgeCheck 23-1

- Name three ways a drug may be classified.
- List at least four ways a drug could be named.

WHAT MECHANISMS PROMOTE DRUG QUALITY AND SAFETY?

Before the 20th century, the United States did not have mechanisms for publishing drug ingredients, regulations to govern the contents of drugs, or limitations regarding drug sales. People could buy medicines containing potent and dangerous ingredients, such as opium. Now, reliable sources of drug information, state and federal regulations and standards controlling drug administration, and a variety of systems for storing and distributing medications in healthcare agencies all work together to protect consumers.

Drug Listings and Directories

Key Point: *When in doubt, look it up!* As a nurse, you are professionally, ethically, legally, and personally responsible for every dose of medication you administer. Always use current information when researching a medication. The following references have become the official standards for the healthcare industry:

- **Pharmacopoeia and formularies.** The *USP-NF* is the official recognized directory for drugs approved to be marketed in the United States. It contains information such as drug substances, composition, dosage forms, therapeutic value, and compounded preparations. Any drug included in this book has met rigorous standards of quality, strength, and purity, and the manufacturer is permitted to use the letters *USP-NF* after the drug name.
- **Nursing drug handbooks.** These commercially published books are a quick resource for drug dosages, side effects, and associated nursing interventions.
- *Physician's Desk Reference (PDR).* This book is commercially compiled by pharmaceutical companies. It lists manufacturers' prescribing information and is a standard resource for professionals prescribing and administering medication. The *PDR* contains information on dosing, routes of administration, and side effects, but it does not include nursing interventions.
- **Pharmacology texts.** A textbook provides more information about physiology, pathophysiology, mechanism of action, and drug classifications than the drug formulary or a handbook. However, it may or may not have detailed information about the specific drug you are administering.
- **Electronic and Internet-based formularies.** The Internet, computer software, personal digital assistants (PDAs), and other handheld devices offer convenient access to formulary databases.
- A **clinical pharmacist** can assist you with medication-related concerns (e.g., dosage calculations, compatibility).
- **Medication package inserts** are packaged with most medications. The insert provides information identical to that found in the drug formulary and specific to that particular drug.
- **Institutional medication policies and procedures.** You should know the policies and protocols for medication administration for each institution in which you practice.

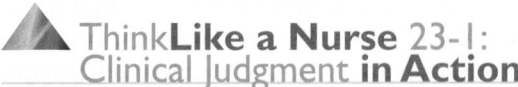

ThinkLike a Nurse 23-1: Clinical Judgment in Action

Mr. Pearson (Meet Your Patients) has a medication, metoprolol (Lopressor), due at 0800. You are not familiar with this medication.

- What do you need to know before giving the drug?
- What resources can you use to learn about this medication?
- Which is the generic and which is the brand name of this medication?
- Select a nursing drug handbook and research this medication. What kinds of information are available to you in the book?
- Now look up the drug in a pharmacology text. How is that information similar to and different from the information in the handbook?

Legal Considerations

Federal, state, and local laws control drug administration. Standards of nursing practice, state nurse practice acts, and organizational policies and procedures define your roles and responsibilities in administering medications. You must be familiar with them to know what you can and cannot do, as well as limitations based on your own experience, skills, and knowledge.

The U.S. Food and Drug Administration (FDA) of the U.S. Department of Health and Human Services regulates the testing, manufacture, and sale of all medications. This agency also monitors the safety and effectiveness of medications available to consumers. This process helps to ensure that ineffective or unsafe drugs are not marketed or are recalled if later found unsafe. However, some medicinal products (e.g., herbal remedies, naturopathic supplements) are *not* regulated by the FDA. Considered "food products," they are advertised as providing health benefits.

Nurse Practice Acts

In most states, a nurse cannot prescribe or administer medications without an authorized provider's (e.g., physician, advanced practice nurse) prescription. State boards of nursing also regulate the types and routes of medications that can be administered by the various levels of nurses. For example, a licensed practical nurse (LPN) in some states cannot administer IV medications, whereas other states require additional education and experience before LPNs can perform this skill. You should refer to your state's nurse practice act for your scope of practice. If you violate the nurse practice act (e.g., by giving medications without a prescription), your state's nursing board could take disciplinary action (e.g., reprimand, suspend, revoke) against your license to practice nursing.

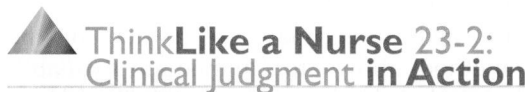

ThinkLike a Nurse 23-2: Clinical Judgment in Action

Obtain a copy of the nurse practice act for the state in which you work. To find a copy,

 Go to the National Council of State Boards of Nursing Web site at https://www.ncsbn.org.

What does your state's nurse practice act tell you about administering medications?

U.S. Drug Legislation

Each state must conform to guidelines of the various federal agencies that regulate the manufacture and sale of medications to protect consumers. Examples include the following:

- **Harrison Narcotics Act**—regulates the manufacture, sale, and use of drugs that cause dependence (e.g., opium, cocaine, marijuana).

- **Durham-Humphrey Amendment**—specifies which drugs require a prescription and mandates the appropriate labeling.
- **Comprehensive Drug Abuse Prevention and Control Act**—regulates the manufacture, distribution, and sale of controlled substances.

In addition, states may institute additional controls. Local governments may enact regulations for the use of alcohol and tobacco.

Regulation of Controlled Substances

Controlled substances are drugs considered to have either limited medical use or a high potential for abuse or addiction. Under the Controlled Substances Act (CSA) of the Comprehensive Drug Abuse Prevention and Control Act of 1970, it is illegal to possess a controlled substance without a valid prescription. Controlled substances are classified by schedules:

- **Schedule I** identifies drugs that have a high potential for abuse and no acceptable medical use (e.g., heroin, LSD, Ecstasy, peyote, mescaline).
- **Schedule II** identifies drugs that have an acceptable medical use but a high potential for abuse (e.g., opium, morphine, cocaine, oxycodone [OxyContin]).
- **Schedule III** identifies medically acceptable drugs that may cause low physical but high psychological dependence (e.g., paregoric, codeine < 90 mg [Tylenol with codeine]; hydrocodone < 15 mg [Vicodin]).
- **Schedule IV** identifies medically acceptable drugs that may cause mild physical or psychological dependence (e.g., diazepam [Valium], alprazolam [Xanax], triazolam [Halcion]).
- **Schedule V** identifies medically acceptable drugs with limited potential to cause dependence (e.g., Robitussin AC, hydrochloride with atropine sulfate).

Controlled substances must be stored, handled, disposed of, and administered according to regulations established by the U.S. Drug Enforcement Agency (DEA):

- Only prescribers with a *National Provider Identifier (NIP)* have the authority to prescribe controlled substances.
- Controlled substances must be **double locked**—stored in locked drawers within a second locked area.
- The facility must keep a record of every dose administered. A count of all controlled substances is performed at specified times, usually at change of shift.
- To facilitate counting and tracking of inventory, drug manufacturers package many narcotics in sectioned containers, with each tablet separately and consecutively numbered (Fig. 23-1).

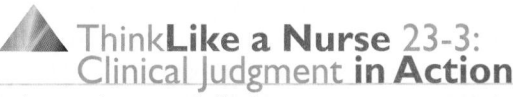

ThinkLike a Nurse 23-3: Clinical Judgment in Action

Locate the controlled substance area on your nursing unit.
- Is a double-locking system in place?
- Does the unit have a system that requires narcotics keys or one that is completely digital?

FIGURE 23-1 To facilitate counting, many narcotics are packaged in sectioned containers, with each tablet numbered consecutively.

- What is the process if there is a discrepancy between a narcotic sign-out sheet and the actual number of narcotic doses present?

Systems for Storing and Distributing Medications

Most inpatient healthcare facilities have specific areas designed for the preparation of medications. Usually, this is a central room ("medication room") or mobile cart. Some nursing units store drugs and supplies in a locked cabinet in or near patient rooms. Whatever the method, all drugs are secured in designated areas accessible only to nurses.

Stock Supply

Medications used most frequently may be kept in **stock supply** (bulk quantity), labeled, and in a central location. For example, acetaminophen elixir and cough syrups may be kept in large multidose bottles from which you measure doses for more than one patient. Stock supplies require you to measure the dose each time a patient needs it, so the potential for measurement error occurs more frequently. However, a bulk supply of medication is often very cost-effective.

Unit-Dose System

A locked mobile cart is used, with drawers containing separate compartments for each patient's medications (Fig. 23-2). Extra drawers contain supplies, such as medication cups, syringes, and alcohol swabs. The pharmacy staff refills the drawers each shift or every 24 hours. Limited amounts of **prn** (give according to patient need) medications and stock medications are also kept in the mobile cart.

A **unit dose** is the prescribed amount of drug the patient receives at a single time. For example, if 800 mg of ibuprofen (Motrin) is prescribed to be given every 8 hours, the unit dose is 800 mg. Each unit dose (usually one tablet) is individually packaged and labeled with the drug name, dose, and expiration date.

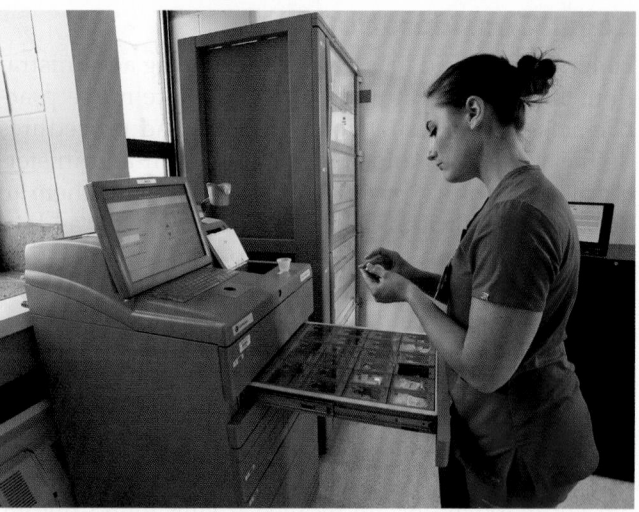

FIGURE 23-2 Medications may be kept in locked, mobile carts with a drawer for each client. Nurses must adhere to the rights of medication administration.

The pharmacist checks each unit dose before sending the drug to the nursing unit. **Key Point:** *Nevertheless, you must recheck the drug and dose when preparing it for administration.* The unit-dose system not only saves nursing time but also is the safest method because of the double-check system.

Automated Dispensing System

An automated dispensing system is a computerized system similar to a unit-dose system. The locked cart contains all the medications frequently used on a particular nursing unit. The computer database contains prescriptions, records, and counts of the medications for each patient on the unit. Each nurse uses a password to access the machine and enters the data about the needed drug, after which the machine dispenses the medication, usually packaged in unit doses.

Some bulk medications may also be kept on the cart. This method allows for immediate availability and administration of newly prescribed and prn medications.

Self-Administration

At times while in the hospital, patients may self-administer medications (SAM). For example, sublingual nitroglycerin (used for chest pain) is self-administered in the outpatient setting, and some patients can continue self-administration of the drug while in the hospital. Drugs prescribed for self-administration are supplied in individual containers and stored at the bedside. Remind the patient to tell you when they take a dose. This method promotes independence and allows you to evaluate the patient's ability to manage medications safely and accurately before discharge. Check the policy in your institution to determine whether self-administration is allowed.

KnowledgeCheck 23-2

- What legislation defines controlled substances in the United States?
- How is medication quality managed?

WHAT IS PHARMACOKINETICS?

Pharmacokinetics refers to the absorption, distribution, metabolism, and excretion of a drug (Fig. 23-3). These four processes determine the intensity and duration of a drug's actions. Each drug has unique pharmacokinetic characteristics. As you study these concepts, relate them to each other and to the key concepts, pharmacology, and medication administration and safety.

What Factors Affect Drug Absorption?

Absorption refers to the movement of the drug from the site of administration into the bloodstream. The rate of absorption determines when a drug becomes available to exert its action; thus, absorption also influences metabolism and excretion. Absorption depends on the route of administration, the form of the drug, drug solubility, the effects of pH, blood flow to the area, and body surface area.

Bioavailability is a subcategory of absorption. It refers to the proportion of a drug that enters the circulation and is able to have an active effect.

Route of Administration

Drugs are manufactured for a specific route of administration and are absorbed at different rates depending on the route. Table 23-1 summarizes the preparations and the advantages and disadvantages of the various routes of administration. Drugs are given for either local or systemic effects.

- The **local effects** of a drug occur at the site of application (e.g., certain topical applications of drugs to the skin), so little if any absorption occurs.
- **Systemic effects** require the drug to be absorbed into the bloodstream before it can be distributed to a distant location. A drug may enter the circulation either by injection into a vein or by absorption from other areas (e.g., muscle, stomach lining, mucous membranes). **Key Point:** *The choice of route is crucial in determining the suitability of the drug for a particular patient.* For example, if your patient is vomiting, an oral drug will not be absorbed effectively in the stomach and would likely be expelled during vomiting. If the patient has diarrhea, rapid motility of the gastrointestinal (GI) tract would decrease absorption. If your patient Cary Pearson (Meet Your Patients) has a prescription for an oral medication, would you question the route? Why or why not?

Solubility of the Drug

Solubility refers to the ability of a medication to be transformed into a liquid form that can be absorbed into

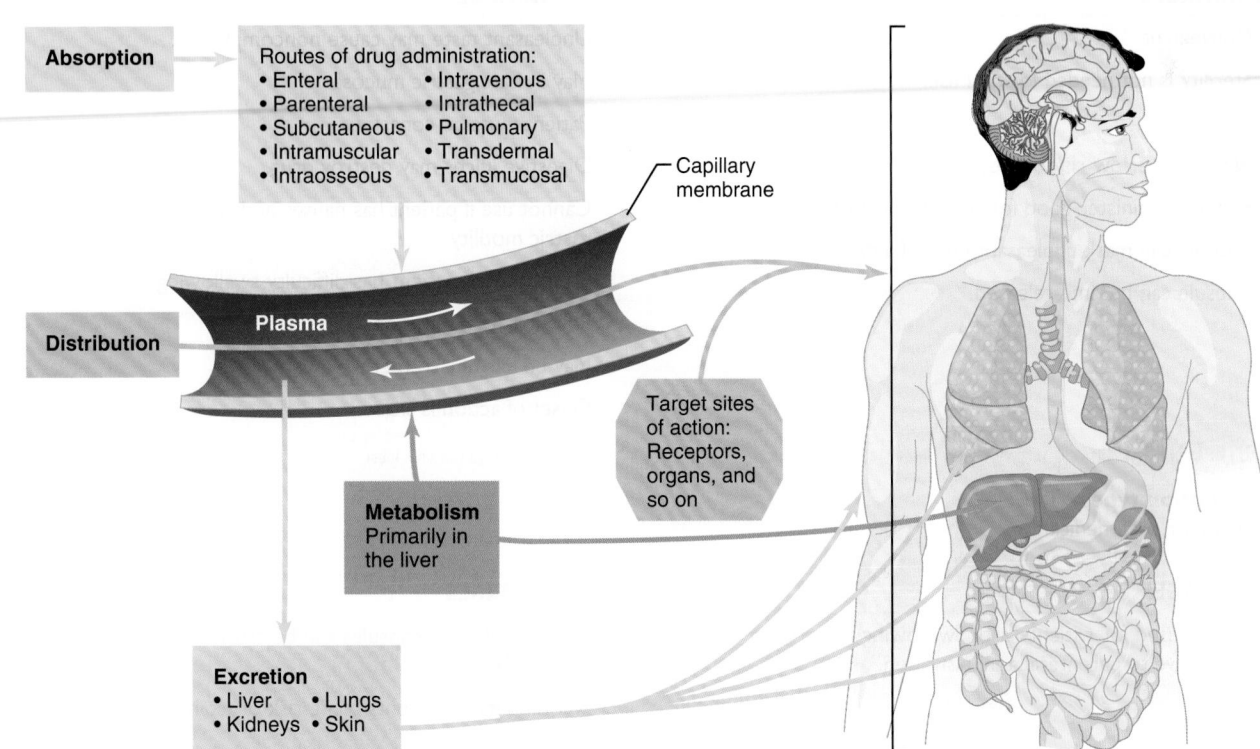

FIGURE 23-3 Pharmacokinetics is the study of drug absorption, distribution, metabolism, and excretion, which determine the intensity and duration of a drug's actions in the body.

Table 23-1 ➤ Advantages and Disadvantages of Routes of Administration

ROUTE: ORAL The drug is swallowed and absorbed from the stomach or small intestine.

Preparation Types

- **Capsule**—A gelatinous container that holds the liquid, powder, or oil form of the drug. When swallowed, the gelatin container dissolves in the gastric juices.

- **Tablet**—A powdered drug is compressed into a hard, compact form (e.g., round, oval) that is easy to swallow and then breaks up into a fine powder in the stomach. The tablet is the most common oral preparation. *Enteric-coated tablets* have an acid-insoluble coating to keep them from dissolving in the stomach; they disintegrate in the alkaline secretions of the small intestine.

- **Time-released tablet or capsule**—A tablet or capsule formulated so that it does not dissolve all at once but gradually releases medication over a few hours.

- **Elixir**—A liquid containing water and about 25% alcohol that is sweetened with volatile oils (e.g., aromatic elixir); not as sticky or as sweet as syrups.

- **Extract**—A very concentrated form of a drug made from animals or vegetables; may be a syrupy liquid or a powder.

- **Fluid extract**—An alcohol-based solution of a drug from a vegetable source (e.g., belladonna); the most concentrated of the fluid preparations.

- **Spirits**—A concentrated alcohol-based solution of a volatile (easily evaporated) substance or oil (e.g., ammonia, peppermint oil, orange oil); contains larger amounts of the substance than can be dissolved in water.

- **Syrup**—An aqueous solution of sugar, used to disguise unpleasant taste of drugs.

- **Tincture**—An alcohol or water-and-alcohol (with a high percentage of alcohol) solution made by extracting potent plants; may also be used externally (e.g., tincture of iodine).

- **Powder**—Finely ground drug(s), usually mixed with a liquid before ingesting; some are used internally, others externally. (Some are mixed with diluents for parenteral injection.)

- **Solution**—Drug(s) dissolved in a liquid carrier. *Aqueous solutions* are medications dissolved in water. May be used orally, externally, and parenterally.

- **Suspension**—Drug(s) that are suspended (not completely dissolved) in a liquid. *Aqueous suspensions* are suspended in water. *Never* used for IV or intra-arterial routes.

ADVANTAGES	DISADVANTAGES
- Convenient	- Unpleasant taste may cause noncompliance.
- Sterility is not needed for oral use.	- May irritate gastric mucosa
- Economical	- Patient must be conscious.
- Noninvasive, low-risk procedure	- Digestive juices may destroy drug.
- Easy to administer, good for self-administration	- Cannot use if patient has nausea and vomiting or decreased gastric motility
- Capsule can mask unpleasant taste of a drug.	- Cannot use if patient has difficulty swallowing
- Capsule can be time-released.	- Potential for aspiration
	- May be harmful to teeth
	- Onset of action is slow.

ROUTE: ENTERAL The drug is given directly into the stomach or intestine (e.g., through a nasogastric [NG] or gastrostomy tube).

Preparation types
Same as for oral medications.

ADVANTAGES	DISADVANTAGES
- Can be used for patients with Swallowing Impairment as an alternative to parenteral administration.	- Not all tablets or capsules can be crushed; medications can clog the NG tube.
	- NG tube itself presents some risk of aspiration.

Table 23-1 ➤ Advantages and Disadvantages of Routes of Administration—cont'd

ROUTE: SUBLINGUAL (a variation of transmucosal administration)—The drug is held under the tongue and absorbed across the sublingual mucous membrane.

Preparation types

Lipid-soluble lozenge (troche)—A flat, round preparation that dissolves when held in the mouth. May act locally or be absorbed through mucosa for systemic effect.

Tablet—See oral route.

ADVANTAGES	DISADVANTAGES
▪ Used for local or systemic effects	▪ May inadvertently be swallowed in the saliva
▪ Convenient	▪ Not useful for drugs with unpleasant taste
▪ Sterility not needed	▪ May irritate the oral mucosa
▪ Quick delivery to general circulation	▪ Patient must be conscious.
▪ Bypasses stomach and intestines; absorbed directly into bloodstream	▪ Useful only for highly lipid-soluble drugs
	▪ Patient must hold the drug in place until it is dissolved, which may take a few minutes.
	▪ Limited period of effectiveness, requiring frequent redosing

ROUTE: BUCCAL/TRANSMUCOSAL ADMINISTRATION Medication is held against the mucous membrane of cheek until it dissolves.

Preparation types

Lipid-soluble lozenge or tablet (See oral and sublingual routes.)

Spray—Can be dispersed to the nasal or pharyngeal mucosa for rapid absorption.

ADVANTAGES	DISADVANTAGES
▪ Same as sublingual	▪ Same as sublingual
▪ Rapid, convenient, portable	

ROUTE: TOPICAL (SKIN) The drug acts locally or is absorbed directly through skin (transdermal or percutaneous absorption).

Preparation types

Gel or jelly—A clear or translucent semisolid substance that liquefies when applied to the skin.

Liniment—An oily liquid to rub into the skin.

Lotion—An **emollient** (softening or soothing agent) for use on the skin; may be a clear solution, suspension, or emulsion.

Ointment—A semisolid, fatty substance (usually petroleum jelly or lanolin based) for skin or mucous membranes; usually not water soluble.

Paste—Similar to an ointment, but thicker and stiffer.

Tincture (See oral route.)

Transdermal patch—Releases constant, controlled amounts of medication for systemic effect.

Aerosol spray or foam—A liquid or foam that is sprayed by air pressure onto the skin.

Cream—A nonoily, semisolid substance applied to the skin.

ADVANTAGES	DISADVANTAGES
▪ Continuous dosing	▪ Effective only for lipid-soluble drugs and must be specially formulated
▪ Sterility not needed	▪ May cause local irritation, especially if the patient is allergic to latex or tape.
▪ For local or systemic effects	▪ Discarded patches may pose danger of poisoning.
▪ Long-acting systemic effect	▪ Leaves residue on skin
▪ Useful if patient is unable to take oral medications	▪ Accurate doses can be difficult to obtain when the drug is in a tube or jar.
▪ Acceptable to most patients	

(Continued)

Table 23-1 ➤ Advantages and Disadvantages of Routes of Administration—cont'd

ROUTE: TOPICAL: INSTILLATIONS The drug is placed into a body cavity (e.g., urinary bladder, rectum, vagina, ears, nose, eye).

Preparation types
Solutions (for nose, ears, and eyes; enemas per rectum)—Drug(s) dissolved in a liquid carrier.
Suppositories (for bladder, vagina, rectum)—Drug(s) mixed with a glycerin-gelatin or cocoa butter base and shaped for insertion into the body. They dissolve gradually at body temperature.
Jellies, creams (for vagina and rectum)—See skin route.

ADVANTAGES	DISADVANTAGES
▪ Continuous dosing	▪ May be embarrassing for the patient
▪ Sterility not needed	▪ Absorption from the rectum is slow, and if stool is present, there is local irritation, or if the patient defecates before the suppository melts, absorption may be further reduced.
▪ Useful if patient is unable to take oral medications; when the oral drug has an unacceptable taste or odor	
▪ Preferred when the patient is vomiting or unconscious	▪ Pain, if the patient has hemorrhoids
▪ May be used for local or systemic effects	▪ As a rule, contraindicated when there is active rectal bleeding

ROUTE: TOPICAL: INHALATION A device (e.g., nebulizer, face mask) breaks the drug into finely dispersed particles, which are breathed into the respiratory passages. Some drugs are intended for local effects in the respiratory passages; others (e.g., anesthetic gases) are for systemic effects, especially in the brain.

Preparation types

Aerosols—Aerosols are liquids in very fine particles that can be inhaled into the lungs; they are sprayed under air pressure.

Gases—Gas is a basic form of matter (i.e., solid, liquid, and gas). A gas must be kept in a closed container; otherwise, the fast-moving molecules escape into the air. Examples are oxygen, nitrogen, carbon dioxide, and anesthetic gases.

ADVANTAGES	DISADVANTAGES
▪ Quick and efficient local and systemic route through the lungs	▪ Requires special equipment
	▪ May irritate lung mucosa
▪ May be given to unconscious patient	▪ Useful only for drugs that are gases at room temperature
▪ Allows continuous dosing; dosage can be easily modified.	▪ May have unexpected systemic effect when only local effect is desired

ROUTE: ALL PARENTERAL ROUTES Drug taken into the body other than through the digestive system.

Preparation types
Depend on route

ADVANTAGES	DISADVANTAGES
Patient may be conscious or unconscious.	▪ Requires sterile procedures
	▪ Poses risk for infection because skin is broken
	▪ Requires skill
	▪ May cause some pain
	▪ Produces anxiety
	▪ More expensive than oral administration

ROUTE: PARENTERAL: IV The drug is injected directly into the vein, either by bolus or slow infusion.

Preparation types
Aqueous solutions—Drug(s) dissolved in water.

Table 23-1 ➤ Advantages and Disadvantages of Routes of Administration—cont'd

ADVANTAGES	DISADVANTAGES
■ Rapid effect because absorption is bypassed; therefore, good for emergency situations ■ Patient needs only one needlestick, even for multiple doses.	■ Poses risk of transient drug concentrations if drug is injected too rapidly ■ Limited to highly soluble medications ■ Poses risk for sepsis because pathogens may be introduced directly into the bloodstream ■ The patient must have usable veins. ■ Cost of supplies and medications

ROUTE: PARENTERAL: INTRAMUSCULAR The drug is injected into the muscle mass.

Preparation types
Primarily aqueous solutions (see IV route), although some preparations (e.g., penicillin) are suspensions.

ADVANTAGES	DISADVANTAGES
■ Rapid absorption, except for oily preparations or suspensions ■ Allows use of drugs that are not stable in solution ■ Causes less pain (than do subcutaneous injections) from irritating drugs because they are deep in the muscle ■ Allows administration of a larger volume than does subcutaneous administration ■ Allows more rapid absorption than does subcutaneous or oral administration	■ May cause irritation and local reactions ■ Poses risk for tissue and nerve damage if site is improperly located ■ Cannot be used where tissue is damaged (e.g., bruised) or peripheral circulation is decreased.

ROUTE: PARENTERAL: SUBCUTANEOUS The drug is injected into the subcutaneous tissue under the skin.

Preparation types
Primarily solutions—Drugs dissolved in a liquid carrier.

ADVANTAGES	DISADVANTAGES
■ Allows faster action than does oral administration ■ Allows better absorption of lipid-soluble drugs than does intramuscular administration	■ Only very small amounts can be given. ■ Absorption is relatively slow and often confined to the injected area.

ROUTE: PARENTERAL: INTRADERMAL The drug is injected under the skin, into the dermis. Most commonly used for diagnostic testing or screening or for injecting local anesthetic.

ROUTE: PARENTERAL: OTHER

Preparation types

Intraspinal—Injection of drug into the spinal canal.

Intrathecal—Injection of drug into the subarachnoid space around the spinal cord.

Epidural—Injection of drug between the vertebral spines into the extradural space. Most commonly used for regional anesthesia and pain control.

ADVANTAGES	DISADVANTAGES
■ Most rapid absorption ■ Highly effective	■ Some patients may be anxious about administration method. ■ Spinal route can produce hypotension, nausea, urinary retention, or headache.

the bloodstream. Drugs must reach the desired blood concentration to achieve their intended therapeutic response. Typically, the more highly soluble the drug, the more rapid the absorption rate.

- **Water-soluble drugs**. Drugs must be water soluble to dissolve in the *aqueous* (watery) contents of the GI tract. Therefore, these drugs are more rapidly absorbed from the GI tract and take effect faster.
- **Lipid-soluble drugs.** Lipid-soluble drugs can penetrate lipid-rich cell membranes and enter the cells, whereas water-soluble drugs (e.g., penicillin) cannot. That is why a highly fat-soluble drug (e.g., nitrous oxide) can easily pass through the blood–brain barrier and induce sedation. Lipid-soluble drugs are preferred when a much longer-acting effect is desired because they are more slowly released into the circulatory system. Lipid solubility depends partly on the drug's chemical structure and the environment at the site of absorption.

    Some lipid-soluble drugs are prepared as a *lozenge (troche)*, a flat, round preparation that dissolves when held in the mouth. Some act locally, and some are absorbed through mucosa for systemic effect.

- **Enteric-coated** drugs cannot be broken down by gastric acids because the coating prevents the medication from being diluted before it reaches the intestines. In this way, the coating delays the action of the drug, which decreases the irritating effects on the stomach. **Timed-release (sustained-release)** medications are formulated to dissolve slowly, releasing small amounts for absorption over several hours. ✚ You should never crush or break enteric-coated and time-released medications; to do so would destroy their protective coatings.

Which of your patients (Meet Your Patient) is most likely to receive a water-soluble medication?

Effects of pH and Ionization

The pH (relative acidity or alkalinity) of the local environment also affects the absorption of a drug. The acidic content of the stomach aids in transporting the medication across the mucous membranes, so *acidic* medications, such as aspirin, are more readily absorbed in the stomach than are *basic* (alkaline) medications, such as sodium bicarbonate, which are readily absorbed in the more alkaline environment of the small intestine. For best absorption, should Mr. Pearson's (Meet Your Patient) medications be acidic or alkaline preparations?

   In solution, some of a drug's molecules are in *ionized* (electrically charged) form, and others are *nonionized* (neutral or noncharged). The ionized molecules are lipid insoluble and thus cannot pass easily through the phospholipid layer of cell membranes. Drug molecules can be easily converted from one form to the other, depending primarily on the pH of the environment. For example, when aspirin is dissolved in stomach acid, most of its molecules remain nonionized because of the low pH, so they easily pass through the membranes of the gastric

mucosa and enter the bloodstream. If the person ingests an antacid before taking aspirin, the pH increases, and the aspirin will become more ionized, which will likely reduce the absorption and effect of the aspirin.

Blood Flow to the Area

Medications are absorbed rapidly in areas where blood flow to the tissue is greatest (e.g., oral mucous membranes). Areas with poor vascular supply (e.g., the skin, scarred areas) experience delayed absorption. Consider the following examples:

- Excessive exercise draws blood away from the stomach and intestines to the muscles. Which route would promote absorption for a person who has just exercised heavily: oral or intramuscular (IM)? Why?
- A person in shock has poor peripheral circulation. Which route would promote faster absorption: IM or IV? Why?

   For the first question, the IM route would be better for the person who has recently engaged in heavy activity. This is because medication injected deep into the muscle where there is a rich blood supply would be absorbed more readily, whereas medication administered orally must first dissolve and be absorbed in the GI tract.

   For the second question, the IV route is more efficient for the person with poor circulation because drugs act more rapidly when injected directly into the bloodstream and do not have to be absorbed. Even in healthy people, the IV route allows for an immediate effect.

KnowledgeCheck 23-3

- Define *absorption*.
- How are drugs absorbed?
- What factors affect absorption?

How Are Drugs Distributed Throughout the Body?

Distribution is the transportation of a drug in body fluids (usually the bloodstream) to the various tissues and organs of the body. Because blood goes to all parts of the body, theoretically, a drug can produce effects (intended or unintended) anywhere. The rate of distribution is influenced by:

- Adequate local blood flow in the **target area** (the site where the drug effects occur)
- The permeability of capillaries to the drug's molecules
- The protein-binding capacity of the drug.

   Local Blood Flow The blood supply of the target site affects the distribution of a drug. For example, it is difficult to deliver a systemic medication to the skin and toes, where the blood vessels are very small.

- Factors that cause vasodilation in an area (e.g., application of warmth to an injection site, fever, and rest) increase circulation to area tissues.

- Factors that cause vasoconstriction (e.g., shock and chilling of the body) decrease circulation to the target tissue.

Membrane Permeability Drug molecules must leave the blood and cross capillary membranes to reach their sites of action. The capillary networks in some organs consist of tightly packed endothelial cells that prevent some drugs from crossing them. For example, the blood–brain barrier allows distribution into the brain and cerebrospinal fluid of only those drugs that are (1) lipid soluble (e.g., anesthetics and barbiturates) and (2) not tightly bound to plasma proteins. This barrier can be bypassed by injecting medications intrathecally (via the spinal canal) into the cerebrospinal fluid.

Protein-Binding Capacity For a given amount of a drug, some molecules bind to plasma proteins, and the remainder will be "free." Only free (unbound) drug molecules can produce pharmacological effects because only free molecules can be metabolized or excreted. For example, nearly all acetaminophen (Tylenol) molecules are free in the bloodstream and are therefore pharmacologically active. By contrast, about 99% of the anticoagulant warfarin (Coumadin) is bound in the blood; therefore, its effects are produced by only the 1% of warfarin molecules that are free.

A drug's tendency to bind to plasma proteins depends mostly on its chemical structure. Some medical conditions also affect protein binding. For example, malnourishment and liver disease reduce the amount of protein (serum albumin) available for binding.

KnowledgeCheck 23-4

- Define *distribution*.
- What factors affect the distribution of drugs in the body?

How Are Drugs Metabolized in the Body?

Metabolism (or **biotransformation**) is the chemical inactivation of a drug through its conversion into a more water-soluble compound or into metabolites that can be excreted from the body. Once a medication reaches its site of action, it is metabolized (changed into the inactive form) in preparation for excretion. **Key Point:** *Metabolism takes place mainly in the liver, but medications can also be detoxified in the kidneys, blood plasma, intestinal mucosa, and lungs.*

If *liver function* is impaired (e.g., liver disease or aging), the drug will be eliminated more slowly, and toxic levels may accumulate. Disease states also affect drug metabolism. For example, patients with diabetes do not metabolize sugar effectively, so they should not take elixirs, which are high in sugar content.

First-Pass Effect Oral medications are absorbed from the GI tract and circulate through the liver before they reach the systemic circulation. Many oral medications will be almost completely inactivated when passing through the liver. This inactivation is known as the **first-pass effect.** For this reason:

- Oral medications are formulated with a higher concentration of the drug than are parenteral medications.
- Some medications can be given parenterally, allowing the drug to be distributed directly to target sites before it passes through the liver. For example, nitroglycerin undergoes this first-pass effect when taken orally; therefore, it is given sublingually or intravenously so that it can bypass the stomach and liver and reach therapeutic levels in the blood.

KnowledgeCheck 23-5

- Define *drug metabolism*.
- Where are drugs metabolized?
- What factors affect drug metabolism?

How Are Drugs Excreted From the Body?

A drug continues to act in the body until it is excreted. For **excretion** to occur, drug molecules must be removed from their sites of action and eliminated from the body. Drugs may be metabolized completely, partially, or not at all when they are excreted. The following are common organs of excretion.

Kidneys The kidneys are the primary site of excretion. Adequate fluid intake facilitates renal excretion. If your patient has decreased renal function (e.g., as indicated by an elevated creatinine level), you should monitor for medication toxicity. Obtain a prescription for adjusted dosing, such as with digoxin, if signs of toxicity are present.

Liver and GI Tract Some drugs broken down by the liver are excreted into the GI tract and eliminated in the feces. Others (e.g., fat-soluble agents) are reabsorbed by the bloodstream, distributed to the target site, and returned to the liver. This is called **enterohepatic recirculation.** The kidneys later excrete these compounds. Anything that increases peristalsis (e.g., diarrhea, laxatives, enemas, chronic bowel disease) accelerates drug excretion via feces. Inactivity, poor diet, and decreased peristalsis delay excretion, increasing the effects of a drug.

Lungs Most drugs removed by the lungs are not metabolized first. Gases and volatile liquids (e.g., general anesthetics) administered by inhalation usually are removed through exhalation. Other volatile substances, such as ethyl alcohol and paraldehyde, are highly soluble in blood and are excreted in limited amounts by the lungs. Examples include the following:

- *Strenuous exercise and deep breathing* increase pulmonary blood flow and thereby promote excretion.
- *Decreased cardiac output* (as in shock) and hypoventilation prolong the period of time for drug elimination.

Exocrine Glands Drug excretion through the **exocrine** (sweat and salivary) **glands** is limited. The elimination of metabolites in sweat is frequently responsible for such side effects as dermatitis. Drugs excreted in the saliva are usually swallowed and absorbed as other orally administered agents.

 ThinkLike a Nurse 23-4:
Clinical Judgment in Action

You are notified that 79-year-old Hattie Banks, admitted 2 days ago to the intensive care unit (ICU) for digoxin toxicity, is being transferred to your unit.

- What theoretical knowledge do you have about the metabolism and excretion of digoxin (Lanoxin)?
- What assessments are important to make for Ms. Banks?

Other Concepts Relevant to Drug Effectiveness

In addition to the processes of absorption, distribution, metabolism, and excretion, you need to understand four other concepts related to a drug's effectiveness: (1) onset, peak, and duration of drug action; (2) therapeutic range; (3) bioavailability of the drug; and (4) concentration of the drug at target sites. As you read about them, try to relate these concepts to the key concepts of medication administration and medication safety.

Onset, Peak, and Duration of Action

- **Onset of action**—The time needed for drug concentration to reach a high enough blood level for its effects to appear. This is the **minimum effective concentration.**
- **Peak action**—When the concentration of medication is highest in the blood.
- **Duration of action**—That period of time in which the medication has a pharmacological effect (before it is metabolized and excreted) (Fig. 23-4).

If the serum level of a medication falls below the minimum effective concentration, then the drug is not effective during that time. If the drug level exceeds the peak level, toxicity occurs.

 ThinkLike a Nurse 23-5:
Clinical Judgment in Action

Refer to Table 23-1. James Bigler (Meet Your Patients) is having right arm pain and needs relief quickly.

- Would it be better to give him oral acetaminophen with codeine or an IM injection of a similar-strength medication? Why?
- Do you have enough information to be completely sure your choice of route will bring the quickest onset of action? Explain.

Therapeutic Range

Even after absorption stops, distribution, metabolism, and excretion continue. When giving multidose medication

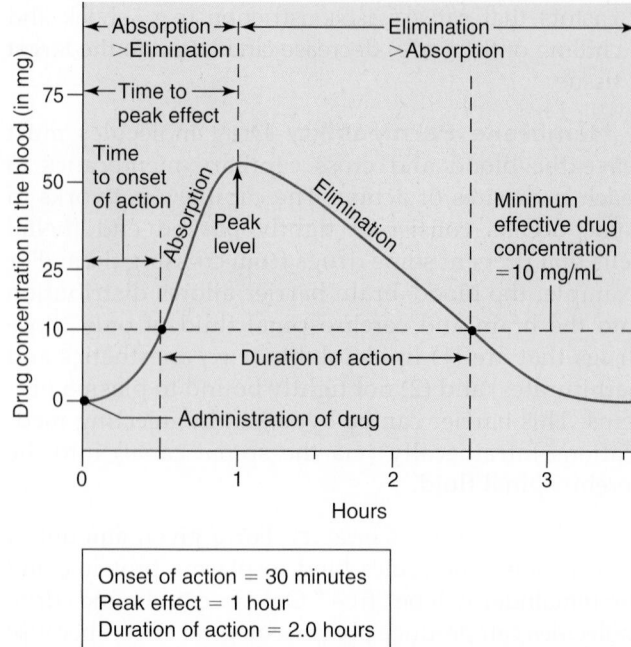

FIGURE 23-4 Once the drug is administered and absorption begins, blood levels begin to rise. When the *minimum effective concentration* is reached, drug effects begin (*onset of action*). *Maximum effect* occurs at peak blood level.

(e.g., an antibiotic), the goal is to achieve a constant, therapeutic blood level. Because a fraction of the drug is constantly being excreted, repeated doses of the medication are given to achieve and maintain a constant therapeutic concentration.

- The **therapeutic range** of a drug is a range of therapeutic concentrations. At the onset of action, the serum drug level is minimal.
- The **therapeutic level** is the concentration of a drug in the blood serum that produces the desired effect without toxicity.
- The **peak level** occurs when the drug is at its highest concentration (when the rate of absorption is equal to the rate of elimination). After that, metabolic and excretory processes begin to remove the drug from the tissues and blood.
- The **trough level** occurs when the drug is at its lowest concentration, right before the next dose is due.

The provider may prescribe a test called a *peak and trough* to ensure the safety and effectiveness of certain drugs. The results are used to adjust the drug dose and timing. The peak and trough are measured at specified times:

- The peak level must be measured when drug absorption is complete and the drug is at its highest level in the patient's bloodstream. This, of course, depends on all the factors that affect absorption.
- The trough level is typically measured about 30 minutes before the next dose of the drug is due,

when the drug is expected to be at its lowest level in the patient's blood. The drug's half-life (see next section) and the time between doses affect the trough level.

Biological Half-Life

A medication's **biological half-life** is the amount of time it takes for half of the drug to be eliminated.

> *Example:* Tramadol, a narcotic-like pain reliever, has a half-life of approximately 6 hours. This means if you take a 50-mg dose at 0800, by 1400, half of that dose (25 mg) will still be left in your body. In 12 hours, one-fourth (12.5 mg) of the initial dose will be left in your body.

Half-life is affected by drug composition and distribution. Liver and kidney disease, aging, absence of food, and slowed metabolic rate prolong half-life because of their effects on metabolism and excretion.

ThinkLike a Nurse 23-6: Clinical Judgment in Action

Rebecca Jones (Meet Your Patients) received tramadol 50 mg for pain at 0800. The prescription allows her to have the drug every 6 hours. At 1400, you give her another dose of tramadol 50 mg. The drug is metabolized in the liver and excreted mainly in the urine.

- When this medication reaches onset of action, about how much tramadol does Ms. Jones now have in her body?
- If the "normal" half-life of tramadol is 6 hours, you would expect that Ms. Jones would still have about 25 mg of her first dose left in her body at the time of the second dose. Given her age, though, do you think she probably has more or less than 25 mg left at 6 hours? Why?

Concentration of Active Drug at Target Sites

The effectiveness of a medication depends ultimately on its concentration at the intended site. For example, a medication such as nitrofurantoin may be prescribed to treat a urinary tract infection. This drug is used because it is highly soluble in urine and therefore tends to accumulate and concentrate in the bladder and kidneys, where the infection exists.

What Factors Affect Pharmacokinetics?

A drug's pharmacokinetics and, therefore, its effectiveness and safety are affected by the following factors:

- **Age.** Infants and young children need smaller doses because of their smaller body mass and immature body systems. Older adults may have declining liver and kidney function and are therefore at higher risk for drug toxicity.
- Table 23-2 summarizes life-span variations in pharmacokinetics.
- **Body mass (weight).** The final concentration of a drug in the body depends on the patient's body mass. The average adult dose is based on the drug quantity that will produce a particular effect in 50% of people 18 to

65 years of age and weighing 150 lb. Obviously, a person who is much larger or smaller than this "average" requires an adjusted dose.
- **Sex.** Men and women absorb drugs differently because women usually have lower muscle mass, a different hormone profile, and different fat and water distribution.
- **Pregnancy.** Most drugs are contraindicated during pregnancy because of their possible adverse effects on the embryo or fetus. Drugs known to cause developmental defects are called **teratogenic** drugs (e.g., alcohol; the anticonvulsant phenytoin [Dilantin]).
- **Environment.** Heat and cold affect peripheral circulation. A noisy environment may interfere with a person's response to antianxiety, sedative, or pain medications.
- **Route of administration.** The route of administration influences the amount of a drug absorbed into the circulatory system and the distribution to the sites of action.
- **Timing of administration.** The presence or absence of food in the GI tract affects an oral drug's pharmacokinetics. Biorhythms and cycles (e.g., drug-metabolizing enzyme rhythms, blood pressure cycles) also influence drug action.
- **Fluids.** Insufficient fluid intake affects the absorption of solid dosage forms.
- **Pathological states.** Intense pain decreases the effect of opioids. Diseases causing circulatory, hepatic, or renal dysfunction interfere with pharmacokinetic processes.
- **Genetic factors.** Abnormal susceptibility to certain chemicals is genetically determined. Enzyme deficiencies and altered metabolism change a patient's responses to a drug.
- **Psychological factors.** Some patients have the same response to a placebo—a pharmacologically inactive substance—as they do to the active drug. If a person has faith that a drug will help them, a *placebo effect* similar to the effect of an active drug may occur. Emotional states, such as anxiety, may cause resistance to tranquilizing drugs.

WHAT IS PHARMACODYNAMICS?

Pharmacodynamics, another subconcept of pharmacology, is the study of *how* medications achieve their effects at various sites in the body—how specific drug molecules interact with target cells and how biological responses occur. You will use pharmacodynamics concepts to help you administer medications safely and to evaluate patient outcomes.

What Are Primary Effects?

Primary or **therapeutic effects** of medications are those that are predicted, intended, and desired. The primary effects are the reason the drug was prescribed.

- **Palliative effects** relieve the signs and symptoms of a disease but have no effect on the disease itself. For

Table 23-2 ➤ Drug Therapy Across the Life Span

PHARMACOKINETIC PROCESS	CHILDREN	OLDER ADULTS
Absorption	■ Exaggerated in infants because of lack of gastric acidity and shorter intestines ■ More complete topical absorption results from a larger body surface and thinner epidermis. ■ Enteral route is unpredictable. ■ Decreased muscle tone makes absorption of parenteral drugs unpredictable. ■ Gastric pH is higher, so medications absorbed in acid environments are absorbed much more slowly.	■ Delayed but more complete ■ Gastric pH is less acidic because of decreased acid production in the stomach. ■ Decreased gastric pH delays absorption of medications absorbed in acid environments. ■ Because of decreased intestinal motility, drugs remain in the system longer, allowing for more absorption.
Distribution	■ Protein binding may be a problem. ■ Greater chance of toxicity because of low albumin levels. ■ Water content in the child's body is higher than in the adult's body, so water-soluble drugs are less concentrated in the child and fat-soluble drugs are more highly concentrated.	■ Low albumin level could create a problem with plasma protein binding. ■ Increased risk of toxicity owing to multiorgan slowdown. ■ Altered because of less lean mass ■ Less body water, greater body fat ■ Dehydration, poor nutrition, and electrolyte imbalances decrease absorption.
Metabolism	■ Metabolism may be altered because of immature liver. ■ Best practice is to base dosage on body weight to avoid toxicity.	■ Presence of diseases may decrease metabolism of the drug. ■ Changes from age, higher blood concentration, and less excretion cause greater chances of toxicity. ■ Some drugs interfere with the liver's ability to metabolize another drug.
Excretion	■ Excretion is delayed because of immature kidneys. ■ Repeat dosing may cause problems.	■ Decreased glomerular filtration rate inhibits excretion from the kidneys. ■ Diminished renal function inhibits excretion, thereby increasing the risk of toxicity.

♥ iCare 23-1

Medicating Patients

■ Medicating patients is routine for nurses, but remember that receiving medications can be anxiety producing for patients.
■ Listen to the message the patient is giving you with their questions, observations, knowledge, or fears.
■ **STOP** if there is any uncertainty.
■ Verify and validate all aspects of the medication process before administration. This helps ensure safe medication practices. Being safe is one aspect of caring.

example, morphine sulfate may be given to a patient with cancer to manage pain, but it does not destroy cancer cells. The goal of palliative therapy is to make the patient as comfortable as possible when treatment options have been exhausted.

■ **Supportive effects** support the integrity of body functions until other medications or treatments can become effective. A patient with a bacterial infection may receive acetaminophen to control fever until blood levels of the prescribed antibiotic are effective in combating the infection causing the fever.
■ **Substitutive effects** replace either body fluids or a chemical required by the body for improved functioning. For example, you may administer insulin to a patient with diabetes to replace the insulin no longer produced by the pancreas.
■ **Chemotherapeutic effects** destroy disease-producing microorganisms or body cells. Two examples are (1) antibiotics, used to treat infections by killing or limiting the reproduction of certain bacteria, and (2) antineoplastic drugs, used to treat cancer by limiting cell reproduction and destroying malignant cells.

■ **Restorative effects** return the body to or maintain the body at optimal levels of health. For example, vitamin and mineral supplements are administered to many patients recovering from surgery.

KnowledgeCheck 23-6

- Name and define the four pharmacokinetic processes.
- How does absorption differ in children and older adults?
- What factors affect excretion?
- You are to administer the following drugs to Cyndi Early (Meet Your Patients): (1) insulin subcutaneously for her diabetes and (2) morphine intravenously to relieve her pain. For which primary effect is each of these drugs being given?

What Are Secondary Effects?

Secondary effects are unintended or nontherapeutic effects—that is, all effects other than the intended effect for which the drug was prescribed. All medications can cause secondary effects (e.g., side effects, adverse reactions, allergic reactions), which can either be harmless or cause injury that may sometimes be predicted.

Side Effects

Side effects are unintended, often predictable, physiological effects of the medication to which patients usually adapt. They occur at the usual prescribed dose and may be immediate (e.g., dizziness) or delayed (e.g., constipation). For hospitalized patients, you will most often see side effects caused by analgesics, antibiotics, antipsychotics, and sedatives. The most common side effects are nausea, vomiting, diarrhea, dizziness, drowsiness, dry mouth, abdominal distention or distress, and constipation.

Key Point: *As a primary nurse, your role includes teaching the patient what side effects to anticipate and how to manage them.*

Adverse Reactions

Adverse reactions are harmful, unintended, usually unpredictable reactions to a drug administered at the normal dosage. They are more severe than side effects and often require discontinuation of the drug.

- **Dose-related** adverse reactions result from the known pharmacological effects of the medication. For example, a patient with diabetes treated with insulin may develop a very low blood sugar if too much insulin is administered.
- **Patient sensitivity** adverse reactions occur because the patient is unusually susceptible to the effects of the drug. Box 23-1 lists patients at high risk for adverse reactions.

The FDA defines **severe adverse reactions** as those that (1) are life threatening; (2) require intervention to prevent permanent impairment or death; or (3) lead to congenital anomaly, disability, hospitalization, or death.

BOX 23-1 ■ Risk Factors for Adverse Drug Reactions

Behavioral and Situational Factors

- History of allergies or previous adverse drug reactions
- Receiving treatment from two or more providers at the same time
- Taking multiple prescription drugs in addition to over-the-counter preparations and herbal remedies and supplements. This is also called *polypharmacy.*
- Taking a drug inconsistently
- Long-term use of a drug (may promote accumulation, leading to toxicity)

Physical Factors

- Concurrent illnesses (e.g., diabetes and renal failure)
- A change in the ability to absorb, metabolize, or excrete the drug (e.g., impaired hepatic or renal function)
- Confusion/cognitive impairment
- Very old or very young age
- Obesity or extreme thinness
- Dehydration or rapid change in hydration status

Health professionals must document serious adverse reactions according to agency policy and report them to the FDA MedWatch program. To make a report, contact the FDA by calling 1-888-463-6332 or visiting the **FDA Medwatch Web site** at **https://www.accessdata.fda.gov/scripts/medwatch/index.cfm.**

You can also contact the Institute for Safe Medication Practices (ISMP) to report errors, close calls, or hazardous conditions, using this URL: https://www.ismp.org/report-medication-error. ISMP guarantees the confidentiality and security of the information received.

Toxic Reactions

Toxic reactions are dangerous, damaging effects to an organ or tissue. They are more severe than adverse reactions, sometimes even causing permanent damage or death. It may help to think of toxicity as poisoning. Antidotes are available for some medications; for example, naloxone (Narcan) is given for opiate toxicity. Toxicity may be caused by any of the following:

- **Overdosing** (administrating a dose that exceeds the prescribed amount). Examples are respiratory depression from excessive morphine and hypoglycemia from too much insulin.
- **Accumulation of the drug in the tissues** (related to long-term use or incomplete metabolism/excretion)
- **Abnormal sensitivity** or allergic response to the drug

Toxic reactions can be:

- **Localized** to a particular tissue or organ, or they can also affect several organ systems.

- **Reversible** (e.g., tinnitus caused by aspirin) **or permanent** (e.g., hearing loss caused by aminoglycoside antibiotics).
- **Immediate and evident** soon after administration, although they can take months or even years to develop (e.g., drug-induced cancers).

ThinkLike a Nurse 23-7: Clinical Judgment in Action

- You have just looked up the antihypertensive drug lisinopril and found the following side effects: neutropenia, dizziness, headache, fatigue, depression, somnolence, paresthesia, hypotension, chest pain, nasal congestion, diarrhea, nausea, dyspepsia, impotence, rash, cough, muscle cramps, angioedema, lethargy, hypokalemia, decreased libido.
- What strategy could you use to help you remember all these side effects?
- You have checked the MAR for Margaret Marks (Meet Your Patients) and prepared her next dose of IV antibiotic. The MAR also indicates that she is receiving morphine for pain and that her last dose was given 1 hour ago. When you enter the room, you find her apparently sleeping. You are not able to awaken her to verify her identity. What do you suspect is happening, and how should you respond? (If you need information about antibiotics and morphine, look it up in an appropriate reference.)

Allergic Reactions

In an **allergic reaction,** the immune system identifies a medication as a foreign substance that should be neutralized or destroyed. The patient experiences no problems with the first dose of the medication, but it acts as an antigen, activating the formation of antibodies against the drug. When the drug is again administered, the antigen–antibody-binding complex prompts an allergic reaction.

Allergic reactions range from minor to serious; however, even a small amount of a medication can cause a severe reaction. Urticaria (hives), pruritus (itching), edema of soft tissue and mucosa, and rhinitis (inflammation of the nasal mucosa) usually occur within minutes to 2 weeks after exposure and are considered mild. Such reactions often disappear after the medication is discontinued and the blood level of the drug falls. Medications most frequently implicated in allergic reactions are antibiotics, biological agents, and diagnostic agents. See Table 23-3.

Key Point: *An anaphylactic reaction is a life-threatening allergic reaction that occurs immediately after medication administration.*

- Anaphylaxis produces sudden constriction of the bronchioles, edema of the larynx and pharynx, severe shortness of breath, wheezing, and severe hypotension (low blood pressure).
- Immediate treatment includes discontinuing the medication and giving epinephrine, IV fluids, steroids, and antihistamines. Respiratory support (e.g., oxygen, intubation, ventilation) may also be required.

Table 23-3 ➤ Medications Frequently Triggering Allergic Reactions

DRUG CLASSIFICATION	EXAMPLE DRUGS	
Analgesics, Anesthetics, and Anti-Inflammatory Agents	Aspirin Codeine Morphine NSAIDs (ibuprofen, acetaminophen, naproxen) Indomethacin Tranquilizers	Local anesthetic agents, such as tetracaine, phenylbutazone, procaine, lidocaine, cocaine, benzocaine, general anesthetics
Antiseizure Drugs	Carbamazepine	Phenytoin
Antibiotics	Cephalosporins Erythromycin Neomycin Penicillin	Streptomycin Sulfonamides Tetracycline Vancomycin
Biological Agents	Allopurinol Antitoxins Corticotropin (ACTH) Enzymes	Gamma globulin Insulin Vaccines
Diagnostic Agents	Iodinated media contrasts Intravenous pyelogram (IVP) dye	
Other Drugs	Dextran Histamines Iodines	Iron Phenothiazides Quinidine

- A patient who is allergic to one drug may also be allergic to other medications in the same class. For example, many patients who are allergic to penicillin are also allergic to cephalexin, a synthetic penicillin.
- Always ask the patient about allergies and their reaction to the medications.
- Remember to document allergies in the patient's medical records, on the care plan, and on the MAR.
- People with severe allergic reactions should wear a Medic Alert bracelet (Fig. 23-5) that identifies the person and the allergen, and they should carry epinephrine for emergency injection.

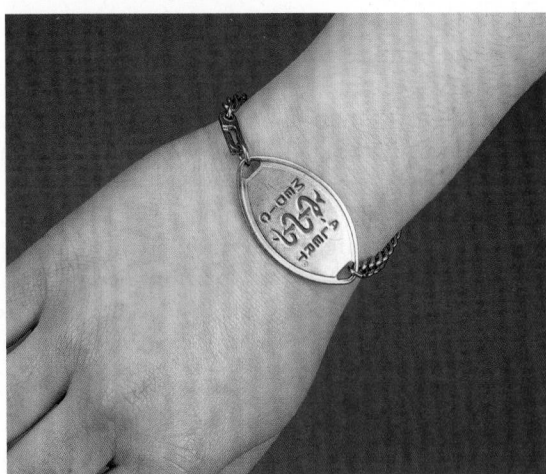

FIGURE 23-5 People with severe allergies to a medication should wear a Medic Alert bracelet.

▲ ThinkLike a Nurse 23-8: Clinical Judgment in Action

You are administering medications to your assigned patients (Meet Your Patients). What should you do in each of the following situations? Which patient should you attend to first? Explain your thinking.

- Ms. Jones has ibuprofen prescribed for her back pain. She tells you she cannot take this medication because it makes her feel nauseated.
- Mr. Bigler had an open reduction and internal fixation (ORIF) of his arm performed yesterday and is receiving an antibiotic, cefazolin 500 mg IV every 8 hours. He has already received three doses of this medication, and you initiated his 0800 dose about 10 minutes ago. He tells you that he thinks his throat is closing shut.

Idiosyncratic Reactions

An **idiosyncratic** reaction is an unexpected, abnormal, or peculiar response to a medication. It may take the form of extreme sensitivity to a medication, lack of a response, or a paradoxical (opposite-of-expected) response, such as agitation in response to a sedative.

Cumulative Effect

A **cumulative effect** is the increased response to repeated doses of a drug that occurs when the rate of administration is greater than the rate of metabolism and excretion (e.g., liver or kidney disorders). Unless the dose is changed, the medication accumulates in the system until a toxic level is reached. Opiates and barbiturates are known for their cumulative effects.

KnowledgeCheck 23-7

- Differentiate between primary and secondary effects of medications.
- List one adverse reaction for each of the following systems: blood, gastrointestinal, neurological, cardiovascular, hepatic, and renal.

- What are some of the symptoms you will see in an anaphylactic reaction?
- What type of patient is most likely to experience an allergic reaction?

How Do Medications Interact?

The more drugs a patient takes, the higher the risk of a drug interaction. Drugs may also interact with certain foods. There are several types of medication interactions:

- **Drug interaction** occurs when one drug alters or modifies the action of another.
- An **antagonistic drug relationship** happens when one drug interferes with the actions of another and decreases the resultant drug effect. For example, an antacid can decrease the effectiveness of aspirin.
- A **synergistic drug relationship** is an additive effect. The effect of both drugs together is greater than the individual effects. For example, the antimicrobials ampicillin and gentamicin are used to treat bacterial heart infections because they target different parts of the organism, leading to better outcomes (Fraser, 2021).
- **Drug incompatibilities** occur when two or more drugs are mixed together, causing a chemical deterioration of one or both drugs. ✚ You can usually recognize an incompatibility when the mixed solution takes on a changed appearance. However, you should always consult medication resources and compatibility charts before mixing medications. Then, after mixing, double-check the medication for changes in appearance. If an incompatibility occurs, do not administer the drug; instead, discard it. You should know and follow your agency policy regarding mixing medications.
- **Drugs may also interact with certain foods.** For example,
  - *High-fat foods and those low in fiber* will delay stomach emptying and medication absorption by up to 2 hours.
  - *Acidic citrus fruits and juices* enhance the absorption of iron. Some citrus fruits, such as grapefruit, interact with medication in an antagonistic manner. For example, grapefruit can decrease the metabolism of atorvastatin (Lipitor), which can lead to higher blood levels of the drug and an increased risk for side effects.
  - *Carbonated soft drinks* can cause medications to dissolve faster, be neutralized, or experience a change in absorption rate in the stomach.
  - *Dairy products* taken with an antibiotic, such as tetracycline, decrease the absorption of the drug in the stomach.
  - *Foods containing tyramine* (e.g., aged, dried, or fermented products), when consumed while taking monoamine oxidase (MAO) inhibitors, may produce a hypertensive crisis.

KnowledgeCheck 23-8

- What type of interaction occurs when one drug interferes with the action of another?
- What interactions occur when one drug has an additive effect on another drug?
- What is drug incompatibility?

What Should I Know About Drug Abuse or Misuse?

- **Tolerance** is a decreasing response to repeated doses of a medication. The person then requires more of the drug to achieve the desired effect.
- **Dependence** is a person's reliance on or need for the drug. It leads to compulsive patterns of drug use wherein the user's lifestyle centers on procuring and taking the drug.
- **Drug misuse** is the nonspecific, indiscriminate, or improper use of drugs, including alcohol, OTC, and prescription drugs. In performing self-care, people frequently misuse laxatives, aspirin, acetaminophen, ibuprofen, cough and cold remedies, and sleep-inducing drugs. Older adults are especially prone to misuse of laxatives in the self-treatment of constipation. Continued use of laxatives can lead to dependence and other medical problems.
- **Drug abuse** is the inappropriate intake of a substance by amount, type, or situation, continuously or periodically. For example, consuming alcohol at work is considered abuse, but having a glass of wine with dinner is not. Drug abuse may or may not lead to drug dependence.
- **Illicit drugs,** also known as *street drugs,* are drugs sold illegally. Many are prescription drugs (e.g., hydrocodone) sought for their mood-altering effects. Prescription drugs can be abused when taken for purposes other than medically intended.

HOW DO I MEASURE AND CALCULATE DOSAGE?

Medications are not always available in the exact dosage the patient needs. Therefore, you must be proficient in calculating drug dosages to be sure your patients receive the correct amount of medication.

Medication Measurement Systems

Medications are usually prescribed and measured using the metric system; however, a few are still dispensed using the apothecary and household systems. You will sometimes need to make conversions from one measurement system to another.

- **Metric system.** The metric system is the preferred system to measure drug dosage because it promotes accuracy by allowing for the calculation of small drug dosages. A disadvantage of this system in the United States is that many people outside the healthcare system are not familiar with it.
- **Apothecary system.** The British apothecary system of measurement (Roman or Arabic numerals) has been used in the United States since colonial times. Only a few medications (e.g., aspirin) are measured using this system because it is less convenient and less precise. For example, *5 grains* might be written as *grains V* or *gr V.*

  To avoid a dosage error, write out the intended unit of measurement (The Joint Commission, 2019). For example, write *grains* so that *gr* (grains) is not mistaken for *gm* (grams).

- **Household system.** Although it is easier to teach a patient about home medications using this system (e.g., teaspoons, ounces, cups), nurses do not often use it because drug dosages are less precise, which can lead to medication dosing errors.

Special Measurements: Units and Milliequivalents

Key Point: *Note that units and mEq cannot be directly converted to the apothecary, metric, or household system.*

Units Units are used to measure insulin, a drug used by people with diabetes to help control their blood sugar (glucose). The standard-strength preparation of insulin is 100 international units (U100). At this strength, 1 mL of the fluid medication contains 100 units of insulin. A prescription for insulin may read: "NPH insulin 14 units subcutaneously every morning."

Heparin (an anticoagulant) and penicillin (an antibiotic) are also prescribed in units.

Key Point: *Be aware that not all units are the same.* For example, 1 mL of heparin does not contain 100 units of heparin. You must always read the container label to know the number of units per milliliter.

Milliequivalents (mEq) Used to indicate the strength of the ion concentration in a drug, a milliequivalent is the number of grams of a solid contained in 1 mL of a solution. Electrolytes, such as potassium chloride (KCl), are measured in mEq. A prescription using mEq may read: "KCl 40 mEq in 1000 mL D_5W administered every 8 hours."

Calculating Dosages

You should be able to calculate accurately using several different methods and formulas. Inaccurate calculations result in incorrect dosages and could harm the patient. For expanded instructions on calculating dosages for adults and children,

 Go to **Chapter 23, Measuring and Calculating Dosages,** in Volume 2.

WHAT MUST I KNOW ABOUT MEDICATION PRESCRIPTIONS?

Before administering any medication, you must obtain a **prescription** from the licensed care provider with prescriptive authority and verify that it is complete, correct, and legible.

- *For inpatients,* prescriptions for medications are usually entered into an electronic health record for automated dispensing. In some cases, the prescription will be written in the medical prescriptions section of the paper medical records. This was traditionally referred to as an "order."

 For outpatients and for medications that will be filled by the patient (instead of the agency pharmacy), the prescription is transmitted electronically to the retail pharmacist that the client selects or written and given to the patient or family. See Figure 23-6 for an example of a prescription. It should contain the following essential elements:

- Patient's full name (some agencies and some states require the address of the patient)
- Name, address, and telephone number of the prescriber, including relevant credentials and legal registration number
  - The NPI is needed for Medicaid, Medicare, and durable equipment prescriptions.
  - Providers who prescribe controlled substances must register with the federal DEA. The prescriber's **DEA number** must be included on the prescription.

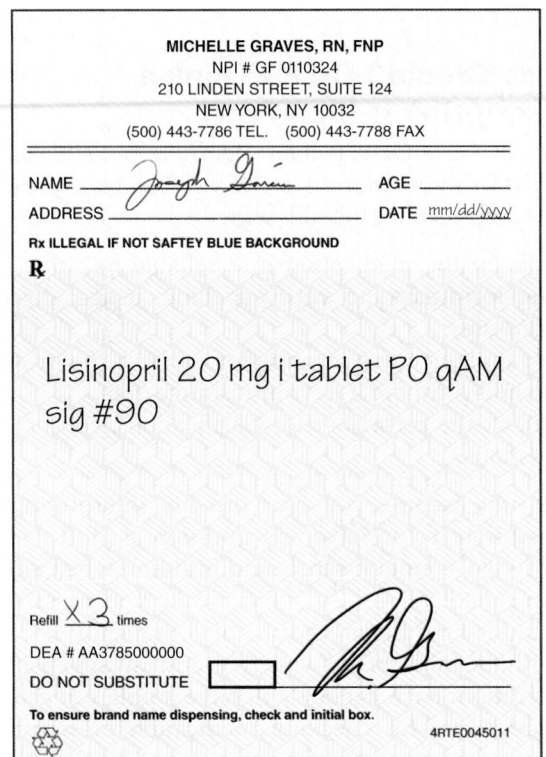

FIGURE 23-6 Example of a written prescription.

- Date and time prescription was written
- Name of medication, dosage (including size, frequency, and number of doses), and route of administration
- Signature of prescriber

 Key Point: *The term prescription is now used to refer to both the traditional inpatient prescription and the outpatient prescription.*

KnowledgeCheck 23-9

- What are the essential parts of a medication prescription?
- How does an inpatient prescription differ from an outpatient prescription?

What Abbreviations Are Used in Medication Prescriptions?

For a list of medication-related abbreviations you may see when reviewing and documenting medications,

 Go to **Chapter 23, Tables, Common Medications-Related Abbreviations**, in Volume 2.

  Because abbreviations can be easily misread, you should write out drug names in full. However, some abbreviations are used in medication administration (e.g., mL, mEq), so you should be familiar with them and your facility's approved list of abbreviations.

 Consult The Joint Commission's official Do Not Use list (see Table 17-1). Also,

 Go to **Chapter 23, Tables, Institute for Safe Medication Practices (ISMP) List of Error-Prone Abbreviations, Symbols, and Dose Designations,** in Volume 2.

Types of Medication Prescriptions

Common types of medication prescriptions are based on the duration, frequency, and/or urgency of the prescription.

- **Standard written prescriptions** apply without a renewal date until the prescriber writes a prescription to alter or discontinue the medication or indicates a specific stop date on the original prescription. For example, "Give furosemide 20 mg IVP twice a day for 5 days." After 5 days, the prescription is discontinued unless the provider renews it.
- **Automatic stop dates** are protocols that hospitals use for discontinuing medications after a certain length of time. Most narcotics are prescribed for only 7 days. If the medication is needed after the automatic stop date, the provider must write another prescription.
- A **STAT** prescription means that a single dose of medication is to be given immediately and only once. For example, "Give furosemide 20 mg IV push STAT," or "Give lorazepam 1 mg IV push now."

- A **single** (or one-time) prescription indicates that the medication is to be given only once at a specified time, usually before surgery or diagnostic procedures. For example: "Give Versed 25 mg intramuscularly on call for when surgical staff requests premedication to be administered."
- **Standing prescriptions** occur when a unit has a standard population of patients and the primary care provider develops a set of *standing prescriptions* for treating a particular disease or set of symptoms (e.g., coronary care, postpartum patients). These are officially accepted sets of prescriptions to be applied routinely by nurses for the care of patients. For example, "Give nitroglycerin 0.4 mg sublingually q3–5 min for chest pain, to a maximum of 3 doses in 15 minutes" may be a standing prescription in coronary care units.
- A **prn prescription** means the provider may prescribe a medication to be given whenever the patient requires (prn). A prn prescription requires the nurse to determine, within the established parameters and in collaboration with the patient, when the medication is to be given. The prescription specifies (1) the condition for which the medication is to be given and (2) the minimum time intervals between doses—for example, "Morphine sulfate 10 mg intramuscularly q3–4hr prn incisional pain." **Key Point: *The medication cannot be given more frequently than prescribed, even if symptoms persist.*** Pain medications, antiemetics (antinausea medications), antipyretics, and laxatives are usually given prn.

How Are Medication Prescriptions Communicated?

Providers communicate medications prescriptions in writing (including electronically) and verbally (orally). The nursing implications are slightly different for each. The provider usually must cosign oral and telephone prescriptions within 24 hours or according to agency policy.

Written Prescriptions You will find written prescriptions either handwritten on a prescription form or on preprinted standard medication order sheets and protocols. Agencies may accept medication prescriptions transmitted electronically or via facsimile from the prescriber to the nurse, with the original copy provided later.

Verbal Prescriptions A prescriber may sometimes give a verbal prescription, which is an oral order spoken to the nurse. When you receive a verbal prescription, you, as the nurse, will then write the prescription and sign it with the provider's name, followed by your name and credentials. Medication names that sound the same can be confusing and lead to administering the wrong drug (Box 23-2). ✚ Repeat the prescription to the provider and spell the medication name to ensure accuracy. Verbal prescriptions increase the risk of miscommunication and errors and should only be used in urgent situations.

BOX 23-2 ■ Medications With Similar-Sounding Names

Alprazolam—lorazepam	NovoLog—Humalog
Baclofen—Bactroban	NovoLog—Novalin R
Cefzil, Keflin—Keflex	Ophthalgan—Auralgan
Celebrex—Celexa, Cerebyx	Percocet—Percodan
Cytoxan—Ciloxan	Phenergan—Phenaphen
Demerol—dicumarol	Procardia—Procardia XL
Digoxin—digitoxin	Quinine—quinidine
Glyburide—glipizide	Ranitidine—amantadine
Humalog—Humulin R	Serzone—Seroquel
Keflex—Kantrex	Taxotere—Taxol
Lamictal—Lamisil—Ludiomil—Lomotil	Zantac—Xanax
Lodine—iodine	Zantac—Zyrtec
Morphine—meperidine	Zostrix—Zestril

Telephone Prescriptions A provider may give you a verbal prescription via telephone, usually in response to a call you have placed to report a change in the patient's condition or the results of laboratory or other tests. The provider usually must cosign the prescription within 24 hours. You should know and follow agency policy on telephone prescriptions. Many providers can send an e-prescription directly to the pharmacy department.

What Should I Do if I Think a Prescription Is Incorrect?

Key Point: *As a nurse, you are legally responsible for the medications you administer.* If you believe a prescription is incorrect, do the following:

- Look up the medication in a reliable resource (e.g., drug formulary) to verify spelling, usage, dosages, and routes.
- Ask another nurse or provider to check the prescription and compare it to your resource data.
- Contact the prescriber for clarifications, concerns, or questions.

Do not assume you are correctly interpreting the prescription if you have any question at all. Use your knowledge, common sense, and intuition when administering medications. To avoid errors, you must know and understand the procedures at your facility, be familiar with the medications you give, and always check the prescription. Each agency will have a policy specifying the procedure for checking medication prescriptions. For example, a unit secretary may transcribe the original prescription onto an MAR, but the nurse must check the accuracy of the transcription.

Most medication errors occur during the prescribing process; however, double-checking prescriptions helps detect errors before the medication reaches the patient (Schwappach et al., 2018). Thus, this double-check system is imperative.

ThinkLike a Nurse 23-9: Clinical Judgment in Action

Find the errors in these medication prescriptions. Use a drug formulary or nursing drug handbook to check dosages, spelling, and so on.

- Ancef 10 g q6hr IV
- Capatril 25 mg orally twice a day
- Digoxin 0.125 mg daily
- Lasix 400 mg by mouth
- NTG gr 1/150 prn chest pain
- Tylenol orally prn fever

MEDICATION ERRORS

A **medication error** is any preventable event that may cause or lead to inappropriate medication use or harm to a patient. Each year, medication errors account for 7,000 to 9,000 patient deaths in the United States, and the total cost of medication-associated patient care exceeds $40 billion annually (Tariq et al., 2021). Medication errors are preventable.

The most common medication errors made by nurses are related to confusion caused by similar drug names, lack of knowledge of the drug (e.g., incorrect dosages or mixing), and lack of information about the patient (e.g., allergies, medical condition). Box 23-3 describes several causes of medication errors by nurses. For a list of high-alert medications that can have devastating consequences when erroneously administered,

 Go to the ISMP Web site at **https://www.ismp.org/sites/default/files/attachments/2018-08/highAlert2018-Acute-Final.pdf.**

How Can I Avoid Errors?

To ensure patient safety, begin by following the "three checks" and the six-plus "rights" found in the Ensuring Safe Medication Administration section later in this chapter. You also must be familiar with and follow the various system-wide measures designed to prevent medication errors in your healthcare agency. For example, The Joint Commission recommends standardizing protocols for prescribing, administering, and documenting medication.

BOX 23-3 ■ Why Do Medication Errors Occur?

The following are several factors associated with medication errors:

Lack of Knowledge or Information

- Lack of knowledge of the drug (e.g., incorrect dosages, incorrect mixing, overly rapid infusion, drug interaction, adverse effects) is the most common factor contributing to medication errors.
- Lack of information about the patient (e.g., allergies, other medications, laboratory results, medical condition for which the medication is contraindicated). This is the second-most-frequent cause of errors.
- A drug is given by the wrong route.

Faulty Communication

- The written prescription is unclear or transcribed incorrectly, resulting in administering the wrong drug or dosage (e.g., confusion between drugs with similar names).
- The telephone prescription is taken incorrectly.
- Protocol is not understood or is violated.
- A drug prescription is entered into the wrong patient's medical records.
- The wrong dosage is prescribed (e.g., by misplacing a zero or decimal point).
- Abbreviations are misunderstood or are incorrect.
- Poor, or no, documentation can result in error. For example, a nurse administers a medication yet fails to record it immediately afterward. A second nurse checking the patient's medical records thinks the drug has not been given and so administers a dose. The patient receives a double dose.

Equipment Errors

- Wrong equipment is used to administer the drug.
- Equipment malfunctions or is not used properly.

Calculation and Measurement Errors

- An error in calculating the dosage is made, so the patient receives the wrong dose.
- There is confusion in the unit of measurement; for example, a drug is prescribed based on kilograms and dispensed or administered based on pounds (and vice versa).

Other

- Medication is improperly handled or stored.
- Failure to follow the six rights of medication administration
- The patient's identity is not checked, and the wrong patient receives the medication.
- Lighting is inadequate.
- The nurse is fatigued, distracted, or interrupted.

Sources: Durham et al. (2016); Kavanagh (2017); MacDowell et al. (2021); Mion & Sandhu (2016); Stefanacci & Riddle (2016); Tariq et al. (2021, 2022).

Critical thinking may be your best way to avoid errors and improve patient care and safety. You need to learn from your mistakes and the mistakes of others, and you also need to think defensively. Ask "are we," "what if," and "why" questions:

- Are we following standardized protocols for prescribing, administering, and documenting medication?
- What will happen if I don't do something or if I do something wrong?
- What assessments are required before and after I give this medication?
- Why am I hanging this IV bag or giving this medication?"

Error-Prevention Technology

Technology has been integrated throughout the medication management process to decrease errors by improving access to information and communication among health professionals. Laptops and handheld mobile devices allow nurses to access detailed information about diseases, similar-sounding drugs, interactions, and side effects.

- **Computerized prescriber order entry (CPOE)** helps prevent errors in orders and transcription resulting from incomplete and illegible handwritten prescriptions. Electronic prescribing systems are safer when combined with clinical decision-support systems (CDSSs) that automatically alert prescribers to possible interactions, allergies, and other potential problems.
- **Barcode medication administration,** especially when combined with CPOE, provides a highly effective system for identifying the right patient. It transfers data electronically, eliminating the error-prone paper transcription process. When used correctly, barcoding at the unit-dose level prevents nurses from selecting an incorrect medication.
- **Smart pumps** are IV infusion technologies used at the point of care to help you avoid programming errors

---

PICOT

Medication Safety

Situation: The student is preparing to administer medications to two clients in the subacute nursing setting. There are several medications to be administered to each client. The student has researched the medications and knows that there are oral, subcutaneous, and IV medications to administer. Before preparing the medication, the student reviews the medications and calculates the doses to ensure accuracy.

PICOT Components:

P	Population/client	=	Nursing students
I	Intervention/indicator	=	Medication administration simulation
C	Comparator/control	=	Math testing only
O	Outcome	=	Safe medication administration skills
T	Time	=	Initial practice after graduation

Searchable Question: Do _____ (P) who receive _____ (I) demonstrate _____ (O) compared with _____ (C) during _____ (T)?

Example of Evidence: Medication errors were identified as a cause of 3% of all sentinel events in 2021 (The Joint Commission, 2022). They result in increases in hospitalization, with costs associated with post–medication errors exceeding $40 billion each year (Tariq, 2022).

> Nursing students often lack confidence in the skill of administering medications. Research showed that a multifaceted simulation approach that included a test before the simulation, video recording of the performance, and the use of a structured form during both observation and debriefing increased students' knowledge (Haukedal et al., 2018). In addition, research revealed very positive results with using simulation to teach professional skills needed for medication administration (Pol-Castañeda et al., 2022).

> Latimer et al. (2017) noted that psychomotor and cognitive skills needed to be integrated. Simulations that included calculating a pediatric dosage (mg/kg/day), administration of the medication, documentation, and evaluation of the efficacy allowed the skills to be practiced in an environment that did not expose clients to harm. Areas for remediation were identified and discussed in the debriefing and reflection session.

> **Practice Change.** Simulation allows students and new graduates to gain the knowledge and confidence to work through medication problems and arrive at accurate results (Pol-Castañeda et al., 2022; Latimer et al., 2017; Marchi et al., 2019).

References: Avraham, R., Shor, V., & Kimhi, E. (2021). The influence of simulated medication administration learning on the clinical performance of nursing students: A comparative quasi-experimental study. *Nurse Education Today, 103*(104947). https://doi.org/10.1016/j.nedt.2021.104947; Haukedal, T., Hedeman, H., & Torunn Bjørk, I. (2018). The impact of a new pedagogical intervention on nursing students' knowledge acquisition in simulation-based learning: A quasi-experimental study. *Nursing Research and Practice,* Article 7437386, https://doi.org/10.1155/2018/7437386; The Joint Commission. (2022). *Sentinel events data released for 2021.* https://www.jointcommission.org/resources/news-and-multimedia/newsletters/newsletters/joint-commission-online/march-9-2022/sentinel-event-data-released-for-2021/#.YrfgsHbMKUk; Latimer, S., Hewitt, J., Stanbrough, R., & McAndrew, R. (2017). Reducing medication errors: Teaching strategies that increase nursing students' awareness of medication errors and their prevention. *Nurse Education Today, 52,* 7–9. https://doi.org/10.1016/j.nedt.2017.02.004; Pol-Castañeda, S., Carrero-Planells, A., & Moreno-Mulet, C. (2022). Use of simulation to improve nursing students' medication administration competence: A mixed-method study. *BioMedical Central, 21,* Article 117. https://doi.org/10.1186/s12912-022-00897-z

and to ensure the correct dose is delivered to the patient. Once programmed, the delivery rate does not change. An alarm will sound or the pump will stop if a nurse attempts to program outside dosing limits or the flow is interrupted (e.g., blocked line). You should promptly investigate the reason for the system alarm.

- **Automated dispensing cabinets (ADCs)** are computerized storage and drug distribution systems that minimize human handling of drugs in the pharmacy. They are known to reduce medication errors when the built-in safety features are used. See the accompanying Safe, Effective Nursing Care box for examples of errors that can occur when technologies for administering medication are misused.

Technology complements other safety regimes and cannot substitute for the need to adhere to all guidelines in medication administration. The death of a premature infant after receiving an IV medication that contained 60 times the normal dose of sodium resulted in a pretrial settlement of $8.25 million (Rubin et al., 2012). A $1.4 million verdict was rendered for the death of a 23-year-old due to nursing errors of failing to administer the prescribed doses of IV potassium (Nurses Service Organization [NSO], n.d.). In these examples, the numerous systems in place failed to detect human errors that led to the death of patients.

What Should I Do if I Commit a Medication Error?

As a nurse, you have a duty to do no harm. If you make a medication error, even though you might be anxious about having put your patient at risk, be embarrassed to admit that you made a mistake, or fear you could lose your job, you must immediately assess the patient's vital signs and physical status and then report your findings to the patient's primary care provider. For detailed guidelines about actions to take if you commit a medication error,

 Go to **Clinical Insight 23-1: Taking Action After a Medication Error** in Volume 2.

Follow your institution's policy regarding incident reporting and other actions. Although an error does not actually occur until the patient has *taken* a medication, you may be required to file a report for a "near miss." These are errors detected during the checking procedure before drug administration (e.g., you discover that the pharmacy sent the wrong medication for a patient).

PracticalKnowledge
knowing how

Regardless of the type of medication or the route of delivery, when giving a medication, you should perform a medication-focused assessment, follow procedures for safe administration, and perform related interventions (e.g., explaining that a certain drug should be taken with food). The rest of this chapter explains these

---

Understanding the Limitations of Technologies for Medication Safety

Chapter Key Concept: Medication Safety

Competencies: Provide safe, quality client care (Thinking); Embrace/incorporate technological advances (Thinking, Doing, Caring)

It is important to understand the limitations of safety-enhancing technologies so that you can apply them correctly (Incorporate Technological Advances) and reduce the risk of patient harm (Safety).

Computerized provider order entry (CPOE). **CPOE** was hailed as the answer to prescribing errors, and it has had many positive effects. When combined with a clinical decision support system (CDSS) and used correctly, it provides safeguards against prescription and dispensing errors. Factors contributing to CPOE errors include:

➤ "Alert fatigue": the tendency for users to ignore frequent interruptions from warning messages.

➤ System and technology issues. These encourage users to bypass decision points.

➤ The origin of the system—commercial versus designed in-house.

➤ Learner cognitive overload associated with learning new systems and tasks.

Barcode-assisted medication administration (BCMA). **Research** shows a high association between workarounds and medication administration errors. A workaround is a method of achieving the task by misusing or not using the appropriate technology. Some of the reasons for workarounds include malfunction of scanning equipment, poor wireless connectivity, medication not labeled, and patient armband not readable. Workarounds greatly increase the risk of error and constitute negligence.

Smart-pump problems. These include software limitations and practitioner misuse (e.g., turning off the pump's dose-checking feature and bypassing alerts), especially with high-alert medications. Such actions are ethically and legally indefensible and do not meet standards of care.

➤ How does the Incorporate Technological Advances competency relate to the Provide Safe, Quality Care competency?

➤ How can you avoid risky behaviors; contribute to the redesign of safety technologies; and put safe, quality patient care first when administering medications?

Sources: Agency for Healthcare Research and Quality (2019); Elshayib & Pawola (2020); Godshall (2018); Kavanagh (2017); Marwitz et al. (2019).

Toward Evidence-Based Practice

Asensi-Vicente, J., Jimenez-Ruis, I., & Vizcaya-Moreno, M. (2018). Medication errors involving nursing students: A systematic review. *Nurse Educator, 43*(5), E1–E5.

A literature synthesis revealed the reported medication error rate of nursing students ranged from 18.8% to 32.1%, with medication omission and wrong doses as the most frequent types. Errors were unreported because of administrative barriers or fear of receiving a lower course grade. Factors contributing to errors included workload inexperience, distraction, and absence of supervision. Students identified feelings of shame, fear, guilt, and anxiety.

Treiber, L., & Jones, J. (2018). After the medication error: Recent nursing graduates' reflection on adequacy of education. *Journal of Nursing Education, 57*(5), 275–280.

A survey of recent graduates revealed that 75% felt adequately prepared for medication administration but not for the real-world issues of time management, multiple distractions, competing demands, and handling stress. Fifty-five percent of respondents had made medication errors because of individual (e.g., fatigue, omitting the six rights because of time pressures) and systemic factors (e.g., wrong medication in dispensing system) leading to the error. Twenty-four percent failed to report it because of time-consuming paperwork, fear, and institutional requirements (e.g., taking classes).

Dennison, S., Freeman, M., Giannotti, N., & Ravi, P. (2022). Benefits of reporting and analyzing nursing students' near-miss medication incidents. *Nurse Educator, 47*(4), 202-207. https://doi.org/10.1097/NNE.0000000000001164

Researchers analyzed near-miss reports involving nursing students to identify the type and contributing factors. A total of 236 near-miss medication reports identified five major areas of incidents. Accounting for 81.4% of the incidents were one or a combination of these factors: (1) dosage errors, (2) omitted dose, (3) wrong time, and (4) wrong drug. The top factors contributing to the near misses were communication failures (47.9%), competency and education (44/1%), environmental and human limitations (35.2%), and policies and procedures violations (29.2%). Analyses of near misses provide insight into strategies and processes that prevented an error from reaching the patient.

Wagner, E. (2022). Engaging nursing students in quality improvement: Teaching safe medication administration. *Journal of Nursing Education, 61*(5), 268–271. https://doi.org/10.3928/01484834-20220303-01

Sophomore nursing students participated in a real-world quality improvement project in which they collected data on interruptions and management during medication administration by their registered nurse (RN) mentors. A common theme was how often interruptions occurred during medication administration, with many being avoidable. Nurses prioritized activities viewed as necessary (e.g., answering call lights, laboratory calls reporting critical values) over continuing with medication administration. After the interruption, nurses used a variety of processes to refocus on medication administration (e.g., starting over, separating scanned and unscanned medications). Data collected and discussed promoted insight into developing strategies to remain focused during medication administration.

1. What consistent themes in these studies were associated with medication errors or near misses?

2. What factors prevented nurses and nursing students from reporting the errors?

3. Which study, if any, justifies not reporting a medication error or near miss?

4. What strategies could help nursing students better prepare for the real world?

---

activities to you. You should become familiar with the guidelines, and

 Go to **Chapter 23, Medication Guidelines: Steps to Follow for All Medications (Regardless of Type or Route),** in Volume 2.

 Think**Like a Nurse** 23-10: Clinical Judgment **in Action**

Mr. Pearson (Meet Your Patients) refuses to take his 1400 dose of antibiotic, stating that he has just taken it. What actions should you take to ensure sound decision making and maintain patient safety?

ASSESSMENT/RECOGNIZING CUES

During your initial patient assessment, you will gather data that you need to administer medications safely.

The following are highlights of medication-related assessments.

- **Before medicating patients:**
  - Measure vital signs.
  - Assess whether the patient's general condition is appropriate for the medication.
  - Evaluate your knowledge of the medication.
  - Identify biological factors that affect drug metabolism.
- **While administering medications,** assess:
  - Mental status
  - Coordination
  - Ability to self-administer the drug
  - Swallowing (for oral medications)
- **After medicating patients,** assess:
  - Effectiveness of the drug
  - Side effects
  - Signs of adverse reactions or toxicity

Medication History When taking a medication history, explore the patient's allergy history (e.g., medication and food allergies). You should also ask about the patient's history of illness, medications, attitudes toward medications, learning needs, and whether the patient is pregnant or breastfeeding. Also check relevant laboratory test results and obtain a list of current medications (prescribed and OTC) and the names of the prescribing providers. Ask the patient about their ability to have their prescriptions filled. Some patients are noncompliant because they cannot afford the medications.

Physical Examination The physical examination helps you to identify potential problems and the need for adapting medication administration procedures. For example, laboratory test results are used to monitor serum drug levels and evaluate proper dosages for the patient. You will also assess relevant body systems and vital signs to confirm the need for the drug (e.g., apical pulse before administering digoxin) and to provide a baseline for evaluating the patient's responses. For oral medications, assess the patient's ability to swallow; for IM medications, assess muscle mass.

▰ NURSING DIAGNOSIS/ANALYZING CUES

The following are some NANDA-I and Clinical Care Classification (CCC) nursing diagnoses that might be useful when medicating patients:

Aspiration
Constipation
Diarrhea
Ineffective Family Health Management
Ineffective Health Management
Nonadherence
Poisoning Risk
Risk for Allergic Reaction

The following are some examples of nursing diagnostic statements you might write for patients receiving medications:

Knowledge Deficient related to lack of motivation to learn about medications
Ineffective Family Health Management related to anxiety over child's health status
Risk for Aspiration related to Impaired Swallowing

A few nursing diagnoses represent medication side effects. However, because a wide range of adverse effects is possible, no attempt was made to include them all. The following sections discuss Risk for Injury and Ineffective Health Management (nonadherence).

Risk for Injury
Risk for Injury may be related to polypharmacy and misuse, overuse, or underuse of medications.

Polypharmacy **Polypharmacy** is the ingestion of numerous medications in an attempt to treat many conditions simultaneously. Many people self-prescribe or rely on OTC medications for symptom relief (e.g., insomnia, headaches, joint pains, indigestion). They may continue taking them in combination with prescribed medications. Polypharmacy increases the potential for adverse reactions and dangerous drug and food interactions.

🍁 In older older adults, the likelihood of increased sensitivity to medications, drug interactions, and adverse drug effects increases as the number of medications taken increases (Nguyen et al., 2020; Rochon et al., 2021). You should carefully assess older adults' medication history to identify combinations that can be especially dangerous to them.

Misuse, Overuse, Underuse Some patients misuse, overuse, or underuse drugs or use them inconsistently. They may even use them when contraindicated. For example, a person takes an antibiotic, "feels better" after a few days of the medication, and then stops taking it when symptoms are gone. The inconsistent dosage schedule hinders the body's ability to achieve a therapeutic blood level of the medication to treat the infection. Some drugs (e.g., beta blockers) can be dangerous or even life threatening when taken inconsistently.

Nonadherence
Nonadherence to the medication regimen is the failure to follow the treatment plan (e.g., not taking a prescribed medication, skipping doses). As you assess the patient's reasons for nonadherence, be prepared to address numerous reasons, such as a lack of symptoms, intolerable side effects, forgetfulness, inability to afford the medication, disagreement with the treatment plan, or a lack of knowledge. Some patients, particularly older adults, have visual and motor deficits that limit their ability to read labels and manipulate access (e.g., bottle caps, syringes).

♥ **iCare** Take actions to help address the patient's reason for not complying with the medication regimen (e.g., providing education on medications, contacting social services to obtain assistance).

Knowledge Check 23-10
- What are the risks involved for patients who engage in polypharmacy?
- List at least three reasons for nonadherence to a medication regimen.

▰ PLANNING/PRIORITIZING HYPOTHESIS AND GENERATING SOLUTIONS

Nursing Outcomes Classification (NOC) standard outcomes depend on the specific nursing diagnoses you choose. The following are examples of NOC outcomes.

Knowledge: Medication, Treatment Regimen
Adherence Behavior

Bowel Elimination
Comfort Status
Compliance Behavior
Knowledge: Medication
Knowledge: Treatment Regimen
Medication Response
Motivation
Risk Control: Drug Use
Self-Care: Non-Parenteral Medication
Self-Care: Parenteral Medication
Swallowing Status

Individualized goals/outcome statement you might write for a client should be stated so that their achievement reflects a resolution of the problem (NANDA-I label). The following are examples:

After explanation, and within 1 week, describes the expected actions and side effects of the medications.
Self-administers the medications in the correct amounts and on the prescribed schedule.

IMPLEMENTATION/TAKING ACTION

Nursing Interventions Classification (NIC) standardized interventions depend on the patient's nursing diagnoses, especially on the etiologies. Examples include:

Precautions
Behavior Modification
Diarrhea Management
Discharge Planning
Health Education
Health System Guidance
Medication Management
Mutual Goal Setting
Self-Responsibility Facilitation
Surveillance
Teaching: Prescribed Medication
Teaching: Psychomotor Skill

Specific individualized nursing activities include preparing and administering medications and teaching clients to self-administer their medications. You will use specific, step-by-step procedures for these activities. However, only the general principles are presented in this section.

TEACHING PATIENTS ABOUT MEDICATION SELF-ADMINISTRATION

Teach the following information to patients to help them safely administer their own medications.

Know and Understand What You Are Taking Take your drugs safely and effectively by knowing and understanding what you are taking and the reasons.

■ **When you are prescribed a new medication, ask why you are taking it,** how long you should take it, what side effects to expect, whether you should take it with food, and whether there are any special precautions.

■ **Ask what each drug is for and what it does.** This can prevent taking two medications that do the same thing, as can occur when you are seeing multiple providers (e.g., a podiatrist and an internist may both prescribe a medication to treat toenail fungus).
■ **Keep a list of your medications,** including doses and times taken. Take this list with you when you visit any healthcare provider or emergency department.

Take the Drug as Prescribed
■ **Take the drug for the entire length of time** to receive its full benefit (e.g., some patients may take only part of an expensive antibiotic, hoping to "save it for later.") This can lead to infection, or an antibiotic resistance may develop, leading to "superinfection," such as methicillin-resistant *Staphylococcus aureus* (MRSA).

 ■ Older adults may forget to take their medications. A simple plan you can follow at home, such as a written schedule, a meds calendar, or setting an alarm on a smartwatch, might help, especially if the drugs are taken other than at mealtimes and bedtime.
■ If you cannot see well, ask a family member to write the schedule in large, black letters. Display it in a highly visible place.
■ Some older adults may take the medication, only to forget shortly thereafter that they did so. Use a divided pill container or a small glass filled with the medications for each dosage time during the day. If the a.m. container is empty, you will know you have taken the morning drugs and won't accidentally repeat them.

Communicate With Your Prescriber Notify your prescriber if you have side effects, adverse reactions, or questions. If you become pregnant, notify your primary care provider as soon as possible so that your medications can be discontinued or adjusted.

✚ **Think About Safety** Be aware of your safety and the safety of others.

■ **Wear a Medic Alert bracelet or necklace** if you have diabetes, take anticoagulants, or have allergies to any medication.
■ **Do not take medications prescribed to others,** and do not share your medications with others.
■ **If you take a variety of medications,** post a list of them in a prominent place that is easy to see in the event of an emergency.
■ **Use childproof caps** if children have access to your medications. If no children are in the home, replace with a simple-closure cap for older patients who might have difficulty opening the containers. Families with young children visiting the homes of older adults need to be alert to the risk of accidental ingestion of medication.
■ **Dispose of expired medications safely.** Do not place them in the trash. Disposing of drugs in the sink or toilet is not environmentally sound (e.g., they can appear in the community water supply). Your community may sponsor a "discard medications day" or provide a place to discard drugs. Check with your local pharmacy.

Administer Your Drugs Correctly The following are steps to administer your drugs correctly:

- **Read the label carefully on the bottle each time** you take the medication so that you take the correct medication in the prescribed dose. Many tablets look alike.
- **Take only the amount and dose prescribed.** If you have questions, call your prescriber.
- **To measure liquids, use kitchen measuring spoons** rather than tableware, which can vary in volume.
  - **If you have difficulty opening containers and administering your medications** because of pain or stiffness in the hands and fingers, ask family members and friends to help you. Ask the pharmacy and the primary care provider *not* to put childproof safety lids on containers for easier handling. Older adults are allowed to sign a release with their pharmacy to do this.

Store Your Drugs Safely

- Do not store a drug in a different container from the one it came in. The medication may lose its strength, or you may take the wrong medication.
- Store all your medications in a dry place, out of the sunlight, and away from the heat.
- If a medication requires cold storage, be sure you return it to the refrigerator immediately after use.

Maintain Your Supply Your drugs need to be up to date and available when you need them.

- **Monitor your prescription amounts, and get refills before you run out.** If you get medications by mail, be sure you order them in plenty of time.
- **Check expiration dates** and properly discard any outdated medications.
- **Do not take expired medications**; they may have lost their strength.

ENSURING SAFE MEDICATION ADMINISTRATION

Medication errors are the most common type of healthcare adverse events.

- **Sources of error.** Errors include giving the dose at the wrong time, omitting doses, giving the wrong dose, and giving the dose without authorization. Many errors occur as a result of interruption or distraction.
- **Safe zones.** One recommendation is to create a "safe zone" when preparing or administering medication. You can do this by putting up "do not disturb" signs, using the medication room, or wearing a bright-yellow apron to alert people not to disturb you when you are preparing or giving medication.
- **Preventing errors.** To help prevent errors, perform "three checks" and the "rights of medication" when giving medication. Also be sure to follow the guidelines you will find in

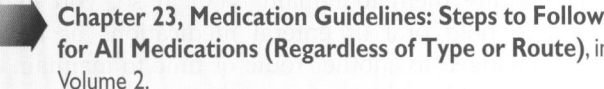
Chapter 23, Medication Guidelines: Steps to Follow for All Medications (Regardless of Type or Route), in Volume 2.

Three Checks

Check each medication three times:

1. *BEFORE you pour*, *mix, or draw up a medication*, check its label against the entry on the MAR. Be sure that the name, route, dose, and time match the MAR entry.
2. *AFTER you prepare the medication*, and before returning the container to the medication cart or discarding anything, check the label against the MAR entry again.
3. *AT THE BEDSIDE*, *check the medication again* before actually administering it.

Observing the "three checks" rule will help you to practice the "rights of medication."

Rights of Medication

Following the **rights of medication** means that you will give the (1) right **medication** to the (2) right **patient** in the (3) right **dose** using the (4) right **route** at the (5) right **time** with the (6) right **documentation** of the medication administration. This system helps you to prevent medication errors.

Right Drug

Obviously, you must always administer the correct medication. That is one reason for reading each label three times (see the "three checks"). Other ways to ensure giving the correct drug are to:

1. **Think critically.**
   - Adhere strictly to the guidelines for taking verbal prescriptions. If you must take a verbal prescription, always repeat it back to the prescriber to be sure you have heard correctly.
   - Always check the MAR to ensure it is the right patient, drug, dose, time, and route.
   - Know the drugs you administer. If you are unsure or do not know, look it up.
   - Ask yourself whether the medication prescription is suitable for the patient's condition. If not, question the prescriber.
   - Participate in daily patient rounds so that you will be better informed about the plan of care and why the medications are prescribed. This ensures you understand the reason the medication is prescribed and its expected benefits.
2. **Be aware of the pitfalls in abbreviations, units of measurement, and handwriting.**
   - Double-check all prescriptions transcribed by hand to the MAR.
   - Do not attempt to decipher illegible handwriting, confusing abbreviations, or units of measurement (e.g., mg and mL, or IU and IV). When in doubt, ask the prescriber to clarify.
   - Be alert for names that look very similar (e.g., Keflex and Keflin). It may be impossible to differentiate them when they are handwritten. Do not

administer a drug prescribed by a nickname; be sure it is written out in full.

3. **Perform the "three checks" of the label against the MAR.** Include all of the following as part of the process:

   - Read the label before and after you prepare the medication, then again at the bedside to verify that you selected the correct product name and strength.
   - Select the prescribed medication from the patient's drug drawer (unless it is a stock drug). Do not "borrow" from another patient's drawer.
   - Do not substitute one medication for another.
   - Even when using a unit dose, read the label. Avoid selecting medications based on size and color because many medications are the same size, shape, and color as others.
   - Be alert for similar-looking labels. If you are accustomed to withdrawing oxytocin (given intravenously to stimulate uterine contractions) from a small vial with a green label, you might be surprised to find that the small green-label vial in your hand is actually a different drug that would be harmful if given intravenously.
   - If a label is hard to read or comes off the container, return the container to the pharmacy. Never give a medication that is not labeled properly. Also, do not transfer medications from one pharmacy container to another.

4. **Take special care with heparin.** Physically separate the highly concentrated heparin sodium (10,000 units/mL in 1-mL vials) from the more diluted 1-mL vials for flushing intermittent IV locks. There is a risk of fatal hemorrhage if the highly concentrated heparin solution is mistakenly used to flush an IV line. Note the FDA-approved labeling that includes new colors and designs to distinguish the various heparin concentrations in the vials.

Right Dose

The right dose is the dose prescribed for the particular patient. Be sure the dose is within the recommended range for the patient's age, weight, and condition. The following are suggestions for avoiding dose errors:

- **Perform the "three checks"** of the container against the MAR. If the pharmacist has sent a dose different from the one prescribed, you will need to calculate how much of the medication to administer. It is a good idea to have another nurse check your calculations. Also, you should know the drug's dosage range.
- **For IV medications, use smart infusion pumps** to help ensure that the correct dose is delivered.
- **Prepare the medications with precision** because how you prepare it can affect the dose the patient

receives. When you must break a tablet, use a knife or approved cutting device. If the tablet does not break evenly, discard and account for it. ✚ When crushing a tablet to mix with liquid or food, clean the crushing device completely before and after use to remove any pieces of a previously crushed drug. This will prevent patients who may have allergies from receiving unintended medications.

- **Read and write measurements carefully.** It is easy to misread "mg" instead of "mL." There is a significant difference between 1 mg and 1 mL of IV morphine.
- **Write out "international units"** instead of abbreviating as "IU." *IU* can be confused with *IV*.
- **Know how and when to use a zero.** Always write a zero *before* a decimal point. It is easy to mistake *.15* for *115* if the decimal point is written large or the *1* is written small (e.g., write "Lanoxin 0.125 mg," not "Lanoxin .125 mg"). Conversely, never write a decimal point and a zero *after* a whole number. The decimal point may be mistaken for a *1* or missed (e.g., write "5 mg," not "5.0 mg").
- **Question prescriptions for multiple tablets or vials** as a single dose. Most doses are one or two tablets or one single-dose vial.
- **Question abrupt and excessive increases in dosage;** most dosages increase gradually.
- **Question prescriptions that are not consistent with the standard (protocol) dosage range** for the patient's age, weight, and condition.
- **Examine the standards of care and practice in your institution** to see if they comply with The Joint Commission's National Patient Safety Goal for high-risk medications.

Right Time

- Check the prescription against the time to give the drug, and document the exact time of administration on the MAR. ✚ If the drug is not documented, never assume the patient received it. If you do, the patient may not receive an essential medication. If you assume the medication has not been given and administer it, the patient may receive an overdose.
- As a rule, you can give scheduled medications within a "window" of one-half hour before and one-half hour after the scheduled time.
- Time oral medications in relation to food. Give drugs that are irritating to the stomach (e.g., potassium, aspirin) with food. Give drugs that absorb better on an empty stomach (e.g., tetracycline, iron supplement) before meals.
- Determine whether your patient is scheduled for any diagnostic procedures, surgery, or blood tests that require them to remain NPO. If so, you may need to hold oral or enteral medications or have them changed to another route or time to maintain a therapeutic blood level.

Right Route

Recall that drug absorption is highly dependent on the route of administration. The following are suggestions for ensuring the right route:

- **Do not guess.** If the prescription does not specify a route, do not guess; clarify with the prescriber. Many medications are available in multiple forms; others are made for one specific route. For example, cephalexin, an antibiotic, comes in capsules, suspensions for oral use, and injectable forms for IM and IV administration. By contrast, the antibiotic penicillin G procaine is prepared for IM injection and is *not* to be given intravenously.
- **The right route also includes the right site.** If an intramuscular injection is prescribed, be sure the site is appropriate, considering the age of the patient and the medical condition.
- **Use an oral syringe to draw up oral liquids** to avoid inadvertent IV administration.

Right Patient

- **Always double-check the patient's identification (ID)** bracelet just before giving the medication. This helps ensure that you have the correct patient. Always use two methods of patient identification; thus, you should also ask the patient to state their name. It is best to say, "Please tell me your name," because patients with hearing impairment or confusion might respond "yes" incorrectly when asked, for example,

"Are you Mary Smith?" Never skip this step, even if you are familiar with the patient. If you are busy and distracted, it is possible to enter the wrong room.

- **Do not leave medications at the bedside.** Suppose you are taking an oral tablet to a patient's room and find him in the bathroom. If you leave it on the table, how would you know whether he really took it? Someone else could come in and take or discard the medication.
- **Be alert for patients with the same last names.** It is common to have two patients with the same or similar last names (e.g., Williamson, Wilkinson, Wilson, Wilkerson). Look for and place special alerts on medical records and MARs to call attention to names that look or sound similar.
- **Ensure that the entry of prescriptions is made in the correct patient's medical record.** CPOE and barcode medication administration transfer data electronically and provide a nearly, but not 100%, foolproof system for identifying the right patient, when used correctly.

Right Documentation

Most nurses consider documentation the sixth right. After administering a medication, document it immediately on the patient's MAR, as in Figure 23-7. To see an electronic MAR, refer to Chapter 17. Be sure to document the following information:

- Name of medication given
- Dose of medication given

HOSPITAL MEDICATION ADMINISTRATION RECORD

Codes For Injection Sites

A - Left Anterior Thigh	H - Right Anterior Thigh
B - Left Deltoid	I - Right Deltoid
C - Left Gluteus Medius	J - Right Gluteus Medius
D - Left Lateral Thigh	K - Right Lateral Thigh
E - Left Ventral Gluteus	L - Right Ventral Gluteus
F - Left Lower Quadrant	M - Right Lower Quadrant
G - Left Upper Quadrant	N - Right Upper Quadrant

Mary Smith 086432

age 46   John Miller, M.D.

ALLERGIES: PCN, Sulfa

				mm/dd/yyyy	mm/dd/yyyy	mm/dd/yyyy
mm/dd/yyyy		Lanoxin 0.25mg po Q D	0900	09 JW		
mm/dd/yyyy		Rocephin ÷ 1 gm IV Q D	1200	1200 JW		
mm/dd/yyyy		Zinacef ÷ 1 gm IV Q 8 hr	0800	08 JW		
			1600			
			2400			

	7-3	JW		
SIGNATURE / SHIFT INDICATES				
NURSE ADMINISTERING MEDICATIONS	3-11			
J Wilson, RN	11-7			

FIGURE 23-7 After administering a medication, immediately document the date, time, dose, route, and person administering the medication on the MAR.

- Route of administration and injection site for parenteral medications
- Date and time administered
- Your name or initials as administering nurse

Most MARs are preprinted with the patient's name, name of the medication, dosage, and route administered (e.g., IM, oral, or IV). If so, you need only to write the time you actually administer the medication, initial each medication, and sign the form one time. Write legibly in ink.

If for some reason you do not administer a prescribed medication (e.g., patient refusal, NPO for diagnostic tests), document that information on the MAR and write a nurse's note explaining why it was not given.

When giving a PRN medication, in addition to recording on the MAR, write a nursing note documenting your assessment and the time the drug was given. Then, after allowing time for the medication to be absorbed and take effect, evaluate and document the patient's responses.

Key Point: *You are responsible for documenting the client's responses to all medications, including therapeutic effects, side effects, and unexpected or adverse reactions.* Never document a drug before you give it. Never document a medication given by someone else. Do not ask someone else to document medications you administered.

Other Rights

In addition to the rights already discussed, patients also have the following rights about medications they receive:

- **Right Reason.** This includes the right not to receive unnecessary medications. For example, a tranquilizer or sleeping pill should be given because the patient is very anxious or cannot sleep, not for the convenience of caregivers who are weary of the patient's incessant demands.
- **Right to Know.** You should tell the patient the name of the medication, why it is being given, its actions, and potential side effects.
- **Right to Refuse.** The patient has the right to refuse a medication regardless of their reasons and regardless of the consequences, except under certain circumstances (e.g., incompetency).

KnowledgeCheck 23-11

- What are the rights of medication?
- Give an example of each one.
- How many times, and when, should you check the medication against the MAR?

ADMINISTERING ORAL MEDICATIONS

The oral route is the one most used for medications. Recall what you already know about oral medications: Where are they absorbed? What are their advantages and disadvantages? What assessments should you

make? If you cannot answer these questions, review Table 23-1 and the discussions of drug preparations and routes of administration. For an overview of administering various types of oral medications, see the Highlights of Procedures box. To see detailed procedural steps,

 Go to **Chapter 23, Procedure 23-1: Administering Oral Medication**, in Volume 2.

Pouring Liquid Medications

Liquid medications are frequently used for children and older adults. They usually come in multidose bottles, so you will need to pour individual doses into a disposable, calibrated cup.

You should use the unit of measurement specified in the prescription. The measurement cup for liquids may have teaspoon, tablespoon, milliliter, and fluid ounce markings. These different measurement volumes can lead to medication errors (ISMP, 2022).

When pouring, hold the bottle so that the liquid does not run over the label, which would make it difficult to read. Place the label inside your palm. Hold the cup at eye level when measuring (Fig. 23-8). Read the dosage where the lowest part of the concaved surface (meniscus) of the fluid is on the line.

Buccal and Sublingual Medications

Although placed in the mouth, buccal and sublingual medications are rapidly absorbed in the mucous membranes rather than in the GI tract.

- **Buccal medications** are held in the cheek.
- **Sublingual medications** are held under the tongue (see Procedure 23-1). Some soluble forms of medications and enzyme preparations are administered by this route and absorbed within seconds.

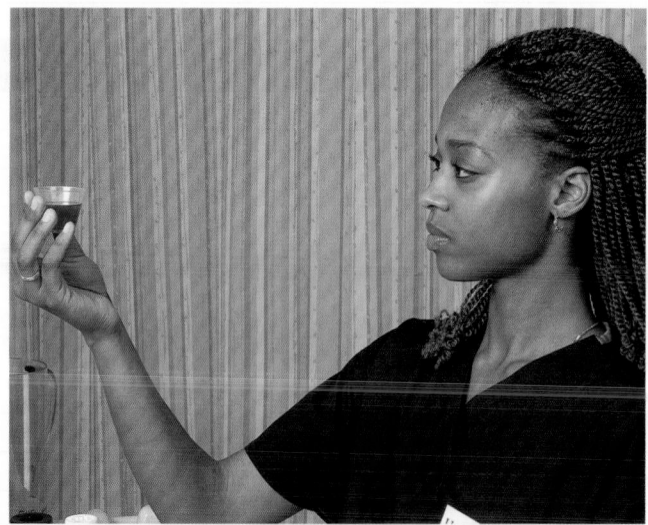

FIGURE 23-8 When pouring a liquid medication, measure the dose while holding the calibrated cup at eye level.

Enteral (Nasogastric and Gastrostomy) Medications

For patients who cannot swallow or who have feeding tubes, you can give oral medications through nasogastric (NG), gastrostomy, or jejunal tubes. Observe the following special considerations when administering enteral medications:

- *Hydrophilic medications*, such as psyllium (Metamucil)—Do not administer these through feeding tubes because they attract water and will solidify in the tube.
- *Crushing tablets*—Some tablets (e.g., enteric-coated or extended-release medications) should not be crushed because crushing can change their action. Always check your drug reference sources.
- *Continuous tube feedings*—Disconnect and flush the tubing before giving medications.
- *Enteral tube suction*—Discontinue the suction for 30 minutes after administration and keep the tube clamped to allow time for the drug to be absorbed, if applicable.

For other procedures related to gastric and enteral tubes,

 Go to **Chapter 24, Procedure 24-2: Inserting Nasogastric and Nasoenteric Tubes, Procedures 24-3: Administering Feedings Through Gastric and Enteric Tubes Using an Open System: Syringe, and Procedure 24-4: Removing a Nasogastric or Nasoenteric Tube**, in Volume 2.

Special Situations

Offer immediate oral hygiene for oral medications that discolor or damage tooth enamel, have an objectionable taste, are difficult to swallow, or cause the patient to gag. Also, follow these tips:

- **Medications that discolor the teeth.** Mix such drugs with liquid, have the patient drink the solution through a straw, and have the patient drink a liberal amount of flavored liquid (e.g., juice) or water afterward to dilute the medication.
- **Medications with an objectionable taste.** Have the patient suck on ice chips for several minutes before taking the medication to numb the taste buds. Unless contraindicated, you can store the medication in the refrigerator. The smell and taste are less objectionable when chilled, especially for oily liquids. When administering, place the medication on the back of the patient's tongue because there are fewer taste buds.
- **Contraindications to oral medications.** Do not give the drug to patients who are NPO, comatose, at risk for aspiration, or experiencing nausea or vomiting. Obtain a prescription for an alternative route or request permission to give the medication with small sips of water.

- **Patients who have difficulty swallowing medications.** Crush soluble tablets and place them in liquids or in a small amount of applesauce or pudding. ✚ Remember that some forms (e.g., time-released tablets) should not be crushed. Always check your drug reference sources to be certain.

KnowledgeCheck 23-12

- Describe two ways to ensure an accurate dosage when pouring liquid medications.
- What instructions should you give to a patient who is taking a sublingual medication?
- Explain the special step required when administering enteral medications to a patient who is receiving continuous tube feedings.
- Describe three methods for disguising the taste of objectionable-tasting drugs.
- For which patients are oral medications contraindicated?

Administering Oral Medication to Children

Children are not motivated by logic. They do not grasp the cause and effect of "Take this; it will make you feel better." If they do not like the taste, they simply will not swallow the medication. Be aware that young children may not be able to swallow tablets and capsules. Therefore, most oral medications for children are prepared as sweetened and flavored liquids or chewable tablets. Always take special care to prevent choking and aspiration. Ask parents how they get their child to take medicines. You may also need to teach techniques for administering medications at home (see the accompanying Self-Care box, Teaching Parents About Medicating Children).

 ## Administering Oral Medications to Older Adults

Many interventions for older adults (e.g., facilitating swallowing) are the same as those discussed in the preceding section on Teaching Patients About Medication Self-Administration and in Procedure 23-1.

However, because of physiological changes associated with aging (see Table 23-2), older adults usually require smaller dosages of drugs, and physical responses to some medications are unpredictable. Therefore, you must carefully observe for both therapeutic and undesired effects. **NOTE:** The following interventions for medications administered by the nurse (also see Box 23-4) and are not included in the self-administration discussion.

- **Address swallowing difficulties.** As the desire to drink decreases with age, the mouth often becomes drier, making it difficult to take large tablets. Crush tablets (if acceptable) or give drugs in liquid form. Try gently massaging the area just below the chin to initiate swallowing. Collaborate

Self-Care

Teaching Parents About Medicating Children

1. Mark each bottle or syringe containing medication with a different color of tape or adhesive label. This makes each clearly distinguishable because many medication bottles look alike.

2. You can reuse syringes for oral medications until the markings or tape begins to wear off or the plunger becomes difficult to move. Wash syringes with warm, soapy water, then rinse well and allow to air dry.

3. Take your time when giving medication, and find a quiet environment. Don't rush the process. It can be frustrating to struggle with a young child who is resisting taking a medication, especially if your time is limited.

4. Give the medication at the same time each day so that it becomes a matter of routine. It is easier to remember when a pattern is established.

5. If the child is old enough to understand, warn them when a medication has an unpleasant taste (e.g., "John, this doesn't taste very good, but you can have a big drink of juice as soon as you swallow it"). You may lose their trust if you surprise them with a bad-tasting medicine.

6. Give the child a frozen fruit bar or frozen flavored ice pop just before the medication. This helps to numb the taste buds to weaken the taste of the medication.

7. To mask bad-tasting medicines, you can crush tablets or empty the contents of a capsule and mix it with soft foods, such as applesauce, hot cereal, or pudding. This is helpful for children who might aspirate liquids. (**Caution:** Check a drug reference book or with the prescriber before crushing a tablet or emptying a capsule. Some medications should not be crushed.)

8. Do not use essential foods in the child's diet (e.g., milk or orange juice) to mask the taste of medications. The child may later refuse a food they associate with the medicine.

9. To prevent choking or aspiration when giving liquids to infants and toddlers, hold the child in a sitting or semisitting position. Use a medicine dropper or syringe to place the medication between the gum and cheek. Instill the medication; avoid giving too much, too fast.

10. Always praise the child after they swallow the medication.

---

with an occupational or speech therapist for other strategies.

- **Accommodate slower reflexes and reasoning ability.** Allow more time to explain and administer medications. When teaching, keep instructions simple and repeat them often. Always reinforce the need to take the medication as prescribed. Some patients may think, "I don't feel any better when I take all this stuff." In the hospital, patients may refuse to take medications, or they may put the tablets in their mouths and spit them out when you leave the room. Stay with the patient until you see that they have swallowed the medications.

KnowledgeCheck 23-13

- What is the chief danger when administering oral medications to children?
- How can you help a person who has some difficulty swallowing oral medications?
- How can you be sure that patients are not spitting out their medications after you leave the room?

ADMINISTERING TOPICAL MEDICATIONS

Topical medications are applied directly to a body site or placed in body cavities by irrigation or instillation. Their action depends on how the drug is prepared:

- *Local effects*—Examples are zinc oxide ointment to protect the skin against irritation associated with bowel and bladder incontinence and corticosteroid creams for itching.

- *Systemic effects*—These are absorbed through the skin and mucous membranes (e.g., estrogen patches; also see Transdermal Medications, following).

Lotions, Creams, and Ointments

Before applying medications to the skin, assess for contraindications (e.g., skin irritation, open lesions). Use a cotton swab, tongue blade, or gloved finger to apply these types of medications so that your skin does not absorb them. For step-by-step procedure,

 Go to **Chapter 23, Procedure 23-7A: Applying Lotion, Cream, and Ointment**, in Volume 2.

Transdermal Medications

Designed to be absorbed through the skin, transdermal medications are prepared as patches made of a special membrane. Patches allow constant, controlled amounts of medications to be released over 24 hours or more, giving a prolonged systemic effect (e.g., nitroglycerin to control angina or chest pain; scopolamine to treat motion sickness; nicotine to control smoking urges). Most patches are prepared with the correct dose already applied and should not be cut; however, some can be cut and are self-adherent (e.g., lidocaine). Check the package insert or ask a pharmacist about proper handling, application, and disposal of patches. Wear gloves when applying, removing, and discarding transdermal patches (Fig. 23-9). For more information, see the Highlights of Procedures box and

Go To **Chapter 23, Procedure 23-7D: Applying Transdermal Medication**, in Volume 2.

BOX 23-4 ■ Reducing Medication Errors for Older Adults

- **Be alert to unnecessary drug therapy.** It is not unusual for prescribers to be reluctant to stop a medication or simply forget to do so. The likelihood of a poor outcome increases as the number of drugs prescribed increases.
- **Request the indication for use** on all medication prescriptions.
- **Suggest nonpharmacological interventions** (e.g., warm massage, guided imagery) before prescribing medication for new symptoms.
- **Consider the "snowball effect."** This occurs when the provider prescribes a drug to counter the side effects of the initial treatment drug. A third drug is then prescribed to counter the side effect of the second drug, and so on. To interrupt this phenomenon, the prescriber can discontinue the medication, reduce the dose, or substitute one that the patient tolerates better.
- **Verify that a newly prescribed medication** does not have a documented drug–drug interaction. Check that the prescribed dosage is correct within the desired range.
- **When titrating drug doses, start low and go slow.** It is best to start with the lowest possible dose when starting a medication because adverse drug effects are dose related, and older adults tend to be more sensitive.
- **Assess urinary status.** Many drugs are cleared through the renal system. Some have toxic effects on the kidneys, particularly for older adults.
- **Recommend safer drugs** if the provider prescribes medication associated with adverse outcomes for older adults. The benefit must exceed the risk to the patient.

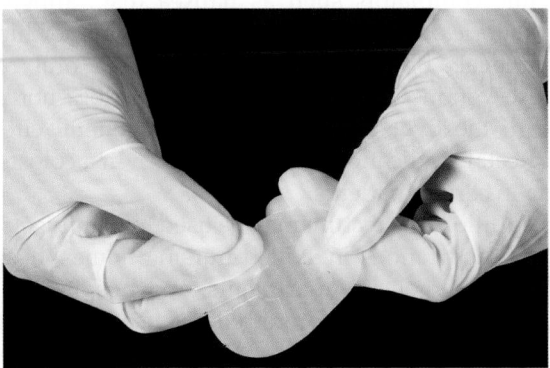

FIGURE 23-9 Patches allow constant, controlled amounts of medications to be released over a 24- to 72-hour period, giving a prolonged systemic effect. Wear gloves when removing and applying them.

PERFORMING IRRIGATIONS AND INSTILLATIONS

Irrigation is the washing out of a body cavity with a steady stream of fluid. Sterile water, saline, or antiseptic solutions are flushed into the eyes, ears, throat, vagina, rectum, or urinary tract to wash out the cavity.

Instillation is the insertion into a body cavity (e.g., eye drops) of medication for retention or absorption. Some medications need to remain in the body cavity for a period of time for maximum absorption and effect. Irrigations and instillations are performed to:

- Remove discharge or foreign bodies (e.g., from the eye or ear)
- Apply heat and cold to an area
- Apply medications (e.g., antiseptics)
- Prepare an area for surgery (e.g., an enema for cleansing the bowels).

You will usually not use sterile technique unless there are breaks in the skin.

Specific types of syringes are used for irrigating and instilling medications and fluids. Each is calibrated to allow you to control the amount and speed of solution delivered into the cavity (Fig. 23-10). For eye irrigations, the Morgan Lens is used to keep the eye closed while delivering the solution to the eye.

Ophthalmic Medications

Ophthalmic ointments or solutions are used for their local effects; to treat eye infections and glaucoma; to lubricate to counter dryness; or to irrigate the eye to remove foreign bodies, secretions, or harmful chemicals.

Ophthalmic medications are packaged in small bottles or tubes with a label that states, "For ophthalmic use only." Do not place any medication in the eye unless that statement appears on the container. Damage to the eye can result in permanent blindness. The **cornea** (the transparent part of the sclera in front of the iris and pupil) is easily injured, so you

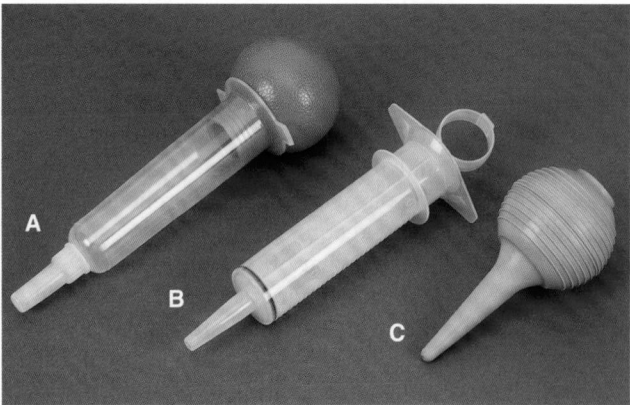

FIGURE 23-10 Syringes for administering enteral medications and performing irrigations and instillations. A, Asepto syringe: Plastic syringe with rubber bulb. B, Toomey (piston) syringe: Calibrated plastic syringe with removable tip that fits into the end of a tube (e.g., urinary catheter or enteral tube). For deep wound and bladder irrigations and administration of enteral medications. C, Rubber bulb syringe for ear irrigations.

should not place medications directly onto the eyeball. Do not touch the tip of the dropper or tube to the eye or conjunctiva; this may lead to bacterial growth on the container or damage the eye. See Chapters 19 and 27 for information about the structure and function of the eyes. For a summary of key points, see the Highlights of Procedures box. For a step-by-step procedure,

 Go to **Chapter 23, Procedure 23-2: Administering Ophthalmic Medication,** in Volume 2.

Otic Medications

Medications or solutions may be dropped into the ear to treat internal and external ear infections, to apply heat to the area, and to soften and remove earwax. Use solutions at room temperature because a solution that is too hot or too cold may cause vertigo, nausea, and pain. You will use clean technique when administering otic medications. ✚ To prevent infection, use sterile technique if the tympanic membrane (eardrum) has been ruptured or a surgical procedure has been done.

See Chapters 19 and 27 for information about the structure and function of the ear. The Highlights of Procedure box provides guidelines for performing otic instillations. For the complete procedure,

 Go to **Chapter 23, Procedure 26-3: Administering Otic Medications,** in Volume 2.

Nasal Medications

Clients usually self-administer nasal drops and sprays, many of which are available without a prescription. The most common nasal medications are used in the treatment of nasal congestion from colds and sinus infections. Nasal decongestants are used to shrink swollen mucous membranes and allow for better airflow and drainage of mucus.

- **Rebound effect.** Caution your patient that long-term use of decongestants may cause a rebound effect that requires continual use of the drug to achieve nasal decongestion. The nasal congestion is relieved immediately after use but recurs and even increases when the effects of the drug wear off.
- **Systemic side effects.** Frequent use of or swallowing excess decongestant can also cause systemic side effects (e.g., increased heart rate, increased blood pressure). These effects can be serious in children; saline drops are safer for them.
- See Chapters 19 and 27 for information about the structure and function of the nose. The Highlights of Procedures box provides guidelines for performing nasal instillations. For the complete procedure,

 Go to **Chapter 23, Procedures 23-4: Administering Nasal Medications,** in Volume 2.

Vaginal Medications

Vaginal medications come in various forms, including foams, jellies, liquids (douches), creams, tablets, and suppositories. They are used for several purposes: contraception, to destroy bacteria before gynecological surgery, to reduce dryness, to treat itching or infection, or to induce labor. To keep suppositories firm, store them in the refrigerator before use. Foams and jellies are inserted using an applicator or inserter. Provide a clean perineal pad to absorb drainage.

A **douche** is a vaginal irrigation using low pressure. Douches are used to administer antimicrobial solutions, remove irritating discharge, or apply heat or cold to reduce inflammation.

Key Point: *Teach patients that douching may be harmful because it disturbs the normal pH and healthy balance of microorganisms in the vagina. Research has shown a connection between douching and ovarian cancer and vaginal infections (Gonzalez, 2016; Hamoonga, 2019; Occupational Safety and Health Administration [OSHA], 2021).*

The Highlights of Procedures box provides guidelines for administering vaginal medications. For the complete procedure,

 Go to **Chapter 23, Procedure 23-5: Administering Vaginal Medications,** in Volume 2.

Rectal Medications

Rectal suppositories and liquid instillations **(enemas)** are used to encourage bowel movements or to treat systemic complaints such as nausea (e.g., antiemetic suppositories). The rectal route may provide for higher blood levels of the medication than the oral route because venous blood from the rectum does not pass through the liver before entering the general circulation. Rectal medication can also be given in a colostomy stoma in certain patients.

In addition, the rectum may be used to administer fluids and medications in skilled nursing homes, hospice settings, emergency departments, and hospitals when rapid hydration or symptom relief is needed and other routes are not available. The Macy Catheter is inserted in the rectum by a registered nurse (RN)/LPN/licensed vocational nurse (LVN) and can remain in place for up to 28 days. A prescription from a provider is required for placement.

For advantages and disadvantages of the rectal route, see Table 23-1.

See the Highlights of Procedures box. For the complete procedure for administering rectal medications,

 Go to **Chapter 23, Procedure 23-6: Inserting a Rectal Suppository** and **Chapter 26, Procedure 26-3: Administering an Enema,** in Volume 2.

ADMINISTERING RESPIRATORY INHALATIONS

Nebulization is the production of a fine spray, fog, powder, or mist from a liquid drug. The patient inhales the medication mixture by breathing deeply through a mouthpiece attached to the nebulizer. Absorption is rapid because of the vascularity of the airways and alveoli.

Types of Nebulizers

The following are four types of devices for achieving nebulization:

1. **Atomizers** disperse the medication in the form of large droplets.
2. **Aerosol sprayers** suspend the droplets of medication in a gas (e.g., oxygen).
3. **An ultrasonic (handheld) nebulizer** mixes a small volume of medication, usually less than 1 mL, with 3 mL of normal saline. The device forces air through the nebulizer and delivers medication and humidity as a fine mist that can be inhaled deep into the lungs.
4. **A metered-dose inhaler (MDI)** (Fig. 23-11) is a type of nebulizer that delivers measured doses of a nebulized drug.

No matter which device is used, the smaller the droplets, the farther the medication can be inhaled into the respiratory tract.

Metered-Dose Inhalers and Dry Powder Inhalers

Metered-Dose Inhaler An MDI is a pressurized container prefilled with several doses of a drug and an eco-friendly substance, called hydrofluoroalkane (HFA), to propel the medication forward. The patient inhales while pushing the canister's pump to release a measured dose of medication through a mouthpiece (see Fig. 23-11a). Sometimes an extender (spacer) is attached to the mouthpiece to enhance the delivery of medication into the respiratory tract (see Fig. 23-11b). Medication is pumped into the extender instead of directly into the patient's mouth. The patient inhales the drug from the chamber.

The **advantage** of MDIs is that high doses of medication can be rapidly instilled in the lungs, producing local effects directly in the airway while avoiding systemic side effects. The **disadvantage** is that the person must have the manual dexterity and skill to coordinate the inhalation of the medication while pushing the canister to administer the dose. These skills are often compromised in older adults and young children. The patient must also be able to inhale and exhale deeply enough to allow penetration of the medication in the more distal bronchioles

Dry Powder Inhaler A dry powder inhaler (DPI) is activated by a pump rather than by inhalation. Once the

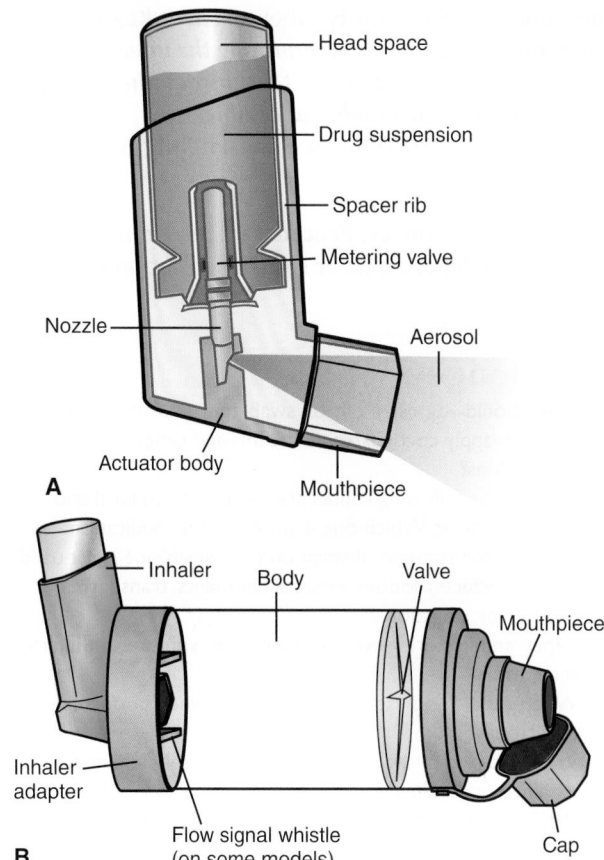

FIGURE 23-11 Inhalers. *A*, Metered-dose inhaler. *B*, Inhaler with a spacer.

dose is loaded, the patient simply takes a deep breath. DPIs are not designed to be used with a spacer. Patients frequently self-administer inhalations (most often bronchodilators or steroids) using an MDI. Teach your patient how to (1) coordinate the inhalation of the medication and the pushing of the canister, (2) inhale and exhale deeply to correctly administer the dose (Fig. 23-12) and (3) track the number of puffs used to avoid the canister

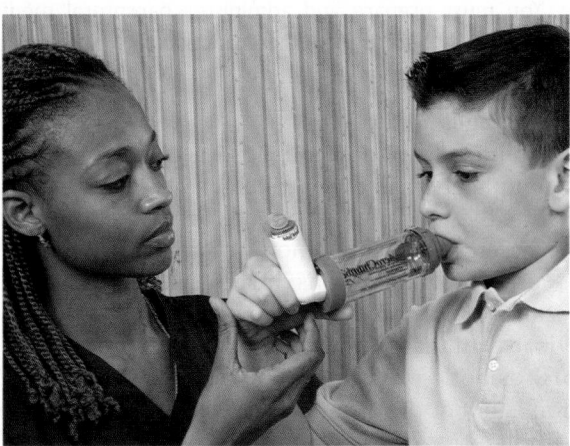

FIGURE 23-12 Child using a metered-dose inhaler with an extender.

being unexpectedly empty when needed. **Key Point:** *The only reliable method for determining the number of doses remaining in the canister is to subtract the number of doses used from the number available.*

For more information, see the Highlights of Procedures box. Also,

 Go to **Chapter 23, Procedure 23-8, Administering Metered-Dose Inhaler (MDI) Medication,** in Volume 2.

KnowledgeCheck 23-14

- Why should you use a cotton swab, tongue blade, or gloved finger to apply corticosteroid creams and other topical medications?
- Most of the following routes are used for both local and systemic effects. Which one is used *only* for medications intended for systemic absorption (i.e., which one is *not* used for local effects): lotions, creams, ointments, transdermal patches, or irrigations?
- When administering eye drops, how can you prevent injury to the cornea?
- When should you use sterile technique when performing otic instillations?
- What are two of the undesired effects of self-administered nasal decongestants?
- What possible harm can result from vaginal douching?
- When is rectal instillation of a drug preferred over oral administration?
- When, as a rule, are rectal medications contraindicated?
- Define *nebulization*.
- What is the best way to determine if an MDI is empty?

ADMINISTERING PARENTERAL MEDICATIONS

Parenteral medications include those that are injected or infused into body tissues or into the bloodstream via the intradermal, subcutaneous, IM, or IV routes. Because the body's first layer of defense against microorganisms, the skin, is broken, administration of parental medications requires the use of aseptic techniques. ✚ You must prepare and administer parenteral medications accurately because the medications, once given, cannot be retrieved.

- **Advantages**
  - Parenteral injections are absorbed faster and more completely than drugs given by other routes; therefore, the results are more predictable, and the dosage can be measured more accurately.
  - Parenteral medications can be used for patients who cannot take oral medications.
- **Disadvantages:** Tissue damage may result if the pH, osmotic pressure, or solubility of the medication is not appropriate to the tissue where the medication is given. For example, medications intended for injection into muscle may damage subcutaneous tissue.

Equipment for Parenteral Medications

When administering injectable (parenteral) medications, you must know about various kinds of needles and syringes. You will need to decide, based on each situation, what size and type of needle and syringe to use. For a summary of the sites and equipment used for parenteral administration, refer to Table 23-4.

Reusing Equipment at Home Many people (e.g., those who have diabetes) must give themselves repeated injections, perhaps several each day. Supplies for home use are expensive. Insurance may or may not cover the cost, or the person may not have insurance. Teach your patient that the Centers for Disease Control and Prevention (CDC) recommends that both the needle and syringe are discarded after a single use (CDC, 2019). Therefore, patients who are experiencing financial difficulties that affect their ability to obtain needed supplies should seek advice from their provider or social worker.

Needles

Needles are disposable, stainless-steel sheaths that attach to a syringe. Figure 23-13 shows the parts of a needle. Needles are made in various lengths and gauges and with different bevel sizes.

Gauge The inside diameter of the needle lumen is the gauge. Needle gauges are numbered 14 through 30. **Key Point:** *The smaller the gauge, the larger the diameter (i.e., a 16-gauge needle has a larger diameter than does a 20-gauge needle).*

- **Choose the gauge** based on the (1) patient's size and skin condition, (2) viscosity of medication used, and (3) speed of administration desired.
- **Smaller needles** (25 to 30 gauge) cause less pain and trauma to the tissue, so they are useful for patients who must have frequent or long-term injections (e.g., insulin and heparin).
- **Larger needles** (14 to 18 gauge) are used for blood and more viscous medications, to mix IV medications, or for rapid infusion of IV medications.

Bevel The bevel is the sharp slanted tip of the needle that creates an opening to administer medications or withdraw blood.

- **A long bevel tip** is sharper and narrower and therefore causes less discomfort during injection. Long bevels are used for subcutaneous and IM injections.
- **Short bevels** are used for intradermal or IV injections. For an illustration of a bevel,

 Go to **Chapter 23, Procedure 23-11: Administering Intradermal Medication,** in Volume 2.

Needle Length The distance from the hub (bottom) of the needle to the tip is the needle length. Lengths usually range from 3/8 inch to 3 inches.

- **Key Point:** *Choose the length according to the (1) thickness of the patient's muscle, (2) amount of*

Table 23-4 ➤ Parenteral Injections: Comparison of Sites and Equipment*

ROUTE	SITE	MAX VOLUME (mL)	NEEDLE GAUGE	NEEDLE LENGTH (inch)	SYRINGE SIZE (mL)	ANGLE OF INJECTION (degree)
Intradermal	Inner aspect of forearm	0.1	26–28	⅜–¾	1.0	5°–15°
Subcutaneous Insulin	Fatty area over triceps, abdomen, anterior thigh	0.3, 0.5, and 1.0	28–31	³⁄₁₆–1 (max ⅝ for upper arm)	0.3, 0.5, 1 (0.3–0.5 for upper arm)	45°–90°
Subcutaneous Other	Fatty area over triceps, abdomen, anterior thigh	0.5–1	25–27	⅜–⅝	1.0–3.0	45°–90°
Intramuscular	Deltoid	0.5–1	22–25	⅝–1 (infants and children) 1–1½ (adults)	1.0	90°
	Rectus femoris *(not recommended)*	2	22–25	1½–3	1.0	90°
	Vastus lateralis	1.0 (infants younger than 12 months) 1–2 (infants and children 1–12 years) 3–5 (adults, depending on muscle size)	22–25	1 (infants younger than 12 months) 1–1¼ (infants 12 to 24 months) 1½–3 (adults, depending on if obese)	1.0–3.0	45°–90°
	Ventrogluteal	2.5–3	20–25	½–3	3.0	90°
Intravenous	Cephalic veins	Continuous infusion	18–25	1–1½		N/A
	Basilic veins	Continuous infusion	18–25	1–1½		N/A

*Dependent on weight and physical condition

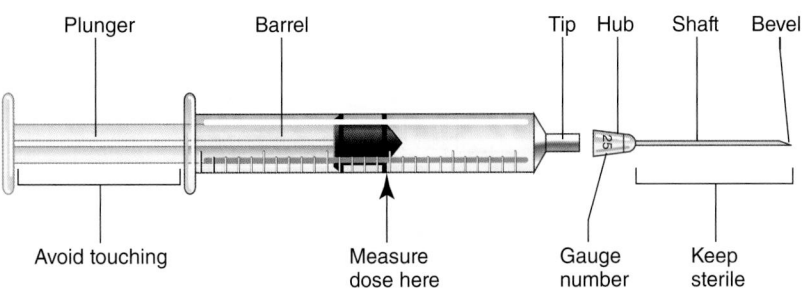

FIGURE 23-13 Parts of a needle and syringe.

adipose tissue, and (3) site in which the drug is to be injected. For example:

- A 1½-inch needle is common for IM injections.
- A shorter ⅜- to ¾-inch needle is used for intradermal injections.

Filter Needles and Filter Straws Filter needles and filter straws are used to trap particles or glass fragments when drawing up a reconstituted medication or a medication from an ampule. ✚ Do not push fluids through a filter needle or straw. You must replace the filter needle with a regular needle before injecting the medication into the patient or into the IV solution.

Safety Needles Many safety needle devices are available. Examples include:

- A resheathing system with a sliding barrel that shields the needle
- Syringes with retractable needles
- Needles with attached covers that reduce the risk of accidental puncture with contaminated needles (Fig. 23-14)

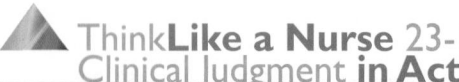

ThinkLike a Nurse 23-11: Clinical Judgment in Action

- You are to administer an IM injection of 1 mL of a thin, watery medication to a frail patient with very little muscle mass (5 ft 5 in. tall, weighs 96 lb). You have these needle sizes available: 16 gauge, 20 gauge, 25 gauge. Which would you use, and why?
- For the same patient, you have needles available in 1-inch and 1½-inch lengths. Which would you use, and why?

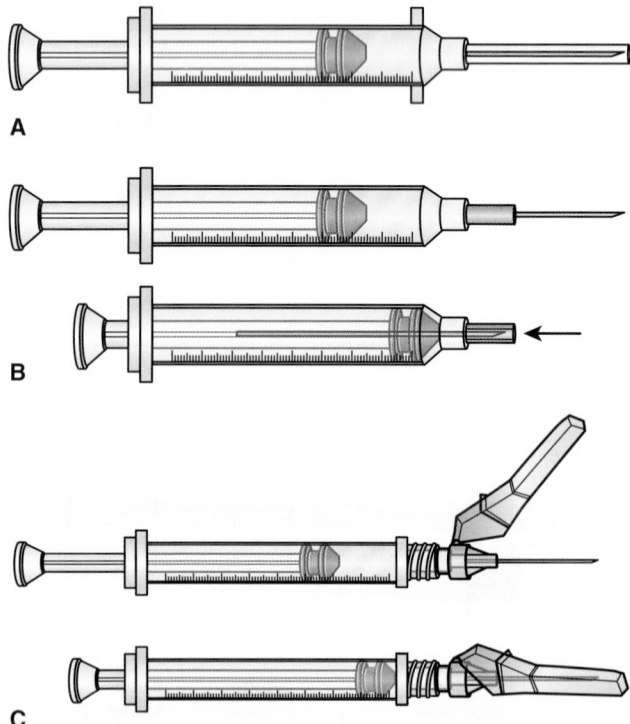

FIGURE 23-14 Needle safety features. *A,* Self-sheathing safety feature: Sliding needle shields attached to disposable syringes and vacuum tube holders. *B,* Syringe with retractable needle. *C,* Needles with covers.

Syringes

A syringe consists of a barrel, plunger, and syringe tip (see Fig. 23-13). Because (a) injections require strict sterile technique and (b) research has not definitively established that the design of the two-part syringe prevents contamination of the plunger and inner barrel (Kelley, 2014; Smith & Szlaczky, 2014), you may touch the outside of the barrel and end of the plunger but not the inside of the barrel, hub, shaft of the plunger, or needle.

Syringes are usually made of plastic and are disposable. Some have the needle attached; others do not. The syringe tip, either **luer-lock** (twist on) or **non-luer-lock** (slip on), fits into the needle hub (Fig. 23-15). Syringes are made in various sizes, from 0.5 to 60 mL. The larger sizes are used for instillations and irrigations. You will usually use a 2- or 3-mL syringe for intramuscular injections (see Fig. 23-15). Three syringes are shown in Figure 23-16.

- **Standard syringes** are supplied in 3-, 5-, and 10-mL sizes. They are commonly supplied without needles

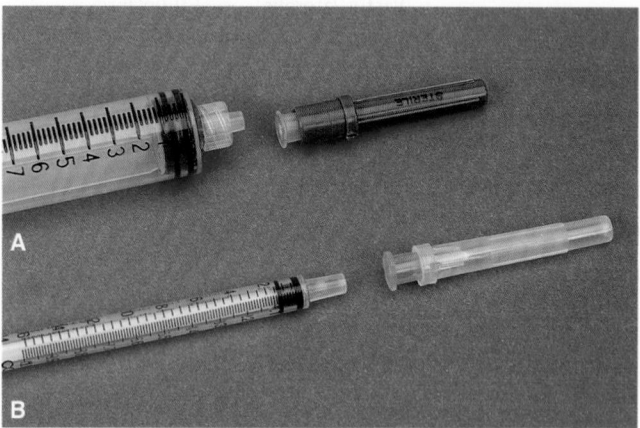

FIGURE 23-15 Syringe tips. *A,* Luer-lock (twist-on) tip. *B,* Nonluer-lock (slip-on) tip.

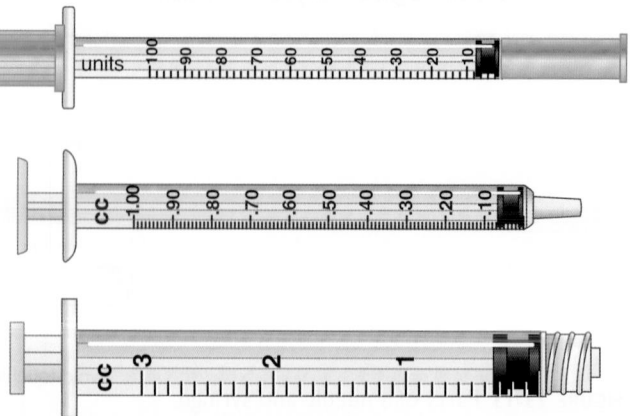

FIGURE 23-16 Syringe types. *A,* 100-unit insulin syringe marked in units. *B,* 1-mL tuberculin syringe marked in increments of 0.01 mL. *C,* 3-mL standard syringe marked in increments of 0.1 mL.

or with 18-, 21-, 23-, or 25-gauge needles that are 0.5 to 3 inches long. To ensure accurate measurement of drugs, syringes are calibrated and marked in 0.1-mL and 1- or 2-mL increments.

- **Tuberculin syringes** have a 1-mL capacity and are calibrated in 0.01-mL increments. They come with a small (usually 25- to 28-) gauge, short (½- to ⅝-in.) needle. Use tuberculin syringes to administer small, precise doses of medication (e.g., to infants or children); for allergy tests; or when administering potentially dangerous medications (e.g., as heparin).

- **Insulin syringes** are calibrated in units and are used to administer insulin. **Key Point: *Insulin syringes are marked in 100 units per milliliter.*** They are made in 0.3-, 0.5-, or 1-mL sizes with very small-gauge needles (26 to 30 gauge).

- **Prefilled unit-dose systems** are reusable syringe holders that hold disposable, single-dose, prefilled medication cartridges. No medication preparation is necessary, but ✚ you must check each cartridge and dose carefully because many of the cartridges look alike. You simply insert the cartridge into the holder and lock it in place. After administering the medication, dispose of the cartridge; clean and keep the holder for reuse.

- **Disposable prefilled, self-contained systems** are available for hospitals, office practices, nursing homes, and self-administration. The injection plunger is attached to the medication barrel and twists in directly. This ready-to-use syringe reduces the risk of constituting or dosing errors. Because you do not need to remove the cartridge from the holder after using it, the risk of a needlestick injury is reduced (Fig. 23-17). To learn more about using prefilled systems,

> ▶ Go to **Chapter 23, Clinical Insight 23-2: Using Prefilled Unit-Dose Systems**, in Volume 2.

- **Safety syringes** come in various types, including devices featuring a resheathing system with a sliding barrel that shields the needle (Fig. 23-18), syringes with retractable needles that spring back into the barrel of the syringe, and needles with attached covers that reduce the risk of accidental puncture with contaminated needles.

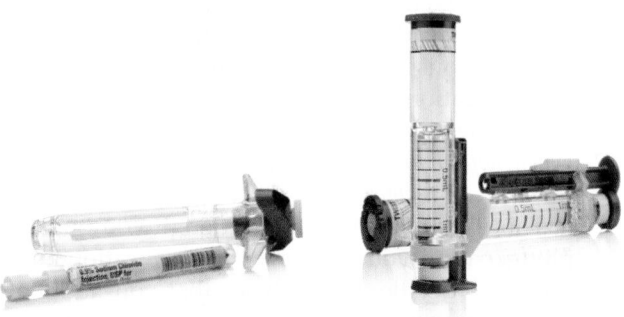

FIGURE 23-17 (*Left*) Prefilled unit-dose system. (*Right*) Disposable, prefilled, self-contained system.

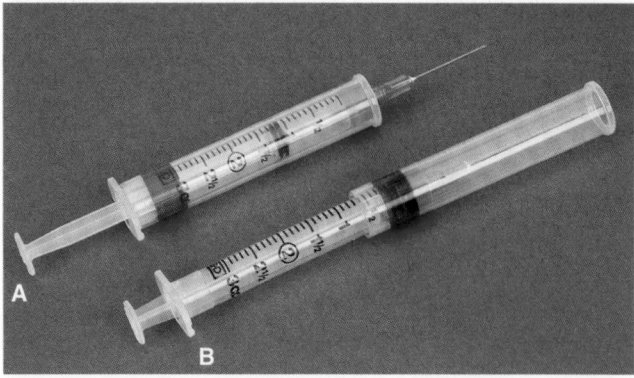

FIGURE 23-18 Safety syringe. A, Needle guard position before injection. B, Needle guard position after injection.

KnowledgeCheck 23-15

- What does the term *parenteral* mean?
- What are two disadvantages of the parenteral route?
- To maintain sterile technique, which part of a syringe must you *not* touch?
- You need to irrigate a wound. Which syringe size do you need: 0.5 mL, 3 mL, 5 mL, or 50 mL?
- Which syringe, as a rule, would you use for an IM injection: tuberculin, 50-mL, 5-mL, or 3-mL syringe?

Drawing Up and Mixing Medications

Most injectable medications are packaged in single-dose or multidose ampules and vials. You will use slightly different techniques, depending on the container.

Drawing Up Medications From an Ampule

An **ampule** is a thin-walled, disposable glass container with a narrow neck that you must snap off to access the medication. Each ampule holds a single dose of a liquid medication, usually 1 to 10 mL, but some hold 50 mL. To learn how to use ampules, see Procedure 23-9A.

- ✚ To prevent injuries, use an ampule opener to snap the glass (Fig. 23-19).

- ✚ Because glass fragments may be introduced into the medication, most agencies require you to use a filter needle or filter straw to draw up the medication.

See the Highlights of Procedures box. Also,

> ▶ Go to **Chapter 23, Procedure 23-9A. Drawing Up Medications From Ampules**, in Volume 2.

Drawing Up Medications From a Vial

A **vial** is a single-dose or multidose plastic or glass container with a rubber stopper that reseals the top after each needle introduction. A plastic or metal cap covers the rubber stopper to protect it until it is used (Fig. 23-20).

- The vial is a closed system, so you must inject air into it to withdraw the solution. Otherwise, a vacuum is

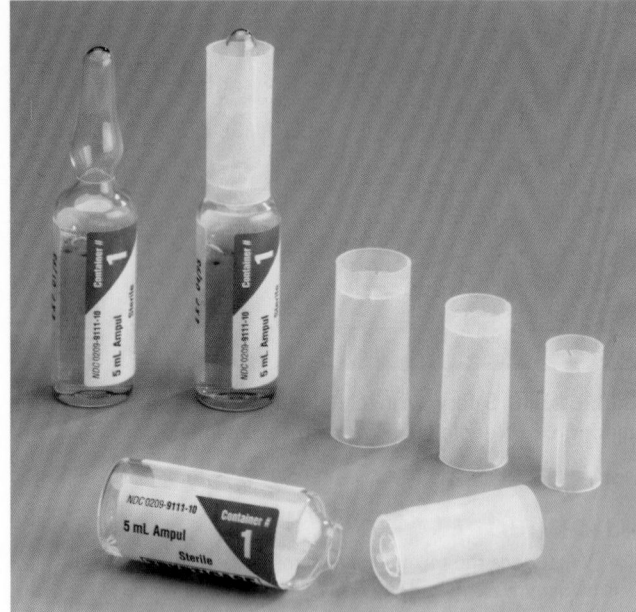

FIGURE 23-19 Safety device for opening glass ampules.

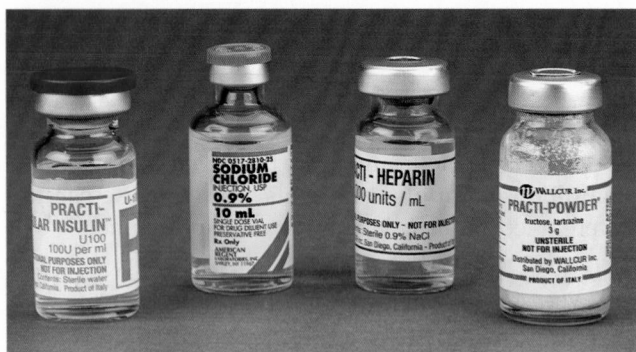

FIGURE 23-20 Vials containing medications.

created in the vial that makes withdrawal difficult. To learn how to use vials, see Procedure 23-9B.

- Nurses traditionally wipe the rubber stopper with alcohol after removing the cap, even on a single-dose vial. The practice removes dust and rubber particles from the top of the vial. Always follow your institution's policy.

Reconstituting Medications

Medications that are not stable in solution are dispensed as powders in vials. You must add a diluent or solvent to the powder to create a solution for injection. The diluent is usually sterile water or saline; however, each packaged vial includes the manufacturer's instructions for the amount and kind of solvent to add. ✚ For safety, use a plastic vial access cannula instead of a needle when possible. For guidelines,

 Go to **Chapter 23, Clinical Insight 23-3: Reconstituting Medications,** in Volume 2.

Mixing Medications in the Same Syringe

You can mix two medications in the same syringe (1) if they are compatible, (2) if the total dose is within accepted limits, and (3) if they are both prescribed by the same route. This technique allows for efficient use of supplies and fewer patient injections.

Medications are compatible if they can be mixed without affecting their constituents or actions. Package inserts and medication references usually include compatibility information.

✚ Always check the compatibility before mixing medications together. If the contents of the syringe become discolored, there are visible particles in the solution, or there is a change in consistency, do not administer the medications.

When mixing medications in one syringe, you must follow these principles:

- Maintain sterile technique (as with all parenteral medications).
- Do not contaminate one container with medication from the other container. In most cases, you must use a separate needle to withdraw from each vial.
- Ensure the total, final dosage is correct by adding the volumes of the two medicines together before administering (see Procedure 23-9C).

Key Point: *A single-dose vial should only be used one time for one patient, using a sterile needle and sterile syringe.*

Accounting for Needle "Dead Space"

Research has not provided evidence-based guidance on the practice of adding 0.2 mL of air to the syringe after measuring a medication for IM injection.

- Some believe a small amount of the patient's medication remains in the needle when an injection is given; therefore, adding 0.2 mL of air clears the needle of medication, ensuring that the patient receives the entire dose.
- Others believe that air should not be added because syringes are calibrated to account for medication left in the needle. We recommend that you add air only in the following situations:
  1. *When the medication is irritating to subcutaneous tissues,* add 0.2 mL of air after measuring the proper dose. The air drives the medication deep into the subcutaneous tissue and creates an air lock above the medication, preventing it from tracking through subcutaneous tissue.
  2. *When you change needles after drawing up the medication (e.g., replace a filter needle).* The new needle has air in it instead of medication. If you push the plunger until you see a drop of medication at the tip of the needle, you will see that you no longer have a complete dose in the syringe. Pulling in 0.2 mL air before changing the needle and then pushing the plunger until you see a drop of

medication at the tip of the new needle will prevent the loss of medication with the needle change.

3. *Agency policy requires adding 0.2 mL of air.*

 Go to **Chapter 23, Clinical Insight 23-4: Measuring Dosage When Changing Needles**, in Volume 2.

Preventing Needlestick Injuries

Workplace injuries from needles and other sharps put healthcare workers at risk for bloodborne diseases (e.g., hepatitis B, hepatitis C, HIV) (see Chapter 21). Needleless systems reduce the risk of needlestick injuries. Figure 23-21 shows three such devices. Also,

 Go to **Chapter 23, Clinical Insight 20-2: Providing a Clean Clinical Environment; Clinical Insight 20-3: Following CDC Standard Precautions;** and **Chapter 23, Procedure 23-10: Recapping Needles Using a One-Handed Technique,** in Volume 2.

The CDC and OSHA recommend the use of "needleless" systems. Most involve adapters for use with regular IV tubing and medication vials, allowing access through a valve system without a needle.

Jet injectors are needle-free systems that drive liquid medication into the intradermal, subcutaneous, or IM tissues by creating a narrow stream under high pressure that penetrates the skin. They are often used for immunizations. Local reactions or injury, such as redness, bruising, and pain, occur more often with jet injectors than by use of a needle.

 Always dispose of needles, glass, and other "sharps" in clearly marked, usually red, puncture-proof containers (Fig. 23-22). Never force a needle into an already full container; you may be injured by sharps protruding from the top. Never put a needle or other sharp in a wastebasket or in your pocket, and never leave it at the patient's bedside.

For tips to prevent needlestick injury,

 Go to **Chapter 23, Clinical Insight 21-2: Preventing Needlestick Injuries,** in Volume 2.

Recapping Contaminated Needles You should never recap a contaminated needle (e.g., after giving an injection). Place it uncapped, needle pointing downward, directly into a sharps-disposal container. However, you may occasionally find that you cannot avoid recapping a contaminated needle. The U.S. Food and Drug Administration (2018) requires using a one-handed technique, although needle removal using a mechanical device is an alternative. For step-by-step instructions, refer to Procedure 23-10.

Recapping Sterile Needles If safety systems (e.g., needleless systems) are not available, we suggest that you not use the one-handed "scoop" technique to recap a sterile needle because the risk of contaminating it is high. Consider one of the other methods described in Procedure 23-10.

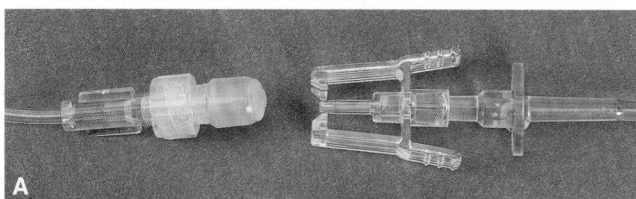
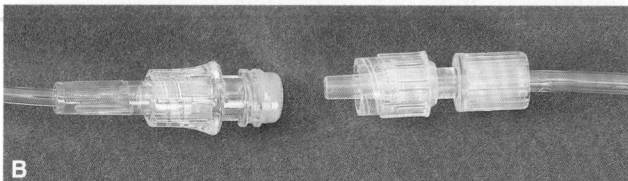
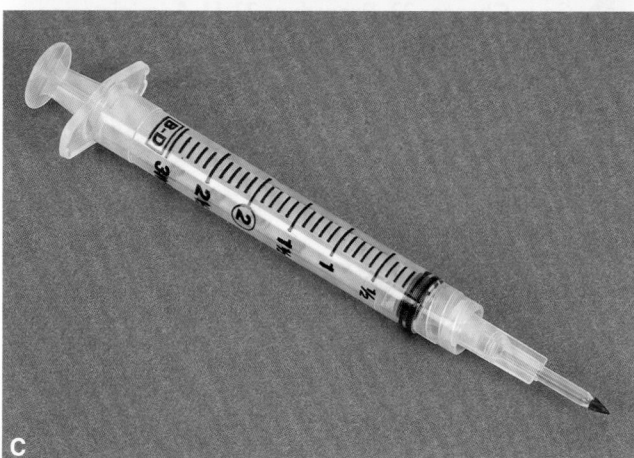

FIGURE 23-21 Needleless systems. *A,* Lever-lock cannula. *B,* Threaded lock cannula. *C,* Blunt-tipped syringe for drawing up medication.

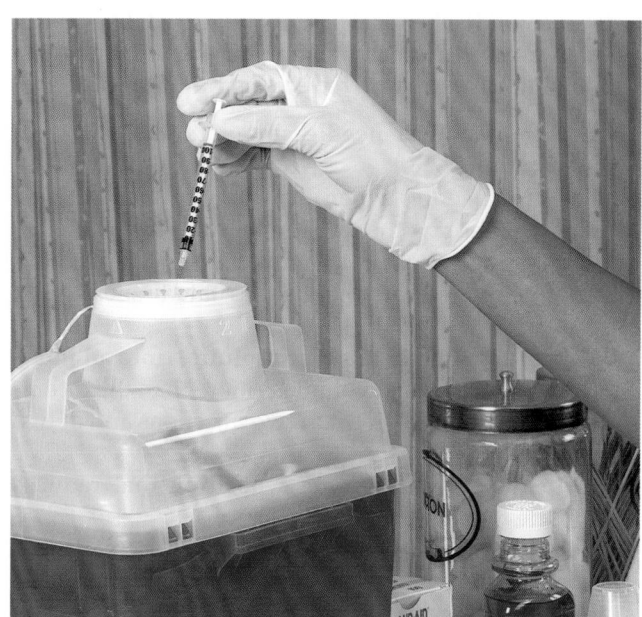

FIGURE 23-22 Disposal system for sharp objects, such as needles and glass. The container must be clearly marked, is usually red, and is puncture-proof.

Comfort and Safety Considerations

Parenteral techniques are invasive. They carry the potential for tissue trauma and provide a portal of entry for pathogens through the skin. You must maintain strict aseptic (sterile) technique to minimize the risk of infection. Moreover, your injection technique and choice of injection site are critical to patient comfort and safety. When choosing a site, consider:

- **Type, viscosity, and volume** of the medication to be administered
- **The anatomical landmarks** underlying injection sites
- **Patient's situation** (e.g., the condition of the tissues at the injection site, the accessibility of certain sites)

The following are **examples of judgment and technique errors** and their consequences:

- **Injecting a large volume of medication into a small muscle** causes pain and may damage the tissues.
- **Injecting into the wrong tissue** (e.g., giving an intramuscular medication too shallowly into the subcutaneous tissue) may (1) accelerate or delay the rate of absorption and (2) cause tissue injury and pain.
- **Incorrectly locating an injection site** may result in bone or nerve injury when you insert the needle.
- **An unsteady needle and syringe** while injecting the drug could lead to pain and tissue trauma.
- **Failing to follow guidelines** before injecting potentially dangerous drugs risks could result in an adverse, even fatal, effect.

Minimizing Discomfort

♥ **iCare** The discomfort associated with an injection comes from three sources: (1) the prick of the needle, (2) the pressure of the volume of the drug in the tissues, and (3) chemical irritation caused by certain drugs. Fear and anxiety magnify discomfort. Use the following techniques to reduce discomfort:

- **Use the smallest needle suited for the site and medication.**
- **Use two needles when drawing up medications:** one to withdraw the medication from the container, and the second one for the injection. If the needle is not free of medication, it may irritate tissues as it is inserted.
- **Do not administer too much solution into an injection site.** If the total volume is more than the recommended amount, give it in two injections and at two sites.
- **Help the patient assume a position that reduces muscle tension** for IM injections.
- **Use the Z-track technique** for intramuscular injections to minimize pain and tissue irritation. The Z-track method is discussed later in this chapter.
- **Pull the skin taut and insert the needle quickly** to avoid pulling the tissues. Remove the needle quickly and at the same angle you inserted it.

- **Steady the syringe** with one hand while injecting the medication.
- **Inject the medication slowly.**
- **Distract the patient** from the procedure by talking to them.
- **Apply gentle pressure** (not massage) after injection unless contraindicated.
- **Acknowledge that the patient will feel some pain** (e.g., "This may hurt a little bit."). Especially with children, if you deny or minimize the pain, the patient might lose trust in you and be even more anxious about future injections.
- **Pat or hug a child after injection,** speak softly, and perhaps play with the child so that they do not associate you only with pain.
- **Use other methods to decrease pain,** such as cooling the skin (e.g., applying ice) or flicking or tapping over the injection area before injecting. Both send distracting signals to the brain so that it can't process the stimuli as easily when the needle is injected.

Intradermal Injections

Intradermal injections are given into the **dermis,** which is the layer of the skin located beneath the skin surface. The intradermal route is commonly used for allergy or tuberculosis (TB) testing.

- Most nurses use the patient's nondominant arm for TB screening and the dominant arm, chest, or upper back for all other tests (Fig. 23-23).
- Give only small amounts of medication by this route—about 0.1 mL.
- Use a 1-mL syringe and a short, small (26- to 28-gauge) needle.
- Insert at an angle of 5° to 15° (Fig. 23-24).

 Do not apply pressure or massage the injection site because the capillaries in the dermal tissue will quickly absorb the medication. Refer to the Highlights of Procedures box for critical elements of intradermal injections. Also,

Go to **Chapter 23, Procedure 23-11: Administering Intradermal Medications**, in Volume 2.

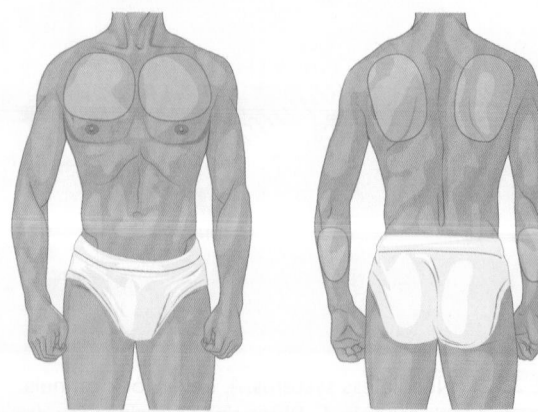

FIGURE 23-23 Sites commonly used for intradermal injection.

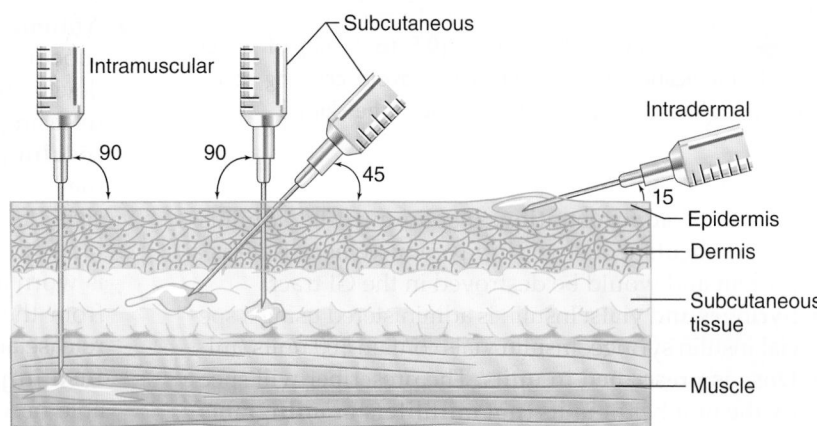

FIGURE 23-24 Standard angles of insertion for intramuscular, subcutaneous, and intradermal injections.

Subcutaneous Injections

Subcutaneous (SUBQ) injections are given into the subcutaneous tissue, the layer of fat located below the dermis and above the muscle tissue. You do not need to aspirate for blood return when giving a subcutaneous injection because of the shallow depth of the needle into the subcutaneous layer under the skin.

- **SubQ absorption is slower than it is through the IM route** because, as a rule, subQ tissue does not have as rich of a blood supply as muscle.
- **Speed of absorption varies with the subcutaneous site selected,** however.
  - **Absorption is fastest** in sites on the abdomen and arms.
  - **Absorption is slower** on the thigh and upper buttocks.
  - **Medication is absorbed more evenly** from the abdomen than from the thighs and buttocks because it is affected less by activity.

The Highlights of Procedures box contains critical elements of the procedure. For a full procedure,

 Go to **Chapter 23, Procedure 23-12: Administering Subcutaneous Medications,** in Volume 2.

Choosing a Subcutaneous Site

See Figure 23-25 for sites to use for subcutaneous injections.

- **Avoid these sites:** (1) areas in which the subcutaneous tissue lies beneath burns, birthmarks, scars, or inflamed tissue; (2) sites with lesions; (3) sites over bony prominences; and (4) sites with large underlying vessels or nerves.
- **When using the abdominal site,** do not inject any closer than 5 cm (2 in. horizontally and vertically) from the umbilicus.
- **For repeated injections,** each injection should be at least an inch apart.
- **Rotate sites for repeated injections** to minimize scarring and hardening of fatty tissue that will interfere with the absorption of medication.

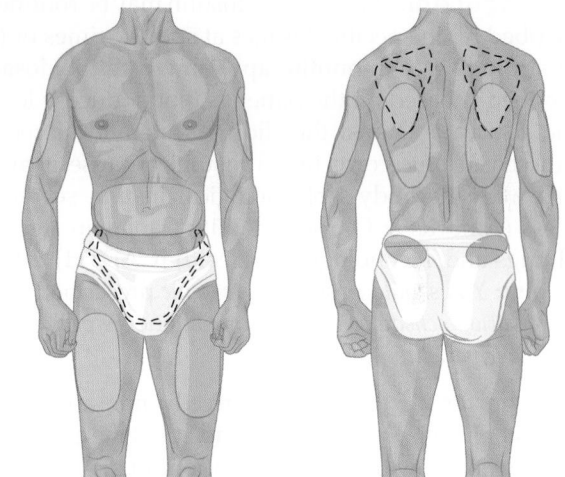

FIGURE 23-25 Sites used for subcutaneous injections.

Choosing a Subcutaneous Needle

Key Point: *As a general rule, use a syringe with a small-gauge, short needle that is long enough to penetrate into the fatty subcutaneous layer but not into the muscle.*

- **Needle length** will vary depending on the amount of adipose tissue that the patient has and the type of injection needed (e.g., insulin, immunization). For most subcutaneous injections, a ⅜- to ⅝-inch needle is preferred. However, shorter needles (e.g., ³⁄₁₆ to ⁵⁄₁₆ inch) are more comfortable for some insulin users.
- The **needle gauge** for subcutaneous injection is typically 25 to 27 gauge.
  - **Insulin users** often prefer finer needles (e.g., 28 to 31 gauge).
  - **For children** and persons with little or average subcutaneous fat, insert a standard-length needle (⅝ in.) at a 45° angle; however, when using a shorter needle, inject at a 90° angle.
  - **Obese patients** will need a longer needle (e.g., 1 in.) and a 90° angle for injection (see Fig. 23-24), and the nurse needs to spread the skin taut rather than pinching.

✚ Inject only small amounts (0.5 to 1 mL) of water-soluble medication subcutaneously to avoid creating sterile abscesses (hardened, painful lumps under the skin).

Administering Insulin

- **Routes of administration:** Insulin must be administered subcutaneously or intravenously because it is a protein and would be destroyed in the GI tract.
- **Syringes and vials:** Insulin is administered using a special insulin syringe. Insulin vials contain 100 units/mL.
- **Dose is prescribed in units.** The prescriber will specify the number of units (**not milliliters or milligrams**) of insulin to administer.

Timing of Administration Insulin may be routinely prescribed (a) in specific dosages at specific times or (b) on a **sliding scale (monotherapy)**, in which the dosage prescribed is based on the patient's blood glucose level. Some advocate against the sliding scale and advocate for the basal plus correctional insulin because it more aligns with the body's physiological insulin secretion process (Ambrus & O'Connor, 2019; Canadian Agency for Drugs and Technologies in Health [CADTH], 2017). **Key Point:** *You should closely adhere to the* prescribed *insulin medication schedule,* follow your agency's policy, *and monitor the patient's blood glucose.*

Categories of Insulin To correctly mix and safely administer insulin, you need to understand the categories of insulin and how they are used to control blood sugar.

- **Basal insulin** is given to cover the body's energy needs without taking the diet into account. Common basal insulins are NPH, insulin glargine (Lantus), and insulin detemir (Levemir).
- **Prandial** (mealtime) and **preprandial insulins,** such as regular insulin (e.g., Humulin R, Novolin R), are given to prevent high blood sugar after eating a meal. However, analogs with a more rapid-acting onset than regular insulin may be prescribed (Slattery et al., 2018). Examples of rapid-acting insulins are Insulin lispro (Humalog), Insulin aspart (NovoLog/NovoRapid), and Insulin glulisine (Apidra).
- **Combination insulins** are manufactured mixtures of a fast-acting and long-lasting insulin. These types of insulin result in fewer injections but require careful monitoring. Although it is less commonly needed because of combination insulins, you can mix two different insulins in the same syringe so that the patient can receive only one injection. For guidelines for mixing insulins,

▶ Go to Chapter 23, **Clinical Insight 23-5: Mixing Two Kinds of Insulin in One Syringe,** in Volume 2.

Insulin Injectors. Insulin can be administered in a variety of ways.

- **Disposable syringes** for subcutaneous injection are the most common.

- **Automatic injectors** are used by some patients for subcutaneous dosing. By pressing a button on the device, the injector releases the needle into the skin, releasing the insulin dose.
- **Insulin pumps** maintain glycemic control because of the benefit of fine-tuning the dosing. The pump consists of a tube with a needle on the end of it that is taped to the abdomen and a computerized device that is worn at the waist. Insulin is received continuously from the pump. A button is pressed at mealtime to release an extra insulin dose.
- **Insulin pen devices** contain a cartridge and disposable needles to deliver certain doses with each injection. They are convenient and may help patients to avoid medication errors. ✚ Incorporating best practices with insulin pens can counter their known risk of cross-contamination and wrong-patient errors in inpatient settings (Haines, 2016; Grissinger, 2017).
- **Nondisposable syringes** (glass syringe and metal needle) may be used repeatedly if they are sterilized after each use.
- **Spray injectors** forcefully spray the insulin dose into the skin. This involves a wider area of skin than would a regular injection.

✚ Always ask patients with diabetes about the type of insulin equipment they use because new products are continuously being developed to facilitate ease of use, achieve better blood glucose control, and incorporate technology (e.g., smartphone, mobile applications). Technology falls into three primary categories: (1) insulin syringes, pens, and pumps; (2) meter or continuous blood glucose monitoring; and (3) hybrid products that combine monitoring and insulin delivery (American Diabetes Association [ADA], 2020). If you are unsure of or unfamiliar with a new device, ask the patient how it operates and look it up.

KnowledgeCheck 23-16

- List three errors in technique that can occur when giving parenteral injections. State their possible consequences.
- Describe at least four ways to minimize the discomfort of an injection.
- Name two reasons for giving an intradermal injection.
- As a rule, what gauge and length of needle would you use for a subcutaneous injection?
- Why should people rotate injection sites when they must have repeated injections over a long time?

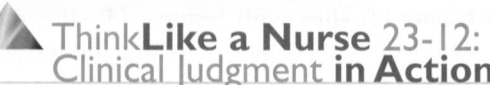

ThinkLike a Nurse 23-12: Clinical Judgment in Action

- What do intradermal and subcutaneous injections have in common?
- How are intradermal and subcutaneous injections different?

Administering Heparin

Heparin is a fast-acting medication that interrupts the blood-clotting process. It may be used for patients at risk for harmful clot formation (e.g., immobility after surgery; cerebrovascular accident [stroke, brain attack]; myocardial infarction [heart attack]).

- **Heparin dosage is based on the patient's weight and results of blood coagulation studies, so always check laboratory values for coagulation studies before giving heparin.**

- **Heparin is administered intravenously or subcutaneously** because it is poorly absorbed from the GI tract. If mistakenly given intramuscularly, it will cause hematoma and pain.
- **Administer the injection deep into the subcutaneous tissue of the abdomen**, at least 5 cm (2 in.) away from the umbilicus, and rotate sites.
- **You will need to modify your injection technique** because of the anticoagulant properties of heparin. For detailed guidelines, refer to Clinical Insight 23-6: Administering Anticoagulant Medication Subcutaneously.

Intramuscular Injections

IM injections (injections into muscle tissue) **are absorbed faster than subcutaneous medications** because of the rich blood supply in the muscles. Large muscles (e.g., vastus lateralis, ventrogluteal) can tolerate 3 to 5 mL of liquid. The smaller the muscle, the less fluid it can tolerate. For example, you should usually give no more than 0.5 to 1 mL in the average-sized deltoid muscle.

When Should You Aspirate Before Injecting Medication The technique of aspiration is used to ensure that the tip of the needle is in the muscle and not in a blood vessel. The literature varies on the advantages and disadvantages of aspiration during an injection. However, you should aspirate when administering medications that would cause harm if accidentally administered intravenously.

- **Key Point:** *You should determine the safety of the drug in deciding whether to aspirate. If the drug has potentially fatal consequences if administered systemically (e.g., immunotherapy), then extra precautions must be taken, including aspiration, to prevent an intravenous injection (Sepah et al., 2017).*
- In addition, you should follow your institution's policies and procedures for IM injections.
- *Aspiration is not recommended for:*
  - **The vastus lateralis and deltoid muscles** because there are no large blood vessels at these sites (CDC, 2022)
  - **Children** because the idea is to give the injection quickly in order to minimize pain (Sepah et al., 2017).

Choosing an Intramuscular Site

When selecting an IM site, you should look for a site that is:

- A safe distance from nerves, large blood vessels, and bones

- Free from injury, abscesses, tenderness, necrosis, abrasion, or other pathology
- Large enough to accommodate the volume of medication to be administered

Muscles commonly used are the vastus lateralis, ventrogluteal, and deltoid.

- **Key Point:** *Because of their proximity to major nerves and vessels, the rectus femoris and dorsogluteal are no longer recommended sites (Arslan & Ozden, 2018).* For a summary description of IM injection sites, refer to the Highlights of Procedures box. For the complete procedure,

Go to **Chapter 23, Procedure 23-13: Locating Intramuscular Injection Sites**, in Volume 2.

Ventrogluteal Muscle—Site of Choice This is the preferred IM site for adults and young children who are able to walk because of the following:

- There are no major vessels or nerves in that area.
- It is a large muscle mass that can tolerate up to 5 mL of medication.
- There tends to be less pain at this site.
- It is less likely to be contaminated when the client is incontinent.

However, some medications (e.g., vaccines) may recommend the deltoid. The ventrogluteal site, located on the lateral hip, involves the gluteus medius and gluteus minimus muscles (Fig. 23-26).

When learning to locate this site, many students notice that it feels "hard" when they palpate it. They worry the needle will hit the bone. In part, the muscle feels hard because there is little subcutaneous tissue over it. To reassure yourself it is safe, examine a skeleton model with the muscles attached. Notice that the ilium is concave (curves in), and the muscle lies deep down in the "cup" it forms. If you are sure you have located the

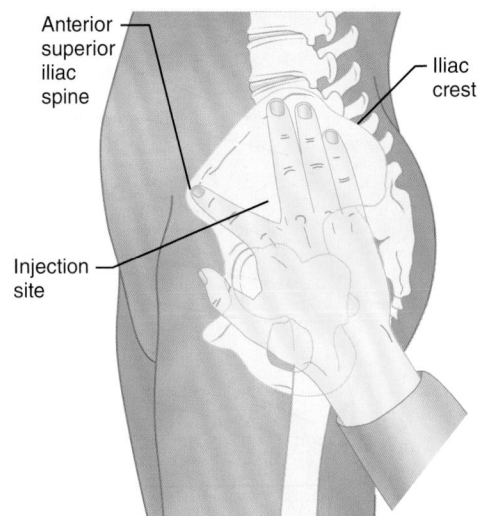

FIGURE 23-26 Locating the ventrogluteal site.

anterosuperior iliac spine and if you follow the procedure steps, you will not hit a bone. In fact, you are less likely to do so than if you use other sites. For guidelines in locating the ventrogluteal site, refer to the Highlights of Procedures box and Procedure 23-13A in Volume 2.

Dorsogluteal Site—Site to Avoid The dorsogluteal site consists of the gluteal muscles of the buttocks. ✚ Avoid using the dorsogluteal site for IM injections because its close proximity to the sciatic nerve and superior gluteal artery increases the risk of (1) injection into a major blood vessel and (2) damage to the sciatic nerve. Furthermore, the site is difficult to identify accurately in older adults and in people with flabby skin.

You may observe some nurses continuing to use the dorsogluteal site because of tradition, ease of use, or lack of knowledge. Your avoidance of the dorsogluteal site gives you the opportunity to role model patient safety by demonstrating correct technique for locating the preferred site.

Deltoid Site The deltoid site is located in the middle third of the upper arm. It is small and lies close to the radial nerve and brachial artery (Fig. 23-27). The area has a small muscle mass with little subcutaneous tissue, so medications are absorbed rapidly. This muscle is easily accessible but is not well developed in many older adults. ✚ You should use the deltoid site only for small amounts of up to 1 mL or when other sites are inaccessible. Avoid using the deltoid site in infants and assess children for adequate muscle mass before use. Some medications (e.g., vaccines, flu shot) may specify the deltoid muscle.

When locating the deltoid, do not merely roll up the sleeve. You must fully expose the entire upper arm and shoulder. Otherwise, you may miss the muscle mass and injure a nerve or blood vessel. For a guide to locating the deltoid site, see the Highlights of Procedures box and Procedure 23-13B in Volume 2.

Vastus Lateralis Site The vastus lateralis muscle, located in the anterolateral thigh (Fig. 23-28), is the preferred site for young infants, particularly before walking age (CDC, 2022). **Advantages of this site are:**

- It is usually the best developed in infants.
- It contains no large nerves or blood vessels, thus minimizing the risk for injury.
- Drugs are rapidly absorbed from this area.
- It can accommodate a larger volume of medication than can the deltoid.
- It is a convenient site for those who self-administer injections.

Disadvantages are:

- The patient can see you administer the injection, and the psychological effect may create some discomfort.
- An ambulatory patient may notice more residual soreness because the muscle is used in walking.

✚ For children and adult patients with small muscle mass, you should grasp ("pinch up") the body of the muscle during injection to be sure that the medication reaches muscle tissue and the needle does not penetrate to the underlying bone (Strohfus et al., 2018). For a guide to locating the vastus lateralis site, refer to the Highlights of Procedures box and Procedure 23-13C in Volume 2.

Rectus Femoris Site—For Adults Only ✚ The rectus femoris site, located in the anterior thigh, is no longer recommended for infants and children. You will use this site for adults only when other sites are inaccessible and the medication needs to be administered intramuscularly. The rectus femoris is often used by patients who self-administer their intramuscular injections because it is easy for them to reach. A disadvantage is that it is usually painful. For a guide to locating the rectus femoris site, refer to the Highlights of Procedure box and Procedure 23-13D in Volume 2.

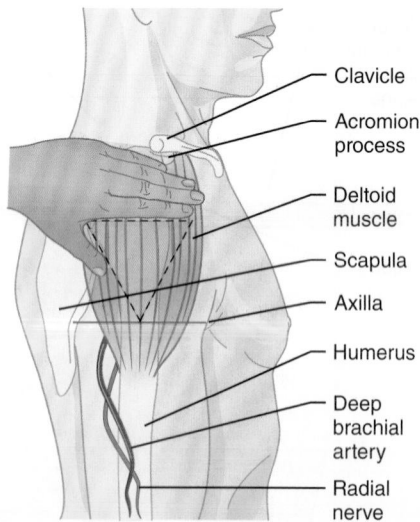

FIGURE 23-27 Locating the deltoid site.

Clavicle
Acromion process
Deltoid muscle
Scapula
Axilla
Humerus
Deep brachial artery
Radial nerve

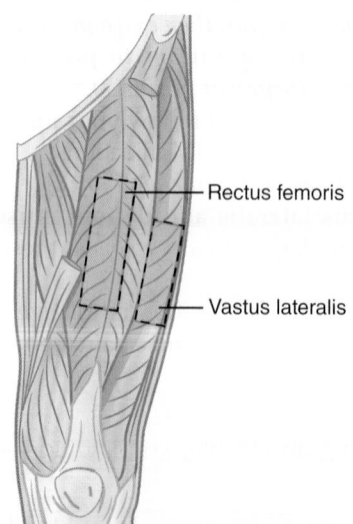

FIGURE 23-28 Locating the vastus lateralis.

Rectus femoris
Vastus lateralis

Choosing an Intramuscular Needle

Although a 1½-inch needle is considered "standard" for IM injections, you should choose the needle gauge and length, as well as the angle of insertion (as a rule, the angle of insertion is 90° [see Fig. 23-24]), based on the following:

- Site
- Size of the muscle
- Amount of medication to be given
- Amount of adipose tissue over the muscle

Consider these examples:

- **In the deltoid muscle,** you might use a 23- or 25-gauge, 1-inch needle. But if the solution is viscous, you would need a larger-bore needle (e.g., 20 gauge).
- **For a very thin person,** you could use a 1-inch needle, even when injecting into the larger muscles.
- **For a person with obesity,** you might need a needle as long as 3 inches to penetrate adipose tissue and reach the muscle (unfortunately, long needles may not be available in some settings). See Table 23-5 for needle length recommendations for immunizations. The Highlights of Procedures box presents the key elements for IM injections. For the complete steps, including the Z-track technique,

 Go to Chapter 23, **Procedure 23-13: Administering an Intramuscular Injection,** in Volume 2.

Z-Track Technique

The Z-track technique seals the needle track and prevents medication from leaking out of the muscle up through the needle track and into the subcutaneous tissues after the needle is withdrawn. The Z-track method is recommended for all IM injections because it is less painful and helps to prevent irritation of subcutaneous tissues. It is also useful for irritating medications (e.g., iron preparations) that irritate or discolor subcutaneous tissue and for older adults who have reduced muscle mass. For this technique, it is best to use the larger muscles: the ventrogluteal and the vastus lateralis.

KnowledgeCheck 23-17

- Name three sites for giving IM injections.
- What is the preferred IM injection site for adults? Why?
- From which route is medication absorbed more rapidly: subcutaneous or IM? Why?

Table 23-5 ➤ Appropriate Needle Size Based on Age and Site for Vaccinations

AGE		NEEDLE LENGTH	SITE
Newborns (first 28 days)		⅝"*	Anterolateral thigh
Infants (1–12 months)		1"	Anterolateral thigh
Toddlers (1–2 years)		1–1¼"	Anterolateral thigh
		⅝–1"*	Deltoid
Children (3–10 years)		⅝–1"*	Deltoid
		1–1¼"	Anterolateral thigh
Children and Teens (11–18 years)		⅝–1"*	Deltoid
		1–1½	Anterolateral thigh
Adults (19 years and older)			
Male or Female	Less than 130 lb	⅝–1*"	Deltoid
Male or Female	130–152 lb	1"	Deltoid
Male	152–260 lb	1–1½"	Deltoid
Female	152–200 lb	1–1½"	Deltoid
Male	260+ lb	1½"	Deltoid
Female	200+ lb	1½"	Deltoid

*A ⅝" needle may be used with the skin stretched tight and injection given at a 90° angle.
Source: Adapted from Centers for Disease Control and Prevention. (2022). *Vaccine administration.* https://www.cdc.gov/vaccines/hcp/acip-recs/general-recs/administration.html#t6_2

- For an "average" adult, what is the standard needle length for IM injections?
- Why is the dorsogluteal site *not* recommended?
- What are the disadvantages of the deltoid site?
- When using the vastus lateralis to give an IM medication to a person with small muscle mass, how can you ensure the medication reaches muscle tissue and the needle does not penetrate to the underlying bone?

Intravenous Medications

IV medications are given through a catheter, or cannula, inserted into a vein. The onset of medication action takes place within seconds, so IV administration is especially useful in emergencies. Without a known antidote, there is no way for you to stop its action if an adverse reaction occurs. Review Table 23-1 for advantages and disadvantages of using the IV route. The following sections explain various methods for administering IV medications. See Chapter 35 for procedures for initiating and maintaining IV fluids.

IV Push Medications

IV push (bolus) medications are injected directly into a vein and enter the systemic circulation immediately. **Key Point:** *Many IV push medications are irritating to vein walls and can cause damage (sloughing, pain, abscesses) if accidentally injected into the tissues (Fig. 23-29).* To prevent these complications, you should:

- Assess the patient before, during, and after giving the medication.
- Determine the compatibility of the drug with the IV fluid that is infusing and the plastic IV bag and tubing. Consult a pharmacist as needed.
- Use sterile technique.
- Administer the medication slowly.
- Observe the patient carefully for signs of adverse reactions.

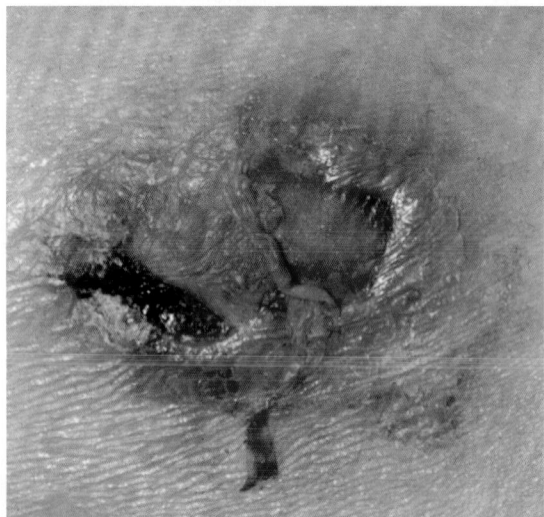

FIGURE 23-29 Tissue and skin injury after IV medication leaks into an infiltrated site.

- Have an antidote on hand if the drug has potentially serious side effects. Be aware, though, that many drugs do not have an antidote.
- If your patient shows signs of a serious allergic reaction, you will need to prepare to support the patient's airway, deliver oxygen, and administer medication to reduce the reaction.

How Fast Can I Push a Drug? Read the package insert or consult with the pharmacist or prescriber for specific guidelines on how fast the drug can be pushed (usually incrementally over 1 to 3 minutes, or longer). One minute can seem like a very long time when you are pushing a medication, so don't guess—look at your watch! "IV push" does not mean the same thing as "give rapidly." If given too rapidly, IV drugs—particularly potassium—can be quite dangerous. Because you cannot retrieve the medication once it is injected, there is no margin for error. Safety is essential.

To learn how to administer IV push drugs, refer to the Highlights of Procedures box, and

Go to **Chapter 23, Procedure 23-16: Administering IV Push Medications**, in Volume 2.

Adding Medications to IV Bags

One way to administer a drug intravenously is to mix it into a bag of IV fluid and administer it through a port on the primary IV line. Although the drug is usually premixed with the fluid in the pharmacy, in some facilities, the nurse may need to add the drug to a small IV bag of fluid.

Use and Advantage: This method is useful when the drug can be infused continuously to achieve the desired effect. Vitamins, potassium chloride, oxytocin, and several blood pressure and cardiovascular drugs are commonly administered this way.

Disadvantage: The main disadvantage is the danger of infusing too much fluid, especially for children, older adults, and people with cardiac or renal disease.

- **Adding medications from multidose vials**—One safe method for adding medication to IV fluids when using multidose vials, while providing sterile air filtration, is to use a reconstitution device. A reconstitution device is designed with a sharp, thin, piercing spike to minimize coring and permit easy penetration of the rubber top of a vial (Fig. 23-30). The luer-lock port maintains a secure closure between the device and the syringe. The hinged cap and the sheath over the spike help maintain sterility before use, minimize "touch" contamination, and ensure a closed system for disposal.
- **Using a transfer needle**—Another safe method for adding medications to an IV container is to use a **transfer needle** or **cannula**—a blunted plastic needle with a double-beveled tip (Fig. 23-31). One end is inserted into the powdered or liquid medication, and the other end is inserted into a port of the IV bag. Solution is transferred from the IV bag into the medication vial, which you shake lightly to mix the medication. Then the medication is transferred back into the IV bag for administration.

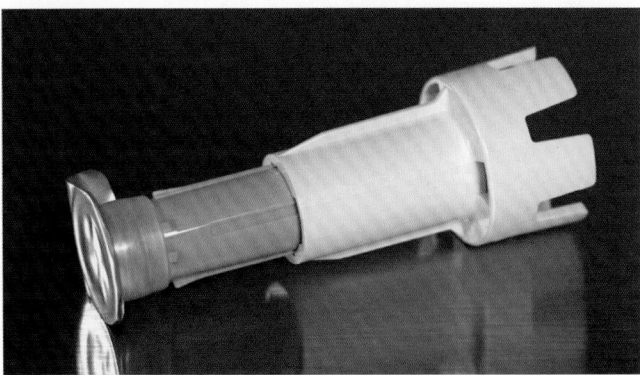

FIGURE 23-30 A reconstitution device is used to add medication from multidose IV vials while providing sterile air filtration.

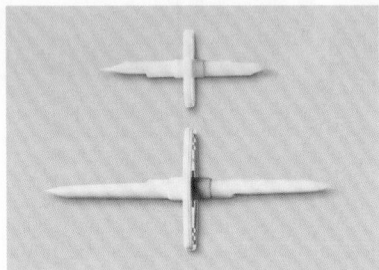

FIGURE 23-31 Transfer needles.

Refer to the Highlights of Procedures box. Also,

 Go to Chapter 23, **Procedure 23-15: Adding Medication to IV Fluid**, in Volume 2.

Intermittent Infusion

Many medications, such as antibiotics, are administered intravenously by intermittent infusion. Intermittent infusions may be given (1) through the port of an infusing IV line or, (2) if the patient does not need the IV fluids, through an intermittent injection port, also called a *saline* or *heparin lock* (Fig. 23-32).

Infusion Setup. Most intermittent infusion medications are supplied in bags containing 50 to 250 mL of 5%

dextrose in water (D_5W) or normal saline (0.9% NaCl). The drug is given over a period of time, usually 30 to 60 minutes, and at regular intervals (e.g., every 6 hours). The small bag of diluted medication (the "secondary" bag) is attached to the primary IV infusion line for administration, usually with a **piggyback setup** (Fig. 23-33). The smaller (secondary) container is connected to the primary (continuous) infusion line at the upper primary port. This setup allows for intermittent use only and the infusion of one solution at a time (see Procedures 23-17A and B).

Needleless Connections. Traditionally, the secondary tubing was attached to the primary set tubing by inserting a needle into the port and taping it in place. However, most agencies now use needleless systems (see Fig. 23-21), which use a threaded or lever-type lock to make the connection. A needleless system:

- Decreases needlestick injuries
- Prevents contact contamination at the IV connection site

You can help prevent catheter-related bloodstream infections by scrubbing the needleless IV connector for 15 seconds. Remember: "Scrub the Hub." When the secondary tubing is no longer needed, a disinfection cap containing either alcohol or chlorhexidine/alcohol solution is placed over the port (Fig. 23-34).

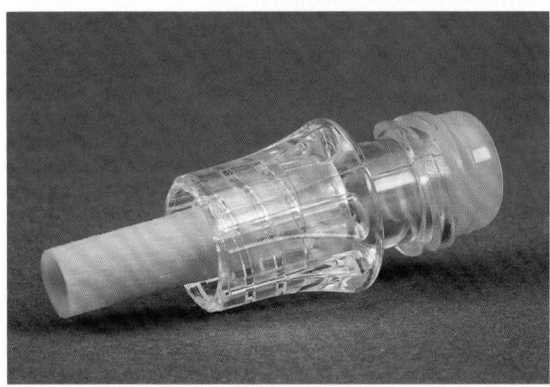

FIGURE 23-32 Intermittent injection port.

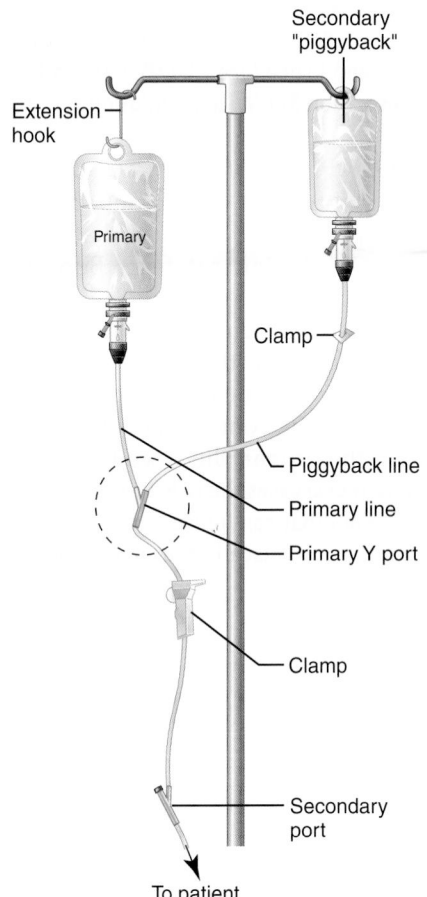

FIGURE 23-33 Piggyback setup is attached to the primary (continuous infusion) IV line at the upper port, allowing for intermittent infusion only.

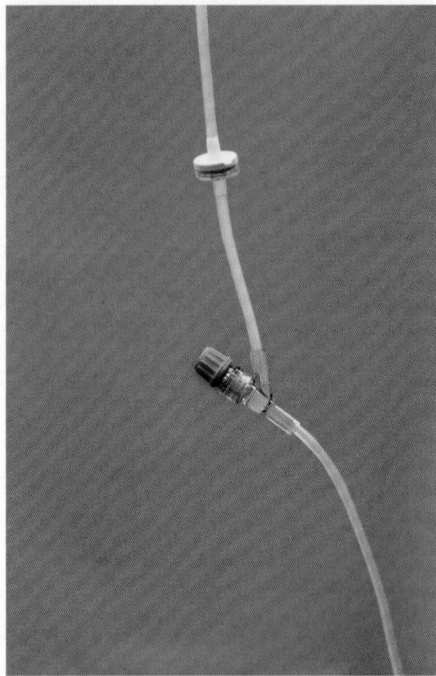

FIGURE 23-34 Disinfection cap for luer-lock needleless hubs.

The Highlights of Procedures box provides guidelines for administering intermittent infusions. Also,

 Go to **Chapter 23, Procedure 23-17A: Using a Piggyback Administration Set With a Gravity Infusion, and Procedure 23-17B: Using a Piggyback Administration Set With an Infusion Pump,** in Volume 2.

Volume-Control Infusion Sets

To effectively control the infusion of smaller amounts of solutions, particularly with pediatric patients, a **volume-control infusion set** (e.g., Buretrol, Soluset, Volutrol, or Pediatrol) may be used (Fig. 23-35). These are small fluid containers (100 to 150 mL) that are attached directly below the primary fluid container. The medication and the desired amount of IV fluid are added to the volume-control container and administered through the primary line (see Procedure 23-17C). This system decreases the risk of overhydration because the amount of fluid that can infuse into the patient is limited to the amount that you place in the small container.

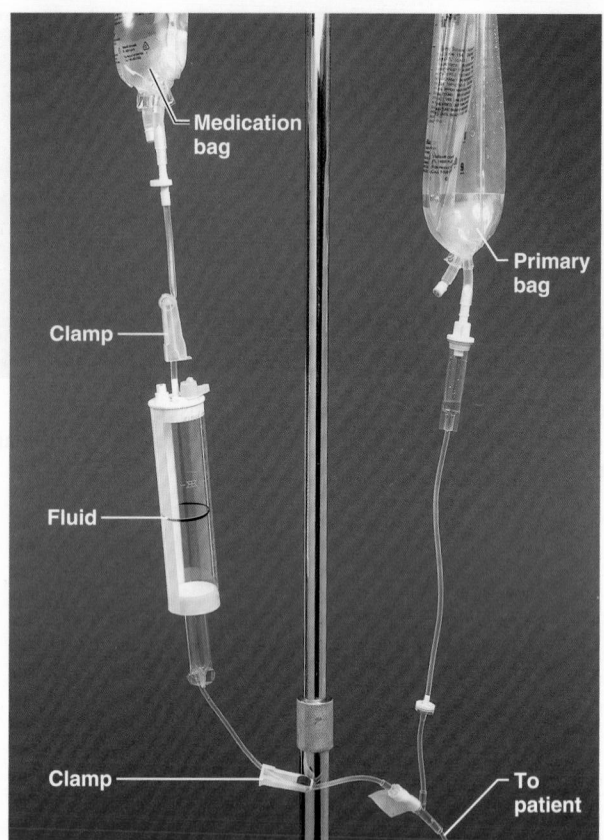

FIGURE 23-35 Volume-control infusion set for intermittent infusion administration; used when the fluid volume is critical and must be carefully monitored.

The Highlights of Procedures box provides guidelines for using volume-controlled infusion sets. Also,

 Go to **Chapter 23, Procedure 23-17C: Using a Volume-Controlled Infusion Set,** in Volume 2.

Central Venous Access Devices

IV medication can be delivered through a central or peripheral vein. The most common reasons for a patient to have a central venous access device (CVAD) are to:

- Give long-term IV therapy
- Provide total parenteral nutrition (TPN) when the patient cannot eat normally

- Have blood drawn without the trauma and complications of repeated venipunctures
- Provide vascular access when peripheral IV placement is difficult

External CVADs can be either tunneled or nontunneled.

- **Tunneled devices** are surgically implanted peripherally and tunneled to a central vein, typically the superior vena cava.
- **Nontunneled catheters** are inserted near the destination site. This category includes **peripherally inserted central catheters (PICCs)**, which are inserted into the central circulation via a peripheral vein and can remain in place for months. For short-term use, the nontunneled central catheter can be inserted into the jugular, subclavian, or femoral veins.

An internal, or implantable, port The internal or implantable port is a CVAD that can remain in place and be functional for years. Access is gained through the skin via a hollow port with a self-sealing silicone cap. These devices are inserted when long-term IV medication is needed or the medication is too irritating for a peripheral site (see Procedure 23-18). See Figure 23-36A for an example of a port for injecting medication into the subclavian vein.

Catheter Lumens Catheter lumens for central venous delivery can be single-lumen or multilumen devices (Fig. 23-36B). Although they are more convenient for administering different medications and fluids, some types of multilumen catheters have a higher infection rate than single-lumen catheters.

To learn how to administer medications through a CVAD, see the summary in the Highlights of Procedures box. Also,

 Go to **Chapter 23, Procedure 23-18: Administering Medication Through a Central Venous access Device,** in Volume 2.

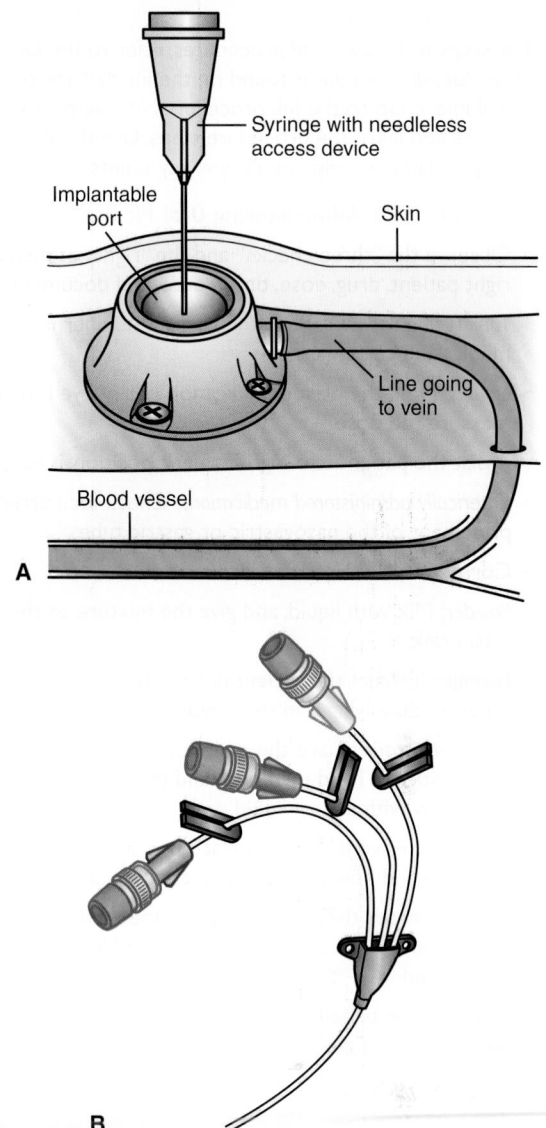

FIGURE 23-36 Central vascular access device: A, Implantable device. B, Multilumen catheter with blunt cannula, split-septum, needleless access device.

For steps to follow in *all* procedures, refer to the Universal Steps for All Procedures found on the inside back cover of Volume 2. Go to the full procedures in Volume 2 to practice and learn the procedure steps. Use these procedure highlights later to help you review key points.

Procedure 23-1: Administering Oral Medication

➤ Observe the "three checks" and the "rights of medication": right patient, drug, dose, time, route, and documentation.
➤ *Tablets and capsules:* Pour the correct number into the medication cup.
➤ *Liquids:* Hold the plastic medication cup at eye level to measure the dose.
➤ Assist the patient to a high-Fowler's position, if possible.
➤ *Enterically administered medications:* Check for correct placement of the nasogastric or gastric tube.
➤ Correctly administer the medication.
  Powder: Mix with liquid, and give the mixture to the patient to drink.
  Lozenge: Instruct the patient not to chew or swallow it before dissolving it in the mouth.
  Tablet or capsule: Place the tablet or medication cup in the patient's hand or mouth and instruct the patient to swallow with sips of liquid.
  Sublingual: Have the patient place the tablet under the tongue and hold it there until it is completely dissolved.
  Buccal: Instruct the patient to place the tablet between the cheek and gums and hold it there until it is completely dissolved.
➤ Stay with the patient until medications have been swallowed or dissolved.

Procedure 23-2: Administering Ophthalmic Medication

For instillations

➤ Use a high-Fowler's position, with the head slightly tilted back.
➤ Work from the inner to outer canthus when cleansing or instilling medication.
➤ Apply the medication into the conjunctival sac.
➤ Do not apply the medication to the cornea.
➤ Do not let the dropper or tube touch the eye.
➤ For eye drops, press gently against the same side of the nose for 1 to 2 minutes to close the lacrimal ducts. For an eye ointment, ask the patient to gently close their eyes for 2 to 3 minutes.

For irrigations

➤ Use a low-Fowler's position, with head tilted toward the affected eye, if possible.
➤ Check the pH in the conjunctival sac, if indicated.
➤ Use a Morgan lens or IV tubing to irrigate the eyes.
➤ For direct-flow irrigation, irrigate from the inner canthus to the outer canthus.
➤ Irrigate for 20 minutes or until the desired pH is reached.

Procedure 23-3: Administering Otic Medication

➤ Warm the solution to be instilled to body temperature.
➤ Assist the patient to a side-lying position, with the appropriate ear facing up.
➤ Straighten the ear canal. For an adult patient, pull the pinna up and back; for a child younger than 3 years, pull it down and back.
➤ Instill the prescribed number of drops into the ear canal.
➤ Do not force the solution into the ear or occlude the ear canal with the dropper.
➤ Instruct the patient to remain on their side for 5 to 10 minutes.

Procedure 23-4: Administering Nasal Medication

➤ Determine head position based on the sinuses targeted for the medication and the patient's ability to assume the position.
➤ Explain to the patient that the medication may cause some burning, tingling, or unusual taste.
➤ Have the patient gently blow their nose and wash their hands afterward.
➤ **For nasal sprays,** position the patient with the head down and forward. Remember: "To spray your nose, look at your toes."
➤ **For drops,** assist the patient to a supine position with the head back.
➤ Place the tip of the sprayer into the right nostril, pointing the tip toward the outside of the nose (toward the outside corner of the right eye). Never point the tip toward the middle of the nose (the septum) or straight up (toward the sinus).
➤ Squirt the spray into the nose while the patient inhales.
➤ Have the patient breathe out through the mouth.
➤ Repeat for the other nostril.
➤ If the patient tastes the medicine, the head was not down or they did not inhale long enough. Advise them to put their head down again and sniff again without the medicine.
➤ If nose drops are used, ask the patient to stay in the same position for 1 to 5 minutes (depending on manufacturer's guidelines).

Procedure 23-5: Administering Vaginal Medication

For instillation

➤ Position the patient in a dorsal recumbent or Sims' position.
➤ Inspect and cleanse the vaginal area before administering the medication.
➤ Use a water-soluble lubricant.
➤ Insert the suppository or applicator along the posterior vaginal wall about 8 cm (3 in.).
➤ Instruct the patient to maintain the position for 5 to 15 minutes after the medication is inserted.

Highlights of Procedures 19-1 through 19-20

For irrigation (douche)

➤ Warm the irrigation solution to approximately 105°F (40.6°C).

➤ Hang the irrigation solution approximately 30 to 60 cm (1 to 2 ft) above the level of the patient's vagina.

➤ Position the patient in a dorsal recumbent position on a waterproof pad and bedpan.

➤ Lubricate the end of the irrigation nozzle.

➤ Insert the nozzle approximately 8 cm (3 in.) into the vagina, and start the flow of irrigation solution.

Procedure 23-6: Inserting a Rectal Suppository

➤ Before inserting the suppository, assess for contraindications, such as rectal surgery, rectal bleeding, or cardiac disease.

➤ Position the patient in the Sims' position.

➤ Don gloves.

➤ Lubricate the suppository with a water-soluble lubricant.

➤ Insert the suppository past the internal sphincter about ½ to 1 inch in infants and 1 to 3 inches in adults. Never force the suppository during insertion.

➤ Instruct the patient to stay on their side for at least 10 minutes and retain (not expel) the suppository for about 15 to 20 minutes or longer

Procedure 23-7: Applying Medication to the Skin

➤ Wear gloves to avoid absorbing the medication through your own skin and to avoid cross-contamination.

➤ Before applying topical medication, cleanse the skin with soap and water.

➤ Do not apply medication to skin with open lesions, irritation, or known hypersensitivity.

➤ Use gentle technique when applying topical medication to fragile skin, which is typical in older adults.

➤ Take care not to overapply the medication.

➤ (Assess for adverse skin reactions (e.g., hypersensitivity, redness, itching, or local irritation).

➤ For transdermal patches, wear gloves when applying and removing; dispose of the patch in an appropriate receptacle, away from children and pets.

Procedure 23-8: Administering Metered-Dose Inhaler (MDI) Medication

➤ Identify the number of remaining inhalations in the canister. The "float method" is no longer recommended.

➤ Assist the patient to a seated or high-Fowler's position. Shake the inhaler. Remove the mouthpiece cap of the inhaler and insert the mouthpiece into the spacer while holding the canister upright.

➤ Remove the cap from the spacer.

➤ Ask the patient to breathe out slowly and completely.

➤ If a patient is unable to use the MDI independently, time the use of the device with the patient's own respirations.

➤ Place the spacer's mouthpiece into the patient's mouth and ask them to seal their lips around the mouthpiece. Press down on the inhaler canister to discharge one puff of medication into the spacer.

➤ Ask the patient to inhale slowly and then hold their breath for as long as possible.

➤ If a second puff is needed, wait at least 1 minute and repeat.

Procedure 23-9: Preparing, Drawing Up, and Mixing Medication

➤ Maintain sterile technique.

➤ Recap the needle or vial access device (VAD) using a needle safety device or the one-handed method.

➤ Change the needle, if indicated.

Procedure 23-9A: Drawing Up Medication From Ampules

➤ Tap the ampule to remove medication trapped in the top of the ampule or shake it with a quick snap of the wrist.

➤ Use an ampule opener to break the ampule neck. Alternatively, with a 2-by-2 gauze pad or an unopened alcohol swab around the neck of the ampule, snap the ampule away from you.

➤ Use a filter needle or filter straw to withdraw the medication.

➤ Withdraw all the medication from the ampule by inverting or tipping the ampule.

➤ Remove the filter needle and replace it with an appropriate-size needle.

➤ Dispose of the broken ampule and filter needle in a sharps container.

Procedure 23-9B: Drawing Up Medication From Vials

➤ Scrub the rubber top of the vial with an alcohol prep pad or a chlorhexidine gluconate (CHG)–alcohol product.

➤ Draw air into the syringe equal to the amount of medication to be withdrawn.

➤ When inserting the needle or VAD through the rubber top of the vial, insert at a 45° to 60° angle, bevel up. Puncture the rubber top at that angle and raise to 90° as you insert the needle.

➤ Keeping the needle above the fluid line, inject air into the vial before inverting the vial and withdrawing the medication.

➤ Remove bubbles from the syringe, hold the vial at eye level, and check that the dose is correct before removing the needle.

Procedures 23-9C, D, and E: Mixing Medication From Two Vials, Mixing Medication From One Ampule and One Vial, and Using a Prefilled Cartridge and Single-Dose Vial—For Intravenous Administration

➤ Make sure the medications are compatible.

➤ Before beginning, determine the total volume of all medications to be put in the syringe and whether that volume is appropriate for the administration site.

Continued

➤ Maintain the sterility of the needles and medication.

➤ Avoid contaminating a multidose vial with a second medication.

➤ Carefully expel air bubbles.

➤ Withdraw the second medication very carefully because the medications are mixed as you pull back the plunger; therefore, you must withdraw the *exact* amount. If there is any excess, you must discard the contents of the syringe and start over.

➤ When opening ampules, protect yourself from injury.

➤ Use a filter needle or straw to withdraw medication from ampules; change to a needle of the proper length and gauge for administering the medication.

➤ When drawing up from a single-dose vial and ampule, draw up from the vial first.

➤ Do not use prefilled cartridges unless they have a safety needle; transfer the medication to a syringe with a safety device before administering.

➤ Always recap a sterile needle using a safety capping process or the one-handed scoop method.

Procedure 23-10: Recapping Needles Using One-Handed Technique

Procedure 23-10A: Recapping Contaminated Needles

➤ Recap a contaminated needle **only if you cannot avoid it.**

➤ Do not place your nondominant hand near the needle cap when recapping the needle or engaging the safety mechanism.

➤ If you are using a safety needle, engage the safety mechanism to cover the needle.

➤ Place the needle cap in a mechanical recapping device if one is available.

➤ If recapping devices are not available and you must recap the needle for your own and/or the patient's safety, use the one-handed scoop technique or one of the methods in Procedure 23-10B.

Procedure 23-10B: Recapping Sterile Needles

➤ Be sure to keep the needle and cap sterile.

➤ Do not place your nondominant hand near the needle cap when recapping the needle or engaging the safety mechanism.

➤ Use one of the following methods:

  ➤ Place the needle cap in a medication cup, and insert the needle into the cap.

  ➤ Place the cap on a clean surface so that the end of the needle cap protrudes over the edge of the counter or shelf, and scoop with the needle.

  ➤ Use a hard syringe cover: Stand it on end; insert the needle cap into the cover, and then insert the needle.

  ➤ Place the needle cap on a sterile surface, such as on open alcohol prep pad, and use the one-handed scoop technique. This is the least desirable method.

Procedure 23-11: Administering Intradermal Medication

➤ Have appropriate antidotes for certain injections readily available before beginning the procedure.

➤ Know the location of resuscitation equipment in case of a life-threatening adverse reaction.

➤ Maintain sterile technique and standard precautions.

➤ Use a 1-mL syringe and a 25- to 28-gauge, ¼- to ⅝-inch needle with a short bevel.

➤ Be aware that an intradermal dose is small, usually about 0.01 to 0.1 mL.

➤ Administer the injection on the ventral surface of the forearm, upper back, or upper chest.

➤ Hold the syringe parallel to the skin at a 5° to 15° angle, with the bevel up.

➤ Stretch the skin taut to insert the needle.

➤ Do not aspirate.

➤ Inject slowly, and create a wheal (bleb).

➤ Do not wipe the site with alcohol, massage the site, or bandage the site.

Procedure 23-12: Administering Subcutaneous Medication (Non-Insulin)

➤ Maintain sterile technique and standard precautions.

➤ Use a 1-mL syringe and a 25- to 27-gauge needle that is less than 1 inch long (usually ⅜ to ⅝ in.).

➤ A subcutaneous dose is typically no more than 1 mL.

➤ Most common injection sites: Use the outer aspects of the upper arms, abdomen (at least 2 inches from the umbilicus), anterior aspects of the thighs, and high on the buttocks near the waist.

➤ Pinch the skin to inject, as a general rule.

➤ For an average-weight or thin patient, pinch up the skin and inject at a 45° angle. Inject at a 90° angle if the adipose tissue pinches 2 inches or more, as a general rule. Use a longer needle and spread the skin taut instead of pinching.

➤ Do not aspirate.

➤ Do not massage the site.

Procedure 23-13: Locating Intramuscular Injection Sites

➤ Always palpate the landmarks and the muscle mass to ensure correct placement.

Procedure 23-13A: Locating the Ventrogluteal Site

➤ On adults, a triangle is formed between your fingers when you place your palm on the head of the trochanter, index finger on the anterior superior iliac spine, and middle finger pointing toward or on the iliac crest. This is the preferred site for adults and children older than 7 to 12 months.

Procedure 23-13B: Locating the Deltoid Site

➤ The injection site is an inverted triangle on the upper arm. The base is the lower edge of the acromion process, and the tip is even with the top of the axilla. In healthy adults, this is a good site for small-volume injections, especially when other sites aren't easily accessible because of drains or dressings.

Procedure 23-13C: Locating the Vastus Lateralis Site

➤ Midlateral thigh: On adults, one handbreadth below the head of the trochanter and one handbreadth above the knee. The site is the middle third of this area. This is the preferred site for infants who are not walking.

Procedure 23-13D: Locating the Rectus Femoris Site

➤ Middle third of the anterior thigh: Use this site only if no others are accessible. It is more painful than other sites.

Procedure 23-14: Administering an Intramuscular Injection

➤ Maintain sterile technique and standard precautions.

➤ Use a 1- to 5-mL syringe and a 21- to 25-gauge, 1-inch needle for deltoid site; 1 ½-inch needle for adults; 3-inch needle if the patient is obese.

➤ The usual volume is no more than 3 mL per injection. If the volume for injection is more than 3 to 5 mL, divide the dose into separate injections. Note that up to 5 mL can be administered in a large, well-developed muscle.

➤ Select an appropriate injection site, and identify the site using anatomical landmarks:

  ➤ The ventrogluteal site is preferred except in special circumstances (e.g., for many adult immunizations).

  ➤ The deltoid site is acceptable for IM doses of 1 mL or less.

➤ Insert the needle at a 90° angle.

➤ Follow agency procedure regarding aspiration. If appropriate, aspirate before injecting. If blood appears, withdraw the needle, discard it, and start over.

➤ Press the plunger slowly to inject the medication (5 to 10 sec/mL).

➤ Z-track technique is recommended. Mnemonic:

Deliver	**D**isplace
All	**A**spirate (if required by agency's policy)
Injections	**I**nject (wait 5–10 seconds)
With	**W**ithdraw
Responsibility	**R**elease

Procedure 23-15: Adding Medications to IV Fluid

➤ Check the compatibility of the IV solution and medication.

➤ Assess the patency of the IV site.

➤ Maintain the sterility of IV fluids and medication admixture.

➤ Affix the medication label to the bag, with the name and amount of medication, date and time administered, and your name or initials.

Procedure 23-16: Administering IV Push Medication

➤ Determine the type and amount of dilution needed for the medication.

➤ Determine how fast the medication may be administered.

➤ Ensure the patency of the line before administration.

➤ Flush the line before and after administering the medication with the flush solution.

➤ Maintain sterility.

Procedure 23-17: Administering Medications by Intermittent Infusion

➤ Ensure the compatibility of the IV solution and medication—both the solution in the primary IV system and in the secondary system.

➤ Assess the IV site and the patency of the line.

➤ Determine the type and amount of IV solution needed to administer the medication

➤ Calculate the amount of medication to add to the solution.

➤ Use the correct rate of administration and the period of time over which the solution should be infused.

➤ Determine the correct primary line port in which to infuse the medication.

➤ Affix the correct label to the secondary bag identifying the infusate, patient name, start date and hour, discard date and hour, and your initials.

Procedure 23-18: Administering Medication Through a Central Venous Access Device

➤ First verify that the medication can safely be administered through a central site.

➤ Check the compatibility of the medication with the existing IV infusion.

➤ Draw up the medication using a needleless device or needle with a filter. Then change to a sterile safety needle or needleless device for administering the medication.

➤ Scrub all surfaces of the catheter port, including the extension "tail," using an alcohol or CHG-alcohol combination product every time you enter the line.

➤ Flush the line before and after administering medication. Use saline or heparinized flush solution, according to agency policy.

➤ For multilumen catheters, flush all lumens.

➤ Clamp the line between the IV infusion set and the medication port. Open the clamp after medication is administered.

To explore learning resources for this chapter,

Go to Davis Advantage and find:

Answers and Suggested Responses for all questions in this chapter

Concept Map

Knowledge Map

References and Bibliography

Supporting Physiological Function

CHAPTER 24

Nutrition

Learning Outcomes

After completing this chapter, you should be able to:

➤ Identify the types, functions, metabolism, and major food sources of (1) energy nutrients, (2) vitamins, (3) minerals, and (4) water.

➤ Differentiate among the various sources of nutritional information (e.g., U.S. Department of Agriculture [USDA] dietary guidelines, ChooseMyPlate, Dietary Reference Intakes [DRIs], Nutrition Facts labels).

➤ Identify the primary nutritional considerations for various developmental stages.

➤ Discuss how the following factors impact nutritional health: age, lifestyle, body mass, diabetes and other health conditions, immobility and functional limitations, pregnancy, diet, and culture.

➤ Describe tools and techniques for gathering subjective data about nutritional status.

➤ Perform various anthropometric measurements.

➤ Calculate a client's basal metabolic rate.

➤ Calculate the body mass index for a client and explain its significance.

➤ List at least five physical assessment findings that indicate nutritional imbalance.

➤ Identify laboratory values that are indicators of nutritional status.

➤ Discuss the need for and advisability of vitamin and mineral supplementation.

➤ Describe nursing interventions for patients with special nutritional needs: impaired swallowing, NPO, older adults, and nausea.

➤ Identify and discuss at least six nursing interventions for each of the following diagnoses:
Imbalanced Nutrition: Less Than Body Requirements
Obesity
Overweight

➤ Safely provide enteral and parenteral nutrition for patients.

Key Concepts

Energy
Metabolism
Nutrition

Related Concepts

See the Concept Map on Davis Advantage.

Example Client Conditions

Overweight and Obesity
Underweight and Malnourished

Meet Your Patients

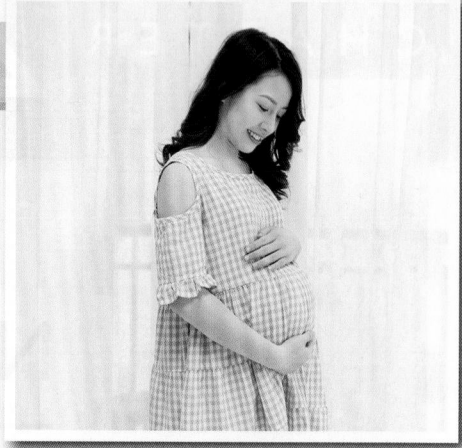

As part of a class assignment, you are to assist a local business with its wellness program. You will complete health risk appraisals and gather the following data on the employees: height, weight, medical and nutritional history, and lifestyle practices. Today you will screen two employees, and then each will have blood drawn for a complete blood count (CBC), comprehensive metabolic panel, and lipid panel:

- **Isaac Schwartz,** a 65-year-old accountant, works long hours. He describes a sedentary lifestyle, no tobacco use, infrequent alcohol use, no medical problems, and a nutritional history of skipping meals and daily consumption of restaurant food. You measure his height as 69 in. and weight as 245 lb.
- **Sujing Lee,** a 29-year-old project manager, regularly works 65 hours per week. Sujing is 30 weeks pregnant. She does not smoke or drink and has never been hospitalized or had surgery. She has gained a total of 25 lb since becoming pregnant. Her diet consists mainly of traditional Asian food. She eats three meals a day and always brings lunch from home. Lately she has felt "tired all the time." At the screening, she weighs 126 lb and measures 63 in. tall.

At the end of your clinical day, you need to compile a report on the clients you have seen. How would you interpret the data on height, weight, and nutrition? What, if any, additional information do you need to help you evaluate their nutritional status? In this chapter, you will read about dietary recommendations, energy balance, and nutritional concerns across the life span. You will gain the theoretical knowledge to answer these questions, as well as practical knowledge about managing nutritional problems.

TheoreticalKnowledge
knowing why

Organic, natural, gluten-free, non-GMO, dairy-free … these are just a few of the numerous labels on packaged foods. With so many options and different recommendations about what's healthy or not, it's no wonder that many people are confused about what to eat.

ABOUT THE KEY CONCEPTS

Nutrition is the study of food: how it affects the human body and influences health. **Metabolism** is the process by which the body converts food into energy. Good nutrition is essential to wellness, and poor nutrition contributes to disease; that is why clients need accurate, current, and appropriate nutritional information. Before you can give effective individualized advice, you need to know about the nutrients found in foods. In this chapter, you will learn about concepts related to energy—for example, **energy** balance, macronutrients, micronutrients, and factors that influence nutritional status.

WHAT ARE SOME RELIABLE SOURCES OF NUTRITION INFORMATION?

Standards and guides provide credible nutrition information.

- **Standards** are a reference for nutrient intake thought to meet the nutritional needs of most healthy population groups. They list nutrient amounts in measurements, such as grams and milligrams, and are not intended to indicate individual requirements or therapeutic needs.
- **Food guides** are more practical tools that you can use to educate patients and families. They specify the number of daily servings of foods needed so that nonprofessionals can use them in making healthful meal choices.
- **Key Point:** *In general, standards and guides provide recommendations for healthy individuals; they are not specific to the needs of people with metabolic or other medical problems.*

Dietary Reference Intakes

The Food and Nutrition Board of the National Academies of Sciences, Engineering, and Medicine (2011) established nutrition standards to promote the consumption of micronutrients (vitamins, minerals, and trace elements) and macronutrients (carbohydrates, proteins, fats) and other substances (fiber) to prevent deficiencies and lower the risk of chronic disease. The Dietary Reference Intakes (DRIs) are used for planning and assessing diets for healthy individuals.

The DRIs encompass four types of nutrient reference values for males and females in different age-groups:

- **Estimated Average Requirement (EAR)**—the amount of a nutrient that is estimated to meet the requirements of half of all healthy individuals within a given age and gender group.

- **Recommended Dietary Allowance (RDA)**—the average daily dietary intake of a nutrient that is sufficient to meet the nutritional requirements of approximately 98% of healthy people.
- **Adequate Intake (AI)**—the amount of a nutrient consumed by a group of healthy people.
- **Tolerable Upper Intake Level (UL)**—the maximum daily intake of a nutrient that is likely to be without adverse health effects for almost all individuals.
- **Acceptable Macronutrient Distribution Range (AMDR)**—the percentage of protein, fat, and carbohydrate associated with reduced risk of chronic disease, provided there is an intake of other essential nutrients. (U.S. Department of Agriculture [USDA], 2002–2005; U.S. Department of Health and Human Services [USDHHS], 2020).

USDA Dietary Guidelines

The USDA developed the *Dietary Guidelines for Americans 2020–2025* to help people improve their nutritional habits. The guidelines do not specify daily amounts of food and nutrients (Box 24-1).

These USDA dietary guidelines are intended as a primary source of health information for nutrition educators, policy makers, and healthcare providers. They are based on scientific evidence and provide information about choosing a nutritious diet, maintaining a healthy weight, achieving adequate exercise, and food safety. The dietary guidelines are updated every 5 years.

MyPlate

MyPlate (Fig. 24-1) is a food guide that visually illustrates a healthy meal—red for fruits, green for vegetables, orange for grains, and purple for protein, as well as a separate blue section for dairy on the side. The MyPlate Web site promotes healthy nutrition based on the USDA *Dietary Guidelines for Americans 2020–2025* and provides guidance on food choices and variety, portion size, and activity, as well as tools for a healthy, nutritional lifestyle.

Adapted Versions of MyPlate

- **MyPlate in Spanish.** The Spanish version is available on the ChooseMyPlate Web site.
- **MyPlate for Older Adults.** This visual food guide illustrates healthy food choices and portions specific to the nutrition and hydration needs of older adults.

It is consistent with the *Dietary Guidelines for Americans 2020–2025*. Both recommend limiting foods high in *trans*- and saturated fats, salt, and added sugars and emphasize the intake of whole grains, foods enriched with vitamin B_{12}, and calcium-rich foods and beverages (USDA, 2020). It also stresses the importance of fluids and promotes physical activity (at least 150 minutes/week) (USDHHS, 2018, p. 68).

Other Food Guides

- **Traditional Asian, Latin American, Mediterranean, and African heritage and vegetarian/vegan diets.**

BOX 24-1 ■ *Dietary Guidelines for Americans 2020–2025:* Key Points

Healthy nutrition and an active lifestyle help to maintain recommended body weight and reduce the risk of chronic disease. The U.S. Department of Agriculture and U.S. Department of Health and Human Services (2020) recommend the following:

Adopt a balanced eating pattern to provide healthy nutrition, maintain recommended body weight, and reduce the risk of chronic disease.

- Limit fats:

  Total fat intake—less than 20% to 35% of total calories

  Saturated fats—less than 10% of total calories

  ***Trans*-fats**—less than 1% of calories

  Cholesterol—less than 300 mg

- **Sources**—Most fats should come from foods such as fish, nuts, and vegetable oils.
- **Include fat-free or low-fat dairy,** including yogurt, milk, and cheese. Avoid processed cheese products and dairy with added sugars.
- **Choose a variety of fruits and vegetables, preferably fresh,** each day—at least 2½ cups of dark green, red, and orange vegetables and legumes (beans and peas).
- **Choose whole grains** often. At least half of complex carbohydrates should come from whole grains.

- **Choose nutrient-dense foods and beverages** in appropriate portions, avoiding those with empty calories and excessive sugar and caffeine. Take in the right calories for you (one size does *not* fit all) based on age, sex, height, weight, and physical activity level.
- **Be physically active each day.** Balance calorie intake based on activity level. Engage in a minimum of 300 min/week of moderate-intensity physical activity (U.S. Department of Health and Human Services, 2020).

Avoiding the "Bad Stuff"

- Limit salt to less than 1,500 mg per day for all African Americans and those with hypertension, diabetes, and chronic kidney disease (including children), as well as persons older than 50. For everyone else, 2,300 mg is the recommended daily limit.
- **Alcohol only in moderation**—Up to one drink per day for women and two per day for men.
- **Practice food safety** by preparing, cooking, chilling, and storing foods to keep them free from harmful microorganisms. Clean hands, food contact surfaces, and fruits and vegetables. Do not wash or rinse meat and poultry. (Also see Chapter 21 for food safety.)

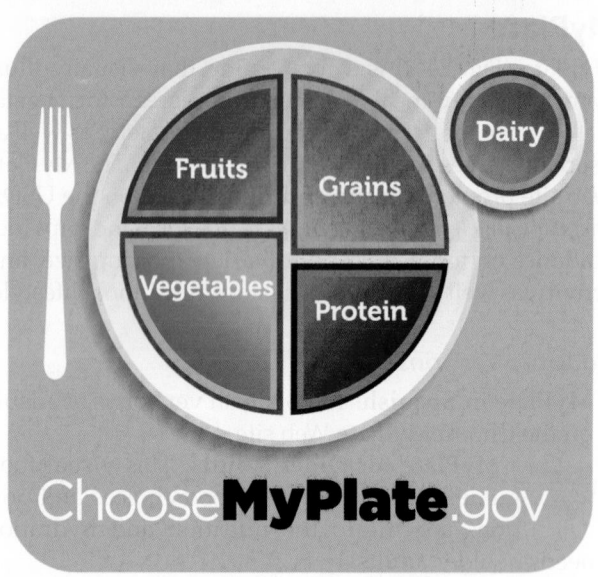

FIGURE 24-1 Build a healthy eating style using the U.S. Department of Agriculture (USDA) ChooseMy Plate.gov.

Although recipes are seasoned with culturally specific ingredients, these different diets similarly emphasize eating fresh local and seasonal foods. These diets avoid excess sugar, salt, and solid fats. For healthy living, portion sizes are moderate. Fish and seafood are staples, with red meat typically eaten twice per week.

- **Diabetes Food Plate.** The American Diabetes Association offers an online interactive tool called *Create Your Plate* to help individuals with diabetes manage blood glucose with correctly portioned meals and a healthy balance of vegetables, protein, and carbohydrates. With the diabetes food plate, half the plate is nonstarchy vegetables. A quarter of the plate is lean protein foods. The other quarter is carbohydrate (American Diabetes Association, 2020).

Nutrition Facts Label

You are likely familiar with the **Nutrition Facts label** shown in Figure 24-2 because the U.S. Food and Drug Administration (FDA) requires this label on all packaged

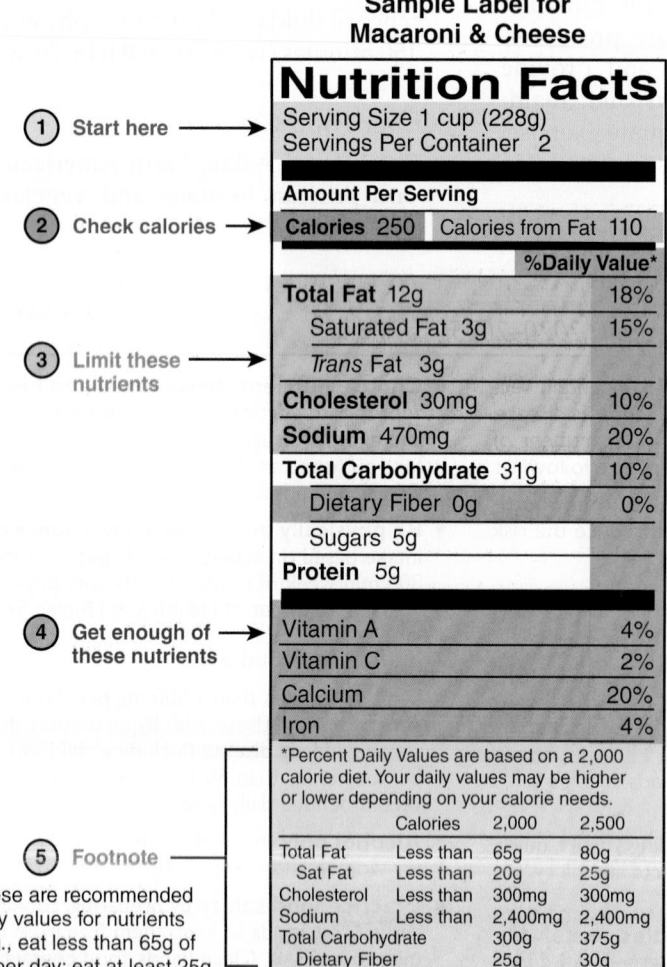

FIGURE 24-2 A Nutrition Facts label.

foods sold in the United States. The Nutrition Facts panel contains important information about serving size, number of servings per package, and total calories and calories from fat per serving; a list of the key nutrients in the food and their amounts; and the *percent daily values* (% DV) for the nutrients listed on the panel. The % DV identifies the percentage that a serving of the food contributes to a consumer's daily intake of the nutrient listed. Teaching your patients how to use these labels will help them to make wiser dietary choices.

KnowledgeCheck 24-1

- What are the DRIs?
- List the current USDA dietary guidelines for Americans.

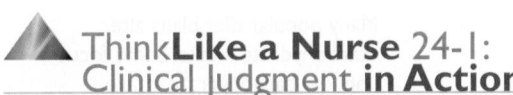

ThinkLike a Nurse 24-1: Clinical Judgment in Action

How might you use the various sources of nutritional information to evaluate the nutritional status of the clients introduced in the Meet Your Patients scenario?

WHAT ARE THE ENERGY NUTRIENTS?

The cells and tissues of the body depend on nutrients for growth, maintenance, and functioning. Any one food may contain a variety of nutrients; for instance, cheese contains carbohydrates, protein, fats, sodium, vitamins, and minerals.

- **Macronutrients** supply the body with energy (kilocalories). Table 24-1 lists the sources of and requirements for macronutrients.
- **Micronutrients** help manufacture, repair, and maintain cells.

Through the process of **metabolism,** the body converts food into complex forms of chemical energy and then into usable energy, which is then carried to individual cells. Metabolism encompasses all the ways in which the body changes and uses nutrients for vital processes and bodily functions. Most metabolic reactions are triggered by enzymes; each is specific and catalyzes only one type of reaction. Two types of metabolic reactions, anabolism and catabolism, occur continually and are adjusted according to the needs of the body.

- **Anabolism** involves the formation of larger molecules from smaller ones. For example, if protein is needed for tissue repair, amino acids are recombined to form proteins. This process requires energy.
- **Catabolism** involves the breakdown of larger molecules into smaller components. This process releases energy.

Carbohydrates

Carbohydrates are the primary energy source for the body.

Types of Carbohydrates

- **Simple carbohydrates,** commonly called *sugars*, are named according to the number of sugar (or *saccharide*) units making up their chemical structure.
    Monosaccharides (simple sugars) consist of a single unit.
    Disaccharides are molecules made up of two saccharides.
- **Complex carbohydrates** consist of long chains of saccharides called **polysaccharides.**

Dietary fiber, a polysaccharide, is the indigestible "fibrous skeleton" of plant foods. Humans do not have the enzymes to digest fiber; thus, it provides no usable glucose.

Functions of CHOs

1. **Supply energy for muscle and organ function.** Carbohydrates are more easily and quickly digested than proteins and lipids. They fuel strenuous, short-term skeletal muscle activity and provide nearly all the energy for the brain. Humans store glucose in liver and skeletal muscle tissue as **glycogen.** Glycogen is converted back into glucose to meet energy needs. This process is called *glycogenolysis.*
2. **Spare protein.** If glycogen stores are low (e.g., in an undernourished person), physical activity causes the body to catabolize stores of protein (*gluconeogenesis)* and lipids (fats) to use for energy. However, when proteins are used for energy, they are not available for their primary functions of tissue growth, maintenance, and repair. Fats are then converted directly into an alternative fuel called *ketones.*
3. **Play a role in nutrition and metabolism.**
    - Enhance insulin secretion. **Insulin** is a pancreatic hormone that promotes the movement of glucose into the cells for use.
    - Increase *satiety* (feeling of fullness and satisfaction).
    - Improve absorption of sodium and excretion of calcium.

Proteins

- **Proteins** are complex molecules made up of *amino acids*. Every amino acid consists of a central carbon atom connected to a hydrogen atom, an acid, an *amine* (a region of the molecule containing nitrogen), and a side chain. Just 20 different amino acids are the building blocks of most of the proteins in the human body.
- **Essential amino acids** must be supplied by food or nutritional supplements because they are not produced within the body.
    Examples: Arginine, histidine, isoleucine, leucine, lysine, methionine, phenylalanine, threonine, tryptophan, and valine
    Note: Some consider arginine to be nonessential because it cannot be synthesized at a rate that will

Table 24-1 ➤ Energy Nutrients

NUTRIENTS	SOURCES	ENZYMES INVOLVED IN DIGESTION	REQUIREMENTS
Carbohydrates	*Simple sugars* occur mainly in corn syrup, honey, milk, table sugar, molasses, sugar cane, sugar beets, and fruits. *Complex carbohydrates* occur in vegetables, breads, cereals, pasta, grains, and legumes.	Salivary amylase (mouth) Ptyalin (mouth and stomach) Pancreatic amylopsin Intestinal: Sucrase, lactase, maltase	Dietary Reference Intake (DRI) requirements for healthy adults are 45%–65% of calories from carbohydrates, or 130 grams per day (g/day). Body size and activity level affect the amount of carbohydrate used by the body. There is debate about the amount of dietary carbohydrate needed. Many popular diet plans alter carbohydrate intake. Some focus on low carbohydrate intake; others recommend a high intake of complex carbohydrates.
Proteins	*Complete proteins* come mostly from animal sources: meat, poultry, fish, eggs, and milk products. *Incomplete proteins* are supplied by plant sources (e.g., grains, nuts, legumes, seeds, vegetables). They can be combined to make complete proteins.	Stomach: Pepsin Pancreas: Trypsin, chymotrypsin, carboxypeptidase Intestine: Aminopeptidase, dipeptidase	10%–35% of the adult diet should be calories from protein, or 0.8 g/kg of body weight (46–56 g/day for an "average" person). Protein needs depend on age, body size, and physical state. Needs are increased during growth periods, such as childhood and pregnancy.
Fats	*Saturated fats* occur in pork, beef, poultry, seafood, egg yolk, dairy, coconut oil, and palm oil. *Unsaturated fats (from plants)* occur in olives, olive oil, vegetable oils (peanut, soybean, cottonseed, corn, safflower), nuts, and avocados. *Essential fatty acids (linoleic acid [omega-6] and alpha-linolenic acid [omega-3])* occur in polyunsaturated vegetable oils and in fatty fish (e.g., salmon). *Trans-fats* occur in hydrogenated oils, some margarines, packaged baked goods, and many processed foods.	Lingual: Lipase Gastric: Lipase, triacylglycerol lipase, bile salts Pancreatic lipase (steapsin)	Healthy adults should get 20%–35% of their calories from fat; children, 25%–40%. The American Heart Association (AHA) recommends that people obtain <30% of their calories from fat; 5%–6% of calories should come from saturated fats and limited *trans*-fat (AHA, 2016, 2017, 2018). People with increased risk for heart disease may need stricter control.

Sources: Institute of Medicine. (2005). *Dietary Reference Intakes for energy, carbohydrate, fiber, fat, fatty acids, cholesterol, protein, and amino acids.* National Academies Press. https://doi.org/10.17226/10490

support growth; it is essential for children but not for adults.

- **Nonessential amino acids** can be synthesized in the body, so we do not need to obtain them from food.

  Examples: Alanine, asparagine, aspartic acid, cysteine, glutamic acid, glutamine, glycine, proline, serine, and tyrosine

Note: Cysteine is considered essential in some situations, such as in immaturity or severe stress.

For protein synthesis to occur, every amino acid necessary to build that protein must be available.

- **Complete proteins** contain all the essential amino acids necessary for protein synthesis. These usually come from animal sources.

- **Incomplete proteins** (e.g., nuts, grains) do not provide all the essential amino acids. However, by combining two incomplete proteins, a complete protein can be made. For instance, peanut butter on whole-grain bread constitutes a complete protein.

Protein Metabolism and Storage

Although protein digestion begins in the stomach, it occurs mostly in the small intestine, where enzymes break it down into amino acids.

- The body continually breaks down and rebuilds protein into tissues, adjusting as needed to maintain the overall protein balance.
- The body also maintains a balance between tissue protein and plasma protein.

Nitrogen Balance occurs when the intake and output of nitrogen are equal.

- A **positive nitrogen balance** exists when nitrogen intake exceeds output, making a pool of amino acids available for growth, pregnancy, and tissue maintenance and repair.
- A **negative nitrogen balance** exists when nitrogen loss exceeds nitrogen intake. This occurs in illness, injury (e.g., burns), and malnutrition.

Functions of Protein

Dietary proteins perform the following functions:

- **Tissue building.** Protein is the structural material of every cell in the body. In fact, except for water, protein makes up the biggest part of the body. It is essential for the growth, maintenance, and repair of body cells and tissues.
- **Metabolism.** Proteins are essential for building body tissue. For example, proteins are precursors to digestive enzymes and hormones (e.g., thyroxine). *Enzymes* facilitate cellular reactions throughout the body. In addition, proteins combine with iron to form hemoglobin, the oxygen carrier in red blood cells.
- **Immune system function.** *Lymphocytes* (specialized white blood cells [WBCs]) and *antibodies* (components of the immune system that defend against foreign invaders) are proteins.
- **Fluid balance.** Because they attract water, proteins in cells and the bloodstream help to regulate fluid balance.
- **Acid–base balance.** Blood proteins function as buffers, helping to regulate acid–base balance.
- **Secondary energy source.** As noted earlier, proteins can be broken down to provide energy when stores of fats and carbohydrates are inadequate (Thompson & Manore, 2018).

Protein needs vary according to age, sex, weight, and health. Lean meat is nourishing and healthy if it is consumed in modest amounts, is low in saturated fat, and is not processed. Many North Americans eat more protein than they need, especially in the form of red meat. Animal proteins high in saturated fat increase the risk for certain cancers and coronary artery disease.

Lipids

Lipids are organic (carbon-containing) substances that are insoluble in water. They are made up of carbon, hydrogen, and oxygen—the same basic elements that make up carbohydrates.

- **Fats** are solid at room temperature.
- **Oils** are liquid at room temperature.

For example, butter is a fat even when it is melted because it would be solid at room temperature. You will hear the terms *lipids* and *fats* used interchangeably.

Fat is an essential nutrient for brain and nerve function, but certain types, when consumed in excess, can also be a health hazard. Lipid metabolism occurs in the small intestine, where bile and pancreatic enzymes begin splitting the fatty acids from their glycerol backbone. Lipids are stored as adipose tissue.

Types of Lipids

The three types of lipids found in foods are glycerides, sterols, and phospholipids.

Glycerides Also called **true fats,** glycerides consist of one molecule of glycerol attached to one, two, or three fatty acid chains.

- **Glycerol** is an alcohol composed of three carbon atoms.
- **Fatty acids** are long chains of carbon and hydrogen atoms ending in an acid.
- **Triglycerides** are the main glycerides found in foods. They are compounds consisting of a glycerol molecule attached to three fatty acids.

Sterols Sterols are lipids but are not made of fatty acids. The most important sterol in the body is **cholesterol,** a waxlike substance needed for the formation of cell membranes, vitamin D, estrogen, and testosterone. Cholesterol is synthesized in the liver, and it is also found in animal foods.

Phospholipids Phospholipids are a key component of **lipoproteins,** which consist of phospholipids and a protein. Because they are water soluble, lipoproteins are the major transport vehicles for lipids in the bloodstream. By "wrapping" triglycerides with water-soluble phosphates and proteins, lipoproteins deliver these substances to body cells.

- **Low-density lipoproteins (LDLs)** transport cholesterol to body cells. Diets high in saturated fats increase the level of LDLs circulating in the bloodstream and may result in fatty deposits on vessel walls, causing cardiovascular disease. As a result, LDL is often known as the "bad cholesterol."

- **High-density lipoproteins (HDLs)** remove cholesterol from the bloodstream, returning it to the liver, where it is used to produce bile. Thus, a high blood level of HDL is considered protective against cardiovascular disease. It is often known as the "good cholesterol."

Saturated and Unsaturated Fatty Acids Fatty acids are classified as saturated, unsaturated, or *trans*-fats (Table 24-2). *Saturation* means that a substance is holding all that it can hold (e.g., think of a wound dressing saturated with blood).

- An **unsaturated fatty acid** is not filled with all the hydrogen it can hold. Therefore, it is lighter and less dense.
- **Monounsaturated fat** molecules have one unfilled spot where hydrogen is not attached.
- **Polyunsaturated fatty acids** contain two or more unfilled spots for hydrogen. At the spot(s) where no hydrogen is attached, the molecule becomes kinked

and does not pack together. This is why fats are liquid at room temperature. Dietary fat should mainly be polyunsaturated and unsaturated to reduce the risk of heart disease and stroke.

- **Saturated fatty acids** are those in which every carbon atom is fully bound to (or "saturated" with) hydrogen. The molecules pack tightly together at room temperature and are dense, solid, and heavy.
- ***Trans*-fatty acids** are saturated fats created when food manufacturers add hydrogen to polyunsaturated plant oils, such as corn oil, to break the double-carbon bonds and straighten out the molecules. This process solidifies the fat and extends the shelf-life of the food. *Trans*-fats are found in processed foods containing *hydrogenated vegetable oils.*

Saturated fats and *trans*-fats are the main dietary factors in increasing blood cholesterol levels. They raise LDL cholesterol levels. The FDA mandates that *trans*-fat content be listed on all food labels. The Word Health Organization (WHO, 2018) released a plan for countries

Table 24-2 ➤ Dietary Fats

TYPE OF FAT	SOURCES	EFFECT ON BLOOD CHOLESTEROL
Monounsaturated	Olives; olive oil, canola oil, and peanut oil; cashews, almonds, peanuts, and most other nuts; avocados	Lowers LDL and raises HDL
Polyunsaturated	Corn, soybean, safflower, sesame, sunflower, and cottonseed oils; fish, nuts, and seeds	Lowers LDL and raises HDL
Saturated	Whole milk, butter, cheese, and ice cream; red meat; chocolate; coconuts, coconut milk, and coconut oil; palm oils; cocoa butter; processed foods	Raises LDL and HDL
Trans-fats	Most margarines; vegetable shortening; partially hydrogenated vegetable oil; deep-fried chips; many fast foods (e.g., French fries, donuts); most commercial baked goods	Raises LDL
Dietary Cholesterol	Foods from animals: meats, egg yolks, dairy products, organ meats (e.g., heart, liver), fish, and poultry	Raises cholesterol

American Heart Association (AHA) Recommendations

Limit foods high in saturated fat, *trans*-fat, and/or cholesterol. Instead, choose foods low in saturated fat, *trans*-fat, and cholesterol. Here are some helpful tips:

- Limit intake of whole-milk dairy products, fatty meats, tropical oils, partially hydrogenated vegetable oils, and egg yolks.
- Include a variety of fruits and vegetables in the diet.
- Eat a variety of grain products; include whole grains.
- Eat fish, particularly fatty fish, at least twice a week.
- Include fat-free and low-fat milk products and legumes.
- Choose skinless poultry and lean meats.
- Choose fats and oils with 2 g or less saturated fat per tablespoon (e.g., olive oil, canola oil, sunflower oil).
- Limit tropical oils (e.g., palm oil, coconut oil); they are high in saturated fats (AHA, 2020, last reviewed; 2018, last reviewed).
- Use healthy cooking methods (e.g., grilling, broiling, steaming).

HDL, High-density lipoprotein; *LDL*, low-density lipoprotein.

worldwide to eliminate or restrict those *trans*-fatty acids from foods and replace them with healthier fats and oils.

Essential and Nonessential Fatty Acids A fatty acid is considered essential if (1) the body cannot manufacture it and (2) its absence creates a deficiency disease. The essential fatty acids, linoleic acid (omega-6) and alpha-linolenic acid (omega-3), help protect against heart disease.

Functions of Lipids

Lipids perform the following functions:

1. **Supply essential nutrients.** Food fats supply the essential fatty acids and aid in the absorption of fat-soluble vitamins.
2. **Energy source.** The body burns fat for energy when engaging in sustained light activity, when glycogen stores are exhausted, and when at rest. During strenuous physical activity, carbohydrates are the primary energy source.
3. **Flavor and satiety.** Lipids give food its creamy taste and texture and promote satiety (the feeling of being "full"). Fats are digested more slowly than carbohydrates, so stomach emptying time slows.
4. **Other functions.** Body fat provides insulation, protects vital organs, aids in thermoregulation, and enables accurate nerve-impulse transmission. In addition, lipids are a component of every cell membrane and are essential to cell metabolism.
5. **Cholesterol functions.** Cholesterol is a component of every cell in the body, where it lends suppleness and support. It is also an ingredient of bile, which helps digest fats, and serves as a precursor to all steroid hormones, including sex hormones. When lipid metabolism is "disordered," cholesterol contributes to atherosclerosis.

ThinkLike a Nurse 24-2:
Clinical Judgment in Action

Review the information you collected on the two employees (Meet Your Patients).

- What conclusions, if any, can you make about their intake of carbohydrates, protein, and fats?
- How might you gather additional data on their intake of the energy nutrients?

WHAT ARE THE MICRONUTRIENTS?

Vitamins and minerals are called *micronutrients* because they are required by the body in only very small amounts. Although they provide no energy, they are critical in regulating a variety of body functions.

Vitamins

Vitamins are organic substances that are necessary for metabolism or preventing a particular deficiency disease. Vitamins are critical in building and maintaining body tissues, supporting our immune systems so that we can fight disease, and ensuring healthy vision. They also help our bodies to break down and use the energy found in carbohydrates, proteins, and lipids. Vitamins are especially critical during periods of rapid growth, pregnancy, lactation, and healing. Some evidence supports the claim that certain vitamins prevent chronic illness. Because the body cannot make vitamins, they must be supplied by the foods we eat.

Table 24-3 summarizes the specific functions of vitamins and lists their DRIs. *Note:* Although The Joint Commission includes the abbreviation *IU* on its "do not use" list, the abbreviation is used in other settings (e.g., on vitamin labels).

Allowances (RDAs) represent the daily dietary intake that is adequate to meet the needs of men, women, infants, and older adults.

Fat-Soluble Vitamins The fat-soluble vitamins are A, D, E, and K. They are stored primarily in the liver and adipose tissues, although vitamin E is deposited in all body tissue.

- **Stored in the body.** Because the body can store these vitamins, we do not need to consume them every day if we are consuming them in adequate amounts. However, diets extremely low in fat and disorders affecting fat digestion and absorption can lead to a deficiency of fat-soluble vitamins.
- **Not readily excreted.** Because they are not readily excreted, excessive supplementation with fat-soluble vitamins can lead to toxicity.
- **Some need more vitamin D.** Those with very little sun exposure, dark skin, osteoporosis, or impaired ability to absorb dietary fat (e.g., inflammatory bowel disease); people who are obese or have undergone gastric bypass surgery; and those who are taking medicines that interfere with vitamin D absorption may require more than the daily recommendation (Institute of Medicine, 2011).

Water-Soluble Vitamins The water-soluble vitamins include vitamin C and the B-complex vitamins (Table 24-3). Because these vitamins are soluble in water, excess amounts are regularly excreted in the urine. Thus:

- Toxicity is rare except in people with renal disease.
- The body cannot store these vitamins, so they need to be consumed every day.

Minerals

Minerals are inorganic elements found in nature. They occur naturally in foods, as food additives, and in supplements.

- **Major minerals (macrominerals)** are minerals that the body needs in amounts of 100 mg/day or greater.
- **Trace minerals** are essential but are needed in a lower concentration.

Text continued on page 678

Table 24-3 ➤ Vitamins: Adult Dietary Reference Intakes (DRIs)

VITAMIN	FUNCTION	RDA/AI*	SOURCES	EFFECTS OF DEFICIENCY/ AT RISK FOR DEFICIENCY	SYMPTOMS OF EXCESS
Fat-Soluble Vitamins					
A	Night and color vision Cellular growth and maturity Maintaining healthy skin and mucous membranes Growth of skeletal and soft tissues Reproduction Antioxidant (protects cells from the effects of free radicals that play a role in heart disease, cancer, other diseases)	*Females:* 9–13 yr— 600 mcg/day; 14 yr and older— 700 mcg/day (equivalent to 2,333) *Males:* 9–13 yr— 600 mcg/day; 14 yr and older— 900 mcg/day (equivalent to 3,000 IU)	Fish liver oil, liver, butter, cream, egg yolk, yellow fruit, green leafy vegetables, fortified milk	Night blindness, xerosis, xerophthalmia, keratomalacia, skin lesions, anemia *At risk for deficiency:* Uncommon in the U.S.	*Short-term:* Nausea and vomiting, vertigo, headache, blurred vision *Long-term:* Bone thinning and pain in the bones and joints, poor muscle coordination, skin irritation, birth defects
D†	Regulates blood calcium levels and the rate of deposit and resorption of calcium in bone Anti-inflammatory, antioxidant properties Supports immune health, muscle function, brain cell activity	Ages 1–70— 600 IU/day After age 71— 800 IU/day	Fish liver oil, fatty fish, fortified milk and yogurt, sunlight exposure	Bone and muscle pain, weakness, softening of bone, fractures, rickets *At risk for deficiency:* Persons with dark skin Persons with obesity Older adults Persons with lack of exposure to sunlight (or excessive sunblock)	Fatigue, weakness, loss of appetite, headache, confusion, and disorientation, kidney stones, cardiac arrythmias
E	Antioxidant (protects cells against the effects of free radicals) Protects red blood, skin, muscle, and tissue cells	Age 14 and older— 15 mg/day	Vegetable oils, nuts, milk, eggs, muscle meats, fish, wheat and rice germ, green leafy vegetables	Nerve pain (neuropathy) and hyporeflexia, ataxia, hemolytic anemia, myopathy	Insufficient blood clotting, impaired immune system, intestinal cramping, blurred vision, gonadal dysfunction

Table 24-3 ➤ Vitamins: Adult Dietary Reference Intakes (DRIs)—cont'd

VITAMIN	FUNCTION	RDA/AI*	SOURCES	EFFECTS OF DEFICIENCY/ AT RISK FOR DEFICIENCY	SYMPTOMS OF EXCESS
	Important to vision, reproduction, brain health			*At risk for deficiency:* Uncommon but supplementation may have neuroprotective effects in slowing progression of Alzheimer disease	
K	Synthesis of clotting factors Bone development	*Females:* Age 19 and older— 90 mcg/day (Adequate Intake [AI]) *Males:* Age 19 and older— 120 mcg/day (AI)	Green leafy vegetables, liver, dairy products Intestinal bacteria synthesize a form of vitamin K, so deficiency is unlikely.	Increased bleeding *At risk for deficiency:* Persons with a clotting disorder, breast cancer, or diabetes; the reversing anticoagulant effects of warfarin; after athletic performance	Jaundice and hemolytic anemia in infants
Water-Soluble Vitamins					
Thiamin (vitamin B_1)	Breakdown of carbohydrates for energy Nervous system function Gastrointestinal system function Cardiovascular system function	*Females:* Age 19 and older— 1.1 mg/day *Males:* Age 14 and older— 1.2 mg/day	Whole grain, brown rice, enriched cereal, beef, pork, liver, peas, beans, nuts	Peripheral neuritis, loss of muscle strength, depression, memory loss, anorexia, constipation, dyspnea, decreased alertness and reflexes, fatigue, irritability, beriberi (also known as *Wernicke-Korsakoff syndrome*)	Unlikely; readily excreted

(Continued)

Table 24-3 ➤ Vitamins: Adult Dietary Reference Intakes (DRIs)—cont'd

VITAMIN	FUNCTION	RDA/AI*	SOURCES	EFFECTS OF DEFICIENCY/ AT RISK FOR DEFICIENCY	SYMPTOMS OF EXCESS
				At risk for deficiency: After bariatric surgery; persons with HIV/AIDS, burns, chronic diarrhea, overactive thyroid, chronic stress, chronic alcohol abuse, or long-term diuretic furosemide (Lasix) use	
Riboflavin (vitamin B₂)	Antioxidant Breakdown of carbohydrate, protein, and fats Tissue health and growth Brain health	*Females:* 1.1 mg/day *Males:* 1.3 mg/day	Dairy products, meat, poultry, fish, eggs; nuts, green vegetables; whole grain, enriched cereals, bread	Tissue inflammation and breakdown; sore throat, stomatitis, swollen tongue, facial dermatitis, anemia; poor wound healing *At risk for deficiency:* Persons with alcoholism, burns, cancer, chronic diarrhea, chronic stress, overactive thyroid, or who have had bariatric surgery; infants with high bilirubin	Unlikely; readily excreted
Niacin (vitamin B₃)	Cellular metabolism to produce energy Controls cholesterol	*Females (nonpregnant):* 14 mg/day *Males:* 16 mg/day	Enriched breads and cereals, chicken, tuna, liver, peanuts, dairy products	*Short-term:* Weakness, poor appetite, indigestion, itching, diarrhea, headache, dizziness, insomnia *Long-term:* Central nervous system damage (confusion, neuritis, dementia), pellagra, gout, liver damage, birth defect if deficient during pregnancy	Facial flushing, itching, nausea, liver damage (especially when taking niacin with alcohol)

Table 24-3 ➤ Vitamins: Adult Dietary Reference Intakes (DRIs)—cont'd

VITAMIN	FUNCTION	RDA/AI*	SOURCES	EFFECTS OF DEFICIENCY/ AT RISK FOR DEFICIENCY	SYMPTOMS OF EXCESS
				At risk for deficiency: Uncommon in the U.S.	
Pantothenic acid (vitamin B₅)	Breakdown of fat, protein, and cholesterol Amino acid activation Heme formation Healthy skin	*All adults:* 5 mg/day; 6 mg/day during pregnancy; 7 mg/day while lactating	Occurs widely in most foods Best sources: Meats, eggs, whole-grain cereals, legumes	Deficiency is unknown. At *risk for deficiency:* Rare in the U.S.	Unlikely; readily excreted
Pyridoxine (vitamin B₆)	Protein (and some carbohydrate) metabolism Red blood cell production Brain development and nerve transmission	*Females:* Age 50 and younger— 1.3 mg/day Age 51 and older— 1.5 mg/day *Males:* Age 50 and younger— 0.3 mg/day, Age 51 and older— 1.7 mg/day	Meats, poultry, fish, potatoes, bananas, beans, nuts, seeds, dairy products, enriched cereals	Rash, stomatitis, seizure, peripheral neuritis, depression At risk for deficiency: Persons with kidney disease, malabsorption diseases, on epilepsy medication, or experiencing alcohol dependence	Irreversible nerve damage, including extremity numbness, walking difficulties Sensitivity to light Reduced ability to sense pain or extreme temperatures
Folate (folic acid, vitaminB₉)	Cellular metabolism Neurotransmitter synthesis Cell division DNA synthesis Hemoglobin formation	400 mcg/day (folic acid); 600 mcg/day when pregnant Females capable of becoming pregnant should take a daily supplement of 400–800 mcg.	Green leafy vegetables, asparagus, liver, yeast, eggs, beans, oranges, lemons, melons, strawberries, enriched cereals	Megaloblastic anemia, neural tube defects At risk for deficiency: Rare deficiency in the U.S. Indicated during pregnancy	Loss of appetite, confusion and irritability, hives, respiratory distress
Cyanocobalamin (vitamin B₁₂)	Cellular metabolism Maintain myelin sheath Hemoglobin synthesis	2.4 mcg/day	Dairy products, meat, poultry, fish, liver, dairy products, cheese, eggs	Anemia, muscle weakness, irreversible nerve damage, memory loss, dementia, mood disturbances	Uncommon because it is readily excreted Tingling sensation in hands and feet

(Continued)

Table 24-3 ➤ Vitamins: Adult Dietary Reference Intakes (DRIs)—cont'd

VITAMIN	FUNCTION	RDA/AI*	SOURCES	EFFECTS OF DEFICIENCY/ AT RISK FOR DEFICIENCY	SYMPTOMS OF EXCESS
	Formation of DNA			*At risk for deficiency:* Persons following a vegetarian or vegan diet; older adults; persons with digestive tract disorders	
C (ascorbic acid)	Collagen synthesis "Cementing" substance for capillary walls Antioxidant Iron absorption Immune protection and healing	*Females:* 75 mg/day *Males:* Age 19 and older— 90 mg/day Additional 35 mg/day for those who smoke	Citrus fruits, berries, tomatoes, potatoes, green vegetables, cauliflower, cabbage, peppers, broccoli, spinach	Anemia, tissue bleeding, easy bone fracture, gingivitis, petechiae, poor wound healing, joint pain, scurvy *At risk for deficiency:* Persons using tobacco; persons with gastrointestinal conditions, cancer, or eating a diet with limited fruits and vegetables	Stomach inflammation, diarrhea, oxalate kidney stones

Note: 1 mcg = 40 International Units (IU).
• **Recommended Dietary Allowances (RDAs)**—Intake sufficient to meet the needs of 97%–98% of individuals in a group.
• **Adequate Intakes (AIs)**—Recommended intake believed to cover the needs of all individuals in the group. These are used when RDAs can't be determined.
• **Upper Intake Levels (ULs)**—The maximum daily intake likely to pose no risk of adverse effects.
*RDAs are usually less than adult values for infants and children, more for pregnant women, and highest for lactating individuals. RDAs for some vitamins (e.g., vitamin A) are higher for older adults and higher for male individuals than for female individuals.
†The American Academy of Pediatrics recommends 10 mcg/day of vitamin D for infancy through adolescence (Wagner et al., 2008). Other clinicians and researchers have suggested that the RDA for adults should be dramatically increased as well, to 20–25 mcg (800–1000 IU) for adults aged 50 and older (Jockers, 2007).
Sources: Institute of Medicine (1998, 2001, 2011); Institute of Medicine (U.S.) Standing Committee on the Scientific Evaluation of Dietary Reference Intakes (2000); National Institutes of Health, Office of Dietary Supplements (n.d.); U.S. Department of Agriculture and U.S. Department of Health and Human Services (2018).

Minerals assist in fluid regulation, nerve-impulse transmission, and energy production; they are essential to the health of bones and blood and help rid the body of by-products of metabolism. Evidence also shows that minerals play key roles in disease prevention and treatment. For example:

1. **Calcium in adequate amounts throughout the life span decreases the likelihood of *osteoporosis* (a condition marked by porous bones). The recommended daily intake is difficult to achieve by diet alone. In the United States, calcium deficiency is one of the most common mineral deficiencies (Table 24-4).**

2. **Iron deficiency causes *anemia* (low hemoglobin), the most common nutritional problem worldwide.**
3. **Magnesium deficiency increases the risk of hypertension and coronary artery disease in women.**
4. **Sodium, consumed in high amounts (>2,500 mg/day), increases the risk for high blood pressure, heart attacks, and stroke.**

If the body is deficient in a mineral, it absorbs more; if the body has enough, it absorbs less and excretes more in the feces. Minerals interact with other minerals, vitamins, and other substances to accomplish absorption and metabolism and perform their functions. For example, iron absorption is enhanced in the presence

Table 24-4 ➤ Minerals: Adult Dietary Reference Intakes*

MINERAL	FUNCTION	RDA†	SOURCES	EFFECTS OF DEFICIENCY	SYMPTOMS OF EXCESS
Macrominerals					
Calcium (Ca)	Bone and teeth formation, blood clotting, nerve conduction, muscle contraction, cellular metabolism, heart action	Age 1–3 years: 700 mg/day (Adequate Intake [AI]) Age 4–8 years: 1,000 mg/day (AI) Age 9–18 years: 1,300 mg/day (AI) Age 19–70: 1,000 mg/day *Females:* Age 51–70 years: 1,200 mg/day Adults 70 years and older: 1,200 mg/day	Dairy products, sardines, green leafy vegetables, broccoli, whole grains, egg yolks, legumes, nuts, fortified products	Bone loss, tetany, rickets, osteoporosis	Kidney stones, constipation, intestinal gas
Magnesium (Mg)	Aids thyroid hormone secretion; maintains normal basal metabolic rate; activates enzymes for carbohydrate and protein metabolism, nerve and muscle function, cardiac function	*Females:* Age 19–30 years: 310 mg/day (AI), *Males:* Age 19–30: 400 mg/day (AI), Age 31 years and older: 420 mg/day	Whole grains, nuts, legumes, green leafy vegetables, lima beans, broccoli, squash, potatoes	Tremor, spasm, convulsions, weakness, muscle pain, poor cardiac function	Weakness, nausea, malaise
Phosphorus (P)	Bone and tooth strength, overall metabolism, formation of enzymes, acid–base balance	Age 19 and older: 700 mg/day (AI)	Dairy products, beef, pork, beans, sardines, eggs, chicken, wheat bran, chocolate	Bone loss, poor growth	Tetany, convulsions
Potassium (K)	Intracellular fluid control, acid–base balance, nerve transmission, muscle contraction, glycogen formation, protein synthesis, energy metabolism, blood pressure regulation	4.7 g/day (AI)	Unprocessed foods, especially fruits, vegetables, meats, potatoes, avocados, legumes, milk, molasses, shellfish, dates, figs	Muscle weakness (including weakness of heart and respiratory muscles), weak pulse, fatigue, abdominal distention (Rarely occurs as a result of inadequate dietary intake.	Cardiac dysrhythmias, cardiac arrest, weakness, abdominal cramps, diarrhea, anxiety, paresthesia

(Continued)

Table 24-4 ➤ Minerals: Adult Dietary Reference Intakes*—cont'd

MINERAL	FUNCTION	RDA†	SOURCES	EFFECTS OF DEFICIENCY	SYMPTOMS OF EXCESS
				More likely due to losses from prolonged vomiting, diarrhea, or some diuretic drugs.)	
Sodium (Na)	Water balance, acid–base balance, muscle action, nerve transmission, convulsions	Age 19–50 years: 1.5 g/day (AI) Age 50–70 years: 1.3 g/day Age 70 years and older: 1.2 g/day	Table salt (NaCl), milk, meat, eggs, baking soda, baking powder, celery, spinach, carrots, beets	Dizziness, abdominal cramping, nausea, vomiting, diarrhea, tachycardia, convulsions, coma	Thirst, fever, dry and sticky tongue and mucous membranes, restlessness, irritability, convulsion
Trace Minerals					
Copper	Aids in iron metabolism, works with many enzymes in protein metabolism and hormone synthesis	Age 19 years and older: 900 mcg/day (AI)	Liver, seafood, cocoa, legumes, nuts, whole grains	Rarely occurs; anemia, low white blood cell count, poor growth	Vomiting, nervous system disorders
Fluoride	Increases resistance to dental caries	*Females:* Age 14 years and older: 3 mg/day (AI) *Males:* Age 19 years and older: 4 mg/day (AI)	Fluorinated water, toothpaste, dental treatment, seaweed, fish, tea	Increased dental caries	Stomach upset, staining of teeth, bone pain
Iodine	Synthesis of the thyroid hormone, thyroxine	Age 14 years and older: 150 mcg/day	Iodized salt, saltwater fish, dairy products, enriched white bread	Goiter, poor infancy growth, cretinism, hypothyroidism	Skin lesions, thyroid malfunction
Iron	Synthesis of hemoglobin, general metabolism (e.g., of glucose), antibody production, drug detoxification in the liver	*Females:* Age 19–50 years: 18 mg/day, Age 50 years and older: 8 mg/day *Males:* Age 19 years and older: 8 mg/day	Meats, eggs, spinach, seafood, broccoli, peas, bran, enriched breads, fortified cereals	Small, pale red blood cells; anemia	Hemochro-matosis

Table 24-4 ➤ Minerals: Adult Dietary Reference Intakes*—cont'd

MINERAL	FUNCTION	RDA†	SOURCES	EFFECTS OF DEFICIENCY	SYMPTOMS OF EXCESS
Zinc	Cofactor for many enzymes involved in growth, insulin storage, immunity, alcohol metabolism, sexual development, and reproduction	*Females:* 8 mg/day *Males:* 11 mg/day	Primarily lean meats, eggs, poultry; oysters; legumes, peas, and whole grains	Skin rash, diarrhea, decreased appetite, hair loss, poor growth and development, poor wound healing, taste abnormalities, mental lethargy	Reduced copper absorption, altered iron function, diarrhea, cramps, depressed immune function

*Dietary Reference Intakes (DRIs) represent:
• **Recommended Dietary Allowances (RDAs)**—Intake set to meet the needs of 97%–98% of individuals in a group.
• **Adequate Intakes (AIs)**—Believed to cover the needs of all individuals in the group.
• **Upper Intake Levels (ULs)**—The maximum daily intake likely to pose no risk of adverse effects.
• Values in table are RDAs unless marked "(AI)."
†RDAs are usually less than adult values for infants and children, more for pregnant individuals, and highest for lactating individuals. RDAs for some minerals are higher for older adults and different for male and female individuals.
Sources: Food and Nutrition Board, Institute of Medicine, National Academies (2011); Institute of Medicine (1997, 1998, 2000, 2001, 2005, 2011, 2019); National Institutes of Health, Office of Dietary Supplements (2020, 2021); U.S. Department of Agriculture (2020).

of vitamin C, and vitamin D deficiency inhibits calcium absorption.

WHY IS WATER AN ESSENTIAL NUTRIENT?

Water is made up of hydrogen and oxygen and constitutes about half of the total body weight—55% to 65% in men and 50% to 55% in women. This is because men have greater muscle mass, and muscle contains a relatively large amount of water. Water is distributed in two body compartments:

■ **Intracellular fluid** is the water contained within each living cell. It makes up about 40% of the total body weight.
■ **Extracellular fluid** is external to the cell membrane (e.g., in the fluid portion of blood and lymph and in the gastrointestinal [GI] tract); it accounts for 20% of body weight.

Water is critical to the body because its functions are essential to life:

■ **Solvent.** Water is the basic solvent for the body's chemical processes.
■ **Transport.** As a component of blood, water serves as a medium for transporting oxygen, nutrients, and metabolic wastes.
■ **Body structure and form.** Water "fills in the spaces" in body tissues (e.g., in blood, lymphatic material, and muscle), and by way of diffusion and osmosis, it transports ions into and out of cells.

■ **Temperature.** Water helps maintain body temperature. When body temperature rises, evaporation of sweat helps to cool the body.
■ **Lubricant.** Fluid reduces friction between moving surfaces, such as in joints, and in the thoracic and abdominal cavities, where organs need to move freely.
■ **Catalyst.** Water is a part of many biochemical reactions, such as the conversion of carbohydrates and proteins into energy during the digestive process.

The amount of water a person requires varies according to the environmental humidity and temperature, activity level, age, and metabolic needs. The AI is about 2.7 L of water per day for adult women and 3.7 L for men (Mazur & Litch, 2019; Sawka et al., 2005). The overall fluid balance is maintained when fluid intake in liquids, foods, and metabolic reactions matches fluid output through urine, feces, respiration, and sweat. Fluid and electrolyte balance is discussed in Chapter 35.

KnowledgeCheck 24-2
■ What is the body's most usable energy source?
■ Which nutrient's primary function is the growth and repair of tissue?
■ Identify five functions of adipose tissue (body fat).
■ Which type of vitamin requires daily consumption to maintain appropriate levels?
■ What distinguishes a major mineral from a trace mineral?
■ Identify at least four functions of water.

Fluid Balance

Situation: The nurse working in the emergency department is reviewing an older client's intake and output (I&O) with them. The I&O are out of balance. The nurse begins to question the client further about other potential consequences of dehydration. How might the nurse phrase a question to design a personalized patient teaching plan before discharge to home?

Searchable Question: Do _____ (P) who are _____ (I) demonstrate _____ (O) compared with _____ (C) during _____ (T)?

PICOT Components

P	Population/patient	=	Older inpatients
I	Intervention/indicator	=	Dehydration
C	Comparator/control	=	Older community dwellers
O	Outcome	=	Complications of dehydration
T	Time	=	During hospitalization

Searching for the Evidence: The overall fluid balance is affected by diet, hydration, activity, environmental factors, illness, and medication. Older people are also more susceptible to dehydration because of cognitive, sensory, and motor impairments, which affect their activities of daily living. They tend to take more medications and have more illnesses that can increase the risk for fluid imbalance. For example, the frail older person with activity intolerance related to chronic pain may become easily dehydrated. If that person becomes ill, it is even more likely that the client will be unable to take in sufficient amounts of fluid independently. It is important to encourage elderly people, both inpatients and in the community, to consume small amounts of fluids throughout the day to maintain adequate fluid balance. Assessment questions that might point to a fluid imbalance would include those regarding intake, activity, and elimination patterns.

Boltz, M., Capezuti, E., Zwicker, D., & Fulmer, T. (Eds.). (2020). *Evidence-based geriatric nursing protocols for best practice* (6th ed.). Springer.

WHAT MUST I KNOW ABOUT ENERGY BALANCE?

The energy in carbohydrates, proteins, and lipids is measured in terms of **calories** or, more precisely, **kilocalories (kcal).** A kcal is the amount of heat required to raise the temperature of 1 kg of water by 1° centigrade. To maintain a stable weight, the number of kcal consumed must equal the number of kcal burned.

- A diet with **too few kcal** results in weight loss and is likely to lack essential nutrients, causing weakened immunity, stunted growth, and hormonal disruption.
- A diet with **too many kcal** can cause weight gain and obesity, which increases the risk for chronic diseases.

The amount of energy liberated from the metabolism of 1 gram of energy nutrients is as follows:

Carbohydrates = 4 kcal/g
Protein = 4 kcal/g
Fat = 9 kcal/g

Key Point: *In determining total energy (kilocalorie) needs, consider the client's basal metabolic rate and the duration and intensity of daily physical activity.*

KnowledgeCheck 24-3

Imagine that you have just eaten a food consisting of 4 g of protein, 18 g of carbohydrate, and 1 g of fat.
- What would your total kcal intake be?
- What percentage of your kcal is from carbohydrates? Protein? Fat?

What Is Basal Metabolic Rate?

The **basal metabolic rate (BMR)** is a measure of the energy used while at rest in a neutral temperature environment—the energy required for vital organs, such as the heart, liver, and brain, to function.

Direct measurement of BMR requires the use of a **calorimeter:** an insulated unit that measures temperature changes of water that are produced by exposure to a fasting individual at rest. Although it is very accurate, it is rarely used because most institutions do not have calorimeters and because the test requires a controlled environment and a 12-hour fast. Direct measurement of BMR is used primarily by researchers.

Indirect calculation of BMR, sometimes called the *resting energy expenditure,* includes the following:

- Measuring oxygen uptake per unit of time. This can be done in an exercise laboratory or with portable machines at the bedside. It is most often done for patients in intensive care units. Not all facilities have this capability.
- Serum thyroxine levels (a blood test).
- A formula for calculating BMR when precise measurement is not required (Box 24-2).

What Factors Affect Basal Metabolic Rate?

When interpreting test results, consider the following factors that influence the BMR:

- *Body composition.* Lean body tissue has greater metabolic activity than fat and bones. This explains why women, who have, on average, more adipose tissue than men, also have lower BMRs.

BOX 24-2 ■ Calculating Basal Metabolic Rate (BMR)

Females:	0.9 kcal/kg of body weight per hour
Males:	1.0 kcal/kg body weight per hour
Example:	Isaac Schwartz (Meet Your Patients) weighs 245 lb.

1 g = 2.2 lb.

Divide 245 by 2.2 to convert pounds to kilograms:

$$245 \div 2.2 = 111.3$$

Now complete the calculation:

1.0 kcal/kg/hr × 111.3 kg × 24 hours = 2,671.2 kcal/day

- *Growth periods.* BMR increases during periods of growth, such as the first 5 years of life, adolescence, pregnancy, and lactation.
- *Body temperature.* The BMR increases by 7% for each 1°F (0.83°C) rise in body temperature.
- *Environmental temperature.* Cold weather, especially temperatures below freezing, causes a slight rise in the BMR to generate body heat and maintain normal body temperature.
- *Disease processes.* Diseases and injuries involving increased cellular activity result in BMR elevation (e.g., cancer, anemia, cardiac failure, hypertension, asthma, severe burns, traumatic injury).
- *Prolonged or high-intensity physical exertion.* Glucose homeostasis preserves or enhances function during this kind of physical stress response (Institute of Medicine, Committee on Military Nutrition Research, 1994).

How Do I Calculate a Client's Total Energy Needs?

A person's total daily energy requirement is the number of kcal necessary to replace those used for basic metabolism plus those used in physical activities. The following are simple, general estimates based on activity level and age:

- Sedentary women and older adults generally need 1,600 kcal/day.
- Children, teenage girls, active women, and most men typically need 2,200 kcal/day.
- Teenage boys, active men, and very active women may need 2,800 kcal/day.

To calculate energy, you need to know the person's age, weight, and physical activity, including the intensity and duration of the activity. Heightened emotional states may also increase energy needs because they increase the catecholamine response, resulting in increased heart rate and muscular activity in the form of muscle tension, restlessness, and agitated movements.

KnowledgeCheck 24-4

You have already calculated the expected BMR for Mr. Schwartz (Meet Your Patients) for a 24-hour period.

- If Mr. Schwartz describes himself as working at a desk for 8 to 10 hours per day, lawn mowing manually every other week during the summer, and playing an occasional game of golf, how would you classify his general activity level?
- After interviewing Mr. Schwartz, you estimate his average caloric intake to be approximately 3,000 kcal per day. Determine whether his kcal intake is sufficient or insufficient to maintain his present activity level.

What Are Some Body Weight Standards?

Weight standards have been established to correlate weight with good health and longevity and to help determine a client's ideal body weight.

General Ideal Weight Guide This approach uses a formula to determine a reasonable weight based on height:

Men: 106 lb (47.7 kg) for the first 5 ft (150 cm), and then add 6 lb/in. (2.7 kg/2.5 cm).
Women: 100 lb (45 kg) for the first 5 ft (150 cm), and then add 5 lb/in. (2.25 kg/2.5 cm).
Add 10% for large body frame; subtract 10% for small body frame.

Height and Weight Tables WHO child growth standards are based on statistical estimates and often include variations for age, sex, weight, length/height, and body frame.

Body Composition Analysis This technique is used to quantify lean body mass versus percentage body fat. Lean body mass includes muscle, bone, and connective tissue. Lean tissue weighs more than fat; thus, a person who engages in regular weight-bearing exercise may weigh more than an individual of similar appearance who is sedentary. Various methods to assess body composition, known as *anthropometric measurements,* are provided in the Assessment section later in the chapter.

ThinkLike a Nurse 24-3: Clinical Judgment in Action

Examine your dietary intake for the next 3 days to determine how balanced your diet is.

- How does your diet compare with the USDA MyPlate in terms of:
  a. Servings of bread, cereal, rice, and pasta? _____
  b. Servings of vegetables? _____
  c. Servings of fruits? _____
  d. Servings of milk, yogurt, and cheese? _____
  e. Servings of meat, poultry, fish, dry beans, eggs, and nuts? _____
  f. Servings of fats, oils, and sweets? _____
- From what you have learned from this activity, what habits could you change in your patterns of eating to achieve optimal nutrition?

WHAT FACTORS AFFECT NUTRITION?

Several factors influence nutritional needs and choices. Some can be modified; some cannot. The most influential factors are development, knowledge, lifestyle, culture, disease processes, and functional limitations. Parents and caregivers are the most important influences on the eating habits of children.

Developmental Stage

At specific developmental stages, nutritional needs and eating patterns vary according to physiological growth, activity level, metabolic processes, disease prevention, and other factors.

Infants to 1 Year

Humans grow most rapidly during the first year of life. Nutritional needs per unit of body weight are greater than at any other time.

Calories and Protein The infant needs adequate protein for tissue building and enough carbohydrates to furnish energy and "spare" the protein. **Key Point: *The period from conception into the second year of life is most critical to brain development; therefore, the baby needs optimal nutrition.*** Severe protein-calorie deficiency in the last trimester of pregnancy or the first 6 months of life may decrease the number of brain cells by 20%.

Vitamins and Minerals Fetal iron stores are depleted at 4 to 6 months, so intake of iron becomes important. The infant also needs calcium for bone growth and the development of teeth, calcium and vitamin C for iron absorption, and vitamin D for calcium regulation.

Fluids Compared with adults, infants have a higher metabolic rate. Infants need proportionately more fluid than adults because infants:

- Have greater water loss through the skin, and skin makes up a greater proportion of the infant body.
- Have immature kidneys.

To meet nutritional and fluid needs, the infant requires 1.5 to 2 oz of breast milk or formula per pound of body weight per day.

Infant Feedings Safe choices for meeting fluid and nutrient needs in the first months of life are breast milk and commercially prepared formulas. Breast milk is the ideal nutrition for infants and is sufficient to support healthy growth and development in infancy (American Heart Association, 2018). Breastfeeding has the following benefits:

- **Enhances maturation of the infant's immune system.** Infants receive secretory immunoglobulin A (IgA) in breast milk. IgA provides a protective coating to the infant's respiratory and GI tracts to prevent microbes (bacteria, viruses, fungi, and parasites) from entering

the lungs, gut, and bloodstream. Colostrum contains high levels of immunoglobulins (Igs) IgE, IgG, IgM, and IgD, which protect against milk allergies, eczema, and respiratory infections (Palmeira et al., 2016).
- **Lower risk of sudden infant death syndrome (SIDS)** (American Academy of Pediatrics [AAP], Task Force on Sudden Infant Death Syndrome et al., 2016).
- **May decrease the risk of developing diabetes mellitus later in life, obesity, asthma, and childhood leukemia** for infants receiving breast milk in the first 6 months of life (AAP, 2012; Endocrine Society, 2018; Uwaezuoke et al., 2017; Wu et al., 2020).

The American Heart Association recommends breastfeeding for 12 months, with the addition of solid foods for micronutrients beginning at 4 to 6 months of life (American Heart Association, 2018). When breastfeeding is contraindicated or the mother chooses not to breastfeed, numerous commercial formulas are available. The most used formula is iron-fortified cow's milk protein, which is available as a powder, liquid concentrate, or ready-to-use liquid. Other types include iron-fortified soy and protein hydrolysate formulas.

- **Infants younger than 1 year should not receive cow's milk** because it may cause GI bleeding and may stress the infant's kidneys. It also can contribute to iron-deficiency anemia. Children between the ages of 1 and 5 years should avoid plant-based milk. Unless a child has dietary restrictions, cow's milk is recommended for children aged 12 months and older to help supply appropriate amounts of protein, calcium, vitamin D, folate, and other nutrients (AAP, 2019].
- **Honey and corn syrup should not be used** as a source of carbohydrates when preparing infant formula. They are potential sources of botulism toxin, which can be fatal in children younger than 1 year of age (Centers for Disease Control and Prevention [CDC], 2021).
- **Whether to boil water before reconstituting infant formula** depends on the water quality of the tap supply. When in doubt, consult the local health department. If unsure, the FDA recommends boiling rapidly for a minimum of 1 full minute and cooling completely before adding it to infant formula.
- **Infant formula should not be diluted.** Watering down formula can lead to nutritional imbalances and potentially serious health problems.
- **Goat's milk is not approved in the United States for infant nutrition** due to excessive protein content and insufficient vitamins and minerals. However, there are goat milk–based baby formulas that may be safe.
- **Plant-based milk alternatives are not recommended for babies under 1 year of age** or infants with certain medical conditions requiring specialized formulas. Soy milk–based formula may be an option for lactose intolerance. Almond milk or other plant milks are too low in protein and minerals to meet infants' needs for nutrition and health.

- **Fluoride might also be prescribed** for infants without a fluoridated water supply. Water that is purified or bottled for use in infant formulas does not contain fluoride. Healthy infants born at term have sufficient iron for their first 4 months. **Iron supplements** are usually given beginning at 4 to 6 months (depending on whether breast- or formula-fed), and they may continue after 12 months if iron needs are not being met (Baker & Greer; AAP, Committee on Nutrition, 2010). Solids foods are generally introduced, beginning with cereal, at 4 to 6 months of age.

Toddlers

Toddlers grow more slowly in comparison with infants and have fewer energy demands. Toddlers generally require about 1,000 kcal and 1,250 mL of fluid per day, depending on body weight. As the GI system matures, they can eat most foods and adjust to the adult pattern of three meals a day. By age 3, most children have all their deciduous teeth and can chew adult food.

- **Food should be cut into small pieces** to avoid choking in toddlers, who sometimes are too active to chew food sufficiently.
- **Sometimes young children "chipmunk" their food** and can later choke on it.
- **Do not give food when the child is in a car seat or bouncy chair,** where choking is more likely and can occur without a parent's noticing.
- **Toddlers' diets are often deficient in nutrients,** commonly iron, calcium, and vitamins A and C. One- and 2-year-old children should drink reduced-fat (2%) milk or, in some cases, whole milk to provide adequate essential fatty acids for the still-growing brain.
- **Parents need to offer a variety of foods to provide essential nutrients.** Each meal should contain at least one fruit or vegetable; juice intake should be limited. This can be a challenge because toddlers often refuse foods to assert their autonomy or manipulate their parents. They may take a long time to eat or refuse to eat.
- **Parents should not turn mealtime into a battle of wills or use foods to punish or reward;** such reactions may affect the child's attitude toward food or magnify problem feeding behaviors. To encourage the child to eat, you may offer parents the suggestions in the accompanying Home Care box, Tips for Encouraging Toddlers to Eat.

Preschoolers

Between ages 4 and 6, caloric needs are typically 1,200 to 1,400 kcal/day. Dietary fat should provide only 25% to 350% of the child's intake (American Heart Association, 2018). Children's appetites naturally regulate food intake, depending on physical needs for energy and nutrition. It is important that parents and caregivers do not overfeed. Preschoolers are similar to toddlers in their growth and nutritional needs; however,

Home Care

Tips for Encouraging Toddlers to Eat

- Be a good food role model. Children don't learn as much by listening to what you say but rather by watching what you do.
- Keep only nutritious foods in the house.
- Serve foods in a child-friendly way; for example, arrange tortillas, cheese, tomato slices, and beans as a smiling face.
- Do not use dessert as a reward for eating other foods (e.g., "You can't have cookies until you eat your meat"). Reward with attention (hugs, kind words) instead of food.
- Include your child in food shopping. Let your child help select nutritious foods and serve them at home.
- Commit to family mealtimes to connect with each other. Turn off the TV and cell phones. Get everyone involved.

their eating patterns typically improve. Preschoolers commonly:

- Form responses to specific foods, such as refusing green vegetables or drinking less milk.
- Eat only one food for several days (called *food jags*).
- Require nutritious between-meal snacks to meet nutritional needs during this time of rapid growth and activity.

Lifelong food habits are developed during this stage, so encourage families to widen the variety of foods offered to preschoolers and investigate the quality of the diet provided by their child's day care or preschool. A variety of foods is essential for children to get enough carbohydrates, protein, and other nutrients.

School-Age Children

In the school-age period, growth and body changes occur gradually. Permanent teeth erupt, and the digestive system matures. Sedentary school-age children need about 1,600 to 1,800 kcal/day; active children typically require an additional 200 to 400 more kcal per day (American Heart Association, 2018).

- **Nutrients.** An adequate supply of vitamins and minerals is critical because the body is still growing and preparing for the demands of adolescence. Foods should be low in saturated fat, *trans*-fat, cholesterol, salt (sodium), and added sugars.
- **Eating behaviors.** Parental control over food intake declines because advertising influences the child's food choices. The child eats away from home and may buy junk food with their lunch money or choose less nutritious foods in the school cafeteria. Even if the child brings lunch from home, they may trade their food or not eat lunch at all. Parents should encourage their children to eat breakfast

to provide nutrients and energy to fuel problem-solving skills, memory, and sports and playground activities.

Adolescents

Adolescence is a time of rapid growth and development of the reproductive system. Boys experience an increase in muscle tissue and bone length and density. At menstruation, girls experience fat deposition. The needs of the adolescent body for energy, vitamins, and minerals approach those of the infant. Adolescents need protein, calcium, iron, and B and D vitamins.

Adolescents have active lifestyles and snack often, often preferring foods of little nutrient value. Adolescents are responsible for their own food decisions, so the best approach for parents is to keep healthful snack foods (e.g., cheese, fruit, raw vegetables) in the home and role model a positive attitude toward healthy eating.

Eating disorders are a concern for some in this age-group. One-third to two-thirds of adolescent girls engage in crash dieting, fasting, self-induced vomiting, diet pills, or laxatives (National Association of Anorexia Nervosa and Associated Disorders, n.d.). Commonly, those with eating disorders exhibit their first symptoms before age 20, some as early as age 10. The majority of those with eating disorders are female.

Young and Middle Adults

- **Young adults** require adequate amounts of protein, vitamins, and minerals, but not at the same levels as in adolescence. If adults continue unhealthful behaviors developed in earlier stages, repercussions will begin to show up in adulthood. Calcium, vitamin D, folic acid, and iron continue to be critical, especially in women, for bone and reproductive health.
- **Middle adults.** The BMR decreases in middle age, potentially causing weight gain if dietary intake and activity level are unchanged. Individuals may begin to experience chronic illnesses such as diabetes, hypertension, obesity, hyperlipidemia, and certain types of cancer as a result of heredity or lifestyle choices. Dietary modification and exercise are essential to control these diseases.

Pregnant and Lactating Patients

Nutritional requirements increase dramatically during pregnancy as a result of the nutritional needs of the fetus.

- **Folate (folic acid)** intake is critical in the first trimester of pregnancy (the first 13 weeks) to prevent neural tube defects. The CDC (2022, September 9) recommends a daily supplement of 400 mcg in addition to the consumption of food containing folate from a varied diet for childbearing patients and during pregnancy.
- **Adequate protein and calcium** are important for the growth of muscle, brain, and bone tissues; iron is essential to maintain maternal and fetal blood supplies and stores during pregnancy.
- **Supplements**—It is almost impossible to consume the recommended amount of dietary *iron,* so supplements are commonly prescribed, as are supplements of *folic acid* and *calcium.*
- **Calories**—Pregnant patients need about 300 additional kcal/day in the second and third trimesters of pregnancy. Patients who are breastfeeding need 500 additional kcal per day. They continue to need additional protein and calcium, as well as increased fluid, to make adequate amounts of breast milk. The nutritional quality of the milk remains the same even if dietary intake is not adequate.
- **Glucose.** Pregnant patients also need to be screened for gestational diabetes (GDM) using the glucose challenge test or the oral glucose tolerance test (OGTT). Complications of uncontrolled GDM include fetal congenital heart defects and other malformations, fetal macrosomia with associated birth trauma, and neonatal hypoglycemia.

Older Adults

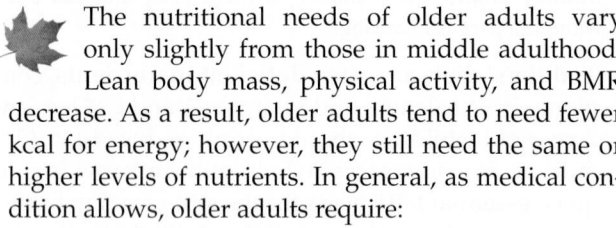

The nutritional needs of older adults vary only slightly from those in middle adulthood. Lean body mass, physical activity, and BMR decrease. As a result, older adults tend to need fewer kcal for energy; however, they still need the same or higher levels of nutrients. In general, as medical condition allows, older adults require:

- Slightly more calcium (e.g., dairy group) and slightly less of all other groups, especially the bread/cereal group.
- Complex carbohydrates (i.e., fiber) to maintain bowel function.

Plenty of hydration. Older adults should be sure to drink at least 64 oz of water or other fluids (e.g., soups) per day, but that amount can increase depending on heat and humidity and can change based on various medications (diuretics) and health conditions. Choose primarily green leafy vegetables and brightly colored fruits to help prevent constipation and dehydration.

Factors Affecting Nutrition The changes of aging often make it difficult for the older adult to achieve good nutrition.

- It is not unusual for older adults to lose interest in eating and to experience a decreased sensation of thirst.
- Older adults with chronic diseases may need to adjust to therapeutic diets low in salt, simple sugars, or fat. Unfortunately, the ability to taste and smell

diminishes with age, and many clients find these diets unappealing.

- Other sensory changes, such as diminished vision or hearing, limit mobility and interaction, making it more difficult to purchase and prepare food.
- Tooth loss and gum disease limit chewing ability, forcing many older adults to eat only soft food.
- Arthritic hands may create difficulty in preparing and eating food, and when they are no longer able to drive, many older adults must rely on local markets, where food choices may be limited and expensive.
- Other physical problems that may affect nutrition include gastroesophageal reflux, decreased gastric secretions, decreased intestinal peristalsis, and glucose intolerance.

Dietary Supplements Many older adults may need supplements of calcium, vitamin D, and vitamin B_{12}. For example, (1) as bone density decreases, calcium requirements increase, especially in women at risk for *osteoporosis*, and (2) low concentrations of vitamin B_{12} and vitamin D have been linked to cognitive decline in older adults (Health Quality Ontario, 2013; Jatoi et al., 2020; Toffanello et al., 2014).

Frail Elderly Syndrome With advancing age, older adults face many losses (e.g., institutionalization). As a result, depression and social isolation are common. Both negatively affect appetite. **Frail elderly syndrome** is a complex disorder characterized by weight loss, decreased activity and interaction, and increasing frailty.

EXAMPLE CLIENT CONDITION: Overweight/Obesity

Definition

- **Overweight or Obesity:** Weight higher than considered healthy for a given height
- **Body measurements:** Body weight 20% > ideal for height and frame
- **Body mass index (BMI)**
  Normal 18.5 to <25
  Overweight 25 to <30
  Class I obesity 30 to <35
  Class II obesity 35 to <40
  Class III obesity 40 or higher
  (Centers for Disease Control & Prevention, 2021; World Health Organization, 1995, 2006).
- **Percentage of body fat:**
  Obesity:
  Men: >25%
  Women: >33%
  Overweight:
  Men: 21%–25%
  Women: 31%–33%

Prevalence

Youth under age 20	18.5%
Men over age 20	37.9%
Women over age 20	41.1%
Total over age 20	39.6%

(Hales et al., 2020)

Risk Factors

- *Genetic factors/family predisposition*
- *Dietary intake*—poor quality, high-calorie, high-fat, high-salt, sugary, and processed foods; larger portions; habit of overeating and binging; snacking
- *Sedentary lifestyle*—high screen time, low physical activity
- *Medical condition*—Prader-Willi syndrome, endocrine and neurological disorders

RECOGNIZING COMPLICATIONS

Physical

- Type 2 diabetes
- Heart disease, hypertension, hyperlipidemia, stroke
- Metabolic syndrome
- Cancer
- Breathing problems, increased asthma, shortness of breath
- Sleeping problems, sleep apnea
- Gallbladder disease
- Joint pain and injuries, osteoarthritis
- Erectile dysfunction, infertility, irregular menstruation
- Skin ulcers, heat rash, fungal infection, acne
- Greater risk of death

Emotional

- Poor self-esteem, shame, guilt
- Loneliness and social isolation
- Depression, anxiety, obsessive–compulsive disorder (binge eating)
- Hormonal changes, slowing metabolism, menopause
- Medication—steroids, some psychiatric drugs
- Learned behaviors/emotional eating—conflict, depression, reward for good behaviors; comfort when feeling sad or lonely; expression of love

(continued)

EXAMPLE CLIENT CONDITION: Overweight/Obesity—cont'd

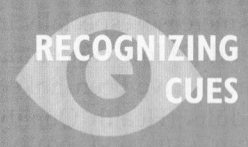

RECOGNIZING CUES

See **Focused Nutritional Assessment.**
See **Clinical Insight 24-1: Measurements to Evaluate Body Composition.**

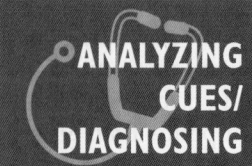

ANALYZING CUES/ DIAGNOSING

Problem Labels

Obesity
Overweight
Body Nutrition Excess
Risk for Body Nutrition Excess

Examples of Diagnostic Statements

- Overweight r/t insufficient physical activity, high-fat and high-sugar diet
- Obesity r/t metabolic disorder

GENERATING SOLUTIONS

NOC Outcomes

Weight
Body Mass
Weight Loss Behavior
Weight Maintenance Behavior
Nutritional Status: Food and Fluid Intake
Nutritional Status: Nutrient Intake

Individualized Goals/Outcome Statements

- Progressively gains weight toward desired goal.
- States factors contributing to weight gain.
- Designs dietary plan for long-term weight control.
- Reaches desired weight loss in an achievable time frame.
- Incorporates physical activities into daily life.

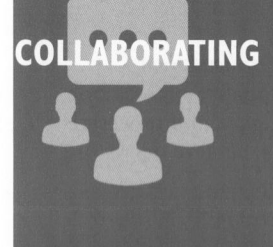

COLLABORATING

Weight-loss options for body mass index (BMI) >40

- Appetite suppressant on an individual basis
- Consult with a dietitian for weight management.

- Refer for appropriate counseling as needed.
- Surgical options: gastric bypass, laparoscopic adjustable gastric banding, gastric sleeve, biliopancreatic diversion with duodenal switch, vagal nerve blockade.

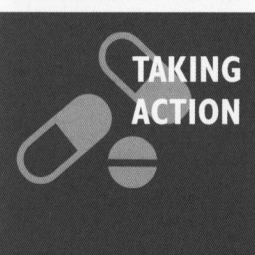

TAKING ACTION

Weight control

- Set realistic expectations for weight loss and physical activity goals.
- Encourage regular exercise, beginning gradually with low-impact activities. Minimum 300 min/week.
- Suggest that the client keep a record of food intake or use a diet tracker mobile application or blogs.

- Weigh the client weekly at the same time. For children, recommend:
  5 servings of fruits and vegetables each day
  2 hours or less of screen time per day
  1 hour of physical activity per day
  0 servings of sweetened beverages

EXAMPLE CLIENT CONDITION: Overweight/Obesity—cont'd

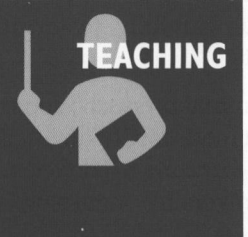

TEACHING

- Teach nutrition strategies that support flexible food choices:

  Healthful eating—Restrict high-carbohydrate, high-fat, sweetened, and refined foods and sugary beverages; eat whole grains, fruits and vegetables, and lean protein.

  Portion control—Adhere to serving sizes. May need to measure portion size when consuming foods.

  Plate method—Half the plate is for vegetables; one-quarter is for protein; the other quarter is for starch or carbohydrates. A glass of water or milk and fruit serving may be added.

  Carbohydrate tracking—Reducing carbohydrate intake is effective for weight loss.
  - Ketogenic low carb: <20 gm/day
  - Moderate low carb: 20–50 gm/day

- Liberal low carb: 50–100 gm/day
- Typical Western diet: 250+ gm/day

  Intermittent fasting:
  - Fast every other day.
  - Fast for 2 days (600 kcal/day), followed by 5 days of unrestricted intake.
  - Fast for 16 hours; consume daily intake over 8 hours.

- Advise clients to avoid fad diets.
- Suggest weight-loss support group or accountability partner.
- Emphasize that quality sleep, managed stress, active lifestyle, self-care, and positive mindset are essential to weight control.

  See **Self-Care Box: Teaching Weight Control Tips.**

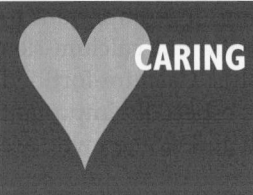

CARING

- ♥ **iCare** • Be encouraging and nonjudgmental, especially when there are setbacks.
- Be aware of weight bias that can lead to depression, low self-esteem, anxiety, and low school or work performance.

- Use sensitive language and neutral terms (e.g., "high BMI" or "unhealthy weight" instead of "obese" or "morbidly obese").

KnowledgeCheck 24-5

- Why is breast milk an ideal food source for infants?
- Why are an infant's nutritional needs per unit of body weight greater than at any other period of development?
- Why is it sometimes a challenge to meet the nutritional needs of toddlers?
- What is the challenge in meeting the nutritional needs of school-age children?
- Which age-group experiences a growth spurt second only to that of infants?
- Why are energy (kcal) requirements less for older adults?

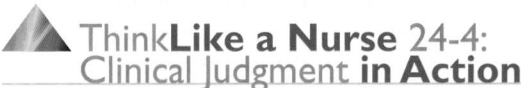

ThinkLike a Nurse 24-4: Clinical Judgment in Action

Make a list of food products you have seen advertised in the media. What are the implications for the nutritional status of the public?

Lifestyle Choices

Nutrition-related lifestyle choices include the following:

- **Dietary patterns.** The type of food consumed is equally important as the amount of food to a person's overall health.
- **Work environment.** Physically demanding work can cause fatigue and affect access to a quality diet and the choices of foods consumed. When time pressure makes it difficult to prepare and eat healthy food during a short lunch break, some workers may rely on convenience foods to save time.
- **Cooking methods and food storage.** Water-soluble vitamins, especially vitamin C, folic acid, and thiamin, can be destroyed with boiling. Steaming is a better cooking method to preserve nutrients. Heat, light, moisture, air, and alkalinity reduce the longevity of vitamins in food. The fresher the food is, the richer the vitamin quality.
- **Oral contraceptive use.** This method of family planning lowers the serum level of vitamin C and several B vitamins, as well as some minerals, such as magnesium and zinc. Patients with poor-quality nutrient intake may need vitamin supplements (Fenasse & McEwen, 2019; Maduforo et al., 2016).
- **Food to relieve stress.** Food is commonly used to cope with stress, depression, loneliness, or boredom. Skipping meals, binge eating, or consuming too much of a single food (e.g., snack foods, chocolate) can result in poor nutrition, obesity, and low self-esteem.
- **Tobacco use.** Smokers use their stores of vitamin C, an antioxidant, faster than nonsmokers. The more a person smokes, the more vitamin is lost. Low levels of vitamin C also are linked to iron deficiency. Vitamin C could provide some protection against tobacco-related lung damage. Smoking cessation is best, but if the person cannot

quit, a vitamin C supplement (2,000 mg/day) offers an antioxidant effect to reduce damage to the lungs (Aghdassi et al., 1999; Ekenedilichukwu et al., 2018; Gupta et al., 2016; Preston et al., 2003).

- **Alcohol.** Heavy alcohol use often leads to excessive caloric intake, contributing to overweight and obesity. In addition, alcohol significantly decreases the rate of fat metabolism. Excessive alcohol use interferes with adequate nutrition by (1) replacing the food in the person's diet, (2) depressing the appetite, (3) decreasing the absorption of nutrients by its toxic effects on the intestinal mucosa, and (4) impairing the storage of nutrients. People who use alcohol heavily need multivitamin supplements, especially B vitamins and folic acid.
- **Caffeine.** Many of our accepted beliefs about the danger and benefits of coffee are myths. Coffee does not create a risk for dehydration, heart disease, or cancer and has little role in hypertension. Caffeine may be associated with bone loss; however, its negative effect can be offset by a small amount of milk. In high doses, it can sometimes cause anxiety and stomach upset. Moderate caffeine consumption (200 mg/day or less) can boost mood and mental and physical performance. It aids the ability to burn fat for fuel instead of carbohydrates and has been linked to a lower risk of Parkinson disease, type 2 diabetes, stroke, liver and endometrial cancer, and dementia (Ding et al., 2014).

Vegetarianism

People choose vegetarian diets for many reasons. Ethical considerations related to the humane treatment of animals also cause some people to adopt a vegetarian diet. However, many people adopt a vegetarian diet simply as a health choice, noting the abundant research indicating that vegetarianism reduces the risk of cardiovascular disease, obesity, diabetes, and various forms of cancer (e.g., colon, stomach, lung, breast, esophageal). A vegetarian diet is rich in fiber, thereby promoting bowel motility and preventing constipation.

Types of Vegetarian Diets All vegetarian diets exclude red meat and poultry but vary in the foods they include and exclude.

- A **lacto-ovo vegetarian** diet excludes meat, fish, and poultry. Dairy products and fish are included.
- **Lacto-vegetarians** consume only dairy and plant-based foods.
- A **pescatarian** diet does not allow meat, poultry, dairy, or eggs but does include fish.
- **Vegans** eat only foods of plant origin.
- **Fruitarians** only consume fruits, nuts, honey, and vegetable oils.

Obtaining Nutrients Soybeans, soy milk, tofu, and processed protein products can be used by all except

fruitarians to enhance the nutritional value of the diet. Although ovo-lacto vegetarians do not have a higher rate of nutrient deficiencies than the meat-eating population, they must choose foods carefully to include enough of the following nutrients:

- **Vitamin B_{12}** is found only in animal products, such as eggs and milk. Vegans must eat foods fortified with B_{12} or take B_{12} supplements. Long-standing B_{12} deficiency can result in severe and irreversible neurological impairment.
- **Vitamin D** may be inadequately supplied by vegetarian diets, so vitamin D–fortified foods or supplements should be included. Soy milk and dairy milk are usually vitamin D fortified. Adequate sun exposure also helps to compensate for a lack of dietary intake.
- **Iron.** The iron from plant foods is not absorbed as well as that from animal sources. However, iron is easier to absorb when it is eaten with foods containing vitamin C, so eating fruit or vegetables containing vitamin C with meals helps to compensate.
- **Calcium.** Vegans, especially, may find it difficult to obtain enough dietary calcium. It is important to include fortified nut and oat milk and calcium-rich vegetables (e.g., kale, broccoli). Calcium-fortified cereals are also available. This is especially important for the growth of vegan children and women who are pregnant or lactating.
- **Zinc.** Normally found in beef and chicken, zinc is also readily available from various seed and bean sources, such as pumpkin, sesame, squash, and watermelon seeds; wheat; chickpeas (hummus); wheat germ; dark chocolate; and garlic.
- **Protein** needs can be met through a diet that includes a variety of plant foods to supply adequate amounts of essential amino acids, such as beans and peas, nuts, and soy products (e.g., tofu) (FDA, n.d.-b) Complementary proteins should be eaten throughout the day, but careful meal-by-meal balance of amino acids is usually not necessary. Review Table 24-1 and the discussion of complete and incomplete proteins earlier in the chapter.

Client Resources To ensure adequate nutrients, it may be wise for vegetarians to consult a qualified nutrition professional, especially during periods of growth, breastfeeding, pregnancy, or recovery from illness. For recommended servings of vegetarian food groups, see MyVeganPlate (Fig. 24-3). This is presented in a similar manner to the ChooseMyPlate.gov nutritional guidelines. MyVeganPlate includes recommendations for food from each food group for those following a vegetarian diet.

Eating for Health and Athletic Performance

In recent decades, the consumption of processed foods, grains, and beverages—which include *trans*-fats, preservatives, and chemical additives—has been linked to

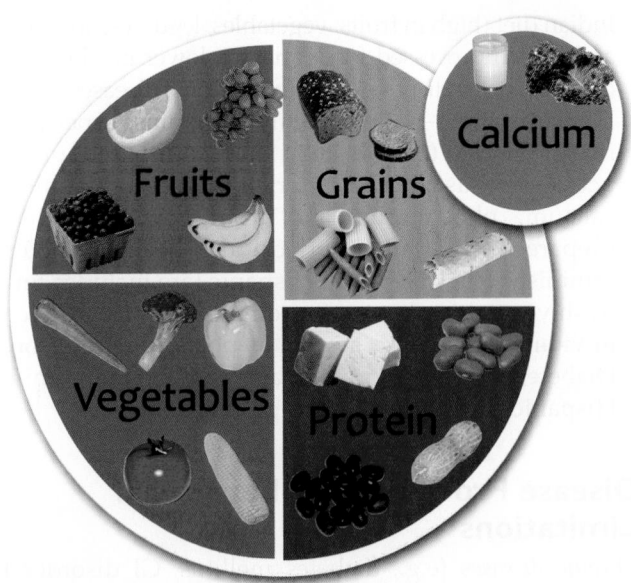

FIGURE 24-3 MyVeganPlate. Nutrition guide for vegetarians.

type 2 diabetes and obesity, heart disease, and cancer. The consumption of organic foods may reduce exposure to pesticide residues and antibiotic-resistant bacteria (Smith-Spangler et al., 2012).

A diet high in meats and fish, fresh fruits and vegetables, nuts and seeds, eggs, and other natural whole foods is biologically healthier than the modern diet. Proponents of the Paleolithic (paleo) diet advocate returning to a "caveman" diet for improved health, nutrition, and athletic performance. Foods to avoid in the paleo diet include all processed foods, grains containing gluten, dairy, refined sugar, legumes, potatoes, processed oils, and caffeine.

Eating for Weight Loss

Many diets, including the Dietary Approaches to Stop Hypertension (DASH) diet, the American Heart Association diet, and others, are nutritionally sound, but many others are fad diets. You can recognize fad diets by the following characteristics. They:

- Promise quick and dramatic weight loss, which is usually only temporary because it results from the loss of body fluids.
- Limit the range of foods from which the dieter can select (e.g., only fruits and vegetables for the first week), leading to an imbalance in nutrients.
- Often recommend the purchase of supplements and/or specially packaged meals; in many cases, these are brands that they endorse or produce.
- Fail to include practical strategies that help dieters permanently change eating and activity patterns.

Individuals who follow such diets often revert to their former eating habits and regain the weight soon after achieving their weight-loss goal.

In contrast, more moderate calorie-restriction diets, such as the American Heart Association diet, have the following characteristics:

- Describe food selection and preparation tips and other behavior modifications that can lead to slow, sustained weight loss.
- Promote a diet that includes a variety of food choices and a balance of nutrients.
- Encourage healthy habits (e.g., physical activity, sleep, reduced stress) as a cornerstone of weight loss.
- Emphasize self-monitoring, cognitive strategies, and behavior modification.

Ethnic, Cultural, and Religious Practices

Religion and culture can have a major impact on diet and lifestyle (see Chapters 12 and 13).

- **Language barriers** may make it difficult for a client to understand nutritional information. For those patients, simple visual aids may be useful.
- **Ethnic/cultural food choices** often reflect the foods that are plentiful in the region of origin (e.g., fish in coastal communities), as well as foods that are readily grown in the native soil.
- **Food preservation needs** influence some diets. For instance, people from various geographic regions without accessible refrigeration eat salted meats and dried fruits and cook with spices to combat microbes.
- **Certain religions** may require fasting or abstaining from certain foods. For example, some Roman Catholics don't eat meat on certain days of the religious calendar; kosher dietary laws prohibit eating pork.
- **Obesity is more common in some ethnic groups.** For example, rates of obesity have been increasing the fastest among non-Hispanic Black people (49.6%), followed by Hispanic people (44.8%), non-Hispanic Whites (42.2%), and non-Hispanic Asians (17.4%) (CDC, 2021, June 7; Hales et al., 2020).
- **Cultural beliefs, perceptions, and attitudes about weight** often may not match those of health providers. Certain cultures may place value on different body types.

Traditional Diets The traditional diets of many cultures are healthful and should not be discouraged; in fact, contemporary adaptations made to these diets may compromise their nutritional quality.

- **Mediterranean diet**—Rich in olive oil, fish, fruits, vegetables, and nuts and low in dairy foods, processed foods, saturated fats, and red meat; includes a glass of red wine per day. Linked to weight loss and a reduced risk of death due to cancer, coronary artery disease, hypertension, and high blood cholesterol (American Heart Association, 2020; Estruch et al., 2013; Panagiotakos, 2014; Salas-Salvado et al., 2011).
- **Asian diet**—A plant-based diet high in fiber, vitamins and minerals, and antioxidants and low in dietary

fat. The diet consists of rice, fresh fruit (e.g., melons, bananas, tangerines), cabbage, and green leafy vegetables. Protein intake primarily consists of beans, nuts, and seeds, with occasional poultry, shellfish, and eggs. The health benefits of this diet include a lower incidence of cardiovascular disease, diabetes, colon cancer, and obesity. Green and black teas contain antioxidants that may lower the risk of cancer. On the other hand, a diet with white rice as a staple is a high-glycemic-index diet, which can contribute to insulin resistance (obesity and type 2 diabetes) (Chan et al., 2009). In recent years, there has been an influx of sugar and unhealthy oils added to traditional cooking and food preparation methods.

- **Indian diet**—The traditional diet contains fresh, home-cooked foods containing a wide array of spices. Meat selection is based on religious preference (e.g., traditionally, people who are Muslim don't eat pork, people who are Hindu aren't permitted to eat beef, and people who are Buddhist are vegetarian). People who eat a traditional Indian diet (high in fruits, vegetables, legumes, and nuts and low in processed foods) have a lower incidence of diabetes, heart disease, and other chronic diseases.

- **Hispanic diet**—Relies heavily on grains, especially rice; legumes (e.g., beans); and corn-based products. Beans, as a staple, are rich in fiber, B vitamins, calcium, phosphorus, and iron; however, when prepared with lard (refried), the health benefits diminish. The traditional Hispanic fare includes few fresh vegetables, except for tomatoes, which are rich in vitamins A and C, as well as potassium and iron. Diabetes type 2 is more prevalent among non–White Hispanics because of their high rate of obesity.

Disease Processes and Functional Limitations

Chronic diseases (e.g., diabetes mellitus, GI disorders) can alter nutrient intake, digestion, absorption, use, and excretion. *Any illness,* especially when accompanied by

Toward Evidence-Based Practice

De Cabo, R., & Mattson, M. P. (2019, December 26). Effects of intermittent fasting on health, aging, and disease. *New England Journal of Medicine, 381*(26), 2541–2551. https://doi.org/10.1056/NEJMra1905136

Evidence supports intermittent fasting, which is limiting food intake within a 6-hour period and fasting for 18 hours, as a method to trigger a metabolic switch from glucose-based to ketone-based energy. The result of this altered metabolism is increased stress resistance, increased longevity, and a reduced incidence of diseases, including cancer and obesity.

Mohorko, N., Cernelic-Bizjak, M., Poklar-Vatovec, T., Grom, G., Kenig, S., Petelin, A., & Jenko-Pražnikar, Z. (2019, February). Weight loss, improved physical performance, cognitive function, eating behavior, and metabolic profile in a 12-week ketogenic diet in obese adults. *Nutrition Research, 62,* 64–77. https://doi.org/10.1016/j.nutres.2018.11.007

In a study involving sedentary obese adults following a ketogenic diet for 12 weeks, researchers found various significant weight loss, reduced appetite, less emotional eating behavior, improved body image satisfaction, and improved physical performance. Laboratory values for blood glucose and insulin, low-density lipoprotein cholesterol, and adiponectin improved with implementation of the 12-week ketogenic diet.

Wachsmuth, N. B., Aberer, F., Haupt, S., Schierbauer, J. R., Zimmer, R. T., Eckstein, M. L., Zunner, B., Schmidt, W., Niedrist, T., Sourij, H., & Moser, O. (2022, January 18). The impact of high-carbohydrate/low fat vs. low-carbohydrate on performance and body composition in physically active adults: A cross-over controlled trial. *Nutrition, 14*(3), 423. https://doi.org/10.3390/nu14030423

In a study examining the effects of consumption of a high-carbohydrate (HC) diet compared with a low-carbohydrate (LC) diet, 24 physically active, nonobese adults were given each diet over a 3-week period. After a 3-week period of rest, those studied switched to the opposite diet for another 3 weeks. Physiological indicators showed higher physical performance and a longer time to exhaustion in the HC-diet consumers. Both groups experienced a significant reduction in body mass and fat mass but not in skeletal muscle mass. Resting metabolic rate was not different between the groups. The HC diet led to a significant reduction in total and low-density lipoprotein cholesterol, whereas triglycerides significantly increased.

1. You are planning nutritional interventions for your client with obesity who is seeking a healthful dietary plan for weight loss. Which of these studies support an approach you might recommend? Why?

2. In counseling this client, what other recommendations might you make to reduce body fat while preserving muscle mass? Explain your thinking.

3. Discuss barriers to adhering to each of the approaches (ketogenic, low-fat diet, low-carbohydrate diet, intermittent fasting). What dietary strategy would you advise your client to consider to improve success?

fever, increases the need for protein, water, and kcal to meet the demands of increased metabolism. A variety of other physical and psychological disorders and/or their treatments can adversely affect a client's nutrition:

- **Traumatic injury** (e.g., burns, surgery) requires extra protein and vitamin C for wound healing and tissue rebuilding.
- **Long-term insufficient calorie intake** (e.g., patients with cancer) causes *protein-calorie malnutrition,* which is characterized by weight loss and muscle wasting.
- **Alcoholism.** Poor appetite, common in alcoholism, results in a reduced intake of nutritious food. Alcohol can also interfere with the function of some vitamins.
- **Cognitive function.** A person with a developmental delay, severe mental illness, head trauma, confusion, or memory loss may be unable to remember what, when, or whether they have eaten. Cognitive dysfunction contributes to poor decision making for healthy selections.
- Ability to Obtain and Prepare Food.
    Paralysis or hemiplegia (e.g., from a stroke and other medical and physical conditions) can cause functional limitations and impaired mobility, limiting the ability to shop for and prepare food.
    Social factors may also limit the ability to purchase food. People with limited income may be forced to choose between buying food or paying for medication or household utilities.
    A person with severe dyspnea or *fatigue* may not have the stamina or time to prepare a nutritious meal. Instead, they may eat prepared foods that are high in sodium. Dyspnea and fatigue are associated with chronic obstructive pulmonary disease (COPD), advanced chronic disease, severe anemia, pregnancy, depression, and excess work.
- **Chewing and swallowing.** Decayed or missing teeth and ill-fitting dentures make chewing difficult. The person often resorts to eating only soft foods or liquids, many of which lack fiber. Acute disorders affecting the throat, such as pharyngitis, make swallowing painful. Oral cancer and esophageal strictures also make swallowing painful or difficult and frequently lead to the avoidance of food.
- **Stomach function.** Heartburn, indigestion, and other stomach disorders are common. People may eat only bland foods or avoid certain foods to prevent the pain or burning sensation that follows eating.
- **Peristalsis.** The wavelike action that propels food through the intestinal tract is called **peristalsis.** Bowel inflammation or infection, diverticula (outpouchings of the intestine), or tumors may increase peristalsis, thereby decreasing the absorption of nutrients. In addition, high stress levels may either speed or slow transit time. If peristalsis is slow, the stomach may not empty properly (gastroparesis). This could lead to early satiety, nausea, or vomiting and affect nutrient intake.

- **Intestinal surface area.** When the amount of intestinal surface area is diminished by surgery or disease, the absorption of nutrients is decreased. This may result in malnutrition even though the patient is consuming adequate calories and protein.
- **Enzyme secretion.** Liver, gallbladder, or pancreas problems affect the secretion of digestive enzymes. Lactose intolerance is prevalent in the United States and worldwide, primarily among people of Native American, Black, and Asian descent (National Institute of Diabetes and Digestive and Kidney Diseases, 2018).
- **Bariatric surgery** alters digestion to achieve rapid weight loss.
    Restrictive procedures (sleeve gastrectomy, adjustable gastric banding) limit the stomach's capacity to hold food and reduce the time of passage through the GI tract.
    Malabsorption surgeries (intestinal bypass) are done to impair the uptake of food nutrients and fats. A combined approach uses stomach restriction and a partial bypass of the small intestine.
    Bariatric weight-loss procedures increase the risk of nutrient deficiency, especially iron, copper, zinc, selenium, thiamine, folate, and vitamins B_{12} and D.

Medications

In addition to the direct effects of diseases and disorders, nutrition may be affected by the drugs and therapies used to treat them, as in the following examples:

- **Some medications directly decrease appetite,** for example, dextroamphetamine (Adderall), aspirin, diphenhydramine (e.g., Benadryl), and lithium carbonate (e.g., Lithobid).
- **Chemotherapy and radiation therapy** may cause oral ulcers, intestinal bleeding, or diarrhea—which interfere with eating and absorbing nutrients from food.
- **Certain drugs alter nutrient metabolism;** some increase or decrease nutrient excretion, whereas others may also alter taste, resulting in changes in overall nutrient intake.
- **A drug may affect specific nutrients.** For example, acetylsalicylic acid (aspirin) decreases folate levels and increases the excretion of vitamin C, laxatives may cause calcium and potassium depletion, and thiazide diuretics decrease the absorption of vitamin B_{12}.
- Almost all oral medications have the potential to cause nausea or vomiting, thereby decreasing appetite.

KnowledgeCheck 24-6

- List at least three nutrients that may be more difficult to supply through a vegetarian diet.
- When selecting a program for weight loss, what factors should a person consider?
- Why should you encourage clients from various cultures to follow their traditional diets?
- Describe the effects on nutrition of (1) tobacco and (2) heavy alcohol use.

Special Diets

Many people must follow a modified diet to assist in managing their illness. In addition, all inpatients at healthcare facilities must have a diet prescribed by their primary care provider. The following sections cover the most prescribed diets.

Regular Diet A regular diet, also called the "house diet," is appropriate for clients without special nutritional needs. This diet is a balanced meal plan that supplies 2,000 kcal per day. Many facilities provide vegetarian and ethnic variations. Typically, inpatients choose each meal from a list of menu choices.

Have you ever heard someone complain that hospital food is bland? There is some justification for that complaint. House diets must accommodate the varied tastes of all patients, so they are usually lightly seasoned. Selections are limited to avoid unpopular items and restrict fatty, fried, or gas-producing foods, which many patients tolerate poorly. However, you should refrain from making negative comments to patients about the food.

NPO *NPO* means no food or fluid (including water) by mouth. This may be ordered before surgery or an invasive procedure to limit the risk of aspiration. A common example is "NPO after midnight." Most well-nourished, well-hydrated patients easily tolerate short-term NPO status. However, no one can tolerate prolonged periods of NPO. IV fluids may be given to provide hydration, and clients who must remain NPO for a lengthy period need enteral (through a stomach tube) or parenteral (IV) nutrition to prevent nutritional deficiency.

Diets Modified by Consistency Patients undergoing surgery, bowel procedures, or acute illness may, for a short period of time, need a diet modified by consistency (see Table 24-5). Patients with chronic health concerns that affect their ability to chew or swallow (e.g., Impaired Dentition and Impaired Swallowing) may need long-term changes in the consistency of their diet.

Diets Modified for Disease Some health conditions require modification of dietary intake. The following are the most common diets:

- **Calorie-restricted**—For clients requiring weight reduction.
- **Sodium-restricted**—For clients with hypertension, Ménière's disease (inner ear problem), or fluid-balance problems.
- **Fat-restricted**—For clients with elevated cholesterol or triglyceride levels; may also be prescribed for general weight loss.
- **Diabetic**—To manage calories and carbohydrate intake for clients with diabetes mellitus.
- **Renal diet**—To manage electrolytes and fluid for clients with renal insufficiency.
- **Protein-controlled diet**—To manage liver and kidney disease.
- **Ketogenic diet**—To treat difficult-to-control epileptic seizures in children. Effective for weight loss and insulin

Table 24-5 ➤ Diets Modified by Consistency

DIET DESCRIPTION AND FOODS INCLUDED	COMMENTS
Clear Liquids. Provides fluids to prevent dehydration and supplies some simple carbohydrates to help meet energy needs. *Foods:* Water, tea, coffee, broth, clear juice (usually apple, grape, or cranberry juice), popsicles, carbonated beverages, and gelatin.	■ Does not supply adequate calories, protein, and other nutrients, so timely progression to more nutritious diets is recommended. ■ If clear liquids are required for more than 3 days, commercial clear liquid supplements are usually prescribed.
Full Liquids. Contains all the liquids included in the clear liquid diet plus any food items that are liquid at room temperature. *Foods:* Add to clear liquid diet: soups, milk, milkshakes, puddings, custards, juices, some hot cereals, and yogurt.	■ Difficult to obtain a balanced diet on a full-liquid plan; use for a short time only. ■ If needed for a longer time, a professional dietitian should be involved in planning of the diet. ■ High-calorie, high-protein supplements are often added.
Mechanical Soft Diet. The diet of choice for people with chewing difficulties resulting from missing teeth, jaw problems, or extensive fatigue. *Foods:* Add to the full-liquid diet: soft vegetables and fruits; chopped, ground, or shredded meat; and breads, pastries, eggs, and cheese.	■ This diet can supply a full range of nutrients but is quite low in fiber. As a result, constipation is a risk. ■ Many food items can be added to this diet by cooking them extensively or blending or grinding to alter their texture.
Pureed Diet. A pureed diet is a blended diet. Some foods may or may not be excluded.	Liquids are often added to the food to create a texture that may be scooped onto serving plates.

control and may have a role in treating cancer and neurological disorders (e.g., migraines, Alzheimer).

- **Antigen-avoidance diets**—For clients allergic to or intolerant of certain foods.

  Gluten-free diet for clients with celiac disease.

  Low-FODMAP diet; FODMAP stands for *fermentable, oligosaccharides, disaccharides, monosaccharides,* and *polyoils.* This type of dietary meal plan may be used to ease digestive symptoms (e.g., pain, bloating, diarrhea) related to irritable bowel syndrome (IBS) or other GI disorders.

- **Calorie-protein push**—Used when there is a need to heal wounds, maintain or increase weight, or promote growth. If the person cannot consume enough kcal by adding fats and proteins to their regular diet, high-calorie, high-protein supplements may be used.

 ThinkLike a Nurse 24-5: Clinical Judgment in Action

Analyze the following diets. Which nutrients are missing or difficult to obtain from these diets?

- Clear liquid
- Full liquid

PracticalKnowledge knowing **how**

Good nutrition is essential for health and disease management. In the rest of this chapter, you will learn about assessing nutritional status and diagnosing and planning care for common nutrition problems.

More than just a physical necessity, nutrition also has emotional associations. We eat when we are hungry, but we also eat for pleasure because the food tastes good! Food has become a part of most social events and activities. A certain food may symbolize one's cultural or religious affiliation or even be a political statement. When supporting patients' nutritional needs, it is wise to keep in mind that personal beliefs, habits, and preferences are as important as nutritional knowledge in determining what a person eats.

ASSESSMENT/RECOGNIZING CUES

There are two kinds of nutritional assessments: (1) screening assessments and (2) thorough, focused nutritional assessments. Usually, you will perform a screening examination. If you identify nutritional risk factors, you then perform a focused nutritional assessment.

HOW DO I SCREEN CLIENTS FOR NUTRITIONAL PROBLEMS?

Key Point: *All hospitalized patients, especially those with obesity and patients at risk for nutritional deficiency, should receive a nutritional screening support*

plan within 48 hours of inpatient admission (Choban et al.; American Society for Parenteral and Enteral Nutrition, 2013). **Cursory screening** consists of the evaluation of height, weight, and BMI, coupled with a brief dietary history.

Clients who are found to have risk factors should be evaluated more fully with one or more of the following methods:

- *The subjective global assessment (SGA)* is a commonly used screening method that makes use of information from the overall medical history and physical examination to evaluate a client's nutritional status.

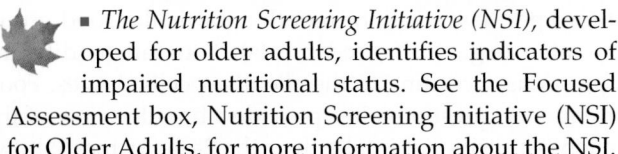 - *The Nutrition Screening Initiative (NSI),* developed for older adults, identifies indicators of impaired nutritional status. See the Focused Assessment box, Nutrition Screening Initiative (NSI) for Older Adults, for more information about the NSI.

 - *The Mini Nutritional Assessment (MNA),* developed for older adults, can be used with clients of all ages (DiMaria-Ghalili & Guenter, 2008). It is a quick and easy method for identifying clients with nutritional risks or malnutrition. The first part screens for nutritional risk. The second part is completed only if the person is found to be at risk. The total of both parts determines whether malnutrition exists and requires multidisciplinary follow-up.

For more information and to see the screening tools for the SGA, NSI, and MNA,

 Go to Chapter 24, **Screening for Nutritional Problems,** in Volume 2.

FOCUSED NUTRITIONAL ASSESSMENT

If screening reveals nutritional problems, perform a more thorough, focused nutritional assessment to evaluate the client. It is especially important to assess nutritional status in older clients carefully to ensure that you detect marginal deficiencies before major problems occur. The nutrition component of a focused nutritional assessment includes both subjective (history) and objective (physical examination) data.

Go to Chapter 27, **Focused Nutritional Assessment,** in Volume 2.

Dietary History

You can obtain a dietary history during any routine assessment. Whether you use a self-administered form or an interview, you will collect general information on the client's basic eating habits, food attitudes and preferences, cultural factors, and use of dietary supplements. A dietary history creates a picture of the client's food habits and eating behaviors. To collect detailed data on what the client is eating, ask them to keep a food diary. Three types of food diaries are described next.

24-Hour Recall A 24-hour recall requires the client to name all foods eaten within a day. Simply ask questions such as "Yesterday, what did you eat for breakfast/lunch/dinner/snacks?" A 24-hour recall is simple; however, the accuracy of the data may be questionable because some people have difficulty remembering all they ate the previous day, and any single day may be atypical. Sometimes, a family member can help the client recall intake more accurately, particularly when the client is ill.

Food Frequency Questionnaire A food frequency questionnaire asks the client to identify the number of times per day, week, or month a particular food group is eaten (e.g., fruits, red meats). You can modify the questions according to the client's specific issues. Food frequency questionnaires provide a broader view of the client's nutritional intake than the 24-hour recall; however, accuracy may still be a problem.

Food Record A food record is the most accurate food diary. It provides information on the quantity and the types of foods eaten. You ask the client in advance to keep a record of measured and weighed amounts of all foods they eat in a 7-day period. From the detailed information collected, you can analyze the total kcal and nutrient content for the recorded period. Although the food record provides meaningful results, it requires cognitive and psychomotor skills that not all clients have. It also requires commitment to the process for 7 days, which may be difficult for some people. You might remind some patients that there are Web sites and apps that can help with journaling their diets and tracking nutritional intake, goals, weight management, and so on.

Physical Examination

You should correlate physical examination findings with other assessments, such as nutritional and medical history, dietary intake, anthropometric measurements, and laboratory results. Refer to Chapter 19 as needed for a review of physical examination techniques. For guidelines in performing a nutrition-focused physical examination,

 Go to Chapter 24, **Focused Assessment: Nutritional Assessment,** in Volume 2.

Assessing Body Composition

You will use **anthropometric measurements** when assessing body composition (the proportion of fat in the body). These are noninvasive physical examination techniques to determine body dimensions such as height and weight. Anthropometric measurements are used to:

- Assess growth rate in children.
- Indirectly assess adults' protein and fat stores.
- Assess overweight, obesity, and underweight.

To obtain accurate data, you must use standardized equipment and procedures and compare the data with existing reference standards for men and women. **Key Point:** *Body weight measurement alone is insufficient for assessing body composition.*

Skinfold Measurements

Approximately half of body fat is located subcutaneously. Therefore, skinfold thickness provides an estimate of a person's body fat content. It reveals information about current nutritional status as well as long-term changes in fat stores. For specific instructions on measuring skinfold thickness, see Clinical Insight 24-1.

Circumferences

Another method of estimating the percentage of body fat is to use girth, or circumference, measurements.

- The *midupper arm circumference* is routinely measured as part of screening.
- The *abdominal circumference,* measured at the iliac crest, is a simple and inexpensive method to assess body fat distribution. This method is highly accurate and should accompany the BMI measurement for assessing adiposity. Abdominal girth helps to estimate **visceral fat,** which forms around the organs. A high level of abdominal fat is associated with an increased risk for hypertension, type 2 diabetes, heart disease and high blood pressure (WHO, 2008), high cholesterol, and Alzheimer disease.
- The *waist-to-hip ratio (WHR)* can indicate obesity by estimating abdominal fat. It is calculated as follows:
  waist circumference (in.) ÷ hip circumference (in.) = WHR
  Example: Robert's waist measurement is 42 inches, and his hip measurement is 45 inches. His WHR is 42 ÷ 45 = 0.93.

The deposition of body fat varies depending on sex, reproductive status (pregnancy), age, and ethnicity. For instance, people of Asian descent typically have a lower WHR than other demographic groups (Amad et al., 2016). Men have a higher ratio than women. A WHR of greater than 0.90 in men and greater than 0.85 in women indicates obesity (WHO, 2008, p. 27).

For specific instructions on measuring midupper arm circumference and WHR, see Clinical Insight 24-1.

KnowledgeCheck 24-7

- What are the most reliable locations for skinfold measurement?
- What are the implications of an increased WHR?

Body Mass Index

BMI is another method of assessing body composition. It is a simple index of the weight-to-height ratio that is commonly used to classify weight in adults (WHO, 1995,

2000, 2004). It can be precisely measured using scanning devices that measure bioelectrical impedance—the conduction of a harmless electrical charge through the client's body. Lean tissue readily conducts the charge, whereas adipose tissue does not.

BMI is computed by taking weight in kilograms (kg) and dividing by the square of the height in meters (m²) (Box 24-3). You may also consult tables with precalculated values based on height and weight (National Heart, Lung, and Blood Institute, n.d.). For an example of a height and weight BMI table, see Procedure 19-1: Performing the General Survey in Volume 2. You can also find BMI calculators on the CDC and National Heart Lung and Blood Institute Web sites.

The normal BMI for adults ranges from 18.5 to 24.9 (although this may vary slightly among professional organizations). The usefulness of BMI values is limited for:

- Athletes—because of their larger muscle mass.
- Pregnant and postpartum women—because they have a higher fluid composition.
- Older adults—values are often inaccurate because adults lose height with age. They are typically less active and lose muscle mass. Because BMI is calculated based on height and weight, the index can be a less sensitive measure of weight status.

Despite these limitations, BMI is generally useful in identifying underweight and obese individuals.

BOX 24-3 ■ Calculating Body Mass Index (BMI)

BMI = weight in kilograms ÷ (height in meters)²

Example:

Robert weighs 165 lb. Convert his weight to kilograms:

165 ÷ 2.2 = 75 kg

He is 71 in. tall. Convert his height to meters.

1 m = 39.37 in.

Divide 71 in. by 39.37 in.; he is 1.8 m tall (rounded off)

His BMI is 75 kg ÷ (1.8)² = 23.

The normal BMI (adults) ranges from 18.5 to 24.9.

Classification of Body Mass Index Values

Classification	BMI (kg/m²)
Underweight	<18.5
Healthy weight	18.5–24.9
Overweight	25.0–29.9
Obese class I	30.0–34.9
Obese class II	35.0–39.9
Obese class III	>40.0

Source: Adapted from World Health Organization (2006); National Heart, Lung and Blood Institute (n.d.).

KnowledgeCheck 24-8
- What is the most accurate type of food diary?
- Compare and contrast four nutritional screening approaches: cursory screening, subjective global assessment, Mini Nutritional Assessment, and Nutrition Screening Initiative.
- Identify three nutritional risk factors.

 ThinkLike a Nurse 24-6: Clinical Judgment in Action

1. Calculate your waist-to-hip ratio (WHR).
2. Use Box 24-3 to calculate your BMI. Evaluate the result.
   - How useful are these data?
   - Do you feel you need to pursue a program of weight loss? Why or why not?

Underwater Weighing

Hydrodensitometry, or underwater weighing, is another method of determining body composition. It requires total submersion of the patient in a tank of water. Because fat readily floats, the person's buoyancy will vary depending on their percentage of body fat. This method is considered the gold standard for body composition measures. However, clinical use of this method is limited because it is impractical to use with children, older adults, or individuals who are severely ill.

What Physical Examination Findings Are Cues to Nutrient Imbalance?

To detect nutritional abnormalities, such as diabetes, you should assess and correlate physical findings, lifestyle, nutritional and medical history, dietary intake, anthropometric measurements, and laboratory testing. Refer to Chapter 19 as needed for a review of physical examination techniques. For guidelines in performing a nutrition-focused physical examination, see the Focused Assessment box, Nutritional Assessment.

 Go to Chapter 24, Focused Assessment 24-3: Nutritional Assessment in Volume 2.

KnowledgeCheck 24-9
- Identify at least 10 physical examination findings that would lead you to suspect nutritional problems.
- What factors would lead to poor wound healing?

What Laboratory Values Reflect Nutritional Status?

Various laboratory or biochemical indicators provide information about nutritional status. These include blood glucose, serum protein level and associated indices, total lymphocyte count, and hemoglobin. To see the norms for these laboratory tests, see the Diagnostic Testing box, Tests Reflecting Nutritional Status: Norms.

Blood Glucose

The blood glucose level indicates the amount of fuel available for cellular energy.

- **Levels above normal** trigger the release of insulin, which causes the glucose to move into body cells and to be stored in the liver and muscles.
- **Levels below normal** signal for the release of glucagon, leading to the release of glucose from storage.

Hypoglycemia (blood glucose of less than 50 mg/dL) limits the fuel supply to the body, resulting in symptoms ranging from weakness to coma. The cause is often insufficient food intake, excessive physical exertion, or a disproportionate number of hypoglycemic agents.

Hyperglycemia (blood glucose greater than 109 mg/dL fasting or greater than 127 mg/dL at random) may be a sign of diabetes mellitus, an endocrine problem, which may develop because of either insufficient insulin production or resistance to the existing supply of insulin (Box 24-4). A characteristic of diabetes is that although there is more than enough glucose in the blood, it cannot enter and be used by the cells. Repeated blood glucose measurements are required before diagnosing diabetes mellitus because glucose levels may be temporarily elevated due to excessive carbohydrate intake or emotional and physical stressors.

- **Symptoms and sequelae.** A rise in blood sugar may produce weakness or fatigue. Prolonged elevations

lead to weight loss, blurred vision, **polyphagia** (excessive hunger), **polydipsia** (excessive thirst), increased urination, **ketosis** (metabolism of fat due to inability to use carbohydrates as fuel), renal failure, and **peripheral neuropathy** (damage to nerves due to prolonged exposure to high glucose levels).

- **Monitoring.** Patients with diabetes usually monitor their own blood sugar levels, but you may need to do it for some. Usually this is done by a fingerstick to obtain capillary blood for testing. Some glucometers can use blood from alternative sites, such as the upper arm, forearm, base of the thumb, or thigh. Other types of monitors include the following:

   Disposable sensor, placed just under the skin. The sensor communicates with a receiver that reads the levels.

   Sensor, worn like a watch, pulls tiny amounts of fluid from the skin without puncturing it.

For complete fingerstick steps,

Go to Chapter 24, **Procedure 24-1: Checking Fingerstick (Capillary) Blood Glucose Levels** in Volume 2.

Serum Protein Levels and Other Laboratory Indices

Protein molecules dissolve in blood to form plasma proteins. Tissue proteins are a combination of albumin and globulin, so serum protein levels are indicators of **protein stores**.

- **Albumin** is synthesized in the liver and constitutes 60% of total body protein. Low levels of albumin are associated with malnutrition; malabsorption; acute and chronic liver disease; and repeated loss of protein through burns, wounds, or other sources. The half-life of albumin is 18 to 21 days. As a result, there is a lag in detecting nutritional problems based on serum albumin. Albumin is also affected by fluid status and, therefore, is not an accurate measure in the patient with fluid imbalance. For example, a patient with positive fluid balance (taking in more than excreted) will have a falsely low albumin level.
- The **prealbumin** level fluctuates daily and is considered a better marker of acute change than albumin.
- **Transferrin** is a protein that binds with iron. Because it has a half-life of only 8 to 9 days, it allows for faster detection of protein depletion than does measuring albumin. Transferrin can be measured directly or indirectly (by a total iron-binding capacity test [TIBC]). It also reflects iron status. In a person with iron deficiency, the TIBC will be increased; in a person with anemia, the TIBC will be decreased.

Other markers are used to monitor protein metabolism:

- **Urea** is formed in the liver as a by-product of protein metabolism and is excreted through the kidneys. As such, the serum blood urea nitrogen (BUN) level is

---

BOX 24-4 ■ When to Assess for Diabetes

- Adults with body mass index (BMI) > 25
- Physical inactivity
- High-risk ethnicity for obesity (e.g., Native Americans, Alaskan Natives)
- First-degree relative with diabetes
- Women diagnosed with gestational diabetes during pregnancy or who have delivered a baby weighing more than 9 lb
- Hemoglobin A_{1c} >5.7% (test for glucose control over a 2- to 3-month period)
- High-density lipoprotein (HDL) cholesterol < 35 mg/dL and/or triglyceride > 250 mg/dL
- History of cardiovascular disease and/or hypertension
- Physical signs indicating low blood sugar (sweating, shakiness, anxiety, confusion, irritability, dizziness, difficulty speaking, lethargy, or loss of consciousness)
- Physical signs indicating high blood sugar (flushed skin, confusion, weakness, labored breathing, sweet or fruity breath, nausea, loss of consciousness)
- Clinical conditions associated with insulin resistance (e.g., foot ulcers that are slow to heal)

If diabetes testing is normal, the American Diabetes Association (2019) recommends repeat evaluation every 3 years or more frequently, depending on risk factors.

an indicator of liver and kidney function. An elevated BUN level is seen with impaired kidney function, dehydration, excessive protein breakdown (often seen with diabetes mellitus, hyperthyroidism, or starvation), or excessive dietary protein intake. Low levels are seen with impaired liver function, fluid overload, and low protein intake.

- **Creatinine,** a by-product of skeletal muscle metabolism, is excreted through the kidneys and is an excellent indicator of renal function. Increased levels may indicate impaired kidney function or a loss of muscle mass.
- **Lymphocytes,** or white blood cells (WBCs), are the body's first line of defense against microorganisms. For a detailed discussion of the role of WBCs in infection control, as well as a discussion of the types of WBCs and their normal values, see Chapter 23. A decrease in total lymphocytes, known as **leukopenia,** is associated with malnutrition, protein deficiency, alcoholism, bone marrow depression, and anemia.
- **Hemoglobin** is composed of **heme,** an iron-rich compound, and **globulin,** a serum protein. Adequate iron intake is required to produce heme. Therefore, low hemoglobin levels may indicate inadequate iron intake or chronic blood loss. Globulin forms the backbone of hemoglobin, as well as antibodies, glycoproteins, lipoproteins, clotting factors, and a variety of key enzymes. A decreased globulin level indicates insufficient protein intake or excessive protein loss.

 Go to Chapter 24, Diagnostic Testing, Tests Reflecting Nutritional Status: Norms, in Volume 2.

May I Delegate Nutritional Assessments?

You may safely delegate to unlicensed assistive personnel (UAP) the measurement of weight, height, and intake and output (I&O); other nursing staff can collect a nutritional history. However, the registered nurse (RN) is responsible for reviewing and interpreting these findings.

KnowledgeCheck 24-10
- What are the likely causes of hyperglycemia?
- Why is it important to identify the serum albumin level?

 ThinkLike a Nurse 24-7: Clinical Judgment **in Action**

The Nutrition Screening Initiative (NSI) is completed for a 70-year-old patient.
- What major indicator on the NSI would indicate impaired nutritional status?
- What minor indicator would you likely see?
- What would malnourishment look like in the adult?
- What type of anthropometric findings would be typical of an older adult with poor nutrition patterns?
- What type of laboratory values would support impaired nutritional status?

 NURSING DIAGNOSIS/ANALYZING CUES

For clients who have no symptoms of or risk factors for nutrition problems, use the diagnostic label Readiness for Enhanced Nutrition. NANDA International (NANDA-I) defines this as "a pattern of nutrient intake, which can be strengthened" (2021, p. 215).

Nutrition as the Problem

To describe nutrition problems, you can use the following diagnoses:

- For the nutritional problems of obesity, overweight, underweight, and malnutrition, refer to Example Client Condition: Overweight and Obesity and Example Client Condition: Underweight and Malnutrition. Also, to see a sample care plan and care map for Obesity and Overweight,

Go to Davis Advantage, Resources, Chapter 24, **Nursing Care Plan, Overweight and Obesity,** and **Care Map, Obesity.**

Nutritional problems can also be the etiology of problems in other functional areas, for example:

- Ineffective Breastfeeding r/t insufficient breast milk production 2° insufficient intake of calories and fluids
- Constipation r/t insufficient intake of fluids and fiber
- Impaired (or Risk for Impaired) Skin Integrity r/t inadequate intake of protein and/or vitamin A
- Disturbed Sleep Pattern r/t excessive caffeine intake or eating fatty and spicy foods near bedtime
- Impaired Social Interaction r/t low self-esteem secondary to Obesity

PLANNING/PRIORITIZING HYPOTHESES AND GENERATING SOLUTIONS

The overall *Healthy People 2030* nutrition goal for the U.S. population is to "promote health and reduce chronic disease through diet and weight control" (USDHHS, n.d.).

NOC Standardized Outcomes directly linked to nutritional problems include the following:

Applicable to most nutrition problems:
Appetite
Nutritional Status
Nutritional Status: Food and Fluid Intake
Nutritional Status: Nutrient Intake
Self-Care: Eating

In addition to these, the following are outcomes for more specific diagnoses:

For Frail Elderly Syndrome:
Behavior: Will to Live
Knowledge: Health
Nutritional Status: Food and Fluid Intake
Self-Care Status

For Obesity and Overweight:

Adherence Behavior	Weight: Body Mass
Eating Disorder	Weight Loss Behavior
Healthy Diet	Self-Control
Knowledge: Healthy Diet	

For Underweight/Malnutrition:

Same as for Obesity/Overweight, except for Weight Loss Behavior

You could choose other NOC outcomes based on the patient's nursing diagnosis. For example:

For Situational Low Self-Esteem related to obesity, you might use Self-Esteem.

Individualized Goals/Outcome Statements you might identify for a patient with nutrition-related problems include the following:

Loses 2 lb per week until ideal weight is attained.
Follows the prescribed modified diet that, at a minimum, meets the DRIs.

IMPLEMENTATION/TAKING ACTION

NIC Standardized Interventions directly linked to nutrition problems include the broad interventions that could probably be used for most nutrition problems, regardless of the etiologies. Examples are:

Nutrition Management	Nutrition Therapy
Nutritional Monitoring	Teaching: Individual

For other nutrition-related nursing diagnoses, the following NIC interventions are appropriate:

For Frail Elderly Syndrome:

Cognitive Stimulation	Hope Inspiration
Nutrition Therapy	Self-Care Assistance

For Overweight/Obesity:

Behavior Modification	Nutrition Management
Nutritional Monitoring	Weight Management
Exercise Promotion	Weight Reduction
Nutritional Counseling	Assistance

For Underweight/Malnutrition:

Eating Disorders	Self-Care Assistance:
Feeding	Management
Enteral Tube Feeding	Swallowing Therapy
Fluid/Electrolyte	Weight Gain Assistance
Management	Weight Management
Nutrition Management	

Individualized Nursing Actions These are determined by the patient's nursing diagnosis. Examples are discussed in the following sections.

Teaching Clients About Vitamin and Mineral Supplementation

Noncredentialled nutrition "experts" recommend, and sell, many kinds of vitamin and mineral supplements to prevent cancer and heart attacks, improve sexual drive, prevent aging, and offer more energy. Yet conservative health professionals may be skeptical of high-dose vitamin supplements on the basis that a nutritious diet provides the essential micronutrients. However, a growing body of research suggests that certain supplements provide health benefits. Remember, too, that RDAs are for average needs; individual needs for micronutrients vary. Given the modern diet of processed foods, it may be difficult to get enough nutrients from diet alone during periods of increased nutrient demands.

NIC Intervention—Nutritional Counseling

Supplements of specific vitamins and minerals may be needed during growth periods (i.e., pregnancy, lactation, and adolescence). However, as a rule, healthy adults eating balanced diets do not need supplements. When teaching clients about supplements, keep the following principles in mind:

1. **Dietary supplements may be appropriate for people whose diet does not provide the recommended intake of specific vitamins or minerals. With a few exceptions, taking nutritional supplements in appropriate amounts is not harmful.**
2. **Individual needs vary, and those needs should determine the specific nutrients and amounts used. For example:**
   - *Vitamin K.* Newborns are given a vitamin K injection to prevent hemorrhage because they do not yet have bacterial flora in the gut to synthesize enough vitamin K.
   - *Vitamin D.* Breastfed infants may need a vitamin D supplement if the breastfeeding patient does not have an adequate diet or if the baby does not receive enough exposure to sunlight.
   - *Iron.* At 4 to 6 months of age, iron stores are depleted, so breastfed infants need iron supplementation at that age.
   - *Folic acid.* Supplementation is recommended for patients of childbearing age and those taking methotrexate (a drug used to treat certain types of cancer).
   - *Calcium.* People who do not eat dairy products, especially postmenopausal patients and those with a family history of osteoporosis, benefit from calcium supplements.
3. **Supplements do not replace the need to eat a nutritious diet. Specific supplements are more effective if the person also has an adequate diet.**
4. **Read supplement labels carefully. They provide information about toxicity levels, dosage, and side effects.**
5. **Encourage patients to ask their primary care provider's advice before taking vitamins.**
6. **Advise patients to follow the DRI or RDA dosages.**
7. **Be certain that any health claims made for a supplement are based on sound research.**

NIC Intervention—Referring Clients to Resources for Nutritional Support

Various subsidized programs are available to assist qualified people in obtaining nutritious foods. You might refer them to the following:

- **Supplemental Nutrition Assistance Program (SNAP).** For low-income households, this program issues coupons that can be used to buy food to cover the household's needs.
- **Commodity Supplemental Food Program (CSFP).** This program is designed to improve the health of low-income older persons of at least 60 years of age by supplementing their diets with nutritious USDA foods.
- **Women, Infants, and Children (WIC).** This federal program aims to safeguard the health of persons of low income who are pregnant or breastfeeding and infants and children younger than age 5 who are at nutritional risk. WIC provides nutritious foods to supplement diets, offers information on healthy eating, provides support for breastfeeding, and makes referrals to healthcare as needed.
- **National School Lunch and Breakfast Programs.** These federally assisted programs subsidize schools that provide free or reduced-rate breakfasts and/or lunches to low-income children. Lunches must supply about one-third of the child's DRIs for energy and nutrients.

Interventions for Impaired Dietary Intake

Nutritional health is related to the type and amount of food patients consume. Physical illnesses that alter appetite, taste, and smell impair dietary intake. Medical restriction in intake, such as NPO, also affects nutritional status. Other factors leading to poor nutritional health include impaired ability to purchase and prepare nutritious food and feed self.

Nausea First, identify the cause of the nausea (e.g., anxiety; pain; constipation; cough; dehydration; electrolyte disorders; treatments, such as surgery, radiotherapy, or chemotherapy; disease processes, such as peptic ulcer or pancreatitis).

♥ iCare 24-1

Caring for Your Patient's Nutritional Status

To promote health and healing, you need to perform a keen assessment of a person's physical status, food and fluid intake, weight changes, and response to treatment. How do you do this?

- Document daily weights, intake and output, food preferences, consumption, tolerances, and intolerances at every meal.
- Be supportive of a patient's/family's wishes regarding artificial hydration and nutrition.
- Realize that different cultures have different beliefs.

To relieve nausea and provide comfort:

- Apply a cool compress on the back of the neck. This may ease nausea, especially if the patient has an elevated temperature.
- Instruct the patient to wear loose clothing.
- Avoid wearing perfume. Discourage scented candles and other aromatic items while the patient is nauseated.
- Provide or assist with frequent oral hygiene. Keep facial tissues and water handy at the bedside for the patient to rinse the mouth as needed.
- Ask the patient to sit in an upright position for 30 to 45 minutes after eating, unless contraindicated. When the patient is lying flat, gastric juices may contribute to feelings of nausea.
- Open a window for cool air or turn on a fan to help move air and reduce odors that contribute to nausea.
- Apply pressure while using a circular motion on the inner wrist approximately 2 ½ inches down in between the two large tendons.
- Help your patient to shift focus to something else. Distraction can help a lot. Deep breathing or meditation can help in coping with nausea.
- Recommend antiemetics if nausea is severe or does not respond to other methods. Some research suggests that CBD oil from a reputable commercial source may also reduce symptoms (Rock et al., 2012).

When serving food or drinks to the patient with nausea:

- Add fresh-squeezed lemons to cool water to ease nausea. The citric acid can settle the stomach and aid in digestion (Wilson, 2017).
- Try serving bland foods. Avoid greasy, warm, spicy, or aromatic foods. In some cases, cold food is better tolerated. The sight and smell of hot food can induce nausea.
- Provide cool (not cold or iced) cola to drink. Suggest the patient suck on an ice cube, popsicle, sorbet, or even a piece of frozen fruit.
- Offer chamomile tea. It also has a sedative effect that can help the patient to sleep when experiencing nausea. Peppermint tea is another good choice for soothing the stomach.
- Instruct the patient to keep crackers by the side of the bed to eat before getting up if nausea occurs upon wakening. It can also help to eat lean meat or cheese before going to bed.
- Offer small snacks instead of larger meals.
- Avoid carbonated beverages, especially those with high sugar content. Bubbly drinks can worsen nausea, cause bloating, and aggravate reflux.

Certain psychological techniques may be effective when the nausea is related to anxiety, stress, or the anticipation of nausea:

- Maintain a calm environment.
- Use distraction, relaxation techniques, guided imagery, systematic desensitization, self-hypnosis, biofeedback, and music therapy.

If nausea persists:

- Administer antiemetics as prescribed or per hospital protocol.
- Arrange a dietary consultation if nausea and vomiting persist.
- For patients with compromised nutrition, consult a dietitian.
- Consider dietary supplements; however, these are often poorly tolerated and may sometimes trigger more nausea.
- Assess for dehydration; if nausea and vomiting are severe or persistent, the patient may need parenteral fluid and electrolytes.

Loss of Appetite; Diminished Sense of Smell and Taste Refer to the Intervention Stimulating Appetite in the Example Client Condition: Underweight/Malnourished.

Nothing by Mouth (NPO) Patients who are NPO for prolonged periods must receive glucose and electrolytes through either IV fluids or total parenteral nutrition and IV lipid infusion to meet the body's fluid and nutritional needs. Provide comfort measures for patients who cannot take food and fluids orally:

- Assist the patient with or provide oral hygiene. If allowed, provide ice chips, hard candy, chewing gum, or sips of water for rinsing the mouth.
- Advise family or visitors not to eat or drink around the patient; try to schedule other activities for the patient at mealtimes.
- Schedule patients who must be NPO for tests or procedures early in the day to decrease the length of time the patient must be NPO. If testing must be late in the day, ask the primary care provider whether the patient can have an early breakfast.

    ■ Remember that remaining NPO for more than 3 days puts the patient at risk for malnutrition. When older adults must be NPO for tests or procedures, schedule them early in the day to decrease the length of time the patient must be NPO. If testing must be late in the day, ask the primary care provider whether the patient can have an early breakfast.

Unwise Food Choices Advise clients to eat nutrient-dense foods and to eat essential foods first.
    Because the sense of taste is decreased, older adults may prefer concentrated sweets; because they may also have a poor appetite, once they eat high-sugar foods, they may not be hungry enough to eat other foods.

Limited Income for Food You can select from the following suggestions to help you teach patients to plan and buy food wisely. See the Self-Care box, Teaching Your Patients to Buy Nutritious Foods with a Limited Budget.

Teaching Your Patients on a Limited Budget to Buy Nutritious Foods

Plan Ahead

➤ Meal planning will help you to control impulse buying and extra trips to the store.

➤ Avoid eating at fast-food restaurants. Meals are more expensive and less nutritious than those you can prepare at home.

➤ Try planting a garden; you can use pots if you live in the city.

Buy Wisely

➤ Buy generic instead of more expensive and widely advertised brands.

➤ Watch for sales of nutrient-dense items. Stock up on and freeze them for later use if you do not need them right away.

➤ Buy in quantity—if it results in real savings and if you can use that amount of food before it spoils.

➤ Limit convenience foods (e.g., frozen dinners), breads, canned goods, chips, and many cheeses; they are often high in fat and sodium.

➤ Buy foods when they are in season; for example, fresh tomatoes are less expensive and better tasting in the summer than in the winter.

➤ Purchase oatmeal and cream of wheat instead of cold, sugared cereals. Buy in bulk rather than single-serving packages, but do not buy so much that food spoils.

➤ Avoid shopping at convenience stores. Items are usually more expensive than in supermarkets.

➤ Buy inexpensive cuts of meat but not high-fat grades; avoid processed lunchmeats and hot dogs.

➤ Buy frozen concentrated or fresh-squeezed fruit juices instead of juice in plastic jugs and cardboard boxes.

➤ Substitute dairy products, beans and lentils, and peanut butter for more expensive meat. Substitute powdered milk for whole milk.

➤ Read the Nutrition Facts panels on prepared foods to be sure you obtain the most nutrition for the money.

Interventions for Patients With Impaired Swallowing

Swallowing Impairment is "the inability to move food from the mouth to stomach" (Clinical Care Classification [CCC], 2020) (Fig. 24-4). It may be caused by mechanical obstruction (e.g., tumor), neuromuscular impairment (e.g., facial paralysis), stroke, cerebral palsy, or a host of other anatomical or physiological defects. Nutritional support for patients with Impaired Swallowing includes activities from the NIC intervention Swallowing Therapy (Butcher et al., 2018, p. 370).

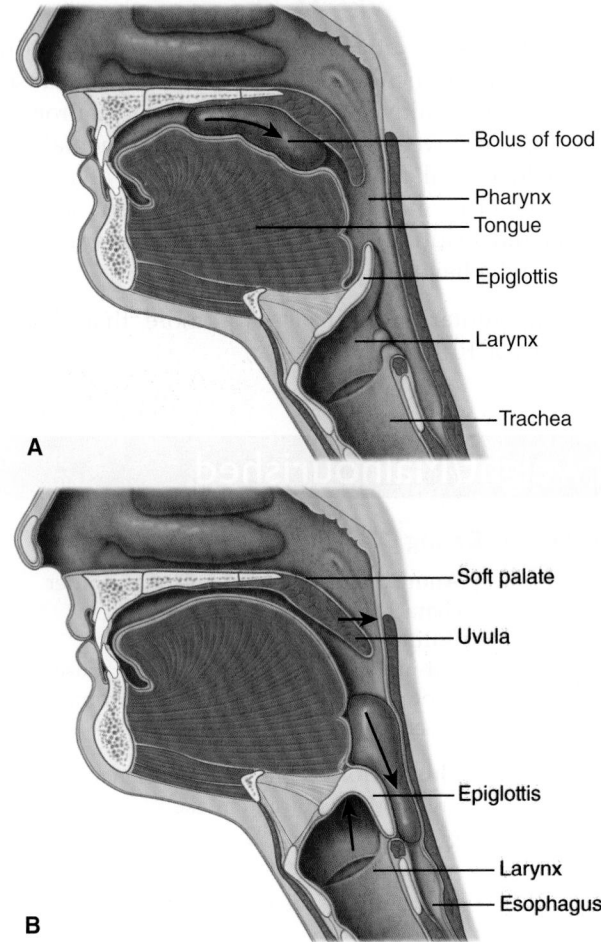

FIGURE 24-4 A. After food is moistened and chewed, the tongue moves it to the back of the mouth. B. As food moves to the pharynx, the epiglottis closes over the tracheal opening.

Provide Nutritional Support

- Provide/use assistive devices, as appropriate.
- Avoid the use of drinking straws.
- Assist the patient to position [their] head in forward flexion in preparation for swallowing (chin tuck).
- Assist patient in placing food at the back of the mouth and on the unaffected side.
- Monitor the patient's tongue movements while they are eating.
- Check mouth for pocketing of food after eating.
- Monitor body weight.
- Monitor body hydration (e.g., intake, output, skin turgor, mucous membranes).

Take Precautions to Prevent Aspiration

- Monitor level of consciousness, cough reflex, gag reflex, and swallowing ability.
- Position the patient upright 90° or as far as possible.
- Keep suction setup available.
- Feed in small amounts.
- Cut food into small pieces.
- Inspect oral cavity for retained food or medications.
- Keep head of bed elevated for 30 to 45 minutes after feeding (Butcher et al., 2018, p. 75).

You will sometimes also offer a special dysphagia diet, depending on the degree of difficulty the patient has with swallowing: dysphagia puree, dysphagia mechanically altered, dysphagia advanced, and regular. Liquid diets vary in *viscosity*, or thickness, based on the degree of swallowing impairment. Clinicians are encouraged to prescribe the minimal level of thickness needed for swallowing safety.

Interventions for Patients With Impaired Digestive Function

Nutritional health is due in part to digestive function, from mastication (chewing) all the way through passing stool. Dysfunction of the GI tract can reduce the transport, absorption, and elimination of food nutrients.

- **Dry mouth.** This is typically an age-associated change. Advise clients to avoid caffeine; alcohol; tobacco; and dry, bulky, spicy, salty, or highly acidic foods. Offer sugarless hard candy or chewing gum to stimulate salivation (unless the patient has dementia). Use lip moisturizer and encourage frequent sips of water.
- **Gastroesophageal reflux.** Advise clients not to eat just before bedtime and to elevate the head of the bed 30° to 40°. It is also important for them to avoid overeating, to avoid bending over, and to take their prescribed medications. They should also avoid fruit juices, fatty foods, chocolate, alcohol, and tobacco use; all of these stimulate reflux. If the client with reflux is also overweight, losing weight can prevent pressure on the diaphragm.
- **Decreased gastric secretions.** People with this problem should eat regularly scheduled meals, chew their food thoroughly, and take prescribed medications. They should be certain to eat foods rich in vitamin D to ensure calcium absorption.
- **Glucose intolerance.** Obviously, patients with glucose intolerance should avoid concentrated, refined sugars (e.g., candy, ice cream, desserts), unless they have been told to use them to treat hypoglycemia. Complex carbohydrates (e.g., whole-grain cereals, vegetables) are better tolerated. Smaller, more frequent meals may also be necessary.
- **Constipation.** To prevent problems with bowel elimination, advise patients to consume foods high in fiber. Soluble fiber allows more water to remain in the stool, which makes it softer and easier to pass. Insoluble fiber adds bulk to the stool for easier defecation. Patients should drink plenty of water—at least 64 oz daily. Also, encourage exercise because physical activity aids in the GI motility needed to pass stool.

Caring for Patients With Underweight and Malnutrition

Some patients are at risk for nutritional deficits because of limited or no ability to feed themselves, which may be caused by loss of cognitive, musculoskeletal, or neuromuscular function; weakness; pain; or environmental barriers. Older adult patients, especially, are at risk for underweight or malnourishment in inpatient settings.

You should institute special nutrition interventions in patients who have one of the following:

- Unintentional weight loss of more than 5% in 30 days or 10% in 180 days.
- A BMI of 18.5 or less.

For information about and nursing care for patients who are undernourished or malnourished, see the Example Client Condition: Underweight and Malnutrition.

Assisting Patients With Meals

Some patients are at risk for nutritional deficits due to a Self-Care Deficit (Feeding), which may be caused by a loss of cognitive, musculoskeletal, or neuromuscular function; weakness; pain; or environmental barriers. Older adult patients, especially, are at risk for underweight or malnourishment in inpatient settings. You should institute special nutrition interventions in patients who have one of the following:

- An involuntary weight loss of more than 5% in 30 days or 10% in 180 days.

EXAMPLE CLIENT CONDITION: Underweight/Malnourished

THEORETICAL KNOWLEDGE

Definition: Intake of nutrients insufficient to meet metabolic needs, based on activity, sex, height, and weight. BMI < 18.5; involuntary weight loss of more than 5% in 30 days or 10% in 180 days. For patients with serious illness, increased mortality is associated with a BMI of <21.

- BMI:
  Severely underweight: <16
  Moderately underweight: 16.00–16.99
  Mildly underweight: 17.0–18.49
  Underweight (World Health Organization, 1995, 2000, 2006a): <18.5

Risk Factors

Most common in:
- Underdeveloped nations; children, older adults
- People with chronic illnesses (cancer, HIV, COPD, GI absorption disorder

Others at risk:
- Serum albumin level < 3.5 g/dL
- Clear liquid diet or NPO for >3 days
- Increased nutritional requirements (wound healing, burns)
- Unplanned loss of 10% or more of patient's usual weight
- Nausea or vomiting lasting 3 days or more
- Chewing and swallowing impairment
- Difficulty feeding self

Eating Disorders

- **Anorexia nervosa**—psychiatric disorder characterized by self-starvation.
- **Bulimia nervosa**—binge eating with self-induced vomiting or laxative abuse to purge food; more common in women; onset before the age of 20.

Malnutrition—Long-term deficiency in energy and/or nutrient intake

- **Kwashiorkor**—severe deficiency of dietary protein
- **Marasmus**—severe protein and overall caloric deficit

COMPLICATIONS

Emotional
- Reduced self-esteem, shame, guilt
- Loneliness and social isolation
- Depression, anxiety

Physical
- Underweight adults have a higher risk of early death—1.8 times greater than that of people of a healthy weight (Cao et al., 2014).
- Osteoporosis, increased risk for fractures
- Reduced resistance to infection

- Metabolic disorders
- Cardiac dysrhythmia
- Organ failure
- Death

Other diseases develop as a result of specific vitamin and mineral deficiencies:
- Beriberi (neurological deficits)
- Scurvy (delayed wound healing, poor bone growth)
- Pellagra (diarrhea and dementia)

EXAMPLE CLIENT CONDITION: Underweight/Malnourished—cont'd

ASSESSMENT

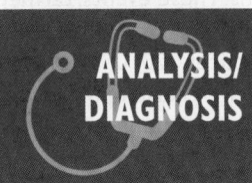

Malnutrition

- **Physical signs**—Reduced physical activity, weight loss, reduced height, abdominal enlargement, hair loss

Eating Disorders

- **Physical signs**—Hair loss, abnormal weight loss, cold intolerance, absent or irregular menstruation, low blood pressure, weakness, atrophy of breasts, iron deficiency anemia, and in adolescents, a delay of stages of sexual maturation

- **Emotional behaviors**—Intense fear of gaining weight, often overachieving or type A personality
- **Body image behaviors**—Wears baggy clothes; perceives self as fat
- **Food behaviors**—Takes only tiny portions; skips meals. Will not eat in front of others. Always has an excuse not to eat. Often has a diet soda or coffee in hand. Eats only food that is low in fat or sugar. Deliberate self-starvation.

ANALYSIS/ DIAGNOSIS

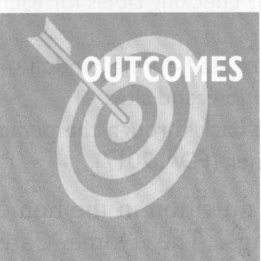

Problem Labels

Body Nutrition Deficit (Clinical Care Classification [CCC], 2020)
Risk for Body Nutrition Deficit (CCC, 2020)

Examples of Diagnostic Statements

Underweight r/t eating disorder
Underweight r/t digestion and absorption disorders

OUTCOMES

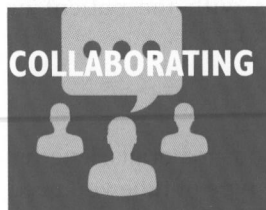

NOC Outcomes

Weight
Body Mass
Weight Gain Behavior
Weight Maintenance Behavior
Nutritional Status: Food & Fluid Intake

Individualized goals/outcome statements

- Progressively gains weight toward goal.
- Verbalizes willingness to take action for weight gain.
- Laboratory values, body mass, and weight within normal limits (WNL).
- Recognizes factors contributing to underweight.

COLLABORATING

- Appetite stimulants on an individual basis.
- Consult with a dietitian about strategies to increase the nutritional content of foods.

- For eating disorders, refer for appropriate counseling.
- Suggest community resources for access to food.

INTERVENTIONS

Stimulating Appetite

- Offer frequent, small, nutrient-dense meals when the person is most likely to be hungry.
- Offer high-protein supplements between meals.
- Restrict liquids with meals to prevent feeling full before patient eats sufficient nutrients.
- Control pain; avoid painful treatments before meal.
- Provide or assist with frequent oral hygiene.
- Keep environment neat, clean, and free of unpleasant sights, odors, and medical equipment.
- Order a late food tray or warm the food if patient is not in their room during mealtime.

- Suggest smokers refrain for 1 hour before a meal.
- Position patient comfortably for mealtime; arrange the tray within easy reach.
- Determine need for tube feedings or IV fluids. Refer to Providing Enteral Nutrition section in the chapter.
- Teach patient and caregiver how to promote healthy eating and vitamin and mineral supplementation. (See content in the Teaching Clients About Vitamin and Mineral Supplementation section.)
- Also see the content in the Providing Enteral Nutrition section.

(continued)

EXAMPLE CLIENT CONDITION: Underweight/Malnourished—cont'd

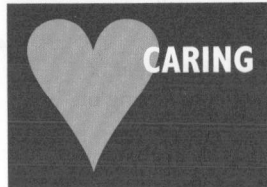

CARING

♥ **iCare** • Encourage others to bring foods the patient likes to eat.
• Vary food textures, colors, and flavors; serve attractively.

• For those who live alone, encourage meals with family or friends or meals at a senior center.

- Leaving more than one-fourth of their food in the past 7 days or two-thirds of meals (based on a 2,000-kcal diet).
- A BMI of 18.5 or less.

NIC Interventions for this situation are Feeding and Self-Care Assistance: Feeding. Important nursing actions include assisting patients with meals. To assist with meals, including care of patients with dementia,

 Go to **Clinical Insight 24-2: Assisting Patients With Meals**, in Volume 2.

Providing Enteral Nutrition

If a patient cannot meet their nutritional needs through an enhanced diet and measures to stimulate the appetite, you may need to use an alternative feeding method, either through the intestinal tract as enteral nutrition or intravenously as parenteral nutrition. **Enteral nutrition** *(tube feeding)* refers to the delivery of liquid nutrition into the upper intestinal tract via a tube. Tube feeding may be used in addition to or instead of oral intake. It is the preferred method of feeding for a patient who has a functioning intestinal tract but needs nutritional support (e.g., patients with swallowing disorders, certain bowel diseases).

Risks Associated With Enteral Feedings Tube feedings are preferred to parenteral (i.e., intravenous) nutrition because they maintain peristalsis and have a lower incidence of infections. However, there are associated risks:

- **Aspiration.** If enteral formula is aspirated into the lungs, it can lead to infection, pneumonia, abscess formation, adult respiratory distress syndrome (ARDS), and in some cases, death.
- **Bacterial growth.** The high glucose content of enteral formulas provides a medium for bacterial growth.
- **Other complications.** Diarrhea, nausea and vomiting, nasopharyngeal trauma, alterations in drug absorption and metabolism, and various metabolic disturbances.

For more about the safe use of parental nutrition, see the Safe, Effective Nursing Care box. For complete instructions on tube feedings,

See **Procedure 24-3, Administering Feedings Through Gastric and Enteric Tubes**, in Volume 2.

✚ **Preventing Tubing Misconnections** There have been some instances in which enteral feedings have been mistakenly connected to intravascular lines and feeding solutions have been infused into veins. These events, termed *tubing misconnections*, are potentially fatal to the patient (Institute for Safe Medication Practices, 2010; The Joint Commission et al., 2007). To prevent catastrophic injury resulting from medical device misconnection errors, the FDA recommends:

Assessing equipment by carefully checking labels for each device.

Communicating with healthcare staff during handoff or transfer about all infusion solutions and sites.

Tracing tubing from the patient back through the pump to the feeding solution container. (FDA, 2017).

Patients may receive enteral nutrition in the home as well as in inpatient settings. The Home Care box, Home Nutritional Support, reviews teaching related to alternative feeding methods in the home. You should review these topics with the patient or caregiver.

Using Enteric Tubes

Enteric tubes are available in various materials, lengths, diameters, and types. Choose the type of tube you need based on the intended use and the length of time you anticipate it will be left in place. This chapter focuses on the use of enteric tubes as a route for feeding; however, they are inserted for other reasons, as well:

- **To lavage the stomach** (e.g., when there is disease, surgery or bleeding in the GI tract, poisoning, or medication overdose)
- **To collect a specimen** of stomach contents for laboratory tests
- To prevent nausea, vomiting, and gastric distention postoperatively

Selecting a Feeding Tube

Short-term (less than 6 weeks) enteral feedings are usually delivered through a nasogastric (NG) or a nasoenteric (NE) tube. The **lumen** (inside diameter) of a feeding tube is measured using the **French (Fr) scale:** the larger the lumen, the larger the diameter. Most feeding tubes for adults are 8 to 12 Fr and 90 to 108 cm (36 to 43 in.) long.

Self-Care

Teaching Weight-Loss Tips

Getting Ready

Make a commitment.
- ➤ Promise yourself; promise others. "I will do this."

Set realistic goals.
- ➤ Aim to lose 1 to 2 lb/wk. To do this, you need to burn 500 to 1,000 calories more than you consume. Losing weight faster usually means losing water weight or muscle tissue rather than fat.
- ➤ Set "process" rather than "outcome" goals. For example, "I will exercise for at least 30 minutes every day" instead of "I will lose 10 pounds this month." Changing your habits (your "processes") is the key to weight loss.
- ➤ Write your goals, your plan for achieving them, and your start date. This makes it reality, not just a thought.
- ➤ Review your goals each week. Readjust them as needed. If you are exercising more than you thought, adjust your goal upward, for example.

Plan for setbacks.
- ➤ Identify situations that might trigger eating or interfere with exercise; plan specific actions you will take to overcome them.

Eat healthier foods.
- ➤ Create a meal plan with whole foods, including more fruits; nonstarchy, fiber-rich vegetables and legumes; nuts; whole grains; and lean meat and fish.
- ➤ Limit foods with added sugar and refined grains.

Get active and stay active.
- ➤ If you have not been exercising, start to do so slowly.
- ➤ Work up to at least 300 min per week to lose weight and maintain the loss.

Get adequate sleep.
- ➤ For most people, this is 7 to 8 hr a night.
- ➤ Sleep deprivation can affect levels of the appetite-regulating hormones leptin and ghrelin (Knutson, 2007).
- ➤ Sleep loss can affect the type of food you crave. When you are tired, you are less able to cope with stress and emotional triggers for eating and more likely to crave comfort foods such as chocolate and ice cream.

Keep a food diary.
- ➤ This can double your weight loss.

Decide what and when to eat.
- ➤ Decide what foods you will eat as well as when you will eat. For example, "I will eat only at the table, three meals and two snacks daily."
- ➤ Make a conscious effort to take small bites and eat slowly.
- ➤ Serve your food on small plates.

Shop wisely.
- ➤ Shop for food on a full stomach.
- ➤ Read food labels when purchasing food (for information about calorie and fat content).

Find ways to exercise.
- ➤ Lay out your workout clothing ahead of time (e.g., at night if you exercise in the morning).
- ➤ Use the stairs instead of the elevator; park in the back of the parking lot, as far from the door as possible.
- ➤ Walk or bike to work when possible.

Get emotional support.
- ➤ Avoid negative self-talk.

Each Fr unit is about 0.33 mm, so a 12-Fr tube is about 4 mm in diameter.

- **Small-bore NG tubes.** As a nurse, you may be asked to place a small-bore **NG feeding tube.** The tube is inserted through one naris, passed through the nasopharynx into the esophagus, and then into the stomach.

  See Procedure 24-2, Inserting Nasogastric and Nasoenteric Tubes, in Volume 2.

- **An NE tube** is longer than an NG tube, extending through the nose down into the duodenum or jejunum (if it extends into the jejunum, it is called an *NJ tube*). A small, flexible tube is preferred for feeding (see Fig. 24-5). An NE tube may be used instead of an NG tube for patients at risk for aspiration (e.g., decreased level of consciousness, absent or diminished gag reflex, or severe gastroesophageal reflux).

- **Large-bore (larger than 12-Fr) NG tubes,** such as the Salem sump (Fig. 24-6), are occasionally used for

Safe, Effective Nursing Care

Safe Use of Parenteral Nutrition

Chapter Key Concept: Nutrition

Competency: Collaborate with the interdisciplinary healthcare team; validate evidence-based research to incorporate in practice; provide safe, quality client care

Clinicians at Memorial Hospital theorized that their poor processes and variation in methods in the use of parenteral nutrition (PN) were producing inconsistent patient outcomes, thus increasing patient risk. The following is a description of how they set out to correct this by identifying the root causes of the problems and standardizing care:

➤ **Problems identified:** Clinicians first organized a multidisciplinary team to collect and analyze data, develop better practices, and evaluate outcomes. They found several problems: inappropriate use of PN, poor glycemic control in patients on PN, inconsistent and confusing ordering practices, insufficient calorie replacement, and insufficient laboratory monitoring.

➤ **Corrective interventions:** Implementing the American Society for Parenteral and Enteral Nutrition's (ASPEN) guideline for PN, revising the PN order form, educating providers and nurses, and establishing twice-weekly PN rounds. The group measured specific quality indicators before and after implementing the new procedures. Changes in the top-four measures over a 2-year period included the following:

1. Compliance with 10 Mandatory Components of an ASPEN PN Order Form

2. Appropriate use of parenteral nutrition
3. Baseline labs ordered before initiating PN
4. Calories delivered within 10% of estimated need

Results/Conclusions: In addition to improving compliance, the new procedures resulted in significant cost savings.

Think about it: Parenteral nutrition is a high-risk treatment associated with serious complications, including death.

➤ Do the previously described measures mean that patient outcomes are improved?

➤ In what specific ways does this quality improvement project demonstrate the QSEN competencies of Quality Improvement, Safety, and Evidence-Based Practice?

➤ Which specific knowledge, skills, and attitudes does it address?

Source: Ayers, P., Adams, S., Boullata, J., Gervasio, J., Holcombe, B., Kraft, M. D., Marshall, N., Neal, A., Sacks, G., Seres, D. S., & Worthington, P. (2014, March). A.S.P.E.N. Parenteral nutrition safety consensus recommendations. *Journal of Parenteral and Enteral Nutrition, 38*(3), 296–333. https://doi.org/10.1177/0148607113511992; Boitano, M., Bojak, S., McCloskey, S., McCaul, D. S., & McDonough, M. (2010). Improving the safety and effectiveness of parenteral nutrition. *Nutrition in Clinical Practice, 25*(6), 663–671.

Home Care

Home Nutritional Support

To assist the client or caregiver with the management of home nutritional therapy, teach the following aspects:

1. *Formula.* Review the type of formula the patient should receive. Enteral or IV solutions are clearly marked with their contents. Emphasize that the caregiver must double-check that the correct solution is being used and that the expiration date and time have not been reached before administering any feeding.

2. *Administration.* Carefully review how to administer the feeding. Emphasize the need for hand washing before hanging the infusion. After a period, the client may be able to tolerate delivering 1 to 3 L of enteral feeding at night. The rate must be increased at the beginning and decreased when ending the delivery. If parenteral nutrition is administered at home, be sure that the client or caregiver is aware of proper technique.

3. *Access device.* Review the care required for the access device, including site care, dressing changes, and flushing.

4. *Storage.* Stored enteral and parenteral nutrition must be refrigerated to prevent bacterial contamination.

5. *Monitoring.* Instruct the client or caregiver to report a rise in temperature, weight loss, change in bowel movements, decrease in urine output, or change in condition.

6. *Follow-up.* Arrange for the client to be weighed and assessed regularly to monitor the adequacy of the feedings. Often clients weigh at home and report to the primary care provider's office or the nutrition support team for ongoing monitoring of progress and review of laboratory work.

feeding but are converted to a smaller tube within the first 2 days. They are less flexible, less comfortable, and more commonly used if it is necessary to empty (lavage) the stomach. Figures 24-5 and 24-7 show three types of feeding tubes.

■ **Tubes for long-term feedings**. A gastrostomy tube (G-tube), percutaneous endoscopic gastrostomy tube (PEG) (Figs. 24-8, 24-9), jejunostomy tube (J-tube, PEJ), or gastrostomy button (G-button) (Fig. 24-10) is preferred for long-term feedings. These are placed

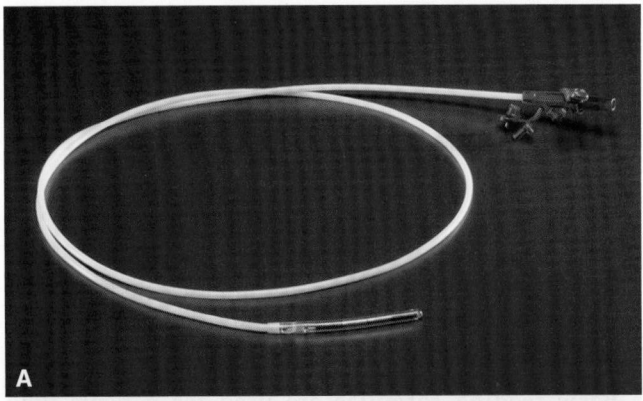

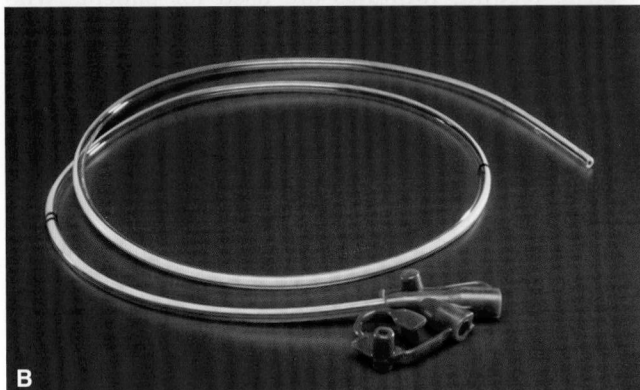

FIGURE 24-5 A. A double-lumen, weighted (Dobhoff) feeding tube. B. A nonweighted (kangaroo) feeding tube.

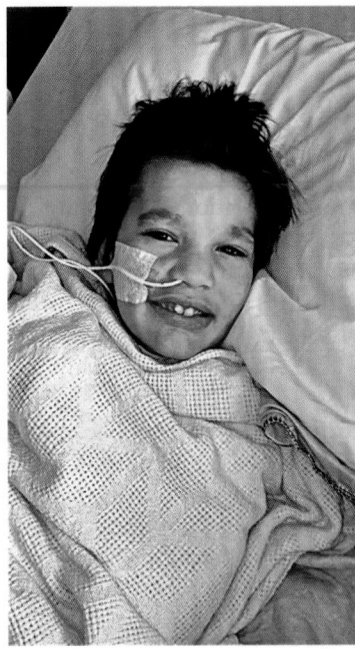

FIGURE 24-6 A small-lumen, flexible nasoenteric feeding tube provides continuous nutrition to patients with impaired swallowing.

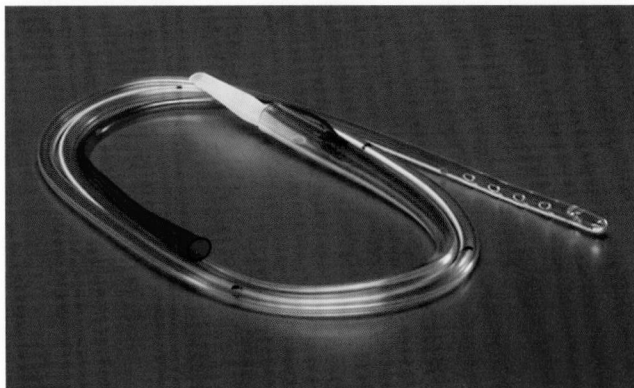

FIGURE 24-7 A large-bore, polyvinyl-chloride (PVC) Salem Sump tube used for gastric lavage.

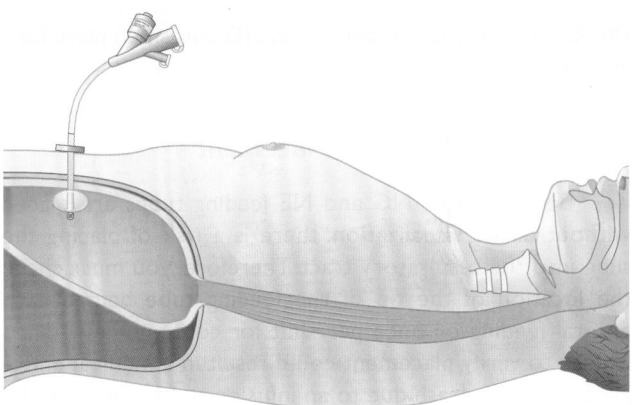

FIGURE 24-8 A percutaneous gastrostomy (PEG) tube for feeding.

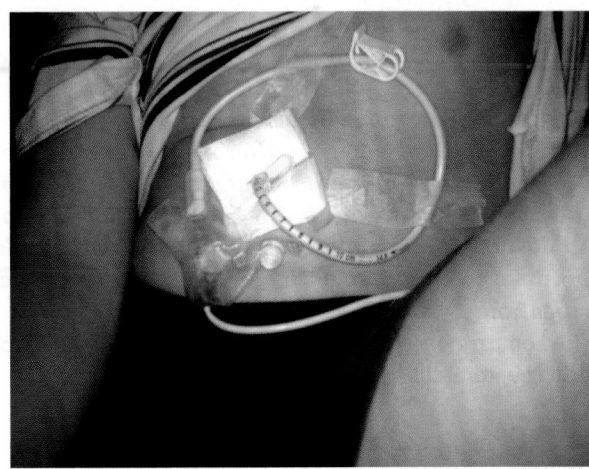

FIGURE 24-9 A percutaneous gastrostomy (PEG) feeding tube is more convenient and comfortable than a nasogastric tube.

surgically or laparoscopically through the skin and the abdominal wall into the stomach or jejunum. The surgical incision is sometimes sutured tightly around the tube to hold it in place and prevent leakage. A gastrostomy tube can be converted to a G-button once healing has taken place. The G-tubes and G-buttons, which can be capped off flush with the abdominal wall when not in use, are the most comfortable of all for long-term use. Patient comfort and improved technology leading to ease of insertion have made PEG or PEJ an option even for short-term use.

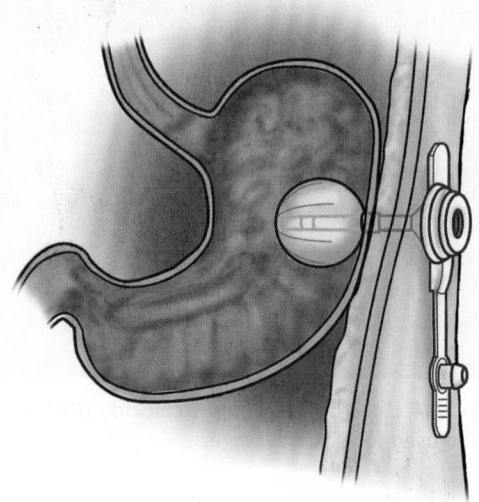

FIGURE 24-10 A gastrostomy button (G-button) in place for feeding.

Checking Feeding Tube Placement

 Because most NG and NE feeding tubes are placed without direct visualization, there is a risk of placing the tube into the respiratory tract. Therefore, you must check the location of the tip of the feeding tube before each enteral feeding or once per shift for continuous feedings. Failure to verify placement could result in a medical emergency or even death due to an infusion of formula into the lungs.

Key Point: *Radiographic verification is the most reliable method for confirming tube placement and must be performed before the first feeding is administered. All feeding tubes contain markings that can be detected by radiographic films. Ongoing bedside assessment is necessary because even when the tube is initially placed correctly in the stomach (or intestine), it may later move upward. If at any time after the initial x-ray you are in doubt about tube placement, obtain a radiograph to determine tube location. No single bedside method reliably verifies tube placement, so you must use the aspirate in combination with other methods for bedside verification.*

To compare methods, see Box 24-5. For guidelines on checking enteral tube placement,

➤ See **Procedure 24-2: Inserting Nasogastric and Nasoenteric Tubes in Volume 2.**

No longer recommended: Adding dye to enteral feedings as a method for identifying the aspiration of gastric contents is not recommended. This is because the dye has been associated with several adverse effects, including gastric bacterial colonization, diarrhea, systemic dye absorption, and death, and it is not effective in detecting aspiration (Metheny & the American Association of Critical-Care Nurses, 2016, updated 2020).

KnowledgeCheck 24-11

- When is enteral nutrition the preferred alternative feeding method?
- Identify and describe the types of enteral nutrition tubes.
- List four tube placement verification techniques.

Administering Enteral Feedings

Types of Enteral Feeding Solutions

The type of enteral feeding formula selected depends on the patient's health condition. Products vary in nutritional components and caloric concentration.

- **Basic feeding formulas** are used for patients who have no significant nutritional deficits but are unable to eat or drink sufficiently. They provide 1 kcal/mL of solution and meet the needs of most clients. A standard formula contains 12% to 20% of kcal from protein, 45% to 60% of kcal from carbohydrates, and 30% to 40% of kcal from fat and also contains vitamins and minerals. They are usually lactose-free and contain complex forms of carbohydrates, fats, and proteins. Therefore, they require digestion and absorption.
- **High-protein formulas** are for patients who have a substantial need for protein, such as those with burns, open wounds, or malnutrition.
- **Elemental formulas** do not contain complex proteins; instead, they contain amino acids or peptides. They are reserved for patients with severe small bowel absorptive dysfunction. These formulas are fiber-free and highly osmotic.
- **Diabetic formulas** are for patients who require tube feedings to meet nutritional needs but have type 1 or type 2 diabetes mellitus. These formulas control carbohydrate intake.
- **Renal formulas** are for patients who require tube feedings to meet nutritional needs but have renal failure or renal insufficiency. These formulas limit potassium, sodium, and nitrogen intake.
- **Pulmonary formulas** provide 55% of the calories as fat so that less CO_2 is produced per unit of oxygen consumed. They are used, for example, for patients with lung disease.
- **Fiber-containing formulas.** Because fiber has a potential protective effect for multiple disease states, including diverticulosis, colon cancer, diabetes, and heart disease, fiber-containing formulas may be used for patients in long-term care facilities or patients who require enteral feedings for a prolonged period.

Feeding Schedules

- **Continuous feedings** provide a constant flow of formula and an even distribution of nutrition over 24 hours. Continuous infusions are usually administered into NG, NJ, PEG, or PEJ tubes, or G-buttons, to patients who require intensive nutritional support. Feedings may be interrupted for periodic instillation of medications or flushing with water. Continuous feedings allow the lowest possible hourly feeding rate

BOX 24-5 ■ Comparison of Methods for Checking Nasogastric Tube (NGT) Feeding Tube Placement

Method	Benefits	Drawbacks
Observation for signs of respiratory distress (difficulty breathing, coughing, choking, oxygen desaturation, cyanosis)	■ Ongoing clinical assessment reveals immediate problems.	■ Tube position in the trachea can occur without signs of apparent distress.
Chest x-ray	■ Considered to be the most accurate method ■ Recommended for infusing feedings or medication	■ Not practical before each feeding or administration of medication through the NGT ■ Time-consuming ■ May be difficult to obtain x-ray in some patients ■ Exposes the patient to radiation ■ Costly ■ Cases of misread x-rays
pH testing of gastric aspirates 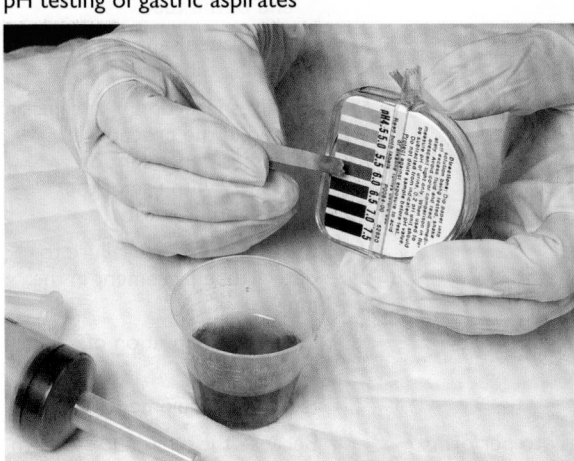	■ Easy to perform ■ Not costly ■ Low pH (1–5.5) indicates the tube is in the stomach. ■ When pH is approximately 6, the tube is likely to be positioned in the intestine. ■ Respiratory secretions have a pH of >7.	■ May be difficult to differentiate between respiratory and gastrointestinal placement based on the visual characteristics of feeding tube aspirates ■ Many variables can make the gastric pH results unreliable (e.g., blood in the stomach, antacid medications). Before measuring the pH of the aspirate, first flush the feeding tube with air or water. This also helps keep a small-bore tube from collapsing when you aspirate.
Capnometry (carbon dioxide detection monitoring) 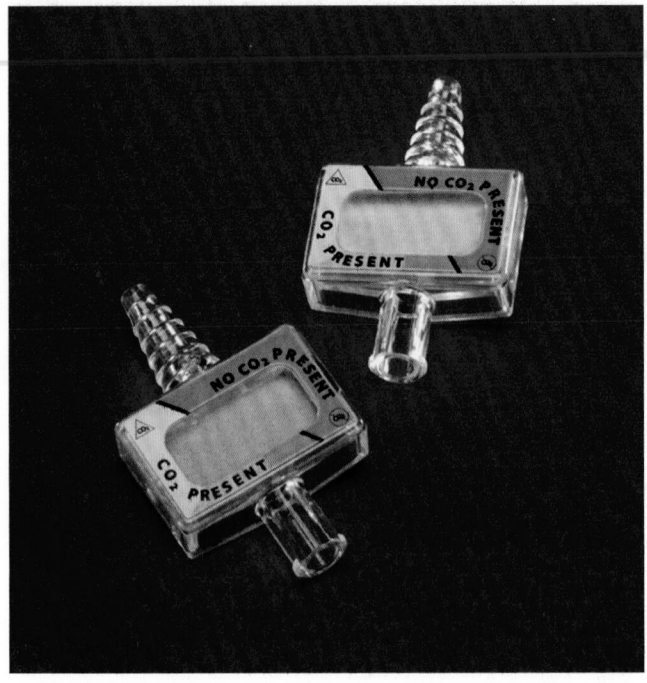	■ Highly accurate ■ Suggests tube placement in the tracheobronical tree rather than stomach	■ Carbonated beverages or certain medications can result in the detection of carbon dioxide in the stomach, leading to a false result. ■ CO_2 sensing does not distinguish tube position in the esophagus vs. stomach.

(Continued)

BOX 24-5 ■ Comparison of Methods for Checking Nasogastric Tube (NGT) Feeding Tube Placement—cont'd

Method	Benefits	Drawbacks
Biochemical markers (measuring bilirubin, trypsin, pepsin in the gastric aspirate)	■ Improve the accuracy of pH testing	■ Expensive ■ Not foolproof because of the time delay between obtaining the aspirate and obtaining the test result (tube could move)
Enteral access device (EAS)	■ Aids in enteral tube placement	■ Transmits real-time positional information visible to an external monitor during insertion ■ Technologies to track the position of the tube include: 　■ Electromagnetic sensor in the stylet 　■ Small camera in the distal end of the tube 　■ Impedance sensor within the feeding tube ■ Requires insertion by a clinician trained in the procedure; success is dependent on familiarity with use of the device and dexterity. ■ Cases of clinician's failure to detect tube placement in the lung ■ Cases of perforation of intestine ■ Expensive equipment
Auscultation of air through NGT	■ Easy to perform ■ Not costly	■ Because the lungs and stomach are positioned close together, the sounds created by sending air through the tube can cause errors in determining placement. ■ **Not recommended** (Bourgault et al., 2015)
Air bubbling method (holding tube under water)	■ Easy to perform ■ Not costly	■ Inaccurate method ■ *False negative:* When tube position is against the wall of the airway, no air releases through the tube. ■ *False positive:* Air is commonly in the stomach. ■ **Not recommended** (Bourgault et al., 2015)

Sources: Emergency Nurses Association, Killian, M., Reeve, N. E., Slivinski, A., Young Bradford, J., Horigan, A., Barnason, S., Foley, A., Johnson, M., Kaiser, J., MacPherson-Dias, R., Proehl, J. A., Stapleton, S. J., Valdez, A. M., Vanhoy, M. A., Zaleski, M. E., ENA Board of Directors Liaisons, Gillespie, G., Proehl, J. A., . . . Gates, L. (2019, May). Clinical practice guideline: Gastric tube placement verification. *Clinical Practice Guideline, 45*(3), e306. https://doi.org/10.1016/j.jen.2019.03.011; Hodin, R. A., & Bordeianou, L. (2018). Inpatient placement and management of nasogastric and nasoenteric tubes in adults. *UpToDate.* https://www.uptodate.com/contents/inpatient-placement-and-management-of-nasogastric-and-nasoenteric-tubes-in-adults; Metheny, N., & Association of Critical-Care Nurses. (2016, April). AACN practice alert. Initial and ongoing verification of feeding tube placement in adults. *Critical Care Nurse, 36*(2), e8–e13. http://dx.doi.org/10.4037/ccn2016141; Peijin Fan, E. M., Tan, S. B., & Ang, S. Y. (2017). Nasogastric tube placement confirmation: Where we are and where we should be heading. *Proceedings of Singapore Healthcare, 26*(3), 189–195. https://doi.org/10.1177/2010105817705141.

to meet nutritional requirements, which can be better tolerated by some patients. Additionally, continuous infusion can lead to better control of blood glucose in patients with diabetes.

Pump-controlled infusions for jejunal and gastrostomy feedings given by continuous infusion can decrease gastroesophageal reflux (American Gastrointestinal Association, 1995). A feeding pump ensures a steady flow rate.

Gravity feedings can also be used for continuous infusions, but the rate of delivery is not precise. The risk of gastroesophageal reflux, diarrhea, and aspiration is greater with this method. You regulate the drip rate by adjusting a clamp on the tubing, much the same as adjusting an IV rate.

- **Cyclic feedings** are administered regularly; however, the infusion time is less than 24 hours per day. The cyclic feeding schedule is more physiological, which is useful in the transition from continuous feedings to eventual oral intake.

    Nocturnal feedings are a form of cyclic feeding. The patient can eat meals and participate in activities throughout the day but receives an infusion of enteral formula at night while at rest.

    A *20-hour infusion* is another variant, during which a 4-hour break allows time for the feeding pump to be disconnected for hygiene and other activities.

- **Intermittent feedings** are given to supplement oral intake or for patients who want greater mobility to take part in activities such as physical therapy. Feedings are given on a regular or periodic basis several times a day, usually over 30 to 60 minutes.

    Periodic feedings are often based on oral intake and are more physiologically similar to normal eating patterns. For example, if a patient consumes a sufficient diet, no additional enteral feeding is given. The less they consume, the more formula is given after the meal.

    The **bolus method** is sometimes used for intermittent feedings. In this method, you use a syringe to deliver 300 to 400 mL of formula through the tube over a 5- to 10-minute period. This is the easiest method to teach family members for home care, and it frees the patient from mechanical devices that limit activity. But because the fluid is given more rapidly by this method, it increases the risk for respiratory aspiration and stomach distention. You can use bolus feeding only with gastric tubes, never with intestinal tubes.

Open and Closed Feeding Systems

- **An open system is exposed to the environment.** One example is to open cans of formula and use a syringe to inject the formula into the tube; alternatively, you can pour it into a reservoir (a bag).

    Flush and clean the system after each delivery.

    Most agencies require that an open-system feeding not hang for more than 4 hours.

- **A closed system is a prefilled system** (bag or a bottle) that functions much like IV fluid. The nurse spikes the container with tubing that is attached to the feeding pump or run through a manually controlled drip chamber.

    Closed systems decrease the risk of contamination.

    A prefilled closed-system container can safely hang for 24 to 48 hours if you use sterile technique.

    You can measure out the specified amount in the drip chamber, allowing the remainder of the container to be used later in the day.

Monitoring Patients Receiving Enteral Nutrition

For patients receiving enteral nutrition, you will need to monitor tube placement, skin condition, laboratory values (especially blood glucose, BUN, and electrolytes), feeding residual, and GI status. This will allow you to detect complications that affect metabolism or fluid and electrolyte balance and assess responses to enteral feeding. Feedings may need to be increased or decreased, depending on the patient's changing clinical condition.

 See **Clinical Insight 24-4: Monitoring Patients Receiving Enteral Nutrition,** in Volume 2.

Contamination of Enteral Feedings

Enteral feeding solutions provide an ideal medium for bacterial growth. Contamination of the feeding can have serious consequences for a patient. To reduce the risk:

- Check dates on feeding solutions and supplies. Do not use any that are outdated.
- Use sterile equipment and supplies; once you have opened them, handle them as little as possible.
- Disposable feeding equipment is meant for one-time use. Do not wash and reuse.
- Use meticulous hand hygiene; wear nonsterile gloves.
- Store opened feeding solutions in the refrigerator in covered and labeled containers. Allow the solution to return to room temperature before giving it to the patient. Discard after 24 hours.
- Keep unopened solutions at room temperature.
- Follow agency policy regarding how long a solution may be left hanging. Usually:

    Sterile feedings may be hung for up to 24 hours (or per unit policy).

    Nonsterile feedings (i.e., reconstituted powder feedings) may hang for up to 4 hours (or per unit policy).

- Label the feeding containers with the patient's name and the date and time hung, and document the time in the patient record.
- Never allow a feeding to hang below the height of the patient's stomach.
- Do not transfer sterile feedings into a second container.
- Replace feeding tubes and equipment according to the manufacturer's recommendations (or agency policy if that is sooner).

■ Use sterile water for (1) patients who are immuno-compromised, (2) patients receiving jejunal feeds, or (3) initially after a gastrostomy insertion.

For more detail,

see **Procedure 24-3A: Administering Feedings Through Gastric and Enteric Tubes With an Infusion Pump**, in Volume 2.

Administering Medication Through Feeding Tubes

Medications given through an enteral tube that are incompatible with this route and those that are constituted incorrectly can lead to patient harm or even death. Improper administration techniques can lead to an occluded feeding tube, reduced drug effect, or drug toxicity (Institute of Safe Medication Practices, 2010).

■ **Before administering any medication** through an NG tube, be sure to check drug compatibility with feeding solutions and other drugs, adverse effects, appropriate dosing, and the drug's risk of clogging the tube. Identify proper tube placement (Boullata et al., 2017).
■ **When giving enteral medication,** always remember "right medication, right patient, right dose, right time, right route, right tube/port, and right dilution." Give one medication at a time. Enteric-coated, extended-release (XR), or slow-release (SR) tablets or capsules cannot be given through the feeding tube.
■ **After medication is given,** flush the tube with 30 to 60 mL of water (Boullata et al., 2017; Memorial Sloan Kettering Cancer Center, 2020).

Removing Feeding Tubes

When a patient's condition has stabilized and they no longer require enteral nutrition, the feeding tube may be removed. A PEG tube is usually clamped if feedings are no longer required. For steps to follow when removing feeding tubes,

Go to **Procedure 24-4: Removing a Nasogastric or Nasenteric Tube,** in Volume 2.

Think**Like a Nurse** 24-8:
Clinical Judgment **in Action**

Your client has dementia and is frequently agitated. She has been progressively losing weight. An interprofessional team recommended enteral nutrition because of poor oral intake; however, the client has repeatedly pulled out her NG tube and had an episode of aspiration pneumonia last month. What recommendations might you consider at the next meeting?

Providing Parenteral Nutrition

Parenteral nutrition (PN) is the delivery of nutrition intravenously into a large central vein. This is the preferred method of feeding for clients who cannot be nourished through the GI tract. Some clients (e.g., those with shortened small bowel secondary to injury or disease) who can partially meet their nutritional needs orally

may supplement with PN to add calories and nutrients. Others (e.g., clients who are severely malnourished, have extensive burns or trauma, or have conditions that require resting the gastrointestinal system) are nourished entirely by PN.

Parenteral Nutrition Solutions These usually contain water, glucose (depending on the patient's calculated energy need), amino acids, essential fatty acids, vitamins, minerals, and trace elements. Standard PN formulas are available at many healthcare facilities; however, PN can be modified to meet individual needs.

Venous Access Devices The type of venous access device used to administer PN will depend on the components of the PN and the anticipated duration.

■ **Large, high-flow vein.** Because PN solutions are hypertonic, they should be administered in a large, high-flow vein through a central venous access catheter. The subclavian vein has been the site of choice (Fig. 24-11); however, the jugular vein is preferred for tunneled catheters and implanted ports.
■ Peripherally inserted central catheter (PICC) lines. PICC lines are also used for PN.
■ **Peripheral vein.** Some types of PN solutions may be infused via a peripheral vein, but this is not common.

Lipid Emulsions These contain essential fatty acids, triglycerides, and supplemental kcal. They are administered weekly for patients who rely on PN to prevent essential fatty acid deficiency. Lipids also add calories to the PN mixture so that lower glucose concentrations can be used, thus reducing the risk of glucose fluctuations. Most IV fats are supplied by safflower or soybean oil and provide 1.1 to 3 kcal/mL.

■ You may administer lipids at the same time as the PN, either through a peripheral line or by Y-connector tubing through a central line.
■ Lipids are also sometimes added to the PN solution (this is called a *3-in-1 admixture*) and administered over a 24-hour period.

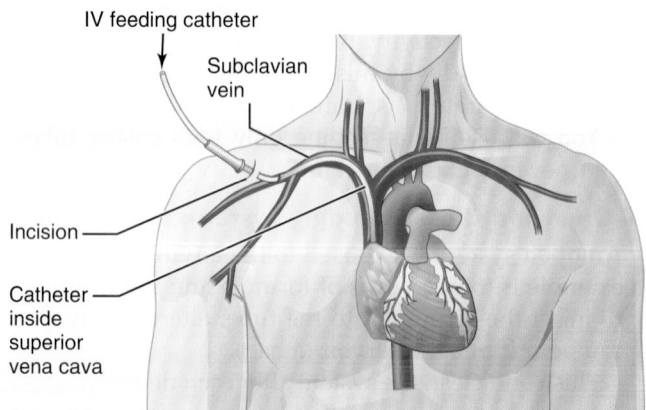

FIGURE 24-11 The subclavian vein is the site of choice for parenteral nutrition.

To learn about monitoring and maintenance of patients receiving parenteral nutrition,

 Go to **Procedure 24-5: Administering Parenteral Nutrition, Procedure 24-6: Administering Lipids,** and **Clinical Insight 24-4: Monitoring and Maintenance Interventions for Patients Receiving Parenteral Nutrition,** in Volume 2.

Complications of Parenteral Nutrition Because PN solutions are high in glucose and administered into the central circulation, complications are possible, including the following:

- **Infection or septic shock** can result from contamination of PN solution or supplies.
- **Blood clots** can occur with chronic IV access in the vascular system. Clots in the central system can result in pulmonary embolism and death.
- **Liver dysfunction,** such as fatty liver or liver failure, is a complication that is not uncommon with long-term PN use.
- **Gallbladder disease,** such as cholecystitis, occurs because of disuse of the GI tract, which leads to bile stasis (sludge) in the gallbladder and biliary ducts.

To explore learning resources for this chapter,

 Go to Davis Advantage and find:

Answers and Suggested Responses for all questions in this chapter

Concept Map

Knowledge Map

References and Bibliography

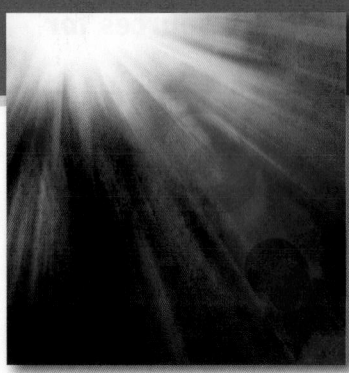

CHAPTER 25

Urinary Elimination

Learning Outcomes

After completing this chapter, you should be able to:

- ➤ Describe the normal structure and function of the organs in the urinary system.
- ➤ Describe the processes of urine formation and elimination.
- ➤ Discuss factors that affect urinary elimination.
- ➤ Conduct a nursing assessment and physical examination focused on urinary elimination.
- ➤ Accurately measure urine output.
- ➤ Describe procedures for collecting various types of urine specimens.
- ➤ Describe diagnostic tests used to identify urinary elimination problems.

- ➤ Discuss common elimination problems: urinary tract infection, urinary retention, and urinary incontinence.
- ➤ Identify nursing diagnoses associated with altered urinary elimination.
- ➤ Describe nursing interventions that promote normal urination.
- ➤ Provide care for clients experiencing urinary problems.
- ➤ Perform urinary catheterizations after accepted procedures.
- ➤ Discuss nursing care appropriate for clients who have a urinary diversion.

Key Concepts

Urinary elimination

Related Concepts

See the Concept Map on Davis Advantage.

Example Client Conditions

Urinary Incontinence

Urinary Retention

Urinary Tract Infection (UTI)

Meet Your Patient

During your clinical experience at University Hospital, you are completing the admission process for Marlena, a 55-year-old female patient who is complaining of frequent, painful urination. As you interview her, Marlena becomes embarrassed. "I really don't enjoy talking about this," she admits. When she asks to use the bathroom, you ask her to give you a midstream clean-catch urine sample. She returns with a small specimen of pink-tinged, strong-smelling urine. "I have a strong urge to go, and then I hardly have any urine. And it burns like crazy when I empty my bladder," she reports.

You close the door and interview Marlena in private about her usual urination pattern and current symptoms. Your calm approach and straightforward manner put her at ease. She confides that she is sexually active and that her symptoms began after spending the weekend with her new partner. You take her vital signs: oral temperature, 99.4°F (37.4°C); radial pulse, 88 beats/min; respiratory rate,

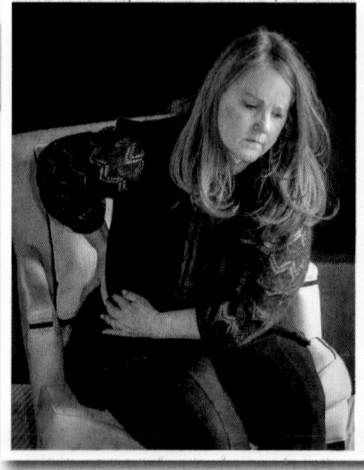

20 breaths/min; and blood pressure, 108/72 mm Hg.

The urgent care provider asks you to perform a dipstick urinalysis on the urine sample and to send the urine sample to the laboratory for culture and sensitivity. They ask: "Well, what do you think we need to do next?" How would you answer this question?

As you gain theoretical and practical knowledge in this chapter, we will return to this case study to discuss how you might answer the provider's question and support Marlena's recovery. You will also have the opportunity to examine your own feelings about giving care that patients may regard as personal or even embarrassing.

TheoreticalKnowledge
knowing **why**

A variety of factors, including personal hygiene, age, nutrition, stress, sexual activity, and medications, play a role in urinary health.

ABOUT THE KEY CONCEPTS

The key concept of **urinary elimination** is important because many of your nursing activities focus on promoting normal elimination. To best care for patients with urinary problems and provide holistic independent and collaborative interventions for them, you must understand the concepts involved in the formation and elimination of urine and how those processes may be altered.

HOW DOES THE URINARY SYSTEM WORK?

The body removes from food and fluids the nutrients necessary for essential bodily functions, such as physical activity, self-repair, and mental operations. The kidneys, ureters, bladder, and urethra help to excrete waste products in the blood and maintain a balance of chemicals and water (Fig. 25-1).

The Kidneys Filter and Regulate

Functions The kidneys are essential for homeostasis.

- **The kidneys filter** metabolic wastes, toxins, drugs, hormones, salts, and water from the bloodstream and excrete

them as urine. If kidney function is impaired, these substances may reach toxic levels and damage body cells.
- **They help to regulate** blood volume, blood pressure, electrolyte levels, and acid–base balance by selectively reabsorbing water and other substances.
- **Secondary functions of the kidneys** are to produce red blood cells, secrete the enzyme renin, and activate vitamin D_3 (calcitriol).

Anatomy The kidneys are **retroperitoneal** (located against the posterior abdominal wall behind the peritoneum). They are positioned under the 11th rib, extending from the T12 to the L3 vertebrae. Each kidney measures approximately 4 inches (10 cm) long by 2 inches (5 cm) wide and 1 inch (2.5 cm) thick. The average kidney weighs about 5 ounces and is the shape of a kidney bean (Thompson, 2020). Figure 25-2 shows the structures of the urinary system and their functions.

The Nephrons Form Urine

The **nephron** is the filtration unit of the kidney that is involved in the formation of urine (Fig. 25-3). Each nephron consists of:

- A **Bowman's capsule** (a double-walled hollow capsule), enclosing a **glomerulus,** a knotty ball of capillaries
- A series of filtrating tubules
- Loop of Henle
- A collecting duct

Together, these structures act as a microscopic filter, controlling the excretion and retention of fluids and

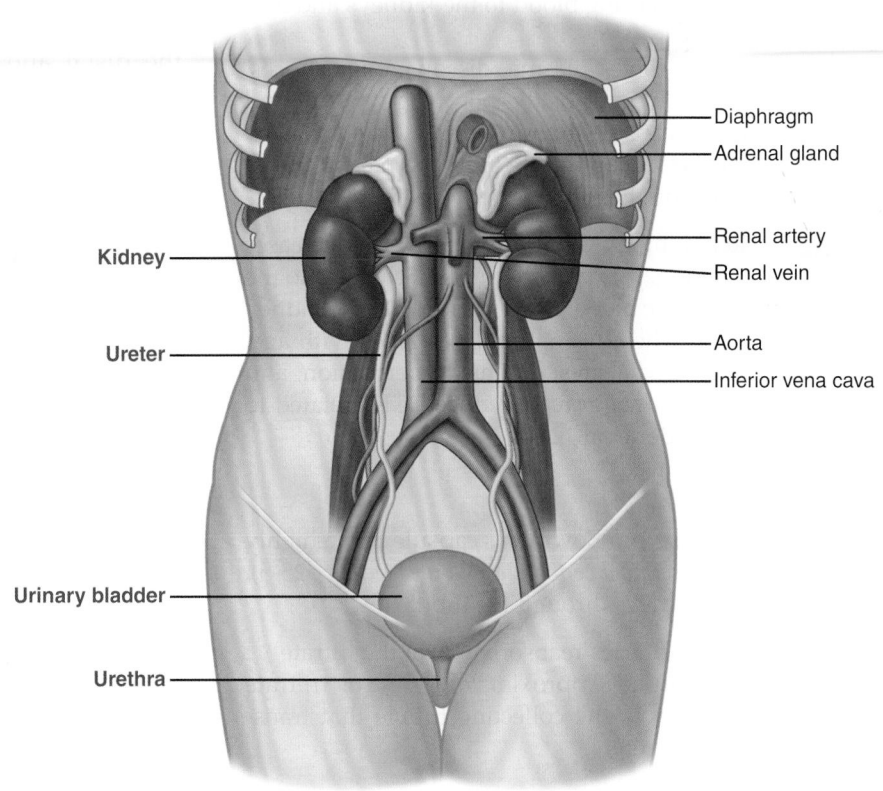

FIGURE 25-1 The organs of the urinary system include the kidneys, ureters, bladder, and urethra.

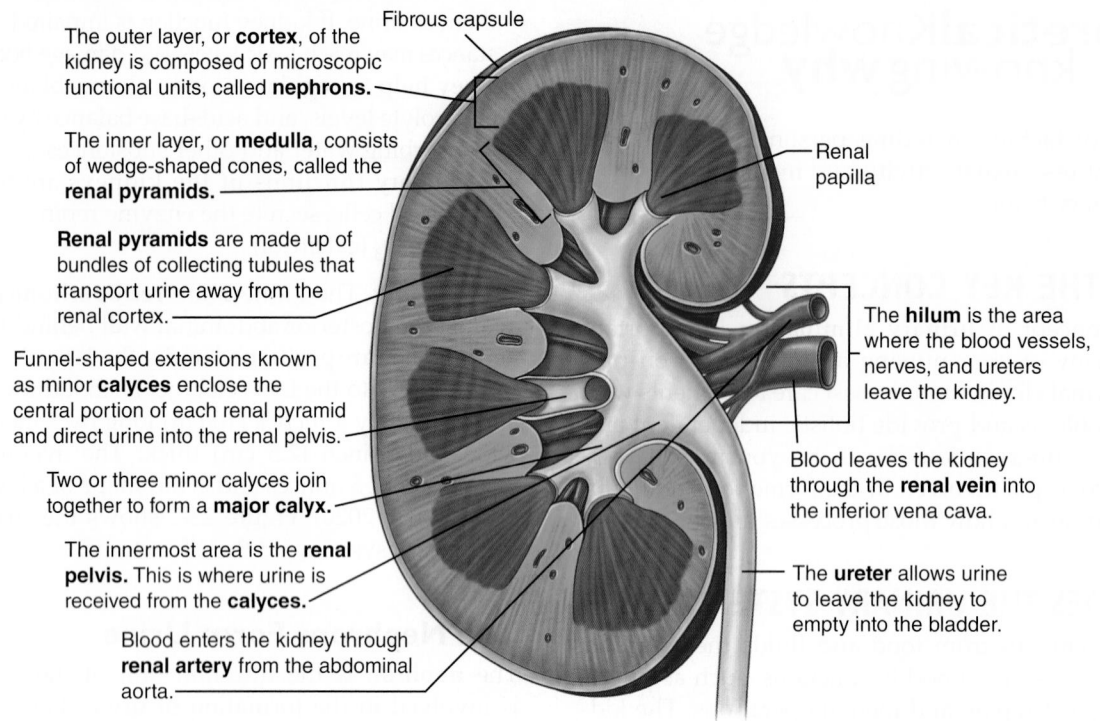

The outer layer, or **cortex**, of the kidney is composed of microscopic functional units, called **nephrons.**

Fibrous capsule

The inner layer, or **medulla**, consists of wedge-shaped cones, called the **renal pyramids.**

Renal papilla

Renal pyramids are made up of bundles of collecting tubules that transport urine away from the renal cortex.

The **hilum** is the area where the blood vessels, nerves, and ureters leave the kidney.

Funnel-shaped extensions known as minor **calyces** enclose the central portion of each renal pyramid and direct urine into the renal pelvis.

Blood leaves the kidney through the **renal vein** into the inferior vena cava.

Two or three minor calyces join together to form a **major calyx.**

The innermost area is the **renal pelvis.** This is where urine is received from the **calyces.**

The **ureter** allows urine to leave the kidney to empty into the bladder.

Blood enters the kidney through **renal artery** from the abdominal aorta.

FIGURE 25-2 A cross section of the kidney showing the renal cortex, medulla, pyramids, and calyces.

solutes to meet the body's needs for fluid and electrolyte balance. Urine is formed by filtration, reabsorption, and secretion (Fig. 25-4).

Glomerular Filtration

Figure 25-5 summarizes the process of urine formation. The first step, **filtration,** occurs in the glomeruli.

- The renal arteries bring blood to the kidneys and into the glomeruli.
- Blood pressure forces plasma, dissolved substances, and small proteins out of the porous glomeruli and into Bowman's capsule to form a liquid called **filtrate.**
- The **glomerular filtration rate** (GFR) is the amount of filtrate formed by the kidneys per minute.

Renal blood flow progressively decreases with aging, primarily because of changes to the microscopic blood vessels leading to the kidney (Shenot, 2021). The GFR naturally declines with age. Diseases such as diabetes, chronic hypertension, and kidney disease can aggravate reduced GFR related to aging (Abdulkader et al., 2017).

Tubular Reabsorption

The filtrate moves from Bowman's capsule into a highly twisted tubule (*proximal convoluted tubule;* see Fig. 25-5). As the filtrate journeys through the tubule:

- **Peritubular capillaries** reabsorb 99% of the filtrate.
- **Collecting tubule**—Approximately 1% of filtrate returns, as urine, to the collecting tubule that transports it into the ureters.

- **Distal and collecting tubules**—Waste and toxins that remain in the blood after filtration are actively transported into the filtrate (reabsorbed). Water and sodium are reabsorbed in these structures when antidiuretic hormone (ADH) and aldosterone are secreted.

When the amount of fluid in the body decreases (e.g., because of low intake or blood loss), the posterior pituitary gland secretes more ADH. This causes the distal and collecting tubules to reabsorb more water into the blood. At the same time, the adrenal cortex secretes more aldosterone, which increases the reabsorption of sodium, and water follows sodium back into the blood. ADH and aldosterone thus have the effect of maintaining normal blood volume and blood pressure.

When the amount of water in the body increases (e.g., as in ingestion of excessive fluids), ADH is suppressed, and the opposite effect occurs. Urine becomes dilute, and water continues to be eliminated until its concentration returns to normal (Scanlon & Sanders, 2018).

Tubular Secretion

As blood flows through the peritubular capillaries:

- **They remove (secrete) metabolic wastes** (e.g., ammonia and creatinine, and some medications) from the blood into the urine.
- **They secrete hydrogen ions** (H^+) to help maintain the normal pH of blood.

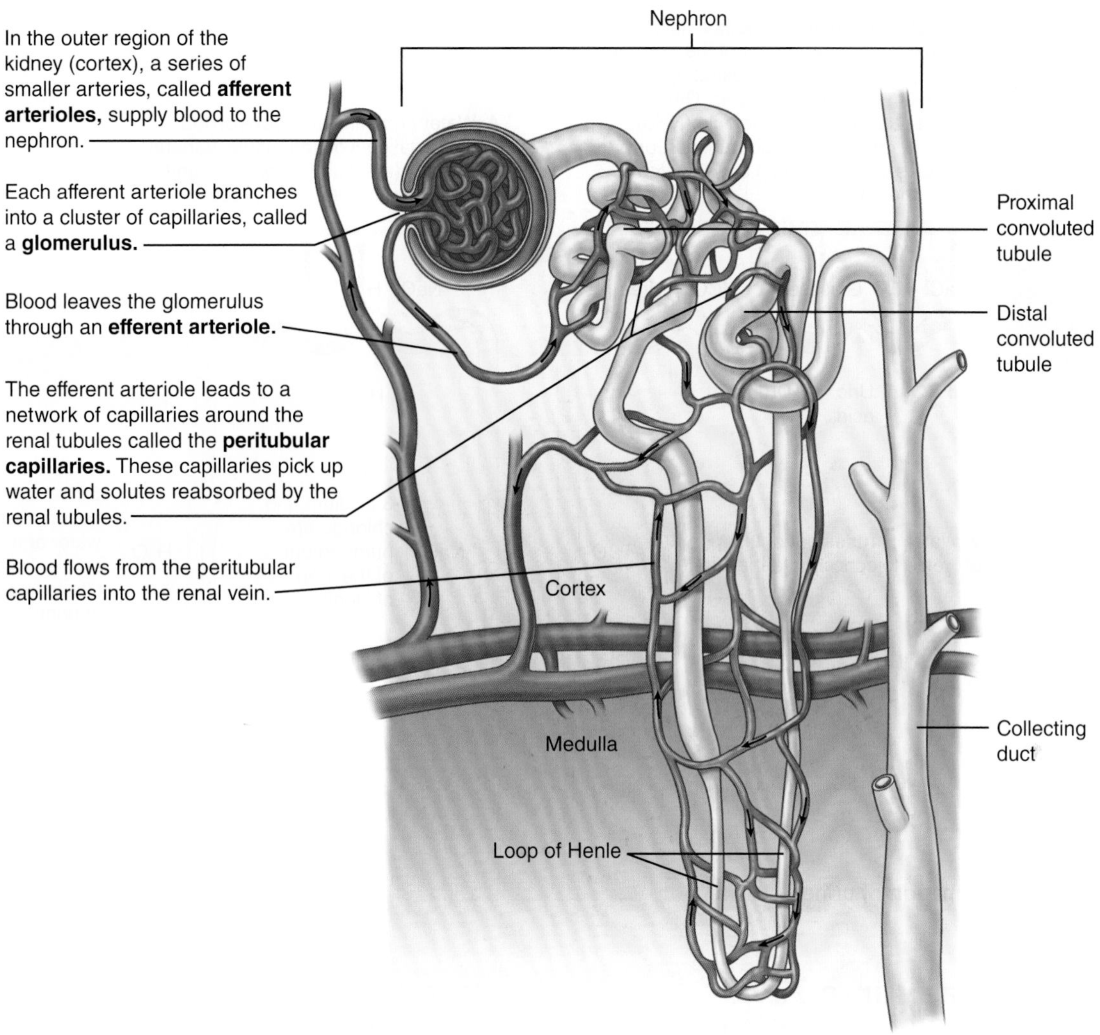

Nephron

In the outer region of the kidney (cortex), a series of smaller arteries, called **afferent arterioles,** supply blood to the nephron.

Each afferent arteriole branches into a cluster of capillaries, called a **glomerulus.**

Blood leaves the glomerulus through an **efferent arteriole.**

The efferent arteriole leads to a network of capillaries around the renal tubules called the **peritubular capillaries.** These capillaries pick up water and solutes reabsorbed by the renal tubules.

Blood flows from the peritubular capillaries into the renal vein.

Proximal convoluted tubule

Distal convoluted tubule

Cortex

Medulla

Collecting duct

Loop of Henle

FIGURE 25-3 The nephron is the basic structural and functional unit of the kidney.

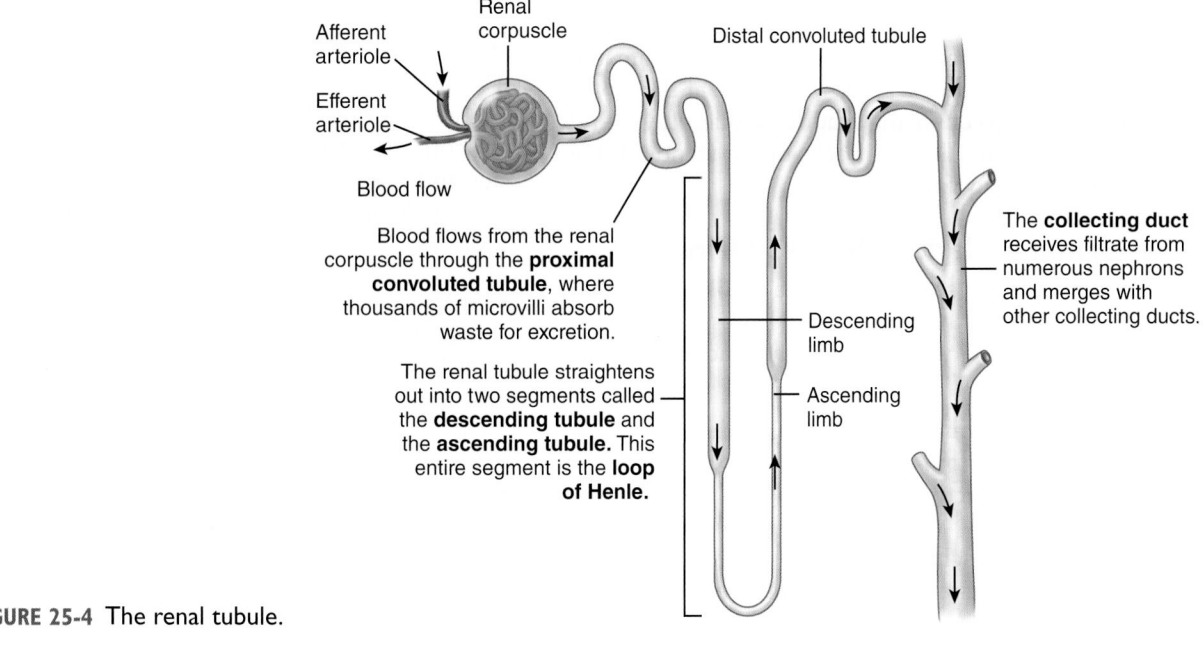

Renal corpuscle

Afferent arteriole

Efferent arteriole

Blood flow

Distal convoluted tubule

The **collecting duct** receives filtrate from numerous nephrons and merges with other collecting ducts.

Blood flows from the renal corpuscle through the **proximal convoluted tubule,** where thousands of microvilli absorb waste for excretion.

The renal tubule straightens out into two segments called the **descending tubule** and the **ascending tubule.** This entire segment is the **loop of Henle.**

Descending limb

Ascending limb

FIGURE 25-4 The renal tubule.

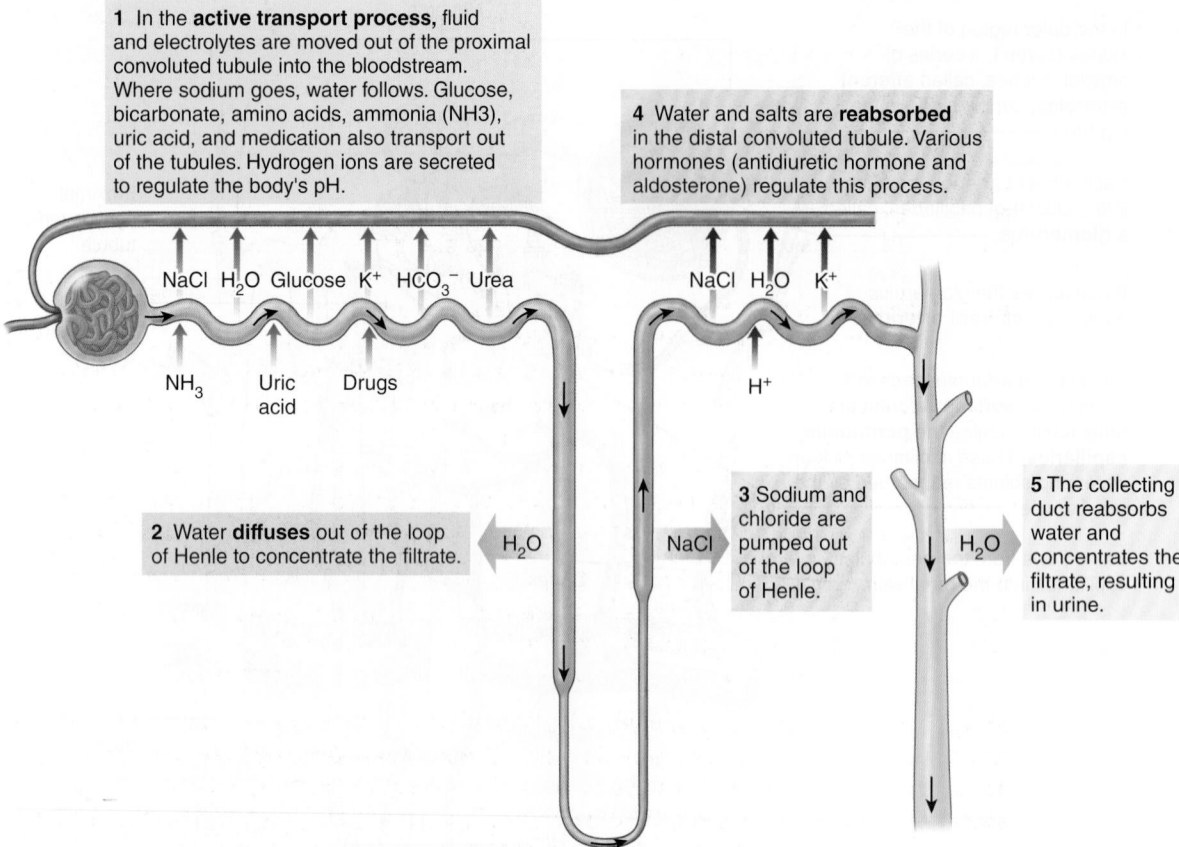

1 In the **active transport process,** fluid and electrolytes are moved out of the proximal convoluted tubule into the bloodstream. Where sodium goes, water follows. Glucose, bicarbonate, amino acids, ammonia (NH3), uric acid, and medication also transport out of the tubules. Hydrogen ions are secreted to regulate the body's pH.

4 Water and salts are **reabsorbed** in the distal convoluted tubule. Various hormones (antidiuretic hormone and aldosterone) regulate this process.

2 Water **diffuses** out of the loop of Henle to concentrate the filtrate.

3 Sodium and chloride are pumped out of the loop of Henle.

5 The collecting duct reabsorbs water and concentrates the filtrate, resulting in urine.

FIGURE 25-5 Formation of urine.

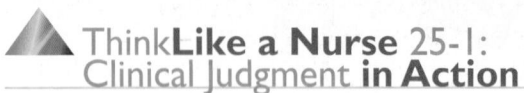

ThinkLike a Nurse 25-1:
Clinical Judgment in Action

If a client is suffering from impaired kidney function, what signs and symptoms might you expect to see?

The Ureters Transport Urine

Ureters are narrow tubes that carry urine from the kidneys to the bladder (see Fig. 25-1). Muscles within the ureter walls tighten and relax, forcing urine from the kidneys into the bladder. A one-way valve at the opening allows urine to enter the bladder while preventing reflux into the ureter. If urine backs up, or stands still, a kidney infection can develop.

The Urinary Bladder Stores Urine

The urinary bladder (see Fig. 25-1) is a saclike organ that receives urine from the ureters and stores it until discharged from the body. The wall of the bladder consists of four layers:

- **An innermost mucous membrane** seals off the remaining layers from exposure to urine.
- **A layer of connective tissue** supports the mucous membrane.
- **The detrusor muscle** is composed of three layers of longitudinal and circular smooth muscle fibers.
- **An outermost layer of fibrous connective tissue** covers the detrusor layer.

An average, normal bladder can store 500 mL (1 pint) of urine but may distend when needed to a capacity twice that amount. You cannot palpate an empty bladder, but you can feel a full or distended bladder in the area above the pubis. It is smooth, firm, and oval-shaped.

The Urethra Transports Urine

The **urethra** transports urine from the bladder to the body's exterior. The mucous membrane of the urethra (in both men and women) is continuous with the bladder and the ureters. Therefore, infection in the urethra can easily spread through the bladder and up into the kidneys.

- *In females,* the urethra is about 3 to 4 cm (1.5 in.) long; it opens at the **urinary meatus** between the clitoris and vaginal opening. Because the female urethra is so short, women are especially prone to urinary tract infection (UTI) from microorganisms residing in the vagina and rectum.
- *In males,* the urethra extends about 20 cm (8 in.) from the bladder to the urinary meatus at the distal end of the penis. As it leaves the bladder, the male urethra passes through a surrounding gland known as the **prostate.** In addition to urine, the male urethra also carries semen.

- Identify the major structures of the urinary system.
- What are the functions of the kidneys?
- Briefly describe how urine is formed.
- What role do the ureters, bladder, and urethra play in urinary elimination?

HOW DOES URINARY ELIMINATION OCCUR?

Where the bladder connects to the urethra is a thickening of smooth muscle, called the **internal urethral sphincter.** When closed, the internal sphincter keeps urine in the bladder from entering the urethra. When the bladder contains 200 to 450 mL of urine (50 to 200 mL in children):

1. **Distention** activates stretch receptors in the bladder wall.
2. **Stretch receptors** send sensory impulses to the *voiding reflex center* in the spinal cord.
3. **Motor impulses** then cause the detrusor muscle to contract and the internal sphincter to relax for **voiding** (also called **urination** or **micturition**). This triggers the conscious urge to void.
    1. The **internal sphincter** is not under voluntary control.
    2. Voiding may be voluntarily delayed by inhibiting release of a second, **external urethral sphincter.**
4. **When the person is ready to urinate,** the brain signals the external sphincter to relax, and urine flows through the urethra. Further contraction of the detrusor muscle normally forces out any urine remaining in the bladder.
5. **After the detrusor muscle relaxes,** the bladder begins to fill with urine again.

In addition to normal functioning of the bladder and urethra, the brain, spinal cord, and nerves supplying the bladder and urethra must be intact. The person must be aware of the need to urinate and able to respond by either inhibiting the reflex or allowing the release of urine.

Normal Urination Patterns

- **The kidneys produce about 50 to 60 mL of urine per hour,** or 1,500 mL per day. Output may fluctuate by 1,000 to 2,000 mL.
- **Most people void about five or six times per day**—typically after awakening, after each meal, and just before bedtime. When fluid intake is increased, urination will be more frequent.
- **Frequent urination** is sometimes a sign of other medical problems, such as diabetes or UTI.
- **Infrequent urination** may indicate dehydration.

Characteristics of Normal Urine

Specific gravity is a measure of dissolved solutes in a solution. As the concentration of the urine solutes increases, specific gravity increases. The specific gravity of distilled water is 1.000 because there are no dissolved solutes. **Key Point:** *The normal specific gravity range for urine is 1.002 to 1.030.*

- **As fluid intake increases,** urine becomes dilute and lighter in color to almost clear as it approaches a specific gravity of 1.000.
- **If fluid intake is low or there have been fluid losses,** as with diarrhea or vomiting, the urine darkens as the specific gravity rises.

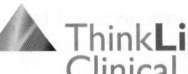 **Think**Like a Nurse 25-2: Clinical Judgment **in Action**

- How does Marlena's (Meet Your Patient) urinary elimination pattern differ from normal?
- What would you expect to find if you measured her specific gravity?
- Marlena's symptoms suggest a UTI. How might this be related to the fact that she is sexually active?

WHAT FACTORS AFFECT URINARY ELIMINATION?

Given the complex structure and physiology of the urinary organs, many of the following variables affect their function.

Developmental Factors: Infants and Children

The normal specific gravity of a newborn's urine is 1.008. Over the first weeks of life, the urine gradually becomes more concentrated, and the well-hydrated infant produces 8 to 10 wet diapers a day. Infants do not have voluntary control of voiding because neuromuscular functioning is immature.

Timing of Toilet Training This is highly variable and is influenced by family and culture (e.g., the presence of older children who can act as role models). In the United States, most parents begin toilet training when their child is between 18 and 36 months of age. Before toilet training can occur, toddlers must be able to control the external urethral sphincter, sense the urge to void, communicate their need to use the toilet, and remove their clothing. However, even after bladder control is achieved, occasional involuntary passage of urine may occur, even in the early school years.

Enuresis, or occasional involuntary passage of urine, is normal in children, even in the early school years—especially when the child is intensely absorbed in an activity. Such events should be accepted calmly.

Nocturnal enuresis, or nighttime bedwetting, occurs in a few children aged 6 to 7 years. However, most children achieve nighttime dryness between 3 and 5 years of age. Nocturnal enuresis is caused by low levels of antidiuretic hormone (ADH), pressure on the bladder, urinary infection, or emotional stress.

The condition tends to run in families and most often resolves without treatment. To manage nocturnal enuresis in children, see the accompanying iCare box and the accompanying Home Care box, Managing Nocturnal Enuresis in Children.

♥ iCare 25-1

Children With Nocturnal Enuresis

- Children, especially older ones, can be embarrassed by *nocturnal enuresis*, not to mention the inconvenience it poses.
- Young children may feel anxious about using the bathroom in a clinic, hospital, or any unfamiliar environment, and they may be especially uncomfortable using a bedpan.
- The stress of an illness or hospitalization may cause a child to regress in their ability to toilet independently.

Developmental Factors: Older Adults

Age-Related Changes in the Kidneys

The size and functioning of the kidneys diminish with age. This results in a decline in filtration rate, which affects the ability to eliminate waste as well as dilute and concentrate urine but does not normally create problems unless an illness alters fluid balance.

- When older adults lose fluids and electrolytes through vomiting and diarrhea, it is difficult for their kidneys to maintain acid–base and electrolyte balances.
- Arteriosclerosis (hardening of the blood vessels), common in older adults, can reduce blood flow and impair the kidney's ability to filter toxins from the blood to excrete into the urine.
- Drug toxicity is a risk as a result of decreased kidney function.

Other Physiological Changes of Aging

- Loss of elasticity and muscle tone in the bladder wall, which can lead to retention of urine or compromised bladder control
- *In females:* Loss of abdominal and perineal muscle tone resulting from childbearing
- *In males:* Prostate gland enlargement, which can lead to blockage of urine

Symptoms Produced by Physiological Changes

- Nocturnal frequency of urine
- Bladder infections resulting from incomplete bladder emptying
- Leakage of urine
- Particularly in males, dribbling, urinary frequency, difficulty starting urination, and reduced force of the urinary stream.
- Retention of urine after voiding, which increases the risk for bladder infections.

Home Care

Managing Nocturnal Enuresis in Children

- **♥ iCare** ➤ Reassure parents that in most cases, loving acceptance and passage of time provide the cure. Shaming, penalties, and taking back rewards are not only ineffective but are detrimental to a child's self-image and relationship with parents at home.
- ➤ Cover the mattress with plastic.
- ➤ Encourage the child to drink most fluids in the morning and early afternoon.
- ➤ Avoid caffeine or carbonated beverages, citrus juices, and sports drinks that irritate the bladder or produce more urine (National Institute of Diabetes and Digestive and Kidney Diseases [NIDDKD], 2017).
- ➤ Have the child empty the bladder twice before bedtime.
- ➤ Use a moisture alarm that wakes the child when wetting occurs. This device helps the child to learn to sense the signal to urinate and gain control over bladder emptying.
- ➤ If bedwetting persists into the school-age years, the child should receive a thorough medical evaluation to rule out underlying disease processes.
- ➤ Parents should plan to bathe the child in the morning rather than at bedtime to minimize urine odor.
- ➤ Anticholinergic medication (oxybutynin) can be effective in calming an overactive bladder unless the child matures and grows out of the problem. Medication is helpful when the child is not sleeping at home.

Personal, Sociocultural, and Environmental Factors

There are many different reasons why people may delay emptying their bladders.

- **♥ iCare ▪ Anxiety.** A person who is anxious and tense may not be able to relax the abdominal and perineal muscles and the external urethral sphincter.
- **Lack of time.** Most people find it difficult to void when they feel rushed; therefore, when helping patients to void, make sure you have scheduled enough time for them to relax fully.
- **Delayed voiding.** Some people wait to empty their bladder while they are working or busy with other activities. This promotes urinary stasis and can lead to bladder infections.
- **Lack of privacy.** Many people require privacy for voiding. Some hospitalized clients may also avoid asking for assistance to the bathroom.

- **Loss of dignity.** Patients who need assistance with toileting may be especially vulnerable to such feelings, especially if they require catheterization or a bedpan. It is important, therefore, to acknowledge such feelings and encourage the patient to participate in other aspects of self-care, such as bathing and dressing.
- **Cultural influences.** Personal, cultural, or religious beliefs regarding toileting may be a reason some patients wait until a visit from a family member to obtain help with voiding.

Lifestyle Factors

Lifestyle factors can also affect kidney function.

- **Activity.** The kidneys conserve water when a person is dehydrated, which results in concentrated urine. During prolonged periods of physical activity, especially in hot weather, the body loses sodium and other electrolytes rapidly through sweat. Electrolyte-replacement beverages may be more beneficial than plain water in helping to prevent dehydration for prolonged, vigorous-intensity activity. For most adults, pale to clear urine indicates adequate hydration.
- **Caffeine** acts as a diuretic and increases urine production.
- **Alcohol consumption.** High alcohol intake impairs the release of ADH, resulting in increased production of urine.
- **Diet.** A high-salt diet causes water retention and decreases urine production.

KnowledgeCheck 25-2

- What quantity of urine in the bladder will stimulate the urge to void?
- Identify at least three methods for determining whether hydration is adequate and urine output is within normal limits.

Medications

Various medications affect urination—for example, by treating pain, increasing urination, relaxing smooth muscles, or causing urinary retention.

- **Analgesics.** Phenazopyridine hydrochloride (Pyridium), a bladder analgesic, turns the urine a deep orange-red color.
- **Diuretics,** sometimes called "water pills," treat blood pressure, fluid retention, and edema by increasing the elimination of urine. Diuretics are classified as thiazide, potassium-sparing, or loop-acting diuretics (Box 25-1).
- **Anticholinergics** promote urine retention by inhibiting involuntary contractions (spasms) of the bladder, increasing bladder capacity, and delaying the urge to void for those with *urge incontinence.* They may be given by oral or transdermal routes. Transdermal medications are commonly used to treat urge

---

BOX 25-1 ■ Common Diuretic Classes

Thiazide diuretics are used to treat high blood pressure by reducing the amount of sodium and water in the body. They also dilate blood vessels, thereby lowering blood pressure.

Potassium-sparing diuretics reduce the amount of water in the body. Unlike other diuretic medicines, these medicines do not cause potassium loss.

Loop-acting diuretics cause the kidneys to excrete more urine by reabsorbing less water. This reduces the amount of water in the body and lowers blood pressure.

Medications that have significant interactions with diuretics include digoxin, antihypertensives, lithium, certain antidepressants (especially when taking thiazide or loop-acting diuretics), and the immunosuppressant cyclosporine, especially when the patient is taking a potassium-sparing diuretic.

Common side effects of diuretics include weakness, muscle cramps, skin rash, increased sensitivity to sunlight (with thiazide diuretics), dizziness, light-headedness, and joint pain.

---

incontinence caused by overactive bladder. The patch relieves symptoms for up to 4 days.

- **Antidepressants** (e.g., duloxetine or imipramine) reduce stress incontinence by relaxing the bladder muscles. Some work by stimulating the nerve that controls the urethral sphincter.
- **Antispasmodics** work to stop bladder muscle contractions (relax the bladder) and prevent urge incontinence. For example, propantheline bromide is prescribed to treat overactive bladder.
- **Muscarinic receptor antagonists** (e.g., tolterodine tartrate) block nerve receptors in the smooth muscle of the bladder. They control bladder contraction and reduce urinary frequency for people suffering from overactive bladder and urge incontinence.
- **Estrogen** is used to improve the blood flow to the urethral tissues and increase the thickness of mucosal and urethral tissues.
- **Botulinum toxin** injections control the spasms of overactive bladder by relaxing the muscles, especially when it occurs from nerve damage, such as with spinal cord injury or multiple sclerosis.

✚ Some medications given for other than kidney conditions are nephrotoxic (damaging to the kidneys). These include some antibiotics, such as gentamicin and amphotericin B, and high doses or long-term use of aspirin and ibuprofen.

Surgery and Anesthesia

Surgery on or in the urinary and reproductive systems can affect urinary function:

- **Urinary tract surgeries** can affect urine solutes, urine characteristics, and the ability to pass urine normally. Manipulation of the urinary tract frequently leads to trauma, bleeding, or the introduction of bacteria into a normally sterile tract. The urine may be tinged with red or pink after any invasive urinary tract surgery or procedure.

- **Diagnostic and invasive procedures and childbirth** can cause swelling and urinary retention.
- **Surgery in the pubic area, vagina, or rectum** is associated with a high incidence of trauma to the urinary organs, lower abdominal swelling, loss of pelvic muscle control, and increased pressure on the kidneys, ureters, or bladder. Postoperatively, patients typically require the use of an indwelling catheter for draining the bladder.
- **Surgery on the reproductive organs,** such as hysterectomy in female patient or transurethral resection of the prostate in male patients, usually requires the use of an indwelling catheter (tube) for draining the bladder postoperatively.
- **Anesthetic agents** can decrease blood pressure and glomerular filtration, thus decreasing urine formation. Spinal anesthesia decreases the patient's awareness of the need to void, which may lead to bladder distention.

Pathological Conditions

Disorders of the Urinary System Disorders of the urinary system that affect urinary elimination include the following:

- **Infection or inflammation** of the bladder, ureters, or kidneys. For information about and nursing care of UTIs, see the accompanying Example Client Condition: Urinary Tract Infection. The most common microorganism is *Escherichia coli* because of the proximity of the fecal excrement with defecation. *Pseudomonas* species, *Enterococcus* species, *Staphylococcus aureus,* coagulase-negative staphylococci, *Enterobacter* species, and yeast can also cause UTI (Brusch, 2021).
- *Renal calculi* **(kidney stones)** *or tumors,* which obstruct the normal flow of urine.
- *Hypertrophy* **(excessive growth)** of the prostate gland, especially in older men, as a result of benign or cancerous lesions, which interferes with the flow of urine from the bladder into the urethra.

Diseases in Other Systems Diseases in other systems can indirectly affect urinary function. For example:

- **Cardiovascular and metabolic disorders** decrease blood flow through the glomeruli and thus impair filtration and urine production.
- **Nervous system** conditions that affect control of the urinary system organs will impair urinary elimination. After a stroke or spinal cord injury, for example, some patients may lose bladder control. **Neurogenic bladder** occurs because of impaired neurological function. The person cannot perceive bladder fullness or control the urinary sphincters. The bladder becomes flaccid or spastic, causing frequent involuntary loss of urine.

- **Systemic infection,** especially when accompanied by a high fever, causes the kidneys to reabsorb and retain water.
- **Immobility and impaired communication** may interfere with the ability to get to the bathroom in time or to communicate the need for assistance. This may result in urination in inappropriate settings or at inappropriate times.
- **Cognitive changes** (e.g., brain changes or severe psychiatric conditions) that alter the perception of the urge to void or severe psychiatric conditions involving altered perception or the ability to manage activities of daily living may lead to **incontinence** (involuntary loss of urine).

KnowledgeCheck 25-3

- What common medications increase the amount of urine voided?
- What types of medications are associated with urinary retention?
- What types of conditions or surgeries are associated with a high incidence of altered urination?

 ThinkLike a Nurse 25-3: Clinical Judgment **in Action**

As you may have concluded, Marlena (Meet Your Patient) has a UTI. What additional history questions would you like to ask Marlena?

PracticalKnowledge knowing **how**

As a nurse, you will monitor and assist clients with urinary elimination, teach them about body functions, and work collaboratively with the healthcare team to facilitate normal urinary function. Also see the Nursing Care Plan and the Care Map.

 Go to Chapter 25, **Nursing Care Plan and Care Map,** in Volume 2.

ASSESSMENT/RECOGNIZING CUES

To assess urinary elimination, you will use data from the nursing history, physical examination, and diagnostic and laboratory reports.

Nursing History

♥ **iCare** Because urination patterns vary among individuals, you will need a nursing history to determine what is normal for a particular person. Customize your assessment to the client's needs, and use language that makes them feel comfortable.
For specific interview questions,

 See Chapter 25, **Focused Assessment Box: Assessment Guidelines and Tools, Urinary Elimination History Questions,** in Volume 2.

EXAMPLE CLIENT CONDITION: Urinary Tract Infection (UTI)

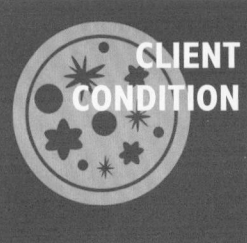

CLIENT CONDITION

Definition: Infection in any part of the urinary system—kidneys, ureters, bladder, and urethra

Transmission: Microorganisms, usually *Escherichia coli,* which normally live harmlessly in the colon, enter the urethra and begin to multiply, overwhelming the normal flora. A urinary tract infection (UTI) is a primary site of infection and cannot be considered secondary to another site of infection (Centers for Disease Control and Prevention, 2022).

Types of UTIs

- **Urethritis**—infection limited to the urethra
- **Cystitis**—bladder infection caused by microbes within the urethra
- **Pyelonephritis**—infection that progresses upward to the ureters or kidneys
- **Catheter-Associated Urinary Tract Infections (CAUTI)**—In otherwise healthy patients, CAUTIs are often asymptomatic and likely to resolve spontaneously with the removal of the catheter.
- **Complications**—UTIs can lead to prostatitis, epididymitis, cystitis, pyelonephritis, and gram-negative bacteremia, particularly in high-risk patients.

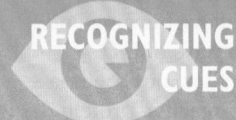

RECOGNIZING CUES

Assess for Risk Factors

- **Sexual activity (female).** During intercourse, perineal pathogens (usually *E. coli*) may enter the urethra. Because the female urethra is short, pathogens can quickly enter the bladder.
- **Use of spermicidal contraceptive gel (women).** Spermicides reduce normal flora in the vagina, allowing pathogens to multiply.
- **Postmenopausal patients.** Estrogen loss leads to drying of the vaginal mucosa and urethra and a reduction in protective normal flora.
- **Pregnant patients.** Hormone changes and pressure of the uterus on the bladder cause urinary stasis and stagnant urine—a good medium for bacterial growth.
- **Enlarged prostate (male patients) and pelvic organ prolapse (female patients).** Pressure from the prostate creates difficulty emptying the bladder, resulting in stagnant urine.
- **Presence of an indwelling catheter.**
  - Pathogens may be introduced into the urethra during catheterization.
  - Failing to maintain a closed drainage system, providing a pathway for bacteria into the urethra.
  - The catheter irritates the urethral mucosa, creating a portal of entry for microbes.
  - The longer the catheter remains, the higher the risk of developing a UTI.
  - The urine collection bag is a closed system, acting as a reservoir for microorganisms.
- For details about diagnostic tests,

 See **Diagnostic Testing** boxes in Volume 2.

- **Kidney stones.** Renal calculi obstruct urine flow, creating stagnation and irritation of the urinary tract as they are passed.
- **Diabetes mellitus.** Glucose in the urine provides nutrients for bacteria to multiply.
- **Immunocompromised.** Neonates, older adults, patients receiving immunosuppressive drugs, and people with a weakened immune system are less able to maintain a healthy balance of normal (resident) and pathogenic microbes in the urinary tract.
- **History of UTIs.** Previous UTIs suggest an increased likelihood of recurrence because the urinary tract is colonized with pathogens.

Symptoms

Bladder spasms
Burning with urination
Chills
Dysuria
Edema
Fever
Flank pain when UTI advances to kidney infection
Foul-smelling urine
Hematuria
Urinary frequency

Diagnostic Tests

- Midstream, clean-catch urine specimen—for culture
- Dipstick urine—for leukocytes, blood, estrace, and nitrates; negative dipstick does not rule out UTI.
- For details about a focused nursing history and physical assessment,

 See the Focused Assessment boxes, **Urinary Elimination History Questions** and **Guidelines for Physical Assessment for Urinary Elimination,** in Volume 2.

(continued)

EXAMPLE CLIENT CONDITION: Urinary Tract Infection (UTI)—cont'd

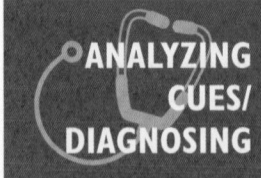

ANALYZING CUES/ DIAGNOSING

Infection Risk
Potential complication: Pyelonephritis

Acute Pain r/t inflammation 2° urinary infection

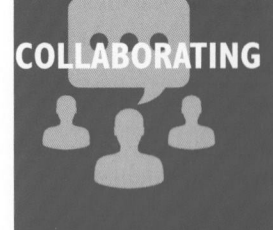

GENERATING SOLUTIONS

Individualized Outcomes Examples
- Resumes normal urinary pattern by [date]
- No pain on urination
- Urine clear (e.g., no blood) within 2 days of starting antibiotics

NOC Standardized Outcomes Examples
- Kidney Function
- Urinary Elimination

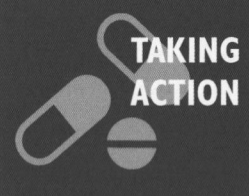

COLLABORATING

Treatment
- Length and type of antibiotic treatment depends on the location and severity of infection
- Cystitis (symptomatic)—oral antibiotics for 1 to 5 days

- Pyelonephritis—IV antibiotics followed by a course of oral antibiotics
- Phenazopyridine to relieve burning and urgency for first 2 or 3 days of UTI
- Liberal fluid intake to flush out bacteria
- Biomarkers, such as C-reactive protein (CRP), document the effectiveness of the antibiotic regimen (Aulin et al., 2021).

TAKING ACTION

Prevention
- Consider alternatives to catheter insertion, when possible.
- After aseptic insertion of the urinary catheter, maintain a closed drainage system.
- Maintain unobstructed urine flow. Clamping the tubing is not necessary before removing it.
- Unless urine obstruction is suspected, do not perform bladder irrigation.
- Preventive antibiotic treatment—not recommended; drug resistance develops easily.

- Leave the catheter in place only as needed. The risk of CAUTI increases the longer the catheter remains in place.
- Use meticulous technique for insertion and care.

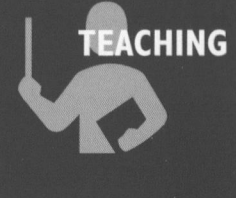

TEACHING

Teaching for Prevention

Teach your patient to:
- **Drink at least 64 ounces of water per day** to keep urine dilute and to flush bacteria from the urinary tract. Although some claim a benefit to drinking cranberry juice, this is unproven.
- **Urinate when you first feel the urge.** Do not postpone urination because bacteria can multiply when holding urine.
- **(Females) Always wipe from front to back** after urination or defecation to minimize the spread of bacteria from the anus to the urethra.
- **Wear cotton underwear.** Nylon and synthetic fabrics prevent evaporation of moisture. Microorganisms grow well in a warm, moist environment.

- **Avoid tight-fitting clothing in the groin area,** for the same reason.
- **Urinate after having intercourse** to flush away bacteria that might have entered the urethra.
- **If you have a history of UTI,** avoid using a diaphragm, spermicidal contraceptive gel, or unlubricated or spermicidal condoms because these can irritate the urethra.
- **Avoid bubble baths** and baking-soda baths if you have a history of UTI because the soap can irritate the urethra.
- **Promptly report any symptoms of UTI** to your healthcare provider. Early treatment speeds healing and helps prevent complications.

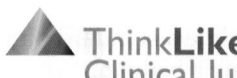

ThinkLike a Nurse 25-4: Clinical Judgment in Action

In the Meet Your Patient scenario, some assessment findings were given for Marlena. What additional physical assessments might you perform to complete this urinary tract assessment?

Physical Assessment

Physical assessment for urinary elimination includes examination of the kidneys, bladder, urethra, and skin surrounding the genitals, as appropriate. For a complete discussion of physical examination of the genitourinary system,

 Refer to **Chapter 19, Procedure 19-17: Assessing the Male Genitourinary System,** and **Procedure 19-18: Assessing the Female Genitourinary System,** in Volume 2.

KnowledgeCheck 25-4

- What should you discuss with your client when performing a nursing history focused on urinary elimination?
- What are the key elements of a physical assessment for a client with urination problems?

ThinkLike a Nurse 25-5: Clinical Judgment in Action

After gathering a focused nursing history pertaining to urinary elimination, you check your patient's vital signs: oral temperature, 99.4°F (37.4°C); radial pulse, 88 beats/min; respiratory rate, 20 breaths/min; and blood pressure, 108/72 mm Hg. What other physical assessment findings might you expect?

Common Diagnostic Procedures

Many diagnostic procedures of the urinary tract are performed in the operating room, procedures suite, or radiology department. Typically, nurses prepare the client for the procedure, assist with specimen collection, deliver aftercare, and sometimes assist the physician.

Blood Studies Blood urea nitrogen (BUN) and creatinine levels are commonly measured to assess renal function and hydration. For normal ranges,

 Refer to **Chapter 25, Diagnostic Testing box, Blood Studies: BUN and Creatinine,** in Volume 2.

Visualization Studies of the Urinary System Direct visualization studies tend to be invasive and therefore require a signed consent form. For associated pre- and post-procedure care of patients having these procedures,

 Go to **Chapter 25, Diagnostic Testing box, Studies of the Urinary System,** in Volume 2.

Assessing the Urine

Urine is an indicator for assessing hydration status as well as detecting or ruling out diseases or infections of the kidneys or urinary tract. When assessing urine, you will first check the color, clarity, and odor of the urine. Be sure to note the ease and frequency of eliminating urine when collecting urine specimens for bedside or laboratory testing.

Interpreting Intake and Output (I&O) Data

The kidneys produce urine at a rate of approximately 50 to 60 mL per hour, or 1,500 mL per day. However, urinary output fluctuates depending on:

- Quantity of fluids the patient drinks
- Ability of the heart to circulate the blood
- Kidney functioning
- Amount of fluid excreted through sweating, urine, stool, and gastrointestinal (GI) losses

Key Point: *To interpret the meaning of fluid data, you must know the intake and output (I&O) and the patient's relevant physical condition.*

- **If the patient's urine output is low,** you might assume their kidneys are not working properly. However, if their intake is also low, they may be dehydrated from sweating excessively or because of vomiting and diarrhea. Reduced output can also be caused by obstruction in urine flow or a high fever.
- **If the patient's intake is high and output is low,** this could mean their kidneys are not functioning well. However, it could also mean that their kidneys are producing urine but that they have urinary retention because something is obstructing flow.

Measuring Intake and Output

Measuring urine output is part of a comprehensive plan to monitor a client's fluid status.

- **Record all fluids** the patient drinks or receives intravenously.
  Fluid intake: oral fluids, semiliquid foods, ice chips, IV fluids, tube feedings, and irrigations instilled and not withdrawn immediately
  Fluid output: urine output, GI fluid loss (e.g., emesis, diarrhea), and drainage (e.g., from suction devices or wounds)
- **Ensure accuracy.** Explain to the client, family members, and caregivers that I&O are being monitored. Post a sign at the bedside or on the door to the room as a reminder. When possible, have the client assist you with monitoring urine output.
- **Measure I&O.** You will usually total I&O at the end of each shift, as well as for each 24-hour period. In intensive care units, you may measure I&O hourly. Most healthcare agencies have standardized I&O forms, either a separate form or part of a flowsheet.

- **Practice asepsis.** When handling urine, observe universal precautions, wear disposable procedure gloves, and avoid splashing the urine on yourself or objects in the room.

Voided Urine

The method you use to measure urine partially depends on the amount of help the patient needs with urination.

- **Ambulatory patients.** Inform them you are monitoring their I&O, and explain how they can help. Place a specimen "hat" (collection container) under the toilet seat to collect urine (Fig. 25-6) or have male clients void into a urinal. Periodically measure the output and empty the urine into the toilet. For clients who can assist with recording the I&O, provide a bedside clipboard.

  ✚ Provide support to patients with poor balance or weakness and encourage them to use safety rails when using the commode. You will also want to be sure a toilet safety frame is in place that accommodates a urinary collection "hat."

- **Patients with mobility problems.** For patients whose movement is restricted or who have difficulty getting out of bed, use a bedpan or urinal to collect urine output. A fracture pan is smaller and flatter than standard-size bedpans and can be positioned more easily for patients who have pelvis, lower back, or leg fractures, casts, splints, or braces or for patients who

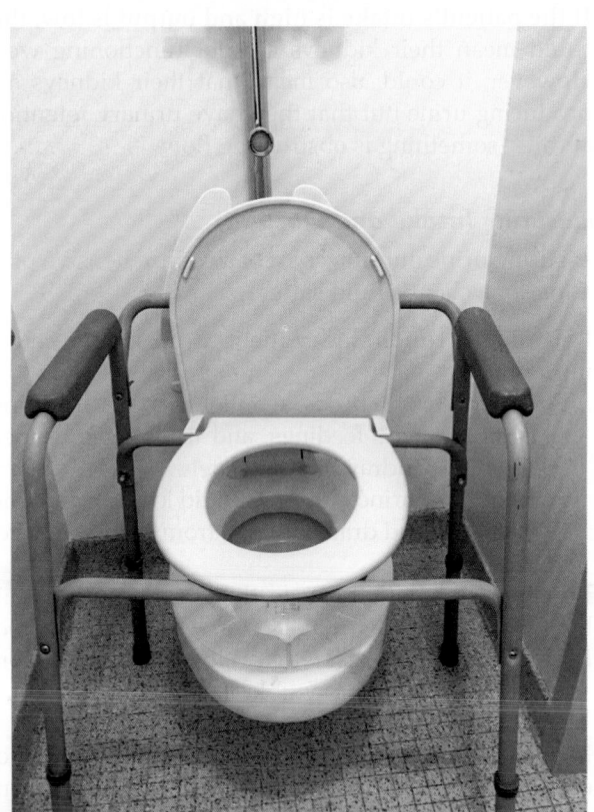

FIGURE 25-6 Toilet safety frame with urinary collection container.

have trouble lifting the pelvis to slide a standard pan underneath. For details about using a bedpan,

 Go to **Chapter 26, Procedure 26-2: Placing and Removing a Bedpan,** in Volume 2.

Urine From a Catheter

An **indwelling urinary catheter** is one that remains in the bladder for continuous drainage. It is held in place by a balloon that is inflated in the bladder above the detrusor muscle. Catheter insertion and ongoing care are discussed in the Planning Interventions/Implementation section of this chapter.

You will usually measure urine output from the indwelling catheter at the end of each shift unless otherwise prescribed. Clients who require close monitoring of I&O will have a special collection bag with a measuring chamber. Often this is used to assess hourly urine output.

Obtaining Samples for Urine Studies

Many disorders of the urinary system can be assessed by examining urine. You will perform some of these tests at the bedside. For others, you will collect a specimen that is analyzed in the lab. Prior to collecting urine, regardless of the type of specimen collection, instruct the patient how to properly clean (or assist with cleaning) the genital area to avoid fecal contamination of the urine specimen.

Freshly Voided Specimen

When collecting a urine sample, pour the urine into a specimen container labeled with the patient's name, patient ID, patient's birthdate, and the date and time of specimen collection. Many facilities require packaging the container in a moisture-proof specimen-handling bag. Follow agency policy on additional packaging. Transport the specimen to the lab as soon as possible (according to agency policies). If there is a delay in getting the specimen to the lab, some agencies recommend refrigeration.

Refer to the Highlights of Procedures box later in this chapter, and

 Go to **Chapter 25, Procedures 25-1: Measuring Postvoid Residual Urine Volume With a Portable Bladder Scanner** and **25-2: Obtaining a Urine Specimen for Testing,** in Volume 2.

Clean-Catch Specimen

Many diagnostic tests require a clean-catch urine specimen. The client must cleanse the genitalia before voiding and collect the sample in midstream because the initial flow of urine may contain organisms from the urethral meatus, distal urethra, and perineum. A midstream sample is free of these contaminants. See the Highlights of Procedures box for a summary of key steps. For the complete procedure,

 Go to **Chapter 25, Procedure 25-2A: Collecting a Clean-Catch Urine Specimen,** in Volume 2.

Sterile Urine Specimen

A sterile urine specimen aids in determining the presence of a UTI. You can obtain a sterile urine specimen by inserting a catheter into the bladder or by withdrawing a sample from an indwelling catheter. Do not take the specimen from the collection bag because that urine may be several hours old.

 Never disconnect the catheter from the drainage tube to obtain a sample. Interrupting the system creates a portal of entry for pathogens, thereby increasing the risk of contamination.

For a description of the steps involved in obtaining a sterile specimen from an indwelling catheter, see the Highlights of Procedures box.

 Go to **Chapter 25, Procedure 25-2B: Obtaining a Sterile Urine Specimen From a Catheter,** in Volume 2.

24-Hour Urine Collection

A 24-hour urine collection may be prescribed to evaluate some renal disorders by showing kidney function at different times of the day and night.

You will need to use a large container and preserve all the urine voided in the 24-hour period. For details about how to collect this type of specimen, see the Highlights of Procedures box.

 Go to **Chapter 25, Procedure 25-2C: Collecting a 24-Hour Urine Specimen,** in Volume 2.

Routine Urinalysis

A routine urinalysis (UA) is commonly used as an overall screening test as well as an aid in diagnosing and monitoring several health conditions. Urinalysis requires a freshly voided sample. Techniques include:

- Urine chemical reagent ("dipstick") testing—usually performed at the bedside
- Microscopic analysis—performed in the lab

Box 25-2 contains several terms used to describe urine characteristics and quantity. For the expected findings and common variants of urinalysis,

 Go to **Chapter 25, Diagnostic Testing, Urinalysis,** in Volume 2.

Chemical Reagent Testing (Dipstick)

Plastic strips immersed in the urine detect specific substances that indicate kidney function, urinary tract health, and other renal abnormalities. Dipstick tests check urine acidity (pH), protein, ketones, bilirubin, leukocyte esterase (a product of white blood cells), and nitrites.

When the reagent on the strips comes in contact with urine, a chemical reaction causes a color change that can then be compared to a color chart (Fig. 25-7). The urine

---

BOX 25-2 ■ Terms Associated With Urination

Acute renal failure (ARF): An acute rise in the serum creatinine level of 25% or more. May be caused by inadequate blood flow to the kidney, injury to the kidney glomeruli or tubules, or obstruction of kidney outflow.

Anuria: The absence of urine, often associated with kidney failure or congestive heart failure. This term is used when urine output is less than 100 mL in 24 hours.

Dysuria: Painful or difficult urination. May be associated with infection or partial obstruction of the urinary tract as well as medications that trigger urinary retention.

End-stage renal disease (ESRD): A chronic rise in serum creatinine levels associated with loss of kidney function that must be treated with dialysis or transplantation. Also known as chronic renal failure (CRF).

Enuresis: Involuntary loss of urine.

Frequency: The need to urinate at short intervals.

Hematuria: Blood in the urine. May be due to trauma, kidney stones, infection, or menstruation.

Micturition: To start the stream of urine; to urinate; release urine from the bladder.

Nephropathy: A broad term meaning disease of the kidney.

Nephrotoxic: A substance that damages kidney tissue. Some antibiotics (gentamicin, tobramycin, and amikacin), NSAIDs, lead, and contrast media have the potential to be nephrotoxic.

Nocturia: Frequent urination after going to bed. May be caused by excessive fluid intake as well as a variety of urinary tract and cardiovascular problems.

Nocturnal enuresis: Involuntary loss of urine while asleep.

Oliguria: Urine output of less than 400 mL in 24 hours. For pediatric patients, oliguria is <0.5–1.0 mL/kg per hour.

Pessary: An incontinence device that is inserted into the vagina to reduce organ prolapse or pressure on the bladder.

Polyuria: Excessive urination. May be caused by excessive hydration, diabetes mellitus, diabetes insipidus, or kidney disease.

Proteinuria: The presence of protein in the urine. May be a sign of infection or kidney disease.

Pyuria: Pus in the urine. May be caused by lesions or infection in the urinary tract.

Urgency: A sudden, almost uncontrollable need to urinate.

---

dipstick should be kept in a closed container and not be exposed to air. Testing with outdated and improperly stored materials can lead to erroneous results (James, 2007). The nurse commonly uses chemical reagent strips in the patient's bathroom.

Specific Gravity

Specific gravity, an indicator of urine concentration, can be measured with a reagent strip. However, when you need to be precise, you should use a refractometer or

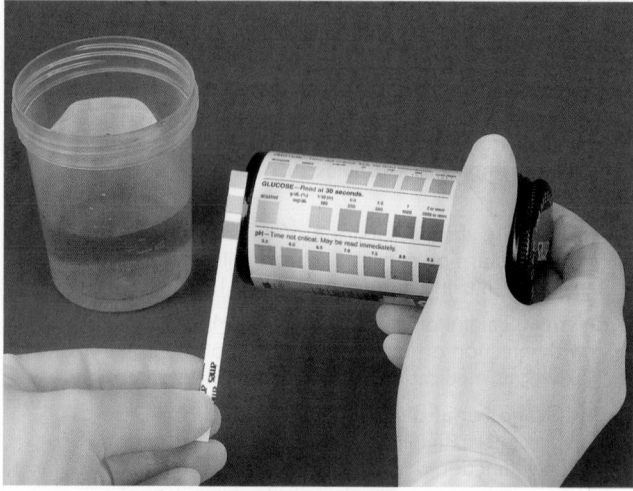

FIGURE 25-7 Chemical reagent strips dipped in urine are a rapid method to detect abnormalities.

send the sample to the laboratory for analysis. A **refractometer** measures the extent to which a beam of light changes direction when it passes through the urine (the *refractive index*). If the concentration of solids is high, the light is refracted more.

KnowledgeCheck 25-5

- Explain how to collect a clean-catch urine specimen.
- You are caring for a patient on a hospital unit from 0700 to 1200. Based on the following information, calculate the I&O and comment on your findings.
  Receiving IV fluid at 125 mL/hr
  0800 breakfast—4 oz juice, toast, scrambled eggs, 8 oz coffee
  0930—3 oz water
  0700 to 1200—wound drainage: 360 mL
  0700 to 1200—urine output per indwelling catheter: 180 mL

ThinkLike a Nurse 25-6: Clinical Judgment in Action

- Why do you think the first voided urine is discarded at the start of a 24-hour urine collection?
- The following are the dipstick findings you obtained on the clean-catch specimen from Marlena (Meet Your Patient).

Urinalysis	Result
pH	8.0
Specific gravity	1.030
Protein	Negative
Glucose	Negative
RBCs	Trace
Nitrite	+1
WBCs	+2
Bilirubin	Negative
Ketones	Negative
Urobilinogen	Negative

a. Identify the abnormal findings.
b. What would you expect the findings of her urine culture and sensitivity to demonstrate?

Safe, Effective Nursing Care

Managing Urinary Incontinence

Competencies: Provide Goal-Directed, Client-Centered Care; Implement Evidence-Based Practice Into Client Care (Thinking, Doing, Caring)

Scenario

Dashondra Simms, registered nurse (RN), works in a urology practice. She asks each female patient how they manage urinary incontinence (UI), where they obtain information, whether the condition has changed their quality of life, and whether they would be willing to participate in a UI support group. Dashondra's notes reveal a population with unmet healthcare needs, so she decides to develop a patient-centered, evidence-based program to increase participants' knowledge and confidence about managing their UI.

- Dashondra goes online to obtain evidence-based guidelines for UI management techniques.

- She searches databases such as MEDLINE and CINAHL for peer-reviewed studies that identify the psychosocial needs of patients and cultural or ethnic differences in managing UI.

- She also consults colleagues for practical strategies for managing this problem.

- Dashondra asks what would be of value to them in a UI self-management program. They suggest education about new treatments; an online discussion forum for members; and phone, text, or e-mail access to Dashondra as components of the program.

- In the support group, Dashondra and the others discuss the emotional impact of living with UI. The participants talk about how it affects their self-worth, dignity, and confidence. Self-image, sexuality, and sense of freedom also emerge as specific issues.

Think About It:

The following questions are for your own reflection or discussion with peers:

- How did Dashondra establish an evidence base for educating group members? How would you find more information about a topic that you are going to present to others?

- How did she make the intervention patient-centered?

- In what ways did Dashondra use information technology to help her design the program?

- How does Dashondra show care for the patients participating in the study group?

Sources: Bedretdinova et al. (2016); Burkhard et al. (2018); Capobianco et al. (2019); Dowling-Castronovo & Bradway (2016); Nambiar et al. (2018).

NURSING DIAGNOSIS/ANALYZING CUES

Urinary elimination problems are described by several nursing and medical diagnoses. NANDA-I and Clinical Care Classification (CCC) diagnoses (CCC, 2012) specific to urinary elimination include the following:

Urinary Elimination, impaired
Urinary Incontinence (functional, overflow, reflex, stress, urge, risk for urge)
Urinary Retention
Urinary Tract Injury, risk for

Urinary problems may also be the etiology of other nursing diagnoses, such as the following:

Anxiety r/t urinary urgency and recent episode of incontinence
Acute Pain r/t bladder spasms and urinary tract infection
Social Isolation r/t frequent periods of incontinence (CCC, 2012)
Fluid Volume Deficit Risk (CCC, 2012)

For a more extensive list of urinary-related nursing diagnoses, refer to the most recent NANDA-I Nursing Diagnoses Definitions and Classification or to other nursing diagnosis handbooks.

PLANNING/PRIORITIZING HYPOTHESES AND GENERATING SOLUTIONS

The general goal related to urinary elimination is that patients will comfortably void approximately 1,500 mL of light-yellow urine in 24 hours. Because normal urine elimination patterns vary, the frequency and amount of urine are based on the individual's pattern, food and fluid intake, medications, and other factors.

Nursing Outcomes Classification (NOC) standardized outcomes for urinary problems, regardless of the specific problem, are the following: Kidney Function, Urinary Continence, Urinary Elimination, Self-Care: Toileting, and Tissue Integrity: Skin & Mucous Membranes (because urinary elimination problems often place the patient at Risk for Impaired Skin Integrity).

Individualized goals/outcome statements you might use to evaluate the effectiveness of interventions for urinary problems can be found in the Example Client Conditions.

IMPLEMENTATION/TAKING ACTION

When Impaired Urination is the patient's problem, you might use *NIC standardized interventions,* such as the following examples:

Bladder Irrigation
Environmental Management
Specimen Management
Tube-Care: Urinary

Fluid Monitoring
Pelvic Muscle Exercise
Prompted Voiding
Self-Care Assistance: Toileting
Urinary Catheterization
Urinary Incontinence Care
Urinary Retention Care

When impaired urination is the etiology of other problems, you might use Nursing Interventions Classification (NIC) interventions, such as Perineal Care, Self-Esteem Enhancement, and Skin Surveillance. The following are examples:

Diagnosis: Risk for Fluid Volume Imbalance
NIC Intervention: Fluid Monitoring, Fluid Management
Diagnosis: Acute Pain r/t bladder spasms
NIC Intervention: Medication Administration

From your chosen intervention(s), use clinical judgment to select the activities that best meet individual patient needs and address problem etiologies.

Specific nursing activities for patients with elimination problems fall into the following categories:

- Promoting normal urination
- Preventing urinary tract infection
- Managing urinary retention
- Managing urinary incontinence
- Caring for patients who have urinary diversions

See Example Client Conditions: Urinary Tract Infection, Urinary Retention, and Adult Urinary Incontinence.

Promoting Normal Urination

♥ iCare *Provide Privacy*

Although urination is a normal physiological process, most people consider it a private matter.

- **Provide privacy** when discussing or providing care related to urination. Excuse visitors from the room, draw the dividing curtains in shared rooms, and close the door to the room.
- **Whenever possible, give the patient privacy** to void. Do not, for example, hover outside the bathroom door asking, "Are you okay?" or "Are you finished?"

If the client is weak and a fall risk, you may need to remain with them.

- **Taking a matter-of-fact approach** confirms to patients that you are comfortable with this aspect of care.

Assist With Positioning

- **Male patients:** Whenever possible, assist the patient to the bathroom to use the toilet and allow him to assume a preferred position to empty the bladder. Alternatively, provide a bedside commode or urinal for the patient to use. To place a urinal, position the patient in a semi-Fowler's position with the legs slightly spread and the penis in the urinal.

   Rationale: Most males stand to void and may have difficulty voiding in other positions.

- **Female patients:** If a female patient must remain in bed, provide a bedpan. Place the patient in a semi-Fowler's position to urinate unless contraindicated. ✚ Raise the siderails or provide an overhead trapeze so that the patient will have grip holds to maneuver themselves onto and off the bedpan. If the patient is weak, you may need an assistant to help you position them on the bedpan, and you may need to stay with them to help maintain the position.

   Rationale: Females generally find an upright seated (semi-Fowler's) or squatting position to be the most comfortable for voiding.

Facilitate Toileting Routines

Most patients void on awakening, after meals or drinking a large volume of fluid, before bedtime, or for some, during the night.

- **Identify your patient's pattern;** stick to it as much as possible.
- **If you anticipate a change in the pattern** for elimination, inform the patient. For example, if the patient is to receive a diuretic, explain that they will need to urinate more often.
- **Similarly, if the patient is scheduled for a diagnostic procedure or activity,** inform them ahead of time so that they may void before the activity begins.
- **Assist patients who have mobility problems** and those who use the bedpan.
- **Discuss with all unlicensed assistive personnel** (UAP) the need to help so that patients experience minimal delays.

Promote Adequate Fluids and Nutrition

Adequate hydration promotes urinary tract function and flushes the system of waste products. Most people should drink eight to ten 8-ounce glasses of fluid daily unless health problems limit the fluid; unfortunately, many do not. Water is preferred because soda, coffee, and tea often contain caffeine or additives that may cause diuresis. However, the amount of fluid is more important than the type. If the patient will not or cannot drink water, provide the fluid they prefer. See Box 25-3 for strategies to increase your patient's fluid intake.

Assist With Hygiene

Urine is irritating to the skin. Therefore, perineal cleansing is an integral part of toileting hygiene. Many patients are unable to do toileting self-care, so you will need to provide perineal care for them. It may include pouring warm, soapy water over the genitals while the patient is seated on the toilet, the bedside

---

BOX 25-3 ▪ Strategies to Increase Patients' Fluid Intake

- For patients with limited mobility, keep water or other liquids in easy reach.
- Remind young children or patients with cognitive or psychiatric disorders to drink fluids.
- For patients who have increased fluid needs, provide goals for intake, and frequently remind them to drink.
- Many foods have a high fluid content.
  - If the patient requires additional fluid for hydration, consider adding soup and watery foods, such as watermelon, to the diet.
  - If the patient requires fluid restriction, you will have to account for these watery foods in the fluid balance.
- Try offering liquids with a straw. Patients tend to drink more this way.
- Chilled drinks might be more appealing, particularly if the patient's mouth is dry. Offer beverages with ice if they are to be served cold.
- Provide good mouth care. Patients will often drink more readily if their mouth feels fresh.

---

commode, or the bedpan. Be sure to rinse with warm water because soap is drying to the genital mucosa. Also offer a moist washcloth or towelette for washing the hands after toileting. If the patient can ambulate to the bathroom, you would simply assist with their usual cleansing routines. **For further information, refer to Chapter 22, Procedure 22-3: Providing Perineal Care, in Volume 2.**

KnowledgeCheck 25-6

- Identify activities that promote normal urination patterns.
- Write at least two nursing diagnostic statements that would be appropriate for a patient with urinary frequency, burning, urgency, and a fever.

Urinary Catheterization

Catheterization, a commonly used intervention, is the introduction of a pliable tube (catheter) into the bladder to allow drainage of urine. Urinary catheterization is performed to:

- **Obtain a sterile urine specimen.**
- **Drain the bladder** for surgical or diagnostic purposes or when emptying is incomplete after urination.
- **Prevent or treat bladder** overdistention and urinary retention (e.g., after surgery) when other measures fail.
- **Measure postvoid residual** (PVR) if a portable bladder ultrasound device is unavailable or if the results are inconclusive.
- **Protect excoriated skin** from contact with urine.
- **Promote comfort** by reducing the need for unnecessary movement of patients who are near death.

Risks and Complications With meticulous nursing technique, complications can be reduced. Indwelling urinary catheterization is associated with *bacteriuria and UTI* because:

- A catheter provides a connection between the external environment and a normally sterile system.
- When the patient has an indwelling catheter in place, microorganisms adhere to the biofilm surface of the catheter. Additionally, bacteria are not flushed along the urethra through voiding.
- There is also the risk of *urethral injury* if the catheter is too large, is forced through strictures, is inserted at an incorrect angle, or is not well lubricated.

Self-Catheterization Patients with spinal cord injuries or neurological disorders use intermittent catheterization to drain the bladder. Many perform intermittent self-catheterization; however, caregivers may assist. Although you will use sterile technique for catheterization, most patients who self-catheterize use clean technique. **Key Point:** *Intermittent catheterization carries a substantially lower risk of infection than does an indwelling catheter (Hooton et al., 2010).*

Refer to **Clinical Insight 25-1: Teaching Clients About Clean, Intermittent Self-Catheterization,** in Volume 2.

EXAMPLE CLIENT CONDITION: Urinary Retention

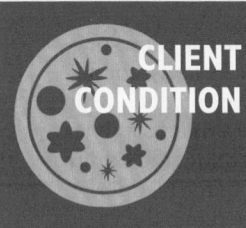 **CLIENT CONDITION**

Urinary retention is the inability to completely empty the bladder; it can be acute or chronic **and is** more common in males and rare in children.

Complications

Urinary tract infection (UTI), bladder damage, kidney damage, urinary incontinence

Etiologies

Obstruction in the Urinary Tract—blockage of urinary outflow:
- Enlarged prostate (benign prostatic hypertrophy)
- Urethra *strictures*
- Scars from previous injury or surgery in the pelvis
- Urinary tract obstruction (tumor, blood clot)
- Fecal impaction
- Inflammation and swelling
- Cystocele, rectocele
- Underactive bladder

Neurological Problems—involving control of the bladder and sphincters:
- Spinal cord or brain tumor; spinal cord injury; herniated disk, stroke or traumatic brain injury, multiple sclerosis, diabetes, pregnancy and vaginal childbirth, Parkinson disease, myelomeningocele, Guillain-Barre syndrome
- Pelvic trauma; bladder overdistention
- Age-related loss of bladder muscle strength
- Viral infections involving perineal nerves

Medications and Anesthesia
- Antihistamines and decongestants, anticholinergics/antispasmodics, tricyclic and selective serotonin reuptake inhibitor (SSRI) antidepressants, antipsychotics, calcium channel blockers, NSAIDs, opioids, amphetamines, some muscle relaxants and antiseizure medications
 • Epidural and spinal anesthetic agents, especially in older adults

Musculoskeletal—Weakened bladder muscles for bladder emptying

Psychological—Anxiety leading to voluntary withholding of urination

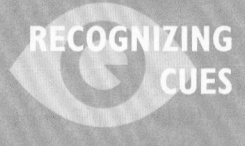 **RECOGNIZING CUES**

Assess for risk factors (see Etiologies) and symptoms of urinary retention.

Acute Retention
- Urinary hesitancy, dribbling, or weak urine stream
- Urgent need to urinate
- Pain, discomfort, bloating in lower abdomen

Chronic Retention
- Urinary retention frequency—urination eight or more times per day

- Trouble beginning a urine stream
- Weak or an interrupted stream
- Urgency, but with little stream
- Feels urination urge, even after voiding
- Mild, constant discomfort in lower abdomen

NOTE: Some may not have symptoms, increasing the likelihood of delaying treatment and leading to complications.

(continued)

EXAMPLE CLIENT CONDITION: Urinary Retention—cont'd

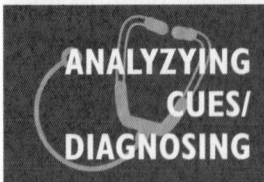

ANALYZYING CUES/ DIAGNOSING

Acute Urinary Retention
Chronic Urinary Retention

Potential complication: UTI

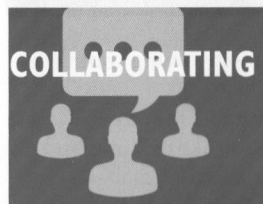

GENERATING SOLUTIONS

NOC Standardized Outcomes

Urinary Elimination

Individualized Outcomes

- Does not delay voiding
- After voiding, patient states they feel they have emptied their bladder completely.
- Postvoiding residual volume < 150 mL
- Bladder not palpable

COLLABORATING

Diagnostic

- Physical assessment
- Postvoid residual (PVR) measurement
- Cystoscopy
- Computed tomography (CT) scan; magnetic resonance imaging (MRI); ultrasound
- Voiding cystourethrogram (VCUG)
- Urodynamic tests—urine flow tests, pressure flow study, cystometry
- Electromyography
- Urinalysis to rule out UTI or other abnormalities

Treatments

- **For mechanical obstruction** to urine flow: surgery, bladder drainage, urethral dilation, urethral stent, laser therapy, prostatic urethral lift, vaginal pessary
- **For loss of bladder tone:** Cholinergic medications stimulate contraction of detrusor muscle to trigger bladder emptying.
- **For poor bladder emptying:** Alpha-adrenergic antagonists reduce urethral resistance.

- **For overactive bladder:** Injections of onabotulinumtoxin A (Botox) into the bladder muscle relax the bladder, which allows it to hold more urine. Sacral nerve stimulator implanted under the skin may relax the muscle wall of the bladder. A removable plug inserted into the vagina also reduces overactive bladder and stress incontinence.
- **For stress incontinence:** Injections of synthetic materials in the tissue surrounding the urethra help to reduce urine leakage.
- **Surgery:** Clients with a mechanical obstruction to urine flow are treated by:
  - Surgery (e.g., resection of the prostate gland, correction of organ prolapse)
  - Sling procedure to keep the urethra closed, especially when coughing or sneezing.
  - Bladder neck suspension supports the urethra and bladder neck.
  - An artificial urinary sphincter is implanted around the bladder to maintain closure when not needed during urination.

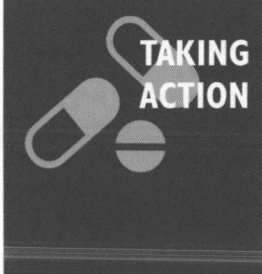

TAKING ACTION

NOC Standardized Interventions

Fluid Monitoring
Tube-Care: Urinary
Urinary Retention Care

Individualized Interventions

- Intermittent urinary catheterization or patient self-catheterization as needed (to drain the bladder)

- Monitor for bladder distention (inspect and palpate).
- Measure PVR with bladder scanner.
- Apply a heating pad to the lower abdomen to relax the muscles near the bladder.
- Run water from the faucet or pour warm (not hot) water over the perineum or sitz bath to stimulate voiding.

EXAMPLE CLIENT CONDITION: Urinary Retention—cont'd

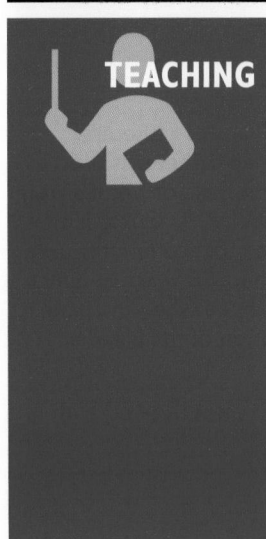

TEACHING

- Teach patient to use Credé's maneuver (manual pressure over the bladder).
- Teach patient to do pelvic floor muscle exercises (PFMEs), bladder training, double voiding (urinating and then reemptying the bladder about 10 minutes later),
- Teach intermittent self-catheterization as appropriate (see Clinical Insight 25-1).

- Advise patient to contact a healthcare professional for symptoms that may indicate infection or blockage in the urinary tract, for example:
  - Complete inability to urinate
  - Intense pain in lower abdomen and urinary tract
  - Fever, vomiting, side or back pain, chills, or passing little urine for 1 to 2 days
  - Blood in the urine, cloudy or foul-smelling urine, frequency or urgency, or discharge from the penis or vagina
- Teach patients to reduce risk by maintaining a healthy weight, avoiding bladder stimulants (coffee, alcohol, acidic foods, nicotine), and eating more fiber to avoid constipation.

Types of Catheter Materials

There are various catheter types and materials to choose from, depending on whether the patient requires catheterization for long-term or short-term use, has product sensitivity, or is at increased risk for infection.

- **Silver-alloy** coated catheters may reduce the risk of catheter-associated UTIs in some populations; however, there is conflicting evidence regarding the effectiveness of the silver-coated catheters in preventing bacterial infection and reducing encrustation for long-term catheterization (Aljohi et al. 2016; Majeed et al., 2019). Patients often report less discomfort with this catheter type compared with standard catheters (Lam et al., 2014).

- ✚ **Teflon-bonded latex-coated** catheters reduce friction and tissue irritation during insertion and while the catheter remains in place. These catheters must not be used in patients with latex sensitivity.

- **Polyvinyl chloride (PVC)** catheters are inexpensive and commonly used for intermittent catheterization. They are more rigid and therefore less comfortable for indwelling use (Wound, Ostomy and Continence Nursing Society [WOCN], 2016).

- **Silicone catheters** are preferable for long-term catheterization. They cause less tissue irritation and prevent encrustation (Gould et al., 2009). They are safe for patients with latex sensitivity.

- **Hydrogel-coated** urinary catheters can be made of either latex or silicone. The lubricating surface of the catheter causes less urethral trauma during insertion, resists encrustation, and can reduce the formation of a biofilm that microorganisms adhere to. Hydrogel-coated catheters remain in place for up to 12 weeks (Turner & Dickens, 2011; Yong et al., 2019). This type of **lubricant and/or antimicrobial coating** helps prevent infection.

- **Antimicrobial-coated** (antibiotics, nitrofurazone) catheters may stop the growth of or kill bacteria on indwelling urinary catheters (Vopni et al., 2021). **Key Point:** *However, the most effective way to reduce catheter-associated infection is short-term use.* Additionally, this type may lead to antibiotic resistance, and catheter materials often cause stinging in the urethra (Al-Qahtani et al., 2019).

Catheter Types and Sizing

Straight Catheter A **straight catheter** (Fig 25-8A) is a single-lumen tube that is inserted for immediate drainage of the bladder (e.g., to obtain a sterile urine specimen, to measure PVR, or to relieve temporary bladder distention). After the bladder is empty or the sample obtained, the catheter is removed, and the patient resumes voiding independently.

Indwelling Catheter An **indwelling catheter,** also known as a *Foley* or *retention catheter,* is used for continuous bladder drainage (e.g., when the bladder must be kept empty or when continuous urine measurement is needed).

- **Double-lumen** (Fig 25-8B)—It is usually a double-lumen tube: one lumen is used for urine drainage, and the second lumen is used to inflate a balloon near the tip of the catheter.
- **Triple-lumen** (Fig 25-8C)—A triple-lumen indwelling catheter is used when the patient requires intermittent or continuous bladder irrigation, for which the third lumen is used.
- **The inflated balloon** holds the catheter in place at the neck of the bladder. The balloon is sized according to the volume of fluid used to inflate it. For most patients you will use a 5-mL balloon; for children, a 3-mL balloon; and for achieving hemostasis after a prostatectomy, a 30-mL balloon.

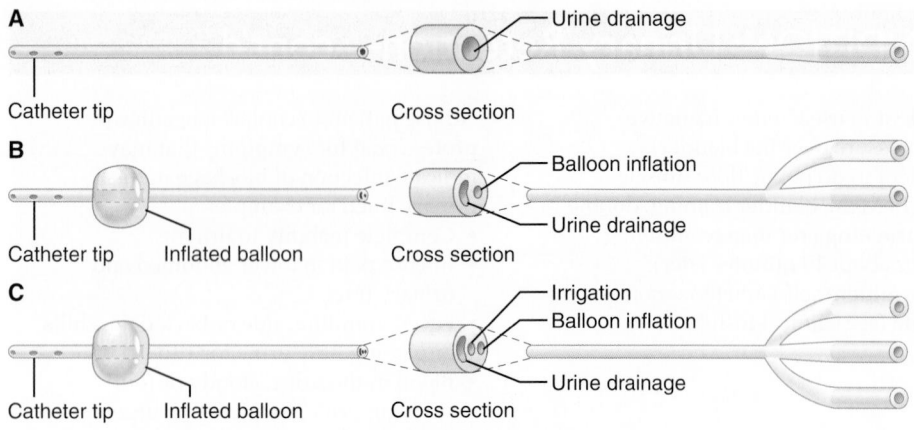

FIGURE 25-8 Types of catheters. *A*, A single-lumen catheter is used to obtain a urine sample or immediately drain the bladder. *B*, A double-lumen catheter is the most commonly used indwelling catheter. *C*, A triple-lumen catheter is inserted when the patient requires irrigation of the bladder.

Suprapubic Catheter A **suprapubic catheter** is used for continuous urine drainage when the urethra must be bypassed (e.g., after gynecological surgery or where there is prostatic obstruction). A suprapubic catheter is inserted through an incision above the symphysis pubis (Fig. 25-9). It may be sutured in place initially. Once the stoma tract has healed, a standard indwelling catheter is usually used and is held in place by inflation of the balloon.

Catheter Sizing Catheters are sized by the diameter of the lumen; the larger the number, the larger the lumen. For example, 8- and 10-Fr catheters are used for children; they are smaller in diameter than the 14- and 16-Fr catheters typically used for adults. Male patients usually need a larger lumen (e.g., 18 Fr) than do female patients. To minimize urethral trauma, use the smallest-diameter catheter possible that provides proper drainage.

Catheters Come in Different Lengths A 22-cm catheter is appropriate for adults who are female, whereas for adults who are male, you will need a 40-cm catheter.

KnowledgeCheck 25-7

- Describe the difference between a catheter used for straight catheterization and one used for ongoing drainage.
- Why is intermittent catheterization preferred for patients who must be catheterized over lengthy periods of time?

Urinary Catheter Insertion

Key Point: *After considering alternatives for bladder drainage, indwelling urinary catheters may be used but should remain in place for only as long as absolutely necessary. The longer the catheter remains in place, the greater the risk of catheter-associated UTI (CAUTI). Maintaining a sterile, closed urinary drainage system is critical to prevent CAUTI.*

To insert a urinary catheter, you will need to:

- ✚ Always check for latex or Teflon and iodine allergies before performing a catheterization.

- Explain to the patient the reason for the catheter insertion, the expected length of time the catheter will be needed, and the sensations they are likely to have. Most patients experience a sensation of pressure and some discomfort (but not pain) when a catheter is inserted. However, if there is swelling or bleeding in the urinary tract, insertion may be painful.
- Explain that when the catheter is inserted, it may feel as though they are voiding, but the urine is going into the tube, not onto the bed.
- Use a dorsal recumbent position for female patients and a supine position for male patients.
  - For female patients, make sure to lower the section of the bed (called the *knee gatch*) so that you can easily visualize the urinary meatus. You may need to place a firm cushion under the patient's buttocks to prevent them from sinking into a soft mattress and obscuring visibility of the meatus.
  - For patients who are unable to assume a dorsal recumbent position, consider Sims' or a lateral position (Fig. 25-10).
- Cleaning around the meatus and perineum is mandatory before insertion of the catheter.

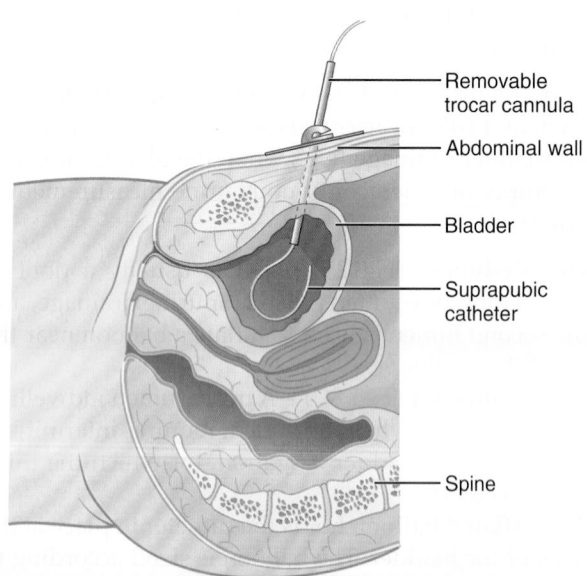

FIGURE 25-9 A suprapubic catheter drains urine from a surgically created opening into the bladder, bypassing the urethra.

Toward Evidence-Based Practice

Urinary catheter insertion is a common procedure and is a major cause of infection in hospitals.

Rimmer, M. P., Henderson, I., Keay, S. D., Khan, K. S., & Al Wattar, B. H. (2020). Early versus delayed urinary catheter removal after hysterectomy: A systematic review and meta-analysis. *European Journal of Obstetrics & Gynecology and Reproductive Biology, 24,* 55–60. https://doi.org/10.1016/j.ejogrb.2020.01.011

Patients with indwelling urinary catheters after hysterectomy surgery for a short duration (less than 6 hours) are less likely to develop catheter-associated urinary tract infections (CAUTI) than those with catheters that are in place for a longer duration.

Basbug, A., Yukel, A, & Kaya, E. (2018). Early versus delayed removal of indwelling catheters in patients after an elective cesarean section: A prospective randomized trial. *Journal of Maternal-Fetal & Neonatal Medicine, 33*(1), 68–71. https://doi.org/10.1080/14767058.2018.1487394

In a study examining the effects of early removal of urinary catheters after elective cesarean section, researchers found that a short duration of catheterization is associated with reduced urethral irritation, improved mobility, and reduced hospital stay.

Leis, J. A., Corpus C., Catt, B., Wong, B. M., Callery, S., & Vearncombe, M. (2016). Medical directive for urinary catheter removal by nurses on general medical wards. *JAMA Internal Medicine, 176*(1), 113–115. https://doi.org/10.1001/jamainternmed.2015.6319

Empowering nurses to remove urinary catheters that were no longer needed resulted in a markedly reduced number of days patients used these catheters. In turn, a reduced duration of catheterization reduces the risk of CAUTI.

Brouwer, T. A., Roon, E. N., Rosier, P. F., Kalkman, C. J., & Veeger, N. (2021, January). Postoperative urinary retention: Risk factors, bladder filling rate and time to catheterization: An observational study as part of a randomized controlled trial. *Postoperative Medicine, 10*(2), Article 2. https://doi.org/10.1186/s13741-020-00167-z

In a study of 936 patients who underwent general surgery, researchers found that bladder volume scanning at least every 3 hours was useful in determining patients' maximum bladder capacity. This practice benefited patients by preventing bladder overdistention, avoiding unnecessary urinary catheterization, and lowering the risk of urinary tract infection and injury.

---

1. The main benefit of reducing the duration of indwelling catheterization in postoperative patients centers around the reduced risk of developing a CAUTI. In addition to reducing the likelihood of CAUTI, what other benefits may occur with early removal of an indwelling catheter?

2. Leis et al. (2016) found that nurses' judgment for removing indwelling urinary catheters contributed to a shorter duration of urinary catheterization. How might you assess your patient after removing the catheter?

3. In these studies, researchers suggested using indwelling urinary catheters for as short of a duration as possible. What other questions might nurses ask about managing urinary catheterization to reduce the risk of infection?

4. Assessment of urinary retention has traditionally been done with either bladder palpation or straight catheterization. What are the advantages of using a portable bladder scanner in assessing urinary retention?

♥ iCare 25-2

Providing Comfort and Privacy During Urinary Catheterization

Many patients feel embarrassed when having a urinary catheter inserted. A professional approach, along with privacy measures, helps relieve discomfort or distress. You can show the patient that you care by placing a warmed blanket over their legs before exposure of the perineum. As you are draping the patient, offer to answer any further questions they may have. To read more about this technique,

 Go to **Chapter 22, Procedure 22-3: Providing Perineal Care,** in Volume 2.

For the complete procedure,

 Go to **Chapter 25, Procedures 25-3: Inserting an Intermittent Urinary Catheter (Straight Catheter),** and **25-4: Inserting an Indwelling Urinary Catheter,** in Volume 2.

Caring for the Patient With an Indwelling Catheter

An indwelling catheter is connected to a drainage tube and collection bag, which constitute a closed system. **Key Point:** *Remember, above all, when providing care for a patient with an indwelling catheter, keep it closed, keep it flowing, and keep it clean.*

Goal 1: Prevent Urinary Tract Infection UTI attributed to the use of an indwelling urinary catheter is one of the most common infections acquired by patients in healthcare facilities.

- **Do not disconnect the tubing** or open the drainage system (e.g., to obtain specimens or measure the urine).
  A closed system minimizes the chance for pathogens to enter the system and infect the urinary tract.
- **Regularly check connections** between the catheter and drainage tubing and the drainage tube and collection bag.
  Loose connections cause leaks and serve as entry points for pathogens.

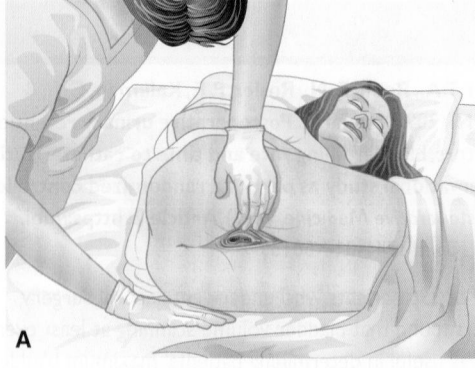

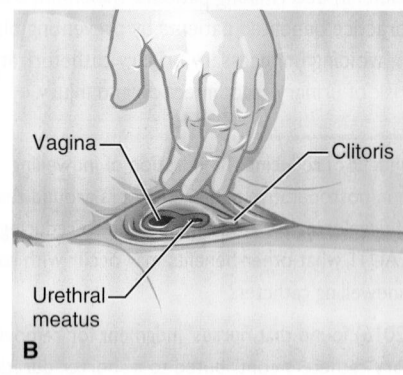

Vagina — Clitoris

Urethral meatus

FIGURE 25-10AB *A,* For women who cannot assume a dorsal recumbent position, you can use the side-lying position. *B,* Lift the superior buttock to expose the urethral meatus.

- **If the system becomes disconnected,** wipe the ends of both tubes with antiseptic (alcohol or chlorhexidine gluconate [CHG]–alcohol combination product) before reconnecting them.
- **After each bowel movement and if the catheter becomes soiled from drainage or feces,** cleanse it with mild soap and water, cleaning from the meatus outward. Rinse the catheter well and pat it dry.
  This removes the medium for the growth of microorganisms.
- **Empty the collection bag** at least every 8 hours and more frequently if urine output is high.
  This prevents stagnation of urine.
- **Do not touch the spout to any surfaces** when emptying the collection bag. If the spout is accidentally contaminated, cleanse it with an antiseptic (alcohol or CHG–alcohol combination product).
- **Keep the collection bag below the level of the bladder, but do not let it touch the floor** (see Goal 2).
  The floor is considered contaminated.
- **Teach the patient to report signs of UTI;** observe for cloudy and strong-smelling urine, chills, or fever.
- **Change the indwelling catheter only when necessary** (e.g., when sediment collects in the tubing or catheter or the urine does not drain well), **and discontinue it as soon as it is no longer necessary**.
  Some agency policies specify that catheters be changed at specific intervals (e.g., monthly). However, this is not advisable because the more often a catheter is changed, the more likely an infection will develop.

- **Routine hygiene is all that is necessary for meatal cleansing.**
  Antiseptic solutions are no more effective than sterile, normal saline for cleansing and may irritate or dry the skin at the urinary meatus.

Goal 2: Maintain Free Flow of Urine Maintaining a free flow of urine prevents backflow of urine into the bladder, which can cause bladder distention and injury. Stasis of urine also provides a medium for the growth of microorganisms.

- **Keep the tubing and bag below bladder level.** Never place the bag on the floor or the bed.
  This prevents backflow of stagnant urine into the bladder. Urine drains by gravity in this system.
- **If the collecting bag must be higher than the bladder** at any time, you must clamp the catheter.
  Clamping prevents backflow of stagnant urine into the bladder.
- **Frequently inspect the tubing** to ensure that the urine flows freely.
  Kinks, coils, or compression of the catheter or tubing may impede flow and cause backup into the bladder.
- **If urine is not flowing,** check to be sure the patient is not lying on the tubing.

Goal 3: Prevent Transmission of Infection
  The urinary collection bag and tubing are unclean surfaces.

- **Be sure you observe standard precautions** when providing catheter care.
- **Wear gloves** when handling the catheter or drainage system.
  Gloving prevents contact with body fluids.
- **Always perform hand hygiene before and after providing care** to any patient, including one with an indwelling catheter.

Goal 4: Promote Normal Urine Production Adequate urine production flushes pathogens out of the bladder, provides natural irrigation of the tubing, and prevents stasis of urine.

- **Encourage oral intake of at least 64 ounces** (approximately 2,000 to 2,500 mL) of fluid per day, unless contraindicated by other health problems (Frellick, 2017; Turner & Dickens, 2011; WOCN, 2009). For patients who are unable to take oral liquid, provide an equivalent amount of parenteral or enteral fluids.
- **Monitor I&O at least every 8 hours** (more frequently if the patient is experiencing fluid and electrolyte imbalance).
- **For accurate determination of output,** empty the urine into a calibrated container.
  Volume markings on the urine collection bag are only approximate.
- **Observe the urine output for color and other characteristics**. Report evidence of blood, sediment, or infection to the primary care provider.

- **Encourage the patient to be active and out of bed** as much as possible.

    This promotes blood flow to the kidneys for better urinary function.

    Goal 5: Maintain skin and mucosal integrity
Perineal skin and mucosa can be irritated by feces and by movement or encrustation of the catheter.

- **Secure the tubing to the patient's thigh** by applying a commercial catheter securement device, such as a catheter tube holder or a Velcro strap (or hypoallergenic tape if a securement device is unavailable).

    Failure to secure the tubing may cause significant injury to the bladder neck and urethra. Although the inflated balloon holds the catheter in the bladder, you must secure the tubing to prevent traction on the bladder and urethral meatus.

- **Assist with routine hygiene care as needed.** Cleanse the area around the meatus with mild soap and filtered tap water or perineal wash solution daily, after each bowel movement, and more often if there is drainage or excessive sweating. Rinse well and pat dry.

    Routine hygiene care normally provides adequate cleanliness. Rinsing helps to avoid skin irritation by soap residue.

- **Avoid using powder or lotions in the perineal area**

    Topical products can be irritating to the skin.

- **Monitor the urethral meatus and upper drainage tube.**

    Encrustation, as evidenced by sandy particles at the meatus, irritates the mucosa and signals the need to change the catheter.

KnowledgeCheck 25-8

- What actions should you take before inserting a catheter?
- When caring for a client with an indwelling catheter, you notice sandy particles (encrustation) around the urethral meatus. What should you do?
- How often should the urine collection bag be emptied?

Bladder Irrigation

You may perform an irrigation to maintain the patency of a urinary catheter, to wash out the bladder (e.g., remove blood clots in the bladder after surgery), and for other urological indications. However, bladder irrigation is not beneficial for the prevention of CAUTI, and in fact, solutions instilled into the bladder may have irritating effects and may lead to resistant microorganisms (Harmon et al., 2017; Loveday et al., 2014).

- **Intermittent irrigation** is most commonly used for medication instillation.
- **Continuous irrigation** is used to maintain patency when blood, clots, or debris is anticipated.
- **Routine intermittent irrigations** (e.g., every shift, every week) are sometimes prescribed to ensure patency; however, these should be avoided (WOCN, 2009).

 A double-lumen catheter system may need to be opened for irrigation and therefore creates a high risk for infection. Although "open" irrigation was used in the past, it is no longer recommended.

For complete procedures,

Go to **Chapter 25, Procedures 25-7A: Intermittent Bladder or Catheter Irrigation,** and **25-7B: Continuous Bladder Irrigation,** in Volume 2.

Removing an Indwelling Catheter

Removing a urinary catheter is a simple task, but you must monitor patients carefully afterward.

- **Note and record the time and amount** of the first voiding and the appearance of the urine.
- **Compare the patient's intake with output** for the next 8 to 12 hours, and palpate the bladder for distention. A portable bladder scanner may also be used to quantify the amount of any retained urine.
- **Monitor regularly for bladder distention** until normal voiding is reestablished. The catheter may have caused some edema of the urethra, which will interfere with voiding at first.

    If a catheter is in place for several weeks, the bladder loses tone, and the patient may require bladder retraining. Agencies have differing procedures for this. One method is to begin clamping the catheter for certain periods of time (e.g., 1 to 4 hours) to allow the bladder to fill and then releasing the clamp to allow urine to drain from the bladder. However, there is limited evidence to support a practice guideline for clamping the catheter before discontinuing it.

    For inpatients who have had a urinary catheter for a short time, it is a good idea to time catheter removal for late at night instead of in the morning. This has been found to lead to a larger and more representative output the first time the bladder is emptied (Griffiths & Fernandez, 2009).

    For guidelines to follow when removing a retention catheter,

Go to **Chapter 25, Procedure 25-6: Removing an Indwelling Catheter,** in Volume 2.

 ThinkLike a Nurse 25-7: Clinical Judgment in Action

- You are caring for a patient who had an indwelling catheter removed 12 hours ago. The patient has not voided. What action should you take?

Clean, Intermittent Self-Catheterization

Self-catheterization to clients is for clients who have compromised ability to spontaneously empty their bladders. In the home setting, this is a clean procedure rather than a sterile one. It is referred to as clean, intermittent self-catheterization (CISC).

Goals of intermittent self-catheterization include:

1. Emptying the bladder
2. Prevention of urinary tract infections
3. Relief of discomfort associated with urinary retention

Teaching Considerations

- In teaching the steps of the procedure, consider the client's physical ability to manipulate the catheter equipment and reach the urethra (e.g., range of motion, fine motor skills, degree of sensation).
- Encourage the client to drink at least 64 oz of fluid without caffeine each day to ensure a quantity of urine adequate to flush the bladder.
- Teach the client to report the signs and symptoms of urinary tract infection: burning, frequency, urgency, dull abdominal ache, fever or malaise, or urine that contains sediment or becomes cloudy.

 Older adults may experience confusion before the other signs and symptoms occur.

- Advise the client to contact a healthcare provider if there is bleeding, pain, or difficulty inserting the catheter.
- Some CISC catheters can be reused; some are disposable.
- Instruct the patient to wash their hands thoroughly before handling the equipment or performing the catheterization.
- Tell the client to catheterize as often as needed. Most patients will need to catheterize 4 to 6 times daily.
- Instruct the client to discard a reusable catheter when it becomes difficult to clean or difficult to insert. A CISC catheter may be reused for up to 7 days.
- Recommendations for cleaning a reusable catheter include washing with soap and water, boiling or microwave sterilization, or soaking in an antiseptic solution. Running tap water forcefully through the catheter may remove encrustation or mucus deposits. The client should follow the specific cleaning recommendations of the catheter manufacturer.

For teaching about self-catheterization,

 See **Clinical Insight 25-1: Teaching Clients About Clean, Intermittent Self-Catheterization (CISC),** in Volume 2.

 ### ThinkLike a Nurse 25-8:
Clinical Judgment in Action

How do you feel about instructing patients about pelvic floor muscle exercises? Do you think a female nurse should always provide this instruction? Explain your thinking.

 ### ThinkLike a Nurse 25-9:
Clinical Judgment in Action

What treatment options for incontinence have you seen used in your clinical experience? What options do you believe should be used more frequently? Less frequently? Explain your thinking.

Urinary Diversion

A **urinary diversion,** or **urostomy,** is a surgically created opening for the elimination of urine, required when the bladder must be removed or bypassed.

- **Uses.** Diversion surgeries are used to treat patients who have conditions such as birth defects, cancer, trauma, or disease of the urinary system.
- **Risks.** The risk of infection and permanent kidney damage are greater with urinary diversion, which can occur from *hydronephrosis* (distention of the kidneys with urine, which results from obstruction of the ureter).
- ♥ **iCare** ▪ **Psychological responses.** Patients with a stoma experience a variety of reactions. Patients with continent urinary reservoirs are usually more comfortable with their stoma because of the control it offers while avoiding the embarrassment, odor, and inconvenience of a conventional urostomy. Your attitude and willingness to discuss the body changes associated with an ostomy will help your patient begin their adjustment. In many communities, the local ostomy association offers counseling to assist patients in coping, discuss the psychological changes associated with a urinary diversion, and help them with physical care of the stoma. They share practical and personal information with patients based on their own experience with similar challenges.

Types of Urinary Diversions

There are four major diversion options, as follows:

- **Cutaneous ureterostomy.** This surgery reroutes the ureter(s) directly to the surface of the abdomen, forming a small stoma. It may be unilateral or bilateral. The procedure has limited use because it provides a pathway for pathogens on the skin to directly enter the kidney. The stomas are small and difficult to fit with a collection appliance.
- **Conventional urostomy (ileal conduit, Bricker's loop, ileal loop).** This is the most common type of urinary diversion (Fig. 25-11) because it is the simplest to perform surgically and eliminates the need for intermittent catheterization. A small piece of ileum is removed, with the blood and nerve supply intact. The remainder of the ileum is reconnected to prevent disruption of flow through the bowel. The free segment of ileum is sutured closed at one end, and the other end is brought out to the abdominal wall to create a stoma. The result is a small pouch into which the ureters are implanted. Urine, along with mucus from the ileum, drains freely into the stoma and is collected in a stoma bag that the patient wears. The downside is that urine can back up into the kidneys, causing infection or stone formation over time.
- **Continent urinary reservoir (ileal reservoir, Indiana pouch).** A continent urinary reservoir (Fig. 25-12)

EXAMPLE CLIENT CONDITION: Urinary Incontinence (UI)

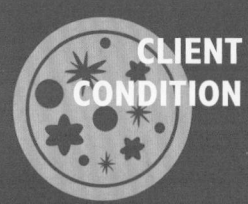

CLIENT CONDITION

Definition: Loss or lack of voluntary control over urination

Types and Causes of UI

Urgency incontinence (overactive bladder)—Involuntary loss of urine with a strong urge to void

Stress Incontinence—Involuntary loss of urine with increased intra-abdominal pressure in the absence of an overactive bladder
    Causes: Pregnancy, childbirth, obesity, chronic constipation and straining, physical activity, laughing, sneezing, coughing, lifting

Mixed incontinence—Combination of urge and stress incontinence; most common in older females

Reflex (unconscious) incontinence—Loss of urine when the person does not realize the bladder is full and has no urge to void
    Causes: Central nervous system (CNS) disease; spinal cord injury; tissue damage from radiation, cystitis, bladder inflammation, or radical pelvic surgery

Functional incontinence—Untimely loss of urine that occurs when a physical or cognitive disability prevents the person from reaching the toilet
    Causes: Immobility, pain, external obstacles, or problems in thinking or communicating

Transient incontinence—Short-term incontinence expected to resolve spontaneously
    Causes: Urinary tract infection (UTI), medications (especially diuretics)

Overflow incontinence—Leakage of urine that occurs when the bladder is too full
    Causes: Fecal impaction, neurological disorders, enlarged prostate

Epidemiology—Who Is Affected?

- UI is common in older adults but is not a normal change of aging.
- Females are twice as likely than males to be affected.
- Current estimates may be low because providers often fail to ask specific questions about incontinence. Many people do not mention leakage of urine to healthcare providers because they are embarrassed, believe nothing can be done, or feel it is an inevitable condition that occurs with age.

Complications

- UTI. Catheter-associated UTIs in healthy patients often resolve spontaneously with the removal of the catheter.
- UI can lead to prostatitis, epididymitis, cystitis, pyelonephritis, and gram-negative bacteremia.
- Emotional distress, intimacy problems, reduced physical activity

Risk Factors

Advanced age
Cigarette use
Diabetes
History of UTIs
Neurological disease (e.g., stroke)
Obesity
Reduced estrogen after menopause
Reduced mobility
Male: Benign prostatic hyperplasia (enlarged prostate) or prostatectomy
Female: Childbirth, specifically vaginal delivery; perimenopause

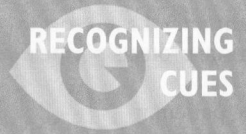

RECOGNIZING CUES

- Assess for risk factors (see Etiologies).
- Ask questions to identify the type of incontinence. For example: "Do you sometimes not make it to the toilet in time?"; "Do you ever dribble urine when you sneeze or cough?"
- Encourage the use of a bladder diary for at least 3–7 days, covering routine, daily activities and atypical situations.

Assess for Symptoms

Back pain, can be on sides or under ribs	Edema	Nausea, vomiting
Bladder spasms	Fever	Pyuria
Chills	Foul-smelling urine	Urgency
Dysuria	Hematuria	Urinary frequency
	Involuntary loss of urine	

Diagnostic Tests

Midstream, clean-catch urine specimen for culture
Dipstick for leukocytes, blood, estrace, nitrates

(continued)

EXAMPLE CLIENT CONDITION: Urinary Incontinence (UI)—cont'd

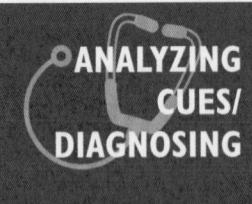
ANALYZING CUES/ DIAGNOSING

Urinary Elimination Alteration
Functional Urinary Incontinence
Overflow Urinary Incontinence
Reflex Urinary Incontinence
Stress Urinary Incontinence
Urge Urinary Incontinence
Risk for Urge Urinary Incontinence

Urinary Retention
Infection Risk
Acute Pain
Renal Alteration

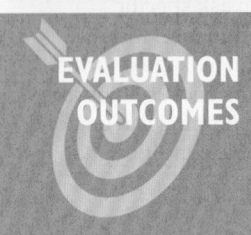
EVALUATION OUTCOMES

- Patient verbalizes improved quality of life, including capacity for physical activity and self-esteem.
- Patient's bladder holds increasingly greater volumes of urine.
- Interval between voidings increases.

NOC Outcomes

Urinary Continence
Urinary Elimination

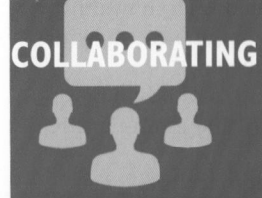
COLLABORATING

Most incontinence is managed with skin care and behavioral interventions, but medications are sometimes used.

Treatments for Urinary Incontinence

- *Medications.* Topical estrogen for women with urogenital atrophy; anticholinergics for involuntary bladder contractions.
- *Botox* injected into the bladder allow more time to get to the bathroom.

Surgical Interventions/Treatments

- *Sling procedures.* Lifts the urethra to relieve pressure.
- *Augmentation of the bladder.* Bladder is surgically enlarged to improve bladder size. Bowel is wrapped around the bladder neck to improve the squeezing action of the bladder.
- *Artificial sphincter.* This patient-controlled device is made up of a pump, pressure-regulating balloon, and cuff that encircles the urethra and prevents urine leakage.
- *Injection of bulking agents.* Collagen is injected alongside of the urethra. Lasts a period of years, with few complications.
- *Sacral nerve stimulator.* A lead wire is placed under the skin near the sacral nerve; it acts like a bladder pacemaker for better control of urge incontinence.
- *Prostate resection.* To relieve pressure of pelvic organs against the bladder.

Devices to Manage Urinary Incontinence

- *Incontinence pessary.* Placed in the vagina; relieves pressure of pelvic organs on the urethra. When used long term, monitor for vaginal infection and ulceration.
- *Vaginal weight training.* Small cone-shaped weight in the vagina for two 15-min periods per day. Contracts the pelvic floor muscles to keep the weight in the vagina.
- *External occlusive device.*
  Female: Urethral meatus covering
  Male: A penis clamp is a reusable, soft, spongy rubber device used to control stress incontinence or dribbling urine, common with enlarged prostate.
- *Internal urethral meatus plug.* Disposable, single-use device for activities that cause stress incontinence; used by male and female patients.
- *Valved catheter.* Urine drained on a schedule.
- *Indwelling urethral catheter.* Last resort to control the flow of urine; protects perineal skin.
- *Bed alarm.* Wakes the patient if incontinence occurs.
- *External collection device.* Condom urinary catheters (urosheaths) for male patients with adequate bladder emptying and intact genital skin.

EXAMPLE CLIENT CONDITION: Urinary Incontinence (UI)—cont'd

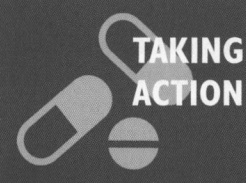

TAKING ACTION

Bladder Training

- Record when emptying bladder (voiding diary).
- Distraction and relaxation strategies help inhibit the urge to void.
- Encourage deep breathing, guided imagery, and pelvic floor contractions to quiet the bladder.

Scheduled Voiding

- Timed voiding (bladder emptying on a schedule), prompted voiding (bladder emptying by suggestion), habit retraining
- Must be mentally and physically capable of self-toileting
- As a pattern develops and the person gains greater control, the length of time between bladder emptying may be increased.

Pelvic Floor Muscle Rehabilitation (Kegel) Exercises (PFME)

- These improve muscle tone by squeezing and relaxing as if stopping urination midstream. Teach the client to hold each contraction for 5 to 10 seconds and then rest for 5 to 10 seconds. However, caution the patient against doing PFMEs while urinating because this may cause backflow of urine.

Intermittent Self-Catheterization

- A straight catheter to drain the bladder for overflow incontinence

Biofeedback

- Electrodes on the abdomen provide feedback about the quality of perineal contraction. Used with PFME.

Supportive Interventions

- Bedside commode, raised toilet seat, bedpan, and urinal make it easier to urinate independently.
- Male patients with UI can use a drip collector—a small pocket of padding worn over the penis, held in place with underwear.

Perineal Skin Care

- Keep skin dry; clean using soap and warm water; rinse well.
- Apply barrier creams and antifungals, as prescribed.
- Use absorbent products for intractable UI.

Complementary Alternative Methods (CAM)

- No CAM cures UI; may reduce symptoms.
- Gosha-jinki gan is a blend of herbs for decreasing urgency, frequency, and nighttime urination.
- Magnesium relieves symptoms by reducing muscle spasms and allowing bladder to empty completely.
- Saw palmetto may be effective for benign prostatic hypertrophy.
- Resiniferatoxin (RTX) and capsaicin block nerve signals between the bladder and brain to help bladder retain urine.
- Pumpkin seed oil strengthens pelvic floor muscles.
- When continence cannot be achieved, consider use of absorbent products with waterproof coverings.
- Acupuncture or percutaneous tibial nerve stimulation may improve symptoms of overactive bladder.

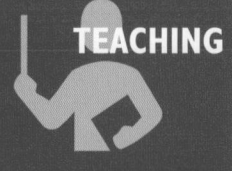

TEACHING

Lifestyle Modification

- **Avoid dehydration.** Although fluid restriction is common, too low fluid intake has not been shown to be useful in preventing UI and increases the risk for UTIs, constipation, and dehydration.
- **Limit caffeine intake** to less than 100 mg daily (i.e., one cup of coffee or two 12-ounce cans of cola). Caffeine is a diuretic and a bladder stimulant.
- **Limiting the intake** of alcohol, artificial sweeteners, spicy foods, and citrus fruits that irritate the bladder.
- **Avoid constipation.** Fecal impaction and chronic constipation, especially in older adults, are associated with an increased risk of UI because they cause pressure on the urinary tract, interfering with flow.

- **Consider low-impact exercise.** High-impact activity (e.g., running, jumping rope) aggravates stress UI.
- **Lose weight** (for persons with a body mass index [BMI] >30). Weight reduction of as little as 5% to 10% may alleviate incontinence symptoms.
- **Stop smoking.** Tobacco use can lead to a chronic cough that puts pressure on the bladder, causing leakage. Nicotine is also a bladder irritant that is linked to stress UI and urge UI among females and to urge UI in males.
- **Take prescribed diuretics early in the morning.** Diuretics taken in the evening can cause nocturia and lead to interrupted sleep.

(continued)

EXAMPLE CLIENT CONDITION: Urinary Incontinence (UI)—cont'd

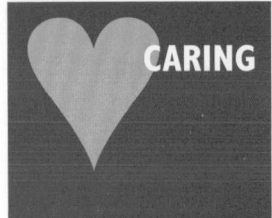
CARING

- **Openly discuss UI with sensitivity and caring.** Be direct and ask about continence using simple questions in a way that will not embarrass the patient, such as "Do you wear a pad to keep your clothes dry?"; "Do you ever experience loss of bladder control?"

- **Reassure that UI is not shameful.**
- **Open discussion about how UI restricts activities** (e.g., social, sexual, and occupational) and how UI can lead to social isolation and low self-esteem.

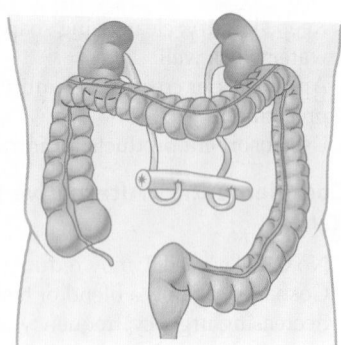

FIGURE 25-11 An ileal conduit is the most common urinary diversion.

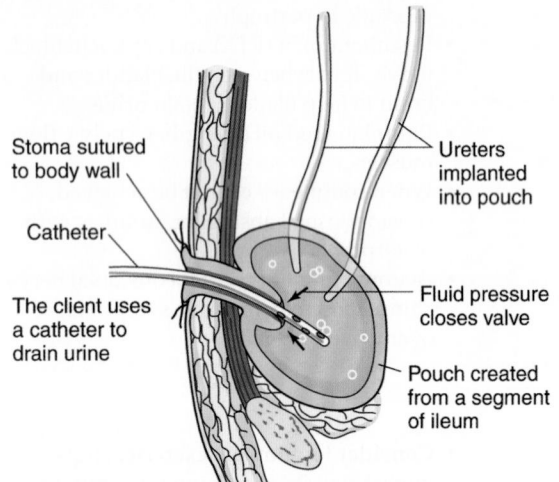

Stoma sutured to body wall

Catheter

The client uses a catheter to drain urine

Ureters implanted into pouch

Fluid pressure closes valve

Pouch created from a segment of ileum

FIGURE 25-12 A continent urostomy allows the client to manage urine without the need to wear an ostomy appliance.

is a variation of the ileal conduit. Urine drains from the ureters into a surgically created ileal pouch. The stoma created on the abdomen contains a nipple valve to keep urine from leaking. Rather than having urine flow constantly, the patient inserts a catheter into the stoma to drain urine through the valve. A second valve prevents reflux of urine back into the kidneys. Unlike the ileal conduit, no external bag is needed; this means minimal risk of leaking and odor.

- **Neobladder.** A neobladder mimics the function of a urinary bladder. A portion of intestine is made into a pouch or reservoir that is connected to the urethra. Urine is then passed through the urethra, similar to the normal passage of urine. For steps in changing an ostomy collection appliance,

Go to **Chapter 26, Procedure 26-6: Changing an Ostomy Appliance,** in Volume 2.

To teach clients how to care for urinary diversions at home, refer to the accompanying Home Care Box, Caring for Urinary Diversion Devices in the Home.

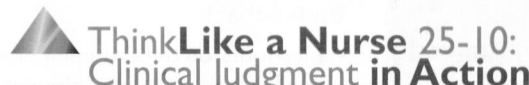
ThinkLike a Nurse 25-10:
Clinical Judgment in Action

What types of challenges or problems do you think a patient with a urinary diversion might experience?

Home Care

Caring for a Urinary Diversion in the Home

A client with a urinary diversion requires physical and psychological care. The long-term goals are for the client to become comfortable with their changed body and to assume self-care.

➤ **Teach the client to perform a thorough assessment of the stoma.** A healthy stoma ranges in color from deep pink to brick red, regardless of skin color, and is shiny and moist. ✚ A pale, dusky, or black stoma often indicates inadequate blood supply. Immediately report such findings to the healthcare provider.

➤ **Teach the client to assess the skin surrounding the stoma for signs of irritation,** such as redness, tenderness, and skin breakdown. **Key Point:** *Skin care is critical. When the normally acidic urine remains in contact with the skin, it becomes alkaline. Encrustations collect on the skin, and the skin becomes macerated and excoriated. Skin breakdown may lead to infection, pain, and leakage.*

➤ **Be certain that the collection device fits** snugly against the skin. A moisture-proof skin barrier is usually placed around the stoma.

Moisture on the skin can lead to irritation and maceration.

➤ **Barrier creams** may be prescribed for irritated skin; if fungal infection develops, nystatin may be prescribed.

➤ **Monitor the amount and type of drainage** from the stoma.

➤ **Empty the device frequently** during the day; connect it to a larger collection bag during the night when the client is sleeping.

♥ **iCare** ➤ **Be available to discuss the client's reaction** to the stoma. Be careful your facial expressions do not convey disgust or disapproval when working with the client and the stoma.

➤ **Provide ample time** to explain stoma care and use of ostomy appliances.

For most clients this is a life-long task; therefore, client teaching is essential.

Continent Urinary Reservoir

These clients will also need instruction about catheterizing their reservoir to drain the urine. Once healed, the reservoir will need to be catheterized four or five times a day.

Neobladder

➤ These clients will not have a stoma but will require bladder training once the postoperative retention catheter has been removed.

➤ Instruct the client to perform pelvic floor muscle exercises three times a day and empty the bladder on a schedule, as often as every 2 hours initially. Once bladder capacity builds, the interval between voiding may be increased.

➤ Teach the client to relax the pelvic muscles and bear down to release urine from the bladder. They may also need to use **Credé's maneuver,** applying manual pressure over the bladder to promote emptying.

➤ If the client is unable to fully empty the bladder with these techniques, they may need to perform intermittent self-catheterization.

For steps to follow in *all* procedures, refer to the Universal Steps for All Procedures found on the inside back cover of Volume 2. Go to the full procedures in Volume 2 to practice and learn the procedure steps. Use these procedure highlights later to help you review key points.

Procedure 25-1: Measuring Post-Void Residual Urine Volume (PVR) With a Portable Bladder Scanner

➤ Assist the patient to a supine position. Uncover only the patient's lower abdomen and suprapubic area.

➤ Select the patient's sex.

➤ Palpate the symphysis pubis and apply ultrasound gel midline on the abdomen above the symphysis pubis.

➤ Position the scanner head in the gel and aim it toward the bladder and slightly downward.

➤ Press and release the SCAN button. Hold the scanner steady until the scan is finished.

➤ Read the bladder volume measurement.

➤ Repeat the scan several times to ensure accuracy.

➤ Press "DONE" when finished. Print the results by pressing PRINT.

Procedure 25-2: Obtaining a Urine Specimen for Testing

➤ Don clean procedure gloves.

Procedure 25-2A: Collecting a Clean-Catch Urine Specimen

➤ Wash with antiseptic solution, then with an antiseptic solution. (For female patients, wash from front to back; for male patients, use a circular motion from the urethra outward.)

➤ Ask the patient to begin voiding. After the stream begins, collect a 30- to 60-mL specimen.

➤ Maintain sterility: Do not touch the inside of the container or the container lid. Avoid getting toilet paper, feces, pubic hair, or anything else in the urine sample.

➤ Place the lid on the container; label the container with the patient's name, the date, and the time of collection.

➤ Follow agency policy on additional packaging.

➤ Transport the specimen to the laboratory as soon as possible. If there is a delay in getting the specimen to the laboratory, most facilities recommend refrigeration.

Procedure 25-2B: Obtaining a Sterile Urine Specimen From a Catheter

➤ Wearing procedure gloves, empty the drainage tube of urine.

➤ Don clean gloves and swab the specimen port with an antiseptic swab.

➤ Insert the needleless access device with a 10-mL syringe into the specimen port and aspirate the amount of urine you need.

➤ Transfer the specimen into a sterile specimen container.

➤ Maintain sterility: Do not touch the needleless access device, the inside of the container, or the container lid.

➤ Label the specimen container with the correct patient identification and transport it to the laboratory in a timely manner.

Procedure 25-2C: Collecting a 24-Hour Urine Specimen

➤ Ask the patient to void. Record the time. Discard this first voiding.

➤ Collect all urine voided during the next 24 hours.

➤ Label the storage container with the patient's name, date, and time the test ended. Transport it to the laboratory after the collection is complete. Otherwise, place the urine in a refrigerator designated for specimen storage per agency policy.

Procedure 25-3: Inserting Intermittent Urinary Catheter (Straight Catheter)

➤ Insertion of an indwelling catheter is a sterile procedure.

➤ Drape the patient for privacy.

➤ Perform perineal care before the procedure; wash your hands; open the kit.

➤ Don sterile gloves and maintain sterile technique while manipulating the supplies in the kit and performing the procedure.

➤ Generously lubricate the catheter before insertion.

➤ Insert the catheter 5 to 7.5 cm (2 to 3 in.) for female patients, 17 to 22.5 cm (7 to 9 in.) for male patients, until urine flows.

➤ Drain the bladder, collect needed samples, measure urine, and then remove the catheter if it is intermittent. If the catheter is indwelling, inflate the balloon and connect the drainage bag.

Procedure 25-4: Inserting Indwelling Urinary Catheter

➤ Insertion of an indwelling catheter is a sterile procedure.

➤ Drape the patient for privacy.

➤ Perform perineal care before the procedure; wash your hands; open the kit.

➤ Don sterile gloves and maintain sterile technique while manipulating the supplies in the kit and performing the procedure.

➤ Generously lubricate the catheter before insertion.

➤ Insert the catheter 5 to 7.5 cm (2 to 3 in.) for female patients, 17 to 22.5 cm (7 to 9 in.) for male patients, until urine flows.

➤ Secure the catheter to the patient's thigh.

Procedure 25-5: Applying an External (Condom) Urinary Catheter

➤ Application of an external (condom) urinary catheter is a clean procedure.

➤ Clean and dry the penis before catheter application.

➤ Apply skin-prep adhesive solution; allow it to dry.

➤ When applying the condom, stabilize the penis with your nondominant hand.

➤ Leave a gap of 2.5 to 5 cm (1 to 2 in.) between the condom and the tip of the penis to prevent skin irritation.

➤ Use only the tape supplied in the application kit to secure the catheter.

➤ For external urinary catheters that contain adhesive material on the inside of the condom, grasp the penis and gently compress the condom onto the shaft.

➤ Be certain that the tubing from the end of the catheter to the drainage bag is free from kinks.

Procedure 25-6: Removing an Indwelling Catheter

➤ Use clean technique. Wash hands before and after removing the catheter. Wear clean procedure gloves.

➤ Be sure to remove the stabilization device or tape securing the catheter to the patient.

➤ Obtain a sterile specimen if needed.

➤ Connect a syringe to the balloon port and allow the balloon to self-deflate or withdraw the fluid slowly. Follow manufacturer's instructions. Check the balloon size on the valve port to verify that all fluid has been removed.

➤ If the balloon does not empty completely, do not pull on the catheter. Report to the charge nurse or the primary care provider before continuing.

➤ Observe the first few voidings after the catheter is removed.

Procedure 25-7A: Intermittent Bladder or Catheter Irrigation

➤ Drape the patient, exposing only the specimen removal port or the irrigation port on a three-way catheter.

➤ Because of the risk of infection, never disconnect the drainage tubing from the catheter.

➤ Use a sterile irrigation solution, warmed to room temperature.

➤ Instill the irrigation solution slowly.

➤ Repeat the process as necessary.

Procedure 25-7B: Continuous Bladder Irrigation

➤ Drape the patient, exposing only the irrigation port of the catheter.

➤ Using aseptic technique, attach the connecting tubing to the irrigation solution container.

➤ Prime the tubing.

➤ Don clean procedure gloves.

➤ Pinch the irrigation port of the catheter and connect the irrigation tubing to the port.

➤ Regulate the flow of the irrigant.

➤ Monitor urine output.

Nursing Care Plan

Client Data

Desmond Washington, a 69-year-old man, comes to the clinic 4 weeks after having a prostatectomy for prostate cancer. He was discharged from the hospital on postoperative day 4 and went home with an indwelling urinary catheter. The catheter was removed at his last visit, 9 days after surgery.

Mr. Washington is meticulously groomed. He is friendly, greeting other patients in the clinic and chatting with the clinic personnel. When his nurse brings him to an examination room and asks how he feels, he says, "I saw the sun come up today. I appreciate that more now. The good Lord has given me a new lease on life, and I intend to use it!" His nurse continues, "That's great, Mr. Washington. How have you been doing since the catheter was removed?" Mr. Washington's smile fades. He lowers his voice and says, "You know, I think that's the worst part of this whole thing. I hate wearing these diapers—they make me feel, well, like an old man. I'm certainly not ready for this."

The nurse continues, "Do you have *any* control of your urine?" Mr. Washington explains, "I may go for hours and stay dry, and then it seems for no reason, I wet myself. Take yesterday, for example. I was sitting on the sofa watching the ball game when someone came to the door. I got up to answer the door, and all of a sudden, I felt wet. I didn't even have anything to drink so that I could make it through the afternoon and stay dry. And if I cough? Forget it. Can something be done so that I can hold my urine again?"

Nursing Diagnosis

Stress Urinary Incontinence related to disruption of the urinary sphincter and related pelvic muscles by surgery as evidenced by client report of involuntary loss of urine with increased intra-abdominal pressure.

NOC Outcomes	Individualized Goals/Expected Outcomes
Urinary Continence (0502) Urinary Elimination (0503)	*By the next visit, Mr. Washington will:* 1. Describe three things he can do that will help regain urinary continence. 2. Explain three interventions to cope with leaked urine. 3. Report that he is drinking adequate amounts of fluids during the day.

NIC Interventions

Urinary Elimination Management (NIC 0590)
Urinary Incontinence Care (NIC 0610)

Nursing Interventions/ Activities	Rationale
1. Obtain midstream voided urine specimen for urinalysis.	Urinary tract infection (UTI) can cause or worsen urinary incontinence (UI) (Lucas et al., 2014; Mayo Clinic Staff, n.d.; Nambiar et al., 2018). Dipstick urinalysis is a rapid, convenient, inexpensive, and easy-to-perform test to detect UTI (BD, n.d.), although it is not always reliable for ruling out UTI (Chu & Lowder, 2018).
2. Identify factors that contribute to Mr. Washington's incontinence by using an incontinence journal for a minimum of 3 days, including variations in his usual activities.	Identifying activities or other factors that cause loss of urine control can guide specific interventions. A journal may help people identify patterns that could otherwise be missed (Lucas et al., 2014; Nambiar et al., 2018; National Institute of Diabetes and Digestive and Kidney Diseases [NIDDKD], 2018A).
3. Use portable bladder scanner to confirm pelvic floor muscle strength.	Pilates exercise program is also effective in recovering continence in men after prostatectomy (Pedriali et al., 2016).

Nursing Care Plan (continued)

Nursing Interventions/Activities	Rationale
4. Teach urgency suppression techniques to delay voiding.	Gradually lengthening the time between voidings can help stretch the bladder so that it can hold more urine (NIDDKD, 2018A; Roscow & Borello-France, 2017).
5. Teach pelvic floor muscle exercises (PFMEs) using a resistance band to strengthen and improve urinary control.	PFMEs strengthen pelvic muscles and enhance sphincter control. Some studies have shown that PFMEs increase UI without side effects in men who have undergone prostatectomy (Appendix C. Sample Bladder Scan Policy, 2017; Campbell et al., 2012; Glazener et al., 2011; Lucas et al., 2014; Nambiar et al., 2018; Pan et al., 2019; Roscow & Borello-France, 2017; Van Kampen et al., 2000).
6. Use surface electromyography (sEMG) biofeedback when needed in conjunction with abdominal training to help Mr. Washington isolate pelvic floor muscles.	Biofeedback allows clients to receive auditory or visual (or both) cues when the proper muscles are contracted to learn how to improve strength of pelvic floor muscles (Hill & Alappattu, 2017; McIntosh et al., 2015; Roscow & Borello-France, 2017; Starr et al., 2016).
7. Teach timed voiding. Have Mr. Washington void on a schedule of every 2 hours.	Bladder training with voiding on a schedule can reduce the amount of urine in the bladder, thus reducing the likelihood of leakage with activities of daily living (Bedretdinova et al., 2014; Davis & Wyman, 2020).
8. Administer prescribed medications.	A variety of medications can increase bladder capacity and decrease frequency of urination (e.g., antimuscarinics, beta-3 agonists, beta-3 adrenergic receptor stimulators, tricyclic antidepressants) (NIDDKD, 2018A). Other medication may be prescribed to reduce urinary leakage.
9. Instruct Mr. Washington to use neuromuscular electrical stimulation.	This treatment is used to retrain and strengthen weak urinary muscles and improve bladder control. A probe is inserted into the anus, and a current is passed through the probe at a level below the pain threshold, causing a contraction. The patient is instructed to squeeze the muscles when the current is on. After the contraction, the current is switched off (Anderson et al., 2015; Roscow & Borello-France, 2017).
10. Explain the need to drink adequate fluids and not limit fluids in an effort to prevent UI. Also avoid drinking fluids at bedtime. Help Mr. Washington identify ways to drink a minimum of 1,500 to 2,000 mL/day.	Adequate fluid intake is important to maintain dilute urine, which is less irritating to the bladder; to maintain systemic hydration; and to reduce the risk for constipation, which can contribute to UI.
11. Advise patient to avoid caffeine, salty, spicy and acidic foods, and alcohol. Encourage a high-fiber diet.	Caffeine and spicy foods increase bladder irritability. Alcohol interferes with signals for urination (Goode et al., 2011; Nambiar et al., 2018). Salty foods can cause the body to retain water, which eventually goes to the bladder. They also increase thirst (WebMD, 2019). Dietary fiber can prevent constipation—a cause of UI (Mayo Clinic Staff, n.d.).
12. Advise the client to keep a healthy weight.	As body mass index (BMI) increases, so does the likelihood of urinary leakage (Gordon et al., 2017; NIDDKD, 2018A).
13. Assist the client in selecting absorbent products that collect urine temporarily while continence management is ongoing.	Incontinence products (e.g., male incontinence guards, underpads, adult incontinence briefs) contain urine, keep skin clean and dry, reduce odor and embarrassment, and reduce the risk for skin breakdown (Davis & Wyman, 2020; Nambiar et al., 2018).

(continued)

Nursing Care Plan (continued)

Nursing Interventions/ Activities	Rationale
14. Help Mr. Washington develop a personal hygiene routine that will maintain skin integrity and control odor.	Conscientious skin care and good hygiene will reduce the risk of skin irritation and infection. Use warm (not hot) water, and pat (do not scrub) the perineal area. A barrier cream repels fluid and reduces skin excoriation. Controlling odor is important in reducing embarrassment and preventing social isolation (Davis & Wyman, 2020).
15. Offer referral to a support group. Encourage the client to speak to family and friends about UI.	Support groups provide a sense of community and enhance the problem-solving skills of members. In sharing their struggle, the patient may find that other people in their life have bladder problems as well (NIDDKD, 2018A).
16. Explain that urinary incontinence is common after prostatectomy but that it may be only temporary.	UI can be a troubling complication of prostatectomy for many men. Fortunately, it often resolves within 6 to 12 months after surgery (McIntosh et al., 2015; Roscow & Borello-France, 2017; Yu Ko & Sawatzky, 2008).

It is important for nurses to understand that the pathophysiology of UI differs between male and female patients and that interventions that are successful in female patients may or may not be equally successful in male patients.

Evaluation

Mr. Washington currently has a positive attitude and is focused on surviving his cancer first and managing the complications of surgery second. Although he previously had been placing folded paper towels in his underwear to collect urine because he thought absorbent products were too expensive, now, with guidance from his nurse, he has identified products he could afford to manage his UI. He liked that they would not be visible through his clothing.

At Mr. Washington's next visit, the nurse will review the initial collaborative goals and stated outcomes and perform a client assessment to determine whether the goals were reached in the stated time frame.

As time passes, incontinence may persist and may become more frustrating for him once he is fully recovered from surgery. Mr. Washington initially declined referral to a support group, but he may be more interested in joining one in the future for help in dealing with the long-term consequences of prostatectomy.

References

Anderson et al. (2015); Appendix C. Sample Bladder Scan Policy (2017); BD. (n. d.); Campbell et al. (2012); Davis and Wyman (2020, February); Glazener et al. (2011); Goode et al. (2011); Gordon et al. (2017); Hill and Alappattu (2017); Lucas et al. (2014); Mayo Clinic Staff (n.d.); McIntosh (2015,); Nambiar et al. (2018), NIDDKD (2018A); Pan et al. (2019); Pedriali et al. (2016); Roscow and Borello-France (2017); Starr et al. (2016); Van Kampen et al. (2000); WebMD (2019); Yu Ko et al. (2008).

Care Map

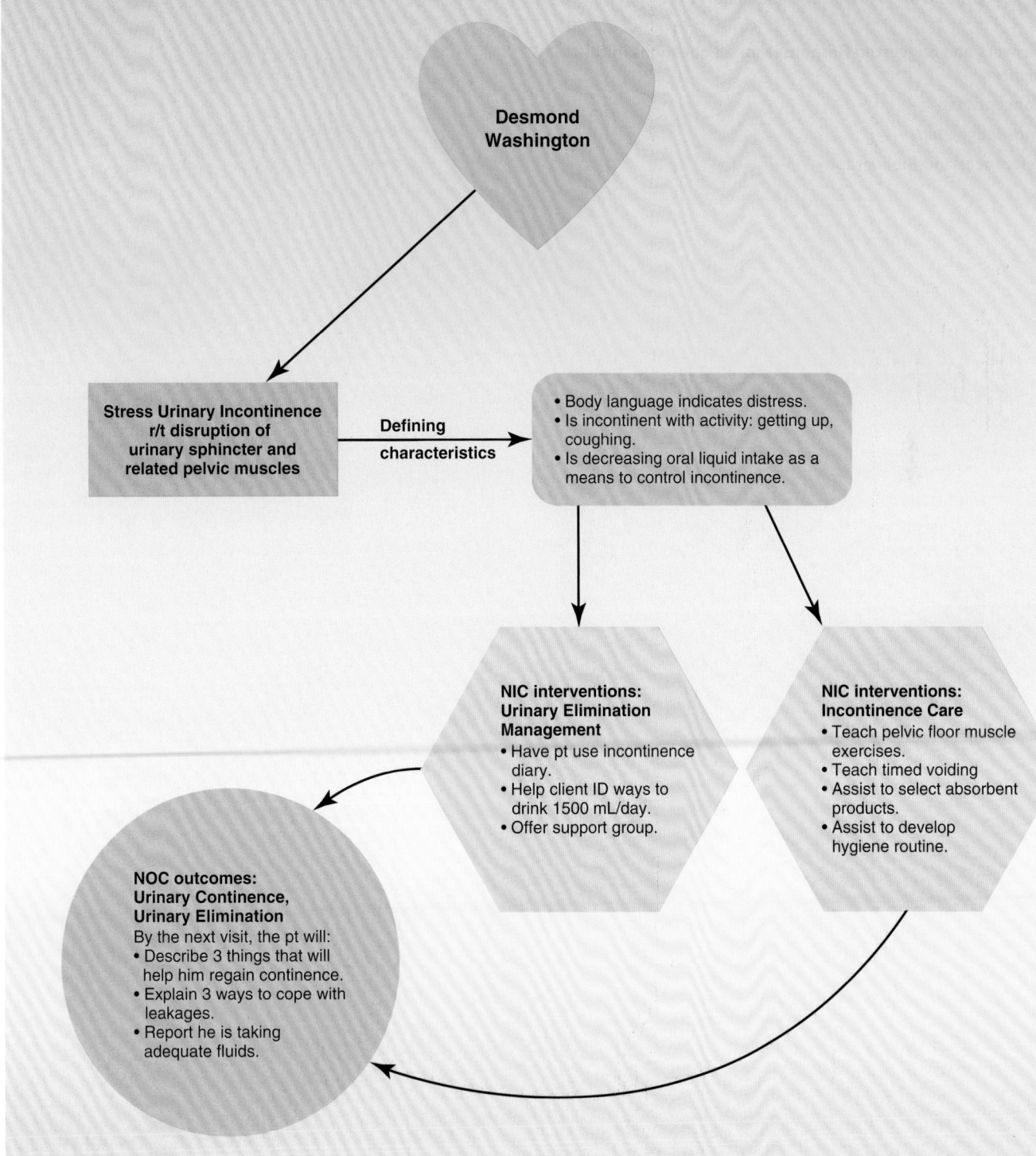

Desmond Washington

Stress Urinary Incontinence r/t disruption of urinary sphincter and related pelvic muscles

Defining characteristics

- Body language indicates distress.
- Is incontinent with activity: getting up, coughing.
- Is decreasing oral liquid intake as a means to control incontinence.

NIC interventions: Urinary Elimination Management
- Have pt use incontinence diary.
- Help client ID ways to drink 1500 mL/day.
- Offer support group.

NIC interventions: Incontinence Care
- Teach pelvic floor muscle exercises.
- Teach timed voiding
- Assist to select absorbent products.
- Assist to develop hygiene routine.

NOC outcomes: Urinary Continence, Urinary Elimination
By the next visit, the pt will:
- Describe 3 things that will help him regain continence.
- Explain 3 ways to cope with leakages.
- Report he is taking adequate fluids.

Key:

- Nursing diagnosis
- Defining characteristics
- NIC interventions and nursing activities
- NOC outcomes

To explore learning resources for this chapter,

Go to Davis Advantage and find:

Answers and Suggested Responses for all questions in this chapter

Concept Map

Knowledge Map

References and Bibliography

CHAPTER 26

Bowel Elimination

Learning Outcomes

After completing this chapter, you should be able to:

➤ Identify the basic structures and functions of the gastrointestinal system.

➤ Discuss factors that affect bowel elimination.

➤ Describe normal bowel elimination.

➤ Differentiate among the various types of bowel diversions.

➤ Discuss common bowel elimination problems.

➤ Identify appropriate nursing history questions to assess bowel elimination problems.

➤ Perform a physical examination focused on bowel elimination.

➤ List and describe diagnostic tests used to identify bowel elimination problems.

➤ Formulate nursing diagnoses associated with altered bowel elimination.

➤ Describe nursing interventions that promote normal bowel elimination.

➤ Provide care for clients experiencing alterations in bowel elimination.

➤ Discuss nursing care associated with the use of bowel diversions.

Key Concepts

Bowel elimination

Motility

Related Concepts

See the Concept Map on Davis Advantage.

Example Problems

Bowel incontinence

Constipation and impaction

Diarrhea

Meet Your Patient

You are assigned to care for Mrs. Zeno, a frail 96-year-old woman who broke her hip last month after a fall at home. Mrs. Zeno was hospitalized for surgical repair of her hip and is now in a skilled nursing facility (SNF) for rehabilitation. The unlicensed assistive personnel (UAP) informs you that Mrs. Zeno has eaten poorly for the past week, only picking at the food on her meal trays and refusing the protein supplements that were added to her diet. Mrs. Zeno tells you she would like to go home: "I have my routine and the foods I like. I think I'd be better there." As you review the chart in preparation for clinical, you note that she has not had a bowel movement (BM) for 3 days. Her last BM was small and very hard.

What additional assessments should you perform? What, if anything, is of concern about her bowel pattern? What actions should you take with Mrs. Zeno?

In this chapter, you will gain theoretical and practical knowledge to help you answer those questions and provide care for clients with bowel elimination concerns.

TheoreticalKnowledge
knowing why

Bowel elimination is a normal process by which we eliminate waste products from our bodies. In this chapter, you will come to understand concepts underlying the function of the gastrointestinal (GI) tract as well as factors that affect bowel elimination.

ABOUT THE KEY CONCEPTS

Bowel elimination is one of the overarching concepts in this chapter—the "hook" on which you hang your theoretical knowledge. The other key concept, **motility,** helps you to understand the processes that occur in normal elimination and in problems such as constipation and diarrhea. Other, more specific, concepts will flesh out your understanding of bowel elimination. For example, when you grasp the concept of bowel diversion, you will understand how it relates to various bowel elimination problems. As you study the chapter, identify the concepts and try to understand how they are connected. This will help you to plan care for clients with any medical diagnosis affecting bowel elimination.

WHAT ARE THE ANATOMICAL STRUCTURES OF THE GASTROINTESTINAL TRACT?

The GI tract is a smooth-muscle tube approximately 10 m (30 ft) long, running through the body from the mouth to the anus. Its major functions are to digest and absorb the nutrients present in food and eliminate food waste products as feces. The structures of the GI tract are the mouth, pharynx, esophagus, stomach, small intestine, large intestine, rectum, and anus (Fig. 26-1).

The Upper Gastrointestinal Tract

The upper part of the GI tract consists of the mouth, pharynx, esophagus, and stomach.

The Mouth This is where mechanical digestion begins, with **mastication,** or chewing. Food is torn into small pieces, mashed, moistened with saliva, formed into a bolus, and then swallowed into the esophagus. The mouth contains glands that secrete enzymes, such as ptyalin and salivary amylase, that begin the digestion of carbohydrates.

The Pharynx The pharynx is the back part of the throat, where food and air pass after chewing. To prevent choking and aspiration, a flap of connective tissue, called the **epiglottis,** closes over the trachea when food is swallowed.

The Esophagus The esophagus is a tube of smooth muscle that alternately contracts and relaxes in waves of

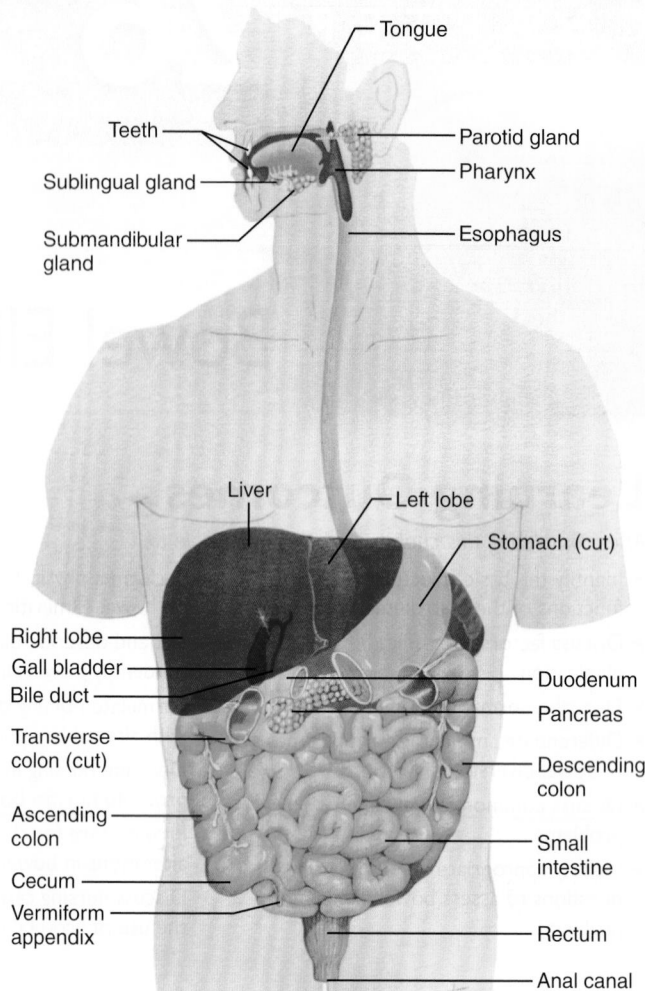

FIGURE 26-1 The gastrointestinal (GI) tract extends from the mouth to the anus. The major functions of the GI system are to digest and absorb the nutrients in food and eliminate food waste products as feces.

peristalsis to push the bolus toward the stomach. The bolus travels the length of the esophagus (about 25 cm, or 10 in.) in about 15 seconds. The *cardiac sphincter* (also called the *gastroesophageal sphincter*) relaxes to allow food to pass into the stomach. When the cardiac sphincter constricts, it prevents acidic stomach contents from flowing back into the esophagus.

The Stomach The stomach is a distensible sac that extends from the esophagus to the small intestine. The stomach stores food while it churns and mixes it, providing further mechanical breakdown. Chemical digestion continues in the stomach, which secretes hydrochloric acid (HCl), a protein-digesting enzyme called *pepsin;* and *gastric lipase,* an enzyme that begins the digestion of lipids. The stomach lining also secretes a mucous coating that protects the stomach from being corroded by HCl. Food remains in the stomach for an average of 4 hours. Food leaves the stomach and enters the small intestine as a liquid, called **chyme.**

The Small Intestine

The small intestine is a folded, twisted, and coiled tube that connects the stomach and the large intestine. About 2.5 cm (1 in.) in diameter and approximately 6 m (20 ft) long if fully extended, it occupies most of the abdominal cavity. Most digestion and absorption of food occur in the small intestine. Chyme travels through it slowly by peristalsis; peristalsis halts periodically to allow for absorption. The small intestine consists of three segments: the duodenum, jejunum, and ileum.

- The **duodenum** is the first section of the small intestine. It is a C-shaped tube that branches off from the stomach, about 30 to 60 cm (1 to 2 ft) long. The duodenum processes chyme by mixing it and adding enzymes. The bile duct and main pancreatic duct both enter the small intestine at the level of the duodenum, providing bile from the liver and gallbladder to digest lipids and pancreatic enzymes to digest lipids, proteins, and carbohydrates.
- The **jejunum** is the coiled midsection of the small intestine. It is about 1.8 to 2.4 m (6 to 8 ft) long and forms the connection between the duodenum and ileum. Its major function is to absorb carbohydrates and proteins.
- The **ileum** joins the small and large intestines. It is responsible for the absorption of fats; bile salts; and some vitamins, minerals, and water. **Key Point:** *However, nutrients are absorbed mainly in the duodenum and jejunum.*

The total length of the small intestine, if it were stretched out, is approximately 6 m (20 ft), but it is much shorter in the body because it is folded to provide a vast surface area for absorption. The inner wall of the small intestine is covered by millions of tiny fingerlike projections called **villi** (Fig. 26-2). The villi are covered with even tinier projections, called **microvilli**. The combination of folds, villi, and microvilli increases the surface area of the small intestine greatly, facilitating the absorption of nutrients.

The Large Intestine

The **large intestine,** also known as the **colon,** is larger in diameter than the small intestine (6.3 cm, or 2.5 in.) but shorter in length—about 1.5 to 1.8 m (5 to 6 ft). It extends from the ileum of the small intestine to the anus. It contains seven segments: the cecum, ascending colon, transverse colon, descending colon, sigmoid colon, rectum, and anus (Fig. 26-3).

- **The cecum.** Undigested food entering the first portion of the large intestine, the **cecum,** consists mostly of cellulose and water.
  - **The ileocecal valve** controls the connection of the ileum to the cecum. Under most conditions, the valve prevents the backflow of chyme from the colon into the small intestine.

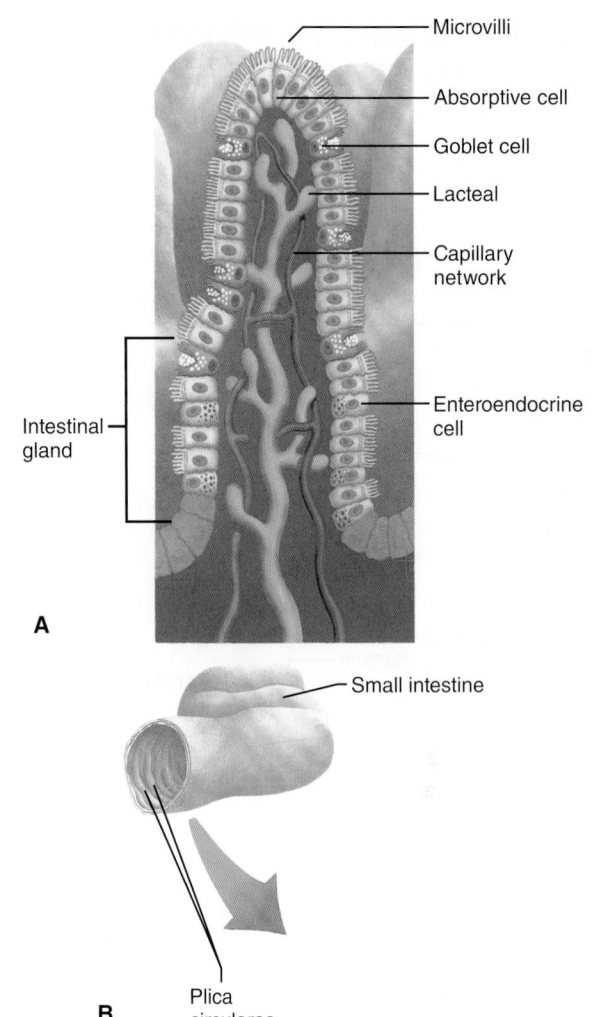

FIGURE 26-2 The small intestine is highly folded, providing a vast surface area for the absorption of nutrients. The microvilli form a brush border, which is the site of most nutrient absorption. A, Microscopic view of a villus showing the internal structure. B, Section through the small intestine showing the plica circulares (circular folds) of the mucosa and submucosa.

- **The appendix** is a small, fingerlike appendage off the cecum. It is believed to be a **vestigial organ**—one whose significance has diminished over time—however, it is lined with lymphatic tissue and may play a role in immune function.
- **The next three segments,** the **ascending, transverse,** and **descending colon,** ring the small intestine.
- **The sigmoid colon** is a final small segment of bowel that twists medially and downward to connect with the rectum and anus.

Functions of the Colon The colon secretes mucus, which facilitates the smooth passage of stool, and absorbs water, some vitamins, and minerals. Approximately 80% of the fluid that enters the colon is reabsorbed along its passage. Normal flora in the colon aid in the digestive process. These bacteria are

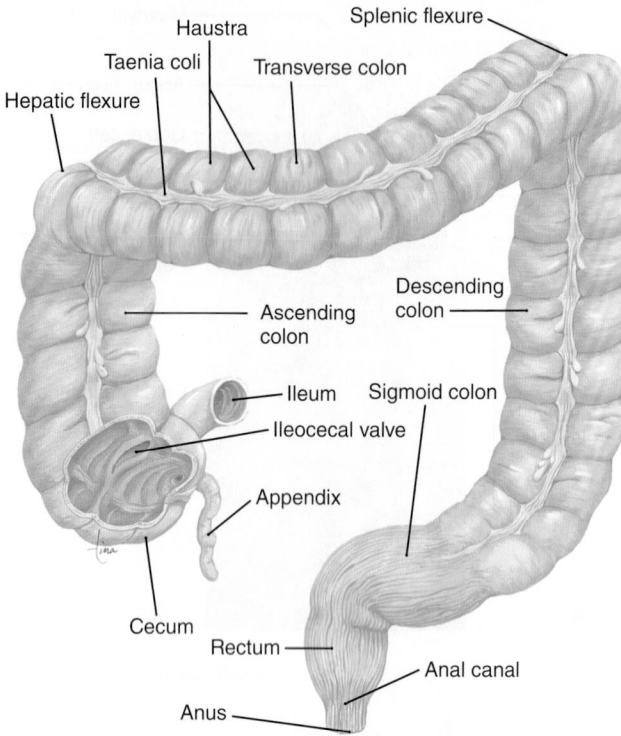

FIGURE 26-3 The large intestine shown in anterior view. The term *flexure* means a turn or bend.

responsible for producing vitamin K and several of the B vitamins.

Peristalsis The large intestine has two sets of muscles that give it a puckered appearance. Longitudinal muscles, known as **taenia coli,** run lengthwise along the colon surface. Tension in these muscles gathers up the colon into pouched segments known as **haustra** all along its length (see Fig. 26-3). In addition, the colon wall contains circular muscles that, together with the taenia coli, cause the colon to expand and contract in length and width to achieve haustral churning, peristalsis, and mass peristalsis.

- **Haustral churning** moves digestive contents around within each haustra. This action promotes reabsorption of water.
- **Peristalsis** continues throughout the length of the large intestine, where it propels intestinal contents toward the rectum and anus.
- **Mass peristalsis** is a powerful contraction along a lengthy segment of bowel. It is facilitated by the **gastrocolic reflex,** which is triggered by food entering the stomach and small intestine. Mass movements usually occur only one to three times each day, and they are responsible for most of the propulsion of the contents in the transverse and sigmoid colon.

The Rectum and Anus

The **rectum** is approximately 15 cm (6 in.) long and is continuous with the **anus,** the last 2.5 cm (1 in.) of the colon. A highly vascular folded tube, the rectum is free

of waste products until just before defecation. The anus has two ringlike muscles that function as sphincters.

- The **internal sphincter** involuntarily relaxes and opens when stool is present in the rectum.
- The **external sphincter** is under voluntary control. Voluntary relaxation of the external sphincter allows stool to be expelled from the body (Fig. 26-4).

The anus is highly vascular. Chronic pressure on the veins within the anal canal, as with prolonged sitting or retained feces, can cause **hemorrhoids** (distended blood vessels within or protruding from the anus).

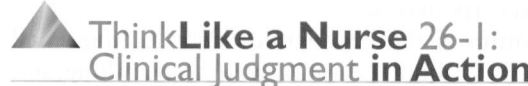

- What are the major functions of the small intestine and large intestine?
- How do the rectum and anus control the elimination of feces from the body?

▲ ThinkLike a Nurse 26-1: Clinical Judgment in Action

Based on your knowledge that hemorrhoids are dilated blood vessels in the anal canal, what symptoms would you expect a patient with hemorrhoids to exhibit?

HOW DOES THE BOWEL ELIMINATE WASTE?

As you have learned, reabsorption of water from chyme in the large intestine results in a semisolid mass known as **feces.** Feces are a mixture of fiber, undigested food,

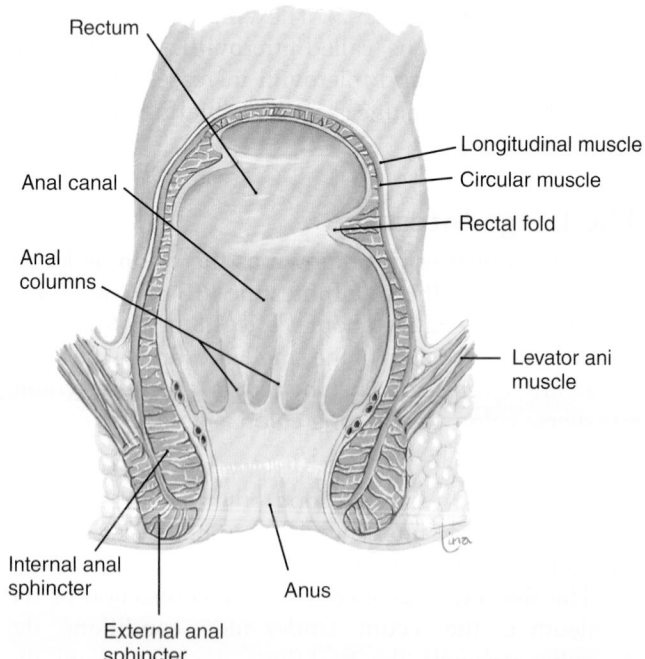

FIGURE 26-4 Internal and external anal sphincters shown in a frontal section through the lower rectum and anal canal.

shed epithelial cells, inorganic material (e.g., calcium and phosphates), bacteria, and water. Small amounts of fat may be present.

Feces are usually brown because **bile salts,** which aid in the digestion of fat, are excreted in the feces. Bile is normally golden yellow, but the action of bacteria in the GI tract changes the color to brown. Bacteria are also responsible for the odor of feces.

Flatus, or gas, is formed in the digestive process. Some is swallowed air that accompanies the intake of food. A small portion diffuses into the GI tract from the blood. However, most of the gas is created by bacterial fermentation in the colon.

The Process of Defecation

The process by which the bowel eliminates waste is called **defecation.** When fecal material reaches the rectum and causes it to distend:

1. Stretch receptors are stimulated to start contraction of the sigmoid colon and rectal muscles.
2. The internal anal sphincter relaxes.
3. At the same time, sensory impulses transmitted to the central nervous system (CNS) produce a conscious urge to defecate.

We respond to this signal by voluntarily contracting our diaphragmatic and abdominal muscles to increase downward pressure while at the same time relaxing the external anal sphincter. These actions allow feces to be propelled through the anus. If we ignore the signal to defecate, the reflexive contractions ease for a few minutes, until mass peristalsis occurs again.

Valsalva Maneuver A person can increase the pressure to expel feces by contracting the abdominal muscles (straining) while maintaining a closed airway (e.g., holding the breath). This is called the **Valsalva maneuver.** Although it assists with the passage of stool, you should caution clients with heart disease, glaucoma, increased intracranial pressure, or a new surgical wound to avoid the Valsalva maneuver because it increases pressure within the abdominal cavity, raises blood pressure, and is associated with an increased risk for cardiac arrhythmias.

Normal Defecation Patterns

The sheer volume of over-the-counter (OTC) products to treat "irregularity" suggests that bowel function problems are common. Nevertheless, many people avoid the topic of bowel elimination, often because they find it embarrassing or do not know the "proper" words to use. As a result, many patients have unanswered questions about their bowel function and may turn to you for information.

Normal Function Part of the confusion about bowel function is that there is a wide range of "normal." The frequency normal of BMs may range from several times per day to once a week. **Key Point:** *As long as the person passes stools without excessive urgency (needing to rush to the toilet), with minimal effort and no straining, without blood loss, and without the use of laxatives, you can regard bowel function as normal.*

Normal Stool Normal stool is a soft, formed semisolid, approximately 75% water and 25% solid when expelled.

- **If passage through the colon is slowed,** more water is reabsorbed from the feces. The stool becomes dry and hard, requiring more effort to pass.
- **If passage through the colon is faster than normal,** less water is reabsorbed, and stools are watery.

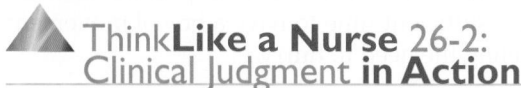

ThinkLike a Nurse 26-2: Clinical Judgment in Action

- Based on your knowledge of normal bowel function, how would you describe Mrs. Zeno's (Meet Your Patient) bowel function? Is it normal or abnormal?
- What additional information, if any, do you need to know to answer this question?

WHAT FACTORS AFFECT BOWEL ELIMINATION?

Each person develops an elimination pattern that is based on several factors, discussed in the sections immediately following.

Developmental Stage

Bowel elimination patterns change throughout the life span.

Infants During the first few days of life, the term newborn passes meconium through the anus. **Meconium** is green-black, tarry, sticky, and odorless. It is formed by swallowed mucus, hair, and amniotic fluid. Stools transition to a yellow-green color over the next few days. After that, breastfed babies pass golden-yellow stools, whereas formula-fed babies pass tan stools. Initially, babies defecate frequently, usually after each feeding. The stools tend to be watery while the large intestine is still immature. Gradually, normal flora develop in the colon, and stools become firmer and less frequent.

Children The ability to control defecation typically develops at about 2 to 3 years of age. Toilet training requires neural and muscular control as well as conscious effort. The child must be aware of the urge to defecate, be able to maintain closure of the external anal sphincter while getting to the toilet, and be able to remove clothing. When toddlers become engrossed in play, they sometimes ignore the need to move their bowels, and soiling is common. As children mature, they gradually learn to gain more control over defecation.

Adults The bowel pattern set in childhood normally continues into late adulthood if the client consumes adequate fiber and fluid and engages in regular physical activity. However, peristalsis, intestinal smooth muscle tone, perineal muscle tone, and sphincter control normally decrease with aging. These physiological processes can contribute to bowel elimination problems among older adults, especially if they decrease their activity and fiber intake.

Personal and Sociocultural Factors

Refer to iCare box 26-1.

Privacy and Time Privacy is important to most people, as is sufficient time to have a bowel movement without feeling the need to hurry.

- Clients working in fast-paced jobs may have difficulty even consciously recognizing the need to defecate, and some habitually ignore the need, promoting bowel dysfunction.
- Parents and caregivers of infants and toddlers may postpone their own toileting needs because of fear of leaving the children alone.
- Some clients are embarrassed by the thought that anyone might realize they are having a bowel movement and will wait until they are entirely alone before even entering the bathroom.

Stress Have you ever heard the following phrase: "He puts his stress in his gut"? Stress has a major influence on the motility of the GI tract. It may cause diarrhea or constipation, and it is a primary risk factor in the development of *irritable bowel syndrome,* a disorder associated with bloating, pain, and altered bowel function.

♥ iCare 26-1

Bowel Elimination

Rob has been a registered nurse (RN) for 6 months. Gladys, 80 years old, is weakened and in need of assistance with her bladder and bowel routine; she is also at risk for falls. She comments that she has a grandson about Rob's age and seems slightly embarrassed that Rob must help her with her elimination needs. Rob is sensitive to her feelings and offers to get a female to assist her. She says, "Yes, please." A few days later, Gladys is getting stronger and can perform her bathroom routine independently, but she remains slightly unsteady on her feet. Rob walks her to the bathroom, makes sure she is safe, and then, while ensuring privacy, stays nearby just outside the door until she is finished. As Rob assists her back to her bed, Gladys thanks him for his good care. She says, "It's hard to depend on someone to take care of private things I've always done for myself. Thanks for being sensitive about that."

Nutrition, Hydration, and Activity Level

Foods and Fiber Regular intake of food promotes peristalsis.

- **A regular schedule for eating.** People who eat on a regular schedule are likely to develop a regular pattern of defecation, whereas irregular eating creates irregular bowel elimination.
- **Adequate intake of fiber.** Fiber promotes peristalsis and defecation. Bulky foods absorb fluids and increase stool mass. The increased mass stretches bowel walls, initiating peristalsis and the defecation reflex. Adults, on average, eat 10 to 15 g of fiber per day, much less than the U.S. department of Agriculture (USDA, 2020) recommendation for adults up to age 50 years (25 g per day for women and 38 g per day for men).
- **Some foods have specific effects in the bowel.** For example:
  - **The active bacteria in yogurt** stimulate peristalsis while at the same time promoting the healing of intestinal infections.
  - **Low-fiber foods,** such as pasta and other simple carbohydrates and lean meats, slow peristalsis.
  - **Foods such as broccoli, onions, and beans** lead to excess gas in many people. Spicy foods may also cause gas, as well as more frequent bowel movements.

Dietary Supplements Dietary supplements can also affect bowel function. For example:

- Calcium may cause constipation.
- Magnesium loosens stools.
- Vitamin C softens stools and, in high doses, may cause diarrhea in sensitive clients.

Fluids Most healthy people can stay hydrated by drinking water and other fluids whenever they feel thirsty. For some people, fewer than eight glasses a day might be enough. But other people might need more.

- **Inadequate fluid intake or excessive fluid loss,** as in diarrhea or vomiting, slows peristalsis and leads to dry, hard stools that are difficult to pass (Emly & Marriott, 2017).
- **Excessive fluid intake** (especially beverages with high sugar content) may lead to rapid passage through the colon and soft or watery stools.
- **Different types of fluids** have varying effects on sensitive individuals. For instance, consuming large amounts of milk may cause constipation in some people. Coffee promotes peristalsis in many clients and may even cause loose stools in sensitive clients.

Activity Physical activity seems to stimulate peristalsis and bowel elimination. In addition, sedentary people are likely to have weaker abdominal muscles. Clients with health concerns that limit activity (e.g., shortness of breath, pain, or required bedrest) often experience constipation.

Medications

Many medications may affect peristalsis. All oral medicines have the potential to affect the function of the GI tract. Examples include the following:

- **Antacids,** often used for heartburn, neutralize stomach acid but may slow peristalsis.
- **Aspirin and other nonsteroidal anti-inflammatory drugs (NSAIDs),** such as naproxen and ibuprofen, irritate the stomach. Repeated use can lead to ulceration of the stomach or duodenum.
- **Antibiotics** given to combat infection decrease the normal flora in the colon. The result is often diarrhea. Bacterial populations can be maintained with supplements of probiotics (e.g., acidophilus) or daily consumption of yogurt (Rosenberg, 2018).
- **Iron,** a common mineral supplement, is available as an OTC medication and is often prescribed for the treatment of anemia. Iron has an astringent effect on the bowel and is notorious for causing constipation and changing stool color to black. It also causes nausea if taken when there is no food in the stomach.
- **Pain medications,** particularly opioids (narcotics), slow peristalsis and are associated with a high incidence of constipation.
- **Antimotility drugs,** such as diphenoxylate (Lomotil), may be used to treat diarrhea. They work by slowing peristalsis.
- **Laxatives** are used to treat constipation. In general, laxatives work by stimulating peristalsis (see Box 26-1). They are frequently abused by people who self-medicate with OTC drugs, who may become dependent on them, requiring ever-increasing dosages until the intestine fails to work properly.

Probiotics

Probiotics are live bacteria or yeasts that have health benefits when taken in sufficient amounts. They are found in foods such as yogurt and dietary supplements. Hundreds of species of microbes live in the human intestines, and nearly all are "good" (normal flora). The key is keeping them all in balance. Significant imbalance can lead to compromised health. Supplementing the diet with specific microorganisms (e.g., *Lactobacillus*) may be a cost-effective way to prevent diseases. For example, probiotics are known to contribute to bowel regularity, may alleviate symptoms of diarrhea and vaginitis, and may also help combat *Clostridium difficile* infections in patients taking antibiotics (Quigley, 2019; Setbo et al., 2019).

As with herbs, there is little regulation, and little attention has been paid to the quality of probiotics. Ongoing research is needed to resolve the following problems (National Center for Complementary and Integrative Health [NCCIH], 2019):

- When you buy a probiotic, you do not know for sure whether (and how long) the bacteria will live and be active.

BOX 26-1 ■ Types of Laxatives

- **Stool softeners** enable moisture and fat to penetrate the stool, thereby softening it and making it easier to pass. The effectiveness of stool softeners in relieving chronic constipation is being questioned, but they are still in use. *Example:* docusate sodium.
- **Osmotic laxatives** work by drawing water into the bowel from surrounding tissue, resulting in bowel distention. *Examples:* polyethylene glycol, lactulose.
- **Lubricant laxatives** coat the stool and the gastrointestinal (GI) tract with a thin waterproof layer. Mineral oil is an example. Because the lubricant coats the entire GI tract, it may interfere with the absorption of nutrients. ✚ Mineral oil is potentially dangerous in debilitated patients. Inhaled droplets can lead to a form of pneumonia.
- **Stimulant laxatives** are bowel irritants. They irritate the intestinal wall, stimulating intense peristalsis. *Examples:* senna, bisacodyl, castor oil.
- **Bulking agents** are soluble fiber or insoluble fiber, which, when taken with water, increase stool bulk and stool frequency. The fiber attracts fluid into the colon, and the increased bulk of the stool stimulates the urge to evacuate. **Key Point:** *These are considered the safest form of laxative, but they may interfere with the absorption of some medicines. They are the drug of choice for chronic constipation. Examples: Metamucil, Citrucel, psyllium, FiberCon.*
- **Chloride channel activators** increase intestinal fluid and motility to help stool pass.
- **Combination laxatives** are laxatives that contain more than one type of laxative ingredient. The most common type is a combination stimulant laxative and stool softener.

- It is difficult to know for certain the types and number of bacteria in the product and whether they are present in the recommended numbers.
- You do not know, for the different bacteria, how long they live under different storage conditions and in different types of products.
- You do not know exactly what protection the product will give you.

Teach patients that up to 1 out of 4 people who take probiotics will suffer diarrhea as a side effect. Teach patients how to read probiotic labels, and urge them to use reputable sources for their information. Remind them to check expiration dates. Probiotics are contraindicated for patients who are immunosuppressed and those taking certain drugs.

Surgery and Procedures

Clients undergoing anesthesia and surgery often experience sluggish bowel elimination. The delay in bowel elimination may be caused by a variety of circumstances.

Anesthesia General anesthesia (which renders the patient unconscious) and analgesics (administered preoperatively and postoperatively for pain) slow bowel motility. Spinal anesthesia and epidural anesthesia are less likely to cause this effect.

Stress Regardless of the type of anesthesia, most clients find surgery a stressful event. As you may recall from Chapter 9, if stress activates the general adaptation syndrome, autonomic nervous system and endocrine responses ensue. Among those responses is a slowing of peristalsis.

Manipulation of the Bowel During Surgery Abdominal or pelvic surgery in which the bowel is manipulated may result in a **paralytic ileus,** a cessation of bowel peristalsis.

- Although peristalsis halts, the bowel continues to produce secretions. The secretions remain stagnant, causing distention and discomfort.
- To decrease the complications of paralytic ileus, patients who have had bowel surgery typically have a nasogastric (NG) tube with low constant or intermittent suction. The NG tube removes secretions until peristalsis returns. To review the insertion of an NG tube or management of a patient with an NG tube,

Go to **Chapter 24, Procedure 24-2: Inserting Nasogastric and Nasoenteric Tubes,** in Volume 2.

Decreased Mobility After surgery, patients often experience discomfort that affects mobility. This further hinders GI motility and increases the risk for constipation.

Perineal Surgery Patients who have had surgical interventions involving the perineal region (e.g., an episiotomy after childbirth) may fear pain or that their sutures will "tear" or "break" during bowel elimination, and therefore they resist the urge to evacuate the bowel.

Anal Sphincter Surgery Patients who have had surgery that disrupts the anal sphincter may experience uncontrolled rectal drainage after surgery.

Pregnancy

In early pregnancy, many women experience fluid loss due to "morning sickness"—periods of nausea and vomiting. As the pregnancy progresses, the growing uterus crowds and displaces the intestines, and the increased level of progesterone slows intestinal motility. As a result, pregnant women often experience constipation, decreased appetite, and irregular food intake. In addition, the increasing pressure of the uterus and the increased blood volume of normal pregnancy increase the woman's risk for hemorrhoids.

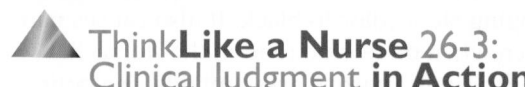

ThinkLike a Nurse 26-3: Clinical Judgment in Action

- Review the case of Mrs. Zeno (Meet Your Patient). What factors may be affecting her bowel elimination?
- What additional information do you need?

Pathological Conditions

Several disorders affect bowel function. Among them are the following:

- Neurological disorders that affect innervation of the lower GI tract
- Cognitive conditions that limit the ability to sense the urge to defecate
- Pain
- Immobility that leads to sluggish peristalsis

Constipation in Pregnancy

Situation: The nurse is interviewing a 27-year-old pregnant client with a history of constipation, gas, and general abdominal discomfort after eating. The client reports increasing their dietary intake of fluid and fiber, but with limited results. Focused assessment reveals hypoactive bowel sounds and a firm abdomen. The client is anxious about taking medication during pregnancy. The nurse wants to learn more about nonpharmacological interventions for constipation.

PICOT Components

P	Population/client	=	Pregnant clients
I	Intervention/indicator	=	Increased physical activity
C	Comparator/control	=	Fiber and liquids only
O	Outcome	=	Relief from constipation
T	Time	=	During pregnancy

Searchable Question: Do _____ (P) who receive _____ (I), compared with _____ (C) demonstrate _____ (O) during _____ (T)?

Example of Evidence: The effect of hormones on the bowel, as well as the increased iron intake in prenatal vitamins, often causes early pregnancy constipation. The increasing size of the uterus and decreased maternal activity can further contribute to constipation. Many clients find relief with increased fiber and fluid intake. A commitment to daily exercise will also increase peristalsis, promoting fecal movement. The client on bedrest can also benefit from thigh-strengthening and ROM exercises.

Application to Practice: The nurse discusses with the client ways in which the client can incorporate increased physical activity into their lifestyle during pregnancy.

Pathological conditions of the GI tract. Additional information about constipation and diarrhea can be found in the Example Problem boxes later in this chapter.

The following are three common disorders that affect bowel function.

Food Allergies The National Institute of Allergy and Infectious Diseases (NIAID) characterizes a **food allergy** as an adverse health effect arising from an immune response that occurs reproducibly on exposure to a given food (NIAID, 2019).

- **Common food allergens** include dairy products, egg whites, shellfish, gluten, peanuts and other nuts, citrus fruits, and soy.
- **Immune responses** to foods manifest as a variety of symptoms, ranging from a mild rash to anaphylactic shock.
- **Common GI symptoms** suggesting food allergy include constipation, diarrhea, a red and blistering rash around the anus, abdominal discomfort, bloating, excessive gas, and intestinal bleeding (Mahdavinia, 2020).

Food Intolerances In contrast to a food allergy, a **food intolerance** is specifically linked to the GI system. It produces such symptoms as GI discomfort, pain, gas, bloating, diarrhea, or constipation after the person consumes the food. Such symptoms can mimic those of a food allergy, but food intolerances are not caused by immune responses. An example is *lactose intolerance,* a deficiency of the enzyme lactase, which is responsible for the breakdown of milk sugar (lactose).

Diverticulosis When the colon must repeatedly move highly compacted fecal material, the longitudinal and circular muscles enlarge over time. This increases the force on the mucosal tissues, causing them to "balloon" out between the muscle layers of the colon wall, forming pouches in which fecal matter becomes trapped. This condition is called **diverticulosis. Diverticulitis** is a condition in which the pouches become infected. Antibiotic therapy or surgery is required. People whose diets are low in fiber or consist mainly of refined foods are especially at risk for diverticulosis. Obesity and red meat intake are also risk factors (van Dijk et al., 2018).

KnowledgeCheck 26-2
- What is a normal defecation pattern?
- Identify the factors that affect bowel elimination.

WHAT IS A BOWEL DIVERSION?

Many pathologies that affect the GI tract can be treated with medication (e.g., laxatives, anti-inflammatory drugs). However, some conditions, such as cancer, ulcerations, trauma, or inadequate blood supply, may require a **bowel diversion:** a surgically created opening for the elimination of digestive waste products.

A client with a bowel diversion does not eliminate via the anus. Instead, the **effluent** (output fecal material) is expelled through a surgically created opening in the abdominal wall, called a **stoma** or **ostomy.** The effluent ranges from liquid to solid, depending on the part of the bowel that is being diverted.

Bowel diversions may be temporary or permanent.

- **Temporary bowel diversions** may be done to allow part of the intestine to rest and heal after a surgical intervention for a benign condition of the bowel. Once healing has occurred, surgical **reanastomosis** (reconnection) of the bowel is performed, and the patient once again has BMs from the anus.
- **Permanent bowel diversions** are performed if the bowel is necrotic (dead) or cannot be salvaged because of severe disease or trauma.

Ileostomy

An **ileostomy** brings a portion of the ileum through a surgical opening in the abdomen, bypassing the large intestine entirely. Because most of the water is absorbed from the feces in the large intestine, drainage at this level is liquid and continuous. The patient must wear an ostomy appliance at all times to collect the drainage. Some variations of an ileostomy are designed to control drainage more effectively and to cause less body image disturbance. However, many clients are not candidates for these procedures because of their underlying disease.

- A **Kock pouch,** or **continent ileostomy,** creates an internal pouch, or reservoir, to collect ileal drainage (Fig. 26-5A). To drain the pouch, the patient inserts a tube through the external stoma into the pouch several times per day. This alternative avoids continuous drainage, so the patient does not need to wear an ostomy appliance.
- A **total colectomy with ileoanal reservoir** is a surgical procedure in which the colon is removed, a pouch is created from the ileum, and the ileum is connected to the rectum (see Fig. 26-5B). The patient evacuates the bowel on the commode in the usual manner. Although this procedure should result in continence of bowel elimination, the feces will still be liquid.

Colostomy

A **colostomy** is a surgical procedure that brings a portion of the colon through a surgical opening in the abdomen. **Key Point:** *The location of the colostomy determines the consistency of the feces eliminated, as well as the need to wear an ostomy appliance (Fig. 26-6).*

- **The closer the colostomy is to the ascending colon and the ileocecal valve** (between the small and large intestine) (see Fig. 26-3), the more liquid and continuous the drainage will be.

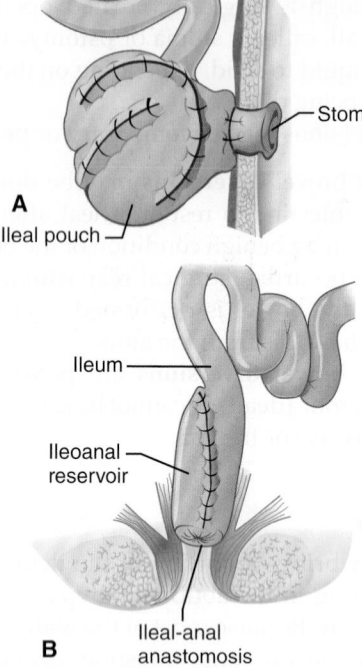

FIGURE 26-5 Ileostomy variations. *A*, Continent ileostomy (Kock pouch). *B*, Ileoanal reservoir.

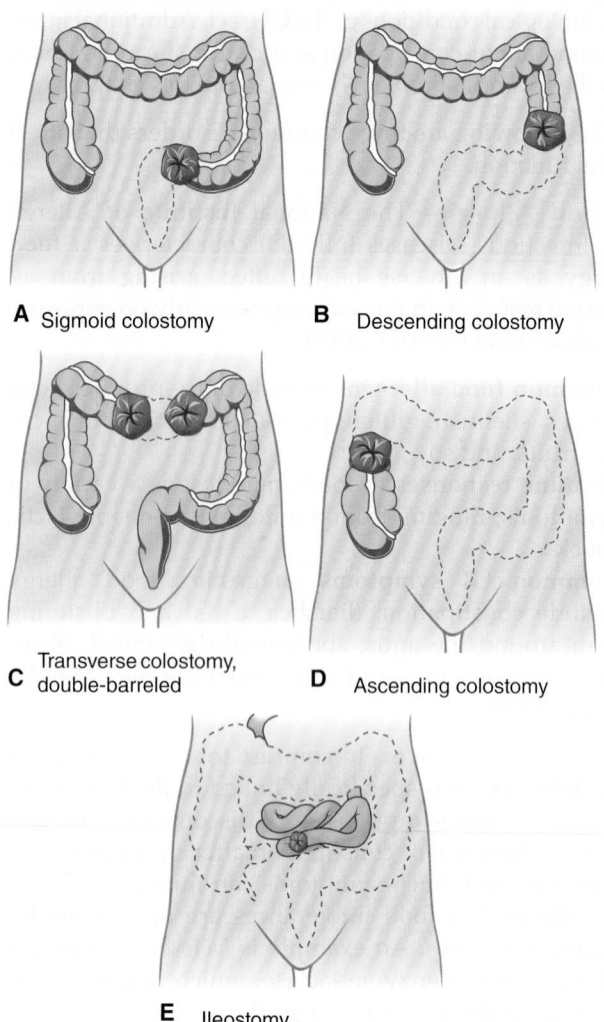

FIGURE 26-6 *A–E*, Location of various bowel diversion ostomies. Shaded areas indicate sections of the bowel that are removed or being "rested."

- **A colostomy close to the sigmoid colon,** in contrast, will produce solid feces.
- **Colostomies near the rectum,** such as sigmoid colostomies, can often be controlled by diet and irrigation. As a result, the client may not need to wear an ostomy appliance to collect drainage.
- A colostomy created in the transverse colon is usually temporary and may be either a double-barreled or loop colostomy.
  - A **double-barreled colostomy** (see Fig. 26-6C) has two separate stomas that externalize the bowel on both sides of the portion that has been removed. The proximal stoma is the functioning end that drains fecal material. The distal stoma may drain mucus and is sometimes called a *mucous fistula.*
  - A **loop colostomy** (Fig. 26-7) consists of a segment of bowel brought out to the abdominal wall. The posterior wall of the bowel remains intact, but a plastic rod is wedged under the bowel to keep it from slipping back into the abdomen. The anterior wall is incised, and the mucosal surface is left visible and open to air. It, too, has a functioning proximal end and limited drainage from the distal end.

KnowledgeCheck 26-3

- What changes in bowel elimination are associated with constipation? With diarrhea?
- Why are bowel diversions performed?
- What determines the nature of the effluent from a bowel diversion?

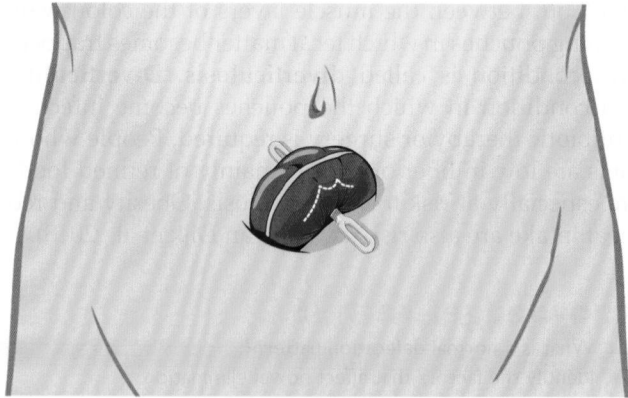

FIGURE 26-7 A loop colostomy.

PracticalKnowledge
knowing **how**

As a nurse, you will work collaboratively with the healthcare team to facilitate normal bowel function in well and ill clients. In the remainder of the chapter, we discuss teaching, monitoring, and assisting clients with bowel function.

▮ ASSESSMENT/RECOGNIZING CUES

For a list of questions to use, as well as complete details of a focused physical assessment of bowel function,

 Go to **Chapter 26, Assessment Guidelines and Tools, Focused Assessment: Bowel Elimination,** in Volume 2.

Focused Nursing History

Because bowel patterns vary, you will need a nursing history to determine what is normal for each client. As you interview clients, pay attention to their reactions to your questions. Many people are embarrassed by discussions of bowel function. Tailor your assessment to the client's needs, and use language that makes the client comfortable. For clients with a bowel diversion, you will also gather data on the client's usual care of the stoma, use of appliances, and adjustment to the ostomy.

Remember to ask the client about medications because many have the potential to cause constipation (e.g., calcium and iron supplements). The following are examples of medications associated with constipation:

Antacids containing aluminum hydroxide or calcium carbonate
Anticholinergic drugs (e.g., belladonna)
Anticonvulsant drugs (e.g., phenytoin)
Antidiarrheals (e.g., loperamide)
Antihistamines (e.g., diphenhydramine)
Antiparkinsonian drugs (e.g., amantadine hydrochloride)
Antipsychotic drugs (e.g., chlorpromazine)
Calcium channel blockers (e.g., verapamil hydrochloride)
Diuretics (e.g., furosemide)
Iron supplements

Lithium
Nonsteroidal anti-inflammatory drugs (e.g., ibuprofen)
Opioids (e.g., morphine, codeine)
Sympathomimetics (e.g., ephedrine)
Tricyclic antidepressants (e.g., nortriptyline)

Focused Physical Assessment

Physical assessment for bowel elimination includes an examination of the abdomen, rectum, and anus, as well as characteristics of normal and abnormal stool (Table 26-1). Observe the size, shape, and contour of the abdomen, and listen to bowel sounds. You might also palpate the anus and rectum for the presence of stool or masses. You may hear the following when auscultating the abdomen:

- **Normal bowel sounds** are high-pitched, with approximately 5 to 15 gurgles every minute.
- **Hyperactive bowel sounds** are very high-pitched and more frequent than normal. They may occur with small bowel obstruction and inflammatory disorders. They indicate hyperperistalsis, which can result in diarrhea.
- **Hypoactive bowel sounds** are low-pitched, infrequent, and quiet. A decrease in bowel sounds indicates decreased peristalsis, which can result in constipation.
- **Absent bowel sounds.** If you hear no bowel sounds after listening in a quadrant for 3 to 5 minutes, you should listen in several areas before describing them as absent. Absent bowel sounds indicate a lack of intestinal activity, which may occur after abdominal surgery and may indicate a paralytic ileus.

KnowledgeCheck 26-4

- What should you discuss with your client when performing a nursing history focused on bowel elimination?
- Describe the physical assessment you would perform for a client with constipation.

Table 26-1 ➤ Normal Characteristics of Feces and Variations			
STOOL CHARACTERISTIC	**CONDITION**	**AGE-GROUP**	**DESCRIPTION**
Frequency	Normal	Infants*	Bottle-fed—1 to 3 stools/day; Breastfed—4 to 6 stools/day
		Adults	Daily; 2 to 3 bowel movements (BMs)/week
	Variations (Hypermotility)	Infants*	>6 stools/day
		Adults	>3 stools/day
	Variations (Hypomotility)	Infants*	Bottle-fed—<1 stool every day or 2 Breastfed—<1 stool/week
		Adults	<1 stool/week

(Continued)

Table 26-1 ➤ Normal Characteristics of Feces and Variations—cont'd

STOOL CHARACTERISTIC	CONDITION	AGE-GROUP	DESCRIPTION
Color	Normal	Infants*	Dark green (1st week); then yellow
		Adults	Brown
	Variations		*Bile* pigment gives feces a brown color. Infant stools are yellow because of their rapid passage.
			White or clay-colored stool may indicate the absence of bile (e.g., as in bile duct obstruction) or the use of some antacids.
			Light-brown stool may indicate a diet high in milk products and low in meat.
			Pale, fatty stool may indicate malabsorption of fat.
			Black, tarry stool (**melena**) may indicate the use of iron medications or upper gastrointestinal (GI) bleeding; eating large quantities of red meat, spinach, and dark green vegetables may cause feces to be almost black.
			Red stool may indicate bleeding in the lower intestinal tract or hemorrhoids.
			Stool darkens the longer it is left standing after defecation.
Quantity	Normal	Adults	Approximately 150 g/day
	Variations		Quantity varies with amount of food eaten, from 100 to 400 g per day.
Shape	Normal		Approximately the diameter of the rectum: about 2.5 cm (1 in.) in diameter
	Variations		Narrow, pencil-shaped stool may indicate intestinal obstruction or constriction or rapid peristalsis.
			Small, marble-shaped stool may indicate slow peristalsis, with a longer time in the large intestine.
Consistency	Normal		Formed, soft, moist
	Variations		Consistency is related to gastric motility and is affected by food and fluid intake.
			Hard stool indicates constipation. The more time spent in the large intestine, the more water is reabsorbed, and the harder the stool. May also indicate dehydration.
			Liquid stool may indicate diarrhea; rapid peristalsis (e.g., from infection).
Odor	Normal		Pungent; affected by foods eaten
	Variations		Normal odor is created by putrefaction and fermentation in the lower GI tract. Odor is also influenced by the pH of the stool, which is normally neutral or slightly alkaline.
			Strong, foul odors may indicate blood in the stool, especially in the upper GI tract, or infection.

*All information about infant stool patterns applies after passage of meconium.

Diagnostic Tests

Several diagnostic tests may be performed to assess for bowel elimination problems (e.g., to screen for colorectal cancer, to diagnose diverticulosis). They may be classified as direct or indirect.

- **Indirect visualization studies** are radiographic views of the lower GI tract. The simplest of the tests is an abdominal flat plate, an anterior to posterior (AP) x-ray view of the abdomen used to detect gallstones, fecal impaction, and distended bowel.
- **Direct visualization studies** are used for diagnostic and treatment purposes. They are invasive procedures and are conducted by a gastroenterologist, who inserts various instruments (e.g., *endoscopes*) to examine the interior of the GI tract. The nurse's role during these studies is to prepare the patient for the test, function as an assistant, and provide aftercare.

For nursing care of patients undergoing such diagnostic tests,

 Go to **Chapter 26, Diagnostic Testing, Direct Visualization Studies of the Gastrointestinal Tract** and **Indirect Visualization Studies of the Gastrointestinal Tract,** in Volume 2.

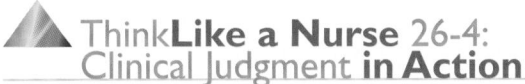 Think**Like a Nurse** 26-4:
Clinical Judgment **in Action**

A client asks you why they must perform a bowel prep with a strong laxative before having a colonoscopy. How might you reply?

Laboratory Studies of Stool

Stool specimens may be analyzed to detect blood, infection, or parasitic infestation. The client must void first and then defecate into a clean, dry bedpan, bedside commode, or special container (half hat) placed under the toilet seat. A small sample is obtained and sent to the laboratory for analysis or analyzed at the bedside. To obtain a specimen from an infant or young child, you will collect freshly passed feces from a diaper.

Handling Stool Specimens

Wear clean gloves when you handle the container or manipulate stool specimens. Use tongue blades to transfer the stool specimen to the container provided by the laboratory. Do not contaminate the outside of the specimen container.

Except when testing for fecal occult blood (see following discussion), you will usually need approximately 2.5 cm (1 in.) of formed stool or 20 to 30 mL of liquid stool. If blood, mucus, or purulent material is present, be sure to include this with the sample. Transport the specimen to the laboratory as soon as possible. If that is not possible, consult the laboratory for appropriate storage.

Usually, you will need to refrigerate the specimen until it can be received in the laboratory.

Testing for Fecal Occult Blood

Blood from the GI tract may be visible to the eye or **occult** (hidden), especially when passed through the stool from higher up in the intestine. You can perform the test for occult blood at the bedside, although some institutions require that it be done in the laboratory. The test is called a *guaiac* or *fecal occult blood test*. It requires the use of a special reagent that detects the presence of **peroxidase,** an enzyme present in hemoglobin. Only a small smear of stool is required. For home testing, remind patients to wash their hands before and after collecting stool. For a summary of the procedure, see the Highlights of Procedures box. For the complete procedure,

 Go to **Chapter 26, Procedure 26-1: Testing Stool for Occult Blood,** in Volume 2.

Screening can detect colorectal polyps so that they can be removed before becoming cancerous. Regular screening for colorectal cancer is key to preventing colorectal cancer. The U.S. Preventive Services Task Force (2021) recommends screening for colorectal cancer using stool for occult blood testing and sigmoidoscopy or colonoscopy for asymptomatic adults age 45 years or older who are at average risk of colorectal cancer and until age 75 years.

Assessing for Pinworms

Pinworms (an intestinal parasite) are small, white, threadlike worms that spread through human-to-human transmission:

- By ingesting (swallowing) infectious pinworm eggs
- By entry through the anus (e.g., when eggs attach to a person's fingers and are transferred to the anal area by scratching or touching the anus)

Once present, the pinworms live in the cecum. They come to the anal area to deposit eggs during the night and migrate back up through the rectum during the day.

- When assessing a child, you can spread the buttocks while the child is sleeping and examine the anus to see whether any pinworms are visible to the naked eye.
- You can also test for the presence of the eggs with tape. In the morning, as soon as the patient awakens, press clear cellophane tape against the anal opening. Remove the tape immediately, and place it adhesive-side down on a slide.
- Alternatively, or in addition, insert a cotton-tipped swab gently into the rectum for not more than 2.5 cm (1 in.). Smear the specimen on a slide for microscopic inspection for parasites and eggs.
- You may also check at night by using a flashlight. The test may need to be repeated on consecutive days.

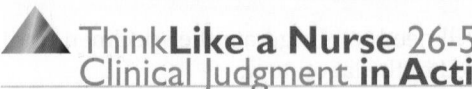

ThinkLike a Nurse 26-5: Clinical Judgment in Action

You are reviewing a client's chart and note that the client was tested for fecal occult blood. The results are as follows:

3/10/xx negative for occult blood
3/11/xx no BM
3/12/xx no BM
3/13/xx no BM
3/14/xx positive for occult blood
3/15/xx negative for occult blood
3/16/xx negative for occult blood

What can you conclude? What questions do these findings raise?

NURSING DIAGNOSIS/ANALYZING CUES

Common nursing diagnoses (Clinical Care Classification [CCC], 2020) related to bowel elimination include the following:

- **Bowel Incontinence** is a change in normal bowel habits characterized by the involuntary passage of stool. It is more common among women and older adults. Other risk factors include neurological diseases, stroke, sphincter damage, inflammatory bowel disease, and functional problems such as a self-care deficit or impaired mobility. (See the Example Problem: Bowel Incontinence, later in this chapter).
- **Constipation**. Because the frequency of bowel elimination varies, constipation is usually defined as a decrease in the frequency of bowel movements resulting in the passage of hard, dry stool. Constipation can be a temporary problem wherein symptoms resolve in a short time. Nearly everyone experiences constipation at some point.
- **Chronic Constipation** typically lasts 3 months or longer and may persist for years.
- **Fecal Impaction.** Unrelieved constipation may eventually result in a fecal impaction, in which dry, hard stools lodged in the rectum cannot be passed. (See the Example Client Condition: Constipation and Impaction, later in this chapter).
- **Risk for Constipation** is an appropriate diagnosis for clients at increased risk because of bedrest, medications such as opioids, or surgery. You might use this diagnosis for a client with a condition or who is taking medications known to decrease peristalsis.
- **Perceived Constipation** is an appropriate diagnosis for a client who makes a self-diagnosis of constipation and uses laxatives, suppositories, or enemas to ensure a daily bowel movement.
- **Diarrhea** is the passage of loose, unformed, or watery stools. (See the Example Client Condition: Diarrhea, later in the chapter).
- **Gastrointestinal Motility Alteration** is a broad label that encompasses increased, decreased, ineffective, or absent peristaltic activity within the GI system. If you use this label, you need to specify whether the GI motility is increased or decreased.

Bowel elimination problems may also form the etiology of other nursing diagnoses and collaborative problems. Examples include the following:

- Social isolation r/t embarrassment secondary to bowel incontinence
- Potential Complication: Electrolyte imbalance secondary to diarrhea. Older adults, very young children, and infants are at especially high risk.
- Skin Integrity Impairment r/t irritating effects of feces secondary to diarrhea
- Anxiety r/t perceived need for a daily bowel movement
- Body Image Disturbance r/t bowel diversion

ThinkLike a Nurse 26-6: Clinical Judgment in Action

- What data do you have about Mrs. Zeno's (Meet Your Patient) bowel function?
- What else would you like to know about her bowel function? What other symptoms often accompany these cues?
- Which nursing diagnosis best describes this cue cluster?
- In addition to this nursing diagnosis, what other cues from the scenario might also be contributing to her infrequent BMs?
- From the scenario data, how would you describe the etiology of Mrs. Zeno's problem?
- What questions do you still have about the etiology?

PLANNING/PRIORITIZING HYPOTHESES AND GENERATING SOLUTIONS

The general bowel elimination goal is that the patient will have soft, formed bowel movements regularly.

NOC standardized outcomes associated with bowel problems include the following:

- **For Bowel Incontinence:** Bowel Continence; Tissue Integrity: Skin and Mucous Membranes
- **For Constipation:** Bowel Elimination; Ostomy Self Care
- **For Perceived Constipation:** Bowel Elimination
- **For Diarrhea:** Bowel Elimination; Bowel Continence; Symptom Severity
- **For Gastrointestinal Motility Alteration:** Bowel Elimination; Gastrointestinal Function

Note that Bowel Elimination is a useful outcome for most bowel problems.

When bowel elimination functions as an etiology, choose outcomes linked to the problem side of the diagnosis. For example, for Skin Integrity Impairment r/t irritating effects of diarrhea stool, you would probably find the relevant NOC outcomes under the diagnosis, Tissue Integrity: Skin and Oral Mucous Membranes.

Individualized goals/outcome statements depend on the nursing diagnosis. Because normal bowel elimination patterns are individualized, regularity is based on the individual's pattern. Examples include the following:

Resumes normal bowel pattern by (date).
Discusses feelings about colostomy.

IMPLEMENTATION/TAKING ACTION

♥ **iCare** Bowel elimination is a normal physiological function. It is important for you to convey an attitude of acceptance and display professionalism when providing care for patients with bowel elimination problems.

NIC *standardized interventions and activities* for patients with bowel elimination problems include the following examples:

Bowel Incontinence Care
Constipation/Impaction Management
Diarrhea Management
Bowel Management
Teaching: Individual

Specific nursing activities to promote normal bowel function and relieve elimination problems are found in the following sections. Both independent and dependent interventions are discussed.

Promoting Normal or Regular Defecation

Six independent nursing activities for promoting regular defecation are covered in the following sections: provide privacy; assist with positioning; consider the timing of defecation; support the healthful intake of food and fluids; encourage exercise; and manage flatulence.

Provide Privacy

Try this exercise. Imagine that your class assignment for today is to stand in front of the classroom and describe to the class your normal pattern of defecation, including frequency, appearance, and other characteristics of the stool. How would you feel about that? Would you do it?

♥ **iCare** Although defecation is a normal physiological function, most patients consider it a very private matter. The following help to minimize embarrassment:

- **Take a matter-of-fact approach.** This confirms to patients that you are comfortable with this aspect of care.
- **Provide privacy** for your patient when discussing or providing care related to bowel elimination. When assisting a patient with bowel elimination, excuse visitors from the room, draw the dividing curtains in shared rooms, and close the door.
- **Control odors** because many patients are embarrassed by the odor of bowel movements and therefore may ignore the urge to defecate. Using an aromatic spray or other odor-reducing product may help to reduce embarrassment.

Assist With Positioning

An upright seated or squatting position is the most comfortable for defecation and decreases the need to strain.

- When possible, assist the patient to the bathroom to use the toilet.

- Place a bedside commode next to the bed for patients who are unable to ambulate to the bathroom.
- A patient who must remain in bed should assume a semi-Fowler's position to use the bedpan. Patients who are unable to assume this position because of surgery, trauma, or other medical conditions must use supine or side-lying positions. These positions are unnatural for bowel elimination and place the patient at risk for constipation.
- Raise the siderails or provide an overhead trapeze so that the patient can grip them to maneuver on and off the bedpan.

For an overview of steps to place a bedpan, see the Highlights of Procedures box; for the complete procedure,

 Go to Chapter 26, **Procedure 26-2: Placing and Removing a Bedpan,** in Volume 2.

Consider the Timing of Defecation

Recall that food entering the duodenum triggers mass peristalsis. As a result, the urge to defecate often occurs after meals. Ignoring this urge may lead to constipation. See the Example Client Condition: Bowel Incontinence, the Example Problem: Constipation and Impaction, and the Example Client Condition: Diarrhea.

Support Healthful Intake of Food and Fluids

- **Diet teaching.** Teach clients the importance of a balanced diet in promoting soft, formed, regular bowel movements.
- **Ample fiber.** Encourage a daily intake of 25 g of fiber for women and 38 g of fiber for men to provide bulk, attract water into the stool, and promote peristalsis. The diet should be rich in fresh fruits, dried fruits, vegetables (especially raw), whole-grain foods, flaxseed, popcorn, dried beans, peas, and legumes.
- **Key Point:** *Adding fiber does not help to relieve opioid-induced constipation unless the patient's current intake is deficient.* In fact, excessive fiber might put the patient at risk for bowel obstruction due to the (1) opioid-induced decreased peristalsis, (2) delayed gastric emptying, and (3) prolonged intestinal transit time of the feces (Star et al., 2018).
- **Adequate fluid.** Without adequate fluid intake, a high-fiber diet can actually cause constipation. Recommend a minimum total fluid intake of 2,700 mL per day (female individuals) and 3,700 mL per day (male individuals) to (1) keep stool soft and (2) aid in the production of mucus to lubricate the colon. At least 80% of fluid intake should come from drinking fluids and the remaining 20% from food and cellular metabolism of food (Mayo Clinic, 2020).
- **Water is preferred.** Water is the preferred fluid because soda, coffee, and tea often contain caffeine or additives that promote diuresis. However, because the diuretic effect of these fluids is minimal, they

are acceptable for clients who simply will not drink enough plain water.

Encourage Exercise

Physical activity increases peristalsis and promotes defecation.

- Encourage patients to exercise three to five times per week and to engage in daily walking or light activity.
- Assist hospitalized or institutionalized patients to ambulate as soon as their condition permits. Even limited activity, such as getting out of bed or walking 10 feet, decreases the risk for constipation.
- Provide range-of-motion (ROM) exercises for patients who must remain on bedrest. Even passive ROM (the joints are moved through ROM by the nurse) promotes peristalsis. Chapter 29 provides additional information about activity and ROM exercises.

For clients who can assist with exercise, the following exercises promote abdominal and perineal strength:

- *Thigh strengthening.* Have the client slowly bring one knee up to the chest, briefly hold it, then lower the leg to the bed. Repeat this pattern, alternating legs. Encourage the client to perform this exercise several times per hour while awake.
- *Abdominal tightening.* Have the client tighten and hold the abdominal muscles for a count of five and then relax. This core exercise works the abdominal muscles used during defecation.

Manage Flatulence

Recall that flatus is a natural by-product of digestion. When gas is excessive or leads to complaints of abdominal distention, cramping, or discomfort, it is known as **flatulence.**

- Some people develop flatulence after eating gas-producing foods, such as beans, cabbage, cauliflower, onions, or highly spiced foods. For others, flatulence occurs when fiber intake is increased.
- Flatulence is one of the cluster of symptoms of irritable bowel syndrome.
- Constipation is often accompanied by flatulence because digestive by-products undergo prolonged fermentation in the colon.

Use the following interventions to help clients manage flatulence:

- Teach clients to be aware of and avoid foods that trigger flatulence.
- Teach clients to follow self-care strategies (identified earlier) for maintaining regular bowel movements.
- Encourage patients who have had surgery with gaseous anesthesia to ambulate and perform bed exercises to stimulate peristalsis and the passage of gas.
- In severe cases, you may need to insert a rectal tube to aid in the elimination of flatus. For a summary, see

the Highlights of Procedures box. To learn the entire procedure,

 Go to Chapter 26, **Procedure 26-5: Inserting a Rectal Tube,** in Volume 2.

Teach Clients When to See a Primary Care Provider

Many GI symptoms are normal and do not require treatment. For example, everyone has excessive flatus and abdominal distention at some time—perhaps as a result of a high-fat, high-sugar meal. And it is common for bowel movements to occasionally become a little irregular. However, clients need to know when a symptom may be signaling a more serious condition.

Teach clients to see their primary care provider for the following if a symptom lasts longer than 3 weeks or is disabling:

- Blood in the stool (unless they have hemorrhoids and this is not an unusual occurrence for them)
- Stomach pain
- Change in bowel habits
- Unintended weight loss
- Constipation that is not relieved after trying fiber, fluids, and exercise

KnowledgeCheck 26-5

Identify at least five independent nursing actions that you can take to encourage regular elimination in a well client.

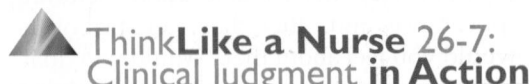 Think**Like a Nurse** 26-7:
Clinical Judgment **in Action**

How could you facilitate regular bowel elimination for Mrs. Zeno (Meet Your Patient)? What information do you need?

INTERVENTIONS FOR EXAMPLE CLIENT CONDITION: DIARRHEA

Nursing interventions focus on treating the causes of the diarrhea, as well as monitoring and treating associated symptoms and defining characteristics. For more information about diarrhea, see the accompanying Example Client Condition: Diarrhea.

INTERVENTIONS FOR EXAMPLE CLIENT CONDITION: CONSTIPATION AND IMPACTION

Many of the nursing strategies to prevent and treat constipation are identical to the activities that promote regular bowel elimination. For more information about caring for patients with constipation and impaction, refer to the Self-Care box Teaching Your Patient About

Laxative Use and the accompanying Example Clint Condition: Constipation and Impaction.

Administering Enemas

An **enema** is the introduction of solution into the rectum to soften feces and distend or irritate the colon, in order to stimulate peristalsis and evacuation of feces. Responses to an enema are governed by the following conditions:

- Height of the solution container
- Speed of flow
- Concentration of the solution
- Resistance of the rectum
  - Muscle tone and history of constipation or other bowel disorders determine the resistance of the rectum.
  - A client with a long history of constipation is more likely to be able to tolerate a large-volume enema because the rectum and colon have become distended over time.
- Hypotonic and isotonic solutions are easier to retain.

The primary care provider generally prescribes the specific type of enema to administer to a patient (e.g.,

Safe, Effective Nursing Care (SENC)

Safe, Effective Nursing Care for Patients in Palliative Care

Competency: *Validate evidence-based research to incorporate in practice:* Incorporate into client care evidence-based findings.

Constipation is one of the most common problems in patients receiving palliative care and can cause extreme suffering and discomfort. Although general principles of prevention should be followed, pharmacological treatment is often necessary. The combination of a softener and stimulant laxative is generally recommended, and the choice of laxatives should be made on an individual basis. An emphasis on evidence-based practice, quality improvement approaches, and further research is required in the assessment, diagnosis, and management of constipation in palliative care.

Competency: *Provide safe quality client care:* Design a "Thinking, Doing, Caring" framework that incorporates a holistic approach to client care.

Recognize the patient or designee as the source of control and full partner in providing compassionate and coordinated care based on respect for the patient's preferences, values, and needs. The key is to strengthen the healthcare provided to include collaboration and improve health outcomes for patients.

Source: Andrews, A., & St Aubyn, B. (2020). Assessment, diagnosis and management of constipation. *Nursing Standard, 36*(9) 59–65. https://doi.org/10.7748/ns.2020.e11512.

cleansing, retention, or return-flow). To learn how to administer various types of enemas,

 Go to Chapter 26, **Procedure 26-3: Administering an Enema,** in Volume 2.

Cleansing Enemas

Cleansing enemas promote the removal of feces from the colon. They have the following uses:

- Treat severe constipation or impaction.
- Clear the colon in preparation for visualization procedures, such as colonoscopy.
- Empty the colon when starting a bowel training program.
- Clear the colon for surgeries of the lower GI tract and for some pelvic surgeries.

"High" and "Low" Enemas A cleansing enema may be given "high" or "low." A "low" enema is given by standard procedure. A "high" enema attempts to clear as much of the large intestine as possible. With a "high" enema, the client receives initial instillation of the fluid in the left lateral position. The client then moves to the dorsal recumbent position and then the right lateral position for the remainder of the instillation. This turning process allows the fluid to follow the shape of the large intestine.

EXAMPLE PROBLEM: Diarrhea

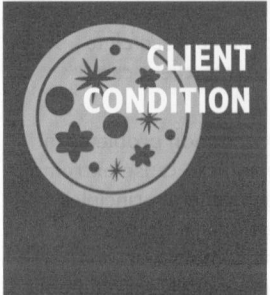
CLIENT CONDITION

Basic Definitions

- **Diarrhea**—the passage of loose, unformed, or watery stools
- **Chronic diarrhea**—persists for more than 1 month
- **Acute diarrhea**—a response to infection or unusual foods

Causes/Related Factors

Contaminated food, viral infection, dietary change, side effect of a medication or dietary supplement, psychosocial and behavioral factors

Potential Complications

- Fluid and Electrolyte Imbalance (especially K+)
- Impaired Skin Integrity

Risk Factors

Key Point: *Infants, young children, and frail elderly are most vulnerable and may require hospitalization and IV fluid replacement therapy.*

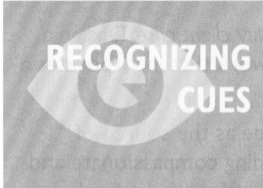
RECOGNIZING CUES

Symptoms/Defining Characteristics

Assess the following:
- Bowel pattern
- Dietary pattern (highly spiced foods, high-fat foods, greasy snacks, or large quantities of raw fruits and vegetables)

- Fever, nausea, vomiting, and abdominal pain (may indicate viral infection)
- Skin and mucous membranes (turgor, moisture/dryness)
- Abdominal cramping

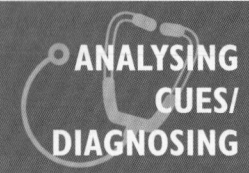
ANALYSING CUES/ DIAGNOSING

Diarrhea
Gastrointestinal Motility Alteration

Risk for Deficient Fluid Volume
Risk for Impaired Skin Integrity

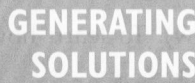
GENERATING SOLUTIONS

- Resumes normal bowel pattern
- Maintains skin integrity

- Maintains fluid and electrolyte balance

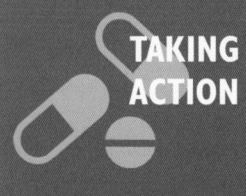
TAKING ACTION

Preventive Interventions

- Teach hand hygiene; stress importance of washing often.
- Provide information about foods that can cause diarrhea (e.g., highly spiced, high-fat, large quantities of raw fruits and vegetables).
- Plain yogurt and other probiotic foods consumed daily may help prevent diarrhea that is a response to antibiotics.

Monitoring Interventions

Monitor:
- Stools (frequency, amount, color, consistency)
- Fluid balance (intake and output, weight, vital signs, skin turgor, mucous membranes)
- Electrolyte levels
- Skin integrity (assess perineum for redness, irritation, and excoriation)

Treatment Interventions

Diet
- Clear liquid diet; electrolyte replacement fluids (e.g., Pedialyte), clear broth, gelatin, popsicles
- Encourage patient to sip liquids.
- Reduce the amount of fiber in the diet when solids are introduced. Resume normal diet gradually.
- Limit caffeine (e.g., coffee, tea, colas).
- Advise a BRAT diet if a client with diarrhea has an appetite (bananas, white rice, applesauce, and toast).
- Breastfed infants should continue on breast milk. It has a protective effect against enteritis.
- Provide prompt hygiene care after any episodes of diarrhea.

EXAMPLE PROBLEM: Diarrhea—cont'd

Toileting
- For patients who are ambulatory, allow some free time after meals to use the restroom.
- Assist those who cannot toilet independently to ambulate to the bathroom or use the bedpan.
- **Key Point:** *Discuss with UAPs the need to offer help without waiting to be asked so that patients experience minimal delays.*

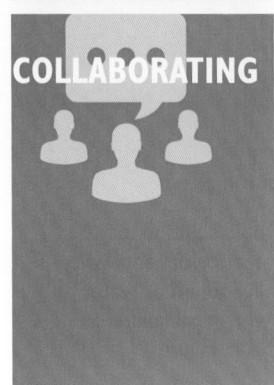

COLLABORATING

Work with the primary provider to administer and monitor effects of prescribed medications.
- *Antidiarrheal medications* (opiates [e.g., paregoric]) and opiate derivatives (e.g., loperamide); these act to slow peristalsis. **Side Effects:** Drowsiness. Advise to use with caution. Review diet, fluid intake, and medicines. Work with the primary care provider to alter the previously listed factors to encourage regular bowel movements.

- *Bismuth subsalicylate (Pepto-Bismol).* An over-the-counter medication. Has antimicrobial and antisecretory properties. Caution to avoid using without instruction from provider.
- **Key Point:** *Antidiarrheal drugs are not used in acute diarrhea. They are usually reserved for chronic diarrhea.*

Enema Solutions Cleansing enema solutions include hypotonic solutions and hypertonic solutions (see Table 26-2).

- **Hypotonic solutions** contain a large volume of fluid that is instilled into the rectum (500 to 1,000 mL for adults, 50 to 150 mL for infants).
- **Hypertonic solutions,** in contrast, are usually smaller in volume (90 to 120 mL, or 3 to 4 oz, for adults).
- **Isotonic solutions.** Refer to Table 26-2.

Retention Enemas

Retention enemas introduce a solution into the colon that is meant to be retained for a prolonged period. Consequently, the volume is small, usually 90 to 120 mL (3 to 4 oz). The following are the most common forms of retention enemas:

- **Oil-retention enemas** instill 90 to 120 mL of oil into the rectum to soften stool and lubricate the rectum. This type of enema may be used to assist a client in passing hard stool or before the digital removal of stool.
- **Carminative enema** is a procedure in which 60 to 180 mL (2 to 6 oz) of solution is instilled into the rectum to help expel flatus and relieve bloating and distention. This procedure is used after abdominal or pelvic surgery when peristalsis is slow to return and the client experiences pressure from gas.

- **Medicated enemas** may be used to instill antibiotics to treat infections in the rectum or anus or to introduce anthelminthic agents for the treatment of intestinal worms and parasites.
- **Nutritive enemas** administer fluid and nutrition through the rectum for patients who are dehydrated and frail. They are most commonly used in hospice care as a means to provide hydration for dying patients.

Return-Flow Enemas

A return-flow enema, known as a *Harris flush*, may be ordered to help a patient expel flatus and relieve abdominal distention. For adults, approximately 100 to 200 mL (3 to 7 oz) of tap water or saline is instilled into the rectum. To learn more,

 Go to **Procedure 26-3D, Administering a Return Flow Enema,** in Volume 2.

Digital Removal of Stool

If fecal impaction does not respond to the use of stool softeners and enemas, you will need to digitally remove feces from the rectum. Digital removal is accomplished by breaking up the hardened mass into pieces and manually extracting the pieces.

Table 26-2 ➤ Solutions Commonly Used in Enemas

SOLUTION	EXAMPLES	ACTION	TIME UNTIL BOWEL MOVEMENT	ADVERSE EFFECTS
Hypotonic	500–1,000 mL of tap water	Large volume distends the colon, thereby stimulating peristalsis; water also softens stool.	15 minutes	Fluid and electrolyte imbalance, especially water intoxication, is possible if enema is not expelled. ✚ Large-volume solutions may be contraindicated in patients who have weakened intestinal walls.
Isotonic	500–1,000 mL of normal saline (0.9% NaCl solution)	Large volume distends the colon, thereby stimulating peristalsis; some softening of stool also occurs.	15 minutes	Fluid and electrolyte imbalance, especially sodium retention
Hypertonic	90–120 mL, or 3–4 oz, of sodium phosphate (e.g., Fleet) for adults; available as a commercially prepared solution	Attracts water into the colon, thereby causing distention and stimulating peristalsis and defecation	Rapid acting: 5–10 minutes	Sodium retention ✚ Hypertonic solution may be contraindicated for patients who tend to retain sodium or water (e.g., those with renal failure of congestive heart failure).
Oil	90–120 mL of mineral oil, cottonseed oil, or olive oil; available as a commercially prepared solution	Softens the feces, lubricates the rectum	Varies widely. An oil-retention enema is often given 1–3 hours before a cleansing enema is administered.	
Soapsuds	Pure Castile soap is added to tap water or saline.	Intestinal irritation stimulates peristalsis.	Varies	Only pure Castile soap is safe. Other soaps and detergents can cause bowel inflammation.
Carminative	For example, 1:2:3 "MGW" solution (e.g., 30 mL magnesium, 60 mL glycerin, and 90 mL water)	Provides relief from abdominal distention caused by flatus.		

Note: Solutions may be commercially prepared or prepared on the unit.

 Aside from discomfort, the pressure generated in the rectum may stimulate the vagus nerve, slowing the heart rate. For that reason, you must have a prescription from the primary care provider.

For a summary of this procedure, see the Highlights of Procedures box. For complete steps,

Go to Chapter 26, **Procedure 26-4: Removing Stool Digitally,** in Volume 2.

KnowledgeCheck 26-6

- Identify the types of enemas available for use.
- How do hypotonic and isotonic enemas differ from hypertonic enemas?
- What actions can you take to make the patient more comfortable when receiving an enema?

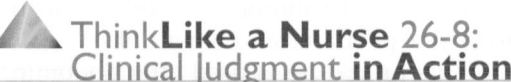

ThinkLike a Nurse 26-8: Clinical Judgment in Action

Mrs. Zeno (Meet Your Patient) begins to pass liquid stool. What actions should you take? Explain your reasoning.

EXAMPLE PROBLEM: Constipation and Impaction

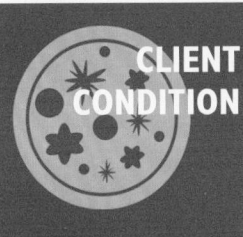
CLIENT CONDITION

Basic Definitions

Constipation:
Decrease in the frequency of bowel movements accompanied by difficult or incomplete passage of stool and/or very hard, dry stool

Short-Term Constipation: Temporary, symptoms resolve in a short period of time.

Chronic Constipation: Lasts for 3 months; may persist for years

Fecal impaction: Presence of a hard, dry fecal mass in the rectum, making it impossible to pass stool from the body in the normal manner. This blockage sets up a cycle of further hardening, with new waste backing up higher in the colon.

Complications of Prolonged Constipation and Fecal Impaction

Hemorrhoids
Tears in the colon wall or anus
Anal bleeding

Causes/Related Factors

Short-term Constipation: Lifestyle factors such as:
- Decreased activity (e.g., prescribed bedrest)
- Medications that slow peristalsis (e.g., opioids)
- Decreased fluid and fiber intake.

Long-Term Constipation:
In addition to the previously noted items, physiological factors such as:
- Dysfunctional anorectal musculature
- Dysfunctional intestinal motility
- Nervous system problems (e.g., spinal cord injury
- Obstruction of the intestinal tract (e.g., tumor)

Fecal Impaction:
Prolonged constipation is the primary cause.

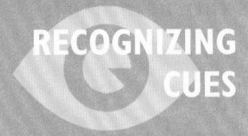
RECOGNIZING CUES

Assess for symptoms, risk factors, and complications.

Symptoms

Subjective
- Abdominal pain, tenderness
- Loss of appetite
- Feeling of rectal pressure
- Fatigue
- Headache
- Indigestion

Objective
- Abdominal distention
- Blood with stool
- Decreased frequency of stools
- Decreased volume of stools
- Hard, formed stools
- Hypo- or hyperactive bowel sounds

Risk Factors

- Bowel pattern
- Dietary pattern (low fiber, processed foods, poor or inadequate fluid intake, large amounts of milk)
- Activity level
- Medications (opioids, laxatives, calcium and iron supplements) and polypharmacy
- Psychological factors (e.g., depression, impaired cognition)

- Behavioral factors (ignoring the urge to defecate)
- Physiological factors
- Lack of privacy for toileting
- Reliance on others for assistance in toileting.

 • Screen all older adults for risk factors, including a history of polypharmacy and taking laxatives.

Note: These risk factors are the same for all ages, but they are more likely for older adults.

Complications

Assess for complications of constipation, such as hemorrhoids or impaction (hardened, dry fecal mass).

Fecal impaction symptoms
- You can detect fecal impaction by digital examination of the rectum.
- Symptoms of constipation are present, along with an inability to defecate, liquid stool, and vomiting.
- Severe symptoms include rapid heart rate, dehydration, fever, agitation, confusion, and urinary incontinence.
- Complications include anal bleeding or tears in the colon wall or anus.

(continued)

EXAMPLE PROBLEM: Constipation and Impaction—cont'd

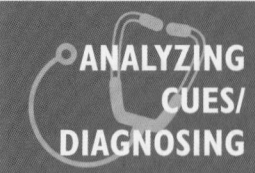

ANALYZING CUES/ DIAGNOSING

Constipation
Perceived Constipation

Risk for Constipation
Decreased GI Motility

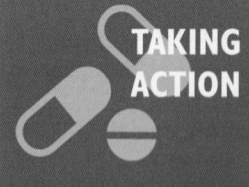

GENERATING SOLUTIONS

NOC Outcomes

Bowel Elimination
Health Beliefs
Knowledge: Health Behavior

Individualized Outcomes

- Ease of stool passage
- Passage of stool without aids
- Describes diet that will more naturally regulate bowel function

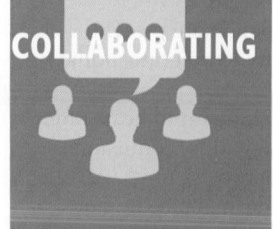

TAKING ACTION

Preventive and Treatment Measures

Notice that many measures for preventing constipation are also used for treating it.
   In general, prevention measures are the same for all ages.

Toileting
- For ambulatory patients, allow uninterrupted time for defecation, especially after meals, when mass peristalsis occurs.
- Provide privacy for using the toilet.
- Advise clients not to ignore urge to defecate because doing so may lead to constipation.
- Assist clients who cannot toilet independently to ambulate to the bathroom or use the bedpan.
- Assist the patient to a seated or squatting position whenever possible. A semi-Fowler's position is preferred for a client on bedrest.
- **Key Point:** *Discuss with UAPs the need to offer help without waiting to be asked so that patients experience minimal delays.*

Diet and Fluids
- Encourage fluid intake: 8 to 10 glasses/day (2,700 mL per day [females] and 3,700 mL per day [males]); minimum should be 1,500 mL or 50 oz per day.
- Increase intake of high-fiber foods if needed (normal adult Recommended Dietary Allowance (RDA)/Adequate Intake (AI) is 25–38 g).
- **Key Point:** *Adding fiber does not help to relieve opioid-induced constipation unless the patient's current intake is deficient.*

Activity
- Increase physical activity.
- For those unable to walk or who are restricted to bed, exercises such as trunk rotation, pelvic tilt, and leg lifts may be helpful.

Monitoring Measures

- Monitor for anal fissures, hemorrhoids, bleeding, and anorexia, which may occur in fecal impaction.
- Monitor for rectal ulcers, fecal seepage, and skin integrity.
- Monitor the pattern of BMs for changes.
- Monitor for severe abdominal pain, which may indicate complications (impaction, obstruction, volvulus, bowel perforation).

COLLABORATING

Chronic Constipation Usually involves some physiological dysfunction. When lifestyle modifications are ineffective in preventing and treating constipation, medications may be prescribed (see Box 26-1).

 • Administer laxative as prescribed. For older adults, osmotic laxatives (e.g., polyethylene glycol [PEG] and lactulose, bulking agents) have been found to be beneficial
- *Note:* Also see the Self-Care box, Teaching Your Patient About Laxative Use.

- Administer enemas as prescribed.

 Go to **Procedures 26-3: Administering an Enema** and **26-5: Inserting a Rectal Tube.**

Fecal Impaction

Treatment
Enemas; digital removal of stool.

Prevention
Once the impaction has been removed, establish a bowel regimen to prevent recurrence of impactions.
   To learn about bowel training regimens, see Example Client Condition: Bowel Incontinence.

INTERVENTIONS FOR EXAMPLE CLIENT CONDITION: BOWEL INCONTINENCE

Clients with persistent bowel incontinence require special nursing care to prevent skin integrity impairment because of the moisture and the activity of enzymes in the stool. In addition, bowel incontinence may be embarrassing. As clients worry about future episodes, anxiety escalates.

For nursing care of patients with bowel incontinence, refer to these resources:

- Accompanying Example Problem: Bowel Incontinence.

Go to Chapter 26, Nursing Care Plan and Care Map for Olivia Grimaldi, in Volume 2.

Fecal Collection and Drainage Devices

Fecal collection and drainage devices are used to (1) prevent impaired skin integrity by keeping feces away from the skin and (2) collect large fecal samples. To learn about fecal drainage devices, see the accompanying Example Client Condition: Bowel Incontinence. Also, see the Highlights of Procedures box, and

Go to Chapter 26, **Procedure 26-8A: Applying an External Fecal Collection System, Procedure 26-8B: Inserting an Indwelling Fecal Drainage Device,** and **Clinical Insight 26-1: Caring for a Patient With an Indwelling Fecal Drainage Device,** in Volume 2.

Bowel Training

A bowel training program assists the patient to have regular, soft, formed stools. It is appropriate for clients who have chronic constipation, impaction, or bowel incontinence. Elements of a bowel training program include the following:

- Plan the program with the patient and caregiver.
- Initiate a designated uninterrupted time for defecation, regardless of last BM or period of incontinence—usually after meals, especially in the morning.
- Provide privacy for the patient during the designated time.
- Develop a staged treatment plan if constipation develops. Usually, additional fiber is added as a first measure. A stool softener is next, followed by a suppository such as bisacodyl (Dulcolax).
- Gradually increase fiber in the diet while monitoring the consistency of the stool.
- Increase fluid intake to at least eight glasses of water per day, if not contraindicated.
- Regularly modify the plan based on the patient's response.

KnowledgeCheck 26-7
- What are the major patient care concerns associated with bowel incontinence?
- What are the elements of a bowel training program?

Caring for Patients With Bowel Diversions

Patients experience a variety of reactions to a bowel diversion, and each person has unique physical and psychological needs. Initially, you will care for the ostomy, but the goal is for the patient to assume self-care. For a full description of the care of an ostomy appliance, including changing and emptying,

Go to Chapter 26, **Clinical Insight 26-2: Guidelines for Ostomy Care;** also see **Procedure 26-6: Changing an Ostomy Appliance,** in Volume 2.

Ongoing Assessment/Recognizing Cues After Diversion

Patients require thorough and ongoing monitoring of the stoma, output, and skin.

Assess the Stoma Key Point: *A healthy stoma (Fig. 26-9) ranges in color from deep pink to brick red, regardless of the patient's skin color, and is shiny and moist. Pallor or a dusky-blue color indicates ischemia, and a brown-black color indicates necrosis.*

- Immediately after surgery, the stoma will be swollen and enlarged. As the inflammation subsides and healing occurs, the stoma will shrink.
- By 6 to 8 weeks, it will be at its permanent size. Stoma size varies according to the size of the person and the part of the bowel that was externalized (see Fig. 26-5).
- The stoma will protrude above the level of the abdomen by approximately 1.3 to 2.5 cm (0.5 to 1 in.)
- An ileostomy stoma is generally smaller than a colostomy stoma.

Assess the Output Monitor the amount and type of drainage from the stoma. Output from an ileostomy stoma is liquid and contains digestive enzymes. An ostomy lower in the GI tract will have more solid output and fewer enzymes. The presence of enzymes in the effluent increases the likelihood of skin breakdown.

Assess the Skin Pay close attention to the skin surrounding a stoma for cues of irritation, such as redness, tenderness, skin breakdown, and/or drainage. Skin breakdown may lead to infection, pain, and leakage.

Helping Patients Adapt to the Diversion

Patients experience a variety of reactions to a bowel diversion, and each person has unique needs. **Key Point: Initially, you will care for the ostomy, but the goal is to have the patient assume self-care and a normal life.**

- **The first step is for the patient to adjust to the presence of an ostomy.** If the patient has been sick before the surgery and the ostomy leads to less pain or discomfort, the transition may be easier. Similarly,

EXAMPLE PROBLEM: Bowel Incontinence

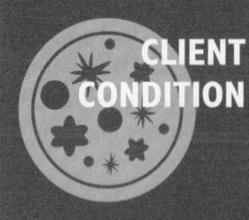

CLIENT CONDITION

Definition

Incontinence is the inability to control the discharge of feces and flatulence.
Key Point: *Because of the moisture and the activity of enzymes in the stool, clients with persistent bowel incontinence need special nursing care to prevent impaired skin integrity.*

Incidence

One-third of critically ill patients have fecal incontinence; it is a leading cause of admission to long-term care facilities in the United States (Pittman et al., 2015).

Causes/Related Factors

- Conditions that affect innervation of the rectum and anus; uncontrolled diarrhea
- Impaction resulting in leakage of stool
- Cognitive or emotional changes that alter the perception of the urge to defecate (e.g., dementia, low level of consciousness)
- Functional limitations (e.g., a client recognizes the need to defecate but cannot get to the toilet independently or on time; Toileting Self-Care Deficit)

External Fecal Collection Devices

- May be used to protect perianal skin or to collect large fecal samples
- A common approach for clients with uncontrolled diarrhea, keeping feces away from the skin
- Pouch systems vary widely. The equipment is similar to that used for patients with an ostomy, which is discussed later in the chapter.

(continues in Column 2)

External Fecal Collection Devices (continued)

- **Advantages:** External collection systems can prevent skin breakdown, minimize odor, track output accurately, and enhance patient comfort.
- **Limitations:** They are not typically used for patients who are ambulatory, agitated, or active in bed because the device may be dislodged, causing skin breakdown.

To learn how to apply and manage an external fecal collection system, see the Procedure Highlights box, and

 Go to **Procedure 26-8A: Applying an External Fecal Collection System.**

Indwelling Fecal Drainage Devices

- Are used to collect liquid stool from bedbound, immobilized ill patients.
- Consist of a soft, latex-free catheter and a collection bag (Fig. 26-8). The tube is inserted, and a balloon on the end is filled with saline or water.
- **Advantages:** Protect perianal skin, protect caregivers from potentially infectious stool, and are thought to decrease urinary tract infections.
- **Disadvantages and Precautions:** They are approved by the U.S. Food and Drug Administration, but:
  - only for 29 consecutive days, and
  - not for pediatric patients.
  Other contraindications include:
  Severe hemorrhoids
  Recent bowel, rectal, or anal surgery or injury
  Rectal or anal tumors
  Stricture or stenosis

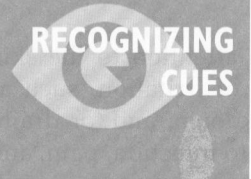

RECOGNIZING CUES

- Bowel pattern
- Factors related to fecal incontinence (medications, diet, activity)
- Skin condition, especially perianal area
- Medical problems

- Psychosocial and behavioral factors (e.g., depression, caregiver problems)
- Other risk factors (e.g., smoking, underweight)
- For more assessment details

 Go to **Focused Assessment: Bowel.**

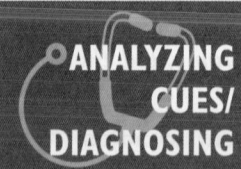

ANALYZING CUES/ DIAGNOSING

Bowel Incontinence
Risk for Skin Integrity Impairment: Excoriation

Gastrointestinal Motility Dysfunction: Increased

EXAMPLE PROBLEM: Bowel Incontinence—cont'd

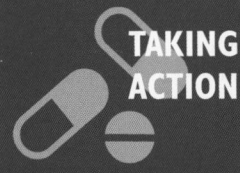

GENERATING SOLUTIONS

NOC Outcomes

Bowel Continence
Tissue Integrity: Skin and Mucous
  Membranes

Individualized Outcomes

Resumes normal bowel pattern
Maintains skin integrity (no excoriation)

TAKING ACTION

Key Point: *The primary goals of nursing care are to promote normal bowel function, preserve skin integrity, and minimize embarrassment to the patient.*

Monitoring

- Monitor pattern of bowel movements (BMs).
- Monitor for skin breakdown, redness, or irritation.

Treatments/Activities

Toileting

- Designate uninterrupted time for defecation,
- Provide the bedpan or assist the patient to the bathroom at regular intervals and at times BMs are most likely to occur.
- For clients who cannot toilet independently, assist to ambulate to the bathroom or use the bedpan.
- **Key Point:** *Discuss with unlicensed assistive personnel (UAPs) the need to offer help without waiting to be asked so that patients experience minimal delays.*

Skin Care

- Change soiled clothing and/or bed linens as soon as possible to prevent skin irritation and embarrassment.
- Provide prompt hygiene care after any episodes of incontinence. Keep the skin scrupulously clean.
- Use state-of-the-art skin protection products, such as perineal cleansers and moisture-barrier products.

Absorbent Products

- Consider absorbent pads and shields to keep from soiling clothing and linens.
- For large quantities, use adult incontinence garments. They may pull on like underwear or fasten like a diaper.
- Place moisture-resistant pads under the patient to help protect bed linens. Change the pad as soon as possible after defecation.
- Never place the plastic side of the pad next to the patient's body. This holds moisture next to the skin, which leads to irritation and breakdown.

  ♥ **iCare** • Never refer to incontinence pads as "diapers" when caring for adults or children who have been toilet trained. This inappropriate reference may cause embarrassment and lower the patient's self-esteem.

TEACHING

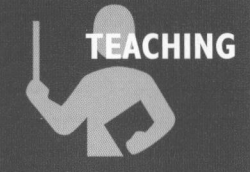

- Review diet, fluid intake, activity, and medicines with patient.

- Teach skin care to patient and caregivers.

(continued)

EXAMPLE PROBLEM: Bowel Incontinence—cont'd

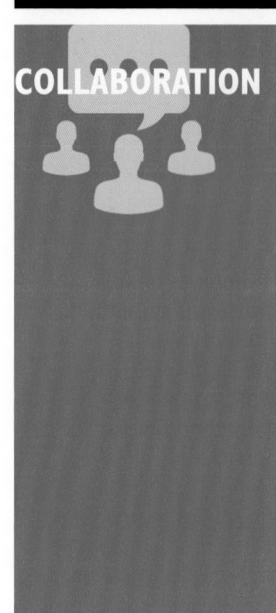

COLLABORATION

- Work with the primary care provider to alter activity, diet, fluids, and medications to encourage regular bowel movements.
- Collaborate with primary care provider to insert and care for fecal drainage devices.

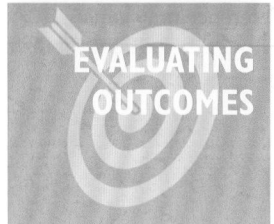

Go to Chapter 26, **Procedure 26-8: Placing Fecal Drainage Devices,** and **Clinical Insight 26-1: Caring for a Patient With an Indwelling Fecal Drainage Device.**

Insertion and Maintenance of Internal Fecal Drainage Device
- Follow the manufacturer's recommendations carefully.
- When the bag is filled, empty or replace it, depending on the type.
- Monitor to confirm placement; you may need to irrigate the device.
- Use external or indwelling fecal collection devices to prevent drainage from soiling clothing.
- **Key Point:** *Do not use external devices if skin is not intact because they will not seal tightly.*
- Research on patient outcomes of most of these methods is limited; they are discussed later in this chapter.

Bowel Training

- Consider a bowel training program (explained later in the chapter; see the section Bowel Training).

EVALUATING OUTCOMES

- Monitor for changes in bowel pattern and resumption of patient's usual pattern of defecation.

- Monitor skin integrity. Skin should be intact and not red.
- Monitor functional ability for toileting and hygiene self-care.

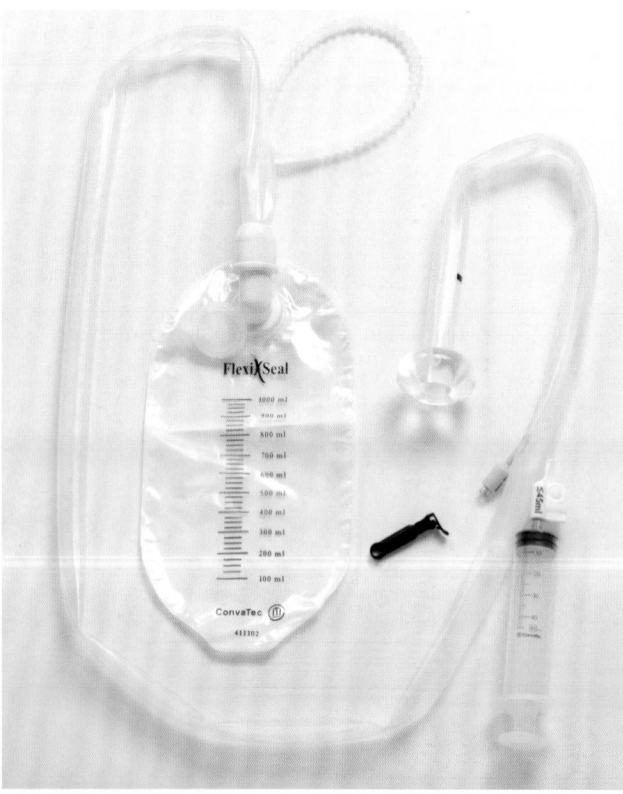

FIGURE 26-8 An indwelling fecal drainage device.

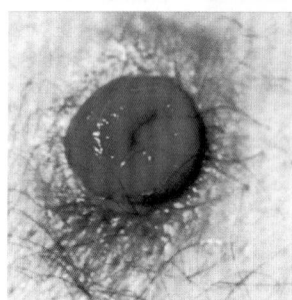

FIGURE 26-9 A healthy stoma is deep pink to brick red and is shiny and moist.

patients with continent ostomies may adapt more easily to their stoma.
- **Ostomy patients no longer have sphincter control, so they may need to modify their diet.** You can promote adaptation by teaching the client about diet modifications. Box 26-2 discusses the effects of some foods on a patient with an ostomy.
- **Ostomy care is a lifelong task,** with the exception of a temporary double-barreled colostomy.
- **Find an enterostomal therapy nurse to assist patients with their ongoing care** and to provide consultation on ostomy appliances. **Enterostomal therapy nurses** are available in many hospitals and large communities.

For steps to follow in *all* procedures, refer to the Universal Steps for All Procedures found on the inside back cover of Volume 2. Go to the full procedures in Volume 2 to practice and learn the procedure steps. Use these procedure highlights later to help you review key points.

Procedure 26-1: Testing Stool for Occult Blood

➤ Persons age 50 or older should be screened every 1 to 2 years for occult (hidden) blood in the stool. Some guidelines suggest annual screening. High-risk groups require initial screening at a younger age.

➤ Patients should avoid foods that may alter the accuracy of the test for 3 days before collecting the stool specimen.

➤ Review the patient's medications. If the patient is taking salicylates, NSAIDs, iron, anticoagulants, or colchicine, consult with the physician.

➤ Take care that the sample is not contaminated by urine or menstrual blood.

➤ Test two small stool samples from separate areas of the large sample.

➤ If the test is being done by laboratory personnel, transfer the specimen to a clean, dry container for transportation to the laboratory.

If the test is being done by the nurse, following the manufacturer's directions, place the correct number and size of drops of developer solution into the "windows" of the opposite side on the Hemoccult slide.

➤ Record a positive result if the slide windows turn blue.

Procedure 26-2: Placing and Removing a Bedpan

➤ Determine whether the patient will need to use a regular bedpan or a fracture pan.

➤ Don clean procedure gloves.

➤ Help the patient to achieve a position on the bedpan that will be most helpful in facilitating elimination. Use a semi-Fowler's position whenever possible. Modify the position based on the patient's condition.

➤ Provide toilet tissue, clean washcloths, and towels for the patient to perform personal hygiene when elimination is complete. Assist if the patient cannot perform these tasks independently.

➤ Stabilize and remove the bedpan, being careful not to spill the contents.

Procedure 26-3: Administering an Enema

➤ Generously lubricate and gently insert the rectal tube.

➤ Instill warm solution at a slow rate.

➤ For best results:

  ➤ Be sure patient is properly positioned (left lateral with knee flexed, if possible).

  ➤ Instruct the patient to retain the solution for 5 to 15 minutes, depending on the type of enema.

➤ Assist the patient in a sitting or squatting position to promote defecation.

➤ Before leaving the bedside, implement fall-prevention measures that are appropriate for your patient.

➤ Use nursing judgment to modify the procedure based on the patient's mobility and ability to follow your instructions.

Procedure 26-4: Removing Stool Digitally

➤ Be aware that this procedure is both painful and embarrassing to your patient.

➤ Trim and file your fingernails so that they do not extend over the ends of your fingertips.

➤ Obtain baseline vital signs, and determine whether the patient has a history of cardiac problems or other contraindications.

➤ Determine whether the procedure will be accompanied by suppository insertion or enema administration.

➤ Use only one or two gloved, generously lubricated fingers, and remove stool in small pieces.

➤ Allow the patient periods of rest, and monitor for signs of vagal nerve stimulation.

➤ Teach the patient lifestyle changes necessary to prevent stool retention.

Procedure 26-5: Inserting a Rectal Tube

➤ A rectal tube may be used to facilitate the passage of gas for clients experiencing intestinal distention.

➤ Attach the collecting device to the end of the tube.

➤ Position the patient on their left side.

➤ Lubricate the tip of the tube; insert 10 to 12.5 cm (4 to 5 in.).

➤ Leave the tube in place for 15 to 20 minutes.

➤ Assist the patient to move about in bed; the knee-chest position is ideal if tolerated.

Procedure 26-6: Changing an Ostomy Appliance

➤ Change the pouch every 3 to 5 days, as a general rule.

➤ Empty the old pouch before removing it, if possible.

➤ Remove the wafer or pouch, pulling down from the top with one hand while holding countertension with the other.

➤ Assess/recognize cues for the stoma and the peristomal skin area (e.g., for discoloration, swelling, redness, irritation, excoriation, bleeding).

➤ Cleanse stoma with skin cleansing agent.

➤ Use a measuring guide to determine the size of the stoma.

➤ Trace the size of the opening onto the back of the wafer, and cut the wafer opening about 2 to 3 mm ($\frac{1}{16}$ to $\frac{1}{8}$ in.) larger.

➤ Apply the new wafer with gentle pressure.

Continued

Note: Some pouches come with the wafer attached, some without. These instructions assume that the wafer is attached.

Procedure 26-7: Irrigating a Colostomy

➤ Consult with the ostomy nurse and/or physician to see if colostomy irrigation is appropriate for your patient.

➤ Determine the patient's normal bowel pattern before surgery.

➤ Prime the tubing before irrigation, using 500 to 1,000 mL, preferably 1,000 mL, of warm tap water.

➤ Position the patient in front of or on the toilet or bedside commode. If the patient is immobile, place in left side-lying (Sims') position, and use a bedpan.

➤ Prepare the new appliance before removing the existing one.

➤ Examine the stoma and peristomal skin.

➤ Lubricate the cone at the end of the tubing and insert it gently.

➤ Open the clamp and slowly infuse fluid, over 10 to 15 minutes.

➤ Remove cone and allow approximately 30 minutes for evacuation.

➤ Remove the sleeve, and rinse, dry, and store it.

Procedure 26-8: Placing Fecal Drainage Devices

Procedure 26-8A: Applying an External Fecal Collection System

➤ Select the fecal management system appropriate for the patient.

➤ Obtain assistance as needed.

➤ Place the patient side-lying.

➤ Cleanse and dry the perineal area; clip hair as needed.

➤ Spread the buttocks and apply the device; avoid gaps and creases.

➤ Hang the drainage bag lower than the patient.

Procedure 26-8B: Inserting an Indwelling Fecal Drainage Device

➤ Select the fecal management system appropriate for the patient.

➤ Obtain assistance as needed.

➤ Place the patient left side-lying.

➤ Remove any indwelling device.

➤ Cleanse and dry the perineal area.

➤ Prepare the device according to instructions (e.g., remove residual air from the balloon).

➤ Lubricate the balloon generously with water-soluble lubricant.

➤ Spread the buttocks and gently insert the balloon end of the catheter.

➤ Inflate the device with water or saline.

➤ Remove the syringe from the inflation port; gently tug the catheter.

➤ Position the tubing, avoiding kinks; position the collection bag lower than the patient.

BOX 26-2 ■ Teaching Dietary Changes Associated With an Ostomy

Note: These are only suggestions. Each person must, by trial and error, discover what works best for them.

General Guidelines for Patients

■ Initially, you may be asked to follow a bland, low-residue, or soft diet for a month or two to prevent obstructions and gastrointestinal (GI) upsets. Advance the diet by adding one new food at a time.

■ Eat three or more meals daily at regular times.

■ Drink additional fluid to keep well hydrated. Those with colostomies need to compensate for the loss of the large intestine, where fluid absorption occurs.

■ Avoid chewing gum because it may cause you to swallow air, causing a noisy stoma.

■ Avoid foods that cause gas, odor, blockage, or loose stools. Eventually introduce them into your diet one at a time and be aware of their effects.

■ Chew your food well to avoid blockage of the stoma.

■ Avoid excessive weight gain.

Foods That May Cause Gas or Odor

Beverages: Alcohol, beer, carbonated beverages

Dairy: Milk, cheese, and other dairy

Fruit: Melon

Vegetables: Asparagus, beans, broccoli, Brussels sprouts, cabbage, cauliflower, cucumbers, garlic, onions, peas, radishes

Other foods: Eggs, fish, cod liver oil, nuts, peanut butter

Foods That May Help Control Gas or Odor

Buttermilk, yogurt

Cranberry juice

Parsley

BOX 26-2 ■ Teaching Dietary Changes Associated With an Ostomy—cont'd

High-Fiber Foods That May Cause Blockage

You can eat some of these foods (e.g., mushrooms, shrimp) if you cut them into small pieces and chew them very thoroughly. As long as blockage does not occur, these foods should not necessarily be avoided, but they should be used carefully.

- Foods with seeds (e.g., raspberries)
- Foods with tough skins (e.g., corn, dried fruits, pears, tomatoes)
- Mushrooms
- Nuts, popcorn
- Raw or minimally cooked fruits and vegetables (e.g., coleslaw, Chinese stir-fried vegetables, oranges, apple skins)
- Shrimp, lobster
- Stringy foods (e.g., celery, coconut, spinach, bean sprouts, green beans, orange pulp)

Foods That May Cause Loose Stools

Alcohol, beer, caffeine, chocolate, licorice

Milk

Baked beans, cooked cabbage, onions

Bran cereal, whole grains

Highly seasoned foods

Large meals

Prunes, raisins

Raw fruits and vegetables

Key Point: *Never restrict fluids in an effort to control diarrhea.*

Foods That May Alleviate Diarrhea

Applesauce

Bananas

Pretzels

Saltine crackers

Tapioca

Yogurt

Starchy foods (e.g., rice, bread, potatoes)

Cheese and creamy peanut butter

Sources: Burgess-Stocks, J. (2022). Eating with an ostomy: A comprehensive nutrition guide for those living with an ostomy. United Ostomy Association of America. https://www.ostomy.org/wp-content/uploads/2022/02/Eating_with_an_Ostomy_2022-02.pdf; Lutz, C., & Przytulski, K. (2018). *Nutrition and diet therapy: Evidence-based applications* (7th ed.). F.A. Davis; United Ostomy Associations of America (2005, updated 2011). *Ostomates food reference chart.* http://www.uoaa.org/ostomy_info/pubs/uoa_diet_nutrition_en.pdf

---

- **Your attitude and willingness to discuss body changes will help your patient begin adapting.**
- For more interventions to promote physical and psychological adaptation,

Go to Chapter 26, **Clinical Insight 26-2: Guidelines for Ostomy Care,** in Volume 2.

Colostomy Irrigation

Colostomy irrigation may be indicated as an occasional intervention for constipation or in a select population of patients. Consult with the ostomy nurse and/or physician to see if colostomy irrigation is appropriate for your patient.

- **Ostomy in descending or sigmoid colon**—The patient may use colostomy irrigation as a means to control bowel evacuation and possibly eliminate the need to wear an ostomy pouch.

- **Ostomy stomas above the descending colon**—These are not irrigated because they usually have liquid output that cannot be controlled.

Colostomy irrigation is similar in some respects to an enema. The nurse or patient inserts a flexible tube into the stoma and instills a traditional enema solution. The patient may use a special plastic sleeve over the stoma or an ostomy appliance to direct the output into the toilet. For the complete procedure,

Go to Chapter 26, **Procedure 26-7: Irrigating a Colostomy,** in Volume 2.

KnowledgeCheck 26-8

- How can you help a patient adapt psychologically to living with a bowel diversion?
- What does a healthy stoma look like?
- Why is skin care around a stoma so important?

Toward Evidence-Based Practice

Mohamed, S. S., Salem, G. M., & Mohamed, H. A. (2017). Effect of self-care management program on self-efficacy among patients with colostomy. *American Journal of Nursing Research*, 5(5), 191–199.

The aim of this pretest/posttest study was to evaluate whether the implementation of a self-management program improved knowledge, self-care practices, and self-efficacy in patients with a colostomy. Twenty adult participants were evaluated, and an individualized self-care management program for colostomy care was developed for each participant. The self-care management program was in the form of handouts and printed material, intended for attracting and guiding patients to independently participate in their self-care colostomy management. Following four 30- to 45-minute sessions, researchers found a significant improvement in knowledge, self-care practices, and self-efficacy management in colostomy patients.

Millard, R., Cooper, D., & Boyle, M. J. (2020). Improving self-care outcomes in ostomy patients via education and standardized discharge criteria. *Home Healthcare Now, 38*(1), 16–23.

The purpose of this quality improvement study was to measure outcomes in four home healthcare patients with new ostomies. Interventions consisted of nurse and patient education. Nurse education included both classroom and hands-on components to promote ostomy care practice change. Patient education included the use of an evidence-based ostomy skills checklist adapted from the Wound, Ostomy, and Continence Nurses Society's ostomy discharge criteria. Analysis of postsurvey data found that the nurses felt more confident managing ostomies after the education sessions. Patient data demonstrated a decrease in the number of weeks patients required home care for a new ostomy diagnosis, a decrease in the number of required visits for patients to reach independence in ostomy care, and a decrease in unscheduled visits.

---

1. Based on these studies, write an education plan you would use to help a patient care for a stoma.

2. The second study included an intervention to educate the home care nurses. Why do you think that teaching nurses about providing stoma care is important? Do you think there is a relationship between the nursing outcome and the patient outcomes in the study? Explain your thinking.

To explore learning resources for this chapter,

Go to Davis Advantage and find:

Answers and Suggested Responses for all questions in this chapter

Concept Map

Knowledge Map

References and Bibliography

CHAPTER 27

Sensation, Perception, & Response

Learning Outcomes

After completing this chapter, you should be able to:

➤ Identify the components of the sensory experience.

➤ Compare and contrast sensory deprivation and sensory overload.

➤ List factors placing clients at risk for altered sensory perception.

➤ Discuss the hazards of sensory deficits in vision, hearing, taste, smell, touch, and proprioception.

➤ Identify factors that affect sensory stimulation.

➤ Assess clients for signs and symptoms of altered sensory perception.

➤ State nursing diagnoses and outcomes appropriate for clients with problems of sensory perception.

➤ Plan and implement nursing interventions to prevent sensory deprivation and sensory overload.

➤ Plan and implement nursing interventions to meet the needs of clients with sensory deficits.

➤ Discuss strategies to enhance communication with clients with sensory deficits.

Key Concepts

Perception

Reception

Sensation

Related Concepts

See the Concept Map on Davis Advantage.

Example Client Conditions

Sensory Deprivation

Sensory Overload

Sensory Deficits

    Visual and Hearing

    Olfactory and Gustatory

    Tactile and Kinesthetic

    Seizures

Meet Your Patients

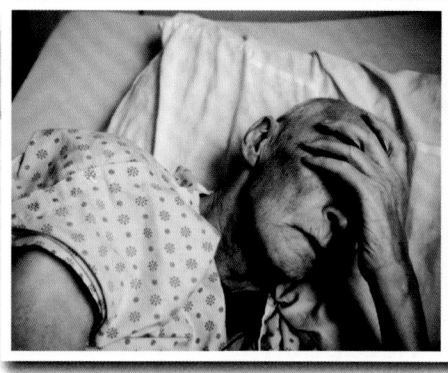

■ Joshua is a 28-year-old patient in the intensive care unit (ICU). He had a car accident 3 weeks ago and has had several surgeries to repair a fractured femur, ruptured spleen, and intracranial bleeding. He was ventilated mechanically for 10 days and has had numerous invasive procedures. The nurses report that he is very confused and has been hallucinating.

■ Richard is a 90-year-old man who has been a resident at a skilled nursing facility for 10 years. He has no visitors, never leaves his room, has no television or radio in the room, and no longer speaks. He does not respond to verbal or tactile stimulation. When staff members try to move him, he moans and howls.

Consider how these patients are similar and how their care might overlap. It seems hard to imagine that these patients could have much in common. What similarities can you see? What differences? As you read this chapter, follow these cases and other examples illustrating the effects of altered sensory or perceptual function.

TheoreticalKnowledge
knowing why

We experience the world through our senses. Vision, hearing, smell, taste, touch, and our sense of our body in space all help us to interpret and interact with our environment in a meaningful way. To grow, develop, and function, we must be able to sense and respond to sensory input.

- **Preexisting sensory deficit.** Many patients who are receiving care for an unrelated condition also have a preexisting sensory deficit (e.g., you may need to teach self-injection to a client with diabetes who is blind).
- **Sensory deficit caused by illness or medication.** Still other patients develop alterations in sensory function as a result of their illness or of medications they are taking.

The Joint Commission (2010) requires that you address the communication needs of patients with vision, speech, hearing, language, and cognitive impairments. You will likely care for patients with sensory deficits wherever you work as a nurse. This chapter will help you provide care for such patients.

ABOUT THE KEY CONCEPTS

To best meet patients' needs, you will need to understand how the concepts of **sensation, reception,** and **perception** influence their sensory experience. In this section, you will also learn about related concepts, including those needed to care for patients who experience sensory deprivation, overload, or deficits.

COMPONENTS OF THE SENSORY EXPERIENCE

The purpose of sensation is to allow the body to respond to changing situations and maintain homeostasis. A sensory experience involves four components in the nervous system: stimulus, reception, perception, and an arousal mechanism.

Stimulus

A **stimulus** may be a sight, sound, taste, touch, pain, or anything that stimulates a nerve receptor. The brain must receive and process it to make it meaningful.

Reception

Reception is the process of receiving stimuli from nerve endings in the skin and inside the body. A receptor converts a stimulus to a nerve impulse and transmits the impulse along sensory neurons to the central nervous system (CNS).

Adaptation Some receptors remain activated for as long as the stimulus is applied. However, most receptors *adapt* to stimuli; that is, their response declines with time. Adaptation explains why, over time, you become unaware of an unpleasant smell or the persistent hum of an air-conditioner.

Specialized Receptors Typically, receptors respond to only one type of stimulus. For example, taste buds in the mouth detect sweet, sour, salty, or bitter, whereas receptors in the retina detect light rays. The following are examples of the many types of sensory receptors in the body:

- **Mechanoreceptors** in the skin and hair follicles detect touch, pressure, and vibration.
- **Hair cells** are receptors for hearing. Located in the cochlea of the ear, they detect sound waves. In the vestibular apparatus of the ear, receptors for equilibrium and balance also detect acceleration of the body and the position of the head.
- **Thermoreceptors** in the skin detect variations in temperature.
- **Proprioceptors** in the skin, muscles, tendons, ligaments, and joint capsules coordinate input to enable us to sense the position of our body in space (proprioception).
- **Photoreceptors** located in the retina of the eyes detect visible light.
- **Chemoreceptors** for taste are in our taste buds. **Olfactory receptors** (chemoreceptors for smell) are in the epithelium of the nasal cavity.

Perception

Perception is the ability to interpret the impulses transmitted from the receptors and give meaning to the stimuli. After the receptors generate nerve impulses, the impulses travel along neural pathways to the spinal cord and brain. They are then relayed to specialized locations in the brain where perception of the stimuli occurs (Fig. 27-1). For example, vision is perceived in the occipital lobes, hearing in the temporal lobes, and touch in the somatosensory area.

- **It is not possible to process all the stimuli that we encounter all the time,** so the brain discards most sensory information as irrelevant and unimportant. For example, you are usually unaware of your clothing touching your body. However, if you focus on it, you can feel it.
- **Perception of a stimulus is affected by past experiences, knowledge, and attitude, as well as the following factors**:
  Location of the receptors and pathway activated
  Number of receptors activated
  Frequency of action potentials generated (which varies according to the intensity of the stimulus)
  Changes in location, number, and frequency

Arousal Mechanism

For the central nervous system to perceive, interpret, and react to incoming stimuli, it must be active. The **reticular activating system (RAS),** located in the brainstem,

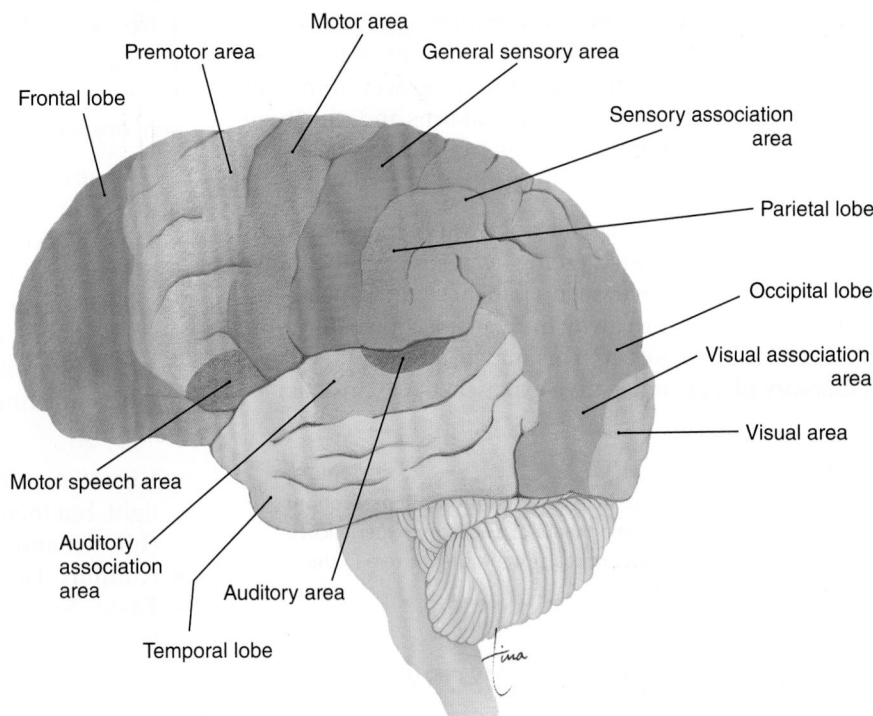

FIGURE 27-1 Special sensory areas of the brain receive and interpret stimuli from the sensory receptors.

controls consciousness and alertness. The neurons of the RAS make connections among the spinal cord, cerebellum, thalamus, and cerebral cortex. These connections relay visual, auditory, and other stimuli that help keep us awake, attentive, and observant.

Without such stimuli, the CNS becomes lethargic, and the person may lose consciousness. Anesthesia, sedatives, opioids, and some other drugs depress the RAS, as does a darkened, quiet environment. Not surprisingly, as you will learn in Chapter 31, sleep is regulated by the RAS.

- **The level of stimuli needed to maintain arousal varies.** Some people feel optimally alert in bright, noisy, active environments, whereas others prefer much lower levels of stimulation.
- **The brain adapts to constant stimuli,** such as a ticking clock or monitor alarms in a busy hospital unit (alarm fatigue) (The Joint Commission, 2018, 2021). Thus, to maintain arousal, some variation in stimuli is required.

Responding to Sensations

Once a stimulus is perceived, the brain (Fig. 27-2) either discards it, stores it in memory, or sends impulses along motor pathways to various parts of the body (e.g., the muscles, the heart, and so on), bringing about a response. Humans respond to sensations when they are alert and receptive to stimulation. For example, a fatigued new mother may wake up to the soft cry of her infant yet sleep through the persistent ringing of the doorbell. The response to a stimulus is based on the factors discussed in the following subsections.

Intensity An intense stimulus excites more receptors, leading to a greater response. For example, a bright, glaring

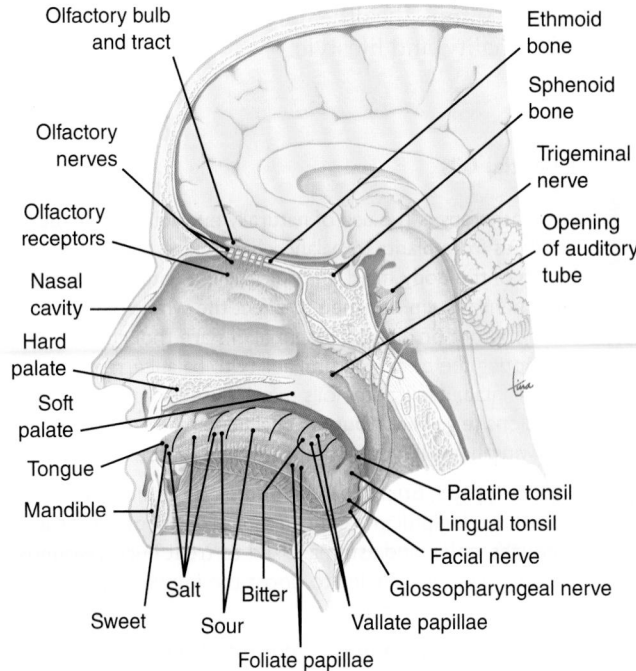

FIGURE 27-2 Structures that aid in olfaction and gustation.

light can cause you to respond by squinting and shielding your eyes, whereas a dim light may cause little reaction.

Contrast Imagine being outside in cold, windy weather. If you enter an unheated garage, you instantly feel warmer because the building blocks the wind. If you then go inside a room with a blazing fireplace, you will need to take off layers of clothing rapidly because the contrast in temperature will make you feel hot.

Adaptation We often take stimuli for granted. Recall your first clinical experience. Did you notice the noise and activity on the unit? Nurses become accustomed to the noise, lights, activity, and even alarms and can "tune them out." These stimuli are new to many patients, so they notice them and may have difficulty resting.

Previous Experience Our previous experience with a stimulus affects our ongoing responses to the same stimulus. Have you ever seen a patient scrunch their eyes, grit their teeth, or turn away from an injection before you are even ready to give it? This may mean that they have a memory of a prior negative experience with injections.

KnowledgeCheck 27-1
- What is the difference between reception and perception?
- What are the four components of a sensory experience?
- What is the role of the reticular activating system in the sensory experience?

FACTORS AFFECTING SENSORY FUNCTION

This section will describe the effects of developmental variations, culture, health status, medications, stress level, personality, and lifestyle.

Life-Span Variations

People have differing sensory perceptual abilities at different stages of life. In addition, the need for and use of sensory stimulation differs throughout life.

Newborns In the first months of life until the autonomic nervous system matures, newborns are easily overstimulated by loud noises, bright light, high-contrast objects, and sensitive areas (back, soles of feet), particularly when more than one sense is involved. Newborns protect themselves from sensory overload by exhibiting avoidance behaviors, such as crying, mottling, poor feeding and sleeping, and even yawning.

- **Visual.** Newborns can track objects and respond to light, but their vision is far less acute than that of older children and adults.
- **Auditory.** Hearing is especially acute at low frequencies.
- **Taste.** Newborns can also discriminate between different tastes, and they prefer sweet over sour.
- **Smell.** Newborns react to odor and seem to be able to discriminate between the smell of their own mother's breast milk and that of another mother.
- **Tactile.** Tactile perception is keenly present at birth. The tongue, lips, fingertips, and soles of the feet are

Holistic Healing

Essential Oils

Aromatherapy is the use of naturally extracted aromatic essences from plants to balance, harmonize, and promote the health of the body, mind, and spirit. It is a natural, noninvasive treatment system designed to affect the whole person, not just the symptom or disease. Essential oils are thought to work by promoting the body's natural ability to balance, regulate, heal, and maintain itself. Some oils may be used topically in certain situations (e.g., minor burns). Beginning research supports the following; however, the evidence base is not strong.

- **Eucalyptus, *Eucalyptus globulus* or *Eucalyptus radiata*.** Helpful in treating respiratory problems, such as coughs, colds, and asthma. Used to treat burns, wounds, and insect bites. Also helps to boost the immune system and relieve muscle tension.
- **Ylang-ylang, *Cananga odorata*.** Promotes relaxation and reduces muscle tension. Good antidepressant. Used for anxiety, hypertension, and stress.
- **Geranium, *Pelargonium graveolens*.** Helps to balance female hormones, good for balancing the skin. Can be both relaxing and uplifting, as well as an antidepressant. Used for acne and oily skin.
- **Peppermint, *Mentha piperita*.** Used in treating headaches; sinusitis; vertigo; muscle aches; asthma; and digestive disorders such as slow digestion, indigestion, nausea, and flatulence.
- **Lavender, *Lavandula angustifolia*.** Promotes relaxation. It is useful in treating wounds and burns and for skin

care. Also used for asthma, itching, labor pains, colic, and dysmenorrhea.
- **Lemon, *Citrus limonum*.** Uplifting, yet relaxing. Helpful in treating wounds and infections and for house cleaning and deodorizing. Sometimes used for athlete's foot, colds, and warts.
- **Clary sage, *Salvia sclarea*.** Natural painkiller, helpful in treating amenorrhea and muscular aches and pains. Relaxing and can help with insomnia. Also helpful in balancing hormones. Used to treat sore throat, stress, and exhaustion.
- **Tea tree, *Melaleuca alternifolia*.** A natural antifungal oil, good for treating all sorts of fungal infections, including vaginal yeast infections, athlete's foot, and ringworm. Used for insect bites, itching, and migraine. Also helps to boost the immune system.
- **Roman chamomile, *Anthemis nobilis*.** Promotes relaxation; can help with sleeplessness and anxiety. Also good for muscle aches, arthritis, and tension. Useful in treating wounds and infection. Used for insomnia, nausea, premenstrual syndrome, and earache.
- **Rosemary, *Rosmarinus officinalis*.** Uplifting and promotes mental stimulation; also used for stimulating the immune, circulatory, and digestive systems. Good for muscle aches and tension.

the most touch-sensitive parts of the body (Polan & Taylor, 2019).

Infants Babies under age 1 require sensory stimulation to grow and develop.

- **Visual.** Lights, color, and contrast allow the infant to observe the world in which they live.
- **Auditory.** Exposure to voices, music, and ambient noise develops the auditory nervous system. By 1 year of age, the child can discriminate between different sounds and often recognizes the source.
- **Tactile.** Cuddling, feeding, and soothing create a bond between infant and caregivers; provide comfort and pleasure; and teach the infant about the external environment.

Children and Adolescents

- **Visual.** In early childhood, visual acuity improves; full depth perception is achieved during the preschool period.
- **Auditory.** Hearing is usually fully developed in young children; however, they may experience reversible hearing loss because of frequent ear infections and cerumen impaction.
- **Psychomotor.** In contrast to toddlers, who often lose their balance when walking, older children are coordinated and can perform more complex motor skills for daily activities and sports.
- **Social.** During the school-age years and adolescence, children are developmentally driven toward interaction with peers, and the increased social interaction provides sensory stimulation that is varied and plentiful. For example, school-age children and adolescents commonly enjoy music (auditory), movies and social media (visual), perfume (olfactory), sweets and treats (gustatory), fashion and toys (tactile), and movement and athletics (kinesthetic).

Adults and Older Adults By early adulthood, senses are at their peak, unless they are affected by illness or injury.

As the adult ages, all the senses are affected. Table 27-1 describes sensory changes associated with aging. Older adults experience a generalized decrease in the number of nerve conduction fibers, resulting in slower reflexes and delayed responses to stimuli. Structural changes also occur in the aging eyes and ears. Sensory acuity declines with aging and may cause social withdrawal and isolation, depression, and hallucinations. Keep in mind that aging is not the only cause of sensory deficits in older adults.

Table 27-1 ➤ Sensory Function Changes With Aging	
SENSE	**CHANGES ASSOCIATED WITH AGING**
Vision	The vitreous humor becomes thinner, and "floaters" appear in the visual field.
	The lens becomes discolored and opaque; the pupil becomes smaller. Therefore, less light reaches the retina, limiting vision.
	The lens becomes less flexible and less able to focus on near objects.
	The ciliary body contracts and the lens thickens, bringing loss of visual acuity, decreased ability to accommodate to distance and sudden changes in illumination, and decreased night vision.
	Peripheral vision decreases.
	Tear production decreases.
Hearing	Cerumen is drier and more solid, creating hearing loss.
	Scarring occurs (e.g., from previous inflammation over the life span).
	Hearing changes commonly include presbycusis (hearing loss of high-frequency tones) and decreased speech discrimination.
Taste	Taste buds atrophy and decrease in number, so there is less ability to perceive tastes, especially sweetness.
	Dry mouth may alter the sense of taste.
Smell	Atrophy and loss of olfactory neurons decrease the ability to perceive smell (may also alter the sense of taste).
Touch	Loss of sensory nerve fibers and changes in the cerebral cortex decrease the ability to perceive light touch, pain, and temperature variations.
Kinesthesia	Kinesthetic changes include a decrease in muscle fibers and diminished conduction speed of nerve fibers, resulting in slowed reaction time, decreased speed and power of muscle contractions, and impaired balance. These changes place older adults at increased risk for falling.

Culture

♥ **iCare** Culture affects the nature, type, and amount of interaction and stimulation that people feel comfortable with. Each person is comfortable with a certain amount of eye contact, personal space, and physical touch. For example, you may consider how your hospitalized patient needs quiet time alone to rest. However, if they are accustomed to being surrounded by a large family, they may rest better amid what seems like chaos to you. **Key Point: *Use touch advisedly and respectfully. For some people, it is comforting; for others, it may be intrusive or even offensive.***

Illness

- **Neurological disorders** (e.g., multiple sclerosis) can slow the transmission of nerve impulses, affecting sensation and perception.
- **Diseases that affect circulation** (e.g., atherosclerosis) may impair the function of the sensory receptors and the brain, thereby altering perception and response.
- **Reduced or lack of oxygen** (anoxia) harms and even destroys cells, causing widespread damage to the neurological system.
- **Some conditions affect specific sensory organs.** For example:
  Diabetic *retinopathy* is the leading cause of blindness among adults.
  Hypertension, too, can damage the retina of the eyes.
  Sickle cell disease, similar to *diabetes,* causes new blood vessels to grow in the eye and pull on the retina, causing a retinal detachment.
  Toxoplasmosis leads to vision loss; the infection may be acquired by the fetus during pregnancy, as well as throughout life.
- **Physiological injury to the brain** may occur from trauma:
  Closed head injury (e.g., acute concussion) occurs when brain tissue is compressed from bleeding, bruising, fluid, or increased pressure inside the skull—for example, after a fall.
  Penetrating injury occurs when a foreign object enters the brain, resulting in damage to the brain tissue or structure.

Medications

Numerous medications can cause a foul or metallic taste. This unpleasant side effect can result from medication taken orally, intramuscularly, or intravenously. Medications that cross the blood–brain barrier affect neurological or sensory function by damaging or killing brain cells. For example:

- **Aspirin and furosemide** (Lasix) can become ototoxic if taken for a long period of time (Ding et al., 2016) and impair function of the auditory nerve.
- **CNS depressants,** such as opioid analgesics and sedatives, reduce the reception and perception of stimuli.

- Some medications (oral, intramuscular [IM], and IV) cause an unpleasant or metallic taste (Table 27-2).

Stress

Physical illness, pain, hospitalization, tests, and surgery are all stressors that can lead to sensory overload—more stimuli than the person can handle. Jason (Meet Your Patients) has been under tremendous physical and emotional stress because of his injuries and surgeries. His situation is one in which you might want to limit unnecessary stimuli (e.g., noise, lights, too many visitors).

Personality and Lifestyle

Are you the kind of person who likes to have people around all the time? Do you thrive on noise and action? Or are you the kind of person who loves to curl up with a book and a cup of tea? Clients, too, vary in their personalities and lifestyles. Some people, by nature, like excitement, change, and stimulation; others prefer a more predictable and quiet life. Clients are at risk for sensory alterations if their previous level of stimuli does not match their current level. Health problems, a change of environment, or the loss of a partner can all create changes in stimuli.

KnowledgeCheck 27-2

- List five major factors that affect sensory function.
- Compare and contrast the sensory changes in childhood with those in older adulthood.

SENSORY ALTERATIONS

Humans are constantly striving to achieve **sensoristasis,** a state of optimal sensory stimulation and alertness. Sensory alterations occur when the body experiences sensory deprivation, sensory overload, or sensory deficits.

Sensory Deprivation

Sensory deprivation occurs as a result of altered sensory reception in which the person does not receive and process enough meaningful sensory input. This may occur when there is disruption or dysfunction with the nervous system (e.g., brain injury) or a deprived environment (e.g., isolation, immobility). This commonly results from understimulation of the senses, common among hospitalized patients, older adults, and ill or injured people in the community. See the Example Client Condition: Sensory Deprivation.

Sensory Overload

Sensory overload occurs when stimuli such as pain or unfamiliar sights, sounds, odors, and routines overwhelm the patient's senses. The complex sensory environment within the hospital contributes to sensory overload. Sensory overload is described further in the Example Client Condition: Sensory Overload.

Table 27-2 ➤ Medications That Cause Smell and Taste Disturbance

DRUG CLASSIFICATION	DRUG	DRUG CLASSIFICATION	DRUG
Anti-infectives	Amoxicillin	CNS drugs/sympathomimetics	Amphetamine and dextroamphetamine, combined
	Azithromycin	Endocrine and diabetes drugs	Glipizide
	Ciprofloxacin		Insulin
Anti-inflammatory, antipyretic, analgesic agents	Aspirin		Metformin
	Diclofenac		Levothyroxine
	Ibuprofen	Gastrointestinal drugs	Omeprazole
	Acetaminophen		Ranitidine
	Tramadol	Psychopharmacologic agents	Amitriptyline
Antihistamines	Loratadine		Bupropion
	Fluticasone		Citalopram
	Prednisone		Fluoxetine
Antihypertensives and cardiovascular agents	Amlodipine		Paroxetine
	Diltiazem		Sertraline
	Enalapril		Trazodone
	Furosemide		Venlafaxine
	Hydrochlorothiazide		Alprazolam
	Lisinopril		Clonazepam
	Losartan		Diazepam
	Metoprolol		Zolpidem
	Propranolol	Pulmonary agents	Albuterol
	Spironolactone	Vitamins	Ergocalciferol
	Triamterene		Potassium
Antilipidemics	Atorvastatin		
	Lovastatin		
	Pravastatin		
	Simvastatin		

CNS, Central nervous system.
Source: Schiffman S. S. (2018). Influence of medications on taste and smell. *World Journal of Otorhinolaryngology—Head and Neck Surgery, 4*(1), 84–91. https://doi.org/10.1016/j.wjorl.2018.02.005

KnowledgeCheck 27-3

- How does sensory deprivation occur?
- Identify five signs of sensory deprivation.
- How does sensory overload occur?
- Identify five signs of sensory overload.

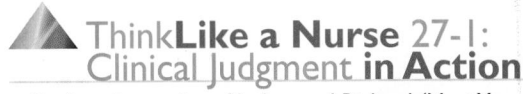

ThinkLike a Nurse 27-1: Clinical Judgment in Action

Review the stories of Joshua and Richard (Meet Your Patients). How are these patients similar? What factors may have contributed to each patient's current concerns?

EXAMPLE CLIENT CONDITION: Sensory Deprivation

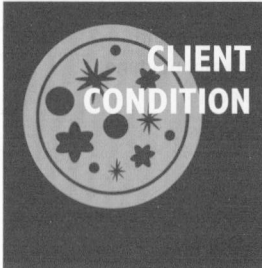
CLIENT CONDITION

Sensory Deprivation—state of depression of the reticular activating system (RAS) caused by less-than-normal or absent sensory input. A silent, dark room or impaired sight, sound, smell, or touch can lead to sensory isolation.

Risk Factors

When external stimuli are severely restricted, the remaining stimuli (e.g., distant noises, minor pain, cold extremities) can become overly noticeable or distorted.
- Bedbound or homebound
- Patients in critical care units
- Hospitalized patent in isolation

Triggers
- Impaired sensory reception (neurological injury, dementia, depression, sleep deprivation, central nervous system [CNS]-depressant medications)
- Nerve or brain injury
- Restricted mobility
- Sensory deficits (blindness, deafness)
- Quiet, monotonous environment
- Inability to interpret language, social cues, and interactions
- CNS disease
- Advanced age

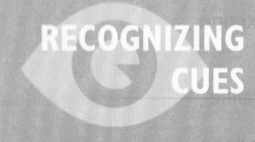
RECOGNIZING COMPLICATIONS

- Depression
- Withdrawal
- Delirium

- Poor patient compliance
- Confusion
- Intensive care unit (ICU) psychosis

RECOGNIZING CUES

Assess for risk factors (see previous list) and symptoms of sensory deprivation:
- Irritability
- Reduced attention span
- Decreased problem-solving skills
- Delusions, hallucinations
- Drowsiness

- Preoccupation with somatic complaints

 See **Focused Assessment** boxes **Nursing History: Overall Sensory Perceptual Status** and **Bedside Assessment of Sensory Function** in Volume 2.

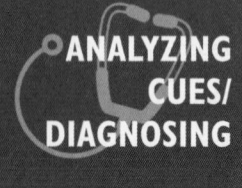
ANALYZING CUES/ DIAGNOSING

Primary Diagnosis
- Sensory Perceptual Alteration

Diagnoses Associated with Sensory Deprivation
- Activity Alteration
- Communication Impairment
- Sleep Pattern Disturbance
- Social Interaction Alteration

GENERATING SOLUTIONS

Outcomes are needed to assess progress of the primary sensory-neuro-response problem and also for diagnoses that may result from it (e.g., Confusion)

NOC Outcomes, Examples
- Cognition
- Cognitive Orientation
- Concentration
- Decision-Making
- Falls Occurrence
- Information Processing
- Memory
- Neurological Status

Individualized Outcomes
- Correctly names the months of the year.
- Communication is clear and appropriate for age and situation.
- Vital signs are within patient's normal limits.
- Recalls recent information accurately.
- Responds to visual and auditory cues.
- Will not fall while in the hospital.

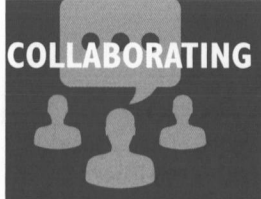
COLLABORATING

- Communicate the plan for care to caregivers and healthcare team.
- Monitor the use of sedatives.

- Music therapy, activities, physical therapy, speech therapy, nutritional therapy, and occupational therapy may all be valuable in the care of the client.

EXAMPLE CLIENT CONDITION: Sensory Deprivation—cont'd

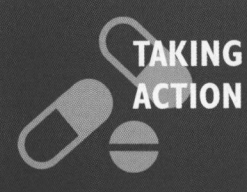

TAKING ACTION

Visual Stimulation

- Help patient to put on clean eyeglasses when awake.
- Put personal items on the walls; place photos or flowers for patient to see.
- Open blinds during the day, except when patient is sleeping.
- Place clock and calendar in view.

Auditory Stimulation

- Help patient with a hearing aid to apply it whenever awake. Be sure it has working batteries and set at an appropriate volume.
- When possible, move to a distraction-free area when communicating important matters with patient.

Olfactory Stimulation

- Offer pleasant scents or aromatherapy to help stimulate appetite.

♥ iCare Tactile Stimulation

- Use touch carefully in patient care activities. People respond differently to physical contact. You might hold the patient's hand while talking or provide a back rub, as tolerated.

Facilitating Communication

- Develop alternative methods of communication for patients with aphasia, those who speak another language, or those who have difficulty hearing (communication board, mobile tablet, writing tools).
- Use a message board in the room; ask family members to post photos, cards, or notes.
- Offer devices for messaging, electronic communication, and social media.

Promoting Adequate Sleep and Rest

- Schedule care to allow for uninterrupted periods of sleep and rest and to provide advance notice of what the client is to expect during the day.

Promoting Social Interaction

- Make regular contact with patient.
- Introduce yourself and address patient by name.
- Provide continuity of care by assigning the same staff whenever possible.
- Encourage patient to participate in scheduled activities.
- Assist acute care patient out of bed for meals or visitors.
- Encourage patient to leave their rooms when possible.
- Patients may play video games with others online.
- Ensure that patient in isolation receives adequate stimulation from healthcare team, family members, or visitors.

Pet Therapy

- Many long-term care and residential facilities allow resident pets or pet visits to promote socialization, lower blood pressure, and reduce loneliness and pain.

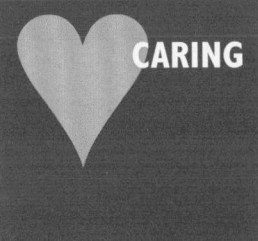

CARING

♥ iCare Minimizing Anxiety & Confusion

- Encourage families to bring familiar objects from home.
- Provide continuity of care when possible.
- Promote orientation (e.g., provide visual cues to place and time).

- Introduce yourself; inform patient of the plan for care using a calm, respectful approach.
- Explain all procedures and care.
- Simplify your communication.
- Maintain a safe environment.

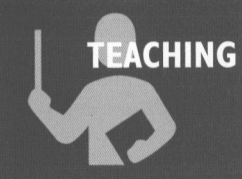

TEACHING

- Teach during times when patient is able to concentrate.

- Provide instruction on stress-reduction techniques.

EXAMPLE CLIENT CONDITION: Sensory Overload

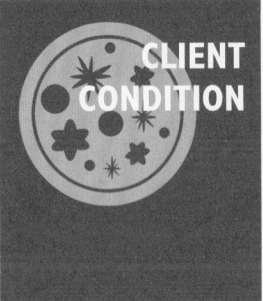

CLIENT CONDITION

Sensory Overload—Environmental stimuli exceed the ability of one or more of the body's senses to process and adapt, especially when stimuli are persistent and nonmeaningful.

Triggers

- Physical discomfort, pain
- Medications that stimulate the central nervous system (CNS; e.g., caffeine, amphetamine)
- Physical conditions that activate the CNS (e.g., hyperthyroidism)

- Neurological or psychiatric disorders (anxiety, psychosis, sensory integration disorder, attention deficit-hyperactivity disorder)
- Sounds such as monitor alarms, talking in halls, paging systems
- Interruptions in rest and sleep by healthcare providers (e.g., for vital signs)
- Invasive medical therapies and procedures
- Lack of privacy
- Unpleasant odors and sights
- Unfamiliar healthcare environment and patient care routines

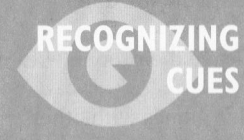

RECOGNIZING CUES

- Irritability, anxiety, restlessness, confusion
- Reduced attention span
- Decreased problem-solving skills
- Drowsiness resulting from insomnia
- Muscle tension
- Inability to concentrate and focus

- Decreased ability to perform tasks
- Disorientation, confusion
- Distractibility

 See **Focused Assessment** boxes **Nursing History: Overall Sensory Perceptual Status and Bedside Assessment of Sensory Function** in Volume 2.

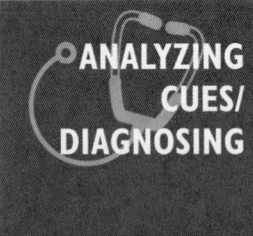

ANALYZING CUES/ DIAGNOSING

Primary Diagnosis

- Sensory Perceptual Alteration

Diagnoses Associated With Sensory Overload

- Anxiety r/t excess sensory stimulation
- Acute Confusion
- Nonadherence to treatments

- Chronic Confusion r/t continuing excess sensory stimulation
- Individual Coping Impairment
- Sleep Pattern Disturbance

GENERATING SOLUTIONS

NOC Outcomes, Examples

- Anxiety Level
- Cognitive Orientation
- Concentration
- Sensory Function

Individualized Outcomes

- Effectively copes with excessive environmental stimuli.
- Reports adequate sleep and rest.
- Identifies correct season.
- Identifies significant others.
- Requests help when needed.

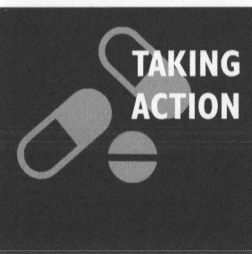

TAKING ACTION

Control Visual Stimuli

- Minimize unnecessary light, especially at night.
- Use a flashlight instead of turning on room lights.

Control Auditory Stimuli

- Minimize unnecessary noise.
- Reduce noise levels, especially at night.
- Speak using a calm and confident voice.
- Consider the use of earplugs for the patient.

Manage Olfactory Stimuli

- Promptly empty commodes and bedpans, remove meal trays, use deodorant sprays, and keep wounds covered.
- Avoid wearing perfume when providing patient care.

Promote Sleep and Rest

- Provide a quiet, restful environment.
- Provide uninterrupted periods of sleep and rest.

EXAMPLE CLIENT CONDITION: Sensory Overload—cont'd

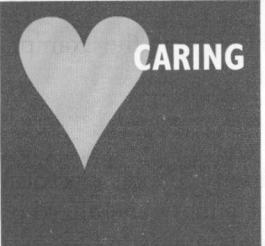

CARING

♥ iCare **Minimize Stress**

- Remove annoying or excessive stimuli when possible.
- Provide a calm presence: do not hurry with care or speak rapidly.
- Offer a private room, if possible, and limit visitors.
- Minimize nonessential tasks.
- Control pain and nausea with prescribed medications and other comfort measures.
- Provide relaxing music.

Minimize Confusion

- Introduce yourself when meeting the patient; address patient by name.
- Encourage families to bring familiar objects from home.
- Provide continuity of care when possible.
- Promote orientation (e.g., provide visual cues to place and time).
- Inform patient of the plan; explain all procedures and care.
- Simplify your communication.
- Maintain a safe environment.

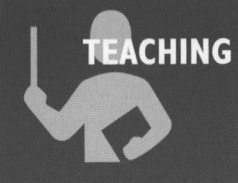

TEACHING

- Avoid screen time for 1 hour before sleep.
- Do not leave the TV or radio on continuously.

- Silence smartphone notification alerts.
- Teach visualization and deep-breathing techniques.

PICOT

Sensory Overload in the Intensive Care Unit

Situation: The nurse is caring for a teen with anxiety disorder who is admitted to the intensive care unit (ICU) after sustaining traumatic injuries from a motorcycle accident. The client has a history of panic attacks and episodes of high anxiety; the nursing team is meeting with a psychiatric social worker to develop an appropriate plan of care.

PICOT Components

P	Population/patient	=	Hospitalized patients with anxiety disorder
I	Intervention/indicator	=	Sensory overload in ICU
C	Comparison/control	=	Patients without a history of high anxiety or panic
O	Outcome	=	Violent behavior
T	Time	=	During hospitalization

Searchable Question: Do _____ (P) who are _____ (I) demonstrate _____ (O) compared with _____ (C) during _____ (T)?

Example of Evidence: Clients with mental health dysfunction who are admitted to the acute medical facility present special challenges for the nursing staff. A priority for care is ensuring safety for this client and others, including healthcare staff. The initial assessment should focus on patterns and types of violent behavior, frequency, and characteristics of targeted victims. The nurse would also assess for possible triggers to agitation. In addition to collecting the client's mental health and medication history, the nurse would also be alert to potential high-stress situations during hospitalization, such as sensory overload coupled with sleep deprivation, that precipitate negative behaviors.

Practice Change: Healthcare staff will modify the environment to avoid exposing clients to excess sensory stimulation, including lights, alarms, and interruptions in sleep and rest.

Sources: Gupta, N., Brown, C., Deneke, J., Maha, J., & Kong, M. (2019, September). Utilization of a novel pathway in a tertiary pediatric hospital to meet the sensory needs of acutely ill pediatric patients. *Frontiers in Pediatrics, 7,* 367. https://doi.org/10.3389/fped.2019.00367; Scheydt, S., Staub, M. M., & Frauenfelder, F. (2017). Sensory overload: A concept analysis. *International Journal of Mental Health Nursing, 26*(2), 110–120. https://doi.org/10.1111/inm.12303

Sensory Deficits

Sensory deficits may stem from impaired reception, perception, or both. They can be visual, auditory, olfactory, gustatory, tactile, and kinesthetic. The two sensory deficits you are most likely to encounter in nursing practice are impaired vision and impaired hearing.

- *Sudden onset* of a deficit may lead to disorientation and anxiety.
- *Gradual changes* allow the person to adapt, often without even realizing the extent of the change.

- *Compensation*—When there is a deficit in one sense, the other senses may become sharper to compensate (e.g., a person who is blind may develop more acute hearing).

Sensory Deficits are described further in the Example Client Condition: Sensory Deficits.

Seizures

Seizures occur because of sudden, chaotic electrical activity in the brain. They may be either generalized or focal. The difference between these types is in how and

---

EXAMPLE CLIENT CONDITION: Sensory Deficits: Visual and Hearing

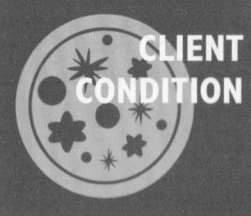

CLIENT CONDITION

Visual

Vision—Light rays on the retina trigger a nerve impulse that is transmitted to the visual area of the brain in the occipital region.

Types of Visual Deficits

Myopia (near-sightedness)—sees close objects clearly but not distant objects. For example, a person with 20/200 vision can see an object from 20 feet away that a person with normal sight could see from a distance of 200 feet.

Hyperopia (farsightedness)—sees distant objects well. A person with hyperopia may have 20/10 vision—they can see an object from 20 feet that a normal eye can see from 10 feet; however, near vision is impaired.

Presbyopia—change in vision associated with aging. The lens becomes less elastic and less able to accommodate to near objects.

Astigmatism—irregular curvature of the cornea or lens that scatters light rays and blurs or distorts the image on the retina.

Cataracts—clouding of the lens, resulting in blurred vision, sensitivity to glare, and image distortion. Can occur in one eye or both.

Glaucoma—increased pressure in the anterior cavity of the eyeball distorts the shape of the cornea and shifts the position of the lens. Results in loss of peripheral vision or blindness. The most common type is open-angle glaucoma.

Macular degeneration—loss of central vision due to damage to the macula lutea, the central portion of the retina. The leading cause of visual impairment in older adults, characterized by slow, progressive loss of central and near vision. Usually present in both eyes. Risk factors include excessive sunlight exposure and smoking.

Auditory

Hearing—Sound waves entering the ear canal are converted to vibrations, then transferred from the middle to inner ear. Vibrations cause hair cells in the cochlea to bend, generating impulses carried by cranial nerve (CN) VIII to the brain. The auditory region in the temporal lobes interprets sound and the direction it is coming from.

Types of Auditory Deficits

- **Conduction deafness**—may be a temporary or permanent condition caused by infection of the middle ear, a punctured tympanic membrane, arthritis of the auditory bones, cerumen impaction, or a foreign object lodged in the ear canal. **Key Point: *A hearing aid may be helpful for conduction deafness.***

- **Sensorineural hearing loss**—nerve deafness that occurs when there is damage to CN VIII or the receptors in the cochlea. It may result from ototoxic medications (e.g., gentamicin), trauma, hereditary causes, and bacterial or viral infections. Chronic exposure to loud noise may also lead to nerve and receptor impairment. **Key Point: *Hearing aids may not help sensorineural hearing loss.***

- **Presbycusis**—progressive sensorineural loss associated with aging. The person experiences diminished ability to hear high-pitched sounds (e.g., *s, z, sh, ch*) and to distinguish sounds in a noisy environment. Presbycusis results from deterioration of the hair cells in the cochlea.

- **Central deafness**—damage to the auditory areas in the temporal lobes. Tumor, trauma, meningitis, or stroke in the temporal lobe may cause this.

- **Tinnitus**—ringing in the ears. Most tinnitus comes from damage to the endings of the nerve in the inner ear caused by trauma, Ménière disease, hypertension, ear infection, medications, otosclerosis, or arthritic changes of the bones of the ear.

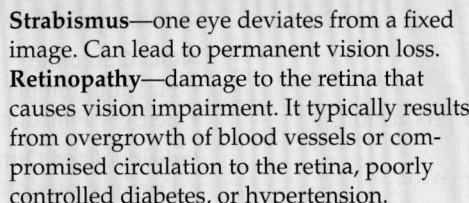

EXAMPLE CLIENT CONDITION: Sensory Deficits: Visual and Hearing—cont'd

Strabismus—one eye deviates from a fixed image. Can lead to permanent vision loss.
Retinopathy—damage to the retina that causes vision impairment. It typically results from overgrowth of blood vessels or compromised circulation to the retina, poorly controlled diabetes, or hypertension.

⊕ **Detached retina**—a separation of the retina from the layer underneath. Occurs from trauma to the eye or failed recent cataract surgery. It presents as a curtain coming down across vision. This is an ophthalmological emergency.

Triggers
- Macular degeneration
- Stroke
- Age-related changes
- Refractive errors
- Orbital trauma
- Cataracts
- Glaucoma
- Diabetic or hypertensive retinopathy

- **Impacted cerumen**—earwax becomes tightly packed in the ear canal, blocking the canal. Patients with impacted cerumen may experience a feeling of fullness or pain, decreased hearing, or tinnitus.
- **Otitis media**—middle ear infection. It is a common childhood illness that may be caused by viruses or bacteria.
- **Otosclerosis**—hardening of the bones of the middle ear, especially the stapes. The stapes becomes fixed, leading to poor sound transmission to the inner ear. The cause of this disorder is unknown.

Causes of Auditory Deficit
- Injury or disease in structures of ear, nerves, or brain—abnormal bony growth or tumor, medication (gentamicin, chemotherapy drugs); problems of the inner ear (Ménière disease), ruptured **tympanic membrane** (eardrum)
- Infection—otitis media, meningitis
- Build-up of **cerumen** (earwax)
- Aging, heredity
- Loud noise

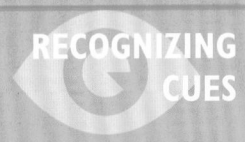 **RECOGNIZING COMPLICATIONS**

Visual Deficit
- Altered activities of daily living, independence, and mobility
- Altered social interactions
- Risk for falls

Auditory Deficit
- Injury resulting from inability to hear warnings
- Depression
- Social isolation

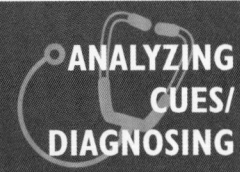 **RECOGNIZING CUES**

Visual Deficit
 Go to **Chapter 19, Procedure 19-6: Assessing the Eyes,** in Volume 2.

Auditory Deficit
 Go to **Chapter 19, Procedure 19-7: Assessing the Ears and Hearing,** in Volume 2.

 See **Focused Assessment** boxes **Nursing History: Overall Sensory Perceptual Status** and **Bedside Assessment of Sensory Function** in Volume 2.

ANALYZING CUES/ DIAGNOSING

Visual Deficit
- Fall Risk r/t impaired vision
- Visual Alteration

Auditory Deficit as a Problem
- Auditory Alteration
- Sensory Perceptual Alteration: Auditory

Auditory Deficit as an Etiology
- Diversional Activity Deficit r/t hearing impairment
- Communication Impairment
- Social Interaction Alteration
- Knowledge Deficit r/t impaired ability to understand instructions
- Injury Risk r/t inability to hear warnings

(continued)

EXAMPLE CLIENT CONDITION: Sensory Deficits: Visual and Hearing—cont'd

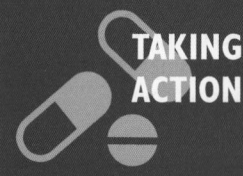

GENERATING SOLUTIONS

Visual Deficit

NOC Outcomes
- Sensory Function: Vision
- Dry Eye (inadequate tear production/evaporation)
- Vision Compensation Behavior

Auditory Deficit

NOC Outcomes
- Hearing Compensation Behavior
- Sensory Function: Hearing

Individualized Outcomes
- Demonstrates proper use of a hearing aid
- Actively communicates with caregiver.

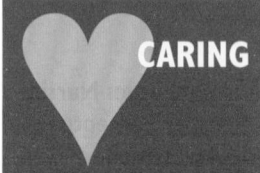

TAKING ACTION

Visual Deficit

NIC Interventions
- Communication Enhancement: Visual Deficit
- Eye Care
- Fall Prevention

For Fear and Anxiety associated with visual deficits:
- Calming Technique
- Emotional Support
- Touch

Individualized Interventions
- Keep the bed in a low position.
- Make sure eyeglasses are clean, in good repair, of proper prescription, and within reach; help patient put them on, if necessary. Assist client in using contact lenses as needed.
- Use soft, diffuse lighting without glare.
- Provide an uncluttered environment. Orient patient to room arrangement, if needed.
- Place call device, phone, self-care items within reach.
- Provide referrals for supportive services (e.g., psychological, social services).

Auditory Deficit

NIC Interventions
- Communication Enhancement: Hearing Deficit
- Environmental Management
- Ear Care

Individualized Interventions
- Inspect ear canals for cerumen impaction.
- Ensure hearing aid batteries are charged.
- Use closed-captioning, voice control for mobile devices and computers.
- Provide written instructions for treatments and self-care.

 See **Procedure 27-1: Performing Otic Irrigation** in Volume 2.

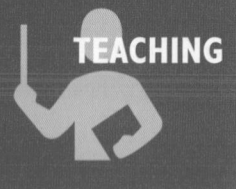

CARING

♥ **iCare** Visual Deficit

 See **Clinical Insight 27-1: Communicating with Clients Who Are Visually Impaired** in Volume 2.

Auditory Deficit

See **Clinical Insight 27-2: Communicating With Clients Who Are Hearing Impaired** in Volume 2.

TEACHING

Vision
- Use magnifying lens, large-print materials, audio, Braille media, as needed.
- Avoid rugs on floors. Keep spaces uncluttered.
- Have regular eye examinations.
  Infants and preschoolers—Screen at routine office visits.
  Young adults—Complete eye examination at least three times between the ages of 20 and 39.

Hearing
- Wear ear protection for those exposed to loud sound.
- Check hearing regularly for those who work in an area with a high noise level.
- Install and use blinking lights that alert an incoming call, door ring, alarm clock, and smoke detector.
- Obtain (and wear) hearing aids, if needed.

EXAMPLE CLIENT CONDITION: Sensory Deficits: Visual and Hearing—cont'd

At age 40—Have a baseline screening, and based on that information, the ophthalmologist will determine how frequently your eyes need to be reexamined.

Age 65 and older—Complete eye examination every 1 to 2 years to check for cataracts and other eye conditions. (American Academy of Ophthalmology, 2015)

- Those at risk for eye disease should have more frequent eye examinations, regardless of age. This includes those who (1) take steroids; (2) are of African ancestry; (3) have a family history of eye disease, diabetes, or high blood pressure; or (4) have any symptoms.
- Call your healthcare provider for prompt examination if you have eye pain, discharge, a change in vision, or bleeding.
- Have prescriptions for glasses or contact lenses reviewed at each screening and updated if needed.
- Ask if visual screening is done at child's elementary school. If not, consult pediatrician or other care provider.
- Work with your primary healthcare provider to control conditions that affect vision (hypertension, diabetes).
- If pregnant, obtain early and adequate prenatal care to prevent the danger of premature birth.
- Insist that children use eye protection when playing sports.
- For children who wear glasses, be sure the lenses are made of shatterproof safety glass.

- If pregnant:
  Obtain early prenatal care.
  Avoid ototoxic drugs.
  Be sure you are tested for syphilis and rubella (German measles).
  Avoid anyone you suspect may have rubella.
- Children with frequent ear infections require evaluation to determine whether hearing loss has occurred.
- Middle and older adults may begin to experience difficulty distinguishing voices in a crowd or hearing the television or radio. These are indications of hearing loss and should be evaluated; hearing loss is not a natural part of aging.

---

where they originate in the brain. Recurrent seizures may be due to a brain disorder, called *epilepsy,* or may result from a brain tumor, head trauma, or a variety of other causes. For more information and nursing care, refer to the Example Client Condition: Seizures, later in the chapter.

Social and psychological factors in epilepsy, such as perceived stigma and societal prejudice, may affect health outcomes in epilepsy. Physical restrictions are put into place when seizures occur, which can affect a person's ability to drive, which, in turn, affects opportunities to maintain employment, access healthcare, and seek social gratification. Other key social determinants

of health, such as low socioeconomic status, are associated with higher adverse effects of epilepsy, including more hospitalization and emergency services, antiepileptic nonadherence, and fewer epilepsy nonpharmacological therapies and surgeries (Szaflarski, 2014).

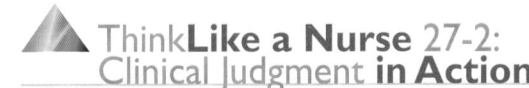

ThinkLike a Nurse 27-2: Clinical Judgment in Action

- Why do you think a person with impaired tactile perception is at risk for injury?
- Speculate as to the possible nature of injuries that might occur.

Text continued on page 802

EXAMPLE CLIENT CONDITION: Sensory Deficits: Olfactory and Gustatory

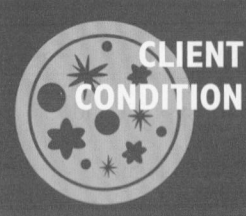
CLIENT CONDITION

Olfaction—Definition

Sense of smell. Specialized sensory cells inside the nose generate impulses that are carried to the brain by the olfactory nerve (CN I). Olfaction plays a role in taste, memory, mood, and safety (see Fig. 27-2).

Triggers
- Cranial nerve damage
- Cocaine and tobacco use
- Concussion
- Zinc deficiency
- Inherited condition (nonpathological)
- Aging
- COVID-19 infection
- Mass in nasal passages
- Neurological condition (Parkinson or Alzheimer disease, multiple sclerosis)
- Dental problems
- Exposure to chemicals (certain insecticides)
- Radiation treatment of the head and neck
- Certain medications (see Table 27-2)

Common Olfactory Disorders
- **Hyposmia** is the reduced ability to smell and detect odor.
- **Anosmia** is the inability to smell.

Gustation—Sense of taste. Taste buds generate nerve impulses that travel along the facial and glossopharyngeal nerves (CN VII and IX) to the taste area in the parietal–temporal cortex of the brain. Taste buds in different areas of the tongue: sweet and salty (tip of tongue), sour (sides of tongue), bitter (back of tongue, soft palate), and savory (see Fig. 27-2).

Triggers
- Xerostomia (excessively dry mouth)
- Low fluid intake
- Poor nutrition
- Inadequate oral hygiene
- Common cold
- Infections of the nose, sinuses, mouth, salivary glands
- Allergies
- Tobacco use
- Vitamin B_{12} or zinc deficiency
- Injury to mouth, nose
- Head injury (concussion); Alzheimer (Yoo, 2018)
- Radiation to head and neck
- Gastrointestinal disturbances (gastric reflux)
- Chemical exposure (lead, pesticides)
- Medications (see Table 27-2)

Common Taste Disorders
- **Phantom taste perception** is an unpleasant taste even though there is nothing in the mouth.
- **Hypogeusia** is the reduced ability to taste flavor (sour, salty, bitter, rancid, metallic).
- **Ageusia** is the rare inability to detect any flavor at all.

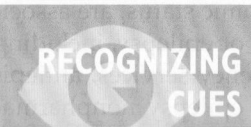
RECOGNIZING COMPLICATIONS

Olfactory Deficit
- Decreased appetite and nutritional deficits. When sense of smell is lost, food tastes different.
- Risk for injury. Smell disorders can compromise the ability to detect fire, toxic fumes, leaking gas, and spoiled food and beverages.

Gustatory Deficit
- Nutritional deficits
- Weight loss

RECOGNIZING CUES

 See **Focused Assessment** boxes **Nursing History: Overall Sensory Perceptual Status** and **Bedside Assessment of Sensory Function** in Volume 2.

Olfactory Deficit

A "scratch and sniff" test uses a paper with scented patches to detect specific odors. For more specific details,

 Go to **Chapter 19, Procedure 19-16: Assessing the Sensory Neurological System**, in Volume 2.

Gustatory Deficit

A "sip, spit, and rinse" test uses chemicals that are applied to the tongue to detect specific flavors. For more specific details,

 Go to **Chapter 19, Procedure 19-16: Assessing the Sensory Neurological System**, in Volume 2.

EXAMPLE CLIENT CONDITION: Sensory Deficits: Olfactory and Gustatory—cont'd

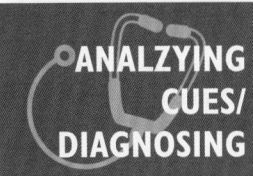
ANALZYING CUES/ DIAGNOSING

Olfactory Deficit

- Olfactory Alteration (describe)
- Injury Risk
- Sensory Perceptual Alteration (describe)

Gustatory Deficit

- Gustatory Alteration (describe)
- Body Nutrition Deficit r/t alteration in taste
- Sensory Perceptual Alteration (describe)

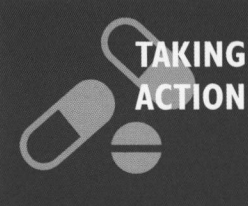
GENERATING SOLUTIONS

Olfactory and Gustatory Deficits

NOC Outcomes

- Appetite
- Nutritional Status: Food & Fluid Intake
- Sensory Function: Taste & Smell

Individualized Outcomes

- Consumes a healthy diet even if sense of smell is altered.
- Maintains a stable weight.

TAKING ACTION

Olfactory and Gustatory Deficits

NIC Interventions

- Environmental Management
- Environmental Management: Safety
- Feeding
- Nausea Management
- Nutrition Management

Individualized Interventions for Olfactory Deficit

- Aromatherapy

Individualized Interventions for Gustatory Deficit

- Check the fit of dentures or dental appliances. Weight changes may affect the fit and make it harder to eat.
- Perform frequent oral hygiene to encourage appetite and enhance the sense of taste.
- Assess for sores on the tongue, palate, and cheeks.
- Teach patient to eat foods one at a time or drink water between bites to enhance flavor.
- Use seasonings, salt substitutes, spices, or lemon to improve the taste of foods, unless contraindicated.

CARING

♥ **iCare** **Olfactory and Gustatory Deficits**

- Serve visually appealing meals.
- Vary food texture, color, temperature.

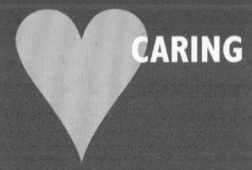
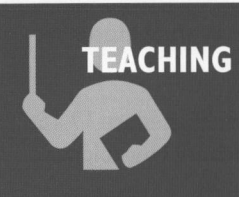
TEACHING

Olfactory Deficit

- Check smoke detectors and replace batteries regularly.
- Do not rely on smell or taste to detect food spoilage; date foods, inspect before eating.
- Arrange regular inspection and maintenance of gas appliances.

Gustatory Deficit

- Dental health is an important aspect of maintaining taste.
- Decayed teeth, gum disease, and other disorders of the mouth may affect the ability to taste.
- Advise clients to have teeth cleaned and examined at least annually.
- Additional dental care may be necessary to promote oral health.

EXAMPLE CLIENT CONDITION: Sensory Deficits—Tactile and Kinesthetic

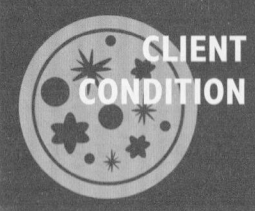

Tactile Deficit

Tactile deficit (or tactile disorder) is a change or alteration in the ability to feel and/or interpret touch, pressure, and temperature.

Physiology

The dermis contains receptors for cutaneous sensations of light touch, pressure, heat, cold, and pain. Information is transmitted to the sensory areas in the parietal lobes. The hands and face have the most receptors and the largest area in the sensory cortex.

Triggers

- Stroke, brain tumor, spinal tumor
- Brain or spinal injury
- Peripheral nerve damage caused by diabetes, Guillain-Barré syndrome, chronic alcoholism, peripheral vascular disease

Types of Tactile Disorders

- **Tactile defensiveness**—diminished tolerance for touch sensations; hypersensitivity
- **Tactile hyposensitivity**—diminished perception of touch sensations
- **Tactile apraxia**—disturbance of hand movements when handling objects
- **Tactile aphasia or agnosia**—reduced or lack of ability to recognize objects by touch
- **Phantom sensation**—hypersensitive nerve conduction involving agitated nerve endings that conduct sensation for a limb that is not there

Kinesthetic Deficit

Kinesthesia, or muscle sense, is the ability to sense position, movement, and one's body in space.

Physiology

- **Proprioception**—Movement stimulates the sensory organs (proprioceptors) and the muscles and bones to sense the position of the head and body when transmitting impulses to the brain. Conscious muscle sense occurs in the parietal lobes, unconscious in the cerebellum.
- **Vestibular function**—The body's ability to maintain equilibrium and balance with movement.

Triggers

- Mismatch between the position or acceleration of the head and the visual field
- *Neurological disorders*—Parkinson disease, tumor, medication, stroke, problems of the inner ear (Ménière disease)

Types of Kinesthetic Disorders

- **Hyperkinetic**—often with repetitive, involuntary motor activity (dystonia, tremors, myoclonus, opisthotonos, chorea, tardive dyskinesia, restless leg movement, tics, rigidity, cramps, spasm)
- **Hypokinetic**—small movements (parkinsonian movement)
- **Bradykinetic**—slow movements
- **Akinetic**—lack of movement

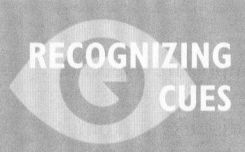

RECOGNIZING COMPLICATIONS

Tactile Deficit

- Failure to detect wounds and injury, increasing the risk of infection

Kinesthetic Deficit

- Pressure injury r/t hypokinesis
- Contracture r/t hyperkinesis
- Injury from falls

RECOGNIZING CUES

 See **Focused Assessment** boxes **Nursing History: Overall Sensory Perceptual Status** and **Bedside Assessment of Sensory Function** in Volume 2.

Tactile and Kinesthetic Deficits

A person's ability to perceive touch is often measured in terms of **2-*point discrimination*,** which is perceiving 2 close but separate points of pressure.

- Discrimination on lips and fingertips is normally at points <4 mm apart
- On the torso, it is wider, at >2 cm.

 Go to **Chapter 19, Procedure 19-16: Assessing the Sensory Neurological System,** in Volume 2.

EXAMPLE CLIENT CONDITION: Sensory Deficits—Tactile and Kinesthetic—cont'd

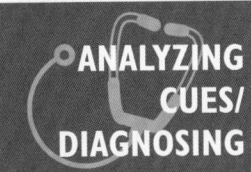

ANALYZING CUES/ DIAGNOSING

Tactile Deficit

- Tactile Alteration
- Injury Risk r/t reduced tactile sensation
- Sensory Perceptual Alteration

Kinesthetic Deficit

- Kinesthetic Alteration
- Bathing Hygiene Deficit r/t kinesthetic impairment
- Sensory Perceptual Alteration

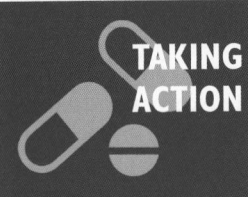

GENERATING SOLUTIONS

Tactile Deficit

NOC Outcomes
- Sensory Function: Tactile
- Heedfulness of Affected Side

Individualized Outcomes
- Recognizes signs and symptoms of peripheral tactile dysfunction
- Remains free of injury

Kinesthetic Deficit

NOC Outcomes
- Sensory Function: Proprioception
- Balance
- Coordinated Movement

Individualized Outcomes
- Walks with effective gait for 12 ft.
- Remains free of falls

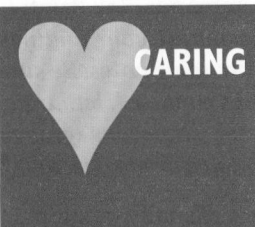

TAKING ACTION

Tactile Deficit

NIC Interventions
- Exercise Promotion: Strength Training
- Exercise Therapy: Balance
- Peripheral Sensation Management

Individualized Interventions
- Change position often to relieve pressure on bony prominences.
- Report signs of impaired circulation (declining motor function, cool, gray-blue coloration).
- Inspect for wounds, abrasions, erythema.

Kinesthetic Deficit

NIC Interventions
- Exercise Therapy: Balance
- Lower Extremity Monitoring
- Neurological Monitoring
- Self-Care Assistance

Individualized Interventions
- Rhythmic movement (tai chi, dance, yoga)
- Aerobic exercise (running, swimming)
- Strength training (light weights)
- Flexibility activities (stretching)
- Balance conditioning (standing on one foot)
- Perform full range of motion (ROM) and rotational movements.
- When helping the patient walk, ask which side patient prefers.

CARING

♥ iCare **Tactile and Kinesthetic Deficits**

- If the patient consents, provide touch by brushing their hair or giving a back rub. You may need to use firm pressure.
- Turn and reposition frequently.

Key Point: *There are wide differences in how touch is perceived among both patients and nurses. Use touch carefully, considering personal and cultural preferences and observing the patient's reaction.*

- Use a bed cradle and keep bed linens loose.

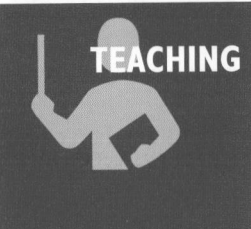

TEACHING

Tactile Deficits

- Use a bath thermometer to monitor water temperature and prevent burns.
- Use properly fitting shoes and socks.
- Report signs of circulatory impairment (cool temperature, discoloration).
- Inspect daily for open areas, cuts, abrasions, or redness.

Kinesthetic Deficits

- Perform activities that tone muscles and improve coordination.
- Move joints through full ROM, especially rotational movements.

KnowledgeCheck 27-4

- Discuss the difference between myopia and hyperopia.
- What is the difference between conduction deafness and nerve deafness?
- Identify three factors that may impair the sense of taste.
- How is the sense of smell triggered?
- What areas of the body have the greatest number of tactile receptors?
- What type of health concerns may be generated by kinesthetic deficits?

ThinkLike a Nurse 27-3: Clinical Judgment in Action

Imagine that you are experiencing sensory deficits. Which deficits would you find most challenging?

PracticalKnowledge
knowing how

Sensory deficits, excess, and overload influence a person's safety and quality of life and may be especially troublesome for those requiring inpatient healthcare.

ASSESSMENT/RECOGNIZING CUES

For details and instructions related to physical examination of sensory-neurological status,

Go to **Chapter 19, Procedure 19-16: Assessing the Sensory-Neurological System, Procedure 19-6: Assessing the Eyes,** and **Procedure 19-7: Assessing the Ears and Hearing,** in Volume 2.

Overall Sensory-Perceptual Assessment Assessment of overall sensory-perceptual status includes both a history and a physical examination.

- **Nursing interview.** As a part of the patient history, you will assess the client's usual and current state of overall sensory function and gather a history of sensory problems and the use of sensory aids. In addition to interviewing the client and family, assess the environment and client situation for factors that may alter sensory function. For sample interview questions,

See the **Chapter 27 Focused Assessment box, Nursing History: Overall Sensory Perceptual Status,** in Volume 2.

- **Physical assessment.** Physical assessment of sensory function requires assessment of the six senses. Perform a focused examination of vision, hearing, taste, smell, touch, balance, ability to respond to stimulation, muscle tone, and coordination.

Assess Usual Sensory Function Obtain a history of the client's usual sensory function, in addition to information about the client's current status. Include in your assessment the client's use of sensory aids—devices that assist with sensory function. These include glasses, contact lenses, hearing aids, canes, and walkers.

Assess Risk Factors for Impaired Sensory Perception You should perform a comprehensive assessment for any patient at increased risk for sensory alterations:

- Older adults
- People who are bedbound or homebound
- Patients in intensive care units
- Those with acute or chronic brain injury, limited mobility, or known sensory deficits, especially if the change has been acute

Routinely assess developmental level, health status, medications, stress and coping mechanisms, personality, history of head trauma, and lifestyle in relation to sensory alterations.

Assess Mental Status Sensory alterations may trigger changes in mental status; altered mental status can interfere with sensory perception. A check of mental status includes an assessment of behavior, appearance, response to stimuli, speech, memory, and judgment. Normal findings include an ability to express and explain realistic thoughts with clear speech, follow directions, listen, answer questions, and recall significant past events. In addition, you must specifically assess the client's level of orientation. Chapter 19 presents additional discussion of mental status screening and orientation.

Assess Level of Consciousness (LOC) As an indicator of cerebral function, LOC includes *arousal* (from alert to deeply comatose) and *orientation* (to time, place, person, and situation). An alert patient will respond to auditory stimuli. If the patient does not respond, progress to tactile and then painful stimuli. Remember, however, that if your client does not speak your language, they may not respond to questions or commands. **Key Point: If you are not using a coma scale, document your findings specifically and objectively in your nursing notes. Be sure to assess whether the patient is alert, confused, lethargic, obtunded (reduced level of alertness), stuporous (groggy or lethargic), or comatose (unresponsive or unconscious).**

Assess the Support Network Usually, a support network is beneficial for a client with a sensory deficit or overload. Support persons may help the client to adapt to deficits by assuming tasks that the client can no longer perform or by providing comfort to relieve the stress associated with sensory losses.

A support network can also be influential when clients are experiencing sensory deprivation or overload. Recall that Richard (Meet Your Patients) has no visitors. What influence do you think frequent visits by family members would have on Richard? If you said that Richard would receive more stimulation and may have less sensory deprivation, you are correct. Family members can also help clients who are confused as a result of sensory alterations by reorienting and calming the client.

Assess the Environment As part of your assessment, observe how the client is responding to the conditions of the environment. Consider how different the environment is for Joshua and Richard (Meet Your Patients). Joshua is in a crowded space with lights and noise 24 hours per day. He has had a number of invasive procedures and is most likely receiving pain medication. In contrast, Richard is in a quiet room with little exposure to light, noise, or touch. As Joshua's and Richard's situations demonstrate, a healthcare environment can have too many or too few stimuli.

- **Compare the patient's personality and lifestyle with the current environmental situation.** In healthcare facilities, patients are subjected to lights, noises, and odors that cause them anxiety. They may hear others who are crying out in pain. A patient from a small family and a quiet environment may develop sensory overload as a result of overstimulation in a hospital setting. Even someone used to a rapid-pace lifestyle may experience overload, particularly when experiencing pain, nausea, dizziness, or other illness symptoms. Additionally, a patient with a busy lifestyle may have difficulty coping with confinement in the hospital.
- **Assess the effect of the environment on sensory deficits.** For a patient with age-related hearing changes, the background noise of the healthcare environment may make it difficult to hear higher-tone or low-volume voices. A patient with visual deficits or impaired balance will often modify their home environment to improve function in the home; however, when the patient is hospitalized or moved to a long-term care facility, these aids may no longer be feasible. **Key Point:** *To assist the patient, you must determine which environmental conditions worsen sensory deficits and which help to compensate.*

For a guide to bedside physical assessment of sensory function,

 See the **Chapter 27 Focused Assessment box, Bedside Assessment of Sensory Function,** in Volume 2.

KnowledgeCheck 27-5

- Identify six areas you should assess for a client with known or suspected sensory alterations.
- What factors must be evaluated when it is known that a client uses a sensory aid?
- Identify at least two ways that you can assess vision and hearing deficits at the bedside.

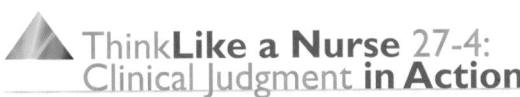

ThinkLike a Nurse 27-4: Clinical Judgment in Action

How would you assess Joshua and Richard (Meet Your Patients) for sensory alterations? You may need to review the Meet Your Patients scenario at the beginning of this chapter to answer this question.

Promoting Adaptation to the Hospital Environment

Changes in any aspect of the sensory experience can be unsettling for patients. Simple changes in approach and environment demonstrate a caring attitude, promote patient trust, and help to minimize the stress of the hospitalization.

- Approach the patient in a calm and reassuring manner.
- Promote a stress-free environment: limit noise, adjust lighting, eliminate clutter, and avoid multiple people gathering or multiple tasks to complete at one time.
- Assist persons with any assistive devices, such as eyeglasses, eye shades, dentures, hearing aids, or gloves, to facilitate optimal sensory perception experiences.
- Control temperature to patient's preference.
- Allow the patient time to speak and express concerns.
- Explore therapeutic touch if the person is receptive.
- Consider using alternative therapies, such as music therapy, that may be soothing and comforting to the patient.

DIAGNOSIS/ANALYZING CUES

The Clinical Care Classification System 2.5 (CCC, n.d.) identifies the following diagnostic labels to describe sensory-perceptual problems:

> Confusion
> Memory Impairment
> Home Maintenance Alteration
> Peripheral Alteration
> Unilateral Neglect

Disturbances and deficits in sensory perception may also be the etiology of other nursing diagnoses. Examples include the following:

> Fall Risk r/t impaired vision
> Injury Risk r/t reduced tactile sensation
> Bathing/Hygiene Deficit r/t kinesthetic deficit
> Body Nutrition Deficit r/t loss of appetite secondary to impaired taste
> Social interaction alteration r/t embarrassment about memory impairment

PLANNING/PRIORITIZING HYPOTHESES AND GENERATING SOLUTIONS

Examples of *Nursing Outcomes Classification (NOC) standardized outcomes* associated with sensory perception and deficits depend on the specific problem identified. Following are examples:

For Sensory Deficits: Sensory Function: Vision; Sensory Function: Hearing; Appetite
For Confusion: Cognitive Orientation, Information Processing
For Memory Deficit: Cognition, Memory
For Unilateral Neglect: Heedfulness of Affected Side; Body Positioning: Self-Initiated

For other outcomes, refer to the Example Client Conditions for sensory deprivation, sensory overload, and sensory deficits.

Individualized goals/outcomes statements you might write for a client with sensory-perception problems include the following:

- Compensates for visual impairment by maximizing the use of touch and hearing.
- Effectively copes with excessive, environmental stimuli.
- Demonstrates proper use of hearing aid.
- Participates in at least one activity daily.

▰ IMPLEMENTATION/TAKING ACTION

Nursing Interventions Classification (NIC) standardized interventions for sensory-perceptual deficits include the following examples:

For Sensory Deficits: See Example Client Condition: Sensory Deficits

For Acute Confusion: Cognitive Stimulation, Reality Orientation

For Chronic Confusion: Anxiety Reduction, Dementia Management

For Impaired Memory: Memory Training, Neurological Monitoring, Surveillance

For Unilateral Neglect: Self-Care Assistance, Unilateral Neglect Management

Specific nursing activities to address sensory perception problems are based on the nursing diagnosis chosen, especially on its etiology, and on the particular client's needs. Common nursing activities are discussed in the following sections and in the Example Client Condition features.

Promoting Optimal Sensory Function

Optimal sensory function requires periodic health screening, along with early identification and treatment of health problems. Comprehensive healthcare is the ideal approach because sensory problems are often related to other health disorders. For example, to protect their vision, a client with hypertension needs to have periodic eye examinations and control their blood pressure.

 Think**Like a Nurse** 27-5: Clinical Judgment **in Action**

Which of the strategies to treat sensory deprivation would be most appropriate for Richard (Meet Your Patients)?

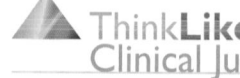 Think**Like a Nurse** 27-6: Clinical Judgment **in Action**

Review the scenario of Joshua, the young ICU patient with sensory overload (Meet Your Patients).

- Which strategies to prevent sensory overload would be most appropriate for an ICU patient?

- Which would be least likely to be successful or not feasible based on the setting?

Provide rationales for your choices. You may need to visit an ICU or talk with classmates who have been to an ICU to answer this question.

KnowledgeCheck 27-6

- Identify three safety measures that may be used with clients with visual impairment.
- Identify three safety measures that may be used with clients with hearing impairment.

Protecting Brain Health

To protect cognitive health in individuals of all ages:

- Be physically active.
- Be intellectually active and continually seek opportunities to learn, remember, or solve problems.
- Engage in personal and social relationships and activities.
- Consume a healthy diet to avoid nutrient deficiency, although dietary supplements might not prevent cognitive decline.
- Reduce risk factors for cardiovascular disease, including hypertension, diabetes, and tobacco use.
- Avoid mind-altering medication, if possible.
- Get adequate sleep; seek professional treatment for sleep disorders, if needed.
- Avoid heavy alcohol consumption. (Blazer et al., 2015).

Caring for Patients With Confusion

Confusion interferes with the ability to interpret stimuli accurately. It can be temporary or permanent. Confusion is an aspect of both delirium and dementia.

- **Delirium** is an acute, reversible state of mind caused by medications and a variety of physiological processes, such as hypoxia, metabolic disturbances, infection, or sensory alterations. It may be accompanied by confusion, restlessness, illusions, incoherence of thought and speech, and changes in the LOC.
- **Dementia** is a chronic and progressive deterioration in cognitive functioning caused by physical changes in the brain and is not associated with changing LOC. A person with dementia has problems with thinking, remembering, learning, and reasoning. Changes in language skills, visual perception, and personality 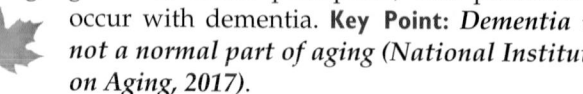 occur with dementia. **Key Point: *Dementia is not a normal part of aging (National Institute on Aging, 2017).***

Sensory deprivation, overload, and deficit can all contribute to confusion; therefore, the following interventions may apply to any of the Example Client Conditions.

Promote Orientation

- Introduce yourself and state the client's name each time you meet with them.
- Wear a readable name tag (large, plain type) to reinforce your introduction.
- Identify the day, date, and time as you interact.
- Provide visual clues to time, such as opening the drapes during the day and closing them at night and placing calendars and clocks where they are easy to see.
- Place personal objects, photos, and mementos in the immediate environment, and discuss them with the client.
- Encourage the patient to participate in familiar activities, such as bathing.

Simplify Your Communications A confused patient cannot interpret stimuli accurately and may not understand what you say.

- Speak slowly and allow adequate time for the client to answer any questions you raise.
- Face the client and speak calmly, simply, and directly.
- Provide simple explanations for all care and treatments.
- Use short sentences with few words: "It's bath time," rather than, "Let's go have a bath and get you all nice and clean for visitors."
- Do not offer too many choices.

♥ **iCare Relieve Anxiety** People with dementia (a common cause of confusion) are often anxious and fearful. Find ways to make the person feel more secure and comfortable before you focus on the content of your conversations.

- Gently hold or pat the patient's hand, but use touch cautiously.
- Realize that the person is probably distressed and is doing the best they can. Be affectionate, reassuring, and calm, even when the things they say make no sense.
- Try to respond to the person's feelings instead of the content of their words. This helps to reassure them. For example, if a patient is constantly searching for their husband, don't say, "Your husband is not here." Rather, say, "You must miss your husband" or "Tell me about your husband."
- If the person has difficulty finding the right word, supply it for them unless it upsets them. This can help control their frustration.
- If you do not understand what the patient is trying to say, ask them to point to it or describe it (e.g., "What does a *zishmer* look like?").
- Consider using alternative therapy, such as music therapy.

Provide for Safety Recognize that the client's decision making may be poor. Maintain a safe environment. For example, store medications away from the patient's reach, keep doors and windows closed securely, and use bed or chair monitors to prevent wandering.

♥ **iCare Provide Continuity of Care When Possible** Establish a routine for care and assign the same caregivers each day when possible. Continuity of care has a positive impact on patients' clinical condition (Yakusheva & Costa, 2017).

KnowledgeCheck 27-7

- What are the major concerns associated with loss of smell and taste?
- What safety measures should be taught to a client with tactile impairment?
- How can you best assist a client who is confused?

Caring for Patients With Altered Level of Consciousness

Consciousness is the state of being wakeful and aware of self, time, and the surroundings. **Unconsciousness** is an abnormal neurological state resulting from disturbance of sensory perception to the extent that the patient is not aware of what is happening around them, is not responsive, and is not oriented. Unconscious patients are dependent on the nurse for patent airway, nutrition and hydration, comfort, elimination, range of motion, skin care, sensory stimulation, and family support and education, as well as the following:

- **Safety measures.** Nurses have a responsibility to protect patients from injury, falls, and medical complications (aspiration, pneumonia, pressure ulcers, urinary retention). Keep the bed in a low position when you are not at the bedside, and keep the siderails up.
- **Eye care.** If the patient's blink reflex is absent or their eyes do not close totally, you may need to give frequent eye care to keep secretions from collecting along the lid margins. On the other hand, you might need to cover the eyes or apply lubricating drops to prevent corneal drying.
- **Oral care.** Patients with lower LOC need oral care because they cannot take fluids by mouth and the oral mucosa can dry out.
- **Pressure injury prevention.** Patients need frequent turning, positioning, and skin care to prevent pressure injuries.
- **Immobility.** Range of motion is necessary for immobile patients to prevent muscle shortening and contractures.

Caring for Patients at Risk for Seizures

Seizures place the patient at high risk for injury from falls and airway obstruction. Institute seizure precautions for patients with any of the following:

- A new diagnosis of a seizure disorder or any seizure activity within the past 12 months
- Frequent seizure activity
- History of head trauma (including surgery) within the past 3 years

Toward Evidence-Based Practice

Sommerlad, A., Sabia, S., Singh-Manoux, A., Lewis, G., & Livingston, G. (2019, August 2). Association of social contact with dementia and cognition: 28-year follow-up of the Whitehall II cohort study. *PLOS Medicine, 16*(8), e1002862. https://doi.org/10.1371/journal.pmed.1002862

In a study involving 10,228 participants who were tested six times over 28 years, researchers found that more frequent social contact during early and midlife helped to preserve cognitive function, which delays or prevents the onset of dementia.

Wood, E. B., Halverson, A., Harrison, G., & Rosenkranz, A. (2019, July). Creating a sensory-friendly pediatric emergency department. *Journal of Emergency Nursing, 45*(4), 415–424. https://doi.org/10.1016/j.jen.2018.12.002

Children with autism spectrum disorder (ASD) and sensory-processing disorder (SPD) are at risk for sensory overload, especially when receiving care within a noisy and chaotic setting, such as an emergency department setting. Researchers studied the effect of modifying the patient care environment and patient-flow process for patients with ASD and SPD. They found that such measures resulted in calmer, safer, and more effective healthcare visits for children with unique sensory needs.

Sargolzaei, K., Shaghaee Fallah, M., Aghebati, N., Esmaily, H., & Farzadfard, M. T. (2017). Effect of a structured sensory stimulation program on the sensory function of patients with stroke-induced disorder of consciousness. *Evidence-Based Care, 7*(2), 7–16. https://doi.org/10.22038/ebcj.2017.23807.1505

Nearly half of stroke patients experience sensory deprivation. Researchers implemented a 14-day sensory stimulation program consisting of the following components:

- Auditory—verbal communication, music, recorded voices
- Visual—flashlight, photos, objects, mirror
- Olfactory—pleasant scents
- Gustatory—oral rinse, gum massage, lemon swabs
- Tactile—massage, washing with cold and warm water
- Motor—passive range of motion

Using the Sensory Modality Assessment and Rehabilitation Technique (SMART) instrument, researchers found that sensory stimulation improved sensory function for patients suffering sensory deprivation after a stroke and also reduced sensory deprivation.

Sollami, A., Gianferrari, E., Alfieri, M., Artioli, G., & Taffurelli, C. (2017). Pet therapy: An effective strategy to care for the elderly? An experimental study in a nursing home. *Acta Bio Medica Atenei Parmensis, 88*(1-S), 25–31. https://doi.org/10.23750/abm.v88i1-S.6281

Researchers studied the effectiveness of pet therapy as an intervention to improve the quality of life for elderly residents in long-term skilled-care facilities who experience sensory deficits, social isolation, impaired communication, and depression. Using measures of well-being, the researchers found a significant improvement in mood and reductions in anxiety, loneliness, and apathy in residents who spent time with dogs in the nursing home. The human–dog interaction led to positive behaviors (e.g., smiles, willingness to communicate, and spontaneity in interaction) that are consistent with other measures representing quality of life.

1. What ideas do you have for maximizing cognitive health for a patient at risk for dementia?

2. The nurse is caring for a child with sensory processing disorder (SPD) who comes to the emergency department for a deep laceration to the foot. The child's behavior is combative while the provider is suturing the injury. What action might the nurse take to deescalate the intensity of the situation and reduce sensory input?

3. When caring for a patient in a comatose state, what strategies would you recommend for reducing sensory deprivation? How might you teach families to interact with their loved one who is unresponsive?

4. How might pet therapy be effective in reducing deprivation in elderly residents in a long-term care facility?

- Withdrawal of antiseizure medication or adjustment of the medication regimen

Key Point: *The goal of seizure precautions is to protect the patient from injury and prevent serious complications.*

For a comprehensive discussion of nursing care for patients with a seizure disorder, see Example Client Condition: Seizures.

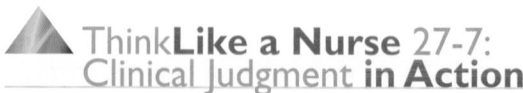

ThinkLike a Nurse 27-7: Clinical Judgment in Action

What types of interventions would be most appropriate for Joshua and Richard (Meet Your Patients)—that is, interventions for sensory deficits, sensory deprivation, sensory overload, or confusion?

EXAMPLE CLIENT CONDITION: Seizures

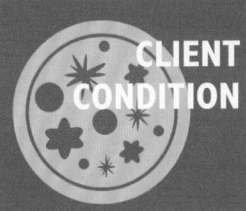

CLIENT CONDITION

Seizures—the abrupt onset of disturbance in electrical activity in the brain; neurons fire abnormally.

- Motor symptoms: rhythmic jerking of the limbs
- Decreased level or a loss of consciousness Symptoms and the duration of the seizure vary, depending on the area of the brain affected.

Duration

- Short in duration—30 seconds to 3 or 4 minutes but may be a medical emergency if lasting more than 5 minutes or if breathing stops.

Incidence

- Most prevalent in children < age 10 and those > age 65
- More common among male individuals, especially in children
- Children with seizures commonly outgrow the condition.

General Types of Seizure

- **Generalized seizures**—widespread electrical activity on both sides of the brain at once
- **Focal seizures (partial seizures)**—electrical discharge from one side in a limited area of the brain
- **Recurrent seizures**—due to a brain disorder called **epilepsy**

Common Causes

- Epilepsy
- Brain tumor
- Brain injury (concussion, hematoma, edema)
- Low oxygen at birth
- Meningitis, encephalitis
- Hypoglycemia
- Stroke
- Genetic conditions (tuberous sclerosis)
- Medication; drug overdose
- Abnormal formation of the brain before birth
- Electrical shock
- Sometimes no cause can be identified.

Common Triggers

- Sleep deprivation
- Stress
- Illness
- Hormone fluctuations (menstruation, puberty)
- High or rapid-onset fevers (especially children 3 months to 6 years)
- Heavy alcohol use
- Drug interactions with seizure medication or missing doses
- Ingesting mood-altering substances
- Rapidly flashing, bright light or certain visual patterns
- Vitamin B_6 deficiency
- Low serum calcium, magnesium, and sodium

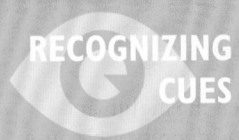

RECOGNIZING COMPLICATIONS

- Respiratory depression or arrest
- Tongue biting, bleeding, avulsion
- Social stigma, withdrawal, and isolation
- Impact on the family, stress, fear of recurring episodes

- Medications can cause anhedonia (lack of sexual pleasure)
- Some types of epilepsy can lead to underemployment, learning differences/delays, and memory lapses.

RECOGNIZING CUES

Specific Seizure Types

- **Tonic-clonic (grand mal)**—general body stiffening, rhythmic jerking of limbs, loss of consciousness, loss of bladder or bowel control
- **Clonic**—spasms of face, neck, or arm muscles
- **Tonic**—brief spasms of arms, legs, or trunk, often during sleep
- **Atonic**—sudden loss of muscle tone. Also called *drop seizures*.
- **Myoclonic**—muscle spasms that resemble the sensation of a shock
- **Absence (petit mal)**—brief disconnection, such as blank stare, eyes rolling back, or fluttering lids

Nursing Assessments

- Assess for triggers and risk factors (see Etiologies).
- Assess the airway during and after a seizure.
- Observe for nystagmus, drooling, confusion, motor activity, staring, breathing quality.
- Observe postseizure behavior: muscle strength, ability to speak, memory, and orientation.

(continued)

EXAMPLE CLIENT CONDITION: Seizures—cont'd

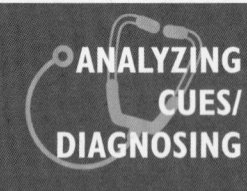

ANALYZING CUES/ DIAGNOSING

NANDA-I Nursing Diagnoses

- Activity Alteration
- Airway Clearance Impairment
- Caregiver Role Strain
- Cerebral Alteration
- Confusion
- Fear
- Injury Risk
- Memory Impairment
- Noncompliance of Medication Regimen
- Impaired Verbal Communication
- Decreased Diversional Activity
- Self Concept Alteration
- Socialization Alteration
- Thought Process Alteration
- Sleep Pattern Disturbance

GENERATING SOLUTIONS

NOC Outcomes

- *Seizure Self-Control* (e.g., avoids seizure triggers and risk factors)
- *Seizure Severity* (rate from "none" to "severe"), preferably using a seizure severity scale

Individualized Outcomes

- Remains seizure-free
- Remains injury-free
- Practices habits of healthy living, with good sleep, healthy diet, minimal alcohol use, minimal video gaming
- Complies with medication regime

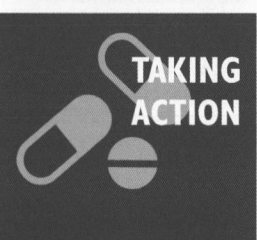

COLLABORATING

Diagnosing Seizures

- **Electroencephalogram (EEG)** records brain wave activity.
- **Magnetic resonance imaging (MRI) or computed tomography (CT) scan** to rule out tumor or other causes
- **Lumbar puncture (spinal tap)** to detect meningitis

Treating Seizures

- **Antiseizure medication**—carbamazepine, diazepam, lorazepam, clonazepam, brivaracetam
- **Vagal nerve stimulation** (VNS)—device under the skin to activate a response from vagal nerve to stop seizure activity
- **Diet**—ketogenic diet with very low carbohydrate and high fat intake can reduce the frequency and/or duration of seizures.

TAKING ACTION

Seizure Precautions

The goal of seizure precautions is to protect the patient from injury and prevent serious complications.

Before a Seizure Event

- Explain to the patient the reasons for the precautions.
- If the patient has frequent or prolonged seizures, establish IV access for diazepam if hospitalized. For intermittent episodes, use rectal diazepam, lorazepam, or midazolam.
- Obtain a bed with full-length siderails.
- Cover the headboard, footboard, and siderails with commercial pads or bath blankets. Tape the blankets in place.
- Keep the rails raised and the bed in low position.
- Place oral or nasal suction equipment at the bedside. Test to be certain it is working.
- Place an airway at the bedside or tape to the wall, depending on your agency protocol.
- Make sure the family knows how to summon help when a seizure occurs.

- Assign the patient to a room in close proximity to the nurses' station.

When a Seizure Occurs

- If you are present when the patient reports having an aura, help them into bed, lower the head, and raise the siderails. If it occurs in another location, help them to the floor; put something soft under their head.
- Provide privacy.
- Turn the patient on their side.
- Stay with the patient.
- Do not attempt to open the mouth and insert a padded tongue depressor because:
  - *This can push the tongue back into the pharynx, causing airway obstruction.*
  - *The patient might bite your fingers.*
  - *If you are anxious, you could break the patient's teeth trying to insert the depressor.*
- Loosen restrictive clothing.
- Move hard or sharp objects out of the way.
- Do not try to restrain the patient or control their movements.
- If the seizure is prolonged, administer oxygen.

EXAMPLE CLIENT CONDITION: Seizures—cont'd

- Administer prescribed antiseizure medication if seizure is prolonged, typically >6 minutes.
- You cannot delegate care of the patient who is having a seizure because nursing assessments and interventions are required. Ask unlicensed assistive personnel to obtain help.
- Usually little nursing action is required beyond preventing physical injury and maintaining a patent airway. The exception is with status epilepticus, in which the patient has repeated seizures without regaining consciousness. **Key Point: *Status epilepticus is a medical emergency; notify healthcare provider immediately.***

After the Seizure
- Turn the patient on their side and apply suction, if needed.
- Reorient and reassure the patient and make them comfortable. If the patient was incontinent, change bedding and clothing.
- Examine for injuries.
- Keep the room quiet; dim the lighting.
- Stay with the patient because they may be sleepy or confused.

- Do not give any food or drink until the patient is fully conscious and alert.
- Monitor vital signs and mental status every 15 to 30 minutes for 2 hours.
- Observe postseizure behavior: evaluate muscle strength, ability to speak, memory, and orientation.
- Pad the siderails, if not already done.
- Ask the patient whether they experienced an aura and what activities preceded the seizure.
- Document characteristics of the seizure:
  How it started
  Location and duration of motor activity
  Type of movements (e.g., stiffening, jerking, twitching, loss of muscle tone)
  Crying out
  Visual and auditory symptoms
  Tachycardia
  Pupil dilation
  Change in level of consciousness
- Note the first symptom and how the seizure progressed.
- You may need to perform suctioning after the episode to prevent aspiration of oral secretions.

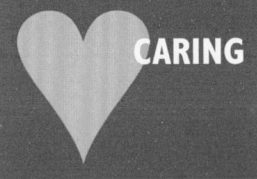

CARING

♥ iCare • Listen empathetically to stresses, concerns, fears, and intrapersonal issues the person may be experiencing.
- Encourage self-help groups to boost self-esteem and coping skills.

- Provide support for those dealing with restrictions in driving, recreational activities (e.g., swimming), or employment.

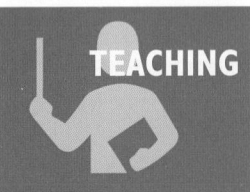

TEACHING

Lifestyle Management
- Get sufficient rest; eat a healthy diet.
- Avoid video gaming and flashing lights.
- Visit primary care provider regularly or epileptologist as needed.

- Take prescribed antiseizure medication on time.
- Avoid excess alcohol and drugs that interact with antiseizure medications.
- Consider use of a seizure dog trained to alert to seizures.

To explore learning resources for this chapter,

Go to Davis Advantage and find:

Answers and Suggested Responses for all questions in this chapter
Concept Map
Knowledge Map
References and Bibliography

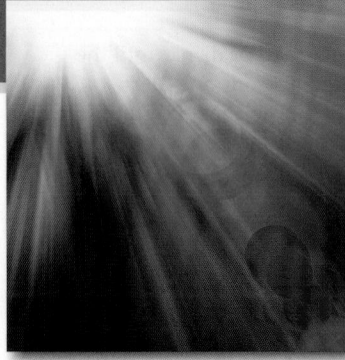

CHAPTER 28

Pain

Learning Outcomes

After completing this chapter, you should be able to:

➤ Define *pain*.
➤ Classify pain according to origin, cause, duration, and quality.
➤ Describe the physiological changes that occur with pain.
➤ Discuss two physiological mechanisms involved in pain modulation.
➤ Discuss factors that influence pain.
➤ Identify the effect of unrelieved pain on each of the body systems.
➤ Discuss nonpharmacological pain relief measures.
➤ Describe pharmacological measures, including nonopioid analgesics, opioid analgesics, and adjuvant analgesics.
➤ Describe chemical and surgical pain relief measures.

➤ Explain why pain should be considered the fifth vital sign.
➤ Identify the steps involved in creating a pain management program for a client.
➤ Individualize goals and interventions for clients with a nursing diagnosis of Acute Pain (Clinical Care Classification [CCC], n.d.).
➤ Individualize goals and interventions for clients with a nursing diagnosis of Chronic Pain (CCC, n.d.).
➤ Explain how to use a patient-controlled analgesia (PCA) system.
➤ Describe a method for evaluating the effectiveness of a pain management program.

Key Concepts

Pain
Pain management

Related Concepts

See the Concept Map on Davis Advantage.

Meet Your Patient

As a special experience, your instructor has arranged for you to spend a clinical shift in the intensive care unit (ICU). As you enter the ICU, you are a little apprehensive. You walk into the room with your clinical instructor to meet your patient, Ms. Eunice Chu Ling, a 23-year-old woman of Asian descent who was in a motor vehicle accident yesterday and sustained chest and abdominal injuries. She was taken to surgery during the night to have her spleen removed. She is intubated (meaning she has an endotracheal tube in her airway that is connected to a ventilator), has IV fluids infusing, and has a chest tube on the left side that is draining blood-tinged fluid. Her parents and siblings are in the room, sitting rigidly in the chairs, smiling at you. Ms. Chu Ling is awake and grimacing. You want to ask her whether she is in pain, but she cannot speak.

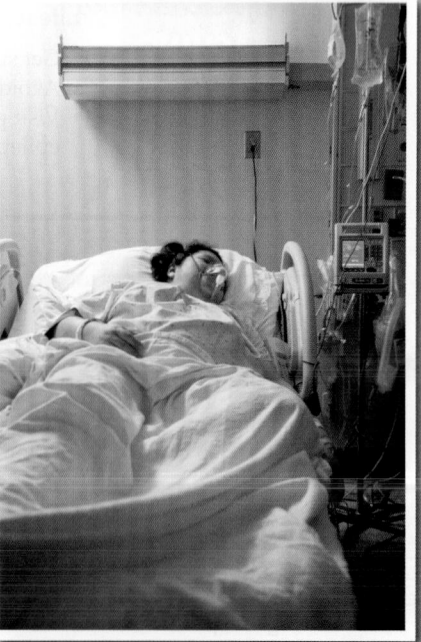

Theoretical Knowledge
knowing **why**

Pain is one of the most distressing symptoms nurses deal with, and it is the most frequent reason people seek healthcare (Santos Torres et al., 2015). The most common causes of death, such as heart disease, cancer, and chronic lower respiratory diseases, are associated with pain. The following are some facts about the incidence of pain:

■ More than 1 in 5 American adults experiences chronic pain; a majority of adults with chronic pain report poor sleep quality (National Sleep Foundation, 2015; Pacheco & Rehman, 2022).

■ Approximately 60% of all community-dwelling adults over the age of 65 and up to 80% of older adults in long-term care facilities report pain that interferes with normal functioning (Herr & Garand, 2001).

■ In spite of measures to relieve pain, more than half of all hospitalized patients experience moderate to severe pain in their last week of life (Tolle et al., 2000).

■ The most commonly reported types of pain are headaches, facial aches, joint pain, lower back, and neck pain.

ABOUT THE KEY CONCEPTS

In this chapter, you will begin to understand the key concepts of **pain** and **pain management.** Related concepts, such as **transduction, transmission, perception,** and **modulation,** will help you to know what pain is and why it occurs, how to better assess it, and how to manage patients' experience of acute and chronic pain.

WHAT IS PAIN?

The following are two descriptions of pain:

■ "**Pain** is an unpleasant sensory and emotional experience association with actual or potential tissue damage or described in terms of such damage" (American Pain Society [APS], 1994, p. 16; Merskey & Bogduk, 1994, p. 971).

■ **Pain** is "whatever the person says it is, and existing whenever the person says it does" (McCaffery, 1968, p. 95). In other words, pain is a subjective experience. Unlike a pulse or blood pressure, you cannot measure pain objectively. In addition, your expectations of your patients' pain will be influenced by your own values, ideals, and life experiences. As McCaffery's definition indicates, you will need to put aside your personal beliefs about pain and focus on the *patient's* experience.

The following are a few facts you should remember about pain:

■ **The pain experience can significantly interfere with a person's quality of life** and affect nearly every aspect of daily living. For example, severe pain can affect job performance, coping skills, engagement in social activities, sexual intimacy, sleep and rest, ability to exercise, and ability to perform activities of daily living; thus, it can be destructive to both the patient and family.

■ **Although we usually think of pain in this negative context, pain is also protective,** warning us of potential injury to the body. Pain can also prompt us to change our actions: after you have been sitting at the computer for a while, muscle pain may prompt you to get up and stretch or go out for a walk, or the thought of pain with an injury may motivate you to be careful when handling sharp objects.

■ **You will be able to manage pain more effectively if you can recognize the type of pain** the patient is experiencing. But remember that patients often experience more than one kind of pain.

Pain can be classified by its origin, cause or type, duration and onset, and quality (which includes intensity and pattern of occurrence).

Origin of Pain

The *origin* of pain refers to the site where pain is felt, not necessarily the source of pain.

Cutaneous or **superficial pain** arises in the skin or the subcutaneous tissue (e.g., a burn or an abrasion). Although the injury is superficial, it may cause short-term pain.

Visceral pain is caused by the stimulation of deep internal pain receptors. It is most often experienced in the abdominal cavity, cranium, or thorax. Visceral pain is not well localized and can be described as tight, pressure, or crampy pain. The description of the quality and extent of the pain often serves as a strong clue to the cause. Menstrual cramps, labor pain, gastrointestinal (GI) infections, bowel disorders, and organ cancers all produce visceral pain.

Deep somatic pain originates in the ligaments, tendons, nerves, blood vessels, and bones. Deep somatic pain is localized and can be described as achy or tender. A fracture or sprain, arthritis, and bone cancer can cause deep somatic pain.

Radiating pain starts at the origin but extends to other locations. For instance, the pain of a severe sore throat may extend to the ears and head. Or the pain of an episode of gastroesophageal reflux (heartburn) may radiate outward from the sternum to involve the entire upper thorax.

Referred pain occurs in an area that is distant from the original site. For example, the pain from a heart attack may be experienced down the left arm, through the back, or into the jaw. See Figure 28-1 for other examples of referred pain.

Phantom pain is pain that is perceived to originate from an area that has been surgically removed.

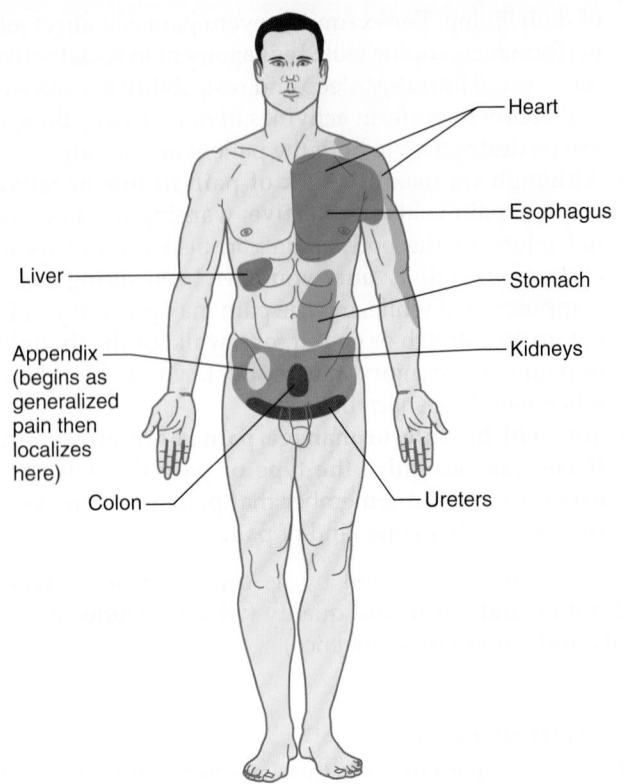

- Heart
- Esophagus
- Liver
- Stomach
- Kidneys
- Appendix (begins as generalized pain then localizes here)
- Colon
- Ureters

FIGURE 28-1 Most common areas of referred pain.

Patients with amputated limbs may still perceive that the limb exists and experience burning, itching, and deep pain in that area.

Psychogenic pain refers to pain that is believed to arise from the mind. The patient perceives the pain despite the fact that no physical cause can be identified. Psychogenic pain can be just as severe as pain from a physical cause. See the discussion of somatoform pain disorder in Chapter 9 if you would like more information.

Cause of Pain

Physical pain is either nociceptive or neuropathic. These two types, or sources, of pain differ in the way they affect the patient as well as in how they are treated.

Nociceptive Pain **Nociceptive pain** is the most common type of pain. It occurs when pain receptors **(nociceptors)** respond to stimuli that are potentially damaging, for example, as a result of noxious thermal, chemical, or mechanical stimuli. Nociceptive pain results from injury to body tissues (e.g., trauma, surgery, or inflammation). It is most commonly described as aching. Two types of nociceptive pain are:

- **Visceral pain** (i.e., pain originating from internal organs)
- **Somatic pain** (i.e., pain originating from the skin, muscles, bones, or connective tissue)

Neuropathic Pain **Neuropathic pain** is a complex and often chronic pain that arises when injury to one or

more nerves results in repeated transmission of pain signals, even in the absence of painful stimuli. Neuropathic pain is described as burning, numbness, itching, and "pins and needles" prickling pain. Nerve pain may be described as stabbing or feeling like an electrical shock or even hypersensitivity to light touch or temperature. Pain may affect a large part of the body or be localized to small areas.

The nerve injury may originate from any of a variety of conditions, such as poorly controlled diabetes, a stroke, a tumor, alcoholism, amputation, injury, or a viral infection (e.g., shingles). Some medications, such as chemotherapeutic agents, can trigger nerve injuries that may cause neuropathic pain even after the medication is discontinued.

Duration of Pain

Acute Pain **Acute pain** has a short duration and is generally rapid in onset. It varies in intensity and may last up to 6 months (APS, 1994). This type of pain is most frequently associated with injury or surgery. It is protective in that it indicates potential or actual tissue damage. Although acute pain may absorb a patient's physical and emotional energy for a short time, it is helpful for the patient to know that it will generally disappear as the tissues heal.

Chronic Pain **Chronic pain**, also called *persistent pain*, lasts 3 to 6 months or longer and often interferes with daily activities. Often, persistent pain is related to a chronic illness (e.g., neuralgia related to diabetes), cancer, or musculoskeletal issues (e.g., osteoarthritis, traumatic injury, torn cartilage, fibromyalgia). Patients with chronic pain may experience periods of remission and exacerbation. People experiencing chronic pain fall more often, have sleep disturbances and poor appetite, and experience other impairments in activities of daily living (ADLs). It may lead to emotional distress, withdrawal, depression, anger, frustration, dependence, fatigue, and catastrophizing (Vlaeyen & Linton, 2000). Persistent pain is the most feared aspect of cancer or other progressive diseases (American Geriatrics Society, Panel on Persistent Pain in Older Persons, 2009).

Intractable Pain **Intractable pain** is both chronic and highly resistant to relief. This type of pain is especially frustrating for the patient and care provider. It should be approached with multiple methods of pain relief.

Quality of Pain

The words patients use to describe the quality of their pain help care providers to determine the probable cause and most effective treatment.

- **Pain quality** may be described as *sharp* or *dull, aching, throbbing, stabbing, burning, ripping, searing,* or *tingling*.
- **Pain periodicity** may be referred to as *episodic, intermittent,* or *constant*.

■ **Pain intensity** is described with a variety of terms, such as *mild, distracting, moderate, severe,* or *intolerable.*

KnowledgeCheck 28-1

How would you classify the pain that the following patients are experiencing? Consider origin, cause, duration, and quality.

■ A patient with metastatic cancer
■ A patient with back pain that was the result of an automobile injury a year ago
■ A patient who had bowel surgery yesterday
■ A patient with a fractured leg
■ A patient who just had their leg amputated but feels as though the leg is still there
■ A patient who just received a paper cut while turning the pages of a book

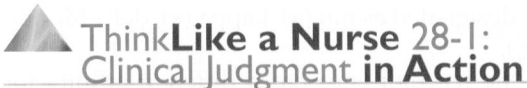 **ThinkLike a Nurse** 28-1: Clinical Judgment **in Action**

How would you expect a patient with neuropathic pain to appear?

WHAT HAPPENS WHEN SOMEONE HAS PAIN?

Review the story of Eunice Chu Ling in the Meet Your Patient scenario. Eunice had been in an auto accident that caused severe injuries. She has had surgery and requires monitoring and invasive devices, such as a ventilator and IV line. You can see that she is grimacing. Consider these aspects of Eunice's experience as we explore the physiology of pain.

Transduction

Pain-sensitive *nociceptors* (sensory nerve cells) are found in the skin, subcutaneous tissue, joints, walls of the arteries, and most internal organs. The skin has the highest density of nociceptors, and the internal organs the least. Painful stimuli prompt the release of substances that trigger the release of inflammatory chemicals. These cause an injured area to become red, swollen, and hot. Inflammation is the most frequent cause of pain.

In the process of **transduction,** nociceptors become activated by the perception of potentially damaging mechanical, thermal, and chemical stimuli.

Mechanical Stimuli Mechanical stimuli are external forces that result in pressure or friction against the body. They involve stretching of tissue in joints and body cavities related to bleeding and swelling, in addition to compression of body tissues caused by the force of the accident. Other types of mechanical stimuli are surgical incisions, friction, or skin shearing (e.g., sliding down in bed or pressure from a mechanical device, such as a cast or brace).

Thermal Stimuli Thermal stimuli result from exposure to heat or cold. If you've ever touched a hot object

and rapidly pulled away or suffered an earache when outdoors on a cold day, you have experienced pain from thermal stimuli.

Chemical Stimuli Chemical stimuli can be internal or external. An example of *external* chemical stimuli is lemon juice or any acidic substance that, when in contact with an open area in the skin, causes sharp, sudden pain. In contrast, the chest pain experienced during a myocardial infarction (heart attack) is caused by *internal* chemical stimuli, specifically, the chemical changes that result from tissue ischemia.

Transmission

Peripheral nerves carry the pain message to the dorsal horn of the spinal cord in a process known as **transmission** (Fig. 28-2).

Transmission to the Spinal Cord Pain messages are conducted to the spinal cord along either of two types of fibers:

■ **A-delta fibers** are large-diameter myelinated fibers that transmit impulses at 6 to 31 meters per second. These fibers transmit *fast pain impulses* from acute, focused mechanical and thermal stimuli. For instance, when you bump your knee, the initial sharp pain is carried by A-delta fibers. Pleasurable stimuli to skin receptors, such as from massage, also stimulate A-delta fibers.

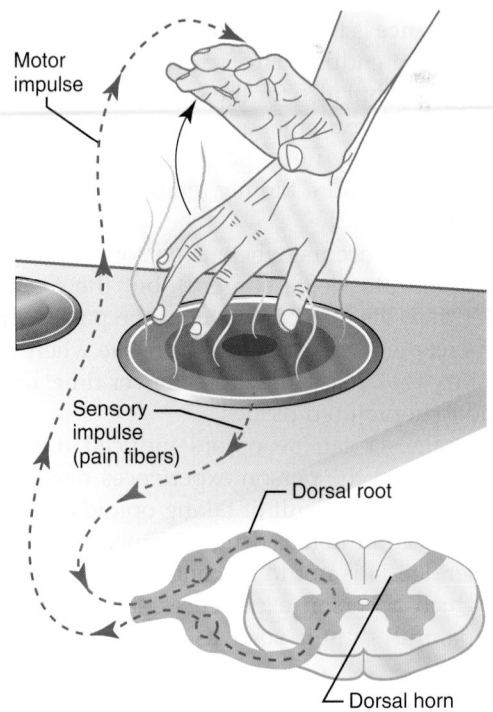

FIGURE 28-2 After nociceptors are activated, pain is transmitted along A-delta fibers or C fibers to the dorsal horn of the spinal cord. From there, the pain message is sent to the brain for perception.

- **C fibers** are smaller unmyelinated fibers that transmit *slow pain impulses,* that is, dull, diffuse pain impulses that travel at a slow rate. C fibers conduct pain from mechanical, thermal, and chemical stimuli. If you bump your knee, the lingering ache in the tissue will be carried by C fibers.

Transmission to the Brain   Pain transmission from the spinal cord involves endogenous chemicals called **neurotransmitters.** Most pain impulses are sent to the thalamus of the brain, which acts as an integrating center to direct the impulses to three regions of the brain:

1. The **somatosensory cortex** perceives and interprets physical sensations.
2. The **limbic system** is involved in emotional reactions to stimuli.
3. The **frontal cortex** is involved in thought and reason. This is when the person perceives pain.

Pain Perception

Perception involves the recognition and definition of pain in the frontal cortex.

- **Pain threshold** is the point at which the brain recognizes and defines a stimulus as pain. The number and intensity of stimuli necessary to produce pain, as well as the duration and characteristics of the pain produced, vary from patient to patient. Although the pain threshold usually remains fairly constant for an individual over time, repeated experience with pain can reduce a patient's threshold.
- **Pain tolerance** is the **duration** or intensity of pain that a person can endure. This varies not only from person to person but also for the same person in different situations. For example, a parent donating a kidney to their child may not report as much postoperative pain as if they had a kidney removed because it was cancerous.
- **Hyperalgesia** occurs when a person experiences a painful stimulus (e.g., surgery), but the response is greater than the expected level of the pain. Increased pain perception may occur in the tissue where the initial injury took place and worsen over time, or it may spread to noninjured tissues.
  - Hyperalgesia can be opioid induced (OIH). This occurs when the person experiences new or worsening pain as a result of taking opioids. OIH is not the same condition as drug tolerance.
  - Hyperalgesia is not to be confused with **allodynia,** in which a person experiences significant pain to nonpainful stimuli such as brushing against the skin.

Pain Modulation

A process called **modulation** changes the perception of pain by either facilitating or inhibiting pain signals through the endogenous analgesia system and the gate-control mechanism.

The Endogenous Analgesia System

In the **endogenous analgesia system,** neurons in the brainstem activate descending nerve fibers that conduct impulses back to the spinal cord. These impulses trigger the release of endogenous opioids and other substances to block the continuing pain impulses and provide pain relief. **Endogenous opioids** are naturally occurring analgesic neurotransmitters (enkephalins, dynorphins, and beta-endorphins) that inhibit the transmission of pain impulses.

- Endogenous opioids bind to opiate receptor sites in the central and peripheral nervous systems at four receptor sites, designated as mu (μ), kappa (κ), delta (δ), and sigma (Σ).
- Each of the receptor sites has a different affinity for various medications.
- Nonpharmacological measures can also prompt the release of endogenous opioids.

The Gate-Control Theory

Pain impulses can also be modulated at the spinal level. In explaining the mechanism of pain perception, the **gate-control theory of pain modulation** suggests that the perception of pain does not occur by direct stimulation of only nociceptors (pain-producing fiber). Instead, pain is perceived by the interplay between two kinds of fibers—those that produce pain and those that inhibit pain.

C (Small, Slow) Fibers   C fibers produce pain. As slow pain impulses travel along C (small) fibers from the periphery to the brain, they encounter a "gate" that either allows or blocks the transmission of the pain sensation to the brain. If the source of stimulation is nonpainful, the gate will be blocked to feeling pain. Likewise, noxious stimulation keeps the gate open to pain.

A-Delta (Large, Fast) Fibers   A-delta fibers inhibit pain. Imagine that you've just hit your arm against a hard surface. Almost without thinking, you reach down and rub the area. Your massage stimulates skin receptors. These send sensory impulses along fast A-delta (large) fibers, which quickly excite inhibitory neurons at the "gate." These neurons in turn block some of the pain signals being carried along the slower C fibers (Fig. 28-3).

The gate-control theory is the basis for:

- Using a Sitz bath after childbirth to produce relief from pain at the perineum. The warm water and gentle pressure block the gate to the perception of pain in the brain.
- Development and use of transcutaneous electrical nerve stimulation (TENS) to relieve pain

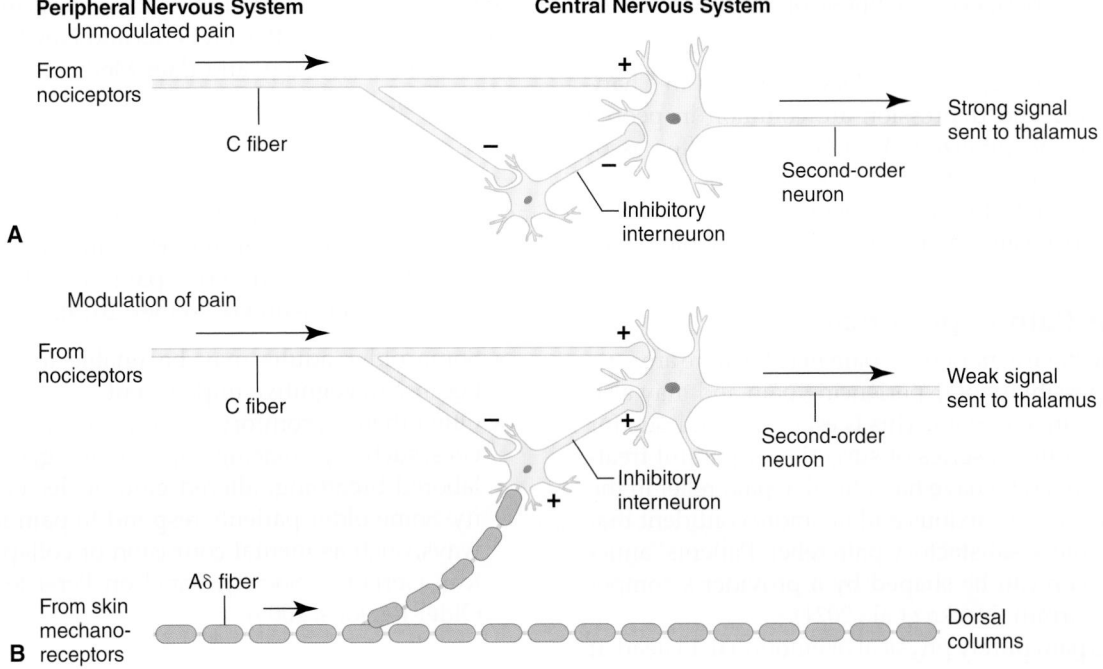

FIGURE 28-3 The gate-control theory of pain modulation. *A*, Normally, C fibers carrying slow pain signals block inhibitory interneurons and transmit their signals across the synapse unimpeded. *B*, A-delta fibers carrying pleasurable signals (e.g., from touch) excite inhibitory interneurons, which then block the transmission of slow pain signals. +, transmission; −, no transmission.

The following are some conditions and strategies thought to open or close the gate. They are discussed in more depth later in the chapter.

- **Descending impulses from the brain,** including impulses related to mood or emotion, are also thought to open or close the gate. For this reason, medications for depression are sometimes used for patients with persistent pain.
- **Nonpharmacological therapies,** such as meditation, exercise, relaxation techniques, and laughter, may also compete with C-fiber impulses and block the gate. These strategies are discussed later in this chapter.

KnowledgeCheck 28-2

- What must occur to generate pain?
- What are the four physiological steps involved in the pain process?

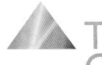 Think**Like a Nurse** 28-2:
Clinical Judgment **in Action**

Based on what you have learned about pain modulation, what nursing interventions might help Eunice (Meet Your Patient) be more comfortable?

WHAT FACTORS INFLUENCE PAIN?

On a purely physiological basis, pain is simply transduction, transmission, perception, and modulation. However, our experience of pain involves far more than these four processes. Think back to the last time you experienced significant pain. Was it obvious to others that you were in pain? Were you demonstrative? Quiet? Withdrawn? Did you moan or cry out? Now recall Eunice Chu Ling's reaction (in Meet Your Patient). What accounts for these different responses to pain?

Key Point: *Pain is universal, yet each person experiences and responds to pain differently as a result of the influence of emotions, age, sociocultural factors, and communication and cognitive impairments.*

Emotions

The most common emotions associated with pain are fear, guilt, anger, helplessness, and loneliness. In Meet Your Patient, imagine how Eunice Chu Ling must be feeling. How might her feelings affect and be affected by her pain?

Fear Some patients (e.g., Eunice in Meet Your Patient) fear that pain means an illness or injury is life-threatening. Others fear the pain will eventually become intolerable. Many others fear that if they ask for pain relief, they will be judged as weak or that they will become dependent on pain medications. When such fears remain unresolved, they can prolong or increase the patient's pain.

Confusion and Helplessness Eunice (Meet Your Patient) is also probably experiencing confusion and helplessness. Depending on her role in the accident, she may also feel angry or guilty. When she is by herself,

Eunice may experience loneliness or even a sense of abandonment.

Anxiety and Depression As you learned in Chapter 10, anxiety and depression are common in people who are ill or hospitalized. Anxiety is most often associated with acute pain, but the anticipation of pain may also trigger anxiety. In contrast, depression is most often linked with persistent pain, especially intractable pain.

Previous Pain Experience

People who have experienced pain may be more anxious about the possibility of experiencing pain and may also be more sensitive to pain. This is especially an issue for those who require a series of surgeries or painful treatments. Patients who have had effective pain relief in the past tend to be less anxious and are more confident that they will achieve satisfactory pain relief. Patients' anticipation of pain can be shaped by a provider's competence and warmth (Necka et al., 2021).

Rarely is pain purely physical or emotional. Instead, it is usually a combination of both. Interventions to relieve pain may relieve feelings of fear and helplessness, and interventions addressing these emotions, such as reflective listening and gentle touch, often aid in pain relief.

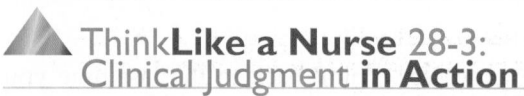
Think Like a Nurse 28-3:
Clinical Judgment in Action

Imagine being in a situation similar to that of Eunice Chu Ling (Meet Your Patient). What emotions might you experience?

Life Stage

Nurses assess and manage patients' pain based on the neurodevelopmental, emotional, cultural, and pain experiences that occur throughout the life cycle from birth to the end of life.

Infants and Children

Newborns in the first month of life can be subjected to painful procedures, with the most immature infants receiving the highest number of painful events (e.g., immunization). **Key Point:** *Term newborns have a similar sensitivity to pain as older infants and children; preterm infants may have a greater sensitivity (McCaffery & Pasero, 1999).*

- **Infants and small children usually respond to pain by crying.** However, in premature and term newborns, the experience of pain does not always evoke a recognizable behavioral response.
- **Indicators of pain in neonates may be subtle,** such as skin mottling, grimacing, twitching, crying, poor feeding, increased or decreased activity, averting gaze, temperature fluctuation, elevated blood pressure, and decreased oxygen saturation.

As a result, even though an infant has a low pain score based on behavioral assessment tools, they may not be pain-free (Anand et al., 2021; American Academy of Pediatrics, Committee on Fetus and Newborn, & Section on Anesthesiology and Pain Medicine, 2016; Slater et al., 2008).

Older Adults

More than half of the older adult population (age 65 and older) reports pain that occurs daily. Most of these describe pain that interferes with ADLs (Galicia-Castillo & Weiner, 2019).

- Some older adults may be unable to report pain because of cognitive impairment.
- Often their discomfort is evident only in nonverbal cues, such as grimacing, rapid blinking, withdrawal, labored breathing, altered gait, or decreased activity. Some older patients respond to pain in atypical ways, such as mental confusion or collapse (American Geriatrics Society, Panel on Persistent Pain in Older Persons, 2009).

Sociocultural Factors

We learn our responses to pain through interaction with family and social support groups. Beliefs about the value of expressing pain or minimizing it are often tied to personal beliefs and customs. As you care for individual clients, you may notice patterns of behavior. Some patients may gain comfort from crying or moaning when they are in pain, whereas other patients silently endure their pain. **Key Point:** *Do not assume that patients will react in the same as others of the same ethnic or cultural group. Each patient is unique.* For example, do you respond to pain in exactly the same way as your parents and siblings?

- **Those suffering from pain have individualized responses** that are often influenced by culture, family, and past experiences. In the Meet Your Patient scenario, recall how Eunice Chu Ling's family is responding. Although you may think it odd that they are smiling, they may be doing so because they want to make a favorable connection with you, the nurse, because you are responsible for providing care to Eunice.
- **Nurses, too, are affected by their culture.** Most nurses respond compassionately to those in pain. However, if you fail to recognize that pain is a unique, multidimensional experience, you may misjudge a patient's reaction to injury, surgery, or other discomforts.
 ♥ **iCare** Nurses have a duty to provide culturally competent care and adequate pain control to every patient.

Communication and Cognitive Impairments

One of your challenges as a nurse will be caring for patients in pain who have impaired cognition or communication (e.g., from stroke or dementia, intubation, or limited fluency in the local language). Adults with cognitive impairments are not less sensitive to pain but rather may:

- **Fail to interpret sensations** as painful
- **Be unable to effectively communicate** their pain to others
- **Be unable to recall their pain,** but they nonetheless still experience it (Horgas et al., 2016)

These patients are at risk for underassessment of pain and inadequate pain relief. You will need to consider their behavioral cues as a form of self-report.

Indicators of Pain Common nonverbal cues of pain include:

- Decreased activity
- Grimacing
- Frowning
- Crying
- Moaning
- Irritability

Less obvious indicators you may see in patients with cognitive impairment include the following:

- **Facial expressions** (e.g., a sad or frightened expression, rapid eye blinking)
- **Vocalizations** (e.g., noisy breathing, profanity, verbally abusive language)
- **Changes in physical activity** (e.g., fidgeting, increased pacing or rocking, disruptive behavior)
- **Changes in routines** (e.g., refusing food, difficulty sleeping)
- **Mental status changes** (e.g., increased confusion)
- **Physiological cues,** including elevated blood pressure, respiration, and pulse
- **Self-injurious behavior** (e.g., self-biting, head banging) (Doody & Valkenburg, 2021)

Key Point: *The absence of these cues does not mean that pain is absent.*

KnowledgeCheck 28-3

- What are the most common emotional responses to pain?
- What factors influence behavioral responses to pain?

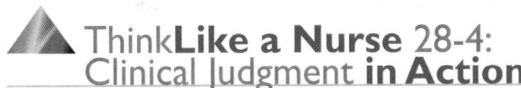

ThinkLike a Nurse 28-4: Clinical Judgment in Action

Eunice Chu Ling (Meet Your Patient) is unable to communicate verbally because of her intubation. She is grimacing in pain. After you medicate her for pain, how would you determine whether her pain has been relieved?

HOW DOES THE BODY REACT TO PAIN?

Pain triggers a variety of changes in the body, depending on the intensity, duration, and quality of the pain.

- **The onset of acute pain activates the sympathetic nervous system.** As discussed in Chapter 9, this fight-or-flight (stress) response is protective. It minimizes blood loss, maintains perfusion to vital organs, prevents and fights infections, and promotes healing.
- **If the pain continues, the body adapts, and the parasympathetic nervous system takes over.** However, the pain receptors continue to transmit the pain message so that the person remains aware of the tissue damage. This, too, is largely protective. For example, the pain you feel for several days after you sprain your ankle reminds you to stay off it until it is fully healed.

The severity and duration of the pain significantly affect how the person continues to respond to it. Often the person is able to ignore mild pain, but pain that is severe and unrelieved can consume thoughts and change daily living patterns. Box 28-1 identifies common pain responses.

Unrelieved Pain

Unrelieved pain can produce harmful effects in various body systems.

Endocrine System Ongoing pain triggers excessive release of hormones, including adrenocorticotropic hormone (ACTH), cortisol, antidiuretic hormone (ADH), growth hormone (GH), catecholamines, and glucagon. Insulin and testosterone levels decrease. These hormone shifts activate carbohydrate, protein, and fat catabolism (breakdown); hyperglycemia; and poor glucose use. The inflammatory process, combined with these endocrine and metabolic changes, can result in weight loss, tachycardia, fever, increased respiratory rate, and even death.

Cardiovascular System Unrelieved pain leads to hypercoagulation and an increase in heart rate, blood pressure, cardiac workload, and oxygen demand. The combination of hypercoagulation and increased cardiac workload may lead to unstable angina (chest pain), intracoronary thrombosis (clot formation in the vessels that supply the heart), and myocardial ischemia and infarction (heart attack).

Musculoskeletal System Uncontrolled pain causes impaired muscle function, fatigue, and immobility. Poorly managed pain can prevent the patient from performing ADLs and engaging in physical therapy.

Respiratory System Patients in pain tend to breathe shallowly—to limit thoracic and abdominal movement in an effort to reduce pain. This is called **splinting.** Splinting reduces tidal volume (air exchanged with each breath) and increases inspiratory and expiratory pressures. These changes can lead to pneumonia and atelectasis, as well as underventilation (retained carbon dioxide, also called *hypercarbia*) and respiratory acidosis.

Genitourinary System Unrelieved pain causes the release of excessive amounts of catecholamines,

BOX 28-1 ■ Common Pain Responses

Physiological (Involuntary) Responses

Sympathetic Responses (Acute Pain)

Dilated blood vessels to the brain, increased alertness

Dilated pupils

Impaired gastrointestinal motility

Increased heart rate and force of contraction

Increased respiratory rate, shallow breathing

Increased systolic blood pressure

Reduced urinary output

Pallor

Parasympathetic Responses (Deep or Prolonged Pain)

Changeable breathing patterns

Constricted pupils

Decreased pulse rate

Decreased systolic blood pressure, feeling faint, possible syncope

Withdrawal

Behavioral Responses (Voluntary)

Agitation, striking out, fidgeting

Grimacing, frowning, fearful facial expression, grinding teeth

Guarding, bracing, or rubbing the painful area

Moaning, groaning, crying, sighing

Rapid speech (acute pain); slow, monotonous speech (persistent pain)

Withdrawing from painful stimuli, resisting certain movements with care

Eating and sleeping poorly

Reduced energy, reduced interest in others, reduced activity level and mobility

Change in gait

Psychological (Affective) Responses

Anger

Anxiety

Depression

Exhaustion

Fear

Hopelessness

Irritability

aldosterone, ADH, cortisol, angiotensin II, and prostaglandins. These hormones lead to decreased urinary output, urinary retention, fluid overload, hypokalemia, hypertension, and increased cardiac output.

Gastrointestinal (GI) System In response to pain, intestinal secretions and smooth muscle tone increase, and gastric emptying and motility decrease.

KnowledgeCheck 28-4

- What are the effects of untreated pain on each of the body systems?
- How might untreated pain affect the progress of a patient recovering from a major illness?

PracticalKnowledge
knowing how

As we discussed earlier, a person's *pain threshold* is the point at which that person perceives a stimulus as painful, whereas *pain tolerance* is the amount of pain a person is able to endure. Both differ greatly from person to person. Practical knowledge includes knowing how to assess for and manage patients' pain.

ASSESSMENT/RECOGNIZING CUES

Key Point: *To treat pain effectively, you must first understand the patient's perception of pain.* Begin with a comprehensive pain history and assessment that includes the following:

- Pain location
- Pain quality and intensity
- Aggravating and alleviating factors
- Timing and duration
- Pain relief and expectations for how much pain is realistic
- Questions that reveal the patient's ability to perform ADLs, such as mobility, sleep, self-care)
- Mobility
- Psychological/social factors (e.g., depression or substance abuse)
- A thorough and unbiased pain assessment is necessary for all patients because there may be a linkage between social determinants (primarily socioeconomic and racial factors) and the occurrence and management of chronic pain. Biases in pain assessment, discrepant pain treatment plans, and gaps in patient–provider communication may result in disparate care and contribute to unfavorable outcomes (Knoebel et al., 2021).

For a list of questions that are typically asked,

See **Chapter 28, Focused Assessment box, Pain Assessment,** in Volume 2.

Key Point: *You should make ongoing assessments regularly and, of course, accept the patient's report of pain.*

- **Patient self-report** is the most reliable indicator of pain, except for those who are unable to communicate (e.g., infants, persons with cognitive impairment or advanced dementia, and patients who are critically ill or unconscious or near the end of life). The inability to self-report pain interferes with pain assessment. As a result, the patient is at risk for underrecognition and under- or overtreatment of pain (Herr et al., 2019).

Self-report is especially important for patients with persistent pain. When pain is ongoing, the autonomic nervous system eventually adapts, so physiological and behavioral signs become less evident (Schneider, 2006–2007).

- **Patient satisfaction** with healthcare can be directly related to how effectively pain is managed. Regular, ongoing pain assessments may indicate change in condition or a need for more aggressive pain management. To ensure patient comfort and satisfaction, teach patients about pain management options and expected outcomes as you assess their responses to pain interventions.

Pain, the Fifth Vital Sign

The APS (1996) introduced the idea of "pain as the fifth vital sign" to emphasize the importance of regular and ongoing pain assessment, just as the nurse does with monitoring patients' vital signs. That would mean asking patients to self-rate their pain intensity using a numerical scale or other pain assessment tool whenever taking a full set of vital signs. **Key Point:** *The numerical rating scale is the most common method to assess pain.*

Key Point: *However, to reduce overprescribing of opioids, the American Medical Association, The Joint Commission, and numerous other authority sources have dropped their advocacy of the "pain as the fifth vital sign" approach because it may contribute to overreporting and overprescribing of opioid pain relievers (Levy et al., 2018).*

The nurse would perform pain assessments more or less frequently, depending on the patient's clinical situation, such as:

- On admission to a healthcare facility
- Before and after each potentially painful procedure or treatment
- When the patient is at rest, as well as when involved in a nursing activity
- Before you implement a pain management intervention, such as administering an analgesic drug, and 30 minutes after the intervention
- With each check of vital signs if the pain is an actual or potential problem
- When the patient complains of pain
- With a change in the patient's condition

Culturally Competent Assessments

Three words—*pain, hurt,* and *ache*—seem to be used across many cultures to describe pain (Pasero & McCaffery, 2011). You might also use descriptions of *burning, itching,* and *cramping* when asking patients about their pain experience. For this reason, various pain assessment tools can be successfully translated into various languages. When patients' primary language

spoken is not English, you may benefit from pain assessment tools that have been translated into the languages you are most likely to encounter.

Using Pain Scales

To help you assess the intensity of the pain as well as any changes in the quality of pain, you can choose from among a variety of pain scales. Select a pain scale by considering the patient's age, level of education, language skills, eyesight, and developmental level. Once you choose a particular pain scale for a patient, use it consistently to prevent confusion and allow for comparison.

 See **Chapter 28, Focused Assessment box, Using Pain Scales,** in Volume 2.

If your patient speaks a different language than you do, ask an interpreter to explain to the patient that it is important to manage pain and that you will be using a pain scale regularly to assess their pain. Ask the interpreter to translate; write out the explanation and directions for the pain scale so that you can refer to these when you assess your patient. Patients can point to a face or numeric line to tell you about their pain when no one is present to translate.

Assessing Pain in Infants and Children

You can assess pain in children through self-report, behavioral observation, or physiological measures. Inaccurate pain assessment can lead to a more intense response to pain and the development of chronic pain. When pain is not assessed and managed properly, the child's sleep suffers, and performance in school, extracurricular activities, and day-to-day behavior may be affected as well (Contrada, 2019).

- Be sure to consult the parents about the child's stress signals and reaction to pain.
- Use art and play as a way to assess the child's understanding of pain and the pain management plan.
- Choose age-appropriate toys to engage the child in acting out feelings.

Tools that combine behavioral and physiological indicators of pain in premature and term infants include the Neonatal Infant Pain Score (NIPS) (Lawrence et al., 1993); the Neonatal Pain, Agitation, and Sedation Scale (N-PASS; Hillman et al., 2015); and others. You can also use a pain rating scale consisting of simple illustrations of faces for children to use a number rating to express the severity of their pain experience—the FACES Pain Scale (Bieri et al., 1990).

Patients Who Are Difficult to Assess

Key Point: *"The inability to communicate verbally does not negate the possibility that an individual is experiencing pain and is in need of an appropriate* *pain-relieving treatment" (International Association for the Study of Pain, 2010).*

For patients who are difficult to assess, you will need to use the patient history and current environment to help you judge the intensity and quality of pain. Does the patient have an underlying painful condition? What is the likely source of pain? Are there physical signs that indicate the patient has increased pain with movement, turning, or other motions?

When using a pain scale, allow sufficient time for the patient to respond. Some examples of tools for patients who are difficult to assess include:

- **Patients with dementia** or cognitive and expressive deficits are also a challenge when assessing the extent of pain. It may not be possible to elicit a reliable self-report for pain, and their behavioral cues might not accurately reflect the pain experience. The lack of initiation of pain assessment and the use of pain assessment tools may contribute to inadequate pain management by nurses (I-Pei, et al., 2018). A good option for assessing pain in this population is the Pain Assessment in Advanced Dementia (PAINAD) Scale (Warden et al., 2003), a five-item observational tool specifically geared toward older adults with dementia (Table 28-1).
- **Patients with delayed development, impaired cognition, or impaired communication** (e.g., brain injury). Techniques to assess pain in individuals with cognitive impairment or developmental delay include: (1) the caregiver's description of pain cues; (2) behavioral pain checklists, assessment tools, and

pain scales; (3) reports from healthcare team, especially a clinical pain nurse expert (Silverman, 2019).

Well-validated tools for cognitively or developmentally delayed patients and those too young to respond to pain assessment include the Noncommunicating Children's Pain Checklist-Revised (NCCPC-R; Breau et al., 2002); and the revised FLACC (Malviya et al., 2006).

- **Patients receiving mechanical ventilation.** The COMFORT Scale is used to evaluate pain in mechanically ventilated pediatric patients (Ambuel et al., 1992).
- **Patients who are under anesthesia or those receiving sedation** are difficult to assess for pain. The Critical Care Pain Observation Tool (CPOT) can assess acute pain in sedated patients (Pereira-Morales et al., 2019).

Nonverbal Signs of Pain

In addition to the patient's verbal report of pain, you must recognize other responses that may signal pain. Is the blood pressure or pulse elevated? Does the client appear pale and clammy? These are signs of sympathetic nervous system stimulation. You will see these signs if the pain is acute. If the pain is unresolved or chronic, the blood pressure and pulse may be lower than normal, and the patient may report feeling faint. These are signs of parasympathetic nervous system stimulation.

Physical Indicators

- **Facial expression, posture, and body position are reliable indicators of the intensity of pain.** Basic and

Table 28-1 ➤ Pain Assessment in Advanced Dementia (PAINAD) Scale

ITEMS	0	1	2	SCORE
Breathing independent of vocalization	Normal	Occasional labored breathing. Short period of hyperventilation.	Noisy labored breathing. Long period of hyperventilation. Cheyne-Stokes respirations.	
Negative vocalization	None	Occasional moan or groan. Low-level speech with a negative or disapproving quality.	Repeated troubled calling out. Loud moaning or groaning. Crying.	
Facial expression	Smiling or inexpressive	Sad. Frightened. Frown.	Facial grimacing.	
Body language	Relaxed	Tense. Distressed pacing. Fidgeting.	Rigid. Fists clenched. Knees pulled up. Pulling or pushing away. Striking out.	
Consolability	No need to console	Distracted or reassured by voice or touch.	Unable to console, distract, or reassure.	
			TOTALS	

Source: Warden, V., Hurley, A. C., & Volicer, L. (2003). Development and psychometric evaluation of the Pain Assessment in Advanced Dementia (PAINAD) Scale. *Journal of the American Medical Directors Association*, 4(1), 9–15. Copyright 2003, with permission from American Medical Directors Association.

common facial expressions that signal pain are lowering the brow, wincing, clenching the jaws, and closing the eyelids. Guarding a painful site or maintaining a tense position is also a sign of pain.

- **Changes in vital signs last only a short time.** The body seeks equilibrium; thus, after an hour or so, the vital signs typically return to baseline even though the patient may still be in pain. Continuous, severe pain may elevate the vital signs again from time to time, but they rarely remain elevated.
- **Key Point:** *Vital signs that are within normal range do not mean that the patient is free of pain.*
- **Patients may be in pain even if they don't "act like" they are.** Unfortunately, it has been well documented that healthcare professionals fail to assess pain and tend to underrate the pain the patient is experiencing (American Geriatrics Society, Panel on Persistent Pain in Older Adult, 2009; McCaffery & Pasero, 1999). They expect to see frowning, crying, or scowling. Patients who use laughter, distraction, or even sleep to cope with their pain are often undertreated.

Emotional Indicators

Beyond what a patient says about pain or how they physically respond to pain, the patient's attitude, mood, and mental and emotional state also affect the expression of pain.

- **Assess for stoicism.** Some patients feel that they are being "bad" or "weak" if they express pain. Such ♥ **iCare** patients may withdraw or become stoic. It is important that you establish a trusting relationship with them. Convey your concern and acknowledge the person's pain. If the patient trusts you, they are more likely to verbalize thoughts and feelings.
- **Assess for depression** (see Chapter 9 if you need to review). Patients with persistent pain are four times more likely to have depression than those without pain (Hooten et al., 2017). If depression is not treated aggressively, efforts to manage the pain may not be successful. **Key Point:** *Likewise, co-occurring pain and depression create a vicious cycle whereby persistent pain can lead to or worsen symptoms of depression, anxiety, and irritability, and then the resulting emotional responses worsen the pain experience.*

KnowledgeCheck 28-5

- How often should you assess the patient for pain if pain is a potential problem for the patient?
- What are some of the common pain scales used?
- Who should determine whether the patient is in pain?

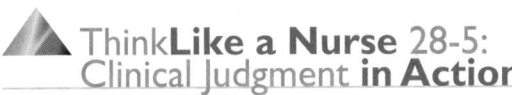

ThinkLike a Nurse 28-5: Clinical Judgment in Action

What pain rating scale would you use to assess Eunice (Meet Your Patient)? Why?

■ NURSING DIAGNOSIS/ANALYZING CUES

Pain as Problem The following Clinical Care Classification (n.d.; CCC 2.5) labels are commonly used when pain is the focus of the problem:

> *Acute Pain.* Pain with an anticipated or actual duration of <6 months.
> *Chronic Pain.* Pain with an anticipated or actual duration of >6 months.

Notice that only duration, not speed of onset or severity, is used to differentiate between Acute Pain and Chronic Pain.

Pain as Etiology Pain affects many areas of functioning. Therefore, it is often the etiology of other nursing diagnoses. The following few examples of such diagnoses are from CCC (n.d.):

- Activities of Daily Living (ADLs) Alteration
- Physical Mobility Impairment
- Home Maintenance Alteration

The following are samples of diagnostic statements you might write for problems caused by pain:

> *Sexuality Pattern Alterations* related to back pain
> *Sleep Pattern Disturbance* related to chronic back pain of more than a year's duration

When writing a pain nursing diagnosis, specify the location of the pain and any etiological or precipitating factors that you are aware of. For example:

> Acute Pain (headache) related to changes of position and secondary to increased intracranial pressure

Also identify any knowledge deficits, fear of addiction, or any other fears or beliefs that may interfere with effective pain management. Focusing on the specific nature of pain enables you to choose the most useful interventions.

■ PLANNING/PRIORITIZING HYPOTHESES AND GENERATING SOLUTIONS

The overall objective when working with a client in pain is to prevent pain whenever possible or, if it is present, to reduce or eliminate it.

Examples of *Nursing Outcomes Classification (NOC) standardized outcomes* are:

For Acute Pain—Pain Control, Pain Level, and Comfort Status: Physical
For Chronic Pain—In addition to those for acute pain: Depression Level, Pain: Adverse Psychological Response, and Pain: Disruptive Effects

Individualized goals/outcome statements you might write for a client with pain include the following:

- By day 2 postop, will require only oral analgesics for pain management.

Assessing and Treating Pain in Patients with Cognitive Impairment

Competency: Provide Goal-Directed, Client-Centered Care

Scenario: Mr. Fagin, who has dementia, has been hospitalized for prostate cancer that has metastasized to his pelvis, femur, and ribs. Mr. Fagin seems confused and is loudly singing hymns and banging his hands against his table in rhythm. The registered nurse (RN) goes to Mr. Fagin's room, observes him carefully, and speaks with him. When asked if his bones hurt, he nods his head "yes." She also asks Mrs. Fagin about her husband's usual responses to pain. Mrs. Fagin states that her husband has always been very religious and often sings hymns when upset. She also says that he never complained about aches and pains in the past and that she believes he is now having "quite a bit of pain." She says, "I can't stand to see him suffer."

The nurse checks the medication administration record (MAR) and obtains the prescribed prn opioid analgesic. While Mrs. Fagin speaks gently to her husband, the nurse administers the opioid analgesic. She documents the medication in the MAR, noting Mr. Fagin's behaviors before being medicated. Thirty minutes later, the nurse observes Mr. Fagin eating dinner with his wife. His body and facial expression are relaxed, and he has stopped singing. Before leaving, the nurse asks Mr. and Mrs. Fagin whether they would like a visit from the hospital chaplain.

Think about it: A central nursing duty in the patient-centered care competency is alleviating pain and suffering. (1) How is Mr. Fagan's situation different from that of a patient with normal cognitive function? (2) What knowledge, skills, and attitudes did the nurse apply that demonstrate competency in pain management (and therefore in patient-centered care), particularly for the patient with dementia? As you think about it, consider the following:

➤ Why was it important to ask Mrs. Fagin about her husband's usual behavior?

➤ Was it appropriate to ask the Fagins whether they wanted a visit from pastoral services?

➤ How did the nurse show respect for Mr. and Mrs. Fagin's preferences, values, and needs?

➤ Singing loudly doesn't seem to be an obvious indication of pain; what other factors let the nurse know Mr. Fagin was in pain?

➤ How is pain assessment modified for patients with cognitive impairment?

➤ Do you see how the nurse recognized Mr. Fagin and his wife as full partners in care?

■ Within 15 minutes of patient-controlled analgesia (PCA) injection, reports pain is <3 on a scale from 0 to 10.
■ Reports that persistent pain does not prevent them from performing ADLs.

■ Pain Control: Uses pain relief diary (4: Often demonstrated) (NOC).

■ IMPLEMENTATION/TAKING ACTION

To alleviate or reduce pain to an acceptable level, you would develop pain treatment strategies that include not only prescribed analgesic but also nonpharmacological options. Pain management should reflect a patient-centered approach that considers the risk and benefits of the strategy, including the potential risk of dependency, abuse, and addiction. When planning care, remember the following:

■ **Each situation is unique.** For example, one patient with terminal illness may request complete relief of pain even if this leads to heavy sedation. Another patient with the same diagnosis and prognosis may prefer that the pain be kept at a just manageable level so that they can interact with their family or complete unfinished business.
■ **The most effective and least invasive method** of pain control is generally preferable.
■ **Remember to include nonpharmacological interventions,** especially when the pain is chronic.
■ **The overall care of the patient depends on** the cause of the pain, whether the pain is acute or chronic, and the patient's unique situation and response to pain-relieving measures.
■ **There are some nursing interventions and activities that address pain,** both acute and chronic, and regardless of its cause, despite the preceding statement.

Nursing Interventions Classification (NIC) standardized interventions for Pain include the following examples:

For Acute Pain—Analgesic Administration, Pain Management: Acute and Chronic, Medication Management
For Chronic Pain—Cognitive Restructuring, Pain Management, Coping Enhancement, Mood Management

Specific, individualized nursing activities (including focused assessments) for clients with Acute Pain and Chronic Pain include the following (adapted from Butcher et al., 2018, pp. 281–282):

■ Perform a comprehensive assessment of pain, function, and quality of life. Include location, onset, duration, frequency, and intensity of pain. Also ask about factors that alleviate or cause the pain. Assessment includes comorbidity history. Reassess periodically and whenever there is a lack of improvement.
■ Explore the patient's knowledge and beliefs about pain.
■ Involve the patient in the development of the pain management plan. Include various treatment methods while avoiding using medication as the sole focus of treatment.
■ Consider cultural influences on the patient's pain responses.

- Monitor pain using a validated tool appropriate for the patient's age and ability to communicate.
- Centers for Disease Control and Prevention in the United States and the Canadian Guideline for Opioid Use in Chronic Non-Cancer Pain recommend nonopioid treatment as the preferred treatment for chronic pain (Agency for Healthcare Research and Quality [AHRQ], 2020).
- Administer analgesics before the pain becomes severe or before pain-inducing activities.
- Administer analgesics using the least invasive route available. Avoid the intramuscular route when possible.
- Use combination analgesics to control severe pain.
- Modify pain control measures as needed by the patient's response to treatment.
- Monitor sedation and respiratory status before administering opioids.
- Monitor sedation and respiratory status at regular intervals when opioids are administered.
- Observe for, prevent, or manage medication side effects.
   - Use analgesics cautiously with older adults; watch carefully for side effects, especially respiratory depression, thought and memory issues, dizziness, constipation, and nausea.
- Notify prescriber if pain control is not satisfactory.
- Keep the family informed about the patient's pain experience.
- Reduce anxiety and fear by offering explanations about care and medications, by allowing the patient to be in control of their pain management, and by providing competent care.
- Collaborate with the healthcare team about complex pain management issues.

See Box 28-2 for a list of strategies for nonpharmacologic pain relief that may be delegated to unlicensed assistive personnel (UAPs).

Nonpharmacological Pain Relief Measures

Nonpharmacological measures offer an alternative for people with mild to moderate pain who want to reduce their use of analgesic drugs for pain relief (The Joint Commission, 2018; Zeidan et al., 2016). Holistic therapies can prompt the release of endogenous opioids. Integrating nonpharmacological measures, including complementary and alternative modalities (CAM), into a pain management plan may help ease persistent pain and reduce the need for traditionally prescribed drugs.

When providing nonpharmacological pain relief measures,

- Assess your patient for openness to the therapy.
- Assess your patient thoroughly and often to determine whether the therapy is effective.
- Modify the pain management plan when the patient does not experience relief.

BOX 28-2 ■ Pain Management Tasks That May Be Delegated to Unlicensed Assistive Personnel

Unlicensed assistive personnel (UAP) may assist you in caring for patients with pain. Your responsibility is to assess the patient's pain, administer prescribed analgesics, monitor the patient's response to pain management strategies, and evaluate the pain management plan.

♥ **iCare** The following tasks may be delegated to UAP:
- Repositioning, using pillows for support
- Back rub or massage
- Providing darkness and quiet in the room for sleep
- Straightening sheets
- Mouth care
- Soft music of the patient's preference
- Using distraction (talking or setting up a favorite game for the patient) and other nonpharmacological treatment

---

Holistic Healing

Natural Supplements for Pain Management

Boswellia—a tree residue; reduces arthritic pain

Cannabidiol (CBD)—inhibits pain pathway signals and reduces inflammation, arthritis, and fibromyalgia

Caffeine—combined with acetaminophen or ibuprofen to relieve headaches

Capsicum/capsaicin—comes from chili peppers; cream soothes back pain, and oral supplement lessens diarrhea and cramping

Comfrey extract—cream eases back pain

Ginseng—fibromyalgia

Glucosamine and **chondroitin**—help to ease joint pain

Magnesium-rich Epsom salt—natural painkiller for bone and joint pain and muscle soreness

Omega-3 fatty acids—lower inflammation; can help with joint pain and stiffness, back pain, and menstrual cramp discomfort

Probiotics—live bacteria in the gut that lesson bowel inflammation; can help reduce gastrointestinal cramping, bloating, and pain

St. John's wort—helps ease pain from sciatica and arthritis and neuropathic pain

Turmeric—related to ginger root; reduces inflammation

White willow bark—known as *nature's aspirin* for headaches or low back pain; can take as tea or capsule

Although these supplements may be natural, they can nonetheless interact with other prescribed medications. Healthcare professionals need to ask patients if they take complementary and alternative medicine (CAM) substances and advise patients to contact the provider if unusual symptoms occur.

- Determine whether there is access to materials needed to perform nonpharmacological pain relief activities.
- Do not withhold analgesics when nonpharmacological methods are being used. In the case of mild pain, alternative therapy may be sufficient.
- Ensure patients and their families receive education about options for nonpharmacologic pain-relieving options. Providing thorough patient education often helps to improve compliance with ongoing treatment and reduce unrealistic expectations of treatment outcomes (The Joint Commission, 2018).

Cutaneous Stimulation

Cutaneous stimulation is a pain relief method based on the gate-control theory. As discussed earlier, skin stimulation sends impulses along the large sensory fibers, which in turn excite inhibitory interneurons in the spinal cord to "close the gate." This process diminishes the patient's perception of pain. Cutaneous stimulation works best on pain that is localized and not diffuse.

TENS Units A **transcutaneous electrical nerve stimulator (TENS)** is a battery-powered device that is worn externally. A TENS unit consists of electrode pads, the connecting wire, and the stimulator. The pads are directly applied to the painful area. Once activated, the unit stimulates A-delta sensory fibers. It can be worn intermittently or for long periods of time, depending on the patient's pain.

PENS Units **Percutaneous electrical stimulation (PENS)** combines a TENS unit with percutaneously placed (through-the-skin) needle probes to stimulate peripheral sensory nerves. PENS is effective in the short-term management of acute and persistent pain. For some, PENS therapy promotes physical activity, increases the sense of well-being, reduces the use of nonopioid medication, and improves sleep.

Holistic Healing

Spinal Cord Stimulator Intractable spinal or limb pain may be treated by a surgically implanted **spinal cord stimulator (SCS).** The SCS produces a tingly sensation that interferes with the perception of pain.

Acupuncture Application of extremely fine needles to specific sites in the body to relieve pain is called **acupuncture.** It is believed to stimulate the endogenous analgesia system. Acupuncture is documented to provide relief from joint, skeletal, myofascial, and a broad range and sources of pain and dental discomfort. It is used after surgery and chemotherapy to treat nausea.

✚ Acupuncture may lead to light-headedness, which may be a concern for patients who are at risk for falls. Assess these patients carefully after the treatment.

Myofascial Trigger Point Dry Needling Myofascial trigger point dry needling, also known as

intramuscular stimulation, is the use of fine needles along trigger points in the muscles to reduce the pain sensation and restore normal muscle and joint function. Similar to acupuncture, dry needling elicits an involuntary twitch response that interrupts the communication of pain from the source to the brain.

Acupressure Acupressure has roots in ancient Chinese healing and wellness therapy—much like acupuncture but without the use of needles to relieve pain, cure disease, induce relaxation, or restore balance. Firm, gentle pressure is applied to points along any of the 12 energy meridians (channels) or acupoints to produce a calming effect through the release of endorphins. Patients can be readily taught acupressure points to stimulate so that they can self-administer acupressure when needed.

Myofascial Release Therapy Myofascial release therapy, also called **active release therapy** (ART), is manual pressure applied to overused or injured muscles and nerves. Direct pressure loosens the adhesions that develop from overuse. ART releases adhesions that cause numbness, tingling, and radiating pain and limit muscle and joint movement. Some common conditions that can benefit from ART are tendonitis ("tennis elbow"), repetitive motion syndrome, back pain, plantar fasciitis, shin splints, and strained muscles.

Massage By providing cutaneous stimulation and relaxing the muscles, **massage** helps to reduce pain. **Effleurage** is the use of slow, long, guiding strokes to relax muscles, promote comfort, and reduce pain. **Key Point:** *For most patients, superficial massage is soothing and relaxing, both mentally and physically. However, some patients do not like to be touched; therefore, always obtain verbal permission from the patient before massage.*

Low-Level Laser Therapy Low-level laser therapy **(LLLT)** (also known as *cold laser therapy*) is a noninvasive technique using low-wattage light to penetrate deeply into tissue. This helps to reduce acute or persistent pain by repairing tissue and minimizing inflammation caused by injury or arthritis. LLLT is an alternative to the use of analgesics or surgery, especially for joint pain.

Temperature Therapy The application of cold causes vasoconstriction and can help prevent swelling and bleeding. The cold sensation helps to numb sharp pain and reduce inflammation, and it can be especially effective in reducing the amount of pain that occurs during procedures. A cold pack to the site before and after a procedure reduces pain. Heat promotes circulation, which speeds healing. It helps to soothe stiff joints and relaxes muscles.

✚ Use caution with these temperature therapies, however, because the skin may be injured by extremes of either hot or cold. The addition of moisture to heat or cold amplifies the intensity of the treatment, so take extra precautions when applying moist heat or cold.

- Avoid direct contact with the heating or cooling device. Cover the hot or cold pack with a washcloth, towel, or fitted sleeve.
- Apply heat or cold intermittently, for no more than 15 minutes at a time, to avoid tissue injury.
- Check the skin frequently for extreme redness, blistering, cyanosis (blue color), or blanching (white color).
- If any of these occur, discontinue the treatment immediately and notify the patient's provider.

Contralateral Stimulation Why does a patient experiencing pain in the right arm experience some relief when lotion is applied and rubbed into the left arm? The principle involved is called **contralateral stimulation**—stimulating the skin in an area opposite to the painful site. Stimulation may be in the form of scratching, rubbing, or applying heat or cold. This intervention is especially helpful if the affected area is painful to touch, under bandages, or in a cast. It has provided some relief to patients who have phantom pain after an amputation.

Oral Sucrose

Sucrose by mouth, alone or in combination with other analgesic measures, can be effective for pain control in newborns exposed to mild or moderately painful procedures (Anand et al., 2022; Committee on Fetus and Newborn, & Section on Anesthesiology and Pain Medicine, 2016; Sharara-Chami et al., 2017).

Immobilization and Traction

- **Immobilizing** a painful body part (e.g., with splints) may offer some relief. It is particularly helpful with

arthritic joints. You must remember to remove the splints at regular intervals so that the patient can exercise the area to strengthen the site and prevent further injury. Patients in severe pain have the tendency to immobilize a painful area by limiting its use.
- **Intermittent mechanical or manual traction** reduces pain resulting from the compression of nerve tissue, especially in the spine.

Cognitive–Behavioral Interventions

Cognitive–behavioral therapy attempts to alter patterns of negative thoughts and encourage more adaptive thoughts, emotions, and actions. It is used to decrease depression and anxiety, both of which play a role in pain. Cognitive therapy helps patients to deal with their pain by fostering a sense of control over their illness and decreasing feelings of helplessness.

♥ **iCare** Be sure to obtain the patient's permission before using these methods because psychological or spiritual distress may occur if they consider them inconsistent with their belief system.

Distraction You can use distraction as a method of drawing the patient's attention away from the pain by focusing on something other than the pain. It is based on the belief that the brain can process only so much information at one time. When distraction works, the patient has only a peripheral awareness of pain. You may have responded to this strategy in the past. Have you ever had a headache or muscle pain go away when you became busy with other activities?

Although distraction can be used for severe pain, it is most effective for mild to moderate pain and for brief periods of time (e.g., for a short procedure such as an injection or infusion). Some patients experience an increase in pain and may become fatigued and irritable when they are no longer distracted. Distraction is useful with all ages.

Distraction can be visual, tactile, intellectual, or auditory. The usefulness of the different methods varies among patients.

- **Visual** tactics, such as watching a football game on TV, serve as effective distraction for some patients.
- **Tactile** distraction, such as massage, hugging a favorite toy or soft blanket, holding a loved one, or stroking a pet, is effective for other patients.
- **Intellectual** distraction includes activities such as becoming engrossed in a crossword puzzle or playing a challenging game.
- **Auditory** distraction in the form of music therapy has been shown to reduce anxiety during acute and persistent pain. Patients' self-reports show that pain is reduced, mood improves, and relaxation is achieved more easily. Physiological measures, such as respirations, heart rate, blood pressure, and muscle tension, indicate a less intense pain experience (Ettenberger et al., 2021; Monsalve-Duarte et al., 2022). Music therapy can also reduce opioid requirements postoperatively and for those suffering from cancer pain

---

Holistic Healing

Nonpharmacological Therapies to Reduce the Pain Experience

Examples of nonpharmacological options that help patients to cope with pain and its effects on lifestyle, mood, and activities of daily living:

➤ Transcutaneous electrical nerve stimulation (TENS)

➤ Acupuncture, acupressure

➤ Chiropractic therapy

➤ Osteopathic manipulative treatment (OMT)

➤ Physical therapy, massage therapy

➤ Myofascial release therapy; trigger point dry needling

➤ Relaxation therapy, visual imagery

➤ Prayer, meditation

➤ Music therapy

➤ Pet therapy

➤ Cognitive behavioral therapy

➤ Therapeutic touch, energy fields

(Cole & Lobiondo-Wood, 2012; Gallagher & Cellini, 2018; Hanser & Mandel, 2012; Richards et al., 2007).

Relaxation Techniques Relaxation techniques reduce pain in a variety of medical conditions, especially persistent pain. In **sequential muscle relaxation (SMR),** or progressive relaxation, the person sits comfortably and tenses a group of muscles for 15 seconds while inhaling and then relaxes the muscles while exhaling. After a brief rest, this sequence is repeated using another set of muscles. Patients often start at the facial muscles and work downward to the feet.

Guided Imagery Using directed words and music, this technique evokes positive, calm imaginary scenarios that lead to relaxation and a positive, focused state of mind (Carpenter et al. (2016). Guided imagery is a holistic technique that creates harmony between the mind and body to promote feelings of well-being, elicit hope, and cope with pain.

Diaphragmatic Breathing Patients can be taught to use the diaphragm (large, dome-shaped muscle at the base of the lungs that is the most efficient muscle of breathing) to intentionally take slow, even breaths when inhaling and exhaling at the rate of five to eight breaths per minute. The technique invokes relaxation and improves tissue oxygenation for managing pain and promoting comfort.

Hypnosis Hypnosis involves the induction of a deeply relaxed state. Once the person is in this state, the hypnotist offers therapeutic suggestions to provide reduction of symptoms (Elkins, 2012). For example, the hypnotist may suggest to a patient with arthritis that the pain can be turned down, like the volume of a radio. Special training in hypnotherapy is required.

Therapeutic Touch Despite its name, therapeutic touch (TT) does not require physical contact. TT focuses on the use of the hands to direct energy fields surrounding the body. Although research studies on its effect are not consistent, some patients become relaxed and require less pain medication after a session of TT.

Humor This method has positive effects on a patient's physical and emotional health (Matz & Brown, 1998). For most people, laughter is positive and indicates mental well-being. Humor may boost the immune system as well. It is especially helpful when used before a painful procedure because it lessens anxiety and serves as a form of distraction. Humor therapy can be used to lessen chronic pain in children and adults. It also works to increase endurance and quality of life in older adults who are cared for in nursing homes (Yusnaeni, 2019).

Some institutions have humor carts and even humor rooms containing humorous videos, books, and playful items, such as bubbles, paints, and puppets. Humor is helpful for both children and adults, but it must always be in good taste and age appropriate. Involve the patient in choosing the humorous material because what one person considers funny, another person may not.

Expressive Writing Journaling, blogging, and storytelling can help the patient cope with persistent pain. Some recommend structured writing sessions in which the patient describes stressful events for a specified period of time over consecutive days. Others benefit from frequent journaling in an informal way, expressing feelings, fears, or what comes to mind.

Animal-Assisted Therapy Animals (typically dogs), trained to be obedient, calm, and comforting, provide therapeutic benefits to people with persistent pain (e.g., fibromyalgia) and other health problems (e.g., cancer, epilepsy). Patients' serum cortisol (stress hormone) levels decrease when they are exposed to therapy animals. In a study involving patients after knee replacement surgery, those with animal-assisted therapy postop required lower doses of pain medication and reported greater well-being after surgery (Havey et al., 2014; Rodrigo-Claverol et al., 2019).

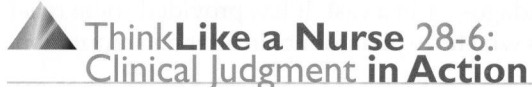

ThinkLike a Nurse 28-6: Clinical Judgment in Action

What has been your experience with using nonpharmacological pain relief measures to manage your own pain? How would you incorporate these methods into your nursing practice?

Pharmacological Pain Relief Measures

Analgesics (pain relievers) are classified into three groups: nonopioids, opioids, and adjuvants. To administer analgesics, you must know and do the following safely, correctly, and effectively:

- Assess for pain and monitor the pain management plan regularly and continuously.
- Titrate medication based on a valid and reliable pain assessment tool and according to the patient's response.
- Know the interactions and side effects of drugs recommended at each step.
- Understand that choice of treatment is based on the level of pain the patient is experiencing.
- If the patient's pain is not controlled, adjust the pain management plan accordingly.

Dosage and Administration **Key Point:** *Analgesics work best if given before pain becomes too severe. "Keeping ahead of the pain" reduces suffering and helps patients to cope better and perform ADLs more independently.*

- Administer analgesics at regular times throughout the day if the patient has pain that lasts throughout the day.
- Determine the dosage that relieves pain at the patient's desired level.
- Assess how long the first dose lasts.
- Administer the next dose before the last dose wears off. Around-the-clock (ATC) dosing is believed to control pain better than prn (as-needed) dosing (Pasero & McCaffery, 2011).

- Avoid administering small, frequent, ineffective, partial doses within a range; this leads to underdosing.

Nonopioid Analgesics

Nonopioid analgesics include a variety of medications that relieve mild to moderate pain. Many also reduce inflammation and fever. A dose of 650 mg of aspirin or acetaminophen (nonopioids) may relieve as much pain as 50 mg of oral meperidine or 3 to 5 mg of oxycodone, both of which are opioid analgesics.

Nevertheless, nonopioid analgesics are often compounded with opioids. This allows for a lower dose of opioid to be administered and reduces the incidence of side effects.

Nonsteroidal Anti-Inflammatory Drugs The largest group of nonopioid analgesics is made up of NSAIDs. These include aspirin, ibuprofen, naproxen, and celecoxib. NSAIDs act primarily by interfering with the production of prostaglandins. Prostaglandins sensitize pain receptors and are involved with inflammation.

Toward Evidence-Based Practice

Because prescription medication misuse and addiction increase the risk of overdose and death, alternative and adjunctive therapies are essential for pain management.

Ettenberger, M., Maya, R., Salgado-Vasco, A., Monsalve-Duarte, S., Betancourt-Zapata, W., Suarez-Cañon, N., Prieto-Garces, S., Marín-Sánchez, J., Gómez-Ortega, V., & Valderrama, M. (2021). The effect of music therapy on perceived pain, mental health, vital signs, and medication usage of burn patients hospitalized in the intensive care unit: A randomized controlled feasibility study protocol. *Frontiers in Psychiatry, 12*(714209), 1–9. https://doi.org/10.3389/fpsyt.2021.714209

Researchers conducted a study to examine the effect of music therapy on pain responses in adult patients in the intensive care unit suffering burn injuries. The Music Assisted Relaxation (MAR) protocol intervention (self-selected music, guided relaxation, imagery) was implemented over 2 weeks (six interventions). Using the Visual Analog Scale (VAS), findings indicated a reduction in patients' perception of pain. Anxiety and depression, vital signs, and use of analgesic medication were also reduced. The researchers concluded that music therapy may be considered as part of a pain management plan to reduce pain intensity and aid in coping with the pain experience.

Blackburn, L. M., Abel, S., Green, L., Johnson, K., & Panda, S. (2019, February). The use of comfort kits to optimize adult cancer pain management. *Pain Management Nursing, 20*(10), 25–31. https://doi.org/10.1016/j.pmn.2018.01.004

As a measure of pain relief for patients with cancer, nurses prepared comfort kits containing tools for complementary therapy for home use. The kits included handheld massagers, audio-guided imagery, and aromatherapy essential oils. Patients using comfort kits to supplement pain medication rated pain intensity 2.25 points lower (on a scale of 0–10). They had a decrease in the use of pain medication and an increase in ambulation, and they reported more satisfaction with overall pain management.

Moore, M., Schuler, M., Wilson, S., Whisenhunt, M., Adams, A., Leiker, B., Butler, T., Shankweiler, C., Jones, M., & Gibson, C. (2019). More than pills: Alternative adjunct therapies to improve comfort in hospitalised patients. *BMJ Open Quality, 8*(2), e000506. https://doi.org/10.1136/bmjoq-2018-000506

In a study examining the effectiveness of alternative therapy for promoting comfort in hospitalized patients with pain or nausea, 88% of patients using aromatherapy or visual relaxation experienced improvement, and 47% of those using heat or cold reported feeling more comfortable. The researchers concluded that the alternative therapy should be an integral part of a comprehensive treatment approach with less emphasis on prescribed analgesic medications.

Palermo, T. M., Law, E. F., Topazian, M. D., Slack, K., Dear, B. F., Ko, Y. J., Swaroop Vege, S., Fogel, E., Trikudanathan, G., Andersen, D. K., Conwell, D. L., Yadav, D., & Consortium for the Study of Chronic Pancreatitis, Diabetes, and Pancreatic Cancer (CPDPC). (2021, June). Internet cognitive-behavioral therapy for painful chronic pancreatitis: A pilot feasibility randomized controlled trial. *Clinical and Translational Gastroenterology, 12*(6), e00373. https://10.14309/ctg.0000000000000373

Researchers studied the effectiveness of Internet-based cognitive–behavioral pain therapy (CBT) for managing pain related to chronic pancreatitis (CP). Their intervention, called the Pain Course, was a five-lesson program delivered over 8 weeks. This program used techniques involving thought channeling, relaxation, and activity pacing. Pain interference, pain intensity, and quality of life were assessed at pretreatment, posttreatment, and the 3-month follow-up. Researchers found a 50% reduction in pain intensity and pain interference in those receiving Internet-based CBT compared with a 13% improvement for those who did not receive the treatment.

1. For patients using alternative or integrative therapies, such as guided imagery, music, and CBT, to manage pain in various situations, why do you think these techniques might be effective?

2. When teaching alternative or integrative therapies for managing pain, how might you best prepare the setting to maximize the effectiveness of the technique?

3. Can you think of reasons patients might resist trying alternative or integrative methods for managing chronic pain? What would you do to encourage patients who seem to oppose the idea of practicing nonpharmacological pain management?

One of the most common side effects of NSAIDs is gastric irritation and bleeding. Because of the risk of GI bleeding, the long-term use of nonselective NSAIDs is generally not recommended in older adults. Additionally, they can lead to renal failure, high blood pressure, and heart failure in geriatric patients (Levenson et al., 2021).

To administer NSAIDs safely, you should know the following:

- Taking NSAIDs with food, lowering the dose, or using enteric-coated pills can reduce the incidence of GI bleeding.
- NSAIDs should be used with caution in patients who are taking anticoagulants (blood thinners) or who have impaired blood clotting, renal disease, and GI bleeding or ulcers. **Key Point: Aspirin is a unique NSAID. In addition to reducing inflammation, fever, and pain, it can also inhibit platelet aggregation (clumping), the first step in clot formation. For that reason, aspirin should be used with caution. Consult a provider about using other NSAIDs.**
- Some of the newer NSAIDs are less irritating to the GI system, so they cause less gastric irritation and bleeding. However, some are available only by prescription.
- Combining two NSAIDs is not often recommended because it increases the risks of side effects and may not be more effective.
- Regular use of aspirin prolongs clotting time, so teach patients who use aspirin that they will bruise easily and will bleed more if cut.

KnowledgeCheck 28-6

- How do NSAIDs induce pain relief?
- What is the main side effect of NSAIDs?
- In which patients are NSAIDs contraindicated?

Acetaminophen Unlike most nonopioid analgesics, acetaminophen has little anti-inflammatory effect. However, it:

- Has analgesic and fever-reducing properties.
- Has fewer side effects and is probably the safest of the nonopioids.
- Does not affect platelet function, rarely causes GI problems, and can be used in patients who are allergic to aspirin or other NSAIDs.
- Acetaminophen can cause severe hepatotoxicity (liver damage) in patients who take excessive quantities, those with high alcohol intake, or those who have liver disease.

Adjuvant Analgesics

Adjuvant analgesics reduce the amount of opioid the patient requires. Drugs in this category include anticonvulsants, antidepressants, local anesthetics, topical agents, psychostimulants, muscle relaxants, neuroleptics, corticosteroids, and others. Adjuvant analgesics are used:

- As a primary therapy for mild pain
- In conjunction with opioids for moderate to severe pain

- Especially by patients experiencing significant side effects from increased doses of opioids
- To manage neuropathic pain

Opioid Analgesics

Opioids are natural and synthetic compounds that relieve pain, although they vary in potency. To some degree, opioids work by binding with pain receptor sites to block the pain impulse. The process of achieving analgesia is more complex than this, however, because there is more than one kind of receptor.

Types of Opioids

Opiate receptors include mu (μ), delta (δ), kappa (κ), and sigma (Σ) receptors; however, mu receptors are most effective in relieving pain.

- **Mu (μ) agonist opioids** stimulate mu receptors and are used for acute, chronic, and cancer pain. They include codeine, hydrocodone, morphine, hydromorphone, fentanyl, methadone, and oxycodone. This class of medication works for **breakthrough pain,** which is pain that occurs when the patient is already receiving an analgesic for pain control. Mu agonist opioids are used in that case for a rescue, extra, or catch-up dose.
  - Drugs used for breakthrough pain should have a rapid onset and short duration.
  - Whenever possible, use the same drug as that given for ongoing pain relief.
  - Increased dosing may be necessary for unrelieved pain.
  - There is no maximum daily dose limit and no "ceiling" to the level of analgesia from mu agonists; you can steadily increase the dose to achieve pain relief, as long as adverse effects do not occur.
- **Agonist–antagonists** are opioids that stimulate some opioid receptors but block others.
  - They are appropriate for moderate to severe acute pain.
  - They should not be given to patients taking mu agonists (e.g., morphine) because they may act as antagonists at the mu receptor sites and reduce or reverse the analgesia from the mu agonist.
  - Commonly used medications include *mixed agonist–antagonists,* such as pentazocine and nalbuphine, and *partial agonists,* such as buprenorphine.

Opioid Effectiveness

The effectiveness of opioids for pain relief can vary depending on individual differences in metabolism. Body mass alone is not the sole factor for appropriate opioid dosing (D'Arcy, 2008b). For instance, an adult patient with class 3 obesity may not achieve a therapeutic effect with the same dosage that effectively treats a frail older adult.

- **Opioids are most effective for certain types of pain.** For instance, visceral pain, which is more generalized, is most responsive to opioid treatment, whereas pain of neurological origin tends to be resistant to opioids, requiring that they be given as an adjunct to other therapies.

- **For acute pain, immediate-release opioids should be prescribed** using the lowest effective dose and for no longer than necessary.
- **Opioids are not the first-line option for relief of persistent pain.** If they are prescribed for pain management, they should be used in conjunction with nonopioid pain relievers or other nonpharmacological therapies (Dowell et al., 2016).
- **Long-term use of opioids can create other hazards,** including overdose, physical dependence, sedation, and cognitive impairment.

Side Effects of Opioids

Most opioids share the same general side effects, but there are some differences among the specific drugs.

You should know, or look up, the side effects of the specific opioid you are to administer.

- **The most common side effects** are nausea, vomiting, constipation, and drowsiness. These side effects tend to improve after a few doses. See Box 28-3 for strategies to prevent common side effects.
- **Large doses** may lead to respiratory depression and hypotension (Jarzyna et al., 2011).
- **Other side effects of opioids** include difficulty with urination, dry mouth, sweating, tachycardia, palpitations, constipation, bradycardia, rashes, urticaria (hives), or pruritus (itching).
- **Sedation is common at the beginning** of opioid therapy or when the dose is increased. Excessive sedation will precede respiratory depression. Monitor postoperative patients who receive opioids for sedation and respiratory depression every 1 to 2 hours during the first 12 to 24 hours after surgery.

BOX 28-3 ■ Preventing and Treating Side Effects From Opioids

Before deciding to add another medication to treat a side effect, consider changing the dose or frequency of the current opioid or changing to another opioid.

Constipation

- Add more fruits, vegetables, and fiber to the diet. Keep in mind, though, that this does not help relieve opioid-induced constipation unless the patient's current fiber intake is deficient. Excessive fiber might even put the patient at risk for bowel obstruction as a result of the opioid-induced decreased peristalsis (refer to Chapter 26, as needed).
- Increase exercise routine. Even walking short distances will help.
- Increase oral fluid intake to eight 8-ounce glasses of water per day.
- If needed, administer stool softeners.
- If the previous steps are not effective, administer a mild laxative.
- If constipation continues, soften stool with glycerin suppository and follow up with a soapsuds enema.

Nausea and Vomiting

- Reduce opioid dose by combining nonopioid or adjuvant drugs.
- Teach patients that nausea will usually subside after several doses.
- Premedicate or medicate consecutively with an antiemetic. Be aware that this may increase sedation, depending on the antiemetic chosen.
- Teach relaxation techniques.

Pruritus

- Reduce opioid dose by combining with nonopioid or adjuvant drugs.
- Use cool packs, lotion, or topical anesthetics.

- Administer antihistamines, such as diphenhydramine (Benadryl). Be aware that this may increase sedation.
- Teach the patient that they can generally expect to develop a tolerance to pruritus.
- Use distraction techniques, which frequently work well.

Respiratory Depression

- Assess the patient's respiratory status *before* administering the opioid and frequently afterward.
- Reduce the opioid dose by combining with nonopioid or adjuvant drugs.
- Reduce the opioid dose by 25% when you observe signs of oversedation.
- If the patient is not responsive or is only minimally responsive, stop the opioid and administer an antagonist, such as naloxone (Narcan), diluted and very slowly. After dosing with an opioid antidote, reassess the patient for respiratory depression. Naloxone is metabolized more quickly than opioids, and therefore repeat dosing might be needed.

Drowsiness

- Assess the patient to ensure that the drowsiness is a result of opioid administration and not from another cause.
- Teach the patient that drowsiness will generally subside after a few days as they develop tolerance.
- If analgesia is adequate, reduce the opioid by 25%.
- Discontinue all other nonessential central nervous system depressant medications.
- During the daytime, offer simple stimulants, such as caffeine.
- Offer a lower dose more frequently to decrease peak concentration.
- Consider another opioid or route of administration.

- **A paradoxical reaction to opioids** occurs when the patient's pain increases despite receiving increasing doses of opioids (Lee et al., 2011).

For an example of an agitation sedation rating scale, see **Focused Assessment box, Richmond Agitation-Sedation Scale,** in Volume 2.

KnowledgeCheck 28-7

- What are the most common side effects of opioids?
- Identify at least three things that you should monitor when administering opioids.
- What is the risk of addiction to opioids for patients with acute pain?

Equianalgesia

Equianalgesia refers to the approximately equal analgesia that a variety of opioids will provide. Equianalgesic dose calculations provide a starting point when changing from one opioid to another or from one route of administration to another. For example, in terms of the analgesic effect produced:

- A parenteral dose of 5 mg of morphine is equivalent to 60 mg of parenteral codeine or 100 mg of oral codeine.
- A parental dose of 5 mg morphine is the equivalent of 15 mg of oral morphine.

Note: These doses are approximate and vary according to the number of doses, the variety of opioids the patient has received, and the needs of the patient.

Opioid Administration Routes

Use the safest and least invasive route to relieve pain using opioids.

Oral The oral route is convenient and generally safe. It is the preferred route of administration unless a rapid onset of analgesia is desired.

- Oral administration produces steady analgesic levels.
- Use the oral route to provide relief for mild to severe pain.
- Oral PCA is being used in some hospitals to eliminate the delay between the patient's request for medication and the nurse's administration of it.

Nasal A rich supply of blood in the intranasal area provides the drug with easy access to the systemic circulation.

- The mixed agonist–antagonist opioid butorphanol and the mu agonist sufentanil can be administered intranasally.
- One drawback to this route is that it may cause burning or stinging.

Transdermal Transdermal administration is a convenient alternative for a patient who requires constant opioid treatment for pain; however, it does not provide immediate relief.

- The transdermal route delivers a continuous release of the drug for up to 72 hours.

- Fentanyl (Duragesic) is commonly given as a transdermal patch.
- ⊕ Use with care on patients who are febrile (increased body temperature increases absorption of the drug). Inform the patient and family about safe storage and proper disposal of transdermal patches. Proper dating and removal of patches after doses are complete can prevent confusion and dosing errors.

Rectal Suppositories are an excellent alternative to the oral route, especially in infants and young children.

- Effective when the patient is vomiting, has a GI obstruction, or is at risk for aspiration
- May be contraindicated in patients with neutropenia or thrombocytopenia because of the potential to cause rectal bleeding while inserting the suppository

Subcutaneous Subcutaneous administration may be used for intermittent injections and continuous administration of opioids.

- Continuous subcutaneous infusion (CSCI) is appropriate for people who cannot tolerate oral opioids or who have dose-limiting side effects from oral administration (e.g., nausea) and who also have limited venous access.
- Frequently, CSCI of opioids is used for chronic cancer pain and in palliative care because it enables at-home pain control that improves the patient's quality of life without the need for IV access (Jin et al., 2015). Hydromorphone and morphine are the drugs most commonly used.
- Absorption and distribution vary based on the injection site, medications, adiposity, age, patient's circulation, hepatic and renal status, and other health factors.
- Small portable medication pumps allow the patient to be mobile. ⊕ Teach patients and their families how to use the pumps, needles, syringes, and other equipment. Because of the small volume of drug (2 to 3 mL per hour) that can be absorbed, two sites may be needed if higher doses are required.

Intramuscular Intramuscular (IM) injections are painful, the onset of action is slow, and absorption is unreliable.

- With repeated administration, sterile abscesses and fibrotic tissue can result.
- The IM route should be avoided if possible, but especially in children because they often refuse pain medication to avoid having an injection.

Intravenous IV administration produces immediate pain relief and is desirable for acute or escalating pain.

- Most commonly used for short-term therapy and for hospitalized patients who can be monitored

- Also used in the home care setting for patients with cancer and other pain who are unable to tolerate oral opioids
- Methods of IV delivery include continuous infusions, bolus, and PCA.
- Patients receiving a continuous infusion can deliver a bolus for breakthrough pain or procedures, such as wound care.
- Drawbacks include the need for venous access and the need to maintain a patent line.
- Patients who previously used oral opioids may find the IV equipment inconvenient, but they typically report less pain and fewer side effects than with the oral route.

Intra-Articular A pain pump is implanted into a joint during arthroscopic surgery as a measure to control postsurgical pain. The pump provides relief to patients by delivering a continuous infusion of local anesthetic directly to the surgical site.

Intraspinal (Intrathecal and Epidural) Analgesics
- **Intraspinal analgesia:** An anesthesiologist or a certified registered nurse anesthetist (CRNA) places a catheter in (a) the **subarachnoid space** (for intrathecal analgesia) or (b) the **epidural space** (for epidural analgesia).
- The epidural space is preferred because it poses less risk of complications, although they can occur (e.g., dural puncture, infection, hematoma, and nerve damage). See Figure 28-4.
- Placement of the catheter, as well as the type and concentration of medication, determines the area affected by the medication.

- Higher doses are needed for epidural than for intrathecal administration.
- The most used opioids for epidural administration are morphine sulfate, fentanyl citrate, and hydromorphone.
- Local anesthetics are frequently combined with opioids to reduce the total amount of drugs necessary to produce analgesia.
- For nursing care activities associated with caring for a client with an epidural catheter for pain management,

See **Chapter 28, Clinical Insight 28-1: Caring a Patient With an Epidural Catheter,** in Volume 2.

Peripheral Nerve Catheter Infusion of regional anesthesia directly to nerves through a catheter provides pain relief during and for the first few days after certain surgeries (e.g., knee, shoulder, ankle).

Patient-Controlled Analgesia (PCA)
PCA is a method for pain management in which the patient self-administers analgesic medication using a programmable infusion pump. The patient presses to self-administer a dose (Fig. 28-5).

Benefits of PCA Compared with requesting medication from the nurse, patients who have control over their analgesic dosing:

- Experience faster and greater pain relief (i.e., lower pain scores) and reduced anxiety
- Report greater satisfaction with pain management
- Those who use PCA for pain management become active participants in their own recovery.
- The use of PCA can reduce or eliminate the need for intramuscular injection.
- Do not experience the peaks and valleys of intermittent opioid use. This may be because they are better able to

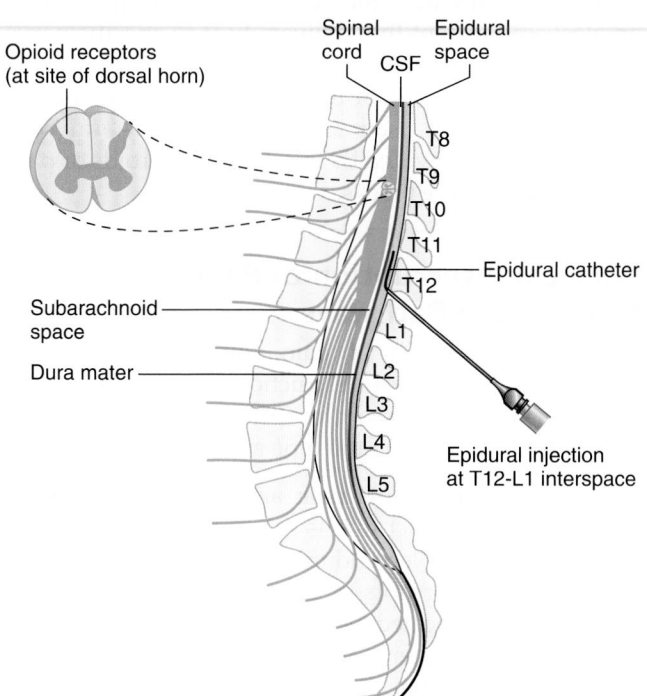

FIGURE 28-4 Placement of an epidural needle and catheter.

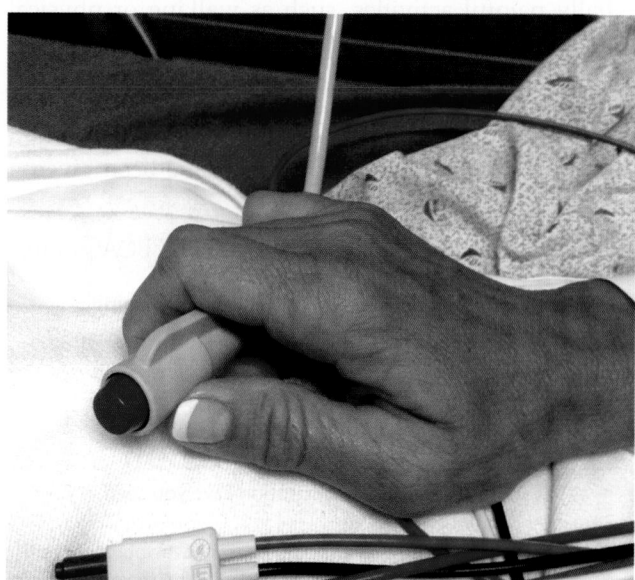

FIGURE 28-5 Dosing button for patient-controlled pump.

self-administer for sufficient pain relief while avoiding dosing that produces undesirable side effects, such as nausea and vomiting, sedation, and hallucinations.

- Use less opioid than when having to wait for the nurse to bring the medication.
- Can move more easily, walk sooner, and breathe deeper because pain is better controlled. This reduces postoperative complications such as pneumonia or blood clots.

Nursing Considerations When Using PCA

- The pump has a built-in computer that is programmed to administer a safe amount of medication over a specific amount of time. Safeguard mechanisms will sound an alarm if the settings are incorrect or if the pump malfunctions.
- Only nurses who are trained in PCAs should set up the pump and the program. As a safety check, another nurse should do an independent verification of the setup before patient use.
- The PCA pump is locked and can only be opened by the nurse or physician. PCA pumps require a special key to unlock them or change the settings.
- PCA pumps are programmed with a 1- or 4-hour maximum lockout interval to prevent overdosing. Even if the patient pushes the button for delivering the dose too many times, the pump will only administer the prescribed amount of medication.
- Nurses assess patients using PCA for signs of excessive sleepiness, changes in mental status, or other signs of the patient being overly medicated.

- Tell patients not to let other people push the button for them, even when they are sleeping. The patient is best at monitoring and administering their own dose.

- Advise patients to always call for help before getting out of bed because dizziness and weakness can occur with opioids.

- Use pulse oximetry to monitor oxygenation while patients are receiving opioid analgesics by PCA. A side effect of opioids can be respiratory depression.
- Encourage patients to administer a dose before potentially painful activities, such as walking or physical therapy.
- If you are teaching the patient about the use of the PCA pump in the postoperative period, before offering your explanation, make sure they are alert enough to understand the directions and have been given a hearing aid or glasses, if needed.

For detailed instructions on the use of a PCA pump,

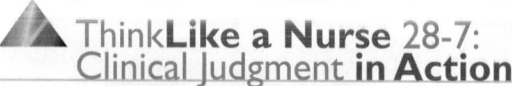

See **Procedure 28-1: Setting Up and Managing a Patient-Controlled Analgesia by Pump,** in Volume 2.

ThinkLike a Nurse 28-7: Clinical Judgment in Action

- What routes of opioid administration have you seen in your clinical rotation?
- What types of pain relief and side effects have you observed?
- What routes of administration would you like to see? Why?

Chemical Pain Relief Measures

Nerve blocks and **epidural injections** are types of regional anesthesia. An anesthetic agent is injected into or around the nerve *(plexus)* that supplies sensation to a specific area of the body. Nerve blocks may be used for short-term pain relief after surgical procedures or for long-term management of persistent pain.

Local Anesthesia Local anesthesia is the injection of local anesthetic into relatively small areas of body tissues for numbing.

- Short-acting agents, such as lidocaine, and long-acting agents, such as Marcaine, may be used.
- Local anesthetic is injected into subcutaneous tissue for minor surgical procedures.
- They may also be injected into joints and muscles for pain relief.
- Pumps are commonly used to administer local anesthetic at surgical sites for postoperative pain relief.

Topical Anesthesia Topical anesthesia involves applying an agent that contains cocaine, lidocaine, or benzocaine directly to the skin, mucous membranes, wounds, or burns. Topical anesthesia is quickly absorbed and provides pain relief for mild to moderate pain. For children, topical anesthetic cream or gel should be applied before vaccination to reduce pain associated with injection (MacDougall et al., 2019; Taddio et al., 1997, 2015) and also before circumcision (Benini et al., 1993; Taddio et al., 1997, 2017) when also used with a ring block and oral sucrose (MacDougall et al., 2019; Sharara-Chami et al., 2017).

Radiofrequency Ablation

Radiofrequency ablation reduces pain by generating an electrical current that delivers heat to specific nerve tissue. By *ablating* (burning) the nerve that is causing pain, the transmission of the pain sensation is blocked. This procedure is used to provide longer-term pain relief than that provided by injections of steroids or pain relievers and nerve blocks.

Surgical Interruption of Pain Conduction Pathways

Surgical interruption of pain conduction pathways results in a permanent destruction of nerve pathways and is used as a last resort for intractable pain. The various options depend on the type and location of pain.

- **Cordotomy** interrupts pain and temperature sensation below the tract that is severed. This is most frequently done for leg and trunk pain.
- **Rhizotomy** interrupts the anterior or posterior nerve route that is located between the ganglion and the cord. Anterior interruption is generally used to stop spastic movements that accompany paraplegia, and posterior interruption eliminates pain in the area

innervated. This procedure may be safely performed at any level along the spine but is most often used for head and neck pain produced by cancer.

- **Neurectomy** is used to eliminate intractable localized pain. The pathways of peripheral or cranial nerves are interrupted to block pain transmission.
- **Sympathectomy** severs the paths to the sympathetic division of the autonomic nervous system. The outcomes of this procedure are improvement in vascular blood supply and the elimination of vasospasm. It is used to treat pain from vascular disorders, such as Raynaud disease.

Surgical therapies disrupting pain pathways are not widely used because of advances in oral and transdermal opioid therapies.

KnowledgeCheck 28-8

- Identify three types of chemical pain relief measures.
- What type of patient might be suitable for surgical interruption of a pain pathway?

Misconceptions That Interfere With Pain Management

Patient Misconceptions Patients sometimes have beliefs about pain or pain management strategies that interfere with the treatment plan. For instance:

- One older patient may fear that severe pain is a sign of weakness and try to endure it.

  - Some older adults might perceive pain with the physical declines that accompany aging, whereas others see it as an acute situation that requires treatment.
- An athlete might believe "no pain, no gain," although actually, pain can signal an injury, strain, or misalignment.

- A family member may worry that pain medication may make the patient nonfunctional.
- A patient might fear addiction to pain medication even though they are taking nonopioid analgesics, which are not addictive.

Clinician and Caregiver Misconceptions The beliefs of healthcare providers and caregivers can also interfere with pain management. For example, nurses and other caregivers sometimes doubt the patient's report of pain because:

- Most people don't have pain from that particular illness or procedure.
- There is no obvious, physical cause for the pain.
- They are concerned about drug-seeking behavior and patient addiction.

As you care for patients in pain, remain open to the patient's description of pain and work with the patient and caregivers to provide pain control. Pain is invisible to others, but it exists even when there are no sure signs of pain or an apparent cause. Table 28-2 highlights some of the most common misconceptions and truths about pain.

Managing Pain in Older Patients

Pain, particularly persistent pain, is common among older adults, especially those suffering from degenerative spine conditions, arthritis, nightly leg pain, or pain as a result of cancer. Undertreated pain and inadequate pain management can result in falls, poor sleep, reduced appetite, delayed healing, reduced activity, mood changes (depression and anxiety), and prolonged hospitalization. It can lead to other problems that diminish the quality of life, such as social isolation, anxiety, fear, and depression (American Geriatrics Society Panel on the Pharmacological

Table 28-2 ➤ Common Misconceptions Among Patients and Caregivers About Pain

FALLACY	TRUTH
The caregiver is more objective than the patient about the amount of pain experienced.	*The patient's report is the "gold standard," and the patient is the authority.*
You should wait until the pain is severe before taking medication.	*You should take pain medication before the pain becomes severe and on a scheduled basis to keep pain under control.*
Pain is a normal component of aging.	*Pain is a symptom that something is wrong and should be treated.*
Complaining of pain will label the person as a "bad patient."	*The patient should report pain so that it can be treated.*
Patients should have severe pain only if they have had major surgery.	*Even minor surgery and injury can produce severe pain.*
Patients will have visible physical or behavioral signs if they are really in pain.	*Even when patients are in severe pain, they may not exhibit physical or behavioral signs.*

Management of Persistent Pain in Older Persons, 2009; Horgas, 2007).

Pain management among older patients is especially complex for the following reasons:

- **Multiple medications.** Most older adults have at least one chronic condition and take multiple medications. Adding analgesics to a complex medication regimen increases the likelihood of drug interactions.
- **Physical changes of aging.** Drug distribution is altered in older patients because of changes in blood flow to the organs, protein binding, renal clearance, liver metabolism, and difference in body composition.
- **Provider reluctance to administer analgesics.** Older adults are at great risk for undertreatment of pain because they and their caregivers may be reluctant to administer analgesics for fear of producing confusion, excessive sedation, drug interactions, and respiratory depression (American Geriatrics Society, Panel on Persistent Pain in Older Persons, 2009).
- **Provider failure to recognize ineffective pain management.** Healthcare providers often fail to recognize poor pain management because of the patient's dementia, coexisting medical conditions, sensory impairment, or inability to verbally communicate the quality or intensity of pain.
- **Giving more analgesics than needed.** With aging and declining renal and liver function, the peak effect of medications is longer, which can lead to giving more pain-relieving medication than needed (American Geriatrics Society, Panel on Persistent Pain in Older Persons, 2009).

Administering Opioids to Older Adults Key Point: *Persistent pain is not a normal part of aging and should not be ignored.*

- **Consider oral opioid therapy** for older adults with severe pain or diminished quality of life because of pain (American Geriatrics Society, Panel on Persistent Pain in Older Persons, 2009).
- **Start low and go slow,** as a general rule—meaning, start with the lowest effective recommended dose and increase the dose slowly if needed (Kaye et al., 2010). Take caution with opioid use because older adults may not clear the medication as effectively as younger adults. Older adults tend to take multiple medications, which increases the likelihood of drug-to-drug and drug-to-disease interactions, compounded side effects, and unpredictable responses to medication.
- **Risk for falls increases.** Be aware that opioid use in older adults increases the risk of falls.

Administering Nonopioid Analgesics to Older Adults Nonopioids have been discussed as an intervention under the heading "Pharmacological Pain Relief Measures." To summarize their use in older adults:

- **Acetaminophen** is a first-line treatment for mild pain, particularly musculoskeletal pain, and is often used as an adjuvant therapy for older persons with recurring pain.
- **NSAIDs** are a good option for those with compromised kidney or liver function.
- **Gabapentin** has few side effects and can also be used in combination with nonopioid analgesics to relieve neuropathic pain.

ThinkLike a Nurse 28-8: Clinical Judgment in Action

- Which groups of patients are most at risk for inadequate pain management?
- What can you do to assist each group?
- How do past pain experiences affect the present pain experience?

Managing Pain in Patients With Substance Misuse and Abuse

Misuse of prescription drugs means taking a medication in a manner or dose other than prescribed, taking someone else's prescription, or using a medication to feel euphoria (National Institutes of Health [NIH], National Institute on Drug Abuse, 2020). **Addiction** is a state of psychological dependence in which a person uses a drug compulsively and will engage in self-destructive behavior to obtain the drug, even when they cause harm to themselves or others.

Screen for Abuse Potential Assessing for abuse is important for all patients who use prescribed opioids and those with chronic, nonmalignant pain.

♥ **iCare** When caring for clients with active addiction, try to remain nonjudgmental.

When devising a pain management plan for patients struggling with substance abuse or misuse, you may assess for the following factors:

- Illegal drug use; prescription drug use for nonmedical reasons
- History of substance use disorder or overdose
- Mental health conditions (e.g., depression, anxiety)
- Sleep-disordered breathing
- Concurrent benzodiazepine use

Key Point: *Healthcare professionals often fail to recognize substance abuse unless they actively screen for it. You can't rely on the normalcy of behavior to indicate opioid abuse. Random drug screening will show opioid use even when unusual behavior is not obvious.* To screen for abuse, use a validated risk assessment tool, such as the following:

- The **Opioid Risk Tool (ORT).** This is a yes/no self-report designed to predict a patient's tendency for aberrant behaviors when prescribed opioid analgesia.

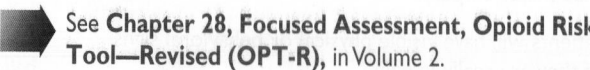

See **Chapter 28, Focused Assessment, Opioid Risk Tool—Revised (OPT-R),** in Volume 2.

- The **Screener and Opioid Assessment for Patients With Pain (SOAPP®).** This is more detailed than the

ORT and is a reliable tool used for assessing patients who are experiencing persistent pain and might be helped with long-term opioid treatment.

- The **Current Opioid Misuse Measure (COMM™)** is used to identify opioid misuse among patients currently taking long-term opioid medication.

Monitor for Substance Abuse Behaviors If you observe the following behaviors, assess the patient carefully because the signs may also indicate untreated withdrawal or increased pain resulting from a complication:

- Repeated requests for opioids or atypical high dosing when pain should normally be diminishing with recovery from an injury or surgery
- Refusal to try oral medication for pain relief
- "Doctor shopping"—moving from provider to provider in an effort to obtain multiple prescriptions for the drug(s) they abuse
- "Pharmacy shopping"—using multiple pharmacies to dispense controlled substances

For more in-depth information about the assessment and treatment of patients with substance abuse and addiction, refer to Substance Abuse and Mental Illness in Chapter 9.

Monitor for and Minimize Suicide Risk Greater opioid dose is a marker for increased suicide risk (Ilegn et al., 2016). To help reduce the risk of overdose and death among patients receiving opioids:

- Refer to a mental health professional for evaluation and therapeutic intervention.
- Check the patient's opioid prescriptions using a drug-monitoring program.
- Arrange for random urine drug testing.
- Ensure the patient has a prescription for naloxone in cases of opioid overdose (U.S. Department of Veterans Affairs, 2017).

- ✚ Opioids should not be prescribed when there is a risk for suicide (U.S. Department of Veterans Affairs, 2017).

Other Interventions
- For those at moderate risk for opioid abuse, maximize appropriate nonopioid medications and other nonpharmacological therapies to reduce pain.
- When analgesics are no longer needed, taper the dose to prevent withdrawal symptoms from occurring (Pasero & McCaffery, 2011).

Key Point: *As a nurse, you have a duty to maintain the balance between providing adequate pain relief and protecting against inappropriate drug use.*

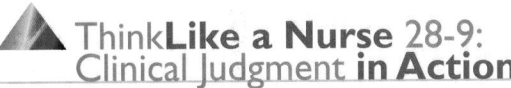

ThinkLike a Nurse 28-9:
Clinical Judgment **in Action**

You are preparing to give your patient a bath. When you remove their bath equipment from under the bedside table, you find illicit drugs mixed in with the bath equipment. What would you do?

Pain Relief From Placebos

A **placebo** is any medication, procedure, or surgery that leads to analgesia or other desired outcome, even if lacking active substances or other actions that contribute to pain relief. Clearly, placebos can relieve pain for some patients. How they do so is not well understood. Theories include operant conditioning, faith, anxiety reduction, and endorphin release. **Key Point:** *Although the use of placebos may be appropriate in clinical trials, they are not suitable for pain management.*

- Occasionally, patients experience less pain after receiving a placebo. However, if the patient responds to a placebo, it does not mean that the patient did not have pain.
- There is no way to determine in advance which patients will experience pain relief from a placebo and which ones will not. Even in the same patient, placebos may relieve pain at one time and not at another.
- Ethically, the most important reason for not using placebos is that their use involves deceit. If discovered, and it frequently is, the patient is likely to lose trust in healthcare professional's care.

Teaching the Patient and Family About Pain

Educate patients about what they can expect for pain outcome and their options for managing pain. When patients and caregivers are well informed, they tend to cope more effectively and tend to be more involved in their care. This helps to fine-tune pain management regimens and improve patient comfort and satisfaction. Because pain can interfere with a patient's learning, be sure to include the patient's family in your teaching. If the patient is discharged from the facility with a prescription for pain-relieving medication, especially one for opioids, you have a responsibility to discuss the following topics with patients and caregivers:

- The cause of pain if it is known
- The normal duration of the pain, if known (e.g., postoperative pain generally decreases every day as tissues heal)
- How to use the selected pain scale; ask for a demonstration of use
- The overall pain management plan
- Information about the analgesic prescribed—dose, interval, and route of administration
- If appropriate, explanation that opioids can be managed carefully to minimize the risk of addiction and that they do not need to suffer unnecessarily
- Nonpharmacological ways to treat pain
- Possible side effects and how to assess for them
- The impact on ADLs
- The need to alter the treatment plan if relief is not achieved

- How the family can contact the healthcare team regarding side effects, missed doses, change in condition, or ineffective pain management
- Safe storage and disposal of opioids when prescribed (The Joint Commission, 2022)

Documentation

Documentation may be narrative, in either nursing or interprofessional notes, or recorded on a pain management flowsheet. Although documentation varies from facility to facility, it typically reflects the entire spectrum of the nursing process:

- The expected outcome for pain management
- The patient's pain level
- The patient's response to interventions for pain
- Adverse reactions that may have resulted from the analgesic
- Planned interventions to improve the pain relief if needed

Typically, pain management records include a field for time, pain ratings, and analgesic used, including dose and route, vital signs, and side effects. They are tailored to the patient population, the type of pain being monitored, and the clinical setting. Documentation is important because typically, pain recall is poor, and patients often underestimate their pain after the fact.

EVALUATION

Evaluation is critical to pain management. Your patient evaluation should include the following:

- Are the patient's pain scores consistently at or better than the desired level? Are they improving?
- Is the patient's behavior, mobility, range of motion, mood, sleep, and/or affect consistent with pain relief?
- What is the quality of the patient's life, according to the patient's standards?

Evaluate the Effectiveness of the Interventions In addition to evaluating the extent to which the pain was relieved, you need to determine which interventions were or were not effective, as well as any adverse reactions to these interventions. Close examination of the patient's pain relief diary should provide most of the data you need for evaluation. For a sample of a client diary,

 See **Chapter 28, Focused Assessment box, Pain Relief Diary,** in Volume 2.

It Is Important to Reassess the Patient's Pain Regularly An increase in pain may be a sign of inadequate pain management, but it may also be a sign of developing complications. Before implementing a change in the treatment plan, you should determine whether the pain management plan was carried out correctly. If the decision of the healthcare team is to make a change, remember to reevaluate the effect of this change. Do not assume your intervention will provide adequate pain relief.

NURSING PROCESS IN ACTION

Mary Jean Thompson, 30 years old, was admitted to the hospital with severe abdominal pain and underwent an appendectomy yesterday. The surgeon has prescribed hydromorphone 2 mg tablet PO q4 hr prn for pain. Ms. Thompson doesn't like the idea of taking pain medication and waits until she rates her pain a 9 or 10 on a scale of 0 to 10 before requesting medication. Even after the medication, her pain never drops below a 7 on a scale of 0 to 10, and she is unwilling to turn or ambulate because of the pain.

When you perform your assessment, she tells you she does not want to be sedated. "I hate that groggy, drugged feeling. I'm willing to have some pain to avoid that." After you discuss the importance of pain management to aid in healing and the ability to participate in activities and therapy, Ms. Thompson states that she would like to have a pain score of 2 to 3 today. See the accompanying plan for her pain management.

Nursing Care Plan

Pain Management: Nursing Care

Nursing Diagnosis

Acute Pain (surgical incision) related to possible inadequate analgesia (drug and dosing) because of reluctance to take pain medication, as manifested by not requesting medication until her pain is at a score of 9.

Expected Outcomes	Nursing Interventions	Rationale
On a scale of 0–10, the patient will verbalize pain relief at a score of 3 or below while in bed and 4 or below while ambulating at all times.	Assess and document the patient's verbal and nonverbal expressions of pain relief with each check of vital signs, with every procedure and ambulation, and when the patient is at rest.	Assessment is necessary to determine the effectiveness of the prescribed medications. Assessment and documentation are legal responsibilities for the nurse as well.
	Discuss with the prescriber the need to modify medication dose or type if pain relief measures are ineffective. Recommend patient-controlled analgesia (PCA).	Ineffective pain management will cause the patient increased stress and can lead to further complications because the patient will be unwilling to move.
	When you obtain new pain orders for a PCA morphine pump, educate the patient about the pump.	A patient using PCA requires instruction about safe use of the pump.
	Provide nonpharmacological interventions, such as a back rub or other techniques described in this chapter, before rest or sleep, with any exacerbation of pain, and after painful procedures such as ambulation.	Nonpharmacological interventions are synergistic and enhance the relief the opioid gives.
The patient will demonstrate pain relief by participating in ambulation and turning within 24 hours.	Teach the patient to deliver the self-administered pain medication using the PCA before activities.	Peak blood levels enable the patient to ambulate, cough and deep-breathe, and perform activities of daily living.

Care Map

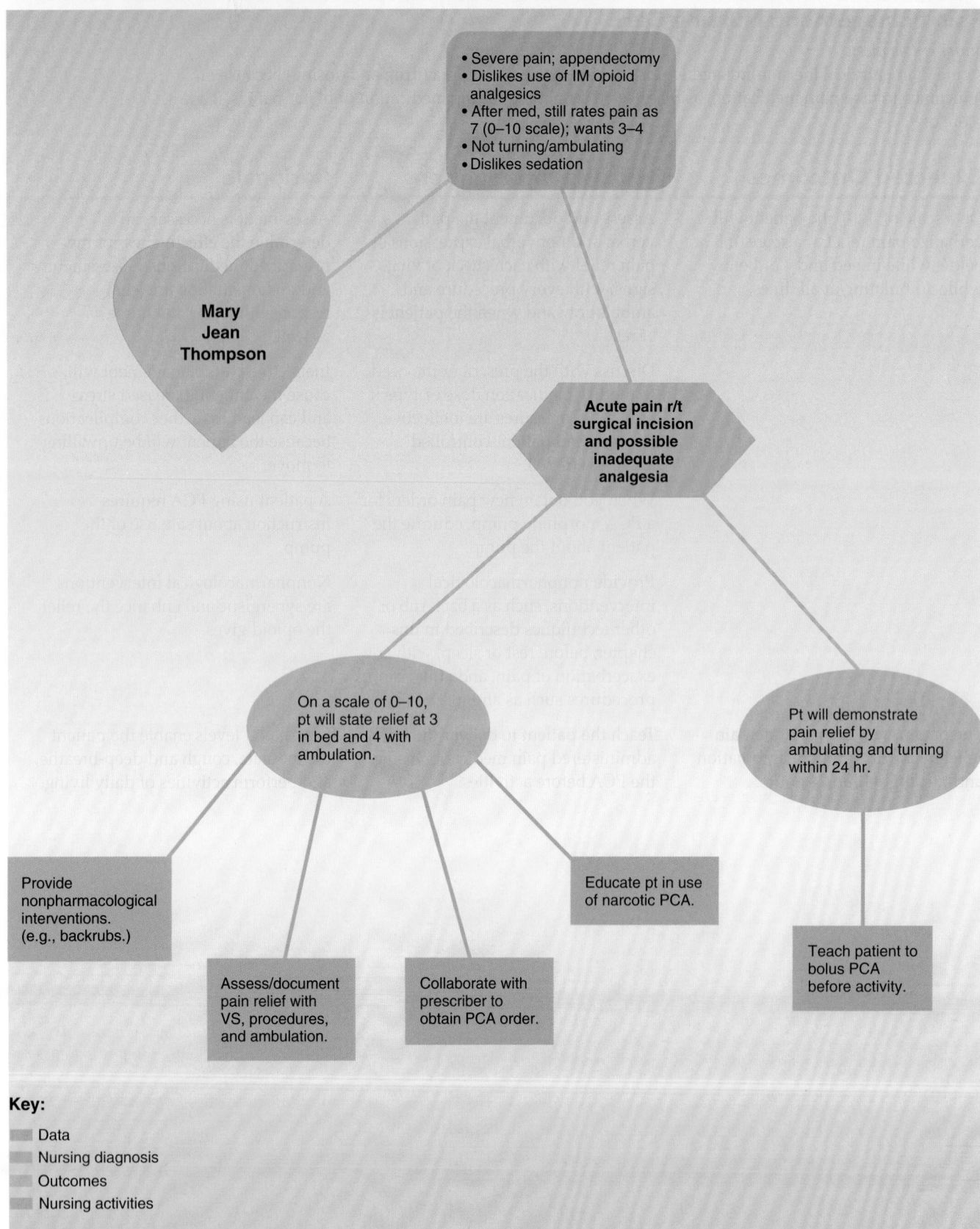

- Severe pain; appendectomy
- Dislikes use of IM opioid analgesics
- After med, still rates pain as 7 (0–10 scale); wants 3–4
- Not turning/ambulating
- Dislikes sedation

Mary Jean Thompson

Acute pain r/t surgical incision and possible inadequate analgesia

On a scale of 0–10, pt will state relief at 3 in bed and 4 with ambulation.

Pt will demonstrate pain relief by ambulating and turning within 24 hr.

Provide nonpharmacological interventions. (e.g., backrubs.)

Assess/document pain relief with VS, procedures, and ambulation.

Collaborate with prescriber to obtain PCA order.

Educate pt in use of narcotic PCA.

Teach patient to bolus PCA before activity.

Key:

- Data
- Nursing diagnosis
- Outcomes
- Nursing activities

To explore learning resources for this chapter,

Go to Davis Advantage and find:

Answers and Suggested Responses for all questions in this chapter
Concept Map
Knowledge Map
References and Bibliography

CHAPTER 29

Physical Activity & Immobility

Learning Outcomes

After completing this chapter, you should be able to:

➤ Discuss the physiology of movement.
➤ Use proper body mechanics when providing patient care.
➤ Discuss the concept of fitness.
➤ Describe the five types of exercise discussed in this chapter.
➤ Compare the effects of exercise and immobility on the body.
➤ Describe the physical activity recommended for health promotion, cardiovascular fitness, and maintenance of healthy weight.
➤ Discuss factors that affect body alignment and activity.
➤ Identify patients who are at risk for immobility or activity intolerance.
➤ Develop a plan of care for patients with decreased activity tolerance.
➤ Implement care related to a patient's mobility problems.

Key Concepts

Fitness
Mobility
Physical Activity

Related Concepts

See the Concept Map on Davis Advantage.

Example Client Condition

Prolonged Immobility

Meet Your Patients

You are attending a health promotion series at the local hospital in order to fulfill the requirement in your state for continuing nursing education. For the next 4 weeks, the topic is exercise. In the group, you meet the following people:

■ **Phillip Flanders** is a 40-year-old accountant. He works long hours in an office setting doing work that is sedentary and requires concentration. Although he is not physically active, he often feels tired. He does not exercise regularly. Many of his friends have suggested that he begin an exercise program to improve his energy and health. Phillip would like to learn how to get started with an overall fitness program that works with his job and family life. Before getting started, he makes an appointment with his primary care provider for a thorough health evaluation.

■ **Peter Phan** is 28 years old and a marathon runner and triathlete. On average, he runs 35 miles per week and cycles at least twice per week. Peter has had plantar fasciitis in the past that was painful and caused him to

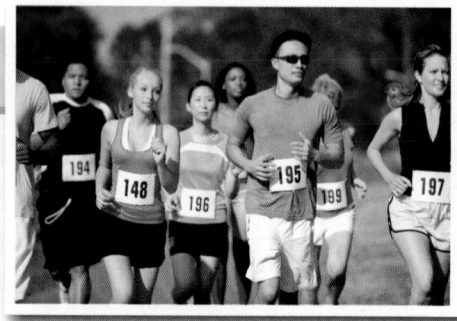

take a break from his training. Peter would like to learn what he can do to prevent other injuries.

■ **Helen Jillian** is 72 years old. She has hypertension and high cholesterol levels, for which she takes four medications. She is 5 ft 1 in. tall and weighs 340 lb. Recently she began having chest pain when starting a brisk walk. Her provider prescribed nitroglycerin for the chest pain, and after a thorough cardiac evaluation, her provider advised her to enroll in a cardio fitness program. She does not understand why she is being asked to do these things because activity seems to trigger her chest pain.

In this chapter, you will find answers to each of these patient questions about activity and exercise. In addition, you will learn more about assisting patients with mobility problems.

Theoretical Knowledge
knowing why

Primitive nomadic people were active just meeting their daily needs. Tribes commonly journeyed to hunt for game; people were on foot, gathering roots, fruits, and other edible plants. Survival depended on physical activity, such as changing locations to find food or escape a dangerous situation. Later, the shift to an agrarian society reduced the need for most people to hunt and gather food. However, farming itself was hard work, and people were physically active most of the year.

Today, with modern grocery distribution systems, we expend minimal physical energy to obtain food. In addition, there are many occupations in which people spend hours in front of a computer screen. Many of today's leisure activities (e.g., watching television, playing video games) are also sedentary. Even though fitness equipment and health clubs are popular among some people, the overall level of fitness in the United States is declining. Only about half of adolescents engage in regular, moderate to vigorous activity on a regular basis. And fewer than a third of adults achieve the recommended amount of physical activity needed for health and fitness. To get enough exercise, most people need to make a conscious effort to build exercise and activity into their lives. This chapter will help you to understand why that is important.

ABOUT THE KEY CONCEPTS

Three concepts are widely used to describe human movement, mobility, physical activity, fitness, and exercise.

- **Mobility,** simply, is body movement.
- **Fitness** (or **physical fitness**) is the ability to carry out activities of daily living (ADLs) with vigor and alertness, without undue fatigue, and with enough energy for leisure pursuits and to respond to emergencies (U.S. Department of Health and Human Services [USDHHS], 2018).
- **Physical activity** is bodily movement produced by the contraction of skeletal muscle that increases energy expenditure above a baseline level (USDHHS, 2018).
- **Exercise** is a subconcept of physical activity. It is planned, structured, and repetitive and is engaged in to improve or maintain physical fitness, physical performance, or health (Caspersen et al., 1985).

As you read this chapter, you will learn how the key concepts of physical activity, fitness, and mobility are related and how they relate to subconcepts such as exercise and body mechanics. Once you have a grasp of these concepts, you should be able to apply them to any patient, regardless of their particular health problem or medical diagnosis.

PHYSIOLOGY OF MOVEMENT

Activity and exercise require body movement **(mobility).** Mobility depends on the successful interaction among the skeleton, the muscles, and the nervous system.

Skeletal System

The skeletal system includes bones, cartilage, ligaments, and tendons. The skeleton forms the framework of the body, protects the internal organs, produces blood cells, and stores mineral salts (e.g., calcium) and fat.

Bones Bones consist of a hard outer shell with a spongy interior (Fig. 29-1). There are 206 bones in the human body:

Long bones—femur and humerus
Short bones—phalanges and metacarpals
Flat bones—sternum and cranial bones
Irregularly shaped bones—vertebrae and tarsal bones

Bone is made up of both spongy **osseous** (bone) tissue and hard, durable **compact** bone.

- Bone is made up of a latticework of bone tissue, called **trabeculae,** that adds strength without extra weight (Fig. 29-1A).
- Bone marrow is within the spongy bone.
- Compact bone consists of layers of onion-like rings, called **lamellae** (Fig. 29-1B).
- Microscopic passageways (**Volkmann canals** and **canaliculi**) provide a way for blood vessels and nerves in the center of the bone to supply the bone matrix with oxygen and nutrients.
- These canals also provide a way for **osteocytes** (bone cells) to move in and out of the bone matrix for the healing and strengthening of bone that occurs with growth, stress to the bone, and repair after injury.

Bones feel strong, so it is easy to forget that they are composed of living tissue that is constantly building and remodeling. **Osteoclasts** are specialized cells that function as housekeepers in the bone by breaking down old or damaged tissue. **Osteoblasts** repair damaged bone and build new bone to keep the skeleton strong. A delicate balance exists between the actions of the osteoblasts and the osteoclasts.

Joints When two bones come close together **(articulate),** a joint is formed. Body movement occurs at the joints. Joints are classified based on the amount of movement they permit:

- **Synarthroses** are immovable joints (e.g., the sutures between the cranial bones). In youth, these joints have some flexibility to allow growth, but they gradually become rigid.

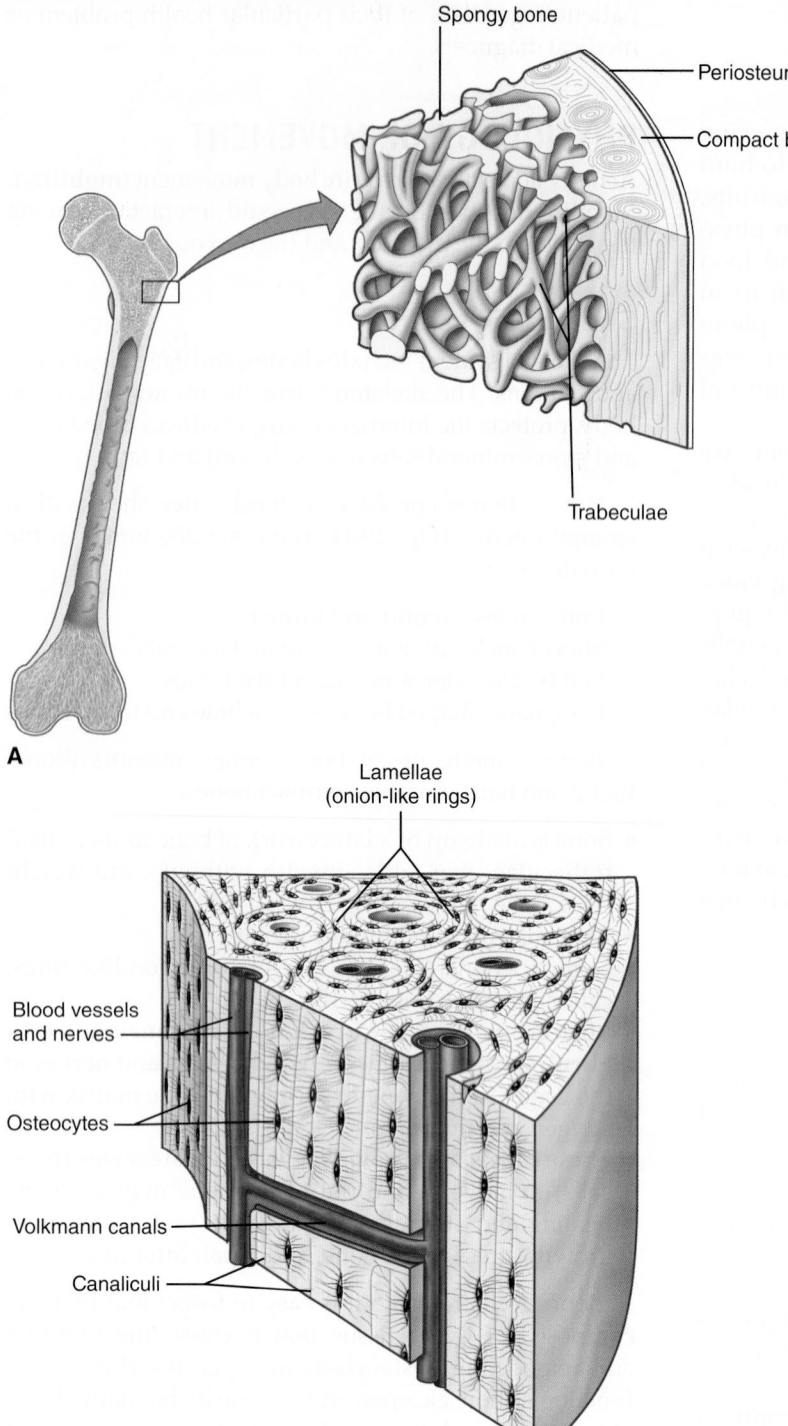

FIGURE 29-1 *A*, Spongy bone. *B*, Compact bone.

- **Amphiarthroses** allow for limited movement. Examples are the joints between the vertebrae and pubic bones.
- **Diarthroses,** or **synovial joints**, are freely movable because of the amount of space between the articulating bones. Synovial joints are filled with **synovial fluid**, and the joint surfaces of the articulating bones are covered with smooth **articular cartilage** (connective tissue found in the joints and skeleton). The synovial fluid and articular cartilage prevent friction as the

bones move. Table 29-1 identifies the types of movable joints in the body.

Cartilage, Ligaments, and Tendons Cartilage, ligaments, and tendons serve as the interface between the skeleton and the muscles.

- **Ligaments** are fibrous tissues that connect most movable joints. Ligaments are flexible to allow freedom of movement but strong and tough so that they do not yield under the force of movement.

Table 29-1 ➤ Types of Synovial Joints

TYPE	DESCRIPTION	EXAMPLES
Ball-and-socket	A rounded head (ball) fits into a cuplike structure (socket) to allow movement in all planes in addition to rotation.	Shoulder and hip joints
Condyloid	An oval-shaped bone fits into an elliptical cavity to allow movement in two planes at right angles to each other.	Wrist
Gliding	Two flat plane surfaces move past each other.	Intervertebral joints
Hinge	A convex surface fits into a cavity, allowing flexion and extension.	Knee and elbow
Pivot	The joint is formed by a ringlike object that turns on a pivot. Motion is limited to rotation.	The atlas and axis of the first vertebrae and base of the skull
Saddle	One bone surface is concave in one direction and convex in the other. The other surface has the opposite construction so that the bones fit together. Movement is possible in two planes at right angles to each other.	Carpal–metacarpal joint of the thumb

- **Tendons** are fibrous connective tissues that attach muscles to the bone. Muscles span a joint and attach by tendons to two different bones.
- **Cartilage** is smooth, elastic connective tissue that acts as a cushion around the joints and other parts of the body (rib cage, ear pinnae, nose, bronchial tubes, vertebral disks). Although cartilage is strong and flexible, it is relatively easy to damage.

Muscles

Muscles make up about half of body weight. When they contract, they cause movement. The type of movement depends on the type of muscle: skeletal, smooth, or cardiac.

- **Skeletal muscle** moves bones and joints.
- **Smooth muscle** occurs in the digestive tract and other hollow structures, such as the bladder and blood vessels. Smooth muscles produce movement of food through the digestive tract, urine through the urinary tract, and blood through the circulatory system.
- **Cardiac muscle** is a unique form of muscle that has the ability to contract spontaneously. It is responsible for the beating of the heart.

Muscles span a joint and attach by tendons to two different bones. They attach at two points: (1) at the **point of origin,** to the more stationary bone, and (2) at the **point of insertion,** to the more movable bone. The "belly" (thickest part) of the muscle lies between these two points. When a skeletal muscle contracts, it shortens, thus causing one bone to move at the joint.

Key Point: *Muscles work in pairs.* For example, the biceps brachii contracts to flex the forearm (bend the elbow joint). When the biceps contracts, the opposing muscle, the triceps brachii, relaxes. Similarly, contraction of the triceps is associated with relaxation of the biceps (Fig. 29-2).

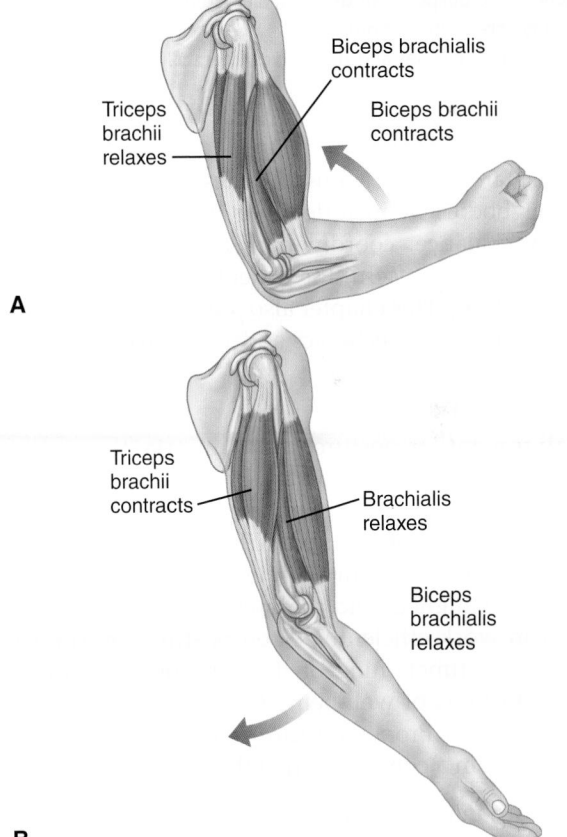

FIGURE 29-2 Antagonistic muscles. A, Flexion of the forearm. B, Extension of the forearm.

Motor Nervous System

The nervous system controls the movement of the musculoskeletal system. Motor nerves are either autonomic or somatic.

- The **autonomic nervous system** consists of the sympathetic and parasympathetic nervous systems that control involuntary muscles, such as the heart, blood vessels, and glands.

■ The **somatic nervous system** controls the voluntary skeletal muscles.

When you make a conscious decision to bend your elbow, the thought originates in the motor area of your cerebral cortex. The upper motor efferent nerves communicate with the lower motor neurons that conduct impulses to the muscles. When the muscle receives sufficient stimuli, it contracts the biceps as the triceps relaxes and moves the elbow.

Movement also occurs through reflex mechanisms. Common reflexes include the knee-jerk reflex and corneal reflex. Reflexes are discussed at length in Chapter 19.

A muscle contraction, whether conscious or reflexive, stimulates afferent nerves that convey information to the cerebral cortex and the cerebellum. This information helps control and coordinate movements.

KnowledgeCheck 29-1

■ Name three purposes of the skeletal system.
■ Identify three types of muscle.
■ How do the muscles and the nerves interact?

BODY MECHANICS

Body mechanics is a term used to describe the way we move our bodies. It includes four components: body alignment, balance, coordination, and joint mobility. These concepts are useful for patient teaching and safe patient handling. This chapter also presents some guidelines for good body mechanics and safe movement.

Body Alignment

Body alignment, or posture, is an important aspect of body mechanics. Proper posture places the spine in a neutral (resting) position. Proper posture maintains the natural curves of the spine (Fig. 29-3) because it allows movement to occur with less stress and fatigue; the bones are aligned, and the muscles, joints, and ligaments can work efficiently. Good posture contributes to the normal functioning of the nervous system and improves feelings of well-being (see the Self-Care box, Tips to Maintain Proper Posture). Most posture problems result from a combination of the following:

Accidents, injuries, and falls
Careless sitting, standing, or sleeping habits
Excessive weight
Foot problems or improper shoes
Negative self-image
Occupational stress
Poor sleep support (mattress)
Poorly designed workspace
Visual difficulties
Weak muscles or muscle imbalance
Skeletal misalignment or malformation (e.g., scoliosis, kyphosis, lordosis)

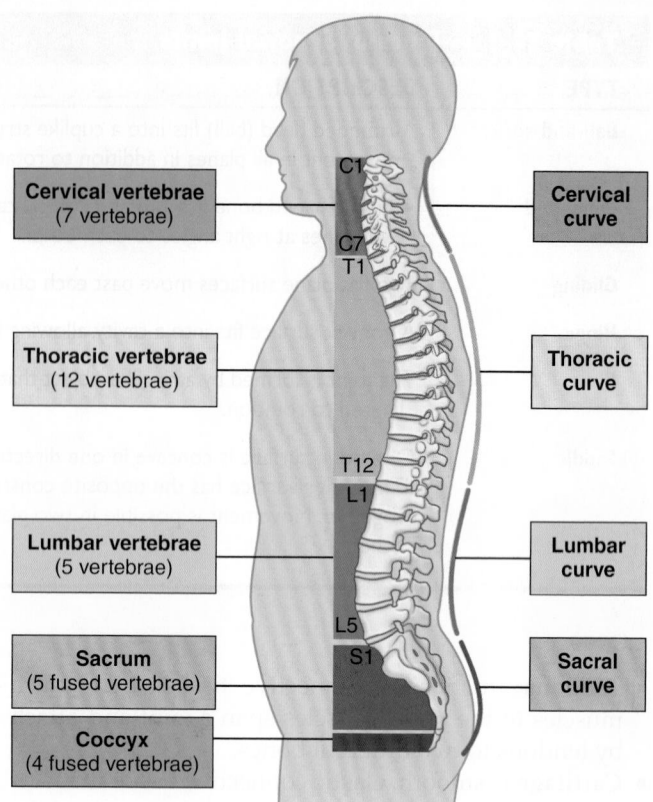

FIGURE 29-3 Natural curves to the spine.

For an illustration,

 See **Chapter 19, Procedure 19-12: Assessing the Chest and Lungs** and **Procedure 19-15: Assessing the Musculoskeletal System,** in Volume 2.

Balance

The body achieves balance when it is in alignment. For your body to be balanced, your line of gravity must pass through your center of gravity, and your center of gravity must be close to your base of support.

■ The **line of gravity** is an imaginary vertical line drawn from the top of the head through the center of gravity.
■ The **center of gravity** is the point around which mass is distributed. In the human body, the center of gravity is below the umbilicus at the top of the pelvis.
■ The **base of support** is what holds the body up. The feet provide the base of support.

To avoid injury when moving objects, place your center of gravity closest to your base of support and stand with your head erect, buttocks pulled in, abdominal muscles tight, chest high, shoulders pulled back, and feet wide (Fig. 29-4).

Use a wide stance, with feet apart and one foot forward, when standing for a long period of time. **Key point:** *The broader the base of support, the lower the center of gravity and the easier it is to maintain balance.*

Tips to Maintain Proper Posture

➤ Avoid standing in one position for a lengthy period. If you cannot change positions, elevate one foot on a stool or box, and alternate foot placement frequently.

➤ Avoid locking your knees when standing upright.

➤ Keep your core muscles tight to support your back.

➤ Do not bend forward at the waist or neck when you are working in a low position.

➤ When you are seated at your desk, work at a comfortable height, with a proper ergonomic chair and equipment.

➤ Do not wear high-heeled or platform shoes for long periods of time.

➤ Maintain good posture when you sit.

➤ Sit close to your work.

➤ Use a chair that supports your back in a slightly arched position.

➤ Sit with your feet flat on the floor and your knees below your hips.

➤ Sleep on a mattress that is firm but not extremely hard. Use pillows between the knees for proper alignment and support.

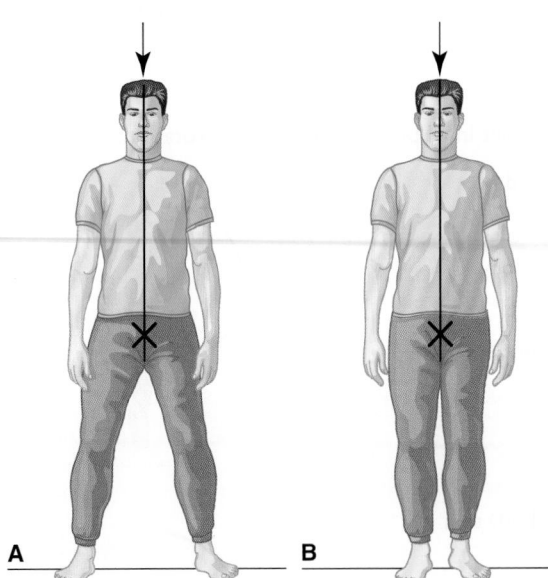

FIGURE 29-4 *A,* With a wide stance, the center of gravity (x) is closer to the base of support. *B,* With a narrow stance, the body is less stable.

Coordination

Smooth movement requires coordination between the nervous system and the musculoskeletal system.

■ **Cerebral cortex**—Initiates voluntary movement.
■ **Cerebellum**—Coordinates movements; largely responsible for controlling *proprioception,* the awareness of posture, movement, and position sense.

■ **Basal ganglia**—Located deep in the cerebrum, assist with coordination of movement.

Damage to the motor cortex, cerebellum, or basal ganglia affects coordination of movement. For example, a stroke affecting the motor cortex alters gait and changes posture.

Joint Mobility

The key concept of **mobility** refers to a person's ability to move within the environment. Joint movement allows us to sit, stand, bend, walk, and perform other activities.

■ **Range of motion (ROM)** is the maximum movement possible at a joint.
■ **Active range of motion (AROM)** is movement of the joint performed by the individual without assistance.
■ **Passive ROM (PROM)** involves moving joints through their ROM when the patient is unable to do so for themselves.

For other terms describing body movement, see Table 29-2.

Body Mechanics Guidelines

✚ Principles of body mechanics are the rules that allow you to move your body while reducing your risk for injury, especially when assisting patients with moving and ambulating. Patient characteristics, as well as the patient care environment, make it difficult to rely on body mechanics alone to prevent injury.

Think about it. A patient's weight may be unevenly distributed or may be positioned awkwardly. They might be combative, which makes moving the patient more difficult and increases the nurse's risk for injury. For guidelines to help you assess patients' transfer abilities and use good body mechanics,

➤ Go to **Chapter 29, Clinical Insight 29-1: Applying Principles of Body Mechanics,** in Volume 2.

KnowledgeCheck 29-2

■ Identify the four components of body mechanics.
■ Give at least five guidelines for good body mechanics.
■ Define the following movements: *abduction, adduction, flexion, extension, circumduction, internal rotation, supination,* and *pronation.*

ThinkLike a Nurse 29-1: Clinical Judgment in Action

While you are attending the health promotion class, Helen Jillian (Meet Your Patients) develops chest pain and must be assisted to a wheelchair for transport to the emergency department.

■ Based on what you know about body mechanics, how would you be able to assist Ms. Jillian?
■ What additional information do you need to know?

Text continued on page 851

Table 29-2 ➤ Range of Motion at the Joints

JOINT	ILLUSTRATION

Neck (Pivot Joint)
The joint is formed by a ringlike object that turns on a pivot. Motion is limited to rotation.

Flexion—Move the head from upright midline position to the chin, resting the head on the chest.

Normal Range: 45° from midline

Extension—Move the head from flexed to upright midline position.

Normal Range: 45° from midline

Hyperextension—Move the head from upright midline position to as far back as possible.

Normal Range: 10°

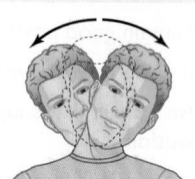

Lateral flexion—Tilt the head laterally from midline position toward the shoulder.

Normal Range: 40° from midline

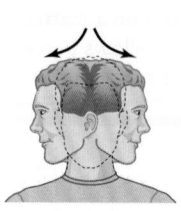

Rotation—Rotate the head in a circular motion from upright midline position to as far right or left as possible.

Normal Range: 180°

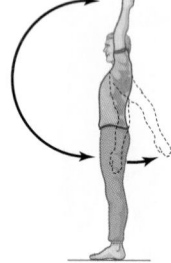

Shoulder (Ball-and-Socket Joint)
A rounded head (ball) fits into a cuplike structure (socket) to allow movement in all planes in addition to rotation.

Flexion—Raise the arm from a neutral position at the side to alongside the head.

Normal Range: 180°

Extension—Move the arm from flexed to a neutral position at the side of the body.

Normal Range: 180°

Hyperextension—Move the arm, keeping the elbow straight, from a neutral position at the side of the bed to behind the body.

Normal Range: 45°–60°

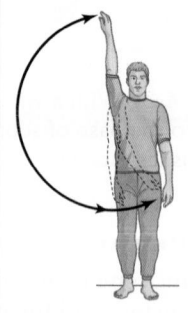

Abduction—Raise the arm laterally from a neutral position at the side of the body to a position at the side of the head, palm facing outward.

Normal Range: 180°

Adduction—Move the arm downward from a position beside the head to across the front of the body as far as possible.

Normal Range: 230°–290°

Table 29-2 ➤ Range of Motion at the Joints—cont'd

JOINT	ILLUSTRATION
Circumduction—Circle the arm from the shoulder. *Normal Range: 360°*	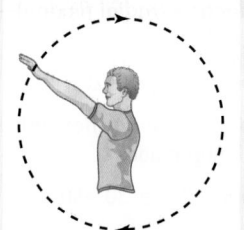
External rotation—Keeping arm held out to the side at shoulder level and bent to a right angle, fingers pointing down, move the arm upward so that the fingers point upward and are above the shoulder. *Normal Range: 90°* **Internal rotation**—Move the arm forward and down to return to the starting position, fingers pointing down. *Normal Range: 90°*	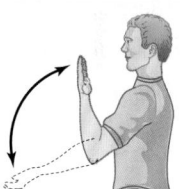
Elbow (Hinge Joint) A convex surface fits into a cavity, allowing flexion and extension.	
Flexion—Bend at the elbow to move the forearm from a straightened position up toward the shoulder. *Normal Range: 150°* **Extension**—Straighten the arm by bringing the lower arm forward and down. *Normal Range: 150°*	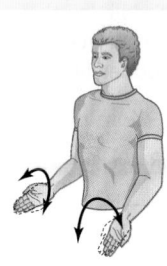
Rotation (for supination)—With the arm at the side, elbow bent, move the hand and forearm so that the palm is facing upward. *Normal Range: 70°–90°* **Rotation (for pronation)**—With the arm at the side, elbow bent, move the hand and forearm so that the palm is facing downward. *Normal Range: 70°–90°*	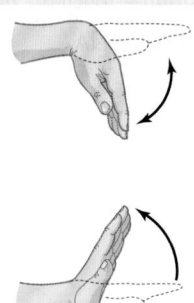
Wrist (Condyloid Joint) An oval-shaped bone fits into an elliptical cavity to allow movement in two planes at right angles to each other.	
Flexion—Bend the fingers of the hand toward the inner aspect of the forearm. *Normal Range: 80°–90°* **Extension**—Straighten the wrist so that it is on the same plane as the forearm. *Normal Range: 80°–90°* **Hyperextension**—Bend the wrist as far back as possible toward the outer aspect of the forearm. *Normal Range: 70°–90°*	

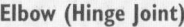
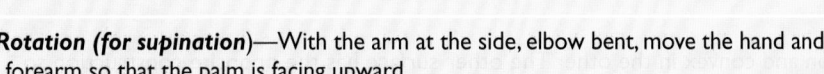

(Continued)

Table 29-2 ➤ Range of Motion at the Joints—cont'd

JOINT	ILLUSTRATION
Abduction (radial flexion)—With the hand supinated, bend each wrist laterally toward the thumb side. *Normal Range:* 0–20° **Adduction (ulnar flexion)**—With the hand supinated, bend each wrist laterally toward the fifth-finger side. *Normal Range:* 30°–50°	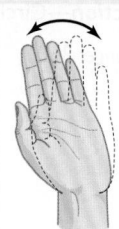

Hands and Fingers (Condyloid Joints: Interphalangeal Joints Are Hinges)

Flexion—Bend the fingers into a fist. *Normal Range:* 90° **Extension**—Straighten the fingers. *Normal Range:* 90° **Hyperextension**—Bend the fingers back. *Normal Range:* 30°	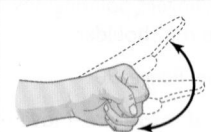
Abduction—Spread the fingers apart. *Normal Range:* 20° **Adduction**—Bring the fingers together. *Normal Range:* 20°	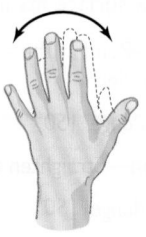

Thumb (Saddle Joint)
One bone surface is concave in one direction and convex in the other. The other surface has the opposite construction so that the bones fit together. Movement occurs in two planes at right angles to each other.

Flexion—Move the thumb across the palm of the hand toward the fifth finger. *Normal Range:* 90° **Extension**—Move the thumb laterally away from the fingers. *Normal Range:* 90°	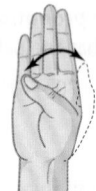
Opposition—Touch the thumb to the top of each finger of the same hand. *Normal Range:* NA	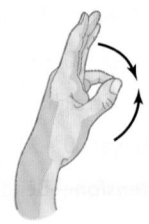

Table 29-2 ➤ Range of Motion at the Joints—cont'd

JOINT	ILLUSTRATION

Hip (Ball-and-Socket Joint)
A rounded head (ball) fits into a cuplike structure (socket) to allow movement in all planes in addition to rotation.

Flexion—Move the leg forward and up.
Normal Range: Knee extended 90°

Extension—Move the leg back down beside the other.
Normal Range: Knee flexed 120°

Hyperextension—Move the leg back behind the body.
Normal Range: 30°–50°

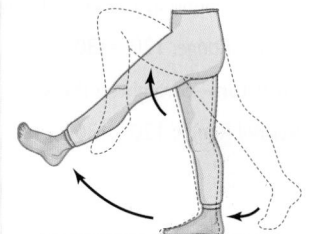

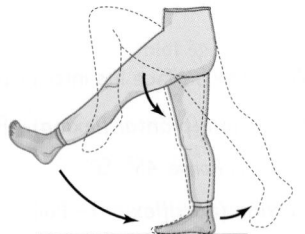

Abduction—Move the leg laterally.
Normal Range: 45°–50°

Adduction—Sweep the leg inward across the midline.
Normal Range: 20°–30° beyond the other leg

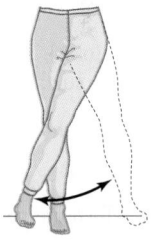

Circumduction—Circle the leg, keeping the knee straight.
Normal Range: 360°

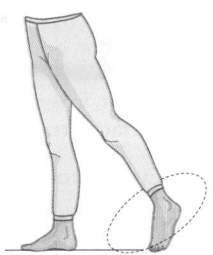

Internal *rotation*—Turn the foot and leg inward toward the other leg.
Normal Range: 90°

External *rotation*—Turn the foot and leg outward, pointing the toes as far as possible away from the other leg.
Normal Range: 90°

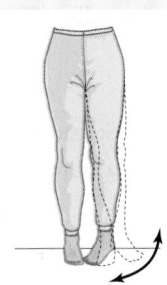

(Continued)

Table 29-2 ➤ Range of Motion at the Joints—cont'd

JOINT	ILLUSTRATION

Knee (Hinge Joint)
A convex surface fits into a cavity, allowing flexion and extension.

Flexion—Bend at the knee, bringing the heel back toward the buttocks.

  Normal Range: 120°–130°

Extension—Straighten the knee, returning the leg to its original position.

  Normal Range: 120°–130°

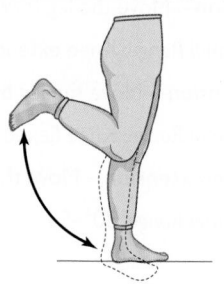

Ankle (Hinge Joint)
A convex surface fits into a cavity, allowing flexion and extension.

Extension (plantar flexion)—Point the toes and foot downward.

  Normal Range: 45°–50°

Flexion (dorsiflexion)—Pull the toes and foot upward.

  Normal Range: 20°

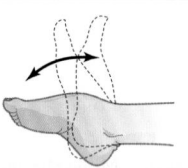

Foot (Gliding Joint)
Two flat plane surfaces move past each other.

Eversion—Turn the sole of the foot laterally.

  Normal Range: 5°

Inversion—Turn the sole of the foot medially.

  Normal Range: 5°

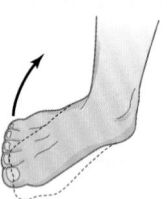

Toes (Hinge Joint, Except Intertarsal Joints, Which Are Gliding Joints)
A convex surface fits into a cavity, allowing flexion and extension.

Flexion—Curl the toes downward.

  Normal Range: 35°–60°

Extension—Straighten the toes.

  Normal Range: 35°–60°

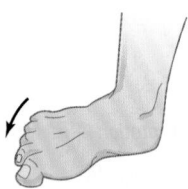

Abduction—Spread the toes apart.

  Normal Range: 0–15°

Adduction—Bring the toes together.

  Normal Range: 0–15°

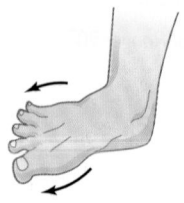

Table 29-2 ➤ Range of Motion at the Joints—cont'd

JOINT	ILLUSTRATION
Trunk	
Flexion—At the waist, bend forward toward the toes. *Normal Range:* 70°–90° *Extension*—Straighten the trunk from the flexed position. *Normal Range:* 70°–90° *Hyperextension*—Bend the trunk backward. *Normal Range:* 20°–30°	
Lateral flexion—Bend the trunk to the side. *Normal Range:* 20°–40°	
Rotation—Turn the upper body from side to side (twist at the waist). *Normal Range:* 30°–45°	

PHYSICAL ACTIVITY AND EXERCISE

Physical activity refers to bodily movement that involves contraction of the skeletal muscles above the basal level and expends energy. Bodily movement can be grouped into two basic categories:

- **Baseline activity** refers to the light-intensity ADLs, such as standing, walking slowly, and lifting light-weight objects.
- **Exercise (health-enhancing physical activity)** is more than baseline to produce health-enhancing benefits

Types of Exercise

Exercise may be classified according to the type of muscle contraction it involves and according to whether it uses oxygen for energy.

Isometric Exercises Isometric exercises exert muscle tension without lengthening or shortening the muscle. There is muscle contraction without motion. This type of static resistance can come from the patient's own body weight (e.g., wall sits), holding an object, using resistance equipment, or pushing against an immovable surface or object. Isometric training is effective for building strength and muscular endurance. Benefits and uses of isometric exercise include the following:

- Often used for rehabilitation because the exact area of muscle weakness can be isolated and strengthening can be administered at the proper joint angle
- Requires no special equipment
- Low risk of joint injury
- Can be used by patients who are bed-bound to maintain or regain muscle strength

Isotonic Exercise Isotonic exercise involves external resistance with movement of the joint during muscle contraction. With this type of moving exercise, weight is used throughout the ROM to build strength and improve performance (e.g., weight training). There are two forms of isotonic exercise: concentric and eccentric movement. **Concentric** exercise occurs when the muscle shortens as it contracts (e.g., curls). **Eccentric** exercise causes the muscle to lengthen even though the muscle is working with contraction (e.g., lowering the weight back down to curl starting position).

Isokinetic Exercise Isokinetic exercise is a type of strength training that uses variable resistance to movement at a constant speed while the muscle moves through the full ROM. Physical therapy uses isokinetic exercises to help patients regain strength and mobility after an injury or illness.

Aerobic Exercise Aerobic exercise is a type of cardiovascular conditioning that acquires energy from metabolic pathways that use oxygen—the amount of oxygen taken into the body meets or exceeds the amount of oxygen required to perform the activity. Aerobic exercise uses large muscle groups, can be maintained continuously, and is commonly rhythmic in nature. It increases the heart and respiratory rates, thereby providing exercise for the cardiovascular system while simultaneously exercising the skeletal muscles. Running, elliptical use, and cycling are common forms of aerobic exercise.

Anaerobic Exercise Anaerobic exercise occurs when the amount of oxygen taken into the body does not meet the amount of oxygen required to perform the activity. Therefore, the muscles must obtain energy from metabolic pathways that do not use oxygen. Rapid, intense exercises such as lifting heavy objects and sprinting are examples of anaerobic exercise.

Planning and Evaluating a Fitness Program

A well-rounded fitness program focuses on flexibility, resistance training, and aerobic conditioning. The concepts of *duration* and *frequency* are used when discussing the amount of activity:

- **Duration** is the amount of time one is exercising.
- **Frequency** indicates how often one is exercising.

See Box 29-1 for physical activity guidelines from the USDHHS. Factors to consider when designing or evaluating an exercise program include the following:

Flexibility Training Stretching before exercise helps warm up the muscles and prevents injury during exercise. Stretching after exercise cools the muscles and limits postexercise stiffness. As we get older, joints and muscles become stiffer. A regular flexibility program helps maintain mobility as aging occurs.

Resistance Training Movement against resistance increases muscular strength and endurance. Perhaps the most common type of resistance training is weightlifting.

> *Exercising for strength*—increase the amount of resistance with each exercise (i.e., lift more weight).
> *Exercising for endurance*—increase the number of repetitions with each exercise.

Aerobic Conditioning Fitness and body composition are improved by aerobic conditioning. Components of aerobic conditioning include intensity, duration, frequency, and mode. Intensity is how hard

---

BOX 29-1 ■ Physical Activity Guidelines for Americans

Children and Adolescents

- Preschool-aged children (ages 3 through 5) should be physically active throughout the day to enhance growth and development.
- Children and adolescents (ages 6 through 17) should engage in at least 1 hour of physical activity daily on at least 3 days a week. Most activity should be aerobic, either moderate or vigorous intensity.
- Physical activity should be enjoyable. A variety of activities will improve adherence.
- At least 3 days/week, children and teens should participate in vigorous-intensity exercise, as well as aerobic and muscle- and bone-strengthening physical activity.

Adults

- **Key Point:** *Adults should move more and sit less. Some physical activity is better than none.*
- Adults should get at least 150 to 300 minutes per week of moderate-intensity aerobic physical activity, or 75 to 150 minutes a week of vigorous-intensity aerobic physical activity, or an equivalent combination of moderate- and vigorous-intensity aerobic activity. More frequent exercise (throughout the week) is even more beneficial.
- Engaging in aerobic activity throughout the week in episodes of at least 10 minutes or longer yields greater health benefits.
- Adults should perform muscle-strengthening activities that involve all major muscle groups on 2 or more days per week.

Specific to Older Adults

- Older adults unable to perform 150 minutes of moderate-intensity aerobic activity per week should be as physically active as conditions allow.
- Physical activity for older adults should include exercises that maintain or improve endurance, balance, tone, flexibility, and muscle strength (Stefanacci, 2022).

Healthy Pregnant and Postpartum Patients

- Consult with the healthcare provider regarding activity level throughout pregnancy. If the pregnancy or postpartum recovery is uncomplicated, patients should do at least 150 minutes of moderate-intensity physical activity. Aerobic activity throughout the week is the best.
- If not already engaged in vigorous-intensity physical activity, while pregnant and after delivery, patients should get at least 150 minutes of moderate-intensity aerobic activity per week, preferably spread throughout the week, after consulting with a healthcare provider.

Adults, Children, and Adolescents With Chronic Conditions or Disabilities

- **Key Point:** *Avoid inactivity and be as physically active as abilities allow with guidance from a healthcare provider.*

Source: Adapted from U.S. Department of Health and Human Services. (2018). *Physical activity guidelines for Americans* (2nd ed.).

one is exercising. Box 29-2 describes three common tests used to evaluate exercise intensity.

Adherence Many people become discouraged because they don't see immediate results from their efforts. However, subtle changes occur long before the person sees changes in weight or body shape. Instructional online fitness videos, trainers, and group exercise make participation more engaging and improve form and safety through the demonstration of proper technique. Tips to help develop an exercise program are included in the Self-Care box, Teaching Clients How to Set Up a Fitness Program.

Key Point: *Anyone with a chronic condition or symptoms of a new health issue should be under the care of a healthcare provider.*

Benefits of Regular Physical Activity

Regular exercise or physical activity, sustained for months and years, produces long-term health benefits, including a lower risk for early death, heart disease, stroke, type 2 diabetes, hypertension, hyperlipidemia, metabolic syndrome, colon and breast cancers, and depression. People who are physically fit can perform ADLs with vigor and alertness and with enough energy to perform work tasks and leisure activities (USDHHS, 2018; Centers for Disease Control and Prevention [CDC], 2022). Cardiorespiratory fitness in the middle-age years promotes healthy aging and may also lead to increased longevity (CDC, 2022; Clausen et al., 2018; Ekelund et al., 2015; Zhao et al., 2020) (Box 29-3). Those with 150 minutes/week or more of physical activity have a lower risk of heart failure and other diseases (Ho et al., 2022). People with disabilities also benefit from physical activity (USDHHS, 2018). See Box 29-1. Even children who engage in vigorous physical activity appear to have a reduced incidence of cardiovascular disease (Fuccenich et al., 2016).

 For older adults, walking is a good form of exercise with a lower risk of injury to joints than other physical activities.

- *Brisk walking* for as little as 30 minutes a day, when done consistently, promotes weight loss and maintenance of normal weight, lowers the risk of disability, reduces loss of bone density, and promotes better heart and lung function and muscular fitness.
- *Moderate-intensity walking* helps to improve strength, balance, and muscle tone, all of which help to prevent falls and improve overall physical stamina. It enhances psychological well-being, reduces depressive symptoms, and improves memory and mental clarity in older adults (Jitramontree, 2010; USDHHS, 2018).

Along with a nutritious diet, social engagement, and mentally stimulating activities, physical activity is associated with a reduced risk of cognitive decline and Alzheimer disease (National Institute on Aging, 2021).

Risks Associated With Exercise

As a nurse, you can help your clients to exercise safely by teaching them realistically about the risks associated

---

BOX 29-2 ■ Tests for Determining Exercise Intensity

Target Heart Rate (THR) Method

The THR is calculated from an estimate of the maximum heart rate (EMHR). The EMHR is calculated using the following formula:

Estimated maximum heart rate (EMHR) = Maximum heart rate (MHR) – age

Example Calculation

The THR is calculated as a percentage of the EMHR. Most people can exercise at 60% to 80% of their maximum heart rate. For a 50-year-old person, using an MHR of 220, exercising at moderate intensity:

- For **EMHR:** 220 (MHR) – 50 (age)
- For **THR,** multiply the EMHR by:

    0.5 for low-intensity exercise

    0.75 for moderate-intensity exercise

    0.85 for high-intensity exercise

Calculation:

EMHR = 220 – 50 = **170 bpm**

THR = 0.75 × 170 = **128 bpm**

For this person, the heart rate during moderate exercise should be 128 beats/min, excluding warm-up and cool-down.

Talk Test

The talk test reflects exercise intensity based on the person's ability to talk while exercising. Short phrases interspersed with breaths or feeling like you can "just respond" is considered an appropriate level of exercise. If you are too short of breath to answer, the level of intensity is too high. An ability to carry on a conversation indicates that you are not exercising vigorously enough.

Borg Rate of Perceived Exertion Scale®

The Rate of Perceived Exertion (RPE) scale is easy to use. The person who is exercising selects the rating based on how difficult the exercise feels at that time. The exerciser selects one of eight categories that best describes the intensity of activity. RPE ratings range from *No Exertion at All* to *Extremely Hard.*

- *Extremely Hard* is associated with exercise that corresponds to almost 100% of maximum heart rate.
- *Somewhat Hard* corresponds with 75% of maximum heart rate. This is the level you should encourage for most individuals.

Source: Borg, G. (1998). *Borg's perceived exertion and pain scales.* Human Kinetics; Foster, C. (2004). "Talk test" measures exercise intensity. *Medicine & Science in Sports & Exercise, 36*(9), 1629–1636.

Teaching Clients How to Set Up a Fitness Program

If you are older than 50, use tobacco or alcohol excessively, are sedentary, are obese, or have a chronic health condition, have a medical evaluation before starting an exercise program.

Getting Started

Customize exercise to you.

➤ Find fun things to do, such as taking a walk through the park or watching your favorite show while riding a stationary bike.

➤ Choose a variety of exercises that you enjoy and feel comfortable doing, such as walking, biking, dancing, or a team sport.

➤ Vary your routine. You may be less likely to get bored or injured.

➤ Choose a comfortable time of day.

Accountability counts.

➤ **Find allies.** Exercising with someone else can make it more fun. If you choose to exercise by yourself, pick a friend with whom you can discuss your exercise progress.

➤ **Find an accountability partner.** A fitness program is not only more enjoyable when shared with someone else but also is more successful when others hold you accountable.

➤ **Consider joining a health club or joining a community fitness program.** The cost gives some people an incentive to exercise regularly.

➤ **Sign a contract** committing yourself to exercise.

➤ **Keep a daily log** of your activities.

Attitude matters.

➤ Don't get discouraged. It can take weeks or months before you notice some of the changes from exercise.

➤ ✚ Forget "no pain, no gain." Although a little soreness is normal after you first start exercising, pain isn't. Stop if you feel pain.

Exercise Tips

➤ Wear good, shock-absorbing footwear. Shoes that do not support your feet will cause stress on bones, joints, and the back and, over time, lead to injury.

➤ Warm up your muscles for 5 to 10 minutes before your main session of aerobic exercise.

➤ Maintain your exercise intensity for 30 to 45 minutes.

➤ Gradually decrease the intensity of your workout (cool down) and then stretch for 5 to 10 minutes at the end of your workout.

➤ Accumulate physical activity throughout the day. For example:

Take the stairs instead of the elevator.

Go for a walk during your breaks or lunch.

Walk all or part of the way to work.

Park your car at the far end of the parking lot.

➤ Alternate easy and hard exercise days, or alternate modes of exercise (e.g., alternate running, swimming, and biking).

➤ Take a day off periodically. The body needs a chance to rest and allow bones, joints, and muscles to rest and repair.

➤ To avoid becoming dehydrated, drink at least 8 ounces of fluid before the exercise, and then pause regularly during the exercise for more. Water is still the best liquid to drink during and after exercise. However, you can't rely on feeling thirsty as a reminder to replace fluid lost through sweating.

✚ Drinking an excess amount of water in a short period of time can cause electrolyte imbalance.

Some sports drinks contain sugar and electrolytes for replacement during endurance activities or prolonged, intense activity.

---

with exercise. Keep in mind that the benefits of exercise far outweigh the risks. Advise clients to follow the tips in the Self-Care box, Teaching Your Patient How to Prevent Back Injury.

Cardiac Injury Fear of triggering a cardiac event prevents some people from exercising. However, physical activity itself is rarely life threatening, especially compared with the health risks related to a sedentary lifestyle and a low level of fitness

Musculoskeletal Injury High-impact exercises may pose a risk for injuries to bones, joints, and muscles. However, you can prevent most such injuries by gradually increasing the activity level or varying activities. Weightlifting using correct form and appropriate

weights markedly builds strength, which can reduce the risk for injury.

Dehydration Fluid and electrolyte loss occurs with prolonged exercise, high ambient temperatures, certain medication, or underlying health problems.

Temperature Regulation Problems

■ **Hyperthermia** can occur when the person exercises in a hot climate. Hyperthermia is often accompanied by dehydration.

■ **Heat exhaustion** is a potentially life-threatening event. Signs of heat exhaustion include light-headedness, nausea, headache, fatigue, hyperventilation, loss of concentration, abdominal cramps, elevated body temperature, and cold and clammy skin.

BOX 29-3 ■ Benefits of Regular Exercise

Cardiovascular System

- ↑ pumping action of the heart
- ↑ circulation by increasing the number of capillaries
- ↑ venous return to the heart
- ↑ blood volume and hematocrit
- ↑ high-density lipoprotein (HDL)
- ↓ low-density lipoprotein (LDL) and total cholesterol
- ↓ risk of thrombophlebitis
- ↓ heart rate, heart rate variability, and blood pressure

Respiratory System

- ↑ pulmonary circulation
- ↑ gas exchange at the alveolar–capillary membrane and ↑ overall aerobic capacity
- Dilates bronchioles to ↑ ventilation

Musculoskeletal System

- ↑ skeletal development in children
- ↑ muscle mass, strength, power, and endurance
- ↑ flexibility
- ↑ coordination
- Helps maintain joint structure and function
- ↑ bone mass and mineral density
- ↑ gait speed, stability, and balance
- ↑ bone mass with aging; reduces risk of osteoporosis
- ↓ risk of falls and helps older adults maintain an independent lifestyle
- ↓ reduces risk of osteoarthritis

Nervous System

- ↑ nerve impulse transmission
- ↑ reaction time
- ↓ sympathetic response to exercise

Endocrine System

- ↑ sensitivity to insulin at the receptor sites
- ↑ efficiency of metabolic processes

- ↑ temperature regulation
- Facilitates weight management
- ↓ adipose surrounding organs

Gastrointestinal System

- ↑ appetite
- ↑ abdominal muscle tone
- ↓ risk of colon cancer

Urinary System

- ↑ efficiency of kidney function

Integumentary System

- ↑ skin tone as a result of improved circulation

Immune System

- ↓ susceptibility to minor viral illnesses
- ↓ systemic inflammation

Mental Health

- ↑ energy level
- ↑ endorphins, which assist with pain control and stress management
- ↑ self-esteem and body image
- ↑ nonpharmacological relief of symptoms of anxiety and depression
- ↑ positive outlook and sense of optimism
- ↑ clearer thinking and improved memory in older adults
- ↑ feelings of well-being and ↓ depressive symptoms
- ↑ social interaction
- ↓ in some stress

Overall Health

- ↑ caloric expenditure to achieve and maintain healthy body weight
- ↑ overall stamina
- ↑ sleep time and improved sleep quality
- ↓ abdominal obesity
- ↓ fatigue

- **Hypothermia** can occur when the person does not wear proper clothing or is exposed to cool water for an extended period. Hypothermia is characterized by fatigue, confusion, and a lack of coordination.

KnowledgeCheck 29-3

- Identify and describe four types of exercise.
- State the components of a fitness program

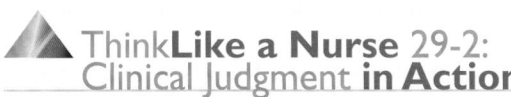

ThinkLike a Nurse 29-2: Clinical Judgment in Action

- How would you address Helen Jillian's (Meet Your Patients) concerns about the risks associated with engaging in a fitness program?

- Peter Phan (Meet Your Patients) has experienced several injuries as a result of his exercise. Based on your knowledge of exercise, what questions would you like to ask Peter about his fitness program?

FACTORS AFFECTING MOBILITY AND ACTIVITY

Mobility refers to a person's capacity for bodily movement, or how well the person is able to move about in the environment. Factors influencing activity and mobility include developmental stage, nutrition, lifestyle, attitudes, external factors, diseases, and physical abnormalities. These factors are discussed in the next sections.

Self-Care

✚ Teaching Your Patient How to Prevent Back Injury

➤ Poor posture is one of the main causes of back pain. Make a conscious effort to maintain good posture at all times.

➤ Use a firm mattress that provides adequate support.

➤ Sit with your knees slightly lower than your hips.

➤ If you must stand for a long period of time, flex your hip and raise one foot on a stool or object 6 to 8 inches off the ground. Periodically switch legs.

➤ Wear comfortable, low-heeled shoes. Avoid high heels as much as possible.

➤ Avoid restrictive clothing that inhibits your ability to use good body mechanics.

➤ Always follow the principles of good body mechanics (e.g., use wide base of support, and do not lift with your back), but keep in mind manual lifting techniques are based on loads that weigh far less than typical patients.

➤ When lifting, be sure the load is stable and held close to the body.

➤ Exercise regularly to maintain your optimal weight and strengthen the muscles of your body.

➤ Include abdominal exercises in your routine. Strong abdominal muscles help support the back.

➤ Avoid lifting excessive weight.

➤ Avoid exercises or movements that cause spinal flexion (e.g., toe-touches, sit-ups with knees extended), excessive flexion of the neck (e.g., abdominal crunches with neck curved to chest), or spinal rotation (twisting).

Developmental Stage

As expected, older adults are the least active age-group but are also the age-group most likely to participate in fitness activities rather than sporting or outdoor activities. See the accompanying Self-Care box, Teaching Older Adults About Increasing Activity and Exercise.

Nutrition

- **Obesity** often leads to health problems, which indirectly reduce activity and can, in turn, contribute to further obesity. Movement becomes more difficult as body size increases. Joint and back injuries and osteoarthritis are more prevalent with obesity, which in turn reduces a person's ability to engage in physical activity for weight loss.
- **Chronic disease** may cause a negative nitrogen balance—that is, inadequate protein stores to maintain or repair body tissue. Muscle wasting and fatigue occur, leading to reduced activity levels and loss of strength and balance.

Lifestyle

Personal values about exercise and fitness determine when, or whether, exercise becomes part of a person's routine. Some people enjoy exercise. Others see it as drudgery or as "something I have to do." A person's culture and support system define what physical activity the person is likely to engage in. Economic and social conditions influence a person's access to fitness amenities, sporting activities, and equipment needed for structured play. Social determinants may influence a person's exercise behavior and weight management.

Sedentary Lifestyle Over recent decades, with the pervasive use of electronic devices for work, entertainment, and social contacts, people are generally more sedentary. In a study by the Physical Activity Council (2022), approximately 24% of Americans reported that in the previous calendar year, they did not once participate in any of 104 listed physical activities (fitness, individual sports, team sports, outdoor sports, racquet sports, water sports, and winter sports); the percentage reporting no participation was higher than in previous years. Some may attribute the inactivity trend to the COVID-19 pandemic and restrictions on other activities and settings. For some, health condition is a deterrent to being active. Others report that having someone to participate might motivate them to begin a new activity.

Environmental Factors

Environmental factors affecting exercise include the following:

- **Weather**—When it is cold, damp, or even hot and humid, people tend to avoid strenuous exercise outside or stay indoors. Encourage patients to choose a variety of activities that they enjoy so that they can exercise regardless of the weather.
- **Pollution**—When air quality is poor, suggest indoor activities to reduce exposure to allergens and pollutants.
- **Neighborhood conditions**—Crime, poor-quality sidewalks and streets, and a lack of parks are examples of conditions that influence attitudes about outside activities. Walking in a closed indoor facility is an example of a successful way to incorporate exercise into daily patterns when neighborhood conditions do not encourage activity.
- **Finances**—Joining a fitness center or engaging in sports might be feasible for some budgets but is not practical for all. However, many activities, such as walking or playing basketball or pickleball in the community park, are inexpensive or free options.
- **Support system**—Family and friends who are active are likely to promote and support your efforts to exercise. Those who are sedentary may not encourage you to be more active or lose weight.

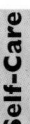

Teaching Older Adults About Increasing Physical Activity and Exercise

What Are the Benefits of Physical Activity for an Older Adult?

➤ Improves and preserves strength so that you can stay as independent as possible.

➤ Maintains balance, increases aerobic capacity, and prevents falls.

➤ Gives you more energy and strength to do the things you want to do.

➤ Helps you to sleep better and feel more rested.

➤ Perks up your mood and enhances sense of well-being.

➤ Prevents or delays some diseases, like diabetes, heart disease, osteoporosis, colon cancer, and cancer (Stefanacci, 2022).

What Kind of Physical Activity Should I Do?

➤ Get at least 150 minutes a week of moderate-intensive activity (brisk walking) or at least 75 minutes a week of vigorous-intensity aerobic activity. Being active on at least 2 days a week is best. Exercise that makes you breathe hard builds muscle strength and endurance.

➤ Wear a physical activity tracking tool to monitor your level of *endurance* activity. Set goals and monitor your progress. If you are taking 10,000 or more steps per day, you are probably getting an adequate amount of physical activity.

➤ Incorporate *resistance* into your exercise; use weight or isometric activity to build strength. Remember that you can do more and are less likely to fall when your muscles are strong.

➤ Do things to work on your *balance* (e.g., standing on one foot). This can help to prevent falls.

➤ Daily stretching will help you be more *flexible* and prevent injury.

Who Should Exercise?

Almost anyone can do some type of physical activity, but before starting a new fitness program, check with your healthcare provider if you experience:

➤ Any change in your health in the past 6 months

➤ Shortness of breath or dizziness

➤ Chest pain or pressure or fluttering heart

➤ Joint pain or swelling

➤ Unexplained weight loss

➤ An infection with fever

➤ Eye problems

➤ Blood clot

➤ Hernia

➤ Recent hip surgery or joint injury

Source: Adapted from the National Institutes of Health, National Institute on Aging. (2020, April 3). *Exercise and physical activity: How older adults can get started with exercise.* https://www.nia.nih.gov/health/how-older-adults-can-get-started-exercise#activity

Diseases and Abnormalities

Diseases and abnormalities in various body systems can negatively influence body alignment, balance, coordination, flexibility, and joint mobility. In the next sections, we describe some disorders that affect activity and exercise.

Congenital Abnormalities of the Musculoskeletal System

The following are common congenital abnormalities that affect appearance, motor function, and mobility:

- **Syndactylism** is the fusion of two or more fingers or toes. Most cases involving the hands are treated surgically at an early age to limit the effect on fine motor development.
- **Developmental dysplasia of the hip (DDH)** is a congenital abnormality of the development of the femur, acetabulum, or both that shows as hip dislocation.
- **Foot deformities,** such as clubfoot (talipes equinovarus), occur in about 4% of all newborns. Serial casts or surgery may be used to correct the defect and preserve function.
- **Scoliosis** is a lateral curvature of the spine. Scoliosis can result from **congenital** (present at birth) bone disorders, neuromuscular impairment, or trauma, but approximately two-thirds of cases have no known cause and are termed *idiopathic scoliosis.*

Diseases Related to Bone Formation or Metabolism

Bone formation abnormalities may be congenital, related to dietary deficiencies, or the result of bone disease.

- **Osteogenesis imperfecta (OI)** is a congenital disorder of bone and connective tissue that is characterized by brittle bones that fracture easily. Infants with OI are often born with fractures and continue to fracture bones with minimal trauma or even spontaneously. Prompt recognition and treatment of fractures help prevent deformities.
- **Achondroplasia,** or dwarfism, occurs when the bones ossify (harden) prematurely.
- **Paget disease** is a metabolic bone disease in which increased bone loss results in pain, pathological fractures, and deformities. This disorder usually affects the skull, vertebrae, femur, and pelvis.
- **Vitamin D and calcium** are needed to form and maintain bone. Deficiencies lead to porous bones. In children, prolonged deficiencies can cause the long bones of the legs to become bowed, retard growth, and lead to frequent fractures.

Diseases Affecting Joint Mobility

Diseases of the joints may be degenerative or inflammatory. Nursing activity for patients with joint mobility problems focuses on assisting with movement, providing comfort, and teaching about medications. If mobility is severely restricted, you will also assist patients with ADLs.

Osteoarthritis Osteoarthritis (OA) is the most prevalent type of degenerative joint disease. OA involves a loss of articular cartilage in the joint, with pain and stiffness as the primary symptoms. Patients may also have decreased ROM and **crepitus,** a creaking or grating sound with joint motion. Symptoms are aggravated by weight-bearing and joint use and are relieved by resting the affected joints. OA is more common in women, older adults, and people who are overweight.

Rheumatoid Arthritis Rheumatoid arthritis (RA) is a systemic autoimmune disease involving chronic inflammation of the joints and surrounding connective tissue, frequently resulting in difficulty in performing ADLs. RA causes joint pain, deformity, and loss of function; patients may also experience fever, fatigue, weakness, and weight loss. RA occurs most frequently in the fingers, wrists, elbows, ankles, and knees. The illness usually begins in midlife and more often affects women. Unlike OA, RA does not improve with rest. Pain is most intense when the person rises from bed. Pain and joint deformities may so severely affect mobility that patients cannot care for themselves.

Ankylosing Spondylitis Ankylosing spondylitis is a chronic inflammatory joint disease characterized by stiffening and fusion of the spine and sacroiliac joints. The inflammation occurs where the ligaments, tendons, and joint capsule insert into the bone. The disease usually develops in young adults, equally in the male and female populations. Patients with ankylosing spondylitis have low back pain and stiffness and decreased ROM of the spine. The convex lumbar curve is lost, and the upper spine curve increases, causing kyphosis (see Chapter 19 for review).

Gout Gout is an inflammatory response to high levels of uric acid. Crystals form in the synovial fluid, and small white nodules, or *tophi,* form in the subcutaneous tissues. An acute episode of gout can occur suddenly. The affected joint is so hot, swollen, and painful that even the weight of a bedsheet may seem intolerable (Fig. 29-5). Symptoms are typically most severe in the first 4 to 12 hours after onset but can develop into a chronic form that progresses to immobility of the joints. Gout usually affects the joint of the great toe but can occur in the feet, ankles, knees, hands, and wrists.

Problems Affecting Bone Integrity

Loss of bone integrity may occur from an imbalance in bone production, infection, or tumors.

Osteoporosis Osteoporosis is a decrease in total bone density, which occurs when osteoclast activity outpaces that of the osteoblasts. The internal structure

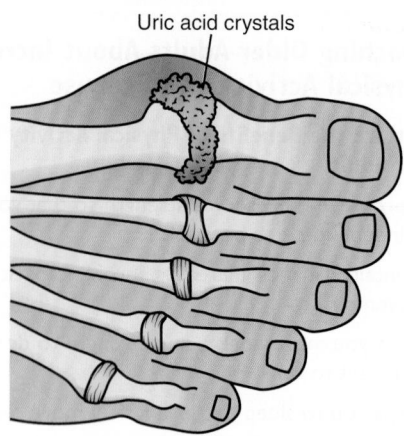

Uric acid crystals

FIGURE 29-5 Painful, swollen joint with the onset of a gout episode.

of the bone diminishes, and the bone collapses in on itself. Normally, bone mass continues to increase up to the third decade of life. After age 30, bone loss begins. Female individuals experience a rapid decline in bone mass at menopause. In male individuals, a gradual loss continues. As bones become porous, they become weak, leading to vertebral collapse or fractures of the long bones of the arms and legs. Fractures may occur spontaneously or with slight trauma.

Genetics, body frame, menopausal status, chronic disease, and lifestyle choices also play a role. The most common risk factors for osteoporotic fracture are advanced age, low bone mineral density, and previous fracture as an adult. Smoking, low calcium and vitamin D intake, excess alcohol use, and sedentary lifestyle also increase the risk (Rosen et al., 2021).

Osteomyelitis Osteomyelitis is an infection of the bone that may develop after bone injury or surgery. It can be difficult and expensive to treat and can leave the patient with permanent disability. Bone contains microscopic channels that are impermeable to most of the natural defenses of the body. Once bacteria enter these channels, they multiply rapidly.

Bone Tumors Bone tumors may also affect form and function. Tumors in the bone cause considerable pain and severely limit activity. Nursing responsibilities for patients with osteomyelitis or bone tumors include collaborative treatments, patient education about the treatment plan, and providing comfort.

Trauma

Trauma can affect bones, ligaments, muscles, and joints.

- A **fracture** is a break in the bone. Signs and symptoms of a fracture include tenderness at the site, loss of function, deformity of the area, a line of bruising along the fracture, and swelling of the surrounding tissues. However, x-ray is required for definitive diagnosis. Fractures are classified according to the type of damage (Fig. 29-6). The type and severity of the fracture determine whether casting, traction, or surgical repair is necessary. To learn about caring for a cast in the home, refer to the Home Care box, Teaching Care of a Cast at Home.

- **Sprains** and strains are more common than fractures.
  - A **sprain** is a stretch injury of a ligament that causes the ligament to tear. A partial tear can usually heal with rest, but a complete tear often requires surgery to stabilize the joint.
  - A **strain** is an injury to muscle caused by excessive stress on the muscle.
- Both strains and sprains cause pain at the site of injury, swelling, and loss of function. The signs and symptoms are the same as those of a fracture. As a result, x-ray studies are used to distinguish these injuries. Think of the initial treatment of fractures, sprains, and strains using the RICE acronym:
  - **R**est
  - **I**ce
  - **C**ompression
  - **E**levation

- **Stretching and tearing injuries** to the meniscus (kneecap), lateral knee ligaments, and Achilles tendon are also common. Magnetic resonance imaging (MRI) studies are done to determine the extent of injury. Rest and ice are necessary, but for some, surgical repair may be needed to achieve full healing.

Disorders of the Central Nervous System

Any disorder that affects the motor centers of the brain or the transmission of nerve impulses will affect mobility:

- Cerebrovascular accident (stroke)
- Head or spinal cord injury
- Multiple sclerosis (a disorder affecting nerve transmission)
- Myasthenia gravis (a disease caused by antibodies to the acetylcholine receptors at the neuromuscular junction)

Progressive degenerative disorders of the neurological system also affect mobility and coordination. For example,

---

Home Care

Teaching Care of a Cast at Home

Keep the Cast Clean and Dry

- Before bathing, cover the cast with a plastic bag and tape the opening shut, or use a commercial cast cover with hook and loop straps with Velcro© brand fasteners.
- Do not place the cast into water unless it is made of water-repellent material.
- Waterproof casts are not for all types of fractures. They can't be used for recently manipulated fractures or when skin pins are used.
- If the cast gets wet enough that the skin gets wet under the cast, it may break down, and infection may occur. ✚ Dry it immediately with a blow dryer on the cool setting. Be careful—skin can be burned when using the hot setting.
- If you have any trouble getting the cast dry, the cast may need to be replaced. Call the healthcare provider if the cast doesn't dry properly.
- Sweating under the cast enough to make it damp may cause mold or mildew to develop. **Key Point:** *Call the healthcare provider if you notice odor coming from the cast. This is a sign of infection.*

Protect Your Circulation and Skin

✚ Never put anything inside the cast. Do not try to scratch the skin under the cast with any sharp objects, such as a hanger or pencil. *This may break the skin under the cast and cause it to become infected.*

- Do not use powders, ointments, or lotions inside the cast.

- Sometimes when swelling goes down, the cast can become loose and rub on the skin. If this is the case, call the primary provider to look at the cast.
- Check the circulation by gently squeezing a finger or toe below the cast. It should blanch (turn lighter) and quickly return to a pink color. The fingers and toes should be warm to the touch, able to move freely, and not tingling or numb. If they are not, notify a healthcare provider immediately.
- Do not trim the cast or break off any rough edges. This may weaken or break the cast. If a fiberglass cast has a rough edge, use a metal file to smooth it or call the healthcare provider.

Support and Protect the Injured Extremity

- A sling may be needed for support if the cast is on the hand, wrist, arm, or elbow. It is helpful to wrap soft sheepskin or padding behind the neck to protect the skin and make it feel more comfortable.
- If the cast is on the foot or leg, do not walk on or put any weight on the injured leg, unless the doctor allows it.
- If the primary care provider allows walking on the cast, be sure to wear the cast boot. The boot is to reduce wear and tear on the bottom and has a tread to prevent slipping and falling.
- Crutches may be needed to walk if a cast is on the foot, ankle, or leg. Make sure the crutches are adjusted properly before leaving the hospital or the provider's office or clinic.

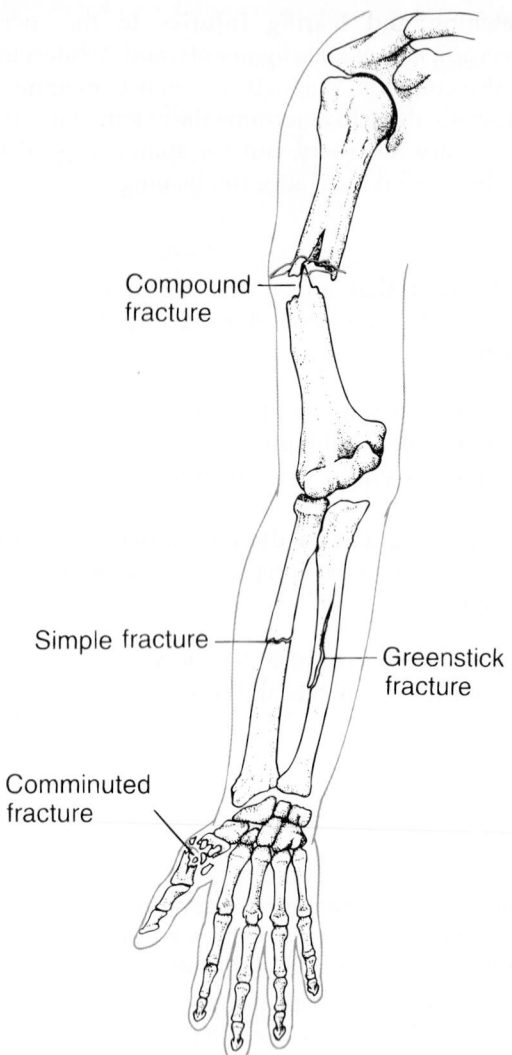

Compound fracture

Simple fracture

Greenstick fracture

Comminuted fracture

FIGURE 29-6 Types of fractures.

Parkinson disease is a progressive degeneration of the basal ganglia. It produces tremor, rigidity, and difficulty coordinating movement.

Diseases of Other Body Systems

Diseases affecting other body systems may affect mobility and activity tolerance, as in the following examples:

- **Respiratory disorders.** Any disorder that affects oxygenation limits exercise tolerance. Chronic obstructive pulmonary disease, asthma, and pneumonia are associated with shortness of breath, which becomes worse with increased activity.
- **Circulatory disorders.** Impaired arterial circulation limits oxygen delivery to the tissue. As activity increases, skeletal muscle pain develops. Impaired venous circulation causes leg swelling and discomfort, which are relieved by elevating the legs. As a result,

patients may become relatively sedentary to relieve the pain and discomfort.

- **Fatigue.** Acute illnesses, such as influenza, produce fatigue and limit activity for short periods of time. Disorders that produce long-standing fatigue include anemia, anorexia nervosa, cancer, depression, and grief.
- **Bedrest.** For certain health conditions or after surgery, bedrest may be prescribed, although infrequently.

KnowledgeCheck 29-4

- In which age-groups are you more likely to see health concerns that affect mobility?
- What types of disorders limit activity or mobility?
- What are the signs and symptoms of a fracture?
- What is the difference between a strain and a sprain?

 ThinkLike a Nurse 29-3: Clinical Judgment in Action

- Your teenage daughter complains when you ask her to take a calcium supplement and encourage her to exercise. What information should you provide so that she understands why these measures are important?
- Phillip Flanders (Meet Your Patients) has never been involved in a regular exercise program. Phillip works as an accountant, and most of his friends are work associates. Phillip's siblings are overweight and do not exercise. Both of his parents died of heart disease. Many of Phillip's friends have suggested that he begin a fitness program to improve his energy and health. What recommendations can you make to Phillip to make it more likely that he will start and continue an exercise routine?

EXAMPLE CLIENT CONDITION: PROLONGED IMMOBILITY

Most people take their mobility for granted until illness, disease, or trauma affects their ability to move. Even short periods of immobility may be difficult. If you've ever had the flu or an illness that sent you to bed, you know that it can take several days to return to your pre-illness state, especially for older adults and people with underlying chronic illness.

To learn about the effects of immobility on various body systems and about a few general interventions, refer to the Example Client Condition: Prolonged Immobility.

KnowledgeCheck 29-5

- Identify the effects of immobility on the cardiovascular, musculoskeletal, and integumentary systems.
- Why might immobility be referred to as a stressor?
- What are three effects of immobility on the gastrointestinal system?
- What changes in mood might be seen with immobility?

EXAMPLE CLIENT CONDITION: Prolonged Immobility

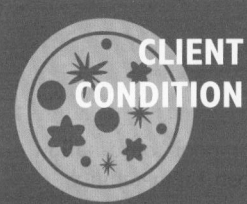

CLIENT CONDITION

Prolonged immobility produces the following effects on body systems:

Musculoskeletal

- **Muscle wasting.** Ten percent loss of muscle strength per week (e.g., gastrocnemius, soleus, and other leg muscles that control flexion and extension of the hip, knee, and ankle)
- **Stiff joints**
- **Contractures.** Strongest muscles (flexors) pull the joints, leading to contractures, or joint ankyloses.

Cardiovascular

- **Venous stasis.** Leads to ↑ cardiac and venous stasis.
- **↓ Cardiac reserve.** Heart rate and stroke volume ↑ to maintain blood pressure. But with immobility, cardiac reserves ↓, which means the heart is less able to respond to the body's demands.
- **Edema.** Without muscle activity, gravity causes blood to pool, which leads to edema. Fluid in the tissue is more prone to pressure injury.
- **Risk for thrombosis.** Leads to compression and injury of the small vessels in the legs and ↓ clearance of coagulation factors, causing blood to clot faster. Stasis, activation of clotting, and vessel injury **(Virchow's triad)** are associated with a ↑ risk for deep vein thrombosis (DVT) formation.
- **Orthostatic hypotension.** Inactivates the baroreceptors involved with vasoconstriction and dilation; less able to regulate blood pressure. Dizziness and light-headedness occur.

Respiratory

- **↓ Ventilation.** ↓ strength of all muscles and ↓ chest wall expansion, which impairs ventilation.
- **Pooling in lungs.** Shallow respirations; secretions pool in lungs.
- **Risk for atelectasis** or pneumonia. Pooled secretions block air passages and alveoli, ↓ air–gas exchange, and often lead to atelectasis (collapse of air sacs) or **pneumonia.**

Integumentary System

- **Pressure injury.** Compresses capillaries; ↓ circulation causes pressure injury.

Metabolism

- **↓ Energy.** ↑ serum lactic acid and ↓ adenosine triphosphate (ATP) (energy).
- **Metabolic rate drops.** Protein and glycogen synthesis ↓; fat stores ↑.
- **Glucose intolerance**
- **↓ muscle mass**
- **Stress response.** Triggers release of thyroid hormones, epinephrine, norepinephrine, and adrenocorticotropic hormone (ACTH) from the pituitary gland and aldosterone from the kidneys.
- **↑ Excretion of calcium.** Immobility alters parathyroid function, calcium metabolism, and bone formation. The result is osteoporosis, calcium depletion in joints, and renal calculi (kidney stones).
- **↑ risk for fractures** with minimal trauma.

Gastrointestinal

- **Slows peristalsis,** leading to constipation, gas, and difficulty evacuating stool from the rectum. **Paralytic ileus** (cessation of peristalsis) can occur.
- **Appetite diminishes and digestion slows,** often leading to ↓ calorie intake.
- **Muscle is broken down** as a fuel source.

Urinary

- **Supine position inhibits drainage of urine** from the kidney and bladder. Urine becomes stagnant—ideal environment for infection.
- **↑ Calcium levels** and stone formation.
- **Urinary retention.** ↓ muscle tone leads to ↓ bladder tone, which leads to urinary retention.
- **Bedpan/urinal.** Many patients have difficulty voiding in a bedpan or urinal.

Psychological Effects

- **Affect.** Moodiness, depression, anxiety, hostility, disturbed sleep, apathy, poor body concept.
- **Cognition.** ↓ concentration, recall, and problem-solving.
- **Self-care.** Reduced ability to perform self-care.

COMPLICATIONS

The following is a summary of common complications of prolonged immobility:
- Pressure injury
- Constipation
- Joint contracture
- Muscle weakness
- Balance problems
- DVT
- Pooling of secretions in lower lobes
- Orthostatic hypotension
- ↑ Risk of mortality

(continued)

EXAMPLE CLIENT CONDITION: Prolonged Immobility—cont'd

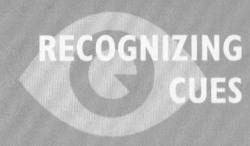

RECOGNIZING CUES

Subjective

Pain or discomfort with movement, exertional dyspnea

Objective

Limited range of motion (ROM), limitations in fine or gross motor movement, poor coordination with movement, difficulty turning, unstable gait, decreased reaction time, postural instability, slowed movement, and difficulty performing activities of daily living (ADLs)

 Go to **Assessment Guidelines and Tools, Focused Assessment: Assessing Activity and Exercise,** in Volume 2.

For a patient on bedrest or with impaired physical mobility, regularly monitor all body systems for indications of complications.
• See Home Care: Home Assessment for a Patient With Mobility Concerns.

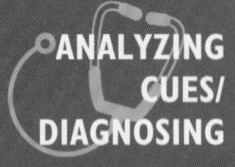

ANALYZING CUES/ DIAGNOSING

Nursing Diagnoses for Mobility as Problem

Impaired Physical Mobility—limitation of independent purposeful movement of the body or of one or more extremities (NANDA International, 2021). Use the following, more descriptive diagnoses when the patient has specific deficits:
• Impaired Mobility: Walking
• Impaired Mobility: Moving in Bed
• Impaired Mobility: Wheelchair Use
• Impaired Mobility: Transfer
• Risk for Disuse Syndrome
• Sedentary Lifestyle
• Potential Complications of Immobility: Pressure injury, DVT, contractures

Etiologies of Impaired Mobility

Neuromuscular, sensoriperceptual, or musculoskeletal impairment; reduced bone mass; obesity; malnutrition; deconditioning due to sedentary lifestyle; lack of motivation for activity and exercise for maintenance of health; anxiety; cognitive impairment or developmental delay; discomfort; limited cardiovascular endurance; medications; pain; prescribed movement restrictions

Mobility Problems as Etiologies of Other Diagnoses

• *Risk for Ineffective Peripheral Tissue Perfusion* (specify) r/t blood flow compromised by reduced mobility
• *Risk for Disuse Syndrome* (NANDA-I, 2021) occurs when there is a risk for deterioration of body systems as a result of musculoskeletal inactivity. Risk factors include prescribed bedrest, severe pain, altered level of consciousness, mechanical immobilization (traction), and paralysis.
• *Acute Pain* r/t musculoskeletal injury
• *Ineffective Health Maintenance* r/t prescribed bedrest
• *Risk for Injury* r/t unsteady gait
• *Self-Care Deficit* (or more specific deficits: *Bathing/Hygiene Deficit, Feeding Deficit, Dressing/Grooming Deficit, Toileting Deficit*) (Clinical Care Classification [CCC], n.d.) r/t Impaired Physical Mobility

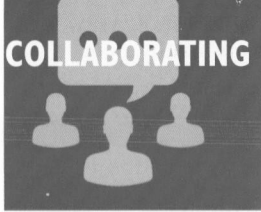

COLLABORATING

• Occupational therapy
• Physical therapy

• Wound specialist
• Dietitian

GENERATING SOLUTIONS

Selected NIC Interventions for Immobility Management

Activity Promotion
Exercise Therapy: Ambulation
Bedrest Care
Positioning
Traction/Immobilization Care
Transfer

EXAMPLE CLIENT CONDITION: Prolonged Immobility—cont'd

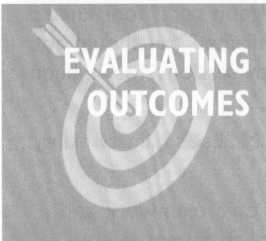

EVALUATING OUTCOMES

NOC Standardized Outcomes

Ambulation
Ambulation: Wheelchair
Body Positioning: Self-Initiated
Coordinated Movement
Immobility Consequences: Physiological

Immobility consequences:
Psycho-Cognitive
Joint Movement (specify)
Joint Movement: Passive
Mobility
Transfer Performance

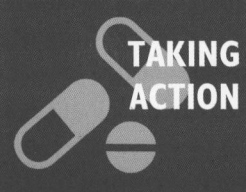

TAKING ACTION

The goal of nursing activities is to prevent complications in all body systems.

Support Oxygenation

- Assist the patient to the orthopneic position to allow for lung expansion and prevent atelectasis and pneumonia.

Support Nutrition

- Offer protein-rich diet to maintain muscle mass.

Support Skin Integrity

- Turn patient every 2 hours to prevent pressure on the skin and minimize edema.
- Keep the bed clean and dry to make it easier to turn the patient and decrease risk of maceration or pressure injury.
- Do not tuck in so tightly as to restrict movement or circulation

Support Cardiovascular Function

- Have patient sit on the edge of the bed before standing to prevent orthostatic hypotension.

Support the Musculoskeletal System

- Assist with conditioning exercises to prepare for ambulation.

 Go to **Clinical Insight 29-3: Assisting with Physical Conditioning** in Volume 2.

- Assist patient to standing position; assist with ambulation as tolerated
- Use positioning devices to maintain body alignment (see Figs. 29-7 through 29-10).
- Encourage active ROM; provide passive ROM as needed.

 Go to Chapter 29, **Clinical Insight 29-2: Performing Passive ROM Exercises,** in Volume 2.

- To see a nursing care plan and care map for the diagnosis Impaired Physical Mobility,

 Go to **Chapter 29, Nursing Care Plan: Impaired Physical Mobility** and **Care Map,** on Davis Advantage.

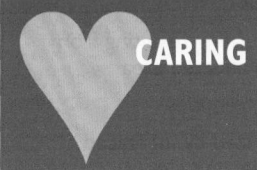

CARING

♥ **iCare** • Provide encouragement and offer praise for making effort for physical activity.
- Help design incentives and rewards to activity.

- Immobility can lead to depression and anxiety. Watch for changes in mood and behavior and seek help immediately.

PracticalKnowledge
knowing **how**

As you have seen in the preceding sections, immobility can result in serious health consequences. In the remainder of the chapter, we discuss nursing activities to promote activity and exercise and eliminate the hazards of immobility.

▮▮ ASSESSMENT/RECOGNIZING CUES

Perform an assessment focused on mobility and exercise for any patient who has musculoskeletal concerns,

is obese, has limited mobility, or is confined to bed or chair. As always, you will validate the nursing history data with physical examination. Box 29-4 defines a variety of terms used to describe problems with muscle mass, strength, or mobility. For a comprehensive, focused assessment tool,

 See **Chapter 29, Focused Assessment box, Assessing Activity and Exercise,** in Volume 2.

To help you with focused mobility assessments in the home, see the Home Care box, Home Assessment for a Patient With Mobility Concerns.

Effects of Teamwork and Collaboration on Activity and Exercise Outcomes

Chapter Key Concepts: Activity, Exercise (Thinking, Doing, Caring)

Competency: Interprofessional Teamwork and Collaboration; Goal-Directed Client-Centered Care

Situation: Mr. Lee underwent surgery to repair a ruptured quadriceps tendon in his left leg. His discharge instructions provided general guidelines about wound care, signs and symptoms to report, and when to follow up with the surgeon.

At his 2-week postop visit, Mr. Lee was making good progress. The surgeon gave him a prescription to begin physical therapy, telling him that the referred therapists knew his protocols. He also told Mr. Lee that he could drive and return to work but that he should "listen to his body" and rest when he was tired or feeling pain. Mrs. Lee mentioned that the drive to work was 1 hour each way and wondered whether that was too much. After the surgeon left, the nurse removed the staples from the incision and talked to Mr. and Mrs. Lee about potential complications and how to perform wound care.

The next day, the physical therapist scheduled Mr. Lee for therapy on Mondays, Wednesdays, and Thursdays. During the first therapy session, Mr. Lee moaned with pain. On the second visit, Mrs. Lee remarked that his knee was swollen, but the therapist disagreed with her, noting that other patients had much more swelling than Mr. Lee had. One week later, Mr. Lee, fearing something was wrong, went to the surgeon's office. He had a fever of 100°F and

a pain rating of 6 out of 10. The surgeon said, "Your knee is not damaged or infected, but it is inflamed. You should not have scheduled back-to-back therapy sessions. You've been overdoing it."

Outcome: It was 2 weeks before Mr. Lee's pain, swelling, and fever subsided.

Think about it: Patient-centered care, teamwork, and collaboration are considered integral to patient safety and quality care. Reflect on this scenario, considering the following questions and concepts:

➤ How would you describe this team's functioning?

➤ What barriers to team functioning do you think might exist in this scenario?

➤ What could the office nurse have done to improve collaboration?

➤ How did teamwork and communication affect Mr. Lee's activity outcomes?

➤ Did the teamwork and communication affect his safety? If so, in what way?

➤ What system changes would you make to improve communication?

➤ Think about client-centeredness. Did the team value Mrs. Lee's input (give examples)? How might outcomes have been different if Mrs. Lee had been recognized as a full partner in planning or providing care? Do you think quality, safety, costs, and patient satisfaction were affected?

BOX 29-4 ■ Terms Used to Describe Problems With Muscle Mass, Strength, or Mobility

Atrophy—a decrease in the size of muscle tissue resulting from a lack of use or loss of innervation

Clonus—spasmodic contraction of opposing muscles resulting in tremors

Flaccidity—a decrease or absence of muscle tone

Hemiplegia—paralysis of one side of the body

Hypertrophy—increase in the size or bulk of a muscle or organ

Paraplegia—paralysis of the lower portion of the trunk and both legs

Paresis—partial or incomplete paralysis

Paresthesia—numbness, tingling, or burning resulting from injury of the nerve(s) innervating the affected area

Quadriplegia—paralysis of all four extremities

Spasticity—motor disorder characterized by increased muscle tone, exaggerated tendon jerks, and clonus

Tremor—involuntary quivering movement of a body part

Focused Nursing History

A nursing history focused on activity and exercise addresses usual activity, fitness goals, mobility problems, underlying health problems, lifestyle, and external factors. When caring for patients with limited activity, assessing the ability to perform ADLs or instrumental activities of daily living (IADLs) may be more appropriate. Recall that ADLs focus on hygiene, feeding, toileting, and transfer out of bed. In contrast,

IADLs focus on tasks that are instrumental in helping a patient maintain independent living status. Assessment tools for ADLs and IADLs are presented in Chapter 3.

Focused Physical Assessment

Important data to include in a physical assessment related to activity and exercise include vital signs, height, weight, body mass index, body alignment, joint

Home Assessment for a Patient With Mobility Concerns

Home Care

Assess the Environment

➤ Are there stairs or other obstacles that the patient must negotiate?

➤ What aspects of the home environment assist with patient care?

➤ What aspects of the home environment hinder patient care?

➤ What is the patient's history of falls or other mobility concerns?

➤ Would the patient benefit from assistive equipment (e.g., hospital bed, walker)?

➤ Can the patient negotiate the distance between the bedroom, bathroom, and kitchen?

Assess the Family's or Caregivers' Abilities and Needs

➤ Who is providing care?

➤ Is the available care sufficient to meet the patient's needs?

➤ Are additional support persons available to assist with care?

➤ Can the caregiver safely move the patient in bed or assist the patient out of bed?

➤ What are the health concerns or physical limitations of the caregivers?

➤ What is the backup plan if the family or caregiver can no longer meet the patient's needs?

Assess Resources

➤ What community resources are available to the patient or caregiver?

➤ Are the patient and caregiver willing to use community resources?

➤ What services are provided by the patient's insurance?

➤ Can the patient or family afford private services? If so, what services are they interested in?

---

function, gait, muscle strength, and activity tolerance. For a description of all the components,

 Refer to the **Focused Assessment box, Assessing Activity and Exercise,** in Volume 2.

Before beginning the examination, be fully aware of the patient's mobility status and any restrictions in movement, pain, injury, or other conditions. As you move through the examination, observe for pain, inflammation, and mobility limitations in all areas.

Gait

The way a person moves communicates a great deal about their general state of health, mood, and risk for falls. You might want to assess abnormal gaits in patients with injury, neurological issues, or the following characteristics:

- **Antalgic gait**—limp to avoid pain when bearing weight on the affected side
- **Ataxic gait**—unbalanced stride. This may be caused by excessive alcohol ingestion, stroke, or certain medications. A walker or other assistive device is helpful for ataxia.
- **Propulsive gait**—a stooped, rigid posture, with the head and neck bent forward; movement forward is by small, shuffling steps with involuntary acceleration; also known as *festinating gait;* common in Parkinson disease.
- **Scissors gait**—legs flexed slightly at the hips and knees, with the thighs crossing in a scissors-like movement; common with cerebral palsy, stroke, or spinal tumor.
- **Spastic gait**—a stiff, foot-dragging walk caused by one-sided, long-term muscle contraction; seen with cerebral palsy, head trauma, or brain tumor.

- **Steppage gait**—an exaggerated motion of lifting the leg to avoid scraping the toes of a foot with footdrop (foot appears floppy, with the toes pointing down); seen with Guillain-Barré syndrome.
- **Waddling gait**—a distinctive rolling motion in which the opposite hip drops; seen in patients with muscular dystrophy or developmental dysplasia of the hip; characteristic gait in late pregnancy.
- **In-toeing and out-toeing**—abnormal gait patterns that occur among some young children. When toes point inward with walking or face outward; can be caused by bowlegs, knock knees, or flat feet.

 For more information, go to **Chapter 19, Procedure 19-15: Assessing the Musculoskeletal System,** in Volume 2.

Activity Tolerance

To promote the benefits of physical activity, people need to pace themselves during exercise, especially those who have been inactive. Health professionals can teach people to rate the perceived level of exertion and monitor target heart rate. Target heart rate requires a pulse check during exercises and staying within 50% to 85% of the maximum heart rate. To figure this out and for more information about optimal target heart rates during exercise, see Box 29-1.

KnowledgeCheck 29-6

- Describe a focused assessment for a patient experiencing mobility concerns.
- Identify the assessment methods (inspection, palpation, percussion, and auscultation) used when performing a physical examination focused on mobility concerns.

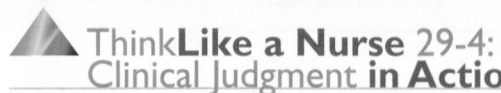

ThinkLike a Nurse 29-4: Clinical Judgment in Action

Review the Meet Your Patients scenario. Which, if any, of the class participants requires a physical examination focused on mobility concerns? Explain your reasoning.

NURSING DIAGNOSIS/ANALYZING CUES

Activity Intolerance is a state in which a patient has insufficient physiological or psychological energy to endure or complete required or desired daily activities (NANDA International, 2021). This is characterized by fatigue, weakness, discomfort on exertion, dyspnea, and verbalization of no interest in activity. When assessing the patient with Activity Intolerance:

Subjective cues: fatigue, weakness, discomfort on exertion, dyspnea, and verbalization of no interest in activity.

Objective cues: changes in heart rate, blood pressure disproportionate to activity, dysrhythmias, or evidence of ischemia on electrocardiogram (ECG), and pallor or cyanosis with activity.

Activity intolerance may occur because of conditions that affect tissue oxygenation (e.g., chronic obstructive pulmonary disease or cardiac disease) and conditions that produce fatigue, such as depression, prolonged immobility, bedrest, and a sedentary lifestyle.

PLANNING/PRIORITIZING HYPOTHESES AND GENERATING SOLUTIONS

Nursing Outcomes Classification (NOC) Standardized Outcomes for mobility diagnoses focus on energy maintenance:

Activity Tolerance	Psychomotor Energy
Endurance	Rest
Energy Conservation	Sleep
Fatigue Level	

Individualized Goals/Outcome Statements depend on the nursing diagnosis used. Because activity and exercise abilities are individualized, goals must consider the patient's current condition, expected condition changes, lifestyle, and values. Examples:

Will independently transfer to the wheelchair by [date].
Will discuss their feelings about the activity restrictions by [date].

IMPLEMENTATION/TAKING ACTION

♥ **iCare**   Because attitudes about fitness and activity vary widely, mobility is often a difficult topic. Some people are devastated by the activity limitations caused by disease or treatment. Others can more easily accept these changes. It is important for you to convey an attitude of caring about the patient's current activity level and provide care that helps the patient achieve their optimal level of function.

NIC Standardized Interventions and Activities   For patients with limitations or restrictions in activity, the following Nursing Intervention Classification (NIC) Interventions promote activity and exercise:

Body Mechanics Promotion	Exercise Therapy: Balance
Energy Management	Exercise Therapy: Joint Mobility
Exercise Promotion	
Exercise Promotion: Strength Training	Exercise Therapy: Muscle Control
Exercise Promotion: Stretching	Teaching: Prescribed Activity/Exercise
Exercise Therapy: Ambulation	

Individualized Nursing Activities   Individualized nursing activities include enhancing mobility, promoting exercise, preventing injury from exercise, positioning patients, moving patients in bed, transferring patients out of bed, performing ROM exercises, and assisting with ambulation.

Caring for Patients With Specific Disease and Abnormalities

In addition, when caring for patients with specific diseases and abnormalities, you will need to add the following interventions:

- **For congenital anomalies**—Nursing responsibilities include early detection and referral for additional treatment, along with parent counseling.
- **For bone formation abnormalities**—Nursing responsibilities include collaborative treatments, providing comfort, and patient education to promote mobility. Also, nurses should teach patients to consume a balanced diet that meets the minimum recommendations for vitamins and minerals.
- **For joint mobility problems**—Nursing activities focus on providing comfort, promoting ROM, and teaching about medications. If mobility is severely restricted, you will also assist patients with ADLs.
- **For osteomyelitis or bone tumors**—Nursing activities include collaborative treatments, patient education about the treatment plan, and providing comfort.

Preventing and Treating Osteoporosis.

Key Point: *The best treatment for osteoporosis is prevention.* Teach adolescents and adults the following measures.

- **A balanced diet** high in calcium, fluoride, and other minerals contributes to strong bones.
  - **Calcium and vitamin D.** The National Institutes of Health, Office of Dietary Supplements (NIHODS) recommends a calcium intake for adults aged 50 and older of 1,200 mg/day (October 6, 2022) and vitamin D 800 to 1,000 IU daily to prevent bone loss (August 22, 2022).

- **Mineral supplements.** Calcium supplementation can also help to prevent demineralization. **Phosphorus** is another important mineral for strengthening bone. But if there is an imbalance of phosphorus compared with the amount of calcium in the diet, bone loss can occur.
  - **Weight-bearing exercise.** Advise older female patients that weight-bearing exercise improves bone density and can reduce the rate of bone loss with aging. People should engage in exercise interventions lifelong.
- **Pharmacological options** for postmenopausal female patients include estrogen-like medication, hormone therapy (estrogen/progestin), parathyroid hormone, calcitonin, denosumab (antibody directed against a specific protein that breaks down bone), and anabolic agents (simulate bone production). Older adults should ask healthcare providers about medications to reduce bone mineral loss (Grossman, 2018). Other medications (bisphosphonates, alendronates, and others) can be prescribed to slow the breakdown of bone for those with the highest risk for fracture (Rosen, 2021).
- **Avoid tobacco use,** particularly among postmenopausal patients. Tobacco reduces the absorption of calcium in the intestine.
- **Limit alcohol** to less than 2 drinks per day to preserve bone density; alcohol decreases the matrix of the bone and reduces the body's ability to absorb calcium. Consuming too much alcohol also increases the risk for falls and poor nutrition (Rosen, 2021).
- **Prolonged use of certain medications can increase bone loss.** For example, glucocorticoids (prednisone), anticoagulants (heparin), and antiepileptics (phenytoin, carbamazepine, phenobarbital) can increase bone loss.

Promoting Exercise

Nurses are in an ideal role to encourage and educate people of all ages to be active for healthy living. Here are some common steps to help people attain and maintain fitness. Also see the Self-Care box, Teaching Clients How to Set Up a Fitness Program.

- **Personalize the benefits of regular physical activity.** In other words, find out what motivates your patient. For instance, your patient might want to lose weight and improve their physical mobility. Yet another patient might be interested in improving the quality of sleep or overcoming periods of low energy during the day.
- **Set personal goals for physical activity.** Simple, realistic goals tend to be best. Be sure to define them so that they are specific and measurable.
- **Include a variety of activities** to keep the patient from feeling bored.
- **Remind your patient to recognize and appreciate success.**

- **Suggest strategies to achieve the patient's goals.** You can also educate your patient about ways to avoid joint injury or falls.
- **Provide encouragement.** For example, offer praise for taking steps toward health and fitness. Support from spouse and significant others can improve compliance and consistency.
- **Promote physical exercise** as an enjoyable activity.
- **Discuss barriers to regular activity** and elicit ways to overcome those obstacles.

People give various reasons for failing to develop a consistent exercise program. See Box 29-5 for suggestions on dealing with such objections.

Exercise for Stress Relief How is your stress level? A high stress level can produce fatigue. Although you may view exercise as one more thing you don't have time for, exercise is energizing and can be used to relieve stress. For example, taking a brisk 20-minute walk during a break may allow you to continue working for several more hours.

You can also use this technique when caring for inpatients. Hospitalized patients and family members often experience a great deal of stress. Helping the patient take a walk in the hallway or to the courtyard or instructing family members on how to handle the wheelchair so that they can take the patient out of the room often will help lessen some of the strain of illness and hospitalization.

Positioning Patients

Healthy people regularly shift position to maintain comfort. However, many patients are unable to move without assistance. They require a change of position at least every 2 hours to prevent skin breakdown, muscle discomfort, damage to superficial nerves and blood vessels, and contractures. People who are immobile are more prone to pressure injury because of reduced circulation, impaired oxygen exchange to the tissues, and edema.

A firm mattress provides support to the patient's body and makes it easier to turn the patient (because they do not sink down into the mattress). Most hospital mattresses are firm. However, when you provide home care, you will find mattresses of various types and conditions. To provide additional support, you can place a piece of plywood under a sagging mattress.

Protecting the Nurse's Back

- **Make sure you have adequate help.** Some lifts and patient care tasks require multiple staff members to accomplish safely, and because low staffing makes this teamwork difficult, nurses often attempt these tasks alone. The amount of help you need depends on the size and shape of the patient, the level of assistance the patient can offer, your size and strength, and the equipment or lines attached to the patient.
- **Avoid manual lifting.** To protect yourself from back injury as you move patients, avoid manual lifting as much as possible.

BOX 29-5 ■ Suggestions for Overcoming Objections to Exercise

Objection	Suggestion
"I hate to exercise."	Pick activities that you enjoy.
"I burn out on exercise."	Plan ahead and build in rest days and varied activities.
"I am self-conscious about going to the gym and don't have the motivation to exercise by myself."	Find a friend to exercise with or develop a reward system for yourself if you continue to exercise. An exercise "buddy" can help increase motivation and consistency in the weekly routine.
"I am too busy with work or family."	Develop a routine that you can do at lunchtime, or exercise with your family.
"I find exercise boring."	Change your routine frequently.
"I can't afford to join a health club, hire a fitness trainer, or buy expensive equipment."	Just get active doing things you enjoy. Go for a brisk walk or play with your (grand)kids. Some of the best core exercises require no equipment at all (e.g., push-ups, planks). You can also use a chair, jump rope, or many things around the house to build into your fitness routine.
"I'm too tired to exercise."	The hardest part is getting started, but after a few minutes or so, you'll feel better and have more energy after you finish.
"Exercise hurts."	Make sure to exercise at your target heart rate and plan a rest day after every weight-lifting session.
"I don't have time."	Schedule your exercise time. If need be, schedule several short 10- to 15-minute sessions throughout the day, and do more as time allows. It all adds up and will benefit you.
"I have pain just about all the time."	Take pain medication an hour or so before starting physical activity. If fatigue is the problem, try to arrange schedule to keep a balance of rest and activity, and avoid stimulants (e.g., caffeine or nicotine) that might interfere with the quality of sleep.
"I have difficulty getting around sometimes."	Stretch adequately before starting exercise, but be careful not to overstretch joints. Also, you will need to walk on smooth, even surfaces.
"I am diabetic and have trouble with my feet. My vision is not very good, either."	Be sure shoes fit properly and the area is well lit.
"I'm too old to exercise."	It's never too late to get active, and any physical activity you do is better than none. Exercises that build strength, stamina, flexibility, and balance improve the quality of life and reduce the risk for falls.

♥ iCare 29-1

Activity & Exercise

Viraj is caring for 82-year-old Mr. Ndiaye, whose physician has ordered Mr. Ndiaye to be out of bed at least three times daily and to ambulate at least 20 feet daily. Mr. Ndiaye is hesitant to ambulate in the hallway because it takes him a while to do so, and he thinks he is a bother to the staff; therefore, he has little to no motivation. During his conversations with Mr. Ndiaye, Viraj learns that Mr. Ndiaye used to run track in high school. Viraj develops signage on the unit to simulate a track with "mile markers" on the wall and floor and takes Mr. Ndiaye for a walk slowly down one side of the hallway and back. This small innovative gesture fosters conversation on the unit among staff and leads to an increase in ambulation among other patients.

- **Use assistive equipment and devices,** as recommended by the American Nurses Association (ANA, 2021).
- **Avoid slippery or wet surfaces** during ambulation or when moving patients.
- **Remove physical obstructions** (e.g., cabinets, toilets) when moving or transferring patients.

- **Arrange a clutter-free environment** that allows for free movement of equipment and personnel.
- **Watch out for uneven floor surfaces or movable rugs.**
- **Lock wheels of furniture and equipment before moving patients.**
- **Avoid moving patients through a path or doorway that is too small.**
- **Wear supportive shoes with nonslip soles.**

Positioning Devices

Devices used to maintain body alignment, prevent contractures, and promote comfort are briefly discussed in the next sections.

Beds

- **Adjustable beds.** Often referred to as a *hospital bed*, an adjustable bed assumes a variety of positions. You can elevate or lower the head of the bed and elevate the foot of the bed. Often, the bed adjusts upward at the knee to keep the patient from sliding down when the head is elevated. You can also adjust the height of the bed. You should raise the bed to waist height when providing care so that you can use proper body mechanics; place the bed in its lowest position before helping a patient get out of bed or if the patient is at risk for falling.

- **Specialized beds.** Several types of specialized beds are used in treating and preventing pressure injury. These include alternating, low-air-loss, immersion (air-fluidized), and oscillating beds. The mattresses may be composed of air, water, or gel. A circular bed and Stryker frame are used in the care of patients with severe mobility restrictions. Both can rotate a patient from supine to prone. With the advent of low-pressure specialized beds, these latter two types of beds are now in limited use. Special beds are discussed later in this chapter.

Pillows Pillows are the most common devices used to assist with positioning, provide support, and elevate body parts (Fig. 29-7). They help position a patient by molding to the body and expanding the weight-bearing area. You will need a variety of sizes to position patients who are unconscious, paralyzed, or frail and those who have had surgery. To obtain the right size or type (e.g., abductor pillows), or if pillows are not available, you can use folded blankets or towels. Foam wedge pillows are useful for elevating the upper body when an adjustable bed is not available and for abducting the hips after hip surgery.

Siderails Most hospital beds are equipped with siderails. The rails may run the full length of each side of the bed or consist of an upper or lower rail on each side. ✚ Siderails are designed to ensure patient safety. They serve as a reminder that the patient should call for assistance before getting out of bed and provide a grip for patients who are able to reposition themselves in bed. Although siderails are designed to protect patients, they can be a source of injury. Patients can get tangled in the railing or fall between the bed and rail, and confused patients may injure themselves by trying to climb over the rails. Siderails may also be considered a form of restraint, so follow your agency's policy for use, and be sure to discuss their purpose with patients and family. See Chapter 21 if you need to review restraint use.

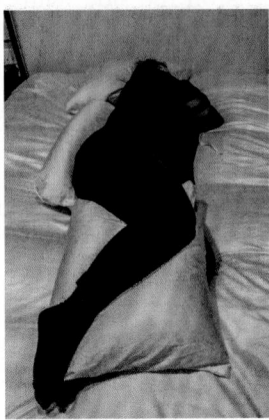

FIGURE 29-7 Pillows assist with neutral positioning and support.

Trapeze Bar A trapeze bar is a triangular-shaped device that is attached to an overhead bed frame. The patient can use the base of the triangle as a grip bar to move up in bed, turn, and pull up in preparation for getting out of bed or getting on and off the bedpan. Patients can use the trapeze to move about in bed and to exercise their upper extremities. Frail patients may not be able to use a trapeze bar because of the amount of effort it requires.

Other Positioning Devices When a person is supine, the toes tend to point downward toward the bed **(footdrop),** and the feet are in plantar flexion. Able-bodied persons usually shift position throughout the night, so the foot and leg muscles are periodically contracted and relaxed. In contrast, the patient who is unable to move independently will experience a shortening of the gastrocnemius muscle and may have difficulty walking again if prolonged plantar flexion occurs.

- A **footboard** is a device placed at the end of the bed to prevent footdrop and outward hip rotation, but it does not relieve heel pressure. For the footboard to be effective, the heels must be touching it. Each time you turn the patient, you may need to reposition the footboard to ensure proper position.
- **Cradle boots** made of spongy rubber with heel cutouts and ankle cushioning prevent footdrop, skin breakdown, and external hip rotation (Fig. 29-8). ✚ If any part of the boot is made of a latex product, be sure the patient does not have a latex allergy before applying.
- **Foot cradles** are metal or plastic devices that are secured at the foot of the bed to hold bedding up off the toes and feet, allowing for free movement.
- **Trochanter rolls** are placed snugly adjacent to the hips and thighs to prevent external rotation of the hips (Fig. 29-9). They are commonly used with hip fracture or after hip replacement surgery.
- **Hand and wrist splints** hold the wrist and hand in a neutral, resting position. **Hand rolls** prevent hand contractures. Most are commercially made. Otherwise, you can make a hand roll from a tightly rolled washcloth (Fig. 29-10).
- **Hip abduction pillows** prevent internal hip rotation and hip adduction when the patient is in a supine position. These wedge-shaped pieces of spongy material are used after femoral fracture, hip fracture, or

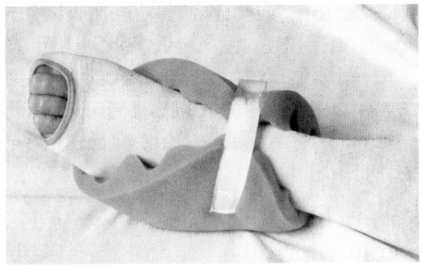

FIGURE 29-8 A foot-positioning boot is placed around the foot to prevent foot drop.

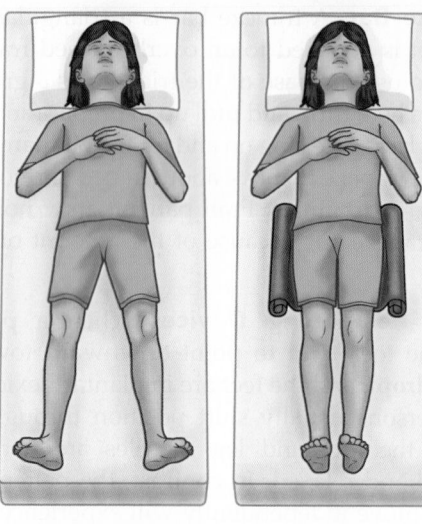

FIGURE 29-9 Proper alignment using a trochanter roll

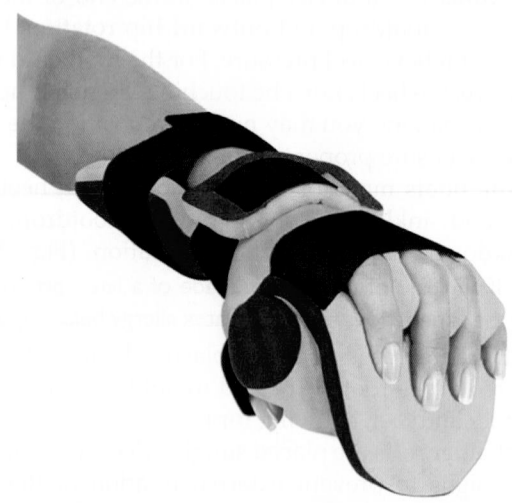

FIGURE 29-10 A wrist splint with hand roll maintains a neutral, resting position.

surgery (Fig. 29-11). Lateral indentations and straps that wrap around the patient's thighs hold the patient in the correct position.

■ **Sandbags** are small fabric bags filled with sand. They are used in the same manner as pillows and trochanter rolls; however, they provide firmer support.

Positioning Techniques

In the next section, we briefly describe the various ways to position patients. Table 29-3 illustrates these positions, identifies potential problems associated with them, and offers solutions to prevent the problems. The positions are also described and illustrated in Chapter 19, Table 19-1.

Fowler's Positions Fowler's position is a semisitting position in which the head of the bed is elevated 45° to 60°. This position promotes respiratory function by lowering the diaphragm and allowing the greatest

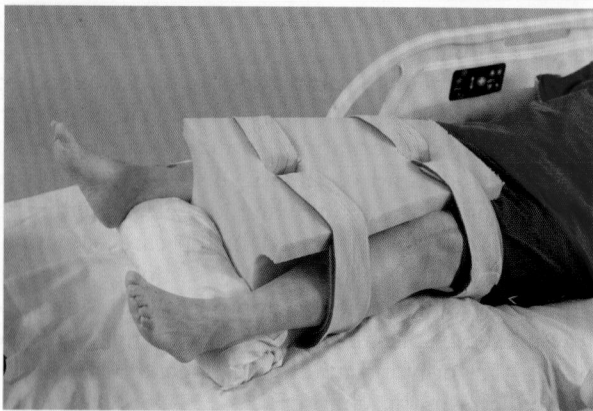

FIGURE 29-11 Hip abduction pillow designed for use after hip surgery when immobilization or postoperative positioning is required.

chest expansion. It is also an ideal position for some patients with cardiac dysfunction. Common variations include:

■ **Semi-Fowler's position**—the head of the bed is elevated only 30°.
■ **High-Fowler's position**—the head of the bed is elevated 90°.
■ **Orthopneic position**—the head of the bed is elevated 90°, and an overbed table with a pillow on top is positioned in front of the patient (Fig. 29-12). Have the patient lean forward, resting their arms and head on the pillow. This position is more comfortable for patients with shortness of breath.

Lateral Positions The **lateral position** is a side-lying position with the top hip and knee flexed and placed in front of the rest of the body. The lateral position creates pressure on the lower scapula, ilium, and trochanter but relieves pressure from the heels and sacrum.

■ The **lateral recumbent position** is side-lying, with legs in a straight line (see Table 29-1).
■ The **oblique position** is an alternative to the lateral position that places less pressure on the trochanter. The patient turns on the side, with the top hip and knee flexed; however, the top leg is placed behind the body (Fig. 29-13).

Prone Position The patient lies on their abdomen with their head turned to one side. This is the only position that allows full extension of the hips and knees. It also allows secretions to drain freely from the sinuses and mouth; thus, it is helpful for an unconscious patient.

✚ However, this is the most difficult position for safely moving an unconscious or frail patient.

The prone position creates a significant lordosis (inward curving of the spine in the lower back) and rotation of the neck.

■ Avoid the prone position for patients with cervical or lumbar spine problems.

Table 29-3 ➤ Positioning a Bed-Bound Patient

POSITION	POTENTIAL PROBLEM	SOLUTION
Fowler's	Hyperextension of the neck	Use a small pillow under the head and neck.
	Posterior flexion of the lumbar curvature	Use a firm mattress. Position the patient so that the angle of elevation begins at the hip.
	Dislocation of the shoulders	Position a pillow under the forearms to prevent pull on the shoulders.
	Flexion contracture of the fingers and abduction of the thumbs	Use hand splints if appropriate; or provide a large roll in the palm of the hand.
	Flexion contracture of the wrist and edema of the hands	Position the hands on pillows in alignment with the forearms.
	External rotation of the legs	Place sandbags or rolls alongside the trochanters and upper thighs
	Hyperextension of the knees	Place a small pillow under the lower legs from the ankles to below the knees. Do this for short periods only; avoid pressure on the popliteal area.
	Footdrop	Use a footboard, positioning boot, or high-top sneakers to hold the foot in position.
Lateral	Lateral flexion of the neck	Place a pillow under the head and neck to provide alignment.
	Internal rotation and adduction of the upper shoulder and limited respirations	Place a pillow under the upper arm, and comfortably flex the lower arm.
	Internal rotation and adduction of the femur	Support the upper leg from groin to foot with pillows.
	Twisting of the spine	Align the shoulders with the hips.
	Flexion of the cervical spine	Place a pillow under the head and neck to provide alignment, unless drainage from the mouth is desired.
Prone	Hyperextension of the lumbar curvature, pressure on the breasts in female patients or genitals in male patients, impaired respirations	Place a small pillow under the abdomen.
	Footdrop	Move the patient down in bed so that the feet extend over the edge of the mattress, or place a small pillow under the shins so that the toes do not touch the bed.
	Lateral flexion of the neck	Place a pillow under the head and neck to provide alignment, unless drainage from the mouth is desired.

(Continued)

Table 29-3 ➤ Positioning a Bed-Bound Patient—cont'd

POSITION	POTENTIAL PROBLEM	SOLUTION
Sims' 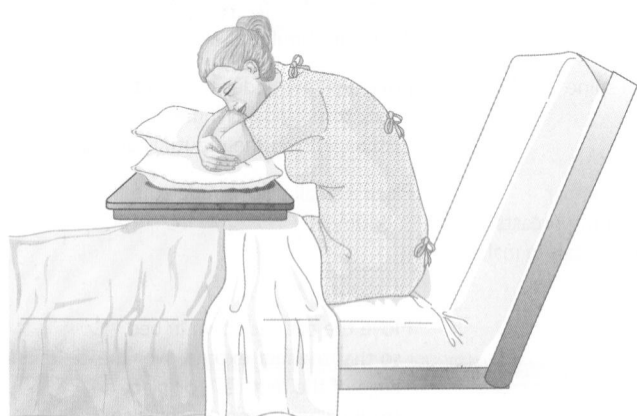	Internal rotation and adduction of the upper shoulder and limited respirations	Place a pillow under the upper arm, and comfortably flex the arm at the elbow.
	Pressure on the shoulder and axilla of the inferior arm	Position the lower arm behind and away from the back.
	Twisting of the spine	Align the shoulders with the hips.
	Footdrop	Support the feet in dorsiflexion with sandbags.
	Hyperextension of the neck	Place a pillow under the head and neck to provide alignment.
Supine	Internal rotation of the shoulders and extension of the elbows	Position the upper arms next to the body. Place pillows under the forearms; position the wrists in slight pronation.
	Flexion of fingers and abduction of the thumbs	Use hand splints if appropriate, or provide a large roll in the palm of the hand.
	Flexion of the lumbar curvature and hips	Provide a firm mattress, or place a small pillow under the lumbar curvature.
	External rotation of the legs	Place sandbags or rolls alongside the trochanters and upper thighs.
	Hyperextension of the knees	Place a small pillow under the lower legs from the ankles to below the knees.
	Footdrop	Use a footboard, cradle boots, or high-top sneakers to hold the feet in dorsiflexion.

FIGURE 29-12 The orthopneic position helps a patient with shortness of breath.

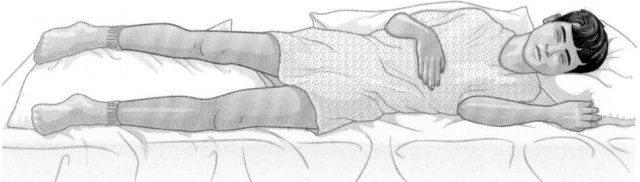

FIGURE 29-13 The oblique position is a modified lateral position that places pressure on the trochanter.

■ Do not use the prone position for patients with cardiac or respiratory difficulty because it inhibits chest wall expansion and, therefore, oxygenation. As a rule, you can use this position only for short periods of time.

Sims' Position This is a semiprone position where the lower arm is positioned behind the patient, and the upper arm is flexed. The upper leg is more flexed than the lower leg. The Sims' position facilitates drainage from the mouth and limits pressure on the trochanter and sacrum. This is an ideal position for administering an enema or a perineal procedure.

Supine Position Also known as the **dorsal recumbent position,** in the supine position, the patient lies on their back with head and shoulders elevated on a small pillow. The spine is aligned with the arms, and the hands comfortably rest at the side.

KnowledgeCheck 29-7

- Describe the following positions: Fowler's, lateral, prone, Sims', and supine.
- What is the advantage of the oblique position versus the lateral position?
- Identify and describe six positioning devices.
- What are three uses for siderails?

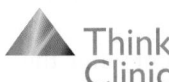

ThinkLike a Nurse 29-5: Clinical Judgment in Action

You are providing care for a young patient who is recovering from Guillain-Barré syndrome, which produces a reversible paralysis after viral illness. They have been healthy until this present illness. How would you position this patient? Explain your reasoning.

Moving Patients in Bed

To position patients, you must be adept at moving and lifting them in bed. This involves positioning the patient in the length of the bed, as well as turning with as little friction and shearing on the skin as possible. Moving patients in bed is a common intervention to help minimize the risk for the Example Client Condition: Prolonged Immobility.

- **Moving up in bed.** Frail patients tend to slide down in bed because of gravity and their inability to correct their position. Elevating the head of the bed accentuates the slide and places the patient in an awkward position. If the patient is light in weight or able to provide aid, you will be able to move them independently. For a summary of these procedures, see the Highlights of Procedures box. For the complete steps,

 See **Chapter 29, Procedure 29-1A: Moving a Patient Up in Bed,** in Volume 2.

- **Turning in bed.** Turn patients at least every 2 hours to protect their skin and prevent other complications of immobility. For efficient use of time, try to time turning to coincide with moving the patient up in bed. Use pillows and other positioning devices to help the patient maintain the new position. For a summary of this procedure, see the Highlights of Procedures box. For the complete steps,

 Refer to **Chapter 29, Procedure 29-1B: Turning a Patient in Bed,** in Volume 2.

- **Logrolling.** Logrolling is a special turning technique used when the patient's spine must be kept in a straight alignment. You will need at least two nurses for this procedure, possibly more if the patient is large. Logrolling moves the patient's body as a unit.

For a summary of this procedure, see the Highlights of Procedures box. For the complete steps,

 Refer to **Chapter 29, Procedure 29-1C: Logrolling a Patient,** in Volume 2.

- **Friction-reducing devices.** You can use one of a variety of friction-reducing devices when moving a patient in bed.
  - **Transfer roller sheets** are thin, low-friction fabric sheets that may be placed beneath the drawsheet to facilitate moving the patient in bed (Fig. 29-14).
  - **A scoot sheet** is also a thin, low-friction fabric sheet that is often positioned under the drawsheet of the patient, but it is attached to a mechanical crank (Fig. 29-15). By turning the crank, a single person can move a patient up in bed. Transfer roller sheets are relatively inexpensive and are widely available on clinical units.
  - A **roller tray** with disposable absorbent underpads can also be used to reduce low back stress when moving patients (Bacharach et al., 2016).

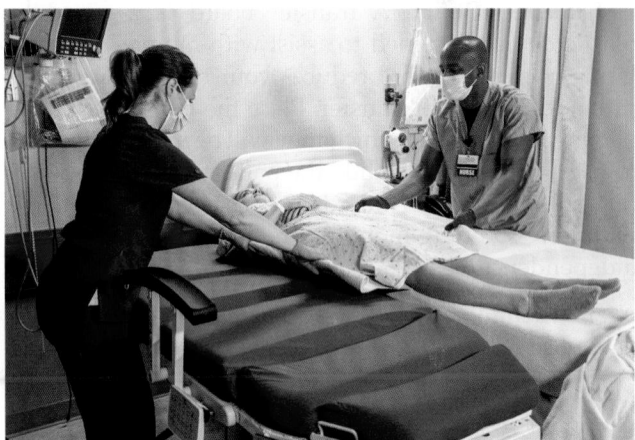

FIGURE 29-14 A transfer sheet reduces friction and facilitates movement.

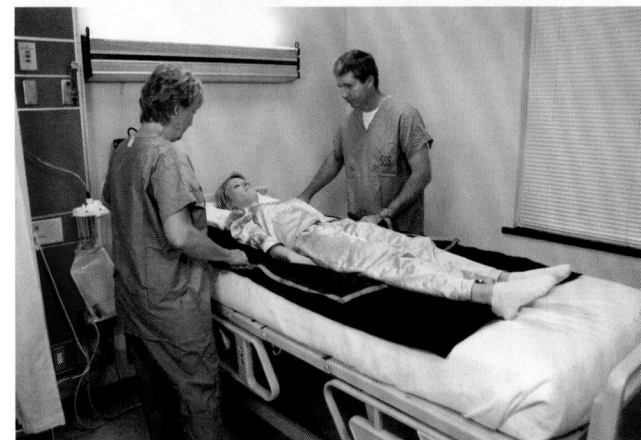

FIGURE 29-15 A scoot sheet allows a single person to move a patient up in bed.

Transferring Patients Out of Bed

Stretchers and wheelchairs are used to transport patients between units and to tests or procedures. A stretcher is usually reserved for the patient who is weak, is sedated, or has a condition that does not permit safe transfer by wheelchair. In addition, you may move patients to a stationary chair to increase their general activity level. For a summary of these procedures, see the Highlights of Procedures box. For the complete steps,

 Refer to **Chapter 29, Procedure 29-2A: Transferring a Patient From Bed to Stretcher, Procedure 29-2B: Dangling a Patient at the Side of the Bed,** and **Procedure 29-2C: Transferring a Patient From Bed to Chair,** in Volume 2.

To know what type of assistive device is appropriate for patient safety and to prevent back injury to the nurse,

 See **Chapter 29, Clinical Insight 29-1: Applying Principles of Body Mechanics,** in Volume 2.

Transfer Board A transfer board is a wood or plastic device designed to assist with moving patients. Using a transfer board reduces your risk of injury and promotes a smooth transfer. Place the board under the patient on the side to which they will be moved. It is best to use a drawsheet to slide the patient across the board (Fig. 29-16). Transfer boards are also used by patients with long-standing mobility problems to increase their independence.

A Mechanical Lift A mechanical lift is a hydraulic device used to transfer patients. Place a fabric sling under the patient, and attach chains or straps from the sling to the lifting device (Fig. 29-17).

- A mechanical lift is especially useful when providing care for patients with obesity or immobility.
- Lifts are often used in home care because they allow one person to transfer the patient safely.
- Most lifts position patients in a seated position and thus are ideal for assisting the patient into a chair.
- Others suspend the patient in a supine position; they may be used to transfer the patient from bed to stretcher or to suspend the patient while the bed is made.
- Many include scales that weigh the patient while they are suspended in the sling.
- Some mechanical lifts are mounted on the ceiling to reduce caregiver back injuries and increase patient safety (Fig. 29-18).

Standing Assist Devices Standing assist devices are mechanical lifts that help the patient move from a sitting to a standing position or support a patient in the standing position (Fig. 29-19). A sling is positioned around the back and under the arms of the patient. Specialized chairs and wheelchairs are also available. Each has a mechanical lift in the seat that rises to assist the patient to a standing position. Mechanical lift devices reduce the risk of back and musculoskeletal injury.

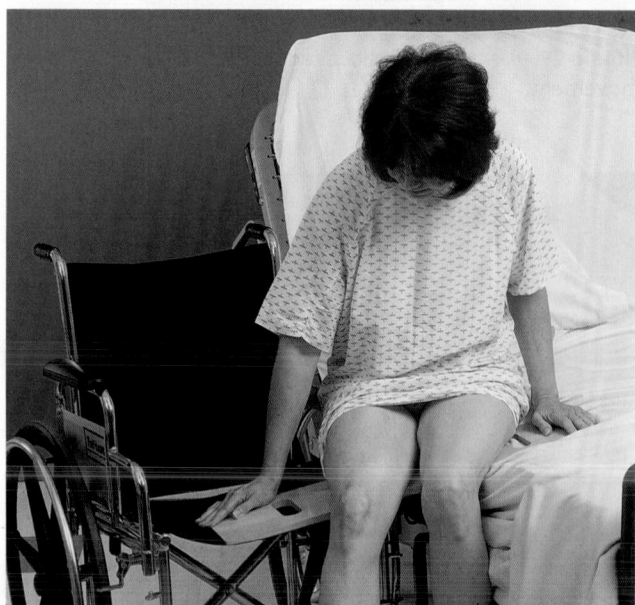

FIGURE 29-16 Transfer boards are used for patients with restricted mobility to increase independence.

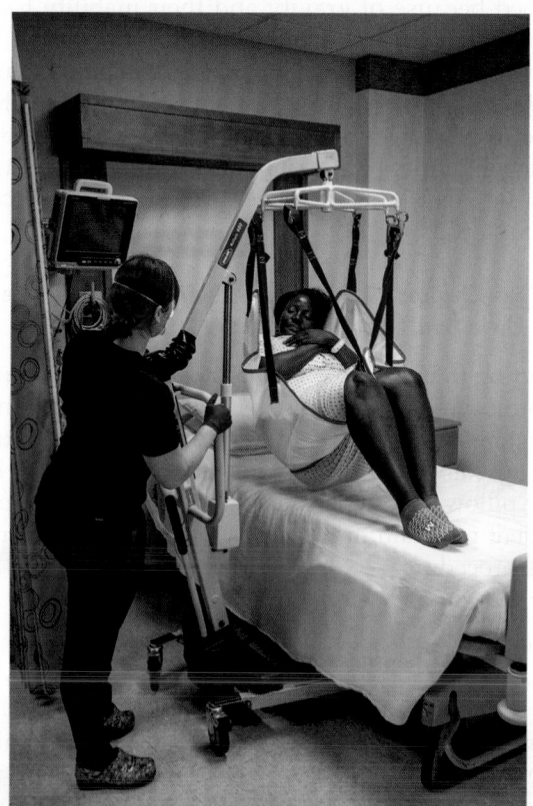

FIGURE 29-17 A mechanical lift is useful when providing care to patients with impaired mobility.

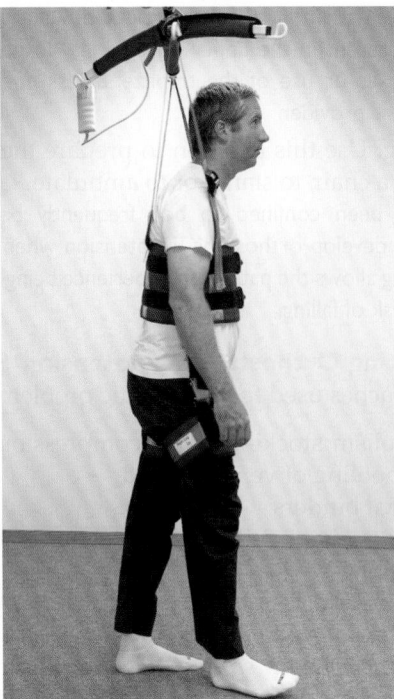

FIGURE 29-18 A ceiling-mounted mechanical lift is used to support patients in the standing position.

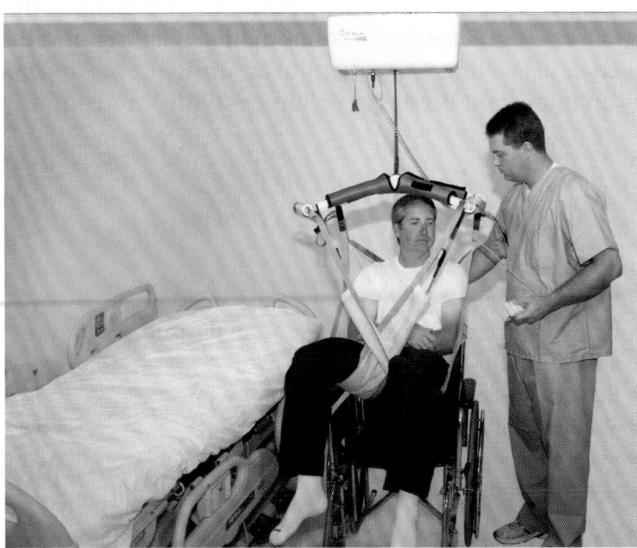

FIGURE 29-19 A mechanical lift with a sling chair is used to safely transfer an immobile patient into a wheelchair.

A Transfer Belt A transfer belt is a heavy belt that is used to facilitate transfer or provide a secure mechanism to hold the patient when ambulating (Fig. 29-20).

- ✚ Apply the belt around the patient's abdomen, close to the patient's center of gravity. The belt may have external grip holds, or you may grip the entire belt with your hand.
- The fit should not be overly tight or cause the patient discomfort. You should be able to easily place your hand under the belt.

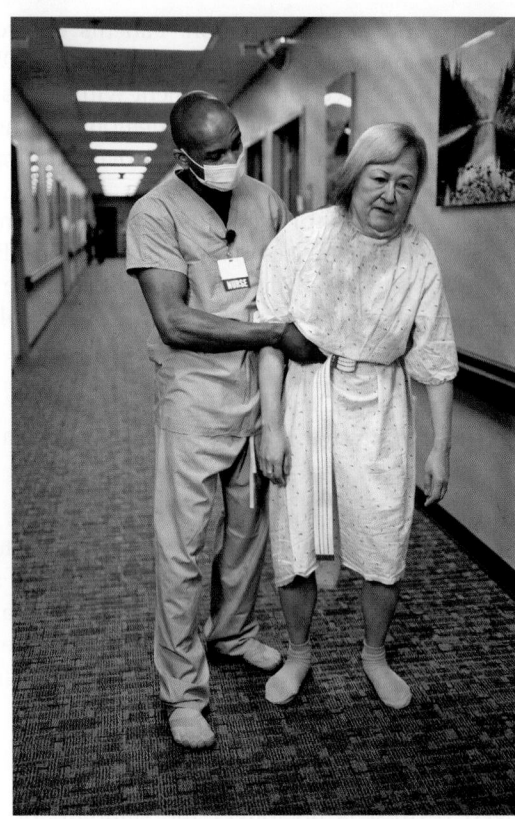

FIGURE 29-20 A transfer belt is placed close to the patient's center of gravity. External grips provide security for the patient who needs assistance ambulating.

- Do not place it over the rib cage because this could compromise breathing.
- Do not use a transfer belt around the patient's hip. This could cause unsteadiness and lead to a patient fall.
- You would not use a transfer belt after abdominal surgery or with other abdominal wounds, a colostomy, or internal organ contusion or other injury.

KnowledgeCheck 29-8
- What criteria determine whether your patient should be logrolled when they are repositioned?
- How often should you turn and reposition a patient?
- Identify the most appropriate device for the following activities:
  Transferring a patient with obesity from a bed to a stretcher
  Assisting a patient with immobility to a recliner chair
  Helping a weak patient from bed to chair

Performing Range-of-Motion Exercises

For patients with limited mobility, nursing interventions focus on preventing complications of disuse, such as muscle atrophy, joint stiffness, and contractures. For a thorough discussion of the physical assessment of the musculoskeletal system, see Chapter 19. For an illustration of joint ROM, see Table 29-1.

- **AROM** occurs when the patient independently moves their joints through flexion, extension, abduction, adduction, and circular rotation. Patients recovering from illness, injury, or surgery often perform AROM as a rehabilitation procedure. Movement with ADLs also helps to improve joint mobility, circulation, and muscle strength and tone. AROM also improves respiratory and cardiac function.

- **PROM** is movement of the joints through their range of motion by another person. Both AROM and PROM improve joint mobility, increase circulation to the area exercised, and help maintain function. For an explanation of how to perform PROM,

 See **Chapter 29, Clinical Insight 29-2: Tips for Performing Passive Range-of-Motion Exercise,** in Volume 2.

- **Continuous passive motion,** also called *CPM,* is a device that repetitively but gently flexes and extends the knee joint. The CPM device is often used after knee replacement or other knee procedures to allow the joint to improve its ROM; eliminate the problem of stiffness; and prevent the development of adhesions, which can limit motion further.

Assisting With Ambulation

Prolonged bedrest is no longer the standard of care. However, as a nurse, you will provide care to patients whose illnesses and injuries curtail their ability to walk and be active. This involves assisting patients with and preparing them for physical activity. For a summary of this procedure, see the Highlights of Procedures box. For the complete steps,

 See **Chapter 29, Procedure 29-3: Assisting With Ambulation,** in Volume 2.

Physical Conditioning

Patients who have been confined to bed for more than a week or who have sustained major injury require conditioning before they are able to resume walking. The following conditioning exercises are summarized here; for a detailed explanation,

 See **Chapter 29, Clinical Insight 29-3: Assisting With Physical Conditioning Exercises to Prepare for Ambulation,** in Volume 2.

- **Quadriceps and gluteal drills.** The quadriceps muscle group and the gluteal muscles are the largest muscles of the body. Patients who are confined to bed can perform isometric exercises to prepare them for walking.
- **Arm exercises.** Patients use the biceps and triceps muscles when getting out of bed and for crutch walking. Exercises to help prepare the patient for ambulation include using a trapeze bar and doing push-ups off the mattress or a chair.
  Be mindful of any cardiac or musculoskeletal precautions that restrict arm movement or weight-bearing on the hands

and wrists, in addition to other upper body injuries. If lymphedema is present in the upper extremities, do not encourage arm exercises or use of the trapeze, unless directed by the primary care provider.

- **Dangling.** Use this position to prepare the patient to get up in a chair, to stand, or to ambulate. 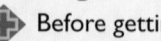 Patients who have been confined to bed frequently become lightheaded or develop orthostatic hypotension when first getting up. Dangling allows the patient to experience being upright with a limited risk of falling.

Preventing Orthostatic Hypotension Some common approaches used for orthostatic problems include:

- Antiembolism stockings with compression wraps to prevent pooling of venous blood
- Abdominal binders
- Medication is available to control orthostatic hypotension.
- **Key Point:** *Patients with spinal cord injury who are experiencing autonomic dysfunction need a high-back reclining wheelchair so that the back of the chair can be lowered (and someone might even have to lift their legs for a few minutes) until blood pressure stabilizes. Tilt-table therapies are also used.*

Daily Activities Moving around in bed and performing ADLs (e.g., brushing hair) exercise many of the muscle groups needed for ambulation. Getting up into a chair accustoms the patient to an upright posture and is an important predictor of success with ambulation.

Assisting the Patient to Walk

Before getting the patient out of bed:

- Assess their readiness to walk.
- Obtain the appropriate equipment and assistance.
- Move floor rugs and loose objects from the path of the patient and caregiver.
- Be sure the floor is not slippery.
- When possible, use a transfer belt.
- Have a chair or additional assistance available on the first few attempts at ambulation.

If the patient becomes faint or begins to fall, do not attempt to hold them up by yourself. Instead, protect the patient as you guide them to a seated or lying position. Create a wide base of support, and project forward the hip closest to the patient. Help the patient slide down your leg as you call for help (Fig. 29-21). Protect the patient's head as their body descends.

For a summary of these procedures, see the Highlights of Procedures box. For the complete steps,

 See **Chapter 29, Procedure 29-3A: Assisting With Ambulation (One Nurse),** and **Procedure 29-3B: Assisting with Ambulation (Two Nurses),** in Volume 2.

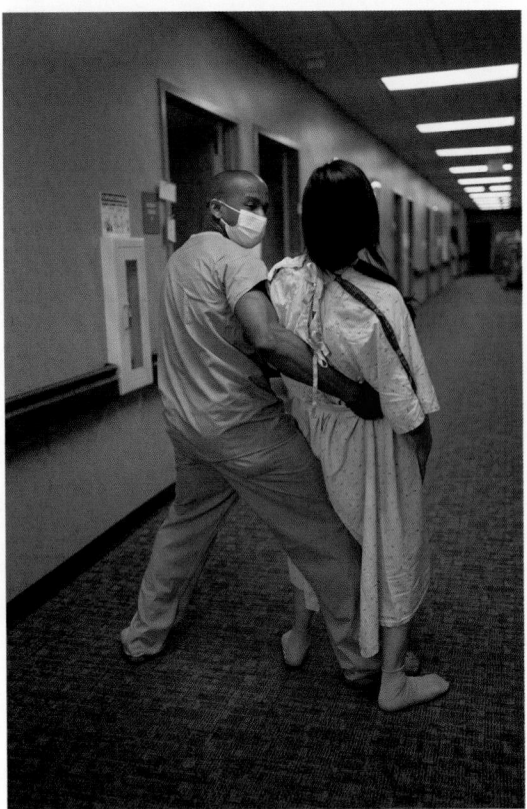

FIGURE 29-21 If the patient begins to fall, the nurse guides the patient gently to the floor or to a chair.

![leaf icon] **Assisting Older Adults** When assisting older adults to ambulate, find out how much assistance, if any, the patient typically requires and modify support as needed. Consider the following nursing interventions:

- **Observe constantly for weakness and fatigue.** Plan for periods of rest during ambulation, if needed. The older adult might become fatigued more quickly and recover more slowly from the physical demands of walking, especially if a heart or lung condition is present.
- **Move the patient gradually** to a sitting position and allow them to dangle at the bedside before coming to a standing position. Observe for dizziness or light-headedness.
- **Assess for fall risk factors**, for example, neurological or cognitive disorders (e.g., Parkinson or Alzheimer disease) and medications that cause dizziness or lethargy. For more information about assessing a patient's risk for a fall, see Chapter 21.
- **Assistive devices,** such as walkers, canes, and transfer belts, can be useful for older adults or others who require additional support.
- **Be cautious when using a transfer belt** for the patient with osteoporosis or back pain. Too much pressure from the belt can cause injury or pain.

KnowledgeCheck 29-9
- Identify four principles to be followed when performing PROM.
- Describe activities that can promote a patient's readiness for ambulation.
- What action should you take if a patient begins to fall when ambulating?

Mechanical Aids for Walking

Several types of aids are available to promote stability and independence when walking. Some patients consider the use of aids a sign of weakness or an inconvenience. As a result, they avoid using the aid and increase their risk of falls. Moreover, most people are likely to be concerned about loss of independence, so you can promote the use of walking aids by stressing their importance in helping the person maintain stability, mobility, and self-reliance.

Canes The following are three basic types of canes used (Fig. 29-22):

- **Single-ended cane with a half-circle handle** for the patient who needs minimal support and can negotiate stairs.
- **Single-ended cane with a straight handle** for the patient with hand weakness who has good balance.
- **Multiprong canes** usually have three or four prongs, and all types have a straight handle. These canes provide a wide base of support and are useful for patients with balance problems.

Walkers A walker is a lightweight metal frame device with four legs that provides a wide base of support as a patient ambulates. Some models have wheels that allow the walker to be rolled forward; others have a seat that allows the patient to rest periodically (Fig. 29-23).

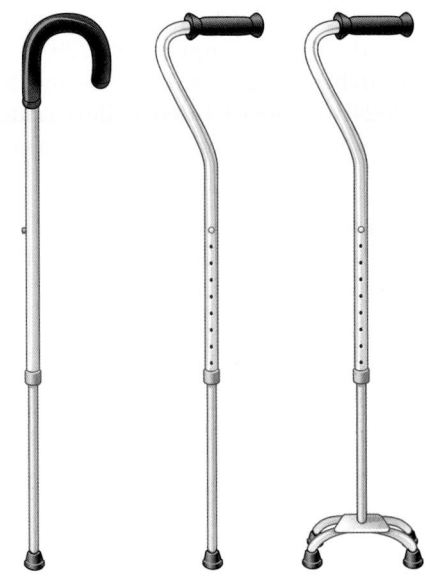

FIGURE 29-22 Types of canes.

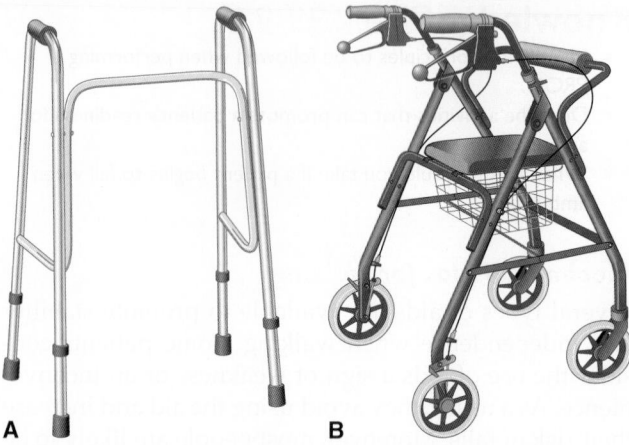

FIGURE 29-23 Walkers. *A,* The basic walker is picked up and advanced as the patient steps ahead. *B,* Some walkers have wheels and seats that allow the patient to rest periodically.

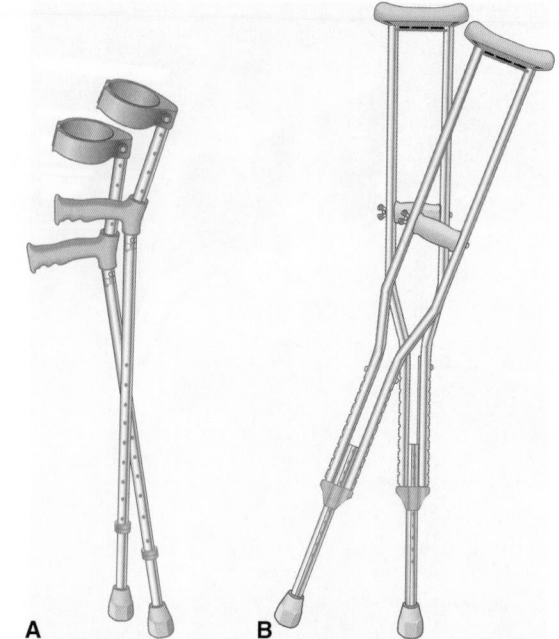

FIGURE 29-24 Crutches. *A,* Forearm support. *B,* Axillary.

These walkers are best for patients whose compromised mobility is related to fatigue or shortness of breath rather than gait instability.

Braces Braces support joints and muscles that cannot independently support the body's weight. They are most often used for the lower extremities. Nursing responsibilities include assisting the patient into and out of the brace and monitoring the condition of the skin under the brace.

Crutches Crutches are commonly used for the rehabilitation of an injured lower extremity. The purpose of using crutches is to limit or eliminate weight-bearing on the leg(s) by forcing the user to rely on strength in the arms and shoulders for support.

- **Forearm support crutches** are more likely to be used by a patient with permanent limitations. They are usually constructed of lightweight aluminum, with a handhold and a forearm support (Fig. 29-24A).
- **Axillary crutches** are for both short- and long-term use (Fig. 29-24B). Properly fitted axillary crutches support the body weight in the hands and arms, not the axilla.

Crutch walking taxes the arms and hands and may cause discomfort to the axillae, arms, and palms where the patient is bearing weight.

- Three-point gait—used when weight-bearing must be avoided
- Four-point gait—used for partial weight-bearing
- Swing-to gait—used when weight-bearing is permitted
- Swing-through gait—used when weight-bearing is permitted.

To learn more about sizing walking aids, basic gaits, and guidelines for teaching patients to use walking aids,

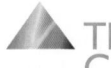 See **Chapter 29, Clinical Insight 29-4: Teaching Patients to Use Walking Aids,** in Volume 2.

Knowledge Check 29-10
- What type of cane should a patient with significant balance problems use?
- When are forearm support crutches used?
- Identify five crutch gaits.

▲ Think Like a Nurse 29-6: Clinical Judgment in Action
Discuss crutch walking with your peers and family. What instruction would facilitate the best understanding of proper crutch-walking technique?

Practical Knowledge clinical application

In Volume 2, you will learn about procedures and techniques for positioning, moving, turning, transferring, and ambulating patients safely. Although the ANA (2021) recommends that you use assistive equipment for all patient lifting and transferring, you may encounter situations in which equipment is not available or you do not have time to get it (e.g., in an emergency). In such situations, using good body mechanics may help you lessen the risk of injury to you and the patient.

For steps to follow in *all* procedures, refer to the Universal Steps for All Procedures found on the inside back cover of Volume 2. Go to the full procedures in Volume 2 to practice and learn the procedure steps. Use these procedure highlights later to help you review key points.

Procedure 29-1A: Moving a Patient Up in Bed

➤ Use a friction-reducing device to move the patient if the patient can assist with movement. Use a full-body sling if the patient cannot assist.

➤ Remove the pillow. Have the patient flex the neck, fold their arms across their chest, and place their feet flat on the bed.

➤ Position a nurse on either side of the patient.

➤ Use a wide base of support.

➤ Have the patient, on the count of three, push off with their heels as you shift your weight forward.

Procedure 29-1B: Turning a Patient in Bed

➤ Use a friction-reducing device and drawsheet to move the patient. Position at least one nurse on each side of the bed.

➤ Place the patient's near leg and arm (e.g., the left arm and leg when turning to the right) across their body; abduct and externally rotate the far shoulder.

➤ Each nurse places one arm at the level of the patient's shoulders and the other at the level of the patient's hips. Each nurse shifts their weight as both simultaneously roll the patient in the intended direction.

Procedure 29-1C: Logrolling a Patient

➤ Move the patient as a unit to the opposite side of the bed; raise the siderail on that side.

➤ Move to the side of the bed that the patient will be turning toward; lower the siderail.

➤ Each staff member evenly distributes their arms across the patient's length. One nurse is responsible for moving the head and neck as a unit.

➤ Shift your weight backward as you roll the patient toward you.

Procedure 29-2A: Transferring a Patient From Bed to Stretcher

➤ Move the patient to the side of the bed where the stretcher will be placed.

➤ Position the stretcher next to the bed; lock it in place.

➤ Keep the destination device (i.e., bed to stretcher, or vice versa) situated a little lower than the surface the patient is on.

➤ Using the drawsheet, roll the patient away from the stretcher.

➤ Place the transfer board against the patient's back halfway between the bed and stretcher. Position a friction-reducing device over the transfer board. Turn the patient to their back and onto the transfer board with the drawsheet.

➤ On a count of three, use the drawsheet to slide the patient across the transfer board and onto the stretcher.

Procedure 29-2B: Dangling a Patient at the Side of the Bed

➤ Place the patient in a supine position; raise the head of the bed to 90°.

➤ Apply a gait transfer belt; place the bed in a low position.

➤ Stand facing the patient with a wide base of support. Place your foot closest to the head of the bed in front of the other foot.

➤ Position your hands on each side of the gait transfer belt.

➤ Rock onto your back foot as you move the patient into a sitting position, and pivot to bring the patient's legs over the side of the bed.

➤ Stay with the patient as they dangle.

Procedure 29-2C: Transferring a Patient From Bed to Chair

➤ Ask the patient to wear nonskid footwear.

➤ Place the bed in the low position; lock the wheels.

➤ Assist the patient to dangle at the side of the bed (see Procedure 29-2B).

➤ Brace your feet and knees against the patient. Bend your hips at the knees; hold on to the transfer belt.

➤ If two nurses are available to assist with the transfer, one nurse should be on each side of the patient.

➤ Instruct the patient to place their arms around you, between your shoulders and waist. Ask the patient to stand as you move to an upright position by straightening your legs and hips.

➤ Instruct the patient to pivot and turn with you toward the chair.

➤ Ask the patient to flex their hips and knees as they lower themselves into the chair. Guide their motion while maintaining a firm hold.

➤ If the chair is a wheelchair, lock the wheels.

Procedure 29-3: Assisting With Ambulation

➤ Ask the patient to wear nonskid footwear.

➤ Place the bed in low position; lock the wheels.

➤ Assist the patient to dangle at the side of the bed (see Procedure 29-2B).

➤ If two nurses are available, each nurse should stand facing the patient on opposite sides of the patient.

➤ Brace your feet and knees against the patient. Bend your hips at the knees; hold on to the transfer belt. Pay attention to any known weakness.

➤ Instruct the patient to place their arms around you between your shoulders and waist (the location depends on the height of the patient and the nurses). Ask the patient to stand as you move to an upright position by straightening your legs and hips.

➤ Allow the patient to steady themselves for a moment.

➤ One nurse: Stand at the patient's side, placing both hands on the transfer belt. If the patient has weakness on one side, position yourself on the weaker side.

Continued

➤ Two nurses: One nurse stands on each of the patient's sides, grasping hold of the transfer belt.

➤ Slowly guide the patient forward. Observe for signs of fatigue or dizziness.

➤ If the patient must transport an IV pole, allow the patient to hold on to the pole on the side where you are standing. Assist the patient to advance the pole as you ambulate together.

To explore learning resources for this chapter,

Go to Davis Advantage and find:

Answers and Suggested Responses for all questions in this chapter

Concept Map

Knowledge Map

References and Bibliography

CHAPTER 30

Sexual Health

Learning Outcomes

After completing this chapter, you should be able to:

➤ Identify the female and male reproductive organs.

➤ Describe the physical, emotional, social, and spiritual aspects of human sexuality.

➤ Explain how gender, gender identity, and sexual orientation contribute to expression of sexuality throughout the life cycle.

➤ Differentiate various forms of sexual expression.

➤ Explore physical and psychological issues that affect sexuality and sexual functioning.

➤ Complete a sexual history as part of a comprehensive nursing assessment.

➤ State nursing diagnoses to describe sexuality problems.

➤ Explain how sexual health is challenged by high-risk sexual behaviors, sexually transmitted infections (STIs), menstrual problems, infertility, negative intimate relationships, sexual harassment, rape, and disorders of the sexual response cycle.

➤ Provide nursing interventions that enhance sexual well-being.

➤ Discuss strategies to increase your personal comfort and confidence in providing holistic nursing care.

➤ Describe approaches for dealing with inappropriate sexual behavior from patients or in the work environment.

Key Concepts

Sexual dysfunction

Sexual health

Sexuality

Related Concepts

See the Concept Map on Davis Advantage.

Meet Your Patients

■ **Jocelyn Carter.** Two days after undergoing a fine-needle aspiration to evaluate a small breast mass, Ms. Carter's surgeon informed her that the mass was malignant. He recommended a mastectomy (removal of the breast). Today, she arrives alone at the surgery registration area. You ask how she is feeling, and she tells you that the last week has been a whirlwind of activity. "I had to arrange childcare, cancel a business trip, and organize the house so that I could take a few days off to have the surgery. My husband is working overseas this fall, so he couldn't be here to help me. Honestly, I don't know how I'm feeling. I haven't had time to think about it." A few minutes later, as she waits in the surgery holding area, she begins to cry. You hold her hand and ask whether she would like to talk. She asks you, "Do you

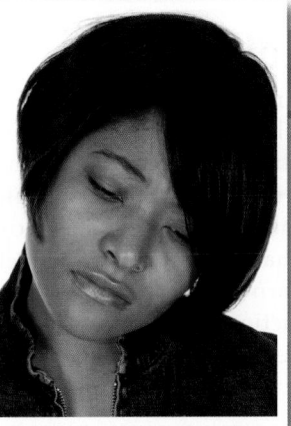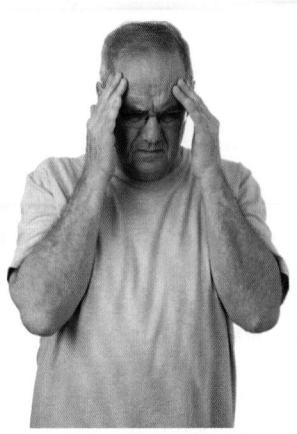

think my husband will still want me? I'm afraid he will be turned off when he looks at me."

■ **Gabriel Thomas.** Mr. Thomas comes to the outpatient clinic complaining of a throbbing headache for the past 3 days. He explains that he has tried several

(Continued)

Meet Your Patients (continued)

over-the-counter medicines without any relief. You check his blood pressure and measure the reading at 240/130 mm Hg. When you ask whether he has ever been treated for high blood pressure, he replies, "Are you another one of these people trying to get me to take drugs that will ruin my sex life?"

- **Frank Thanee.** Mr. Thanee, who has heart disease, had a mitral valve replacement 3 days ago. He has been transferred to the cardiology unit for an additional day of observation. His partner, Greg, has spent the past 3 days at the hospital and has just left to check on the apartment and feed their cat. Frank confides that he is worried about his parents' expected visit. "I've never been able to tell them about Greg. They wouldn't be able to understand our relationship, much less approve of it based on their religion. I don't know how to handle this. What do you think I should do?"

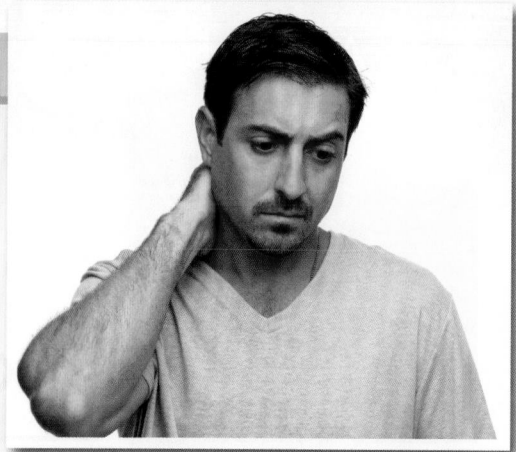

Although each of these patients has a different medical diagnosis, all are experiencing a concern related to sexuality. In this chapter, we explore the relationship between health and sexuality and the nurse's role in promoting sexual health.

Theoretical Knowledge
knowing why

Many parents want to know the gender of their baby early in the pregnancy at the first ultrasound. Hopes and dreams of future parent–child relationships often begin to form even during the first months of pregnancy. As you will learn, sexuality encompasses much more than gender. It includes how we perceive ourselves, how we relate to others, and how we express ourselves as sexual beings.

ABOUT THE KEY CONCEPTS

Like some people, you may have been socialized to avoid talking openly about **sexuality.** As a nurse, though, you will find that you must discuss a variety of issues pertaining to sexuality that are vital for patients' optimal wellness. Some of these discussions may include **sexual dysfunctions,** infections, or behaviors. As you learn about concepts related to sexuality and sexual function, you will be challenged to confront and set aside your own biases to address your clients' **sexual health** needs comfortably and competently.

SEXUAL AND REPRODUCTIVE ANATOMY AND PHYSIOLOGY

The role of the reproductive system in human life extends far beyond its basic function of producing children. It influences body image, sexual desire, and sense of sexual identity. To explore human sexuality, you will need to understand the basics of reproductive anatomy and physiology.

Female Reproductive Organs

The female reproductive system consists of a pair of ovaries and fallopian tubes, the uterus, vagina, and external genital tissues (Fig. 30-1).

- **Ova** (eggs) are produced in the ovaries and travel through the **fallopian tubes** to the **uterus.** If fertilization occurs, the embryo embeds in the wall of the uterus for further development.
- The **vagina** is a muscular tube that receives sperm during sexual intercourse, allows the exit of menstrual flow if fertilization does not occur, and serves as a birth canal at the end of pregnancy.
- The external mons pubis and the genitalia are a source of pleasurable sensations.
  - The **mons pubis** is a pad of fatty tissue over the symphysis pubis. It is covered with coarse hair and contains sensitive nerve endings.
  - The external genitalia, or **vulva,** consist of the clitoris, labia majora, labia minora, Bartholin's glands, urinary meatus, and vaginal introitus. The **clitoris** contains erectile tissue, blood vessels, and nerves. It is extremely sensitive and reacts to pleasurable stimuli. The **labia minora** also engorge and become sensitive during sexual stimulation. External genitalia organs, such as the clitoris, are protected by the **labia majora.**
  - The **breasts** are important to female sexual arousal; in fact, some people can be brought to orgasm solely by caressing the breasts and nipples. The **mammary glands,** enclosed within the breasts, are also part of

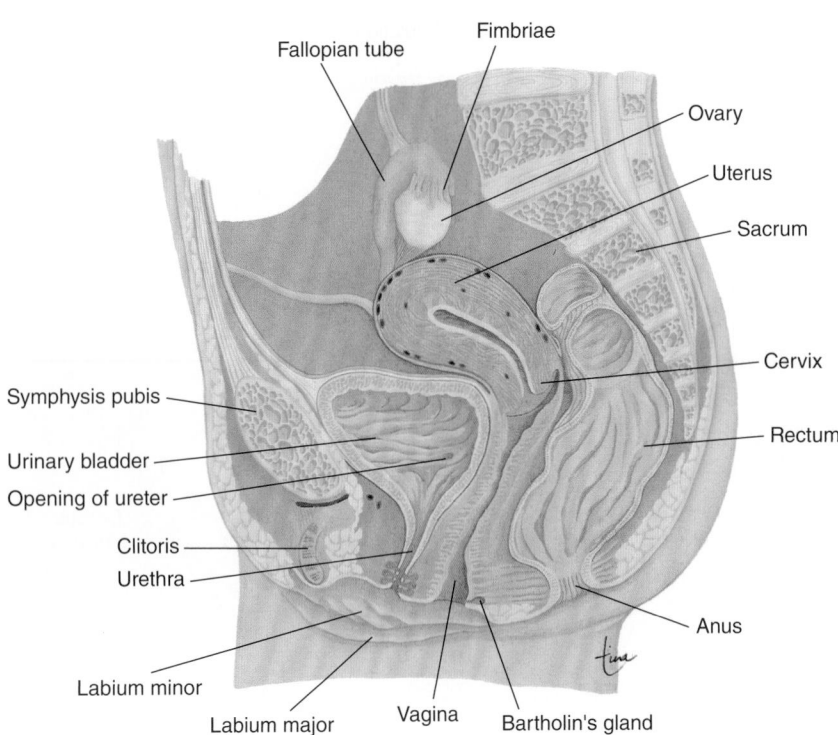

Fallopian tube

Fimbriae

Ovary

Uterus

Sacrum

Cervix

Rectum

Symphysis pubis

Urinary bladder

Opening of ureter

Clitoris

Urethra

Anus

Labium minor

Labium major

Vagina

Bartholin's gland

FIGURE 30-1 The female reproductive system.

the reproductive system. Their function is to produce milk to provide nourishment for an infant after birth.

The Menstrual Cycle

Menstruation begins with puberty and involves hormone changes that prepare the body for pregnancy. The phases of the menstrual cycle are triggered by hormonal changes (Fig. 30-2).

- **Menstrual phase**
  - Menstruation usually lasts 3 to 7 days, averaging 5 days.
  - During this phase, the uterus sheds the endometrial lining, and several ovarian follicles develop.
  - Follicle-stimulating hormone (FSH) from the anterior pituitary gland begins to increase during this phase, leading to a rise in estrogen levels.
- **Follicular phase**
  - This phase begins on the first day of the menstrual cycle.
  - It is associated with the growth of ovarian follicles and the regrowth of the endometrium of the uterus.
  - This phase ends with **ovulation,** or the release of the ovum from the mature follicle, around day 13 or 14 of the menstrual cycle.
  - Luteinizing hormone (LH) levels from the anterior pituitary gland rise, as does the estrogen level.
- **Ovulatory phase**
  - A surge in LH and FSH occurs, lasting about 16 to 36 hours.
  - The follicle then ruptures, and the egg is released for fertilization.

- Estrogen peaks and progesterone rises, which stimulates growth of the endometrium.
- **Luteal phase**
  - If fertilization occurs, the endometrium thickens to support an embryo.
  - The pregnancy hormone, called *chorionic gonadotropin,* is produced. Pregnancy tests are based on detecting levels of this hormone.
  - If fertilization does not occur, progesterone levels drop, and menses begins.

Male Reproductive Organs

The male reproductive system consists of the testes and a series of ducts and glands that transport sperm.

- The **testes** produce sperm, which are transported through the *epididymis, ductus deferens, ejaculatory duct,* and *urethra* (Fig. 30-3). Along the path, the **reproductive glands** (*seminal vesicles, prostate,* and *bulbourethral glands*) add secretions that mix with the sperm to produce semen.
- The **penis** functions in the urinary system to transport urine from the bladder to the outside of the body. It also has important functions in the reproductive system.
  - Within the penis are three sections of **erectile tissue**: the corpus cavernosum and sections of corpus spongiosum above and below the urethra.
  - During sexual arousal, these erectile tissues fill with blood, making the penis erect.
- **Ejaculation** (the expulsion of semen) is brought about by peristalsis of the reproductive ducts and contraction of the prostate and muscles of the pelvic floor.

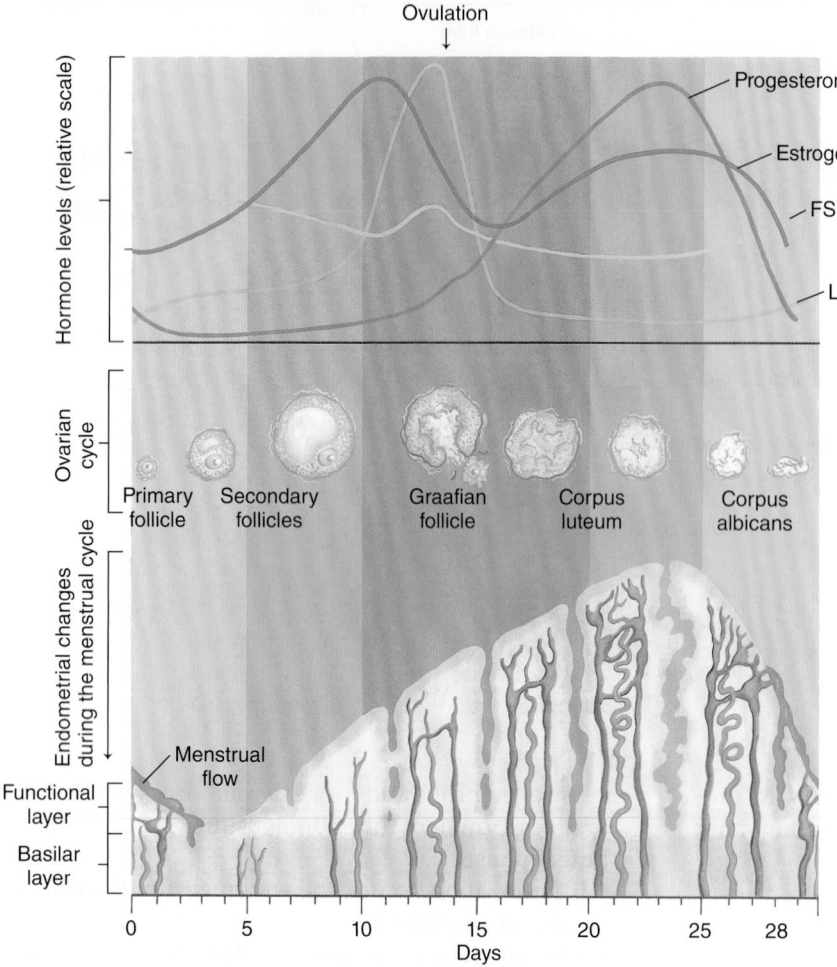

FIGURE 30-2 The menstrual cycle. Hormone levels and endometrial thickness throughout the cycle are shown.

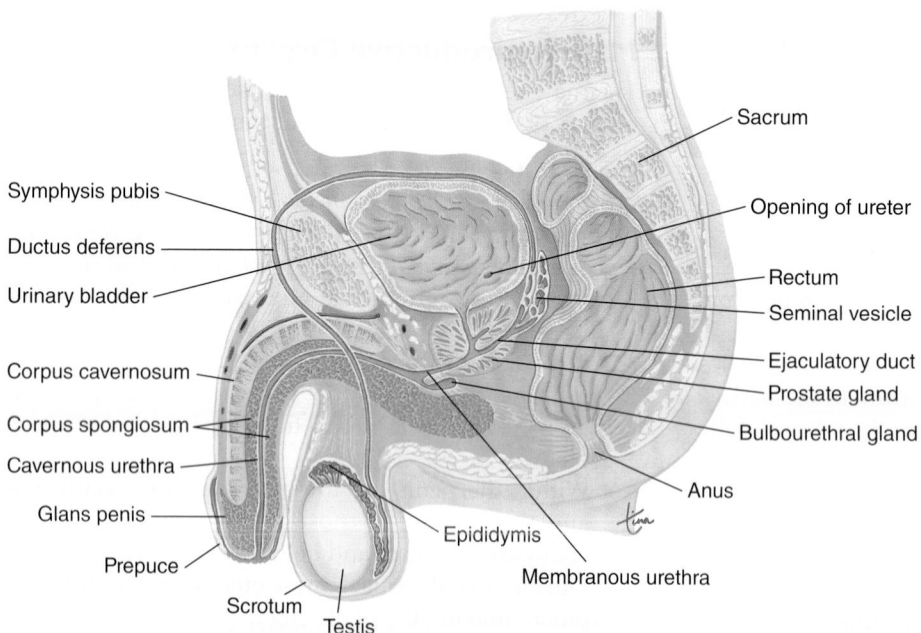

FIGURE 30-3 The male reproductive system.

With each ejaculation, approximately 100 million sperm cells are expelled in 2 to 4 mL of semen.

SEXUALITY

People often think of *sexuality* as a synonym for *sex*. This is inaccurate. In fact, even the word *sex* has multiple meanings. For example, *sex* is used to describe intimate pleasurable activity (e.g., "We had sex yesterday") or to indicate whether an individual is male or female (e.g., "What sex is your baby?"). In this chapter, we use the term **sex** to indicate biological sex status (male or female) and follow the definition of sexuality given by the World Health Organization (WHO).

- **Sexuality** is defined by the WHO (2006) as a "central aspect of being human throughout life and encompasses sex, gender identities and roles, sexual orientation, eroticism, pleasure, intimacy and reproduction." Similarly, the American Sexual Health Association (ASHA) identifies sexuality as essential to physical and emotional health, defining it as "the ability to embrace and enjoy our sexuality through our lives" (ASHA, n.d.).
- **Gender identity** is a person's perception of their gender, gender identity, and gender role, whereas **sexual identity** is a person's perception of their sexuality and their sexual orientation. All of these are also a part of the person's overall self-concept (see Chapter 6 to review self-concept).

   Key Point: *Sex is determined at the moment of conception, when an ovum is fertilized by a sperm. The ovum always provides an X chromosome.* The sperm may contribute either a second X chromosome, which results in a female offspring, or a Y chromosome, resulting in a male offspring (Fig. 30-4).

What are Gender Roles?

Gender roles are the societal norms for gender-appropriate behavior. There are social expectations for men and women—expectations for behavior, communication style, occupation, family responsibilities, and almost every other aspect of life. Although modern society has become more egalitarian in these expectations, many of the values underlying historical social norms remain embedded at some level within our contemporary culture (Dicke et al., 2019).

   Historically in Western culture:

- **People expected men to be strong and control their feelings.** Boys received positive reinforcement for "masculine" behaviors, such as competitiveness, and

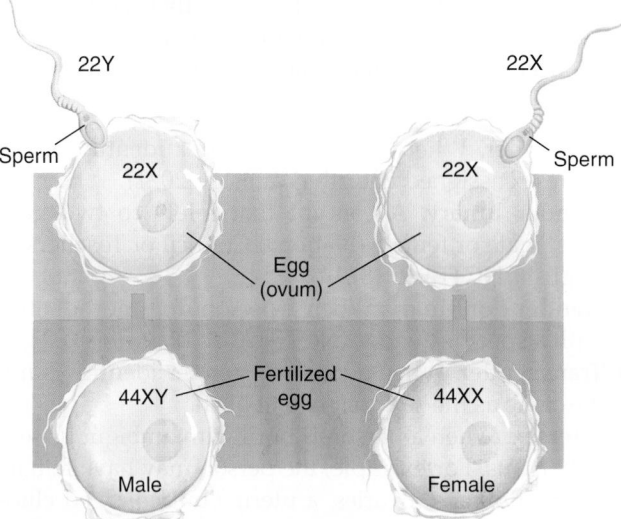

FIGURE 30-4 The female provides the X chromosome, and the male may contribute either a second X chromosome, which results in a female offspring, or a Y chromosome, resulting in a male offspring.

ridicule or teasing for showing emotions or being passive.

- **Women were expected to be gentle and to express their feelings.** In girls, "feminine" behaviors, such as cooperation and passivity, were reinforced, whereas assertiveness was often labeled as unacceptable aggression.

   Over time, social expectations regarding gender roles have changed and expanded. Women now perform jobs formerly thought to be "for men only" (e.g., physician, police officer), and men are active in professions once dominated by females (e.g., teaching, nursing).

   Today, many parents encourage some **androgyny** in their children. The word *androgyny* is a combination of the Greek words for male, *andro*, and female, *gyn*. By one of its definitions, *androgyny* refers to a blending of traditional masculine and feminine roles. It means that everyone has some skills, traits, and behaviors that may be classified as masculine and some that may be feminine. Androgyny is a positive trait in that it gives an individual greater adaptability in life situations.

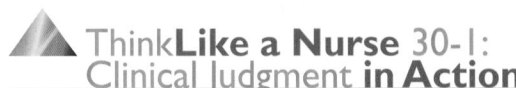

ThinkLike a Nurse 30-1: Clinical Judgment in Action

- Provide at least three examples of nonconformity to traditional gender-role expectations.
- As a parent, how might you encourage androgyny in your children, if you wished to do so?

What Is Gender Identity?

Gender identity is the image we have about our gender. For some people, their gender identity does not fit into the classification of "man" or "woman"; for others, their gender identity may not fit the sex of their body. One's sense of gender identity is an internal experience.

Concepts used to understand gender identity are as follows:

- **Cisgender.** When a person's gender identity aligns with sex assigned at birth (Wamsley, 2021).
- **Gender binary.** A concept that refers to two genders, male or female (National Council of Teachers of English [NCTE], 2018).
- **Gender nonbinary.** When a person does not identify with a specific gender (NCTE, 2018; Wamsley, 2021).
- **Transgender.** When a person's gender identity is not the same as the sex assigned at birth.
- **Intersex.** When a person is born with ambiguous sexual organs. For example, the person may have female internal organs (ovaries, a uterus) but enlarged clitoral tissue resembling a penis. Initially, a developing embryo is in an undifferentiated sexual state until about the seventh week of pregnancy, when the gonads form into either testes or ovaries. A mutation of any of the genes during this process may result in altered genitalia. Parents must decide whether to have the child undergo surgery to make the assigned sex consistent with the physical appearance or to delay assignment and allow the child to choose at a later time.
- **Gender transition.** A period in which a person undertakes activities to better reflect the gender with which they identify (e.g., appearance, clothing, official documents, hormone therapy, medical procedures) (Wamsley, 2021).

Key Point: *Although there are numerous and different terms associated with the concepts of gender and sexual identity, you must focus on providing nonjudgmental and quality client care. Barriers to care result from healthcare providers having limited awareness of the client's communication, social, and healthcare needs (Clark et al., 2018).*

♥ **iCare** You should also ask the client what they prefer to be called and communicate any information to the healthcare team verbally or in the medical records to minimize repetitive questions to the client.

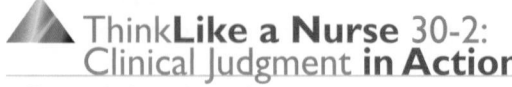

KnowledgeCheck 30-2
- How is sex determined?
- Distinguish *sex*, *gender role*, and *gender identity*.
- What is *androgyny*?

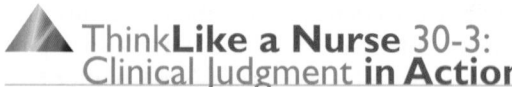

ThinkLike a Nurse 30-2: Clinical Judgment in Action
Do you believe that androgyny is a positive attribute? Explain your thinking.

What Is Sexual Orientation?
Sexual orientation refers to the general tendency of a person to feel attracted to another person. The attraction can be emotional, romantic, or sexual (Wamsley,

2021). With increasing research on the biological aspects of sexual orientation (Roselli, 2018), more professionals are concluding that it is more important to focus on the needs of the patient, create a welcoming environment, and treat every person with respect.

A focus on the patient's needs will facilitate a therapeutic nurse–patient relationship, which is important to individualize care. The literature attributes health disparities in the lesbian, gay, bisexual, transgender, and queer (LGBTQ+) population to societal stigmas, discrimination, and various other factors (*Healthy People 2030* [Office of Disease Prevention and Health Promotion, n.d.]). Relationships between people of the same gender or diverse genders, although not readily accepted by some religions, are being integrated into the dominant U.S. culture. The landmark ruling by the U.S. Supreme Court has created a freedom of sexual expression in the LGBTQ+ community and recognized legitimacy in relationships and marriage (*Obergefell v. Hodges*, 2015). More individuals from the LGBTQ+ community now share this aspect of their lives with employers, colleagues, family, and friends, as well as with researchers and pollsters. However, some individuals, like Frank Thanee (Meet Your Patient), may still experience conflicts in sharing with others.

Key Point: *The focus in any client encounter is creating a therapeutic nurse–patient relationship to identify healthcare needs and concerns.*

KnowledgeCheck 30-3
- What is meant by *sexual orientation*?
- What is the key focus in working with all patients?

ThinkLike a Nurse 30-3: Clinical Judgment in Action
- Would you have difficulty working with clients whose sexual orientation is different from your own?

How Does Sexuality Develop?
We are sexual beings from birth to death. The expression of our sexuality evolves throughout the life span. If you require additional discussion on sexuality and developmental stages, see Chapters 6 and 7.

Birth Through Preschool
Beginning at birth, parents, caregivers, and others respond to the infant with preconceived thoughts of what that gender role entails. The first 2 years of life can be highly sensual; as infants are nursed, stroked, bathed, and massaged, they develop their first attachment experiences through bonding with the parent or caregiver (Fig. 30-5). It is not unusual for children in this age-group to touch their genitals and enjoy being nude. This behavior is part of their exploration of their bodies and is a normal part of child development. By age 3, most children recognize gender differences and know the names of body parts. Toddlers are interested in their bodies and curious to see the genitals of others.

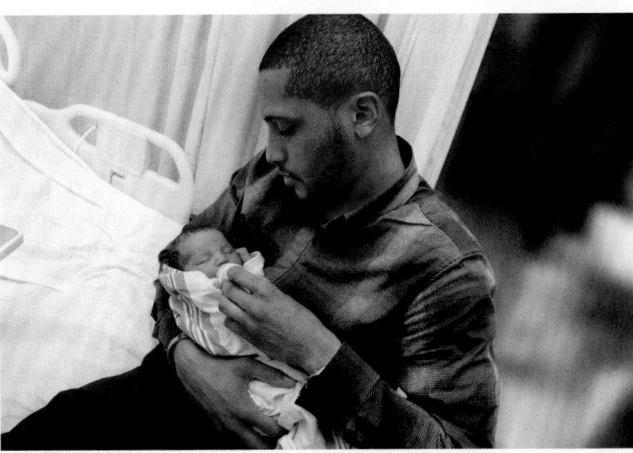

FIGURE 30-5 Parent–infant attachment occurs through daily contact and care through activities such as feeding, bathing, and holding.

By age 5, children mimic adults by holding hands or hugging. Adults, who find these actions amusing or endearing, frequently reinforce such behaviors. Young children also may practice getting married, playing house, or playing doctor. It is not unusual for preschool children to masturbate and ask questions about "where babies come from." Parents should give factual answers without offering additional information.

School Age Through Puberty

The school-age child strongly usually identifies with their parent of the same gender and has mostly same-gender friends. Through interaction at home, school, and other activities, children gain awareness of gender roles and emerging gender identity. From age 8 to 12, the child is in transition between childhood and puberty. Secondary sex characteristics become apparent.

- In females, breast buds form, and pubic hair appears. For a significant portion of the female population, **menarche** (beginning of menstruation) occurs.
- Male individuals become more muscular, the voice deepens, facial and axillary hair develop, and the genitals begin to increase in size.
- The first attraction may occur during this stage, and the child may begin to masturbate more frequently but privately.
- For information on the Tanner stages of sexual development in children,

 Go to **Chapter 19, Procedure 19-17: Assessing the Male Genitourinary System** and **Procedure 19-18: Assessing the Female Genitourinary System,** in Volume 2.

Many school-age children are curious and may ask explicit questions about sexual activity, reproduction, and sex roles. Parents and nurses should answer with facts and follow up with age-appropriate resources. When children reach ages 10 to 12, parents

should begin teaching them basic information about body changes, menstruation, sexual intercourse, and reproduction.

Adolescents

Adolescence is a time of heightened sexual interest and activity, primarily because of the following:

1. Hormonal changes accompanying puberty
2. The cultural emphasis on sex

Masturbation is a common, safe, and comforting sexual activity that has neither interpersonal nor disease risks. However, some adolescents may encounter parental, cultural, or religious disapproval of masturbation.

Further sexual exploration usually begins with kissing, moves on to fondling, and can lead to genital contact. This progression may occur over a period of years, or there may be an early initiation of oral, vaginal, or anal intercourse.

Incidence of Sexual Activity in Adolescence The nationwide **Youth Risk Behavior Surveillance System (YRBSS)** provides data on the health practices and experiences among high school students. Results showed that from 2015 to 2019, there was an overall decline in high school students who:

- ever had sexual intercourse
- had sexual intercourse before age 13
- had sexual intercourse with ≥4 persons
- are sexually active
- did not use any birth control method

In contrast, the percentage of high school students who were tested for HIV went from 10.2% in 2015 to 8.4% in 2019, whereas only 8.6% were tested for sexually transmitted infections (STIs) in 2019 (Centers for Disease Control and Prevention [CDC], 2020).

Similarly, the **National Survey of Family Growth (NSFG)** data on sexual activity and contraception for teenagers revealed an overall decline in sexual activity from previous surveys and a rise in responsible sexual behaviors (Martinez & Abma, 2020). For example, results show that 78% of females and 89% of males aged 15 to 24 who experienced their first sexual intercourse before age 20 used a birth control method. Common methods of contraception used by teenage girls include condoms, withdrawal, and birth control pills.

The decline in sexual intercourse for teenagers coincides with a drop in teenage pregnancies. In 2021, the number of babies born to girls and women aged 15 to 19 declined by 6% in 2021 (Hamilton et al., 2022), continuing the trend of a record-low birth rate for U.S. teens.

Health Risks of Sexual Activity in Adolescence Sexual activity is known to have unintended health consequences, most commonly STIs (CDC, 2021).

- There were 1.58 million cases of chlamydia in 2020. A 15% decline occurred among females aged 15 to

19 years. At least two-thirds of cases occurred in adolescents and young adults aged 15 to 24 years.

- In 2020, there were over 677,769 reported cases of gonorrhea. Females had a larger percentage increase (15%) compared with males (6.6%). At least two-thirds of cases occurred among men having sex with men (MSM).
- Overall, there were 134,00 reported cased in 2020, a 6.8% increase from 2019. Among women, rates increased 21%, whereas MSM accounted for 53% of male cases.

Key Point: *Sexuality education at home and at school dispels myths and prepares teens for adult roles. To make informed choices as they move toward adulthood, adolescents need information about body changes, interpersonal relationships, contraception (birth control), and preventing STIs.*

Gender and Sexual Identity in Adolescence A major developmental goal in adolescence is identity development. Adolescents may engage in a number of activities to explore and define their gender and sexual identity. A nationwide survey of U.S. high school students revealed behaviors and risks grouped by sexual identity (CDC, 2021):

- A higher percentage (45%) of lesbian, gay, or bisexual students had engaged in sex, compared with 38% of heterosexual students.
- A higher percentage (19%) of lesbian, gay, and bisexual students reported being forced to have sex compared with heterosexual students (6%).
- Students who identify as lesbian, gay, and bisexual reported more illicit drug use (28%) compared with their heterosexual counterparts (13%).
- A significantly higher percentage of lesbian, gay, and bisexual students (66%) reported feeling persistently sad or hopeless, compared with 32% of their heterosexual counterparts.
- Of major concern is the percentage of high school students seriously considering suicide: 40% of lesbian, gay, and bisexual students had made a suicide plan, compared with 12% of heterosexual students.

Key Point: *Little is known about how gender identity and gender variance evolve. Therefore, it is important for adolescents to have open, accepting, nonjudgmental discussions about their feelings, thoughts, and concerns (Kaltiala-Heino et al., 2018).*

To review the physical changes of adolescence, see Chapters 6 and 19.

Young Adults

During early adulthood, people continue to define their sexual identity, sexual orientation, and self-concept. Young adults commonly engage in sexual activity within and outside of committed relationships, even though many also practice **serial monogamy,** in which partners are mutually faithful. During this time, young adults may find a life partner and make long-term plans, which may include marriage and parenting.

However, some adults continue to struggle with their sexual identity, sexual orientation, or ability to form or commit to intimate relationships. Young adults often wonder whether their sexual behaviors and responses are normal (e.g., "How often do most people have intercourse?"; "Do other women have an orgasm every time they have sex?"). Information about birth control, prevention of STIs, and sexual expression, along with effective communication, is still needed.

Middle Adults

In their middle years, adults experience life changes that may enhance physical and emotional intimacy. Some may have more privacy and time to spend together because their children are now young adults who no longer rely on parental support. Others may still be engaging in child-rearing activities. Regardless, middle age is a time of transition, with various factors affecting sexual patterns. These include physical changes, the emergence of chronic diseases, caring for aging parents, and parenting demands. In addition, middle-aged adults are often seriously affected by economic downturns.

Female Transitions Female adults transition through **menopause** (cessation of menstruation), a process that varies widely. Some are relieved that the prospect of childbearing has ended, whereas others may mourn the loss of the ability to give birth. Normal physiological changes include decreased vaginal secretions and vaginal wall thinning, which result from decreased levels of estrogen and progesterone. These changes may result in painful intercourse and decrease the desire for sexual activity. Some female adults also experience hot flashes, sleep disturbances, and mood changes.

Male Transitions Because of the aging process or health conditions (e.g., type 2 diabetes or hypertension), male adults may experience erectile difficulty in middle age. Some may perceive this problem as a threat to their masculinity and sexual attractiveness, and their self-image may suffer. Male adults also experience a decrease in the sex hormone testosterone. Many male adults remain fertile into old age, although sexual desire and the ability to achieve and maintain erection decrease gradually with aging.

It may be a challenge for you to view middle adults as individuals who engage in and enjoy sexual relations. Patients of this age may remind you of your parents, and thus it may be difficult for you to see them as persons who have sexual relationships. Holistic nursing care requires you to assess and formulate strategies to address their sexual concerns.

Older Adults

Most older adults are sexually active and regard sexuality as an important part of life. Research supports the premise that age-related changes can result in decreased sexual relationships, but many older adults adapted to remain sexually active and are satisfied with their sex lives (Erens et al., 2019). **Key Point:** *Your assessment and planning should consider the importance of sexual activities in their lives and their sexual needs (e.g., reassurance from a sexual partner or sexual stimulation), preferences, lifestyle, and self-identified limitations.*

Sexual problems are more likely to result from failing physical health and medication side effects than from age alone. For example, as noted earlier, male adults with diabetes are more likely to have difficulty achieving and maintaining an erection. Common obstacles to sexual expression include the absence of a partner or the strength of the relationship (Erens et al., 2019).

Some problems that may occur as a result of age-related changes are:

- **Postmenopausal female adults report less sexual stimulation and reduced desire,** so they tend to need more foreplay and direct clitoral stimulation for sexual enjoyment. They may have fewer orgasms or orgasms that are weaker in intensity. Nevertheless, some people "rediscover" sexual desire after menopause.
- **Older female adults may complain of pain during intercourse,** caused by loss of vaginal lubrication, thinning, and dryness. You can help your patients by suggesting water-soluble lubricants to counteract vaginal dryness and enhance pleasurable sensations during sexual activity.
- **Some male adults report erectile difficulty** and need more time and more direct genital stimulation to achieve erection. It may take longer to ejaculate, and the orgasmic contractions may be less intense. When penetration is not possible (e.g., because of male erectile dysfunction), many couples find satisfaction with alternate forms of sexual stimulation and expression.

In the past, many healthcare providers have hesitated to offer sexual counseling to older adults out of fear that such intimate discussion might offend their patients. Older adults may also hesitate to discuss their sexual problems with healthcare providers unless encouraged to do so. Address the topic as you would any other area (e.g., "We have discussed your medical needs and your dietary needs; let's now discuss your sexual needs"). Once you introduce the subject, your patients may feel comfortable discussing their sexuality and welcome your input.

You can help older clients to understand that sexual feelings do not necessarily disappear with age, and sexual expression need not stop (Fig. 30-6). For example, sexual expression may include kissing, hugging, caressing, oral sex, and mutual manual stimulation. In addition, you may suggest ways to adapt coital positions to accommodate bodily changes, for example, when a partner has joint immobility.

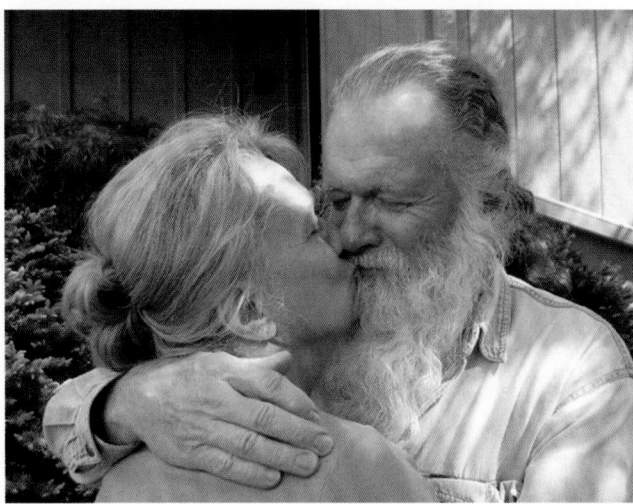

FIGURE 30-6 Healthy older adults maintain sexual intimacy.

KnowledgeCheck 30-4

- Why is it important to consider sexuality throughout the life cycle?
- What factor contributes to adolescents' heightened sexual interest, and what activity do some engage in?
- What aspects of human sexuality are associated with young and middle adulthood?
- What challenges to sexuality may older adults encounter?

What Factors Affect Sexuality?

Various factors affect our attitudes toward sexuality, sexual behaviors, and intimate relationships. This section will help you to provide nonjudgmental, holistic care to people who have a wide range of values, lifestyles, and states of well-being.

Culture

Culture influences our ideas about gender roles, gender identity, sexual identity, marriage, sexual expression, and social responsibilities. However, it is not unusual for people to be **ethnocentric**—that is, to see their own culture and sexual behaviors as the norm for all. Because the United States is a multicultural country, beliefs and practices related to human sexuality vary widely.

Culture, both social and personal, determines what is acceptable and what is not. In some societies, **polygamy** (marriage to more than one partner) may be acceptable. Many cultures have special rites of passage at puberty, such as the Jewish bar mitzvah for boys and bat mitzvah for girls or the vision quest in certain Native American cultures. **Key Point:** *Generally, you should honor cultural practices unless they are harmful, illegal, or unethical.*

Female Genital Mutilation Formerly known as **female circumcision,** female genital mutilation (FGM) is an example of a practice viewed as harmful by many. It is illegal in most countries, and the United States has taken a zero-tolerance attitude (U.S. Department of

Toward Evidence-Based Practice

Sexual relations and activities, when voluntary, are forms of leisure and pleasure that contribute to individual well-being. Stringent contact limitations imposed by the COVID-19 pandemic affected the sex lives of many people.

> Gleason, N., Banik, D., Braverman, J., & Colem, E. (2021). **The impact of the COVID-19 pandemic on sexual behaviors: Findings from a national survey in the United States.** *Journal of Sexual Medicine, 18*(11), 1851–1862. https://doi.org/10.1016/j.jsxm.2021.08.008

In total, 1,051 participants were included in this research that examined sexual behaviors (frequency of partnered and solitary sexual behavior, sexual functioning, satisfaction, and intimate partner violence) during the pandemic. The results revealed that most participants indicated that the frequency of sexual behaviors remained the same during the pandemic: sex with their current partner (54.7%), masturbation (64.7%), porn use (65.6%), use of sex toys (59.7%), and sending sexual messages or photos (49.6%). A large majority of participants also reported that sexual desire (57.6%), sexual enjoyment/pleasure (66.5%), and relationship satisfaction (68.0%) stayed the same. Higher depression scores were seen with decreased sexual enjoyment/pleasure. However, decreases were seen in many areas requiring close contact (e.g., hook-ups, sex with casual partner). Increases were seen in the use of webcam/cybersex (37.8%). The long-term impact of contact restrictions on sexual health remains unknown.

> Lehmiller, J., Garcia, J. R., Gesselman, A. N., & Mark, K. P. (2020). **Less sex, but more sexual diversity: Changes in sexual behavior during the COVID-19 pandemic.** *Leisure Sciences, 43*(1–2), 295–304. https://doi.org/10.1080/01490400.2020.1774016

The researchers conducted an anonymous survey to gather information on participants' (n = 1,559) sexual behaviors during the restrictions imposed by the pandemic. The results revealed that only a small percentage (13.6%) of participants reported an improvement in their sex life, whereas 43.5% reported a decline. Similarly, a small percentage reported declines in solo and partnered sexual behaviors during the pandemic (e.g., masturbation, oral sex, intercourse). However, 20% of participants reported adding a new element to their sex life (e.g., sexting, cybersex). The new additions: trying new positions; bondage, discipline, sadism, masochism (BDSM); massages; and acting on fantasies were strongly correlated with reported improvements in the sex life of participants. Stress and loneliness were linked to engaging in new activities. SexTech (sexting, sharing nude photos) was not associated with improving the sex life of participants.

1. What common factors were seen in both studies?

2. Based on these studies, what would you include in a teaching plan for a couple separated by distance to promote sexual health?

Justice [DOJ], 2021). In this procedure, the labia majora, labia minora, and clitoris are excised, and/or the vagina is sutured closed **(infibulation).** Infibulation may be done to ensure virginity, whereas clitoral excision is meant to reduce sexual desire and ensure that a partner remains faithful to their spouse **Key Point:** *In addition to its psychosocial consequences, the procedure carries a high risk of infection and can cause the development of scar tissue that makes vaginal birth impossible.*

The U.S. Congress passed a law in 1996 making FGM for individuals younger than 18 a federal offense. However, in *United States v. Nagarwala* (2018), the court ruled the federal law unconstitutional, indicating that such a law properly belongs at the state level. As of 2022, only 10 states had not made the practice illegal (Equality Now, 2021).

Religion

Religion also has a powerful influence on a person's perception of their sexual identity and their sexuality. Consider the following:

- Religious practices restricting premarital sex, birth control, same-sex relationships, abortion, extramarital relationships, and masturbation are common.

- Some religions restrict opposite-gender healthcare providers and have rules about body coverings and modesty.
- Some religions govern education about the structure and function of the human body.

When the sexual values of the broader social culture conflict with a person's traditional religious values, anxiety and sexual dysfunction may result. To review the influence of religion on health, see Chapter 13.

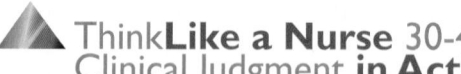

ThinkLike a Nurse 30-4: Clinical Judgment in Action

How have religion and culture influenced your views on sexuality?

Lifestyle

Life experiences encompass our interactions with others and the environment. Family, socioeconomic status, employment factors, and interpersonal relationships shape, but do not fully determine, our lifestyle. Consider the following examples:

- Having a beloved brother reveal to you that he is gay might alter your perception of sexual orientation.

Similarly, being raised by a same-sex couple might affect your view of gender roles.

- Working a high-stress job and meeting family demands might leave you too exhausted to desire sex with your spouse.
- Being in an abusive relationship could affect how you feel about yourself and might cause you to avoid intimacy in the future.

Lessons learned through day-to-day experience create powerful impressions on our views and often modify cultural and religious influences.

Sexual Knowledge

Although sexuality and family life are part of the curriculum in many public schools, you cannot assume that patients have adequate sexual knowledge. Community values play a large role in determining how sexuality is viewed and taught. For example:

- State-mandated sex education as a part of the curriculum usually includes provisions for opting out with parenteral consent.
- Schools may limit discussion on reproduction, STIs, birth control, intimacy, exploitive relationships, domestic abuse, or rape, believing that these topics are best addressed by the family or church.
- Children who are home-schooled or taught in private or church-affiliated schools may not have class time allocated to sex education.

Key Point: *Do not let your clients' age, level of education, or life experiences lead you to make assumptions about their knowledge of sexuality.* For example:

- A married person may not be sexually active.
- A female patient with several children may not know what is involved in a pelvic examination, the phases of the menstrual cycle, or how conception occurs.
- A highly educated person may be uninformed regarding their body structure and function.

It is difficult for most people to admit to a professional that they lack knowledge. Therefore, you must assess each client's knowledge and understanding of sexual terms. At times, you may need to use vernacular terms or basic terminology to be understood. You can then introduce medically specific terminology.

KnowledgeCheck 30-5
- What sexual knowledge would you expect a male adult with children to have?
- What sexual knowledge would you expect a nursing student to have?

Health and Illness

Sexuality involves the body, mind, and spirit, so it is not surprising that health status affects sexuality. Certain health issues can have an impact on both the physical and emotional aspects of sexuality, and you must be open to discussing any sexual issues with your patients.

Physical Illness Diseases, injuries, and medical treatments may result in lifestyle changes, including sexual functioning.

- **Heart disease or respiratory disease** may cause people to restrict sexual activity because of fatigue, dyspnea, or fear of overstressing the heart.
- **Diabetes mellitus** leads to neurological changes that may cause male erectile dysfunction. Female patients may experience vaginal dryness and loss of orgasmic ability. In addition, vaginal yeast infections are common with diabetes, causing itching and painful intercourse.
- **Cancer** may be accompanied by body image changes, fatigue, treatments that create nausea, and fear of death—all of which may lead to feeling unattractive, with a reduced desire for sexual activity.
- **Spinal cord injury** may make it impossible for the person to feel physical stimulation. Depending on the level of the injury, the person may experience changes in psychogenic or reflexogenic genital arousal. Some male adults may achieve erection and ejaculation and are fertile; others may have no genital response.

Surgeries Surgery may alter a person's body image. This can range from a surgical scar to the removal of a body part. When the body part is perceived as important to sexual functioning (e.g., a breast, a testicle), the client may experience sexual esteem issues (e.g., feeling unattractive, concern about partner's reaction).

- **Hysterectomy** (surgical removal of a uterus) may enhance the sexual experience if it relieves pain and bleeding that were present before surgery. In contrast, some female patients report difficulty becoming aroused or having less intense orgasms after a hysterectomy. These problems may be related to trauma to nerves in the pelvic area, to the absence of uterine contractions during orgasm, or to anxiety because the patient's personal gender identity is tied to childbearing.
- **Mastectomy** (surgical removal of a breast) can have a significant influence on a patient's self-esteem and may negatively affect sexuality.
- **Prostatectomy** (removal of the prostate gland, usually to treat prostate cancer) may be accompanied by erectile and other sexual dysfunction.
- **Orchiectomy** (removal of the testicle) is usually performed for testicular cancer. Male patients can experience infertility, which is associated with a loss of self-concept, sexual identity, and intimacy.
- A **colostomy** is a surgical procedure that brings a portion of the colon through a surgical opening in the abdomen (see Chapter 26 for review). The patient must usually wear a pouch to expel feces. Ostomy surgery profoundly affects sexuality. Patients with ostomies often experience body image difficulties, loss of desire for intercourse, fears about leakage, pain, and concern about how their partners will react (American Cancer Society [ACS], 2019).

If a person becomes disabled while in a marriage or other committed relationship, the strain can threaten the relationship. In contrast, a person who is single or has a lifelong disability may have trouble establishing an intimate relationship because of physical limitations, social isolation, poor self-image, or discrimination.

♥ **iCare** The human need for intimacy still exists even when people lose interest in sexual activities. Communication about sexual needs and desires may be difficult for couples, but as a nurse, you can support and facilitate discussions of your patients' concerns. You can also make referrals to holistic rehabilitation programs that offer comprehensive services and promote discussions regarding sexuality and relationship issues.

Mental Health Disorders Psychiatric disorders can lead to interpersonal disruptions and difficulty with sexual expression.

- **Depression.** A person experiencing depression can have a significant loss of interest in activities that previously brought pleasure. Thus, it is common for people with depression to avoid engaging in interpersonal activities, including sex.
- **Hypermania or mania.** Conversely, a person with hypermania or mania may be preoccupied with pleasurable activities and display increased sexual activity, as well as verbalization and acting out. Both extremes are disruptive to a relationship.

- **Psychosis.** For a person with psychosis, interpersonal relationships and sexual patterns are disrupted by a lack of contact with reality or frank delusions.

Key Point: *Counseling for the couple is important when symptoms are controlled. During times of acute illness, it is vital that the partner have medical and psychological support.*

Medication Many medications used to treat health problems have unwelcome sexual side effects. Gabriel Thomas (Meet Your Patients) clearly illustrates the concern some clients have about commonly prescribed medications. Table 30-1 lists a number of drugs and their effects on sexual function.

- **Medications may be prescribed to enhance sexual function,** particularly for patients experiencing erectile dysfunction (ED), patients with diabetes mellitus, or those who are taking beta-adrenergic blocking agents to treat high blood pressure. Three oral drugs are available for impotence: sildenafil, vardenafil, and tadalafil. These drugs generally work within 1 hour of administration, but they have no effect without sexual stimulation. They increase blood flow to the corpus cavernosum of the penis.
- ✚ Sildenafil (Viagra) should be used with caution in patients with cardiovascular disease because of its vasodilation effects, and it is contraindicated in patients receiving nitrate drugs. You should conduct a careful medication history and provide the appropriate patient teaching.

Table 30-1 ➤ Effects of Drugs on Sexual Function

MEDICATION	POSSIBLE EFFECT
Alcohol	In limited quantities, alcohol may enhance desire and function. However, heavy or chronic use may lead to decreased libido, orgasmic dysfunction, and erectile dysfunction.
Antianxiety agents	Decreased libido, delayed ejaculation
Anticonvulsants	Decreased libido, prolonged painful erections, difficulty achieving orgasm
Antidepressants	Decreased libido, difficulty achieving orgasm
	Bupropion (Wellbutrin) and trazodone (Desyrel) are least likely to cause sexual side effects.
Antihistamines	Decreased libido, decreased vaginal lubrication
Antihypertensives	Decreased libido, erectile dysfunction, delayed ejaculation
	Calcium channel blockers are least likely to cause sexual difficulties.
Chemotherapy	Fatigue, decreased libido
Hormones	Decrease sexual arousal
	Leuprolide (Lupron), goserelin (Zoladex)
Opioids	Decreased libido, erectile dysfunction
Stimulants (cocaine, methamphetamines)	Initially, stimulants cause increased intensity of the sexual encounter; however, with continued use, sexual dysfunction develops.

KnowledgeCheck 30-6

- Identify four factors associated with physical illness or surgeries that may affect sexuality or sexual functioning.
- What determines our sexual attitudes?

SEXUAL HEALTH

The WHO defines **sexual health** (a key concept in this chapter) as a state of physical, emotional, mental, and social well-being related to sexuality; it is not merely the absence of disease, dysfunction, or infirmity. Attaining and maintaining sexual health requires the following:

- A positive and respectful approach to sexuality and sexual relationships
- An openness and opportunity to have pleasurable and safe sexual experiences, free of coercion, discrimination, and violence
- The respected, protected, and fulfilled sexual rights of all persons (WHO, 2006)

To promote sexual health effectively, you will need theoretical knowledge about sexual responses, modes of sexual expression, and problems affecting sexuality.

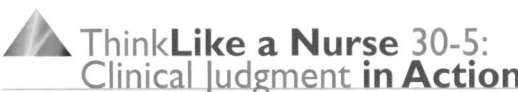 **ThinkLike a Nurse 30-5: Clinical Judgment in Action**

Examine your own beliefs about sexuality. Identify areas of concern you have regarding sexuality. How do you think this will affect your ability to assist patients with sexual health concerns?

What Is the Sexual Response Cycle?

The **sexual response cycle** is the sequence of physiological events that occurs when a person becomes sexually aroused. Based on research conducted in the 1950s, Masters and Johnson (1966) identified a four-stage sexual response: excitement, plateau, orgasm, and resolution (Fig. 30-7). Some scholars have suggested that the stage of desire be added to the original Masters and Johnson model. In some people, desire can either precede or follow excitement (Basson, 2001, 2008). The degree to which individuals experience each cycle and the changes/responses varies.

Although it is most intense in the genitals, **sexual response** is a total-body response involving many physiological changes (e.g., increased heart rate, flushing). The emotional and mental aspects of sexual activity are equally important to the person's satisfaction. The body has many **erogenous zones** (areas that cause sexual arousal when stimulated): the genitals, the skin, lips, ears, breasts, buttocks, and thighs. Table 30-2 shows normal physiological changes in sexual response that occur with aging.

Desire

Desire is a stage of varying length characterized by an interest in sexual intimacy, either in anticipation of sexual activity or with physical stimulation. Desire occurs in the mind and is communicated either verbally or through body language. This communication may be subtle and easily misread. Desire increases in proportion to the level of sex hormones (e.g., a patient with low testosterone is not as interested in sex). For patients who have a menstrual cycle, desire reaches a peak each month near the time of ovulation, when estrogen levels are high.

Libido is an individual's typical level of desire (Basson, 2001, 2008). What is considered "sexual" or "attractive" can vary greatly because societal, cultural, and personal values influence the range of stimuli that provoke sexual desire. Desire may last only moments or be ongoing for years. Transient sexual thoughts are fleeting moments of desire that might be triggered by exposure to sexually explicit media or erotic thoughts, words, or actions.

Excitement

Excitement is the body's physical response to desire; **sexual arousal** is desire that occurs with erotic stimuli, such as sights, sounds, and fantasies. During excitement, the following bodily changes occur: heart rate, blood pressure, and respiratory rate increase; muscles tense **(myotonia);** nipples become erect; and genital and pelvic blood supply increases **(vasocongestion).**

- **In female adolescents and adults,** vasocongestion leads to vaginal lubrication, swelling of the breasts, rise of the uterus, and swelling of the labia and clitoris.
- **In male adolescents and adults,** erection begins as the penis increases in length and diameter. The testes rise closer to the body, and the scrotum thickens.

Excitement may lead to further sexual activity, but this is not inevitable. For both sexes, the person may lose and regain initial physical excitement many times without advancing to the next stage. Excitement may be communicated verbally or through body language.

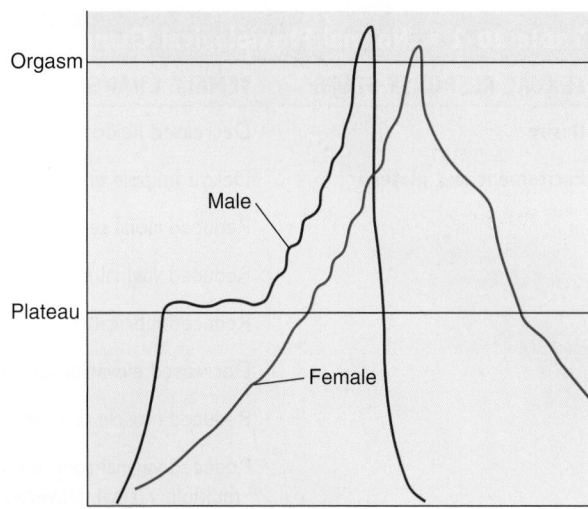

FIGURE 30-7 The sexual response cycle.

Table 30-2 ➤ Normal Physiological Changes in Sexual Response That Occur With Aging

SEXUAL RESPONSE STAGE	FEMALE CHANGES	MALE CHANGES
Desire	Decreased libido	Decreased libido
Excitement and plateau	Delayed nipple erection	Delayed nipple erection
	Reduced labial separation and swelling	Delayed and less firm erection
	Reduced vaginal expansion	Longer excitement stage
	Reduced lubrication	Decreased preejaculatory emissions
	Decreased elevation of the uterus	Reduced muscle tension
	Reduced muscle tension	Reduced lifting of the scrotum and testes
	Reduced vaginal tone (in those who have had multiple vaginal deliveries); results in less stimulation during intercourse	Shorter phase of impending orgasm
		May require more direct stimulation to achieve and maintain an erection
Orgasm	Reduced spread of sexual flush	Shorter ejaculation time
		Fewer ejaculatory contractions
		Reduced volume of ejaculate
Resolution	No cervical dilation	More rapid loss of erection
		Longer refractory period
		Nipple erection lasts longer after orgasm

Sources: SexInfo.online. (2018). *Aging and the sexual response cycle*. University of California, Santa Barbara. https://sexinfo.soc.ucsb.edu/article/aging-and-sexual-response-cycle; Cash, J., & Glass, C. (2019). *Adult-gerontology practice guidelines* (2nd ed.). Springer; U.S. Health and Human Services, National Institute on Aging. (2017). *Sexuality in later life*. https://www.nia.nih.gov/health/sexuality-later-life

Plateau

If stimulation continues, the person reaches the **plateau** phase. Plateau is associated with continued increases in pulse, respiratory rate, blood pressure, and muscle tension. Some people flush around the face, neck, and chest in this phase. The person may achieve, lose, and regain the plateau phase several times without experiencing orgasm.

- **In female adolescents and adults,** the areolae become firmer, the clitoris retracts into the clitoral hood, Bartholin's glands lubricate, and the lower vagina swells and narrows. With a male partner, the vagina tightens around the penis, increasing sexual stimulation.
- **In male adolescents and adults,** the ridge of the glans penis becomes more prominent, preejaculate (two or three drops of fluid) is emitted, and the testes rise closer to the body.

Orgasm

Orgasm occurs at the peak of the plateau phase. At the moment of orgasm, the sexual tension that has been building is released. The heart rate, respiratory rate, and blood pressure reach their peak, and there is a loss of voluntary muscle tone.

- **In female adolescents and adults,** spinal cord reflexes cause powerful rhythmic contractions of the vagina,

uterus, anus, and pelvic floor muscles; feelings of warmth spread through the pelvic area. The cervical canal dilates, allowing easy transport of the sperm to the uterus. Orgasm may last for a few seconds or up to nearly a minute.
- **In male adolescents and adults,** spinal cord reflexes cause the urethra, anus, and pelvic floor muscles to contract, followed by **ejaculation** (the expulsion of semen through the urethra). Orgasm usually lasts no more than 30 seconds.

The intensity of orgasm varies among individuals and in each individual from one sexual experience to another. Orgasm may involve intense spasms associated with an intense focus on the sexual pleasure, or it may be signaled by as little as a sigh or subtle relaxation.

Resolution

Resolution is the period of time after orgasm. The muscles relax, and the body returns to its preexcitement state.

- **Male adults,** immediately after orgasm, experience a **refractory period,** during which they cannot achieve an erection. The duration of this period varies among individuals and increases with age.
- **Female adults** experience no refractory period—they can either enter the resolution stage or return

to the excitement or plateau stage immediately after orgasm.

KnowledgeCheck 30-7

Identify the phase of the sexual response cycle described.

- This phase is reached if there is ongoing stimulation. This stage may be achieved, lost, and regained several times without the occurrence of orgasm.
- This stage occurs in the mind and may be communicated between potential sexual partners either verbally or through body language.
- This phase is associated with the release of sexual tension.

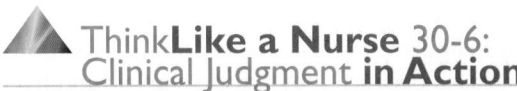

ThinkLike a Nurse 30-6: Clinical Judgment in Action

Critique the theory of Masters and Johnson, as represented in the preceding discussion of the sexual response cycle. How would you respond to the statement that the theory does not adequately address variation among individuals and even within an individual's sexual response?

What Are Some Forms of Sexual Expression?

People express their sexuality and gain sexual satisfaction in different ways. Although opinions vary, a range of behaviors is socially acceptable and therefore considered "normal" by most people in our society. These behaviors are discussed in the next few sections.

Developing Intimate Relationships A willingness to take risks and offer trust is involved in developing intimate relationships. Intimacy involves openness, mutual respect, caring, commitment, protection, honesty, and devotion. Although we often think of intimate relationships as sexual, they are not necessarily so. Furthermore, in our society, many sexual relationships occur without intimacy.

Fantasies and Erotic Dreams Most people have sexual fantasies. They may be related to past experiences, dreams, or desires or to stories heard, seen, or read. Sexual fantasies serve to increase self-esteem and sexual arousal and serve as an outlet to explore sexual desires. People in long-term monogamous relationships may fantasize to bring variety and excitement into a routine sexual encounter. Erotic dreams are also common. Nocturnal (nighttime) orgasm may or may not occur with the dream.

Masturbation Masturbation is self-stimulation of the genitals. A person may hold and stroke the shaft of the penis or manually stimulate the clitoris to achieve orgasm.

- **Young children** touch their genitals as a part of body exploration, but they quickly learn either that touching certain areas is not acceptable or that it should be done in private.
- **Adolescents,** particularly male adolescents, may masturbate frequently.

- **Adults** may masturbate for sexual release when a partner is not available or for variety in a partnered relationship.
- **Sex therapists** often recommend masturbation as a means to resolve orgasm difficulties and ejaculatory problems.
- **Religious and social taboos** discouraging masturbation are common.
- **Misconceptions:** Some people mistakenly believe that masturbation is harmful, causing acne, warts, blindness, or insanity. More commonly, some people consider masturbation a "dirty," shameful, or perverted act.

Shared Touching Also called *mutual masturbation,* shared touching may be an alternative to sexual intercourse. This is particularly appealing to individuals who seek to maintain their virginity or decrease the risk of STIs and those who have mobility or other physical problems that make intercourse difficult. Mutual masturbation is recognized as a form of safer sex because body fluids are not likely to be exchanged. This behavior can be satisfying because it allows for a significant level of sexual intimacy and for participants to experience orgasm.

Sexual Intercourse and Coitus These terms are used to describe penile penetration of the vagina. People use a variety of positions for intercourse, depending on preference, mobility, cultural and religious influences, the relationship, and other personal beliefs. For some people, manual stimulation of the clitoris is also necessary to achieve orgasm. Partners typically do not reach orgasm at the same time, despite the romantic preoccupation with this phenomenon.

Unprotected intercourse may lead to conception and pregnancy. Because body fluids are exchanged, sexual intercourse may also lead to the transmission of infections. Using a lubricated condom decreases this risk, but it is not a foolproof measure to prevent STIs.

Oral–Genital Stimulation Couples practice oral–genital stimulation (oral sex) for sexual variety or as foreplay. Oral sex provides intimacy and cannot result in pregnancy; therefore, some people consider their virginity status protected. For the latter reasons, oral sex has become prevalent among adolescents. **Key Point: Oral–genital contact may, however, lead to STIs.**

Cunnilingus is the oral stimulation of the female genitals. **Fellatio** is the stimulation of the male genitals by a partner's mouth. Although swallowing semen is not a health issue, it may be a matter of personal preference as to whether the recipient ejaculates in the partner's mouth. Dental dams, plastic wrap, or latex condoms can be used to prevent the transmission of STIs.

Anal Stimulation or Anal Intercourse Couples can engage in oral–anal stimulation (called **anilingus**). Objects for sexual stimulation, or the partner's finger, tongue, and mouth, may be used to stimulate the anus. **Anal intercourse** is the insertion of the penis into the partner's rectum.

When a couple engages in anal intercourse, lubrication is essential to lessen the chance of tiny tears to the rectal mucosa or damage to the anal sphincter. A lubricated latex condom can be used to decrease the risk of STIs. The condom must be changed before vaginal penetration to avoid the transfer of *Escherichia coli* bacteria from the rectum to the vagina. Couples should follow the same precaution when using objects for sexual pleasure.

Celibacy Sometimes referred to as *abstinence,* **celibacy** is a state in which an individual refrains from sexual activity. Traditionally, a person who chooses to be celibate remains unmarried, often for religious reasons, and sublimates sexual desire through prayer, meditation, and service. There are numerous other reasons a person may remain celibate:

- Fear of or lack of desire for intimate relationships
- Childhood sexual trauma
- A developmental or physical disability that limits opportunities for meeting prospective partners, limits privacy, or interferes with the ability to communicate or act on desires
- The desire to focus energies elsewhere because of a low libido
- The need to regain balance after the loss of a relationship, whether through separation, divorce, or death

Married couples may be happily celibate in a stable relationship. Other people might be celibate after the loss of a relationship, whether through separation, divorce, or death. Some may feel a considerable void, whereas others may feel differently.

KnowledgeCheck 30-8

- What are aspects of an intimate relationship?
- Identify solitary types of sexual expression and those that may be conducted with a partner.

What Problems Affect Sexuality?

Sexual well-being is a complex mesh of physical, emotional, cognitive, social, and spiritual components. Therefore, it is not surprising that many people experience challenges to their sexual health. Difficulties can arise in loving, healthy relationships, as well as in dysfunctional relationships. Sexual dysfunction may be temporary and situational, or it may be a long-standing issue.

Sexually Transmitted Infections (STIs)

- **Transmission**—An STI may be caused by bacteria, viruses, fungi, or parasites.
  - STIs are spread through direct sexual contact with an open wound or with body fluids, such as semen, vaginal secretions, or blood that contains pathogens.

- **Key Point:** *Contrary to many myths, STIs are not transmitted by casual touching, coughing, or other indirect means.*
- **Key Point:** *Because many STIs have few or no initial symptoms, an infected person can unknowingly transmit the infection*
- **Incidence**—More than 20 different STIs have been identified, and STIs affect millions of men and women each year. The incidence of STIs, including HIV, among older adults has increased because many sexually active adults are exposed to the same risk factors as are their younger counterparts (Shaw, 2020). A sexual history should be a component of the assessment in older adults.
- **Mandatory reporting**—STIs are **reportable** (or **notifiable**) **diseases** because they have a significant effect on public health. When healthcare providers diagnose STIs, mandatory reporting laws require that the CDC be notified.
  - **STI cases continue to increase sharply**—Over 2.4 million cases of chlamydia, gonorrhea, and syphilis were reported in 2018, with each infection showing an increase in cases since 2017 (CDC, 2021).

The following are examples of commonly reported STIs:

Chlamydia Trachomatis
- Most common transmitted bacterial STI in the United States
- Also known as the "silent infection" because the infected person may not have symptoms
- Can cause serious damage to a female's reproductive system if untreated and may cause urethral infections and testicle changes in males

Gonorrhea
- Caused by a bacterium
- Common STI among sexually active teenagers and young adults
- A reported 111% increase in cases since 2009 (CDC, 2021)

Syphilis
- Caused by a bacterium
- Transmitted from person to person by direct contact with the syphilis sore, which can occur on the external genitalia, vagina, lips, mouth, or anus and in the rectum
- If left untreated, long-term neurological complications and even death may occur.

Genital Human Papillomavirus Genital human papillomavirus (HPV) is the most common STI in the United States.

- Many people with HPV do not know they are infected, and the HPV infection can go away without intervention.
- HPV can cause bumps/warts in the genital area and certain types of cancer (e.g., cervical, vagina, penis, anal).

- The HPV vaccine is recommended to protect against cancers caused by common strains of HPV (CDC, 2022a).

Detection of STIs To determine whether a patient has an STI, you must obtain a culture, that is, a swab of secretions from the genitals.

- Male—Insert the swab into the urethral opening.
- Female—Use the swab to obtain secretions from near the cervix.
- Obtain a culture of the throat or rectum if the person has had oral or anal sex.

Many STIs can be treated fairly easily with antibiotics. However, if left untreated, they may cause serious problems. In female patients, the pathogens can travel up through the uterus and into the fallopian tubes and cause pelvic inflammatory disease (PID). Untreated PID may cause sterility.

The best ways to prevent STIs are to practice abstinence or to participate only in a mutually monogamous sexual relationship with someone who has never had or is at low risk for an STI.

The following increase the risk for an STI:

- Unprotected sex
- More than one sexual partner
- Alcohol and drug use
- Sharing needles
- Nonadherence to the STI treatment regimen

To read about various STIs and their symptoms, treatment, and effects on sexual functioning, fertility, and childbearing, see Table 30-3.

Dysmenorrhea

Dysmenorrhea is painful menstruation caused by strong uterine contractions that cause ischemia of the uterus.

- **Physical symptoms:** Cramping, lower abdominal pain, back and upper thigh pain, headache, vomiting, and diarrhea.
- **Treatments:** Bedrest; application of heat to the back and abdomen; and analgesics such as aspirin and other NSAIDs, for example, ibuprofen or naproxen.

Premenstrual Syndrome

Premenstrual syndrome (PMS) is characterized by physical and emotional changes occurring 3 to 14 days before the onset of the menstrual period.

- **Physical symptoms** include headaches, constipation, breast tenderness, and weight gain associated with bloating, abdominal swelling, or swelling of the hands and feet.
- **Emotional and social symptoms** often occur. Some may feel as though they are on an emotional roller coaster, with periods of depression, anxiety, irritability, tension, and an inability to concentrate. Some have difficulty maintaining social interactions because of severe emotional symptoms.
- **Premenstrual dysphoric disorder (PMDD)** is a more severe form of menstrual cycle dysfunction that can cause serious depression for a week or more before the menstrual period.
  - PMS is shorter, is usually milder, and involves more physical symptoms than PMDD.
  - A person can suffer from both PMS and PMDD at the same time or may have only one.

KnowledgeCheck 30-9

- Identify three methods to decrease the transmission of STIs.
- What are physical and emotional symptoms of premenstrual syndrome (PMS)?

Negative Intimate Relationships

Many couples have satisfying sexual relationships. However, some intimate relationships are not mutually satisfying based on a variety of factors (e.g., stress, physical and mental illness, hormones, fatigue, distractions, low self-esteem). Couples may be involved in a nonsexual intimate relationship (celibate or loveless union) for several reasons, including:

- Financial security, social status, parenting obligations, or cultural or religious restrictions regarding divorce.
- **Domestic violence** (also called *intimate partner violence*), which may include physical and/or emotional intimidation, assault, and rape. Women are the most common victims of domestic violence, although men are also victims of abuse. Victims may hesitate to admit the cause of their injuries, even in hospital settings. Many abused individuals are either emotionally or financially dependent on their partner and believe staying in the relationship is their only option. If you wish to learn more about abuse and violence, see Chapter 6.

Sexual Harassment and Sexual Assault

- **Sexual harassment** occurs when a person in power makes unwanted sexual advances that implicitly or explicitly relate to the victim's employment, academic status, or success (e.g., sexual comments or behaviors, such as touching). Because of the power imbalance, the victim may keep silent and suffer physically and psychologically.
- **Sexual** harassment may take two forms:
  1. In *quid pro quo*, the employer makes the employee feel that they must engage in unwelcome sexual advances to maintain employment.
  2. In *hostile environment* situations, the sexual advances are more subtle, but persistent, and create an intimidating environment.
- **Sexual assault** includes contact with or without penetration, sexual touching of intimate parts, and any unwanted sexual activity.

Table 30-3 ➤ Common Sexually Transmitted Infections (STIs)

Chlamydia

SYMPTOMS	TREATMENT AND LONG-TERM EFFECTS
Female: Usually asymptomatic **Male:** Occur 1–2 weeks after infection: thin, clear urethral discharge; mild discomfort with urination	**Treatment:** Antibiotics ***Long-Term Effects*** *Females:* Invasion of the uterus and fallopian tubes, resulting in pelvic inflammatory disease (PID), which may lead to pain, sterility, and ectopic pregnancy *Pregnant persons:* In utero transmission to fetus; newborn may have pneumonia; may be fatal *Males:* Epididymitis (may lead to sterility), proctitis (with anal intercourse)

Trichomoniasis

SYMPTOMS	TREATMENT AND LONG-TERM EFFECTS
Female: Cheesy, frothy, irritating, odorous vaginal discharge **Male:** Usually asymptomatic	**Treatment:** Amebicide and antibiotic ***Long-Term Effects*** May be passed back and forth between partners if the male is not treated Untreated, it may damage cervical cells

Gonorrhea

SYMPTOMS	TREATMENT AND LONG-TERM EFFECTS
May be asymptomatic in both men and women **Female:** Usually no early symptoms **Male:** Thick white or yellowish urethral discharge, burning, frequent/painful urination	**Treatment:** Antibiotics **Key Point:** *Some strains are becoming resistant.* ***Long-Term Effects*** *Females:* Invasion of the uterus and fallopian tubes resulting in PID, which may lead to pain, sterility, and ectopic pregnancy *Pregnant persons:* Blindness and pneumonia in the newborn *Males:* Infertility, arthritis

Human papillomavirus (HPV)

SYMPTOMS	TREATMENT AND LONG-TERM EFFECTS
Female: Genital warts on the vulva, cervix, vaginal walls, anus, or mouth; cauliflower-like appearance **Male:** Genital warts on the urethra, shaft of the penis, scrotum, anus, or mouth; cauliflower-like appearance	**Treatment:** Antibiotics ***Long-Term Effects*** Warts appear months after genital contact. Greatest risk factor for cervical cancer; associated with cancer of the penis and anus

Genital herpes (HSV-2)

SYMPTOMS	TREATMENT AND LONG-TERM EFFECTS
Female: May be asymptomatic Small, painful blisters on the genitals; pain with burst blisters as they become wet sores for several weeks; may include fever **Male:** Same as female	***Treatment*** No cure Vaccine currently under investigation Antiviral (may minimize the duration and severity of an initial infection or later flare of symptoms; reduce the likelihood of transmission to a partner) ***Long-Term Effects*** Increased risk of HIV and cervical cancer Transmission to infant during vaginal delivery, with serious, even fatal sequelae Lifelong transmission risk, especially during flare-ups

Table 30-3 ➤ Common Sexually Transmitted Infections (STIs)—cont'd

Syphilis

SYMPTOMS	TREATMENT AND LONG-TERM EFFECTS
Female - *Primary Stage:* Chancre (painless, ulcer-like sore at site of contact; will disappear in about 14 days without treatment; cervical chancres will be undetected by the female) - *Secondary Stage:* Generalized, nonitchy, painless rash; sore throat; low-grade fever; aches and pains **Male** - *Primary Stage:* Chancre (painless, ulcer-like sore at site of contact, will disappear in about 14 days without treatment) - *Secondary Stage:* Generalized, nonitchy, painless rash; sore throat; low-grade fever; aches and pains	**Treatment**: Antibiotics **Long-Term Effects** If untreated: *Latent Stage:* Bacteria continue to attack internal organs. *Late (tertiary) Stage:* Damage to the heart, blood vessels, and central nervous system. May lead to death

Hepatitis B (HBV)

SYMPTOMS	TREATMENT AND LONG-TERM EFFECTS
Female: May be asymptomatic Flu-like symptoms (low-grade fever, fatigue), decreased appetite, dark urine, and jaundice **Male:** May be asymptomatic Flu-like symptoms (low-grade fever, fatigue), decreased appetite, dark urine, and jaundice	**Treatment** Vaccine for prevention Rest, good nutrition Avoidance of alcohol and drugs **Long-Term Effects** Liver cancer Death

HIV

SYMPTOMS	TREATMENT AND LONG-TERM EFFECTS
Female: Asymptomatic carrier state Low T4 cell count Weight loss, fatigue, diarrhea, fever Vulnerability to bacterial, viral, and fungal infections **Male:** Asymptomatic carrier state Low T4 cell count Weight loss, fatigue, diarrhea, fever Vulnerability to bacterial, viral, and fungal infections	**Treatment** No cure (research is being conducted) Viewed as a chronic disease with treatment Nucleoside inhibitors, nonnucleoside inhibitors, protease inhibitors **Long-Term Effects** Opportunistic infections

Rape

- Rape is nonconsensual vaginal, anal, or oral penetration. It occurs through force, by the threat of bodily harm, or when the victim is incapable of giving consent.
- Rape is a crime of violence rather than of sex. We discuss it here because it often involves the sexual organs and usually has negative effects on the victim's sexuality.
- **All states consider rape, even within a marriage, to be a crime**.

Key Point: *Victims of rape range from infants to older adults and may be either gender, although women are more likely to be victims.* The number of self-reported incidents of rape or sexual assault was 2.6 million in 2020 (Morgan & Thompson, 2022).

Types of Rape

- **Group rape** (gang rape) occurs when more than one person sexually assaults a victim. Group rape usually occurs when drugs and alcohol are involved.
- **Statutory rape** is sexual activity between an adult and a person under the "age of consent" (this ranges from 16 to 18 years of age, depending on state regulations). This charge may be filed even when the sex is consensual.
- **Date rape** is rape by an acquaintance when the assault occurs during an agreed-upon social encounter or date. Although date rape is not a lesser violation, our society tends to wrongfully blame the victim when date rape occurs.

Why Many Rapes Go Unreported

The incidence of rape is probably higher than published statistics because many individuals do not report the crime to law enforcement. Rape is an assault that involves significant psychological and physical injury; therefore, the police often become involved because the victim requires medical attention. After a rape or other forms of sexual assault, care may be delayed for various reasons:

- Involvement of alcohol or drugs (particularly for teens)
- Fear of the assailant or fear of consequences to the assailant
- Knowledge of the low conviction rate for rapists
- Desire to avoid a trial and exploration of past sexual history
- Shame, embarrassment, and self-blame
- The wish to deny the event and its possible consequences and move on

Effects of Rape

Rape can result in both physiological trauma and long-lasting psychological effects (e.g., anxiety, depression, suicidal thoughts). In addition, rape victims have a risk for STIs and, for females, the risk of pregnancy. The economic costs of rape is estimated at $122,461 per victim based on medical costs, criminal justice activities, lost work productivity, and other costs (CDC, 2022b).

Key Point: *Referral of the patient to a local sexual assault support group is critical. A sexual assault nurse examiner (SANE) is a registered nurse who has received special training in the immediate care of sexual assault victims.* To learn about providing care to sexual assault victims, see the accompanying iCare Box and,

 Go to **Chapter 30, Clinical Insight 30-1: Providing Care After Sexual Assault,** in Volume 2.

Sexual Response Cycle Disorders

Disorders in various stages of the sexual response cycle may affect desire, arousal, excitement, and orgasm.

Low Libido Hypoactive sexual desire, or low libido, manifests as a significant decrease in or absence of both sexual fantasies and sexual activity. Low libido can affect anyone and can be transient or long term. The person may experience low libido only with one particular partner, or the lack of desire can extend to all sexual activity. Persons with low libido may reluctantly engage in sexual encounters or avoid all sexual contact. However, once sexual activity has been initiated, the person is usually able to achieve orgasm.

Factors contributing to hypoactive sexual desire include the following:

- Sexual trauma
- Negative attitude toward sex
- Negative relationships
- Biological factors (e.g., hormone deficiencies, perimenopause)
- Side effects of various medications

♥ iCare 30-1

Sexual Health

The topic of sexual health is one of the most private topics a nurse can discuss with a person. Be compassionate, but take a matter-of-fact and accepting approach. Remember, the patient may want information but may not know how to bring up the topic. The following are tips for showing that you care:

- Confidentiality is paramount.
- Be available to listen. Sit down face to face, approach the topic unhurriedly, and make eye contact.
- Provide privacy and help the person feel comfortable. Pull the curtain; close the door.
- Be observant for both verbal and nonverbal cues that may indicate a concern.
- Be empathetic to the person's situation or concern, whatever it may be.
- Be aware that people can be very vulnerable when discussing sexual health topics.
- Be prepared to accept a wide range of emotions, from withdrawal to outbursts of anger.

PICOT

Sexuality, Dementia, and Competency

Situation: The adult children of a widow with early-onset Alzheimer disease are concerned about their mother's sexual advances directed at another resident at the assisted living facility. Although the residents are, legally, consenting adults, the children are concerned about their mother's judgment and sexual appropriateness.

PICOT Components:

P	Population/client	=	Adults with early onset Alzheimer's disease
I	Intervention/indicator	=	Nonpharmacological behavior modification
C	Comparator/control	=	No sexual relationships
O	Outcome	=	Appropriate, consensual sexual relationships
T	Time	=	Late adulthood

Searchable Question: Do _____ (P) who receive/are exposed to _____ (I) demonstrate _____ (O) compared with _____ (C) during _____ (T)?

Example of Evidence: All people have needs for intimacy, companionship, and touch. Clients with dementia pose a particularly difficult situation for both family and professionals, who may consider sexual behavior to be inappropriate based on the client's age, setting, situation, or health issues. The central question for you to answer is whether the client is competent. The family and staff need to carefully and sensitively assess the following areas: Is the client's mental status suited to engaging in a consensual sexual relationship? Who is initiating sexual contact? Is the client able to consent to sexual intimacy? Is the client aware of emotional and physical potential risks, such as the relationship ending? Is the sexual activity consistent with behavior the client exhibited before the onset of the dementia? Although there are no established treatment guidelines, various nonpharmacological plans may help to ensure appropriate expression of sexuality.

Practice Change: After obtaining a thorough sexual assessment, the nurse may plan nonpharmacological behavior modifications for the client to demonstrate appropriate sexual behaviors and meet the client's intimacy needs.

Source: Dhingra, I., DeSousa, A., & Sonavane, S. (2016). Sexuality in older adults: Clinical and psychosocial dilemmas. *Journal of Geriatric Mental Health, 3,* 131–139; Rector, S., Stiritz, S., & Morley, J. (2020). Sexuality, aging, and dementia. *Journal of Nutrition, Health & Aging, 24,* 355–370. https://doi.org/10.1007/s12603-020-1345-0

Low sexual desire sometimes responds positively to testosterone administration.

Arousal Disorders Arousal disorders can be experienced by anyone. In female patients, arousal disorders manifest as minimal or absent pelvic congestion and vaginal lubrication even though desire may be present.

- **Dyspareunia,** or painful intercourse, further decreases sexual desire.
  - **In female patients,** dyspareunia is often caused by vaginal dryness resulting from hormonal changes, the aging process, tampon use, and medications (e.g., antihistamines). A water-based lubricant or saliva helps to resolve vaginal dryness. Other causes of female dyspareunia include vaginal or urinary tract infections, pelvic inflammatory disease, and endometriosis.
  - **In male patients,** dyspareunia most commonly results from urinary tract infection or **phimosis,** a condition in which the foreskin of the penis is too tight. **Balanitis,** inflammation of the penis, is another cause of dyspareunia in men.
- **Vaginismus** is a rare disorder affecting desire and arousal. It is characterized by intense involuntary contractions of the perineal muscles, which close the vaginal opening and prevent penile penetration. Vaginismus may be associated with psychological disorders (e.g., negative attitudes toward sex, history of sexual abuse or trauma) or physiological disorders (e.g., trauma during childbirth).
- **Erectile dysfunction (ED),** formerly known as *impotence,* is the persistent or recurring inability either to achieve or to maintain an erection sufficient for satisfactory sexual performance. Causes of ED include the following:
  - Diseases of the blood vessels (e.g., hypertension, high cholesterol, or diabetes) are the most common cause.
  - Neurological problems (e.g., spinal cord injury, Parkinson's disease, stroke)
  - Endocrine problems (diabetes)
  - Common psychological problems, such as performance anxiety, childhood sexual abuse, relationship issues, or mental illness
  - Certain medications, such as antihistamines, antidepressants, antipsychotics, and antihypertensives

Orgasmic Disorders These are conditions with a delay in or absence of orgasm after a normal sexual excitement phase.

- **Female orgasmic disorders**
  - More prevalent in younger patients who have not had adequate sexual experience to learn how to reach orgasm
  - Manual clitoral stimulation may be required to reach orgasm; many people cannot achieve orgasm through intercourse alone.
  - Loss of the ability to achieve orgasm is often caused by sexual trauma, poor sexual communication, a conflicted sexual relationship, a mood disorder, a medical condition, or direct physiological effects from a drug.

- **Male orgasmic disorders**
  - If orgasm cannot be achieved during intercourse, it may be possible through masturbation or manual or oral stimulation by a partner.
  - **Premature ejaculation** occurs when orgasm and ejaculation occur before, at the time of, or shortly after penetration. Any related disappointment may lead to issues with self-esteem, sexual avoidance, and ED. There are sexual techniques as well as medications that can help to delay ejaculation.
  - **Retrograde ejaculation** occurs when the semen empties into the bladder instead of being ejaculated through the urethra. Normally, this cannot occur because the internal bladder sphincter closes in the orgasmic phase. However, some medications, prostate surgery, and spinal cord injuries may lead to retrograde ejaculation, resulting in sterility.

KnowledgeCheck 30-10

- Identify three forms of sexual victimization.
- In which phases of the sexual response cycle can sexual dysfunction occur?

PracticalKnowledge
knowing **how**

Although you understand the importance of comprehensive client assessment, you may find it difficult to gather information related to sexuality. Students and some nurses may be shy when it comes to talking about sexuality. They may also be concerned that the client will be embarrassed to talk openly about sexual topics because these matters are personal and private, and disclosure can threaten a person's self-esteem.
 ♥ **iCare** Including sexuality as a routine part of your nursing assessment reinforces the concept that sexuality is an integral part of life and provides an opportunity for much-needed client teaching on this topic.

ASSESSMENT/RECOGNIZING CUES

The extent to which you will assess a client's sexual health status varies. For example, a patient with a suspected STI requires a comprehensive health assessment and a focused sexual assessment. Similarly, clients with illnesses that affect their sexual functioning should receive a full assessment. Jocelyn Carter (Meet Your Patients) is an example. Recall that chronic illness can have a profound effect on sexual functioning (e.g., Frank Thanee and Gabriel Thomas, also in the Meet Your Patients scenario).

A focused sexual health assessment is needed in the following situations:

Pregnancy, infertility work-up, request for birth control
Menstrual cycle irregularities or problems
Annual health visit or as part of a comprehensive physical examination

Unusual discharge from or change in genital organs
Urination problems
A known sexual problem (e.g., dyspareunia)
Illness, surgeries, or drugs that may affect sexual function (e.g., arthritis, colostomy, antihypertensives)

Sexual History

Most healthcare facilities use a standard nursing assessment form. Some address sexuality in a comprehensive manner, but most have only a few superficial questions or nothing at all. You will need to be sensitive to your client's verbal and nonverbal cues to identify and explore relevant issues that are not on the form. For topics to include in a sexual history and for suggestions for questions to ask,

 Go to **Chapter 30, Assessment Guidelines and Tools, Focused Assessment: Guidelines and Questions for Taking a Sexual History,** in Volume 2.

♥ **iCare   Tips for Taking a Sexual History** When asking personal questions, always provide privacy. It is one thing to discuss blood pressure in the presence of family but quite another to discuss sexual health issues, which may threaten the very core of a relationship. For example, a wife is not likely to discuss domestic violence with her abusive husband at her side, or an 18-year-old man may not want to discuss his sexual behavior when his father is present. For other suggestions,

 Go to **Chapter 30, Clinical Insight 30-2: Guidelines for Taking a Sexual History,** in Volume 2.

Focused Physical Examination

Sexual health assessment includes a physical examination focused on the reproductive system. For detailed instructions about performing these examinations,

 Go to **Chapter 19, Procedure 19-17: Assessing the Male Genitourinary System,** and **Procedure 19-18: Assessing the Female Genitourinary System,** in Volume 2.

KnowledgeCheck 30-11

What techniques can you use to increase comfort and communication during a sexual history assessment?

 Think**Like a Nurse** 30-7:
Clinical Judgment **in Action**

Review the three case scenarios in the Meet Your Patients discussion. Consider the following questions for each client:

- Would you be comfortable caring for and responding to each of these clients?
- What topics, if any, have been raised by these clients that would be difficult for you to handle?
- How would you answer each of the questions the clients asked in this scenario?

NURSING DIAGNOSIS/ANALYZING CUES

Nursing diagnoses for describing sexual problems focus on the expression of concerns and on actual problems. The following discussion should help you differentiate between them.

- **Sexual Patterns Alterations.** Use this diagnosis when the patient expresses concerns about their sexuality. Examples of such concerns might include conflict about sexual orientation, value conflicts, fear of acquiring an STI, lack of knowledge about how to adapt sexual techniques to altered body function, lack of privacy, not having a partner, or impaired relationship with the partner.
- **Sexual Dysfunction.** Use this label when there is an actual change in sexual function that the patient views as unsatisfying, unrewarding, or inadequate. This includes sexual response cycle disorders, such as low libido, arousal disorders, orgasmic disorders, vaginismus, premature ejaculation, and erectile dysfunction. If these defining characteristics for Sexual Dysfunction do not seem to "fit" the patient, then use the more general diagnosis, Sexual Pattern Alterations.

Defining Characteristics

Each of the two diagnoses has defining characteristics that differentiate them, as described in the following subsections.

Sexual Pattern Alterations A defining characteristic of Sexual Pattern Alterations is that the patient reports difficulties or alterations in sexual behaviors or activities.

- Jocelyn Carter (Meet Your Patients) is not actually experiencing problems with sexual satisfaction or performance. She is expressing a broader concern about her sexuality—about her future desirability as a sex partner. Therefore, the better diagnosis for her is Sexual Pattern Alterations.
- The same is true for Gabriel Thomas (Meet Your Patients), who is expressing fear that he may have sexual problems in the future.
- Frank Thanee will also have this diagnosis. He is experiencing conflict with his sexual orientation.

Sexual Dysfunction Sexual Dysfunction is the more specific diagnosis for physiological problems and for concerns about sexual performance. Thus, it is best to use Sexual Dysfunction when the patient has one or more of the following defining characteristics:

Alteration in sexual activity
Alteration in sexual excitation
Alteration in sexual satisfaction
Change in interest toward others
Change in sexual role
Decrease in sexual desire
Perceived sexual limitation

Seeking confirmation of desirability
Undesired change in sexual function

Etiologies of Sexuality Diagnoses

Several nursing diagnoses may be the cause of sexuality problems. The following are the more common ones:

- *Activity Intolerance* and *Fatigue* (e.g., from cardiac or respiratory disease) may cause the person to alter their lifestyle, including sexual activity, to conserve energy. A lack of energy may decrease the person's interest in sex, or it may require a change in the mode of sexual expression.
- *Physical Mobility Impairment* (e.g., as occurs with arthritis, spinal cord injuries) may affect a person's ability to interact, meet potential partners, and perform sexually (e.g., assume certain positions, make certain movements).
- *Fear* that sexual activity may be dangerous can inhibit desire and the ability to perform (e.g., after heart surgery). This diagnosis may also apply to the client's partner, who may be afraid that sexual activity will hurt the client after surgery or hurt a pregnant partner or the baby.
- *Chronic Pain* may directly affect interpersonal relationships, interest in sex, or comfort during sexual intimacy. It may cause fatigue, indirectly affecting sexuality.
- *Chronic Low Self-Esteem* may result from chronic health problems and their consequences (e.g., loss of employment, inability to perform parenting roles). Sexual expression may also become a challenge, yet the intimacy and reassurance that accompanies sexual encounters can be vital to self-esteem and a sense of wholeness.
- *Self-Care Deficits.* For clients who need assistance with activities of daily living (ADLs)—for example, with toileting—family or caretakers often find it difficult to accept and facilitate sexual relationships. When a person with a physical disability lives in a residential facility, lack of opportunity and privacy may interfere with sexual expression (Fig. 30-8).
- *Growth and Development Alterations.* Relationship challenges also exist for people who are developmentally disabled. Those with very low cognitive functioning may be unable to seek out or understand sexual relationships. Unfortunately, this makes them vulnerable to sexual abuse. Sex education is vital for these individuals to help them understand body structure and function, relationship issues, and ways to avoid exploitation and abuse.

Similarly, sexuality problems can be the etiology of other nursing diagnoses, for example:

- *Disturbed Body Image* related to change in appearance secondary to orchiectomy (removal of a testicle)
- *Pain (during coitus)* related to inadequate vaginal lubrication secondary to aging

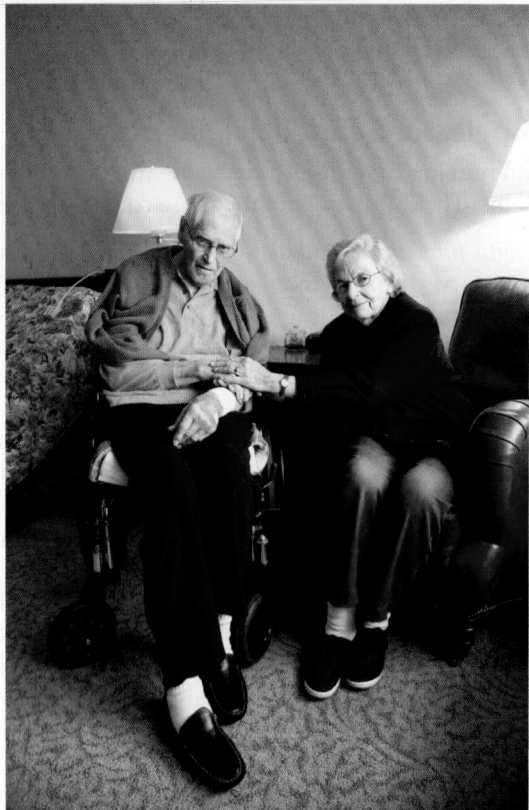

FIGURE 30-8 Adults with physical restrictions or those living within group settings, such as skilled nursing care, can maintain sexual relationships.

- *Fear* related to sexual abuse by others
- *Rape-Trauma Syndrome* (Note that you do not need an etiology for this nursing diagnosis. It is self-explanatory, as are most syndrome diagnoses.)

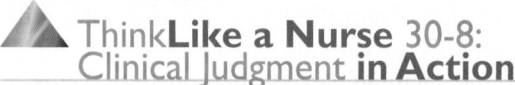

ThinkLike a Nurse 30-8: Clinical Judgment in Action

Give a specific example (client situation) for each of the defining characteristics of Sexual Dysfunction listed in the preceding section.

▰ PLANNING/PRIORITIZING HYPOTHESES AND GENERATING SOLUTIONS

Nursing Outcomes Classification (NOC) standardized outcomes associated with Ineffective Sexuality Patterns and Sexual Dysfunction include the following examples (Moorhead et al., 2018):

Abuse Recovery: Body Image	Role Performance
	Self-Esteem
Physical Aging	Sexual Functioning
Risk Control: Sexually Transmitted Diseases	Sexual Identity

Individualized client outcomes and goals depend on the nursing diagnosis you identify. For Sexual Dysfunction

and Ineffective Sexuality Patterns, you might write the following desired outcomes:

- Expresses comfort with sexual orientation.
- Describes plans for resolving values conflicts about extramarital sex (e.g., will talk to his therapist).
- Describes techniques for preventing STIs.

The following are examples of outcomes that apply specifically to Sexual Dysfunction:

- Communicates sexual needs and preferences to partner.
- Maintains penile erection through orgasm.
- Describes ways to adapt positions for intercourse to accommodate painful knee joints.

▰ IMPLEMENTATION/TAKING ACTION

Specific nursing activities for sexuality problems depend on the etiology of the problem and on the goals selected. Broadly speaking, nursing interventions involve teaching about sexual health and self-care, counseling for altered sexual functioning, and dealing with inappropriate sexual behavior. Those interventions are discussed in the following sections. You will also find a nursing care plan and care map for Ineffective Sexuality Problems on the following pages.

Teaching About Sexual Health

Before you begin teaching, take the time to get to know your client and find out what they already know about sexuality. The time you take putting the client at ease is well spent. When you develop rapport and trust, the client will be more likely to speak openly with you about sensitive or embarrassing topics, retain what you teach, and feel free to ask questions. Offer to include the partner in the discussion if the client wishes. See Chapter 16 for a review of teaching and learning.

As part of teaching about sexual health, you should discuss the prevention of STIs with all clients and discuss contraception with clients of childbearing age. Other common topics are also presented in the next sections.

Body Function and Reproduction

A person's age, experience, and educational level do not ensure knowledge of sexual functioning. Before you begin any teaching, explore your client's knowledge base by asking open-ended questions, such as "What questions do you have about sex?"

Visual Aids Patients often find visual aids (e.g., a diagram of reproductive system anatomy) helpful. For example, drawings and charts illustrating fetal development can be helpful for pregnant clients. Most agencies provide handouts and brochures so that clients can review information at home.

Myths and Misconceptions As part of your general discussion on sexuality and bodily function, you may

Application of Education and Evidence-Based Practice to Client Care

Chapter Key Concepts: Sexuality, Sexual health

Competencies: Provide Goal-Directed, Client-Centered Care (Thinking, Doing, Caring); Validate Evidence-Based Research to Incorporate Into Client Care

Background: *Goal-directed, client-centered care* addresses the client's physical, psychosocial, and spiritual needs. This includes incorporating sexual health into your assessment.

The SENC competency of *goal-directed, client-centered care* directs that nurses provide education to foster informed decisions and involvement in care and to facilitate postdischarge health. Jocelyn Carter (Meet Your Patients) is expressing concern that after mastectomy, her husband will not find her attractive. In addition to measures to show caring (holding her hand, taking the time to listen to her), now is an opportunity to provide information on the effectiveness of postoperative cosmetic advances. This information can help to lessen the degree of loss she may feel.

The SENC competency of *validating evidence-based practice to incorporate into client care* involves keeping abreast of current research and applying findings to promote effective client outcomes. Research literature reveals that satisfaction with cosmetic outcomes was similar between women who had breast-conserving surgery and those who had mastectomy with reconstruction (Jagsi et al., 2015). Ms. Carter may not focus on this information preoperatively, so you must include it in the nursing care plan so that other nurses can reinforce it. In addition, research shows that for patients undergoing treatment for breast cancer and reconstructive surgery, spouses are a significant source of support; however, to better support their partners, spouses need tailored information (Spires, 2017; Carr et al., 2019).

Think about it:

What other resources are available to promote Ms. Carter's sexual health?

wish to discuss common myths and misconceptions about sex. The following list contains several inaccurate statements about sex that provide a good starting point for discussion. **Key Point: *The statements are all false.***

- You can't get pregnant the first time you have sex.
- You can't get pregnant if you are using a condom.
- You can tell the size of a man's penis by the size of his feet.
- You always have symptoms if you have an STI.
- Only "dirty" people have STIs. You will not get an STI if your partner practices good hygiene.
- People over 70 do not have sex.
- A vaginal orgasm is better than a clitoral orgasm.
- If the relationship is good, the sexual partners will achieve simultaneous orgasm.

- It is not healthful to have intercourse during menstruation.
- The only normal position for intercourse is face to face. Anything else is deviant or at least "not nice."
- If a person does not have an orgasm, they do not really love their partner.

Douching

Teach female patients that douching is unnecessary and is associated with significant risks. It can wash away the lactobacilli that clean the vagina and protect it from infection. Douching increases the risk for some STIs and for PID (Office on Women's Health, 2019). Furthermore, douching is essentially useless as a method of contraception.

Some patients douche because they notice an odor. Reassure them that this is normal during certain times of their menstrual cycle. If the odor does not disappear after washing, they should see their healthcare provider.

Menstruation

- **Sexual activity during menstruation.** You may need to provide information to dispel myths about menstruation. It is not dangerous to engage in sexual activity during menstruation. The bloody fluid is from the uterus, not the vagina, so intercourse will not harm the vagina. Menstruation increases the vascularity, warmth, and lubrication in the pelvic region, which can increase pleasurable sensations during sex. Also, an orgasm may relieve menstrual cramps.

  A protective pad placed under the buttocks will protect the bed linen. A diaphragm can be used to prevent the flow from entering the vagina. The use of a menstrual cup during menstruation can help limit excessive bloody fluid during sex (Marquez, 2021).
- **Odor.** Odor prevention requires good perineal hygiene, daily baths or showers, and frequent changes of pads or tampons. Advise patients who use tampons to follow the manufacturer's directions for reducing the risk of toxic shock syndrome. Deodorized pads and tampons are not very effective and can cause irritation to the vulva and vagina. Another option is the menstrual cup, which decreases odor because, unlike with tampons, the bloody fluid is not exposed to air. Menstrual cups are also associated with a healthy vaginal pH (Marquez, 2021; Eijk et al., 2019).
- **Cramping.** For mild cramping occurring before or during menses, aspirin and NSAIDs, such as ibuprofen or naproxen, are effective and can be taken unless contraindicated for other reasons. These drugs inhibit uterine contractions and also have analgesic properties. A warm bath or a heating pad may be comforting; lying supine also keeps the abdomen warm.

Premenstrual Syndrome: Treatments

For patients with PMS, the following may be used:

- **Nonpharmacological treatments.** You might suggest a variety of treatments, such as getting adequate sleep; eating small, frequent meals; reducing dietary intake of sugar, caffeine, alcohol, and salt; taking vitamin and mineral supplements; and exercising.

- **Medications.** Selective serotonin reuptake-inhibiting drugs, such as fluoxetine (Prozac) and sertraline (Zoloft), are commonly used as front-line therapy for managing the symptoms of PMS.

Menopause: Hormone Replacement Therapy

Hormone replacement therapy (HRT) (estrogen-only, progestin-only, or combination) remains the most effective treatment to relieve the symptoms of menopause, such as itching, dryness, discomfort with intercourse, hot flashes, and sleep disturbances.

- **Other benefits of HRT.** Prevention of loss of bone density in menopausal patients, which leads to fewer hip fractures, is one benefit. HRT also reduces the risk of colorectal cancer. HRT can either increase or decrease the risk of heart disease, depending on when hormone therapy is started, how long patients remain on it, and individual differences.
- **Risks of HRT.** In a small number of patients, the risks associated with long-term use include heart disease, blood clots, breast and ovarian cancers, and dementia. Therefore, consumers, healthcare providers, and third-party payers have become more conservative in using HRT or reserving treatment for short-term use.
- **Teaching.** Teach patients to discuss the risks and benefits of HRT with their primary care provider. Also inform them that there are some natural remedies and bioidentical therapies that may provide symptom relief (see the related Holistic Healing box).

Screening Examinations: Guidelines

Breast self-examination and testicular self-examination are vital aspects of sexual health. For more information and for details about the purposes of screening examinations and about these assessments in particular, see Chapter 19.

Breast Examination Any change in how the breasts normally look and feel should be immediately reported to the healthcare provider. The American Cancer Society (2022) guidelines for screening female patients are organized by age, as follows:

- Ages 40 to 44 years—patients should have the opportunity to begin annual screening with a mammogram.
- Ages 45 to 54 years—patients should have an annual mammogram.
- Ages 55 years and older—patients should have a mammogram every other year or have the opportunity to continue screening annually.
- Patients who have a high risk of breast cancer (e.g., genetic markers, family history) should have a combination of magnetic resonance imaging (MRI) and mammogram.
- Patients are encouraged to report changes in the look and feel of their breasts to their healthcare provider.

Holistic Healing

Treatment of Perimenopausal Symptoms

Help, including hormone therapy, is available for perimenopause symptoms. In addition to finding a primary care provider with whom to discuss their symptoms, you might advise women to try the following:

➤ Eat a balanced diet, low in fat and rich in calcium.

➤ Use supplemental vitamins, if necessary.

➤ Take supplemental calcium and magnesium.

➤ Get adequate sleep.

➤ Exercise daily.

➤ Avoid tobacco use.

➤ Limit alcohol and caffeine.

➤ Drink plenty of water to counteract the drying effect of low estrogen levels.

➤ Use soy products (e.g., soy milk, tofu, and soy flour), which are rich in phytoestrogens that are converted to very weak estrogens during digestion.

➤ Try the herbal remedies red clover and black cohosh.

➤ Use natural progesterone cream, which is made from a yam root. A small amount of the cream can be applied for 12 days out of each month.

Testicular Examination The American Cancer Society (2018) advises that screening for testicular cancer should be a part of the annual screening examination for male patients, unless certain risk factors are present (e.g., previous germ cell tumor in one testicle, family history, undescended testicle). A lump in the testicle could be a sign of testicular cancer; however, some cancers may be at an advanced stage before symptoms are present. Monthly examinations are a personal preference; however, checking for lumps after puberty is a good idea to detect changes in the testicles.

Preventing Sexually Transmitted Infections

STIs are a worldwide health concern, and education is a key component of prevention.

- **Key Point:** *The only absolutely safe sex is total avoidance of sexual activity with a partner.* However, sexual intercourse and intimacy are important for most adults.
- The next safest sex occurs within a long-term, mutually monogamous relationship.
- Other safer sex practices involve the consistent, correct use of a condom and limiting the number of sexual partners.
- Be honest about current sexual practices and sexual history, as well as sexual health concerns.
- Avoid the exchange of body fluids, including semen, blood, and vaginal secretions, by correctly and consistently using latex barriers.
- Avoid contact with genital sores or growths.
- Have routine checkups for infection.

- Consult a healthcare provider for diagnosis and treatment of symptoms such as abnormal discharge from the vagina, penis, or rectum; a burning sensation with urination; sores in the genital area; or painful intercourse.

You should also include the following prevention interventions:

- Teach your clients the proper use of condoms. For information about the use of male and female condoms,

 Go to **Chapter 30, Clinical Insight 30-3: Teaching Your Patient to Use a Condom,** in Volume 2.

- Encourage your clients to discuss their sexual feelings, activity, birth control, STIs, and safer sex practices with their partners or potential partners. If individuals are not comfortable talking about these topics, they need to consider whether it is wise to begin a sexual relationship.
- Advise clients to choose a healthcare provider with whom they feel comfortable and free to speak frankly and openly about their sexual health concerns. This is important to their health.
- Assure clients that testing, examination, and treatment for STIs are always confidential, but also explain mandatory reporting requirements.

Contraception

Your sexual health teaching may include methods for preventing unwanted pregnancies. Several family planning strategies are available, each with advantages and disadvantages. For information on several fertility control methods,

 Go to **Chapter 30, Tables, Methods of Contraception,** in Volume 2.

Counseling for Sexual Problems

The PLISSIT model was developed as a guideline for counseling for sexual problems (Annon, 1976). The first three PLISSIT steps have been successfully adapted to address sexual knowledge deficits, which you are qualified to treat. The acronym PLISSIT represents the following:

Permission. Permission means that you communicate an open, accepting attitude so that the client feels free to ask open-ended questions and express concerns and feelings and to engage in sexual behaviors with a consenting partner. For example, you might state, "Many people experience decreased vaginal lubrication after menopause. Tell me how well you have been lubricating."

Limited Information. Supplying limited information may include teaching about normal sexual functioning, expected changes in sexual functioning, medication side effects, and medical and surgical impacts on sexuality. For example, you might

say, "Some people experience decreased vaginal lubrication because of decreased levels of certain hormones."

Specific Suggestions. You might make specific suggestions for self-care, as presented in this chapter. For example, you might say, "Some people have found that using a water-soluble lubricant is helpful."

Intensive Therapy. If these interventions do not relieve the client's concerns, you should refer the client to someone with specialized knowledge of sexual health. For example: "You might consider discussing this with your gynecologist."

Dealing With Inappropriate Sexual Behavior

Nursing involves intimate contact. We see people disrobed, literally touch bodies, and discuss private topics. In most cases, patients recognize this as professional behavior associated with providing healthcare. Occasionally they may respond inappropriately. For example, a client may make sexually suggestive comments, request sexually related care that is not required (e.g., ask you to bathe their genitalia when they can do it adequately themselves), disrobe or expose body parts that are not involved in the care delivered, or touch or grab you as you provide care.

The following are the most common reasons for sexually inappropriate behaviors:

- Confusion
- Neurological disorders, especially those involving the frontal lobe
- Mental illnesses
- Poor impulse control
- Misinterpretation of nursing care
- Desire for power or control over others, especially when the clients feel powerless in other aspects of their lives
- Worries about sexual functioning
- Unrealistic view of nursing based on sexual stereotypes

If you believe a client is demonstrating inappropriate sexual behaviors, immediately tell the client that the behavior is inappropriate. Do not express anger, but use clear statements, such as, "I don't like your comments. They are inappropriate and make me feel uncomfortable. Please stop." Next, let the client know what behavior you expect. Be direct with your comments. If the client is exposing himself, let him know what you expect him to wear ("I expect you to keep your pajama bottoms on"). If the client is attempting to touch you, tell him, "Don't touch me." Refocus the client's attention on the care you are delivering ("I need you to hold still now while I tape your IV"). If you are extremely uncomfortable or the client persists in the comments or actions, leave the room and report the incident to your instructor or the nurse assigned to the client. You may also wish to consider discussing the situation with the client while another person is in the room.

Sexual Harassment Sexual harassment is a unique form of inappropriate sexual behavior (refer to Sexual Harassment and Sexual Assault in the Theoretical Knowledge section).

- If you believe you are being sexually harassed, you should confront your harasser and clearly state your concerns.
- If you feel unable to confront your harasser (e.g., if the harasser is a teacher or supervisor), keep a written record of the events, and report your concerns to the worksite or school official in charge of personnel.
- By law, all worksites and educational environments must have a written procedure for handling cases of sexual harassment that details how to file a grievance, what forms you need to use, to whom to report the incident, and the procedure for a hearing and resolution. For further information, see Chapter 39.

Teaching Children About Sexual Predators

As a nurse, there is important information you can teach parents and caregivers to reduce children's risk of sexual violence, predators, or other unhealthy exposure.

Set the Stage for Open Discussion

- Talk openly and directly with your child about their own development and sexuality. This establishes trust and makes it easier for the child to come to you when they have questions.
- Be open to your child's questions. Acting embarrassed discourages further conversation.
- Assure your child that they won't get in trouble for "tattling" on someone who asks them to keep a secret about sexual or touching encounters.
- Make discussion a natural part of growing up—don't save it "for later."

Know What's Going on

- Be involved in your child's everyday life and ask questions—where they are, who they are with, what they are doing, what their closest friends are doing.
- Know the other adults your child is around. Go to your child's activities and get to know the adults involved.
- Know what your child watches on TV, the tablet, the computer, and the Internet or what media games they play.
- Locate computers in a central area in the home where you can monitor Internet use.
- Activate parental controls to limit access to and monitor Web sites that would expose your child to sexual content or predators.
- Know whether sexual predators live near you. Check out the sexual predators' registry in your area.
- Establish curfew times and contingency communications if curfew is breached. Teach your child

to use a code word that communicates they are in trouble.

Just Say no

- Teach your child about body parts that are private and should not be touched or seen by others—except for medical reasons.
- Teach your child to firmly say no and get away if someone tries to touch or look at them in a way that makes them feel uncomfortable.
- Urge your child to tell you or another trusted adult if someone tries to touch or look at private areas or if the person tries to show the child their own private body parts.
- Teach your child never to get in the car with strangers and never go near a stranger's car for any reason.
- Always use a buddy system to prevent the child from being alone.
- Teach your child to yell, "Help! Stranger!" if anyone tries to follow them, either walking or in a car.
- Do not allow unlimited and unsupervised Internet use.
- Teach children not to disclose personal information in public settings or on the Internet, especially social networking sites.

PUTTING IT ALL TOGETHER

Consider the three patients discussed in the Meet Your Patients scenario. Each situation illustrates how important sexual identity is to the sense of self. Each of the patients is concerned about how their medical problem might affect their sexuality:

- Jocelyn Carter is worried about how surgery will affect her relationship with her husband.
- Gabriel Thomas is concerned that blood pressure medications will impair his sexual abilities.
- Frank Thanee, recovering from open-heart surgery, is focused on explaining his long-term relationship to his family.

The full-spectrum nursing model can help you to find the best approach when dealing with sexual health. In the following sections, we will use the three clients from Meet Your Patients to illustrate how a nurse might use clinical judgment.

Thinking

Theoretical Knowledge A sound knowledge base enables you to teach and respond sensitively to all your clients. You will need theoretical knowledge about sexuality, the common myths and taboos, the effect of health concerns on sexual function and expression, and the treatment of sexual health problems. What knowledge do you already have that would enable you to address Gabriel Thomas' concerns? What knowledge do you still need?

Critical Thinking To help Gabriel Thomas, you will need to focus on what he is experiencing and critically examine his concerns in light of what is known about hypertension and its treatment. You will need to prioritize your concerns about Mr. Thomas, balancing the need to control his blood pressure with his sexual requirements. Encourage him to discuss his concerns with his healthcare provider and explore alternate medications. You can also help him consider and discuss alternative forms of sexual expression.

Doing

Practical Knowledge When dealing with sexuality, your verbal and nonverbal skills demonstrate to patients your comfort with sensitive topics. Consider the situation of Jocelyn Carter. Suppose you responded to Jocelyn's question by telling her, "That's the least of your worries." How do you think she would feel? Now consider what might happen if you responded, "You appear to be worried about your sexual relationship. Tell me a little more about what you're feeling."

Nursing Process To help Mr. Thomas, you will need to assess his knowledge and concerns, clearly identify his problems (elevated blood pressure and Sexuality Patterns Alteration), and develop a plan of care that is acceptable to him. When working with clients with sexual health concerns, tailor your approach to each individual's needs, just as you do in all areas of health.

Caring

♥ **iCare   Self-Knowledge** To help clients identify and resolve sexual health concerns, you will need to examine your own beliefs and values. The self-knowledge gained from examining your own views on sexuality will help you to be open to your clients' sexual concerns. What are your beliefs about sex and sexuality? Are you uncomfortable around people whose sexual orientation is different from yours? Imagine how you would feel if Frank Thanee asked you for help with his family relationships.

Nursing Care Plan

Client Data

Emilio Juarez is a 50-year-old man hospitalized for cardiac monitoring after an acute myocardial infarction (MI; heart attack). He has no history of diabetes or hypertension. Mr. Juarez owns a computer software company and is active in the community (president of the Chamber of Commerce).

After dinner, Mr. Juarez's nurse sits down to teach Emilio and his wife, Luz, about the medications that he will be taking. The nurse also begins to talk to them about a cardiac rehabilitation program. Mr. Juarez asks, "What do you mean by 'activity restriction'? Do I have to stop doing all the things I did before?" The nurse asks, "What things are you thinking about?" Mr. Juarez hesitates, then says, "Oh, like working in the yard, going up the stairs, and, you know, personal things." Mrs. Juarez immediately says, "There is no need to talk about that now. The most important thing is for my Emilio to feel better and get home—there is plenty of time for other things later." The nurse tells the Juarezes that many couples are anxious about resuming sexual activity after a heart attack and says, "I'd like to give you some information about that and answer any questions you might have."

Nursing Diagnosis

Sexuality Pattern Alterations related to lack of knowledge about post-MI sexual activity and reluctance to ask questions, as evidenced by Mrs. Juarez's comment, "There is no need to talk about that now."

NOC Outcomes	Individualized Goals / Expected Outcomes
Sexual Identity (1207) Sexual Functioning (0119) Body Image (1200)	*By discharge, Mr. Juarez will:* 1. Be able to identify two resources he can use to learn more about sexual activity after MI. 2. Commit to attending the cardiac rehabilitation classes offered at the hospital. *During and by the end of the cardiac rehabilitation program, Mr. Juarez will:* 1. Identify stressors in his life related to sexual activity. 2. Report a desire to resume sexual activity to pre-MI levels. 3. Resume previous sexual activity. 4. Discuss any problems encountered.

NIC Interventions/Activities

NIC Interventions	Rationale
Sexual counseling (5248) Body image enhancement (5220) Anxiety reduction (5820)	

Nursing Activities	Rationale
1. Initiate discussions about sexual activity after MI, beginning with general, nonthreatening statements. Reassure Mr. Juarez that sexual activity after recovery from an MI presents no greater risk of another MI.	Clients and significant others are often too embarrassed to ask about sexual matters. ■ The client's perception of his sexuality affects personal and social behavior outside the bedroom (Steinke et al., 2016). ■ Lack of counseling and education on resuming sexual activity was associated with a loss of sexual activity 1 year after MI (Cohen et al., 2022; Lindau et al., 2016). ■ Clients should understand any risks that sexual activity may have on their recovery. Providers must incorporate all factors and tailor the discussion to the client's situation (Steinke et al., 2016).

Nursing Care Plan (continued)

Nursing Activities	Rationale
2. Allow Mr. Juarez the opportunity to bring up concerns regarding sexual activity, but be prepared to include the topic in your teaching if he does not.	■ The subject of sexual activity should be raised with patients within the context of cardiac rehabilitation (Cohen et al., 2022). This shows respect for the client's privacy and his sexuality. ■ Both the provider and patient may expect each other to initiate the discussion on resuming sexual activity (Steinke et al., 2016).
3. Listen carefully to Mr. Juarez's verbal and nonverbal expressions of concerns.	■ Anxiety interferes with patients' return to sexual activity after an acute cardiovascular event (Cohen et al., 2022; Lindau et al., 2016). ■ Some patients may overtly express uninterest in discussing sexual matters; others avoid the topic by joking, avoiding eye contact, or brushing off concerns as not pressing. ■ Patients may avoid verbalizing feelings in this area because of the personal nature and threats to their gender identity. ■ Although depressive symptoms are more common in women after an MI and contribute to higher rates of rehospitalization, men also show depression (Cohen et al., 2022; Lindau et al., 2016).
4. Seek consultation from other members of the healthcare team as needed.	When nurses are uncomfortable talking about sexual matters and do not initiate the conversation, the client may think sexual activity is prohibited after MI. It is imperative that healthcare professionals incorporate sexuality into the plan of care to effectively meet the care needs of their clients (Cohen et al., 2022; Seitzer, 2022).
5. Include Mrs. Juarez in counseling as much as possible, with Mr. Juarez's consent.	■ Marriage and close interpersonal relationships allow each member to support the other and alleviate the negative effects of stress. ■ Sexual activity is a component of quality of life and a healthy marital lifestyle (Cohen et al., 2022; Gök & Demir, 2018). ■ The client and their spouse may have different perceptions of recovery, anticipated needs, sexuality, and other uncertainties that must be addressed to minimize stress (Steinke et al., 2016).
6. Be clear about exploring the Juarezes' specific concerns and correct any misinformation.	■ Anxiety about sexual activity after MI often arises from misconceptions (Gök & Demir, 2018). ■ Regular exercise, such as in a cardiac rehabilitation program, reduces the risk of MI from sexual activity (Boothby et al., 2018). ■ The typical period of maximum risk (which is still very low) is within 4 weeks of the MI (Lindau et al., 2016). ■ Exercise training after acute MI improves cardiovascular efficiency and reduces myocardial oxygen demand during customary activities, including sexual activity. ■ For some cardiac patients, sexual problems begin before a heart attack. Erectile dysfunction, the consistent inability to sustain an erection, affects more than 50% of the male population older than 60 and is a recognized symptom of cardiovascular disease (Steinke et al., 2016).
7. Discuss the risks of using drugs for erectile dysfunction together with nitrates.	An unsafe drop in blood pressure can occur when erectile dysfunction medication is taken with nitrates (Lee & Gerriets, 2022). Patients should be taught to contact their prescribers if they experience an erection lasting more than 4 hours or if a change in vision occurs.

(continued)

Nursing Care Plan (continued)

Evaluation

After Mrs. Juarez left for the evening, the nurse returned to bring Mr. Juarez a medication. He said, "Thanks for bringing that up and for leaving the booklet. I love my wife, and I was worried. I sure didn't want to have another heart attack. She was embarrassed to let on that it is important to her, but we will be sure to make use of the rehab program." The nurse followed up later by giving the Juarezes a link to a video and other resources that discuss sexual issues, which they can access at home and watch in privacy and comfort when they are ready to do so.

References

Boothby, C., et al. (2018). The effects of cardiac rehabilitation attendance on sexual activity outcomes in cardiovascular disease patients: A systematic review. *Canadian Journal of Cardiology, 34*(12), 1590–1599. https://doi.org/10.1016/j.cjca.2018.08.020

Cohen, G., Nevo, D., Hasin, T., Benyamini, Y., Goldbourt, U., & Gerberet, Y. (2022). Resumption of sexual activity after acute myocardial infarction and long-term survival. *European Journal of Preventive Cardiology, 29*(2), 304–311, https://doi.org/10.1093/eurjpc/zwaa011

Gök, F., & Demir, F. (2018). Sexual counseling provided by cardiovascular nurses. *Journal of Cardiovascular Nursing, 33*(6), E24–E30. https://doi.org/10.1097/JCN.0000000000000535.

Lee, P., & Gerriets, V. (2022). Nitrates. *StatPearls.* https://www.ncbi.nlm.nih.gov/books/NBK545149/

Lindau, S., D'Onofrio, G., Lichtman, J. H., Lorenze, N. P., Mehta Sanghani, R., Spatz, E. A., Spertus, J. A., Strait, K. M., Wroblewski, K., Zhou, S., & Krumholz, H. M. (2016). Sexual activity and function in the year after an acute myocardial infarction among younger women and men in the United States and Spain. *Journal of American Medical Association Cardiology, 1*(7), 754–764. https://doi.org/10.1001/jamacardio.2016.2362

Steinke, E. E., & Jaarsma, T. (2015). Sexual counseling and cardiovascular disease: Practical approaches. *Asian Journal of Andrology, 17*(1), 32–39. https://doi.org/10.4103/1008-682X.135982

Steinke, E., Johansen, P. P., & Dusenbury, W. (2016). When the topic turns to sex: Case scenarios in sexual counseling and cardiovascular disease. *Journal of Cardiopulmonary Rehabilitation and Prevention, 36*(3), 145–156. https://doi.org/10.1097/HCR.0000000000000155

Care Map

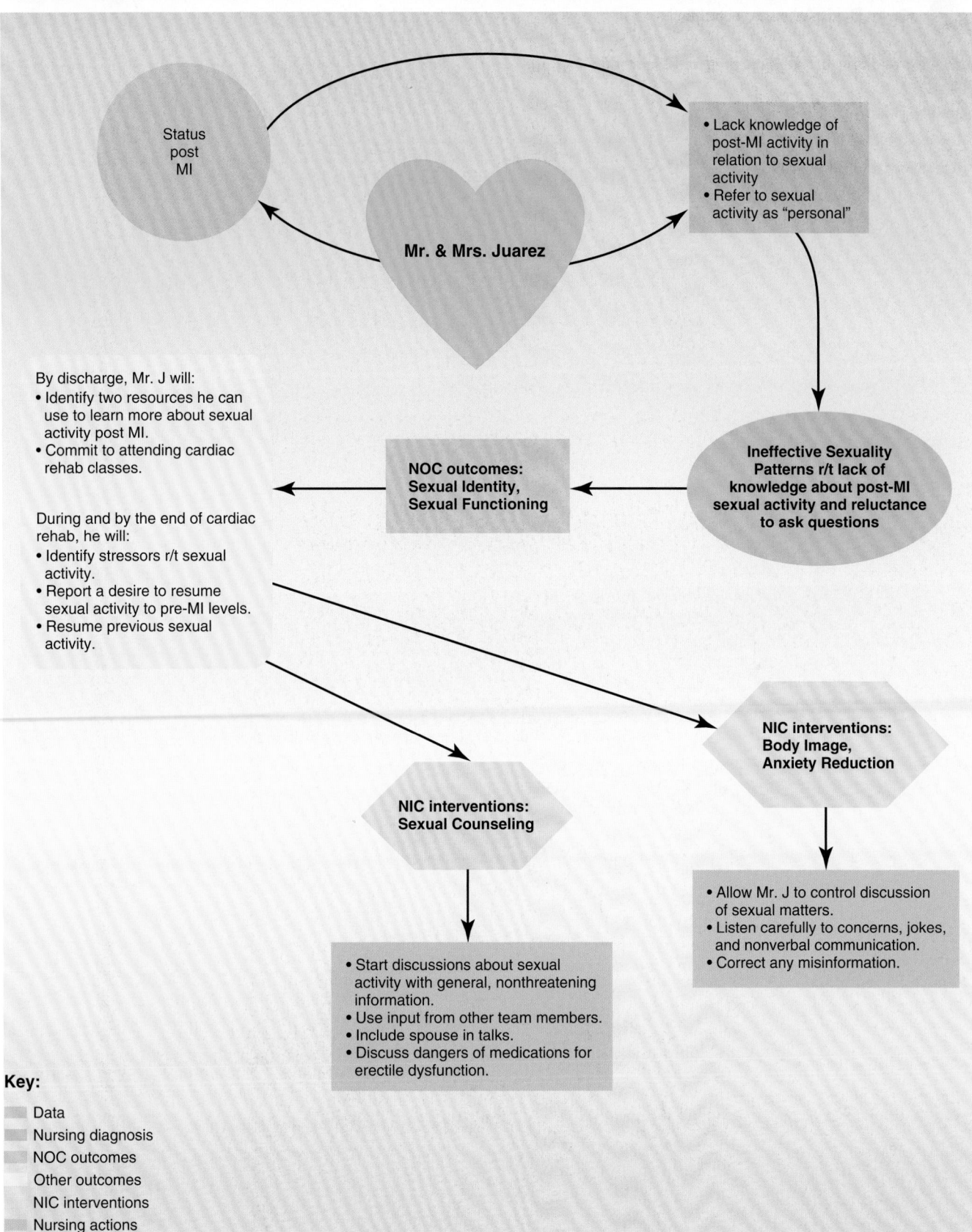

Status post MI

Mr. & Mrs. Juarez

- Lack knowledge of post-MI activity in relation to sexual activity
- Refer to sexual activity as "personal"

By discharge, Mr. J will:
- Identify two resources he can use to learn more about sexual activity post MI.
- Commit to attending cardiac rehab classes.

During and by the end of cardiac rehab, he will:
- Identify stressors r/t sexual activity.
- Report a desire to resume sexual activity to pre-MI levels.
- Resume previous sexual activity.

**NOC outcomes:
Sexual Identity,
Sexual Functioning**

Ineffective Sexuality Patterns r/t lack of knowledge about post-MI sexual activity and reluctance to ask questions

**NIC interventions:
Body Image,
Anxiety Reduction**

**NIC interventions:
Sexual Counseling**

- Allow Mr. J to control discussion of sexual matters.
- Listen carefully to concerns, jokes, and nonverbal communication.
- Correct any misinformation.

- Start discussions about sexual activity with general, nonthreatening information.
- Use input from other team members.
- Include spouse in talks.
- Discuss dangers of medications for erectile dysfunction.

Key:

- Data
- Nursing diagnosis
- NOC outcomes
- Other outcomes
- NIC interventions
- Nursing actions

To explore learning resources for this chapter,

Go to Davis Advantage and find:

Answers and Suggested Responses for all questions in this chapter

Concept Map

Knowledge Map

References and Bibliography

CHAPTER 31

Sleep & Rest

Learning Outcomes

After completing this chapter, you should be able to:

➤ Explain why rest and sleep are important.

➤ Describe the functions and physiology of sleep.

➤ Explain circadian rhythms and how they relate to sleep.

➤ Identify factors that influence rest and sleep.

➤ Discuss how sleep affects physical, mental, and spiritual well-being.

➤ Describe nursing implications for age-related differences in the sleep cycle.

➤ Identify at least five common sleep disorders.

➤ Perform a comprehensive sleep assessment using appropriate interview questions, a sleep diary, and a sleep history.

➤ Formulate nursing diagnoses that identify sleep problems that may be treated through specific nursing interventions.

➤ Plan, implement, and evaluate nursing care related to specific nursing diagnoses addressing sleep problems.

Key Concepts

Rest

Sleep

Related Concepts

See the Concept Map on Davis Advantage.

Example Client Condition

Sleep Apnea

Meet Your Patient

You are a nurse working on a surgical unit. Today you are meeting with Anna for preoperative teaching. She is scheduled for a complete hysterectomy next Monday. She has a secondary diagnosis of fibromyalgia, a chronic disorder characterized by widespread muscle pain and nonrestorative sleep.

Anna is a 49-year-old married woman with three children. She works full time and manages the family with her husband. She says, "I'm a little nervous about the surgery, but I know I need it. But I haven't been sleeping well because of thinking about it." Anna tells you that she has had trouble sleeping for the last 20 years. "I take an Ambien pill, 10 mg, every night to help me sleep. Will I be able to get that in the hospital? I really can't sleep at all without it," explains Anna.

As you continue the interview, Anna explains that she suffered from physical and emotional abuse as a young woman and has had sleep problems ever since. She has been to counseling, but that did not improve her sleep. Recently, her sleep has been even more troublesome. In addition to her upcoming surgery, she has been coping with the recent death of her father. You realize that sleep-promoting measures will be an important part of her nursing care.

What clues would cause you to suspect that Anna will have difficulty sleeping while in the hospital? What characteristics of the hospital environment might interfere with Anna's sleep? You may not have enough theoretical knowledge and experience to feel confident about your answers to these questions, but use your present knowledge and your life experiences to think about them.

TheoreticalKnowledge
knowing why

Have you felt tired after waking up from a night's sleep? Have you ever been tired, but not sleepy, and after relaxing for a while, felt your normal energy return? How do you think sleep and rest are different? How are they alike? This chapter will help you to make those distinctions and explain why both are important to health and wellness.

ABOUT THE KEY CONCEPTS

In this chapter, we will examine the concepts of rest and sleep, along with related concepts (e.g., stages of sleep, sleep disorders).

Rest is a condition in which the body is inactive or engaging in mild activity, after which the person feels refreshed. A person at rest is calm, at ease, relaxed, and free of stress and exertion (Fig. 31-1). People rest by doing things that they find calming and relaxing.

Sleep is a cyclically occurring state of decreased motor activity and perception (Fig. 31-2). Body functions slow, and metabolism slows considerably to conserve energy for bodily restoration and healing. Sleep is characterized by altered consciousness: a sleeping person is unaware of the environment and responds selectively to external stimuli. For example, an alarm clock, bright light, or other meaningful stimuli usually awaken a sleeper, but low-volume background noises and soft light do not.

Although necessary and beneficial, rest without sleep is inadequate. **Key Point:** *At rest, the body is affected by exterior stimuli, whereas in sleep, it is screened from them by altered consciousness. Thus, sleep replenishes the body; rest alone is not as restorative as sleep.*

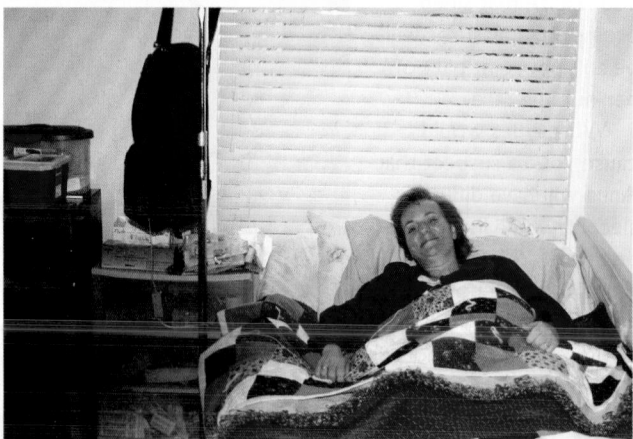

FIGURE 31-1 Patient receiving hospice care resting comfortably.

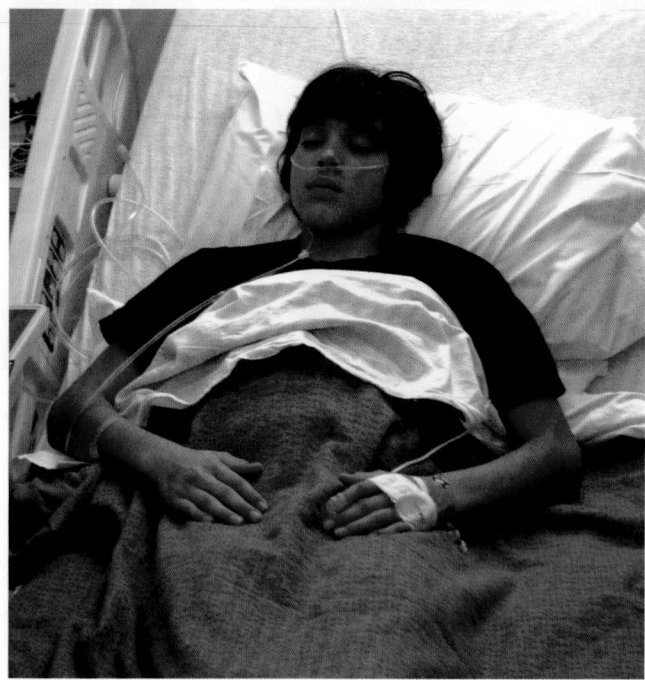

FIGURE 31-2 Child sleeping in hospital setting.

WHY DO WE NEED TO SLEEP?

We spend more time sleeping than in any other activity. So why is sleep so important? Before you try to answer, think back to the last time you slept poorly. Remember the mental fogginess, the physical fatigue, the feeling of slight nausea? Poor-quality sleep or an insufficient length of sleep for even one night can reduce mental performance and affect mood; long periods of sleep deprivation can result in stress-related illnesses. Sleep deprivation is a major cause of fatal sleepiness-related motor vehicle accidents (Kalsi et al., 2018).

- **Sleep affects almost every tissue in our bodies.** Sleep isn't essential just for the brain; it also affects growth and stress hormones, and even hormones that affect appetite and control body weight. Sleep also strengthens the immune system to help the body fight infection (Ackermann et al., 2012; Cohen et al., 2009; Irwin & Opp, 2017). A lack of sleep increases the risk of heart disease and stroke (Bhagavan, 2021; Fan et al., 2020; Javaheri et al., 2019; Tobaldini et al., 2017) and suppresses the immune system, which increases the susceptibility to viral infections (Ragnoli et al., 2022) and possibly even cancer (Chen et al., 2018; Hakin et al., 2014).
- **Sleep is an important regulator of energy metabolism.** Despite the fact that some regions of the brain are more active during sleep than when we are awake, total energy output is reduced during sleep, giving the body the opportunity for restoration and repair. However, sleep fragmentation may lead to changes in glucose metabolism involving leptin, ghrelin, and appetite-regulating hormones (Mosavat et al., 2021; Stamatakis & Punjabi, 2010). The body is less

able to tolerate glucose and yet responds with insulin resistance (Huang & Redline, 2019). Additionally, not enough sleep leads to reduced energy expenditure, obesity, and an increased risk of type 2 diabetes (Broussard et al., 2012; Lee et al., 2016; Parameswaran & Ray, 2021). On the other hand, too much sleep is often related to depression and anxiety, a sedentary lifestyle, habitual late sleeping, and poor dietary habits (Tan et al., 2017).

- **Sleep may improve learning and adaptation.** It gives the person a chance to mentally repeat and rehearse facts and situations before they are encountered in wakeful life. Sleep and dreaming may facilitate the storage of long-term memory by assisting the brain in reorganizing and storing information. Adequate sleep helps to improve processing of information, increase attention and creativity, and aid in decision making.
- **Sleep also appears to reduce stress and anxiety,** improving coping and concentration on activities of daily living.
- **More sleep also lessens the body's sensitivity to pain** (Roehrs et al., 2012; Simonelli et al., 2019). Similarly, nonrestorative sleep lowers pain tolerance (Sivertsen et al, 2015; Staffe et al., 2019), which is common in older adults (McBeth et al., 2014).
- **Sleep/rest and illness are interrelated** (Fig. 31-3). Illness and injury increase the need for sleep and at the same time make it difficult to sleep. In turn, a lack of sleep increases the susceptibility to illness by compromising the immune system (Hui et al., 2007). People who are ill or experience pain need more sleep to restore the energy needed for tissue repair and healing. However, they often have difficulty resting or sleeping because of pain and other symptoms of their illness.

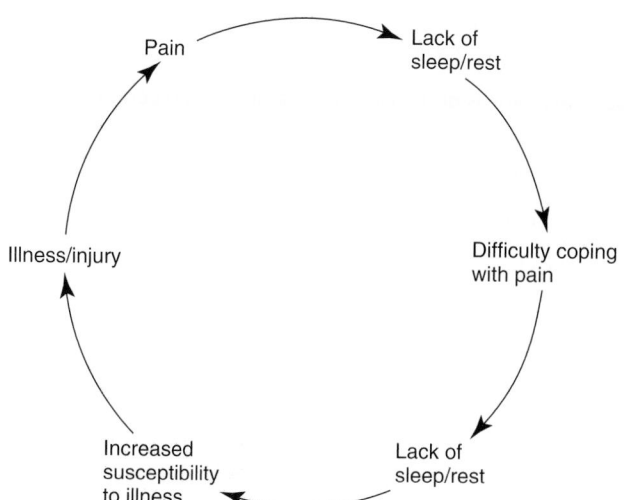

FIGURE 31-3 Relationship between sleep/rest and illness. Lack of sleep and rest increases susceptibility to illness. Likewise, the pain and stress of illness disturb sleep.

KnowledgeCheck 31-1

- Compare and contrast sleep and rest. How are they different? Alike?
- Why is promoting sleep an important nursing intervention?

 ThinkLike a Nurse 31-1: Clinical Judgment in Action

What effect do you think surgery will have on Anna's sleep (Meet Your Patient)? Why?

PICOT

Acupuncture for Neuropathic Pain

Situation: The nurse is caring for a client with peripheral neuropathy secondary to type 2 diabetes with poor glucose control. The client is showing signs of daytime drowsiness, irritability, and restlessness. They state they have trouble sleeping but do not want to take medication for pain.

PICOT Components

P	Population/client	= Sleep-deprived adults with chronic pain
I	Intervention/indicator	= Exercise
C	Comparator/control	= No exercise
O	Outcome	= Decreased pain and increased sleep
T	Time	= (none needed)

Searchable Question

Do _____ (P) who receive/are exposed to _____ (I) demonstrate _____ (O) compared with _____ (C)?

Example of Evidence

Persistent neuropathic pain can interfere with quality of life and impair sleep. Intensive lifestyle interventions are emerging as effective treatment strategies to reduce pain caused by peripheral nerve dysfunction. Patients with type 2 diabetes who engaged in an exercise intervention (supervised aerobic exercise with or without resistance training) reported a reduction in diabetic nerve pain. Therefore, the client with neuropathic pain who engages in a regular exercise program rests more comfortably and can minimize the sleep disturbances that impair the sleep–rest cycle.

Application to Practice

The client who reports unsatisfactory sleep requires a more in-depth sleep history, including questions about the quality of sleep, sleep hygiene, napping, and bedtime routines. A complete medication and pain history should be obtained. Because sleep disturbance may increase a patient's pain, the nurse may decide to explore with the healthcare team the possibility of suggesting an exercise regime to a patient who is dealing with chronic pain.

Ang, L., Cowdin, N., Mizokami-Stout, & Pop-Busui, R. (2018, August). Update on the management of diabetic neuropathy. *Diabetes Spectrum, 31*(3), 224–233. https://doi.org/10.2337/ds18-0036

HOW MUCH SLEEP DO WE NEED?

Key Point: *Sleep needs vary widely among individuals. Even though the accepted standard has been 7 to 9 hours per night for adults, there is no definitive amount or pattern of sleep that is best suited for all people.* Some people are refreshed after napping for 20 minutes;

others feel groggy after napping; others cannot nap at all. Many people routinely awaken several times a night and do not report being tired, whereas others report fatigue and loss of mental clarity if their sleep is even minimally interrupted. Despite individual variations, however, different sleep patterns are characteristic of different age-groups (Table 31-1).

Table 31-1 ➤ Typical Sleep Requirements and Characteristics

AGE-GROUP	HOURS PER DAY	SLEEP-RELATED ONSIDERATIONS
Newborns (birth–4 wk)	15–18	▪ Sleep occurs in short periods of 2 to 4 hours at a time. ▪ Sleep cycles are not related to circadian rhythm. ▪ Premature infants sleep more. Infants with colic sleep less.
Infants (4 wk–1 yr)	12–16	▪ Sleep–wake patterns begin about 6 weeks of age. ▪ Day–night confusion ends. ▪ In the first year, most will nap in the morning and afternoon.
Toddlers (1–2 yr)	11–14	▪ By 18–21 months, most take only one nap per day. ▪ Most infants sleep several hours during the overnight period, with a morning and afternoon nap each day.
Preschoolers (3–6 yr)	10–13	▪ Naps gradually get shorter.
Middle and late childhood (6–12 yr)	9–12	▪ Children with insufficient sleep experience problems with behavior, coping, and school performance, as well as health risks (e.g., headaches, hypertension, obesity, depression). ▪ Children who do not get enough sleep are more likely to show less interest in learning new things, have higher odds of not doing homework, and care less about doing well in school (Gordon, 2019).
Adolescents (13–18 yr)	8–10	▪ Screen time and technology use commonly interfere with sufficient sleep. ▪ Sleepier teens are more likely to fail to stay calm when faced with a challenge. They are also less likely to complete homework and show curiosity in a learning situation (Gordon, 2019). ▪ Sleep-deprived adolescents commonly experience health issues, especially shoulder and neck pain, fatigue, and dizziness (Paiva et al., 2015).
Young and middle adults (18–64 yr)	7–8	▪ In some cultures, total sleep time is divided into an overnight sleep period and a midafternoon nap. ▪ Hormone changes with menopause commonly interfere with quality sleep.
Older adults (65 years and older)	7–9	▪ Sleep may be more fragmented with rest or naps during the day. ▪ About half of those 60 years or older take longer to fall asleep, wake up too often, or have a hard time staying asleep. ▪ Frequent waking is commonly a result of physical discomfort, anxiety, and nocturia. ▪ If sleep is interrupted, older adults may experience fatigue, irritability, and impaired cognition. ▪ Older adults are more likely than younger people to suffer from obstructive sleep apnea, restless legs syndrome, or periodic limb movement disorder.

Sources: Centers for Disease Control and Prevention. (2017, March 2). *How much sleep do I need?* http://www.cdc.gov/sleep/about_sleep/how_much_sleep.html; Paruthi, S., Brooks, L. J., D'Ambrosio, C., Hall, W.A., Kotagal, S., Lloyd, R. M., Malow, B.A., Maski, K., Nichols, C., Quan, S. F., Rosen, C. L., Troester, M.W., & Wise, M. S. (2016, May 25). Recommended amount of sleep for pediatric populations: A statement of the American Academy of Sleep Medicine. *Journal of Clinical Sleep Medicine, 12*(6), 785–786. https://doi.org/10.5664/jcsm.5866; American Academy of Pediatrics. (2016, June 13). *American Academy of Pediatrics supports childhood sleep guidelines.* https://blog.summit-education.com/wp-content/uploads/AAP-sleep-norms.pdf

ThinkLike a Nurse 31-2: Clinical Judgment in Action

- How much sleep might Anna (Meet Your Patient) need on a normal night?
- How will a good night of sleep benefit Anna while she is in the hospital?
- If you were preparing for an important test, would it be better to stay up all night studying, or should you try to get a good night of sleep?
- How many hours of sleep do *you* need to feel rested and function well the next day? Compare notes with family members, friends, and classmates. Do they all need the same amount of sleep as you?

PHYSIOLOGY OF SLEEP

Our environment plays a role in the physiology of our sleep, so let's begin with an exploration of circadian rhythms, by which the body maintains synchronicity with nature. **Synchrony** occurs when something happens at the same time or works or develops on the same time scale as something else.

How Do Circadian Rhythms Influence Sleep?

Biorhythms are "biological clocks" that are controlled within the body and synchronized with environmental factors (e.g., gravity, electromagnetic forces, light, and darkness). Biorhythms influence many physical and mental functions.

> *Examples:* (1) Body temperature is typically lowest when the person wakes up in the morning. (2) Female menstruation follows an approximately 28-day cycle, like the lunar cycle on which our calendar months are based.

Do you feel sleepy at about the same time each night? Do you often awaken before the alarm clock goes off? If so, that's because the timing of sleeping and waking is influenced by your circadian biorhythm. A **circadian rhythm** is a biorhythm based on the day–night pattern in a 24-hour cycle. A person's circadian rhythm is regulated by a cluster of cells in the hypothalamus of the brainstem that responds to changing levels of light. Circadian rhythm affects our overall level of functioning:

> *Example:* Most people have a higher energy level in the daytime and less energy at night. However, some people are more alert and active in the morning, and others function at a higher level in the afternoon or evening.

Key Point: *Sleep quality is best when the time at which you go to sleep and wake up is in synchrony with your circadian rhythm* (Kim & Duffy, 2018), as in the following examples:

- **People who work evening and night shifts** can suffer significant sleep deprivation until their bodies adjust to the new pattern (see the accompanying Self-Care box, Fatigue and Sleep Deprivation Among Healthcare Workers).
- **Changing time zones** can also disrupt sleep–wake cycles and can thus be troublesome for people who travel frequently.
- **Hospitalization** can also interfere with a patient's circadian rhythm. Noises, lights, waking the patient for vital signs or medications, altered normal bedtime rituals, absence or presence of family members, homesickness, recent losses, worry, fear of the unknown, and pain may compromise the patient's quality of sleep and the ability to fall and stay asleep (Astin et al., 2020; Auckley, 2022).

ThinkLike a Nurse 31-3: Clinical Judgment in Action

What may upset Anna's (Meet Your Patient) circadian rhythm?

Self-Care

Fatigue and Sleep Deprivation Among Healthcare Workers

 Extended hours and rotating shift work significantly increase fatigue and impair on-the-job performance and safety.

Impact of Fatigue

➤ Lapses in attention and memory; poor concentration

➤ Irritability

➤ Reduced motivation, apathy, and indifference

➤ Diminished reaction time

➤ Impaired judgment and decision making

➤ Altered communication

➤ More errors, needlestick and sharp-related injuries, and adverse events to patients

Fight Sleepiness on the Job

➤ Be honest with yourself about how you tolerate rotating shifts, night shifts, and longer shifts (e.g., 12 hours), and schedule accordingly. Plan rest days in between consecutive workdays.

➤ Engage in conversation with others; do not just listen and nod.

➤ Do something that requires physical action periodically, even if it means just getting up and moving around.

➤ Take frequent breaks (e.g., every 1 to 2 hours) during the night shift, if possible.

➤ Be smart about your caffeine use; that is, don't take caffeine when you don't need it to stay awake, and avoid caffeine at the end of your shift before sleep.

➤ Practice good sleep hygiene measures during your off hours. See the Self-Care box, Teaching Your Patients About Sleep Hygiene.

Source: The Joint Commission. (2011; 2018, May 14, addendum). Health care worker fatigue and patient safety. *The Joint Commission Sentinel Event Alert, 48,* 1–4.

How Is Sleep Regulated?

What makes us fall asleep? What happens in the brain during sleep? The mechanisms of sleep are complex and poorly understood, but we know that sleep is controlled by the lower part of the brain that produces sleep by actively inhibiting wakefulness. As just noted, a major factor in regulating sleep is the amount of light received through the eyes. The increasing light of the sky at dawn signals the hypothalamus (Fig. 31-4) to induce gradual arousal from sleep.

Reticular Activating System A collection of nerve cell bodies within the brainstem, called the **reticular formation,** is responsible for maintaining wakefulness. The reticular formation is activated by stimuli from the cerebral cortex. Together, these reticular and cortical neurons are called the *reticular activating system* (RAS). Neurotransmitters associated with excitatory and inhibitory sleep mechanisms include catecholamines, acetylcholine, serotonin, histamine, and prostaglandins.

An **electroencephalogram (EEG)** is used to record the electrical activity of the neurons in the brain. Electrical impulses are transmitted from the brain through electrodes attached to the scalp. These impulses create five different wave patterns, or *brain waves.* Figure 31-5 shows examples of different types of brain waves during sleep:

- **Alpha waves** are high-frequency, medium-amplitude, irregular waves. These occur in the drowsy stage.
- **Beta waves** are high-frequency, low-amplitude, irregular waves. These occur during periods of wakefulness.
- **Spindles** or **K-complexes** are peaked, irregular waveforms that occur in the earlier phases of non–rapid eye movement (NREM) sleep.

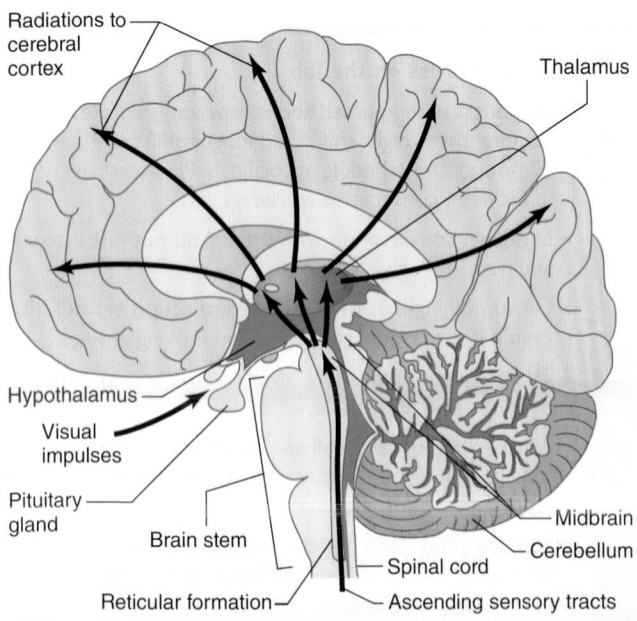

FIGURE 31-4 The reticular activating system works to regulate sleep and wakefulness.

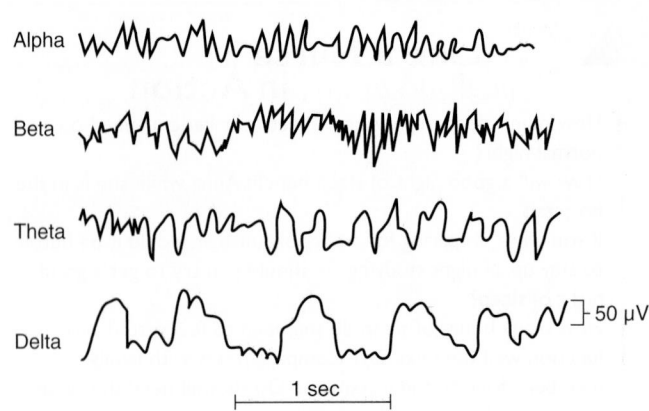

FIGURE 31-5 Types of brain waves.

- **Theta waves** are high-amplitude waves that are common in children but rare in adults. These occur with delta waves when transitioning to a deeper sleep stage.
- **Delta waves** are low-frequency, high-amplitude, regular waves common in deep sleep.

The EEG of a waking person differs greatly from that of a sleeping person. In general, the greater the brain activity is, the more rapid will be the brain waves on the EEG.

- **While the person is awake,** brain waves are very rapid, irregular, and low in amplitude, mostly alpha and beta waves. Many neurons are firing at different intervals, at different times, and with different strengths.
- **When a person is relaxed,** without intense stimulation of the senses, the EEG records mostly alpha activity.
- **During sleep,** alpha waves disappear. They are replaced by slower, higher-amplitude delta waves.

What Are the Stages of Sleep?

Key Point: *There are two distinct types of sleep, NREM and rapid eye movement (REM). The body moves between them during the sleep cycle.*

NREM Sleep

NREM sleep is generally the restful phase of sleep in which physiological function is slow. NREM sleep is also called *deep* or *slow-wave sleep (SWS)* because it is characterized by the presence of delta waves.

- Cortisol (stress hormone) is lowest during this phase.
- NREM is divided into three stages, each deeper than the one preceding it. The parasympathetic branch of the autonomic nervous system becomes progressively more dominant during each NREM stage.
- During NREM sleep, muscles relax; body temperature lowers; and heart rate, respirations, and blood pressure decrease.
- This phase is thought to be important for *memory consolidation;* this is when information or skills move into long-term memory.

REM Sleep

During **REM** sleep, the brain becomes highly active, and the brain waves resemble those of a person who is fully awake. Rapid eye movements occur, which can often be detected even though the sleeper's eyelids are closed.

- More spontaneous awakenings occur during the REM stage than any other.
- Most dreams occur during REM sleep.
- REM sleep is essential for mental and emotional restoration.
- Loss of REM sleep impairs memory and learning.

A person who is deprived of REM sleep for several nights will usually experience *REM rebound*; that is, the person will spend a greater amount of time in REM sleep on successive nights, keeping the total amount of REM sleep constant over time.

Sleep Cycles

Key Point: *Cycling between REM and NREM sleep produces restorative rest.* The American Academy of Sleep Medicine identifies four stages of sleep (three NREM stages and the REM stage), based on brain activity and other physiological characteristics (Table 31-2). The NREM/REM sleep cycle repeats four to six times throughout the night, depending on the total amount of time spent sleeping (Fig. 31-6). Each cycle lasts, on average, 90 to 100 minutes. The first REM period may last only about 20 minutes, but with each cycle, the REM period lengthens until, in the last cycle of a typical 8-hour sleep period, REM may last as long as 60 minutes. The amount of time spent in each sleep stage varies over the life span.

KnowledgeCheck 31-2

- List the stages of sleep.
- Describe the progression of a typical sleep cycle for a young adult.
- Describe the physiological activity characteristic of each stage of sleep.
- What is the stage that must be "made up" if not enough time is spent in it?

Table 31-2 ➤ Characteristics of Stages of Sleep

Stage: W (Wakefulness)

TYPICAL BRAIN-WAVE TYPE	CHARACTERISTICS
Beta waves with some alpha waves	Ranges from full alertness to the early stages of drowsiness
	Reading eye movements
	Eye blinks with eyes open or closed

Stage: Non–Rapid Eye Movement I (NREM)

TYPICAL BRAIN-WAVE TYPE	CHARACTERISTICS
Alpha waves with occasional low-frequency theta waves	Transition between wakefulness and sleep (falling asleep)
	Slow eye movements
	Light sleep; can be awakened easily
	Relaxed but aware of surroundings
	Groggy, heavy-lidded
	Regular, deep breathing; eyelids open and close slowly
	Accounts for about 5% of total sleep
	Dreams are usually not remembered

Stage: Non–Rapid Eye Movement II (NREM)

TYPICAL BRAIN-WAVE TYPE	CHARACTERISTICS
Theta waves, K-complexes, and sleep spindles	Light sleep
	Easily roused
	Temperature, heart rate, and blood pressure decrease slightly
	Accounts for about 50% of total sleep

(Continued)

Table 31-2 ➤ Characteristics of Stages of Sleep—cont'd

Stage: Non–Rapid Eye Movement III (NREMIII)

TYPICAL BRAIN-WAVE TYPE	CHARACTERISTICS
Delta waves; sawtooth waves	Deep sleep
	Difficult to rouse; if awakened in this stage, may be confused
	Parasympathetic nervous system predominates: temperature, pulse, respirations, and blood pressure slow even more.
	Skeletal muscles are very relaxed.
	Snoring may occur.
	Some dreaming may occur, but dreams are less vivid than those that occur in rapid eye movement (REM) sleep. This sleep stage is especially important for restorative processes such as healing, growth, and muscle and tissue repair.
	Makes up 20%– 25% of total sleep time

Stage: Rapid Eye Movement (REM)

REM	TYPICAL BRAIN-WAVE TYPE	CHARACTERISTICS
	5–30 minutes (usually at least 20–30)	Highly active sleep with spontaneous awakenings
		Less restful than NREM sleep
		Eyes move rapidly, and small muscles twitch.
		Essential for mental and emotional restoration
		Metabolism, temperature, pulse, and blood pressure increase.
		Pulse may be rapid and irregular.
		Apnea may occur.
		Gastric secretions increase.
		Deep-tendon reflexes are depressed.
		Dreaming occurs.
		If awakened, person will react normally.
		Accounts for about 25% of total sleep

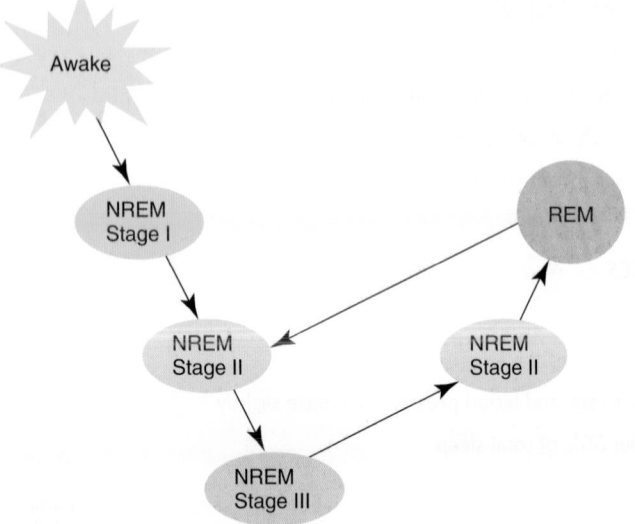

FIGURE 31-6 The normal adult sleep cycle.

ThinkLike a Nurse 31-4: Clinical Judgment in Action

- Anna's (Meet Your Patient) provider has prescribed zolpidem (Ambien) for her. Ambien is a sedative–hypnotic (nonbarbiturate) used in the short-term treatment of insomnia. Why do you think the provider prescribed medication to induce sleep even though Anna is physiologically and psychologically dependent on it?
- Anna will likely receive narcotic analgesics after surgery. How do you think they will affect her sleep?

WHAT FACTORS AFFECT SLEEP?

People vary not only in the amount of sleep they need but also in their sleep patterns. **Sleep quality** has both subjective and objective components. It is related to (1) the total amount of sleep, (2) how well the person slept, and (3) whether the person obtained the needed amounts of NREM and REM. Several factors affect the amount and quality of sleep.

Age

Age is an important factor affecting the duration of sleep (see Table 31-1). But sleep *patterns* are also affected by age.

Toddlers and Preschoolers Children in this age-group often have trouble falling asleep and may experience frequent awakenings, nightmares, and heavy snoring. They may have difficulty "winding down" after hectic activities in the late afternoon and early-evening hours.

School-Age Children and Adolescents Children and adolescents may suffer sleep disturbances related to stress, excitement, or social concerns, such as anticipating a school event or sports competition.

Adolescents Adolescents may not sleep well because of:

- Normal shifts in circadian rhythms that occur with puberty
- Increased demands at school or staying up late to complete assignments
- Evening use of electronic devices and sleeping with smartphones near their beds. The light produced by such devices disrupts circadian rhythms and suppresses naturally occurring melatonin, which results in difficulty falling asleep (Owens & Weiss, 2017; Pacheco & Vyas, 2022).
- Caffeine, alcohol, nicotine, or drugs

College Students College students may stay up all night to study for examinations or may experience difficulty falling asleep or staying asleep because of stress about grades or future career choices. Many have a preference for a late-night schedule, yet they have schedules requiring them to attend an early class.

Young Adults Young adults may:

- Drive themselves too hard to succeed, prompting late nights at work or sleep loss as a result of hectic travel schedules or work-related stress
- Not obtain enough sleep because of social and personal entertainment
- Work an evening or night shift

Parents of Young Children Parents with young children often experience sleep interruptions. Parents of toddlers often wake up to care for a child who is having a nightmare, is ill, or needs to use the bathroom.

Middle-Aged Adults Middle-aged adults may experience sleep difficulties because of depression, anxiety, and tension that result from stress and competing demands on time, such as:

- Work and family responsibilities
- The need to care for a parent

- Marital discord
- Worry about children
- Financial problems

The lack of sleep compounds the problem, leading to reduced ability to cope and again contributing to further difficulty achieving quality sleep.

Menopausal Patients Patients experiencing menopause may have trouble falling and staying asleep because of hormonal fluctuations. Obstructive sleep apnea (OSA) also plays a role in insufficient sleep.

Older Adults Older adults may experience sleep disturbances because of:

- Side effects of medications
- Underlying illnesses
- Depression
- Discomfort
- Nocturia
- Pain
- Declining levels of melatonin, which occur in the latter decades of life

Lifestyle Factors

Lifestyle factors influencing sleep include work, exercise, nutrition, and use of medications and drugs. For example, people who cross time zones frequently because of travel may experience difficulty falling asleep, early wakening, or daytime fatigue.

Physical Activity If exercise occurs at least 2 hours before bedtime, exercise promotes sleep. Fatigue from a normal physically active day is thought to promote a restful night's sleep. However, the more tired a person is, the shorter the first period of REM sleep will be. Also, a sedentary lifestyle is a factor in sleep disorders.

Diet Foods can either promote or interfere with sleep.

- **A meal high in saturated** fat near bedtime may interfere with sleep.
- **Dietary L-tryptophan and adenosine** are essential amino acids (meaning the body does not produce its own) found in milk, cheese, and animal products that may help to induce sleep by converting into serotonin.
- **Carbohydrates** seem to promote relaxation through their effects on brain serotonin levels. In general, satiation induces sleep, whereas many people, especially infants and children, have difficulty falling asleep when they are hungry.

Nicotine and Caffeine Central nervous system stimulants, such as nicotine and caffeine, interfere with sleep.

- **Nicotine**—Smokers tend to have more difficulty falling asleep and are more easily roused than non-smokers. People who stop smoking often experience temporary sleep disturbances during the withdrawal period.

- **Caffeine**—Caffeine blocks adenosine and thereby inhibits sleep. However, individuals vary greatly in their sensitivity to caffeine.

Alcohol
- **Disrupts REM.** Consumption of alcohol, especially if heavy, may hasten the onset of sleep; however, it disrupts REM and slow-wave sleep and may cause spontaneous awakenings with difficulty returning to sleep.
- **Vivid dreams in REM.** In some people, heavy alcohol consumption can prompt dreams that can lead to awakening during REM sleep.
- **Nocturia.** Because alcohol is a diuretic, it can interrupt sleep by inducing nocturia.

Medications Many of the medications people take cause either sleeplessness or excessive grogginess and sedation. Medications to induce sleep (i.e., hypnotics) tend to increase the amount of sleep while decreasing the quality.

- *Zolpidem tartrate* (Ambien) promotes normal REM sleep and appears to influence sleep quality less than other hypnotics.
- *Amphetamines, tranquilizers, and antidepressants* reduce the amount of REM sleep; barbiturates, in addition, interfere with NREM sleep.
- *Opioids,* such as morphine, suppress REM sleep and cause frequent awakening.
- *Beta blockers* are reported to cause sleep disorders and nightmares.

Illness

Illness increases the need for sleep and rest. At the same time, its associated mental and physical distress can cause sleep problems.

- **Disease symptoms,** such as fever, pain, nausea, and respiratory conditions (e.g., shortness of breath, dyspnea, sinus congestion), can also interfere with sleep.
- **Specific disease conditions** altering the quality of sleep include allergies, hyperthyroidism, and Parkinson disease.
- **Anxiety** increases gastric secretions, intestinal motility, heart rate, and respirations, all of which contribute to a restless night. Anxiety also stimulates the sympathetic nervous system, increasing the level of norepinephrine. This decreases stage III and REM sleep and leads to more awakenings.
- **Depression** may be associated either with too much sleep or with difficulty sleeping.
- **Fear of the unknown outcome** of an illness and **role changes** associated with hospitalization can cause anxiety and interfere will falling or staying asleep.

Environmental Factors

Environmental factors can promote or inhibit sleep. Some people need a cool room, whereas others need

warmth. Some prefer heavy blankets, and others like to sleep with just a light sheet.

Noise Noise can also inhibit sleep, but a person can become habituated to noise over time and be less affected by it. Any change in the usual environmental stimuli can affect sleep.

- Some people routinely fall asleep to music or while listening to the radio or television.
- Loud noises may be needed to awaken a person in NREM stages III and REM sleep.
- Equipment noise, the muffled sounds of a busy medical–surgical unit, or the labored breathing or snoring of a roommate can interfere with the patient's ability to sleep.

Light When people who are accustomed to sleeping in a dark room are hospitalized, they may have trouble falling asleep because of light outside their window or filtering into the room from the hallway. However, light can be therapeutic for some patients suffering from sleep problems. Exposure to bright light can alter circadian rhythms in some adults.

KnowledgeCheck 31-3

- For each of the following patients, propose at least two factors that might affect sleep:
  Newborn in the neonatal intensive care unit
  Preschooler being treated for pneumonia
  Adolescent with cancer
  Breastfeeding mother of an infant
  Older man who has fractured his hip
- Identify at least three types of environmental stimuli that can disturb sleep.

WHAT ARE SOME COMMON SLEEP DISORDERS?

Sleep disorders are classified by their signs and symptoms. The more common disorders fall into two groups:

- **Dyssomnias**—Sleep disorders characterized by insomnia or excessive sleepiness. They include insomnia, sleep–wake schedule (circadian) disorders, sleep apnea, restless legs syndrome, hypersomnia, and narcolepsy.
- **Parasomnias**—Patterns of waking behavior that appear during sleep (e.g., sleepwalking).

Insomnia

Insomnia, as defined by the *Diagnostic and Statistical Manual of Mental Disorders,* 5th edition *(DSM-5),* is the predominant complaint of dissatisfaction with sleep quantity, associated with the inability to fall asleep, remain asleep, or go back to sleep.

- **The sleep disturbance causes significant distress** or impairments in social, occupational, academic, behavioral, and other important areas of functioning.

- **True insomnia occurs at least 3 nights per week and is present for 3 months or longer**, even when there is ample opportunity for sleep (American Psychiatric Association, 2013).
- **Sleep difficulty may be** *transient/short term* (less than a month) **or** *chronic* (longer than a month). People with sleep difficulty usually report an insufficient quantity and quality of sleep and wake without feeling refreshed, even though they are often observed to sleep more than they perceive that they do.

Incidence Key Point: *Insomnia is the most common sleep disorder.* It is more prevalent in women and in older adults, those who suffer from chronic illness (e.g., hypertension, obesity, cancer, thyroid disorders [Budhiraja et al., 2011; Institute of Medicine, 2006]), and shift workers (Budhiraja et al., 2011).

In young adults, difficulties with sleep initiation are more common; in middle-aged and older adults, problems of maintaining sleep are more common (Chawla et al., 2022).

Etiologies Insomnia may occur as a result of:

- Illness, depression, anxiety disorders, acute stress, substance abuse
- A side effect of medications (e.g., steroids, central adrenergic blockers, bronchodilation agents)
- Poor sleep hygiene (e.g., watching TV in bed, drinking caffeine-containing beverages before bedtime)

Symptoms
- Daytime consequences of insomnia include symptoms of excessive daytime sleepiness, poor concentration, fatigue, lethargy, and irritability.
- Insomnia can also create an increased risk for depression, anxiety, and possibly cardiovascular disorders.
- Insomnia may be the presenting symptom of other primary sleep disorders, such as restless legs syndrome.

Treatment Primary care providers can diagnose and manage most cases of insomnia. Once underlying medical or psychiatric conditions have been identified and treated, a combination of behavioral and pharmacological therapy may be effective. The use of medication to induce sleep is controversial because some types of medication can become habit forming, can become less effective when taken continuously, and can have serious side effects. However, sedative–hypnotic treatment is justified in short-term insomnia to avoid the negative effects of insomnia on mood and performance. Short-term aggressive treatment may prevent the development of chronic insomnia.

Sleep–Wake Schedule (Circadian) Disorders

Abnormalities in sleep–wake schedules may be caused by rapid time-zone changes (jet lag), shift work (Witkoski Stimpfel et al., 2019), or a change in total sleep time from day to day. Symptoms include decreased vigilance, decreased ability to perform psychomotor tasks, and short sleep episodes *(microsleeps)* that the person is not aware of. People suffering a disruption in sleep–wake schedule can take several days to adjust their sleep pattern.

Restless Legs Syndrome

Restless legs syndrome (RLS) is a disorder of the central nervous system characterized by a strong and often overwhelming urge to move the legs while resting or before sleep onset.

Incidence Cases of RLS:

- Affect 2% to 10% of adults (Pacheco & Wright, 2022)
- Tend to run in families
- Tend to occur more often in women than in men

- Are especially common in older adults, although children and young adults also experience this condition
- Are sometimes associated with low levels of iron (Leung et al., 2022; National Institute of Neurological Disorders and Stroke [NINDS], 2022; Winkelman et al., 2016)
- Are associated with the use of certain antidepressants (Muth, 2017)

Symptoms The unpleasant creeping, crawling, itching, or tingling sensations in the legs are relieved only by moving the legs, which prevents the person from relaxing and falling asleep. People who have RLS also have a condition called **periodic limb movement** disorder (PLMD). PLMD involves repetitive flexing or twitching of the limbs while asleep. Unlike RLS, these movements are uncomfortable, and they occur during sleep, so patients are often not aware of them (Pacheco & Wright, 2022).

Management
Mild to moderate symptoms may be managed with lifestyle changes:

- Decrease alcohol and tobacco use.
- Avoid stimulants, such as caffeine.
- Maintain a regular sleep pattern.
- Follow a program of regular, moderate-intensity aerobic and leg-stretching exercise.
- Walking, massaging, stretching, heat or cold compresses, medication, vibration, and acupressure may all be beneficial.
- Apply a foot wrap with a pad that delivers vibration to the back of the leg and also puts pressure underneath the foot.

Moderate to severe symptoms of RLS may be treated with medication:

- **Dietary iron supplement** if serum ferritin and transferrin saturation levels are low (NINDS, 2022)
- **Dopaminergic** agents (increase dopamine levels) and medication used to treat Parkinson disease (e.g., ropinirole, pramipexole, rotigotine)

- **Anticonvulsants** (e.g., gabapentin enacarbil) to control the creeping and crawling sensation in the legs (Pacheco & Wright, 2022; NINDS, 2022)
- **Benzodiazepines** can help individuals get more restful sleep but should be reserved as a last choice because of side effects (daytime sleepiness, aggravation of sleep apnea).

Sleep Deprivation

Sleep Deprivation is a NANDA-I nursing diagnosis. It is not actually a sleep disorder but, rather, in NANDA-I terms, a human response to prolonged sleep disturbances (e.g., insomnia and parasomnias) involving NREM or REM deprivation or both.

Defining Characteristics Persons experiencing sleep deprivation are likely to:

- Feel drowsy during the day or a have a general feeling of malaise
- Have difficulty performing daily tasks
- Experience impaired cognitive processing, problem-solving, and decision making
- Have mood issues (impatient, irritable, unable to cope with problems, less socially engaged, more likely to experience depression) (Pacheco & Rehman, 2022)
- Exhibit restlessness, perceptual disorders, slowed reaction time, and irritability
- Exhibit somatic (body) complaints (e.g., hand tremors)
- Experience delusions, paranoia, and other psychotic behavior if sleep deprivation is severe and prolonged
- Have diminished body protection against infection

Etiologies Illness and hospital care are common causes of sleep deprivation, especially for patients in critical care units (CCUs). In this environment, lights are on most of the time, and equipment noise, frequent treatments, and assessments all combine with the client's fragile physical condition to create sleep deprivation.

✚ Likewise, healthcare providers who work long and late hours or rotating day–night shifts experience serious fatigue that can lead to reduced work productivity (Yang et al., 2018), medical error, and increased risk of occupational injury and patient injury (The Joint Commission, 2011, 2018; Pacheco & Rehman, 2022).

Hypersomnia

Hypersomnia is excessive sleeping, especially in the daytime.

- **Symptoms.** People with excessive daytime sleepiness doze, nap, or fall asleep at times and in situations when they need or wish to be awake and alert.
- **Etiologies.** Common causes of hypersomnia are OSA and narcolepsy; disorders of the central nervous system, kidney, or liver; and metabolic disorders (e.g., diabetic acidosis and hypothyroidism).
- Hypersomnia can also be a symptom of depression.

Sleep Apnea

Sleep apnea is a common disorder with serious consequences. Many people do not receive treatment because of improper diagnosis or because the idea of wearing a mask and using a machine at night is intolerable. Sleep with numerous pauses in breathing and frequent awakenings can affect quality of life and increase the risk of diabetes, high blood pressure, and cardiovascular diseases.

Narcolepsy

Narcolepsy is a chronic disorder caused by the brain's inability to regulate sleep–wake cycles normally. The distinction between being asleep and being awake is blurred. At various times, the person with narcolepsy experiences a sudden, uncontrollable urge to sleep lasting from seconds to minutes, even though the person sleeps well at night. The person cannot avoid the sleep episodes but awakens easily. Narcolepsy is controlled by central nervous system stimulants, such as methylphenidate (Ritalin), with little evidence of tolerance, dependence, or abuse.

Pseudonarcolepsy Pseudonarcolepsy is a condition characterized by involuntary episodes of sleep, but the episodes are related to acute or chronic sleep deprivation. When the person is well rested, the episodes resolve.

Defining Characteristics Narcolepsy is characterized by:

- Sleepiness, slurred speech, slackening of the facial muscles, a feeling of impending weakness of the knees, paralysis, and hallucinations
- Impaired performance during microsleep episodes
- ✚ Sleep episodes that come on suddenly, even while the person is alert and active. If they occur while the person is driving, working, or operating machinery, they can be dangerous.
- Awakening from episodes of unavoidable sleep feeling refreshed (NINDS, 2022)
- **Cataplexy,** a sudden loss of muscle tone, usually triggered by an emotional event (e.g., laughter, surprise, or anger). However, most patients only have hypersomnia.
- Intolerance of irregular sleep–wake patterns, such as shift work, and difficulty staying awake with passive activity, such as watching television.

KnowledgeCheck 31-4

- What is the most common dyssomnia?
- What factors in the hospital may contribute to sleep deprivation in patients?

Toward Evidence-Based Practice

Benito-González, E., Palacios-Ceña, M., Fernández-Muñoz, J. J., Castaldo, M., Wang, K., Catena, A., Arendt-Nielsen, L., Fernández-de-las-Peñas, C. (2018). Variables associated with sleep quality in chronic tension-type headache: A cross-sectional and longitudinal design. *PLOS ONE, 13*(5), e0197381. https://doi.org/10.1371/journal.pone.0197381

In a study involving 135 people with chronic tension-type headaches, investigators found a positive correlation between sleep quality and headache intensity, headache frequency, and headache duration.

Xu, M., Chattopadhyay, K., Qian, X., Li, X., Sun, J., & Li, L. (2022). Association between nocturnal sleep duration and obesity indicators among people with type 2 diabetes: A cross-sectional study in Ningbo, China. *Diabetes Metabolic Syndrome and Obesity, 15,* 1357–1364. https://doi.org/10.2147/DMSO.S350347

In a study of Chinese adults with type 2 diabetes mellitus, a shorter duration of sleep at night was associated with higher visceral and general obesity indicators (visceral fat area, subcutaneous fat area, waist circumference, body weight, and body mass index) after taking into account sociodemographic factors and health conditions.

Reutrakul, S., & Van Cauter, E. (2018, July). Sleep influence on obesity, insulin resistance, and risk of type 2 diabetes. *Metabolism, 84,* 56–66. https://doi.org/10.1016/j.metabol.2018.02.010

Of those studied, subjects receiving less sleep reported more hunger and had greater caloric intake than energy expenditure, which led to weight gain. The researchers suggest that getting more higher-quality sleep may have beneficial metabolic effects for reducing obesity and type 2 diabetes risk.

Simonelli, G., Mantua, J., Gad, M., St. Pierre, M., Moore, L., Yarnell, A. M., Quartana, P. J., Braun, A., Balkin, T. J., Brager, A. J., & Capaldi, V. F. (2019, February). Sleep extension reduces pain sensitivity. *Sleep Medicine, 54,* 172–176. https://doi.org/10.1016/j.sleep.2018.10.023

Researchers found that additional sleep increased pain tolerance; however, the pain threshold was the same. Increasing the amount of sleep before surgery could be a strategy to manage pain after surgery.

Skarpsno, E. S., Mork, P. J., Nilsen, T. I. L., & Nordstoga, A. L. (2019). Influence of sleep problems and co-occurring musculoskeletal pain on long-term prognosis of chronic low back pain: The HUNT Study. *Journal of Epidemiology & Community Health, 74*(3). http://dx.doi.org/10.1136/jech-2019-212734

People with chronic low back pain and other sites with musculoskeletal pain are more likely to reduce pain intensity when avoiding sleep problems.

Dominguez, F., Fuster, V., Fernandez-Alivra, J. M., Fernández-Friera, L., López-Melgar, B., Blanco-Rojo, R., Fernández-Ortiz, A., García-Pavía, P., Sanz, J., Mendiguren, J. M., Ibañez, B., Bueno, H., Lara-Pezzi, E., & Ordovás, J. M. (2019, January). Association of sleep duration and quality with subclinical atherosclerosis. *Journal of the American College of Cardiology, 73*(2), 134–144. https://doi.org/10.1016/j.jacc.2018.10.060

In a study involving 3,974 adults, researchers found short sleeping times and fragmented sleep to be associated with an increased risk of symptom-free atherosclerosis.

1. Sleep deprivation produces detrimental effects for people of all ages. The studies discussed show an association between poor sleep quality and health problems, such as obesity and type 2 diabetes, atherosclerosis, headaches, low back pain, and general pain sensitivity. In what other ways do you think sleep deprivation creates problems for the body?

2. On the one hand, sleep can be a way for people with headaches to deal with the pain. On the other hand, too much sleep, such as daytime naps, can interfere with good, restful sleep at night. How would you guide patients who experience chronic tension-type headaches and who are dealing with sleep difficulty?

3. People who are sleep deprived often report having a lower quality of life. Describe your own personal experience with sleep deprivation.

4. Considering the negative consequences of sleep deprivation on physical, mental, and emotional health and well-being, what questions might you ask your patients who report getting less than 6 hours of sleep per night?

- What are the clinical signs of sleep deprivation?
- Why are sleep-inducing medications not recommended for chronic insomnia?
- Why is snoring significant?

 Think**Like a Nurse** 31-5: Clinical Judgment **in Action**

Compare and contrast insomnia and hypersomnia. How are they different? How are they alike?

Parasomnias

The parasomnias include sleepwalking, sleeptalking, bruxism, night terrors, REM sleep behavior disorders, and nocturnal enuresis.

Sleepwalking Sleepwalking, or somnambulism, occurs during stage III of NREM sleep, usually 1 to 2 hours after the person falls asleep. The sleeper leaves the bed and walks about, with little awareness of

EXAMPLE CLIENT CONDITION: Sleep Apnea

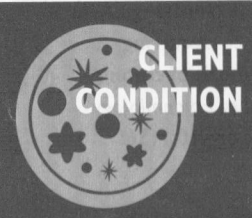

CLIENT CONDITION

Definition

- Sleep **apnea** is a periodic interruption in breathing during sleep—an absence of airflow through the nose or mouth during sleep.
- Pauses that last 10 to 30 seconds. Episodes may occur several or a hundred times a night and may last up to 1 minute or longer.
- During periods of apnea, the oxygen level in the blood drops, and the carbon dioxide level rises, causing the person to wake up.

Types

Obstructive Sleep Apnea (OSA)

- Typically, the soft tissue of the pharynx and soft palate collapse, and the tongue falls into the back of the throat and obstructs the upper airway.
- OSA is diagnosed clinically by reports of at least five witnessed breathing interruptions or awakenings resulting from gasping or choking events per hour.

Central Sleep Apnea (CSA)

- The brain doesn't send proper signals to the muscles that control breathing.
- Only about 10% of sleep apnea is central in origin.
- People with CSA tend to awaken during sleep and, therefore, experience daytime sleepiness.

Mixed Apnea

Combination of the two main types

Causes and Risk Factors

Obstructive Sleep Apnea

- Caused by airway occlusion resulting from a collapse of the hypopharynx or from other structural abnormalities
- More common after age 40, in males, and in Black or Latino individuals
- Overweight, large neck size (17 inches or greater in men, 16 inches or greater in women)
- Large tonsils, large tongue, small mandible (jawbone), enlarged adenoids, enlarged thyroid
- Nasal obstruction (deviated septum, chronic sinus blockage)
- Family history of OSA
- Alcohol use before sleep and use of sleep-inducing medication
- Smoking can increase swelling in the upper airway

Central Sleep Apnea

- Prematurity—immaturity of the respiratory center
- Medication (e.g., opioids, tranquilizers)
- Head trauma
- Problems affecting the brainstem, such as infection, stroke, or cervical spine conditions; severe obesity

---

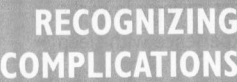

RECOGNIZING COMPLICATIONS

- Cardiac dysrhythmias (irregularities), heart attack, stroke, hypertension
- Job-related injuries, motor vehicle accidents related to sleepiness and fatigue
- Depression, worsening attention deficit-hyperactivity disorder (ADHD)

- Headaches
- May result in accelerated aging (Carskadon et al., 2019; Li et al., 2019)

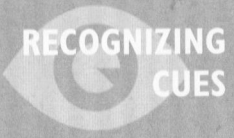

RECOGNIZING CUES

Nursing History

Observe for and ask the patient about the following symptoms:

- Snoring, snorting, gasping, restlessness during sleep (reported by sleep partner). More pronounced when people sleep on their backs.
- Unrefreshed sleep, tired during the day

- Morning headache
- Waking up with dry or sore throat
- Easily falling asleep during sedentary activity
- Forgetfulness, mood changes, decreased interest in sex

Note: Some may experience mild sleep apnea without any symptoms.

EXAMPLE CLIENT CONDITION: Sleep Apnea—cont'd

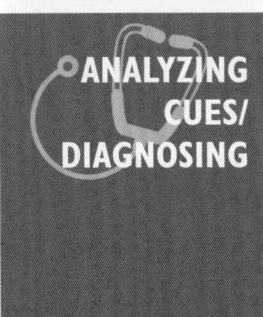

ANALYZING CUES/ DIAGNOSING

Disturbed Sleep Pattern
Sleep Deprivation
Risk for Inadequate Oxygenation

Examples

- Disturbed Sleep Pattern r/t obstructive sleep apnea
- Sleep Deprivation r/t central sleep apnea
- Risk for Infection r/t microbes thriving in a moist environment within the equipment (face mask, tubing)
- Altered Skin Integrity r/t poorly fitting continuous positive airway pressure (CPAP) mask and straps

GENERATING SOLUTIONS

NOC Outcomes

Hours of sleep
Sleep quality
Sleep pattern
Interrupted sleep
Sleep apnea
Snoring
   (Refer to the Collaborating category for definitions of the following.)
Electroencephalogram (EEG) findings
Electromyogram (EMG) findings
Electro-oculogram (EOG) findings

Individualized Goals/Outcome Statements

- Sleeps uninterrupted for at least 6 hours.
- States factors contributing to OSA.
- Designs dietary plan for long-term weight control to reduce OSA.
- Avoids alcohol, tobacco, and sleep-inducing drugs before bedtime.
- Uses CPAP or bilevel positive airway pressure (BiPAP), as prescribed.

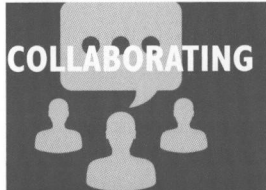

COLLABORATING

Diagnosis

The interprofessional team is involved with the diagnosis of sleep apnea.
- **Nasal airflow sensor**
- **Sleep study**—consists of an EEG, monitoring of arterial oxygen saturation, and an electrocardiogram (ECG)
- **EMG** to record muscle activity (facial twitch, teeth grinding, leg movements) during sleep
- **EOG** to record eye movement during sleep
- **Snore microphone** to record snoring

Treatment

The interprofessional team is involved with the treatment of sleep apnea.
- **Oral appliances** adjust the position of the lower jaw and tongue to prevent obstruction during sleep.
- **CPAP**—device that delivers forced air to keep the airways open. Types include:
  - Nasal mask over the nose
  - Nasal mask with prongs under the nose
  - Full mask covering mouth and nose
  - No mask or straps; instead, a mouthpiece that holds nasal puffs in the nares

- **BiPAP**—similar to CPAP, but airflow changes primarily with breathing in but also with breathing out
- **Nose tapes**
- **Saline sprays,** nose drops, and cortisone sprays are also used—all with mixed success.
- **Surgery** to remove any obstruction (enlarged tonsils, deviated septum)
  - **Uvulopalatopharyngoplasty** is a surgical procedure to remove soft tissue on the back of the throat and palate to increase the width of the airway.
  - **Maxillomandibular** advancement surgery is performed to correct airway obstruction related to the structure of the chin.
- **Implanted upper airway stimulator (Inspire)**—a small pulse generator is placed under the skin in the upper chest, with wires leading to the lungs and to the neck. A mild impulse stimulates the nerves that control airway muscles during sleep.

(continued)

EXAMPLE CLIENT CONDITION: Sleep Apnea—cont'd

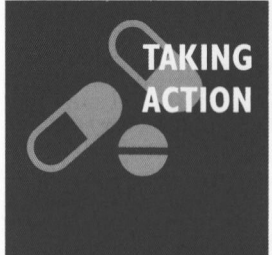

TAKING ACTION

- Keep the skin clean and dry under CPAP or BiPAP mask and straps *to preserve skin integrity.*
- Provide nasal spray for those with CPAP or BiPAP *to relieve dry, stuffy nose.*
- Position patients with OSA on the side to open the airway. Use pillows *to maintain a side-lying position.* (Some people use shirts with tennis balls sewn into the back to keep from rolling flat.)
- Adjust the size and fit of the mask to prevent a loose seal or excess pressure on the skin.

- Ensure the machine is turned on and oxygen tubing (if needed) is connected when in use.
- Observe for leaks in the air hose. *These develop with use over time.*
- Ensure equipment is clean before and after each use.
- Change filter and tubing weekly. Replace water daily.
- Add water to the reservoir *so that air gains moisture as it flows through the machine and into the mask.*

CARING

- ♥ **iCare** • Be empathetic to those who need to use CPAP or BiPAP machines at night to sleep. They are noisy and awkward. Masks, straps, and tubes may be uncomfortable.
- Help the patient who needs to use CPAP or BiPAP to find the best fit, understanding that straps and masks often make the patient's face and nose sore. Extra skin care may be needed.

- Be sensitive to moodiness related to sleep deprivation.
- Be sensitive to the effects of snoring on others and/or the need to sleep with a mask and tubing.

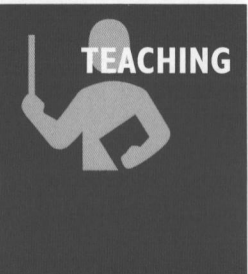

TEACHING

- Teach patients healthy habits for sleep (see the Self-Care box, Teaching Your Client About Sleep Hygiene).
- Stress the importance of daily and weekly cleaning of CPAP and BiPAP equipment, according to the manufacturer's instructions.
- Advise patient requiring CPAP or BiPAP to use equipment every night, even when traveling.
- Advise patients to have their machines calibrated by the provider at the recommended intervals (e.g., annually).

- Advise patients to replace masks and tubing at recommended intervals (about every 6 months).
- Avoid alcohol and smoking, especially before sleep. *These substances relax the muscles in the back of the throat, which can lead to airway obstruction.*
- Lose excess weight *that can lead to compression of the neck and upper airway.*
- ⊕ Caution patients with sleep apnea about driving if drowsy. They are 5 to 7 times more likely to have a motor vehicle accident than those without apnea.

---

surroundings. They may perform what appear to be conscious motor activities (e.g., brushing their teeth, making coffee), but they do not wake up. The person is not aware of sleepwalking and has no memory of the event on awakening. The event may last 3 to 4 minutes or longer. Stress, fatigue, and some drugs can trigger sleepwalking.

⊕ Children sleepwalk more often than adults do. If the child does not outgrow the condition or serious safety risks exist, medication may be given to suppress the deepest stage III sleep.

Sleeptalking Sleeptalking occurs during NREM sleep, just before the REM stage. Speech is often disorganized and hard to understand. It does not usually

interfere with the person's rest but may be disturbing to others.

Bruxism Bruxism is grinding and clenching of the teeth. It usually occurs during stage II NREM sleep. It can eventually erode tooth enamel and loosen the teeth.

Night Terrors Night terrors are sudden arousals in which the person (often a child) is physically active, often hallucinatory, and expresses a strong emotion such as terror. Children experiencing night terrors typically cry or scream in fear, thrash about, and resist all attempts by their parents or other caregivers to hold or console them. The child appears to be fully awake, but they are not; in fact, children experiencing night terrors are extremely difficult to awaken during the episode. They may last from 10 to 30 minutes. However, the child typically returns to sleep without awakening and, in the morning has no memory of the event.

Unlike **nightmares** (unpleasant, frightening dreams), which occur during REM sleep, night terrors occur during stage III (deep NREM) sleep.

REM Sleep Behavior Disorders These disorders are associated with REM (or dreaming period) sleep, in which the sleeper violently acts out the dream. People have actually injured themselves or others without waking.

Nocturnal Enuresis Nocturnal enuresis, or bed-wetting, is nighttime incontinence past the stage at which toilet training has been well established. It has incorrectly been associated with dreaming; however, most incidents occur during NREM sleep, during the first third of the night when the child is difficult to rouse. It may be distressing to the child and family because of the importance society places on continence, the inconvenience of keeping bed linens clean, and the misconception that the child is bed-wetting to act out against parents. **Key Point:** *Because most children outgrow enuresis, the best strategy is patience* (McCance & Huether, 2018). If the problem persists, the child should have a full medical evaluation.

Secondary Sleep Disorders

Secondary sleep disorders occur when a disease causes alteration in sleep stages or in the quantity and quality of sleep. The following are the most common causes:

- **Depression.** Depressed persons may spend a great deal of time in bed. However, in general, they have difficulty falling asleep, experience less slow-wave (deep) sleep, spend less time in REM sleep, awaken early, and have less total sleep time.
- **Hyperthyroidism or hypothyroidism.** An increase in thyroid secretion causes an increase in stage III sleep; hypothyroidism causes a decrease in those stages. Hyperthyroidism increases the metabolic rate, making it difficult for the person to fall asleep.
- **Pain.** Both acute and chronic pain interfere with sleep. Chronic pain affects both the quality and quantity of sleep. Pain delays the initiation of sleep, increases arousals during sleep, and causes longer waking intervals during the night (Mathias et al., 2018).

Disorders That Are Provoked by Sleep

Sleep-provoked disorders are those that occur when signs and symptoms of the disease appear or become worse during sleep.

- **Coronary artery disease.** During REM sleep, dreams may increase the heart rate and provoke angina and ECG changes.

- **Asthma.** People with asthma may experience bronchospasm during REM sleep. In adults, asthma attacks frequently occur during the night as the esophageal sphincter relaxes and reflux results. In children, they occur mostly during the final two-thirds of the night, when there is less stage III sleep.
- **Chronic obstructive pulmonary disease (COPD).** Persons with COPD experience lowered oxygen tension and increased carbon dioxide retention during sleep, especially during REM sleep, when neuromuscular control is normally depressed. This can result in pulmonary spasm and transient pulmonary hypertension.
- **Diabetes.** Blood glucose levels vary during sleep. When diabetes is uncontrolled, it may profoundly affect the blood sugar level during sleep, when the person is not alert enough to deal with it. Therefore, patients with uncontrolled diabetes may need to have blood glucose levels monitored during sleep.
- **Gastric and intestinal ulcers.** During REM sleep, people with duodenal ulcers secrete up to 20 times more gastric acid than do people who do not have duodenal ulcers. Peptic ulcers also contribute to increased acid, often producing nocturnal epigastric pain and sleep loss.
- **Epilepsy.** Seizures are sensitive to sleep patterns. Sleep deprivation can trigger seizures, increase their intensity, or cause seizures to last longer. Some forms of epilepsy are especially reactive to sleep cycles or transitions between sleep states (Schachter et al., n.d.).

KnowledgeCheck 31-5

- List and define at least three parasomnias.
- Describe ways in which depression can affect sleep.
- List two sleep-provoked disorders, and explain how the sleep stage affects the disease.

PracticalKnowledge
knowing **how**

Because sleep enhances wellness and speeds recovery from illness, promoting sleep is an important independent nursing intervention. In this section, you will learn how to assess for signs of sleep disturbance, as well as specific interventions to facilitate sleep for each client.

ASSESSMENT/RECOGNIZING CUES NP

It is important to assess usual sleep patterns and rituals for all patients who are being admitted to the hospital or seeking help for a sleep problem. A brief assessment for all patients should include questions about the following:

- Usual sleeping pattern
- Sleeping environment
- Bedtime routines/rituals

- Sleep aids
- Sleep changes or problems

Key Point: *You would conduct a more in-depth sleep assessment for patients who wake up at least three times a night, for those who take more than 30 minutes to fall asleep, and in cases where the difficulty falling or staying asleep has been going on for more than 30 days. A sleep study is recommended for unexplained daytime sleepiness (Qaseem et al., 2014).*

- A **sleep history** (self-report) includes in-depth questions about the person's usual times for sleep; any preparation, preferences, and routines; quality of sleep; napping habits (if any); and whether they wake early and cannot return to sleep.
- A **sleep log** provides very specific information on your patient's patterns of sleep. This allows you to identify trends in sleep/wakefulness and identify any relationship with sleep habits. You will usually ask the patient to keep the log for 14 days. Remind them that it is important to be diligent in maintaining it.
- **Social history** can reveal habits that can affect sleep quality: use of tobacco, caffeinated products, and recreational drugs. Prescription and nonprescription medication can also interfere with sleep (e.g., beta blockers, clonidine, theophylline, certain antidepressants [fluoxetine], and decongestants).

For examples of a sleep history and a sleep log,

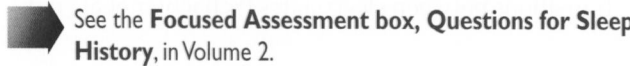 See the **Focused Assessment box, Questions for Sleep History,** in Volume 2.

- An **actigraph** is an application on a mobile device that estimates a person's sleep and wake patterns, including time spent in various sleep stages.
- A **sleep study** is a test that observes what happens in the body during sleep. It is most useful in detecting sleep apnea and other sleep disorders, such as narcolepsy, night terrors, and periodic limb movement disorder.
- **Polysomnography,** one of the most common sleep studies performed in a sleep laboratory, records brain-wave activity, eye movement, oxygen and carbon dioxide levels, vital signs, and body movements during the sleep phases. The American College of Physicians recommends polysomnography for anyone suspected to have OSA (Qaseem et al., 2014).

NURSING DIAGNOSIS/ANALYZING CUES

It is important to determine whether lack of sleep is a problem, is a symptom of a problem, or is contributing to (etiology of) a different problem. For health promotion applications, use the NANDA-I diagnosis Readiness for Enhanced Sleep when a client has no particular sleep problem but wishes to move to a higher level of functioning in the area of sleep.

Sleep as the Problem

When you wish to focus on interventions to promote sleep, use the following NANDA-I labels on the problem side of the nursing diagnosis:

- **Insomnia**—Use for patients who have a disruption in the amount or quality of sleep to the extent that it impairs functioning.
- **Sleep Deprivation**—Use as the nursing diagnosis when the patient's amount, consistency, or quality of sleep is decreased over prolonged periods of time. The defining characteristics of Sleep Deprivation are more severe than those for Disturbed Sleep Pattern, so nursing activities may focus as much on relieving symptoms (e.g., confusion, paranoia) as on sleep promotion.
- **Disturbed Sleep Pattern**—Use as the diagnosis when assessment data point to a time-limited sleep problem caused by external factors (e.g., inability to sleep in the unfamiliar hospital environment).

The problem should be one that can be treated by nursing therapy. Carefully describe the etiologies for sleep problems because they determine your interventions. To help you individualize goals, add modifying words to specify the type of sleep problem, as in these examples:

- *Disturbed Sleep Pattern* (difficulty falling asleep) related to worries about family
- *Disturbed Sleep Pattern* (difficulty falling and remaining asleep) related to noise of hospital environment and need for scheduled treatments
- *Disturbed Sleep Pattern* (premature awakening) related to sleeping aid dependence and lack of knowledge of nonpharmacological aids for insomnia
- *Disturbed Sleep Pattern* (excessive daytime sleeping) related to effects of biological aging and depression
- *Disturbed Sleep Pattern* (altered sleep–wake patterns) related to frequent rotations of shift and overtime work

ThinkLike a Nurse 31-6: Clinical Judgment in Action

In the following nursing diagnoses, how do you think your interventions would be different for each diagnosis? Disturbed Sleep Pattern related to:

- Changes in bedtime routines
- Exercising within 2 hours before sleep
- Drinking caffeinated beverages, eating chocolate, and drinking alcohol within 2 hours before sleep
- Emotional or physical pain
- Drug dependence or withdrawal
- Physical illness

Sleep Pattern as an Etiology

Disturbed Sleep Pattern and Sleep Deprivation affect many areas of functioning, so they often are the etiology of other nursing diagnoses, as in these examples:

- **Risk for Injury or Falls** related to sleepwalking (or REM sleep behavior disorder or narcolepsy)

- **Fatigue (or Activity Intolerance)** related to chronic insufficient quality or quantity of sleep (e.g., secondary to insomnia)
- **Ineffective Coping** related to decreased cognitive functioning and awareness, secondary to lack of sleep
- **Disturbed Thought Processes** related to decreased cognitive functioning, secondary to lack of sleep
- **Anxiety (or Fear)** related to fear of death from sleep apnea

Sleep Pattern as a Symptom

Difficulty sleeping may be one of the symptoms of another problem. For example, a client may have Spiritual Distress related to challenges to belief system *as manifested by nightmares, sleep disturbances, and verbalization of inner conflict about beliefs.* In this instance, you would focus on interventions for Spiritual Distress, assuming that the sleep pattern would improve as the Spiritual Distress is resolved. Other nursing diagnoses that may cause sleep loss include Anxiety, Chronic Sorrow, Death Anxiety, Decisional Conflict, Dysfunctional Grieving, Diarrhea, Gas Exchange Impairment, Nausea, Pain, and Relocation Stress Syndrome.

KnowledgeCheck 31-6

- For a chronic, long-term sleep problem, would you use a diagnosis of Sleep Pattern Disturbance, Sleep Deprivation, or Readiness for Enhanced Sleep?
- Name at least two nursing diagnoses that might have a sleep problem as the etiology.
- Name at least one nursing diagnosis that might have a sleep problem as the defining characteristic.

■ PLANNING OUTCOMES/EVALUATION

Nursing Outcomes Classification (NOC) standardized outcomes linked to the NANDA-I sleep labels are as follows:

- For **Disturbed Sleep Pattern:** Rest, Sleep, and Personal Well-Being
- For **Sleep Deprivation:** Rest, Sleep, and Symptom Severity
- For **Insomnia:** Concentration, Endurance, Fatigue Level, Mood Equilibrium, Personal Health Status, Personal Well-Being, Quality of Life, Rest, and Sleep

When sleep disturbances are the etiology of another nursing diagnosis, you will need to use the NOC outcomes associated with that diagnosis. For example:

Nursing diagnosis: Anxiety related to Sleep Deprivation
NOC outcomes for Anxiety: Anxiety Self-Control, Coping

Individualized goals/outcome statements you might use to evaluate the success of interventions for sleep enhancement include the following:

- Verbalizes feeling rested or feeling less fatigue.
- Falls asleep within 30 minutes; sleeps 6 hours without awakening.

- Maintains a sleep–wake pattern that provides sufficient energy for the day's tasks.
- Demonstrates self-care behaviors that provide a healthy balance between rest and activity.
- Identifies stress-relieving rituals that enable falling asleep more easily.
- Demonstrates decreased signs of sleep deprivation.
- Verbalizes feeling less fatigued and more in control of life activities.

■ PLANNING INTERVENTIONS/IMPLEMENTATION NP

Nursing Interventions Classification (NIC) standardized interventions for Sleep Deprivation and Sleep Pattern Disturbance include the following: Coping Enhancement, Energy Management, Environmental Management: Comfort, Relaxation Therapy, and Sleep Enhancement. Linkages have not yet been established for Insomnia.

Specific nursing activities for clients with sleep problems are described in the next sections.

For a care plan and care map for Sleep Pattern Disturbance,

 Go to **Davis Advantage, Resources, Chapter 31, Care Plan** and **Care Map.**

Schedule Nursing Care to Avoid Interrupting Sleep

♥ **iCare** Use nursing judgment to decide when a procedure must be done and when it is more important for your patient to sleep. Healthcare routines usually allow time for rest periods. In addition, you may consider the following caring interventions:

- Some patients need to rest after a procedure or after meals.
- Give prescribed sleep-inducing medication when providing care to avoid waking them later in the evening.
- You can often alter routines; for example, you can allow the patient to sleep as long as they can in the morning and bring their breakfast later.
- Cluster care to avoid unnecessary interruptions in sleep. Unless the patient is critically ill, do not wake them for morning vital signs if they are sleeping.
- Keep the noise level to a minimum. Be aware that activities, conversation, and equipment, even outside the patient's room, can disrupt sleep.

Create a Restful Environment

Many people find it difficult to sleep in a strange bed, even a comfortable one. Hospital beds are not noted for their luxury, but you can help make them more comfortable.

- Be sure the bed linens are tight on the bottom and loose on top to allow movement.
- Keep linens clean, dry, and free of irritants. Perspiration on the hospital gown or linens can lead to chill.

- Good body alignment also facilitates relaxation (Fig. 31-7). Use extra pillows, a blanket from home, or any other item that may help the patient rest.
- Keep the room dark and quiet unless the patient prefers a light.
- As much as possible, control the temperature of the room and provide good ventilation.

Promote Comfort

Pain, itching, and nausea may all be deterrents to rest and sleep in an ill person. Be sure to offer pain medications at their scheduled times and before the patient's sleep time. Other comfort measures include providing a restful environment (see the preceding intervention) and offering fluids, cool cloths, or a massage or back rub (Mathpati & Dias, 2014).

Support Bedtime Rituals and Routines

Most people have some kind of a routine before bed, be it reading, watching TV, drinking warm milk, praying, or meditating, to allow them to prepare for sleep.

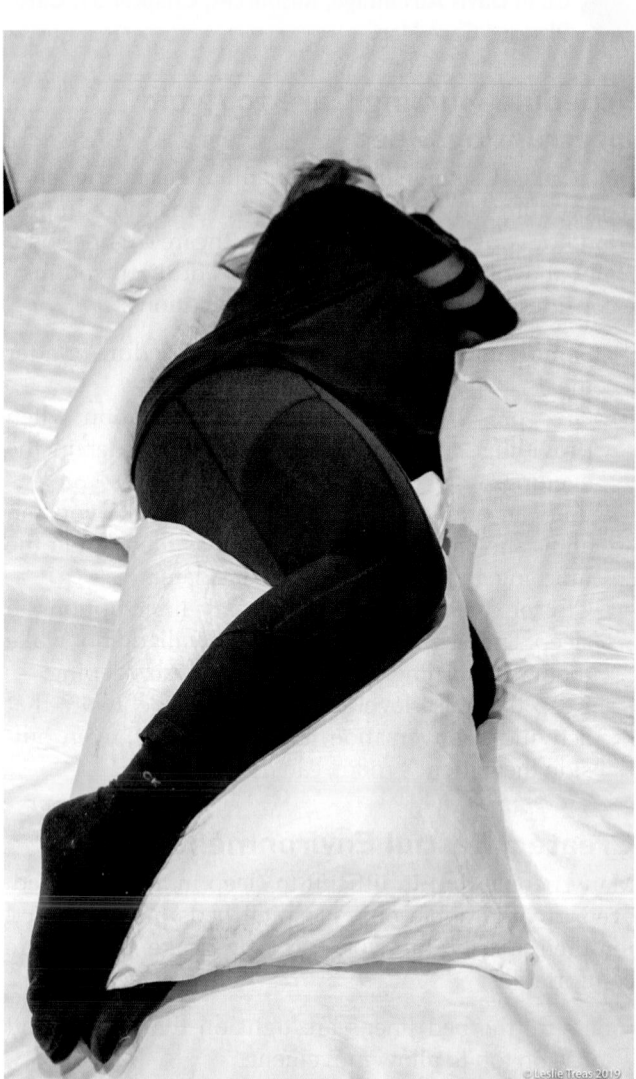

FIGURE 31-7 Good body alignment promotes rest and sleep.

For children, a favorite stuffed animal, blanket, or bedtime story, as well as brushing their teeth, may enhance sleepiness. Be sure to include any routines or rituals in the nursing plan of care to ensure continuity. Advise patients who smoke not to smoke after the evening meal—or at all.

Offer Appropriate Bedtime Snacks or Beverages

- Complex carbohydrates (e.g., bread, cereal) seem to help most people sleep because they likely increase the level of sleep-inducing tryptophan in the blood.
- A small amount of protein (e.g., milk, cheese) with the snack reduces the sugar boost and keeps blood glucose more stable. However, a high-protein food may be more difficult to digest.
- Advise the client to avoid alcohol, especially in the evening. Although it may induce sleepiness at first, alcohol interferes with the deep-sleep cycle.
- The client should avoid consuming caffeine-containing foods and beverages (e.g., tea, coffee, energy drinks, chocolate, colas) after the evening meal.
- Advise the client to drink plenty of fluids during the day but to restrict fluids close to bedtime.
- Nicotine is a stimulant and should be avoided.

Promote Relaxation

Base your choice of relaxation strategies on your repertoire of techniques and on patient preference. Relaxation strategies may include a massage, a warm bath, or one of the following:

- **Guided imagery** can be used to help your patient move their mind to a safe place where relaxation is possible. You may ask the patient what type of place will soothe them and "guide" them there through visualization. See Chapter 9 if you need to review.
- **Progressive muscle relaxation,** relaxing each muscle independently and progressing from head to toe, may help to promote sleep.
- **Music therapy** has been shown to be effective in promoting relaxation. Some patients respond well and can put away their troubles while listening to music, whereas others may find music irritating. Slow, quiet music or a recording of forest or ocean sounds may be soothing.

⊕ Maintain Patient Safety
Sleepwalkers

A person who sleepwalks needs protection from injury because the risk of falling is great (e.g., stairs). Also, IV infusions, catheters, and nasogastric tubes can produce injury if they are pulled out of the body when the person gets out of bed. Guide sleepwalkers back to bed, and remember that they startle easily, so be gentle and quiet.

Safe Sleep for Infants

Infant suffocation is a common cause of death in infants, along with entrapment and strangulation. Some factors include:

- **Infant position and the sleep environment,** such as the use of blankets, pillows, and infant positioners. **Key Point:** *The safest position for infants under 3 months of age is the supine position (not on the side) on a firm sleep surface.* Commercial positioning devices are not recommended unless prescribed (American Academy of Pediatrics Task Force on Sudden Infant Death Syndrome, 2016; Centers for Disease Control and Prevention [CDC], 2012; U.S. Food and Drug Administration [FDA], 2019).
- **Sharing a room but not a bed.** A separate, safe surface in the parent's room lowers the chance of sudden infant death syndrome (SIDS) by 50% (American Academy of Pediatrics, 2016).
- **Soft objects, loose bedding, and hanging window treatments** should be kept away from the infant's sleep surface.

One in five mothers places her infant in a nonsupine position to sleep, more than half share a bed with their infants, and more than one in three uses soft bedding or toys in the sleep area. Clearly, more education and counseling are needed to improve safe sleep practices (American Academy of Pediatrics Task Force on Sudden Infant Death Syndrome, 2016; Bombard et al., 2018; CDC, 2012).

Teach About Sleep Hygiene

Most people with sleep problems manage them at home by creating a restful environment, relaxing, avoiding distractions, and trying various sleep strategies without using sleep-inducing medication. Refer to the Self-Care box, Teaching Your Client About Sleep Hygiene, when teaching clients self-care for sleep.

Administer and Teach About Sleep Medications

When considering sleep medications, it is important for the patient to understand the options, be aware of potential side effects, and know what questions to ask.

- Some medications are habit forming; others may have unpleasant side effects.
- When patients first start taking prescription sleep aids, they should use caution during morning activities until they are sure how the drug affects them.
- **Key Point:** *As a general rule, sleep medications are not recommended for long-term use.* The long-term effects of sleep-inducing medications are not known.
- Some natural or homeopathic aids can promote rest and sleep.

Prescription Sleep Medications

You should be familiar with prescription and nonprescription sleep medications your patients may be taking. Prescription sleep medications are typically classified into the following five categories.

Nonbenzodiazepines These sedative–hypnotics have a short half-life, which means that they are eliminated from the body quickly and do not cause daytime sleepiness. Examples are zolpidem tartrate and zaleplon.

- **Nonbenzodiazepines** are **selective,** meaning that they target specific receptors that are thought to be associated with sleep rather than depressing the entire central nervous system.
- **General side effects** include drowsiness, dizziness, fatigue, headache, and unpleasant taste.
- The **long-term effects** of these medications are not yet known, although an increased risk of fatal overdose has been reported.

Benzodiazepines This class of sedative–hypnotics is the first-line treatment for insomnia. Benzodiazepines have the following characteristics:

- They may be long-acting or short-acting.
- The long-acting ones linger in the body and potentially cause daytime drowsiness. Older adults are particularly at risk for daytime sleepiness and dizziness.
    - They carry a greater risk for rebound insomnia, dependency, and tolerance. This is especially true for older adults.
- They are potentially dangerous when combined with alcohol and some medications.
- Many were originally formulated to treat anxiety. Examples are diazepam, alprazolam, flurazepam, lorazepam, and triazolam.

Selective Melatonin Agonists This class regulates the sleep–wake cycle by targeting melatonin receptors. Ramelteon is used to treat insomnia that is associated with difficulty falling asleep. It is not designated as a controlled substance.

Barbiturates These sedative–hypnotics and anticonvulsants are rarely prescribed for insomnia because of the risk of addiction, abuse, and overdose. Examples are amobarbital, pentobarbital, and secobarbital.

Tricyclic Antidepressants At times, primary care providers prescribe antidepressants to promote sleep. They show clinical benefit for some people with insomnia who also suffer from depression. Examples are amitriptyline, doxepin, imipramine, and nortriptyline.

Nonprescription Sleep Medications

Although nonprescription sleep aids can be helpful to induce restfulness or initiate sleep, when used over a long period of time, they can lose their effectiveness.

Self-Care

Teaching Your Client About Sleep Hygiene

To Do

➤ **Use your bedroom only for sleep;** do not turn your bedroom into the family room.

➤ **Follow a regular routine** for bedtime and morning awakenings.

➤ **Go to bed each night at the same time,** even on days you are off work.

➤ **Keep your bedroom as dark, cool, and quiet as possible.**
  ➤ The ideal temperature for most people is 65° to 69°.
  ➤ Even an illuminated clock is a light source that can be distracting. Replace the clock or block the light with something.
  ➤ Use earplugs to block out noise, if necessary.

➤ **Try a weighted blanket.** Most manufacturers recommend using a blanket that is 10% of the user's weight.

➤ **If you cannot fall asleep in 30 minutes,** get up and do something nonstimulating, but avoid using electronics with illuminated screens. When you feel sleepy, go back to bed. The wavelengths of blue light emitted from the screen arouse the brain into a wakeful state.

➤ **Use relaxation methods;** read a book, pray, or meditate. Try closing your eyes and visualizing something peaceful when trying to fall asleep. Imagining your favorite relaxing place where you find comfort or familiarity can relax you and help you get to sleep.

➤ **Use aromatherapy to relax.** An essential oil diffuser may help to induce sleep. Lavender scent, for example, slows the heart rate and lowers blood pressure.

➤ **Try progressive relaxation to fall asleep.** Follow recorded instructions directing you in a sequence of relaxing certain muscle groups.

➤ **Exercise at the right time.** Ideally, this would be more than 3 hours before bedtime. Exercise stimulates a hormone that makes you more alert (cortisol). However, for some, evening exercise is not associated with worse sleep (Buman et al., 2014).

➤ **Nap the right amount and at the right time.** A short (20-minute) nap can recharge your battery, but longer naps can leave you feeling groggy and make it difficult to fall asleep at night. Naps later in the day disrupt a sleep routine.

➤ **If you take prescription drugs,** ask your prescriber or pharmacist about the side effects.

➤ **You may consider taking a melatonin supplement.** Although it does not induce sleep, it has a calming effect.

➤ **Take a warm, not hot, bath just before going to sleep.** This will raise your body temperature and relax you to help you fall asleep more easily.

➤ **Find your best sleep position,** perhaps with a pillow under or between your knees. A side-lying position is best for someone who snores or has sleep apnea. Using a pillow between the knees keeps the spine in better alignment. A side-lying position also relieves back compression, helping prevent lower backache. Sleeping on your left side is better than the right side if you experience heartburn from acid reflux.

➤ **Try using a sleep tracker** to get a feel for how much movement you have while you are asleep. Even though sleep trackers do not record actual sleep, they can indicate restlessness, which reveals sleep quality.

To Avoid

➤ **Don't try to "catch up" on sleep.** Rise at your regular time, even if you went to bed later than usual.

➤ **Limit screen time before going to sleep.** Too much "blue light" given off by your cell phone, computer, or tablet can interfere with sleep quality.

➤ **Don't depend on sleeping aids;** be aware of the potential dangers of sleeping medications.

➤ **Avoid cold medications that contain stimulant ingredients** (e.g., pseudoephedrine).

➤ **Avoid caffeine, alcohol, tobacco products, and heavy meals before going to sleep.** Remember that some beverages and foods, such as black tea, chocolate, and cola, contain caffeine. Tobacco is also a stimulant. Alcohol interferes with the transition to deeper phases of sleep. Heavy alcohol consumption can contribute to breathing impairment during the night.

➤ **Avoid eating carbohydrates** (e.g., crackers, cereal, or bread) before bed. They boost blood glucose levels, so a few hours later, the rapid drop in sugar will wake you.

➤ **Don't overhydrate before bedtime.** Although you don't want to awaken thirsty, too much water can cause you to awaken to empty your bladder during the night.

➤ **Avoid going to bed angry or frustrated;** stay clear of emotional discussions before going to sleep.

Nonprescription sleep medications usually contain an antihistamine.

Antihistamines Diphenhydramine may induce drowsiness, although because of the long half-life of the drug, grogginess commonly lasts into the next day.

■ It is important to check the ingredient label of any over-the-counter (OTC) medication to see whether it contains an antihistamine.

■ Advise clients that OTC sleep medications can interact with other medicines they may be taking, so they should consult their prescriber or pharmacist before using them.
■ Diphenhydramine can also cause constipation and urinary retention and may impair memory over time.

For more information about natural sleep aids, see the Holistic Healing box, Natural Sleep Aids.

Natural Sleep Aids

Melatonin is a natural hormone produced by the pineal gland to modulate sleep. Although generally safe for short-term use, melatonin is unregulated and varies in strength and purity across manufacturers. In addition, melatonin may interfere with anticoagulants, birth control pills, antidiabetic medication, and other drugs that suppress the immune system. Tart cherries are a natural source of melatonin to improve sleep quality.

Herbal remedies produce a calming effect that can help with relaxation and falling asleep. **Key Point:** *These herbal remedies have not undergone extensive testing for benefits and safety and have not been proven to be effective sleep aids.*

Some examples include:

➤ **Chamomile** relaxes muscles for transitioning to sleep. This herb has a calming effect but can also interact with certain medications.

➤ **Valerian root** (known as "poor man's Valium") reduces the time it takes to fall asleep. It also improves sleep quality.

➤ **Hops** have an aromatic quality that helps with relaxation, leading to sleep.

➤ **Passionflower** is known for its calming properties because it contains gamma-aminobutyric acid (GABA), a chemical in the brain that affects mood and sleep.

➤ **Kava** plant is used to ease insomnia caused by stress; however, it has been linked to liver damage.

➤ **Magnolia bark** has a compound, called *honokiol*, that keeps the body from releasing the stress hormone adrenaline.

➤ **Cannabidiol (CBD) oil** is extracted from marijuana and hemp plants. It can help to induce sleep by taking the edge off tension and anxiety at sleep time.

➤ **Magnesium** supplements may improve sleep in older people and those with restless legs syndrome. Too much magnesium can lead to nausea and cramping.

KnowledgeCheck 31-7

- What is the classification of zolpidem tartrate? Why is it an especially desirable medication for sleep?
- What are two other classes of medications that are sometimes prescribed for sleep?
- Describe three independent nursing interventions to promote sleep.
- Why should people contact their prescriber before taking nonprescription sleep aids?

PUTTING IT ALL TOGETHER

Anna (Meet Your Patient) has arrived back on the surgical unit after her surgery. She has a urinary catheter, oxygen mask, IV line, and morphine by patient-controlled analgesia (PCA) for pain control. She is nauseated from the anesthesia and moaning in pain. Her husband, Eric, is at the bedside, looking worried. He tells you that Anna didn't sleep at all the night before surgery. "She was nervous and didn't want to take a sleeping pill because we were supposed to be at the hospital by 5:30 a.m.," he explains.

In your initial assessment, Anna's vital signs are as follows: blood pressure, 118/74 mm Hg; pulse, 88 beats/min and regular; respirations, 26 breaths/min; temperature, 99.4°F. Her lungs are clear, the dressing is dry and intact, and a small amount of light-yellow urine is draining from the urinary catheter. The electronic health record (EHR) indicates that Anna has not received medication for pain in more than 90 minutes. The PCA is connected, but the pump supplies analgesia only when the patient triggers the device. Anna has been sedated and does not remember that she must push the button to obtain pain medication. You trigger a bolus of morphine and show Anna and Eric how the PCA works. You realize that she may not remember what you have taught her, but Eric assures you that he will be staying for the day and will reinforce your instruction.

Several minutes later, Anna is calm. Her respirations have slowed to 20 breaths/min, and she is lightly snoring. Eric sighs in relief. "I guess she'll sleep for a while now," he says. You explain that she will sleep with the pain medication but that "with the morphine, she will wake frequently and not get much REM sleep—that's a type of sleep we all require for health."

You gathered data preoperatively from Anna about her sleep habits and routines. You are also aware that Anna has had chronic insomnia. In the nursing care plan, you have written the diagnosis "Disturbed Sleep Pattern related to pain (secondary to fibromyalgia), dependence on Ambien, anxiety, grief, stresses of surgery, and unfamiliar environment." You ask Eric to bring Anna's pillow and personal items from home that are part of her usual bedtime ritual. Eric says, "She sometimes listens to music before bed," so you suggest that he also bring her a small wireless speaker for her favorite music. When you make your rounds, you report that you would like to keep her usual bedtime routine and that she will be getting Ambien this evening. Anna is visibly relieved by your reassurance.

This scenario demonstrates full-spectrum nursing and shows how a nurse can make a difference for patients and their families by recognizing the need for sleep and providing appropriate interventions.

To explore learning resources for this chapter,

   Go to Davis Advantage and find:

Answers and Suggested Responses for all questions in this chapter
Concept Map
Knowledge Map
Care Plan
Care Map
References and Bibliography

32

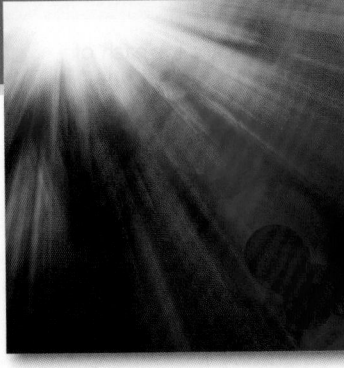

Skin Integrity & Wound Healing

Learning Outcomes

After completing this chapter, you should be able to:

➤ Discuss the factors that affect skin integrity.

➤ Identify wounds based on accepted classification schemes.

➤ Describe the three phases of wound healing.

➤ Distinguish primary intention healing, secondary intention healing, and tertiary intention healing.

➤ Describe the three types of wound drainage.

➤ Review the major complications of wound healing.

➤ Explain the factors involved in the development of pressure injury.

➤ Use the Braden scale to assess risk for pressure injury.

➤ Assess and categorize pressure injuries based on the staging system.

➤ Provide nursing care that limits the risk of pressure injury development.

➤ Differentiate the kinds of chronic wounds.

➤ Accurately chart an assessment of a wound.

➤ Demonstrate appropriate techniques for irrigating a wound.

➤ Describe care of a wound with a drain.

➤ Differentiate the five forms of wound débridement.

➤ Discuss the different kinds of tissue found in wounds.

➤ Discuss when and how to use absorbent dressings, alginate dressings, collagen dressings, gauze dressings, transparent films, hydrocolloids, hydrogels, and foam and antimicrobial dressings.

➤ Describe guidelines to follow when applying heat or cold therapy.

➤ Demonstrate bandage and binder application.

Key Concepts

Skin integrity

Wound

Wound healing

Related Concepts

See the Concept Map on DavisAdvantage.

Example Client Condition

Pressure Injury

Meet Your Patient

William Harmon is a 78-year-old man who fell and fractured his left hip 3 days ago. After being admitted to the hospital, he underwent an open reduction and internal fixation (ORIF) of the left hip. Today is his second postoperative day. He is unable to roll or pull himself up in the bed.

Mr. Harmon's weight on admission was 140 lb (63.64 kg). His height is 73 in (185.42 cm). His family reports that he has been steadily losing weight. He expresses little interest in eating and says he has suffered depression since his wife died last year.

A large dressing covers the incision on Mr. Harmon's left hip. During your assessment, you loosen the dressing and see that the staples are intact at the incision site, and there is a minimal amount of serosanguineous drainage on the bandage. As you

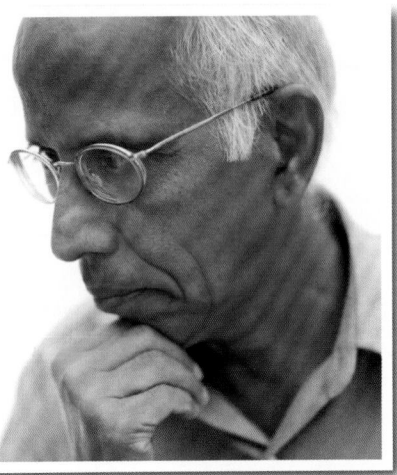

(Continued)

Meet Your Patient (continued)

turn him in bed, you see a 10-cm by 6-cm reddened area on his coccyx and a 2-cm by 3-cm purple bruiselike area on his left heel. Mr. Harmon now has three wounds, an intentional surgical wound and two pressure injuries that have resulted from his impaired mobility. How will you care for each of these wounds? What factors contributed to each of the wounds? How will you promote healing?

Theoretical Knowledge
knowing why

The integumentary system consists of the skin, hair, nails, sweat glands, and subcutaneous tissue below the skin. The skin is the largest organ of the body (covering about 20 square feet). The major functions of the skin include protection of the internal organs, unique identification of an individual, thermoregulation, metabolism of nutrients and metabolic waste products, and sensation.

ABOUT THE KEY CONCEPTS

For optimal function, **skin integrity** must be preserved—that is, all layers of the skin must be intact. A **wound** is a disruption in the normal skin integrity. It is easy to see how the concepts of skin integrity and wound are related; they are opposites. You will use your knowledge of both concepts as you protect your patients' skin and promote the physiological process of **wound healing.**

WHAT FACTORS AFFECT SKIN INTEGRITY?

For optimal function, all layers of the skin must be intact. Breaks in the skin (e.g., surgical incisions, injuries) increase the risk of infection. In the following sections, you will learn about factors that influence the ability to maintain intact skin and heal wounds (e.g., age and mobility).

To understand skin integrity, you need to understand the structure of the skin (Fig. 32-1).

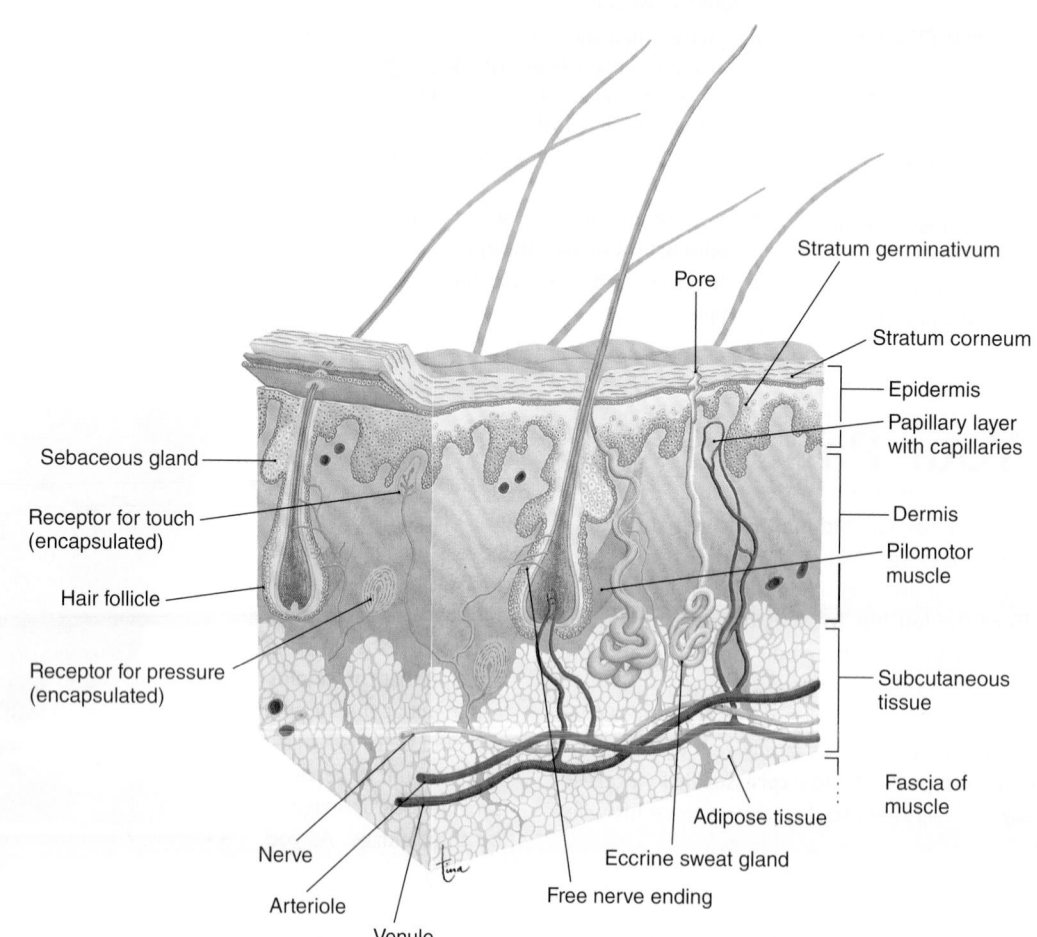

FIGURE 32-1 The structure of the skin.

Epidermis The **epidermis** is the outer portion of the skin that functions as protection from the environment. The epidermis is made up of four layers, of which the most important are the inner and outer layers.

- The **stratum corneum,** the outermost layer, is composed of numerous thicknesses of dead cells. Functioning as a barrier, it restricts water loss and prevents fluids, pathogens, and chemicals from entering the body.
- The **stratum germinativum,** the innermost layer of the epidermis, continually produces new cells, pushing the older cells toward the skin surface. In the dermal layer, the **keratinocytes** are protein-containing cells that give the skin strength and elasticity. Deeper in the epidermis are **melanocytes,** which produce melanin, a pigment that gives skin its color and provides protection from ultraviolet light. **Langerhans cells** are mobile. Their function is to phagocytize (engulf) foreign material and trigger an immune response.

Dermis The **dermis** lies below the epidermis and above the subcutaneous tissue. It is made of irregular fibrous connective tissue that provides strength and elasticity to the skin and is generously supplied with blood vessels. Within the dermis are sweat glands, sebaceous (oil) glands, ceruminous (wax) glands, hair and nail follicles, sensory receptors, elastin, and collagen. This layer contains nerves that sense pain, touch, and temperature.

Subcutaneous Tissue The **subcutaneous layer** is composed primarily of connective and adipose tissue. It provides insulation, conserves the body's heat, protects the inner organs, and reserves calories in the case of severe malnutrition. This layer varies in thickness in different body sites. Sex hormones, genetics, age, and nutrition also influence the distribution of subcutaneous tissue.

Age-Related Variations

Age affects the condition and structure of the skin.

Infants and Children Infants are born with varying amounts of *vernix caseosa,* a creamy substance that protects their skin. Their skin is thinner and more permeable than that of adults, which predisposes infants to skin breakdown (e.g., diaper rash). Infant skin is at higher risk for fluid loss and greater systemic absorption of topical agents applied to the skin, especially with prematurity (McNichol et al., 2021). The subcutaneous layer (brown fat) and sweat glands are not fully developed, especially for preterm infants. As a result, in the first few weeks of life, thermoregulation is immature, and the infant must be swaddled to maintain body heat for the first days to weeks of life.

Infant skin has other unique characteristics:

- **Milia**—small, pearly white, firm, raised bumps on the face. They disappear after a few weeks.
- **Erythema toxicum**—a common, harmless skin rash that occurs 1 to 3 days after birth and disappears by a week. It looks like small *pustules* (pimples) on a red base, often on the face, trunk, and arms.
- **Newborn acne**—mild acne caused by the mother's hormones passed to the baby. This rash most often clears in a few weeks.
- **Congenital nevi**—birthmark that is darkly pigmented skin at birth, resembling a mole. They range in size, but larger nevi carry a greater risk of developing into a type of skin cancer.
- **Mongolian spots**—blue-gray spots seen deep within the skin of the lower back and upper buttocks. They are most common on dark-skinned babies.
- **Café-au-lait spots**—light-tan, flat marks on the skin that resemble the color of coffee with milk. They are often noted at birth but can also develop in the first few years of life. Café-au-lait markings indicate a condition called *neurofibromatosis.*
- **Port wine stains**—flat, purplish markings on the skin caused by overgrowth of blood vessels under the skin. They are commonly seen on the face but can occur anywhere on the body.
- **Hemangiomas**—raised overgrowth of *capillaries* (tiny blood vessels) that commonly appear in the first few months of life.
- **Stork bites**—harmless flat red patches on the baby's forehead, eyelids, and base of the neck. They are caused by stretching of the blood vessels under the skin.

Adolescents and Adults Sex hormones released during puberty increase sebaceous and sweat gland activity, which leads to perspiration, odor, and sometimes acne. In female individuals, especially during pregnancy, high estrogen levels may contribute to the softening of connective tissue and cause striae and darkening of the skin, usually on the face, areolae, nipples, vulva, and umbilicus, particularly in people with dark skin.

 Older Adults As adults age, the activity of the sebaceous and sweat glands diminishes, resulting in drier skin. **Xerosis** (itchy, red, dry, scaly, cracked, or fissured skin) is a problem for up to 85% of older adults and can be a threat to the integrity of their skin.

With aging, especially in people with a lean body mass, the subcutaneous tissue layer thins. As the strong bond between the epidermal and dermal layer weakens, the dermal layer loses elasticity as a result of changes in its collagen fibers. These changes make the skin prone to breakdown and prolong wound-healing time. Regeneration of healthy skin and healing of wounds is significantly slower in older adults than in young adults.

Furthermore, some older adults have chronic diseases that interfere with healing. Diabetes, for instance, predisposes a person to infection. Immune deficiency leads to slower wound healing, and liver dysfunction interferes with the synthesis of blood-clotting factors.

Impaired Mobility

A healthy person moves and shifts position unconsciously when they sense pressure or discomfort. However, for people who are unable to move independently or lack sensation in a body area, the weight of the body on the bed or chair causes an increase in pressure that can lead to skin tissue injury. Examples of conditions that increase the risk for immobility-related pressure injury include paralysis, extreme fatigue, high-risk pregnancy, sedation, casts, traction, and altered sensory perception.

KnowledgeCheck 32-1

- Identify the major functions of the skin.
- What is the function of the stratum corneum, the outermost layer of the skin?
- What is the function of the subcutaneous layer?
- What effect does aging have on the skin?
- What effect does immobility have on the skin?

Nutrition and Hydration

Skin condition reflects a person's overall nutritional status because nutritional intake affects the skin. Adequate intake of protein, cholesterol, calories, fluid, vitamin C, and minerals is essential to maintaining skin integrity.

Protein Healthy skin depends on adequate protein levels to maintain the skin, repair minor defects, and preserve intravascular volume. As protein levels decline:

- Skin injury is slow to heal, and minor defects cannot be repaired.
- Fluid leaks from the vascular compartment of dependent areas, and **edema** (excess fluid in the tissues) develops.
- Edema decreases skin elasticity and interferes with the diffusion of oxygen to the cells. Therefore, the skin becomes prone to breakdown.

Cholesterol Low cholesterol levels predispose patients to skin breakdown and inhibit wound healing. Patients on low-fat tube feedings may experience deficiencies in cholesterol, fatty acids, and linoleic acid. Together, these fats aid in providing fuel for wound healing and maintain a waterproof barrier in the stratum corneum.

Calorie Intake If calorie intake is inadequate, the body uses proteins for energy **(catabolism);** they are then unavailable for building and maintenance functions **(anabolism)** (see Chapter 24 as needed). With prolonged malnutrition, the person experiences weight loss, loss of subcutaneous tissue, and muscle atrophy. As a result, padding between the skin and the bones decreases, predisposing the skin to a pressure injury.

Ascorbic Acid, Zinc, and Copper Vitamin C (ascorbic acid), zinc, and copper are involved in the formation and maintenance of collagen. A deficiency of any of these elements can delay wound healing.

Hydration Poor skin turgor may occur because of dehydration, whereas edema may result from overhydration. Both dry, dehydrated skin and edematous, overhydrated skin are prone to injury, especially when exposed to pressure, shearing, friction, and moisture. For further discussion on fluid requirements, see Chapter 35.

Diminished Sensation or Cognition

If you've ever touched a hot surface and quickly pulled back your hand, you know the importance of tactile sensation. Patients with peripheral vascular disease, spinal cord injury, diabetes, cerebrovascular accident, trauma, or fractures often have diminished

---

PICOT

Pressure Injury and the Effect of Nutritional Support on Healing

Situation: While caring for an emaciated patient after surgery, the nurse notes two new wounds on the patient's bony prominences. Pressure injury has developed secondary to the patient's immobility, friction, shear, and postoperative drainage.

PICOT Components:

P Population/patient	=	Malnourished adults
I Intervention/indicator	=	Nutritional supplements
C Comparator/control	=	Diet without supplements
O Outcome	=	Improved (or faster) healing time
T Time	=	

Searchable Question: Do _____ (P) who receive/are exposed to _____ (I) demonstrate _____ (O) compared with _____ (C) during _____ (T)?

Example of Evidence: Protein intake has been associated with improved wound healing. To prevent pressure wounds, many acute and long-term care facilities recommend that patients' diets have increased protein content. To examine the effect of nutritional intervention in pressure injury care, researchers reviewed seven research studies on the use of oral nutritional supplementation enriched with arginine (an amino acid), vitamin C, and zinc for pressure injury care. Results showed improved pressure injury healing and reduced risk of developing a pressure injury.

Practice Change: The nurse caring for patients at risk for pressure wounds needs to address the patients' nutritional needs, including a diet high in protein.

Sources: Munoz, N., Posthauer, M. E., Cereda, E., Schols, J., & Haesler, E. (2020). The role of nutrition for pressure injury prevention and healing: The 2019 international clinical practice guideline recommendations. *Advances in Skin and Wound Care, 33*(3), 123–136. https://doi.org/10.1097/01.ASW.0000653144.90739.ad

tactile sense. They are therefore more prone to skin breakdown.

- *Patients with diminished sensation* are less able to sense a hot surface and more likely to suffer a burn. A cut or wound in an area with limited sensation may go unnoticed and therefore untreated. They are also unable to feel pressure in an affected area. As a result, they may not shift position to relieve pressure over bony prominences or be aware that footwear or clothing are constricting.
- *Patients with impaired cognition* (i.e., Alzheimer disease, dementia, altered level of consciousness) are at higher risk for pressure injury because they are not aware of the need to reposition. Cognitive impairment can be subtle and difficult to recognize. Talk to your patients' families or caregivers and review the patient's health history so that the plan of care can be adjusted.

Impaired Circulation

The vascular system brings oxygen-rich blood to the tissues and removes metabolic waste products.

- *Impaired arterial circulation* restricts activity, produces pain, and leads to muscle atrophy and thin tissue that can lead to tissue death.
- *Impaired venous circulation* results in engorged tissues containing high levels of metabolic waste products that make the tissue susceptible to edema, ulceration, and breakdown.

Both forms of circulatory impairment interfere with tissue metabolism and delay wound healing. **Key Point:** *Circulatory impairment is one of the main causes of chronic wounds.*

Medications

Any medication that causes pruritus (itching), dermatoses (rashes), photosensitivity, alopecia (hair loss), or pigmentation changes can result in changes that impair skin integrity or delay healing (Fig. 32-2). The following are examples:

- *Blood pressure medications* decrease the amount of pressure required to occlude blood flow to an area, creating a risk for ischemia.
- *Anti-inflammatory medications,* such as over-the-counter (OTC) NSAIDs and steroids (e.g., prednisone), inhibit wound healing.
- *Anticoagulants* (e.g., heparin, warfarin) can lead to extravasation of blood into subcutaneous tissue. As a result, even minimal pressure or injury can cause a hematoma (large bruise).
- *Chemotherapeutic agents* (e.g., methotrexate) delay wound healing as a result of toxicity to rapidly growing cells.
- *Certain antibiotics, psychotherapeutic drugs, and chemotherapy agents* increase sensitivity to sunlight, increasing the risk for sunburn.

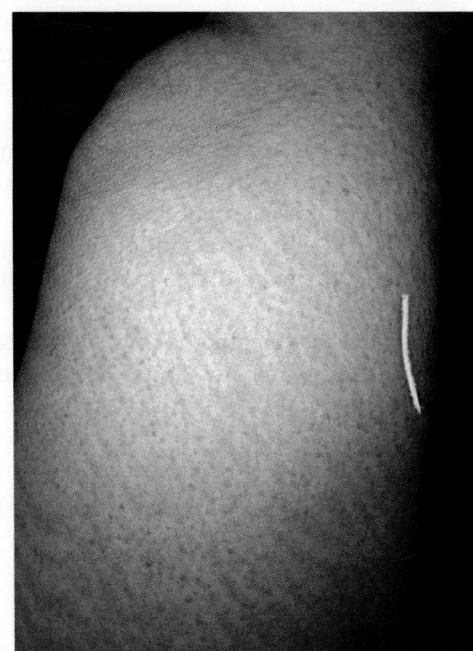

FIGURE 32-2 Skin reaction to medication.

- *Certain antibiotic, antifungal, anticonvulsant, and psychotherapeutic drugs* can trigger a severe rash and skin peeling (known as *Stevens-Johnson syndrome*).
- *Several herbal products,* such as those containing lavender and tea tree oil, cleanse but dry out the skin.

Moisture on the Skin

Excessive exposure to moisture leads to **maceration** (softening of the skin) and increases the likelihood of skin breakdown. Incontinence and fever are the most common sources of moisture. Bowel incontinence is particularly troublesome because feces contain digestive enzymes and microorganisms that can readily lead to **excoriation** (denuding) of superficial skin layers. This can lead to **moisture-associated skin damage (MASD), dermatitis** (inflammation of the skin), pressure injury, and infection.

Fever

Fever leads to sweating, which can cause skin maceration if ongoing. Fever also increases the metabolic rate, thereby raising the tissue demand for oxygen. An increased oxygen demand is especially difficult to meet if there is circulatory impairment or pressure-induced tissue compression.

Contamination or Infection

- **Contamination** of a wound refers to the presence of microorganisms in the wound. **Key Point:** *All chronic wounds are considered contaminated.*
- **Colonization** occurs as microorganisms begin to increase in number but are causing no harm. Wounds

are colonized from the surrounding skin and local skin organisms, the external environment, and internal sources, usually from the mucous membranes of the gastrointestinal system.

- **Critical colonization** occurs when the bacteria begin to overwhelm the body's defenses. You may be able to detect this event by noticing an increase in drainage, a new foul odor, a change in color of the wound bed, new tunneling of the wound, or absent or friable granulation tissue.
- **Infection** implies that the microorganisms are causing harm by releasing toxins, invading body tissues, and increasing the metabolic demands of the tissue. Infection of the skin makes it more vulnerable to breakdown and impedes the healing of open wounds. If not stopped, bacteria can gain access to the systemic circulation.

Lifestyle

- *Sun exposure* helps the body to produce vitamin D, a necessary nutrient for health. However, too much exposure to the sun can injure the skin and retina of the eyes. It also increases the risk of skin cancer. The damaging ultraviolet (UV) rays cause drying and *photoaging* (premature aging of the skin).
- *Skin cleansing* that is either excessive or insufficient may impair skin integrity. Frequent bathing and use of soap remove skin oils and may lead to drying, which compromises the skin's barrier function. Infrequent cleansing of the skin contributes to excessive oiliness, clogged sebaceous glands, and inadequate removal of microbes on the skin, which can then infect a wound or lesion.
- *Regular physical activity* improves circulation, which is necessary for skin integrity and wound healing.
- *A nutritious diet* provides the nutrients needed to maintain skin integrity, as already discussed.
- *Tobacco use* compromises the oxygen supply to the tissues, making skin more prone to breakdown and delaying wound healing. It also interferes with vitamin C absorption, which is needed for collagen formation.
- *Body piercings and tattoos* present a risk for infection and scarring. The most common complications of tattooing are local inflammation (irritation at the site), allergic reaction to the ink, and skin infection (cellulitis). Unsterile conditions can lead to a systemic infection, such as hepatitis C.

  Bacterial infections at or near the site of body piercings are most commonly *Staphylococcus* and *Pseudomonas* strains. Endocarditis can occur in new piercings (Armstrong et al., 2008). A pierced nipple is more likely to get infected and form an abscess than other types of piercings. Healing time is longer when piercing occurs in the nipple tissue. Nipple piercing can interfere with breastfeeding because scar tissue or nipple jewelry can block the release of milk. Infant

latch-on may be a problem. There is also a risk of swallowing or choking on a loose nipple ring.

  Oral piercings can result in gingivitis, damage to teeth and gums, choking, difficulty eating, and changes in speech. Prolonged bleeding can result with piercing of the tongue if a blood vessel is punctured (Meltzer, 2005). Advise patients to become informed about the procedure and about aftercare and to find reputable piercers.

KnowledgeCheck 32-2

- Identify the factors that affect skin integrity.
- What nutritional components are essential to maintain skin integrity?

ThinkLike a Nurse 32-1: Clinical Judgment in Action

- Review the case of William Harmon (Meet Your Patient). What risks, if any, does Mr. Harmon have for skin breakdown or delayed healing?
- What additional information do you need to know to fully evaluate his risk?
- What risks do you have for impaired skin integrity? What actions can you take to protect your skin?

WOUNDS

Wounds are a disruption in the normal integrity of the skin. Wounds may be intentional, such as a surgical wound, or unintentional, such as a cut or a pressure injury.

Types of Wounds

Wounds are classified according to the length of time the wound has existed, as well as the condition of the wound (e.g., contamination, severity).

Skin Integrity The simplest wound classification system is based on the integrity of the skin.

- A **closed wound** exists when there are no breaks in the skin. Contusions (bruises) or tissue swelling from fractures are common closed wounds.
- An **open wound** occurs when there is a break in the skin or mucous membranes. Open wounds include abrasions, lacerations, puncture wounds, and surgical incisions. A compound fracture may also lead to an open wound caused by the projection of bone through the skin. Several open and closed wounds are described in Table 32-1.

Length of Time for Healing The length of time for wound healing varies according to the skin integrity and the factors affecting it, discussed in the previous section.

- **Acute wounds** are expected to be of short duration. In a healthy person, these wounds heal spontaneously without complications through the three phases of wound healing (inflammation, proliferation, and maturation).

Table 32-1 ➤ Types of Wounds

TYPE	DESCRIPTION
Abrasion	A scrape of the superficial layers of the skin; usually unintentional but may be performed intentionally for cosmetic purposes to smooth skin surfaces (also see *excoriation*)
Abscess	A localized collection of pus resulting from invasion from a pyogenic bacterium or other pathogen; must be opened and drained to heal
Contusion	A closed wound caused by blunt trauma; may be referred to as a *bruise* or an *ecchymosis*
Crushing	A wound caused by force leading to compression or disruption of tissues, often associated with fracture. Usually there is minimal or no break in the skin.
Excoriation	Superficial wound, usually self-inflicted as a result of excessive scratching or mechanical force
Incision	An open, intentional wound caused by a sharp instrument
Laceration	The skin or mucous membranes are torn open, resulting in a wound with jagged margins.
Penetrating	An open wound in which the agent causing the wound lodges in body tissue
Puncture	An open wound caused by a sharp object; often, there is collapse of tissue around the entry point, making this wound prone to infection
Tunnel	A wound with an entrance and exit site

- **Chronic wounds** are wounds that exceed the expected length of recovery, usually because the natural healing progression has been interrupted or stalled because of infection, continued trauma, ischemia, or edema. Chronic wounds include pressure injuries, or arterial, venous, and diabetic ulcers (Fig. 32-3). These wounds are frequently colonized with several types of bacteria, and healing is slow because of the underlying disease process. Unless the type of wound is properly diagnosed and the underlying disease process is treated, a chronic wound may linger for months or years (Table 32-2).

Level of Contamination

- **Clean wounds** are uninfected wounds with minimal inflammation. They may be open or closed and do not involve the gastrointestinal, respiratory, or genitourinary tracts (these systems frequently harbor microorganisms). There is little risk of infection in a clean wound.
- **Clean-contaminated wounds** are surgical incisions that enter the gastrointestinal, respiratory, or genitourinary tracts. There is an increased risk of infection for these wounds, but there is no obvious infection.
- **Contaminated wounds** include open, traumatic wounds or surgical incisions in which a major break in asepsis occurred. The risk of infection is high for these wounds.
- **Infected wounds** are those in which the bacteria count in the wound is above 100,000 organisms per gram of tissue. **Key Point:** *Keep in mind that the presence of beta-hemolytic streptococci, in any number, is considered an infection.* Signs of wound infection include

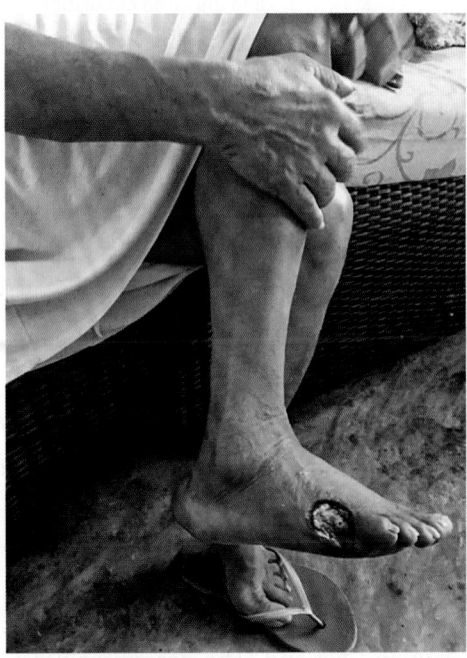

FIGURE 32-3 Diabetic foot ulcer.

erythema and swelling around the wound, fever, foul odor, severe or increasing pain, large amount of drainage, or warmth of the surrounding soft tissue.

Depth and Location of the Wound Major determinants of healing time are the depth of the wound and its location. **Key Point:** *The deeper the wound, the longer the healing time. Wounds located at points of pressure or movement are also slower to heal. Wounds in areas*

Table 32-2 ➤ Chronic Wounds

TYPE	ETIOLOGY	CHARACTERISTICS
Pressure injury	Caused by pressure, shear, and friction, resulting in tissue ischemia and injury	■ Appearance depends on the stage or tissue layers involved. ■ Pressure injuries tend to be located over bony prominences or related medical device (National Pressure Injury Advisory Panel [NPIAP], 2019). ■ Can cause serious tissue damage
Arterial ulcers	Caused by inadequate circulation of oxygenated blood to the tissue, which leads to tissue ischemia and damage	■ Commonly found over the lower leg, especially the ankles, toes, side of the foot, and shin ■ Ulcer appears "punched out," small and round with smooth borders. ■ Wound base is usually pale, with or without necrotic tissue. ■ Surrounding skin is shiny, thin, and dry and is cool to the touch. ■ Loss of hair in the surrounding area ■ Delayed capillary refill time in the area ■ Very painful, especially at night and with increased activity
Venous stasis ulcers	Caused by incompetent venous valves, deep vein obstruction, or inadequate calf muscle function, resulting in venous pooling, edema, and impaired circulation of the skin	■ Usually located around the inner ankle or in the lower part of the calf ■ Surrounding skin is reddened or brown and edematous. ■ Usually shallow, with irregular wound margins ■ Wound bed appears "ruddy" or "beefy" red and granular. ■ Drainage may be moderate to heavy, depending on amount of edema. ■ Pain usually occurs with leg dependence and dressing changes.
Diabetic foot ulcer	Caused by narrowing of the arteries, which leads to reduced oxygenation to the feet, resulting in delayed wound healing and tissue necrosis	■ Often painless; often with drainage, swelling, redness, and ulceration ■ Occurs mainly on the plantar surfaces and toes (balls of the foot or underside of the toes) ■ Highly susceptible to wound infection because of the poor sensation, circulation, and immune protection

of poor circulation are more difficult to heal (e.g., feet for those with diabetes or congestive heart failure).

- **Superficial wounds** involve only the epidermal layer of the skin. The injury is usually the result of friction, shearing, or burning.
- **Partial-thickness wounds** extend through the epidermis but not through the dermis.
- **Full-thickness wounds** extend into the subcutaneous tissue and beyond. The descriptor *penetrating* is sometimes added to indicate that the wound involves internal organs.

KnowledgeCheck 32-3

- Explain the difference between an acute and a chronic wound.
- Describe the wound categorization system based on the level of contamination.
- How does wound depth affect healing?

Wound Healing Process

All wounds heal through a physiological process in which epithelial, endothelial, and inflammatory cells, platelets, and fibroblasts (cells in connective tissue that produce fibrin) migrate into the wound to bring about tissue repair and regeneration. The process is essentially the same regardless of the type of injury or the type of tissues involved.

Types of Healing

Wounds may heal by regeneration or by primary, secondary, or tertiary intention.

- **Regenerative/epithelial healing.** This takes place when a wound affects only the epidermis and dermis. No scar forms, and the new (regenerated) epithelial and dermal cells form new skin that cannot be distinguished from the intact skin. Partial-thickness wounds heal by regeneration.
- **Primary (first) intention healing.** This occurs when a wound involves minimal or no tissue loss and has edges that are well approximated (closed) (Fig. 32-4A). Little scarring is expected. A clean surgical incision heals by this method. Even so, a scar is only 80% as strong as the original tissue (Mercanetti, 2021).

Primary intention

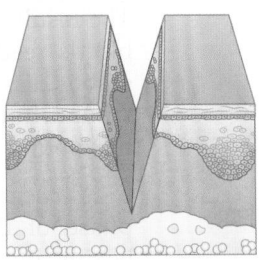 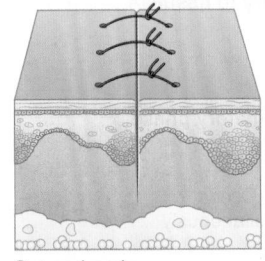 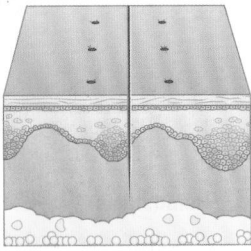

A Clean wound   Sutured early   Results in hairline scar

Secondary intention

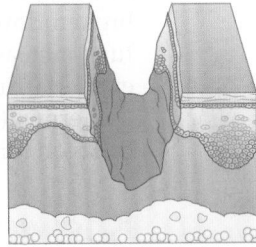 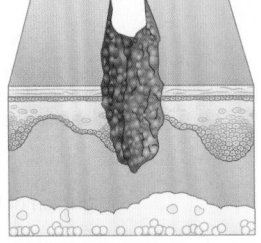 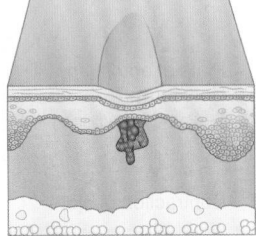

B Wound gaping and irregular   Granulation occurring   Epithelium fills in scar

Tertiary intention

FIGURE 32-4 *A,* In a wound with minimal tissue loss, the edges may be sutured together, resulting in rapid healing and minimal scarring. *B,* A wound that heals by secondary intention heals from the inner layer to the surface. Healing takes longer, and there is scarring. *C,* A wound that heals by tertiary intention is initially healed by secondary intention and later sutured.

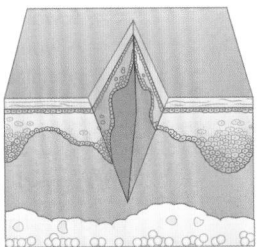 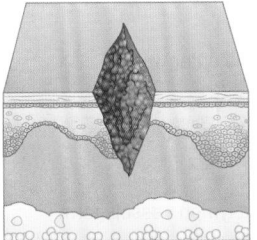 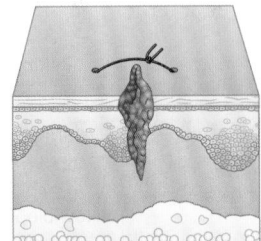

C Wound not sutured   Granulation partially fills in wound   Granulating tissue sutured together

- **Secondary intention healing.** This occurs when a wound (1) involves extensive tissue loss that prevents wound edges from approximating or (2) should not be closed (e.g., because of infection). Because the wound is left open, it heals from the inner layer to the surface by filling in with beefy-red **granulation tissue** (a form of connective tissue with an abundant blood supply) (Fig. 32-4B). Healing epithelial tissue may appear in the wound as small pink or pearl-like areas. **Key Point:** *Wounds that heal by secondary intention heal more slowly, are more prone to infection, and develop more scar tissue.*
- **Tertiary intention healing.** Also called *delayed primary closure,* this occurs when two surfaces of granulation tissue are brought together (Fig. 32-4C). This technique may be used when the wound is clean-contaminated or contaminated. Initially, the wound is allowed to heal by secondary intention. When there is no evidence of edema, infection, or foreign matter, the wound edges are closed by bringing together the granulating tissue and suturing the surface. Such wounds require strict aseptic technique during all dressing changes because they are prone to infection.

Tertiary intention healing creates less scarring than secondary healing but more scarring than primary intention healing.

Phases of Healing

Wound healing occurs in three stages: inflammatory, proliferative, and maturation (Fig. 32-5).

Inflammatory Phase—Cleansing This phase lasts from 1 to 5 days and consists of two major processes: hemostasis and inflammation.

- *Hemostasis.* At the time of injury, tissue and capillaries are destroyed, causing blood and plasma to leak into the wound. Area vessels constrict to limit blood loss. Platelets aggregate (clump together) to slow bleeding. At the same time, the clotting mechanism is activated to form a blood clot.
- *Inflammation.* The inflammatory reaction is characterized by edema, erythema, pain, temperature elevation, and migration of white blood cells into the wound tissues. Within 24 hours, macrophages begin engulfing bacteria (**phagocytosis**) and clearing debris. Along with plasma proteins and fibrin, they form a

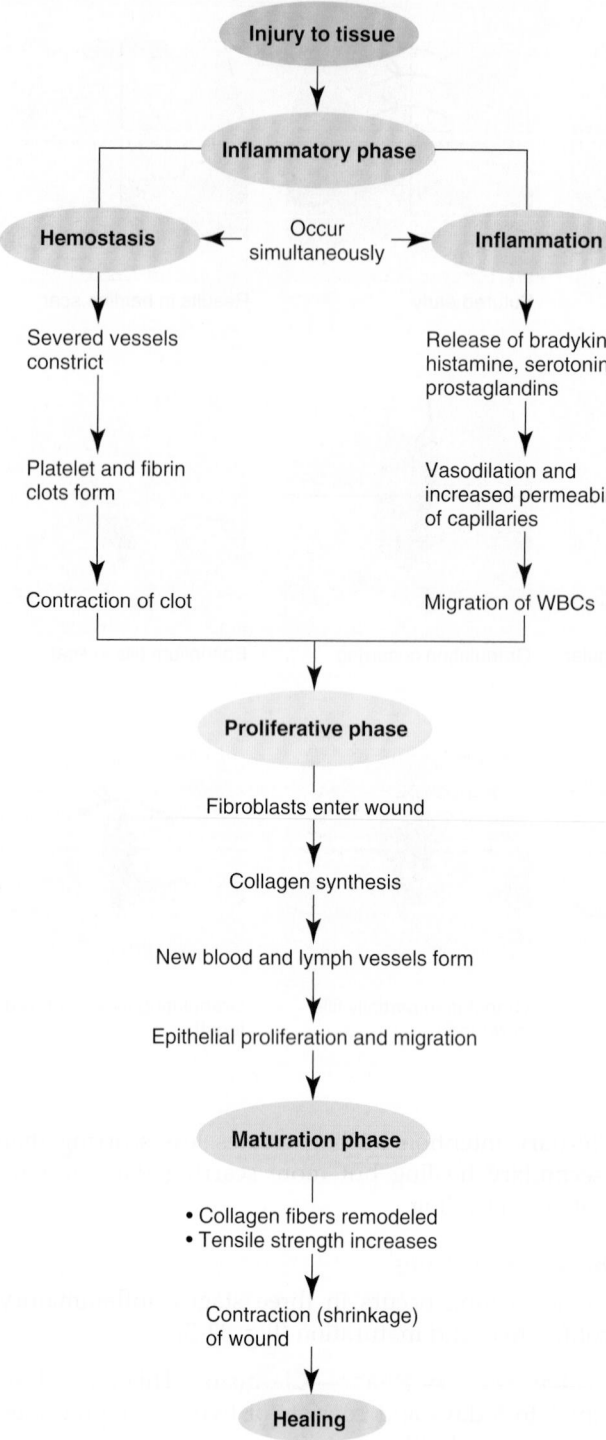

FIGURE 32-5 Stages in the wound-healing process.

scab on the wound surface, which seals the wound and helps prevent microbial invasion.

Proliferative Phase—Granulation This phase occurs from days 5 to 21. Cells develop to fill the wound defect and resurface the skin. **Fibroblasts** (connective tissue cells) migrate to the wound, where they form **collagen,** a protein substance that adds strength to the healing wound. New blood and lymph vessels sprout

from the existing capillaries at the edge of the wound. The result is the formation of granulation tissue, which bleeds readily and is easily damaged. As the clot or scab is dissolved, epithelial cells begin to grow into the wound from surrounding healthy tissue and seal over the wound **(epithelialization).**

Maturation Phase—Epithelialization The final phase of the healing process, known as *remodeling,* begins in the second or third week and continues even after the wound has closed. During the next 3 to 6 months, the initial collagen fibers that were laid in the wound bed during the proliferative phase are broken down and remodeled into an organized structure, increasing the tensile strength of the wound. However, scarring can result when the keratinocytes in the epidermis (outer layer of the skin) produce too much collagen for healing.

KnowledgeCheck 32-4

Identify the type of wound healing (primary, secondary, or tertiary intention):

- A wound that heals from the inner layer to the surface
- A wound with approximated edges
- A wound that heals by approximating two surfaces of granulation tissue
- A wound that is sutured and has minimal or no tissue loss

Wound Closures

Wounds that heal by primary and tertiary intention may be closed in several ways.

Adhesive Strips In the following situations, adhesive strips are used for wound closing by:

- Closing superficial low-tension wounds, such as skin tears or lacerations
- Closing the skin on a wound that has been closed subcutaneously to aid in healing and reduce scarring
- Giving additional support to a wound after sutures or staples have been removed

Adhesive strips are often kept in place until they begin to separate from the skin on their own. For complete instructions,

 See **Chapter 32, Procedure 32-9, Placing Skin Closures,** in Volume 2.

Sutures The traditional wound closures are sutures ("stitches"). Suturing creates small puncture wounds along the track of the laceration or incision. Several types of suture materials are available.

- *Absorbent sutures* are used deep in the tissues—for example, to close an organ or **anastomose** (connective) tissue, or with fine facial sutures. Because they are made of material that will gradually dissolve, there is no need to remove absorbent sutures.

■ *Nonabsorbent sutures* are placed in superficial tissues and require removal, usually by the nurse. For complete steps,

 See **Chapter 32, Procedure 32-12A, Removing Sutures and Staples,** in Volume 2.

Surgical Staples Made of lightweight titanium, surgical staples provide a fast, easy way to close an incision (Fig. 32-6). They are also associated with a lower risk of infection and tissue reaction compared with sutures. The downside of staples is that some wound edges are more difficult to align. The most common sites for wound stapling are the arms, legs, abdomen, back, scalp, and bowel. **Key Point: *Wounds on the hands, feet, neck, or face should not be stapled.***

Surgical Glue This is safe for use in clean, low-tension wounds. It is an ideal wound closure method for skin tears.

Collaborative Wound Treatments

Collaborative treatments are necessary for wounds that will not heal despite aggressive care. Such treatments include the following:

■ **Surgical options,** such as extensive débridement, skin grafts, secondary closure of the wound, and flap techniques (partially detached tissue placed over a wound), are used for complicated wounds.
■ **Hyperbaric oxygen therapy (HBOT)** is the administration of 100% oxygen under pressure to a wound site. HBOT increases the oxygen concentration in the tissue, stimulates the growth of new blood vessels, and enhances white blood cell (WBC) action. HBOT also promotes the development of fibroblasts for wound healing.
■ **Platelet-derived growth factor** augments the inflammatory phase of wound healing and accelerates collagen formation in the wound.

Types of Wound Drainage

Drainage that oozes from a wound or cavity is referred to as **exudate.** Exudate is formed from inflammation and may take several forms:

■ **Serous exudate** is watery in consistency and contains very little cellular matter. Serous exudate consists of *serum,* the straw-colored fluid that separates out of blood when a clot is formed. Clean wounds typically drain serous exudate.
■ **Sanguineous exudate** is bloody drainage. It indicates damage to capillaries. You will often see sanguineous exudate with deep wounds or wounds in highly vascular areas. Fresh bleeding produces bright-red drainage, whereas older, dried blood is a darker, red-brown color.
■ **Serosanguineous drainage** is a combination of bloody and serous drainage. It occurs most commonly in new wounds.
■ **Purulent exudate** is thick, often malodorous, drainage that is seen in infected wounds. It contains pus, a protein-rich fluid filled with WBCs, fibrin, bacteria, and cellular debris. It is commonly caused by infection with **pyogenic** (pus-forming) bacteria, such as streptococci or staphylococci. Normally, pus is yellow in color, although it may take on a blue-green shade if the bacterium *Pseudomonas aeruginosa* is present.
■ **Purosanguineous exudate** is red-tinged pus. It indicates that small vessels in the wound area have ruptured.

Complications of Wound Healing

Recall that wounds heal by moving through the phases of inflammation, proliferation, and maturation. At times, this process is interrupted by complications, such as hemorrhage, infection, dehiscence, evisceration, and fistulas.

Hemorrhage

Hemorrhage implies a profuse or rapid loss of blood. Whenever a capillary network is interrupted or a blood vessel is severed, bleeding occurs. **Hemostasis** (cessation of bleeding) usually occurs within minutes of the injury. Hemostasis can be delayed when large vessels are injured, a clotting disorder exists, or the patient is on anticoagulant therapy. If bleeding begins again after initial hemostasis, something is probably wrong. Possible causes include a slipped suture, erosion of a blood vessel, a dislodged clot, or infection. **Key Point: *The risk***

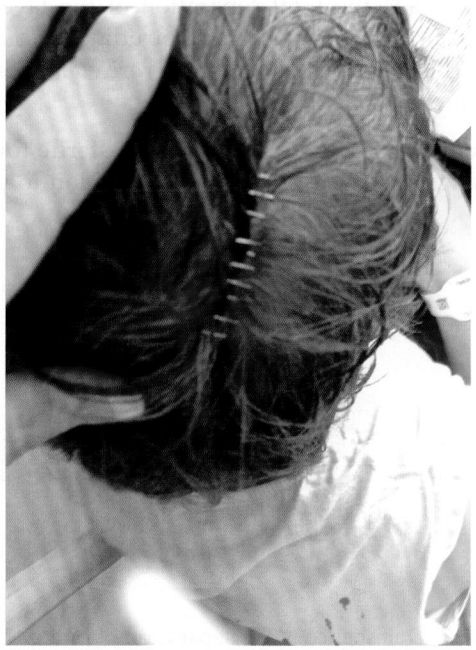

FIGURE 32-6 Surgical staples in the scalp.

of hemorrhage (both internal and external bleeding) is greatest in the first 24 to 48 hours after surgery or injury.

Internal Hemorrhage Swelling of the affected body part, pain, and changes in vital signs (i.e., decreased blood pressure, elevated pulse) may indicate internal bleeding. In this chapter, the term *internal bleeding* refers to a **hematoma,** a red-blue collection of blood under the skin, which forms because of bleeding that cannot escape to the surface. A large hematoma causes pressure on surrounding tissues. If the hematoma is located near a major artery or vein, it may impede blood flow.

External Hemorrhage External hemorrhage is relatively easy to recognize. You will see bloody drainage on the dressings and in the wound drainage devices. When there is a brisk hemorrhage, blood often pools as the dressings become saturated. To be sure that you are aware of the full extent of the bleeding, remember to look underneath the patient.

Infection

Early recognition of infection is crucial to wound management.

- **Suspect infection if a wound fails to heal.** Other symptoms suggesting infection are:
  - Localized swelling
  - Redness
  - Heat
  - Pain
  - Fever (temperatures higher than 38°C [100.4°F])
  - Foul-smelling or purulent drainage
  - A change in the color of drainage
- **In a contaminated or traumatic wound,** the symptoms are likely to occur within 2 to 3 days.
- **In a clean surgical wound,** you will usually not see signs and symptoms of an infection until the fourth or fifth postoperative day.

Distinction between infection in the superficial tissues and those in deeper compartments is important for guiding treatment plans. Typically, superficial infections respond to topical antimicrobials; deep infection requires the use of systemic antimicrobial agents.

For identifying superficial infection, think of the acronym NERDS:

- "**N**onhealing wounds
- **E**xudative wounds
- **R**ed and bleeding wound surface granulation tissue
- **D**ebris (yellow or black necrotic tissue) on the wound surface
- **S**mell or unpleasant odor from the wound" (Sibbald et al., 2006, p. 452)

For deep infection, consider the acronym STONES:

- "**S**ize is bigger
- **T**emperature increased
- **O**s [probe to or exposed bone]

- New or satellite areas of breakdown
- **E**xudate, erythema, edema
- **S**mell" (Sibbald et al., 2006, p. 452).

Dehiscence

Rupture (separation) of one or more layers of a wound is called **dehiscence** (Fig. 32-7). Wound dehiscence is most likely to occur in the inflammatory phase of healing, before large amounts of collagen have been deposited in the wound to strengthen it. An increased risk of dehiscence occurs from incisions that begin draining within 5 to 7 days after surgery.

Common causes of wound dehiscence are:

- Poor nutritional status
- Inadequate closure of the muscles
- Wound infection
- Increased tension on the suture line (e.g., coughing, lifting an object)
- Obesity because fatty tissue does not heal readily, and increased tissue mass puts additional strain on the suture line.

Dehiscence is usually associated with abdominal wounds. Patients often report feeling a "pop" or tear, especially with sudden straining from coughing, vomiting, changing positions in bed, or standing. Usually, there is an immediate increase in serosanguineous drainage. Nursing interventions include the following:

- Maintaining bedrest with the head of the bed elevated at 20° and the knees flexed
- Applying a binder, if necessary, to prevent evisceration
- Notifying the provider of the dehiscence immediately

Evisceration

Evisceration is the total separation of the layers of a wound with internal viscera protruding through the incision (Fig. 32-8). **Key Point: *This rare complication is a surgical emergency.***

- **Immediately cover the wound with sterile towels** or dressings soaked in sterile saline solution to prevent

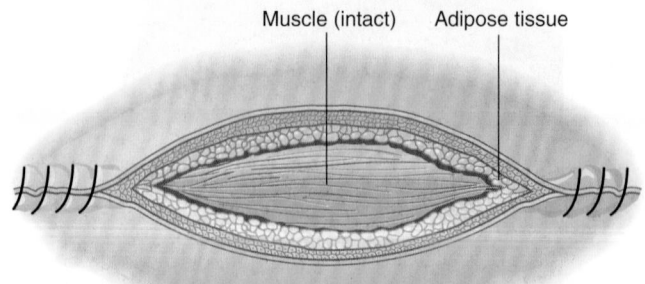

Muscle (intact)   Adipose tissue

FIGURE 32-7 Dehiscence is the separation of one or more layers of a wound. It is most common in the inflammatory phase of healing.

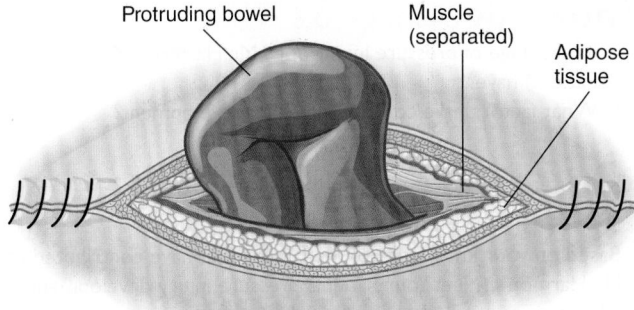

FIGURE 32-8 Evisceration is a total separation of the layers of a wound, with internal viscera protruding through the incision.

the organs from drying out and becoming contaminated with environmental bacteria.

- **Have the patient stay in bed with the knees bent** to minimize strain on the incision.
- **Do not put a binder on the patient.**
- **Notify the surgeon** and ready the patient for surgery (see Chapter 36 for care of the surgical patient).

Fistulas

A **fistula** is an abnormal passage connecting two body cavities or a cavity and the skin. Fistulas often result from infection or debris left in the wound. Fistulas can occur after bowel surgery, especially in compromised patients. It can also occur spontaneously and is associated with certain diseases, such as inflammatory bowel disease (IBD) and cancer (McNichol et al., 2021). An abscess forms, which breaks down surrounding tissue and creates the abnormal passageway. Chronic drainage from the fistula may lead to skin breakdown and delayed wound healing. The most common sites of fistula formation are the gastrointestinal and genitourinary tracts. Figure 32-9 illustrates a fistula between the rectum and vagina.

KnowledgeCheck 32-5

- Describe four types of wound closures.
- Identify five types of wound complications.
- Describe three signs of internal hemorrhage.
- Compare dehiscence and evisceration.

 ThinkLike a Nurse 32-2:
Clinical Judgment **in Action**

Recall the case of Mr. Harmon (Meet Your Patient). What form of wound healing (primary, secondary, or tertiary) is he undergoing? How long would you expect it to take before his wounds heal?

CHRONIC WOUNDS

A chronic wound is one that has not healed within the expected time frame. Wounds that do not heal within

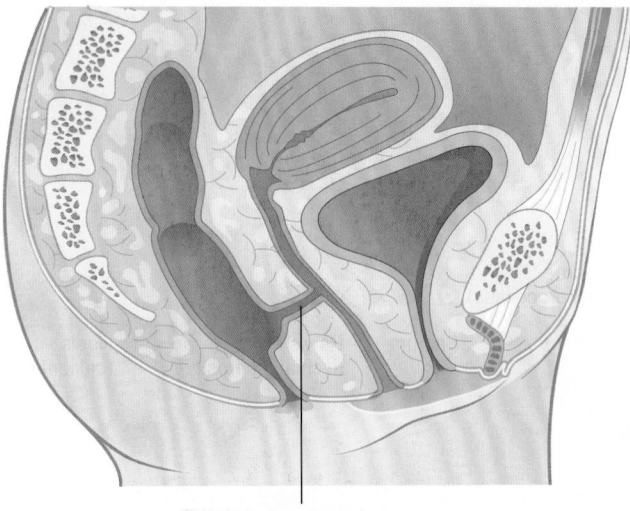

Fistula between rectum
and vagina (enterovaginal)

FIGURE 32-9 A fistula is an abnormal passage connecting two body cavities or a cavity and the skin. Fistulas are most common in the gastrointestinal and genitourinary tracts.

2 to 4 weeks may be considered chronic. A pressure injury is a type of chronic wound. To learn about pressure injuries, see the Example Client Condition: Pressure Injury and Figures 32-10 and 32-11.

PracticalKnowledge
knowing **how**

As a nurse, you will care for many patients who have wounds or who are at risk for skin breakdown. The remainder of the chapter explains how to

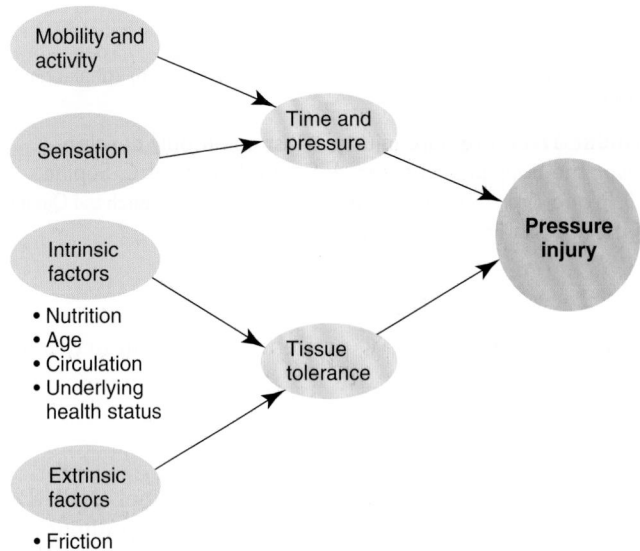

FIGURE 32-10 Several factors contribute to the development of a pressure injury.

A

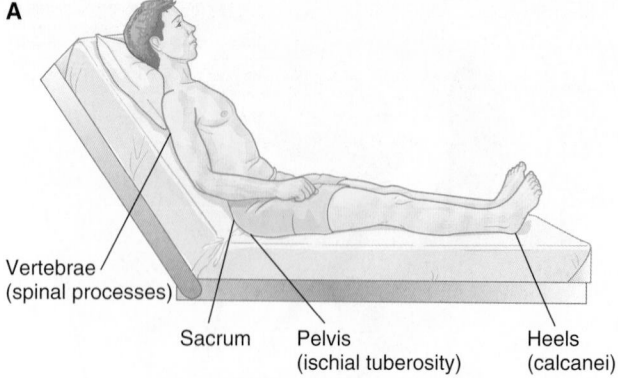

Vertebrae
(spinal processes)

Sacrum   Pelvis   Heels
          (ischial tuberosity) (calcanei)

B

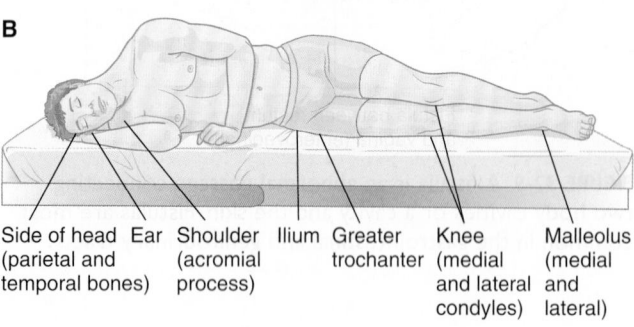

Side of head Ear   Shoulder   Ilium Greater   Knee   Malleolus
(parietal and (acromial   trochanter (medial   (medial
temporal bones) process)   and lateral and
                                       condyles)   lateral)

C

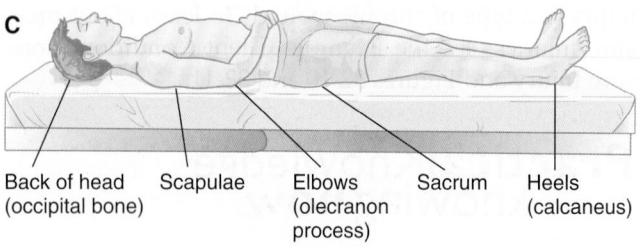

Back of head Scapulae   Elbows   Sacrum   Heels
(occipital bone)   (olecranon   (calcaneus)
                         process)

D

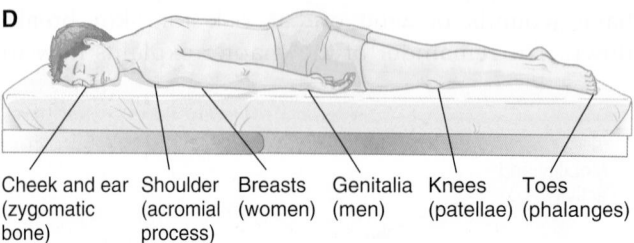

Cheek and ear Shoulder   Breasts   Genitalia Knees   Toes
(zygomatic   (acromial (women)   (men)   (patellae) (phalanges)
bone)   process)

FIGURE 32-11 Pressure injuries most commonly develop over the bony prominences. *A,* Sitting. *B,* Lateral. *C,* Supine. *D,* Prone. (*Source:* Adapted from Agency for Healthcare Research and Quality [AHRQ] Clinical Practice Guidelines.)

maintain skin integrity, prevent pressure injury, and treat wounds.

ASSESSMENT/RECOGNIZING CUES

The National Pressure Injury Advisory Panel (NPIAP) recommends that nurses perform a comprehensive wound assessment while identifying other health problems and their impact on wound healing. A thorough skin evaluation includes a nursing history, physical examination, and diagnostic testing.

KnowledgeCheck 32-6

- What stage of pressure injury does Mr. Harmon (Meet Your Patient) have?
- What factors have contributed to its development?

ThinkLike a Nurse 32-3: Clinical Judgment in Action

Based on your knowledge of the factors that have contributed to Mr. Harmon's (Meet Your Patient) pressure injury development, what actions may lead to healing of the pressure injury?
Note: To answer this question, you do not need to know about wound care (e.g., irrigation) for a pressure injury.

Focused Nursing History

To assess wound-healing ability and the risk for skin breakdown, you will need to gather data on factors that affect skin integrity (discussed previously): age, mobility, nutrition, hydration, sensation, circulation, medications, moisture, lifestyle, underlying health and disease status, and the presence of microorganisms (Fig. 32-10). Also consider the psychosocial issues related to coping with chronic wounds. Bolstering coping strategies and increasing resilience can help with increasing feelings of well-being; likewise, improving well-being can improve wound healing (Dudfield et al., 2019).

♥ **iCare**   You will need to assess with care and compassion how the patient:

- Copes with the pain of a chronic wound
- Handles the loss of control and independence
- Is adapting to changes in body image
- Deals with the financial burden of caring for complex wounds
- Adjusts to the social isolation that comes with impaired mobility and chronic illness

For history questions to help you assess these factors,

 See **Chapter 32, Focused Assessment, History Questions for Skin and Wound Assessment,** in Volume 2.

Focused Physical Examination

Physical assessment of skin integrity focuses on skin inspection, mobility, and activity assessment.

Assessing the Skin   Assess all areas of the body routinely for skin color, integrity, temperature, texture, turgor, mobility, moisture, lesions, and hair distribution. Check pressure points for erythema, tenderness, or edema. Assess all bony prominences of individuals at risk for skin breakdown routinely (Fig 32-11). Examine skin under special garments such as shoes, heel elevators, and antiembolism stockings. Also assess vulnerable pressure points for bed- or chair-bound patients. See Chapter 19 for more details on skin assessment.

Assessing Mobility and Activity Level Patients who have some degree of immobility are at a higher risk for developing pressure injury and should be closely monitored to detect early signs of the formation of pressure-related wounds. See Chapter 29 for more details about physical activity and immobility.

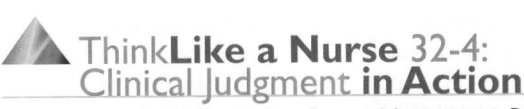

ThinkLike a Nurse 32-4: Clinical Judgment in Action

Review the Braden scale (see Focused Assessment, Braden Scale for Predicting Pressure Sore Risk in Volume 2). Apply this risk assessment scale to Mr. Harmon (Meet Your Patient).

- What additional information, if any, do you need to complete these assessments?
- Calculate a Braden score based on Mr. Harmon's risk factors if he had also been incontinent of urine twice that day.

Assessing Treated Wounds

All wounds require a focused assessment. Assessment frequency depends on the condition of the wound, the work setting, the patient's overall condition and underlying disease process, the type of wound, and the type of treatment used for the wound. If you are providing wound care, you will assess the wound with every treatment (Table 32-3). For a wound assessment summary,

 See **Chapter 32, Focused Assessment, Physical Examination: Wound Assessment,** in Volume 2.

Location Describe the wound location in anatomical terms. For example, describe an incision from cardiac surgery as a midsternal incision extending from the manubrium to the xiphoid process. An accurate description of the location is important because:

- *Location influences the rate of healing.* Wounds in highly vascular regions, such as the scalp or hands, heal more rapidly than wounds in less vascular regions, such as the abdomen or a heel.
- *Location affects movement.* Wounds that can be readily stabilized heal more rapidly than those in areas that are affected by the constant stress of movement.
- *Location can give you clues to the wound etiology.* A wound over a bony prominence could be related to pressure, whereas one on the bottom of the foot could be a diabetic foot ulcer.

Type of Wound Is it an acute wound? If the wound is sutured, examine the closure. Are the wound edges approximated (together)? Is there tension on any aspect of the wound? Are the stitches intact? Or is this a chronic wound?

Size Place the patient in a neutral position to measure the wound. Variations in positioning can distort soft tissue, causing you to obtain a larger or smaller measurement. Use a consistent method to measure the length, width, and depth of the wound in centimeters. To measure wound depth, gently insert a sterile cotton-tip applicator into the deepest part of the wound. Measure the applicator from the tip in the wound bed to the skin level.

Serial photographs with grids showing the wound's dimensions, especially if the wound has an irregular border, are useful for documenting the baseline and wound healing (European Pressure Ulcer Advisory Panel [EPUAP] et al., 2019).

Undermining or Tunneling Assess the wound edges for any undermining or tunneling. Pay close attention to any tissue that appears to have a separation in either tissue type or plane because tunnels may frequently be found. Measure the depth and location of any undermining or tunneling using the face of a clock as a guide.

Periwound Examine the skin surrounding the wound. Skin discoloration may indicate a hematoma or additional injury to the surrounding tissue. Look for the following conditions:

- **Maceration** is caused by excessive moisture from pooled drainage on intact skin for periods of time or when a moist dressing is inappropriately applied, is left on too long, or overlaps onto healthy skin. The skin may appear pale and wrinkled ("pruned") and may flake and peel.
- **Undermining** (tunneling) will produce a boggy feel around the wound.
- **Crepitus** is gas trapped under the skin. If you palpate the surrounding skin and feel a crackling sensation, this is crepitus. Crepitus may be due to air leaking from the lung in a chest wound or may also indicate the presence of gas-producing bacteria.
- **Erythema**, **swelling,** or other signs of irritation indicate that the surrounding tissue is in jeopardy.
- **Epibole** is closed or rolled wound edges. Examine wound edges for epithelial tissue and contraction. Epibole may indicate that epithelial cells have moved down and rolled under the wound edges. The edges tend to be lighter in color than surrounding tissue and may feel *indurated* (hardened). Once the cells reach the wound bed, they will stall wound healing.
- **Slough,** which is often soft, stringy, and pale yellow or gray, is moist necrotic tissue that needs to be removed from the wound bed.
- **Eschar** (also known as an *unstageable pressure injury*) is dry necrotic tissue that appears thick, hard, and black or brown in the wound bed.

Extent and Type of Tissue in the Wound Base Assessment of the types of tissue and their amounts can give you an idea of the severity of the wound, treatment options, and/or healing of the wound. Table 32-4 outlines different types of tissue you might see in a wound bed.

- **Key Point:** *Viable (living) tissue must be distinguished from nonviable tissue.*

Table 32-3 ➤ Staging Pressure Injury

STAGE	CLINICAL FINDINGS	DISCUSSION
Stage 1 Pressure Injury 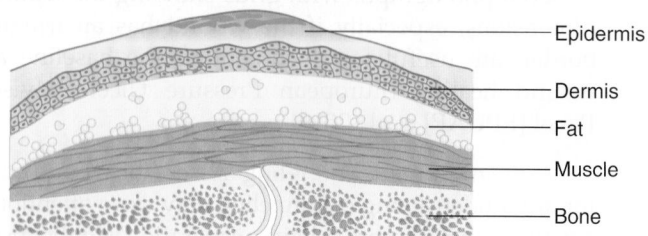 **Stage I** 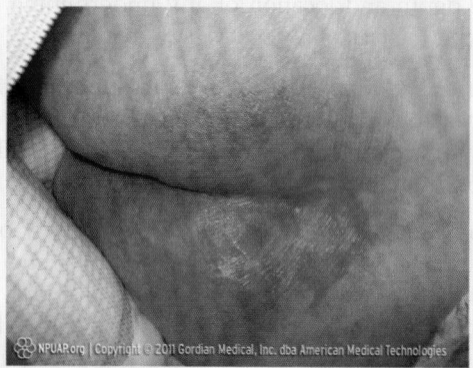	Localized area of intact skin with nonblanchable redness (does not become pale under applied light pressure), usually over a bony prominence, but not maroon or purple discoloration The area may be painful, firm, soft, or warmer or cooler compared with adjacent tissue. Discoloration will remain for more than 30 minutes after pressure is relieved.	Dark skin may not have visible blanching (becomes pale when light pressure is applied); its color may differ from that of the surrounding area. Therefore, stage I may be difficult to detect.
Stage 2 Pressure Injury 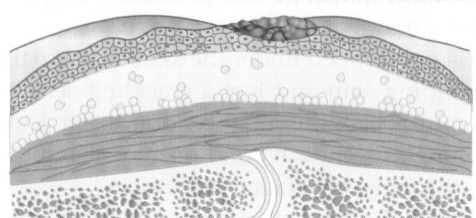 **Stage II** 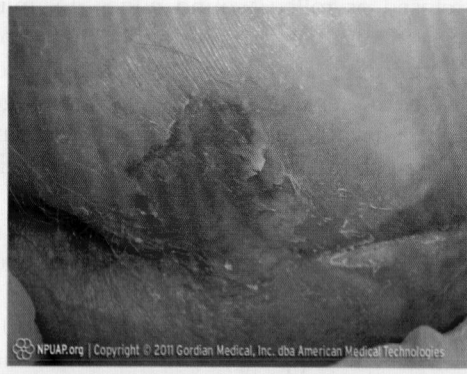	Involves partial-thickness loss of dermis Stage 2 pressure injury is open but shallow and with a reddish-pink wound bed. There is no *slough* (tan, yellow, gray, green, or brown necrotic tissue). May also be an intact or open/ruptured serum-filled blister or a shiny or dry shallow ulcer without slough or bruising	Do not use this stage to describe skin tears, tape burns, perineal dermatitis, maceration, or excoriation. Do not mistake moisture-associated skin damage or fungal infections for stage 2 pressure injury. Stage 2 pressure injury does not involve sloughing or bruising.

Labels on Stage I diagram: Epidermis, Dermis, Fat, Muscle, Bone

Table 32-3 ➤ Staging Pressure Injury—cont'd

STAGE	CLINICAL FINDINGS	DISCUSSION
Stage 3 Pressure Injury 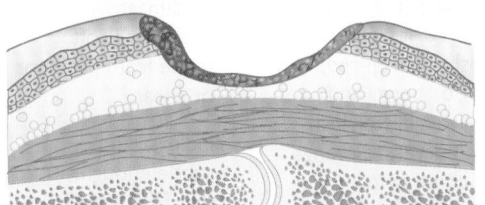 **Stage III** 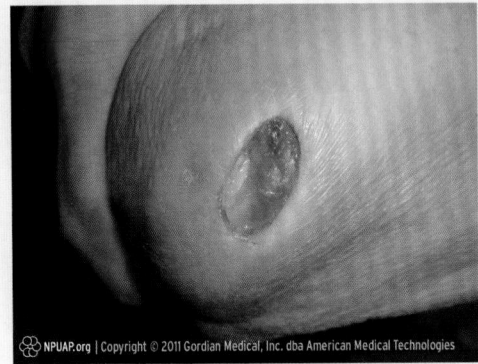 NPUAP.org | Copyright © 2011 Gordian Medical, Inc. dba American Medical Technologies	A deep crater characterized by full-thickness skin loss with damage or necrosis of subcutaneous tissue. Adipose is visible. May extend down to, but not through, underlying fascia Undermining (deeper-level damage under boggy superficial layers) of adjacent tissue may be present. Bone/tendon is not visible or directly palpable.	Some stage 3 pressure injuries can be extremely deep when located in an area with significant adipose layers.
Stage 4 Pressure Injury 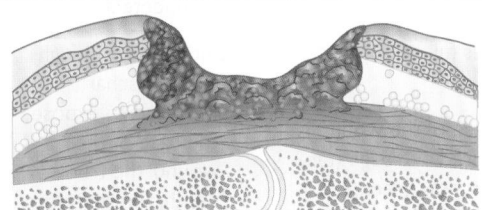 **Stage IV** 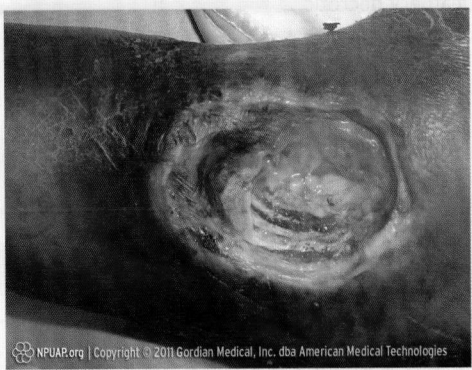 NPUAP.org | Copyright © 2011 Gordian Medical, Inc. dba American Medical Technologies	Involves full-thickness skin loss, with extensive destruction, tissue necrosis, or damage to muscle, bone, or support structures Exposed bone/tendon is visible or directly palpable. Slough or *eschar* (tan, black, or brown leathery necrotic tissue) may be present. *Epibole* (rolled edges), undermining, and sinus tracts (blind tracts underneath the epidermis) are common.	The depth of a stage 4 pressure injury varies by location. They can be shallow on the bridge of the nose, ear, occiput, and malleolus because these areas do not have subcutaneous tissue. Stage 4 injuries can extend into muscle and supporting structures (e.g., fascia, tendon, or joint capsule). Often requires a full year to heal. Even once healed, the site remains at risk for future injury because the scar tissue is not as strong as the original tissue.

(Continued)

Table 32-3 ➤ Staging Pressure Injury—cont'd

STAGE	CLINICAL FINDINGS	DISCUSSION
Deep Tissue Pressure Injury (DTI) NPUAP.org | Copyright © 2011 Gordian Medical, Inc. dba American Medical Technologies	An area of skin that is intact but persistently discolored. It might be purplish or deep red, painful, or boggy and may have a blister. Pain and temperature change often come before changes in skin color.	Occurs as a result of damage of underlying soft tissue from pressure or shear Findings can be subtle enough that DTI often is not recognized until after severe tissue damage has occurred. May heal or evolve further and become covered by thin eschar, rapidly exposing additional layers of tissue, even with optimal treatment. In individuals with dark skin, discoloration might go undetected.
Unstageable Pressure Injury NPUAP.org | Copyright © 2011 Gordian Medical, Inc. dba American Medical Technologies	Involves full-thickness skin loss The base of the wound is obscured by *slough* (tan, yellow, gray, green, or brown necrotic tissue) or *eschar* (tan, black, or brown leathery necrotic tissue).	Until enough slough and/or eschar is removed to expose the base of the wound, the true depth, and therefore stage, cannot be determined. *Stable eschar* is dry, adherent, and intact, without erythema or fluctuance. Do not remove or soften a stable eschar because it serves as "the body's natural cover."

Source: Reprinted with permission. Edsberg, L. E., Black, J. M., Goldberg, M., McNichol, L., Moore, L., & Sieggreen, M. (2016). Revised National Pressure Ulcer Advisory Panel Pressure Injury Staging System: Revised pressure injury staging system. *Journal of Wound Ostomy Continence Nursing, 43*(6), 585–597. https://doi.org/10.1097/won.0000000000000281

- **Many wounds may have different types of tissue** at the same time. Describe each type with percentages. For example, "80% of the wound bed contains granulation tissue, and 20% remains necrotic."
- **Granulation tissue** is evidence of healing.
- **A pale color or dry texture** may indicate a delay in healing.

- **Necrotic tissue** of any type will delay wound healing and should be removed. The exception is stable eschar on a heel that is firmly attached to the healthy wound edges without signs of infection.

Drainage Determine whether exudate is present. If so, describe the amount, color, consistency, and odor.

Table 32-4 ➤ Types of Tissue in the Wound Bed

TYPE OF TISSUE	DESCRIPTION	NURSING GOAL
Slough	Soft, moist, devitalized (necrotic) tissue; may be white, yellow, tan; may be stringy, loose, or adherent to bed	Débride the wound.
Eschar	Necrotic tissue; dry, thick, leathery; may be black, brown, or gray depending on moisture level	Débride the wound.
Granulation Tissue	Pink to red, moist tissue; made of new blood vessels, connective tissue, and fibroblasts; surface is granular or pebble-like	Cleanse, protect. Promote epithelialization (epithelial growth).
Clean, Nongranulating	Absence of granulation tissue, but bed is pink, shiny, and smooth	Cleanse, protect. Promote growth of healthy tissue.
Epithelial	Regenerating epidermis; may appear pink or pearly white as it crosses the wound bed; may begin as a ring around the wound or from epithelial cells lining hair follicles	Cleanse, protect.

Compare changes in the exudate with the patient's previous status.

- *Amount.* Describe the amount as none, light, moderate, or heavy. Drainage amounts vary according to the type of wound (i.e., venous stasis ulcers usually produce more drainage than arterial ulcers).
- *Drains.* If a drain is present, measure the amount of fluid in the collection container.
- *Color.* Describe the color or consistency as serous or clear, serosanguineous, sanguineous, purulent, or seropurulent (composed of serum and pus).

- *Odor.* Describe odor as absent, faint, moderate, or strong.
  - Clean the wound of all exudate or foreign material before assessing for odor because odor characteristics vary depending on wound moisture, organisms present, amount of nonviable tissue, and types of dressings used.
  - Odor may indicate fistula formation or bacterial contamination. For example, if a patient has an abdominal wound that was odorless but begins to smell of bile or feces, you should carefully assess for the presence of a fistula. If confirmed, notify the provider.

Safe, Effective Nursing Care

Improving Wound Care With Interprofessional Teams

Key Concept: Wound Healing

Competency: Collaborate with the interprofessional healthcare team

Interprofessional collaboration is essential to providing quality patient care and strengthening the healthcare system. The use of a team approach in treating both acute and chronic wounds, including diabetic foot ulcers, venous stasis ulcers, and pressure injuries, has been a topic of research. Within this model, the patient remains central, with care efforts being provided based on patient needs and desires. Characteristics such as trust, effective communication, role clarity, and mutual respect are needed to create high-functioning teams.

The World Health Organization suggests a "wound navigator" as a wound care team leader. The navigator functions as a patient advocate, focusing on patient-perceived needs and involving the expertise of healthcare professionals. The wound navigator collaborates with other professionals to determine the best plan of care for each patient, using a referral and follow-up system. For example, the wound navigator could provide each patient with a list of care/

service providers, including names and contact information, that are appropriate resources for the patient. Having easily accessible information about reliable care would lessen the burden on the patient.

Think about it.

➤ What considerations are important when building an interprofessional team?

➤ What practical challenges may need to be addressed within the context of a wound care team?

➤ How can technology play a role in effective implementation of wound care teams?

Source: Buggy, A., & Moore, Z. (2017). The impact of the multidisciplinary team in the management of individuals with diabetic foot ulcers: A systematic review. *Journal of Wound Care, 26*(6), 324–339. https://doi.org/10.12968/jowc.2017.26.6.324;
Moore, Z., Butcher, G., Corbett, L. Q., McGuiness, W., Snyder, R. J., & van Acker, K. (2014). AAWC, AWMA, EWMA position paper: Managing wounds as a team. *International Journal of Wound Care, 23*(5), S1–S38. https://doi.org/10.12968/jowc.2014.23.Sup5b.S1

Wound and Tissue Pain Routinely ask your patients about pain or discomfort related to the wound or wound care. You will need to develop a pain management plan if the patient is uncomfortable. **Key Point:** *Always take the patient's complaint of pain seriously, especially if there is a sudden increase. Pain is often an early symptom of infection—in the immunocompromised patient, pain may be the only symptom of infection.*

Nutritional Status Screen and assess the nutritional status of each patient admitted with a pressure injury and whenever there is a change in the patient's condition. A referral to the dietitian for early assessment and intervention may be necessary if nutritional problems are present. Sufficient calories are needed for wound healing. This plan may involve adding oral supplemental meals or even enteral or parenteral nutrition.

Assessing Untreated Wounds

For an untreated wound, make the same assessments as for a treated wound. Make additional assessments that allow you to determine the immediate treatment needed. For example, assess for bleeding. If bleeding is profuse, apply direct pressure to the site. If bleeding continues after you apply pressure for 5 minutes or if blood is spurting from the wound, call the provider immediately. Severe pain, numbness, or loss of movement below the wound also requires immediate, comprehensive evaluation. For a description of focused assessment for an untreated wound,

 See the **Chapter 32, Focused Assessment, Physical Examination: Wound Assessment,** in Volume 2.

Tetanus Immunization Determine whether the patient needs a tetanus immunization. Tetanus-prone wounds include compound fractures, gunshot wounds, crush injuries, burns, punctures, foreign object injuries, wounds contaminated with soil, and wounds neglected for more than 24 hours. An immunization should be given if:

- The last immunization was 10 or more years ago (Centers for Disease Control and Prevention [CDC], 2020; Havers et al., 2020).
- The wound is contaminated with dirt or debris or is a burn, and the most recent tetanus immunization was given more than 5 years ago.
- It is uncertain when the patient last received an immunization.

Laboratory Data

You should integrate laboratory data with your history and physical assessment findings. The most common laboratory assessments related to skin integrity are protein levels, complete blood count, erythrocyte sedimentation rate, glucose, thyroid and iron levels, coagulation studies, and wound cultures. To learn more about these tests and see the normal ranges,

 See **Chapter 32, Diagnostic Testing, Tests for Assessing Wounds,** in Volume 2.

Wound cultures may be ordered to determine the types of bacteria present. Local or systemic signs of infection, suddenly elevated glucose levels, pain in a neuropathic extremity, or lack of healing after 2 weeks in a clean wound may indicate the need for a wound culture. Cultures may be obtained by swab, aspiration, or tissue biopsy.

Swabbing The most common and most noninvasive method to obtain a culture is with a swab. Swab specimens have been shown to be acceptably accurate in representing bacteria counts biopsied from a wound (Haalboom et al., 2018). The use of swab cultures is a reasonable alternative to biopsy in the clinical setting, except when antibiotic-resistant bacteria are suspected (Copeland-Halperin et al., 2016).

To see the complete procedure,

 Go to **Chapter 32, Procedure 32-1: Obtaining a Wound Culture by Swab,** in Volume 2.

Needle Aspiration Specifically trained providers (e.g., physicians, advanced practice nurses) may perform needle aspiration of a wound. This procedure involves the insertion of a needle into the tissue to aspirate tissue fluid. Organisms present in the tissue fluid can then be detected. Needle aspiration is an invasive procedure with the risk of inadvertent needle damage to tissue and underlying structures.

Tissue Biopsy The most accurate method for culturing a chronic wound is *tissue biopsy*. It has long been considered the "gold standard." A specially trained provider removes tissue from the wound edge and sends it to a pathology laboratory or other specialized diagnostic center. This invasive procedure creates a risk of sepsis, causes pain, and disrupts the wound bed, sometimes causing delayed healing.

KnowledgeCheck 32-7

- What should be included in a wound assessment?
- What is the preferred method of wound culture that may be performed by a registered nurse (RN)?
- Identify three types of laboratory data that may be associated with a delay in wound healing.

What Assessments Can I Delegate?

Initial assessment of a wound, as well as ongoing evaluation of a wound that requires treatment, must be done by the RN. You may delegate the following to unlicensed assistive personnel (UAP):

- **Inspection of the skin for evidence of skin breakdown.** Instruct the UAP to notify you of redness, tissue warmth, or drainage observed during care of the patient.

- **Turning and position changes.** You must provide the UAP with the times for the turning and instructions for how they should position the patient at each turn. Turning and movement prevent tissue damage from ischemia, thereby preventing pressure injury.

NURSING DIAGNOSIS/ANALYZING CUES

The following nursing diagnoses are appropriate for patients who are at risk for skin breakdown or for patients who have wounds:

- *Risk for Impaired Skin Integrity* is appropriate for patients who have one or more risk factors for skin breakdown (e.g., immobility, incontinence, extremes of age, impaired circulation, impaired sensation, undernutrition, emaciation). Use a risk assessment tool (e.g., Norton or Braden scale) to evaluate the patient's risk.
- *Impaired Skin Integrity* is appropriate for patients who have experienced damage to the epidermis or dermis—for example, patients who have superficial wounds or a stage 1 or 2 pressure injury.
- *Impaired Tissue Integrity* is appropriate for patients with wounds that extend into the subcutaneous tissue, muscle, or bone. Use this diagnosis for patients with deep wounds or a stage 3 or 4 pressure injury.
- *Risk for Impaired Tissue Integrity* is appropriate for patients with Impaired Skin Integrity who are at risk for delayed healing. For example, Mr. Harmon (Meet Your Patient) has a stage 1 pressure injury but is at risk for further progression of the injury because of his age, his nutritional state, and the presence of another wound.

Skin problems and wounds can be the etiology for other nursing diagnoses as well, for example:

- *Risk for Infection* is an appropriate diagnosis if the patient has a traumatic wound or is immunosuppressed, undernourished, or immobile.
- *Pain* is a diagnosis that may be used for patients who are experiencing discomfort from the wound or from the treatments required to heal the wound.
- *Disturbed Body Image* should be used if the patient is experiencing distress about the wound. Consider this diagnosis even if the patient is expected to make a complete recovery. Some patients experience extreme distress about wounds. You will certainly want to consider this diagnosis if the patient experiences an injury that is expected to result in disfigurement.

PLANNING/PRIORITIZING HYPOTHESES AND GENERATING SOLUTIONS

Examples of associated Nursing Outcomes Classification (NOC) standardized outcomes for skin and tissue integrity diagnoses include the following:

Infection
Immobility Consequences: Physiological
Nutritional Status: Food & Fluid Intake
Tissue Integrity: Skin & Mucous Membranes
Wound Healing: Secondary Intention

Individualized goals/outcome statements should address the need to maintain intact skin or heal the wound. For patients who have a diagnosis of Risk for Impaired Skin Integrity, you might write a goal such as the following:

Maintains intact skin throughout treatment, as evidenced by good skin turgor with no erythema, edema, or breaks in the skin.

For patients who have a wound (actual Impaired Skin Integrity or Impaired Tissue Integrity), you might write a goal such as the following:

Wound will heal by May 1, as evidenced by a progressive decrease in the size of the wound, a decrease in drainage from the wound, improvement in the condition of the surrounding skin, and no evidence of infection (erythema, purulent drainage, or odor).

IMPLEMENTATION/TAKING ACTION

Examples of Nursing Interventions Classification (NIC) standardized interventions for skin and tissue integrity problems include the following:

Bedrest Care
Infection Protection
Pressure Injury Prevention
Pressure Management
Skin Surveillance
Nutrition Management
Positioning
Wound Care
Wound Irrigation

Specific nursing activities directed at maintaining skin integrity or healing wounds focus on preventing and treating pressure injuries (see Example Client Condition: Pressure Injury) and other chronic wounds, providing wound care, and applying heat and cold therapies.

What Wound Care Competencies Do I Need?

Care planning to meet the complex, individualized needs of a patient with a chronic wound involves the entire multidisciplinary team (e.g., dietitians, infection control specialist, wound specialist). Your wound assessment will guide your choice of interventions, which depend on the nature of the wound. Consider these two examples:

- **A patient with a diabetic foot ulcer** must have all the pressure taken off that area because every step traumatizes healing tissues. The appropriate dressing must be selected; in addition, this patient will need to wear a special shoe that is specially made for patients with neuropathy.
- **Patients with a venous stasis ulcer** commonly wear compression garments (e.g., elastic hose, stocking, or multilayer compression wrap). These provide continuous pressure to the veins, which improves venous

return and helps the ulcer to heal. You will need to keep the following in mind:

- Before applying elastic compression, be sure the limb is not increasing in size because of edema.
- Lower extremity arterial disease must be ruled out before applying compression because it can compromise arterial circulation.

To see the complete procedure,

 See **Chapter 36, Procedure 36-2: Applying Antiembolism Stockings,** in Volume 2.

The rest of the chapter will assist you in obtaining various wound care competencies.

KnowledgeCheck 32-8

If you need to review content to answer these questions, see the Interventions in the Example Client Condition: Pressure Injury.

- Identify the major interventions for preventing pressure injury.
- What nursing diagnosis is most appropriate for a patient at risk for pressure injury development?

Cleansing Wounds

Cleansing removes exudate, slough, foreign materials, and microorganisms from the wound. This helps promote healthy tissue healing. Always clean a wound initially and with each dressing change. To cleanse a wound, gently pat the surface with gauze soaked with saline or other prescribed wound cleanser. If there is granulation tissue, be careful not to disrupt it. The ideal solution should be isotonic, easy to sterilize, inexpensive, and available. It should not irritate or damage tissue or cause bleeding.

- **Antiseptic solutions** include Dakin's solution, acetic acid, hydrogen peroxide, povidone-iodine, chlorhexidine, and alcohol. Historically, these solutions have been used to cleanse all types of wounds. However, some of these antiseptic solutions can damage granulating tissue and should not be used on healing tissue. Although controversial, betadine may be nontoxic and effective in cleansing chronically infected wounds (National Institute for Health and Care Excellence [NICE], 2016). Antiseptic solutions should be reserved for:
  - New wounds
  - Wounds that won't heal
  - Wounds in which the bacterial burden is more harmful than the solution itself
- **Normal saline** is *isotonic* (same concentration as the blood and other cells in the body); it is safe, and it will

---

EXAMPLE CLIENT CONDITION: Pressure Injury

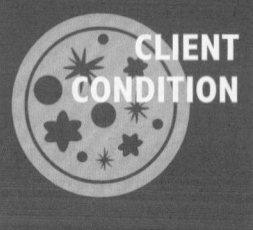

Definition

Pressure Injury: Localized injury to the skin and underlying tissue, usually over a bony prominence (see Fig. 32-11). Formerly called *decubitus ulcers, pressure ulcers, bedsores*.

Stages

Staged by degree of tissue involvement (see Table 32-3)
- Become progressively shallow by filling with granulation tissue
- Reduced muscle, subcutaneous fat
- Dermis not replaced
- Healing pressure injuries are not "reverse" staged. A stage 4 pressure injury does not become a stage 3; it is described as "stage 4 pressure injury: healing."

Risk Factors

- Impaired circulation, such as patients with diabetes, atherosclerosis, or low blood pressure
- Reduced oxygen supply in the blood, such as patients who use tobacco or have anemia
- Limited mobility or reduced sensation to feel pressure points:
  - nerve damage
  - head injury, stroke, spinal cord injury
  - contractures
  - diabetes

Contributing Factors

- **Pressure**—Compresses small blood vessels, hindering blood flow and nutrient supply. Tissues become ischemic or injured.
- **Friction**—When skin is moist, fragile, or rubbed against another surface (wrinkled sheets).
- **Shear**—When one layer of tissue slides horizontally over another, compressing adipose and muscle tissue and reducing normal blood flow. Shear is friction plus the force of gravity (e.g., when patient slides down in the bed).
- **Moisture**—Urine, stool, and sweat macerate the skin.

Patient Health History

Patient's health condition combined with unrelieved pressure increases the risk (see Fig. 32-10):
- Immobility
- Poor nutrition
- Fever
- Infection
- Dehydration
- Edema
- Impaired sensation (spinal cord injury, stroke)

EXAMPLE CLIENT CONDITION: Pressure Injury—cont'd

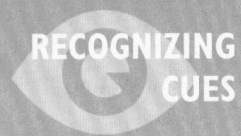 **RECOGNIZING CUES**

Physical Findings

When ischemia first occurs, the skin over the area is pale and cool. When pressure is relieved (by turning the patient), vasodilation occurs, extra blood goes to the area, and the area flushes bright red **(reactive hyperemia).** If the redness does not disappear quickly, tissue damage has occurred.

Inspecting Skin Daily

1. Begin skin care with regular assessment of the skin for appearance, temperature, texture, and color.
2. Ensure adequate light to detect subtle, early skin changes.
3. Check pressure points for erythema, tenderness, or edema (see Fig. 32-11).
4. Instruct caregivers on how to detect early signs of skin problems.
5. Look for skin breakdown under breasts, in abdominal folds, and where there is skin-to-skin contact in patients with obesity.

Assessing for and Evaluating Pressure Injury

• The **Braden scale** rates sensory perception, moisture, activity, mobility, nutrition, friction, and shear. The lower the score, the more likely the patient will develop a pressure injury. The Braden Q is for children.

 Go to **Chapter 32, Focused Assessment: The Braden Scale for Predicting Pressure Sore Risk Assessment Scale,** in Volume 2.

• The **Norton scale** assesses risk based on the patient's physical condition, mental state, activity, mobility, and incontinence. The lower the score, the higher the risk is for pressure injury.

 See **Chapter 32, Focused Assessment: Norton Pressure Sore Risk Assessment Scale,** in Volume 2.

• The PUSH tool reports the progression of a pressure injury. Surface area, exudate, and type of wound tissue are scored and totaled. As the injured area heals, the total score falls.

 See **Chapter 32, Focused Assessment: PUSH Tool for Evaluation of Pressure Injuries,** in Volume 2.

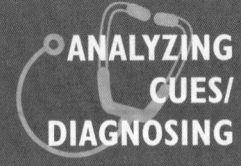 **ANALYZING CUES/ DIAGNOSING**

• Impaired Skin Integrity, Actual or Risk for
• Impaired Tissue Integrity, Actual or Risk for

• Infection, Actual or Risk for
• Pain
• Altered Body Image

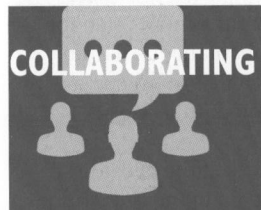 **COLLABORATING**

Adjunctive Wound Care Therapies

• **Surgery.** Excision and débridement, skin graft, drains, and flaps close wounds and promote healing.
• **Electrical stimulation.** Stimulates cellular growth through development of fibroblasts and new collagen; increases blood flow and tissue oxygenation.
• **Hyperbaric oxygen therapy (HBOT).** High oxygen under pressure accelerates healing. HBOT also enhances white blood cell activity to improve healing.
• **Tissue growth factors.** Naturally occurring proteins that cause specific cells to grow and replicate; platelet-derived growth factor for chronic wound healing for diabetic and other nonhealing wounds; used for clean wounds without necrotic tissue and that have good blood supply.

• **Ultrasound.** Sound waves that pass into tissue cause vibration and heat. This stimulates movement of fluid within and between cells, aids in debridement, and increases cell metabolism.
• **Bioengineered skin substitutes.** Aid in temporary or permanent closure of partial- and full-thickness wounds. Made of human epidermis or dermis, animal cells, or synthetic material.
• **Nitric oxide (NO).** Enhances wound healing by improving circulation to the wound bed. Additionally, NO promotes the growth of fibroblasts and collagen for repair of skin and tissue. NO has high antibacterial effects and thus decreases infection (Saidkhani et al., 2016).
• **Maggot therapy.** More precise débridement method because irradiated maggots eat only necrotic tissue.

(continued)

EXAMPLE CLIENT CONDITION: Pressure Injury—cont'd

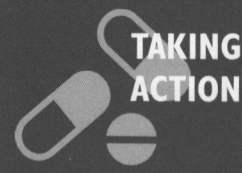

TAKING ACTION

PREVENTION Is the Priority INTERVENTION!

For at-risk patients, use visual cues (stickers on charts, dots on ID bands, colored armbands) to remind staff to implement prevention strategies.

Pressure Injury Monitoring

- Reassess hospitalized patient daily, at transfer or discharge, and if condition changes.
- Assess at-risk patients more often, typically every 8–12 hours.
- Reassess nursing home residents weekly for first 4 weeks, then quarterly or if condition deteriorates.
- Monitor home patient with every visit. Inform the healthcare provider of the patient's risk.

Manage Moisture

Incontinence Care

- Provide skin care with gentle cleansing soon after each incontinence episode.
- Apply moisture barrier cream to protect perineal skin.
- Use absorbent products that wick moisture away from the skin.
- For persistent bowel incontinence, consider using a pouching system or fecal containment device to protect the skin from the moisture.

Bathing

- Diaphoretic patients may need frequent bathing; sweat can irritate sensitive or injury-prone skin.
- Older adults don't usually require daily bathing because of ↓ sebaceous oil and sweat production.
- Gently bathe fragile skin, using a minimum of force and friction; washcloths can be abrasive.
- Use a mild, emollient cleansing soap only as needed; be sure to rinse thoroughly and gently pat the skin dry. Some soaps remove oils from the skin.
- Use warm water; hot water dries the skin.

Barrier Cream

- Consider using a barrier cream to prevent skin damage in adults at risk for pressure injury (incontinent, edematous, or inflamed skin).

Lotion and Massage

- Use a gentle massaging motion to promote circulation and wound healing.
- Do not massage over bony prominences; this can irritate the area and lead to tissue injury.

Linens

- Keep the linens soft, clean, dry, and free from wrinkles by changing them frequently.

Dressings

Also refer to Table 32-5: Types of Wound Dressings.

- **Hydrating dressing.** Use hydrocolloid or foam dressings to reduce wound size.

 See Procedure 32-8 in Volume 2.

- **Negative pressure wound therapy.** Placed on a wound packed with foam or gauze dressings to create a vacuum. Subatmospheric pressure reduces edema from swollen tissues, promotes granulation tissue formation, removes exudate and infectious material, and stimulates blood vessel growth to improve wound perfusion.

 See Procedure 32-6 in Volume 2.

- **Silver dressing.** Acts as barrier to bacteria in wound bed, eliminates bacterial biofilms, and can reduce prophylactic antibiotic use (therefore preventing antibiotic resistance).
- **Transparent dressing.** Apply the clear film or drape free of wrinkles. The occlusive dressing creates a seal to help create negative pressure within the wound.

 See Procedure 32-7 in Volume 2.

Minimize Pressure: Turn and Reposition

- Most patients who are at risk for pressure injury have mobility problems.
- **Key Point:** *Must provide frequent position changes to prevent tissue damage from ischemia.*

Turning Frequency

- Turn at least every 2 hours, more often for fragile skin or little subcutaneous tissue.
- Turn every hour for chair-bound patient; teach patient to shift weight every 15 minutes.
- Place a turning schedule at the bedside so that all caregivers can aid in the prevention strategy.

The "Rule of 30": Guide to Positioning

- Elevate the head of the bed (HOB) to a 30° angle or less.
- When side-lying, position at a 30° angle to avoid direct pressure on the trochanter.
- If the HOB is up to more than a 30° angle, limit time in this position to minimize pressure and shear.
- ✚ Use lift devices or drawsheets, heel and elbow protectors, sleeves, and stockings. Never drag a patient up in bed.

EXAMPLE CLIENT CONDITION: Pressure Injury—cont'd

Support Surfaces

- Specialty mattresses, integrated bed systems, mattress overlays—consist of air, gel, foam, water
- Various sizes and shapes for beds, chairs, and examination and surgical tables
- These surfaces and systems redistribute pressure and moisture to prevent bacterial growth on the skin.
- Use products that raise the heels off the bed. Pillows may not redistribute the weight of the patient's foot.
- Use pressure-redistributing devices for chairs and wheelchairs. Avoid foam rings and donut-type devices.

Optimize Nutrition and Hydration

Patients at risk: rapid weight loss, ↑ metabolic demands, limited intake, or ↓ serum albumin

1. Monitor hydration status and offer water (if appropriate) whenever you reposition the patient.
2. Provide adequate calories (30–35 kcal/kg/day) and protein (2 g/kg in an under-nourished patient with a wound). Add protein or amino acid supplementation to reduce wound size.
3. Consider the consistency of the diet (soft diet for a patient who is frail or missing teeth).
4. Tube feeding or parenteral nutrition to supplement oral intake; dietary referral as needed.

TEACHING

Teach the at-risk patient and family the following measures for preventing pressure injury:

- Characteristics of healthy skin
- Appearance of skin that has experienced unrelieved pressure
- Protection of the skin and prevention of pressure injury
- Skin care and hygiene
- Importance of adequate nutrition
- Techniques for turning and positioning
- Importance of frequent position changes
- Use of pressure-redistributing devices
- Healthy diet with adequate calorie and protein intake
- Skin changes that should be reported to healthcare professionals

HOME CARE

W-O-U-N-D

Tips for taking care of wounds at home:

Wet → Dry it
Open → Cover it
Unclean → Clean it
Necrotic → Don't scrub it
Dry → Moisten it

---

not harm injured or healing tissue. It will cleanse most wounds if enough is used to thoroughly flush the wound. *Note:* Normal saline should be used within 24 hours of opening the container to avoid bacterial growth within the solution.

- **Sterile water** and **distilled water** are clean, contain no additives, and are less expensive than normal saline. However, they are *hypotonic* (lower concentration of solute than the blood and other cells in the body), which means they can cause fluid shifts to damaged cells. When large volumes of sterile water are used, water toxicity to an open wound can occur.

- **Potable (drinkable) tap water** can also be used to cleanse wounds, especially in the community setting. Studies have shown that tap water is as effective for cleansing as saline (Fernandez & Griffith, 2012; Chan et al., 2016; Burch & Köpke, 2018). **Key Point:** *However, the decision to use tap water should be based on the nature and complexity of the wound and the patient's general condition, including the presence of comorbid conditions (e.g., diabetes) and immunological status (Burch & Köpke, 2018; Chan et al., 2016; Fernandez & Griffiths, 2012).*

- **Purified water** (instead of tap water) should be used for cleansing wounds to reduce the risk of microbial

♥ iCare 32-1

Skin Integrity and Wound Healing

- *Scenario 1*—Mary is caring for Mrs. Skylar, a 62-year-old patient with diabetes and venous stasis ulcers on her legs. Since developing these venous stasis ulcers, Mrs. Skylar has become very self-conscious and embarrassed about her legs. When taking Mrs. Skylar to x-ray, Mary covers Mrs. Skylar's legs with a bath blanket for comfort and privacy. Mary was not only providing comfort and protecting privacy. She was also aware of Mrs. Skylar's feelings and cared enough to respond to them.
- *Scenario 2*—Mr. Robert Brown is an 18-year-old paraplegic who has developed a stage 4 sacral pressure ulcer with a foul odor. He is expecting some of his friends from school for a visit. Ken, his nurse, while nonchalantly cleaning up the room, makes sure to remove the garbage liner with the old dressings in it. He also brings in some fresh-cut flowers and a cup of wet coffee grounds. Both the flowers and the coffee grounds are natural odor eliminators. Mr. Brown has a great visit with his friends from school.

contamination from biofilm in the hospital setting and in patients with a higher risk of acquiring infection (compromised immune system, other comorbidities). **Biofilm** (a coating of bacteria that adheres to a surface) forms in hospital water delivery systems. Biofilms impede wound healing by reducing the effectiveness of fibroblasts in repairing the wound bed. This substance also reduces the effectiveness of antimicrobials.

- **Liquid or foam skin cleansers** that are pH balanced may be used to cleanse periwound skin or incontinence effluent. They are not for use inside wounds.

Key Point: *The most important thing to remember is to use universal precautions to minimize the risk of cross-contamination when cleansing periwound or other nonwound skin.*

Irrigating Wounds

Nurses commonly use irrigation **(lavage)** to:

- **Cleanse wounds** by flushing debris and bacteria on the surface.
- **Hydrate** the site.
- **Remove debris** for better visual inspection of the wound and periwound surface.
- **Facilitate progression** from the inflammatory to the proliferative phase of healing.
- **Improve wound healing** from the inside tissue layers to the skin surface.
- **Reduce infection** by preventing premature surface healing, especially over an infected area of a wound.

Selecting Irrigation Solution. Irrigation solutions include topical cleansers and antiseptics to clean wounds, antibiotics and antifungals to prevent or treat wound infection, and anesthetics and analgesics for

pain. **Key Point:** *The most used wound irrigation solution is normal saline.* Bacterial growth in saline may occur as soon as 24 hours after opening the saline bottle. Sterile water may also be used for irrigation, particularly when other solutions are not available.

Ideally, the irrigation solution should be:

Isotonic to prevent injury to healing tissue.
Nonhemolytic to prevent bleeding.
Nontoxic to healing tissue. Cytotoxic solutions may impair wound healing.
Transparent to allow visualization of the wound bed.
Inexpensive for frequent irrigation using a sufficient volume of solution.
Warmed to room temperature to prevent hypothermia.

Selecting an Irrigation Delivery Method. The following are common methods of delivery.

- **Piston syringe for irrigation.** This larger, sterile, disposable syringe has a thumb ring designed to minimize hand slippage and prevent contamination. The elongated tip is able to better direct the stream of irrigation fluid.
- ✛ The use of a bulb **syringe** is not advised because it increases the risk of aspirating the drainage and disrupting healing granulation tissue.
- **Commercial irrigation systems,** such as whirlpool agitators, whirlpool hose sprayers, pressurized canisters, and pulsed lavages. **Continuous irrigation** is an uninterrupted stream of irrigation solution to the wound's surface. **Pulsed** irrigation is the intermittent delivery of irrigation solution.

Choosing Safe and Effective Pressure

- **To remove debris from a wound,** introduce the irrigation solution with a gentle amount of force. Ideal irrigation pressures range from 4 pounds per square inch (psi) to 15 psi.
- **To remove material adhering to the wound bed,** use a 35-mL syringe attached to a 19-gauge angiocatheter to deliver the solution at approximately 8 psi (Lewis & Pay, 2022).
- ✛ Pressures **above 15 psi increase the risk** of driving bacteria into the tissues, as well as causing mechanical damage to the wound and increasing the risk of infection (Gabriel & Schraga, 2021). Closely evaluate the amount of pressure commercial irrigation systems deliver before you use these devices. High-pressure irrigation systems (35 to 70 psi) may (1) dislodge healing granulation tissue and new epithelial cells, especially in chronic wounds, (2) cause pain, and (3) drive bacteria deeper into the wound compartment, leading to an increased risk of infection (Gabriel & Schraga, 2021).

Using Appropriate Volume for Irrigation A sufficient volume of irrigation solution for flushing is necessary for proper cleansing of the wound. The ideal volume is 50 to 100 mL per centimeter of length of the laceration (Gabriel & Schraga, 2021). However, more irrigation volume would be needed if the wound is highly contaminated. Chemical burns also require more irrigation.

Preventing Infection When Irrigating

- You need to use gowns, masks, and goggles because there is a risk of splattering when irrigating.
- A plastic shield at the end of the irrigating syringe reduces splashing, particularly for IV sites and other open areas.
- Sterile technique is used for acute surgical wounds, for wounds that have recently undergone sharp débridement, or when prescribed by the provider.
- Most wound irrigations use clean technique.

For the complete steps,

 See **Chapter 32, Procedure 32-2: Performing a Sterile Wound Irrigation**, in Volume 2.

Caring for Wounds With Drainage Devices

A variety of drains may be inserted into wounds to allow fluid and exudate to exit. Drains prevent excessive pressure from building up in the tissues. Drains are usually placed during a surgical procedure. Some are sutured into place, whereas others are simply placed into the cavity.

Types of Drains

A Penrose drain is a flexible, flat latex tube that is placed in the wound bed but usually not sutured into place. A clamp or pin may be attached to the drain at the insertion site to keep it from slipping into the wound. You may be asked to advance the drain by gradually removing it from the wound bed, or it may be removed all at one time. For complete guidelines,

 See **Chapter 32, Procedure 32-13: Shortening a Wound Drain,** in Volume 2.

Some drains are attached to a collection device, such as the Hemovac and Jackson-Pratt drains (Fig. 32-12). The provider may order a device to be "placed to suction." This means you will compress the device to create suction and facilitate the removal of drainage (Fig. 32-13). For complete guidelines,

 See **Chapter 32, Procedure 32-14: Emptying a Closed Wound Drainage System,** in Volume 2.

If a specific pressure is to be applied, some drains can be connected to wall suction. The provider will prescribe the amount of suction. For example: "Place Hemovac to 20 mm Hg suction at all times."

Nursing Activities for Maintaining Drains As a nurse, you are responsible for monitoring wound drains.

- **The provider will describe the number and type of drains present.** Describe drain placement using the drain's position on a clock face. Consider the patient's head to be at the 12 o'clock position.

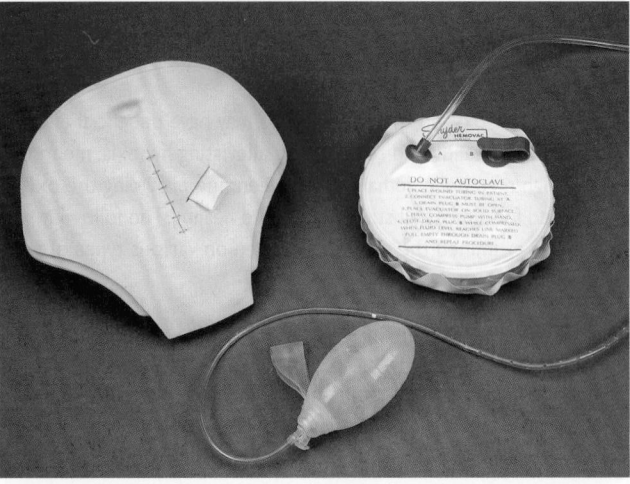

FIGURE 32-12 *(Left)* Penrose drain. *(Center)* Jackson-Pratt device. *(Right)* Hemovac drainage system.

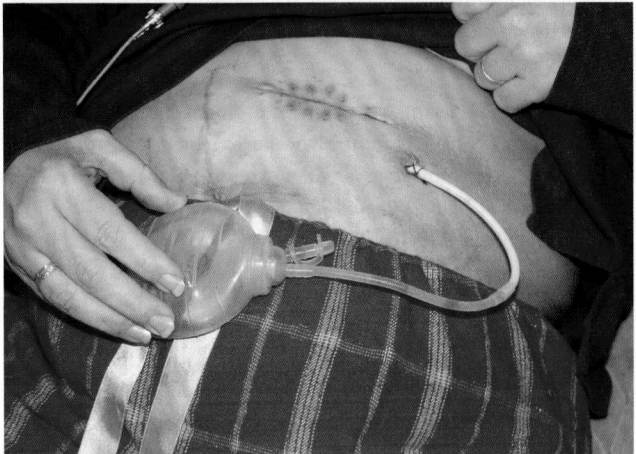

FIGURE 32-13 Compress the bulb of the Jackson-Pratt drain to create suction and remove wound drainage.

- **Some patients have more than one drainage device in a wound.** Label the drains numerically with a marker or by placing tape on the collection apparatus so that each caregiver provides consistent care.
- **When removing dressings or irrigating wounds, be careful to avoid dislodging the drain.** Remember, many drains are not sutured in place.
- **Monitor the amount and character of the drainage,** and record this information in your nursing notes as well as on the intake and output (I&O) record.
- **Report to the provider any significant change** in the amount or character of the drainage.
- **If you suspect a drain is occluded, check the drain line** from the insertion site to the collection device. Remove any kinks in the tubing. If this does not correct the problem, notify the provider of the blockage.
- **You need to empty the collection apparatus at a designated volume to maintain suction.** As the device fills, suction pressure decreases. If there is significant drainage, you may need to empty the device several times during your shift.

Toward Evidence-Based Practice

Hyperbaric Oxygen Therapy

Hyperbaric oxygen therapy (HBOT) may have beneficial effects on wound healing and recovery by alleviating hypoxia, meeting the high metabolic demand for oxygen, and providing the oxygen needed for almost all stages of wound healing. The following studies examined the effects of oxygen on various types of skin injuries.

> Huang, E., Heyboer, M., & Savaser, D. J. (2019, May 29). Hyperbaric oxygen therapy for the management of chronic wounds: Patient selection and perspectives. *Chronic Wound Care Management and Research, 6,* 27–37. https://doi.org/10.2147/CWCMR.S175721

Researchers investigated the impact of HBOT on other types of wounds besides diabetic foot ulcers. The findings indicate that HBOT could improve wound healing in all chronic wounds, although more rigorous studies are needed to evaluate the effectiveness of HBOT for chronic wounds that are not diabetic foot ulcers.

> Hatibie, M. J., Islam, A. A., Hatta, M., Moenadjat, Y., Susilo, R. H., & Rendy, L. (2019, March). Hyperbaric oxygen therapy for second-degree burn healing: An experimental study in rabbits. *Advances in Skin & Wound Care, 32*(3), 1–4. https://10.1097/01.ASW.0000553110.78375.7b

In laboratory rabbits with second-degree burns, those that received HBOT showed more active inflammatory cells for healing and greater epithelization for repair of injured tissue. Researchers found no improvement in blood supply to the burn injury using HBOT.

> Chen, C., Wu, R. Hsu, M., Hsieh, C., & Chou, M. (2017). Adjunctive hyperbaric oxygen therapy for healing of chronic diabetic foot ulcers. *Journal of Wound, Ostomy and Continence Nursing, 44*(6), 536–545. https://doi.org/10.1097/WON.0000000000000374

Chen and colleagues compared the results of the use of HBOT to standard wound care for patients with diabetic foot ulcers. In this study, HBOT significantly reduced the risk of amputation of the affected limb. The study also showed that at least 20 HBOT sessions are required to be effective.

> Lalieu, R. C., Brouwer, R. J., Ubbink, D. T., Hoencamp, R., Bol Raap, R., & van Hulst, R. A. (2019, October 31). Hyperbaric oxygen therapy for nonischemic diabetic ulcers: A systematic review. *Wound Repair and Regeneration, 28*(2), 266–275. https://doi.org/10.1111/wrr.12776

Based on current evidence, researchers were not able to demonstrate accelerated healing in patients with diabetic foot ulcers who received HBOT for wound care. The rate of amputations was not lower in those receiving HBOT. Therefore, Lalieu and colleagues could not recommend routine clinical use of this therapy for the treatment of diabetic foot ulcers.

---

1. How does HBOT improve wound healing?

2. What are some benefits of using HBOT on chronic wounds?

3. Why is HBOT not used often in wound care?

KnowledgeCheck 32-9

- Identify goals for wound care before applying a dressing to a wound.
- What solutions are used to cleanse a wound?
- How can you control the amount of force applied for wound irrigation?
- Identify three nursing responsibilities when caring for a patient with a wound drain.

 ThinkLike a Nurse 32-5: Clinical Judgment in Action

- Describe the percentage and type of tissue found in Mr. Harmon's (Meet Your Patient) wounds.
- What are the goals of treatment for each of Mr. Harmon's wounds?

Débriding a Wound

Débridement is the removal of devitalized tissue or foreign material from a wound (Manna & Morrison, 2022). It also helps remove cells that are alive but not functioning **(senescent)** from the wound bed and edges. Removal of necrotic tissue, exudate, and infective material helps stimulate wound healing and prepare the wound bed for advanced therapies or biological agents. **Key Point:** *Keep in mind that there are reasons not to débride a wound. It is critical not to remove eschar if the wound has poor circulation at the ulcer site. You would also not débride a stable heel eschar. Additionally, débridement would not benefit the patient who is critically unstable or those with a grave prognosis.* There are five types of débridement: sharp (surgical), mechanical, enzymatic, autolytic, and biotherapy (maggot) therapy.

Sharp Débridement This is the use of a sterile, sharp instrument, such as a scalpel or scissors, to remove devitalized tissue. This method provides an immediate improvement of the wound bed and preserves granulation tissue.

- A physician, nurse, or physical therapist may perform this procedure at the bedside if they have received specialized training.
- If a wound requires extensive débridement, it may be performed in the operating room.

■ Many stage 4 pressure injuries extend into the bone, so a bone biopsy is often performed at the same time. The biopsy will detect **osteomyelitis,** extension of the infection into the bone.

Mechanical Débridement   This may be performed via lavage (discussed in a preceding section), the use of wet-to-damp dressings, or hydrotherapy (whirlpool).

■ **Wet-to-dry dressings** are coarse gauze moistened with normal saline packed into the wound, allowed to dry, and then removed several times a day. This form of débridement was common once, but its use has declined because it causes pain and provides only **nonselective débridement**. That is, it removes not only debris but also healing granulation tissue. If you must use this method, medicate the patient beforehand with opioid analgesics. Rewetting the gauze aids in its removal and decreases the pain, but it also may eliminate the débriding action of the dressing change.

■ **Hydrotherapy or whirlpool treatments** are a vigorous form of nonselective débridement reserved for wounds with a large amount of nonviable tissue, such as burns. Hydrotherapy is usually performed in the physical therapy department once or twice per day. The wound is placed in a whirlpool containing tepid water for a prescribed amount of time (perhaps 5 to 15 minutes). The wound should not be exposed directly to the water jets. Risks include the following:

■ Increased risk for periwound maceration, contamination by waterborne infectious agents, and cross-contamination; strict adherence to infection control measures is essential.

■ Vasodilation, which may increase edema and congestion in patients with venous stasis; use hydrotherapy with caution.

■ Increased risk for burns in persons with diabetic neuropathies due to a decrease in sensory abilities.

Enzymatic Débridement   This uses proteolytic agents to break down necrotic tissue without affecting viable tissue in the wound. Enzymatic débridement is used for the removal of eschar in burn-related wounds and for taking off slough in pressure injuries, diabetic foot ulcers, and other complex and chronic wounds. It is less painful than traditional sharp débridement.

To use an enzymatic product, clean the wound with normal saline, apply a thin layer of the enzyme, and cover the wound with a moisture-retaining dressing. This procedure may be done once daily, depending on the product. Apply the product only to devitalized tissue because it might cause some local irritation. Certain cleansing agents can inactivate or slow the action of the enzymes.

Autolytic Débridement (Autolysis)   This is the use of an occlusive, moisture-retaining dressing and the body's own enzymes and defense mechanisms to break down necrotic tissue. This process takes more time than the other techniques, but it is better tolerated. The procedure involves applying the dressing and observing the fluid that collects under it (wound fluid may be tan in color). The dressing is normally changed every 72 hours, or sooner if drainage breakthrough occurs. At that time, the wound is cleansed before a new dressing is applied. Observe the wound closely and regularly for signs of infection, such as an increase in pain or a foul odor. **Key Point:** *Autolysis is contraindicated in the presence of infection or immunosuppression.*

Biotherapy (Maggot) Débridement Therapy   This is the use of medical-grade larvae of the greenbottle fly to dissolve dead and infected tissue from wounds. The larvae secrete enzymes that break down dead tissue. The enzymes are neutralized when they contact normal tissue, so healthy tissue is unharmed. The larvae also digest bacteria from the wound. This therapy is effective and simple to use, although containing the larvae within the dressing can be problematic. Larvae are usually changed every 48 to 72 hours and disposed of as biohazardous medical waste. Patients are likely to feel a nipping or picking sensation at the application site. This can be painful.

♥ **iCare**   The use of maggots can be emotionally disturbing to both patients and nurses, so take this into consideration and discuss it with the patient (King, 2020).

Providing Moist Wound Healing

A physiological wound environment is one that maintains the right amount of moisture for cells to flourish. The skin maintains the necessary balance of moisture by allowing moisture to evaporate as needed. With damage to the skin, body cells can dehydrate, so wound dressings must function as a barrier to water vapor loss.

Choosing a Dressing

When choosing a dressing, ask yourself whether it will achieve the purposes listed in the foregoing sections. Also consider how long the dressing should stay in place, how often it needs to be changed, and whether it can be removed without damaging fragile skin or the wound itself (Table 32-5). The type of dressing used on a wound depends on the characteristics of the wound and the goals of treatment. The dressing of choice should:

■ Prevent drying of the wound bed.
■ Absorb drainage.
■ Keep the surrounding tissue dry and intact.
■ Protect from contamination and infection.
■ Aid in hemostasis.
■ Débride the wound.
■ Eliminate dead space.
■ Prevent heat loss.
■ Splint the wound site.
■ Provide comfort to the patient.
■ Control odor.
■ Minimize scarring

Table 32-5 ▶ Types of Wound Dressings

DRESSING TYPE AND DESCRIPTION	USE	CAUTIONS	WOUND SIZE
Absorbent Dressings ■ Made from highly absorptive layers of fibers such as cellulose, cotton, or rayon ■ May or may not have an adhesive border See Procedure 32-4 and Procedure 32-5 in Volume 2.	■ Can be used as a primary or secondary dressing to manage drainage from partial- or full-thickness wounds ■ Highly absorptive. Used for wounds with moderate to large amounts of drainage.	■ Do not use to pack undermining wounds. ■ Do not use if the wound is not draining. This can dry out the wound bed and damage tissue.	Moderate to large
Alginates ■ Fibers derived from brown seaweed and kelp ■ Available in pad or rope form.	■ Very high absorbency (20 to 40 times their weight) ■ Promote a moist environment ■ Facilitate autolytic débridement ■ Ideal for wounds that have depth, tracts, tunneling, or undermining	■ Will adhere to the wound bed if there is no drainage ■ When the alginate comes in contact with exudate, a nonadhesive gel is created. Must irrigate this gel from the wound before placing the next dressing. ■ Allergy to antibiotic components, seaweed, or kelp	Large
Antimicrobials (Antibiotic and Antifungal) ■ Available as ointments, impregnated gauzes, pads, gels, foams, hydrocolloids, and alginates ■ Commonly contain silver and iodine	■ Reduce exudate and prevent infection by reducing bacteria in the wound ■ Promote collagen deposition ■ Can be used on partial- or full-thickness wounds, malodorous wounds with little to large amounts of drainage, or highly contaminated or infected wounds	■ Allergy to silver or iodine	Large
Collagens ■ Made from bovine (cow) or porcine (pig) sources and made into sheets, pads, powders, and gels	■ Use with partial- and full-thickness and contaminated or infected wounds ■ Absorb exudate ■ Promote a moist wound bed for healing ■ Stimulate wounds to produce collagen fibers and granulation tissue in the wound bed ■ Do not stick to the wound bed and are easy to apply and remove	**Key Point:** *If using porcine dressings, check that your patient has no religious practices that would forbid this use.*	Minimal to large
Foams ■ Made from semipermeable hydrophilic foam that forms an impermeable barrier over the wound	■ Absorbent; for wounds with moderate to heavy exudates ■ Thermal insulation ■ Promote a moist environment	■ Do not use with wounds that have tunneling or tracts. ■ Not recommended for dry, desiccated wounds ■ May macerate periwound skin, if dressing becomes oversaturated	Moderate to large

Description	Uses	Considerations	Exudate
■ Made into wafers, rolls, and pillows; have film coverings; and are adhesive or nonadhesive	■ Do not stick to wound bed ■ Used under compression ■ Protect friable periwound skin ■ Can be shaped around body contours ■ May be used in combination with alginates or films	■ Opaque, with inability to see wound bed for assessment ■ High probability of bacterial invasion	Minimal to large
Gauze ■ Simplest and most widely used dressings ■ Made of woven and nonwoven fibers of cotton, rayon, polyester, or a combination of these ■ Some are impregnated with antimicrobial agents, medications, or moisture, and others contain petrolatum to keep the wound moist.	■ Cleansing ■ Protection ■ Used for packing large wounds, cavities, or tracts; deep or dirty wounds; or heavily draining wounds ■ Used in combination with amorphous hydrogels, saline, or medications ■ May be packed as sterile or nonsterile, in bulk or in smaller packages ■ Affordable and easily available	■ Labor intensive ■ Can stick to wound tissue and damage new, regenerated cells with gauze removal ■ Does not ensure a moist wound environment because it allows for fluid evaporation ■ May be applied incorrectly because it must be fluffed to avoid pressure or overpacking of a wound ■ Dressing change interval is dependent on the amount of fluid saturation of the gauze. Frequent dressing changes disrupt the wound bed and cause the wound to become hypothermic (cold), which physiologically impairs cell growth for healing.	
Hydrocolloids ■ Wafers, pastes, or powders that contain hydrophilic (water-loving) particles See Procedure 32-8: Applying a Hydrating Dressing (Hydrocolloid or Hydrogel), in Volume 2.	■ Hydrophilic particles interact with water to form a gel that keeps the wound moist. ■ Provide a protective layer against friction/caustic agents and bacteria. Also reduce pain ■ Ideal for wounds with minimal exudates (e.g., partial thickness wounds, stage 2 pressure injury) ■ Promote autolysis ■ Used under compression ■ Mold to the shape of the body, making them useful for difficult areas, such as heels or between buttocks ■ Use around stomas to create an even surface on which to place the ostomy appliance ■ Do not require a secondary dressing	■ Not the dressing of choice for wounds that require frequent dressing changes ■ Opaque—do not allow the wound to be visualized ■ Not recommended for wounds surrounded by friable or sensitive skin (difficult to remove) ■ Should not be used on infected wounds because they are impermeable to oxygen, moisture, and bacteria ■ When an exudate comes in contact with the hydrocolloid material, it can produce an odor that might be confused with a malodorous wound. Clean the wound bed first before determining whether it is malodorous. ■ May facilitate the growth of anaerobic bacteria ■ Should not be used on wounds with tunneling or tracts because these wounds must be packed and allowed to drain. Wound should be shallow enough that the hydrocolloid touches the wound bed.	Light to moderate

(Continued)

Table 32-5 ▶ Types of Wound Dressings—cont'd

DRESSING TYPE AND DESCRIPTION	USE	CAUTIONS	WOUND SIZE
Hydrogels ▪ Sheets, granules, or gels with a high water content, creating a jelly-like consistency that does not adhere to the wound bed ➤ See Procedure 32-8: Applying a Hydrating Dressing (Hydrocolloid or Hydrogel), in Volume 2.	▪ Enhance epithelialization to promote a moist environment ▪ Rehydrate the wound bed ▪ Seal or reconnect disrupted tissue without sutures or staples and protect the wound bed (Annabi et al., 2017) ▪ Promote autolysis ▪ Soft, cooling texture promotes comfort. ▪ Soften slough or eschar in necrotic wounds	▪ Have limited absorptive capabilities (not practical for wounds with significant exudate). Require a secondary dressing ▪ Easily macerate periwound skin because of high moisture content	Minimal
Skin Sealants and Moisture Barriers ▪ Skin sealants—made from liquid transparent copolymer ▪ Moisture barrier ointments—petrolatum, dimethicone, or zinc-based products that can be applied to skin to protect it from exudate, moisture, urine, and feces	▪ Simple and fast to use, and if needed, should be used with each dressing change ▪ Can be wiped or sprayed on skin to protect it from wound exudate and moisture, friction, and skin stripping from adhesives ▪ Provide a barrier of protection over vulnerable skin from the effects of moisture and mechanical and chemical skin injury	▪ Ointments impair the adhesion of wound dressings or tapes.	Any
Transparent Films (see Fig. 32-15) ▪ Clear and semipermeable ➤ See Procedure 32-7: Applying and Removing a Transparent Film Dressing, in Volume 2.	▪ Promote a moist environment ▪ Occlusive with oxygen permeability ▪ Promote autolysis ▪ Often used to dress IV sites ▪ Prevent external bacterial contamination ▪ Allow wound assessment without removing or disturbing the dressing ▪ Can be placed over joints without inhibiting movement	▪ If used over wounds that are draining, the tissues will become macerated. ▪ Adhere to the skin, so not for use on friable skin	Minimal to none

Primary dressings are those that are placed in the wound bed and physically touch the wound. A **secondary dressing** is one that covers or holds a primary dressing in place. Many dressings can act as both, touching the wound bed and securing themselves to the wound with some type of adhesive. Figure 32-14 shows various sizes of gauze dressings. Figure 32-15 shows a transparent film dressing over an IV site.

There is no single "recipe" for healing a wound. Each wound must be treated and dressed individually based on the patient history and assessment. Many wound materials are available, and new products are continually introduced. The "newest" type of dressing is not necessarily the best for the wound that you are treating. Choose the dressing based on what the wound needs and not the manufacturer's brand name. Perform ongoing reassessment of your dressing choice every time you assess the wound, modifying dressings and treatments as the wound evolves.

KnowledgeCheck 32-10

- What should you consider when choosing a dressing?
- Describe the five types of wound débridement.
- Identify the purposes of a wound dressing.
- Differentiate between the different categories of dressings.
- What types of dressings may be used for wounds with a large amount of exudate?
- What form of dressing is appropriate for a wound with eschar that needs to be eliminated?

Securing Dressings

What you will use to secure a dressing depends on wound size, location, and amount of drainage; frequency of dressing changes; the patient's activity level; and the type of dressings used. Tape, ties, bandages, secondary dressings, and binders are among the choices.

Tape is most often used. It is available in several forms:

- **Adhesive tape** provides stability to a dressing. It is durable and can be used if you need to apply pressure

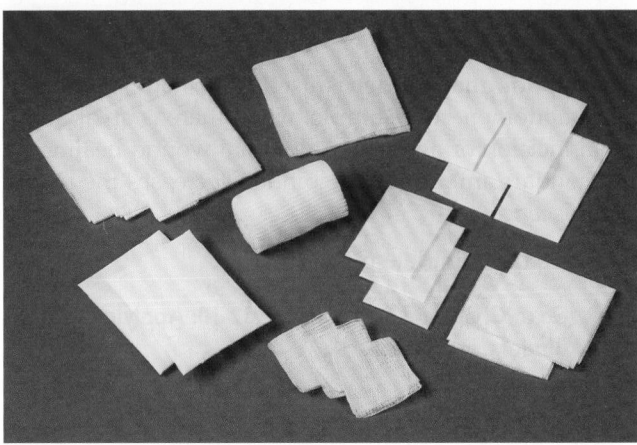

FIGURE 32-14 Gauze dressings are available in a variety of shapes and forms.

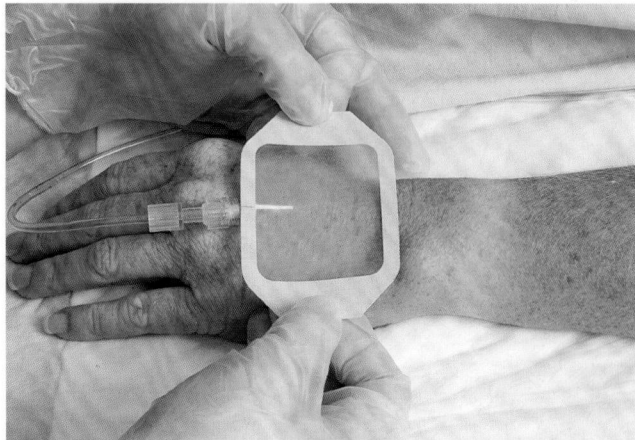

FIGURE 32-15 IV sites are commonly dressed with transparent film dressings.

to a wound. It leaves a residue on the skin and can cause trauma to the surrounding intact skin when it is removed. However, commercial adhesive removers can dissolve the residue and can be used to loosen the tape as it is removed. Adhesives in the tape can cause allergic skin reactions in some patients. Monitor for this complication.
- **Foam tape** readily molds to the contours of the body and is ideal for dressings over joints.
- **Nonallergenic tape and paper tape** are best for sensitive skin. Ask patients whether they have any history of tape allergies or irritation; use a tape that the patient has tolerated well in the past.

To tape a dressing, place strips of tape at the ends of the dressing, and space them evenly over the remainder of the dressing. For the fragile skin of older adults or infants, use porous tapes and avoid unnecessary tape use. Consider using thin hydrocolloids, low-adhesion foam dressings, or skin sealants under the tape to further help prevent skin tears. To see the complete procedure,

Go to **Chapter 32, Procedure 32-3: Taping a Dressing,** in Volume 2.

If a dressing requires frequent changes, you can use Montgomery straps with ties to secure the dressing (Fig. 32-16). Montgomery straps decrease the amount of pulling and irritation of the skin around a wound. Apply the adhesive part of the straps to the skin at the ends of the dressing and at evenly spaced intervals. Lace the cloth ties between the straps to secure the dressing. Change the ties whenever they become soiled. Keep the straps in place until they begin to loosen from the skin.

Controlling Infection

A wound provides a portal of entry or exit for microorganisms. When caring for patients with closed wounds, follow CDC Standard Precautions. For patients with open or draining wounds, follow CDC Tier

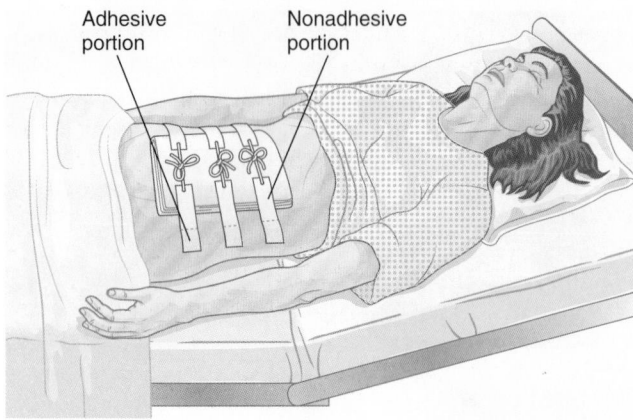

Adhesive portion   Nonadhesive portion

FIGURE 32-16 Montgomery straps with ties may be used to secure a dressing that requires frequent changing.

Two: Contact Level Precautions in addition to Standard Precautions.

 See Chapter 20 and **Chapter 20, Clinical Insight 20-4: Following Transmission-Based Precautions,** in Volume 2.

Several nursing activities also aid in preventing and controlling wound infections.

Asepsis Measures If the patient has an infection, place them in a private room or in a room with a patient who has an active infection caused by the same organism and no other infections. Follow any additional specific precautions for the microorganism identified. Most importantly, wash your hands frequently and thoroughly with soap and warm water.

- Use clean gloves when caring for the patient with a wound.
- Remove gloves and wash your hands before physical contact with another patient.
- Change your gloves after removing a soiled dressing and before applying a clean dressing.
- If a patient has multiple wounds, treat the least contaminated wound first, and then progress to the most contaminated. Wash your hands and change gloves between each wound.

Sterile Technique for Sharp Débridement To prevent infection, use sterile instruments for sharp débridement. Monitor the patient for signs and symptoms of sepsis (e.g., fever, tachycardia, hypotension, and altered level of consciousness) after sharp débridement. Remember, only specially trained providers can do sharp débridement. See the content under the heading Sharp Débridement if you need to review.

Dressings and Supplies

Acute wounds may require sterile dressings.
Chronic wounds require clean dressings. However, even a chronic wound may require sterile dressings if the patient is immunocompromised.

Disposal of Dressings
- Carefully dispose of contaminated dressings in biohazard waste receptacles.
- Discard unused dressings if they become contaminated.

Storage of Dressings
- Store patient dressing supplies in a clean and dry area.
- Do not share supplies among patients.
- Access only the number of supplies you need for the dressing change.

Protection of Dressings
- Do not touch the supply of dressings with gloves that have touched the wound.
- Discard unused dressings if they have become contaminated.

 ThinkLike a Nurse 32-6: Clinical Judgment **in Action**

What would be the best method to secure dressings for Mr. Harmon (Meet Your Patient)?

Supporting and Immobilizing Wounds

Binders and bandages are used to hold a dressing in place, apply pressure to a wound to impede hemorrhage, and support and immobilize an injured area, thereby promoting healing and comfort. Before applying a bandage or binder, determine the purpose of the application and assess the part being bandaged.

Binders

Binders may be used to keep a wound closed when there is a danger of dehiscence or to immobilize a body part to aid in the healing process. They are typically used on large areas of the body and are designed for a specific body part. They may be made of cloth or elasticized material and fasten with straps, pins, or Velcro. The most common binders are the following:

- A **triangular arm binder or sling** is used to support the upper extremities. Because commercial slings are readily available, you will rarely use a triangular sling.
- A **T-binder** is used to secure dressings or pads in the perineal area.
- An **abdominal binder** is used to provide support to the abdomen, for example, when there is an abdominal incision or an open abdominal wound healing by secondary intention. The binder decreases the risk of dehiscence.

To see the complete procedure,

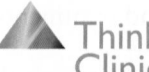 Go to **Chapter 32, Procedure 32-10: Applying Binders,** in Volume 2.

Bandages

A bandage is a cloth, gauze, or elastic covering that is wrapped in place. Except for slings, most bandages come in rolls and in various widths, commonly 1.5 to 7.5 cm (0.5 to 3 in.). Use a narrow width on small body parts, such as a finger, and wider bandages on the arms and legs.

- **Cloth bandages** are most used as slings to immobilize an upper extremity or to hold large abdominal dressings in place.
- **Gauze** is the most frequently used type of bandage. It is available in many sizes and forms and readily conforms to the shape of the body. It may also be impregnated with medications for application to the skin or with plaster of Paris, which, when dried, hardens to form a cast.
- **Elastic bandages** are used to apply pressure and give support (e.g., to improve venous circulation in the legs). Ace bandages are the most common form of elasticized bandage.
- A **rolled bandage** is a continuous strip of gauze, stretchable gauze, or elastic webbing that you unroll as you apply it to a body part. To learn how to apply roller bandages,

 See **Chapter 32, Procedure 32-11: Applying Bandages,** in Volume 2.

Using Heat and Cold Therapy

Local application of heat or cold has been used for therapeutic purposes for centuries. Temperature-sensitive nerve endings respond readily to temperatures between 59°F and 113°F (15°C and 45°C). The response to heat or cold depends on the area being treated, the nature of the injury, the duration of the treatment, patient age and physical condition, and the condition of the skin.

When heat or cold is first applied, the thermal receptors react strongly, and the person feels the temperature most intensely. Over about 15 minutes, the receptors adapt to the new temperature, and the person notices it less. Caution patients not to change the temperature when this occurs because doing so can cause tissue injury. Monitor the patient especially carefully in the following situations:

- **Extremes of age.** The very young and the very old are the least tolerant of heat and cold therapies.
- **Sensory impairment.** Patients with sensory impairment are at increased risk for injury related to the use of heat and cold therapy because they may not perceive temperature changes, burns, or ischemia.
- **Highly vascular areas.** Highly vascular areas, such as the fingers, hand, face, and perineum, are very sensitive to temperature changes and thus are at high risk for injury from heat and cold.
- **Application to a large area.** Application of cold or heat to a large body surface area decreases the patient's tolerance of the treatment. Application to a small area is best tolerated.
- **Injured skin or wounds.** Intact skin tolerates heat and cold therapy better than skin that has been injured or has open wounds.

Applying Heat Therapy Local application of heat is used to relieve the stiffness and discomfort associated with musculoskeletal problems. It may also be used for patients with wounds. When heat is applied to a large area of the body, vasodilation may cause a drop in blood pressure and a feeling of faintness. Warn patients to be alert for this effect if they will be administering heat at home.

- **Increases blood flow to an area** through the mechanisms of vasodilation, increased capillary permeability, and reduced blood viscosity. Increased blood flow brings oxygen and white blood cells to the wound and aids in the healing process.
- **Promotes the delivery of nutrients and removal of waste products** from the tissue.
- **Promotes relaxation** and decreases stiffness and muscle tension.

Either moist heat or dry heat may be used, depending on the patient situation and the goal of therapy.

- **Moist heat.** Adding moisture to heat amplifies the intensity of the treatment. Moist heat can be applied in several forms, depending on the skin condition.
    Washcloth or towel. If heat is being applied for relaxation and the skin is intact, you can soak a washcloth or towel in warm water and wring out the excess moisture before applying to the skin. Do not microwave moistened towels to warm them. This causes unequal heat distribution and may cause burns to the patient.
    Gauze compress. If there are any open areas, you still need to use a sterile gauze compress.
    Soaks. A **soak** involves immersion of the affected area. Soaking helps cleanse a wound and remove encrusted material.
    Baths. A **bath** is a modification of a soak in which a special tub or chair may be used. The most used bath is a sitz bath (Fig. 32-17). A **Sitz bath** soaks the patient's perineal area. Disposable sitz baths are often used to help prevent infection.
- **Dry heat.** You may use electric heating pads, disposable hot packs, or hot-water bags to apply dry heat. Caution patients to place the heating pad or device over the body area and never to lie on it. The pad or bag should be covered with its own cover or a towel.
    Electric heating pads have the advantage of providing a constant temperature, but the risk of burns is high.
    Aquathermia pads (Fig. 32-18) may also be used for dry heat application. Aquapads are plastic or vinyl pads that circulate water in the interior of the pad to create a constant temperature.
    Disposable hot packs and hot-water bags or bottles are also available. Hot-water bags are common for in-home use but not for healthcare agencies because of the danger of burns from improper use.

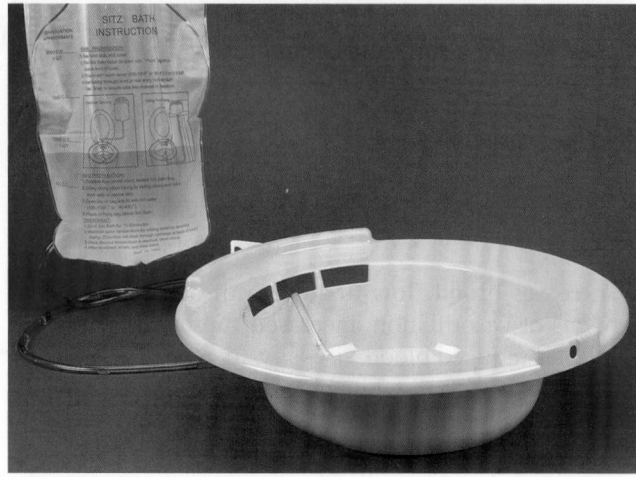

FIGURE 32-17 A Sitz bath soaks the patient's perineal area.

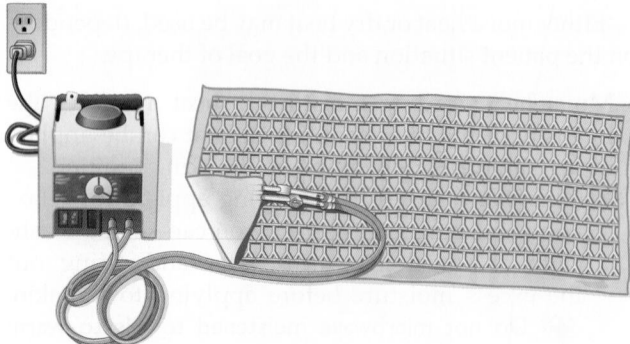

FIGURE 32-18 Aquathermia pads circulate water in the interior of the pad to create a constant temperature.

For guidelines (including water temperatures) for applying moist and dry heat,

See **Chapter 32, Clinical Insight 32-1, Using Heat Therapy,** in Volume 2.

Applying Cold Therapy The application of moist or dry cold causes vasoconstriction and decreases capillary permeability. It produces local anesthesia, reduces cell metabolism, increases blood viscosity, and decreases muscle tension. It also slows bacterial growth. Applications of cold are used to:

- Prevent or limit edema.
- Reduce inflammation and pain.

- Reduce oxygen requirements.
- Help control bleeding.
- Treat fevers.
- Treat musculoskeletal injuries (e.g., sprains, strains, fractures, and contusions).
- Prevent or reduce swelling after surgery (e.g., an ice pack may be applied to the perineum after childbirth; an ice collar may be applied to the throat after a tonsillectomy).

Applications of cold have the following side effects:

- **Elevated blood pressure.** Because cold causes vasoconstriction, cold therapy may increase the patient's blood pressure.
- **Shivering.** Prolonged cold may cause shivering, a normal response as the body attempts to produce heat.
- **Tissue damage.** Prolonged exposure to cold may cause tissue damage from impaired circulation.

For guidelines in applying cold therapy,

 See Chapter 32, **Clinical Insight 32-2 Using Cold Therapy,** in Volume 2.

KnowledgeCheck 32-11

- What is the effect of adding moisture to heat or cold treatments?
- How long should heat or cold be applied to an area?
- What precautions should you take before using heat or cold therapy?

 To explore learning resources for this chapter,

 Go to Davis Advantage **and find:**

Answers and Suggested Responses for all questions in this chapter

Concept Map

Knowledge Map

References and Bibliography

Care Plan

Care Map

CHAPTER 33

Oxygenation

Learning Outcomes

After completing this chapter, you should be able to:

➤ Describe the structure and function of the respiratory system.

➤ Identify individual, environmental, and pathological factors that influence oxygenation.

➤ Assess/identify cues for oxygenation, breathing, and gas exchange.

➤ Interpret diagnostic testing related to oxygenation, breathing, and gas exchange.

➤ Analyze cues and develop nursing diagnoses related to oxygenation, breathing, and gas exchange.

➤ Plan outcomes and generate solutions for maintaining and improving oxygenation.

➤ Safely and correctly perform common nursing actions related to oxygenation, breathing, and gas exchange.

➤ Evaluate adequacy of oxygenation, breathing, and gas exchange, and modify nursing activities appropriately based on outcomes.

➤ Recognize medications used to enhance pulmonary function.

Key Concepts

Oxygenation

Respiration

Ventilation

Related Concepts

See the Concept Map on Davis Advantage.

Example Client Conditions

Pneumonia

Upper Respiratory Infection and Influenza

Meet Your Patients

In a pulmonary clinic, your student assignment is to (1) perform a focused assessment related to breathing and oxygenation, (2) perform common therapeutic interventions related to breathing and oxygenation, (3) identify desired outcomes and evaluate achievement of those outcomes, and (4) plan for follow-up and home care needs. During your clinical day, you care for the following clients:

■ **Mary** is a 4-year-old patient with a history of asthma. Her mother, Ms. Green, has brought her in because of an "asthma attack." Mary is sitting on her mother's lap and breathing rapidly through an open mouth. Her cough sounds congested and wheezy. The nurse practitioner has prescribed a nebulized treatment containing albuterol (Proventil) and ipratropium bromide (Atrovent).

■ **Mr. Chu** is a 78-year-old patient complaining of cough, sore throat, fatigue, and weakness. His temperature is

100.4°F (38°C), pulse is 90 beats/min, respirations are 26 breaths/min, and blood pressure (BP) is 166/82 mm Hg.

■ **William** is a 19-year-old male patient who has had a sudden onset of right-sided chest pain and shortness of breath. His chest x-ray revealed a right pneumothorax, and he is currently receiving 35% oxygen by face mask while waiting for an ambulance to transport him to the hospital for further evaluation.

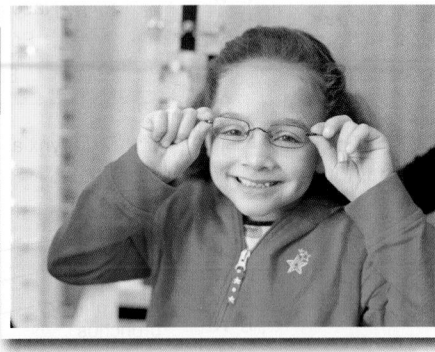

Each of these patients is experiencing an oxygenation problem. In this chapter you will learn a variety of assessment techniques and interventions to support breathing, oxygenation, and gas exchange for patients such as these.

Theoretical Knowledge
knowing why

The pulmonary, cardiovascular, musculoskeletal, and neurological systems work together to achieve oxygenation. The musculoskeletal and neurological systems regulate the movement of air into and out of the lungs. The lungs oxygenate the blood, and the heart circulates the blood throughout the body and back to the lungs. In this chapter, we focus on the pulmonary system; Chapter 34 presents the cardiovascular system. Remember, however, that the two systems work together. Changes in one system create changes in the other.

ABOUT THE KEY CONCEPTS

The concept of **oxygenation** refers to how well the cells, tissues, and organs of the body are supplied with oxygen. The concepts of **respiration** and **ventilation** are the two major processes that occur in the pulmonary system to oxygenate the blood. All of the problems and interventions in this chapter relate in some way to oxygenation, respiration, or ventilation. Knowledge of these concepts will help you to understand the rationale

for interventions such as airway suctioning, oxygen, mechanical ventilation, and chest tubes.

THE PULMONARY SYSTEM

The pulmonary system has two major components: the *airway* and the *lungs.* The following presents a brief review of the anatomy and physiology of the pulmonary system and explains how breathing is controlled. For more in-depth information, consult anatomy and physiology texts.

The Airway

The airway consists of the nasal passages, mouth, pharynx, larynx, trachea, bronchi, and bronchioles (Fig. 33-1). Air flows through these structures into and out of the lungs. In addition, the airway structures do the following:

- *Moisten the air*—A moist mucous membrane lining adds water to inhaled air.
- *Warm the air*—Blood flowing through the vascular airway walls transfers body heat to the inhaled air.
- *Filter the air*—(1) Specialized cells in the lining of the airways secrete sticky mucus to trap foreign particles.

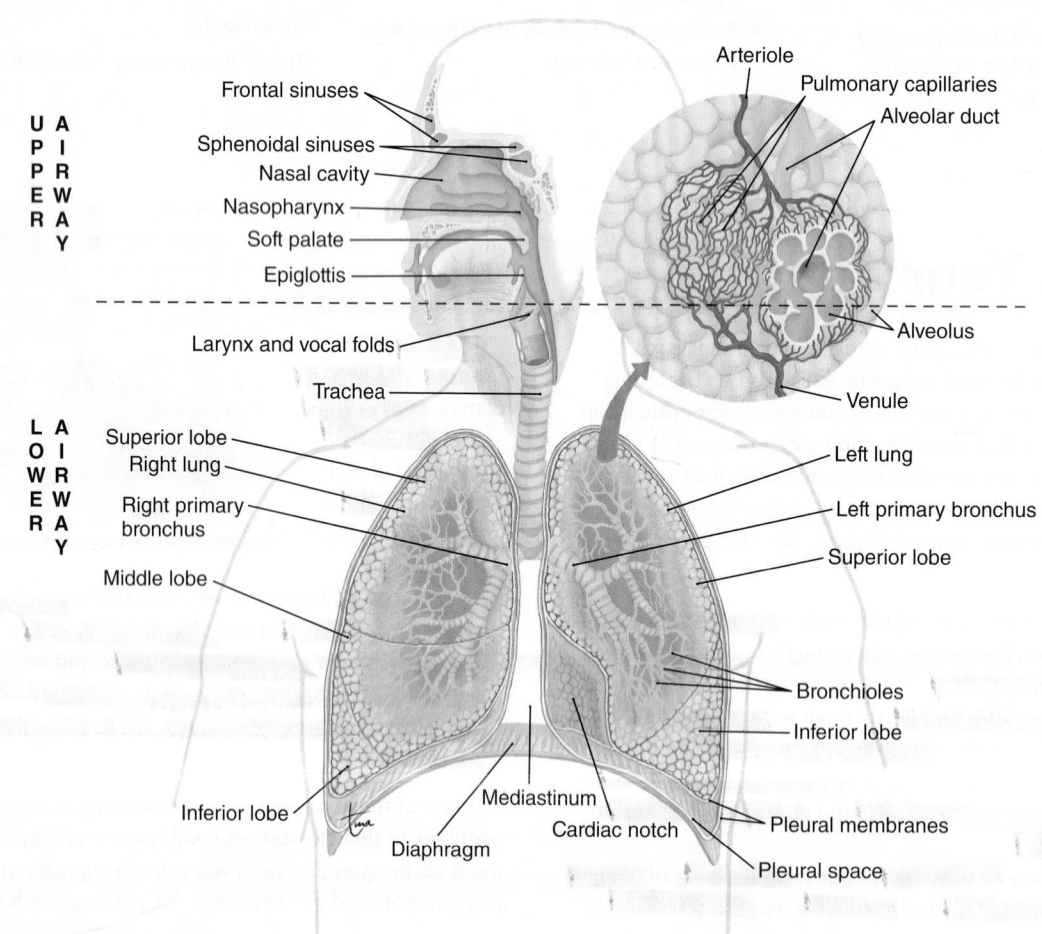

FIGURE 33-1 An anterior view of the respiratory system. The upper airway lies above the larynx. The lower airway, located below the larynx, is considered sterile.

(2) **Cilia,** tiny hairlike projections from the walls of the airways, move rhythmically to sweep trapped debris up and out of the airway.

Upper Airway Located above the larynx, the upper airway includes the nasal passages, mouth, and pharynx.

- The *pharynx* (throat) contains the openings to the esophagus and trachea.
- The *trachea* lies just in front of the esophagus.
- The *epiglottis* is a small flap of tissue superior to the larynx.
  - It closes off the trachea during swallowing so that food and fluids do not enter the lower airway.
  - It opens during breathing to allow air to move through the airway.

Lower Airway Located below the larynx, the lower airway includes the trachea, bronchi, and bronchioles. The lower airway is considered sterile. The **trachea,** sometimes called the "windpipe," extends from the larynx to the point at which it divides to form the right and left mainstem bronchi. As the airways branch and become smaller, they have progressively thinner and less cartilage, until it disappears completely in the smaller bronchioles. The walls of the bronchi and bronchioles contain layers of smooth muscles. Spasm of the layers of smooth muscles in the bronchi and bronchioles **(bronchospasm)** narrows the airway and obstructs airflow.

The Lungs

The **lungs** are soft, spongy, cone-shaped organs. They are separated by the **mediastinum,** which contains the heart and great vessels. The right lung has three lobes; the left lung has two lobes.

- **Apex.** The upper portion of each lung, the *apex,* extends upward above the clavicle.
- **Base.** The lower portion of each lung, the *base,* rests on the diaphragm.
- **Alveoli.** The lungs are composed of millions of *alveoli*—tiny air sacs with thin walls surrounded by a fine network of capillaries. Gases (oxygen and carbon dioxide) easily pass back and forth between the alveoli and capillaries. See Figure 33-2 for an illustration of the alveolar structure.
  - *Type I alveolar cells* are the gas-exchange cells.
  - *Type II alveolar cells* produce **surfactant,** a lipoprotein that lowers the surface tension within alveoli to allow them to inflate during breathing.

Key Point: *Knowing the location of lung tissue beneath the chest wall helps you to perform a complete and accurate assessment of the lungs.*

KnowledgeCheck 33-1

- What happens to inhaled air in the airways? How does this occur?
- In which structures of the lung does gas exchange take place?
- What does surfactant do for alveoli?

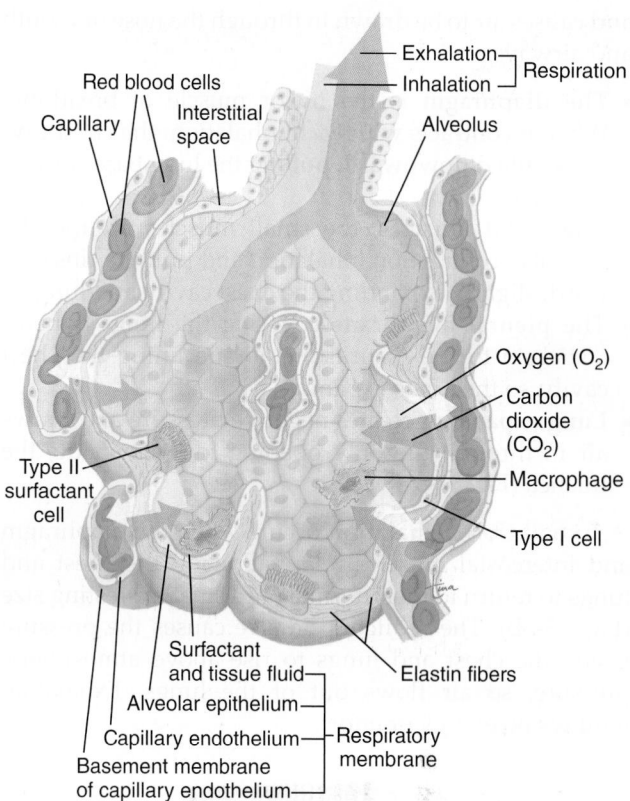

FIGURE 33-2 Alveolar structure showing type I and type II cells. Type I cells are the gas exchange cells. Type II cells produce surfactant.

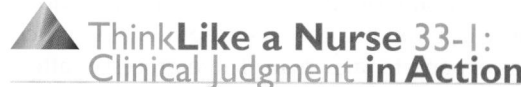

ThinkLike a Nurse 33-1: Clinical Judgment in Action

You are assigned to care for an adult patient who has a medical condition with which you are not familiar. You look it up and find that the condition causes a dramatic loss of surfactant. Based on your knowledge of the function of surfactant, what problems is this patient at high risk for developing?

WHAT ARE THE FUNCTIONS OF THE PULMONARY SYSTEM?

Two of the key concepts in this chapter are major processes that occur in the pulmonary system:

- **Ventilation** is the movement of air into and out of the lungs through the act of breathing.
- **Respiration** is the exchange of the gases oxygen and carbon dioxide in the lungs.

Pulmonary Ventilation

Key Point: *Oxygenation of the blood, and ultimately of organs and tissues, depends on adequate ventilation.* Ventilation must move enough air through the lungs to make adequate oxygen available to the alveoli. Ventilation is accomplished through cycles of inhalation and exhalation.

Inhalation Inhalation is the expansion of the chest cavity and lungs with negative pressure inside the lungs and causes air to be drawn in through the nose or mouth and airways.

- **The diaphragm** is the major muscle of breathing. When it contracts with each inhalation, the chest cavity is pulled downward, pulling the lung bases downward with it.
- **Intercostal muscles,** the small muscles around the ribs, also contract on inhalation and pull the ribs outward, slightly expanding the chest cavity and lungs.
- **The pleural membrane** covering the lungs adheres ("sticks") to the pleural membrane lining the chest cavity, so the lungs expand.
- **Lung expansion** creates negative pressure and draws air in through the only opening to the outside, the trachea (Fig. 33-3A).

Exhalation Exhalation occurs when the diaphragm and intercostal muscles relax, allowing the chest and lungs to return to their normal (and smaller) resting size (Fig. 33-3B). The reduction in size causes the pressure inside the chest and lungs to rise above atmospheric pressure, so air flows out of the lungs. Exhalation requires no energy or effort.

What Factors Affect Ventilation?

The adequacy of ventilation is affected by the rate and depth of respirations, lung compliance and elasticity, and airway resistance.

- **Respiratory rate and depth** are almost self-explanatory. **Rate** is how fast you breathe, and **depth** is how much your lungs expand to take in air. These processes affect oxygen and carbon dioxide levels in the blood.
  - **Hyperventilation** occurs when a person breathes fast and deeply to move a large amount of air through the lungs, causing too much carbon dioxide to be removed by the alveoli.
    - *Severe hyperventilation* is usually triggered by medication, central nervous system (CNS) abnormalities, high altitude, heat, exercise, panic, fear, or anxiety.
    - *Mild hyperventilation* can occur in response to **hypoxemia** (a low level of oxygen in the blood). When blood oxygen is low, ventilation increases to draw additional air (and oxygen) into the lungs. However, as ventilation increases, carbon dioxide levels fall.
- **Hypoventilation** occurs when a decreased rate or shallow breathing moves only a small amount of air into and out of the lungs. Hypoventilation can lead to hypoxemia because less air (carrying oxygen) reaches the alveoli. The concern is that hypoxemia will progress to **hypoxia** (an oxygen deficiency in the body tissues).
- **Lung elasticity** (or elastic recoil) refers to the tendency of the elastin fibers to return to their original position away from the chest wall after being stretched (think of stretching a rubber band, then letting go of it). Alveoli that have been overstretched, as with emphysema, lose their elastic recoil over time. This loss of elasticity allows the lungs to inflate easily but inhibits deflation, leaving stale air trapped in the alveoli.
- **Lung compliance** refers to the ease of lung inflation. Normally the lungs inflate easily. Lung compliance is reduced by increased lung water (edema), loss of surfactant, or conditions that cause elastin fibers in the lungs to be replaced with scar tissue (collagen).
- **Airway resistance** is the resistance to airflow within the airways. The larger the diameter of the airway, the more easily air moves through it. However, even small decreases in airway diameter (as might occur with secretions in the airway or mild bronchospasm) markedly increase airway resistance. Mary, the young patient with asthma (Meet Your Patients), is undoubtedly experiencing airway resistance.

KnowledgeCheck 33-2

- What is the difference between ventilation and respiration?
- Describe how the diaphragm, accessory muscles, and pressure changes within the lungs create inhalation and exhalation.
- How does hypoventilation affect the risk for hypoxemia and hypoxia?

Respiration (Gas Exchange)

Respiration refers to gas exchange, that is, the oxygenation of blood and elimination of carbon dioxide in the lungs. Although nurses commonly use the term *respirations* to mean "breaths" in an assessment of vital signs, strictly speaking, this is not accurate: **Key Point: You cannot measure gas exchange by counting breaths per minute. Gas exchange occurs at two equally essential levels: external (in the lungs) or internal (in other body tissues).**

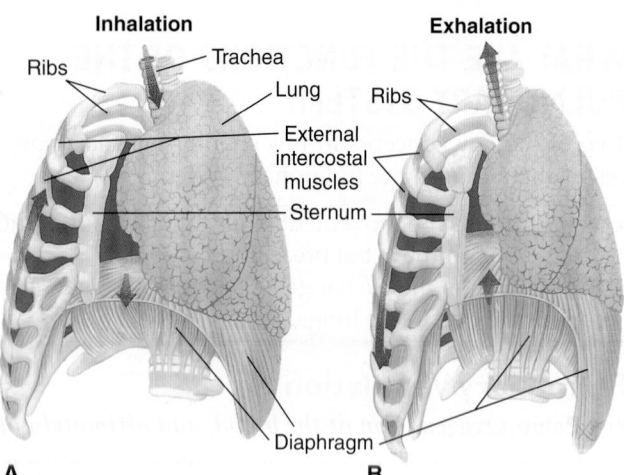

FIGURE 33-3 A, During inhalation, the diaphragm contracts, pulling the chest cavity and lung bases downward; the intercostal muscles pull the rib cage up and outward. B, In exhalation, the diaphragm relaxes, the lung bases move upward, and the ribs and intercostal muscles move down and in, resulting in lung compression.

External Respiration External respiration (alveolar–capillary gas exchange) occurs in the alveoli of the lungs:

- **Oxygen (O_2)** diffuses across the alveolar–capillary membrane into the blood of the pulmonary capillaries.
- **Carbon dioxide (CO_2)** diffuses out of the blood and into the alveoli to be exhaled (Fig. 33-4).
- **The rate of diffusion** depends on the thickness of the membrane and the total surface of lung tissue available for gas exchange.
- **Conditions that slow diffusion** include:
  Pleural effusion (fluid around the lungs)
  Pneumothorax (lung collapse)
  Asthma (bronchospasms)

If blood is not adequately oxygenated in the alveoli, **hypoxemia** (low blood-oxygen levels) occurs. Getting oxygen into the blood as it flows through the lungs is only the first step in oxygenation.

Internal Respiration Internal respiration (or capillary–tissue gas exchange) occurs in body organs and tissues:

- **Oxygen diffuses from the blood** through the capillary–cellular membrane into the tissue cells, where it is used for metabolism.
- **CO_2, a waste product of cellular metabolism, diffuses from the cells** through the capillary–cellular membrane into the blood, then is transported to the lungs and exhaled.

Key Point: *Tissue oxygenation requires both adequate external respiration and adequate peripheral circulation.*

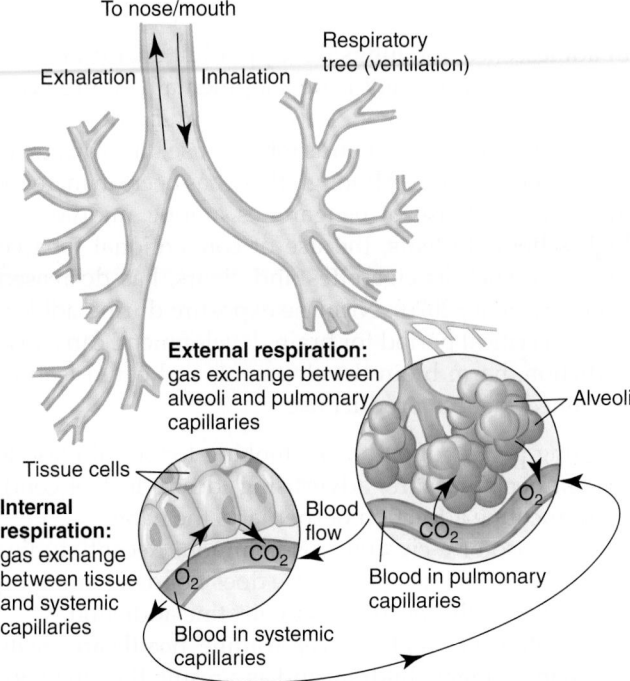

FIGURE 33-4 External respiration occurs at the alveolar–capillary membrane. Internal respiration occurs at the tissue–capillary membrane.

Limitations in either function may lead to hypoxia (oxygen deficiency in body tissues). In addition, if tissue cells are using more oxygen for metabolism than normal (e.g., during a high fever), hypoxia will occur unless more oxygen is made available to the tissues.

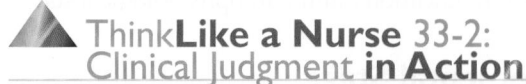

ThinkLike a Nurse 33-2: Clinical Judgment in Action

William (Meet Your Patients) has a right pneumothorax. Which of the two factors affecting the rate of gas diffusion is causing William to be hypoxemic? If you do not know what a pneumothorax is, look it up.

How Is Breathing Controlled?

Voluntary control from the **motor cortex** can override the involuntary respiratory centers but only temporarily. This allows a person to continue breathing while doing activities such as talking, singing, swallowing, whistling, and blowing. The respiratory centers in the brainstem control breathing using feedback from chemoreceptors and lung receptors.

Chemoreceptors Chemoreceptors, located in the medulla of the brainstem, the carotid arteries, and the aorta, detect changes in blood pH, O_2, and CO_2 levels and send messages back to the central respiratory center in the brainstem. In response, the respiratory center increases or decreases ventilation to maintain normal blood levels of pH, O_2 (Po_2), and CO_2 (Pco_2).

- High blood CO_2 levels stimulate breathing to eliminate the excess CO_2. **Key Point:** *Normally, the blood CO_2 level provides the primary stimulus to breathe.*
- **Low blood O_2 levels** stimulate breathing to get more oxygen into the lungs. Therefore, hypoxemia is a secondary, although important, drive to breathe.

Lung Receptors Lung receptors, located in the lung and chest wall, are sensitive to breathing patterns, lung expansion, lung compliance, airway resistance, and respiratory irritants. The respiratory center uses feedback from the lung receptors to adjust ventilation. For example, if the lung receptors sense respiratory irritants such as dust, cold air, or tobacco smoke, the respiratory center triggers airway constriction and a more rapid, shallow pattern of breathing.

KnowledgeCheck 33-3

- Describe two ways in which breathing is controlled.
- The level of which gas (oxygen or carbon dioxide) is the primary stimulant for breathing?

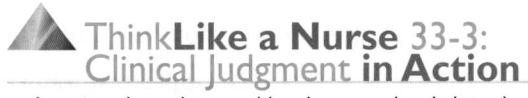

ThinkLike a Nurse 33-3: Clinical Judgment in Action

A patient has adequate blood oxygen levels based on a pulse oximeter reading of 98%. Can you conclude that organ and tissue oxygenations are adequate? Explain your thinking.

WHAT EXTERNAL FACTORS INFLUENCE PULMONARY FUNCTION?

Factors that influence pulmonary function include developmental stage, the environment, individual and lifestyle factors, medications, and pathophysiological states.

Developmental Stage

Normal development influences lung, heart, and circulatory function, all of which affect oxygenation. Developmental factors have less effect on function in young and middle adults than in older adults.

Infants

Premature Infants Premature infants (less than 35 weeks' gestation) are at high risk for **respiratory distress syndrome (RDS),** which is characterized by widespread **atelectasis** (collapse of alveoli). This risk exists because premature infants:

- Do not have a fully developed alveolar surfactant system. Surfactant is the substance that keeps air sacs inflated for effective respiration.
- Have immature pulmonary circulation. Together with hypoventilation, this leads to **hypercarbia** (high CO_2 blood levels) and hypoxemia.

Infants Born at Term Term infants are also at risk for oxygenation problems (e.g., infection and airway obstruction) for the following reasons:

- The newborn's lower airway structures are immature and small, allowing an infectious agent to spread rapidly.
  - The infant's airways are quite narrow in diameter and, therefore, easily obstructed by edema, mucus, or a foreign body, such as meconium passed at birth.
  - In preterm infants and even in some full-term infants, the CNS is immature, leading to periodic breathing patterns and apnea.
  - The immune system of infants is immature in the first few months of life. Although at birth, infants enjoy the benefit of some maternal immunoglobulin circulating in their systems, this protection is limited and not sufficient for fighting certain infections.
  - By age 6 months, infants are at risk for choking on small objects. This is because at that age, in addition to their existing small airway diameter, infants can grasp small objects and put them in their mouths.

Toddlers

As the toddler's respiratory and immune systems mature, the risk for frequent and serious infections diminishes.

Upper Respiratory Infections **Upper respiratory infections** (URIs), however, remain common because:

- The tonsils and adenoids are relatively large, predisposing toddlers to tonsillitis.

- Many children are exposed to new infectious agents in preschool and day care.

Most children recover from URIs without difficulty.

Other Respiratory Problems Toddlers actively explore the environment and often put objects in their mouth, which puts them at risk for other respiratory problems, for example:

- *Acquiring and transmitting infections* through toys and other objects
- *Airway obstruction* from aspiration of small objects (e.g., candy, buttons, coins, peanuts, grapes). The toddler's airway is still relatively short and small and may be easily obstructed.
- *Drowning* in very small amounts of water around the home (e.g., in a bucket of water or toilet bowl).

Preschool and School-Age Children

Preschool and school-age children have mature lungs, a fully developed heart, and a circulatory system that can adapt to moderate stress and change.

- *URIs.* Healthy children typically have bouts of tonsillitis or URIs, which usually resolve without difficulty.
- *Viral infections,* such as croup and pneumonia, are common, especially in preschoolers and younger school-age children.
- *Asthma.* Exercise-induced (and other) asthma is also a problem.
- *Tobacco use.* Unfortunately, as early as middle school, children may begin social habits, such as tobacco use, that can have long-term adverse effects on oxygenation in both the pulmonary and cardiovascular systems.

Adolescents

In adolescence, the lungs develop adult characteristics. The average adolescent is developmentally at little risk for lung diseases. Some, however, may be developing behaviors and habits, such as tobacco use, that can create risk throughout life. Although there has been an increase in the current use of e-cigarettes among middle and high school students, the use of conventional tobacco products, such as cigarettes and cigars, has decreased (Gentzke et al., 2020). Nicotine exposure during adolescence, a critical period for brain development, can cause addiction, harm brain development, and could lead to sustained tobacco product use.

- Young people often begin smoking for social reasons (e.g., peer pressure, advertising, desire to feel cool), but nicotine addiction perpetuates the habit.
  - The use of e-cigarettes is common. Recent studies indicate that e-cigarette use does not deter smoking and actually contributes to nicotine addiction.
  - Adolescents make fewer routine healthcare visits than younger children, and as a result, they may not receive the recommended influenza vaccines.
  - Exercise-induced asthma is still a problem in this age-group.

Young, Middle, and Older Adults

- *Unhealthy practices* (e.g., smoking and a lack of aerobic exercise) begun during adolescence often continue into adulthood. More than 12% of U.S. adults are cigarette smokers (Centers for Disease Control and Prevention [CDC], 2022a).
- *Changes in the respiratory system* begin in middle age and increase in older adulthood. These may become significant when the person experiences stressors such as infection, surgery, anesthesia, and emotional problems. The number of cells and the efficiency of the organs decline subtly and progressively as a person ages. **Key Point:** *Keep in mind, though, that endurance training and regular exercise minimize the rate of these changes. In fact, an older person who is physically conditioned by regular exercise may have better lung function than will a younger adult who is not well conditioned.*

 Older Adults Older adults tend to experience the following changes:

- *Reduced lung expansion and less alveolar inflation,* especially in the bases of the lungs. This is because:
  1. Costal cartilage begins to calcify, reducing chest wall movement during breathing.
  2. The lungs have less recoil ability.
  3. The alveoli lose elasticity.
- *Difficulty expelling mucus or foreign material* because of a less effective cough reflex, drier mucus, and fewer cilia in the airways.
- *Diminished ability to increase ventilation* when oxygenation demands increase (e.g., with exercise). As diaphragm strength decreases, vital capacity is reduced; therefore, exhalation becomes less efficient, causing progressive air-trapping.
- *Declining immune response,* especially cell-mediated immunity, T-cell activity, and the inflammatory response
- *Gastroesophageal reflux disease* is more common in older adults, creating a risk for aspirating stomach contents into the lungs. This may result in an inflammatory response.
- *Chemoreceptors* respond more slowly to increased O_2 demand or rising levels of CO_2, making hypoxemia more likely when respiratory problems occur.

All of these changes put older adults at risk for respiratory infections. URIs that would be mild and short-lived in a younger person may quickly lead to pneumonia in an older adult.

Environment

Environmental factors can affect oxygenation.

Stress The stress response stimulates the release of catecholamines from the sympathetic nervous system, resulting in (1) increased tendency of blood to clot (e.g., as in pulmonary embolus) and (2) suppression of the immune system and inflammatory response.

A chronically suppressed immune and inflammatory response increases the risk for all infections, including respiratory infections. For additional information on the effects of stress, see Chapter 9.

Allergic Reactions An **allergy** is a hypersensitivity, or overresponse, to an antigen. Pulmonary allergens include such things as dust, dust mites, cockroach particles, pollen, molds, newsprint, tobacco smoke, animal dander, and sometimes foods.

- **Hay fever** is an allergic reaction affecting the eyes, nose, and/or sinuses. It causes the release of *histamine,* which is largely responsible for the symptoms of an accumulation of nasal fluid; swollen nasal membranes; nasal congestion; and itchy, swollen, watery eyes. Antihistamines are effective in combating hay fever.
- **Asthma** is an allergic reaction occurring in the bronchioles of the lungs. *Slow-reacting substance of anaphylaxis* (SRS-A) is released, which causes bronchoconstriction and lower airway edema and spasms, making breathing difficult and ineffective. Because histamine is not a major factor in causing the asthmatic reaction, antihistamines have little effect in the treatment of asthma. **Key Point:** *Asthma is the most common serious chronic disease of childhood, and it can be life threatening.*

Air Quality Air pollution triggers respiratory problems (e.g., lung cancer, carbon monoxide poisoning) that interfere with oxygenation. Even healthy people may experience headache, coughing, and other symptoms when exposed to air pollution. People with existing respiratory disease may become unable to function.

Some sources of air pollution are natural (e.g., forest fires), but the most common and damaging sources result from human activities (e.g., automobile exhaust emissions). Indoor air pollutants include carbon monoxide, nitrogen oxides, radon, and suspended particles (e.g., dust, mold spores, aerosols, and tobacco smoke). Pollutants are most harmful to infants, toddlers, older adults, and people with heart or lung disease.

Altitude Atmospheric pressure falls from 760 mm Hg at sea level to 523 mm Hg at 10,000 feet.

- As the atmospheric pressure decreases, the partial pressure of oxygen also decreases.
- The decreased partial pressure makes it harder for the oxygen molecules to cross the alveolar membrane and get into the bloodstream.
- These changes can cause hypoxemia and hypoxia.

The percentage of molecules of oxygen in the air does not change with altitude, but the molecules are more spread out, so fewer are inhaled with each breath. If a person is suddenly exposed to low oxygen levels, arterial chemoreceptors stimulate ventilation, making more oxygen available in the alveoli and at the tissue level.

Over the long term, people who live at high altitudes undergo physiological changes that facilitate oxygenation, including an increase in the following:

- **Ventilation,** which brings more oxygen into the lungs
- **Production of red blood cells (RBCs),** which aids in the transport of oxygen to organs and tissues
- **Lung volume and pulmonary vasculature,** which results in increased surface area for alveolar–capillary gas exchange
- **Vascularity of body tissues,** which allows for improved oxygen delivery to the tissues
- **Production of hemoglobin,** which readily binds with oxygen so that the tissue cells can use oxygen even when oxygen pressure is low in the environment

Temperature and Humidity When it is very hot or very cold, the body must expend additional energy to maintain a constant body temperature. The additional energy increases the amount of oxygen the body is using. Breathing hot or cold air can also dry and irritate the airway, causing bronchospasm. This decreases the size of the airway and makes it more difficult to move air in and out of the lungs, causing shortness of breath, especially in those with respiratory conditions such as asthma or chronic obstructive pulmonary disease (COPD). High humidity also contributes to shortness of breath.

Lifestyle

The following lifestyle factors affect oxygenation.

Pregnancy During pregnancy, oxygen demand increases dramatically. Maternal metabolism increases by approximately 15% during the last half of pregnancy, increasing the demand for O_2. At the same time, the enlarging uterus pushes upward against the diaphragm, limiting its downward movement. In response, the maternal respiratory rate increases in order to increase *minute ventilation* (amount of air moved into and out of the lungs in 1 minute) (Hall, 2020).

Occupational Hazards Occupational hazards may affect pulmonary function by irritating airways or causing cancer. Toxic agents may be categorized as follows:

- **Chemicals and their fumes** irritate the sensitive membranous lining of the lungs and airways and may lead to lung cancer or leukemia. Even common household cleaners can emit toxic fumes.
- **Products of combustion** (e.g., carbon monoxide) are known causes of lung cancer and chronic lung disease.
- **Microorganisms,** such as viruses, fungi, and mold, may lead to infections and precipitate asthma.
- **Fine particles** (e.g., coal dust and asbestos) suspended in the air can be inhaled into the smallest airways, causing irritation and toxic reactions, including cancer.

Nutrition The body needs an appropriate balance of proteins, carbohydrates, fats, and other nutrients for proper immune function. A healthy diet builds resistance to disease and infection, promotes normal cellular function and tissue repair, and maintains a healthy weight. Poor nutrition, especially in those with pulmonary disorders, can lead to a loss of ventilatory muscle strength, making breathing more difficult.

Obesity Obesity is defined as a body mass index (BMI) above 30. Obesity increases the risk of multiple health problems, many of which affect pulmonary function. The following are two examples:

- **Respiratory infections.** Excess abdominal fat presses upward on the diaphragm, preventing full chest expansion, leading to hypoventilation and dyspnea on exertion. The risk for respiratory infection then increases because the lower lung lobes are poorly ventilated and secretions are not removed effectively.
- **Sleep apnea.** When the person lies down, chest expansion is limited even more. Excess neck girth and fat deposits in the upper airway often lead to obstructive sleep apnea, a condition characterized by daytime sleepiness, loud snoring, and periods of apnea lasting 10 to 120 seconds (Norris, 2018).

Exercise Exercise increases metabolic demands. The body responds by increasing the heart rate and the rate and depth of breathing. Lack of exercise has the opposite effect. A sedentary lifestyle reduces the capacity to increase ventilation in response to exercise.

Substance Abuse People abuse various kinds of substances, including prescription medications.

- **Prescription medications.** Excess use or overdose of respiratory depressants, such as opioids, sedatives, antianxiety agents, and hypnotics, can cause hypoventilation, apnea, and respiratory failure, in some instances resulting in death.
- **Over-the-counter (OTC) medications** and other legally available products, such as alcohol, tobacco, caffeine, glue, aerosols, "bath salts" (a stimulant and hallucinogenic), and other inhalants, also have abuse potential and can be lethal. Large amounts of alcohol, for example, depress the respiratory and vasomotor centers of the brain.
- **Illicit drugs,** including stimulants (e.g., amphetamines, cocaine), hallucinogens (e.g., LSD, PCP), marijuana, and in some states, "bath salts" also have adverse effects on the respiratory system. And of course, an overdose of these substances can depress respirations and increase the risk for aspiration.

Smoking

Tobacco smoke contains tiny particles of tar and approximately 200 known toxic chemicals, more than 60 of which are known to cause cancer. Tobacco smoke:

- Constricts bronchioles
- Increases fluid secretion into the airways

- Causes inflammation and swelling of the bronchial lining
- Paralyzes cilia

These effects lead to reduced airflow and increased production of secretions that are not easily removed from the airways. Lung inflammation stimulates the release of enzymes that break down elastin and other alveolar wall components. Continued smoking leads to chronic bronchitis, obstruction of bronchioles and alveolar walls, and emphysema. Cigarette smoking is estimated to be the cause of more than 80% of cases of lung cancer. **Key Point:** *The longer a person smokes and the more cigarettes they smoke, the greater the risk for cancer and other chronic lung diseases* (CDC, 2021).

However, once a person stops smoking, the body begins to repair the damage. In the first few days, the person will cough more as the cilia begin to clear the airways. Then the coughing subsides, and breathing becomes easier. Even long-time smokers can benefit from smoking cessation (Box 33-1).

E-cigarettes E-cigarettes, also referred to as *e-cigs, vapes, e-hookahs, vape pens,* or *electronic nicotine delivery systems* (ENDS), contain a liquid that is converted into an aerosol by an e-cigarette product. The liquid is typically a mixture of water, food-grade flavoring, nicotine of varying levels, cannabis (THC, CBD), and propylene glycol (PG) and/or vegetable glycerin (VG). PG and

VG are used to produce aerosols that simulate tobacco cigarette smoke.

E-cigarette aerosol is not harmless. It can contain nicotine, heavy metals (e.g., lead), toxic gases, and cancer-causing agents. Although there are many unknowns about e-cigarettes, including what chemicals make up the vapor and how they affect health over the long term, data suggest a link between e-cigarette use and chronic lung disease and asthma, as well as associations between the combined use of e-cigarettes and traditional cigarettes with cardiovascular disease (Selekman et al., 2019; Orimoloye et al., 2019; Osei et al., 2020).

Secondhand Smoke Also known as **environmental tobacco smoke** (ETS), *secondhand smoke* is a general term for any smoke that nonsmokers are exposed to. There are two types of secondhand smoke:

- **Mainstream smoke** refers to the smoke that a smoker inhales and then exhales.
- **Side-stream smoke** refers to the smoke released from the end of a lit cigarette, cigar, or pipe. Side-stream smoke accounts for 85% of the ETS in a smoky room, so although it is no worse for you than mainstream smoke, it makes up the bulk of smoke that nonsmokers may encounter.

The Environmental Protection Agency (EPA) classifies secondhand smoke as a Group A carcinogen, meaning it is a substance known to cause cancer in humans. There is no safe level of exposure to secondhand smoke. Even short exposure can make blood platelets stickier, causing damage to blood vessel lining and disturbing the heart rate. Secondhand smoke leads to death from cancer and heart disease and has been linked to cerebral vascular accidents (stroke). Children younger than 18 months are especially vulnerable to lower respiratory tract infections related to secondhand smoke (American Lung Association, 2020).

KnowledgeCheck 33-4

- What are the major risks to oxygenation related to developmental factors?
- What environmental and lifestyle factors that influence ventilation can be avoided or minimized?

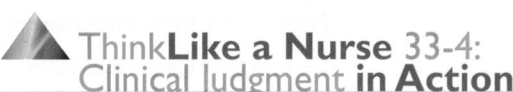

ThinkLike a Nurse 33-4: Clinical Judgment in Action

Review the Meet Your Patients scenario at the beginning of this chapter.

- Which patient(s) may be experiencing developmental, environmental, or lifestyle-related problems with oxygenation?
- Identify any additional information you need to know to answer this question.

Medications

Many drugs can interfere with pulmonary function by depressing respiration. Respiratory depressants generally act by depressing CNS control of breathing or by weakening the muscles of breathing. They include general

---

BOX 33-1 ■ Benefits of Smoking Cessation

- Life expectancy increases.
- Blood pressure and heart rate decrease.
- Circulation to the extremities improves within 2 hours.
- Carbon dioxide levels in the blood begin to drop within 4 hours.
- Oxygen levels in the blood begin to improve within 8 hours.
- Digestion improves.
- Coughing, congestion, and shortness of breath decrease.
- Overall energy increases.
- Lungs increase ability to clean themselves, thereby reducing the risk of infection.
- Risk of heart attack decreases and returns to that of a nonsmoker in 1 year.
- Risk of lung and other cancers, stroke, and chronic obstructive lung disease decreases.

Key Point: Office of Disease Prevention and Health Promotion *(Healthy People 2030, 2020) identified the goal of reducing illness, disability, and death related to tobacco use and secondhand smoke exposure by establishing policies to reduce exposure to secondhand smoke, increase the cost of tobacco, restrict tobacco advertising, and reduce illegal sales to minors.*

anesthetics, opioids (e.g., morphine), antianxiety drugs (e.g., diazepam [Valium]), sedative-hypnotics (e.g., barbiturates), neuromuscular blocking agents, and magnesium sulfate. Drugs that block beta-2 adrenergic receptors (e.g., used to lower blood pressure) have little effect on healthy lungs but can lead to serious bronchiole constriction in people with asthma.

Medications are also used to improve respiratory function. A few examples include bronchodilators, anti-inflammatory agents (e.g., corticosteroids), cough suppressants, expectorants, and decongestants (Table 33-1).

What Pathophysiological Conditions Alter Gas Exchange?

Poor exchange of oxygen and carbon dioxide at the alveolar–capillary membrane or the tissue level alters the levels of O_2 and CO_2 in the blood. Unchecked, it affects oxygenation in tissues and organs and can be life threatening. Box 33-2 describes some alterations in gas exchange.

Alterations in gas exchange are caused by infections, as well as a number of other disorders that affect the structure,

function, and regulation of the pulmonary and cardiovascular systems. Because it is difficult to separate pulmonary and cardiovascular causes and effects, both are included in the following discussion of pulmonary disorders. For a thorough description of these diseases and pathological conditions, consult a medical–surgical nursing text.

KnowledgeCheck 33-5

- What are some indirect indicators of tissue oxygenation?
- How are hyperventilation and hypoventilation related to carbon dioxide levels?
- What are the effects of carbon dioxide levels on the nervous system?

 ThinkLike a Nurse 33-5: Clinical Judgment in Action

You are assessing a very anxious young patient who looks frightened and is complaining of having trouble breathing. The patient's respiratory rate is 32 and deep. The patient states their fingers and hands are numb.

- What is the most likely cause?
- What blood levels would help you clarify what is going on?

Table 33-1 ➤ Respiratory Medications That Promote Ventilation and Oxygenation

CLASS COMMENTS	ACTION	EXAMPLES AND COMMENTS
Bronchodilators	▪ Relax the smooth muscles lining the airways ▪ Can be administered as oral or inhaled medicines	Beta-2 adrenergic agonists Anticholinergics Methylxanthine
Respiratory Anti-Inflammatory Agents	▪ Combat inflammation in the airways ▪ Important in treating and controlling respiratory conditions characterized by hypersensitive airways and airway inflammation (e.g., asthma)	Corticosteroids Cromolyn Leukotriene modifiers
Nasal Decongestants	▪ Relieve stuffy, blocked nasal passages by constricting local blood vessels through stimulation of alpha-1 adrenergic nerve receptors in the vessels ▪ Although the desired effect is on the nasal mucosa, these medications can have systemic adrenergic effects causing elevated blood pressure, tachycardia, and palpitations, especially in those with a history of cardiovascular conditions.	Ephedrine Pseudoephedrine Phenylephrine
Antihistamines	▪ Prevent the effects of histamine release ▪ Used to treat upper respiratory and nasal allergy symptoms	Diphenhydramine Chlorpheniramine Brompheniramine Loratadine Fexofenadine Cetirizine
Cough Preparations	▪ *Antitussives* (cough suppressants) reduce the frequency of an involuntary, hacking, nonproductive cough. ▪ *Expectorants* help make coughing more productive. ▪ The goal is to reduce the frequency of dry, unproductive coughing while making voluntary coughing more productive.	These agents are often found mixed together in one preparation to achieve both desirable effects with one medication.

BOX 33-2 ■ Alterations in Gas Exchange

Hypoxemia—Low Arterial Blood Oxygen Levels

Etiology: Poor oxygen diffusion across the alveolar–capillary membrane into the blood (ineffective external respiration) as a result of lung or pulmonary circulation disorders. Hypoventilation predisposes to the development of hypoxemia and may lead to hypoxia.

Comments: Even if the blood is adequately oxygenated, hypoxia may still occur in the organs and tissues because of poor circulation.

Hypoxia—Inadequate Oxygenation of Organs and Tissues

Etiology: Either hypoxemia or circulatory disorders

Comments: The effects of hypoxia depend on the organs affected. For example:

- Hypoxic central nervous system tissue causes abnormal brain functioning (e.g., altered level of consciousness).
- Hypoxic renal tissue causes abnormal kidney functioning (e.g., poor urine output).
- Hypoxic limb tissue results in abnormal muscle functioning (e.g., muscle weakness and pain with exercise).

Hypercarbia (Hypercapnia)—Excess of Dissolved CO_2 in the Blood

Etiology: Hypoventilation is caused by abnormalities affecting the lungs or chest cavity or by neuromuscular abnormalities that interfere with normal breathing. Hypercarbia can occur suddenly, as in acute airway obstruction or drug overdose, or chronically, as in chronic lung disease.

Comments: Very high blood levels of CO_2 have an anesthetic effect on the nervous system and can lead to somnolence that progresses to coma and death, a syndrome known as *carbon dioxide narcosis.*

Hypocarbia (Hypocapnia)—Low Level of Dissolved CO_2 in the Blood

In most cases (except high altitude), blood O_2 levels remain normal.

Etiology: Hyperventilation

Comments: Severe hypocarbia stimulates the nervous system, leading to muscle twitching or spasm (especially in the hands and feet) and numbness and tingling in the face and lips.

Respiratory Infections

Respiratory infections are any infection of the sinuses, throat, airways, or lungs. Respiratory infections are one of the main reasons why people visit their primary care provider. The common cold is the most widespread. Respiratory infections are usually caused by viruses but can be caused by bacteria.

Example Client Condition: URI and Influenza

URIs are among the most common causes of short-term disability in the United States. Diagnosis is difficult because many other conditions begin with coldlike symptoms (e.g., allergies, measles, and pneumonia). Colds are more common in children and tend to be less frequent in adults. They are rarely dangerous to healthy adults and children. See the Example Client Condition: URI and Influenza.

Infections of the Lower Airways

Lower respiratory tract infections (including acute bronchitis, pneumonia, and tuberculosis) occur more often in children, older adults, and those with impaired immunity or lung function.

Respiratory Syncytial Virus Respiratory syncytial virus (RSV) can affect the upper respiratory tract and the lower airways. Healthy people usually recover from RSV infection in 1 or 2 weeks. However, RSV can be severe in infants, young children, and older adults. Almost all children have had an RSV infection by the age of 2 years (CDC, 2020b). It is spread by airborne droplets and by direct and indirect contact with infected persons, and it can survive on hard surfaces for many hours.

Acute Bronchitis Acute bronchitis is an infection of the bronchi that causes bronchial irritation and inflammation, leading to coughing and mild airway obstruction. The bronchi are inflamed, but the individual shows no evidence of pneumonia, common cold, or asthma. Bronchitis may be viral or bacterial. Symptoms include fever, cough, chills, malaise, and chest wall pain from coughing. In bacterial infections, the cough is productive, with yellow to green sputum. In viral infections, the cough is nonproductive and aggravated by cold, dry, or dusty air and may cause prolonged bouts of continuous coughing.

Tuberculosis Tuberculosis (TB) is an infection caused by the acid-fast bacillus *Mycobacterium tuberculosis.* Although TB is commonly thought of as a respiratory disease, infection may occur anywhere in the body. Historically, TB was a major cause of death and disability in North America. TB was almost eradicated after 1950 because of the use of effective antibiotics. However, the incidence is rising again because of (1) the growing number of drug-resistant strains and (2) the number of people with compromised immune responses (related to aging and disease).

- **Transmission and infection.** Pulmonary TB is transmitted via airborne droplets, which may occur in overcrowded, poorly ventilated living conditions. Once inhaled into the lungs, the TB bacteria are usually walled off through the inflammatory response into granulomatous lesions. Immunity develops, and the bacteria either can remain walled off and dormant

EXAMPLE CLIENT CONDITION: URIs and Influenza

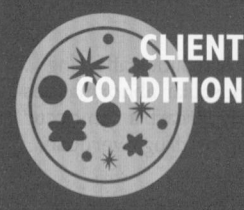

Definitions: Upper Airway Infections (URIs).

Most URIs are caused by viruses and are rarely dangerous to healthy adults and children. The following are some URIs:

- **The common cold**—nonspecific upper respiratory infections caused by viruses.
- **Rhinosinusitis**—inflammation of the nasal mucosa and sinus cavities. Differentiating viral from bacterial sinusitis cannot be done on the basis of clinical findings alone.
- **Pharyngitis**—sore throat. May be viral or bacterial. "Strep" throat, caused by *Streptococcus pyogenes*, is the most common cause of infectious pharyngitis. It cannot be differentiated from a viral sore throat by any one sign or symptom, so pharyngeal cultures or rapid antigen tests are conducted.

Definition: Influenza

- Influenza is a respiratory infection that is usually more severe than the common cold and often involves the airways (nose, throat, and lungs).
- Influenza can cause serious complications. Most influenza fatalities occur in children under age 2 and older adults, especially the frail elderly.

Transmission: URI and Influenza

Key Point: *The flu virus is highly contagious.* Most respiratory and flu viruses are passed from person to person by contact with respiratory droplets. Contact can occur by:
- Direct bodily contact; such as kissing
- Touching something with virus on it: such as shaking hands with someone who is ill and then touching your mouth, nose, or eyes
- Respiratory droplets from a person coughing or sneezing can be propelled into eyes, nose, or mouth over distances of about 3–6 feet.

Flu virus may be able to infect others beginning 1 day before symptoms occur and up to 1 week after symptoms begin. Children can be infectious for up to several weeks.

Pathophysiology

URI:
- Direct invasion of the mucosa and mucous membranes of the upper airway (nasal cavity, sinus, throat) by a virus or bacteria
- Pathogens have varying ability to overcome the body's defense system and cause infections.
- Organisms show variation in time of onset from when they enter the body to when symptoms occur (incubation time).

Influenza:
- When the influenza virus enters the body, it moves into the respiratory tract.
- The respiratory tissues become inflamed, and as the viral cells replicate, they move into the bloodstream, and the first symptoms appear.
- The replication process continues for up to several days, until the body's immune system begins to fight the virus off.

Symptoms

- **URIs**—Coldlike symptoms: stuffy nose, sore throat, cough, sneezing, tearing, and a mild fever
- **Influenza**—In addition to coldlike symptoms, the person with influenza may experience headache, muscle pain, fatigue, weakness, exhaustion, and high fever. Some individuals may also have gastrointestinal symptoms such as vomiting and diarrhea.

Complications

URIs
- Respiratory compromise
- Secondary infection by bacteria (bronchitis, pneumonia)
- Involvement of the ears, resulting in middle ear infections (otitis media)
- Worsening of underlying chronic lung disease (asthma, chronic obstructive pulmonary disease)
- Spread of infection to the heart (pericarditis, myocarditis)
- Muscular pain and rib fractures from forceful coughing

Flu
- Viral or bacterial pneumonia
- Dehydration
- Ear infections or sinus infections, especially in children
- Worsening of underlying chronic medical conditions (congestive heart failure, asthma, or diabetes)
- Increased risk of myocardial ischemia
- Inflammation of the heart (myocarditis) or of the sac around the heart (pericarditis)

EXAMPLE CLIENT CONDITION: URIs and Influenza—cont'd

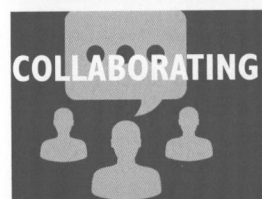

COLLABORATING

Prevention of Influenza

Key Point: *Prevention is key. The most effective strategy for preventing influenza is annual vaccination.*

The Centers for Disease Control and Prevention (2022c) continues to recommend universal vaccination—that is, that all people aged 6 months and older receive annual influenza vaccination.

 Although less effective in preventing the disease in older adults, immunization decreases the severity of the disease, the development of secondary complications, and the incidence of death (Izurieta et al., 2020).

Treatment

Collect swabs for cultures as needed to identify whether the infection is viral or bacterial. This guides treatment.

Prescription Medications (Influenza)
Key Point: *To be effective, antiviral medications must be started within the first 48 hours after symptoms emerge.*
Examples of antivirals:
- Baloxavir marboxil (Xofluza) and oseltamivir (Tamiflu) are oral medications.
- Zanamivir (Relenza) is an inhaled medication.
- Peramivir (Rapivab) is an intravenous medication.

Over-the-Counter Medications (Influenza and URI):
- Fever reducers
- Antihistamines
- Decongestants
- Cough medicines
- Acetaminophen, ibuprofen, or naproxen sodium (for body aches)

Key Point: *Do not give aspirin to anyone under 19 years old. It is linked with Reye's syndrome.*

Alternative Therapy: (Influenza)
Oscillococcinum has been shown to shorten the flu duration and ease your symptoms, but there is no evidence that it prevents the flu.

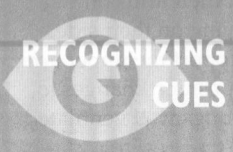

RECOGNIZING CUES

Interview/History

- Assess/recognize cues for risk factors (e.g., contact with an infected person within the past 72 hours).
- Ask about immunization for influenza.
- Assess/recognize cues for history of fever and chills, hoarseness, laryngitis, sore throat, rhinitis, or rhinorrhea.
- Assess for fatigue and malaise.

Physical Examination

- Inspect the patient's throat for redness of the soft palate, tonsils, and pharynx.
- Palpate for enlargement of the anterior cervical lymph nodes.

- Assess/recognize cues for an increase in patient temperature.
- Assess/recognize cues for respiratory rate, which may be increased.
- Assess/recognize cues for skin turgor.
- Monitor fluid intake.
- Auscultate the patient's lungs.

For a focused assessment of oxygenation,

 Go to **Chapter 33, Assessment Guidelines and Tools, Focused Assessment box, Oxygenation,** in Volume 2.

To assess respirations,

 Go to **Chapter 19, Procedure 19-5: Assessing Respirations,** in Volume 2.

(continued)

EXAMPLE CLIENT CONDITION: URIs and Influenza—cont'd

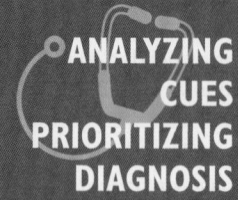

ANALYZING CUES PRIORITIZING DIAGNOSIS

Key Point: *URIs and influenza begin with similar symptoms. It is important to distinguish between them because (1) antiviral medications are available for the flu, but they are not effective for colds, and (2) flu can have serious complications.*

Diagnoses and Collaborative Problems

- Ineffective Airway Clearance related to tracheobronchial and nasal secretions
- Potential Complication of Influenza: Pneumonia

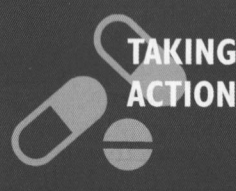

GENERATING SOLUTIONS

NOC Outcomes

- Discomfort Level
- Respiratory Status: Airway Patency
- Rest
- Vital Signs

Individualized Goals

Patient will be free of infection as demonstrated by:

- Breath sounds clear to auscultation
- Abating cough
- Respiratory status parameters with optimal air exchange
- Temperature: 99°F (37°C)
- Improved energy level

TAKING ACTION

Colds

Note: Refer to Collaborating and Teaching categories for more interventions.

Interventions are focused on easing symptoms:

- Provide plenty of fluids.
- Encourage extra rest.
- To ease nasal congestion, suggest saline nasal sprays.
- Suggest staying away from tobacco smoke.
- Provide medications to relieve symptoms (antipyretics, antihistamines, analgesics). See earlier Collaborating section.
- Encourage absence from school or work until fever-free for 24 hours.
- To help prevent the common cold, assess and monitor for healthy behaviors, such as balanced diet, adequate rest, and daily exercise.

For additional interventions, see the Teaching category in the following row.

Influenza

- Encourage fluid intake, up to 3–4 L/day unless contraindicated.
- Encourage deep-breathing exercises and coughing exercises.
- Ambulate as often as possible without creating fatigue.
- Encourage rest.

Position for Maximal Lung Expansion and Comfort

- Patients with impaired respiratory function adopt a tripod position to allow maximum expansion. Provide an overbed table to lean forward and rest their arms on.
- When the patient is lying on their side, provide pillows to support the upper arm.
- Assist with frequent position changes to keep all areas of the lungs well ventilated.

Ongoing Monitoring for Evaluation

- Assess respiratory status for rate, depth, ease, use of accessory muscles, and work of breathing.
- Auscultate the lung fields for the presence of wheezes, crackles (rales), rhonchi, or decreased breath sounds.
- Monitor patient for cough and production of sputum, noting amount, color, character, and patient's ability to expectorate secretions and ability to cough.

Monitor for Complications

- Increased or prolonged fever
- Change in cough or sputum production
- Change in mental status

EXAMPLE CLIENT CONDITION: URIs and Influenza—cont'd

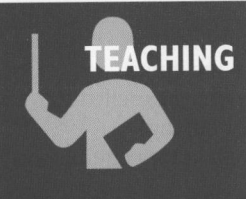
TEACHING

Teach patients and family that:
- There is no cure for the common cold.
- Healthy behaviors (e.g., balanced diet, adequate rest, and daily exercise) increase resistance to pathogens.

Ways to Avoid Infection and Spread of Colds and Flu

- Avoid others who are sick.
- Avoid close contact with others, such as hugging, kissing, or shaking hands.
- Move away from people before coughing or sneezing.
- Cough and sneeze into a tissue and then throw it away, or cough and sneeze into your upper shirt sleeve, completely covering your mouth and nose.
- Wash your hands after coughing, sneezing, or blowing your nose.
- Disinfect frequently touched surfaces and objects such as toys and doorknobs.

Taking Medications

Teaching should include:
- Take prescription medications as prescribed.
- ✚ Antibiotics should be used only as prescribed for diagnosed bacterial infections.
- Antibiotics are not without risks, and they are not effective for treating influenza or the common cold.
- Take the full course of prescribed antibiotics, even if symptoms are no longer present.
- Do not pressure clinicians for prescriptions.
- Do not take antibiotics from previous prescriptions.

EVALUATING OUTCOMES

- Monitor for improved respiratory status.
- Monitor body temperature.

- Monitor for complications (e.g., dehydration, pneumonia).

---

or can escape and cause active tuberculosis, especially in someone with impaired immunity.

- **Symptoms.** Common signs and symptoms include fatigue, weight loss, anorexia, night sweats, and blood-tinged sputum.
- **Diagnosis.** TB diagnosis is made via sputum cultures or chest x-ray changes.
- **Collaborative treatment.** Medications are the cornerstone of tuberculosis treatment. Treating TB takes much longer than treating other types of bacterial infections; antibiotics must be taken for at least 6 to 9 months. The exact drugs and length of treatment depend on age, overall health, possible drug resistance, the form of TB (latent or active), and the infection's location in the body.

Example Client Condition: Pneumonia Pneumonia is an infection of the lungs caused by bacteria, fungi, viruses, or rarely, parasites. It occurs more often during winter months and often follows a recent upper respiratory tract infection or influenza. For more information, refer to the Example Client Condition: Pneumonia.

Other Disorders Affecting Gas Exchange

In addition to respiratory infections, gas exchange may be altered by disorders in the pulmonary system, the pulmonary circulation, the CNS, and the neuromuscular system.

Pulmonary System Abnormalities

The following is a brief discussion of various pulmonary abnormalities that can lead to alterations in gas exchange.

Structural Abnormalities Structural abnormalities include anything that restricts or limits the free movement of the chest wall (e.g., fractured ribs, kyphosis), interruptions in the chest cavity that inhibit inflation of the lungs (e.g., pneumothorax), or a collection of fluid (blood, lymph, pus) in the pleural space that inhibits lung expansion.

Airway Inflammation and Obstruction Allergic reactions (e.g., asthma) or irritation from smoke or other irritants may cause airway inflammation. Obstruction may be mechanical, as with a foreign object or bolus of food, or due to spasm (e.g., laryngospasm). Swollen tonsils and a swollen epiglottis may also cause obstruction.

Alveolar–Capillary Membrane Disorders These disorders are characterized by a change in the consistency of the lung tissue, especially at the alveolar level. The alveoli become stiff and difficult to ventilate, and gas exchange is impaired. Pulmonary edema, acute respiratory distress syndrome (ARDS), and pulmonary fibrosis are examples.

Atelectasis Anything that reduces ventilation (e.g., tumor, obstructed airway) can cause **atelectasis,** or alveolar collapse.

EXAMPLE CLIENT CONDITION: Pneumonia

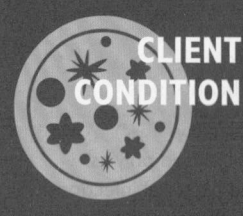
CLIENT CONDITION

Key Point: *Pneumonia is a leading cause of infectious death in the United States.*
Key Point: *Pneumonia has a mortality rate of about 50% in people older than age 65.*

Basic Definitions

Pneumonia
Infection of the lungs caused by bacteria, fungi, or viruses

Healthcare-Associated Pneumonia (HCaP)
Lung infection in nonhospitalized patients who had recent contact with the healthcare system, such as residence in a long-term care facility or outpatient treatment in a hospital or hemodialysis clinic.

Ventilator-Associated Pneumonia (VAP)
Lung infection that develops 48 hours or longer after mechanical ventilation is given by means of an endotracheal tube or tracheostomy through the ventilator tube. Mortality rates are high.

Characteristics/Symptoms of Pneumonia

Cough, malaise, pleural pain from coughing, discolored sputum, fever, chills, dyspnea, elevated white blood cell (WBC) counts

Transmission

Organisms gain entry to the lungs:
- Through the air (after being expelled by coughing, sneezing, or talking)
- From contaminated respiratory equipment, as in VAP
- From spreading to the lung via the blood, or from the nose and throat, as in HCaP

Pathophysiology

Pneumonia
Full-scale inflammatory response triggers edema in the small airways and deposits debris and exudate in the alveoli. The affected area of the lung becomes **consolidated** (solid rather than air filled).

Ventilator-Associated Pneumonia
In VAP, the endotracheal or tracheostomy tube allows passage of bacteria into the lower segments of the lung in a person who is at high risk for infection. Invasion by bacteria initiates the full-scale inflammatory response, leading to lung consolidation.

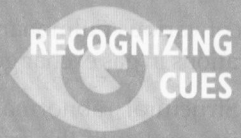
RECOGNIZING CUES

History

- Obtain history of: Immunization, fever and chills, cough, pleural pain, discolored sputum, dyspnea, shortness of breath, malaise

Examination

- Auscultate the lungs.
- Observe sputum for color, consistency, and amount.
- Observe for and describe any cough.
- Obtain the temperature (may be elevated).
- Observe for increased respiratory rate and difficulty breathing.

Diagnostic Tests

- Blood tests
- Chest x-ray
- Sputum culture
- Pulse oximetry

For a focused assessment of oxygenation,

 Go to **Chapter 33, Assessment Guidelines and Tools, Focused Assessment box, Oxygenation,** in Volume 2.

To assess respirations,

 Go to **Chapter 19, Procedure 19-5: Assessing Respirations,** in Volume 2.

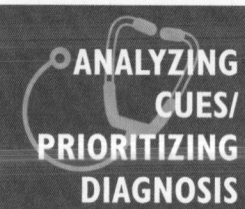
ANALYZING CUES/ PRIORITIZING DIAGNOSIS

- Ineffective Breathing Pattern
- Activity Intolerance

Gas Exchange Impairment (Clinical Care Classification [CCC], n.d.)

EXAMPLE CLIENT CONDITION: Pneumonia—cont'd

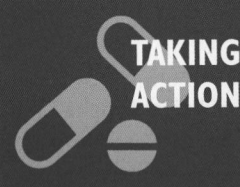

GENERATING SOLUTIONS

NOC Standardized Outcomes

Activity Tolerance
Respiratory Status: Gas Exchange
Respiratory Status: Ventilation
Vital Signs

Individualized Outcomes

- Demonstrates adequate oxygenation (activity tolerance, O₂ saturation, mucous membrane color).
- Respiratory rate and depth at baseline
- Temperature: 99°F (37°C)
- Lungs clear to auscultation

TAKING ACTION

Therapeutic Measures

- Humidity, to moisten inhaled air
- Hydration, to thin secretions
- Rest, to conserve body energy stores
- Perform deep-breathing and coughing exercises. For information about teaching patients to deep-breathe,

 Go to **Chapter 33, Procedure 33-1A: Collecting an Expectorated Sputum Specimen,** in Volume 2.

- Position patient for ease of breathing.
- Patients with impaired respiratory function adopt a tripod position to allow maximum expansion. Provide an overbed table to lean forward and rest their arms on.
- When the patient is lying on their side, provide pillows to support the upper arm.
- Assist with frequent position changes to keep all areas of the lungs well ventilated.
- Ambulate as often as possible without creating fatigue.
- Perform pulmonary hygiene (deep breathing, coughing, and chest percussion and vibration) to move secretions out of the airways. See Figure 33-8.

Prevention Recommendations

Immunization for high-risk groups, including the following (Centers for Disease Control and Prevention [CDC], 2022c):
- Adults aged 65 years or older
- Children younger than age 5 years
- Children aged 6 through 18 years who have certain medical conditions
- People aged 2 through 64 years who have chronic illnesses (e.g., those with heart disease, diabetes, pulmonary disease, alcoholism, HIV infection) or lowered resistance to infection
- Adults aged 19 through 64 years who have asthma or are smokers

Preventing HCaP

Guidelines for preventing healthcare-associated pneumonia include following standard precautions for hand hygiene and gloving.

- Wear gloves when handling respiratory secretions or objects contaminated with respiratory secretions of all patients.
- Change gloves and decontaminate hands:
  - Between contacts with different patients
  - After handling respiratory secretions or contaminated objects and before contact with another patient, object, or environmental surface
  - Between contacts with a contaminated body site and the respiratory tract or respiratory device on the same patient (Andersen, 2019)

Preventing VAP

- Minimize a patient's exposure to and duration of mechanical ventilation.
- Provide routine oral care with chlorhexidine.
- Prevent aspiration of oral secretions with routine oral suctioning.
- Maintain positioning (head of bed at 30–45 degrees) and encourage early ambulation.

For more information about preventing VAP,

Go to **Chapter 33, Procedure 33-10: Caring for Patients Requiring Mechanical Ventilation,** in Volume 2.

Also, see Toward Evidence-Based Practice box.

(continued)

EXAMPLE CLIENT CONDITION: Pneumonia—cont'd

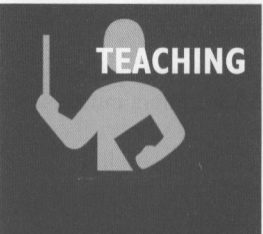

TEACHING

Teaching:

- Eat well-balanced meals.
- Get adequate rest.
- Exercise.
- Avoid smoking.
- Avoid others with upper respiratory infections.
- Get prompt treatment for early symptoms.

- Drink large amounts of fluids to thin secretions and replace fluid loss.
- Avoid spread of infections by washing hands and properly disposing of tissues.
- Wash hands frequently.

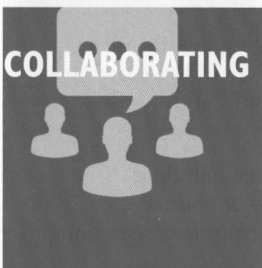

COLLABORATING

As needed and prescribed:
- Antipyretics, for fever
- Expectorants, to enhance mobilization of secretions
- Curative therapy includes appropriate anti-infective agents
- Chest physiotherapy (postural drainage, chest percussion, and chest vibration). See the section Perform Chest Physiotherapy. for more in-depth information.
- Also,

- Oxygen therapy

 Go to **Chapter 33, Clinical Insight 33-3: Oxygen Therapy Safety Precautions,** in Volume 2. Also see, **Administering Respiratory Inhalations** in Chapter 23, and see **Figures 23-11** and **23-12.**

 Go to, **Chapter 33, Procedure 33-3: Performing Percussion, Vibration, and Postural Drainage,** in Volume 2.

Pulmonary Circulation Abnormalities

For gas exchange to occur in the alveoli, there must be adequate blood flow through the pulmonary circulation. The most common causes of impaired pulmonary circulation are pulmonary embolus and pulmonary hypertension.

- A **pulmonary embolus** is an obstruction of pulmonary arterial circulation by a foreign substance (e.g., a blood clot, air, or fat).
- **Pulmonary hypertension** is elevated pressure within the pulmonary arterial system. High pressure increases the workload of the heart. Over time, this causes right-sided heart failure, with a reduced amount of blood pumped into the pulmonary circulation. You will learn about the difference between right-sided and left-sided heart failure in a medical–surgical nursing course.

Central Nervous System Abnormalities

Any condition that injures or alters the function of the CNS can interfere with the regulation of breathing and, therefore, gas exchange.

- **Trauma and stroke** (cerebrovascular accident) are the most commonly seen CNS problems in adults.
- **Spinal cord injuries** interfere with nerve transmission between the brain and the area below the level

of the injury and may, for example, limit diaphragm function.
- **Immature breathing patterns,** such as apnea or periodic breathing, are common in preterm and full-term infants.

Neuromuscular Abnormalities

As the name implies, neuromuscular abnormalities can involve both the muscles and the nerves involved in breathing.

- Neuromuscular abnormalities can affect gas exchange by limiting movement of the muscles involved with breathing. Trauma, stroke, and medications are the most common causes.
- Neuromuscular disorders that affect the nerves involved in breathing interfere with the regulation of breathing, leading to depressed respiratory function (e.g., Guillain-Barré syndrome, amyotrophic lateral sclerosis, and myasthenia gravis).

KnowledgeCheck 33-6

- Identify four pathophysiological conditions that affect pulmonary function. How are they similar? How are they different?
- What types of injuries are most likely to cause oxygenation problems?

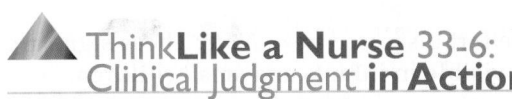

ThinkLike a Nurse 33-6: Clinical Judgment in Action

You are the nursing supervisor on the night shift in a small community hospital. At the beginning of the shift, you have only one critical care bed available. During your shift, you receive calls for assistance on the following patients:

- Patient A has burns on the face, scalp, and chest and is coughing up sputum with black streaks.
- Patient B has pneumonia but has suddenly become confused.
- Patient C is short of breath and complaining that they can't breathe. Their skin is cool and moist, and they are coughing up clear sputum with small bubbles in it.

Which patient would you admit to the critical care bed? Why?

PracticalKnowledge
knowing how

In the remainder of the chapter, we discuss focused respiratory assessment/recognizing cues and the nursing activities to maximize ventilation and gas exchange. In Chapter 19, the section Respiration provides more information about assessing respirations. Also,

 Go to **Chapter 19, Procedure 19-5: Assessing Respirations,** in Volume 2.

ASSESSMENT/RECOGNIZING CUES

An evaluation of overall oxygenation includes a history and physical examination to assess lung, heart, and circulatory function. **Key Point:** *The order of data collection and the priorities of assessment vary with the patient's condition and the purpose of the assessment.* For example:

- **For someone in obvious respiratory distress,** the immediate assessment/recognizing cues focus is to

---

♥ iCare 33-1

Oxygenation

Experiencing **inadequate oxygenation** is very frightening. Anxiety, fear, and panic can set in very quickly.
- Use a calm and confident approach when performing interventions to promote optimal respiratory function.
- Provide emotional support and comfort during episodes of deoxygenation to help alleviate fear.
- Sit down and make eye contact. Speak calmly and keep the patient informed of what you are doing—for example, "Mr. Brown, I realize you are having trouble breathing right now, but you have had a nebulizer treatment. I am here with you. Let's take some deep breaths together and relax. I will recheck your respiratory status and oxygenation level in a few minutes."
- Hold the person's hand, practice therapeutic touch, and sit with the person while providing interventions.

---

ask simple questions about current symptoms while performing a quick examination to determine the adequacy of breathing, circulation, and oxygenation.
- **For a healthy person,** assessment/recognizing cues for risk of respiratory disease might include more extensive questions about occupation, smoking habits, and living environment; a medical history; and an extensive physical examination.
- **For a complete focused respiratory assessment/recognizing cues,** you will need to identify risk factors, perform a physical examination, and be familiar with certain diagnostic tests.

Assessing/Recognizing Cues for Risk Factors

The health history should include questions about the presence of risk factors that affect lung and airway function. Topics to assess include demographic data, health history, respiratory history, cardiovascular history, environmental history, and lifestyle. For a detailed list of interview questions for each of these topics,

 Go to **Chapter 33, Assessment Guidelines and Tools, Focused Assessment: Oxygenation,** in Volume 2.

Key Point: *All patients, not just those with oxygenation problems, should be asked whether they use tobacco and should have their tobacco-use status documented regularly.*

Physical Examination

You will use all four examination techniques to assess respiratory function:

- **Inspect** to observe respiratory patterns, signs of respiratory distress, chest structures and movement, skin and mucous membrane color, presence or absence of edema, sputum characteristics, and overall general appearance. Refer to Chapter 19 to review the details of inspecting the skin and mucous membranes.

 Go to **Chapter 19, Procedure 19-2: Assessing the Skin,** in Volume 2.

- **Palpate** pulses, skin temperature, heart pulsations through the chest wall, and areas of tenderness.
- **Percuss** over the lung fields to screen for areas of consolidation or excess air pockets in the lungs.
- **Auscultate** breath sounds, heart sounds, and vascular sounds. For a step-by-step discussion of how to assess the chest and lungs,

 Go to **Chapter 19, Procedure 19-12: Assessing the Chest and Lungs,** in Volume 2.

- You may also need to use pulse oximetry and capnography to monitor oxygenation and ventilation.

Assessing/Recognizing Cues for Pain

Recall that pain alters the rate and depth of respirations. Patients in pain often breathe shallowly and are at risk for atelectasis.

- Regularly assess all patients for pain.
- Once you have medicated the patient, reassess breath sounds and encourage the patient to breathe deeply and cough.

Assessing/Recognizing Cues for Breathing Patterns

Assess for normal and altered breathing patterns. Most irregular breathing patterns result from brain injury or the effects of drugs on the brain. Irregular patterns are described in the following list; they are illustrated in Table 18-5.

- **Eupnea**—Normal breathing; rate about 12 to 20 breaths/min
- **Tachypnea**—Fast, shallow breathing; more than 24 breaths/min. Generally caused by hypoxemia or increased oxygen demand (e.g., exercise). Rapid, shallow respirations draw limited air into the alveoli and may result in hypoventilation.
- **Bradypnea**—Slow respirations; fewer than 10 breaths/min. Bradypnea may cause poor gas exchange. Causes include sedative and opioid medications and neuromuscular dysfunction.
- **Kussmaul's respirations**—Regular respirations but increased in rate and abnormally deep. These may be a compensatory mechanism for metabolic disorders that lower blood pH, as well as a form of hyperventilation caused by fear, anxiety, or panic.
- **Biot's respirations**—Irregular respirations of variable depth (usually shallow), alternating with periods of apnea. This pattern is often associated with damage to the medullary respiratory center or high intracranial pressure as a result of brain injury.
- **Cheyne-Stokes respirations**—Gradual increase in depth of respirations, followed by a gradual decrease in depth, then a period of apnea. This pattern often results from damage to the medullary respiratory center or high intracranial pressure (e.g., resulting from brain injury).
- **Apnea**—Absence of breathing. Respiratory arrest requires immediate cardiopulmonary resuscitation.

Assessing/Recognizing Cues for Respiratory Effort/Dyspnea

A patient experiencing shortness of breath or dyspnea requires a thorough assessment. However, you must take care not to increase the respiratory effort. Use closed questions that the patient can answer with *yes*, *no*, or only a few words. Ask whether the shortness of breath began suddenly or gradually, how severe it is right now, and whether it is getting better or worse. At the same time, observe for cues of the signs of increased respiratory effort discussed next. *Note:* **These signs are most easily visible in infants and small children.**

- **Nasal flaring**—The visible enlargement of the nostrils with inhalation. It helps reduce resistance to airflow in the nose and keep the nasal passages open to take in more air.
- **Retractions**—The visible "pulling in" of intercostal, supraclavicular, and subcostal tissue, caused by excessive negative pressures generated in the chest, to try to increase the depth of inhalation.
- **Use of accessory muscles** during inspiration—The patient may use the intercostals, abdominal muscles, and muscles of the neck and shoulders when there is an increased demand for oxygen or problems with ventilation.
- **Grunting**—Noisy, difficult breathing. It is caused by forced expiration against a closed glottis and by involuntary muscle contraction during expiration to help keep alveoli open and enhance gas exchange.
- **Body positioning** to facilitate respirations—The patient usually finds an upright posture the most comfortable. In the upright position, gravity pulls the abdominal organs down and allows the diaphragm more room to contract. Most patients with dyspnea cannot tolerate lying down. **Orthopnea** is the term for describing difficulty breathing (shortness of breath) when lying down. Ask how the patient usually sleeps. Some patients may report sleeping in a recliner or chair.
- **Paroxysmal nocturnal dyspnea**—Sudden awakening due to shortness of breath that begins during sleep. The patient feels panic and extreme dyspnea and must sit upright to ease breathing.
- **Conversational dyspnea**—The inability to speak complete sentences without stopping to breathe. The more frequently the patient pauses when speaking, the more severe the dyspnea.
- **Stridor**—A high-pitched, harsh, crowing, inspiratory sound caused by partial obstruction of the larynx or trachea. You can hear it without a stethoscope. ✚ Partial airway obstruction can easily become complete airway obstruction. Therefore, the patient with stridor needs immediate care.
- **Wheezing**—A musical sound produced by air passing through partially obstructed small airways. It is often heard in patients with asthma and lung congestion.
- ✚ **Diminished or absent breath sounds**—In a patient experiencing dyspnea, these are signs of worsening ventilation and oxygenation. Oxygen therapy and measures to restore adequate ventilation may be required.

Assessing/Recognizing Cues for Cough

Everyone coughs from time to time to remove small amounts of mucus and debris from the airways. Coughing is a normal protective response to known respiratory irritants (e.g., cigarette smoke, irritating fumes, dust particles) or when food or fluid accidentally gets into the airways. If a cough persists, is recurring, or is productive, it may indicate ongoing or recurring airway irritation. **Key Point:** *Advise patients to obtain medical evaluation for a cough that lasts more than 3 weeks and cannot be explained.*

Assess/Recognize Cues for the Type of Cough

- Is it dry, productive, or hacking? A cough is described as productive if it raises sputum (mucous and debris) up from the airway.
- When does the cough occur, and how long has the patient been coughing?
- What makes it worse? What seems to help it?
- What has been used to treat the cough, and what were the effects?

Assess/Recognize Cues for Other Clinical Findings Associated With a Cough
This helps determine its cause.

- **Allergies.** A cough associated with nasal congestion, sneezing, watery eyes, or nose discharge is most likely due to allergies and may be successfully treated with OTC remedies.
- **URI.** A cough occurring with fever, chest congestion, noisy breath sounds, and sputum production is more likely to be due to a URI, which may require antibiotics.
- **Airway obstruction/constriction.** A cough associated with dyspnea, chest tightness, and wheezing may be due to an airway obstruction disorder, such as asthma, which requires corticosteroids and bronchodilating medications.

Assess/Recognize Cues for the Sputum
Observe sputum appearance, odor, amount, and timing.

- **Sputum appearance and odor** provide valuable *cues* about the cause and significance of a cough (Box 33-3).
- **Sputum amount** can vary from a teaspoon to pints. In general, sputum production increases with the severity of the underlying condition. However, limited sputum production does not always indicate

that the problem is minor because excess mucus and debris may be trapped in the airways and the patient is unable to cough it up and out of the body.

- **Sputum timing.** Sputum production ranges from constant to once per day. Tobacco smokers often have a "morning cough," which helps clear their airways of mucus and debris accumulated overnight. In contrast, someone with a URI is more likely to produce sputum throughout the day.

KnowledgeCheck 33-7

- What areas should you include in a nursing history for a patient with oxygenation concerns who is undergoing a comprehensive assessment?
- When is a cough significant? What aspects of a cough should be assessed?
- Identify at least five cues that you may observe in a patient experiencing dyspnea.
- A patient has a respiratory rate of 30 breaths/min that is rhythmic and moderate in depth. What term would you use to describe this breathing pattern?

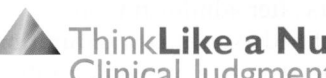

ThinkLike a Nurse 33-7: Clinical Judgment in Action

Review the patients presented in the Meet Your Patients scenario.

- Which patients are experiencing respiratory distress? Identify the cues of distress in these patients.
- Which patients require a comprehensive assessment, and which patients will need a rapid assessment and immediate treatment because of the severity of their symptoms?

Diagnostic Testing

Diagnostic testing helps clinicians identify the causes of impaired oxygenation and monitor patient responses to treatment. You will need to assist with and be familiar with the results of the tests of respiratory function. We discuss several of these tests in the next sections. For others,

 Go to **Chapter 33, Diagnostic Testing: Tests Related to Oxygenation,** in Volume 2.

BOX 33-3 ■ Significance of Sputum Appearance and Odor

Color/Appearance	Significance
White or clear	Usually present in viral infections (e.g., common cold, viral bronchitis), often requiring only supportive care
Yellow or green	A sign of bacterial infection
Black	Caused by coal dust, smoke, or soot inhalation
Rust-colored	Associated with pneumococcal pneumonia, tuberculosis, and possibly the presence of blood
Hemoptysis	The coughing up of blood or bloody sputum. It may range from small streaks of blood to large amounts of frank blood.
Pink and frothy	Associated with pulmonary edema
Foul-smelling sputum	Usually indicates bacterial infection (e.g., pneumonia, lung abscess).

Obtaining Sputum Samples

You may need to collect sputum samples. Sputum is examined microscopically and cultured in the laboratory to identify organisms and test for sensitivity to different anti-infective agents. For a summary of this procedure, see the Highlights of Procedures box. For the complete steps,

 Go to **Chapter 33, Procedure 33-1: Collecting a Sputum Specimen,** in Volume 2.

Skin Testing

- **Tuberculin skin testing** is widely used to detect exposure and antibody formation to the tubercle bacillus.
- **Annual screening** is recommended for low-income populations, residents in congregate living conditions (e.g., dormitories, correctional facilities), immigrants from countries with a high prevalence of TB, and healthcare workers.
- **For the skin test to be effective,** you must administer the antigen intradermally, not subcutaneously. Read the test site 48 to 72 hours after administration.
- **A positive skin test** is defined as an area of **induration** (hardness) at the test site. The size of the induration that indicates a positive result depends on risk factors. Patients with positive TB skin tests must undergo further testing (chest x-ray study and sputum cultures) to determine whether they have merely been exposed to disease or whether they have active disease.
- For guidelines for interpreting test results,

 Go to **Chapter 33, Diagnostic Testing: Reading a Tuberculin Skin Result,** in Volume 2.

- **Allergy testing** uses skin testing to identify antigens that may cause hypersensitivity reactions in susceptible individuals. Testing is performed by scratching antigen samples onto the skin. The area is then observed for allergic skin reactions. Skin testing is performed in facilities with resuscitation equipment and personnel trained in its use because life-threatening airway obstruction sometimes occurs in response to the allergens.

Pulse Oximetry

Pulse oximetry is a noninvasive estimate of arterial blood oxygen saturation (SaO_2). **SaO_2** reflects the percentage of hemoglobin molecules carrying oxygen. The normal value is 95% to 100%. Values below 94% are considered abnormal in healthy people and should be investigated to determine the cause.

Well-oxygenated hemoglobin and deoxygenated hemoglobin absorb light differently. Using a light-emitting diode (LED), the oximeter is able to detect this difference and calculate the percentage of oxygenated hemoglobin.

Pulse oximetry is simple to perform, provides a rapid reading, and can be used intermittently or continuously. The frequency of measurement depends on the clinical condition of the patient. Recent recommendations are that pulse oximetry can be used to screen newborns for critical congenital heart disease (Barreto, 2019; Ewer et al., 2019; Oster et al., 2019).

For a summary of the steps, see the Highlights of Procedures box. For the complete procedure,

 Go to **Chapter 33, Procedure 33-2: Monitoring Pulse Oximetry (Arterial Oxygen Saturation); and Clinical Insight 33-1: Tips for Obtaining Accurate Pulse Oximetry Readings,** in Volume 2.

Capnography

Capnography measures the carbon dioxide (CO_2) in inhaled and exhaled air. Capnography directly measures ventilation and indirectly measures the partial pressure of CO_2 in the arterial blood. Normally, the difference between arterial blood and expired CO_2 is very small.

- One method is to use a device that displays the results digitally and prints out a graph showing CO_2 at various times in the breathing cycle. As a beam of infrared light passes through a sample of respiratory gases, more or less of it is absorbed depending on the amount of CO_2 present.
- A second method is a **nasobuccal sensor** (Fig. 33-5) designed to collect expiratory gas immediately at the airway opening, both at the nose and mouth. To perform the measurement, a sample of gas is transmitted from the patient to the monitor (Fig. 33-6). For each respiratory cycle, the capnogram is displayed on the monitor.

Capnography is often used with pulse oximetry because:

- Capnography provides information about ventilation because it shows accumulation or depletion of CO_2,

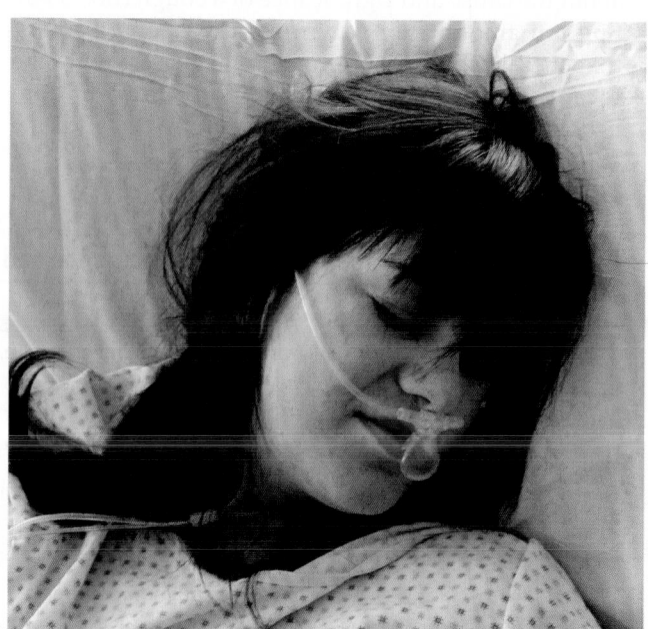

FIGURE 33-5 Nasobuccal sensor.

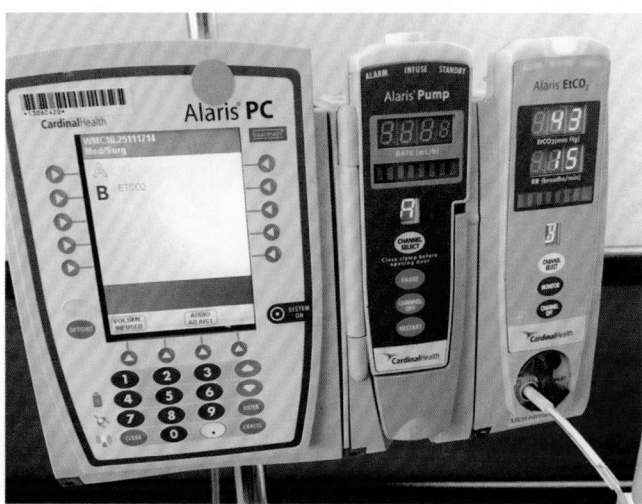

FIGURE 33-6 Nasobuccal monitor. Module B *(far right)* enables continuous respiratory monitoring, including end tidal CO_2 (EtCO₂) and respiratory rate (RR), via a nasobuccal sensor monitor.

whereas pulse oximetry reflects only oxygenation of the blood.

- Capnography is a more reliable indicator of respiratory depression than is pulse oximetry.

A few among the many situations in which capnography is used include the following: when a patient is receiving opioids, during general anesthesia, and for adjusting parameter settings in mechanically ventilated patients.

CO₂ detectors, although they do measure carbon dioxide, are different from capnography. They use chemically treated paper that changes color when exposed to CO_2. They do not give exact readings and can only measure a range of values.

Spirometry

Spirometry is a measure of air that moves into and out of the lungs. To describe the events of pulmonary ventilation, the air in the lungs is divided into four volumes and four capacities. Normal lung volumes and capacities vary with body size, age, and exercise. Men, large people, and athletes have greater lung volume and capacity for ventilation. For a summary of this information,

 Go to **Chapter 33, Diagnostic Testing: Lung Volumes and Capacities,** in Volume 2.

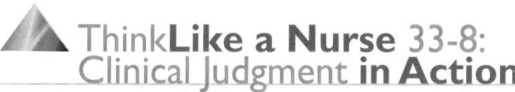 ThinkLike a Nurse 33-8: Clinical Judgment in Action

You hear a pulse oximeter alarm sound in a nearby patient room and find it reading 75%.

- What observations should you make?
- What actions should you take?

Arterial Blood Gases

Arterial blood gas (ABG) analysis measures the levels of oxygen and carbon dioxide in arterial blood. ABG analysis measures pH, partial pressure of oxygen (Po₂), partial pressure of carbon dioxide (Pco₂), saturation of oxygen (Sao₂), and bicarbonate (HCO₃) level. Here, we discuss only Po₂ and Pco₂. For a more thorough discussion of ABG values, see Chapter 35.

A blood sample is obtained from an artery (usually the brachial, radial, or femoral), either by arterial puncture or by withdrawal from an existing arterial line. Arteries are located deep under the skin and alongside nerves, making needle insertion painful. Nurses in critical care units routinely draw ABGs and monitor patients with invasive arterial monitoring; however, you may care for patients on medical–surgical units, or even outpatients, who will undergo periodic ABG evaluation.

Measuring Arterial Blood Oxygen Three values are important when assessing the degree to which the tissues are receiving oxygen:

- **Hemoglobin** is the iron-containing pigment of red blood cells that, as *oxyhemoglobin,* carries oxygen in the blood.
- **Po₂ (partial pressure of oxygen)** is the amount of oxygen available to combine with hemoglobin to make oxyhemoglobin.
- **Sao₂ (saturation of oxygen)** reflects oxygen that is actually bound to hemoglobin.

At sea level, the normal Po₂ range in arterial blood is 80 to 100 mm Hg. After tissues have extracted oxygen from arterial blood and the blood enters the veins to return to the heart, the venous blood Po₂ has fallen to around 40 mm Hg. **Key Point:** *The Sao₂, along with the Po₂ and hemoglobin level, indicates the degree to which the tissues are receiving oxygen.* Small changes in Sao₂ are associated with large changes in Po₂. For blood gas values,

 Go to **Chapter 35, Diagnostic Testing: Assessing Fluid, Electrolyte, and Acid–Base Balance,** in Volume 2.

To fully interpret Po₂ and Sao₂ values, you need to know the percentage of oxygen in the air the patient is inhaling. This is known as the **fraction of inspired oxygen,** or Fio₂. At sea level, atmospheric air (commonly known as *room air*) is 21% oxygen (Fio₂ = 21%). The norms quoted for Po₂ and Sao₂ are based on an Fio₂ of 21%.

- If a healthy patient receives 100% oxygen for a few minutes, the arterial Po₂ will rise to 500 to 600 mm Hg, and the Sao₂ will remain at 100%. The reason is that the Sao₂ measures the oxygen *bound to hemoglobin*—and of course the hemoglobin cannot be "filled" with oxygen to more than 100% capacity.
- When gas exchange is impaired as a result of disease or injury, Po₂ and Sao₂ levels fall. However, they can be kept at normal levels if supplemental oxygen is given.

Measuring Arterial Blood Carbon Dioxide The **partial pressure of carbon dioxide (PCO₂)** is a measure of the CO_2 dissolved in the blood. Normal arterial P_{CO_2} is 35 to 45 mm Hg.

Carbon dioxide readily diffuses across the alveolar–capillary membrane in the lungs, even when there are obstacles such as alveolar fluid or thickened membranes. As a result, P_{CO_2} levels remain normal until a severe disorder interferes with all gas exchange. Once in the alveoli, the amount of carbon dioxide exhaled from the lungs is directly influenced by how well air is moving into and out of the lungs (ventilation).

- **Hypocarbia.** When a person hyperventilates, they exhale large amounts of CO_2, causing arterial P_{CO_2} values to fall. Hyperventilation brings more oxygen into the lungs, so unless it is triggered by hypoxemia, oxygen levels (P_{O_2}) usually remain normal.
- **Hypercarbia.** Conversely, in hypoventilation, less CO_2 moves into the alveoli for exhalation, leaving more CO_2 in the arterial blood. This causes P_{CO_2} values to rise. High P_{CO_2} levels (hypercarbia) suppress the respiratory drive, have an anesthetic effect on the nervous system, and can be toxic. Hypoventilation severe enough to cause hypercarbia is usually associated with hypoxemia because not enough oxygen is inhaled.

KnowledgeCheck 33-8

- What does a pulse oximetry reading tell you?
- What is the relationship between arterial P_{O_2} and SaO_2 levels?
- Identify normal P_{O_2}, SaO_2, and P_{CO_2} levels.
- What effect does ventilation have on arterial P_{CO_2}?
- How is P_{CO_2} related to oxygenation?

 ## ThinkLike a Nurse 33-9: Clinical Judgment in Action

You are caring for two patients, both of whom have a P_{O_2} of 95 mm Hg and an SaO_2 of 99%. Do they have similar lung function? Explain your answer.

Peak Flow Monitoring

The peak expiratory flow rate (PEFR) measures the amount of air that can be exhaled with forcible effort. Patients with asthma use PEFR monitoring to detect subtle changes in their condition, often before symptoms occur. A peak flow meter is used to monitor these changes (Fig. 33-7). Peak flow is expressed in liters per minute. Treatment protocols describe the use and frequency of medications based on individualized peak flow rates. The Home Care box, Home Use of a Peak Flow Meter, describes self-monitoring.

NURSING DIAGNOSIS/ANALYZING CUES

Alterations in pulmonary function may be nursing diagnoses, etiologies of other problems, or merely symptoms of other problems. In analyzing the assessment data, you must determine which because the diagnosis and etiology

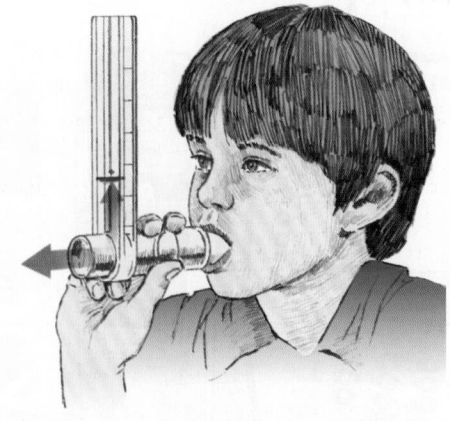
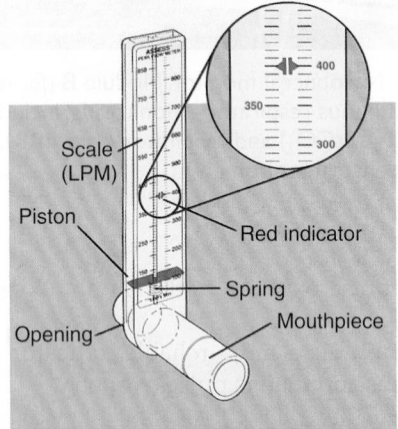
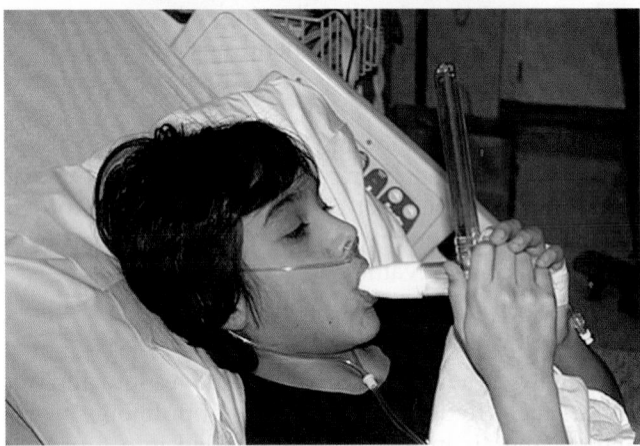

FIGURE 33-7 A patient with asthma using a peak flow meter to monitor peak expiratory flow rate (PEFR).

will guide your choice of interventions. For example, suppose a patient is breathing shallowly and slowly. The pulmonary problem might be one of the following:

- **A nursing diagnosis:** *Ineffective Breathing Pattern (hypoventilation)* r/t pain secondary to rib fractures. In this case, you would provide pain relief; the desired outcome is that the patient will have effective (normal) ventilation. To see a nursing care plan and care map for Ineffective Breathing Pattern,

 Go to Davis Advantage, Resources, Chapter 33, Care Plan and Care Map.

Home Use of a Peak Flow Meter

People with asthma are often asked to monitor their peak flow readings at home and to compare their current readings with their baseline "personal best."

➤ Teach patients that to get an accurate reading, they need to take a deep breath and forcefully exhale.

➤ Teach patients to take a series of three readings and record the highest reading.

➤ Teach patients to maintain or adjust their medication according to their highest reading. They should follow the color-coded treatment protocols prescribed by their physician. These are individualized for each patient. Notice that these correspond to the color-coded markers on the peak flow meter.

Green = _All clear: Baseline peak flow_—*Peak flow is within 80% to 100% of personal best baseline.*

Treatment protocol calls for routine medication use.

Yellow = _Caution: Peak flow is 50% to 80% of usual or "normal" rate._ *Said another way, there is a 20% to 50% reduction in peak flow—This reading signals the onset of airway changes.*

Treatment protocols usually specify an increase in the dosage of maintenance medications, the use of rescue therapies (e.g., fast-acting bronchodilators), or a call to the healthcare provider. These measures are designed to reverse acute exacerbations before they become severe.

Red = _Medical alert: Peak flow is less than 50% of personal best baseline._ *Severe reduction in peak flow.*

Treatment protocols usually specify immediate treatment with rescue medications and to seek emergency treatment if symptoms do not improve.

Source: Adapted from American Lung Association. (2021). *Measuring your peak flow rate.* http://www.lung.org/lung-health-and-diseases/lung-disease-lookup/asthma/living-with-asthma/managing-asthma/measuring-your-peak-flow-rate.html

- **An etiology:** Risk for Ineffective Cerebral Tissue Perfusion (Cerebral) *r/t Ineffective Breathing Pattern (hypoventilation).* In this case, you might address the etiology by administering oxygen; the desired outcome would be effective cerebral perfusion, evidenced by normal speech and alertness.

- **A symptom:** Intracranial Adaptive Capacity Impairment (Clinical Care Classification [CCC], n.d.) r/t brain injury, *as manifested by Ineffective Breathing Pattern (hypoventilation), and baseline ICP ≥ 10 mm Hg.* In this situation, you would, of course, support ventilation (the symptom) until the problem subsides. However, the primary interventions would be directed toward the head trauma and increased intracranial pressure (ICP). Once these etiologies are corrected, the hypoventilation would disappear. The goal would be normal intracranial pressure, evidenced in part by a normal breathing pattern.

Problems of Ventilation and Gas Exchange The following nursing diagnoses directly describe problems with ventilation and gas exchange. Use these diagnoses when they are the central problem and you intend to use interventions to eliminate the cause of the problem.

- *Ineffective Airway Clearance* is the inability to maintain a clear airway.
- *Ineffective Breathing Pattern* is used to describe inadequate ventilation, such as hypoventilation, hyperventilation, tachypnea, or bradypnea.
- *Gas Exchange Impairment* is the appropriate diagnosis if the patient is ventilating adequately but diffusion of gases across the alveolar–capillary membrane is impaired.
- *Ineffective Spontaneous Ventilation* describes a condition in which a patient, as a result of decreased energy reserves, is unable to maintain breathing adequate to support life.
- *Dysfunctional Ventilatory Weaning Response* represents a specific situation in which a patient who is being mechanically ventilated cannot adjust to lower levels of ventilator support, prolonging the ventilatory weaning process.
- *Aspiration Risk* should be used when there is a risk for secretions, solids, or fluids entering into tracheobronchial passages (e.g., for patients who have had head or neck surgery or who have a reduced level of consciousness).

▆ PLANNING/PRIORITIZING HYPOTHESES AND GENERATING SOLUTIONS

Nursing Outcomes Classification (NOC) standardized outcomes appropriate for patients with pulmonary function problems include, for example:

> Mechanical Ventilation Weaning Response: Adult
> Respiratory Status: Airway Patency
> Respiratory Status: Gas Exchange
> Respiratory Status: Ventilation
> Swallowing Status
> Vital Signs

These provide a general guide for care planning. Depending on individual patient needs, other NOC outcomes or Nursing Interventions Classification (NIC) interventions may also be appropriate (Moorhead et al., 2018).

Individualized goals/outcome statements depend on the nursing diagnosis you identify. For diagnoses related to gas exchange, the following are examples of goals you might write:

> Expectorates secretions effectively
> No dyspnea or shortness of breath
> Lungs clear; no adventitious sounds present

▆ IMPLEMENTATION/TAKING ACTION

NIC standardized interventions related to oxygenation are found in the Respiratory Management category. They focus on maintaining a patent airway and promoting gas exchange, and they include Airway Management, Airway Suctioning, Cough Enhancement, Oxygen Therapy, and Respiratory Monitoring.

Specific nursing interventions for patients with oxygenation problems include health promotion, prevention, and treatment activities. They are discussed in the sections that follow.

Administering Respiratory Medications

Respiratory medications promote ventilation and oxygenation by their effects on the respiratory system itself. Some need a prescription; others do not. Medications are also used to improve respiratory function. A few examples include bronchodilators and anti-inflammatory agents such as corticosteroids, cough suppressants, expectorants, and decongestants.

See the accompanying Self-Care box, Cough and Cold Medicines: Tips for Parents, for assistance in

administering such medications to children. Also refer to the accompanying Holistic Healing box for some common alternative cold remedies.

Promoting Optimal Respiratory Function

Deep, regular breathing promotes ventilation and optimizes gas exchange. Other interventions to promote optimal function include preventing and treating URIs, influenza, and pneumonia (including immunizations); supporting smoking cessation; positioning; incentive spirometry; and preventing aspiration.

Prevent Healthcare-Associated Pneumonia

Healthcare-associated pneumonia (HCaP) is pneumonia that is contracted by a patient in a hospital or inpatient facility. It is often caused by bacteria other than *Streptococcus pneumoniae,* which is the organism involved in most cases of pneumonia. HCaP tends to be more complicated and have a higher mortality rate than community-acquired pneumonia. For specific prevention interventions, see the Example Client Condition: Pneumonia.

Self-Care

Cough and Cold Medicines: Tips for Parents

➤ Do not give children medicines labeled for adults only.

➤ Do not give over-the-counter (OTC) cough and cold remedies to children younger than age 4 years. There is a risk of serious and even life-threatening side effects.

➤ The safety and effectiveness of OTC cough and cold remedies for children ages 2 through 11 years are still in question. It is not certain they are safe, and they may not be effective.

➤ Read labels. Some labels are marked "Do not use for children under age 4."

➤ Choose medications with safety caps. Close caps tightly and store out of sight and reach of children.

➤ Check the "active ingredients" on the label. Do not give more than one medicine with the same active ingredient. Your child could be harmed by getting too much of the ingredient.

➤ Carefully follow the directions on the label for how to use the medicine. Overuse or misuse can cause serious side effects (e.g., drowsiness, breathing problems, and seizures).

➤ Measure carefully. Do not use household spoons because they come in different sizes.

➤ Understand that OTC medicines do not cure the cold or cough. They only treat symptoms such as runny nose, congestion, fever, and aches. They do not shorten the length of time your child is sick.

Source: Centers for Disease Control and Prevention. (2020a). *For parents: Young children and adverse drug events. Medication Safety Program.* Retrieved from http://www.cdc.gov/MedicationSafety/parents_childrenAdverseDrugEvents.html; U.S. Food and Drug Administration. (2018). *Use caution when giving cold and cough products to kids.* Retrieved from https://www.fda.gov/Drugs/ResourcesForYou/SpecialFeatures/ucm263948.htm

Holistic Healing

Common Cold Remedies

➤ Cold care products containing *Pelargonium sidoides,* an extract of the South African geranium, have been shown to reduce the duration and intensity of symptoms of the common cold (Riley et al., 2019; Schapowal et al., 2019). In the United States, Zucol products are one example.

➤ A systematic review concluded that honey may be better than no treatment, diphenhydramine, or placebo for the symptomatic relief of cough in children, but it is not better than dextromethorphan (Mani et al., 2019). However, avoid giving honey to children younger than the age of 1 year because it is a reservoir of *Clostridium botulinum* spores and may cause botulism in infants.

➤ Although not fully proven, large doses of vitamin C (1000 to 2000 mg per day) may help reduce how long a cold lasts but do not protect against getting a cold. The likelihood of success varies from person to person. Be aware that in amounts greater than 2,000 mg, vitamin C may cause diarrhea and gas (Mousa, 2017).

➤ A systematic review of research studies found there is no evidence that echinacea preparations are effective for preventing and treating the common cold (David et al., 2019).

➤ Although the evidence is still uncertain, elderberry *(Sambucus nigra),* an herb, may reduce the duration and severity of colds and reduce the duration of influenza. Additionally, some studies found that the use of elderberry-containing products may result in a lower risk of influenza complications and adverse events (Wieland et al., 2021).

Promote Immunization for Influenza and Pneumonia

The most effective strategy for preventing influenza and pneumonia is vaccination. Vaccines for influenza are developed annually to closely match the major known strains of the virus that have evolved. Immunizations given to healthy young adults are 70% to 90% effective. The CDC (2022b) recommends that all adults age 65 years or older receive one dose of the pneumococcal conjugate vaccine PCV15 or the pneumococcal conjugate vaccine PCV20. If PCV15 is used, a dose of the pneumococcal polysaccharide vaccine (PPSV23) should be administered at least 1 year later. If PCV20 is used, a dose of PPSV23 is not required.

Support Smoking Cessation

Smoking cessation is important in preventing and treating all respiratory problems, including URIs, influenza, and pneumonia. **Key Point: *All patients should be asked whether they smoke (tobacco or e-cigarettes), and their use status should be documented regularly (e.g., by chart stickers or computer prompts) (Berry et al., 2019; Selekman et al., 2019)).*** The U.S. Public Health Service guidelines suggest the "5A's" model for treating tobacco dependence (Box 33-4) (Krist et al., 2021).

Motivational counseling includes discussion about the connection between tobacco use and current health status, the risks of continued tobacco use, the rewards of quitting, anticipated barriers to quitting, and strategies for addressing barriers. It may also be important to refer the person to a tobacco cessation program. Most smokers are not able to quit "cold turkey."

A combination of medication and counseling is more effective than either used alone. Encourage patients to contact their primary care provider for nicotine replacement therapy or other medications (e.g., antidepressants, clonidine) to treat tobacco dependence. For pregnant women, smokeless tobacco users, light smokers, and adolescents, medications may be contraindicated or may lack evidence of effectiveness (Hartmann-Boyce et al., 2019; Krist et al., 2021; Pirnia et al., 2019).

Box 33-1 highlights some of the benefits of smoking cessation. Share these and smoking cessation tips with patients (see Self-Care: Smoking Cessation Tips).

BOX 33-4 ■ The 5A's for Treating Tobacco Dependence

Ask about tobacco use and document tobacco use status for every patient at every visit.

Advise to quit. Use a clear, strong, personalized approach to urge the patient to quit.

Assess willingness to make a quit attempt at this time.

Assist in a quit attempt. If the patient is willing, refer for counseling and medication. If the patient is not willing to quit at this time, provide interventions designed to increase future quit attempts.

Arrange follow-up. If the patient is willing to quit, make follow-up contacts beginning the first week after the quit date. If the patient is not willing to quit at this time, address tobacco dependence and willingness to quit at the next clinic (or other) visit.

Source: Adapted from U.S. Preventive Services Task Force. (2021). Interventions for tobacco smoking cessation in adults, including pregnant persons: US Preventive Services Task Force recommendation statement. *Journal of the American Medical Association, 325*(3), 265–279.

Self-Care

Smoking Cessation Tips

➤ Identify several personal reasons to quit smoking, such as "I'll live longer and be able to spend more time with my children and grandchildren" or "My father died of lung cancer and really suffered. I have no desire to experience that."

➤ Make a list of things you enjoy doing. Choose one of these items as a reward for not smoking.

➤ Before smoking, ask yourself, "What can I do instead of smoking this cigarette?"

➤ Identify friends who do not smoke and plan to spend time with them.

➤ Have carrot sticks, celery, gum, or sunflower seeds available to chew instead of smoking a cigarette. These also help you cope with the increased hunger you may feel.

➤ Learn several relaxation techniques, such as meditation or visualization, to help you through the stress of quitting.

➤ Use positive affirmations daily. "I can successfully quit smoking. I am no longer a smoker."

➤ Tell several supportive people of your plan to quit. Ask them to help you be successful.

➤ Plan a time to quit. Choose a time that will not require many additional demands on you.

➤ Talk with friends and coworkers who have successfully quit smoking.

➤ Save the money you would have spent on cigarettes. Treat yourself to an activity or event with the money you have saved.

➤ Tell your healthcare providers that you would like to quit smoking.

➤ When you feel a craving to smoke, breathe deeply, find something to distract yourself, or call a supportive person.

➤ To help cope with irritability, use relaxation exercises or deep breathing, take a hot bath, or do something else you enjoy.

➤ Participate in a structured smoking cessation program, if possible.

➤ Consider asking your healthcare provider about nicotine-replacement therapy, such as gum or patches.

Position for Maximum Ventilation

An upright or elevated position pulls abdominal organs down, allowing maximum diaphragm excursion and lung expansion. Therefore, this intervention is applicable to almost all respiratory problems, including URI, influenza, and pneumonia (see the Example Client Conditions).

- If the patient is short of breath, provide an overbed table to lean forward on. Patients with impaired respiratory function adopt a tripod position to allow maximum expansion. They may need to rest their arms on an overbed table.
- When the patient is lying on their side, provide pillows to support the upper arm.
- Assist with frequent position changes to keep all areas of the lungs well ventilated, and ambulate as often as possible without creating fatigue.

Assist With Incentive Spirometry

Incentive spirometers are designed to encourage patients to take deep breaths by reaching a goal-directed volume of air. It is usually reserved for patients at risk for developing atelectasis or pneumonia (e.g., patients who have had abdominal, chest, or pelvic surgery; are on prolonged bedrest; or have a history of respiratory problems). Incentive spirometers offer various visual cues (e.g., elevation of a ball or piston) to show patients whether they are inhaling deeply enough.

  Delegation As a registered nurse (RN), you can delegate incentive spirometry coaching to licensed practical nurses (LPNs) and qualified unlicensed assistive personnel (UAPs). However, you are responsible for ensuring that incentive spirometry is carried out correctly and at the required frequencies. You must also evaluate patient responses, airway clearance, and ventilation. See Figure 36-6 and the Self-Care box, Teaching Your Patient About Incentive Spirometry, in Chapter 36.

Take Aspiration Precautions

Aspiration is a risk for patients with a decreased level of consciousness, diminished gag or cough reflex, or difficulty with swallowing. Preventing aspiration requires you to have practical knowledge about positioning, enteral and oral feedings, and administering medications. For guidelines to use with at-risk patients,

 Go to **Chapter 33, Clinical Insight 33-2: Guidelines for Preventing Aspiration,** in Volume 2.

  Many of the guidelines involve basic care and can be delegated to qualified LPNs and UAPs. **Key Point:** *The RN is responsible for monitoring for aspiration.* Record in the nursing notes any preventive measures taken.

KnowledgeCheck 33-9

Identify at least three nursing actions to promote optimal respiratory function in a hospitalized patient with chronic lung disease.

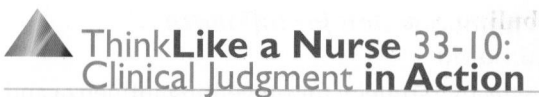

ThinkLike a Nurse 33-10: Clinical Judgment in Action

- Review the Meet Your Patients scenario. For which of these patients should you recommend annual flu or pneumonia immunizations? Why?
- A 24-year-old nursing student has no previous hospitalizations or known chronic health problems, takes no medications, and has no current respiratory symptoms. On routine purified protein derivative, or PPD, testing (tuberculin skin testing), the student has an area of induration measuring 5 mm. How would you interpret these results?

Mobilizing Secretions

Coughing promotes deep inhalation and forceful expulsion of secretions. Interventions that help enhance coughing and mobilize secretions include deep breathing, coughing exercises, and hydration. Mobilizing secretions is useful for many respiratory conditions, including UTI, influenza, and pneumonia.

Teach Deep Breathing and Coughing

Deep breathing promotes ventilation and gas exchange. Coughing after deep breathing mobilizes secretions, which keeps the airways and alveoli open and provides a greater surface area for gas exchange. This intervention is important, for example, in treating pneumonia and preventing stasis pneumonia postoperatively. For information about teaching patients to deep-breathe,

 Go to **Chapter 33, Procedure 33-1A: Collecting an Expectorated Sputum Specimen,** in Volume 2.

  Key Point: *Alter this procedure for patients with chronic lung disease. Have the patient exhale through pursed lips and cough throughout expiration in several short bursts to avoid high expiratory pressures, which collapse diseased airways.*

Maintain Hydration

The following activities are important to keep pulmonary secretions thin and mobile (e.g., in infections such as influenza and pneumonia):

- *Maintain systemic hydration.* Encourage oral fluid intake as much as possible. Supplement oral intake by IV fluid administration if the patient cannot ingest adequate amounts of fluid. For guidelines to use in teaching patients to maintain hydration, refer to the Self-Care box, Teaching Patients to Prevent Fluid and Electrolyte Imbalances, in Chapter 35.
- *Humidify inhaled air.* You can accomplish this with humidification devices or nebulizers.
  - A **humidifier** is a device that delivers small water droplets from a reservoir. Small humidifiers filled with sterile distilled water are attached to oxygen delivery systems to moisten the dry oxygen and keep secretions thin and mobile.

- A **nebulizer** is a device that turns liquids into an aerosol mist that can be inhaled directly into the lungs. Nebulizers are often used to deliver medications to the lungs, but they can also be used to deliver moisture to the airways and lungs.

See Administering Respiratory Inhalations in Chapter 23, and Figures 23-11 and 23-12. Also,

 Go to **Chapter 33, Clinical Insight 33-3: Oxygen Therapy Safety Precautions,** in Volume 2.

Perform Chest Physiotherapy

Chest physiotherapy moves secretions to the large, central airways for expectoration or suctioning (Fig. 33-8). It involves postural drainage, chest percussion, and chest vibration. In many institutions, respiratory therapists routinely perform chest physiotherapy. However, these procedures are briefly discussed in the Highlights of Procedures box. For a detailed discussion,

 Go to **Chapter 33, Procedure 33-3: Performing Percussion, Vibration, and Postural Drainage,** in Volume 2.

- **Postural drainage** is the use of positioning to promote drainage from the lungs. Postural drainage uses gravity to drain the lungs, so you will position the affected area uppermost so that secretions will drain down toward the large, central airways. For example, if the patient has pneumonia of the right lower lobe, you

would place them on their left side and elevate the foot of the bed to allow the right lower lobe to drain.
- *Chest percussion and chest vibration* are used in conjunction with postural drainage to loosen and mobilize secretions. Have the patient assume the desired position for 10 to 15 minutes before percussing and vibrating.
  - **Chest percussion** is the rhythmic clapping of the chest wall using cupped hands.
  - **Chest vibration** is the vibration of the chest wall with the palms of the hands.

 Think**Like a Nurse** 33-11 Clinical Judgment **in Action**

Your patient has pneumonia in the right lower lobe. The patient is mildly dyspneic with any activity. Plan how you would perform chest physiotherapy on this patient. What activities would you consider to make this procedure more tolerable for the patient?

Providing Oxygen Therapy

Oxygen therapy provides oxygen at concentrations greater than the level found in room air. Room air contains only about 21% oxygen. Because oxygen is a medication, it requires a medical prescription for dosage (concentration) and route. Many agencies have protocols with standing orders for oxygen administration in an emergency. (Note that oxygen therapy may be needed for pneumonia.) Oxygen is supplied in several different ways.

- **Wall outlets** connected to a large central tank of oxygen are usually provided in healthcare facilities (Fig. 33-9).

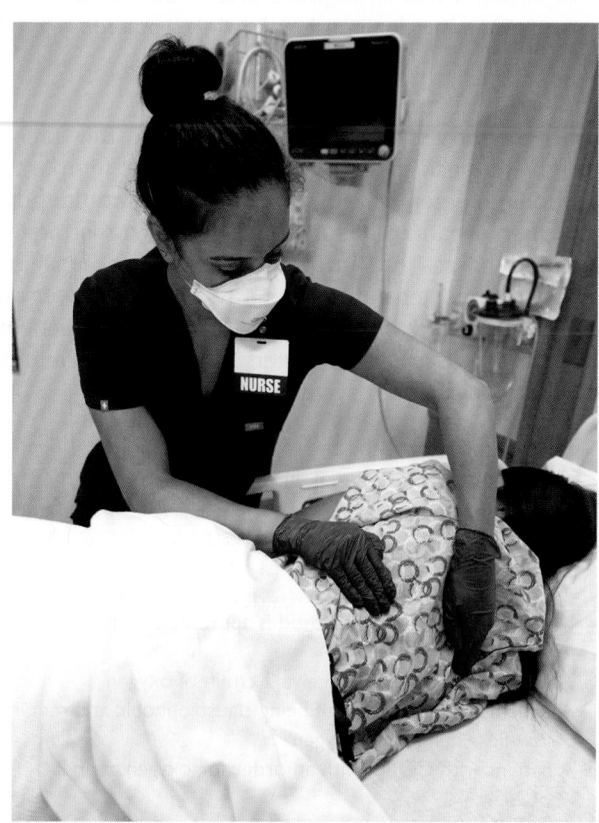

FIGURE 33-8 Patient receiving chest physiotherapy.

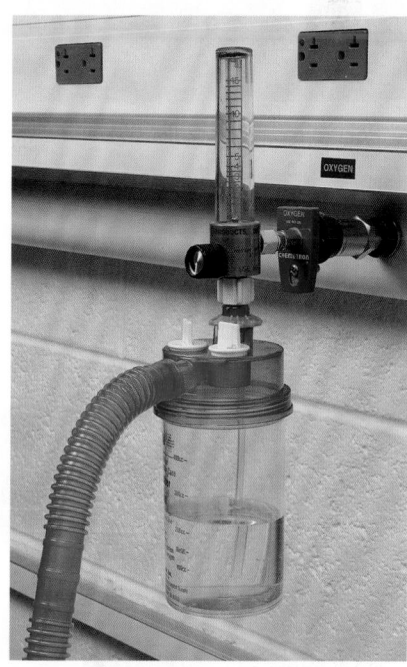

FIGURE 33-9 Healthcare facilities usually have oxygen available through wall outlets connected to a large central tank of oxygen.

- **Compressed O₂ in portable tanks** (Fig. 33-10) may also be available.
- **Liquid oxygen units** are often used for home oxygen therapy (Fig. 33-11).
- **An oxygen concentrator** removes nitrogen from room air and concentrates O₂. It requires a battery pack or electrical outlet for power. These devices eliminate the need to buy oxygen cylinders, relieving clients' anxiety about running out of oxygen. However, they are

expensive, noisy, and not portable; moreover, the client must still have backup oxygen in case of a power failure.

The Highlights of Procedures box summarizes how to set up and apply oxygen therapy. For the complete procedure and to see various types of masks,

 Go to **Chapter 33, Procedure 33-4: Administering Oxygen,** in Volume 2.

Oxygen Hazards

The following risks are associated with oxygen therapy. For guidelines to minimize these risks, see the Highlights of Procedures box, and

 Go to **Chapter 33, Clinical Insight 33-3: Oxygen Therapy Safety Precautions,** and **Procedure 33-4: Administering Oxygen,** in Volume 2.

- **Oxygen toxicity can develop** when O₂ concentrations of more than 50% are administered for longer than 48 to 72 hours. Prolonged use of high O₂ concentrations reduces surfactant production, which leads to alveolar collapse and reduced lung elasticity.
- **Oxygen supports combustion,** although it does not burn. High concentrations of oxygen will turn a small spark or fire into a large fire. Fire prevention precautions must be used near oxygen delivery systems.
- **Oxygen tanks contain oxygen under pressure.** If the tank ruptures or falls, compressed oxygen shoots forcefully from the tank, turning it into an unguided missile. Oxygen tanks have been known to hurtle through walls when ruptured.

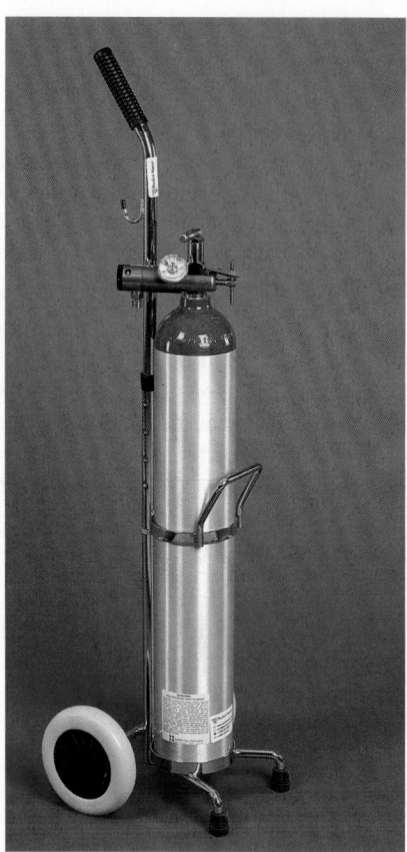

FIGURE 33-10 Portable oxygen tanks come in a variety of sizes.

Transtracheal Oxygen Delivery

A **tracheostomy** is a surgical opening into the trachea through the neck. It may be permanent or temporary. Traditional oxygen is delivered by nasal cannula; however, when a patient has a tracheostomy, **transtracheal oxygen** bypasses the upper airway, which normally warms and moistens air before it reaches the lower airway. Oxygen may be delivered through the tracheostomy via a collar or an adapter. For more information about oxygen delivery systems,

 Go to the table at the end of **Procedure 33-4: Administering Oxygen,** in Volume 2.

KnowledgeCheck 33-10

- Why is oxygen humidified?
- Which oxygen delivery method is appropriate for the following patients?
  - A patient prescribed to receive 2 L/min of oxygen
  - A patient who complains of being claustrophobic and requires low-flow humidified oxygen
  - A patient with COPD with an order for oxygen at an FIO₂ of 24%
  - A patient who wants to avoid intubation but requires an FIO₂ of 100%

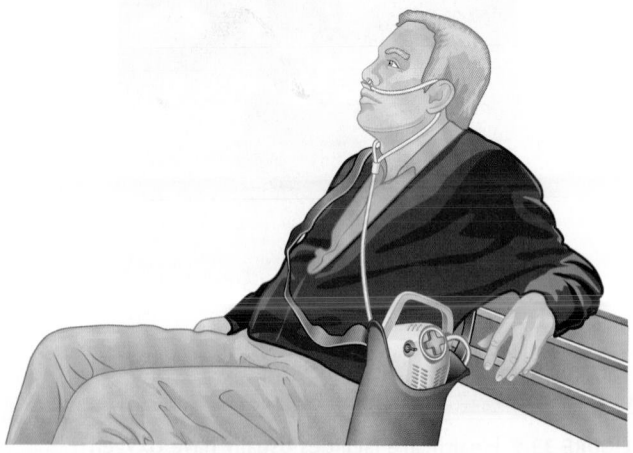

FIGURE 33-11 Liquid oxygen units are small and portable. They are ideal for home use.

Using Artificial Airways

Artificial airways provide an open airway for patients who have or who are at risk for airway obstruction. Airways may be placed into the pharynx or deeper, into the trachea.

Pharyngeal Airways

Pharyngeal airways provide an open air passage by holding the tongue away from the back of the pharynx. When artificial airways are properly placed, air can flow around and through them, and suction catheters can be passed through them. Pharyngeal airways may be placed through the mouth or the nose.

- **Oropharyngeal airways** are C-shaped, hard plastic devices inserted through the mouth into the pharynx. To select the appropriate size, hold the airway next to the patient's face. The length of the airway should extend from the front of the teeth to the end of the jawline. If it is *too short*, it will not keep the tongue pulled forward; if it is *too long*, it may push the epiglottis against the laryngeal opening and completely obstruct the airway.
- **Nasopharyngeal airways** are flexible rubber tubes that are inserted through a nostril into the pharynx. Patients who are semiconscious can tolerate nasal airways because they do not stimulate the gag reflex. Nasopharyngeal airways are available in a variety of pediatric and adult sizes. To learn about inserting a nasopharyngeal airway, see the Highlights of Procedures box and

 Go to **Chapter 33, Procedure 33-13: Inserting a Nasopharyngeal Airway,** in Volume 2.

Endotracheal Airways

Patients who cannot breathe effectively because of airway obstruction or respiratory or cardiac failure need an airway inserted directly into the trachea. **Endotracheal airways** are pliable tubes inserted into the trachea through the following routes:

Orotracheal tube—the mouth
Nasotracheal tube—the nose
Tracheostomy tube—an opening directly into the trachea

There are several types of tracheostomy tubes, made of various materials. They may be cuffed or uncuffed and may have a single or double lumen.

- A cuffed tube is used for patients who are being ventilated or who have difficulty swallowing.
- For self-care at home, a tube with an inner cannula is preferred because the inner tube can be removed and cleaned to avoid tube occlusion, primarily resulting from the accumulation of secretions in the airway.

Because tracheostomy tubes bypass the upper airway, the patient inhales air directly into the lower airway without humidification, filtering, or warming. For this reason, devices that warm and humidify inhaled air are used with endotracheal airways. Figure 33-12A illustrates the parts of an endotracheal airway. Figure 33-12B shows the placement of an orotracheal tube. Nursing responsibilities related to endotracheal airways are to assist in their insertion, maintain stabilization, and provide routine suctioning and management.

Assisting With Endotracheal Airway Insertion

Insertion of endotracheal airways is within the scope of practice of certain specially trained nurses (e.g., nurse anesthetist). As a general-practice nurse, you will assist with insertion by gathering equipment and preparing the patient. On most units, you will find intubation equipment in the resuscitation cart. Intubation must often be done quickly in response to a temporary decline in the patient's respiratory function during a procedure. For more information about assisting with and managing endotracheal airways,

 Go to **Chapter 33, Clinical Insight 33-4: Caring for Patients With Endotracheal Airways,** in Volume 2.

Managing Endotracheal and Tracheostomy Tubes

Managing endotracheal and tracheostomy tubes generally requires the expertise of a respiratory therapist

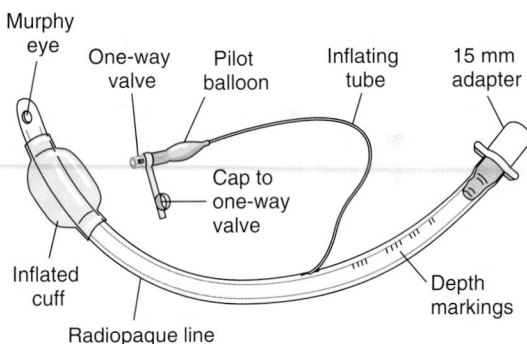

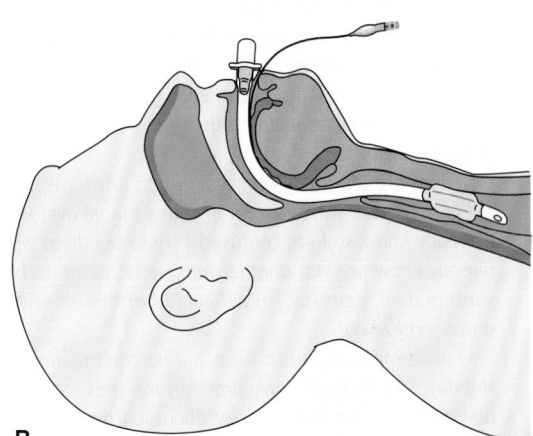

FIGURE 33-12 *A,* An endotracheal tube. *B,* Placement of an orotracheal tube.

or an RN, but you can delegate this activity to specially trained and skilled LPNs, especially in critical care areas. Once the ostomy is well healed, the airway will not collapse if the tracheostomy tube is dislodged. This means a UAP, or even the patient, can reinsert it if necessary. Many patients with permanent tracheostomies perform self-care at home.

Evidence is still mixed about whether to use sterile or clean gloves when performing endotracheal care. The following are the different levels of asepsis currently in use for tracheostomy care:

- **Sterile technique** is the use of a sterile suction catheter and other supplies with sterile gloves. For new tracheostomies, most facilities use sterile technique. However, some use sterile technique only for patients who have increased susceptibility to infection.
- **Modified sterile technique** is the use of a sterile suction catheter and supplies but with nonsterile procedure gloves. For healed tracheostomies, and in many institutions for all tracheostomies, the trend is toward a modified sterile technique.
- **Clean technique** is the use of a clean catheter and clean hands or nonsterile gloves. The portion of the catheter that will be inserted in the tracheostomy tube is protected to avoid contact with unclean surfaces. Clean technique is the usual method in the home setting.

Anyone who is not a family member should wear non-sterile procedure gloves, even in the home setting.

You should follow the technique used in your healthcare facility or school. To learn a procedure and guidelines for tracheostomy care, respectively, see the Highlights of Procedures box, and

 Go to **Chapter 33, Procedure 33-5: Performing Tracheostomy Care Using Sterile Technique** and **Clinical Insight 33-4: Caring for Patients With Endotracheal Airways,** in Volume 2.

KnowledgeCheck 33-11

- In what circumstances would you use an oropharyngeal airway? A nasopharyngeal airway?
- What facts should you record if a patient is intubated?
- Describe seven nursing actions associated with caring for a patient with an endotracheal tube.

Suctioning Airways

Airways are suctioned to remove secretions and maintain patency. Signs that indicate the need for suctioning include:

Agitation
Gurgling sounds during respiration
Restlessness

Safe, Effective Nursing Care

Removing Barriers to Patient and Family Involvement in Care

Provide goal-directed, client-centered care (Thinking, Doing, Caring)

Scenario: Mrs. Yablonski, a 66-year-old former smoker, has recently had a permanent tracheostomy but can speak using an electromechanical device. She needs to learn how to suction herself and change the tracheotomy dressing. For 3 days in a row, different nurses have tried to explain how to perform the care. Each time, she became tearful and frustrated. The nurse manager speaks with her to identify problems that may be occurring. Mrs. Yablonski cites several issues:

Sometimes it's me. I may just feel too overwhelmed, or I may just not have any energy. But the nurses don't always ask me if I feel well enough to learn. None of them really knows me, and they don't take enough time with me. And sometimes my nurse would rather just do it themself and get it over with.

There are too many nurses trying to teach me. They tell me different ways to do it or make me go over what I already know, so I get confused. I try to tell them what I already know or what another nurse told me to do, but they want to do it their way. They should have this all written down somewhere.

I want my husband to learn, but he can't be here during the day, and that's the only time anyone tries to show me how to do it. I asked the doctor about learning about it later on in his office, but he didn't want to talk about it. He said the nurses here would teach me.

Thinking: Including patients or their significant others as equal partners in care is the foundation of patient-centered care. Think about the following questions:

➤ What barriers to participating in her own care does Mrs. Yablonski identify? Would they be applicable to other patients?

➤ How is team communication affecting this situation?

➤ Does Mrs. Yablonski see herself as a valuable partner in her care?

➤ What might the effects be if Mrs. Yablonski felt more empowered?

➤ Does she seem to have a conflict regarding how much care she wants to take over? If so, how should her nurse manage the conflict?

➤ What are the potential negative outcomes if Mrs. Yablonski goes home before she masters her tracheostomy care?

➤ What can the nurse manager do to make Mrs. Yablonski's care more patient centered?

Source: Ward, A., Pandian, V., & Brenner, M. J. (2018). The primacy of patient-centered outcomes in tracheostomy care. *The Patient-Patient-Centered Outcomes Research, 11*(2), 143–145.

Labored respirations
Decreased oxygen saturation (Sao_2)
Increased heart and respiratory rates
Adventitious breath sounds on auscultation.

 Although suctioning helps remove secretions, it also removes air from the airways and causes the patient's O_2 levels to fall. Therefore, suctioning must be done quickly and is often accompanied by supplemental oxygen. Suctioning can also irritate mucous membranes if done too frequently.

Suction catheters may be open tipped or "whistle tipped" (Fig. 33-13A and B). Most suction catheters have a port on the side, over which you place your thumb to control the suction. A Yankauer tube (Fig. 33-13C) is a rigid device for suctioning the oral cavity.

Collaborating and Delegating Both respiratory therapists and nurses are responsible for suctioning and tracheostomy care. The respiratory therapist and the nurse should keep each other informed of changes in the patient's condition. Airway suctioning is usually performed by RNs and LPNs but not by UAPs. UAPs may use a Yankauer tube to suction the oral cavity as part of maintaining hygiene and preventing aspiration of oral secretions.

Suctioning the Upper Airway

Key Point: *Pharyngeal suctioning is performed to prevent oral and nasal secretions from entering the lower airway when the patient is too weak to cough them up.* Suctioning the pharynx triggers a cough, which helps loosen and mobilize secretions.

- The patient's condition determines whether you suction the pharynx through the mouth or nose.

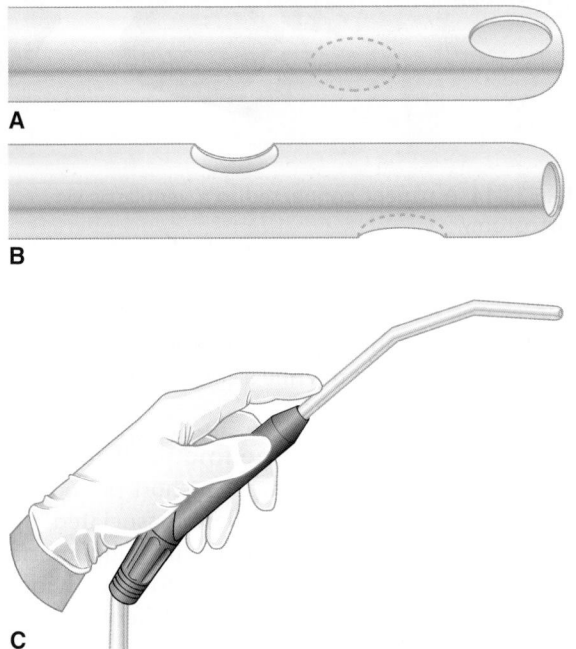

FIGURE 33-13 *A,* Whistle-tipped suction catheter. *B,* Open-tipped suction catheter. *C,* Yankauer (oral) suction tube.

- Most patients find **oropharyngeal suctioning** more comfortable than the nasal approach.
- Nevertheless, you should use a **nasal approach** if the patient is unable to cooperate and automatically bites down when anything is placed in the mouth, or if the jaw is wired.

To learn how to suction the pharynx, see the summary in the Highlights of Procedures box. For the complete steps,

 Go to **Chapter 33, Procedure 33-9: Performing Upper Airway Suctioning,** in Volume 2.

Suctioning the Lower Airway

Key Point: *In tracheal suctioning, a catheter is passed beyond the pharynx and into the trachea to remove secretions from the lower airway.* The trachea may be suctioned through the mouth, nose, or an endotracheal airway. In the healthcare setting, deep tracheal suctioning is a sterile procedure.

Orotracheal or Nasotracheal (NT) Approach When suctioning through the nose or mouth, insert the catheter into the pharynx and advance it into the trachea during inspiration. This prevents the catheter from entering the esophagus and causing the patient to gag or vomit. When the suction catheter enters the trachea, it will stimulate coughing. Except in an emergency, NT suctioning should be done through a nasopharyngeal airway. The Highlights of Procedures box provides a summary of this procedure. For the complete steps,

 Go to **Chapter 33, Procedure 33-8: Performing Orotracheal and Nasotracheal Suctioning (Open System),** in Volume 2.

Endotracheal or Tracheostomy Approach An endotracheal or tracheostomy tube provides a direct path into the trachea. To suction, insert the catheter through the artificial airway and into the trachea. You do not need to insert the catheter as far into a tracheostomy tube because you are bypassing the long upper airway. Before suctioning, make sure the airway is secured so that it is not dislodged by coughing or suctioning. The Highlights of Procedures box summarizes this procedure. For the complete steps,

Go to **Chapter 33, Procedure 33-6: Performing Tracheostomy Suctioning (Open System),** in Volume 2.

KnowledgeCheck 33-12

- Describe the difference between pharyngeal and tracheal suctioning.
- How can you ensure that the suction catheter enters the trachea and not the esophagus?

Toward Evidence-Based Practice

Najafi Ghezeljeh, T., Kalhor, L., Moradi Moghadam, O., Lahiji Niakan, M., & Haghani, H. (2018). The effect of head-of-bed elevation of 45 degree on the incidence of ventilator-associated pneumonia among hospitalized patients in intensive care units. *Iran Journal of Nursing, 31*(111), 65–74.

Eighty (80) patients who were under mechanical ventilation in an intensive care unit (ICU) were randomly assigned to either a control group or an intervention group. The patients in the intervention group were positioned with the head of the bed elevated to 45 degrees, whereas the patients in the control group experienced routine positioning. After 3 days, ventilator-associated pneumonia was found to be significantly higher in the control group. According to the researchers, patients receiving mechanical ventilation should be positioned with the head of the bed at 45 degrees.

Tesoro, M., Peyser, D. J., & Villarente, F. (2018). A retrospective study of non–ventilator-associated hospital acquired pneumonia incidence and missed opportunities for nursing care. *Journal of Nursing Administration, 48*(5), 285–291.

A retrospective chart review was completed to determine the incidence of non–ventilator-associated hospital-acquired pneumonia (NV-HAP) and to assess associated nursing care. The chart review identified 205 patients with NV-HAP (incidence of 0.47 per 1000 patient days) in a 12-month time period. The results revealed that 60.5% of patients with NV-HAP had no documented oral healthcare, and only 8 of the 205 (3.9%) patients received documented oral care at least 4 times a day. The lack of documented oral healthcare demonstrates a missed opportunity for nursing care in potentially preventing NV-HAP. Barriers to the provision of oral care include a lack of time and staffing resources, which may lead to the delegation of oral care to untrained personnel.

1. Based on these study findings, list at least two interventions a staff nurse could implement to help prevent VAP.

2. Which study might you use to convince a hospital administrator to hire more nurses?

Caring for a Patient Requiring Mechanical Ventilation

A **mechanical ventilator** is a machine that assists a patient in breathing. The patient is intubated before they are connected to the ventilator. An endotracheal tube or a tracheostomy tube is connected by oxygen tubing to the ventilator. Mechanical ventilation is indicated for acute or chronic respiratory failure and may be a short- or long-term therapy.

- **Negative pressure ventilators** consist of shells that fit externally around the chest. Negative pressure generated inside the shell pulls the chest outward and forces the patient to inhale air, similar to normal breathing. These ventilators are rarely used for acutely ill patients, but they are occasionally used for chronic conditions, for example, in patients with muscle weakness from neuromuscular disease.

- **Positive pressure ventilators** (also called *mechanical ventilation*) are the most widely used type. They require the patient to have an artificial airway (Fig. 33-14). Positive pressure ventilation carries risks, including *barotrauma* (injury to the airways as a result of pressure changes) and a drop in cardiac output as the positive pressure in the chest decreases venous return to the heart.

To care for a patient receiving mechanical ventilation, you will need to be familiar with the types of ventilators in use. You need a thorough understanding of the ventilator you are using, its settings, and how to troubleshoot problems. In the event of a malfunction, if the

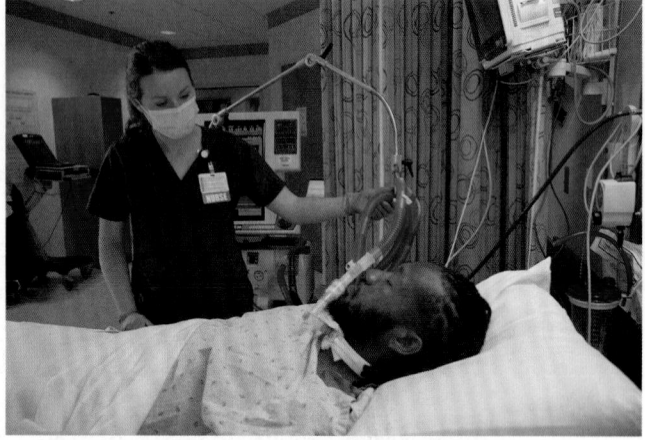

FIGURE 33-14 A patient connected to a ventilator via tracheostomy.

repair is not readily obvious, manually ventilate the patient with an Ambu bag (resuscitation bag) connected to supplemental oxygen while a colleague troubleshoots the problem.

Ventilator-Associated Pneumonia Patients being mechanically ventilated, even for a short period, are at high risk for developing **ventilator-associated pneumonia (VAP).** VAP is associated with high mortality rates. For more information, see the Toward Evidence-Based Practice box and the Example Client Condition: Pneumonia.

The Highlights of Procedures box describes the care of a patient on a mechanical ventilator. For the complete procedure, including ventilator terminology and measures to prevent VAP,

Go to **Chapter 33, Procedure 33-10: Caring for Patients Requiring Mechanical Ventilation,** in Volume 2.

Caring for a Patient Requiring Chest Tubes

Normally, there is negative pressure in the pleural space and only a thin layer of fluid between the membranes.

- **Hemothorax**—Accumulation of fluid and blood in the pleural space interferes with lung expansion, ventilation, and gas exchange.
- **Pneumothorax**—Air in the pleural space creates positive pressure, causing lung tissue to collapse.

The purpose of a chest drainage system is to make room for the lungs to fully expand. This is done by removing air and fluid from the pleural space. A valve in the line or a water-sealed compartment prevents reentry of air and fluid. A chest drainage system is composed of a chest tube inserted into the pleural space and a drainage collection system. The system usually is attached to some form of suction.

The flow of air and fluid must be in one direction: from the patient to the collection system. Think of the chest tube as an extension of the pleural space. To provide negative pressure within the chest tube, the open end of the tube is placed under water. With each exhalation, air is expelled through the chest tube into the water, but no air is drawn in during inhalation (Fig. 33-15). Once all air is expelled from the pleural space, negative pressure is reestablished, and the lung can fully expand. When the lung tissue is reexpanded, the chest tube can be safely removed.

Types of Drainage Systems

Various chest drainage systems are available, including the older, reusable, glass, three-bottle, water-seal system. However, you will most often use a disposable system. These are more compact and lightweight. Disposable systems may be water-seal or dry-seal and may or may not use suction. To learn how to set up disposable chest drainage systems,

Go to **Chapter 33, Procedure 33-11: Setting Up Disposable Chest Drainage Systems,** in Volume 2.

Water-Seal Systems Water-seal systems can consist of one, two, or three chambers (or bottles in the traditional glass bottle system).

- **A one-chamber device** is the simplest chest drainage system. The chest tube connects to one drainage chamber, which serves as both a collector and a water seal. This system can handle only small volumes of fluid or air. As fluid drains through the chest tube, it

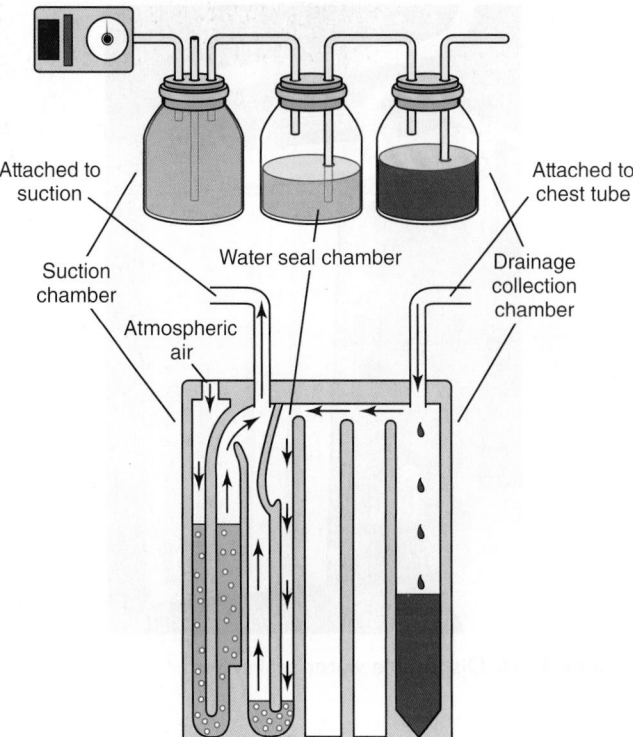

FIGURE 33-15 A disposable chest drainage system.

raises the fluid level in the chamber, making it harder for the patient to exhale. It is important that the device not be tipped over because the vent tube would no longer be below the water, and air would enter the pleural space.

- **A two-chamber system** has one chamber that connects directly with the chest tube and serves as a collection bottle. The second chamber serves as the water seal; it maintains negative pressure as air flows through it. Because the chest drainage never enters the water-seal chamber, you can measure the amount of drainage more accurately. The two-chamber system can handle large amounts of fluid drainage, but its design can still contribute to labored breathing.
- **A three-chamber system** adds a third chamber, which connects to the water-seal chamber and is placed to suction (Fig. 33-16). This creates controlled negative pressure within the system. The suction control chamber has three vent tubes: one connected to suction, one connected to the water-seal chamber, and a long middle tube with one end open to air at the top. The amount of sterile water in the suction chamber determines the maximum suction possible within the system. Suction pressure is expressed in centimeters of water.

For proper functioning, adjust the suction regulator to create gentle bubbling in the suction control bottle.

Dry-Seal Systems Dry-seal systems are fairly new. They are a one-piece device with three chambers: fluid collection, dry seal, and dry suction control. They do

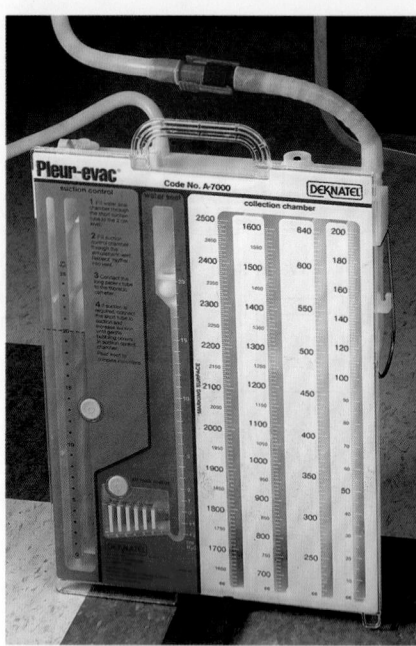

FIGURE 33-16 Disposable water-seal system.

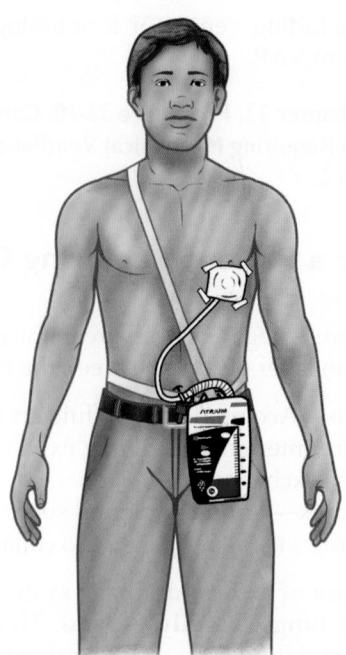

FIGURE 33-17 A one-chamber, dry-seal, portable chest drainage system.

not use water in the suction chamber, relying instead on a mechanical automatic control valve (ACV) and an air leak monitor. The valve allows air to pass out of the patient and prevents it from returning to the patient—even if the system is knocked over. Pressure is set by adjusting the rotary suction dial. The ACV keeps the pressure constant by adjusting to changes in air leaks and fluctuations in the suction source.

Portable Systems Portable or mobile systems consist of a single dry-seal chamber attached to the patient's chest tube (Fig. 33-17). It drains by gravity but can be connected to wall suction.

- **Advantages:** (1) Portable systems improve ambulation and reduce the risk of deep vein thrombosis and pulmonary embolism. (2) Portable systems are thought to decrease the length of time a patient must stay in the hospital.
- **Disadvantages:** The collection chamber holds a maximum of 500 mL, so portable systems are not practical for patients whose drainage is more than 500 mL daily.

For more information on how to set up disposable chest drainage systems, see the Highlights of Procedures box, and

 Go to **Chapter 33, Procedure 33-11: Setting Disposable Chest Drainage Systems,** in Volume 2.

For guidelines to help you manage care for patients with chest tubes,

 Go to **Chapter 34, Clinical Insight 34-5: Managing Chest Tubes,** in Volume 2.

KnowledgeCheck 33-13

- What is the purpose of mechanical ventilation?
- Why is a chest tube inserted?
- What is the advantage of a three-chamber system (compared with a one-chamber or two-chamber system)?
- How does a portable chest drainage system compare to a water-seal drainage system?

For steps to follow in *all* procedures, refer to the Universal Steps for All Procedures found on the inside back cover of Volume 2. Go to the full procedures in Volume 2 to practice and learn the procedure steps. Use these procedure highlights later to help you review key points.

Procedure 33-1: Collecting a Sputum Specimen

Procedure 33-1A: Collecting an Expectorated Sputum Specimen

➤ Use a high- or semi-Fowler's position, or use a sitting position at the edge of the bed.

➤ If the patient has an abdominal or chest incision, have the patient splint the incision with a pillow.

➤ Caution the patient not to touch the inside of the sterile container or lid.

➤ Instruct the patient to breathe deeply for three or four breaths, cough forcefully, then expectorate in the container.

➤ Cover the specimen container immediately, and label the specimen container with the patient's name, test name, and collection date and time.

➤ Place the specimen in a plastic bag with a biohazard label. Follow agency policy.

➤ Send the specimen to the laboratory immediately. If specimen transport is delayed, consult the laboratory; refrigeration may be required.

Procedure 33-1B: Collecting a Suctioned Sputum Specimen

➤ Position patient in a high- or semi-Fowler's position.

➤ Administer oxygen to the patient if indicated.

➤ Don protective eyewear.

➤ Attach the suction tubing to the male adapter of the inline sputum specimen container.

➤ Don sterile gloves.

➤ Attach the sterile suction catheter to the rubber tubing on the inline sputum specimen container.

➤ Lubricate the suction catheter with sterile saline solution.

➤ Insert the tip of the suction catheter through the nasopharynx, endotracheal tube, or tracheostomy tube. Advance into the trachea.

➤ When the patient begins coughing, apply suction for 5 to 10 seconds to collect the specimen.

➤ If an adequate specimen is not obtained, allow the patient to rest for 1 minute, and then repeat the procedure. Administer oxygen at this time, if indicated.

➤ When an adequate specimen is collected, discontinue suction, then gently remove the suction catheter.

➤ Label the specimen container.

➤ Place the specimen in a plastic bag with a biohazard label.

➤ Send the specimen to the laboratory immediately. If specimen transport is delayed, consult the laboratory; refrigeration may be required.

Procedure 33-2: Monitoring Pulse Oximetry (Arterial Oxygen Saturation)

➤ Choose a sensor that is appropriate for the patient's age, size, and weight and for the desired location.

➤ Prepare the site by cleaning and drying it. Remove nail polish if the finger is the desired location.

➤ Remove the protective backing and attach the probe sensor to the site, with photodetector and light-emitting diodes facing each other.

➤ Connect the sensor probe to the oximeter, and turn it on.

➤ Read the SaO_2 measurement on the digital display when it reaches a constant value.

➤ If continuous monitoring is necessary, set and turn on the alarm limits for SaO_2 and pulse rate, according to the manufacturer's instructions, patient condition, and agency policy.

➤ Rotate the site as required.

➤ When monitoring is no longer needed, remove the probe sensor, and turn off the oximeter.

Procedure 33-3: Performing Percussion, Vibration, and Postural Drainage

➤ Help the patient assume the appropriate position based on the lung field that requires drainage.

➤ Keep the patient in the desired position for 10 to 15 minutes.

➤ Using cupped hands, perform percussion over the affected lung area for 1 to 3 minutes while the patient is in the desired drainage position.

➤ Next, perform vibration.

➤ Assist the patient to sit up. Ask the patient to cough at the end of a deep inspiration to clear the airways of secretions.

➤ Repeat postural drainage, percussion, and vibration for each lung field that requires treatment. The entire treatment should not exceed 60 minutes.

➤ Provide mouth care.

Procedure 33-4: Administering Oxygen

➤ Attach the flow meter to the oxygen source.

➤ Assemble and apply the oxygen equipment according to the device prescribed (nasal cannula, face mask, or face tent).

➤ Attach the humidifier to the flow meter.

➤ Turn on the oxygen using the flow meter, and adjust according to the prescribed flow rate.

➤ Double-check that the oxygen equipment is set up correctly and functioning properly.

➤ Assess the patient's respiratory status before you leave the bedside.

Procedure 33-5A: Performing Tracheostomy Care Using Modified Sterile Technique

➤ Position the patient in a semi-Fowler's position.

➤ Don personal protective equipment (PPE; gown, eye protection, and clean procedure gloves).

➤ Hyperoxygenate the patient as needed, and suction the tracheostomy.

➤ Remove soiled dressing; remove gloves; perform hand hygiene.

Continued

- Using clean technique, open and prepare supplies (disposable wipes, one cotton-tipped applicator, new disposable inner cannula, Velcro tracheostomy ties or twill tape).
- Don clean procedure gloves.
- Remove the oxygen source, using nondominant hand, if the patient is receiving supplemental oxygen, and attach to outer cannula if possible. If not possible, have the respiratory therapist set up a blow-by while you clean the inner cannula.
- Unlock and remove the inner cannula with your nondominant hand, and care for it accordingly.
- Clean the stoma under the faceplate with the cotton-tip applicators saturated with filtered tap water or normal saline.
- Clean the top surface of the faceplate and the skin around it with the gauze pads and cotton-tip applicators saturated with filtered tap water or normal saline. Use each wipe once and discard.
- Dry the skin around the faceplate and stoma with dry sterile gauze.
- With the help of an assistant, remove soiled tracheostomy stabilizers.
- Ask the patient to flex their neck, and apply new tracheostomy ties.
- Insert a precut, sterile tracheostomy dressing under the faceplate and new ties.

Procedure 33-5B: Performing Tracheostomy Care Using Modified Sterile Technique

- Position the patient in a semi-Fowler's position.
- Don PPE (gown, eye protection, and clean procedure gloves).
- Hyperoxygenate the patient as needed, and suction the tracheostomy.
- Remove soiled dressing; remove gloves; perform hand hygiene.
- Set up sterile field and prepare the equipment, keeping supplies sterile.
- Don sterile gloves.
- Remove the oxygen source, if the patient is receiving supplemental oxygen, and attach to outer cannula if possible. If not possible, have the respiratory therapist set up a blow-by and clean the inner cannula before proceeding.
- Unlock and remove the inner cannula with your nondominant hand, and care for it accordingly.
- Clean the stoma under the faceplate with the cotton-tip applicators saturated with normal saline solution.
- Clean the top surface of the faceplate and the skin around it with the gauze pads and cotton-tip applicators saturated with normal saline.
- Dry the skin around the faceplate and stoma with dry sterile gauze.
- With the help of an assistant, remove soiled tracheostomy stabilizers.

- Ask the patient to flex their neck, and apply new tracheostomy ties.
- Don a new pair of sterile procedure gloves.
- Insert a precut, sterile tracheostomy dressing under the faceplate and new stabilizers.

Procedure 33-6: Performing Tracheostomy Suctioning (Open System)

- Suction only when necessary.
- Use a suction catheter that is no more than half the internal diameter of the airway tube.
- Position the patient in a semi-Fowler's position.
- Don PPE (face shield or goggles and protective gown).
- Adjust the suction regulator according to agency policy, using the lowest possible suction pressure.

  Adults: 100 to 150 mm Hg

  Children: 100 to 120 mm Hg

  Infants: 50 to 95 mm Hg

- Don a nonsterile glove and test suction equipment by occluding the connection tubing.
- Remove glove, open suction catheter, and maintain sterility of inside of suction kit or gathered supplies.
- Don gloves according to agency policy and prepare sterile saline and suction catheter.
- Don sterile gloves. (Dominant hand is sterile; nondominant is unsterile.)
- Using your dominant hand, attach the suction catheter to the connecting tubing, and suction a small amount of normal saline solution through the suction catheter.
- Hyperoxygenate the patient if desired.
- Lubricate catheter tip with normal saline and insert the catheter gently, without suction.
- Advance the suction catheter, gently aiming downward, no further than the carina tracheae (or a maximum of 6 inches).

  Do not force the catheter.

  Do not apply suction as you enter the airway.

- Apply continuous suction as you withdraw the catheter. Apply suction for no longer than 15 seconds.
- Avoid saline lavage during suctioning.
- Repeat suctioning as needed, allowing intervals of at least 30 seconds between suctioning.
- Hyperoxygenate the patient between each pass.
- Use normal saline to clear secretions from the catheter.
- Replace the oxygen source when finished.
- Provide mouth care and reposition the patient.

Procedure 33-7: Performing Tracheostomy or Endotracheal Suctioning (Inline Closed System)

- Position the patient in a semi-Fowler's position unless contraindicated.
- Don clean procedure gloves.

➤ Unlock the suction control port (if a lock is present).

➤ Adjust the suction regulator according to guidelines or agency policy.

➤ Hyperoxygenate the patient according to agency policy.

➤ Insert the suction catheter within the sterile sleeve, gently, with suction off.

➤ Advance the suction catheter gently, aiming downward, no farther than the carina trachea (premeasure). Do not force the catheter.

➤ Do not apply suction as you enter the airway.

➤ Apply continuous suction as you withdraw the catheter, but for no longer than 15 seconds.

➤ Avoid saline lavage during suctioning.

➤ Repeat suctioning as needed, allowing at least 30 seconds between each suctioning.

➤ Hyperoxygenate the patient between each pass.

➤ Withdraw suction catheter completely into the sleeve, until you see the indicator line.

➤ Use normal saline to clear secretions from the catheter.

➤ Lock the suction regulator port.

Procedure 33-8: Performing Orotracheal and Nasotracheal Suctioning (Open System)

➤ Position the patient in a semi-Fowler's position.

➤ Don PPE (face shield or goggles and protective gown).

➤ Adjust suction pressure according to guidelines or agency policy. Typically:

Adults: 100 to 150 mm Hg

Children: 100 to 120 mm Hg

Infants: 80 to 100 mm Hg

Neonates: 60 to 80 mm Hg

➤ Don procedure gloves and test equipment by occluding the connection tubing.

➤ Prepare the suction equipment. For the nasotracheal (NT) approach, open the water-soluble lubricant.

➤ Don clean nonsterile gloves (sterile gloves in using sterile technique).

➤ Using nondominant hand, pour sterile saline into saline container.

➤ Holding the suction catheter in your dominant hand, attach it to the connection tubing.

➤ Suction a small amount of normal saline solution through the suction catheter.

➤ Preoxygenate the patient, if indicated.

➤ Premeasure the approximate depth to which the suction catheter should be inserted, and insert nasopharyngeal airway if using a nasal approach.

➤ Lubricate and insert the catheter, and advance it to the pharynx as the patient inhales.

➤ Advance the catheter to the predetermined distance as the patient inhales.

➤ Apply suction (no longer than 15 seconds) while you withdraw the catheter, using a continuous rotating motion.

➤ Withdraw the catheter and clear it with sterile saline.

➤ Repeat lubrication and suctioning as needed, allowing intervals of at least 30 seconds between suctioning.

➤ Replace the oxygen source.

➤ Coil the suction catheter in your dominant hand. Pull the sterile glove off over the coiled catheter. Discard in a biohazard receptacle.

➤ Make sure new suction supplies are readily available for future suctioning.

➤ Provide mouth care.

Procedure 33-9: Performing Upper Airway Suctioning

➤ Position the patient in a semi-Fowler's position.

Oropharyngeal: Patient's face turned toward you

Nasopharyngeal: Neck hyperextended

➤ Adjust suction regulator according to agency policy. Typically:

Adult: 100 to 120 mm Hg

Children: 95 to 110 mm Hg

Infants: 50 to 95 mm Hg.

➤ Test the suction equipment by occluding connection tubing.

➤ Open and prepare suction equipment.

➤ If using the nasal approach, open the water-soluble lubricant.

➤ Don PPE (face shield or goggles and gown) and procedure gloves.

➤ Pour sterile saline into sterile container, using nondominant hand.

➤ Using your dominant hand, attach the suction catheter to the connection tubing and suction a small amount of sterile saline through the suction catheter.

➤ Approximate the depth to which the suction catheter should be inserted.

➤ Remove the oxygen delivery device, if necessary.

➤ Lubricate and insert the suction catheter.

➤ Gently and quickly advance the catheter into the naris.

➤ Advance suction catheter, aiming downward, to the premeasured distance. Do not force catheter.

➤ Engage the suction and apply it while you withdraw the catheter, using a continuous rotating motion.

➤ Clear the catheter with sterile saline.

➤ Lubricate the catheter and repeat suctioning as needed, allowing 20-second intervals between suctioning.

➤ Coil the suction catheter in your dominant hand. Pull the sterile glove off over the coiled catheter. Discard in a biohazard receptacle.

➤ Make sure new suction supplies are readily available for future suctioning.

➤ Provide mouth care.

Continued

Procedure 33-10: Caring for Patients Requiring Mechanical Ventilation

➤ Prepare the resuscitation bag; keep it at the bedside.

➤ Respiratory therapists are responsible for setting up mechanical ventilation in most agencies. If you must assume the responsibility, refer to the manufacturer's instructions and:

  ➤ Verify ventilator settings with the medical prescription.

  ➤ Make sure the ventilator alarm limits are set appropriately.

  ➤ Don PPE (gloves, gown, and eye protection).

  ➤ Attach the ventilator tubing to the endotracheal tube or tracheostomy tube, and secure the ventilator tubing.

  ➤ Attach capnography device, if available.

  ➤ Prepare the inline suctioning equipment.

After the initial ventilator setup:

➤ Check arterial blood gases and assess respiratory status about 30 minutes after setup.

➤ Check the ventilator tubing frequently for condensation.

  Drain the condensate into a collection device, or briefly disconnect the patient from the ventilator and empty the tubing into a waste receptacle, according to agency policy.

  Never drain the condensate into the humidifier.

➤ Maintain the patient in a semirecumbent position (head of bed at 30° to 45°).

➤ Check ventilator and humidifier settings regularly.

➤ Check the inline thermometer.

➤ Provide the patient with an alternative form of communication.

➤ Reposition the patient regularly (every 1 to 2 hours).

➤ Moisten the lips with a cool, damp cloth and water-based lubricant. Provide regular antiseptic oral care, including mouthwash twice a day for adult patients.

➤ Ensure the call device is within reach; answer the call device and respond to ventilator alarms promptly.

➤ Monitor tracheostomy tube for proper cuff inflation.

➤ Monitor for gastric distention.

➤ Clean, disinfect, or change ventilator tubing and equipment according to agency policy.

➤ Give sedatives or antianxiety drugs as prescribed.

Procedure 33-11: Setting Up Disposable Chest Drainage Systems

➤ Obtain and prepare the prescribed chest drainage unit (CDU).

➤ Position the patient according to the indicated insertion site.

➤ Set up the sterile field and supplies you will need for dressing the insertion site.

➤ Don PPE (mask, gown, and sterile gloves).

➤ As soon as the chest tube is inserted, attach it to the drainage system.

➤ Set the prescribed suction level on the CDU.

➤ Turn on the suction source (usually −80 cm H_2O).

➤ Don a clean pair of sterile gloves.

➤ Using sterile technique, wrap petroleum gauze around the chest tube at the insertion site, and dress the site with two precut sterile drain dressings covered by a large drainage dressing.

➤ Secure the dressing with wide tape to create an occlusive dressing over the insertion site (cover the dressing completely). Date, time, and initial the dressing.

➤ Using the spiral taping technique, wrap 1-inch silk tape around the connections. Wrap from top to bottom and bottom to top. (Or use locking connections, if available.)

➤ With an 8-inch-long piece of 2-inch tape, secure the top end of the drainage tube to the chest tube dressing.

➤ Make sure the tubing lies with no kinks and no dependent areas, in a straight line to the CDU.

➤ Prepare the patient for a portable chest x-ray examination.

➤ Keep emergency supplies at the bedside in the event of tube dislodgement or system failure.

➤ Maintenance: Prevent tubing kinks, ensure patency of the air vent, and keep the system below the level of the chest tube.

➤ Position patient for comfort, and keep the head of the bed elevated to at least 30°.

Procedure 33-12: Inserting an Oropharyngeal Airway

➤ You will need a variety of sizes of airway, procedure gloves, tongue blade, suction equipment, and possibly a handheld resuscitation bag and oxygen source.

➤ Measured on the outside of the cheek, the airway should extend from the front teeth to the end of the jawline.

➤ Don PPE (face shield or goggles, gown, and procedure gloves).

➤ Clear the mouth of debris and secretions. Suction if needed.

➤ Position patient in supine or semi-Fowler's position, neck hyperextended.

➤ Open mouth and remove dentures, if present.

➤ Hold the tongue down with a tongue blade, as needed, and insert the airway in the upside-down position.

➤ Rotate the airway 180° and continue inserting until the front flange is flush with the lips.

➤ Keep the patient's head slightly tilted and chin elevated.

➤ Verify airway patency by auscultating breath sounds.

➤ Do not tape the airway in place.

➤ Position patient on side.

➤ Provide oral hygiene and remove and cleanse airway at regular intervals.

Highlights of Procedures 33-1 Through 33-13

Procedure 33-13: Inserting a Nasopharyngeal Airway

➤ You will need a correctly sized nasopharyngeal airway, procedure gloves, tongue blade, water-soluble lubricant, suction equipment, and possibly a handheld resuscitation bag and oxygen source.

➤ Measured on the outside of the cheek, the airway should extend from the tip of the nose to the earlobe. It should be slightly smaller than the nares.

➤ Don PPE (face shield or goggles, gown, and procedure gloves).

Position patient in a supine or semi-Fowler's position, neck hyperextended.

➤ Lubricate the airway with water-soluble lubricant.

➤ Advance the airway through the naris until the outer flange rests on the nostril. Do not force.

➤ Visually inspect the top of the posterior pharynx; only the tip of the tube should be visible.

➤ Use your finger to check for air exchange at the naris.

➤ Auscultate the lungs bilaterally.

➤ Remove and clean airway at least every 8 hours and reinsert into other nostril.

To explore learning resources for this chapter,

Go to Davis Advantage and find:

Answers and Suggested Responses for all questions in this chapter

Concept Map

Knowledge Map

References and Bibliography

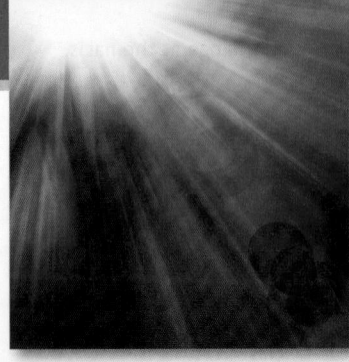

CHAPTER 34

Circulation & Perfusion

Learning Outcomes

After completing this chapter, you should be able to:

➤ Describe the structure and function of the cardiovascular system.

➤ Identify individual, environmental, and pathological factors that influence circulation and perfusion.

➤ Assess/recognize cues for circulation and perfusion.

➤ Interpret diagnostic testing related to circulation and perfusion.

➤ Analyze cues and develop nursing diagnoses related to circulation and perfusion.

➤ Safely and correctly perform common nursing procedures related to circulation and perfusion.

➤ Evaluate adequacy of circulation and perfusion, and modify nursing activities appropriately based on outcomes.

➤ Provide measures to promote peripheral circulation.

➤ Recognize medications used to enhance cardiovascular function.

Key Concepts

Circulation

Perfusion

Related Concepts

See the Concept Map on Davis Advantage.

Example Client Condition

Decreased Cardiac Output

Meet Your Patients

You are scheduled for a clinical placement in an urgent care clinic. For each patient you see, you are to (1) perform a focused assessment related to circulation, (2) perform common therapeutic interventions related to circulation, (3) identify desired outcomes and evaluate achievement of those outcomes, and (4) plan for follow-up and home care needs. One of your clients is Ms. Saunders, a 55-year-old accountant. Ms. Saunders complains of being extremely tired, easily becomes short of breath, and is unable to complete chores without frequent rest breaks. Ms. Saunders is pale and moves slowly. Vital signs are as follows: temperature, 98.4°F (36.7°C); pulse, 86 beats/min; respirations, 24 breaths/min and unlabored; blood pressure, 136/78 mm Hg; and pulse oximetry, 98% on room air. Ms. Saunders is now waiting for laboratory results, which include a complete blood count (CBC).

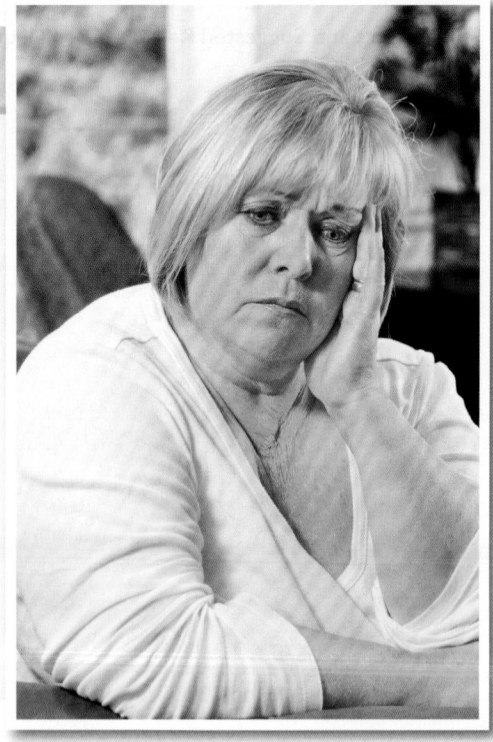

TheoreticalKnowledge
knowing why

As you have learned in Chapter 33, the pulmonary, cardiovascular, musculoskeletal, and neurological systems work together to achieve oxygenation. Changes in one system create changes in the other:

- The lungs oxygenate the blood.
- The heart circulates the blood throughout the body and back to the lungs.
- The circulatory system transports oxygenated blood throughout the body to meet the body's needs.

The theoretical knowledge in this chapter consists of the structures, functions, regulation, and factors affecting the cardiovascular system, as well as factors that affect cardiovascular function.

ABOUT THE KEY CONCEPTS

- **Circulation** refers to flow of blood throughout the heart and blood vessels.
- **Perfusion** describes blood flow to a capillary bed to provide nutrients and oxygen to tissues and organs.

Although the distinction between these two concepts is subtle, they go hand in hand in explaining how a healthy circulatory system contributes to healthy functioning of every organ in the body.

WHAT ARE THE STRUCTURES OF THE CARDIOVASCULAR SYSTEM?

The structures of the cardiovascular system are the heart, the systemic and pulmonary blood vessels, and the coronary arteries.

The Heart

The heart is a four-chambered muscular organ encased in the *pericardium* (a sac of connective tissue) located inside the chest cavity.

- **Atria**—Two thin-walled **atria** receive blood into the heart.
- **Ventricles**—Two thick-walled **ventricles** pump blood out of the heart.
- **Valves** between the heart chambers (a) open widely to allow blood to flow easily and without turbulence from one chamber to another and (b) close tightly to prevent the backflow of blood.
- **The base,** or broadest side of the heart, which houses the atria, faces upward.
- **The apex,** or tip of the heart, which houses the ventricles, faces downward (Fig. 34-1).

A strong, efficient heartbeat keeps blood flowing through the vascular system.

- **Deoxygenated blood** from organs and tissues flows through the venous system and into the right side of the heart and then into the pulmonary circulation.
- **External gas exchange** occurs at the alveolar–capillary membrane.
- **The newly oxygenated blood** then flows from the lungs into the left side of the heart and out into the arterial circulation.

The Cardiac Cycle

The **cardiac cycle** is the sequence of mechanical events that occurs during a single heartbeat. Very simply, it is the simultaneous contraction of the two atria, followed a fraction of a second later by the simultaneous contraction of the ventricles. The electrical activity of the myocardium regulates the cardiac cycle (Fig. 34-2).

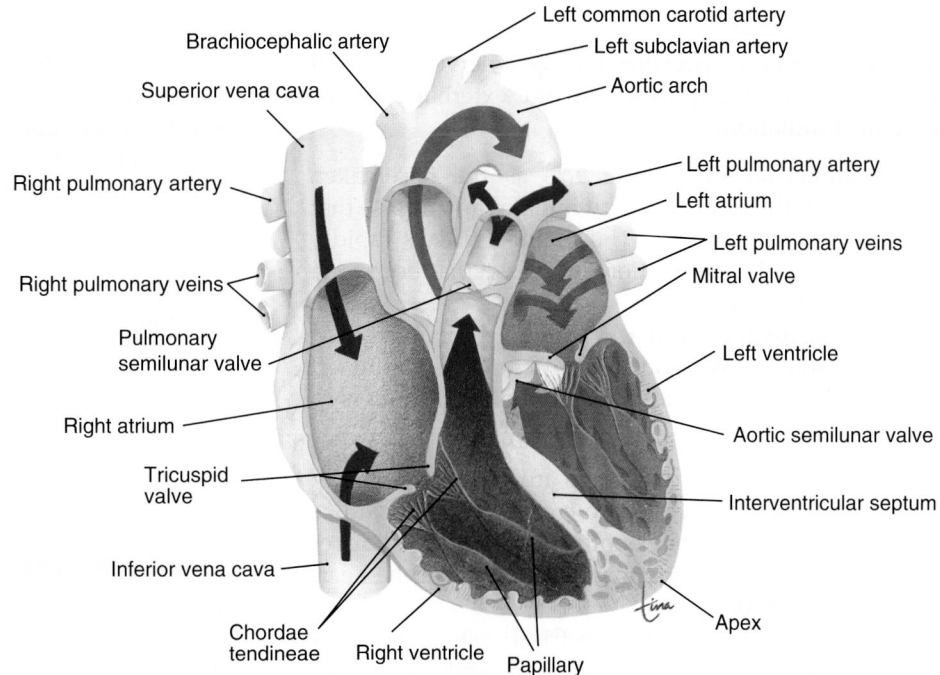

FIGURE 34-1 The atria receive blood into the heart; the ventricles pump blood out of the heart. Valves between the chambers allow blood to flow in one direction from one chamber to another without backflow.

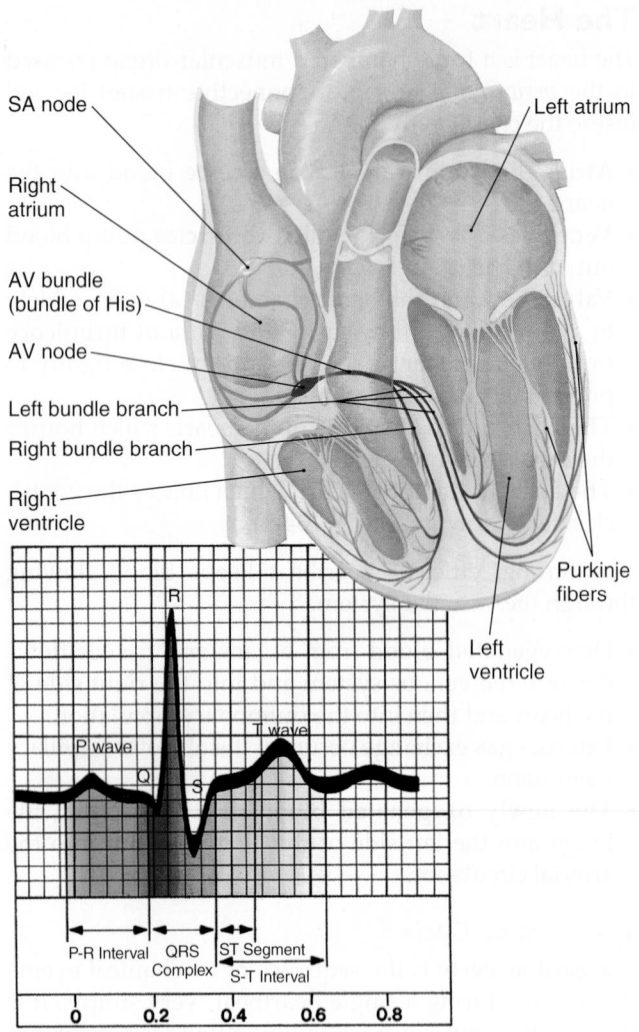

Labels on figure: SA node, Right atrium, AV bundle (bundle of His), AV node, Left bundle branch, Right bundle branch, Right ventricle, Left atrium, Purkinje fibers, Left ventricle. ECG: R, P wave, T wave, Q, S, P-R Interval, QRS Complex, ST Segment, S-T Interval, 0, 0.2, 0.4, 0.6, 0.8

FIGURE 34-2 Conduction pathway of the heart. Anterior view of the interior of the heart. The electrocardiogram tracing is one of a normal heartbeat. See text for description.

Electrical Conduction

The heart contains specialized areas of nerve tissue that initiate electrical impulses without external nervous system stimulation.

- The **sinoatrial (SA) node** acts as the pacemaker. Located in the right atrium, it initiates an impulse that triggers each heartbeat. The impulse travels rapidly down the atrial conduction system so that both atria contract as a unit.
- At the **atrioventricular (AV) node,** there is a slight delay. From the AV node, impulses pass into the left and right *bundles of His* and into the *Purkinje fibers* to the ventricles.

In this way, myocardial fibers are electrically stimulated almost simultaneously to create a unified cardiac muscle contraction strong enough to pump blood out of a heart chamber. This spontaneous rhythm of the heart is called **automaticity.**

If there are defects in this electrical system, impulses travel more slowly through the heart, and some areas

contract before others. This can lead to ineffective heart pumping and decreased cardiac output. For more information, see the Example Client Condition: Decreased Cardiac Output, later in this chapter.

Normally, the SA node is in charge and initiates a rate of 60 to 100 beats/min, depending on the body's oxygen needs.

- *If the SA node fails,* the AV node can take over as the pacemaker, but it generally triggers a slower heart rate.
- *If both the SA and AV nodes fail,* the conduction fibers in the myocardium can initiate impulses. Ventricular conduction generates a very slow rate, usually less than 40 beats/min; however, this can be lifesaving if no other node or fiber is initiating an impulse.

Systemic and Pulmonary Blood Vessels

The vascular system is composed of three types of vessels: arteries, veins, and capillaries. All vessels are lined with a smooth endothelial layer that promotes nonturbulent blood flow and prevents platelets from sticking to the sides of the walls and beginning a clot.

- **Arteries** have thick, elastic walls that allow them to stretch during cardiac contraction **(systole)** and to recoil when the heart relaxes **(diastole).**
- **Arterioles** are smaller branches of arteries.
  - They are primarily smooth muscle and thinner than arteries.
  - They are controlled by the sympathetic nervous system.
  - Arterioles constrict or dilate to vary the amount of blood flowing into capillaries and help maintain blood pressure.
- **Capillaries** are microscopic vessels, created as arterioles branch into smaller and smaller vessels.
  - Capillaries connect the arterial and venous systems and carry blood from arterioles to venules.
  - Because they are only one cell thick, capillaries facilitate the exchange of gases, nutrients, and wastes between the tissue cells and the blood.
  - Billions of capillaries provide blood flow to every cell in the body.
- The **venous system** returns the deoxygenated blood to the heart. **Veins** and **venules** have thin, muscular, but inelastic walls that collapse easily. These walls contract or relax in response to feedback from the sympathetic nervous system: when blood volume is low, the veins contract to provide a smaller space for smaller volume of blood; when blood volume is high, veins relax and enlarge to accommodate the increased volume of blood. Think of the venous system as a holding tank for fluctuations in blood volume.

Coronary Arteries

The heart has its own blood supply through the coronary arteries (Fig. 34-3). The coronary sinus (not shown in Fig. 34-3), located just above the aortic valve, fills with

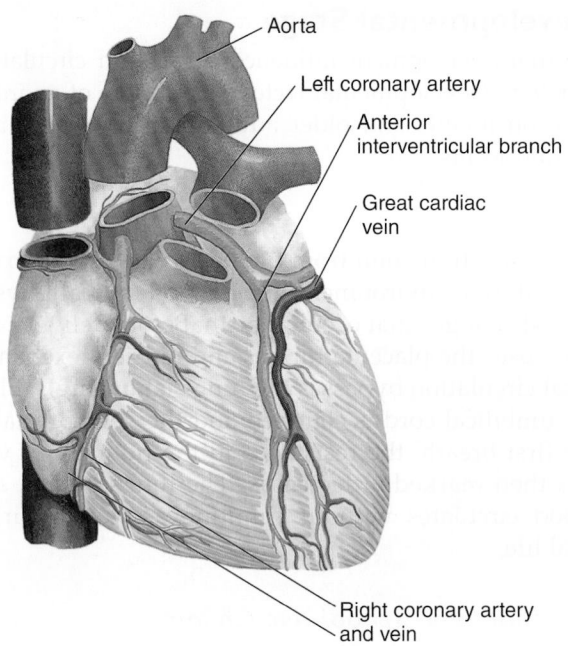

- Aorta
- Left coronary artery
- Anterior interventricular branch
- Great cardiac vein
- Right coronary artery and vein

FIGURE 34-3 Coronary vessels in anterior view. The pulmonary artery has been cut to show the left coronary artery emerging from the ascending aorta.

blood during diastole. From the coronary sinus, blood flows into the two main coronary arteries, which branch into several sections to supply the heart muscle with blood. The coronary arteries are the only arteries in the body that fill during diastole.

KnowledgeCheck 34-1
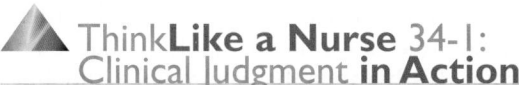

- Describe *oxygenation* and *perfusion*.
- Trace the path of normal electrical impulses in the heart.
- How do the walls of arteries, veins, and capillaries differ?
- What is the importance of diastole to perfusion of the heart?

▲ ThinkLike a Nurse 34-1: Clinical Judgment in Action

Your patient has a condition that has caused the mitral valve to become stiff, with only a narrow opening for blood flow. What type of problems related to oxygenation would you anticipate in this patient?

HOW ARE OXYGEN AND CARBON DIOXIDE TRANSPORTED?

The cardiovascular system circulates oxygenated blood to organs and tissues and returns deoxygenated blood to the heart. Maintaining this blood flow requires (1) adequate circulation and (2) effective regulation of cardiovascular function.

Hemoglobin—A reservoir for oxygen

- Of total blood oxygen, 97% is bound to hemoglobin, the iron-containing protein in red blood cells; only 3% is in a dissolved state.

- At the tissue level, O_2 leaves the hemoglobin, becomes dissolved in the blood, and passes through the capillary membrane into the tissues.
- **Key Point:** *Only the dissolved form of O_2 can pass through capillary membranes.*

Hemoglobin thereby serves as a reservoir for oxygen until it is needed in the dissolved state.

Carbon Dioxide CO_2 is a waste product of normal aerobic tissue metabolism. **Key Point:** *CO_2 diffuses through cellular and alveolar–capillary membranes only in its dissolved state.*

Carbon dioxide can be carried in the blood in three ways. Approximately:

- **7% of CO_2 is dissolved in plasma.**
- **23% attaches to hemoglobin.** The CO_2 bound to hemoglobin eventually detaches and becomes dissolved in the plasma for diffusion into the alveoli of the lungs.
- **70% is converted into bicarbonate ions.** The bicarbonate ions in the plasma are converted back to CO_2, which becomes dissolved, diffuses into the alveoli, and is exhaled.

HOW IS CARDIOVASCULAR FUNCTION REGULATED?

Cardiovascular function is regulated by the autonomic nervous system (ANS) and by control centers in the brainstem.

Autonomic Nervous System

The ANS regulates cardiovascular function through its influence on (a) cardiac rate, (b) cardiac muscle contractility, and (c) vascular tone.

Heart Through branches at the thoracic level of the spinal cord:

- **Sympathetic fibers** stimulate the heart to beat faster and contract more strongly.
- **Parasympathetic fibers** innervate the heart through the vagus nerve. Parasympathetic stimulation results in a slowed heart rate, but it does not influence myocardial contractility.

Vascular System All blood vessels are innervated by *sympathetic fibers*. The *parasympathetic nervous system* has no significant control over blood vessels.

- **Sympathetic control maintains the blood vessels in a constant baseline state of partial contraction (tone).** Vascular tone maintains blood pressure and blood flow even when a person is resting or asleep.
- **Sympathetic stimulation above and beyond baseline tone varies in response to body needs.** Increased sympathetic stimulation causes (a) *constriction* of some vessels (e.g., skin, gastrointestinal tract, and kidneys) and (b) *dilation* of other vessels (e.g., in skeletal

muscle). This shunts blood flow to the skeletal muscles for a fight-or-flight response.

For more complete information, consult an anatomy and physiology text.

Brainstem Centers

The brainstem centers integrate feedback from baroreceptors and chemoreceptors in the body to regulate cardiac function and blood pressure.

- The **vasomotor center** controls sympathetic stimulation of the heart and vascular system.
- The **cardioinhibitory center** controls parasympathetic slowing of the heart rate.

Baroreceptors Baroreceptors located in the walls of the heart and blood vessels are sensitive to pressure changes. The aortic arch and carotid artery baroreceptors are particularly important in the regulation of heart rate and vascular tone. When baroreceptors sense even a small drop in pressure, they send messages to the brainstem centers to stimulate the sympathetic nervous system to increase heart rate and induce vasoconstriction. This mechanism allows us to change positions and maintain blood pressure.

Chemoreceptors Chemoreceptors located in the aortic arch and the carotid arteries are sensitive to changes in blood pH, oxygen levels, and carbon dioxide levels. Their main function is to regulate ventilation, but they also send information to the vasomotor center in response to a lack of oxygen. The vasomotor center responds by activating sympathetic stimulation.

KnowledgeCheck 34-2

- How are oxygen and carbon dioxide transported in the blood?
- How is the cardiovascular system regulated?
- Does poor peripheral perfusion increase the risk for hypoxemia (a low level of oxygen in the blood)?

 ThinkLike a Nurse 34-2:
        Clinical Judgment in Action

You are assigned the care of a 4-year-old with a history of asthma. Your patient is receiving a nebulized treatment containing albuterol and ipratropium bromide. These medications stimulate the sympathetic nervous system.

- What cardiovascular side effects can you anticipate?
- How might these side effects affect oxygenation?
- What do you need to know about the patient's history to safely administer the drugs?

WHAT FACTORS INFLUENCE CARDIOVASCULAR FUNCTION?

Similar to respiratory function, cardiovascular function is influenced by developmental stage, environment, lifestyle, substance abuse, medications, and pathophysiological conditions.

Developmental Stage

Normal development influences heart and circulatory function. Developmental factors exert more of an influence on infants and older adults than on young and middle adults.

Infants

Successful transition from life inside the uterus to the extrauterine environment depends on critical physiological changes that occur at birth. Before delivery, the fetus uses the placenta for gas and nutrient exchange. Fetal circulation bypasses the lungs **(shunting).** When the umbilical cord is clamped and the newborn takes the first breath, the resistance in the pulmonary vessels then markedly decreases. The lungs inflate, and blood circulates without shunting as it did during fetal life.

Preschool and School-Age Children

The heart and circulatory systems of preschool and school-age children are mature enough to adapt to moderate stress and change. However, even school-age children sometimes begin social habits, such as *tobacco use,* that can have long-term adverse effects on the cardiovascular system.

- *A diet high in fats and sugars* contributes to hyperlipidemia and the beginning of plaque lining the walls of blood vessels.
- *Processed foods contain a great deal of salt and fat*, which can contribute to high blood pressure and high cholesterol, even in children.

Adolescents

In adolescence, the heart and blood components develop adult characteristics. The average adolescent is developmentally at little risk for heart or circulatory disorders, although some athletes can be at risk for collapse and sudden cardiac dysrhythmia that is familial. Guidelines for health professionals performing sports assessments call for thorough investigation of the family history for fainting, collapse, or sudden death. Some adolescents adopt behaviors and habits that can create risk throughout life.

- **Tobacco use**—Of adults who use tobacco, 87% were regular smokers by their 18th birthday, and almost half of middle and high school students reported using two or more tobacco products on one or more of the 30 days preceding the survey (American Lung Association, 2020).
- **Obesity**—The overall incidence of childhood obesity in the United States has risen to epidemic levels. As a result, some adolescents exhibit signs of cardiovascular disease (e.g., high blood levels of lipids and cholesterol, a known factor in the development of high blood pressure, heart disease, and blockages in the arteries of the heart).

Young and Middle Adults

Lifestyle in young and middle adulthood can create cardiac risk factors.

- **Poor nutrition**—Some adults become "too busy" to prepare and eat nourishing foods or simply prefer the taste of high-fat, high-sugar foods.
- **Lack of exercise**—A sedentary lifestyle and lack of aerobic exercise contribute to cardiovascular disorders in this group.
- **Substance abuse**—Tobacco use is a risk factor for cardiovascular disorders. Crack cocaine and methamphetamine abuse can lead to sudden cardiac failure.
- **Family history** of cardiovascular disease is yet another risk factor for this age-group.

Older Adults

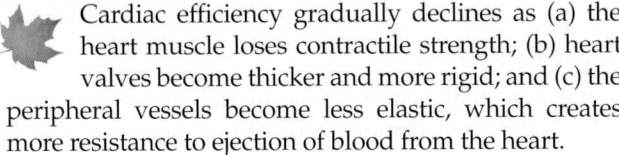 Cardiac efficiency gradually declines as (a) the heart muscle loses contractile strength; (b) heart valves become thicker and more rigid; and (c) the peripheral vessels become less elastic, which creates more resistance to ejection of blood from the heart.

As a result of these changes, the heart becomes less able to respond to increased oxygen demands, and it needs longer recovery times after responding. For example, in response to exercise, an older adult's heart rate does not increase as much as a younger person's, but it does remain elevated longer. Thus, older adults have lower exercise tolerance, need more rest after exercise, and are more prone to orthostatic hypotension.

Key Point: *Keep in mind, though, that endurance training and regular exercise slow the rate of these changes.* In fact, an older person who is physically conditioned by regular exercise may have better heart and circulatory function than a younger adult who is not well conditioned.

Environment

Environmental factors, such as stress, allergic reactions and air quality, altitude, and temperature, affect cardiovascular function.

Stress

The stress response stimulates the release of catecholamines from the sympathetic nervous system. This results in increased heart rate and contractility, vasoconstriction, and increased tendency of blood to clot. **Key Point:** *Sustained stimulation of the sympathetic nervous system can lead to cardiovascular disease.*

In addition, a chronically suppressed immune and inflammatory response increases the risk for all infections. For additional information on the effects of stress, see Chapter 9.

Allergic Reactions and Air Quality

An **allergy** is a hypersensitivity, or overresponse, to an antigen. Inflammatory substances released during an allergic response (e.g., histamine, protease) cause the following cardiovascular events:

- Blood vessels dilate in areas affected (which increases blood flow to the areas).
- Eosinophils and neutrophils are attracted to the reaction site.
- Local tissues are damaged by protease.
- Capillaries become more permeable, resulting in fluid leak into tissues.
- Local (e.g., vascular) smooth muscle cells contract.

Altitude

Oxygen pressure falls proportionally with increased altitude (to review, refer to Chapter 33), making more oxygen available in the alveoli and at the tissue level. Over the long term, people who live at high altitudes undergo physiological changes that facilitate oxygenation. Among the cardiopulmonary changes are the following:

- Increased production of red blood cells (RBCs)
- Increased vascularity of body tissues
- Increased ability of tissue cells to use oxygen even when atmospheric oxygen pressure is low

Heat and Cold

- **Heat generally causes vasodilation,** which increases cardiac output and oxygenation.
- **Heat also increases metabolism.** As a result, people are naturally more sedentary in hot weather.
- **Cold slows cell metabolism,** reducing O_2 demand.
- **Cold also causes vasoconstriction** and slows the heart rate.
  - **Examples:**
    Induced hypothermia is used in some medical and surgical procedures.
    Victims of cold-water near-drowning have been revived after long periods of time, in part because of the reduced O_2 demands associated with hypothermia.
  - **Prolonged exposure to cold** causes frostbite, loss of hypothalamic temperature regulation, and death.

Lifestyle

Lifestyle factors that affect cardiovascular function include pregnancy, nutrition, obesity, exercise, tobacco use, and substance abuse.

Pregnancy

During pregnancy, oxygen demand increases dramatically because of the needs of the fetus. Therefore:

- **Maternal metabolism increases** by approximately 15% during the last half of pregnancy.
- **Maternal blood volume increases** by 30% to compensate.
- **Maternal iron requirements increase** in order to (1) produce the extra blood and (2) meet fetal requirements. Failure to meet these iron demands can result in maternal

anemia, reducing tissue oxygenation to the mother and fetus.

Nutrition

The body needs an appropriate balance of proteins, carbohydrates, fats, and other nutrients for proper immune function, resistance to disease and infection, normal cellular function and tissue repair, and maintenance of a healthy weight.

- **A diet high in saturated fat** predisposes a person to atherosclerosis, coronary artery disease, and hypertension, all of which can compromise circulation and oxygenation. A low-fat, low-cholesterol, low-sodium diet is considered "heart healthy."
- **Vitamins, minerals (especially iron), and protein** are important to prevent anemia, which reduces the oxygen-carrying capacity of the blood.
- **Green tea** consumption has been associated with reduced mortality due to cardiovascular disease (Fang et al., 2019).

Obesity

Obesity is a body mass index (BMI) of 30 or above (see Chapter 24). Obesity can contribute to multiple health problems, many of which affect the heart and circulation.

- Obesity increases the risk of developing atherosclerosis and hypertension.
- Excess fat stores in and around the heart itself reduce its effectiveness as a pump.
- The workload of the heart is increased by the need to perfuse the excess body tissues.

Exercise

Exercise improves blood circulation and delivery of oxygen to tissues and cells. It also increases metabolic demands.

- The body responds by increasing the heart rate and the rate and depth of breathing.
- Like skeletal muscles, the heart muscle is strengthened with regular aerobic exercise. As the heart becomes stronger, it becomes a more efficient pump.
- As a result, the resting heart rate is slower because a higher heart rate is not required to maintain cardiac output.

  Lack of exercise has the opposite effect.

- A sedentary lifestyle reduces the efficiency of the heart and the capacity to increase ventilation in response to exercise. See Chapter 29 for more information about the effects of exercise and activity on cardiovascular health.

Tobacco Use

Key Point: *Tobacco use is a major risk factor in several chronic cardiovascular conditions: stroke, peripheral arterial disease, aortic aneurysm, and heart disease.*

Smoking has been shown to cause atherosclerosis (fatty buildups in the arteries), hypertension, and decreased high-density lipoprotein (HDL) (good) cholesterol—all of which lead to coronary heart disease and heart attack.

- The risk of coronary artery disease is four times higher in cigarette smokers than it is in nonsmokers.
- Cigarette smoking doubles a person's risk for stroke.

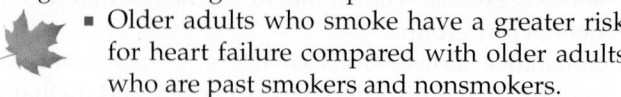

- Older adults who smoke have a greater risk for heart failure compared with older adults who are past smokers and nonsmokers.
- Former smokers' risks are related to how long they have smoked.
- Even light smoking increases the risk of sudden cardiac death.
- Cigar and pipe smoking are also implicated but not to the extent of cigarettes (Rostron et al., 2019).

Substance Abuse

Substances that people abuse include over-the-counter (OTC) and prescription medications, commonly available commercial products, and illegal substances.

- **Large amounts of alcohol** depress the respiratory, cardiac, and vasomotor centers of the brain. Chronic alcohol abuse causes fatty infiltration of the heart muscle, thrombi in the coronary arteries, heart enlargement, and dysrhythmias, all of which can ultimately lead to heart failure.
- **Illicit drugs,** including stimulants (e.g., methamphetamine, cocaine), hallucinogens (e.g., LSD [acid], mescaline [buttons]), and cannabinoids (e.g., marijuana), also have adverse effects on the cardiovascular system (e.g., links to myocardial dysfunction, dysrhythmias, endocarditis, and aortic dissection).

Medications

Various types of medication are used to improve cardiac output and tissue oxygenation. They act to slow the heart rate or reduce the force of myocardial contraction, ease the workload of the heart, dilate blood vessels and reduce blood pressure in the pulmonary circulation and systemically, rid the body of excess fluid accumulation, and block abnormal heart rhythms (American Heart Association, 2020). See Table 34-1.

Aspirin Aspirin blocks the production of prostaglandin, a hormone-like substance that activates the formation of blood clots, signals an injury, and triggers pain. This helps reduce the risk of heart attack or stroke from clot-blocked arteries, decreases pain and inflammation, and reduces the short-term risk of death among people suffering from heart attacks. A low-dose aspirin regimen can help prevent cardiovascular disease in patients aged 40 to 69 years, but current guidelines recommend that patients begin an aspirin regimen only after weighing the risks and benefits with their primary care provider (Arnett et al., 2019).

Toward Evidence-Based Practice

Thurston, R. C., Aslanidou Vlachos, H. E., Derby, C. A., Jackson, E. A., Brooks, M. M., Matthews, K. A., Harlow, S., Joffe, H., & El Khoudary, S. R. (2021). Menopausal vasomotor symptoms and risk of incident cardiovascular disease events in SWAN. *Journal of the American Heart Association, 10*(3), e017416.

A longitudinal study of 3,083 women (48% White, 28% Black, 9% Japanese, 8% Chinese, and 7% Hispanic) aged 42 to 52 years at baseline took place over a 22-year period. Participants were not experiencing clinical cardiovascular disease (CVD) symptoms or history (with the exception of hypertension) at baseline. Participants underwent initial and follow-up assessments, including questionnaires on vasomotor symptom (VMS) frequency, physical measures, blood work, and reported CVD events (myocardial infarction, stroke, heart failure, and revascularization). Over the time period of the study, a subset of events was obtained from individual medical records and death certificates. Researchers analyzed the data to determine whether a relationship existed between baseline VMS or persistent VMS and incidents of nonfatal and fatal CVD and CVD risk factors. Participants experienced 231 CVD events over the study time period (22 years). Women with frequent baseline VMS had a 50% higher risk of CVD events. Women with frequent VMS that persisted over time had a 77% higher risk of a future CVD event. The findings indicated that associations were not explained by standard cardiovascular disease risk factors or by endogenous hormone levels.

1. Women may experience CVD symptoms differently than men. How can the findings in this study be used in the initial assessment of risk factors for CVD in women?

2. What other risk factors do you think the researchers considered when analyzing data for this study?

Table 34-1 ➤ Medications That Promote Circulation

CLASS	ACTION	EXAMPLES AND COMMENTS
Vasodilators	■ Enhance cardiac output, providing increased blood flow and oxygenation to organs and tissues ■ Cause vessel dilation, which eases workload of the heart ■ Control blood pressure ■ Treat heart failure	Angiotensin-converting enzyme (ACE) inhibitors Angiotensin II receptor blockers Nitrates
Beta-Adrenergic Blockers	■ Block norepinephrine and epinephrine (adrenaline) ■ Reduce the workload of the heart and oxygen consumption ■ Control abnormal heart rhythms (dysrhythmias) by slowing conduction through the atrioventricular (AV) node ■ Control blood pressure	Beta$_1$-selective: atenolol, metoprolol Nonselective: carvedilol, metoprolol, propranolol
Calcium-Channel Blockers	■ Block the flow of calcium into the cells of the heart and blood vessels ■ Decrease blood pressure ■ Reduce the strength of myocardial contraction; slow heart rate ■ Dilate the arteries and arterioles	Nifedipine
Positive Inotropic Agents	■ Improve the effectiveness of the heart's pumping action without creating excess cardiac workload and oxygen demand ■ Reduce the heart muscle cells' ability to trigger their own contraction (automaticity) ■ Dilate blood vessels	Cardiac glycosides: digoxin Phosphodiesterase (PSE) inhibitors: PDE3 inhibitors (congestive heart failure) PDE5 inhibitors (erectile dysfunction)

(Continued)

Table 34-1 ➤ Medications That Promote Circulation—cont'd

CLASS	ACTION	EXAMPLES AND COMMENTS
Diuretics	▪ Remove sodium and water from the body through urine ▪ Reduce the volume of circulating blood ▪ Prevent accumulation of fluid in the pulmonary circulation and body tissues	Thiazide diuretics: hydrochlorothiazide (HCTZ), metolazone Loop diuretics: furosemide Potassium-sparing diuretics: spironolactone Bumetanide Metolazone Triamterene

KnowledgeCheck 34-3

▪ What changes occur in the cardiovascular system with aging?
▪ How does smoking affect the cardiovascular system?

Pathophysiological Conditions

Alterations in circulation and perfusion at the tissue or cellular level may be life threatening, particularly when hypoxemia and acidosis occur. Refer to Chapter 33 to review the effect of poor oxygenation on body systems.

Cardiovascular Abnormalities

Alterations in gas exchange are caused by a number of disorders that affect the structure, function, and regulation of the cardiovascular system. Cardiovascular abnormalities interfere with the flow of oxygenated blood to organs and tissues, and they continue to be the number-one cause of death for adults in the United States (Centers for Disease Control and Prevention [CDC], 2022). Major abnormalities are as follows:

▪ **Heart failure** occurs when the heart becomes an inefficient pump and is unable to meet the body's demands. Blood is oxygenated when it passes through the lungs, but it is not well circulated to the organs and tissues. Impaired circulation leads to systemic and pulmonary edema, which further impairs gas exchange.
  ▪ **Right-sided heart failure** occurs when the right ventricle does not pump sufficient amounts of blood to the lungs for oxygenation, and blood backs up into the peripheral veins.
  ▪ **Left-sided heart failure** occurs when the left ventricle does not pump sufficient amounts of blood to body organs and tissues.
  ▪ **Both right-sided and left-sided heart failure** reduce the amount of oxygenated blood available to organs and tissues, resulting in fatigue and organ dysfunction.
  ▪ **Key Point:** *Because the right and left ventricles are part of one circuit, failure of one side of the heart eventually leads to failure of the other side.*

▪ **Cardiomyopathy** is a heart muscle disorder that results in heart enlargement and impaired cardiac contractility.
  ▪ **Primary cardiomyopathy** results from genetic or noncardiovascular causes.
  ▪ **Secondary cardiomyopathy** results from another cardiovascular disease. Secondary cardiomyopathy occurs as previously normal heart muscle enlarges to compensate for the increased workload.
▪ **Cardiac ischemia** occurs when the oxygen requirements of the heart are unmet. Prolonged ischemia leads to myocardial infarction (MI) as parts of the heart *necrose* (die) from inadequate oxygen. **Angina pectoris** is transient chest pain due to myocardial ischemia. The tissue becomes injured but does not necrose.
  ▪ **Stable angina** is a predictable pattern of ischemic chest pain that is precipitated by known triggers (e.g., activity, large meal, temperature extremes, cigarette smoking, stimulants, sexual activity, strong emotion, circadian rhythm patterns). It is alleviated by rest and medications.
  ▪ **Unstable angina** (sometimes called *preinfarction angina* or *crescendo angina*) is ischemic chest pain that has worsened in frequency, severity, or duration and is not relieved by usual measures. When untreated, it may lead to MI.
▪ **Coronary artery disease,** a leading cause of cardiac ischemia, is a condition in which plaque builds up inside the coronary arteries. Plaque narrows the arteries, reducing blood flow to the heart muscle and making it more likely that clots will form and block the arteries.
▪ **Dysrhythmias** (alterations in heart rate or rhythm) can lower cardiac output, decrease tissue oxygenation, and increase the risk of stroke.
▪ **Heart valve abnormalities** create turbulent flow, leading to a decrease in cardiac output and compromised tissue oxygenation. Often there is an audible murmur. The valves most commonly affected are the mitral and aortic valves.
  ▪ **Valve stenosis** (narrowing) refers to blood flow through a narrow, constricted opening. Pumping

blood through a narrow valve increases the workload of the heart and leads to hypertrophy of the chamber that precedes the stenotic valve. The chamber receiving blood through a stenotic valve can be underfilled.

- **Valve incompetence** refers to incomplete closure of a valve, resulting in regurgitation of blood into the chamber from which it came. Regurgitation causes distention and increased work for the chamber ejecting the blood. The chamber ejecting the blood can become weak and ineffective as a pump. The chamber receiving blood through an incompetent valve can be underfilled.

Peripheral Vascular Abnormalities

Disorders of peripheral blood vessels impair blood flow to and from organs and tissues.

- **Arterial abnormalities disrupt the flow of oxygenated blood to tissues.** When arterial blood flow is compromised, signs and symptoms include pallor, pain, weak or absent pulses, poor capillary refill, cool skin, and tissue dysfunction.
- **Venous abnormalities disrupt blood return to the heart.** Clinical signs of compromised venous blood flow include edema, brown skin discoloration, and tissue dysfunction (e.g., stasis ulcers).

Oxygen Transport Abnormalities

Even if the heart is functioning well and arterial blood flow is intact, tissues can become hypoxic if the blood is unable to carry adequate amounts of oxygen. The most common causes are anemia and carbon monoxide poisoning.

- **Anemia** is an abnormally low level of red blood cells, hemoglobin, or both.
- **Carbon monoxide** is a colorless, odorless gas produced by the combustion of flammable materials and fuels. When inhaled, carbon monoxide binds tightly to hemoglobin at the oxygen receptor sites, making it impossible for hemoglobin to carry oxygen.

PracticalKnowledge
knowing **how**

Nursing care for patients with cardiovascular problems is directed at assessing for and maximizing the effectiveness of the heart and circulatory system.

ASSESSMENT/RECOGNIZING CUES

Although this section focuses on cardiovascular assessments, evaluation of overall oxygenation status includes a history and examination that gathers cues about lung, heart, and circulatory function. **Key Point:** *The patient's condition and the purpose of the assessment/recognizing cues determine your priorities for assessment and the order in which you gather information.* For example:

- *For someone with a cardiac emergency,* the immediate assessment focus would be to ask simple questions about current symptoms while performing a quick examination to determine the adequacy of breathing, circulation, and oxygenation.
- *For a healthy individual at risk of coronary artery disease, assessment* might include more extensive questions about occupation and smoking habits, a medical history, and an extensive physical examination.

You will need information about the patient's past and present cardiovascular signs and symptoms, risk factors, medications, activity level, tolerance of activity, and lifestyle factors that affect cardiovascular functioning.

Assessing/Recognizing Cues for Risk Factors

One aspect of improving cardiovascular health and quality of life is the prevention, detection, and treatment of risk factors for heart attack and stroke (*Healthy People 2030,* 2020). A health history related to cardiovascular functioning includes questions about the presence of risk factors that affect the heart and peripheral vascular function. Topics to assess include the following:

- Demographic data
- Health history
- Family history
- Respiratory history
- Cardiovascular history
- Environmental history
- Lifestyle

Women Cardiovascular disease is the leading cause of death of women in the United States and worldwide. Approximately 44% of U.S. women age 20 years or older are living with prevalent cardiovascular disease (Virani et al., 2021). A comprehensive history, including female reproductive history (menarche, menopause, history of preeclampsia, premature menopause, and autoimmune disease) will provide cues of risk-enhancing factors for cardiovascular disease (Wong et al., 2022).

Social Determinants of Health Social determinants of health (SDOH) can have important implications for a person's risk for cardiovascular disease. SDOH include unemployment, lack of health insurance or inability to pay medical bills, low income, psychological distress, delayed care resulting from lack of transportation, food insecurity, and educational attainment. Information on SDOH should always be considered in the assessment of the risk for cardiovascular disease and in assessing a patient's possible access and adherence to lifestyle and medical therapies (Javed et al., 2022).

Anxiety You should also assess the patient's anxiety level. Patients with cardiac or respiratory problems are almost certain to be anxious, and anxiety interferes with achieving good outcomes for these patients. Pay close attention to verbal cues because heart rate and blood pressure changes may not be useful in assessing acutely ill patients for anxiety.

For a detailed list of interview questions for each of these topics,

 Go to **Chapter 34, Assessment Guidelines and Tools, Focused Assessment: Assessing Circulation,** in Volume 2.

Physical Examination

- Obtain the patient's height and weight to start the physical examination.
- Measure BMI and waist circumference; these are indicators of obesity, which is a major risk factor for cardiovascular disease.
- Assessment of heart and peripheral vessels includes inspection, palpation, and auscultation (and occasionally percussion).
  - **Inspect**—Use inspection to observe for signs of distress (e.g., chest pain), skin and mucous membrane color, presence or absence of edema, and overall general appearance.
  - **Palpate**—pulses, skin temperature, edema, heart pulsations through the chest wall, and areas of tenderness.
  - **Auscultate**—heart sounds, vascular sounds, and blood pressure. Auscultate the lungs because adventitious sounds, such as rales, may signal decreased cardiac output.

For a step-by-step discussion of physical assessment of the heart and vascular system,

 Go to **Chapter 19, Procedure 19-13: Assessing the Heart and Vascular System,** in Volume 2.

Also,

 Go to **Chapter 34, Focused Assessment: Assessing Circulation,** in Volume 2.

Assess Pain

Cardiac Pain ✛ If a patient has chest pain, evaluate it immediately because chest pain is the most common heart attack symptom. Ask the patient to describe the pain and its location, duration, frequency, and radiation. Ask the client to rate the pain on a scale of 0 to 10, with 0 representing no pain and 10 representing the worst possible pain.

Chest pain may also be caused by musculoskeletal or respiratory conditions, for example, a fractured rib or pleuritis (inflammation in the pleural space).

Key Point: *You can differentiate cardiac pain because:*
- *It is usually in the center or on the left side of the chest and radiates to the left arm (most often in men).*
- *The pain typically lasts several minutes; it may go away and come back.*
- *The pain typically does not change with inhalation or exhalation.*

Some women have milder (or no) chest pain, and women are more likely than men to experience other symptoms, such as jaw or back pain, nausea, fatigue, and shortness of breath.

See Chapter 28 for pain assessment, as needed.

♥ **iCare** Patients experiencing chest pain are likely to be fearful—most people are aware that chest pain may signal a heart attack. You need to work quickly but calmly to instill confidence in the patient. If the person is experiencing a cardiac event, anxiety and stress can make it worse by increasing oxygen consumption, thereby extending hypoxic damage to the heart.

Assess/Recognize Cues for Fatigue

Fatigue is a subjective experience. The patient feels tired and lacks endurance. Fatigue is a common symptom of various oxygenation problems, including anemia and heart failure. Ask your patient to rate their fatigue on a 0-to-10 scale, as you do for pain.

Assess/Recognize Cues for Dyspnea

Dyspnea (shortness of breath) is discussed in Chapter 33 in relation to respiratory conditions. Recall that dyspnea is a sign of hypoxia, which can be associated with cardiovascular diseases and anemia, as well as with respiratory problems. As with pain, dyspnea provokes anxiety.

Assess/Recognize Cues for Peripheral Circulation

Even if the lungs and heart are functioning well, pathology in the arteries and veins can interfere with tissue perfusion.

- Palpate the peripheral pulses, assess skin color and temperature, and note the distribution of hair on the extremities. Weak pulses, cool feet, lack of hair, and shiny skin on the lower legs and feet usually accompany peripheral vascular disease.
- Look for skin ulcers, which often accompany severe venous or arterial disease.
- Check for edema of the feet and ankles; this is one symptom of heart failure.
- Assess for a clot in the veins **(deep vein thrombosis [DVT]),** deep under the muscles of the leg. Signs of DVT are pain, warmth, redness, and swelling of the leg. Homan's sign (pulling toes forward) and Pratt's sign (squeezing calf to trigger pain) are not reliable in diagnosing DVT. However, these signs may help confirm DVT when also considering the clinical signs of DVT. More accurate and specific diagnostic tests include ultrasound and venography (Kruger et al., 2019).

KnowledgeCheck 34-4

- Why would you auscultate the lungs as a part of your assessment of cardiac function?

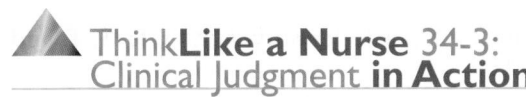

ThinkLike a Nurse 34-3: Clinical Judgment in Action

Why might it be more difficult to recognize heart attack symptoms in women than in men?

Diagnostic Testing

Diagnostic testing helps clinicians identify the causes of cardiovascular symptoms and monitor patient responses to treatment. We discuss several of these tests in the next sections. For others,

 Go to **Chapter 34, Diagnostic Testing: Tests Related to Circulation,** in Volume 2.

Providing Safe Clinical Monitoring

Chapter Key Concepts: Circulation, Perfusion

Competencies: (1) Embrace/Incorporate technological advances: Use technology to deliver safe, effective care. (2) Collaborate with the interprofessional healthcare team: Function as an essential member of the healthcare team (Thinking, Doing).

Because of reported safety issues that have been identified with the clinical monitoring of patients, The Joint Commission has asked hospitals to analyze the safety of hospital-based monitoring devices. Keep in mind that telemetry monitoring is not in and of itself a lifesaving intervention, but it is known to improve mortality in certain conditions in which cardiac dysrhythmia is possible or likely. As a telemetry nurse, you may be asked to participate in evaluating and identifying techniques/processes to avoid medical/nursing errors in the delivery of client care.

Several initiatives have been implemented to improve the safety of cardiac monitoring for patients, including the following:

➤ Updated hospital-specific procedures to include escalation, team empowerment, and alarm management for daily operations

➤ Standardized training course mandatory for all telemetry technicians and telemetry unit nurses (including competency testing)

➤ Four-week preceptor-supervised unit orientation mandatory for all new telemetry nurses, with skills checklist completion

➤ Quarterly lethal dysrhythmia drills on all shifts

➤ Maximum ratio of monitored patients to telemetry technicians

➤ Telemetry policy to emphasize medically indicated telemetry use

Source: Whalen, D.A., Covelle, P. M., Piepenbrink, J. C., Villanova, K. L., Cuneo, C. L., & Awtry, E. H. (2014). Novel approach to cardiac alarm management on telemetry units. *Journal of Cardiovascular Nursing,* 29(5), E13–E22.

Safe, Effective Nursing Care

Tests of Blood Oxygenation

Pulse oximetry, capnography, and arterial blood gases were discussed in Chapter 33. You should understand, though, that the results from all of those tests are pertinent to cardiac conditions. **Key Point:** *Remember: The heart and lungs work together to provide oxygenation; a problem in one creates a problem in the other.* For the complete procedure,

 Go to **Chapter 33, Procedure 33-2: Monitoring Pulse Oximetry (Arterial Oxygen Saturation)** and **Clinical Insight 33-1: Tips for Obtaining Accurate Pulse Oximetry Readings,** in Volume 2.

To review (and use in clinical assignments) arterial blood gas values, see the section Interpreting ABGs, and Table 35-6, in Chapter 35.

Laboratory Testing

Cholesterol, lipid panel, C-reactive protein (CRP), and glucose testing are valuable parts of cardiovascular risk assessment.

- **Lipid Panel.** The National Heart, Lung, and Blood Institute (NHLBI, 2022) recommends testing total cholesterol, HDL and low-density lipoprotein (LDL) levels, and triglyceride levels:
  - **Age 19 years or younger:** Begin screen at ages 9 to 11 years and repeat every 5 years. Screening may be performed as early as age 2 years if there is a family history of high blood cholesterol, heart attack, or stroke.
  - **Age 20 to 65 years:** Younger adults should be screened every 5 years. Men aged 45 to 65 years and women aged 55 to 65 years should be screened every 1 to 2 years.
  - **Older than 65 years:** Older adults should be screened every year.
    - For adults with total cholesterol of >200 mg/dL, a fasting measurement is recommended.
    - In the past, providers relied on specific ranges for LDL and HDL. These ranges are no longer used; rather, LDL levels are considered as one factor of many in evaluating cardiovascular risk.
- **Glucose testing** is indicated, particularly for those at risk for metabolic syndrome, which includes heart disease.
- **C-reactive protein. Key Point:** *The CRP appears to be the most reliable marker for arterial inflammation currently available.*

Screening for Children An Expert Panel appointed by the NHLBI (n.d.) recommended aggressive cholesterol screening for all children, regardless of family history. The panel recommends:

- Routine measurement of length/height and weight beginning in infancy, with calculation of BMI annually beginning at age 2 years to identify growth trends

- Yearly assessment of blood pressure from age 3 years
- Universal screening of triglyceride levels beginning between the age of 9 and 11 years
- Measuring fasting glucose levels to test for diabetes in children 10 years of age (or at the onset of puberty) who are overweight and have other risk factors, including a family history, for type 2 diabetes mellitus

Cardiac Monitoring

Cardiac monitoring is the continuous monitoring of the electrical activity of the heart. Monitoring is done by specially trained nurses or technicians.

- The **electrocardiogram (ECG)** is a rendering of the electrical activity of the heart. Three to five electrodes placed on the skin of the chest display a waveform on a monitor screen or printout (Fig. 34-4).
- **Electrocardiography,** in contrast, uses 12 "leads" (views of the heart).

The ECG illustrates electrical activity but not mechanical activity. In other words, the ECG reflects what the nerves are telling the heart muscle to do but *not* what the heart muscle is actually doing in response.

The purposes of cardiac monitoring are to:

- Identify the patient's baseline rhythm and rate.
- Recognize significant changes in the baseline rhythm and rate.
- Recognize lethal dysrhythmias that require immediate intervention.

Cardiac Cycle The ECG reading illustrates the complete cardiac cycle. Each part of the ECG complex

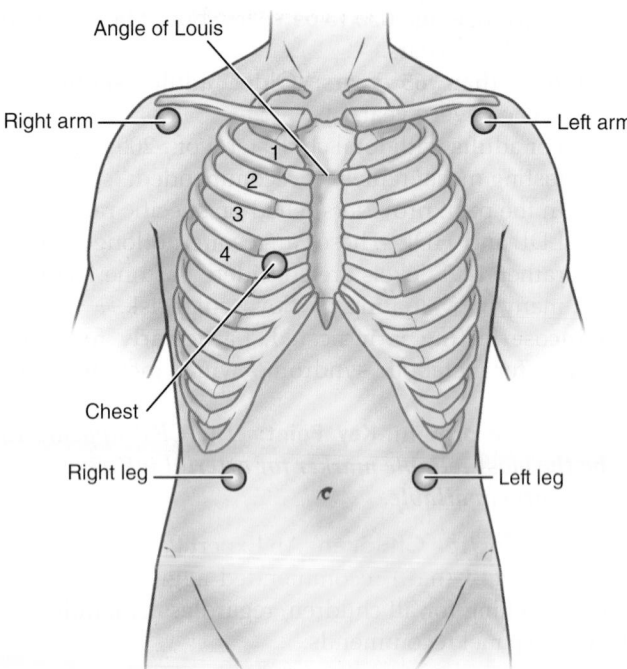

FIGURE 34-4 Electrodes placed for continuous cardiac monitoring.

has been given a letter to identify it: **P, Q, R, S, T, and sometimes U.**

- The **P wave** represents the firing of the SA node and conduction of the impulse through the atria. In a healthy heart, this leads to atrial contraction.
- The **QRS complex** represents *ventricular depolarization* and leads to ventricular contraction.
- The **T wave** represents the return of the ventricles to an electrical resting state so that they can be stimulated again *(ventricular repolarization)*. The atria also repolarize, but they do so during the time of ventricular depolarization; thus, they are obscured by the QRS complex and cannot be seen on the ECG complex.
- The **U wave** is not always seen on the ECG but may be detected with electrolyte imbalance, such as hypokalemia or hypercalcemia. U waves sometimes occur in response to certain medications (e.g., digitalis, epinephrine). An inverted U wave may occur with ischemia to the cardiac muscle.

Cardiac Rhythms Dysrhythmias (abnormal heart rhythms) can be broadly categorized according to type as follows:

Tachydysrhythmias—Rates of >100 beats/min
Bradydysrhythmias—Rates of <60 beats/min
Ectopy—extra beats

Within each of these categories, dysrhythmias can be further classified by their site of origin:

Supraventricular—Above the ventricles
Junctional—Within the AV node
Ventricular—In the ventricles

Note that a tachy- or bradydysrhythmia depends on the patient's baseline heart rate. Some people have a low resting heart rate (fewer than 60 beats/min) without distress. Keep this in mind before assuming that the heart rate is abnormal.

All dysrhythmias have the potential to decrease cardiac output, resulting in hypotension and tissue hypoxia (see Example Problem: Decreased Cardiac Output). Skill in identifying cardiac rhythms (both normal and abnormal) requires study and experience and is beyond the scope of this chapter. The Highlights of Procedure 34-1 box summarizes the activities involved in the care of a patient requiring a cardiac monitor. For the complete procedure,

Go to **Chapter 34, Procedure 34-1: Performing Cardiac Monitoring,** in Volume 2.

KnowledgeCheck 34-5

- What do the P wave, QRS complex, and T wave of an ECG complex represent?
- What kind of dysrhythmia would describe a heart rate of 140 beats per minute that originates in the ventricles?

NURSING DIAGNOSIS/ANALYZING CUES

Several nursing diagnoses address impaired circulation and tissue or organ hypoxia. They are briefly discussed here.

- *Decreased Cardiac Output* is the appropriate diagnosis when the heart is unable to pump adequate amounts of blood to meet the metabolic demands of the body. Definitive interventions for this problem are collaborative.
- *Risk for Impaired Cardiac Tissue Perfusion* is appropriate for a patient who has no symptoms of decreased cardiac perfusion but has risk factors such as elevated CRP, cardiac surgery, use of birth control pills, hyperlipidemia, or substance abuse.
- *Risk for Impaired Cerebral, Gastrointestinal, or Renal Tissue Perfusion* is appropriate for a patient who is at risk for experiencing poor perfusion to those systems (e.g., a patient with a brain tumor, certain heart problems, embolism, substance abuse).
- *Impaired Peripheral Tissue Perfusion* is appropriate for a patient experiencing poor perfusion to the periphery that compromises health.
- *Risk for Shock* should be used for patients who have inadequate blood flow to body tissues that may lead to life-threatening cellular dysfunction (e.g., patients with sepsis and hypovolemia). Alternatively, you could use a collaborative problem, such as *Potential Complication of Sepsis: Shock.*

Cardiovascular functioning can also be the etiology of other nursing diagnoses, such as the following examples:

- *Activity Intolerance Risk* related to decreased oxygen-carrying capacity of the blood secondary to anemia
- *Acute Pain* secondary to myocardial ischemia
- *Anxiety* related to shortness of breath
- *Death Anxiety* related to diagnosis of myocardial infarction (heart attack)
- *Impaired Individual Coping* related to hospitalization for inadequate oxygenation secondary to congestive heart failure

PLANNING/PRIORITIZING HYPOTHESES AND GENERATING SOLUTIONS

Nursing Outcomes Classification (NOC) standardized outcomes and evaluation criteria related to cardiovascular status are included in Domain II: Physiologic Health, in the Cardiopulmonary Class.

Individualized goals/outcome statements depend on the nursing diagnosis you identify. For diagnoses related to cardiac function or circulation, the following are examples of goals you might write:

- No dyspnea or shortness of breath
- Heart rate in expected range
- Peripheral pulses strong and equal bilaterally
- Brisk capillary refill

EXAMPLE CLIENT CONDITION: Decreased Cardiac Output

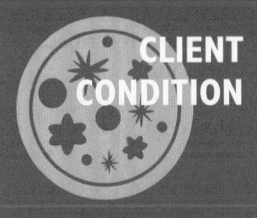

Basic Definition

Decreased Cardiac Output is the appropriate diagnosis when the heart is unable to pump adequate amounts of blood to meet the metabolic demands of the body.

Characteristics/Symptoms

- Fatigue, confusion, agitation, and/or decreased level of consciousness
- Cool, clammy, mottled extremities
- Delayed capillary refill time; diminished peripheral pulses
- Hypotension
- Tachycardia (early) or bradycardia (late)
- Thready pulse
- Raised jugular venous pressure; neck vein distention
- Increased respiratory rate
- Breathlessness and hypoxemia
- Paroxysmal nocturnal dyspnea or orthopnea
- Edema

Etiologies

- Valvular heart disease
- Congenital heart defects
- Chronic hypertension
- Dehydration
- Hemorrhage
- Arterial or venous insufficiency
- Cardiomyopathy
- Diabetes
- Kidney disease

Pathophysiology

Reduced:
- Efficiency of the heart muscle, through damage or overloading
- Force of contraction due to overloading of or damage to the ventricle
- Stroke volume as a result of a failure of systole, diastole, or both
- Circulating blood supply as a result of anemia, dehydration, or blood loss
- Ability of kidneys to dispose of sodium and water, which increases edema

(continued)

EXAMPLE CLIENT CONDITION: Decreased Cardiac Output—cont'd

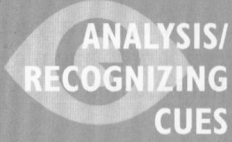

ANALYSIS/ RECOGNIZING CUES

Assess for risk factors for and symptoms of impaired cardiac and peripheral vascular function. Obtain health history and physical examination.

Signs & Symptoms:

Assess/recognize cues for:
- Skin color, temperature, and moisture
- Decrease in level of consciousness
- Heart rate and blood pressure
- Fluid balance
- Weight gain. Weigh patient regularly before breakfast.
- Pedal and sacral edema
- Respiratory rate, rhythm, and breath sounds
- Presence of paroxysmal nocturnal dyspnea (PND) or orthopnea
- Urine output
- Assess/recognize cues for reports of fatigue and reduced activity tolerance.

Diagnostic Tests

Routine blood work can provide cues to the etiology of decreased cardiac output.
- Arterial blood gases
- Complete blood count
- Electrolytes
- Monitor kidney function:
  - Serum creatinine
  - Blood urea nitrogen (BUN) levels
- Cardiac biomarkers: creatine kinase (CK), lactate dehydrogenase (LDH), aspartate aminotransferase (AST)
- Chest x-ray
- Electrocardiogram (ECG)

For a detailed list of interview questions for a focused assessment,

 Go to **Chapter 34, Assessment Guidelines and Tools, Focused Assessment: Assessing Circulation,** in Volume 2.

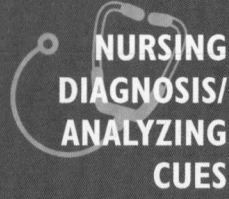

NURSING DIAGNOSIS/ ANALYZING CUES

Primary Diagnosis
- Decreased Cardiac Output

Related Diagnoses
- Activity Intolerance
- Death Anxiety
- Risk for Impaired Cardiac Tissue Perfusion

- Risk for Impaired Cerebral, Gastrointestinal, or Renal Tissue Perfusion
- Risk for Shock
- Tissue Perfusion Alteration: Abdominal, Cerebral, Pulmonary, Peripheral

IMPLEMENTATION/ TAKING ACTION

Definitive actions for this problem are collaborative.

NIC Standardized Interventions

- Bleeding Reduction
- Cardiac Care
- Cerebral Perfusion Promotion
- Circulatory Care: Arterial Insufficiency
- Circulatory Care: Venous Insufficiency
- Hemodynamic Regulation
- IV Therapy
- Shock Management

Individualized Nursing Actions

Monitor and Support Adequate Ventilation
- Record intake and output.
- Limit fluids and sodium as ordered.
- Provide small, frequent meals.
- Auscultate heart sounds; note rate, rhythm, and presence of S3, S4.
- Auscultate lung sounds for crackles or other adventitious sounds.
- Monitor for and control bleeding.
- Closely monitor for symptoms of decreased cardiac output (see Characteristics/Symptoms, earlier).

Maintain Adequate Ventilation and Perfusion
- Position patient in semi-Fowler's to high-Fowler's.
- Administer oxygen therapy as prescribed.
- Administer blood products and medications (i.e., diuretics) as ordered.
- Monitor oxygen saturation continuously using pulse oximeter.
- Coach slow respiratory rate using therapeutic touch, making eye contact, and communicating in a calm and supportive fashion.
- Schedule nursing care to provide rest and minimize fatigue.

Manage Anxiety
- Speak calmly and quietly to the patient and those around you.
- Do not leave the patient alone.
- Provide clear factual information, and keep the patient and family informed about treatments being given.

Also, see the discussion under the heading Manage Anxiety.

EXAMPLE CLIENT CONDITION: Decreased Cardiac Output—cont'd

Promote Circulation and Prevent Clot Formation
- Teach patients to avoid sitting with the legs crossed; doing so interferes with blood flow.
- Encourage and support early and frequent ambulation (e.g., after surgery).
- Encourage or provide range-of-motion (ROM) exercises.
- Apply compression devices.
  - Antiembolism stockings (thrombo-embolic deterrent [TED] hose)
  - Sequential compression devices (SCDs)

COLLABORATING

Medications & Blood Products
- Administer medications as prescribed, noting side effects and toxicity.
- Digitalis therapy
- Diuretics
- Vasodilator therapy
- Antidysrhythmics
- Angiotensin-converting enzyme (ACE) inhibitors
- Inotropic agents
- Anticoagulants

- Monitor blood pressure, pulse, and condition before administering cardiac medications.
- Notify physician if heart rate or blood pressure is low before holding medications.
- Administer blood or blood products.

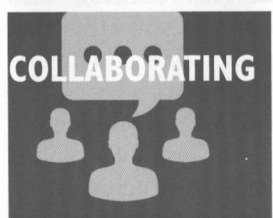

TEACHING

- Explain importance of smoking cessation and avoidance of alcohol intake.

- Educate patient on the need for and how to incorporate lifestyle changes.

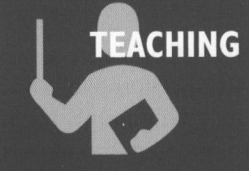
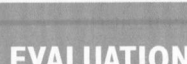

EVALUATION

NOC Standardized Outcomes
- Blood Loss Severity
- Cardiac Pump Effectiveness
- Circulation Status
- Tissue Perfusion: Cardiac
- Tissue Perfusion: Abdominal Organs
- Tissue Perfusion: Cerebral
- Tissue Perfusion: Peripheral
- Tissue Perfusion: Pulmonary
- Vital Signs

NOC Standardized Outcomes, Examples
- Patient demonstrates adequate cardiac output as evidenced by:
  - Blood pressure within normal limits
  - Warm, dry skin
  - Regular cardiac rhythm
  - Clear lung sounds
  - Strong bilateral, equal peripheral pulses
- Patient is able to tolerate activity without symptoms of dyspnea, syncope, or chest pain.

IMPLEMENTATION/TAKING ACTION

Nursing Interventions Classification (NIC) standardized interventions related to the cardiovascular system are found in NIC Domain 2: Complex Physiological Interventions, in the subcategory of Tissue Perfusion Management. Tissue Perfusion Management focuses on optimizing circulation. These provide a general care planning guide. Depending on individual patient needs, other NOC outcomes or NIC interventions may also be appropriate.

Specific nursing interventions for patients with cardiovascular problems focus on relieving anxiety, promoting circulation, administering medications, and performing cardiopulmonary resuscitation (CPR). For interventions specifically for Decreased Cardiac Output, see the Example Problem: Decreased Cardiac Output.

Manage Anxiety

Anxiety activates the sympathetic nervous system and triggers the stress response.

- Hormone changes occur, including the release of aldosterone, which promotes fluid retention and increases blood pressure.
- Heart rate and contraction force increase.
- Peripheral and visceral vessels constrict.
- Blood clots more readily.

All of these make a cardiac or vascular condition more serious. Therefore, anxiety reduction is a priority intervention. You will, of course, need to intervene first to prevent life-threatening situations. However, strive to implement interventions to relieve anxiety (see the interventions under the heading Manage Anxiety in Example Problem: Decreased Cardiac Output). If you need a review of detailed information about assessments and interventions for anxious patients, go to Chapter 10.

Promote Circulation

Adequate circulation ensures that oxygenated blood reaches tissues and organs and that venous blood returns to the heart. Two important nursing interventions are to promote venous return and prevent clot formation.

Promote Venous Return

Measures that promote venous return increase the flow of blood back to the vena cava and the right side of the heart.

- **Elevate the patient's legs above the level of the heart.** Gravity promotes venous return from the feet and legs.
- **Have the patient sit in a recliner that elevates the legs** rather than sitting upright in a chair with the legs

elevated on a stool. Flexion of the hips, legs, and knees constricts the veins and slows venous blood flow.

- **Teach patients not to sit with the legs crossed;** doing so interferes with blood flow.
- **Encourage and support early and frequent ambulation** (e.g., after surgery). Contraction of the muscles in the legs moves blood upward against gravity.
- **Encourage or provide range-of-motion (ROM) exercises,** which increase venous blood flow through rhythmic massaging of the veins by the active muscles (see Chapter 29 to review ROM).
- **Apply compression devices.**
  - **Antiembolism stockings (thrombo-embolic deterrent [TED] hose)** are elastic stockings that compress superficial leg veins and promote venous return.
  - **Sequential compression devices (SCDs),** also called *pneumatic compression devices,* are cuffs that surround the legs and alternately inflate and deflate to promote venous return to the heart.

Antiembolism stockings and SCDs are frequently used in perioperative patients to promote venous return and prevent clot formation (Ritchie et al., 2018). See Chapter 36 for further discussion and instructions on how to apply these stockings and appropriate follow-up care.

 Go to **Chapter 36, Procedure 36-2: Applying Antiembolism Stockings,** in Volume 2.

Promote Peripheral Arterial Circulation

Peripheral artery disease, usually found in the legs and feet, occurs when tissues do not receive enough blood flow to keep up with the demand for oxygen. It is caused by the buildup of fatty deposits and plaque within the arteries (atherosclerosis). Symptoms include:

- **Pain with exercise.** When arteries that supply blood to the legs are narrowed, leg pain occurs, especially with walking. This is called **intermittent claudication.**
- **Pain at rest.** As the blood flow becomes more restricted, pain occurs at rest, as well as numbness or a cold feeling in the leg or foot, especially on one side. Other symptoms are weak pulse, change in color, hair loss or shiny skin on the legs, sores that won't heal, and erectile dysfunction in men.

Patient Teaching Teach the patient and family the following:

- **Do not use tobacco.** Patients with poor peripheral circulation need to quit using tobacco because smoking restricts blood flow.
- **Foot care.** When circulation is poor, healing is slower. It is especially important to take good care of the feet and prevent injury to the feet. Even dry, cracked skin can result in a sore and become infected. Patients need to wear well-fitting shoes with smooth, dry socks.
- **Regular exercise** improves circulation and oxygen delivery to body tissue.

- **Proper positioning** is important. Remind patients that crossing their legs can interfere with blood flow. Additionally, elevating the feet above heart level can slow circulation to the feet, leading to increased pain.
- **Medication** might be needed to control blood pressure, control pain, lower cholesterol, prevent clots, and control blood sugar if the patient has diabetes.
- **Warmth.** Promote vasodilation by preventing long periods of exposure to cold. Keep the affected extremity warm by wearing socks or insulated shoes.
- **Key Point:** *Never apply direct heat to the limb (heating pad, hot water bottle) because it increases the risk of burns.*
- **Graft bypass surgery** or **angioplasty** using a mesh stent might be necessary to create a new path for blood flow to go around the damaged area of the blood vessel. When treated properly, new collateral blood vessels can form, allowing blood to circulate around the damaged area.

Prevent Clot Formation

- A **thrombus** is a stationary clot adhering to the wall of a vessel. Clots can form after injury to vessels or in response to hypercoagulability.
- An **embolus** is a clot that travels in the bloodstream.

Anticoagulant Therapy Patients at high risk for thrombus formation may be prescribed anticoagulant medications to help prevent abnormal clot formation. Anticoagulant medications include heparin and warfarin sodium. Newer anticoagulants (e.g., dabigatran, apixaban, and rivaroxaban) work by inhibiting thrombin or factor X in the clotting chain. They have the advantage of not requiring tests of blood levels. However, unlike heparin and warfarin, they have no specific antidote.

Other Nursing Activities Of course, all the strategies to promote venous return also help prevent clot formation.

- **Turn patients frequently;** teach patients to change positions frequently. This prevents vessel injury from prolonged pressure in one position.
- **Use scrupulous sterile technique** for intravenous therapy. This prevents infection that can damage the vessel lumens.
- **Be sure IV medications are adequately diluted.** This prevents chemical irritation of veins.
- **Promote adequate hydration** (i.e., monitor intake and output, assess hydration, manage fluid intake, teach patients to drink plenty of fluids). Unless contraindicated, adult fluid intake should be approximately 2,000 mL per day to keep urine output at about 1,500 mL per day. Adequate hydration keeps respiratory secretions thin but also keeps the blood from becoming viscous ("thick"). Viscous blood clots more readily.

- **Promote smoking cessation.** Nicotine increases the risk for thrombus formation because of its constricting effects on vessel walls.

Administer Cardiovascular Medications

Cardiovascular medications are used to prevent atherosclerosis and to enhance cardiac output, thus providing increased blood flow and oxygenation to organs and tissues. They include the following:

- **Vasodilators** cause vessel dilation, which eases the work of the heart. Vasodilating agents include angiotensin-converting enzyme (ACE) inhibitors, angiotensin II receptor blockers, and nitrates.
  - *Drugs that dilate arterioles* decrease the resistance against which the heart pumps (afterload).
  - *Drugs that dilate veins* decrease venous return to the heart (preload).

Key Point: *Vasodilators can cause hypotension, especially when the person rises from a sitting or lying position. Patients should be warned of this effect. You will need to monitor the patient's blood pressure and observe for symptoms of hypotension.*

- **Beta-adrenergic agents** block stimulation of beta receptors, which are located primarily in the heart, lungs, and blood vessels. Beta-1 selective agents are used to treat angina, acute myocardial infarction, and congestive heart failure (CHF). They decrease heart rate, slow conduction through the AV node, and decrease myocardial oxygen demand by reducing myocardial contractility.
- **Diuretics** increase the removal of sodium and water from the body by increasing urine output. In patients with congestive heart failure (CHF), diuretics are used to reduce the volume of circulating blood and prevent accumulation of fluid in the pulmonary circulation.
- **Positive inotropes** increase cardiac contractility. They are used therapeutically to make the heart a more effective pump. The goal is to improve pumping effectiveness without creating excess heart work and oxygen demand. The two main classes of positive inotropes are cardiac glycosides and phosphodiesterase inhibitors.
- **Anticholesterol medications (statins)** are a class of drugs that protect against coronary artery disease by lowering the level of triglycerides and reduce the production of cholesterol by the liver. Statins block the liver enzyme that is responsible for making cholesterol. Statins are used for those who have an elevated LDL cholesterol level.

Cardiopulmonary Resuscitation

You must be prepared to perform *CPR* in the event your patient experiences a respiratory, cardiac, or cardiopulmonary arrest.

- **Cardiac arrest** is the cessation of heart function. Signs of cardiac arrest are pale, cool, grayish skin; absence of femoral or carotid pulses; apnea; and pupil dilation. **Key Point:** *In the event of cardiac arrest, you have only 4 to 6 minutes before the brain is damaged by a lack of oxygen.*

- **Respiratory (pulmonary) arrest** is the cessation of breathing. It can be caused by a blocked airway or may occur after a cardiac arrest; it may be sudden or preceded by increasingly labored breathing.

CPR procedures are regularly updated as new knowledge is gained. The American Heart Association provides training sessions for healthcare professionals to become certified in CPR. This is a prerequisite for employment and clinical practice. **Key Point:** *We recommend you obtain CPR training from certified professionals.* However, if you are already trained and just want to review the procedure,

 Go to the American Heart Association website for Guidelines for CPR and emergency cardiovascular care (ECC) at http://eccguidelines.heart.org

Guidelines for Trained Professionals

Key points of the most recent guidelines *for trained professionals* include the following:

- Focus on effective, uninterrupted chest compressions.
- Push hard and push fast in the center of the chest.
- Administer about 100 compressions per minute.
- Perform 30 compressions to 2 breaths—for all victims except newborns.
- Give breaths over 1 second and make the chest rise visibly (American Heart Association, 2015; Olasveengen et al., 2017).

In-Hospital Arrests All agencies have procedures (called a "Code Blue" in many agencies) for announcing cardiac or respiratory arrest; in acute care facilities, there is usually an emergency alert system in the patient rooms. In the event of an arrest:

1. **Activate the alert system** (e.g., by pulling down a handle) to summon a code team trained in CPR.
2. **Begin CPR immediately after activating the alert** because it will take a few minutes for the code team to arrive. Use a defibrillator as soon as one is available.
   - *For an automatic external defibrillator* (AED), follow the visual and audio prompts from the AED.
   - *For a manual defibrillator,* use a dose of 2 joules/kg for the first shock and a dose of 4 J/kg for the second and subsequent shocks.

Key Point: *Before beginning CPR, you are responsible for knowing whether your patient has an advance directive stating whether or not they would want CPR.*

Hands-Only™ CPR The American Heart Association (2022) recommends different responses for laypersons, first responders, and CPR-trained professionals.

The goal of these changes is to make it easier to learn, remember, and perform CPR.

- **Hands-Only™ CPR,** using compressions only, is recommended for people who see an adult collapse suddenly in the community.
- **Traditional CPR,** which combines breaths and compressions, should be used only for:
  Adults found already unconscious and not breathing normally
  Victims of drowning or collapse due to breathing problems
  All infants and children

See the Self-Care box, Teaching Your Client Hands-Only™ CPR for a detailed description of CPR that you can teach to laypersons.

Self-Care

Teaching Your Client Hands-Only™ Cardiopulmonary Resuscitation (CPR) for a Single-Rescuer, Adult-Victim Collapse

Witnessed Collapse

If you see an adult suddenly collapse in an "out-of-hospital" setting:

1. Call 911 (or send someone to do that).
2. Push hard and fast in the center of the chest (100 pumps per minute).
3. Continue until help arrives.

For an Unwitnessed Collapse of an Adult Victim:

1. Establish unresponsiveness (ask, "Are you okay?").
2. Call 911 (or send someone to do it).
3. Obtain an automated external defibrillator (AED), if possible.
4. Start traditional CPR, if you know how, while waiting for the AED.

Traditional CPR

1. When the AED arrives, turn it on for rhythm analysis.
2. After turning on the AED, open the airway (tilt the head, lift the chin).
3. Check for breathing.
4. Give two rescue breaths (each 1 second long). Look for chest movement, listen for breathing, and feel for air coming from the mouth or nose.
5. Administer one shock and wait for the AED to tell you what to do next.
6. When the AED says to continue CPR, start alternating 30 compressions with 2 breaths. Continue until help arrives. Stop only to check the AED for rhythm.

Key Point: *The most important action is to deliver uninterrupted, hard and fast chest compressions.*

Source: American Heart Association. (2022). *Hands-Only CPR.* https://cpr.heart.org/en/cpr-courses-and-kits/hands-only-cpr

KnowledgeCheck 34-6

- Identify three strategies that prevent clot formation.
- How do diuretics affect oxygenation?

Highlights of Procedure 34-1

Procedure 34-1: Performing Cardiac Monitoring

➤ Prepare the monitoring equipment.

➤ Identify electrode sites based on the monitoring system and the patient's anatomy.

➤ If the patient's chest is very hairy, shave the small areas for the electrodes.

➤ With an alcohol pad, clean the areas for electrode placement; allow to dry.

➤ Connect lead wires to electrodes.

➤ Apply the electrodes, pressing firmly.

➤ Secure monitoring equipment based on monitoring system used.

➤ Check the electrocardiogram (ECG) tracing on the monitor. If necessary, adjust the gain (sometimes called *sensitivity*) to increase the waveform size.

➤ Set the upper and lower heart rate alarm limits and turn them on.

➤ Obtain a rhythm strip by pressing the "record" button, interpret and mount appropriately.

To explore learning resources for this chapter,

Go to Davis Advantage **and find:**

Answers and Suggested Responses for all questions in this chapter

Concept Map

Knowledge Map

References and Bibliography

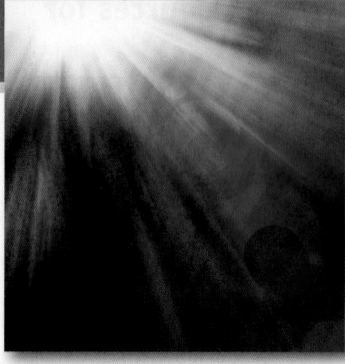

CHAPTER 35

Hydration & Homeostasis

Learning Outcomes

After completing this chapter, you should be able to:

- Identify the fluid compartments within the body.
- Describe the location and function of the major electrolytes of the body.
- Differentiate between active and passive transport, osmosis, diffusion, and filtration.
- Describe the body mechanisms for maintaining fluid and electrolyte balance.
- Summarize the major fluid and electrolyte balance disorders.
- Compare and contrast respiratory and metabolic acidosis and alkalosis.
- Describe compensatory mechanisms for acid-base imbalances.
- Apply the nursing process to clients with fluid, electrolyte, and acid-base imbalances.

Key Concepts

Acid-base balance

Electrolyte balance

Fluid balance

Related Concepts

See the Concept Map on Davis Advantage.

Example Client Condition

Fluids, Electrolytes, and Acid-Base Imbalance

Meet Your Patients

Your instructor assigned you to care for Jackson LaGuardia, a 60-year-old man with end-stage renal disease. You arrived at the hospital to review his medical records to provide care the next day. On the unit, the charge nurse informs you that Mr. LaGuardia is still in the emergency department (ED) waiting to be admitted to the medical-surgical unit. You go to the ED to review his medical records, gather data, and introduce yourself as a student nurse.

The ED charge nurse tells you that five members of the LaGuardia family have all come to the hospital complaining of nausea, vomiting, and diarrhea related to severe gastroenteritis, a viral intestinal disorder. The family members include the following:

- 8-month-old Jason, grandson of Jackson
- 26-year-old Susanna, Jackson's daughter and Jason's mother

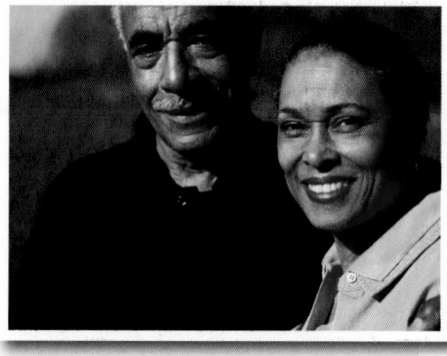

- 58-year-old Gemma, Jackson's wife
- 60-year-old Jackson
- 82-year-old Martha, Jackson's mother

Jason, Jackson, and Martha are being admitted to the hospital. However, Susanna and Gemma have been asked to follow up tomorrow in the urgent care clinic. As you prepare for your clinical day, you think, "If they all have the same disorder, why are only three family members being admitted? What makes these patients different?" In this chapter, we follow the LaGuardias and answer those questions

TheoreticalKnowledge
knowing**why**

When we are healthy, the fluid and chemical state of our bodies is in balance. However, illness can disturb this balance. In this chapter, we examine how fluid, electrolyte, and acid–base balances are maintained, as well as what happens when there are disturbances in each of these areas.

ABOUT THE KEY CONCEPTS

The concepts of **fluid balance** and **electrolyte balance** are intricately related. Usually, when one electrolyte changes, so does another, and often with fluids shifts that can lead to dysfunction. Likewise, disruption of **acid–base balance** can affect overall body functioning. The pH balance (acidity and alkalinity) has a profound effect on overall health.

BODY FLUIDS AND SOLUTES

Body fluid is essential for proper functioning of the body organs. It is made up primarily of water and contains gases (e.g., carbon dioxide and oxygen) and *solid substances,* called **solutes,** that dissolve in body fluids. Solutes are of two types:

- **Electrolytes**—substances (e.g., sodium, potassium) that develop an electrical charge when dissolved in water
- **Nonelectrolytes**—substances (e.g., glucose, urea) that do not conduct electricity

Total body water content varies with the number of fat cells, age, and sex (Table 35-1). Females have less body fluid than males because women have proportionately more body fat. Likewise, people who are obese have less body fluid proportionately than those of lean build. Body fluids perform several important functions:

- Maintain blood volume
- Regulate body temperature
- Transport material to and from cells
- Serve as a medium for cellular metabolism
- Assist with digestion of food
- Serve as a medium for excreting waste

What Are the Body Fluids Compartments?

Most body fluid is contained within two compartments. Figure 35-1 illustrates the distribution of body fluids.

Intracellular Fluid (ICF) ICF is contained within the cells. It accounts for approximately 40% of body weight and is essential for cell function and metabolism.

Extracellular Fluid (ECF) ECF is found outside the cells. ECF carries water, electrolytes, nutrients, and

AGE	TOTAL BODY FLUID (% OF BODY WEIGHT)
Full-term newborn	70%–80%
I-year-old	64%
Young adult	Males: 60%
	Females: 50%–55%
Middle adult	Males: 55%
	Females: 45%–50%
Older adult	Males: 50%
	Females: 45%

Table 35-1 ➤ Total Body Fluid in Relation to Sex and Age

oxygen to the cells and removes the waste products of cellular metabolism. It accounts for 20% of body weight and exists in three main locations in the body.

- **Interstitial fluid** lies in the spaces between the body cells. Excess fluid within the interstitial space is called *edema.*
- **Intravascular fluid** is the plasma within the blood. Its main function is to transport blood cells.
- **Transcellular fluid** includes specialized fluids that are contained in body spaces (e.g., cerebrospinal, pleural, peritoneal, and synovial fluid) and digestive juices.

Third Spacing Certain conditions cause fluid to move into an area that makes it physiologically unavailable, such as into the peritoneal space (in *ascites*), the pericardial space (with *pericardial effusion*), or into the *vesicles* (blisters) with a burn wound. This type of fluid movement is known as **third spacing** because fluid is literally trapped in a third compartment—not within interstitial (cells) or the intravascular spaces (blood vessels).

What Electrolytes Are Present in Body Fluids?

In addition to water, body fluid is composed of oxygen, carbon dioxide, dissolved nutrients, metabolic waste products, and electrolytes. **Electrolytes** are substances that carry an electrical charge, either positive or negative:

- **Cations** carry a positive charge
- **Anions** carry a negative charge

Electrolytes are measured in milliequivalents per liter (mEq/L) of water or milligrams per 100 mL (mg/100 mL or mg/dL). Note that 1 dL, or deciliter, equals 100 mL. **Key Point:** *The milliequivalent is a*

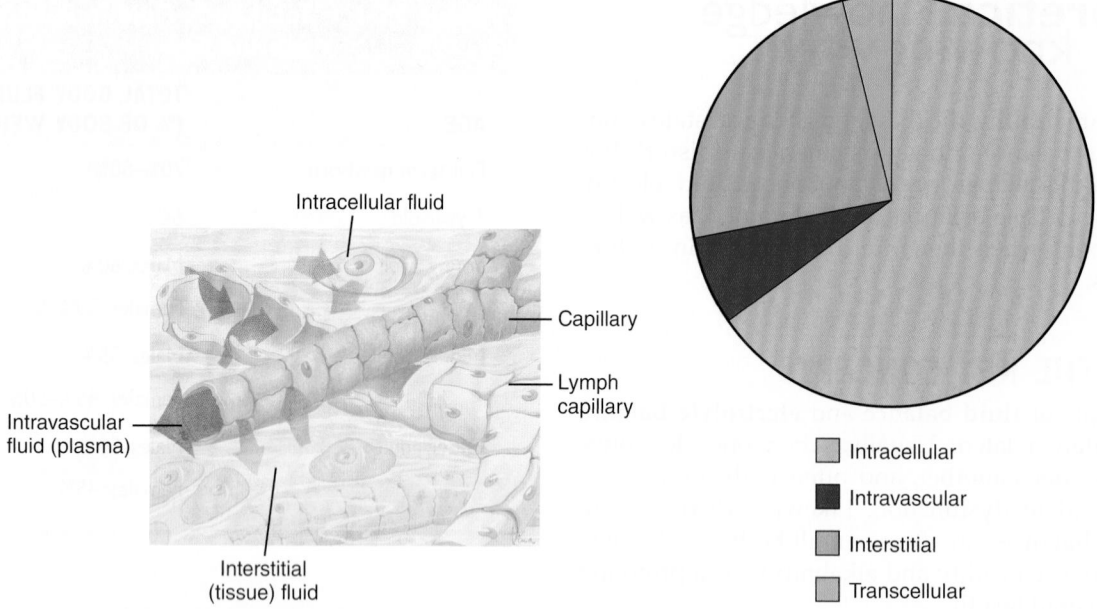

FIGURE 35-1 Normal distribution of body fluids. Transcellular fluid includes specialized fluids, such as cerebrospinal and peritoneal fluid and digestive juices.

measure of chemical combining power, whereas the milligram is a weight measure.

The composition of body fluids varies between compartments.

Intracellular Fluid (ICF)

- **Cations**—The major cations are *potassium* and *magnesium.*
- **Anions**—The major anion is *phosphate.*
- Other electrolytes are present but to a lesser degree.

Extracellular Fluid (ECF)

- The major electrolytes are *sodium, chloride,* and *bicarbonate.*
- *Albumin* is also present in the ECF, mostly in the intravascular fluid.
- *Transcellular fluids,* such as gastric and intestinal secretions, also contain electrolytes.

Severe electrolyte imbalances can occur if electrolytes move into a compartment they do not normally occupy or if they are lost in excess amounts from the body through perspiration, wounds, injury, or illness.

KnowledgeCheck 35-1

- Define *solute, electrolyte, intracellular fluid, extracellular fluid, cation,* and *anion.*
- Identify the major electrolytes in the ICF and ECF.

ThinkLike a Nurse 35-1: Clinical Judgment in Action

- Based on the information presented in the Meet Your Patients scenario, rank the members of the LaGuardia family based on total body water content.
- Does this information help you understand which family members were admitted to the hospital?

How Do Fluids and Electrolytes Move in the Body?

The selectively permeable membranes of cells and capillaries separate ICF and ECF (Fig. 35-1). Fluid and electrolytes move across these membranes by passive and active mechanisms.

- In **active transport,** movement of fluid and solutes requires energy.
- **Passive transport** requires no energy.

Passive Transport

The three passive transport systems are osmosis, diffusion, and filtration.

Osmosis Osmosis involves movement of water (or other pure solute) across a membrane from an area of a less concentrated solution to an area of more concentrated solution. Water moves across the membrane to dilute the higher concentration of solutes (Fig. 35-2).

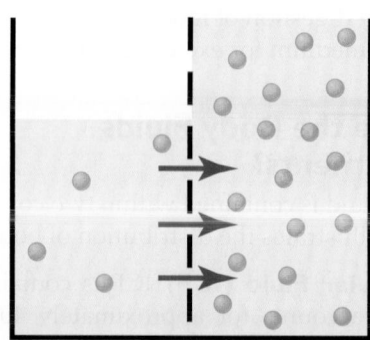

FIGURE 35-2 Osmosis is the movement of water across a membrane from a less concentrated solution to a more concentrated solution.

Recall that a **solute** is a substance dissolved in body fluid. Solutes may be crystalloids or colloids.

- **Crystalloids** are solutes that readily dissolve (e.g., electrolytes).
- **Colloids** are larger molecules that do not dissolve readily (e.g., proteins).

Osmolality (or tonicity) refers to the concentration of solutes creating pressure in body fluid. **Osmols** refers to the number of particles of solute per kilogram of water and is expressed as milliosmoles per kilogram (mOsm/kg). **Key Point:** *Sodium is the greatest determinant of serum osmolality, and potassium is the greatest determinant of intracellular osmolality.* Glucose and urea also contribute to osmolality in the ICF and ECF.

- **An isotonic solution** is of the same osmolality as blood; thus, no osmosis (movement of water) will occur. Isotonic fluids are often given by intravenous (IV) infusion if blood volume is low because the fluid will remain in the vascular space.
- **A hypotonic solution** is of lower osmolality than blood. When a hypotonic solution is infused, water moves by osmosis from the vascular system into the cells.
- **A hypertonic solution** contains a higher concentration of solutes than does blood. When a hypertonic solution is given to a patient, water moves by osmosis from the cells into the ECF.

Diffusion Diffusion is a passive process by which molecules of a solute move through a cell membrane from an area of higher concentration to an area of lower concentration. Movement occurs (Fig. 35-3) until the concentrations are equivalent on both sides of the membrane.

For example, if you add cream to a cup of coffee, the cream is initially concentrated in the area where poured. However, very soon, the cream becomes evenly dispersed throughout the coffee. If you stir the coffee, the cream disperses even more quickly.

Fluids within the human body work on a similar principle; body movement speeds the diffusion of molecules. The rate of diffusion varies according to the size of the molecules, the concentration of the solution, and the temperature of the solution.

- *Small molecules* move more rapidly than larger molecules.
- *Large differences in concentration* require a longer period of time to reach equilibration.
- *Higher temperatures* cause molecules to move faster, so diffusion occurs more rapidly.

Filtration Filtration is the movement of both water and smaller particles from an area of high pressure to one of low pressure (Fig. 35-4).

- **Hydrostatic pressure** is the force created by fluid within a closed system and is responsible for normal circulation of blood. Blood flows from the high-pressure arterial system to the lower-pressure capillaries and veins. As fluid (plasma) moves through the capillary membrane, only solutes of a certain size can flow with it.

  For example, the membrane pores of Bowman's capsule in the kidneys are very small, and only albumin, the smallest of the proteins, can be filtered through the membrane. By contrast, the membrane pores of liver cells are extremely large, so a variety of solutes can pass through and be metabolized.

- **Osmotic pressure** is the power of a solution to draw water. A highly concentrated solution (with many molecules in solution) has a high osmotic pressure and draws water. The plasma proteins in the blood exert osmotic (colloidal) pressure to help maintain fluid in the vascular space. When hydrostatic pressure exceeds osmotic pressure, fluid leaves the vessels.
- **Filtration pressure** is the net pressure created when hydrostatic pressure exceeds osmotic pressure. This pressure difference is the force that moves fluid and solutes. For example, the hydrostatic pressure is higher at the arteriole end of the capillary and lower at the venous end; thus, blood is forced out at the arteriole end and returned at the venule side.

Active Transport

Active transport occurs when molecules (e.g., electrolytes) move across cell membranes against a concentration

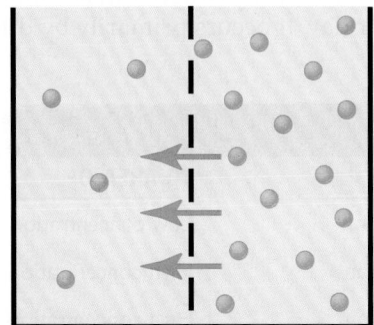

FIGURE 35-3 Diffusion is the movement of molecules of a solute through a cell membrane from an area of higher concentration to an area of lower concentration.

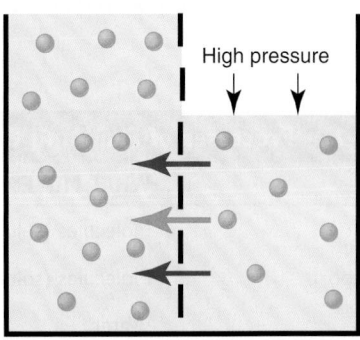

FIGURE 35-4 Filtration is the movement of water and smaller particles from an area of high pressure to an area of low pressure.

gradient (from an area of low concentration to an area of high concentration). Active transport requires energy expenditure (Fig. 35-5).

- **Adenosine triphosphate (ATP)** is released from the cell to enable certain substances to acquire the energy needed to pass through the cell membrane. For example, the sodium concentration is greater in the ECF; therefore, sodium tends to enter by diffusion into the intracellular compartment.
- The **sodium-potassium pump,** which is located on the cell membrane, offsets the tendency of ATP. In the presence of ATP, the sodium-potassium pump actively moves sodium from the cell into the ECF and potassium from the ECF into the cell.

Active transport is vital for maintaining the unique composition of both the extracellular and intracellular compartments. Table 35-2 summarizes the processes of fluid and electrolyte movement.

KnowledgeCheck 35-2

For each of the following, identify the appropriate mechanism: osmosis, diffusion, filtration, or active transport.

- Molecules move across a membrane to equalize concentration.
- Fluid moves across a membrane to equalize concentration.
- Molecules move against a concentration gradient.
- Molecules move to equalize pressure.

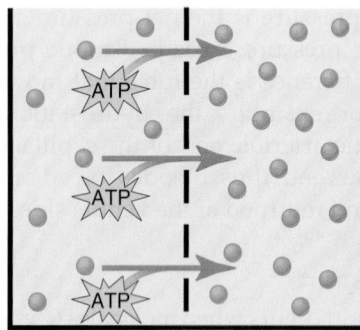

FIGURE 35-5 Active transport is the movement of electrolytes against a concentration gradient. For the movement to occur, active transport requires energy expenditure.

How Does the Body Regulate Fluids?

A balance between fluid intake and output (I&O) is essential to maintain homeostasis. Excesses or deficits of intake or output can lead to severe disorders.

Fluid Intake

You have undoubtedly been told to drink 8 to 10 glasses of water or 1,920 to 2,400 mL of fluid per day. The National Academies of Sciences, Engineering, and Medicine (2019), however, recommends a total fluid intake for adults over age 19 of 2,700 mL per day for females and 3,700 mL per day for males. At least 80% of our intake of water should come from drinking fluids and the remaining 20% from food and cellular metabolism of foods (Mayo Clinic, 2020). Prolonged exercise and heat exposure increase the requirements. No upper limits on fluid intake were set.

> The recommended daily fluid intake is 1,600 mL for older women and 2,000 mL for older men, unless restricted by a medical condition (Volkert et al., 2019; Masot, 2020). To determine the actual amount needed, as with acute illnesses, a formula using 1,500 mL of water as the minimum water intake is then adjusted by adding 15 mL fluid per kg of actual weight minus 20 kg (Faes et al., 2007).

Thirst is the major regulator of fluid intake. Changes in plasma osmolality signal the thirst center in the hypothalamus, which leads to the urge to drink.

- **Situations that increase plasma osmolality,** thereby promoting thirst, include excessive fluid loss, excessive sodium intake, and decreased fluid intake.
- **Situations that inhibit the thirst mechanism** include a high intake of fluids, fluid retention, excessive IV infusion of hypotonic solutions, and low sodium intake.

Fluid Output

Fluid loss occurs throughout the day, creating a constant need to replenish fluid. In a healthy state, fluid losses are equivalent to fluid intake.

- **Sensible fluid loss** is measurable and perceived (e.g., urine, diarrhea, ostomy, and gastric drainage).
- **Insensible fluid loss** is loss that we do not perceive, is not easily measured, but accounts for about 900 mL per day. It occurs primarily by diffusion and

Table 35-2 ➤ Processes of Fluid and Electrolyte Movement			
PROCESS	**WHAT MOVES**	**FROM AREA OF**	**TO AREA OF**
Diffusion	Molecules (solute)	High concentration	Low concentration
Active transport	Molecules (solute)	Low concentration	High concentration
Osmosis	Water	Low concentration	High concentration
Filtration	Water and small particles	High pressure	Low pressure

evaporation through the skin but also from the lungs. Insensible loss increases with open wounds, burns, or other breaks in the protective layer of the skin.

The following are common sources of fluid loss:

- **Urine** (1,500 mL/day). Urine accounts for the greatest amount of fluid loss. Urine output varies according to intake and activity but should remain at least 30 to 50 mL/hr. The volume of urine increases as fluid intake increases, and it decreases to compensate for other fluid losses (e.g., vomiting and excessive perspiration).
- **Feces** (100 to 200 mL/day). Soft stools contain more water than hard stools. As stool frequency increases, water loss also increases.
- **Skin** (about 600 mL/day). Fever, exercise, and some disease processes increase metabolic activity and heat production, leading to increased fluid loss.
  - **Sensible (perceived) loss** through the skin occurs through perspiration. Perspiration varies based on temperature, skeletal muscle activity, and metabolic activity.
  - **Insensible loss** through the skin occurs through evaporation.
- **Lungs** (about 300 mL/day). Insensible loss occurs through the lungs as water is exhaled with each breath. An increase in respiratory rate increases the amount of fluid lost.

Hormonal Regulation

Key Point: *The kidneys are the principal regulator of fluid and electrolyte balance. The following hormones are involved.*

Antidiuretic Hormone Pressure sensors in the vascular system stimulate or inhibit the release of **antidiuretic hormone (ADH)** from the pituitary gland. ADH causes the kidneys to retain fluid.

- **If fluid volume is low** within the vascular system, fluid pressures within the system decrease, and more ADH is released.
- **If fluid volume (and therefore pressure) increases,** less ADH is released, and the kidneys eliminate more fluid.
- **Other:** ADH is also produced in response to a rise in serum osmolality, fever, pain, stress, and some opioids.

Renin–Angiotensin System When extracellular (i.e., intravascular) fluid volume is decreased, receptors in the glomeruli respond to the decreased perfusion of the kidneys by releasing renin.

- **Renin** is an enzyme responsible for the chain of reactions that converts angiotensinogen to angiotensin II.
- **Angiotensin II** acts on the nephrons to retain sodium and water and directs the adrenal cortex to release aldosterone.

Aldosterone When aldosterone is released via the renin-angiotensin system, it stimulates the distal tubules of the kidneys to reabsorb sodium and excrete potassium. Sodium reabsorption results in passive reabsorption of water, thereby increasing plasma volume and improving kidney perfusion. When fluid excess is present, renin is not released, and this process stops.

Other Hormones Other hormones affect fluid and electrolyte balance by their effect on certain organs of the body:

- **Thyroid hormone** affects fluid volume by influencing cardiac output. An increase in thyroid hormone causes an increase in cardiac output, thereby increasing glomerular filtration rate and urine output. A decrease has the opposite effect.
- **Atrial natriuretic peptide (ANP), brain natriuretic peptide (BNP),** and **C-type natriuretic peptide (CNP)** are important in renal and cardiovascular regulation of fluid maintenance. **Natriuresis** (natriuretic) is the discharge of sodium through urine.
  - All three of these peptides are produced by heart cells; in addition, BNP is also released from the brain.
  - In clinical practice, BNP can be measured in the serum to help determine the presence of heart failure with fluid excess and to distinguish heart failure from pulmonary edema. The test can be performed at the bedside.

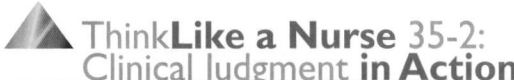

ThinkLike a Nurse 35-2: Clinical Judgment in Action

Apply the information on fluid balance to the LaGuardia family (Meet Your Patients).

- What have you learned that helps you explain why some family members require hospitalization?
- What additional information do you need to be able to predict each person's fluid balance?

How Does the Body Regulate Electrolytes?

To maintain health, the body must balance electrolyte losses and intake. For example, potassium lost through diarrhea and vomiting must be replaced by dietary potassium or potassium supplements. Table 35-3 provides information about the function, regulation, and food sources of major electrolytes in the body. Maintenance of normal serum electrolyte levels also depends on dietary intake, as well as various other mechanisms, discussed in the remainder of this section.

Sodium (Na⁺)

Sodium is the major cation in the ECF. Its primary function is to regulate fluid volume. When sodium is reabsorbed in the kidney, water and potassium are also reabsorbed, thereby maintaining ECF volume. Adults should limit the intake of salt to 2,300 mg/day (U.S. Department of Agriculture and U.S. Department of Health and Human Services, 2020). People who are

Table 35-3 ➤ Major Electrolytes

ELECTROLYTE	FUNCTION	REGULATION	SOURCES
Sodium (Na⁺) Major cation in the ECF Normal serum level is 135–145 mEq/L*	Regulates fluid volume. Helps maintain blood volume. Interacts with calcium to maintain muscle contraction. Stimulates conduction of nerve impulses.	Moves by active transport across cell membranes. Regulated by aldosterone and ADH levels. Reabsorbed and excreted through the kidneys. Minimal loss through perspiration and feces. Low sodium may be caused by excess water intake.	Table salt, soy sauce, cured pork, cheese, milk, processed foods, canned products, and foods preserved with salt.
Potassium (K⁺) Major cation in the ICF Normal serum level is 3.5–5.3 mEq/L	Maintains ICF osmolality. Regulates conduction of cardiac rhythm. Transmits electrical impulses in multiple body systems. Assists with acid–base balance.	Regulated by aldosterone. Excreted and conserved through the kidneys. Lost through vomiting and diarrhea. Loss triggered by many diuretics.	Common food sources include bananas, oranges, apricots, figs, dates, carrots, potatoes, tomatoes, spinach, dairy products, and meats.
Calcium (Ca²⁺) Most abundant electrolyte in the body Normal serum level is 8.5–10.5 mg/dL	Promotes transmission of nerve impulses. Major component of bone and teeth. Regulates muscle contractions. Maintains cardiac automaticity. Essential factor in the formation of blood clots. Catalyst for many cellular activities.	Combines with phosphorus to form the mineral salts of the teeth and bones. Calcium and phosphorus levels are inversely proportional. PTH stimulates release of calcium from bones and reabsorption from kidneys and intestines. Calcitonin (from the thyroid) blocks bone breakdown and lowers calcium levels. Absorption is stimulated by vitamin D.	See Table 35-4 for average daily requirements. Common food sources include milk, milk products, dark green leafy vegetables, and salmon, as well as calcium-fortified foods such as breads and cereals.
Magnesium (Mg²⁺) Present in skeleton and ICF; second most abundant cation in ICF Normal serum level is 1.6–2.6 mEq/L	Involved in protein and carbohydrate metabolism. Necessary for protein and DNA synthesis within the cell. Maintains normal intracellular levels of potassium. Involved in electrical activity in nerve and muscle membranes, including the heart. May have a role in regulating blood pressure and may influence the release and activity of insulin (National Academies of Sciences, Engineering, and Medicine, 2019).	Ingested in the diet and absorbed through the small intestine. Excreted by kidneys. Loss may be triggered by diuretics, poorly controlled diabetes mellitus, and excess alcohol intake.	Average daily requirement is 18–30 mEq. Found in most foods, but high levels are present in green vegetables, cereal grains, and nuts.

Table 35-3 ➤ Major Electrolytes—cont'd

ELECTROLYTE	FUNCTION	REGULATION	SOURCES
Chloride (Cl⁻) Major anion in the ECF Normal serum level is 95–105 mEq/L	Works with Na+ to maintain osmotic pressure between fluid compartments. Essential for production of HCl for gastric secretions. Functions as buffer in oxygen–carbon dioxide exchange in RBCs. Assists with acid–base balance.	Reabsorbed and excreted through the kidneys along with sodium. Levels increase and decrease simultaneously with sodium levels. Regulated by aldosterone and ADH levels. Deficits lead to potassium deficits; potassium deficits lead to chloride deficits.	Found in foods high in sodium.
Phosphate (PO₄⁻) Major anion in the ICF Normal serum level is 2.5–4.5 mEq/L	Serves as a catalyst for many intracellular activities. Promotes muscle and nerve action. Assists with acid–base balance. Important for cell division and transmission of hereditary traits.	Combines with calcium to form the mineral salts of the teeth and bones. Calcium and phosphorus levels are inversely proportional. Regulated by PTH; has inverse response to calcium. Excreted and reabsorbed by the kidneys.	Foods high in phosphorus are meat, fish, poultry, milk products, carbonated beverages, and legumes. Readily available in body as a result of metabolism.
Bicarbonate (HCO₃⁻) Major buffer in the body In ECF and ICF Normal serum level is 22–26 mEq/L	Maintains acid–base balance by functioning as the primary buffer in the body. Levels rise and fall to maintain pH.	Lost through diarrhea, diuretics, renal insufficiency. Excess possible if person ingests quantities of acid neutralizers.	Present in acid neutralizers (e.g., sodium bicarbonate). Not consumed in the diet; produced by the body to meet current needs

*Note that normal ranges may differ among references and in different laboratories.

ADH, Antidiuretic hormone; *ECF,* extracellular fluid; *HCl,* hydrochloric acid; *ICF,* intracellular fluid; *PTH,* parathyroid hormone; *RBC,* red blood cell.

especially sensitive to the blood pressure–raising effects of salt are advised to limit salt intake to 1,500 mg/day. This includes people (including children) with or who are statistically predisposed to a chronic disease (e.g., hypertension, diabetes, kidney disease) and those older than age 51. This limitation applies to nearly half of the U.S. population.

Potassium (K⁺)

Potassium is the major cation of the ICF and a key electrolyte in cellular metabolism. Only 2% of body potassium is found in the extracellular fluid. Adult males 19 years and older should consume at least 3,400 mg of potassium daily, compared with 2,600 for females (National Institutes of Health [NIH], 2022). However, most people do not consume enough potassium. Moderate potassium deficiency is associated with increases in blood pressure, salt sensitivity, risk of kidney stones, and risk of bone turnover (U.S. Department of Agriculture and U.S. Department of Health and Human

Services, 2020). Low intake of dietary potassium is associated with an increased risk of stroke.

In a healthy person, a high potassium intake does not result in hyperkalemia because the kidneys efficiently eliminate excess dietary potassium. However, potassium should, ideally, come from one's diet (e.g., fruit, vegetables) rather than from supplements.

Calcium (Ca²⁺)

Calcium is responsible for bone health and neuromuscular and cardiac function and is an essential factor in blood clotting. About 99% of body calcium is located in the bones and teeth. The remaining 1% circulates in the blood and affects system functions. Because calcium is so vital for cardiac and muscle function, serum levels are tightly regulated. As serum levels drop, calcium leaches from the bones and into the blood to compensate.

Although calcium requirements are highest during childhood, adolescence, pregnancy, and breastfeeding, it should be a regular component of the diet throughout the life span (Table 35-4). Most Americans do not include the recommended amount of calcium in their diets. Prolonged insufficient dietary intake can cause bone loss that leads to osteoporosis. People over the age of 50 are susceptible to osteoporosis, which can lead to fractures. You should teach patients that most calcium should be obtained from naturally calcium-rich foods, such as dairy products; however, calcium-fortified foods and calcium supplements can be used as a secondary source.

Magnesium (Mg²⁺)

Magnesium is a mineral used in more than 300 biochemical reactions in the body. Like calcium, only about 1% of magnesium is found in the blood. The remaining 99% is divided between the ICF and bone (in combination with calcium and phosphorus). Although magnesium deficiency is rare, you may find low levels in individuals who have a high alcohol intake. Some malabsorption disorders may also cause magnesium depletion.

Chloride (Cl⁻)

Chloride is the most abundant anion in the *extracellular* **fluid. It is usually bound with other ions, especially sodium or potassium** (e.g., as sodium chloride, or salt). A healthy adult between the ages of 19 and 50 should consume 2.3 grams of chloride each day along with 1.5 grams of sodium to replace daily losses

and maintain serum blood levels (National Academies of Science, Engineering, and Medicine, 2019).

Phosphorus (Phosphate [PO_4^-])

Phosphate is the most abundant *intracellular* **anion. Phosphate in the ECF is known as phosphorus.** Most phosphorus in the body is combined with oxygen, forming **phosphate**—mostly bound with calcium in teeth and bones as calcium phosphate.

Phosphate and calcium exist in an inverse relationship; as one increases, the other one decreases. As a result, high blood phosphate levels decrease the movement of calcium from the bones.

Bicarbonate (HCO_3^-)

Bicarbonate is present in both ICF and ECF. The kidneys regulate extracellular bicarbonate to maintain acid–base balance. When serum levels rise, the kidneys excrete excess bicarbonate. If serum levels are low, the kidneys conserve bicarbonate. Bicarbonate is not consumed in the diet but is produced by the body to meet current needs.

KnowledgeCheck 35-3

- Identify the major functions of sodium, potassium, calcium, magnesium, chloride, phosphate, and bicarbonate.
- What are the major concerns associated with sodium and potassium intake?

Table 35-4 ➤ Recommended Daily Allowances (RDAs) for Calcium and Vitamin D

AGE	CALCIUM (MILLIGRAMS)	VITAMIN D* (INTERNATIONAL UNITS)
Birth to 6 months	200	400
6–12 months	260	400
1–3 years	700	600
4–8 years	1,000	600
9–13 years	1,300	600
14–18 years	1,300	600
19–30 years	1,000	600
31–50 years	1,000	600
51–70 years, males	1,000	600
51–70 years, females	1,200	600
Older than 70 years	1,200	800
18 years or younger (pregnant or lactating)	1,300	600
19–50 years (pregnant or lactating)	1,000	600

*Adequate intake of vitamin D is necessary for absorption of calcium.

Source: National Academies of Sciences, Engineering, and Medicine. (2019). *Dietary reference intakes for sodium and potassium.* National Academies Press. https://doi.org/10.17226/25353; U.S. Department of Agriculture. (2020). *Dietary guidelines for Americans, 2020–2025* (9th ed.). https://www.dietaryguidelines.gov/sites/default/files/2021-03/Dietary_Guidelines_for_Americans-2020-2025.pdf

- Identify at least five potassium-rich foods.
- Identify the ideal calcium intakes for each member of the LaGuardia family (Meet Your Patients).

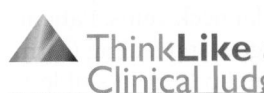

ThinkLike a Nurse 35-3:
Clinical Judgment in Action

Based on the information you have learned about the major electrolytes of the body, which electrolytes are most likely to be out of balance in members of the LaGuardia family? Explain your answer.

How Is Acid–Base Balance Regulated?

Acids and bases are formed in the body as part of normal metabolic processes.

- An **acid** is any compound that contains hydrogen ions (H^+) that can be released. For this reason, acids are referred to as *cation donors* (a **cation** is a positively charged particle). A common strong acid is hydrochloric acid (HCl), which is present in gastric secretions.
- A **base** or **alkali** is a compound that combines with (accepts) hydrogen ions in solution. Therefore, bases are referred to as *cation acceptors*. A strong base has a tendency to bind hydrogen ions, whereas a weak base binds only a small portion of the available hydrogen ions.

pH Measurement **pH is a measure of the amount of acid or base present in a solution.** The pH value is classified on a scale of acid (1.0 to 6.9), neutral (7.0), or alkaline (7.1 to 14). The lower the pH, the more *acidic* the solution. In contrast, an alkaline solution will have a higher pH. **Key Point:** *pH is measured on a logarithmic scale. For example, a pH of 4 is 10 times more acidic than a pH of 5. The body functions normally within a narrow range of pH values.*

- **Normal serum pH**—Arterial blood and tissue fluid normally have a pH of 7.35 to 7.45; therefore, they are slightly alkaline.
- **A serum pH below 7.30 or above 7.52** alters enzymatic activity and creates myocardial irritability.
- **A serum pH below 6.9 or above 7.8** is usually fatal.

Three complex mechanisms maintain acid–base balance: (1) buffers, (2) respiratory control of carbon dioxide, and (3) renal regulation of bicarbonate (HCO_3^-).

Buffers

Buffer systems prevent wide swings in pH. A **buffer system** consists of a weak acid and a weak base. Buffer molecules keep strong acids or bases from altering the pH either by absorbing or releasing free hydrogen ions.

Carbonic Acid–Sodium Bicarbonate System **Key Point:** *Carbonic acid (H_2CO_3) and sodium bicarbonate ($NaHCO_3$) buffer almost 90% of metabolic processes in the ECF.* Blood and tissue fluids depend on this buffer system to maintain a relatively constant pH. During normal metabolism, blood and tissue fluids tend

to become acidic; therefore, more sodium bicarbonate is required than carbonic acid.

- **(Normal) The usual ratio of $NaHCO_3$ to H_2CO_3 is 20:1.** As long as this ratio is maintained, the pH remains within its normal range.
- **(Acidosis) If bicarbonate is depleted** while neutralizing a strong acid, the pH may drop below 7.35, resulting in a condition called **acidosis.**
- **(Alkalosis) If carbonic acid is depleted** (by adding a strong base to extracellular fluid), the pH may rise above 7.45, resulting in a condition called **alkalosis.**

Phosphate System The phosphate system helps regulate acid–base balance in intracellular fluids. The phosphate system works in the same way as the bicarbonate system but converts *alkaline* sodium phosphate (Na_2HPO_4) to *acid* sodium phosphate (NaH_2PO_4).

Protein System Plasma proteins and the globin portion of hemoglobin (in red blood cells) contain chemical groups that can either combine with or free up hydrogen ions. This system helps buffer intracellular fluid and plasma to maintain pH balance.

Respiratory Mechanisms

Key Point: *The lungs are the second line of defense to restore normal pH.* They control the body's carbonic acid supply via carbon dioxide retention or removal to maintain the 20:1 ratio of base to acid.

- **When the serum pH is too acidic (pH is low),** the lungs remove carbon dioxide through rapid, deep breathing. This reduces the amount of carbon dioxide available to make carbonic acid.
- **When the serum pH is too alkaline (pH is high),** the lungs try to conserve carbon dioxide through shallow respirations.

Renal Mechanisms

Key Point: *The last line of defense is the kidneys, which regulate the concentration of plasma bicarbonate.* They can neutralize more acid or base than either the respiratory system or the chemical buffers.

- **If the serum pH is too acidic,** the kidneys conserve additional bicarbonate to neutralize the acid.
- **If the serum pH is too alkaline,** the kidneys excrete additional bicarbonate to lower the amount of base and thereby decrease the pH.
- The kidneys also buffer pH by forming acids and ammonium (a base).

Compensation Although the renal system is very effective at altering pH, it is slow. It may take up to 3 days to return pH to normal limits. This process is known as **compensation.** The pH returns to normal, but the carbon dioxide or bicarbonate level is abnormal. Over time, or when the original problem is corrected, these levels also return to normal.

KnowledgeCheck 35-4

- Briefly describe the three mechanisms used to maintain pH.
- Rank the acid–base balance mechanisms in order from the most rapidly acting to the slowest acting.

IMBALANCES: FLUID, ELECTROLYTE, AND ACID–BASE

Illness or disease may lead to imbalances of fluid, electrolytes, or pH. These are discussed in the next sections. The Practical Knowledge section, later in this chapter, presents some interventions to correct these imbalances.

Example Client Condition: Fluid Imbalances

Fluid imbalances involve a deficit or excess in fluid volume or an alteration in distribution among the fluid compartments. Concepts used to describe fluid imbalances are:

> *Hypovolemia* (fluid deficit); *Hypervolemia* (fluid excess) (*hypo* = low; *hyper* = high; *vol* = volume; *emia* pertains to blood).

Deficient Fluid Volume

Deficient fluid volume (hypovolemia) occurs when there is a proportional loss of fluid and electrolytes from the ECF from various causes (e.g., surgery, trauma, or uterine rupture).

Dehydration

Dehydration describes a state of negative fluid balance in which there is a loss of water (*hydro* = water) from the intracellular, extracellular, or intravascular space. Dehydration can be categorized by three causes:

1. **Insufficient fluid intake** (e.g., as may occur with depression, sedation, or alcohol abuse)
2. **Excessive fluid loss** (e.g., bleeding, vomiting, diarrhea)
3. **Fluid shifts** (e.g., intravascular fluid may leak into body tissues, burns)

When dehydration occurs from the loss of body fluids, electrolytes may also be lost. Fluid loss can also lead to an increase is serum osmolarity.

The first symptom of dehydration is thirst. Patients usually respond by drinking liquids. A fluid deficit occurs if the patient is unable to drink liquid, fluids are not provided, or blood loss exceeds replacement fluids (e.g., hemorrhage). At that point, the heart rate increases and the blood vessels constrict. This increases the blood pressure to help circulate the remaining fluid to meet the body's fluid demands.

Continuing Fluid Loss (Hypovolemic Shock)

As volume loss continues, the heart pumps faster but not as powerfully, resulting in a rapid, weak pulse and orthostatic hypotension. This is known as **hypovolemic**

shock. Water is pulled from the interstitial spaces and the ICF into the vascular system, resulting in dry skin and mucous membranes, decreased skin and tongue turgor, decreased urine output, and flat neck veins. Patients complain of muscle weakness, fatigue, and feeling warm. Temperature increases because the body is less able to cool itself through perspiration. However, body temperatures in older adults may not be elevated above normal.

Assessing for and Preventing Deficient Fluid Volume

Check for the early symptoms of dehydration, mentioned previously. Assess the blood pressure when the patient is lying, sitting, and standing. A drop in the systolic blood pressure (BP) (from lying to sitting or standing) of 20 mm Hg or more is called **orthostatic hypotension**. Other assessments include the following:

- **Key Point:** *Weight is a sensitive measure of fluid loss. A sudden loss of body weight of 5% is clinically significant, severe at 8%, and usually fatal at 15%.*
- The ratio of blood urea nitrogen (BUN) to creatinine and the hematocrit are elevated because there is less water in proportion to the solid substances.
- Urine specific gravity increases as the kidneys attempt to conserve water, resulting in more concentrated urine.

The patients at highest risk for dehydration are older adults, infants, children, and any patients with conditions associated with fluid loss (e.g., diabetes insipidus, vomiting, diarrhea, fever). See the Implementation/Taking Action section for ways to facilitate intake and provide parenteral fluids.

Excess Fluid Volume (Hypervolemia)

Excessive retention of sodium and water in the ECF increases osmotic pressure and causes fluid to shift from the cells into the ECF. **Excess fluid volume (hypervolemia)** can result from excessive salt intake, disease affecting kidney or liver function, or poor pumping action of the heart.

- **Signs of fluid overload**—Elevated blood pressure; bounding pulse; increased shallow respirations; cool, pale skin; and distended neck veins. When excess ECF accumulates in the tissues, especially in dependent areas, **edema** and rapid weight gain occur.
  - **In severe fluid overload,** the patient develops moist crackles in the lungs, dyspnea, and **ascites** (excess peritoneal fluid). Hemodilution causes the BUN, hematocrit, and specific gravity of the urine to decrease.
- **Preventing fluid overload**—Monitor I&O and use electronic pumps to carefully regulate IV infusions to minimize the risk of fluid overload. See the Implementation/Taking Action section for additional measures.

KnowledgeCheck 35-5

- Define *deficient fluid volume* and *excess fluid volume*.
- Identify the signs and symptoms of deficient fluid volume and excess fluid volume.
- Describe dehydration and hypervolemia.

Example Client Condition: Electrolyte Imbalances

Any electrolyte may become imbalanced. Table 35-5 discusses the common causes; signs and symptoms; and treatment of sodium, potassium, calcium, magnesium, and phosphate imbalances.

We can apply the information in Table 35-5 to the LaGuardia family (Meet Your Patients). Jackson LaGuardia has end-stage renal disease (ESRD) and is at risk for electrolyte imbalances. Now he is experiencing nausea, vomiting, and diarrhea. This will further aggravate the imbalance of potassium and sodium. He requires careful monitoring of all of his electrolytes and may need fluid replacement (rehydration). He is a candidate for admission to the hospital. The remaining family members are likely to be experiencing sodium, potassium, and fluid deficits.

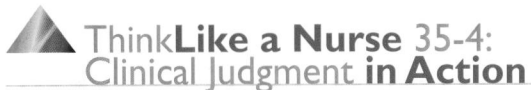

ThinkLike a Nurse 35-4: Clinical Judgment in Action

Martha LaGuardia (Meet Your Patients) takes the following medications: atenolol 50 mg daily at bedtime, alendronate sodium 10 mg daily, furosemide 20 mg every morning, and calcium carbonate 500 mg three times per day. Using your reference books, look up her prescribed medications. Given that Ms. LaGuardia is now experiencing nausea and vomiting, she may be at risk for developing medication-related side effects and problems. Which medications may cause problems? What problems might they cause? Explain why.

Example Client Condition: Acid–Base Imbalances

The two broad types of acid–base imbalance are acidosis and alkalosis:

- **Acidosis** occurs when the serum pH falls below 7.35.
- **Alkalosis** occurs when the serum pH increases above 7.45 (Fig. 35-6).

Arterial blood gases (ABGs) are used to monitor acid-base balance. **ABG analysis** measures pH, partial pressure of oxygen (Po_2), partial pressure of carbon dioxide (Pco_2), saturation of oxygen (Sao_2), and bicarbonate (HCO_3^-) level. **Key Point:** *Acid–base balance is reflected by the pH, PCO_2, and HCO_3 values.*

- **A respiratory disturbance alters the carbonic acid portion** of the buffering system, and the resulting imbalance is labeled *respiratory acidosis* or *respiratory alkalosis*.
- **A metabolic disturbance alters the bicarbonate portion** of the buffering system, so the resulting imbalance would be labeled as *metabolic acidosis* or *metabolic alkalosis*.

Table 35-5 ➤ Electrolyte Imbalances

DISORDER	COMMON CAUSES	SIGNS AND SYMPTOMS	TREATMENT
Hyponatremia Na⁺ <135 mEq/L	Diuretics GI fluid loss Adrenal insufficiency Excessive intake of hypotonic solutions, such as water or D₅W IV fluids Syndrome of inappropriate ADH	Anorexia, nausea, and vomiting Weakness Lethargy Confusion Muscle cramps or twitching Seizures	Monitor I&O. Monitor sodium level. Increase oral sodium intake. Administer IV saline infusion and take seizure precautions, if severe.
Hypernatremia Na⁺ >145 mEq/L	Excessive sodium intake Water deprivation Increased water loss through profuse sweating, heat stroke, or diabetes insipidus Administration of hypertonic tube feeding	Thirst Elevated temperature Dry mouth and sticky mucous membranes If severe: Hallucinations Irritability Lethargy Seizures	Monitor I&O. Monitor sodium level. Monitor vital signs and level of consciousness. Restrict sodium in the diet. Beware of hidden sodium in foods and medications. Increase water intake. Administer IV solutions that do not contain sodium.

(Continued)

Table 35-5 ➤ Electrolyte Imbalances—cont'd

DISORDER	COMMON CAUSES	SIGNS AND SYMPTOMS	TREATMENT
Hypokalemia K^+ <3.5 mEq/L	Diuretics GI fluid loss through vomiting, gastric suction, or diarrhea Steroid administration Hyperaldosteronism Anorexia or bulimia	Fatigue Anorexia, nausea, and vomiting Muscle weakness Decreased GI motility Dysrhythmias Paresthesia Flat T wave on ECG Increased sensitivity to digitalis	Monitor I&O. Monitor potassium level. If the client is taking digoxin, monitor pulse and observe for toxicity. Encourage intake of foods rich in potassium. Administer potassium supplements. (*Note:* IV supplements must be well diluted and administered into a central vein slowly.)
Hyperkalemia K^+ >5.0 mEq/L	Renal failure Potassium-sparing diuretics Hypoaldosteronism High potassium intake coupled with renal insufficiency Acidosis Major trauma Hemolyzed serum sample produces pseudohyperkalemia.	Muscle weakness Dysrhythmias Flaccid paralysis Intestinal colic Tall T waves on ECG	Monitor I&O. Monitor potassium level. Caution about potassium-rich food intake in patients with elevated creatinine levels.
Hypocalcemia Ca^{2+} <8.5 mq/dL	Hypoparathyroidism Malabsorption Pancreatitis Alkalosis Vitamin D deficiency	Diarrhea Numbness and tingling of extremities Muscle cramps Tetany Convulsions Laryngeal spasms Cardiac irritability *Positive Trousseau's and Chvostek's signs	Monitor I&O. Monitor serum calcium. Encourage increased calcium intake. Administer calcium supplements. If severe, monitor patency of airway, institute seizure and safety precautions, and administer parenteral calcium.
Hypercalcemia Ca^{2+} >10.5 mq/dL	Hyperparathyroidism Malignant bone disease Prolonged immobilization Excess calcium supplementation Thiazide diuretics	Muscle weakness Constipation Anorexia, nausea, and vomiting Polyuria and polydipsia Kidney stones Bizarre behavior Bradycardia	Monitor I&O. Encourage fluid intake to prevent stone formation. Encourage fiber to prevent constipation. Eliminate calcium supplements and limit calcium-rich foods. Avoid calcium-based antacids. Renal dialysis may be required.

Table 35-5 ➤ Electrolyte Imbalances—cont'd

DISORDER	COMMON CAUSES	SIGNS AND SYMPTOMS	TREATMENT
Hypomagnesemia Mg^{2+} <1.6 mEq/L	Chronic alcoholism Malabsorption Diabetic ketoacidosis Prolonged gastric suction	Neuromuscular irritability Disorientation Mood changes Dysrhythmias Increased sensitivity to digitalis	Monitor I&O. Encourage foods high in magnesium. Avoid alcohol intake. If the client is taking digoxin, monitor pulse and observe for toxicity.
Hypermagnesemia Mg^{2+} >2.6 mEq/L	Renal failure Adrenal insufficiency Excess replacement	Flushing and warmth of skin Hypotension Drowsiness, lethargy Hypoactive reflexes Depressed respirations Bradycardia	Monitor vital signs and airway. Monitor reflexes. Avoid magnesium-based antacids and laxatives. Restrict dietary intake of foods high in magnesium.
Hypophosphatemia PO_4^- <2.5 mg/dL	Refeeding after starvation Alcohol withdrawal Diabetic ketoacidosis Respiratory acidosis	Paresthesia Joint stiffness Seizures Cardiomyopathy Impaired tissue oxygenation	Monitor serum phosphorus level. Monitor calcium levels as phosphate is replaced. Start TPN slowly to avoid drops in phosphate.
Hyperphosphatemia PO_4^- >4.5 mg/dL	Renal failure Hyperthyroidism Chemotherapy Excess use of phosphate-based laxative	Short term: Tetany symptoms—tingling of extremities and cramping Long term: Calcification in soft tissue	Monitor serum phosphorus level. Monitor for tetany. If severe, administer aluminum hydroxide with meals to bind phosphorus.

*See **Clinical Insight 35-1: Assessing for Trousseau's and Chvostek's Signs,** in Volume 2.

ADH, Antidiuretic hormone; *ECG,* electrocardiogram; *GI,* gastrointestinal; *I&O,* intake and output; *IV,* intravenous; *TPN,* total parenteral nutrition.

Source: Van Leeuwen, A., & Bladh, M. (2021). *Davis's comprehensive handbook of laboratory & diagnostic tests with nursing implications* (9th ed.). F.A. Davis.

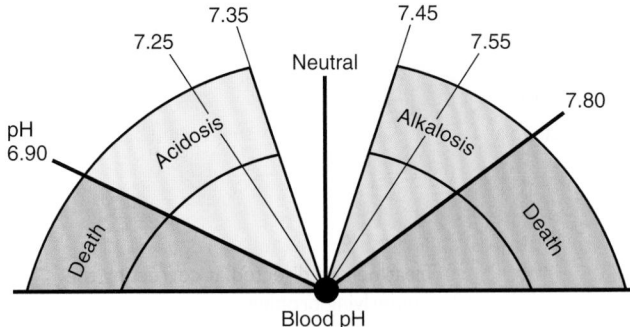

FIGURE 35-6 The pH scale ranges from 1 to 14. Normal blood pH is 7.35 to 7.45.

Metabolic and respiratory problems can coexist, resulting in disturbances of both sides of the buffering system. Compensatory mechanisms may also produce both bicarbonate and carbon dioxide abnormalities.

Interpreting ABGs

To determine acid–base balance, you must examine the ABG results. The pH, Pco_2, and HCO_3^- values are of primary importance (Table 35-6). The partial pressure of oxygen (Po_2) and saturation of oxygen (Sao_2) are also part of the ABG result, but they affect tissue oxygenation (see also Chapter 33). Table 35-7 describes the causes, manifestations, ABG results, and treatments of acid–base imbalances. Use the following steps to interpret acid–base balance of blood.

Step 1: Examine the pH. *Is it acidotic, alkalotic, or normal?*

- If the **pH is low (<7.35),** the blood is *acidic.*
- If the **pH is high (>7.45),** the blood is *alkalotic.*
- If the **pH is between 7.35 and 7.45,** the blood is *normal.*

Key Point: *Don't forget that neutral pH is 7.4. This will be very important when we discuss compensation.*

Table 35-6 ➤ Using ABGs to Assess Acid–Base Balance

EXPLANATION OF CHANGES	ABG COMPONENT	NORMAL RANGE	ACIDOSIS	ALKALOSIS
Indicates acidosis, alkalosis, or normal acid–base balance	pH	7.35–7.45 (7.4 is "neutral")	Low	High
Carbon dioxide ("acid") Signals respiratory cause	PCO_2	35–45 mm Hg	High	Low
Sodium bicarbonate ("base") Signals metabolic cause	HCO_3-	22–26 mEq/L	Low	High

Table 35-7 ➤ Acid–Base Imbalances

DISORDER	CLINICAL MANIFESTATIONS	INTERVENTIONS
Respiratory Acidosis May be caused by conditions or medications that impair gas exchange at the alveolar–capillary membrane, depressed respiratory rate and depth, or injury to the respiratory center in the brain.	**Acute:** Increased pulse and respiratory rate Headache, dizziness Confusion, decreased level of consciousness (LOC) Muscle twitching **Chronic:** Weakness Headache	Provide pulmonary hygiene. Institute measures to improve gas exchange, such as chest physiotherapy, bronchodilators, antibiotics. Provide supplemental oxygen. Maintain hydration.
Respiratory Alkalosis May be caused by hyperventilation resulting from anxiety, fever, sepsis, thyrotoxicosis, lesion in the respiratory center in the brain, or excessive ventilation with a mechanical ventilator.	Confusion, difficulty focusing Headache Tingling Palpitations Tremors	If caused by anxiety, encourage the patient to relax and breathe slowly. For other causes: Identify and treat the underlying disorder.
Metabolic Acidosis May be caused by retained acids in the blood resulting from renal impairment, poorly controlled diabetes mellitus, or starvation. Conditions that decrease bicarbonate, such as excessive GI loss, will also trigger metabolic acidosis. May be caused by excessive intake of acids, which may occur with aspirin poisoning, or by prolonged infusion of chloride-containing IV fluids.	Headache Confusion, drowsiness Weakness Peripheral vasodilation Nausea and vomiting Kussmaul's breathing (rapid and deep) Frequently associated with hyperkalemia	Treatment is directed at correcting the underlying problem. Bicarbonate may be prescribed.
Metabolic Alkalosis May be caused by excessive acid loss due to vomiting or gastric suction, use of potassium-wasting diuretics, hypokalemia, excess bicarbonate intake, or hyperaldosteronism.	Dizziness Tingling of extremities Hypertonic muscles Decreased respiratory rate and depth	Treatment is directed at correcting the underlying problem. Treatment often includes administration of sodium chloride solutions or sodium-rich fluids.

GI, Gastrointestinal; *IV,* intravenous.

Step 2: Check the amount of carbon dioxide in the blood (PCO_2). *Is there too little or too much?*

- If PCO_2 is <35 mm Hg—there is too little acid in the blood (*respiratory alkalosis*).
- If PCO_2 is >45 mm Hg—there is too much acid in the blood (*respiratory acidosis*).
- If PCO_2 is 35 to 45 mm Hg—the cause for the *abnormal pH is not respiratory.*

Step 3: Think about the bicarbonate level (HCO_3^-). *Is there too little or too much?*

- If HCO_3^- is <22 mEq/L—there is too little base in the blood (*metabolic acidosis*).
- If HCO_3^- is >26 mEq/L—there is too much base in the blood (*metabolic alkalosis*).
- If HCO_3^- is 22 to 26 mEq/L—*the cause for the abnormal pH is not metabolic.*

UNCOMPENSATED ABG	pH	$Paco_2$	HCO_3^-
Respiratory acidosis	↓	↑	Normal
Respiratory alkalosis	↑	↓	Normal
Metabolic acidosis	↓	Normal	↓
Metabolic alkalosis	↑	Normal	↑

Step 4: Is there compensation? *If so, is it partial or full?*

Now let's look at what happens when the acid–base imbalance continues for a period of time.

Key Point: *The body will naturally try to correct the unhealthy situation by using the lungs and kidneys to buffer the abnormality and return the pH to a normal range.*

- **If breathing is the reason** for the abnormal pH, then the kidneys will pick up the slack and try to improve the situation.
- **If the problem is metabolic,** then breathing (either faster and deeper or slower and more shallow) is the corrective approach.

No Compensation If the pH is abnormal, no compensation has occurred. The following example shows a low pH level and a high level of carbon dioxide. This is respiratory acidosis with no compensation.

pH = 7.30, PCO_2 = 50 mm Hg, HCO_3^- = 24 mEq/L

Partial Compensation Partial compensation is taking place if all of the following are present:

- pH and one ABG component are abnormal.
- Second ABG value is starting to change.
- pH is moving toward normal.

Now compare no compensation values with the following example of partially compensated respiratory acidosis:

pH = 7.32, PCO_2 = 50 mm Hg, HCO_3^- = 28 mEq/L

In this example, although the pH is increasing, it is still acidotic, and the Pco_2 remains high. Note that the HCO_3^- is increasing to alkalosis to bring the pH closer to normal.

PARTIAL COMPENSATION	pH	$Paco_2$	HCO_3^-
Respiratory acidosis	↓	↑	↑
Respiratory alkalosis	↑	↓	↓
Metabolic acidosis	↓	↓	↓
Metabolic alkalosis	↑	↑	↑

Full Compensation Full compensation occurs when the following are present:

- pH returns to *normal* range.
- The other two ABG components are *abnormal.*

The initial causal component is still abnormal, and the second ABG component (that had the normal values) has changed enough to return the pH to normal.

Note that in the following blood gas values, the pH is now in the normal range, and the Pco_2 is still high. But the HCO_3 is now also high; it has moved enough to raise the pH into the normal range. The problem is now *fully compensated respiratory acidosis.*

pH = 7.35, PCO_2 = 50 mm Hg, HCO_3^- = 30 mEq/L

FULL COMPENSATION	pH		$Paco_2$	HCO_3^-
Respiratory acidosis	Normal, but less than 7.35		↑	↑
Respiratory alkalosis	Normal, but greater than 7.45		↓	↓
Metabolic acidosis	Normal, but less than 7.35		↓	↓
Metabolic alkalosis	Normal, but greater than 7.45		↑	↑

KnowledgeCheck 35-6

Interpret the following ABG results:

pH = 7.53 PCO_2 = 26 mm Hg HCO_3^- = 22 mEq/L
pH = 7.40 PCO_2 = 39 mm Hg HCO_3^- = 25 mEq/L
pH = 7.30 PCO_2 = 70 mm Hg HCO_3^- = 30 mEq/L
pH = 7.48 PCO_2 = 46 mm Hg HCO_3^- = 30 mEq/L

PracticalKnowledge
knowing **how**

In the remainder of this chapter, you will learn to apply theoretical knowledge of fluids, electrolytes, and acid–base balance to patient care.

ASSESSMENT/RECOGNIZING CUES

The purposes of a focused assessment found in the Example Client Condition: Fluid, Electrolytes, and Acid-Base Imbalances are to:

- Identify clients at risk for or already experiencing imbalances.
- Identify the nature of the disorder.
- Evaluate responses to treatments.

The assessment includes a focused nursing history, a physical assessment, and a review of pertinent laboratory tests.

- **A focused nursing history** for fluids, electrolytes, and acid–base balance includes questions about demographic data, past medical history, current health concerns, food and fluid intake, fluid elimination, medications, and lifestyle.
- **A focused physical** assessment requires you to correlate physical assessment data with the nursing history and laboratory studies.

For questions to use in obtaining a focused nursing history,

 Go to **Chapter 35, Assessment Guidelines and Tools: Focused Assessment for Fluid, Electrolyte, and Acid–Base Balance, Nursing History,** in Volume 2.

KnowledgeCheck 35-7

- Identify 10 physical assessment components that can be used to monitor fluid, electrolyte, and acid–base balance (refer to the **Focused Assessment for Fluid, Electrolyte, and Acid–Base Balance, Nursing History,** in Volume 2).
- What aspects should be evaluated in a nursing history focused on fluid, electrolyte, and acid–base balance?

 Think**Like a Nurse** 35-5:
Clinical Judgment **in Action**

What vital sign changes would you expect to find when assessing Jackson LaGuardia (Meet Your Patients)?

Laboratory Studies

Several laboratory tests are performed to evaluate fluid, electrolyte, and acid–base status.

Complete Blood Count Fluid status is reflected in a **complete blood count (CBC),** which is a measure of red blood cells (RBCs), white blood cells (WBCs), and

platelets. Included in the CBC is the **hematocrit,** a measure of the percentage of RBCs in whole blood.

- **As fluid levels decrease,** the hematocrit increases (because the percentage of blood made up by cells increases).
- **As fluid levels increase,** the hematocrit decreases.

Serum Electrolytes Venous blood samples are taken to measure sodium, potassium, chloride, and bicarbonate levels. In many labs, a basic metabolic

---

PICOT

Early Treatment of Metabolic Acidosis

Situation: Several family members are being seen in the emergency department for suspected food poisoning. The grandfather, who has chronic kidney disease (CKD), is diagnosed with metabolic acidosis and admitted for treatment. The nurse wonders about the rationale for the treatments the patient receives.

PICOT Components:

P Population/client	=	Patients with CKD
I Intervention/indicator	=	Early metabolic acidosis treatment
C Comparator/control	=	Late or no treatment for metabolic acidosis
O Outcome	=	Reduced muscle wasting
T Time	=	The course of the disease

Searchable Question: Do _____ (P) who receive/are exposed to _____ (I), compared with _____ (C), demonstrate _____ (O) during _____ (T)?

Example of Evidence: The kidneys regulate fluid, electrolyte, and acid–base homeostasis. When these balances are altered, a client with CKD commonly develops chronic metabolic acidosis. This can lead to acceleration of the CKD, muscle wasting, development of bone disease, resistance to insulin, and increased mortality. Metabolic acidosis can be treated early in renal disease with oral medications or the addition of bases to dialysate. This helps maintain a normal plasma bicarbonate level and prevent chronic CKD.

Practice Change: The nurse acquired new knowledge of the importance of early treatment of CKD and its potential for preventing muscle wasting and other CKD complications.

_____

Sources: Dhondup, T., & Qian, Q. (2017). Acid-base and electrolyte disorders in patients with and without chronic kidney disease: An update. *Kidney Diseases, 3*(4), 136–148. https://doi.org/10.1159/000479968; Lin, J., Cheng, Z., Ding, X., & Qian, Q. (2018). Acid-base and electrolyte managements in chronic kidney disease and end-stage renal disease: Case-based discussions. *Blood Purification, 45*(1), 179–186. https://doi.org/10.1159/000485155; Vaidya, S., Aeddula, N. R., & Doerr, C. (2021). Chronic renal failure (nursing). *StatPearls.* https://www.ncbi.nlm.nih.gov/books/NBK568778/

panel also includes calcium, BUN/creatinine ratio and glucose. BUN and creatinine are sensitive measures of fluid status and kidney function. Physical assessment can also reveal hypocalcemia; for more information,

 Go to **Chapter 35, Clinical Insight 35-1: Assessing for Trousseau's and Chvostek's Signs,** in Volume 2.

Serum Osmolality Serum osmolality is a measure of the solute concentration of the blood, expressed as milliosmoles per kilogram (mOsm/kg). Changes in serum osmolality usually indicate alterations in sodium levels because sodium is the greatest determinant of serum osmolality. Glucose and urea also contribute. Serum osmolality may be directly measured with venous blood or estimated by doubling the serum sodium level.

- In **fluid volume deficit,** serum osmolality rises.
- In **fluid volume excess,** serum osmolality decreases.

Urine Osmolality Urine osmolality measures the solute concentration of urine. The body excretes nitrogenous wastes as well as electrolytes. As a result, urine osmolality is substantially higher than serum levels.

- **Fluid volume deficit** increases urine osmolality.
- **Fluid volume excess** decreases urine osmolality.

This test may require a 24-hour urine specimen or discarding the first-morning specimen and collecting a clean-catch specimen 2 hours later.

Urinalysis The **routine screening urinalysis** includes a measure of urine pH and specific gravity. **Key Point:** *Urine pH normally ranges from 5.0 to 9.0, with an average of 6.0.*

- Urine pH
  - Urine becomes *more acidic* in fluid volume deficit, acidosis, or starvation.
  - Urine becomes *more alkaline* with alkalosis.
- **Specific gravity** rises and falls in opposition to fluid status. **Key Point:** *A normal range is 1.001 to 1.029.*
  - **A low specific gravity** occurs when fluid is plentiful.
  - A **high specific gravity** occurs when fluid levels decrease and urine becomes more concentrated.

Arterial Blood Gases Interpretation of ABGs was discussed earlier in this chapter. For a list of these values, along with other laboratory studies discussed earlier,

 Go to **Chapter 35, Diagnostic Testing: Assessing Fluid, Electrolyte, and Acid-Base Imbalances,** in Volume 2.

NURSING DIAGNOSIS/ANALYZING CUES

Fluid, electrolyte, and acid–base imbalances may constitute nursing diagnoses, or they may form the etiologies of nursing diagnoses.

Imbalances as Diagnoses/Cues *Nursing diagnoses directly related to fluid* include Fluid Volume Deficient [isotonic], Fluid Volume Excess, Fluid Volume Deficient Risk, and Fluid Volume Alteration Risk.

Nursing diagnoses directly related to electrolyte or acid–base imbalances include Electrolyte Imbalance and Gas Exchange Impairment.

Example: Gas Exchange Impairment is appropriate for a client with a disorder affecting gas exchange at the alveolar–capillary membrane in the lungs (see Chapter 33). This condition limits the effectiveness of the carbonic acid–bicarbonate buffer system and alters serum pH, predisposing the patient to acid–base imbalances.

Imbalances as Etiologies Such imbalances (e.g., dehydration, metabolic acidosis, respiratory alkalosis) may also be etiologies of other nursing diagnoses. The following are a few examples:

- Activity Intolerance related to excess fluid and electrolyte loss through Diarrhea
- Oral Mucous Membranes Impairment related to Deficient Fluid Volume
- Cardiac Output Alteration related to hypovolemia

PLANNING/PRIORITIZING HYPOTHESES AND GENERATION SOLUTIONS

The overall goal for a client experiencing the Example Client Condition: Fluid, Electrolytes, and Acid–Base Imbalance is to restore balance.

Outcomes for describing fluid and electrolyte status include:

- **Electrolyte & Acid/Base Balance**—Balance of electrolytes and nonelectrolytes in the intracellular and extracellular compartments of the body
- **Electrolyte Balance**—Concentration of serum ions necessary to maintain equilibrium among electrolytes
- **Fluid Balance**—Balance of the input and output of fluids in the body
- **Fluid Overload Severity**—Severity of signs and symptoms of excess intracellular and extracellular fluids
- **Hydration**—Adequate water in the intracellular and extracellular compartments of the body

Individualized goals/outcome statements you might write for a client include the following examples:

- Maintains fluid balance, as evidenced by balanced 24-hour intake and output; good skin and tongue turgor; blood pressure and heart rate within normal limits; and no adventitious breath sounds.
- Electrolyte balance restored, as evidenced by alertness and cognitive orientation and no muscle cramping, seizures, or electrocardiogram changes.
- Drinks at least 2,500 mL in 24 hours.
- Urine specific gravity within normal limits.

PLANNING/PRIORITIZING HYPOTHESES AND GENERATING SOLUTIONS

Examples of interventions related to the Example Client Condition: Fluid, Electrolyte, and Acid-Base Imbalances include the following:

Acid–base management—Promotion of acid–base balance and prevention of complications resulting from acid–base imbalance

Electrolyte management—Promotion of electrolyte balance, prevention of complications resulting from abnormal or undesired serum electrolyte levels

Fluid management—Promotion of fluid balance and prevention of complications resulting from abnormal or undesired fluid levels

Fluid/electrolyte management—Regulation and prevention of complications from altered fluid and/or electrolyte levels

There are, of course, *specific* Nursing Interventions Classification (NIC) interventions for each type of fluid, acid–base, or electrolyte imbalance, for example:

Acid–Base Management: Metabolic Acidosis
Electrolyte Management: Hypernatremia
Fluid Management

Overall, nursing care focuses on preventing imbalances, modifying oral intake, providing parenteral fluids, and transfusing blood products as discussed in this chapter.

Individualized nursing interventions: The following sections describe nursing interventions and activities for

preventing and treating the Example Client Condition: Fluid, Electrolyte, and Acid–Base Imbalance.

PREVENTING FLUID AND ELECTROLYTE IMBALANCES

It is better to prevent imbalances than to treat them. Use the data obtained from your assessment to plan with your client to avoid imbalances. Common strategies

---

♥ iCare 35-1

Fluids, Electrolytes, and Acid–Base Balance

- Because an alteration in fluids, electrolytes, and acid–base balance encompasses such a wide variety of disease processes, nurses must possess keen assessment skills.
- Constant observation of a person's weight, laboratory values, eating habits/choices, and bowel and bladder habits is essential to proper care and management.
- Consideration of the patient's cultural preferences and religious beliefs concerning fluids and artificial feeding should be explored and honored at all times. You may be involved in some of these conversations with patients/families. You are obligated to share the patient's preferences and beliefs with other members of the healthcare team to provide a unified approach and to respect the patient's wishes—especially if it involves the withholding of fluids/feedings. If appropriate, you can suggest a palliative care consultation to help patients/families and teams.

Self-Care

Teaching Patients to Prevent Fluid and Electrolyte Imbalances

➤ Teach the client about usual fluid needs and circumstances that increase fluid needs: high environmental temperature, fever, gastrointestinal fluid loss, or draining wounds. Base your teaching on the client's current intake and the changes required to meet fluid goals.

➤ Identify medications or conditions that place the client at risk for imbalances. For example, if the client is receiving a potassium-wasting diuretic, they will need to increase potassium intake, either by taking a supplement or by altering the diet.

Also teach clients to do the following:

➤ Drink at least eight to ten 8-ounce glasses of water per day unless your healthcare provider has told you to limit fluids.

➤ Healthy adults use thirst as a guide to fluid intake. However, adults older than age 50 may have diminished thirst sensation and cannot depend solely on thirst for fluid replacement.

➤ Colorless urine is also a guide to adequate hydration, whereas darker urine is associated with dehydration. You can also use a urine color chart to monitor hydration.

➤ Limit consumption of fluids high in salt, sugar, caffeine, or alcohol.

➤ Vigorous exercise may delay the thirst mechanism. Athletes should become accustomed to consuming fluids at regular intervals during training sessions and competitions so that they do not experience dehydration.

➤ Drink water before, during, and after strenuous exercise.

➤ Avoid routine use of laxatives, antacids, weight-loss products, or enemas. These products may cause imbalances of fluids and electrolytes such as sodium and potassium.

➤ Weigh yourself daily if fluid balance is critical or if you are experiencing excessive loss or gain.

➤ Contact a health professional if there is a sudden change of weight, decreased urine output, swelling in dependent areas (e.g., hands and feet), shortness of breath, or dizziness.

➤ Contact a healthcare provider if you experience prolonged vomiting, diarrhea, or inability to tolerate liquids or food.

➤ Eat a well-balanced diet, including dairy products rich in calcium.

are listed in the accompanying Self-Care box, Teaching Patients to Prevent Fluid and Electrolyte Imbalances.

Dietary Changes

Key Point: *To promote fluid and electrolyte balance, most people need to limit their sodium intake and increase their intake of dietary potassium and calcium.* Some may need oral electrolyte supplements as well. Teach clients to:

- Eat foods rich in potassium and calcium daily.
- Avoid sodium-rich foods (e.g., processed foods).
- Read labels to identify the percentage of each (see Chapter 24 to review foods, as needed).

Oral Electrolyte Supplements

Many clients are unable to correct electrolyte disturbances with dietary changes alone. This is especially true for clients who have food intolerances, who rely on prepared meals, or who live in group settings. Such clients may need oral supplements to meet their dietary requirements. Some electrolytes that are commonly supplemented are potassium and calcium. See suggested nursing activities for these supplements in the accompanying Self-Care box, Taking Oral Electrolyte Supplements.

 Most adults, especially older adults, consume less dietary calcium per day than the 1,200 mg recommended amount. This increases their risk for osteoporosis and fractures.

KnowledgeCheck 35-8

- Identify laboratory tests that monitor fluid, electrolyte, and acid–base balance.
- Give at least five strategies to prevent fluid and electrolyte imbalance.

Self-Care

Taking Oral Electrolyte Supplements

➤ Encourage clients to take potassium supplements with juice to mask the taste.

➤ Teach clients to take supplements as prescribed to maintain electrolyte balance.

➤ Remind clients that supplements are medications and should be viewed as part of the treatment plan.

➤ If the client's medications are altered, review the continued need for supplements.

➤ Caution clients that salt substitutes contain potassium. If the client has been advised to use salt substitutes, evaluate the need for potassium supplements.

➤ Encourage clients who take calcium supplements to consume at least 2,500 mL of fluid per day to avoid constipation and reduce the risk of kidney stone formation.

Modifying Oral Fluid Intake

Clients experiencing fluid imbalances may need to restrict or increase their daily oral intake to correct the underlying disorder.

Facilitating Fluid Intake

Clients with actual or potential fluid volume deficit may need to increase their fluid intake. Whenever possible, clients should take fluids by mouth. You may provide replacement through a nasogastric or feeding tube if the client is unable to meet their needs independently but can tolerate fluids in the gastrointestinal tract. Parenteral fluid replacement is used only when enteral replacement cannot meet the client's fluid needs (for review, see Chapter 24).

To increase fluid intake successfully, you must first establish the desired amount of fluid intake for the client. The daily fluid goal reflects the client's current fluid balance and underlying condition. For example, if a prescription for a client with a dehydration reads, "Force fluids: 2,500 mL oral fluids per 24 hours," you can use this to develop a fluid schedule. Typically, people drink more fluid during the day and early evening, when they are more likely to be active, and less in the late evening to avoid sleep interruption. Thus, an example of a fluid distribution is:

0700 to 1500—1,300 mL
1500 to 2300—1,000 mL
2300 to 0700—200 mL

Strategies to increase fluid intake include the following:

- Assess the client's fluid preferences.
- Offer a variety of fluids throughout the day on a regular schedule. Vary hot and cold liquids, and offer a choice of drinks each time you are at the bedside.
- Instruct unlicensed assistive personnel to make "fluids rounds" to offer and help with oral fluids.
- Break daily goals into hourly amounts. For example, in the preceding example, in the 8 hours between 0700 and 1500, have the patient drink 150 mL of fluid every hour.
- Provide a cup with milliliter markings so that the patient will know how much they are drinking.
- Always have fluid readily available for the patient. Keep a pitcher of water at the bedside.
- Encourage family members to participate in offering fluids and tracking the intake amount.
- Schedule procedures to minimize the length of time the patient must fast (be NPO—nothing by mouth).
- For ambulatory patients (e.g., residents in long-term care facilities), schedule "tea time" or other events to promote increased intake.

Facilitating Fluid Restriction

Patients may need to limit fluids for a variety of reasons (e.g., impaired cardiovascular, liver, or renal function).

To facilitate fluid restrictions effectively, teach patients and caregivers the reason for the restriction and the amount of fluid allowed per shift. Fluid restrictions usually include *all* forms of intake. For example, a prescription might read: "Limit total fluid intake to 1,500 mL per 24 hours." If the patient is receiving IV antibiotics in 75 mL four times per day, you must include this 300 mL as a part of the total fluids. You can distribute the remaining 1,200 mL of oral intake to 800 mL on the day shift and 400 mL on the night shift.

Strategies to restrict fluid intake include the following:

- Do not offer liquids with meals. Reserve liquids for between meals.
- Limit intake of foods that increase thirst (e.g., dry, salty, or spicy foods).
- Keep liquids away from the bedside; offer ice chips to help quench thirst.
- Provide frequent oral hygiene.
- Provide diversional activities for the patient.

PARENTERAL REPLACEMENT OF FLUIDS AND ELECTROLYTES

When fluid loss is severe or the client cannot tolerate oral or tube feedings, fluid volume is replaced parenterally.

Replacement fluids and electrolytes should be carefully supervised.

- **Parenteral** refers to any route other than through the alimentary canal (passage from the mouth to the anus).
- **IV therapy** is the administration of fluids, electrolytes, medications, or nutrients by the venous route. IV fluids are used to:
  - Expand intravascular volume.
  - Correct an underlying imbalance in fluids or electrolytes.
  - Compensate for an ongoing problem that is affecting either fluid or electrolytes until oral intake is tolerated.

Martha LaGuardia (Meet Your Patients) is being treated in the emergency department (ED) for gastroenteritis. She is experiencing fluid loss from vomiting and diarrhea, complicated by her use of a diuretic. Mrs. LaGuardia will receive IV fluids to expand her intravascular volume and to maintain hydration, along with replacement electrolytes based on her laboratory results.

Other members of the LaGuardia family are experiencing fluid losses and should increase their fluid intake but may not need IV fluid replacement.

When initiating and maintaining IV infusions, always use careful aseptic technique. Remember that the IV catheter provides a portal of entry for pathogens directly into the bloodstream. You should know that Medicare will not reimburse a hospital for the expenses (e.g., antibiotics, extra hospital days) caused by catheter-related infections that occur during hospitalization. Excellent nursing technique can reduce IV catheter–associated infections.

Types of Intravenous Solutions

Solutions, including IV fluids, are classified according to how they compare to the osmolality of blood serum. To review: IV fluids are classified as isotonic, hypotonic, and hypertonic solutions. To help you remember, here is a summary. When infused:

- **Isotonic** fluids *remain in* the intravascular compartment.
- **Hypotonic** fluids *pull body water out* of the intravascular compartment.
- **Hypertonic** fluids *pull body water into* the intravascular compartment.

Isotonic Fluids

Normal blood serum osmolality is 275 to 295 mOsm/kg. Isotonic solutions have similar tonicity (250 to 375 mOsm/L). Therefore, when infused, they remain inside the blood vessels. **Key Point: As a result, isotonic fluids are useful for clients with hypotension or hypovolemia.** Commonly prescribed isotonic fluids are the following:

- 0.9% sodium chloride (0.9% NaCl), also called *normal saline* (NS)
- Lactated Ringer's (LR)

The solution 5% dextrose in water (D_5W) may be classified as both isotonic and hypotonic. It is isotonic in the bag but is not prescribed for isotonic use because after (rapid) metabolism, it is hypotonic in the body.

Clients at risk for fluid volume excess (e.g., congestive heart failure) must be closely monitored when they receive isotonic fluid replacement because they may easily develop fluid overload.

Hypotonic Fluids

The osmolality of a hypotonic solution is less than that of serum (less than 250 mOsm/L). Therefore, when infused, these solutions pull body water from the intravascular compartment into the interstitial fluid compartment. As the interstitial fluid is diluted, its osmolarity decreases, drawing water into the adjacent cells. **Key Point: Hypotonic fluid is used for hyperglycemic conditions, such as diabetic ketoacidosis, in which high serum glucose draws fluid out of the cells and into the vascular and interstitial compartments.** Examples of hypotonic fluids include:

- D_5W. Recall that D_5W is isotonic in the bag, with an osmolality of 253 mOsm/L, but becomes hypotonic in the body.
- 0.45% NaCl (½ normal saline)

- 0.33% NaCl
- 0.2% NaCl

✛ Administer hypotonic fluids carefully to prevent a sudden fluid shift from the intravascular space to the cells. Never give hypotonic solutions to patients at risk for increased intracranial pressure because they can cause or worsen cerebral edema.

Hypertonic Fluids

The osmolality of hypertonic fluids is higher than that of serum. When administered, they pull fluids and electrolytes from the intracellular and interstitial compartments into the intravascular compartment. **Key Point:** *Hypertonic fluids can help stabilize blood pressure, increase urine output, and reduce edema. Volume expanders (e.g., dextran and serum albumin) are hypertonic and are used to increase blood volume after severe loss of blood or plasma, such as in major burns or hemorrhage.* The following are examples of hypertonic fluids:

- D_5 0.9% NaCl (D_5 NS)
- D_5 0.45% NaCl (D_5 ½ NS)
- D_5 lactated Ringer's
- 3% NaCl and 5% NaCl—highly hypertonic; used only in critical situations
- 10% dextrose in water ($D_{10}W$)
- $D_{20}W$—used as an osmotic diuretic to promote diuresis

Peripheral Vascular Access Devices

IV therapy requires the placement of a vascular access device (VAD). You will choose the type of device based on the client's condition, the type of fluid that will be infused, and the anticipated length of treatment.

Key Point: *IV catheters (and needles) are sized by their diameter, which is called the* **gauge.** *The smaller the diameter, the larger the gauge (e.g., a 16-gauge catheter is larger than a 21-gauge catheter).* Therefore, the smaller the gauge, the more rapidly fluid can be delivered. Various types of catheters are used to access peripheral veins, including the following.

Over-the-Needle Catheters Over-the-needle catheters are also called **angiocaths,** short for *angiocatheters* (Fig. 35-7A). A polyurethane or Teflon catheter is threaded over a metal stylet (needle). You pierce the skin and vein with the needle, advance the catheter into the vein, and remove (or retract) the metal needle. In most cases, the plastic catheter is less than 7.5 cm (3 in.) in length. This type of access device is ideal for brief therapy. However, you cannot give highly irritating or hyperosmolar solutions through this type of catheter because it may cause severe damage to the vein.

Inside-the-Needle Catheters Inside-the-needle catheters are similar to the over-the-needle catheters; however, the polyurethane or Teflon catheter lies inside the

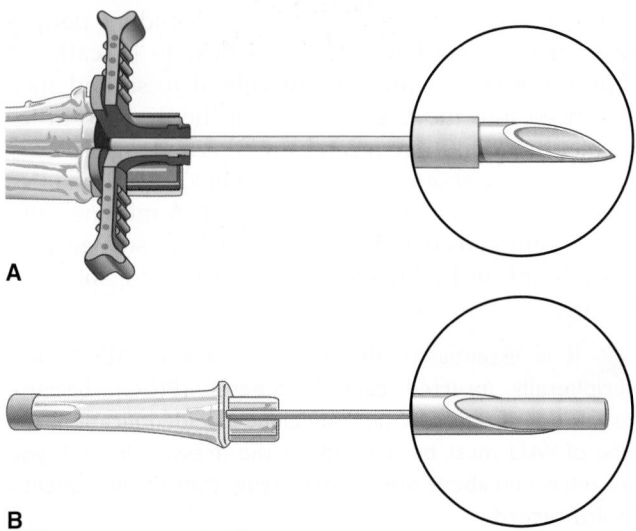

FIGURE 35-7 Typical intravenous (IV) access devices. A, An over-the-needle catheter. B, An inside-the-needle catheter.

metal needle (Fig. 35-7B). After you advance the catheter into the vein, you withdraw the needle.

A Butterfly Needle A butterfly needle is also called a *scalp vein needle* or *wing-tipped catheter.* It is a short, beveled metal needle with flexible plastic flaps attached to the shaft (Fig. 35-8). You can pinch the flaps and hold them tightly together to facilitate insertion. After insertion, flatten them out and tape them against the skin to prevent dislodgement during the infusion process. **Key Point:** *The Infusion Nurses Society (INS, 2021) recommends that the steel wing-tipped catheter is used only for single-dose administration or drawing blood and should not be left in place.* ✛ Because the inflexible metal needle remains in the vein, a butterfly needle is more likely to infiltrate (damage the vein and allow fluid to leak into the interstitial spaces) than a flexible plastic catheter.

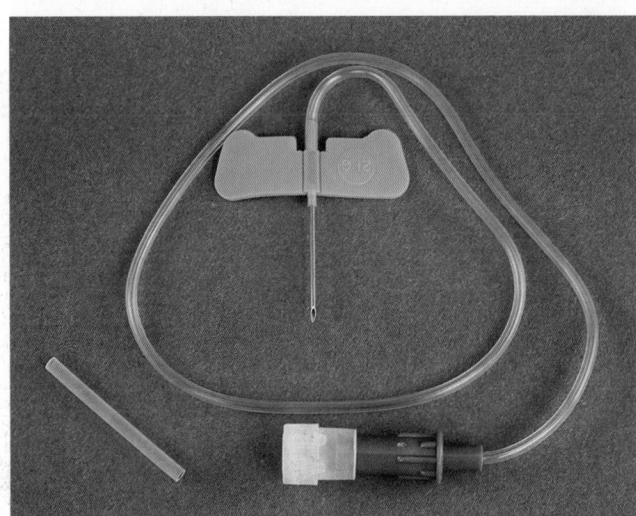

FIGURE 35-8 The butterfly, or scalp vein, needle is commonly used for drawing blood, single-dose medication administration, or administration of small volumes of fluids to infants and older adults.

A Midline Peripheral Catheter A midline peripheral catheter (midline VAD) is a flexible IV catheter, typically inserted into the antecubital fossa and then advanced into the larger vessels of the upper arm for greater hemodilution. It can be used for a longer period of time than a shorter, over-the-needle catheter; the INS recommends 5 to 14 days (INS, 2021). A midline catheter is still considered a peripheral line, so you cannot administer highly osmolar and irritating solutions through it.

✥ It is essential to distinguish a midline VAD from a peripherally inserted central catheter (PICC). Because visual identification is not sufficient for identification, the *type* of VAD must be marked on the dressing label. If you are uncertain about the catheter type, consult the patient's health record.

A Peripheral Intravenous Lock A peripheral IV lock (e.g., saline lock, prn adapter, heparin lock) establishes a venous route as a precautionary measure for clients whose condition may change rapidly or who may require intermittent infusion therapy. A peripheral IV catheter is inserted into a vein, and the hub is capped with a lock port (Fig. 35-9). The patency of the lock is maintained by injecting normal saline or a dilute heparin solution, depending on agency policy (see Procedure 35-6).

Central Venous Access Devices

A **central venous access device (CVAD)** is an intravenous line inserted into a major vein. Typically, the subclavian or internal jugular vein is used. Using surgical asepsis, a catheter is advanced from the insertion

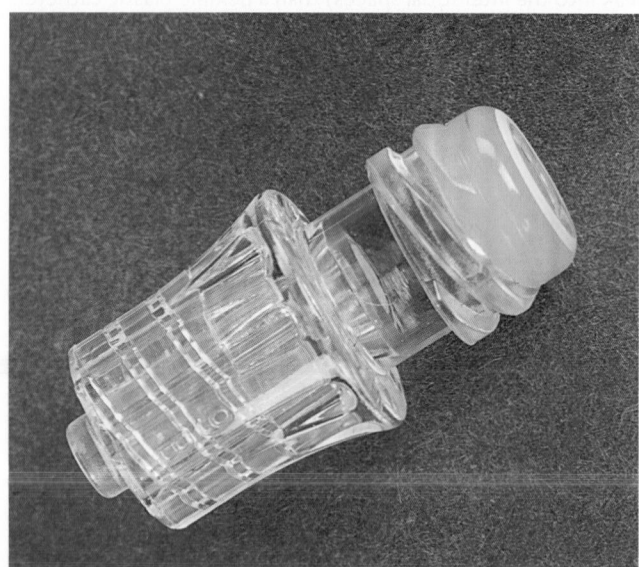

FIGURE 35-9 A peripheral intravenous lock establishes a venous route as a precautionary measure for clients whose condition may change rapidly or who may require intermittent infusion therapy.

site into the superior vena cava. You will likely care for patients with central lines, and you may need to assist with inserting them. To learn how to care for patients with central lines, see the Highlights of Procedures box for a summary, and

 Go to **Chapter 35, Clinical Insight 35-4: Caring for Patients With a Central Venous Access Device, Procedure 35-5B: Central Line Dressings,** and **Procedure 35-9: Assisting With Percutaneous Central Venous Catheter Placement,** in Volume 2.

Advantages of Central Lines A central line offers several advantages:

- A central vein can accommodate highly irritating and hyperosmolar solutions because the blood and solution mix rapidly at the infusion site.
- Central veins are accessible even if the patient is experiencing severe fluid depletion.
- Some types of central lines may also be used to monitor central venous pressure.
- Central lines are recommended for infusions with an anticipated duration of greater than 15 days (INS, 2021).
- Nutrition can be given parenterally.
- Phlebitis, extravasation, and infiltration are less likely to occur with central lines.
- Central lines with extra ports allow you to withdraw blood from a port to use for laboratory tests.

Disadvantages of Central Lines Drawbacks to central lines include:

- Practitioners must have specialized training to insert the catheter.
- Patient consent is required. Placement is treated as a minor surgical procedure.
- Placement must be confirmed by radiography.
- Placement and dressing changes require strict sterile technique.
- Several possible risks (e.g., sepsis, air embolus, ventricular dysrhythmia if the catheter floats to the right side of the heart; pneumothorax when placed though the subclavian vein).
- A greater risk of air embolus and infection exist compared with peripheral IVs.
- Increased risk for catheter-related bloodstream infections and sepsis than for peripheral sites.

Preventing Central Line–Associated Bloodstream Infections Key Point: *To help prevent CVC catheter-related infections, the following measures are recommended:*

- **Education and training**—Regarding proper infection control measures to prevent intravascular catheter-related infections. Encourage patients to report any changes or new discomfort in their catheter site.
- **Hand hygiene**—Wearing gloves does not make hand washing unnecessary.

- **Full barrier precautions for insertion**—Includes sterile drape for patient, head cover, mask, and sterile gown and gloves.
- **Chlorhexidine skin antisepsis**—Use alcohol-based chlorhexidine solution to prep the insertion site.
- **Optimal catheter site selection**—The subclavian vein has the lowest rate of infection. The femoral vein should be avoided if possible.
- **Type of catheter**—To reduce the risk of catheter-related infection, the catheter with the fewest number of ports or lumens needed to manage the patient is best.
- **Daily review of lines**—The CVC should be removed as soon as it is no longer necessary. The risk of infection is closely related to the length of time the CVC is in place (INS, 2021; Hicks & Lopez, 2022).

Types of Central Venous Catheters

There are four types of CVADs: peripherally inserted central catheters, nontunneled CVCs, tunneled CVCs, and implanted ports.

Peripherally Inserted Central Catheters (PICCs)
PICCs are long, soft, flexible catheters inserted at the antecubital fossa through the basilic or cephalic vein of the arm. The catheter is then advanced into the superior vena cava (Fig. 35-10). A qualified provider performs the insertion. PICC lines are most commonly used for prolonged IV antibiotic therapy, parenteral nutrition, and chemotherapy. **Key Point: *A PICC line is intended for intermediate- to long-term use and does not need to be replaced unless the site appears infected or the catheter is no longer patent.***

Nontunneled Central Venous Catheters Nontunneled CVCs are inserted by a qualified provider through the skin into the jugular, subclavian, and occasionally, femoral veins. They are sutured in place.

Often these are referred to as *single-, double-, triple-, or quadruple-lumen catheters,* depending on the number of ports in the line (Fig. 35-11). **Key Point: *These CVADs are intended for shorter use than a PICC line (less than 6 weeks) and should not be routinely replaced.*** Nontunneled CVCs account for the majority of central line–associated bloodstream infections (CLABSIs).

Blood can be drawn from a nontunneled CVAD for diagnostic studies or used to measure central venous pressure (CVP) to obtain information on blood volume.

✚ If parenteral nutrition or blood is running in a port, you cannot use that same port for blood draws.

Example: Imagine that you have a patient who needs two different kinds of IV fluids, parenteral nutrition, and frequent blood draws for laboratory tests. The patient has fragile peripheral veins and is at high risk for infection. With a multiple-lumen central catheter, the patient needs only one insertion site. You can infuse both fluids and the parenteral nutrition fluids and still reserve one port for drawing blood. The patient has less risk for the catheter to become dislodged or infiltrated or for phlebitis to develop.

Tunneled Central Venous Catheters Key Point: *Tunneled CVPs are intended for long-term use.* The catheter is inserted by a surgeon through a 7.5- to 15-cm (3- to 6-in.) subcutaneous tunnel in the chest wall and then into the jugular or subclavian vein (Fig. 35-12). One end of the catheter comes out through the skin and is sutured in place, with the sutures removed when fibrosis has developed around the catheter, or it can be secured with an IV-securing device. CVCs are tunneled through the skin rather than through a vein and therefore have a lower risk of systemic infection.

Implanted Ports Implanted ports are devices made of a radiopaque silicone catheter and a plastic or stainless-steel injection port with a self-sealing silicone-rubber septum. The catheter enters the internal jugular vein in

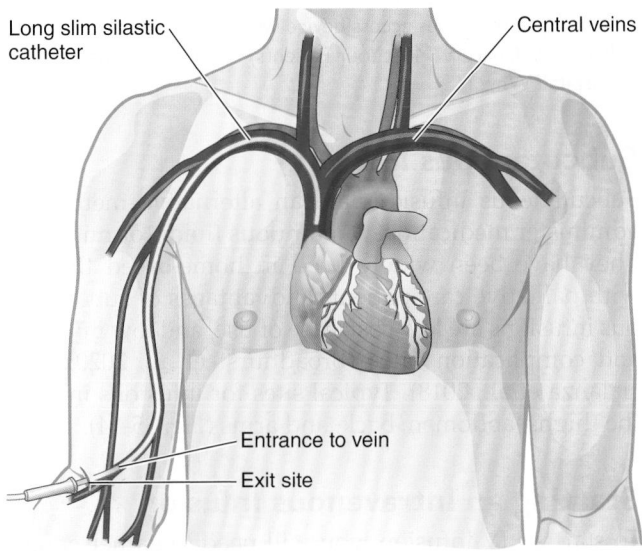

FIGURE 35-10 A peripherally inserted central catheter (PICC) line is a long, soft, flexible catheter inserted through a vein in the arm and threaded into a central vessel.

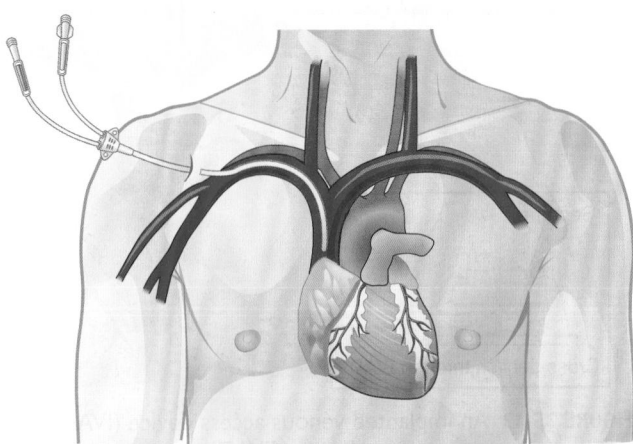

FIGURE 35-11 Nontunneled central venous catheters are inserted into the jugular, subclavian, and occasionally, femoral veins.

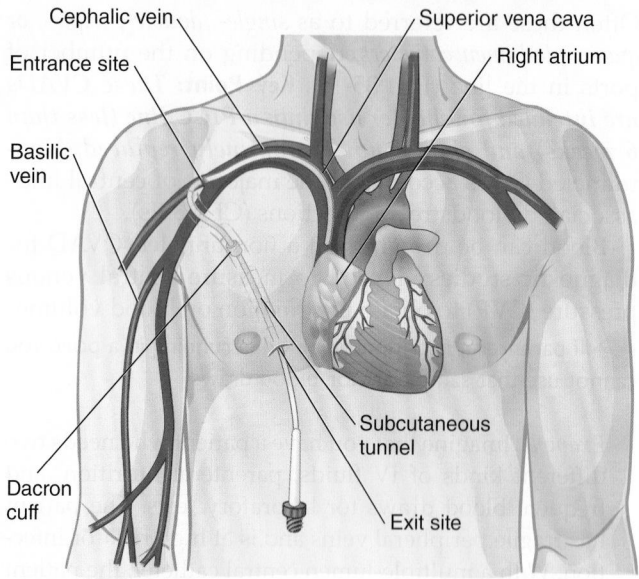

FIGURE 35-12 A tunneled central venous catheter is inserted through subcutaneous tissue in the chest wall into the jugular or subclavian vein.

the neck, and it may be tunneled or untunneled to a completely implanted subcutaneous reservoir (port) in the upper chest (Fig. 35-13). **Key Point: *Implanted ports are also intended for long-term use.*** They are placed by surgeons, and only specially trained nurses are allowed to access an implanted port because of the risk of infiltration into the tissue if the needle placement is not correct.

✚ Avoid taking blood pressures or drawing blood in the extremity on the side of the chest where the implanted port has been placed.

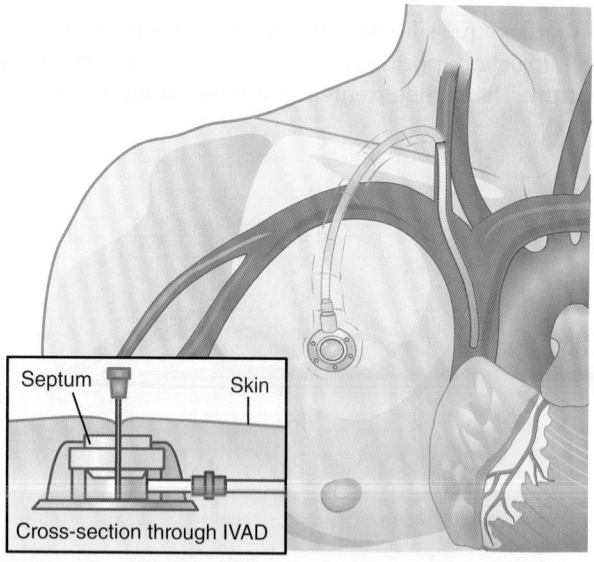

FIGURE 35-13 An implanted venous access device (IVAD) is a central venous access device (CVAD) that enters the internal jugular vein in the neck but is tunneled to a completely implanted subcutaneous reservoir (port) in the upper chest.

The Highlights of Procedures box summarizes steps for assisting with the placement of a percutaneous central venous catheter. For the complete procedure,

 Go to **Chapter 35, Procedure 35-9, Assisting With the Percutaneous Central Venous Catheter Placement,** in Volume 2.

Intraosseous Devices

Designed for immediate access (within seconds) and short-term use (less than 24 hours), intraosseous (IO) access devices are used to administer fluids when a peripheral catheter cannot be inserted or when a central line insertion is not advisable, especially in emergency situations. IOs are placed into the matrix of a bone. The venous sinusoids in the matrix can quickly absorb fluids to send to the central circulation. The most common access site is the proximal tibia in both children and adults. The sternum and the head of the humerus can also be used in adults. Osteomyelitis is a rare complication, occurring in fewer than 1% of cases.

✚ Contraindications for IO use include obesity, fracture, recent surgery, infection, or evidence of poor circulation at the proposed insertion site.

KnowledgeCheck 35-9

- What is the purpose of intravenous fluids?
- Describe the functions of the three types of IV solutions—isotonic, hypotonic, and hypertonic—and identify two commonly prescribed fluids in each category.
- Under what conditions would a central venous access device be preferable to a peripheral device?

 Think**Like a Nurse** 35-6:
      Clinical Judgment **in Action**

What type of venous access device would you expect Martha LaGuardia (Meet Your Patients) to receive in the hospital? Why?

Subcutaneous Infusion

Subcutaneous infusions are an alternative method to administer medications, continuous fluids, or nutrition. They have been widely used in home-based therapy with palliative care patients. Advantages of subcutaneous infusions are low cost, ease of use, and low infection and complication rates (Broadhurst et al., 2020; Caccialanza et al., 2018). Typical sites for infusions include the thighs, abdomen, back, and arms (Fig. 35-14).

Starting an Intravenous Infusion

To start an IV infusion, you will need to gather equipment and supplies, set up the solution and administration set, select a venipuncture site, and perform the venipuncture.

Toward Evidence-Based Practice

Jones, M., Franklin, B. D., Raynor, D. K., Thom, H., Watson, M. C., & Kandiyali, R. (2022). Costs and cost-effectiveness of user-testing of health professionals' guidelines to reduce the frequency of intravenous medicines administration errors by nurses in the United Kingdom: A probabilistic model based on voriconazole administration. *Applied Health Economic Health Policy, 20*(1), 91–104. https://doi.org/10.1007/s40258-021-00675-z

Intravenous medication errors can be attributed to difficulty finding relevant, clear, and comprehensive information in technical documents. User testing is a process that involves several rounds of interviews with participants to identify whether they can find essential information in a document, along with revisions to better guide practice. The results revealed a higher frequency of correct administration of intravenous medication with user-tested guidelines. This research concluded that user testing is a low-cost patient safety intervention that can reduce the costs of and consequences from medication errors.

Wolf, A., & Hughes, R. (2019). Best practices to decrease infusion-associated medication errors. *Journal of Infusion Nursing, 42*(4), 183–192. https://10.1097/NAN.0000000000000329

Researchers conducted a review of infusion-related medication errors and near misses reported to a national database over a 21-year period. Of 534 errors, 60% of errors occurred during the administration phase, followed by 21% during dispensing. Knowledge-based mistakes or planning failures were the most frequent error type (36.5%), followed by skill-based slips and memory lapses or execution failures (35.5%). Improper dose or quantity overdose (28.2%) and wrong drug (25.3%) accounted for the most types of errors. For nurses, two major categories of devices associated with infusion errors were pump-associated malfunctions and provider errors/overrides, along with tubing and catheter-associated errors. Best practices to improve safety included policy changes related to medication storage, use of labels to identify medications and the amount in infusions, and regular in-services on safety.

1. You noticed an increased rate of medication errors associated with a new medication. What process can be implemented to address this problem?

2. You have been assigned to develop a presentation on the prevention of infusion-related medication errors. What factors should you include in your presentation?

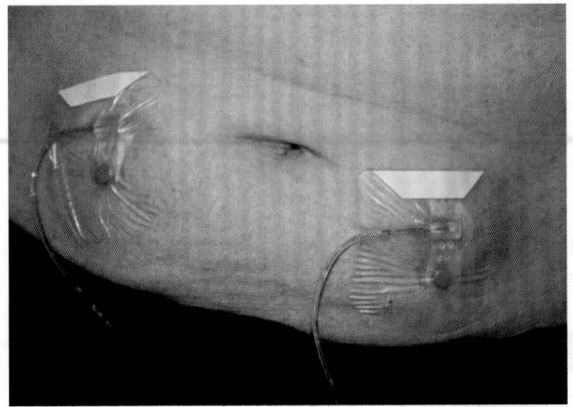

FIGURE 35-14 Subcutaneous infusions of medications, continuous fluids, or nutrition are widely used in home palliative care.

Obtain Equipment and Supplies

Venipuncture supplies and IV infusion equipment are sterile, prepackaged, and disposable. They vary based on manufacturers, so familiarize yourself with what is available in your facility. Set up the solution and administration set before performing the venipuncture.

IV Catheter Select the catheter with the smallest diameter and the shortest length that will accommodate the prescribed therapy. Nurses commonly use a 20- or 22-gauge catheter for adult peripheral infusions. A 20-gauge needle will accommodate adult blood transfusions. You will need the larger 16- or 18-gauge needle for rapid infusions, viscous (thick) fluids, or surgical or trauma patients. The smaller 24-gauge needle is used in geriatric patients and neonates. The following are infusion rates catheters of different gauges are expected to deliver (Elmore, 2019):

18 gauge	4,000 mL/hr
20 gauge	3,500 mL/hr
22 gauge	2,000 mL/hr
24 gauge	1,500 mL/hr

Administration Set (Infusion Kit) The administration set connects the fluid container to the catheter inserted in the patient. The set consists of tubing with a plastic insertion spike, a drip chamber, a roller clamp to regulate the flow, an injection port, and a catheter adapter (hub) (Fig. 35-15).

Both ends of the infusion set (the spike and the hub) must remain sterile. Remove the protective caps just before use. Avoid touching the spike and hub when connecting the tubing to the solution container and the IV catheter in the patient's vein.

The drip chamber is calibrated to allow a predictable amount of fluid to be delivered in each drop. The drop

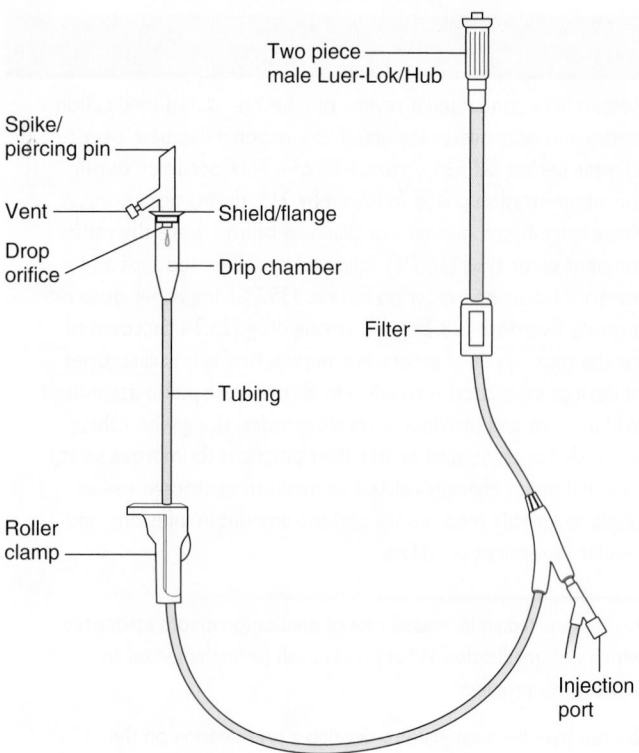

FIGURE 35-15 A basic administration set, or infusion kit.

factor is indicated on the package. A roller clamp on the tubing controls the rate of flow.

- A **macrodrip** delivers 10 to 20 drops per milliliter of solution, depending on the manufacturer. Select a macrodrip for most adult infusions.
- A **microdrip** delivers 60 drops per milliliter. It is used for very slow infusion rates or for infants and children.

Extension Tubing   The end of the IV tubing contains an adapter that attaches to the inserted sterile IV catheter. This should be a locking or screw-on connection, if one is available. You may use extension tubing to lengthen the primary tubing (e.g., for active patients) or to provide additional Y-injection ports for administration of multiple IV solutions or medications.

Filters.   Particulate matter may be generated when glass ampules are opened or from additives or medications that tend to clump. Occasionally, a filter will be used to remove particulate matter from the solution or to filter microorganisms. Filters come in a variety of sizes; the finer the filter, the greater the degree of solution filtration. Some administration sets have built-in filters, or you may attach one to the end of the tubing.

Injection Port.   Use the injection port to administer a secondary IV fluid or medication. For more information,

 Go to **Chapter 23, Procedures 23-15: Adding Medications to Intravenous Fluids, Procedure 23-16: Administering IV Push Medications,** and **Procedure 23-17: Administering Medication by Intermittent Infusion,** in Volume 2.

Solutions   Inspect the solution container to be certain that it contains the desired fluid, the fluid is clear, the container is intact, and the solution has not expired. Most IV containers are plastic, but a few are glass. Plastic containers collapse as fluid infuses, so you can use a nonvented administration set. Glass bottles do not collapse and therefore require a vented administration set.

Fluids for continuous infusions are packed in 1-L or 500-mL bags. Smaller bags (50 mL, 100 mL, and 250 mL) are used for intermittent infusions, such as antibiotics or other medications.

Select a Peripheral Intravenous Site

To select a venipuncture site, consider the following factors:

- **Age.** For adults, use the veins located on the dorsal and ventral surfaces of the upper arm, including the metacarpal, cephalic, basilic, and medial (INS, 2021). Hand veins should only be used for therapy less than 24 hours; for infants, use veins in the forearm or dorsum of the foot (Beecham & Tackling, 2021). Use the scalp as a last resort (INS, 2021).
- **Type of solution.** For hypertonic solutions, viscous solutions, or irritating medications, use a large vein to cause the least amount of trauma.
- **Speed of infusion.** The faster the rate, the larger the vein and the larger the IV catheter you will need. Use the largest vein available, keeping other selection criteria in mind.
- **Duration of infusion therapy.** Vascular access devices are removed when clinically indicated and not based on length of dwell time (INS, 2021). These guidelines should align with your institution's policy.
- **Presence of disease or previous surgery.** For example, avoid areas with scarring or impaired circulation.

For more detailed guidelines for selecting an insertion site,

 Go to **Chapter 35, Clinical Insight 35-3: Guidelines for Selecting a Peripheral Venipuncture Site,** in Volume 2.

Perform Venipuncture

For a successful venipuncture, you need to be able to visualize or palpate the vein before attempting to insert the catheter. Use a vein viewer, if available, to aid in locating the vein. These instruments use infrared light and camera technology to project the patient's superficial veins onto the skin surface. The Highlights of Procedures box summarizes the procedure for venipuncture. For other points of venipuncture (e.g., stabilizing the vein, angle of insertion, other techniques),

Go to **Chapter 35, Procedure 35-1: Initiating a Peripheral Intravenous Infusion,** in Volume 2.

Key Point: *If you are not successful with the venipuncture, you can make a second attempt above the initial site or in the opposite extremity. Do not make more than two attempts to start an IV on a patient. Get help from a more experienced colleague.*

Regulating and Maintaining an Intravenous Infusion

IV fluids can flow by gravity or be regulated by an electronic infusion-control device (pump). You are responsible for maintaining the correct rate of flow and for monitoring the client's response to the infusion. Many factors can influence the flow rate of an IV solution, especially when using gravity flow.

- **Height of the solution container.** The greater the distance between the height of the container and the patient's heart, the faster the flow will be. Check the flow rate each time the client or IV solution is repositioned to ensure that it is correct.
- **Patient position.** Pressure on the IV site decreases flow. If an IV is infusing in the right arm and the patient is positioned on their right side, the pressure on the right arm will be greater than if the patient were positioned supine or on the left.
- **Blood pressure.** As blood pressure rises, more force is required to infuse into the vein.
- **The internal diameter of the IV catheter.** The smaller the diameter (that is, the higher the gauge), the more you must open the roller clamp to achieve the desired flow rate.
- **Condition of the catheter and tubing.** If the catheter is dislodged from the vein, flow may stop entirely or continue at a slowed rate. A knot or kink at any point in the tubing will slow flow.

Gravity Flow

Most IV fluids are administered by a volume-control pump. However, you may still encounter instances when you will need to regulate the rate with the roller clamp on the tubing. You should check gravity infusion rates hourly and adjust the flow as needed.

- **If the fluid is running too slowly,** do not attempt to catch up by administering extra fluid rapidly. If the fluid is running too fast, slow the rate, and assess the client for signs of fluid volume excess.

- **If the client is ambulatory,** attach the fluid container to a pole with wheels. Instruct the client to keep the solution container above the infusion site and to avoid pulling on the tubing or the infusion site.

The Highlights of Procedures box summarizes how to regulate a gravity-flow IV. For the complete procedure,

 Go to **Chapter 35, Procedure 35-2: Regulating the IV Flow Rate,** in Volume 2.

Volume-Control Set

A volume-control set (e.g., Buretrol, Soluset, Volutrol) is another method for regulating an IV infusion (see Fig. 23-17C). You will drain a small amount of fluid from the larger IV solution container into the volume-control container. Typically, the volume placed in the volume-control container is equal to the prescribed hourly infusion rate.

The rate is regulated in the same way as with other administration sets (the drip factor is usually 60 gtts/mL [60 drops/mL]); however, the maximum amount of fluid that can enter a patient is limited to the volume in the volume-control set.

- An advantage of this system is that medications can be added to the volume-control set and diluted with IV fluid for intermittent administration. You may use this type of equipment when the client is at risk for fluid volume excess and for infants and children, who require close supervision of fluid intake. However, more often, the policy will be to use an infusion pump for continuous infusions for such patients.

To learn or review how to use a volume-control set,

Go to **Chapter 23, Procedure 23-17C: Using a Volume-Control Administration Set,** in Volume 2.

Infusion Pump

If you are using an electronic volume-control device (pump), the machine will maintain the infusion rate after you program it. Most infusion pumps sound an alarm when the fluid bag is almost empty, when air is in the line, or when there is resistance to flow. Infusion-control devices save time and prevent accidental delivery of large amounts of fluid. They do not, however, excuse you from regularly monitoring the flow rate and assessing the needle insertion site.

 You should know that absence of an alarm does not mean there is no problem. For example, if the IV is infiltrated, the pump may keep infusing fluid into the tissues.

To find more about how to regulate an IV using an infusion pump, see the Highlights of Procedures box and

Go to **Chapter 35, Procedure 35-3: Setting Up and Using Volume-Control Pumps,** in Volume 2.

KnowledgeCheck 35-10

- What factors should you consider when selecting an insertion site for a peripheral IV line?
- What are the preferred locations for peripheral IV lines?
- What equipment is needed when inserting an IV and starting an IV infusion?
- Identify three ways to regulate the flow rate of IV fluid.

Calculating Flow Rates

As you already know, IV administration sets are sized as microdrips (deliver fluid at a rate of 60 drops/mL) or macrodrips (deliver fluid at a rate of 10 to 20 drops/ mL). To begin calculating, you need the following information:

- Prescribed infusion rate
- Flow rate of the administration set in drops per minute

See Box 35-1 to learn how to calculate flow rates.

Managing Multiple Lines

When a patient has multiple IV solutions and multiple lines, you must label each line to identify the solution that is infusing through it. Label the IV tubing close to the catheter so that it is easy to see which fluid is infusing in the line. This is especially true when using double- and triple-lumen catheters. Multiple lines are often used because solutions are not compatible with each other.

 You can never infuse blood, parenteral nutrition, or lipids through a line with anything else, and you can never draw blood samples from these lines.

- **Record the name of each line in your nursing notes and the intake form.** For peripheral IVs, use *RA* for right arm, *LA* for left arm, and so on, and designate a number for each site because there may be more than one line or site in each arm (e.g., RA-1, RA-2, LA-1). If the lines are in separate arms, it may seem unnecessary to give each one a number; however, over the course of therapy, some lines may need to be discontinued and new ones started.
- **For multiport central lines, label each port, in addition to recording in nursing notes.** For example, with a triple-lumen central catheter, you might have named each lumen as proximal, mid, and distal, or CVAD-1,

CVAD-2, CVAD-3. The finished labeling and nursing record may indicate "CVAD-1—TPN; CVAD-2—$D_5\frac{1}{2}$ NS; CVAD-3—insulin."

- The INS recommends using a visually prominent label that differs from others to identify the site for administration of IV push medications (INS, 2021).

- Always keep the lines untangled and know where your main IV fluid is (e.g., the D_5-$\frac{1}{2}$ NS) so that if a crisis occurs or intermittent infusions are needed, you can quickly identify the correct solution and tubing for use.

Complications of Intravenous Therapy

All IV therapy can have general complications. Inserting an IV catheter breaks the body's first line of defense (the skin) and provides a portal of entry for microorganisms. In addition, trauma roughens the vein wall and predisposes the patient to platelet clumping and thrombus formation. Minimize this effect by swiftly piercing the skin and anchoring the catheter and tubing to reduce tissue trauma.

Complications at the IV site include infiltration, extravasation, infection, thrombus, and thrombophlebitis.

Systemic complications occur less frequently than local complications but may be life threatening. They include fluid volume excess, sepsis, and embolus. Table 35-8 describes the potential complications of IV therapy. For more information on managing infiltration and extravasation,

▶ Go to **Chapter 35, Clinical Insight 35-5, Managing Infiltration and Extravasation,** in Volume 2.

Changing Intravenous Solutions, Tubing, and Dressings

Follow practice guidelines and agency policies for changing IV solutions, tubing, and dressings. As with IV insertion, use meticulous aseptic technique.

Changing IV Solutions Hang a new container of fluid when the present container is nearly empty but fluid still remains at the appropriate level in the drip chamber. The infusion rate dictates how often you need to change the IV solution.

Examples:
A liter of IV fluid infusing at 125 mL/hr must be changed every 8 hours.
A liter infusing at 50 mL/hr will hang for 20 hours.

Evidence-based practice does not provide an exact length of time that an IV solution can hang before it has to be changed (INS, 2021); therefore, you should follow your agency's policy. For full instructions on the procedure for changing solutions, tubing, and dressings,

▶ Go to **Chapter 35, Procedures 35-4A: Changing the IV Solution, Procedure 35-4B: Changing the IV Administration Tubing and Solution, and Procedure 35-5: Changing IV Dressings,** in Volume 2.

BOX 35-1 ■ Calculating IV Flow Rates

Microdrips = 60 drops/mL

Macrodrips = 10 to 20 drops/mL

You need to know drops per minute: the prescribed infusion rate and the flow rate of the administration set.

1. Multiply the hourly rate (number of mL to be infused in 60 minutes) by the drop factor (in drops per milliliter) to obtain the total drops per hour.

2. Then divide by 60 to get the drip rate in drops per minute. For example, an hourly rate of 100 mL multiplied by 15 drops per milliliter and divided by 60 equals the drip rate. Therefore, the drip rate equals 25 drops per minute.

Use this formula to calculate flow:

$$\frac{\text{Hourly rate in mL} \times \text{drop factor (drops/mL)}}{60 \text{ minutes}} = \text{drip rate}$$

Example Calculation:

$$\frac{100 \text{ (mL per hour)} \times 15 \text{ (gtts/mL)}}{60 \text{ minutes}} = 25 \text{ gtts/min}$$

Table 35-8 ➤ Complications of Intravenous Therapy

COMPLICATION	CAUSES	SIGNS AND SYMPTOMS	NURSING RESPONSE
Local Complications			
Hematoma—a localized mass of blood outside the blood vessel	Nicking the vein during an unsuccessful insertion, discontinuing an IV line without holding pressure over the site, or applying a tourniquet too tightly above a previously attempted venipuncture site	Ecchymosis, localized mass, discomfort	Be gentle with venipuncture technique. Apply pressure when discontinuing an IV.
Infiltration*—the seepage of nonvesicant solution or medication into surrounding tissues	IV catheter dislodges or the tip penetrates the vessel wall	Slowed or stopped flow. Swelling, tenderness, pallor, hardness, and coolness at the site. The patient may report a burning sensation in the area.	Stop the infusion immediately. Do not flush the VAD. Do not apply pressure to the area. Restart the IV infusion in a different vein, higher in the extremity or in another extremity. Elevate the affected arm on a pillow to promote absorption of excess fluid.
Extravasation*—seepage of a vesicant substance into the tissues. (A *vesicant* is a solution that causes the formation of blisters and subsequent tissue sloughing and necrosis.)	IV catheter dislodges, or the tip penetrates the vessel wall	Slowed or stopped flow. Pain, burning, and swelling at IV site; blanching and coolness of the surrounding skin. Blistering is a late sign. If extravasation resulted from vasoconstricting medication, may see necrosis (death) of dermis.	Treatment depends on the severity of the infiltration. Stop the IV infusion immediately. Administer an antidote, if one is available. (Antidotes alter the pH, alter DNA binding, neutralize the drug, or dilute the extravasated drug.) Elevate the extremity. The type of compress, if any, depends on the solution and medication.
Phlebitis—inflammation of the vein	May be due to mechanical irritation, infusion of solutions that are irritating to the vessel, or sepsis. Dextrose solutions, potassium chloride, antibiotics, and vitamin C are associated with a higher risk of phlebitis. Trauma to the vessel, compression of the line by client movement, or a low flow rate	Redness, pain, and warmth at the site; local swelling; palpable cord along the vein; sluggish infusion rate; and elevated temperature. Slowed or stopped infusion, localized warmth at the site, inability to restart flow of IV	Discontinue the IV infusion and restart in a new location. Initially, apply cold compresses to the site if the site is warm and tender. Thereafter, use warm compresses. Assess for circulatory impairment. Consult the primary care provider if there is streaking or erythema along the vein or a palpable cord. *Prevention measures:* Use the smallest catheter practical (usually 22-gauge or 24-gauge thin-walled catheter). Use polyurethane catheters instead of Teflon. Stabilize and secure the catheter to minimize movement in the vein. Rotate the site when the catheter is changed; no more frequently than every 72–96 hours, or as clinically indicated.

(Continued)

Table 35-8 ➤ Complications of Intravenous Therapy—cont'd

COMPLICATION	CAUSES	SIGNS AND SYMPTOMS	NURSING RESPONSE
Thrombophlebitis—thrombosis and inflammation	Use of veins in the legs for infusion, use of a hypertonic or highly acidic solution; can be a result of untreated phlebitis	Sluggish flow rate, edema, tender and cord-like veins, warmth and erythema at site	Discontinue the IV infusion and restart in the opposite extremity, using all new equipment. Apply warm, moist compresses. Consult the primary care provider.
Local infection—microbial contamination of the cannula or IV site	Using poor technique when inserting the catheter, leaving the catheter in place for longer than 96 hours, or direct contamination	Redness, swelling, exudate, elevated temperature	Remove the IV line. Apply a sterile dressing over the site. Administer antibiotics, if necessary.
Nerve injury—a nerve is inadvertently injured during venipuncture (direct) or is compressed.	Using veins on inner surface of the wrist and forearm; not anchoring the vein for puncture; using a large needle; advancing the needle across instead of with the vein; "probing" (excessive redirection of the needle at insertion); inserting too deeply and through the back wall of the vein; too many venipuncture attempts; infiltration; extravasation; tourniquet too tight or left on too long	*Direct injury*—sharp, acute pain at the site or up and down the arm; pins and needles or electric shock sensation; pain, numbness, or tingling in fingers; pain that persists after the needle is removed. *Compression injury*—pain and tingling typically appear 24 to 96 hours after venipuncture.	Do not make more than two venipuncture attempts. ***If patient complains of symptoms:*** Stop the procedure and withdraw the catheter. Report to the supervisor and provider. Do not start a new IV in the affected arm. Treat infiltration if it occurs. **Fasciotomy** (incisions around the area to let blood or fluid seep out) is the usual treatment, or fluid may be expressed.
Systemic Complications **Septicemia**—the presence of microorganisms or their toxic products in the circulatory system	A break in aseptic technique or contaminated IV solution	Fluctuating fever, chills, tachycardia, confusion, hypotension, altered mental status, elevated WBC count	Discontinue the IV infusion immediately. Consult the primary care provider. Treatment often involves antibiotics, fluids, and medications to support vital signs.
Fluid overload	Infusing excessive amounts of IV fluids or administering fluid too rapidly	Weight gain, edema, hypertension, shortness of breath, crackles, distended neck veins	Slow the IV flow rate. Place the client in high-Fowler's position. Monitor vital signs. Administer oxygen, if needed. If severe, diuretics may be prescribed.
Air embolus—a rare complication involving the introduction of air into the vascular system	Loose connections, adding a new IV bag to a line that has run dry without clearing the line of air, air in tubing cassette of infusion pump	Palpitations, chest pain, light-headedness, dyspnea, cough, hypotension, tachycardia, sudden change in mental status	Call for help. Place client in Trendelenburg position on the left side. Administer oxygen. Have emergency equipment available.

Table 35-8 ➤ Complications of Intravenous Therapy—cont'd

COMPLICATION	CAUSES	SIGNS AND SYMPTOMS	NURSING RESPONSE
Catheter embolus—a piece of catheter breaks off and travels through the vascular system.	Reinserting a catheter used in an unsuccessful insertion; removing and reinserting a stylet, causing shearing of the catheter; placing the catheter in a joint flexion	Sharp, sudden pain at IV site, jagged catheter end on removal, dyspnea, chest pain, tachycardia, hypotension	Apply a tourniquet above the site. Notify the provider and radiologist. Start a new IV line. Prepare the patient for radiographic examination.

*For more information about interventions for infiltration and extravasation, see Clinical Insight 35-5: Managing Infiltration and Extravasation, in Volume 2.

IV, Intravenous; *VAD*, venous access device; *WBC*, white blood cell.

Source: Gorski, L., Hadaway, L., Hagle, M. E., Broadhurst, D., Clare, S., Kleidon, C., Meyer, B. M. Nickel, B., Rowley, S., Sharpe, E., & Alexander, M. (2021). Infusion therapy standards of practice (8th ed.). *Journal of Infusion Nursing, 44* (1S), S1–224; Phillips, L., & Gorski, L. (2018). *Manual of IV therapeutics* (7th ed.). F.A. Davis.

Changing Administration Sets The INS (2021) recommends the following:

- **If the patient is not receiving blood, blood products, or fat emulsions:**
  - **Continuous infusions**—Change the primary and secondary sets no more frequently than every 96 hours but at least every 7 days, when the system is compromised, or when the VAD is changed. Always follow facility policy or manufacturer's guidance.
  - **Intermittent infusions**—Change the administration sets every 24 hours because the repetitive disconnections and reconnections increase the likelihood of contamination. This also includes a secondary administration set that is detached from a primary continuous infusion.
- **Parenteral nutrition**—Change the administration set with each new solution but at least every 24 hours.
- **Intravenous fat emulsions**—Replace the administration set, if infused separately, every 12 hours.
- **Blood**—Replace the administration set and filter after completion of each unit but at least every 4 hours.

Key Point: *As a rule, if you start an IV at a new site, use a new administration set. Reusing a set from a previous site increases the risk of contamination.*

Changing IV Dressings The INS (2021) recommends dressing changes based on the following:

- **Transparent semipermeable membrane dressing**—At least every 7 days, or earlier as clinically indicated (e.g., when the dressing becomes damp, soiled, or loose).
- **Gauze dressings**—At least every 2 days, even if they are covered by a transparent dressing.
- **Neonates**—As needed or clinically indicated.
- **Regardless of site,** change any dressing when it becomes soiled, damp, or loosened.

Key Point: *It is best to dress both central and peripheral lines with transparent, semipermeable dressings.* These dressings (a) allow direct visualization of the site between dressing changes, (b) permit evaporation of moisture, and (c) provide a secure anchor for the catheter. You may still sometimes see tape securing a catheter at the insertion site; however, the use of a catheter stabilization device is preferred over tape or sutures (INS, 2021).

Converting to a Peripheral Intravenous Lock

The terms *peripheral lock, saline lock,* and *prn adapter* are used interchangeably. Recall that you may need a peripheral IV lock (PIV):

- For intermittent infusions
- For venous access for emergencies
- When clients do not need the additional fluids provided by a constant infusion of solution

A peripheral infusion can be easily converted to a peripheral lock. To do this, you simply remove the tubing from the IV catheter and replace it with a sterile injection cap (see Fig. 35-9). Research shows that a passive disinfection cap that contains a disinfectant agent can reduce contamination (INS, 2021). Once removed, the cap should be discarded. Some IV locks also contain a short segment of tubing.

- **Key Point:** *Each time you give a medication through the lock, you will need to disinfect and flush the lock before and after you administer the medication.* A PIV lock should also be flushed and locked at least every 12 hours when not in use.
- **Disinfecting:** The INS (2021) recommends "a vigorous mechanical scrub" of the needleless connector before access with an acceptable disinfecting agent (e.g., 70% isopropyl alcohol, or alcohol-based chlorhexidine).

- **Flushing:**
    - **Peripheral IV lock**—A preservative-free 0.9% sodium chloride (USP) is recommended.
    - **Midline or CVADs**—Use either a heparin solution (10 units/mL) or 0.9% sodium chloride.

Discontinuing an Intravenous Line

Discontinue the IV line and IV catheter when IV fluids and medications are no longer needed or if the integrity of the line is compromised. Inspect the catheter to ensure that it is intact when you remove it. The Highlights of Procedures box summarizes removal of an IV catheter. For the complete procedure,

 Go to **Chapter 35, Procedure 35-7: Discontinuing a Peripheral IV,** in Volume 2.

KnowledgeCheck 35-11

- A prescription reads, "5% dextrose in water/0.45% saline solution (D_5 ½ NS) with 20 mEq KCl; infuse 1 liter in 5 hours." Calculate the hourly rate and the drip rate using (1) a macrodrip administration set with 15 gtts/mL and (2) a microdrip set.
- Describe the difference between infiltration and extravasation as a complication of IV therapy.
- In general, how often are administration sets changed on peripheral IV lines? How often are administration sets changed when total parenteral nutrition (TPN) is being infused?

REPLACEMENT OF BLOOD AND BLOOD PRODUCTS

Key Point: *IV fluids can replace fluid volume, but they do not restore oxygen-carrying capacity or replace clotting factors.* Blood products are infused when the patient has (a) experienced significant blood loss, (b) diminished oxygen-carrying capacity, or (c) a deficiency in one of the blood components.

The American Red Cross (n.d.) notes that 6.8 million people each year donate blood. Each unit of donated blood is separated into multiple components, such as red blood cells, plasma, platelets, and clotting factors. Thus, 1 unit of donated blood may be used in the care of several clients.

Donating Blood To be eligible to donate blood, a person must be in good health (no cold or flu, uncontrolled hypertension, anemia, or diabetes), at least 16 years of age (although some states permit younger people, with parental consent, to donate), and weigh at least 110 pounds. In addition, each potential donor is screened for travel to certain countries and for a variety of disorders (e.g., hepatitis, HIV, Creutzfeldt-Jakob disease—the human form of mad cow disease).

Blood Groups

Human blood is classified into four main groups (A, B, AB, and O) based on the presence or absence of certain antigens and antibodies. You inherit your blood group from your parents. See Table 35-9 for a description of blood groups.

- **If you belong to blood group A,** you have A antigens on the surface of your red blood cells (RBCs) and B antibodies in your plasma.
- **If you belong to blood group B,** the opposite is true; you have B antigens on the surface of your RBCs and A antibodies in your plasma.
- **If you belong to blood group AB,** you have both antigens on the surface of the red blood cells and no antibodies at all in the plasma.
- **A person in group O,** in contrast, has neither A nor B antigens on the surface of the red blood cells but has both A and B antibodies in the blood plasma (see Table 35-9).
- **Rh factor**—An additional antigen, known as *Rh factor,* is also important with blood typing. If the antigen is present, you are referred to as *Rh-positive* (Rh⁺). If it is absent, you are *Rh-negative* (Rh⁻).

Thus, you can belong to one of the following eight groups:

| A Rh⁺ | B Rh⁺ | AB Rh⁺ | O Rh⁺ |
| A Rh⁻ | B Rh⁻ | AB Rh⁻ | O Rh⁻ |

People who are Rh⁺ may receive blood with or without Rh factor. However, people who are Rh⁻ may receive only Rh⁻ blood.

Blood Typing and Crossmatching

Typing Once blood is donated, several tests are performed on the sample, for ABO and Rh type and for evidence of donor infections.

- **ABO and Rh**—First, the sample is tested for ABO group (blood type) and Rh type (positive or negative), as well as for any unexpected RBC antibodies that may cause problems in a recipient.

Table 35-9 ➤ Blood Transfusions

BLOOD GROUP	ANTIGENS	ANTIBODIES	CAN GIVE BLOOD TO	CAN RECEIVE BLOOD FROM
AB	A and B	None	AB	AB, A, B, and O
A	A	B	A and AB	A and O
B	B	A	B and AB	B and O
O	None	A and B	AB, A, B, and O	O

- **Screening for infection**—Screening tests assess for evidence of donor infection with hepatitis B and C viruses, HIV, human T-lymphotropic viruses, West Nile virus, and syphilis. If all disease screens are negative, the blood is acceptable for transfusion and is placed in the pool of available products.

Crossmatching When a potential donor is identified, crossmatching is performed. **Crossmatching** identifies possible minor antigens that will affect the compatibility of the donor blood in the recipient.

- RBCs from the donor blood are mixed with plasma from the potential recipient. A reagent is added, and the sample is observed for clumping or agglutination.
- If no clumping is observed, the risk of transfusion reaction is low, and it is considered safe to transfuse the sample of blood.

Table 35-9 summarizes blood group matching.

Key Point: *Individuals with the blood type of AB positive are known as the "universal recipient" because the absence of plasma antibodies allows them to receive blood from all blood groups.*

Individuals with a blood type of O negative are known as a "universal donor" because the absence of plasma antigens allows individuals in all blood groups to receive type O negative blood. Patients must receive only blood that is compatible with their own blood group to prevent a hemolytic reaction (see Table 35-10).

Autologous donation When possible, **autologous** (self-donated) units of blood are given instead of blood from a donor. This negates the risk of a mismatch or exposure to undetected disease. The patient's blood is usually collected in the preoperative weeks for possible transfusion during elective surgery. Autologous donation is most often done with orthopedic, cardiac, and vascular surgery. The process of donating autologous blood stimulates the bone marrow to produce new blood cells. Given adequate time for recovery, the collected cells may be wholly or partially replaced before surgery.

Blood Products

Several blood products are available for transfusion:

- **Whole blood** contains RBCs, WBCs, and platelets suspended in plasma.
- **RBCs** are prepared from whole blood by removing the plasma. RBCs can raise the client's hematocrit and hemoglobin levels while minimizing an increase in volume. RBCs are available for transfusion as packed RBCs (PRBCs).
- **Plasma** is the liquid portion of the blood. It is 90% water and makes up about 55% of blood volume. Plasma may be transfused whole or may be separated into specific products, such as albumin, clotting factor concentrates, and immune globulins.
- **Platelets** help the clotting process by sticking to the lining of blood vessels. Units of platelets are prepared by using a centrifuge to separate the platelet-rich

plasma from the donated unit of whole blood. The platelet-rich plasma is then centrifuged again to concentrate the platelets further. Platelets are used to treat clients who have a shortage of platelets or have abnormal platelet function.

- **WBCs,** specifically granulocytes, can be collected by centrifugation of whole blood. They are transfused within 24 hours after collection and are used for infections that are unresponsive to antibiotic therapy.
- **Plasma derivatives** are concentrates of specific plasma proteins prepared from many units of plasma. Plasma derivatives include a variety of clotting factors, immune globulins, and albumin.

Initiating a Transfusion

It is critical to identify the patient and the blood product when transfusing blood. Before beginning a transfusion, verify the written prescription for the blood product.

♥ **iCare** Some patients will refuse a blood transfusion because of cultural, religious, or other beliefs. Be ready to discuss with them any available alternatives to whole-blood administration. You should convey acceptance of their decision and remain nonjudgmental. For more information on working with patients who refuse blood transfusion, see Chapter 5.

- **Obtain a set of vital signs within the 30 minutes before initiating the infusion (INS, 2021).** If the patient's temperature is elevated, inform the primary care provider before hanging the transfusion. Most patients experience a minor temperature elevation after a transfusion is given. A preexisting elevated temperature may exacerbate this response. As a result, premedication may be prescribed.
- **Inspect the IV site to be sure it is patent before obtaining the blood from the blood bank and before hanging the blood product.** Nurses commonly use a 20-gauge catheter to infuse blood and a larger size for rapid flow rates. A 20- to 24-gauge catheter can be used for blood transfusions (INS, 2021). Certainly, for children and the frail elderly, you will need the smaller, 22- or 24-gauge, catheter.

The Highlights of Procedures box summarizes the procedure for initiating and monitoring a blood transfusion. For the complete procedure,

 Go to **Chapter 35, Procedures 35-8A: Administering Blood and Blood Products,** and **Procedure 35-8B: Managing a Transfusion Reaction,** in Volume 2.

Transfusion Reactions

Even when you use perfect technique, transfusion reactions can and do occur. Five types of reactions are possible: allergic, bacterial, febrile, hemolytic reactions, and circulatory overload. Table 35-10 describes each of these reactions. To help prevent transfusion reactions, be extremely careful in identifying the patient and the blood, start the transfusion slowly, remain with

Table 35-10 ➤ Transfusion Reactions

TYPE OF REACTION	SIGNS AND SYMPTOMS	NURSING RESPONSIBILITIES
Allergic—allergy to blood being transfused	Flushing, itching, wheezing, urticaria (hives); anaphylaxis, if severe	Stop the transfusion. Replace with a saline infusion. Notify the provider immediately. Administer prescribed antihistamine.
Bacterial—contamination of the blood	Fever, chills, vomiting, diarrhea, hypertension	Stop the transfusion. Replace with a saline infusion. Notify the provider. Administer antibiotics as ordered. Treat symptoms.
Febrile—temperature elevation due to sensitivity to WBCs, plasma proteins, or platelets	Fever; chills; warm, flushed skin; aches	Stop the transfusion. Replace with a saline infusion. Notify the provider. Treat symptoms.
Hemolytic reactions—destruction of RBCs as a result of infusing incompatible blood; occurs in 1 in 600,000 transfusions	Fever, chills, dyspnea, chest pain, tachycardia, hypotension; can be fatal	Stop the transfusion immediately. Replace with a saline infusion. Notify the provider immediately. Send the remaining blood, including tubing and filter; a sample of venous blood; and the first voided urine to the laboratory for analysis. Treat shock.
Circulatory overload—administering too great a volume or too rapidly	Persistent cough, crackles, hypertension, distended neck veins	Slow or stop the transfusion. Monitor vital signs. Place the client upright. Notify the provider.

RBC, Red blood cell; WBC, white blood cell.

the patient for the first 5 minutes of the transfusion, assess again at 15 minutes, and assess at least every 30 minutes during the transfusion (see Procedure 35-8).

✚ You must assess your patient throughout the transfusion. Research revealed that transfusion reactions can occur 2 hours into the infusion and later (Cortez-Gann et al., 2017; INS 2021).

KnowledgeCheck 35-12

- Identify eight potential blood types.
- Describe the types of blood products that are available for transfusion.
- Identify and describe types of transfusion reactions.

For steps to follow in *all* procedures, refer to the Universal Steps for All Procedures found on the inside back cover of Volume 2. Go to the full procedures in Volume 2 to practice and learn the procedure steps. Use these procedural highlights later to help you review key points.

For all intravenous procedures, maintain scrupulous aseptic technique to prevent infection and possible sepsis.

Procedure 35-1: Initiating a Peripheral Intravenous Infusion

➤ Prepare the IV solution and administration set, including extension tubing and volume-control device if used. Prime the tubing.

➤ Label the IV solution container and place a time tape on it with the infusion rate. Label the tubing with the date and time.

➤ Apply the tourniquet.

➤ Locate a vein. Then loosen the tourniquet. (As a rule, select the most distal vein in an upper extremity.)

➤ Don clean nonsterile gloves and open the catheter package. Keep the catheter sterile.

➤ Reapply the tourniquet and cleanse the site. Allow the antiseptic to dry on the skin.

➤ Inform the patient that you are about to insert the catheter.

➤ Stabilize the vein with your nondominant hand.

➤ Hold the catheter, bevel up, at a 30° to 45° angle and pierce the skin.

➤ Look for a flashback of blood. Lower the catheter so that it is parallel to the skin and advance into the vein.

➤ When the needle is at least halfway into the vein or when a steady backflow of blood occurs, gradually withdraw the needle while advancing the catheter fully into the vein.

➤ While holding the catheter in place with one hand, release the tourniquet with your other hand.

➤ Connect the IV administration set to the IV catheter.

➤ While stabilizing the catheter with your hand, adjust the flow rate according to the provider's prescription.

➤ Secure the connection, stabilize the catheter, and dress the IV insertion site.

➤ Label the dressing.

➤ Loop and tape the tubing to the skin.

➤ Place an arm board as needed.

Procedure 35-2: Regulating the IV Flow Rate

➤ Follow all "checks" and "rights" of medication administration, including:

　➤ Verify the prescription.

　➤ Check the solution to make sure that you have the proper IV fluid with the prescribed additives.

➤ Calculate the hourly rate and the drip rate; verify your calculations.

➤ Apply a time tape to the solution container. Mark the time the infusion was started.

➤ Open the roller clamp so that the IV fluid begins to flow.

➤ Hold a watch beside the drip chamber; count the number of drops for 1 minute.

➤ Adjust the roller clamp, increasing or decreasing the flow until you achieve the prescribed drip rate.

➤ Monitor manually regulated infusion rates closely for the first 15 minutes after you begin the infusion; then monitor the rate hourly.

Procedure 35-3: Setting Up and Using Volume-Control Pumps

➤ Calculate and verify the infusion rate.

➤ Attach the volume-control pump to the IV pole and plug it into the nearest electrical outlet.

➤ Close the clamp on the administration set and spike the port of the solution container. Attach a filter if one is needed.

➤ Label the tubing and solution container.

➤ Hang the solution container on the IV pole.

➤ Fill the drip chamber halfway.

➤ Place the electronic sensor on the drip chamber, if there is one. If not, consult the manufacturer's instructions.

➤ Prime the administration tubing, then close the clamp.

➤ Turn on the pump and load the administration tubing into the pump.

➤ Program the pump with the hourly infusion rate, total hours, and the volume to be infused.

➤ Don clean nonsterile gloves and check the IV site for patency.

➤ Scrub the injection port; allow to dry.

➤ Connect the tubing adapter to the injection port.

➤ Unclamp the administration set tubing and press the start button.

➤ Make sure that the alarms are turned on and audible.

➤ Check the pump regularly to make sure that the correct volume is infusing.

➤ At the end of your shift (or at the specified time), clear the pump of the volume infused and record the volume.

Procedure 35-4: Changing IV Solutions and Tubing

Procedure 35-4A: Changing the IV Solution

➤ Prepare and label your next container of IV solution at least 1 hour before the present infusion is scheduled to finish.

➤ Close the roller clamp on the infusing (empty) administration set.

➤ Wearing nonsterile gloves, remove the old IV solution container from the IV pole. Remove the spike from the bag, keeping the spike sterile.

➤ Spike the new IV solution container.

➤ Hang the new IV solution and inspect the tubing for air.

➤ Adjust the drip rate.

➤ Place the time tape on the new IV solution container. Mark the times.

Continued

Procedure 35-4B: Changing the IV Administration Solution and Tubing

➤ Prepare and hang the new IV solution and tubing.

➤ Close the roller clamp on the old administration set.

➤ Wearing clean nonsterile gloves, stabilize the IV catheter while applying pressure over the vein just above the insertion site.

➤ Remove the protective cover from the distal end of the new administration set and connect the new tubing.

➤ Adjust the drip rate.

➤ Cleanse the IV site.

➤ Resecure the IV catheter and tubing connection; loop and tape the tubing.

➤ Label tubing and solution with date, initials, rate, and time tape.

Procedure 35-5: Changing IV Dressings

Procedure 35-5A: Peripheral IV Dressings

➤ Wearing clean procedure gloves, stabilize the catheter with your nondominant hand, and carefully remove the dressing.

➤ Inspect the insertion site.

➤ Don clean gloves. Cleanse the insertion site, following the manufacturer's guidelines for product use.

➤ Allow the antiseptic to dry on the skin.

➤ Perform hand hygiene and don nonsterile gloves.

➤ Apply a new sterile catheter stabilization device and dressing.

➤ Secure the connection between the catheter and the tubing.

➤ Loop and tape the tubing to the patient's skin.

➤ Label the dressing with the date and time of insertion, catheter size, the date the dressing was changed, and your initials.

Procedure 35-5B: Central Line Dressings

➤ Obtain sterile central line dressing kit (or equivalent supplies if there is no kit) and a mask for the patient, if one is needed.

➤ Place the patient in a semi-Fowler's position, if tolerated.

➤ Ask the patient to turn his head to the opposite side of the insertion site; if unable, place a mask on the patient.

➤ Don mask and clean nonsterile gloves.

➤ Carefully remove the old dressing and stabilization device.

➤ Inspect the site for signs of complications.

➤ Remove gloves and perform hand hygiene

➤ Set up a sterile field, open dressing change kit, and don sterile gloves.

➤ Arrange sterile supplies as needed.

➤ Scrub the insertion site with gentle friction for at least 30 seconds, using the antiseptic swabs contained in the kit.

➤ Scrub the sutures (if any) and the catheter from the insertion site to the hub or bifurcation with an antiseptic swab for at least 15 seconds.

➤ Allow the site to dry completely; do not fan.

➤ Apply the transparent dressing that comes in the kit.

➤ Apply the new catheter stabilization device, if one is used.

➤ Remove drape, if one was used.

➤ Loop the catheter gently and secure it with tape to the skin (do not tape it to the dressing).

➤ Label the dressing with the date changed, time, and your initials.

Procedure 35-5C: PICC Line Dressings

➤ Obtain sterile central line dressing kit (or equivalent supplies if there is no kit) and mask for the patient, if one is needed.

➤ Place the patient in a comfortable semi-Fowler's position.

➤ Explain the procedure to the patient.

➤ Ask the patient to turn their head to the opposite side of the insertion site; if unable, place a mask on the patient, if consistent with agency policy.

➤ Inspect the site for signs and symptoms of infection.

➤ Don mask and nonsterile gloves.

➤ Remove and discard your gloves, along with the old dressing.

➤ Perform hand hygiene.

➤ Set up a sterile field, open dressing change kit, and don sterile gloves.

➤ Arrange sterile supplies, as needed.

➤ Using sterile tape, measure the external length of PICC to compare to base insertion length, if consistent with agency's policy.

➤ Scrub the catheter's insertion site and the surrounding skin that will be covered by the dressing for 30 seconds.

➤ Allow to air dry completely.

➤ Apply the stabilization device, if one is used.

➤ Apply the transparent dressing. Loop the catheter and injection clamp so that it is pointing up.

➤ Label the dressing with the date, time, and your initials.

➤ Loop and anchor the catheter; secure with tape.

Procedure 35-6: Converting a Primary Line to a Peripheral IV Lock

➤ Maintain sterility of equipment throughout.

➤ Don clean nonsterile gloves.

➤ Remove the IV lock from the package and flush the adapter, according to agency policy. Do not contaminate the lock.

➤ Remove the IV dressing and the tape that is securing the tubing.

➤ Close the roller clamp on the administration set.

➤ With your nondominant hand, apply pressure over the vein just above the insertion site; stabilize the catheter hub with your thumb and forefinger.

➤ Disengage the used tubing from the IV catheter.

➤ Quickly insert the lock adapter into the IV catheter and turn it to lock it in place.

➤ Scrub the adapter injection port and flush the lock again with the second syringe.

➤ Apply a sterile transparent semipermeable dressing; do not cover the catheter-tubing connection.

➤ Label the dressing with date and initials.

➤ Discard used supplies.

Procedure 35-7: Discontinuing a Peripheral IV

➤ Place a linen-saver pad under the extremity with the intravenous (IV) catheter.

➤ Don clean nonsterile gloves and close the roller clamp on the administration set.

➤ Remove the dressing, catheter stabilization device, and tape; scrub the catheter–skin junction with an antiseptic pad for 15 seconds.

➤ Place a sterile 2 in. × 2 in. gauze pad above the IV insertion site and gently remove the catheter.

➤ Apply firm pressure with the gauze pad; hold pressure for 1 to 3 minutes, or longer if bleeding persists.

➤ Replace the soiled 2 in. × 2 in. gauze pad with a new sterile one. Secure it with tape or use a transparent dressing.

Procedure 35-8: Administering a Blood Transfusion

Procedure 35-8A: Administering Blood and Blood Products

➤ Verify that informed consent has been obtained.

➤ Verify the provider's prescription, noting the indication and rate of infusion.

➤ Administer any prescribed pretransfusion medications.

➤ Obtain a blood administration set and 250 mL of IV normal saline solution.

➤ Obtain infusion pump, if possible, and blood warmer, if necessary.

➤ Obtain the blood product from the blood bank according to your institution's policy. Verify that the blood matches the prescription. Inspect it for abnormalities.

➤ With another qualified staff member (per agency policy), verify the patient and blood product identification (e.g., date of birth, hospital identification number, blood type). If all verifications are in agreement, both staff members should sign the blood bank form. Contact the blood bank immediately if there are discrepancies, and do not administer the blood product.

➤ Document on the blood bank form the date and time the transfusion is begun.

➤ Close all clamps on the blood administration set. Label the tubing.

➤ Hang the normal saline and prime the tubing.

➤ Gently invert the blood product container several times.

➤ Spike the blood product and hang the blood on the IV pole.

➤ Obtain a set of vital signs.

➤ Scrub the port with an alcohol swab or chlorhexidine/alcohol antiseptic product for at least 15 seconds before connecting to an existing line.

➤ Attach the administration set tubing to the IV catheter.

➤ Slowly open the roller clamp closest to the blood product. Start the infusion rate slowly for the first 15 minutes. Set to the prescribed rate if no reaction occurs after 50 mL has infused.

➤ Remain with or near the patient until 50 mL has infused. Measure vital signs in 15 minutes, then again in 30 minutes. Assess the patient every 30 to 60 minutes throughout the transfusion.

➤ Observe for and ask the patient to immediately report symptoms of transfusion reaction.

➤ When the blood has transfused, flush the line with the normal saline solution.

➤ Disconnect the tubing from the IV catheter and dispose of the blood product container and tubing per agency policy.

➤ If a second unit of blood is to be transfused, the same administration set may be used.

➤ Discard used supplies in a biohazard receptacle.

Procedure 35-8B: Managing a Transfusion Reaction

➤ If there are signs or symptoms of transfusion reaction, stop the transfusion immediately. Do not flush the tubing.

➤ Disconnect the administration set from the IV catheter.

➤ Call for help and prepare for emergency care.

➤ Obtain vital signs, and auscultate heart and breath sounds.

➤ Maintain patency of the IV catheter by hanging a new infusion of normal saline solution, using new tubing.

➤ Notify the primary care provider.

➤ Place the administration set and blood product container, with the blood bank form attached, inside a biohazard bag. Send the bag to the blood bank immediately.

➤ Obtain blood (in the extremity opposite the transfusion site) and urine specimens according to your institution's policy.

➤ Continue to monitor vital signs frequently.

➤ Administer medications, as prescribed.

Procedure 35-9: Assisting With Percutaneous Central Venous Catheter Placement

➤ Explain procedure to the patient and verify informed consent.

➤ Obtain vital signs.

➤ Gather supplies and perform meticulous hand hygiene.

➤ Position the table so that it is easily accessible by the provider.

➤ Prepare sterile field and add supplies.

➤ Position the patient (Trendelenburg with a rolled towel between the shoulders).

Continued

➤ After the physician or advanced practice nurse performs hand hygiene, offer mask, gown, and sterile gloves (and possibly hat, depending on agency policy).

➤ Don mask and then sterile gloves.

➤ Prep an 8 in. × 10 in. area around the site, using alcohol-based chlorhexidine preparation (Infusion Nurses Society [INS], 2021). Follow agency policy.

➤ Place the large sterile drape to cover patient's head and chest.

➤ Have the patient turn their head opposite the direction of insertion.

➤ Observe while the provider inserts and sutures the catheter.

➤ Apply sterile transparent dressing, close any lumen clamps, and place tape across the lumens near the injection caps.

➤ Monitor for complications (especially respiratory distress).

➤ Obtain a chest x-ray, per provider's prescription.

To explore learning resources for this chapter,

Go to Davis Advantage and find:

Answers and Suggested Responses for all questions in this chapter
Concept Map
Knowledge Map
References and Bibliography

Care of the Surgical Patient

Learning Outcomes

After completing this chapter, you should be able to:

➤ Discuss the importance of perioperative safety.

➤ Name and differentiate the three phases of the perioperative period.

➤ Describe the ways in which surgeries can be classified.

➤ Discuss factors that affect the degree of risk of surgery.

➤ Describe nursing actions associated with the preoperative phase, including physical preparations for surgery, preoperative teaching, and surgical consent forms.

➤ Compare and contrast the roles of the circulating and scrub nurse.

➤ Compare and contrast general anesthesia, local anesthesia, regional anesthesia, and conscious sedation.

➤ Discuss common nursing interventions during the intraoperative phase, including skin preparation, positioning for surgery, and intraoperative safety measures.

➤ Describe nursing assessments/recognize cues appropriate for surgical clients on admission to the nursing unit.

➤ Provide nursing care to prevent postoperative complications, including application of elastic and sequential compression devices, use of incentive spirometry, and management of gastric suction.

➤ Analyze cues and use nursing diagnoses appropriately to describe a patient's unique needs during the preoperative, intraoperative, and postoperative periods.

Key Concepts

Intraoperative care

Perioperative nursing

Postoperative care

Preoperative care

Related Concepts

See the Concept Map on Davis Advantage.

Meet Your Patient

Nishad Singh is a 68-year-old patient who came to the emergency department (ED) with sudden onset of rectal bleeding. The patient tells the ED nurse, "I've been really tired and dragging for several months. This morning I felt a little worse than usual. When I went to the bathroom, there was a lot of blood. I've never had that before, and it scared me. I've had to go to the bathroom a couple of times this morning, and it's all blood." The ED nurse collects the following data:

Blood pressure (BP): 138/88 mm Hg
Pulse: 104 beats/min and regular
Respiratory rate: 20 breaths/min
Temperature: 36.7°C (98.0°F)
Oxygen saturation: 98%

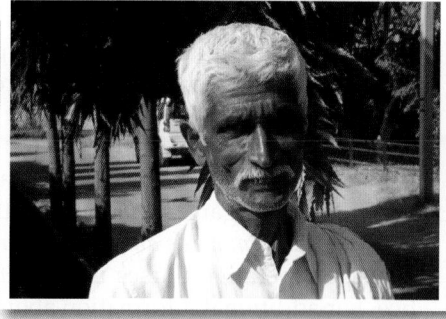

The ED nurse assesses that Mr. Singh is mildly anxious. His breath sounds are clear, but his abdomen is tender in the left lower quadrant (LLQ). The nurse draws blood to be sent to the laboratory. While they are waiting for the laboratory results, Mr. Singh tells the nurse, "My stomach is cramping down low, and I need to go to the bathroom." She provides him with a bedpan. He passes approximately 200 mL of bright-red blood with a small amount of fecal material. He becomes sweaty and light-headed after the

(Continued)

Meet Your Patient (continued)

bowel movement (BM). The nurse rechecks his vital signs and notes that his BP is now 120/76 mm Hg and that his pulse is up to 120 beats/min. The nurse shows the ED physician the bloody bowel movement and updates him on the change in vital signs. When the ED physician examines Mr. Singh, he tells Mr. Singh that he will need to be admitted to the hospital for further evaluation of the bleeding.

You are the nurse assigned to care for Mr. Singh on the medical–surgical unit. Mr. Singh has been sent from the

ED directly to radiology for a computed tomography scan of his abdomen. The scan reveals a tumor in the sigmoid colon. Since leaving the ED, Mr. Singh has had three more bloody BMs. His blood pressure is 100/72 mm Hg, and his pulse rate is now 134 beats/min. The physician prescribes a bolus of 1,000 mL of lactated Ringer's solution and a unit of packed red blood cells as soon as it is available. Mr. Singh is scheduled for colon resection surgery, which will occur as soon as the surgical team can be assembled and the room prepared.

ABOUT THE KEY CONCEPTS

In order to provide care to the surgical patient, you must understand and remember the key concepts of this chapter, which include **preoperative, intraoperative,** and **postoperative care.** We discuss how to prepare a client for surgery and the activities that occur before, during, and after surgery as we follow Mr. Singh (Meet Your Patient) through his perioperative experience. We present definitions and examples of the key concepts, as well as numerous subconcepts that relate to each other in various ways. We begin with perioperative nursing.

PERIOPERATIVE NURSING

Perioperative nursing involves the care of clients before, during, and after surgery and other invasive procedures. Historically, perioperative nursing practice was called *operating room nursing* and was limited to transferring patients into and out of operating rooms and handing instruments to surgeons during surgical procedures. Now nurses in all phases of the operative experience actively provide and manage care, teach, and study the care of perioperative patients.

The Association of perioperative Registered Nurses (AORN) is one of the most well-organized and influential specialty organizations within the nursing profession. AORN *Standards and Recommended Practices* (2020) keep perioperative nurses up to date on current practice. For additional information about AORN,

 Go to the **AORN Web site** at http://www.aorn.org

Perioperative Safety

An important aspect of the perioperative nursing role is to help prevent complications of surgery. Hand hygiene is an important component of prevention (Box 36-1).

Preventable perioperative errors cause surgery-related deaths, have an unfavorable financial impact on healthcare institutions, and result in physical and

BOX 36-1 ■ Recommended Practices for Hand Hygiene

- Perform hand hygiene:
    - Immediately before and after each patient contact
    - After removing gloves. Wearing gloves does not substitute for hand hygiene.
    - Anytime you may have come in contact with blood or potentially infectious substances
    - Before and after eating
    - After using the restroom
- Remove rings, watches, and bracelets before performing hand hygiene.
- It is preferable that you do not wear rings. They have been associated with a significant increase in skin microorganism count.
- Keep fingernails short and clean. They should not extend beyond the fingertips.
- Replace nail polish when it is chipped or at least every 4 days.
- Do not wear artificial nails. Fungal growth often occurs under them.
- Be certain there are no lesions or breaks in skin integrity on your hands.
- For hand-washing and handrub procedures,

 Go to **Chapter 20, Procedure 20-1: Hand Hygiene,** in Volume 2.

Sources: Adapted from AORN. (2020). *Guidelines for perioperative practice;* Boyce, J., & Pittet, D. (2002). Guideline for hand hygiene in health-care settings. Recommendations of the Healthcare Infection Control Practices Advisory Committee and the HICPAC/SHEA/APIC/IDSA Hand Hygiene Task Force. *Morbidity and Mortality Weekly Report (MMWR), 51*(RR16), 1–44. http://www.cdc.gov/mmwr/pdf/rr/rr5116.pdf; Siegel, J., Rhinehart, E., Jackson, M., Chiarello, L., & Healthcare Infection Control Practices Advisory Committee. (2007). *2007 guideline for isolation precautions: Preventing transmission of infectious agents in healthcare settings.* http://www.cdc.gov/hicpac/2007IP/2007isolationPrecautions.html

emotional harm to patients. Various government and private organizations stress the importance of patient safety:

- *The Association of perioperative Registered Nurses (AORN, 2020).* Perioperative Safety is one of the three domains under which AORN organizes its perioperative patient outcomes. Specific safety outcomes include prevention of injury and freedom from infection.
- *The Joint Commission (2022).* The Joint Commission 2022 National Patient Safety Goals applicable to surgery include preventing infection, improving the accuracy of patient identification, using medication safely, and performing a time-out immediately before starting procedures to prevent mistakes in surgery.
- *National Quality Partners Leadership Consortium (2022).* The National Quality Partners (NQP) National Quality Forum established a national priority that includes the aims of achieving better care, providing improved health for people and communities, and making quality care more affordable. One of its priorities and goals is making care safer by identifying the social determinants of health as a means of providing health equity in the delivery of care.
- *The Institute for Healthcare Improvement (n.d., 2011).* This is an independent, not-for-profit organization that works to reduce morbidity and death in American healthcare, including perioperative care. One goal of its 100,000 Lives Campaign and its 5 Million Lives Campaign was to reduce surgical complications and specifically surgical infections. To see the entire list of IHI recommendations,

 Go to the Institute for Healthcare Improvement (IHI) Web site at **http://www.ihi.org**

"Never Events"

"Never events" are serious and costly errors resulting in severe consequences for the patient; they are mostly preventable. Believing these events are reasonably preventable and should never happen in a hospital, Medicare no longer reimburses institutions for care related to such complications (Centers for Medicare and Medicaid Services, 2019). Several of the never events (also called *serious reportable events*) are also targeted by the national organizations listed earlier. Among the never events important to perioperative care are

- Surgery on the wrong body part
- Surgery on the wrong patient
- Wrong surgery on a patient
- Deep vein thrombosis (DVT) or pulmonary embolism (PE) after total knee or hip replacement
- Foreign body left in a patient after surgery (e.g., sponge, clip for draping)
- Surgical site infections after certain elective procedures (e.g., bariatric surgery for obesity). AORN, The

Joint Commission, the NQP, and the IHI extend that to include all infections. The Centers for Disease Control and Prevention (CDC) targeted certain antimicrobial-resistant bacterial infections.

You will see those themes recur in the theoretical and practical knowledge in the remainder of this chapter and in Volume 2.

PREOPERATIVE CARE

The **preoperative phase** begins with the client's decision to have surgery and ends when they enter the operating room. The length of the preoperative period and the extent of the patient teaching depend on the type of surgery to be done and the patient's overall health status.

TheoreticalKnowledge
knowing why

Nursing care during the preoperative phase focuses on identifying existing health concerns, planning for intraoperative and postoperative needs, and providing preoperative teaching. Preoperative nursing care is delivered in a variety of settings. More than two-thirds of surgeries in the United States are performed in outpatient settings, such as endoscopy suites, physicians' offices, and ambulatory surgery centers (Hall et al., 2017).

How Are Surgeries Classified?

Knowing the type of surgery helps you identify the patient's perioperative needs and plan patient care. Surgeries can be classified by body system, purpose, level of urgency, and acuity. The classifications often overlap.

♥ iCare 36-1

Perioperative Care

- Perioperative nursing is a specialized area of nursing with specific, established standards of care. A caring nurse strives to integrate those standards into the nursing process and apply standards to each patient in a caring manner.
- Caring nurses ensure that a person is cognitively and psychologically prepared for surgery.
- Caring nurses advocate for patients. An example is stopping the line and placing a HOLD on surgery when a person identifies an error or a risk in a process or in the surgical procedure. This exhibits *200% accountability* and embraces *high-reliability* behaviors. You can do this by saying to others, *"I have a concern"; "We need to stop and verify"; "I am uncomfortable proceeding";* or even stronger language: *"I cannot send Ms. Brown until the surgeon comes back up and reviews her surgical procedure with her again; she clearly does not understand."*

Key Point: *Preventing errors and "never events" is everyone's responsibility.*

By Body System

The body system classification is useful for determining the postoperative risk of infection. For example, surgical incisions that enter the gastrointestinal, respiratory, or genitourinary tract have a higher risk for infection compared with surgeries of other body systems. However, if an organ ruptures or surgery is required to repair a penetrating injury, the risk of infection is very high regardless of the body system involved. Mr. Singh (Meet Your Patient) will have surgery involving the gastrointestinal system.

By Purpose

See whether you can identify the purpose that describes Mr. Singh's (Meet Your Patient) surgery.

- **Ablative surgery** involves the removal of a diseased body part. For example, a cholecystectomy removes a diseased gallbladder.
- **Diagnostic (exploratory) surgery** is done to confirm or rule out a diagnosis. Examples include biopsies; fine-needle aspiration; and invasive testing, such as cardiac catheterization.
- **Palliative surgery** is performed to relieve discomfort or other disease symptoms without producing a cure. Examples include nerve root destruction for chronic pain.
- **Reconstructive surgery** is performed to restore function, for example, rotator cuff repair (repair of a torn ligament).
- **Cosmetic surgery** is done to improve appearance (e.g., a facelift).
- **Transplant surgery** replaces a malfunctioning body part, tissue, or organ. Joint replacements and organ replacement procedures are included in this category.
- **Procurement surgery** is related to transplant surgery. An organ or tissue is procured or harvested from someone pronounced brain dead for transplantation into another person.

By Degree of Urgency

Based on the following definitions, how would you describe the degree of urgency for Mr. Singh's surgery?

- **Emergency surgery** requires transport to the operating suite as soon as possible to preserve the patient's life or function. The surgical team is summoned and preparations are made rapidly. Internal hemorrhage, rupture of an organ, and trauma are common causes of emergency surgery.
- **Urgent surgery** is scheduled within 24 to 48 hours to alleviate symptoms, repair a body part, or restore function. Removal of a cancerous breast and internal fixation of a fracture are examples.
- **Elective surgery** is performed when surgery is the recommended course of action but the condition is not time sensitive. The client may delay surgery to gather information, consider options, or organize care for the

family. Examples include repair of a torn ligament and removal of rectal polyps.

By Degree of Risk

♥ **iCare** There is an old adage concerning surgery: "The only minor surgery is someone else's surgery." This statement reflects the anxiety that often accompanies surgery. Nevertheless, surgery is defined as major or minor based on the degree of seriousness or risk associated with the procedure. The degree of risk varies with the condition of the client, as well as with the type of surgery and anesthesia.

- **Major surgery** is associated with a high degree of risk—for example, the potential for significant blood loss, a prolonged or complicated procedure, surgery involving vital organs, or a high risk for postoperative complications. Some examples of major procedures are coronary artery bypass graft, nephrectomy (removal of a kidney), and colon resection.
- **Minor surgery,** often performed on an outpatient basis, involves little risk and usually has few complications. Examples include arthroscopy, breast biopsy, and inguinal hernia repair.

What Factors Affect Surgical Risk?

The patient's age, general health, and personal habits can contribute to increased risk during any surgical procedure.

Age   The very young and very old are at greatest risk during surgical procedures.

- **Infants** have the following risk factors:
  - Limited ability to regulate temperature.
  - Immature immune, cardiovascular, liver, and renal systems.
  - Increased risk for infection.
  - Increased risk for excess fluid volume, and deficient fluid volume. Even minor blood loss may represent a substantial portion of the infant's blood.
  - Infants may have difficulty calming. They are unable to understand what is happening, so you cannot use verbal reassurance and explanations for comfort.
- **Toddlers** understand simple explanations but may be anxious about separation from parents or caregivers. Many have fear of the dark.
- **Preschoolers** fear damage to body parts. Fear of pain or needles is common for children of any age.
- **Teens** might fear disfigurement resulting from scars.
- **Young adults** are commonly anxious about the cost associated with hospitalization or surgery.
- **Older adults** are at increased risk because they have less physiological reserve and often have comorbid conditions (other illnesses not related to the surgery). Many of the physiological changes of aging predispose older adults to increased risk. Among these changes are decreased kidney

function, diminished immune function, decreased bone and lean body mass, increased peripheral vascular resistance, decreased cardiac output, decreased cough reflex, and increased time required for wound healing.

Type of Wound Both preexisting wounds (e.g., from trauma) and the wounds (incisions) created by the surgical procedure can pose a risk for infection (Table 36-1).

Risk to the patient increases, along with the risk for or presence of infection. Which type of wound will Mr. Singh (Meet Your Patient) have immediately after surgery?

Preexisting Conditions The ideal surgical candidate is a healthy young adult who takes no medications. Unfortunately, many surgical clients have underlying acute or chronic disorders that increase surgical risk (Box 36-2). Also see the accompanying PICOT box.

Table 36-1 ➤ Wound Type and Potential for Infection

WOUND TYPE	WOUND CHARACTERISTICS	EXAMPLES OF SURGERY ASSOCIATED WITH THE WOUND
Clean Wounds	Uninfected; minimal inflammation; little risk of infection AND Surgery does not involve the gastrointestinal, respiratory, or genitourinary tract.	Facelift, cataract surgery, joint replacement, breast biopsy, tonsillectomy
Clean-Contaminated Wounds	Not infected, but carry increased risk for infection	Surgical incisions that enter the gastrointestinal, respiratory, or genitourinary tracts
Contaminated Wounds	Not infected, but carry high risk for infection	Surgery to repair trauma to open wounds, such as compound fractures; surgery in which a major break in surgical asepsis occurred
Infected Wounds	Evidence of infection, such as purulent drainage, necrotic tissue, or bacterial counts above 100,000 organisms per gram of tissue	A postoperative surgical incision of any type that has evidence of infection

BOX 36-2 ■ Preexisting Conditions That Increase Surgical Risk

Acute Conditions

Acute infections tax the patient's energy and physiological reserves, increasing the risk for various postoperative complications.

Upper respiratory tract infections are associated with increased risk of postoperative pneumonia, especially if the patient receives a general anesthetic.

Chronic Conditions

Cardiovascular diseases (such as hypertension, congestive heart failure, and myocardial infarction) affect the ability of the heart to work as an efficient pump. If these disorders are well controlled (e.g., with blood pressure medications or cardiotonic medications), risk is limited.

Chronic respiratory disorders (such as emphysema, asthma, or bronchitis) decrease pulmonary function, increase the risk of respiratory infection, and may be exacerbated (made worse) by general anesthesia.

Coagulation disorders delay clotting and increase blood loss, placing the patient at risk for hemorrhage and hypovolemic shock. In contrast, a hypercoagulation state increases the risk of stroke, embolism, or intravascular clotting.

Diabetes mellitus delays wound healing and increases the risk of infection and cardiovascular disorders associated with diabetes.

Liver disease affects the body's ability to metabolize amino acids, carbohydrates, and fat; manufacture prothrombin for clotting; and detoxify medications. Therefore, the patient is at increased risk for poor wound healing, hemorrhage, and toxic reactions to anesthetics and medications.

Neurological disorders (such as paralysis or spinal cord injury) increase the risk for vasomotor instability and thus create the potential for wide swings in blood pressure. In addition, patients with seizure disorders are more likely to have a seizure in the perioperative period.

Nutritional disorders can affect surgical outcomes. Patients who are malnourished or obese are at risk for delayed wound healing, infection, and fatigue. Obese clients are also more prone to cardiovascular disorders and impaired pulmonary function.

Renal disease affects the patient's ability to excrete many medications, including anesthetic agents. It also affects the ability to regulate fluid and electrolytes.

PICOT

Older Adults, Comorbidity, and Risk for Surgical Site Infection

Situation: The student is caring for an elderly patient who is 4 days postoperative after a colon resection. The abdominal incision is reddened, with purulent yellow drainage on the dressing. The patient has a history of chronic obstructive pulmonary disease (COPD) and obesity (body mass index of 31).

PICOT Components

P	Population/patient	=	Older adults
I	Intervention/indicator	=	Chronic disease and comorbidity
C	Comparator/control	=	No health problems
O	Outcome	=	Increased risk of incision infection
T	Time	=	After surgery

Searchable Question

Do _____ (P) who receive/are exposed to _____ (I), compared with _____ (C), demonstrate _____ (O) during _____ (T)?

Example of Evidence: Surgical site infections (SSIs) account for roughly 11% of hospital-acquired infections in patients aged 65 and older. Older people who experience SSIs tend to have a worse clinical outcome than younger adults. Researchers evaluated cases of elderly patients with SSIs and identified several independent predictors of SSIs. These include obesity, COPD, congestive heart failure, American Society of Anesthesiologists grade of ≥3, wound class of >2, and socioeconomic factors.

Application to Practice: Patients with these risk factors can be identified preoperatively, and nursing care can be adjusted to decrease the potential for SSIs.

Source: Agodi, A., Quattrocchi, A., Barchitta, M., Adornetto, V., Cocuzza, A., Latino, R., Li Destri, G., & Di Cataldo, A. (2015). Risk of surgical site infection in older patients in a cohort survey: Targets for quality improvement in antibiotic prophylaxis. *International Surgery, 100*(3), 473–479.

Mental Status Patients with altered cognition, from either physical or mental illness, may be unable to comprehend preoperative instructions or give informed consent for surgical procedures. They may also require medications (e.g., antipsychotic agents) that interact with anesthetics and analgesics. Surgery and anesthesia may aggravate preexisting dementia, confusion, and disorientation.

Medications Both prescribed and over-the-counter medications may increase surgical risk (Box 36-3). For example, patients who self-prescribe vitamin E may be at increased risk for bleeding. Certain herbal and alternative medications can have the following effects:

- Increase the risk for cardiac dysrhythmias secondary to potassium loss
- Interfere with metabolism of anesthetics because of their effects on the liver
- Increase the potential for excessive bleeding
- Decrease cerebral blood flow
- Cause hypertension
- Increase the effects of opioids and sympathetic nervous system stimulants

Personal Habits The following are some personal habits that may increase surgical risk.

- Smoking affects pulmonary function.
- Long-term alcohol use contributes to liver disease, increasing the risk for bleeding.
- Alcohol and drugs interact with anesthetic agents and medications to create adverse effects.
- Habitual substance abusers may have a cross-tolerance to anesthetic and analgesic agents, causing them to need higher-than-normal doses.

BOX 36-3 ■ Medications That Increase Surgical Risk

Antibiotics	May potentiate the action of anesthetic agents
Anticoagulants	Increase risk for bleeding
Antidysrhythmics	May impair cardiac function during anesthesia
Antihypertensives	Increase the risk for hypotension during surgery; may interact with anesthetic agents to cause bradycardia and impaired circulation
Aspirin	Increases risk for bleeding
Corticosteroids	Delay wound healing and increase risk for infection
Diuretics	Alter fluid and electrolyte balance (especially potassium balance)
Opioids	Increase the risk of respiratory depression
NSAIDs	Inhibit platelet aggregation, increasing the risk for bleeding
Tranquilizers	Increase the risk of respiratory depression

Allergies Patients may be allergic to medications (e.g., antibiotics, such as penicillins or cephalosporins), analgesics (e.g., codeine), tape, latex, and solutions used in surgery. Reactions range from unpleasant to life threatening.

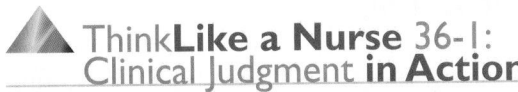

KnowledgeCheck 36-1

- Define *preoperative phase.*
- What are four ways surgery can be classified?
- What factors affect surgical risk?

ThinkLike a Nurse 36-1: Clinical Judgment in Action

How would you evaluate Mr. Singh's (Meet Your Patient) surgical risk? What additional information do you need to answer this question?

PracticalKnowledge knowing how

The nursing focus in the preoperative phase is to prepare the patient for surgery. You will use the nursing process to analyze cues and identify any unique nursing diagnoses a patient might have. However, many perioperative nursing interventions are routine preventive measures that you will use for *all* surgical patients.

Perioperative Nursing Data Set

The Perioperative Nursing Data Set (PNDS) is a standardized vocabulary specifically designed to describe the care of perioperative patients. It is recognized by the American Nurses Association. The latest update of PNDS reflects the nursing process, including nursing assessment, diagnoses, identified nursing-sensitive outcomes, nursing interventions, and implementation and evaluation. The PDNS promotes better communication among nurses and other healthcare providers, increases the visibility of nursing interventions, improves patient care, and standardizes a way to evaluate nursing care outcomes (Westra & Peterson, 2016).

Perioperative Patient-Focused Model The PNDS is derived from AORN's Perioperative Patient-Focused Model (Van Wicklin, 2020). The patient is at the center of the model and the focus of care. The perioperative nurse intervenes within the context of the healthcare system to assist the patient throughout the perioperative experience to achieve outcomes in the Health System domain and the Patient-Centered domains (which include Safety, Physiological Responses to Surgery, and Behavioral Responses to Surgery).

The Health System domain refers to the system in which perioperative care is given. It involves administrative and structural elements necessary for successful surgical outcomes—for example, equipment, supplies, staff, and policies (AORN, 2020).

■ ASSESSMENT/RECOGNIZING CUES

For patient safety, patient data must be correct and complete. To prevent the omission of important information, many organizations have developed a preoperative checklist. Although the forms may vary at each institution, the areas for assessment/recognizing cues are the same and are discussed in the sections that follow.

Focused Nursing History

It is essential to determine whether the client is physiologically, cognitively, and psychologically prepared for the intraoperative and postoperative phases of surgery. For an accurate nursing history, collect assessment data (cues) from the client, significant others, medical records, and other members of the healthcare team. Include the following topics in your preoperative assessment: health history, physical status, allergies, medications (including herbal products and over-the-counter medications), mental status, knowledge and understanding of the surgery and anesthesia, cultural and spiritual factors, access to social resources, coping strategies, and use of alcohol and drugs. It is also important to elicit patients' values and expressed needs (see the accompanying Safe, Effective Nursing Care box).

For an example of a preoperative assessment form developed by AORN,

> Go to **Chapter 36, Assessment Guidelines and Tools, Example of a Preoperative Checklist,** in Volume 2.

Additional assessments may be needed if the client is undergoing outpatient surgery or has a planned short stay after surgery (see the Home Care box, Preoperative Assessment for the Surgical Client Who Will Be Discharged to Home).

Safe, Effective Nursing Care

Surgical Team Communication

Key Concepts: Perioperative Nursing, Preoperative Care, Intraoperative Care, Postoperative Care

SENC Competency: Provide goal-directed, client-centered care

Eliciting each patient's values, preferences, and expressed needs as part of the focused nursing history will assist you in providing goal-directed, client-centered care. You can then communicate patient values, preferences, and expressed needs to other members of the healthcare team to ensure patient-centered care with sensitivity to and respect for the diversity of individual patients.

SENC Competency: Collaborate with the interprofessional healthcare team

To provide for effective collaboration within nursing and interprofessional teams, nurses must engage in open communication, display mutual respect, and share decision making to ensure safe and effective patient care. Two-minute briefings just before surgery, led by the attending surgeon using a standardized format, have been found to improve communication and reduce delays and wrong-site surgery (Lee, 2016). Surgical briefings encourage team members to talk when there is no problem so that they are more likely to speak up when they have misgivings when problems occur (Koleva, 2020).

Home Care Box 36-1

Preoperative Assessment for the Surgical Client Who Will Be Discharged to Home

The type of surgery, the client's condition, and the support system determine whether it is safe to discharge a client to home after surgery. Your assessment should focus on the following questions:

➤ What kind of care will be needed?

➤ Is the client able to take care of themself? If not, who is available to assist with care?

➤ Does the caregiver have the necessary skills to provide care?

➤ If not, can these skills be taught before the client is discharged?

➤ What features in the home environment will facilitate the client's progress? What features will inhibit progress? For example, can the client get to the bathroom? Can the client negotiate the stairs in the house?

➤ How will the client be followed after discharge? That is, how soon should the client visit their physician? Will the client receive home nursing care?

Focused Physical Assessment

If you identify risk factors from the nursing history, focus on these aspects during your brief head-to-toe physical assessment. For example, if the patient states they had a cough last week, perform a focused assessment of the ear, nose, throat, and lungs to determine how the cough may affect the patient's risk. If the patient has lower airway congestion, as evidenced by rhonchi and productive cough, communicate these findings to the surgeon and the anesthesia team; if a general anesthetic is planned, it may be necessary to delay the surgery. For all patients, assess risk factors for thrombophlebitis because venous thrombus is one of the never events that can lead to potentially life-threatening pulmonary emboli.

Recent guidelines state that optimal preoperative assessment of older adults includes the following:

- Cognitive ability
- Capacity to understand the surgery
- Nutritional status
- Risk factors for postoperative delirium and pulmonary complications
- Patient's treatment goals and expectations
- Family and social support system
- Depression
- Cardiac status
- Functional status
- History of falls
- Detailed medication history, including polypharmacy

- Baseline frailty score
- Diagnostic tests specific to elderly patients (Mohanty et al., 2016)

Diagnostic Testing

Preoperative screening tests are usually prescribed before surgical procedures. The type of testing depends on the patient's age, health history, and facility policies.

- **Complete blood count (CBC), urinalysis (UA), and electrocardiogram (ECG).** Most institutions require a CBC and a UA, along with an ECG for patients older than age 50.
- **Routine chest x-ray is *not* recommended** for all patients before surgery. Chest radiology incurs extra costs to the healthcare system and exposes patients to small risks from radiation exposure.
- **Patients** with chronic health problems may require additional testing.

 Go to **Diagnostic Testing: Common Preoperative Screening Tests,** in Volume 2.

KnowledgeCheck 36-2

- List the information you should gather in the preoperative nursing history.
- What type of physical assessment is performed as part of the preoperative assessment?
- What laboratory tests are most commonly prescribed before surgery?

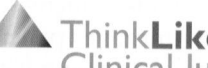 ## ThinkLike a Nurse 36-2: Clinical Judgment in Action

- What factors will affect your preoperative assessment of Mr. Singh (Meet Your Patient)?
- Describe how you might perform the assessment as well as provide physical care. What modifications, if any, should you make in his assessment?

NURSING DIAGNOSIS/ANALYZING CUES

As you learned in Chapter 3, nursing diagnoses/analyzing cues describe the individualized needs of patients. However, preoperative patients share a common set of needs, regardless of their individual differences and the type of surgery they are to have. Consider the following examples:

- All preoperative patients need preoperative teaching, so it's not necessary to write a nursing diagnosis of Knowledge Deficit for every patient. Agency protocols or critical pathways will almost certainly mandate teaching.
- Almost all surgical patients have at least mild anxiety, and many of your routine actions will help to relieve anxiety, so there is no need to always include a diagnosis of Anxiety.

Key Point: *Do not put any nursing diagnosis on the care plan unless you plan to address it with something other than the routine preoperative interventions.*

Individualized Nursing Diagnoses/ Analyzing Cues

Individualized nursing diagnoses for the preoperative patient evolve from your assessment. You should identify an actual nursing diagnosis only if the patient has the defining characteristics for it. **Key Point:** *Identify risk (potential) diagnoses only if the patient has an underlying condition that places them at higher risk than the average surgical patient.* The following nursing diagnoses may be useful for certain preoperative patients:

- *Anxiety* may be mild, moderate, severe, or at a panic level. In the preoperative client, anxiety may be related to the current change in health status or due to concerns about being unable to provide care for loved ones. Make this diagnosis only if the client has symptoms such as restlessness, trembling, increased pulse, and other defining characteristics.
- *Fear* is a common reaction to surgery. Fear may be related to the unknown outcome of the surgery, to learning the diagnosis after a diagnostic procedure, and to the prospect of pain during and after surgery. Fear and Anxiety share several defining characteristics. Many of the routine preoperative interventions help to address Fear.
- *Airway Clearance Impairment* may be used for patients who have a preexisting health problem, such as bronchitis or emphysema.
- *Disturbed Sleep Pattern* often results from anxiety about the upcoming surgery.
- *Ineffective Coping* may be appropriate for a patient with extreme anxiety and concerns about the outcomes of the surgery.
- *Latex Allergy Response* is appropriate for patients who have a known allergy to latex.
- *Risk for Latex Allergy Response* is appropriate for patients who have had multiple surgeries or urinary catheterizations; are in professions with daily exposure to latex; have a history of asthma; or are allergic to bananas, avocados, kiwi, chestnuts, or poinsettia plants. Do not use it routinely for all patients.
- *Deficient Knowledge.* As you know, you do not usually need a Knowledge Deficit diagnosis. If you believe the patient may not learn or that the information is too complex to remember, then identify the problem likely to result from the Deficient Knowledge. For example:
    Nonadherence to Therapeutic Regimen related to Knowledge Deficit of postoperative medications and office visits
    Risk for Infection related to Knowledge Deficit of wound care and asepsis

Special Risks for Older Adults Older adults, especially those older than age 70 and the frail elderly, are likely to need some individualized nursing diagnoses. They present unique risks not only because they often have other illnesses but also because of certain physiological changes that accompany aging. For example, older adults metabolize anesthetic agents differently from younger adults (see Table 36-2), so they may experience Confusion or Gas Exchange Impairment.

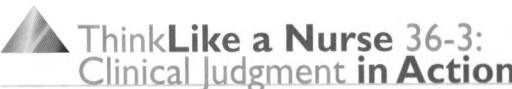

ThinkLike a Nurse 36-3: Clinical Judgment in Action

Which, if any, of the preceding nursing diagnoses would be most appropriate for Mr. Singh (Meet Your Patient)? Do not use the potential complications in Table 36-2. Explain your reasoning.

PLANNING, PRIORITIZING HYPOTHESES, & GENERATING SOLUTIONS

The overall nursing goal in the preoperative phase is to prepare the patient adequately for surgery and deliver the patient to the operating suite in the best condition possible. Outcomes that provide evidence of achieving this goal, and that are appropriate for nearly all preoperative patients, are that the patient:

- Is able to describe the surgical procedure in a basic manner.
- Provides informed consent.
- When asked, states what is expected in the postoperative period.
- States very little anxiety.

Associated Nursing Outcomes Classification (NOC) outcomes for the preoperative nursing client depend, of course, on the nursing diagnoses you identify. You will evaluate the nursing care plan by examining the extent to which the goals have been met.

IMPLEMENTATION/TAKING ACTION

Many preoperative nursing activities are routine interventions to be used for *all* preoperative patients, regardless of their nursing diagnoses. The Nursing Interventions Classification (NIC) has a special Perioperative Care domain (category) for such interventions. The following are the preoperative NIC interventions in that domain:

- *Preoperative Coordination:* Facilitating preadmission diagnostic testing and preparation of the surgical patient. (Activity example: Notify the physician of abnormal diagnostic test results.)
- *Surgical Preparation:* Providing care to a patient immediately before surgery and verifying required procedures/tests and documentation in the clinical record. (Activity example: Complete the preoperative checklist.)
- *Teaching: Preoperative:* Assisting a patient to understand and mentally prepare for surgery and the postoperative recovery period. (Activity example: Correct unrealistic expectations of the surgery, as appropriate.)

Table 36-2 ➤ Special Risks for Older Adults

RISK FACTORS	POTENTIAL COMPLICATIONS (PC) AND NURSING DIAGNOSES
Coronary artery disease. Most older adults have at least some degree of coronary artery disease.	• PC: Hypotension • Risk for Falls r/t orthostatic hypotension
Delirium is one of the most common surgical complications in older adults. Predisposing factors include older age, functional disabilities, and a high number of coexisting conditions. Male sex, poor vision and hearing, depressive symptoms, mild cognitive impairment, laboratory abnormalities, and alcohol abuse may also increase risk (Marcantonio, 2017).	• PC: Delirium • Acute Confusion • Chronic Confusion
Respiratory changes. Age-related respiratory changes, such as decreased chest wall compliance, forced vital capacity, and diaphragmatic strength	• PC: Pneumonia • PC: Atelectasis • Gas Exchange Impairment • Ineffective Airway Clearance
Age-related skin changes: Dry, fragile skin; decreased turgor and elasticity	• Risk for Impaired Skin Integrity Impairment • Risk for Pressure Injury
Age-related musculoskeletal changes: Decreased bone mass and muscle fiber mass	• Risk for Impaired Physical Mobility • Risk for Falls
Comorbidities of the central nervous system are more common in older adults. Some conditions may be aggravated by surgery and anesthesia.	• PC: Dementia • Risk for Acute Confusion
Decreased gastrointestinal motility	• PC: Ileus • Aspiration Risk secondary to vomiting
Decreased genitourinary function: decreased bladder tone, elasticity, and tone; decreased renal function	• PC: Side effects of medications • PC: Renal complications • PC: Urinary tract infection • Risk for Impaired Skin Integrity r/t urinary incontinence

The following sections explain in more detail how to carry out interventions that are "routine," in that they are performed for all preoperative patients (e.g., confirming surgical consent, providing preoperative teaching, communicating with the surgical team).

Confirm That Surgical Consent Has Been Obtained

Before a surgical procedure is performed, professional standards and the law require the surgeon to obtain the patient's informed consent. The signed consent form verifies that the surgeon and patient have communicated adequately about the surgery (Dale et al., 2018). Once signed and witnessed, the consent form is part of the patient's record and accompanies the patient to the operating room.

Key Point: *The surgeon is responsible for (1) giving the patient the necessary information and (2) determining the patient's competence to make an informed decision*

about the surgery. You are responsible for verifying that the surgical consent form is signed and witnessed.

The following two sections are about the "mechanics" of consent. They describe the contents of a consent form and the process for obtaining a patient's signature.

What Is a Surgical Consent Form? A **surgical consent form** includes the following information (The Joint Commission, 2010):

• The type of surgery being performed
• The name and qualifications of the person performing the surgery (e.g., Jason Esmar, MD) and the primary practitioner for the patient's care and treatment
• A statement that the risks and benefits of surgery, as well as reasonable alternatives, have been explained to the patient
• A statement of the relevant risks, benefits, and side effects of the alternatives
• The likelihood of achieving goals

- A statement that the patient has the right to refuse surgery or withdraw consent at any time
- When indicated, any limitations on the confidentiality of information about the patient

How Do I Obtain a Signature? Often, you will obtain the patient's signature and document on the preoperative checklist that you have done so. As a patient advocate, you should:

- **Verify.** First verify with the patient that the physician has explained the procedure and answered all questions. Ask the patient to state what they were told during the consent process.
- **Notify and delay, if necessary.** If the patient has questions or if you have any questions about the patient's competence, notify the surgeon and delay sending the patient to surgery.
- **Document.** Be sure to document these conversations, and document in the patient's record that the surgeon was notified of any additional questions or concerns.

What Is Informed Consent? A signature on a form implies consent. However, you must be certain that the signature represents *informed* consent. **Key Point: Informed consent requires that the patient understood the communication and was not coerced (pressured) to consent.** There are two important requirements:

- The patient must be alert, rational, mentally competent, and not sedated when they sign.
- The information must be given to the patient in a language and vocabulary that the patient can understand.

Patients who are unconscious or have a mental disability; who have been judged insane; who cannot read, write, or hear; and those under the influence of sedative drugs or alcohol are generally not competent to give consent (Buppert, 2012). In most states a family member, conservator, or legal guardian may give consent for the procedure.

- **Informed consent** helps protect patients from having a surgery they do not understand or want.
- **The signed document** protects the healthcare agency and workers from later claims that the patient did not consent to have the procedure.

If you would like more information on *informed* consent, see Chapter 39.

KnowledgeCheck 36-3

- Who is responsible for obtaining informed consent for the surgical procedure?
- What are the nursing responsibilities related to informed consent?

Provide Preoperative Teaching

Preoperative teaching prepares the patient for the surgical experience, allays fears, and decreases the risks of postoperative complications. See Chapter 16 as needed to review patient teaching.

What to Teach

The content of the teaching plan should focus on:

- What will happen before, during, and after surgery
- How the patient or caregiver can participate in the care
- Common feelings and concerns that patients have about surgery. This helps the patient feel supported and less anxious.
- What patients and families can do to prevent surgical site infection (The Joint Commission, 2022). Teach patients the content in the Self-Care box, Teaching Patients How to Help Prevent Surgical Site Infections.

The type of surgery influences the content of your teaching. For example, if the patient is scheduled for an outpatient knee arthroscopy (visualization of the joint) under spinal anesthesia, the teaching plan needs to describe the procedure and the anticipated discharge of the patient within hours after surgery. This is different from the teaching for a patient who will have cardiac

---

Self-Care

Teaching Patients How to Help Prevent Surgical Site Infections

Before Surgery

- If you smoke, stop. Those who smoke are more likely to get infections.
- Discuss your health problems with your surgeon (e.g., diabetes, allergies). These can affect incision healing.
- Ask your surgeon whether you should have antibiotics before surgery.
- Don't shave near where you will have surgery. Not all procedures require hair removal, but if they do, it should be done with electric clippers. If someone starts to use a razor to shave you, speak up.

After Surgery

- Be sure family and friends wash their hands or use alcohol-based handrub before and after they visit you.
- When anyone examines you or checks your incision, ask them if they have washed their hands (or used alcohol-based handrub).
- Wash your hands before and after caring for your own incision.
- Do not allow family and friends to touch your incision or the surgical dressing.
- Be sure you know how to care for your incision before you go home.
- If you have fever or redness, pain, or drainage at the surgery site, call your physician right away.

Source: Adapted from Centers for Disease Control and Prevention. (2020). *What you should know before your surgery.* http://www.cdc.gov/features/SafeSurgery/

surgery and spend a number of days in the hospital. **Key Point:** *In general, preoperative teaching should focus on explaining what will happen before, during, and after surgery.* To find suggested teaching content

 Go to **Chapter 36, Clinical Insight 36-1: Preoperative Teaching,** in Volume 2.

For the complete steps of deep breathing, coughing, moving in bed, and leg exercises, see the summary in the Highlights of Procedures box, and

Go to **Chapter 36, Procedure 36-1: Teaching a Patient to Deep-Breathe, Cough, Move in Bed, and Perform Leg Exercises,** in Volume 2.

How to Teach

You can use written instructions, video presentations, phone contact, or face-to-face discussion to provide preoperative teaching. Teach in a language the patient understands and at a level that is easily understood. Use terms the patient understands clearly; that is, avoid medical jargon. See Chapter 16 if you need to review patient teaching techniques and information about health literacy.

Obtain an interpreter for translation if the patient speaks a language that you do not speak. When possible, avoid using family members as translators to protect the patient's privacy or avoid a bias in translation (see Chapter 12 if you need more information about language differences).

Teaching Children Include family members in the teaching as much as possible and as much as desired by the patient, especially if the patient is a child or dependent adult. Play is an effective way for children to learn (e.g., have the child give medicine to a doll with an empty syringe or listen to its "heart" with your stethoscope). Simple language is a must! For example, you'd say to a young child, "Lie on your tummy, please."

Older Adults Older adults may experience physical, psychological, and/or psychosocial issues that impair their ability to learn. Decreased hearing, vision, and sense of touch may interfere with their ability to understand and remember information. To increase understanding, provide an environment conducive to learning, allow for more time for the patient to process information, and provide written material that clearly conveys the essentials.

When to Teach

- **For elective surgery,** many patients have a scheduled preoperative assessment about a week before the surgery. The session may include preoperative testing, an appointment with the anesthesia staff, signing the consent form, and planned preoperative teaching.

- **Patients undergoing emergency surgery** usually require extensive physical care preoperatively. You may need to give IV fluids, transfuse blood, treat for pain, and administer many medications, as in the case of Mr. Singh (Meet Your Patient). This means that you may have limited time for preoperative teaching. However, you should always teach the patient as much as possible to prepare the patient for the surgical experience.

Prepare the Patient Physically for Surgery

Physical preparation of the patient for surgery involves several nursing concerns.

Maintaining Normothermia Evidence-based guidelines stress that maintaining a normal body temperature helps produce good surgical outcomes (Levin et al., 2016; Pędziwiatr et al., 2018; Rightmyer & Singbartl, 2016). Compared with normothermic patients, hypothermic patients have more frequent wound infections, cardiac complications, and blood transfusions. Hypothermic patients feel uncomfortable, and shivering raises oxygen consumption by about 40%.

- **Core temperature.** The patient's core temperature should be measured 1 to 2 hours before the start of anesthesia and either continuously or every 15 minutes during surgery.
- **Passive thermal care.** You can also provide passive thermal care measures, such as providing blankets, socks, and head coverings and keeping the room temperature at or above 75°F (24°C).
- **Active prewarming** before induction of general anesthesia has been found to be effective in preventing perioperative hypothermia. Prewarming, with forced-air warming gowns or mattresses, should last for 10 to 30 minutes.

Nutritional Status Anxiety and anesthesia reduce gastrointestinal motility. To decrease the risk of nausea and vomiting, patients usually fast, taking no food or liquids (NPO) for 8 hours before surgery. Stress to patients and family the importance of fasting (for the prescribed length of time) to avoid the danger of aspiration.

Key Point: *You should know, though, that years of evidence support shorter fasting times than you will see used in most institutions.* The American Society of Anesthesiologists preoperative fasting guidelines for healthy patients recommends ingesting clear liquids up to 2 hours before surgery—and even a light meal up to 6 hours before surgery (King, 2019; Lambert & Carey, 2015; "Practice Guidelines for Preoperative Fasting," 2011; Regan et al., 2017).

Skin Preparation Preoperative whole-body bathing or showering is considered good clinical practice to make the skin as clean as possible before surgery in order to reduce the number of bacteria on the skin, especially at the site of incision. Patients should bathe or shower with either soap or an antiseptic (e.g., 4% chlorhexidine gluconate, Betadine) the evening before surgery and the morning of the surgery (Link, 2022; World Health Organization [WHO], 2018). Final skin preparation and hair removal, if done, should be completed before taking the patient into the surgical suite.

Bowel Preparation Enemas are now used primarily for surgical procedures of the colon, not for all surgeries. To empty the colon of feces, patients are asked to consume a low-residue diet for several days before surgery and are given a regimen of medications and/or enemas to clear the bowel. Stress the importance of adhering to the regimen to limit the risk of contaminating the operative site with feces.

Urinary Preparation Indwelling catheters are not routinely inserted for surgery. Catheterization may be prescribed in the following situations:

- If it is important to keep the bladder empty during surgery
- If fluid status is being carefully monitored
- If surgery is expected to last for a prolonged period of time

✚ If a catheter is not prescribed, have the patient void before receiving preoperative medications. The patient could fall if they get out of bed to use the bathroom after being sedated or given opioids for pain.

Preoperative Medications The anesthesiologist may prescribe preoperative medications to relax the patient, reduce respiratory secretions, or reduce the risk of vomiting and aspiration (Table 36-3). The medication is prescribed at a prearranged time (e.g., at 0615), or it may be prescribed to give "on call." You will give the on-call medication when the surgical suite staff notifies you it is time to do so.

Antibiotics are often administered prophylactically to help prevent postoperative infections in patients before:

- Clean surgery involving the placement of a prosthesis or implant
- Clean-contaminated surgery
- Contaminated surgery

You will usually administer the antibiotic intravenously, timed so that a bactericidal concentration of the drug will be present in the serum and tissues by the time the incision is made (usually within the hour preceding incision, just as the patient is going to the surgical suite) (Allegranzi et al., 2016; Berríos-Torres et al., 2017). Antibiotics may, instead, be given at the start of anesthesia and repeated if the surgery is longer than the duration of the antibiotic.

Routine Medications Many routine medications are held (not administered) on the day of surgery.

Example: A patient with insulin-dependent diabetes may be instructed to hold the morning injection or

Table 36-3 ➤ Preoperative Medications

TYPE OF MEDICATION	USE	EXAMPLES
Antibiotics	Reduce the microbial burden of intraoperative contamination to a level that cannot overwhelm host defenses	Cephalosporins (e.g., cefazolin, cefoxitin), clindamycin, vancomycin
Anticholinergics (e.g., phenothiazines)	Reduce oral and pulmonary secretions, prevent laryngospasms, prevent bradycardia	Atropine, chlorpromazine, scopolamine, glycopyrrolate
Anxiolytics (e.g., benzodiazepines)	Control anxiety, calming	Alprazolam, clonazepam, diazepam, lorazepam, midazolam
Antihistamines	Provide sedation and antiemetic effects	Hydroxyzine, diphenhydramine
Barbiturates	Provide sedation without significant cardiopulmonary depression	Secobarbital, pentobarbital
H_2 receptor antagonists	Reduce gastric acidity	Cimetidine, ranitidine
Hypnotics	Provide sedation and increase the duration of sleep	Temazepam
Neuroleptics	Provide sedative, antiemetic, and anticonvulsant effects	Droperidol, fentanyl
Opioid analgesics	Provide pain relief and sedation; induce anesthesia	Fentanyl, meperidine, morphine

administer half of the normal dose. The patient needs less insulin because NPO status will keep blood sugar lower than usual. The anesthesiologist will monitor the blood sugar in the operating room and give additional insulin if needed. Some patients may be instructed to stop routine medications several days before surgery.

Example: A client receiving warfarin for anticoagulation may need to stop the medication 7 days before surgery.

Prostheses Before being transported to the operating suite, the patient must remove all artificial body parts, such as dentures, artificial limbs, or contact lenses. Wigs, eyeglasses, makeup, and jewelry must also be removed.

Antiembolism Stockings Antiembolism stockings are also referred to as *thromboembolic disorder hose* (or "TED hose"). They are elastic stockings that compress the veins of the legs and increase venous return to the heart (Fig. 36-1). The stockings may be applied preoperatively to prevent venous pooling during surgery and decrease the risk of thrombus formation. Along with prophylactic medications (antithrombotics), antiembolism stockings aid in the prevention of DVT and PE. However, hospitals are increasingly using sequential compression devices and anticoagulation therapy instead of elastic stockings to prevent DVT (Llau et al., 2018; Shahi et al., 2017).

- **Risk Factors:** Older adults and those with risk factors for venous thromboembolism are most in need of antiembolism stockings. Risk factors include the following conditions (AORN, 2020):
  - *Venous stasis* (such as occurs with bedrest, lengthy surgery, varicose veins, and heart failure)
  - *Vascular wall injury*, which initiates clotting (e.g., surgery, IV catheter, irritating IV drugs, prior DVT, smoking).
  - *Hypercoagulability* (e.g., estrogen therapy, oral contraceptive use, cancer, dehydration, pregnancy)
    - Older adults may be at higher risk for DVT because they have more than one of these risk factors. Safety measures to prevent DVT in older adults include range-of-motion exercises and applying antiembolism stockings to prevent pooling of blood in the extremities (Wolfe et al., 2020).

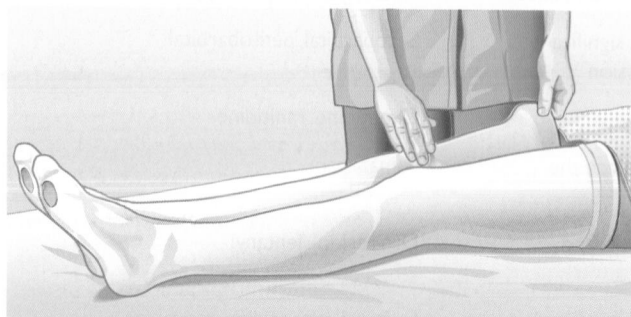

FIGURE 36-1 Antiembolism stockings compress the veins of the legs and increase venous return to the heart.

- **Types.** Antiembolism stockings may extend from foot to knee or foot to thigh, although the Institute for Clinical Systems Improvement (ICSI) suggests that thigh-high stockings be avoided because of their tendency to roll and restrict circulation (Laxa et al., 2016). Some stockings have an opening at the toes that allows you to assess circulation in the feet.
- **Sizing and application.** Stockings must be sized and applied correctly to be effective. Stockings are contraindicated for some patients (e.g., those with peripheral arterial disease) (Wade et al., 2017). The procedure for applying antiembolism stockings is summarized in the Highlights of Procedures box. For complete steps,

 Go to **Chapter 36, Procedure 36-2: Applying Antiembolism Stockings,** in Volume 2.

Take Measures to Prevent Wrong Patient, Wrong Site, Wrong Surgery

The following safety measures will help prevent patient misidentification and wrong-site surgery (The Joint Commission, 2022):

- Use a preoperative checklist to confirm that appropriate documents are available and the appropriate activities have been performed.
- Verify the patient's identity before the patient leaves the preoperative area.
- Mark the surgical site before surgery. Use a permanent marker that will not be removed by the surgical skin prep and involve the patient in the marking process.
- Take a time-out with all team members before starting the procedure (see "Perioperative Safety" near the beginning of this chapter).

Communicate With the Surgical Team

The most common root cause of medical errors is communication failure (Koleva, 2020). For this reason, good communication is essential for patient safety in perioperative care. For successful communication, surgical team members must:

- Receive a summary of the plan of care (e.g., a short briefing by the surgeon) and develop a shared understanding of the plan.
- Speak up and be assertive with concerns about the procedure or decisions.
- Ask questions to clarify confusion.
- Acknowledge that they have heard and understood.
- Ask for and provide feedback (e.g., read back) on critical information.
- **Use standard terminology** (e.g., checklists). In one study, implementation of the WHO's Surgical Safety Checklist was associated with a reduction in morbidity, length of in-hospital stay, and mortality (Scott et al., 2018).

■ **Two-minute briefings** just before surgery, led by the attending surgeon using a standardized format, have been found to improve communication and reduce delays and wrong-site surgery (Lee, 2016). Surgical briefings encourage team members to talk when there is no problem so that they are more likely to speak up when they have misgivings or when problems occur (Collings et al., 2022).

KnowledgeCheck 36-4

- ■ Identify topics that should be discussed in preoperative teaching.
- ■ Describe the typical physical preparation of a client undergoing surgery.

 ThinkLike a Nurse 36-4: **Clinical Judgment in Action**

- ■ What aspects of preoperative teaching should you stress when caring for Mr. Singh (Meet Your Patient)?
- ■ A bowel preparation is typically part of preoperative preparation for a client having colon surgery. Do you think this will be part of Mr. Singh's physical preparation? Why or why not?

Transfer Patient to the Operative Suite

Once you have completed your preoperative care, the patient is ready for transport by stretcher to the operative area, usually to the surgical holding area (Fig. 36-2). Attend to the following:

- ■ *Preoperative checklist and the patient's record*—Must accompany the patient.
- ■ *Valuables*—Lock these up according to agency policy, or have the patient's family keep them.
- ■ *Glasses, hearing aid*—Occasionally, especially if the patient has a significant sensory deficit, the patient can wear their hearing aid or glasses to the surgical suite. You will need to arrange this in advance with the surgical staff or anesthesia team.

Children are often permitted to bring a favorite toy with them to the operating room (OR) to provide comfort. They may fear being separated from their

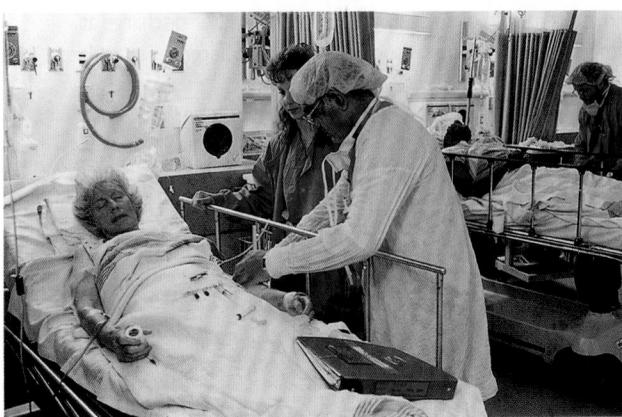

FIGURE 36-2 Surgical holding area.

parents, so arrange for parents to spend time with the child immediately before the surgery and as soon as possible after the surgery. Keep the parents informed, and let them know what to expect.

Prepare the Postoperative Room

If you transfer the patient to the surgical suite from a nursing unit in the hospital, you should prepare the room for the patient's return after surgery. Put clean linens on the bed and arrange the supplies and equipment you will need. Raise the bed to stretcher height and lock the wheels. For complete instructions,

 Go to **Chapter 36, Clinical Insight 36-2: Preparing a Room for a Patient's Return From Surgery**, and **Chapter 11, Clinical Insight 11-1, Preparing the Room for a Newly Admitted Patient**, in Volume 2.

INTRAOPERATIVE CARE

The **intraoperative phase** begins when the patient enters the operating suite and ends when the patient is admitted to the postanesthesia care unit.

TheoreticalKnowledge knowing why

To provide intraoperative care, you will need theoretical knowledge of the roles of the various members of the intraoperative team and the different types of anesthesia that are used.

Operative Personnel

The personnel who attend the client during the surgical procedure are called the *intraoperative team*. The team is divided into members who must use sterile technique and those who use clean technique (see Chapter 20 if you need to review medical and surgical asepsis). During the intraoperative phase, a registered nurse (RN) can function as the scrub nurse, circulating nurse, or registered nurse first assistant (RNFA). Each of these roles contributes to the safe care of surgical clients.

Sterile Team Members of the sterile intraoperative team include the surgeon, surgical assistant, and scrub person. Before beginning the surgery, they perform a surgical scrub of the hands and arms, dry with sterile towels, and don sterile gowns and gloves. To review these procedures, see Chapter 20.

- ■ The **scrub nurse** can be an RN, licensed vocational nurse (LVN)/licensed practical nurse (LPN), or surgical technician. The scrub nurse sets up the sterile field, prepares the surgical instruments, assists with the sterile draping of the patient, anticipates and responds to the surgeon's needs, and maintains the integrity of the sterile field.

- An **RNFA** is an RN with additional education and training in surgical technique. The RNFA serves as an assistant to the surgeon, a role that has historically been filled by physicians. The RNFA may be employed by the surgeon or the hospital.

Sterile team members are the only persons allowed to enter the sterile field. Creation of the operative field is explained in:

 Chapter 36, Clinical Insight 36-3: Creating an Operative Field, in Volume 2.

Clean Team Team members who abide by clean technique (medical asepsis) include the anesthesiologist or nurse anesthetist, the circulating RN, biomedical technicians, and radiology technicians. **Key Point:** *These personnel never enter the sterile field but instead function around and beyond it.*

- Either an **anesthesiologist** or a **nurse anesthetist (CRNA)** induces amnesia, analgesia, and muscle relaxation or paralysis with anesthesia. The role is to continuously monitor and evaluate the patient's responses to the anesthetic agent and the surgical procedure. CRNAs administer more than half of all anesthetics in the United States.

- The **circulating nurse** is a registered nurse who applies the nursing process to coordinate all activities in the operating room. They are a client advocate who continuously monitors the client and the sterile field. The circulating nurse maintains a safe, comfortable environment, communicates with appropriate personnel outside the operating room, and responds to emergencies. An important aspect of the circulating nurse's role is to attend to the patient during the induction of anesthesia.

KnowledgeCheck 36-5

- Identify the intraoperative nursing roles that are part of the sterile intraoperative team and those that are part of the clean intraoperative team.
- Which nursing roles are always held by a registered nurse?

Toward Evidence-Based Practice

Study A:

Karakul, A., Akgül, E. A., Yalınız, R., & Meşe, T. (2022). Effectiveness of music during cardiac catheterization on children's pain, fear, anxiety and vital signs: A randomized, blind controlled trial. *Journal of Pediatric Nursing, 65,* 56–62. https://doi.org/10.1016/j.pedn.2022.02.009

The researchers examined the effectiveness of music during pediatric cardiac catheterization procedures on children's pain, fear, anxiety, and vital signs. Children undergoing a cardiac catheterization procedure were randomly assigned to one of three groups: control, classical music, or self-selected group. Pain, fear, and anxiety levels were measured before and after the procedure. Vital signs were measured before, during, and after the cardiac catheterization procedure. Findings indicated that children in the musical intervention groups experienced less pain, fear, and anxiety and a lower heart rate and blood pressure than the children in the control group. No statistical difference was found in the pain, fear, and anxiety levels of the children in the classical music and self-selected music groups.

Study B:

Laframboise-Otto, J. M., Horodyski, M., Parvataneni, H. K., & Horgas, A. L. (2021). A randomized controlled trial of music for pain relief after arthroplasty surgery. *Pain Management Nursing, 22*(1), 86–93.

The researchers investigated whether surgical patients who listened to music along with prescribed analgesics experienced reduced acute pain and the need for additional pain medication. Participants were randomly assigned to treatment or control groups. The treatment group listened to self-selected music for 30 minutes three times per day postoperatively in the hospital and for 2 days after discharge. Patients in both the treatment group and the control group were given analgesic medication as prescribed. Participants who listened to music after surgery self-reported significantly lower pain intensity and distress in the hospital and after discharge at home. There were no statistically significant differences in analgesic medication use after surgery between groups.

1. Use the following table to identify the similarities and differences between the two studies.

Answer:

	POPULATION	INTERVENTION	MEASUREMENT	OUTCOME
Study A				
Study B				

2. How can the results of the studies be used in the care of postsurgical patients?

Types of Anesthesia

During surgery, anesthesia is used to obtain analgesia (control of pain), muscle relaxation or paralysis, and amnesia (memory loss). Anesthesia is classified as general, conscious sedation, regional, or local.

General Anesthesia

General anesthesia produces rapid unconsciousness and loss of sensation. The anesthesiologist or certified registered nurse anesthetist (CNRA) administers inhaled and intravenous medications that depress the patient's central nervous system and relax the musculature. Muscle relaxants, paralyzing agents, narcotics, barbiturates, and inhaled gases are some of the agents used during general anesthesia.

Advantages of General Anesthesia

- The patient is unconscious and, as a result, experiences no anxiety that might affect cardiac and respiratory functioning.
- The muscles are relaxed, so the patient remains completely motionless during the surgical procedure.
  - Anesthesia can be adjusted to accommodate the length of the procedure and the patient's age and physical condition. For example, an older adult may require less anesthetic than anticipated; if so, the anesthetist can decrease the dosage without interrupting the procedure.
- If complications occur, the anesthesia can be continued for longer than originally planned.

Disadvantages of General Anesthesia

- The respiratory and circulatory muscles are depressed, so mechanical ventilation is needed while the patient is under the effects of the anesthetic agent(s). These effects predispose the patient to pneumonia and thrombophlebitis in the postoperative period.
- General anesthesia creates a risk for death, heart attack, stroke, and malignant hyperthermia. **Malignant hyperthermia** is a rare, often fatal, metabolic condition that can occur during the use of muscle relaxants and inhalation anesthesia. Metabolism increases in the skeletal muscles, and they become rigid. The temperature rises rapidly. Predisposition to this condition is inherited.
- Frequent minor complaints after general anesthesia include sore throat (from intubation), nausea and vomiting (from relaxation of gastrointestinal smooth muscle), headache, uncontrollable shivering, and confusion.

Conscious Sedation

Conscious sedation is an alternative form of anesthesia that provides intravenous sedation and analgesia without producing unconsciousness. During conscious sedation, the patient may feel sleepy but is aware of their surroundings, can be easily aroused by touch or speech, and can talk with the surgical team. Nevertheless, blood pressure, heart rate, respiratory rate, and oxygen saturation are monitored, and the patient usually receives oxygen via nasal cannula during the procedure. Because of the amnesic effect of many of the medications, the patient may not recall aspects of the procedure afterward. Conscious sedation is used for procedures such as bronchoscopy and cosmetic surgery.

> *Advantages:* Pain and anxiety are adequately controlled without the risks of general anesthesia. Recovery is rapid.
> *Disadvantages:* Not practical for highly anxious patients.

Regional Anesthesia

Regional anesthesia prevents pain by interrupting nerve impulses to and from the area of the procedure. The patient remains alert but is numb in the involved area. Regional anesthesia may be administered by infiltration of the surgical site and surrounding tissue with local anesthetics, such as lidocaine or bupivacaine. These medications may also be injected into and around specific nerves to depress the sensory, motor, and/or sympathetic impulses of a limited area of the body.

> *Advantages:* Low in cost, simple to administer, and requires a minimal recovery period. It is especially suitable for minor ambulatory procedures.
> *Disadvantages:* May not be practical if the patient is highly anxious or if adequate pain control cannot be achieved. Many patients are apprehensive about being able to see and hear the procedure.

Techniques for achieving regional anesthesia include the following.

Peripheral Nerve Block A **nerve block** is the injection of an anesthetic into and around a nerve or group of nerves (e.g., the facial nerve).

A **Bier (intravenous) block** is a nerve block technique in which the anesthetist places a tourniquet on an arm or leg and then injects a local anesthetic agent intravenously below the level of the tourniquet. The tourniquet is maintained at a pressure that limits venous return but continues to allow arterial circulation. The patient feels no pain in the extremity as long as the tourniquet is in place.

Advantages of the Bier block
- Onset and recovery time are both rapid.
- The tourniquet decreases bleeding during the surgical procedure and prevents systemic absorption of the local anesthetic.

Disadvantages of the Bier block
- When the procedure is finished, the tourniquet is deflated, and there is potential for systemic absorption of the anesthetic.
- To prevent tissue damage, the tourniquet must not be left in place for more than 2 hours.

Spinal Anesthesia Spinal anesthesia is the injection of an anesthetic into the cerebrospinal fluid (CSF) in the subarachnoid space (Fig. 36-3A). This injection blocks sensation and movement below the level of the injection. Spinal anesthesia is often used for surgical procedures in the lower abdomen, pelvis, and lower extremities.

Advantages:
- Allows the patient to remain conscious during the procedure
- Usually does not depress respirations

Disadvantages and Side Effects:
- Occasionally, a higher level of spinal anesthesia is achieved than intended—that is, the medication may migrate upward in the spinal fluid. This can depress respirations and cardiac rate. Placing the patient in Fowler's position may prevent respiratory paralysis.
- Side effects of spinal anesthesia include hypotension, nausea, vomiting, urinary retention, or a headache from leakage of CSF. A headache after spinal anesthesia must be closely monitored and may require additional treatment by the anesthesia staff.
- The blood pressure may also decrease suddenly due to pervasive vasodilatation—the anesthesia blocks the sympathetic vasomotor nerves, which normally maintain muscle tone in peripheral blood vessels.
- Patients with these complications often require ventilation and support of blood pressure during surgery, so they must be carefully monitored during surgery and in the recovery period.

Epidural Anesthesia Epidural anesthesia requires the insertion of a thin catheter into the epidural space (Fig. 36-3B). Anesthetic agents are infused through the catheter to produce loss of sensation. Epidural anesthesia can be used as a surgical anesthetic and to provide postoperative analgesia.

Advantages and Disadvantages: similar to those of spinal anesthesia.
- Epidural anesthesia is safer than spinal anesthesia because the anesthetic does not enter the subarachnoid space, and the depth of anesthesia is not as great.
- Drugs used for epidural administration are of a higher concentration than those for spinal administration, so if the medication is inadvertently injected too deeply (into the subarachnoid space), hypotension and respiratory paralysis occur, and temporary mechanical ventilation is necessary.
- Epidural anesthesia is ideal for obstetrics procedures (e.g., cesarean birth or pain control with vaginal birth) because the patient is awake to bond with the newborn, and mobility is limited for only a short time.

Local Anesthesia

Local anesthesia produces loss of pain sensation at the desired site (e.g., a wound to be sutured, a skin growth to be removed). It is typically used for minor procedures. However, after finishing a major surgery, the surgeon may infiltrate the operative area with local anesthetics to provide postoperative pain relief.

Local anesthetics may be applied topically or injected. A **topical anesthetic** is applied directly to the skin and mucous membranes. Lidocaine and benzocaine are commonly used because they are rapidly absorbed and rapid-acting.

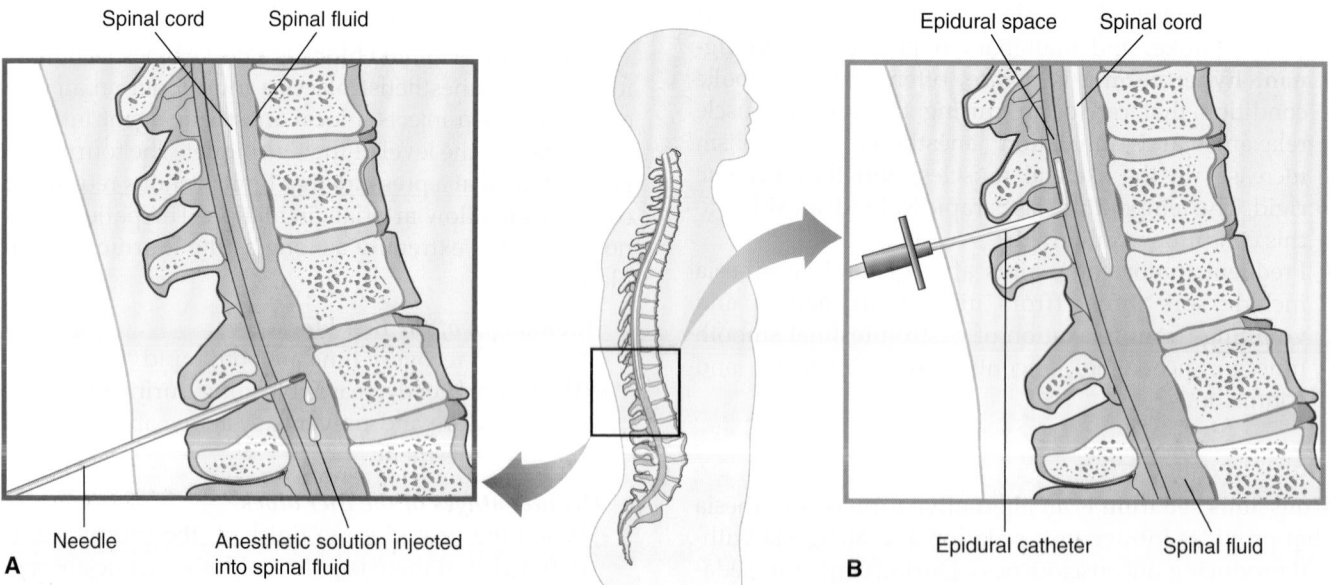

FIGURE 36-3 *A,* Spinal anesthesia is the injection of a local anesthetic into the subarachnoid space to block sensation and movement. *B,* Epidural anesthesia can also be used to provide continuous postoperative analgesia.

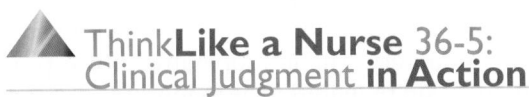

KnowledgeCheck 36-6

- What is the purpose of anesthesia?
- Under what type(s) of anesthesia does the client remain conscious?

Think**Like a Nurse** 36-5:
Clinical Judgment **in Action**

What form of anesthesia is Mr. Singh (Meet Your Patient) most likely to receive? Why?

PracticalKnowledge
knowing **how**

When a patient arrives in the surgical suite, the nurse verifies the information on the preoperative checklist and assesses the patient. The nursing focus is on safe and successful completion of the surgery.

ASSESSMENT/RECOGNIZING CUES

The circulating nurse greets the client in the preoperative holding area and performs a brief assessment by doing the following:

- Verify that the surgical consent has been signed and witnessed and that the preoperative checklist is complete.
- Assess the client's anxiety level and physical condition.
- Measure the vital signs; examine the surgical site; and inspect IV lines, drainage tubes, and catheters. Often the circulating nurse or the anesthetist starts an IV line in the holding area if one is not already present.
- Give preoperative medication in holding area, if prescribed.
- Monitor vital signs often, or even continuously, during the intraoperative period.

For common interview questions to use in the intraoperative period,

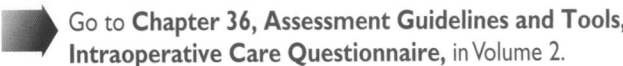
Go to **Chapter 36, Assessment Guidelines and Tools, Intraoperative Care Questionnaire,** in Volume 2.

In addition to the checklist completed in the preoperative period, the surgery team will also complete a surgical safety checklist. The WHO Surgical Safety Checklist covers the three phases of a surgical procedure, commonly referred to as "sign in," "time-out," and "sign out." The three phases of the checklist are reviewed by the checklist coordinator, who verbally checks that each element was done. The goal of using a surgical checklist is to enhance communication, teamwork, and safety by addressing key activities that occur as part of the perioperative process (WHO, 2009).

To see the complete WHO checklist,

Go to **Chapter 36, Assessment Guidelines and Tools, Example of a Surgical Safety Checklist,** in Volume 2.

NURSING DIAGNOSIS/ANALYZING CUES

As in the preoperative phase, most intraoperative nursing care consists of standard activities to be used for all patients.

Potential Complications (Collaborative Problems) Most intraoperative patients, regardless of the surgery, have the following potential complications (collaborative problems) of surgery and anesthesia:

- Potential complications of surgery:
  Hypothermia
  Fluid and electrolyte imbalance
  Excessive bleeding or hemorrhage
  Musculoskeletal injury secondary to positioning
- Potential complications of anesthesia:
  Aspiration
  Vasomotor instability (and resultant hypotension and diminished peripheral perfusion)
  Respiratory depression
  Cardiovascular compromise

Nursing Diagnoses/Analyzing Cues Except in unusual circumstances (e.g., a patient in poor nutritional status, a frail elderly patient), you may not need to identify nursing diagnoses for a patient because the standardized care addresses all the potential complications. However, for nurses who prefer to organize care according to nursing diagnoses, the following potential diagnoses apply to most patients having major surgery:

- *Perioperative Hypothermia* related to exposure in cool environment and administration of cool IV fluids. This applies especially to very young, very old, and very thin patients.
- *Risk for Aspiration* related to depressed respirations and reflexes. For patients who have weak muscles for coughing or a poor gag reflex, this diagnosis is especially relevant.
- *Risk for Fluid Volume Alteration* related to NPO status and blood loss from surgery. Some patients are at higher-than-normal risk, for example, patients with renal or cardiac problems.
- *Risk for Perioperative Positioning Injury* related to patient factors such as edema, emaciation, obesity, and sensory–perceptual disturbances secondary to anesthesia.

Use the following nursing diagnoses only if the patient has the necessary defining characteristics or risk factors. Do not use them for all patients.

- *Risk for Latex Allergy Response* related to multiple exposures (e.g., multiple surgeries, catheterizations) or history of related allergies
- *Latex Allergy Response* (needs no etiology)

PLANNING/PRIORITIZING HYPOTHESES AND GENERATING SOLUTIONS

The overarching goals in the intraoperative phase are that the patient will:

Be free from injury
Remain physiologically stable
Experience optimal surgical outcomes

Notice that the goals are appropriate for nearly all surgical patients.

Individualized goals/outcome statements are formulated from the patient's nursing diagnoses. The following are examples:

- Maintains body temperature within the normal range.
- Has clear lung sounds and patent airway.
- Has urine output of at least 30 mL/hr.
- Will have no skin, tissue, or neuromuscular injury as a result of positioning.
- Will not acquire healthcare-related infection.

IMPLEMENTATION/TAKING ACTION

Intraoperative care focuses on maintaining a safe environment and assisting the surgery team in providing appropriate care for the client. The CNRA manages the interventions for most of the patient's potential problems, for example, fluid volume status, airway protection, and vital signs monitoring.

NIC standardized interventions for the intraoperative period come from the domain of Perioperative Care. They include interventions for all intraoperative patients, regardless of their individual nursing diagnoses. One intervention, Anesthesia Administration, must be performed by an anesthesiologist or CRNA. The nurse assists in implementing a number of interventions:

- Anesthesia Administration
- Autotransfusion
- Infection Control: Intraoperative
- Positioning: Intraoperative
- Surgical Assistance
- Surgical Precautions
- Surgical Preparation
- Temperature Regulation: Intraoperative

Notice, however, that most of the interventions apply to all surgical patients. As in all patient care, you should always be mindful of using hand hygiene. Sterile asepsis is an important focus in the intraoperative period; you can review that in Chapter 20.

The following sections explain in more detail how to carry out "routine" interventions, such as providing skin preparation, positioning, and intraoperative safety measures. **Key Point:** *Note that "routine" in this context means that the activities are planned and performed for all patients. Nursing interventions are never routine in the general sense; they must always be performed with thought and skill.*

Skin Preparation

Surgical skin preparation reduces the risk of postoperative wound infection by reducing the microbial count at the operative site. Skin preparation may begin in the preoperative phase, when the client cleanses the skin with an antimicrobial solution the evening before and the morning of surgery. The intraoperative nurse provides additional skin preparation as follows:

- **Assess skin for signs of infection, rash, or other forms of skin irritation.** Document the condition of the skin on the intraoperative record.
- **Remove hair from the site only if necessary.** Historically, the surgical site was always shaved. Now, however, you will remove hair only if there is a large amount of it in the area of the surgery or if the surgeon specifies a preference for hair removal. Hair removal increases the risk of abrasions or nicks in the skin, which can provide a portal of entry for bacteria. If you do remove hair, you will likely do it in the preoperative holding area immediately before surgery to reduce the time for bacterial growth. Use clippers or depilatory cream to trim hair because they are less likely than a razor to cause skin irritation.
- **Cleanse the surgical site.** In the operative suite, skin preparation precedes draping of the client. Using sterile technique, cleanse the surgical site and a generous part of the surrounding area with the recommended anti-infective solution. Povidone-iodine (Betadine) is commonly used for the scrub; then the skin is painted with Betadine solution. ✚ If the client is allergic to iodine, use an alternative preparation solution.

Positioning

The position of the patient in the OR is determined by the surgical site, access to the patient's airway, the need to monitor vital signs, comfort, and safety. A position that is ideal for accessing the surgical site may not be used if any of the other factors are compromised. If the patient has preexisting injuries or discomfort, factor this information into the decision about how to position. For example, a patient with chronic cervical spine pain may be positioned using a neck roll.

The patient is usually positioned after anesthesia has begun. Use straps, wedges, pillows, and surgical table attachments to maintain the position during the surgery. To prevent shearing, lift—do not slide—the patient into position. In many cases, the surgical team assists with positioning.

The circulating nurse is responsible for preventing positioning injuries. Surgical patients often spend 3 to 4 hours, or even longer, in the same position. This places them at risk for pressure ulcer formation. Some anesthetic agents decrease tissue perfusion, further increasing the patient's risk for sustaining positioning injuries. Padding the bony prominences is one measure to protect the client during surgery.

Intraoperative Safety Measures

Just before starting any surgical or invasive procedure, you should conduct a final verification process to confirm the correct patient, procedure, and site (The Joint Commission, 2022). The circulating nurse is responsible for a variety of other measures that protect the patient in the intraoperative phase. These measures are briefly explained here.

- **Assist the scrub nurse in preparing and maintaining the sterile field.** The circulating nurse gathers surgical supplies and equipment for use during surgery. The circulating nurse then works with the scrub nurse to transfer the supplies to the sterile field.
- **Provide supplies and materials during surgery.** If additional supplies are needed during surgery, the circulating nurse obtains them and opens them on the sterile field. Supplies may include dressings, surgical equipment, medications, irrigating solutions, or sutures.
- **Monitor intake and output of the client.** Together with the anesthetist, the circulating nurse monitors the fluid infused, urine output, drainage, and blood loss.
- **Handle specimens.**
  - *The circulating nurse* handles specimens and sends them to the lab or pathology for evaluation after the surgery is complete.
  - *The surgeon* may sometimes obtain a tissue sample that must be analyzed during the operative procedure.
  - *The circulator* receives the specimen, coordinates with the pathologist to review the sample, and reports the pathology findings to the surgeon.
  - **Perform sponge, sharps, and instrument counts.**

    The circulating nurse and the scrub nurse count the material that is added to the sterile field. As the surgery comes to an end, a repeat count is performed to ensure that no instruments, sponges, or sharps are left inside the client. A retained sponge can lead to infection and additional surgeries. A major surgery, such as a heart surgery, can use several hundred sponges. Once soaked in blood, sponges can blend in with the body cavity and be difficult to see.
  - **Some agencies are now using sponges with barcodes, which the nurse scans before and after use.** The system alerts the surgical team if they are left behind. In another system, the surgical team relies on chip-embedded sponges with radiofrequency identification technology to count sponges and locate any that are left behind.
  - **Document the care provided and the client's response to care on the surgical record.** This is usually a graphic or a checklist form, perhaps with some space for narrative notes about anything the form does not address.

KnowledgeCheck 36-7

- For what activities is the circulating nurse responsible in the surgical suite before the skin incision?
- Describe six intraoperative safety measures performed by the circulating nurse.

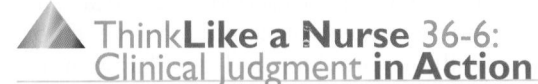

ThinkLike a Nurse 36-6: Clinical Judgment in Action

What special concerns, if any, do you have about Mr. Singh (Meet Your Patient) during the intraoperative phase of care?

POSTOPERATIVE CARE

The postoperative phase begins when the client enters the postanesthesia care unit and ends when the patient has healed from the surgical procedure. This phase consists of two parts: recovery from anesthesia and recovery from surgery.

TheoreticalKnowledge
knowing why

When the surgical procedure is complete, members of the surgical team prepare the client for transfer to the postanesthesia care unit (PACU), also called the *recovery room* (Fig. 36-4).

Recovery From Anesthesia

- **The first postoperative phase** is often known as the *postanesthesia phase* or the *immediate postoperative phase*. This phase begins when the client is transferred from the operating table to a bed (or gurney) for transport to the PACU. During this phase, the client is at high risk for respiratory and cardiovascular compromise. As a precaution, the anesthetist and the circulating nurse accompany the client and attend to the client's needs during transport. They are also responsible for giving a comprehensive report to the PACU nurse.
- **The PACU,** located near the OR, is typically an open unit that allows nurses to observe clients easily. PACU nurses have specialized education and experience in caring for postoperative clients. Commonly, nurses

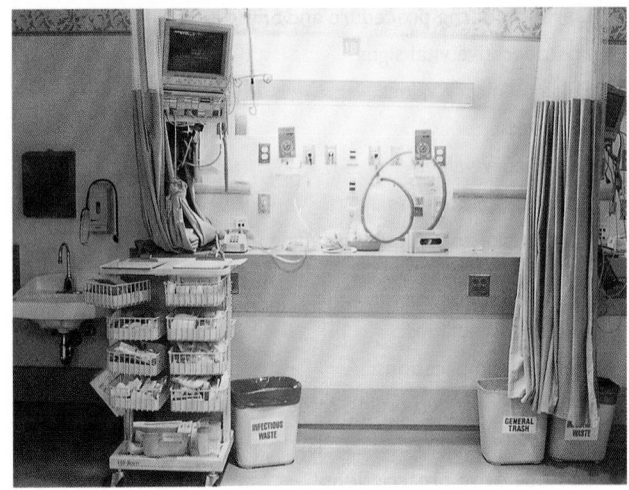

FIGURE 36-4 Postanesthesia care unit.

working in the PACU have experience in critical care. The PACU nurse receives a comprehensive report from the anesthesia provider and circulating nurse (Box 36-4).

Recovery From Surgery

The second phase of postoperative care begins when the patient is discharged from the PACU and admitted to the surgical nursing unit. The patient is transported to the surgical unit only after they have recovered from anesthesia and their condition is stable. The goal of this phase is to facilitate healing and prevent postoperative complications.

PracticalKnowledge
knowing**how**

The next sections discuss nursing care associated with both phases of postoperative care.

Nursing Care in the Postanesthesia Care Unit

- **Initial assessment.** The PACU nurse performs a quick, focused initial assessment of the surgical patient in the presence of the anesthesia provider and circulating nurse.
- **Continuing assessment.** After that, the PACU nurse assesses the patient every 5 to 15 minutes.
  - AORN (2020) has identified the essential elements of assessment in the PACU. For that information,

 Go to **Chapter 36, Assessment Guidelines and Tools, Focused Assessment, Postanesthesia Assessment: Essential Elements,** in Volume 2.

- **Positioning.** An unconscious client is usually positioned on their side to help maintain an open airway. This decreases the likelihood of aspirating mucus or saliva by allowing it to drain out instead of back into the throat. Elevating the superior arm on a pillow allows for good chest expansion so that the patient can breathe deeply and expand the lungs fully.

- *NIC: Postanesthesia Care.* The only postoperative intervention from the NIC's Perioperative Care category is Postanesthesia Care. This NIC intervention encompasses the preceding assessments and adds measures such as providing for safety and administering oxygen.

- **Determining recovery from anesthesia.** Patients may arrive in the PACU with an artificial airway or endotracheal tube in place. The patient remains in the PACU until the PACU nurse determines that they have recovered from the effects of anesthesia (Box 36-5) and are able to maintain their own airway. The PACU nurse then removes the airway and transfers the patient to the surgical unit.

BOX 36-4 ■ Information Contained in the Report From the Surgical Suite

- Procedure performed
- Type of anesthesia
- Medications administered in the surgical suite
- Duration of the procedure and anesthesia
- Postoperative vital signs
- Pulse oximetry values
- Allergies
- Laboratory values
- Estimated blood loss
- Fluid intake and output, including urine, stool, gastric losses
- Preoperative mobility status, skin integrity, and sensory perception abilities
- Surgical complications
- Presence of tubes, drains, catheters
- Existing IV lines
- Postoperative prescriptions

BOX 36-5 ■ Evidence of Recovery From Anesthesia

Airway—The patient is able to maintain a patent airway independently, deep-breathe, cough, and expectorate secretions.

Level of consciousness—The patient is conscious and easily reoriented. Often patients will drift off to sleep between arousals; however, they easily reorient and are generally aware of circumstances and surroundings.

Vital signs—Vital signs are stable and within an acceptable range. The blood pressure (BP) may be markedly different from that taken during the immediate preoperative measures because BP is often elevated preoperatively. This can also be caused by anxiety, pain, and not administering routine BP medications because of NPO status. The patient may require medication to control pain or BP before discharge from the postanesthesia care unit (PACU).

Mobility and sensation—The patient is able to move all extremities that could move preoperatively. The patient regains movement and sensation once spinal or epidural anesthesia has worn off.

Fluid balance (intake and output [I&O])—The patient is urinating at least 30 mL/hr and is in relative fluid balance. Consider blood loss, urine output, gastric drainage, and emesis when calculating fluid balance.

Dressings and drains—Dressings are dry and intact, or wound drainage is considered appropriate for the procedure. The patient should have no overt signs of excessive blood or fluid loss before being transferred to the surgical unit.

Postoperative Nursing Care on the Surgical Unit

The assigned nurse admits the patient to the surgical unit. If the patient is transported by gurney, assist the patient to the bed. As soon as the patient has arrived, perform an assessment, and listen to a summary report from the PACU nurse (see Box 36-4).

ASSESSMENT/RECOGNIZING CUES NP

The initial postoperative assessment is identical to the assessment performed by the PACU nurse. However, the patient has undergone a period of stabilization since surgery, so assessments can be less frequent than in the PACU, where the patient was assessed every 5 to 15 minutes. You may increase the frequency if the patient's condition changes. Of course, agency protocols vary, but a common pattern is to assess the patient:

On arrival to the nursing unit
Every 15 minutes for the first hour
Every 30 minutes for the next 2 hours
Every hour for the next 4 hours
Then every 4 hours

KnowledgeCheck 36-8
- What are the two phases of the postoperative phase of care?
- How often is a patient typically assessed after surgery?
- What assessments are made in the postoperative phase?

NURSING DIAGNOSIS/ANALYZING CUES

If healing proceeds normally and no complications develop, most postoperative patients have a common set of collaborative problems (Table 36-4), regardless of the type of surgery they underwent. You will not need to write potential ("risk for") nursing diagnoses, except in special situations (e.g., patients with comorbid conditions, such as diabetes or asthma).

Potential Nursing Diagnoses/Analyzing Cues Key Point: *Write potential nursing diagnoses/analyze cues (instead of collaborative problems) only if a patient has a higher risk for the problem than the average surgical patient.* For example, you might use:

- *Peripheral Tissue Perfusion Alteration Risk* for patients who have a history of peripheral arterial disease or cardiac insufficiency.
- *Fluid Volume Deficit Risk* for patients who have lost a large amount of blood in surgery or who are dehydrated on admission.
- *Breathing Pattern Impairment Risk* for patients with weak accessory muscles for breathing, with a decreased level of consciousness, or with a respiratory condition such as emphysema.
- *Infection Risk* for patients who have compromised immune status or who may not be capable of managing their own wound care at home.

Actual Nursing Diagnoses/Analyzing Cues Key Point: *Of course, you will use a nursing diagnosis/analyze cues whenever a problem becomes actual instead of merely potential.* Nursing diagnoses/analyzing cues will vary based on the surgical procedure and the client cues. There is no need for a *Knowledge Deficit* diagnosis because patient teaching is a routine intervention for all postoperative patients.

Examples of two common postoperative nursing diagnoses are:

- *Surgical Recovery Delay.* This is appropriate when the patient requires more days to recover than the anticipated length of stay for the surgery.
- *Acute Pain.* Almost every surgical patient experiences pain. There are independent nursing interventions to relieve pain (e.g., teaching the patient to splint the incision). However, they do not usually provide adequate relief in the early postop period. You will nearly always need to administer analgesics, which require a medical prescription.

Other nursing diagnoses/analyzing cues and etiologies that may occur postoperatively include the following:

- *Activity Intolerance* r/t pain, manipulation of tissues in the surgical procedure, stressors of surgery
- *Anxiety* r/t change in health status, unfamiliar (hospital) environment
- *Nausea* r/t manipulation of gastrointestinal tract; decreased peristalsis secondary to anesthesia
- *Constipation* r/t decreased activity, decreased food or fluid intake, decreased peristalsis secondary to anesthesia, pain medication
- *Urinary Retention* r/t anesthesia, preoperative medications (anticholinergics), pain, fear, unfamiliar surroundings, client's position
- *Surgical Recovery Delay* (etiologies will vary with pathology)

PLANNING/PRIORITIZING HYPOTHESES AND GENERATING SOLUTIONS

A comprehensive plan of care for common postoperative nursing diagnoses includes NOC standardized outcomes as well as individualized goals. Because of shortened hospital stays, the postoperative period now extends well past the patient's discharge from the hospital. Often, especially for those who have had major or complex procedures, a home health nurse continues to follow the patient at home to facilitate a smoother transition through the postoperative process.

Examples of *NOC standardized outcomes and individualized goals* for the postoperative period include:

Activity Tolerance	Hydration
Ambulation	Nausea and Vomiting Severity
Anxiety Level	Pain Control; Pain Level
Blood Loss Severity	Post-Procedure Recovery
Bowel Elimination	Urinary Elimination

Circulation Status   Wound Healing: Primary
Energy Conservation   Intention

■ IMPLEMENTATION/TAKING ACTION

Most postoperative interventions focus on prevention and early detection of potential complications (collaborative problems). Many such interventions are done as a part of the preoperative teaching. Others are described in Table 36-4. These are routines that are followed for all postoperative patients, regardless of type of surgery.

Specific nursing activities should be designed to relieve identified nursing diagnoses. In the next sections, we discuss pain management, routine postoperative teaching, and the use of sequential compression devices.

Table 36-4 ➤ Potential Postoperative Complications (Collaborative Problems)

Respiratory System

PC: Aspiration Pneumonia—Airway inflammation caused by inhaling gastric secretions (especially hydrochloric acid from the stomach) because of absent gag reflex secondary to anesthesia

Clinical Signs	Interventions for Prevention and Early Detection
Cough, fever, elevated white blood cell (WBC) count, decreased or absent breath sounds, decreased oxygen saturation (SaO_2), tachypnea, dyspnea, blood-tinged sputum	*Preoperative:* Institute NPO, as prescribed, before surgery. *Postoperative:* Continue NPO until intestinal motility returns; carefully monitor sedated patient and place in side-lying position.

PC: Atelectasis—Collapse of alveoli due to hypoventilation, airways blocked by mucous plugs, opioid analgesics, immobility

Clinical Signs	Interventions for Prevention and Early Detection
Decreased or absent breath sounds, noisy respirations, decreased O_2 saturation (SaO_2), chest asymmetry, sternal retractions, accessory muscle use, trachea deviated from midline, fever, tachypnea, dyspnea, tachycardia, diaphoresis, pleural pain, increased restlessness, anxiety	■ Monitor for clinical signs. ■ Monitor rate, rhythm, depth, and effort of respirations. ■ Monitor ability to cough effectively. ■ Determine need for suctioning by listening for crackles and rhonchi over major airways. ■ Suction, as needed. Auscultate lung sounds after suctioning and other respiratory treatments to determine effectiveness. ■ Encourage deep breathing, coughing, moving in bed, ambulation, use of incentive spirometry. ■ See interventions for NIC category Respiratory Monitoring.

PC: Pneumonia—Inflammation of the alveoli due to infection with bacteria or viruses, toxins, or irritants. Caused by hypoventilation secondary to anesthesia and opioid analgesics and by poor cough effort as a result of aging or weakness.

Clinical Signs	Interventions for Prevention and Early Detection
Productive cough with blood-tinged or purulent sputum, fever, elevated WBC count, decreased or absent breath sounds, decreased SaO_2, chest pain, tachypnea, dyspnea	■ Monitor for clinical signs. ■ Encourage and assist with deep breathing, coughing, moving in bed, ambulation, use of incentive spirometry.

PC: Pulmonary Embolus—A clot that occludes blood flow to a portion of the lungs; usually a result of the formation of a clot in the lower extremities, which breaks loose and migrates to the lungs. May also be due to venous injuries, hypercoagulable state, use of high-dose estrogen, or preexisting circulatory disorders.

Clinical Signs	Interventions for Prevention and Early Detection
Sudden onset of dyspnea, shortness of breath, chest pain, hypotension, tachycardia, decreased SaO_2, cyanosis	■ Prevent thrombophlebitis: Encourage and assist with leg exercises, ambulation, antiembolism stockings, sequential compression devices, hydration. See Procedures 36-2 and 36-3. ■ If thrombophlebitis occurs, position and immobilize the limb; do not massage calves.

Table 36-4 ➤ Potential Postoperative Complications (Collaborative Problems)—cont'd

Cardiovascular System

PC: Thrombophlebitis—Blood clot and inflammation of a vein or artery, usually in the legs. Results from increased coagulability and venous stasis due to immobility during and after surgery.

Clinical Signs	Interventions for Prevention and Early Detection
Superficial: Vein is red, hard, and hot to touch. *Deep:* Limb is pale and edematous; aching, cramping in limb; Homans' sign (pain in calf when foot is dorsiflexed).	Refer to earlier Pulmonary Embolus actions section.

PC: Embolus—Movement of a thrombus or foreign body from its original location.

- Movement in the arterial system results in symptoms in the area affected (e.g., cerebrovascular accident, myocardial infarction, or loss of circulation to an area).
- In the venous system, often results in pulmonary embolus (see earlier Pulmonary Embolus section).

Clinical Signs	Interventions for Prevention and Early Detection
See earlier Pulmonary Embolus section. For arterial emboli, symptoms depend on the location.	■ Monitor for clinical signs. ■ Prevent thrombophlebitis. If thrombophlebitis occurs, position and immobilize the limb. ■ Do not massage calves.

PC: Hemorrhage—Bleeding may be internal or external. May be caused by slipped ligature, uncontrolled bleeding, or infection.

Clinical Signs	Interventions for Prevention and Early Detection
If external: Dressings saturated with bright-red blood; increased output in drains or chest tubes *If internal:* Increased pain, increasing abdominal girth, ecchymosis or swelling around incision, tachycardia, hypotension	Frequently monitor vital signs, dressings, and wound drainage.

PC: Hypovolemia—Decreased blood volume. May be due to blood loss during and after surgery; dehydration; or excess loss through vomiting, diarrhea, or drains.

Clinical Signs	Interventions for Prevention and Early Detection
Hypotension, tachycardia, decreased urine output, fatigue, thirst, dehydration	■ Monitor vital signs and intake and output (I&O). ■ Insert urinary catheter, if appropriate. ■ Monitor skin color, temperature, and moistness; central and peripheral cyanosis. ■ Identify possible causes of changes in vital signs. ■ Administer IV therapy as prescribed. ■ Promote oral intake when tolerated. ■ Prepare to administer blood or blood products, as prescribed.

(Continued)

Table 36-4 ➤ Potential Postoperative Complications (Collaborative Problems)—cont'd

Gastrointestinal System

PC: Nausea and Vomiting—Stomach upset or vomiting related to pain, anxiety, anesthesia, medications, or oral intake before peristalsis returns

Clinical Signs	Interventions for Prevention and Early Detection
Vomiting, retching, stated nausea	■ Have patient remain NPO until return of bowel sounds.
	■ Advance diet slowly.
	■ Treat pain.

PC: Abdominal Distention (Tympanites)—Excess gas within the intestines; may be due to a slow return of peristalsis or from handling of the intestines during surgery.

Clinical Signs	Interventions for Prevention and Early Detection
Abdominal discomfort, bloating, hypoactive or absent bowel sounds	■ Encourage and assist to move in bed and ambulate.
	■ Maintain NPO until return of bowel sounds; avoid drinking with a straw.
	■ Provide fluids at room temperature.

PC: Constipation—A decrease in the frequency of bowel movements, resulting in the passage of hard stool. Usually related to use of opioids, immobility, inadequate fluid intake, or low-fiber diet.

Clinical Signs	Interventions for Prevention and Early Detection
Abdominal discomfort, bloating, hypoactive or absent bowel sounds	■ Encourage and assist to move in bed.
	■ Ambulate.
	■ Increase fluid and fiber intake after bowel sounds return.

PC: Ileus—Loss of the forward flow of intestinal contents due to decreased peristalsis secondary to anesthesia, handling of the intestines during surgery, electrolyte imbalances, infection, or ischemic bowel

Clinical Signs	Interventions for Prevention and Early Detection
Abdominal pain, distention, absent bowel sounds, vomiting	There are few independent preventive measures. Observe for symptoms; notify the surgeon.

Genitourinary System

PC: Renal Failure—Decreased or absent urine output due to hypovolemia, shock, or toxic reaction to medications

Clinical Signs	Interventions for Prevention and Early Detection
Urine output <30 mL/hr; rising blood urea nitrogen (BUN) and creatinine levels	Carefully monitor I&O and laboratory values.

PC: Urinary Retention—Accumulation of urine in the bladder. May result from poor muscle tone as a result of anesthesia and anticholinergic medications, handling of tissues during surgery, or inflammation in the pelvic region.

Clinical Signs	Interventions for Prevention and Early Detection
Bladder distention, suprapubic pain; diminished urine output or output less than fluid intake; inability to void or small, frequent voidings; hypertension; restlessness	■ Monitor for clinical signs.
	■ Provide privacy and adequate time to urinate.
	■ Catheterize if needed.

PC: Urinary Tract Infection—Infection in the urinary tract related to catheterization, stagnant urine in the bladder secondary to immobility or anticholinergic medications, or instrumentation of the urinary tract

Clinical Signs	Interventions for Prevention and Early Detection
Urinary frequency, suprapubic discomfort, burning on urination, cloudy urine	■ Monitor for clinical signs.
	■ Monitor I&O.
	■ Use aseptic technique with catheterization and perineal care.
	■ Provide adequate IV and oral fluids.

Table 36-4 ➤ Potential Postoperative Complications (Collaborative Problems)—cont'd

Surgical Incision

PC: Dehiscence—Separation of one or more layers of the wound due to poor nutritional status, obesity or other strain on suture line, inadequate closure of the muscles, or wound infection

Clinical Signs	Interventions for Prevention and Early Detection
A pop or tearing sensation, especially with sudden straining from coughing, vomiting, or changing positions in bed. Usually an immediate increase in serosanguineous drainage occurs.	▪ Provide adequate nutrition. ▪ Use binders to support the incision. ▪ Have client avoid strain. ▪ Monitor for infection.

PC: Evisceration—Protrusion of organs or tissues through the separated incision. For causes, see earlier Dehiscence section.

Clinical Signs	Interventions for Prevention and Early Detection
Visible protrusion of organs through incision	Same as for Dehiscence.

PC: Wound Infection—Inflammation or drainage from a wound due to growth of microorganisms secondary to inadequate aseptic technique or pathogens already present in surgical area.

Clinical Signs	Interventions for Prevention and Early Detection
Localized swelling, redness, heat, pain, fever >100.4°F (38°C), foul-smelling drainage, or a change in the color of the drainage	▪ Effective skin prep in preoperative period ▪ Surgical scrub according to guidelines in the intraoperative period ▪ Monitor for systemic and localized signs and symptoms of infection. ▪ Inspect incision and drain areas for redness and extreme warmth. ▪ Inspect surgical dressings for drainage and odor. ▪ Monitor vital signs, especially temperature. ▪ Maintain aseptic nontouch technique with surgical dressing changes. ▪ Use and teach good hand hygiene. ▪ Use sterile saline for wound cleansing for up to 48 hours postop (National Institute for Health and Clinical Excellence, 2020). ▪ Limit the number of visitors, as appropriate. ▪ Obtain cultures as needed. ▪ Encourage sufficient nutritional and fluid intake. ▪ Teach client about signs of infection.

Pain Management

The primary goal of postoperative pain management is to minimize the dose of medications (to lessen side effects) while still providing adequate pain management. **Key Point:** *Keep in mind that no one drug is likely to work for every person with pain.*

▪ **Pain control should be individualized,** with consideration of medical, psychological, and physical condition; age; level of fear or anxiety; surgical procedure; personal preference; and response to care. Begin with a validated pain assessment tool and assess the patient's response to pain control measures. Alternative methods of pain relief may be initiated for patients who are at increased risk for analgesia-related complications or side effects (see the Holistic Healing box).

▪ **A multidisciplinary team approach should be used** to formulate a plan for pain relief, particularly in complicated patients, such as those who have medical comorbidities. Potential benefits, possible adverse events, and patient preferences must be weighed in order to decide which pain relief method to use.

▪ **The benefits of adequate pain management** are early mobilization, shorter hospital stay, reduced hospital costs, and increased patient satisfaction.

▪ **Postoperatively, a patient usually receives analgesics via more than one route.** For example, in the immediate postoperative period, the patient may receive IV or epidural medications, progress to oral opioids in a day or two, and then move to nonopioid analgesics (e.g., acetaminophen).

▪ **Key Point:** *Oral opioids should be given preference to IV opioids when possible. intramusclar (IM) injections* *can cause additional pain. Plus, absorption is unreliable postoperatively.*

- **Administer around-the-clock NSAIDs** in addition to other pain control measures if not contraindicated. This helps to keep ahead of the pain.

  - **Providing sufficient pain control for older adults can be a challenge.** Because of concerns about impaired cognition, medical comorbidities, drug interactions, and problems with appropriate dosing, many older adults may be undermedicated and experience unnecessary pain (Gjorgjievski et al., 2019).

- **Monitor for side effects of analgesics,** including respiratory depression, hypotension, and allergic reaction (Hyland et al., 2021).

For a complete discussion of types of pain relief, refer to the section **Opioid Administration Routes** in Chapter 28. Also,

Go to **Chapter 28, Procedure 28-1: Setting Up and Managing Patient-Controlled Analgesia by Pump** and **Clinical Insight 28-1: Caring for the Patient With an Epidural Catheter.**

Single-Use, Continuous-Flow Pump   A single-use, continuous-flow pump administers a continuous, regulated flow of local anesthetic through a thin catheter directly into the patient's surgical site. A dressing holds the tubing in place, and the pump can be carried in a small bag and used after the patient returns home. It reduces the need for opioids, thus reducing complications such as nausea, vomiting, and respiratory depression. It is said to hasten ambulation and the return to normal activities. Depending on the type of pump, it is filled with 65 to 750 mL of medication and can remain in place for up to 5 days, depending on the amount of anesthetic included (Fig. 36-5).

Holistic Healing

Acupuncture for Acute Postoperative Pain

Hsu, H.-C., Fang, H.-Y., Kuo, C.-C., Su, S.-F., Liang, W.-M., & M, W.-F. (2022). The effectiveness of acupressure for managing postoperative pain in patients with thoracoscopic surgery: A randomized control trial. *Journal of Nursing Scholarship, 54(4),* 411–421.

Hsu et al. (2022) collected data from 100 patients who underwent thoracoscopic surgery. Participants were randomly assigned to receive acupressure three times a day for 2 days after thoracic surgery or to receive usual care after thoracic surgery. Patients who received acupressure reported significantly lower pain than that of the control group. Additionally, findings indicated that patients who received acupuncture continued to experience significant symptom relief on day 2. Acupressure may add a nonpharmacologic intervention for symptom management in patients undergoing thoracoscopic surgery. Nurses can use acupressure to help control pain in patients after thoracoscopic surgery.

Postoperative Teaching

Teaching is especially important postoperatively because most patients must perform quite a bit of self-care. Postoperative teaching should reinforce content taught preoperatively. In addition, you should teach the patient about the topics in the Self-Care box, Postoperative Patient Teaching Topics.

- To use time efficiently, try to do some teaching each time you are at the bedside for other care.
- Be sure the patient is comfortable but alert.
- Do not attempt teaching when the patient is in pain, needs to void, or is drowsy from opioid analgesics.

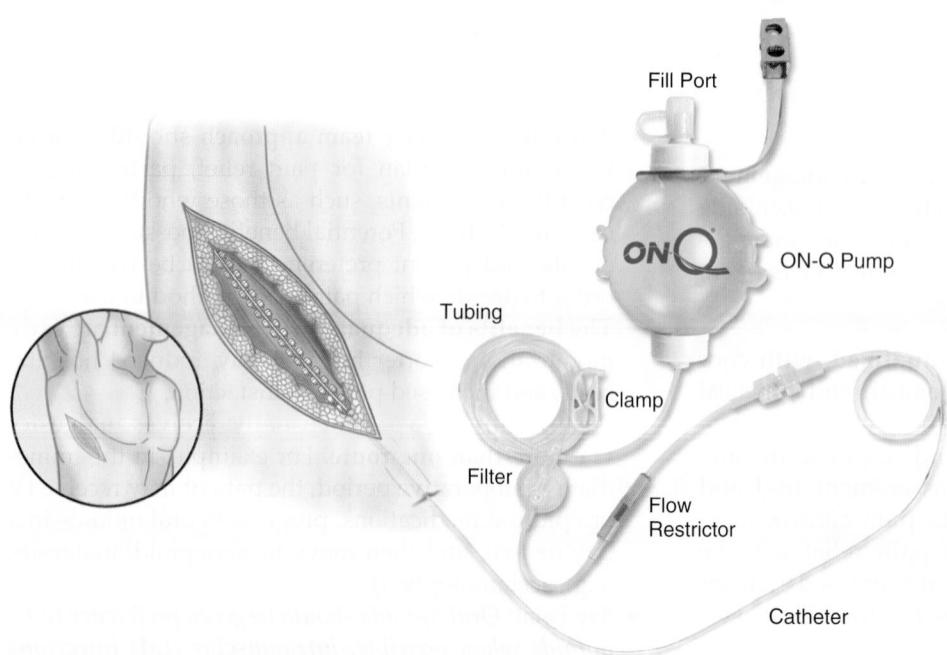

FIGURE 36-5 A single-use pain relief pump delivers a local anesthetic directly into the patient's surgical site.

Postoperative Patient Teaching Topics

➤ Postoperative treatment regimen (e.g., dressing changes, exercises), including rationale for the treatments

➤ Self-management of the treatment regimen

➤ Expected results and effects of the surgery

➤ The prescribed diet and how to select foods on the diet

➤ Prescribed activity

➤ Signs and symptoms of complications that require the patient to notify the surgeon or primary care provider

➤ Return office or clinic visits

➤ Lifestyle changes that may be needed

➤ Community resources available (e.g., Reach for Recovery)

Teaching Your Patient About Incentive Spirometry

➤ Explain to the patient that the machine will enable them to monitor the depth of their breathing.

➤ Patients with abdominal or chest incisions may require pain medication to use the incentive spirometer.

➤ Assist the patient to an upright position in the bed or chair.

➤ Instruct the patient to do the following:

1. Breathe out normally.

2. Place the mouthpiece in the mouth and create a seal.

3. Breathe in slowly and as deeply as possible through the mouthpiece. Monitor the depth of inspiration by viewing the gauge. (Establish goals for the patient so that progress can be monitored.)

4. Hold your breath as long as possible, at least to a slow count of 3.

5. Remove the mouthpiece from your mouth and exhale.

6. Rest for a few seconds.

7. Repeat this process 10 times every hour while awake, if possible.

8. After each set of 10 deep breaths, cough to be sure lungs are clear. Support any incision when coughing by holding a pillow firmly against it.

Incentive Spirometry

Incentive spirometry may be prescribed for patients who are at high risk for atelectasis and pneumonia (e.g., the patient has a history of lung problems or smoking or will experience a prolonged period of inactivity). Incentive spirometry facilitates deep breathing, increases lung volume, and promotes coughing to clear mucus from the respiratory tree. The equipment varies in appearance, but all devices include a gauge to monitor the patient's progress visibly (Fig. 36-6).

If incentive spirometry is prescribed postoperatively, explain its use to the patient (see the Self-Care box, Teaching Your Patient About Incentive Spirometry). If you know in advance that the patient will be using an incentive spirometer postoperatively, include its use in your preoperative teaching.

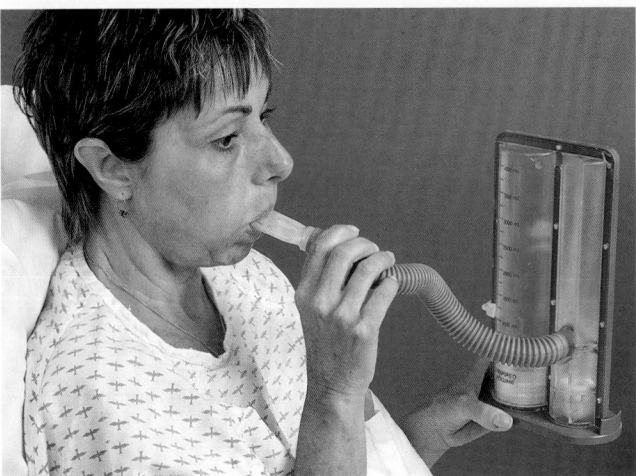

FIGURE 36-6 Incentive spirometry facilitates lung expansion and coughing to clear mucus from airways.

Antiembolism Stockings and Sequential Compression Devices

More than half of all hospitalized patients are at risk for venous thromboembolism, and surgical patients seem to be at higher risk than medical patients. Preventive measures include anticoagulant medications (so-called blood thinners), postoperative exercises, and antiembolism stockings.

Antiembolism Stockings Antiembolism stockings were discussed previously as a preoperative care intervention in preparing the patient physically for surgery. Encourage postoperative patients to ambulate as soon and as much as possible to promote peripheral circulation and prevent thrombophlebitis. **Key Point:** *Antiembolism stockings are not a substitute for activity.*

To learn how to apply antiembolism stockings, see the summary in the Highlights of Procedures box, and

 Go to **Chapter 36, Procedure 36-2: Applying Antiembolism Stockings,** in Volume 2.

Sequential Compression Devices Sequential compression devices (SCDs) may be prescribed for patients at high risk for thrombophlebitis. The SCD is a plastic sleeve with chambers. The sleeve is wrapped around the patient's legs and connected to an air pump that

provides sequential pressure to the chambers of the plastic sleeve. Starting at the ankle, the first chamber is inflated. When the second chamber inflates, the first chamber deflates, and so on. SCDs apply brief pressure to each segment of the leg. This compresses the veins and promotes venous return to the heart. To learn how to apply SCDs, see the summary in the Highlights of Procedures box, and

 Go to **Chapter 36, Procedure 36-3: Applying Sequential Compression Devices**, in Volume 2.

Gastrointestinal Suction

Patients having certain surgeries, such as a laparotomy to close a bowel perforation or surgery to relieve a bowel obstruction, are at high risk for abdominal distention. In addition to causing pain, distention can increase post-operative respiratory problems, place a strain on suture lines, and interfere with wound closure. Such patients will return from surgery with a nasogastric (NG) or nasointestinal tube in place for gastric or intestinal decompression. If prolonged intestinal decompression is anticipated, a gastrostomy may be performed instead of using a nasogastric tube.

Decompression tubes are typically connected to either intermittent or continuous suction to collect excess fluid and gas. Suction is continued until peristalsis resumes, bowel sounds are audible, and the patient is passing flatus. While suction is in place, the patient remains NPO. To review the insertion and care of NG and nasoenteric tubes, see Chapter 24. To learn how to manage gastrointestinal suction, see the summary in the Highlights of Procedures box, and

 Go to **Chapter 36, Procedure 36-4: Managing Gastric Suction**, in Volume 2.

KnowledgeCheck 36-9

- Identify six potential postoperative complications.
- Why are sequential compression devices used?

Highlights of Procedures 36-1 through 36-4

For steps to follow in *all* procedures, refer to the inside back cover of Volume 2. Go to the full procedures in Volume 2 to practice and learn the procedure steps. Use these procedure highlights later to help you review key points.

Procedure 36-1: Teaching a Patient to Deep-Breathe, Cough, Move in Bed, and Perform Leg Exercises

➤ Assess the patient's readiness to learn.

➤ Ensure that the patient is clear about the difference between coughing and merely clearing the throat.

➤ Demonstrate how to splint a potential chest or abdominal incision.

➤ Make sure the patient flexes the knees before turning on their side in bed.

➤ Support the patient who is unable to maintain a side-lying position with pillows.

➤ Teach the patient to alternately flex and extend the knees.

➤ Teach the patient to alternately dorsiflex and plantar flex the foot.

➤ Teach the patient to rotate ankles in a complete circle.

Procedure 36-2: Applying Antiembolism Stockings

➤ Measure the patient's leg to ensure that you select stockings of the correct size.

➤ Inspect the legs and feet for edema, abrasions, lesions, open areas, and circulatory changes.

➤ Elevate the patient's legs for at least 15 minutes before applying stockings.

➤ Insert your hand and turn the stocking inside out to the level of the heel.

➤ Insert patient's foot into stocking. Gradually pull the remaining portion of the stocking up and over the leg.

Keep knee-high stockings 2.5 to 5 cm (1 to 2 in.) below the joint.

Do not apply thigh-high stockings if the thigh circumference is greater than 82 cm (32 in.).

➤ Make sure the stocking is free of wrinkles and is not rolled at the top or bunched.

Procedure 36-3: Applying Sequential Compression Devices

➤ Determine whether elastic stockings are to be used concurrently with the sequential device. If so, apply them (see Procedure 36–2).

➤ Place the regulating pump for the sequential compression in a location that will ensure patient safety.

➤ Place the patient in a supine position.

➤ If you are using SCD and PAS brand thigh-high compression sleeves, measure the thigh.

➤ Place the lower extremity on the open sleeve, ensuring that the compression chambers are located over the correct anatomical structure (e.g., knee opening is at the level of the joint).

➤ Leave one to two fingerbreadths between the sleeve and the extremity.

➤ Set the regulating pump to the correct pressure, as ordered.

➤ Instruct the patient to call for assistance in disconnecting the tubing from the sleeve.

Highlights of Procedures 36-1 through 36-4

Procedure 36-4: Managing Gastric Suction

Procedure 36-4A: Initial Equipment Setup

➤ Connect and secure the suction source, collection container, and drainage tubing.

➤ Don nonsterile gloves.

➤ Connect suction drainage tubing to nasogastric (NG) tubing.

➤ Secure the NG tube to the patient's nose and gown (if not already done).

➤ Turn on the suction.

Procedure 36-4B: Emptying the Suction Container

➤ Don nonsterile gloves.

➤ Turn off the suction; close the stopcock (or clamp the tubing).

➤ Empty the suction container and measure the contents.

➤ Empty and wash the graduated measuring container.

➤ Cleanse the suction container port and close the stopper; place the container back in the holder.

➤ Turn on the suction.

➤ Observe for proper functioning and tubing patency.

Procedure 36-4C: Irrigating the Nasogastric Tubing

➤ Prepare the irrigation set.

➤ Don nonsterile gloves.

➤ Place patient at a 30° to 45° elevation

➤ Check for NG tube placement.

➤ Fill the syringe with 10 to 30 mL of saline.

➤ Turn off the stopcock or clamp the NG tube.

➤ Disconnect the NG tube from drainage.

➤ Drain the suction tubing and turn off the suction source.

➤ Turn on the stopcock or unclamp the NG tube.

➤ Slowly instill and withdraw irrigant into the NG tube until fluid flows freely.

➤ Turn off the stopcock or reclamp the NG tube.

➤ Reconnect the NG tube.

➤ Turn on the stopcock or release the clamp.

Procedure 36-4D: Providing Comfort Measures

➤ Don nonsterile gloves.

➤ Provide mouth care.

➤ Remove nasal secretions.

➤ Apply water-soluble lubricant to nostrils.

➤ Check that tape or tube fixation device is secure.

To explore learning resources for this chapter,

Go to Davis Advantage **and find:**

Answers and Suggested Responses for all questions in this chapter

Concept Map

Knowledge Map

References and Bibliography

Nursing Functions

CHAPTER 37

Community & Home Health Nursing

Learning Outcomes

After completing this chapter, you should be able to:

➤ Define the meaning of community.
➤ Identify at least four factors by which you can recognize a healthy community.
➤ Discuss factors that create vulnerability for a population.
➤ Compare and contrast community-based care, community health nursing, public health nursing, and community-oriented nursing.
➤ Distinguish primary, secondary, and tertiary interventions in regard to a community health scenario.
➤ Discuss at least three strategies that nurses use to gather community data.
➤ Describe the roles of nurses in the community setting.
➤ Identify the primary goal of home care.
➤ Describe ways in which home healthcare differs from hospital nursing.
➤ Categorize the various agencies that deliver home healthcare according to purpose, client served, and funding source.
➤ Describe how the nurse's emphasis differs in hospice care compared with home health nursing.

➤ List at least four criteria clients must meet for home care to be reimbursed by Medicare.
➤ Outline the steps required to prepare for a home visit, including considerations for the nurse's safety.
➤ Discuss ways in which the assessment process is unique for in-home care.
➤ Explain the role of the nurse in helping clients and families manage medications and treatments in the home setting.
➤ Describe how infection control measures differ in the home and in the hospital.
➤ State two important safety concerns in home care that arise out of The Joint Commission 2023 home care safety goals.
➤ Describe the nurse's role in treating caregiver strain.
➤ Apply the nursing process to the care of patients in the home and community.
➤ Use standardized nursing language taxonomies (NANDA-I, Nursing Outcomes Classification [NOC], Nursing Interventions Classification [NIC], Omaha, and Clinical Care Classification [CCC]) to describe care planning in community and home care.

Key Concepts

Community nursing
Home healthcare
Population

Related Concepts

See the Concept Map on Davis Advantage.

Meet Your Patients

Your Neighbor, Tanya

You are nearing completion of your fundamentals course. One night while you are preparing for your next clinical, you receive a text and then a phone call. It is your neighbor, Tanya. Her 7-year-old son, Jacob, came home from school with a notification from the school nurse stating that a classmate tested positive for SARS-CoV-2 (COVID-19, coronavirus) and that other students in the class had been exposed to the disease.

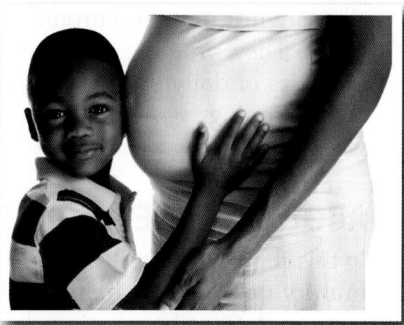

(Continued)

Meet Your Patients (continued)

Tanya is concerned about the risks to Jacob and the rest of the family. Tanya is 8 months pregnant, and the family has no health insurance. She says, "You are a nursing student; do you know what I should do or where I might go for assistance?"

Although you are flattered that Tanya has consulted you, you need to consider whether you have the expertise to answer her questions. This situation requires knowledge from many aspects of nursing (e.g., immunizations, pregnancy, microbiology, pathophysiology). Although you may not have all of the information you need to answer her questions, you should be able to help your neighbor resolve her concerns. You will need to consider the following questions:

- What is going on in the situation that may influence the outcome?
- Who should be involved to improve the outcome?
- What theoretical knowledge do I need to answer my neighbor's questions? Where would I find this information?
- What additional data do I need to collect from my neighbor?
- What suggestions and/or referrals should I offer to my neighbor?

Your Patients, the Escobars

Flora Escobar is 78 years old. She lives at home with her husband, Roland, age 78. Both enjoyed good health until

Roland was hospitalized for a cerebrovascular accident (CVA; or stroke) 3 weeks ago. He then spent 2 weeks in a skilled nursing facility (SNF) that offered physical rehabilitation care. He returned home yesterday and will be followed by the local home health agency for physical therapy and nursing care.

At your initial visit, Mrs. Escobar greets you at the door. She is a frail woman who looks exhausted. Her apron pockets are stuffed with pill bottles. The hallway is partially blocked with a bedside commode, walker, and tray table. Mr. Escobar, wearing pajamas and a robe, is in a hospital bed in the living room. He is a tall, stocky man who is sitting up in bed but is slumped and leaning to the left.

After introducing yourself, you ask an open-ended question to build rapport: "How have things been going since you came home yesterday?" Mrs. Escobar sighs and says, "I'm worried that I'm doing things wrong. I have a hard time helping him move. He is so much bigger than I am, and I don't want to hurt him. He is frustrated with me, but he has difficulty talking and can't tell me what he needs." Tears fill Mrs. Escobar's eyes. Her husband turns away to avoid eye contact with you. To refocus their attention, you suggest that you go over some information and then begin to look at what additional services might be helpful.

Imagine how stressed Mrs. Escobar must feel. How do you think you could best help this family? In this chapter, as you read the section on home health nursing, you should find it easier to answer those questions.

TheoreticalKnowledge
knowingwhy

In the past couple of decades, the population has aged, and in many cases, hospital stays have become shorter in order to reduce costs. As a result, community-based healthcare, including home nursing care, is rapidly expanding. Community and public health nurses regularly provide health screening and interventions for preventing disease. Home care nurses provide care to clients with complex, chronic, or terminal illness in the home. They promote self-care and independence with activities of daily living (ADLs), regardless of the level of functioning.

ABOUT THE KEY CONCEPTS

In this chapter, you will learn about the concepts of **community nursing** and **home healthcare** and how different **populations** have unique healthcare needs. You will understand how these concepts are related to each other and to subconcepts, such as public health nursing, vulnerable populations, and home visits.

UNDERSTANDING THE CONCEPT OF COMMUNITY

The word **community** comes from the Latin term *communis*, meaning the "gift or fellowship of common relations and feelings." Historically, it meant a body of like-minded people or the inhabitants of a town. Then and now, the term suggests a general sense of selflessness, sharing, relationship, and doing good that comes from working together. Most members of a community share a common language, certain rituals, and special customs.

In contrast to community, we tend to think of a **population** as a certain geographic region. But the term *population* has other meanings, as well.

- It can mean the group of people of a particular demographic group in a specified place (e.g., "There are 1,500 Latino people living in Edwards County").
- It can also mean *any* group of people subject to statistical or other study (e.g., all the people who are homeless in Edwards County or all the adolescents who are pregnant and living in Edwards County).

The U.S. Bureau of the Census conducts a survey and a count of the population of the United States every 10 years. The most recent census is the one conducted in the year 2020 (U.S. Bureau of the Census, 2022).

When the census is completed, the U.S. Census Bureau groups the data into sections of 1,200 to 8,000 people (average 4,000), known as **census tracts.** The area of individual census tracts varies according to the density of the population. In urban centers, a census tract covers a small area. Rural census tracts are large. Census tracts are useful to public officials, market analysts, and anyone—including community nurses—who studies the characteristics and concerns of smaller sections of people.

Maps and census tracts show the *geopolitical* boundaries of a community. But as we noted earlier, a community can also be a group of people with a common purpose. They may live in different geographical areas, but they have a "sense of belonging" to their group (community). For a comparison of geopolitical boundaries and census tracts, see Figure 37-1.

An **aggregate** is a group of individuals with at least one shared characteristic, either personal or environmental. For example, a community health nurse may work with a class of high school girls to reduce the incidence of adolescent pregnancy. The shared characteristics of this aggregate are that they are female, of childbearing

age, and attend a particular school. As another example, the nursing students in your school are an aggregate. What characteristics and goals do you share?

KnowledgeCheck 37-1

- Give several examples of a community.
- How is a population different from a community?

 ## ThinkLike a Nurse 37-1: Clinical Judgment in Action

- Why might the boundaries of a census tract change every 10 years?
- How could you figure out what census tract you live or go to school in?

What Are the Components of a Community?

To understand a particular community and its needs, you will need information about its three components: the concepts of structure, status, and process.

Structure *Structure* refers to the general characteristics of a community. These include:

- **Demographic data:** For example, gender, age, ethnicity, and educational and income levels
- **Data about healthcare services:** For example, number of primary care providers or emergency care facilities in the area

Status *Status* describes the biological, emotional, and social outcome components of a community.

- **Biological** data include morbidity (illness) and mortality (death) rates, life expectancy ratios, and risk-factor profiles for the respective age-groups within a community.
- **Emotional** data include general indications of mental health and consumer satisfaction survey results about various aspects of the community compared with other locales.
- **Social** data include crime rates, citizenship involvement in community-wide activities, and general functioning levels of the community members.

Process *Process* describes the overall effectiveness level of the community. For example:

- Do the members of the community perceive that they are part of a group with a common purpose, values, or interests?
- What is the extent of interaction among community members?
- Does the community have an established forum for conflict resolution?

What Makes a Community Healthy?

As with individuals, the meaning and perception of health vary among aggregates. For nurses, it is important to understand what a particular community defines

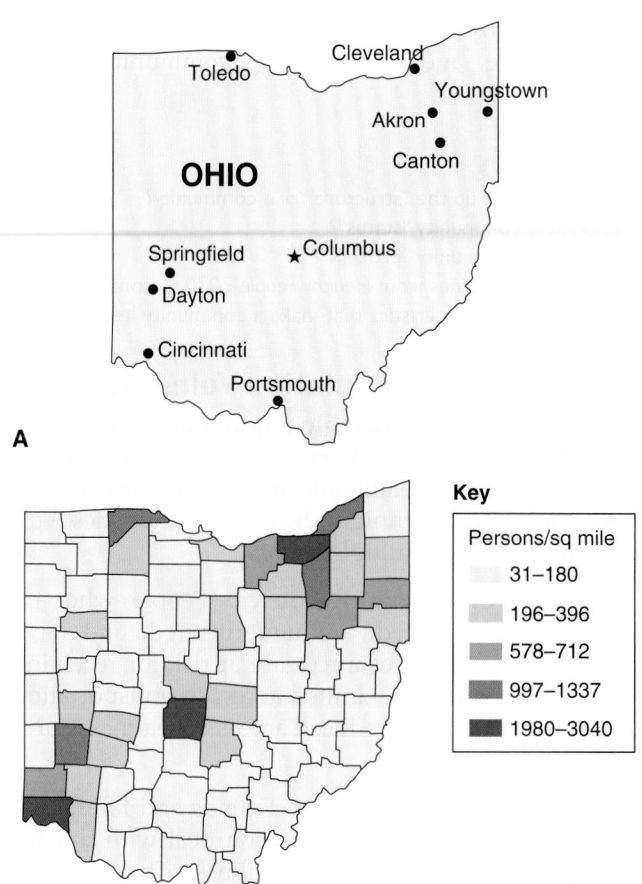

FIGURE 37-1 *A,* Political boundaries. *B,* Population density using census tract data.

(and values) as health rather than relying on personal definitions.

Healthy People 2030 provides useful guidelines for promoting health, with the understanding that many of the health problems of Americans are preventable and can result from social determinants of health (SDOH). The U.S. Department of Health and Human Services (USDHHS) defines SDOH as "the conditions in the environments where people are born, live, learn, work, play, worship, and age that affect a wide range of health, functioning, and quality-of-life outcomes and risks" (USDHHS, n.d.) (Fig. 37-2).

SDOH can be grouped into the following categories:

Economic stability. Those living in poverty can't afford housing, healthcare, and healthy food. The stress of economic uncertainty and food scarcity are more likely to lead illnesses and complications, such as heart disease, diabetes, and depression.

Education access and quality. People with higher levels of education are more likely to be healthier and live longer. Those with low literacy and poor-quality education are more likely to suffer hardships that affect health and access to care.

Healthcare access and quality. Without primary healthcare services, people don't get preventative care, screening and early detection of disease, and necessary care to treat illness.

Neighborhood and built environment. People who live in areas with high rates of violence, unsafe air or water, and exposure to toxins and disease are more likely to experience health problems.

Social and Community Context Those without social support from family, friends, coworkers, and community members are more likely to suffer anxiety and depression and other mental health issues. They may not have help with transportation needed to access healthcare (USDHHS, Office of Disease Prevention and Health Promotion [ODPHP], n.d.).

Some examples affecting community health include:

Physical activity	Mental health
Obesity	Injury and violence
Tobacco use	Environmental quality
Substance abuse	Immunizations
Sexual behavior	Access to healthcare

For the complete list of indicators, see Focus Areas of *Healthy People 2030.*

The four overarching goals of the *Healthy People 2030* initiative are to:

1. Attain high-quality, longer lives free of preventable disease, disability, injury, and premature death.
2. Achieve health equity, eliminate health disparities, and improve the health of all groups.
3. Create social and physical environments that promote good health for all.
4. Promote quality of life, healthy development, and healthy behaviors across all life stages.

These aggregate goals are to be achieved by promoting healthy behaviors, increasing access to quality healthcare, and strengthening community health resources.

KnowledgeCheck 37-2
- What makes up the "structure" of a community?
- What is community "status"?
- What is community "process"?
- Use the guidelines from *Healthy People 2030* to compile a list of several characteristics that make a community healthy.

What Makes a Population Vulnerable?

The concept of **vulnerable population** is defined as a population at increased risk for disparate healthcare access and adverse health outcomes because of common economic, cultural, ethnic, or health characteristics. Vulnerability involves multiple factors.

Limited Economic Resources People who are socially disadvantaged, are underinsured, and have inadequate financial resources are at risk for receiving inadequate healthcare. Limited access to transportation may also contribute to reduced access to healthcare providers or facilities.

Limited Social Resources Friends and family are valuable resources to help a person deal with day-to-day stress and the demands of an illness. They can provide feedback, listen to concerns, and offer emotional and physical assistance. However, not everyone has social resources. Older adults who live alone and people

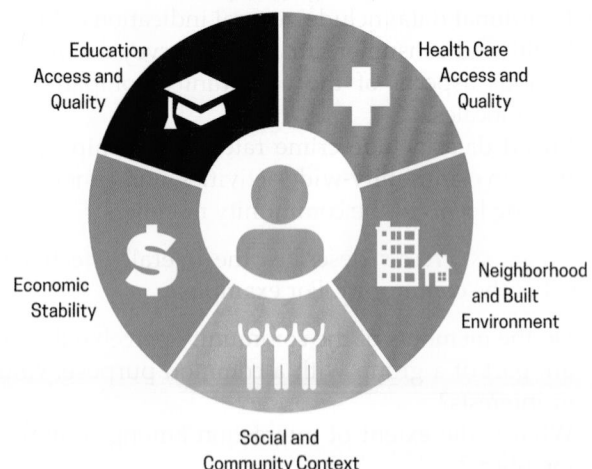

Social Determinants of Health

Education Access and Quality

Health Care Access and Quality

Economic Stability

Neighborhood and Built Environment

Social and Community Context

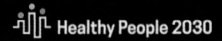

Social Determinants of Health
Copyright-free

Healthy People 2030

FIGURE 37-2 *Healthy People 2030* social determinants of health. (From U.S. Department of Health and Human Services, Office of Disease Prevention and Health Promotion. *Healthy People 2030.* https://health.gov/healthypeople/priority-areas/social-determinants-health)

with cognitive challenges or mental illness are examples of groups at increased risk for poor health outcomes due to social isolation.

Age The very young and the very old are less able to adapt to physiological stress and are at increased risk of disease and complications. They are more prone to infections and may not be able to protect themselves against environmental hazards, such as cold or heat.

Chronic Disease and Obesity People who have chronic diseases are at greater risk of health problems. For example, people with obesity have an increased risk of heart disease, diabetes, impaired mobility, joint pain, and other complications. People with diabetes are at risk for blindness, impaired wound healing, kidney failure, poor peripheral circulation, heart disease, and other complications.

History of Abuse or Trauma People who have experienced abuse or traumatic events often feel they have limited control over their health and circumstances. They may feel powerless or hopeless and be unable to take actions that promote health or lead to early treatment of illness. Abuse and trauma also tax a person's reserves, placing them at risk for mental health problems.

UNDERSTANDING THE CONCEPT OF COMMUNITY-BASED NURSING

A community can be either a *site* for healthcare delivery or a *recipient* of healthcare services. In fact, the first hospitals in the United States were established only in the late 1860s to protect society from contagious disease. Several decades passed before hospitals and other freestanding clinics became the predominant settings for providing healthcare. However, as the technological advances of the past few decades have escalated the costs of delivering health services, efforts to lower costs have resulted in a move back to more community-based care, including complementary and alternative care.

Community-based care refers to healthcare or rehabilitative services performed in clinics, offices, mobile care units, and other facilities in the community—rather than in acute care settings, such as hospitals (although acute care settings also exist within the community).

Example: Many surgeries and diagnostic procedures are now performed in privately owned surgical centers, health clinics, and providers' offices rather than in hospitals. People also receive mental, physical, cardiac, and pulmonary rehabilitation services in outpatient settings. Extended care facilities commonly provide rehabilitative care for patients after acute traumatic injuries, as well as continuous skilled care for older adults and people with chronic illness.

The following sections describe three approaches to community-based nursing care: community health

nursing, public health nursing, and community-oriented nursing.

Community Health Nursing

Although many people use the terms *community health nursing* and *public health nursing* interchangeably, the two are not identical. **Community health nursing** focuses on how the health of individuals, families, and groups affects the community as a whole. Community health nurses strive to promote, protect, preserve, and maintain the health of the population through the delivery of personal health services to individuals, families, and groups.

> *Example:* A community health nurse may work in a prenatal clinic providing services for low-income pregnant patients. The nurse provides a direct service to each pregnant patient, yet they are doing so to improve the general health of the entire community. By providing nutritional counseling, recommendations for physical activity, and education to avoid harmful substances, the nurse improves the health of both the patients and their fetuses and therefore improves the overall health of the community.

Public Health Nursing

Public health nursing focuses on the community as a whole and the eventual effect of the community's health status on the health of individuals, families, and groups. The goal of public health is to prevent individual disease and disability, in addition to promoting and protecting the overall health of the community. Public health nurses who act in a health promotion role need competency in the following areas:

- "Analytical/assessment
- Policy development/program planning
- Communication
- Cultural competency
- Community dimensions of practice
- Public health sciences
- Fiscal planning and management
- Leadership and systems thinking" (Council on Linkages Between Academia and Public Health Practice, 2014, p. 3)

> *Example:* A public health nurse is employed by a county health department to provide surveillance services to monitor for tuberculosis (TB). The nurse helps to protect the entire community by screening for TB at the local school, by testing high-risk individuals for TB, and by identifying and tracking clients with active disease to ensure that they complete the prescribed 6- to 9-month medication regimen.

Because public health focuses on comprehensive programs for the community, government-based agencies often provide these services. The U.S. Public Health Service (USPHS) is an example of a public health agency within the federal government. Some examples of successful public health programs are human papillomavirus (HPV) immunizations for adolescents, smoking cessation for healthcare workers, motor vehicle and infant car-seat safety, the SARS-CoV-2 (COVID-19, coronavirus) public health vaccination program (Fig. 37-3), and obesity prevention programs for adults and children.

Community-Oriented Nursing

Community-oriented nursing combines components of community and public health. It focuses on health promotion, illness prevention, early detection, and treatment provided within the community setting. The practice is evidence based and collaborative with other community health disciplines. The approach is a comprehensive look at the individual, family, group, and community at large.

> *Example:* A nurse with a community-oriented approach might work in an adolescent prenatal program. The nurse provides individual care at the local clinic 2 days per week. While at the clinic, she gathers data from adolescent clients about the schools they attend; their knowledge of birth control, pregnancy, and childbirth; and the issues these young people face with pregnancy. On the remaining 3 days, she meets with school officials to identify pregnant teenagers who need prenatal care, teaches a class about sexuality in the local high school, works with teachers to identify strategies to make sure teenagers who are pregnant stay in school, provides parenting education to adolescents who have children, and advocates changing a bus route so that students can easily get to the local clinic.

Each aspect of care allows the nurse to gather more data about the needs of the individuals and the community as a whole. Figure 37-4 provides a schematic of the relationship among the various community-based nursing approaches identified in this section.

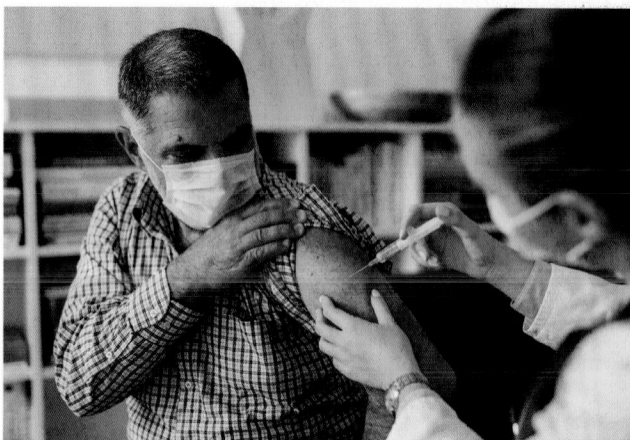

FIGURE 37-3 Nurse showing care when performing client care tasks.

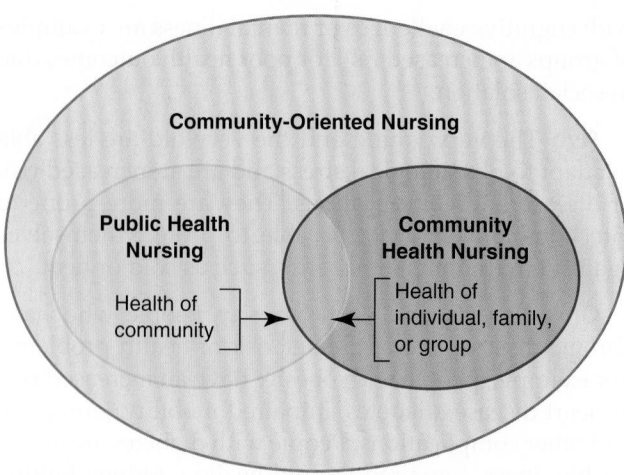

FIGURE 37-4 Schematic relationship of community nursing approaches.

KnowledgeCheck 37-3

- What is the distinction between an aggregate population and a vulnerable population?
- Identify practice differences between a community-based nurse and an acute care nurse.
- How is public health nursing different from community health nursing? How is it the same?
- How is community-oriented nursing related to community health nursing and public health nursing?

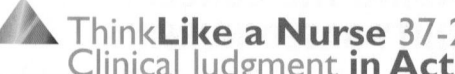 ThinkLike a Nurse 37-2: Clinical Judgment in Action

Review the scenario of Tanya and Jacob (Meet Your Patients). Which form of community-based nursing would be most appropriate to address their concerns?

Who Were Some Pioneers of Community Nursing?

The following are some of the most notable people who have contributed to the development of community-based nursing care.

- *Florence Nightingale*—Established the importance of promoting health by manipulating the environment (e.g., light, warmth, sanitation, cleanliness) and providing nursing care for the whole person.
- *Lillian Wald*—Known as the first community health nurse; founded the first visiting nurse service, the Henry Street Visiting Nurse Service, in New York.
- *Clara Barton*—Founder of the American Red Cross.
- *Margaret Sanger*—Founded the International Planned Parenthood Federation. Pioneered the use of family planning and birth control education.

WORKING WITHIN COMMUNITIES

Community nurses' roles vary depending on the community and its identified needs. Community nursing care is holistic by nature, and it serves a large client population. Therefore, one of the most effective nursing interventions is **empowerment.** This means assisting the client (individual or community) to recognize and use available resources to achieve or maintain the desired level of health, achieve autonomy, and maintain positive self-esteem.

What Are the Roles of Community Nurses?

Community health nurses function as client advocates, educators, collaborators, counselors, and case managers. All of these roles require excellent written and oral communication skills. Although the widespread use of electronic health records, electronic messaging (e.g., text, e-mail), and other applications have made it possible to communicate efficiently with groups of people, access to technology may be a problem in some areas. In addition, there are many people with limited or no computer or technology skills.

Client Advocate 🍀 The effective community health nurse consistently supports the identified or expressed concerns of the client and/or community. Because disparities in health and inequities affect the health of people and the community, the community nurse advocates for health by partnering with other public sectors to improve the conditions in people's environment. Advocating for a community often requires political involvement at the local, state, or national level. The challenge is in knowing whom to approach for political support and how to gain their support. As a community health nurse, you can effect change by getting involved in your local Student Nurses Association, professional nursing organizations, school board, and citizen committees or by attending council meetings.

Educator Because community nursing focuses on wellness and disease prevention, much of what the nurse does involves client education—of individuals, aggregates at risk of disease, politicians, or a community. It is difficult to evaluate the effect of the health education because people may not act on the knowledge for months or years after the teaching moment. When planning teaching, you must be aware of the stage of development, educational level, and learning style of the community group you intend to educate. The best learning programs are short; provide relevant, practical information; and can be easily incorporated into the learner's daily routine. For more information about teaching clients, see Chapter 16.

Collaborator A primary role of a community health nurse is to serve as a collaborator. Consider the following example:

Example: A community health nurse is concerned about poor compliance with recommended immunization schedules for children in a particular community. After surveying some of the parents, the nurse discovers that

the clinic's operating hours are limited. Additionally, the automated call routing system is frustrating for people trying to set an appointment, and the clinic does not offer online scheduling. The nurse also discovers that some offices do not send reminders to clients or follow up to reschedule missed appointments. The nurse schedules a meeting of clinic staff, practice managers, and patients to resolve these issues. At the meeting, some larger issues are revealed, such as the insufficient number of Medicaid providers to serve the community and the failure of state Medicaid agencies to reimburse the providers adequately and in a timely manner.

Counselor Once you have established rapport with a group, members may consult you about a variety of health-related and non–health-related concerns. ✚ Be careful to offer counsel only on topics within your scope of practice and make recommendations that are practical yet meet the needs of the community. It may be that you may need only to serve as a witness to and listen to the group's concerns. **Key Point:** *Allowing clients to discuss or work through issues empowers them and fosters self-reliance.*

Case Manager Community nurses commonly make referrals to or collaborate with various health and social agencies. Be aware when referring clients to these resources that agency policies and financing change frequently. Also, because community agencies often operate on grants and time-limited funding, a program that is available at one time may be dissolved at another. As a community health nurse, you will need to remain informed about the community services in your area.

Example: A local group has established a healthcare program at a minimal charge for low-income families. Providers and nurses volunteer their time to provide the care. Pharmaceutical representatives donate the medical supplies and common medications. Healthcare specialists (e.g., surgeons) provide services to those with complex or specialized needs. However, in such a clinic, the appointment times fill up quickly, and clients often have to wait for more than a month or two for an appointment. Before enrolling families in the program, you would need to be aware of these limitations and share this information with clients.

KnowledgeCheck 37-4
- Give an example of a nursing activity involved in each of the following community health roles: educator, advocate, case manager, counselor, and collaborator.

How Are Community Nursing Actions Classified?

There are three basic levels of care in which nursing interventions can be classified: primary, secondary, and tertiary. Most community-oriented nursing practices are aimed at the primary (prevention) level.

Primary Interventions

The goal of **primary (first-level) interventions** is to promote health and prevent disease. Examples include:

- **Educating** susceptible individuals with no active disease or infection is a routine, primary intervention that community health nurses practice.

  Example: A nurse may educate ninth-grade students about the risk of hepatitis B and HPV, the benefits of vaccination, and strategies to reduce the likelihood of exposure to contaminated body fluids.

- **Collaborating** with local agencies to provide clean and secure temporary housing for migrant farmworkers
- **Lobbying** elected representatives to advocate for the public against dramatic increases in pharmaceutical pricing on medically necessary and life-saving injectable medication indicated for severe allergic reactions.

Secondary Interventions

Secondary (second-level) interventions aim to reduce the impact of the disease process through early detection and treatment. For example, a community health nurse:

- Screens an adolescent patient who is sexually active for hepatitis B and/or HPV. The patient has known risk factors for sexually transmitted infection (STI) but no apparent disease symptoms. The nurse will also teach the patient how to protect themself from STIs, hepatitis B, and HIV in the future.
- Provides outreach screening programs offering mammography, scoliosis screening, lipid testing, or prostate-specific antigen (PSA) testing for prostate cancer (Fig. 37-5).

Tertiary Interventions

The goal of **tertiary (third-level) intervention** is to halt disease progression and/or restore client functioning to the predisease state. Tertiary-level interventions require the nurse to collaborate with other healthcare providers to provide treatment.

Example: A female student reports to a school nurse that she has been involved in unprotected sexual activities. The school nurse refers the student to the public health clinic for a pelvic examination and laboratory testing to detect STIs and screenings for hepatitis B, HPV, and HIV. The student has an abnormal Pap smear, showing cells that suggest exposure to HPV. The clinic nurse, in collaboration with the provider, administers medical treatment. There is no cure for HPV, so the student also needs to learn how to prevent the spread of the disease to others, get immunized with the HPV vaccine, and obtain regular Pap and pelvic examinations to detect cervical cancer and other STIs.

 ThinkLike a Nurse 37-3: Clinical Judgment in Action

What level of intervention is required to address the concerns of Tanya and Jacob (Meet Your Patients)? Discuss your response.

KnowledgeCheck 37-5

For each of the nursing actions listed, identify the level of the nursing intervention as *primary*, *secondary*, or *tertiary*.

- Taking a client's blood pressure at a local health fair
- Administering insulin to an older adult at an extended care facility
- Teaching second-grade students to wash their hands correctly

What Career Opportunities Are Available for Community-Based Nurses?

The following are only a few of the many career opportunities for those who want to practice community-based nursing.

School Nursing

Nursing practice in the school setting began when educators realized that children with health problems had more difficulty learning. School nurses:

- Provide direct care for children with chronic health conditions such as asthma, attention deficit disorder, and diabetes.
- Perform routine procedures for children, such as catheterization, during the school day.
- Administer prescribed medication.
- Ensure that age-appropriate immunizations are documented.
- Offer health education on topics such as nutrition, physical activity, smoking cessation, and sexual and reproductive health.
- Perform health screenings, such as those for vision, hearing, and scoliosis.
- Coordinate referrals with other healthcare providers.

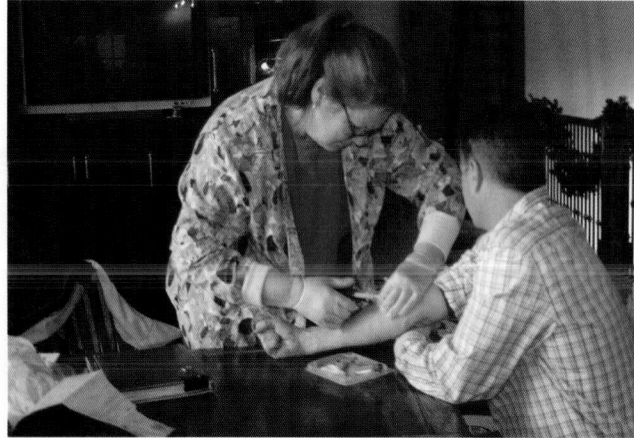

FIGURE 37-5 Secondary interventions. Early detection of heart disease with lipid screening.

- Serve as liaison between school personnel, families, and healthcare providers.
- Advocate for students who lack parental support or who are struggling with peer pressure.

For the most part, a school nurse is autonomous and must be capable of prioritizing and making decisions (American Nurses Association [ANA] & National Association of School Nurses [NASN], 2017; Selekman et al., 2019).

Occupational Health

Occupational health nurses work primarily in industrial or corporate settings. Their work includes the following:

- Provide health promotion programs for employees and their families in an effort to reduce absentee hours, increase productivity, and reduce illness and complications.
- Complete required medical documentation for disability claims or occupational hazardous events.
- Conduct preemployment post-offer assessments and annual screenings.
- Provide care to injured or ill workers.
- Identify hazards in the workplace, including ergonomics, to prevent occupational disease and accidents.
- Obtain random drug testing.
- Assist with filing worker's compensation claims.

To reduce costs, some industries contract a staffing agency to provide trained occupational health nurses. Nursing autonomy and responsibility vary with the employer and the negotiated contract.

Faith Community Nursing

Faith community nursing is a specialized area of nursing practice that focuses on the promotion of health within the context of the values, beliefs, and practices of a faith community. Integrating faith with health, nurses act as educators of holistic health (e.g., parenting issues, use of medications, choosing healthcare providers). In the role of personal health counselor, parish nurses increase awareness of the interrelationship between lifestyle, personal habits, attitudes, and faith. Nurses working in this role develop support groups, provide information through seminars and printed or electronic materials, train volunteers, and act as a liaison to community services as needed (ANA & Health Ministries Association, 2017). The level of autonomy and responsibility of faith community nurses varies, depending on the faith.

Nursing in Correctional Facilities

Nurses in correctional facilities deliver healthcare within the criminal justice system, for example, in juvenile detention, substance abuse treatment facilities, and prisons. The nurse provides primary care services to people of all ages in an unbiased and nonjudgmental manner (ANA, 2020a). Nurses have a high level of autonomy in most correctional or substance rehabilitation facilities. Correctional facilities employ providers who conduct routine examinations and acute and chronic healthcare on a scheduled or as-needed basis. Common interventions in this setting include:

- Performing intake assessments
- Delivering triage care
- Performing primary healthcare services as needed
- Referring patients to specialist care, mental health services, physical therapy, and other providers
- Performing occupational health duties for facility staff

✚ For personal safety, nurses must meet certain physical requirements and complete special weapons training before working in most prisons.

Public Health Clinics

Many community nurses practice within local and state departments of health, including public health clinics. Services offered by health departments can range from basic to comprehensive, based on the needs of the community and funding. Large cities tend to employ nurses who may specialize in an area, such as immunizations, prenatal health, school health, or epidemiological survey. Smaller communities may have only one nurse (or full-time equivalent) providing all services. The autonomy and scope of practice of public health nurses are often limited by the philosophy of the political administration and availability of funding (ANA, 2022).

Disaster Services Nursing

A disaster is any event or catastrophe inflicting widespread loss of life, health, and destruction of property. Features characterizing a disaster typically involve unpredictability, urgency, threat, speed, and uncertainty. They may develop as a sudden-onset or slow-onset event.

- *Human-generated disasters* might be the result of acts such as a terrorist attack, war, or use of nuclear energy to cause harm or fear.
- *Technological disasters* cause damage or disruption on a large scale (e.g., computer systems failure, mass power outage, explosion, or hazardous substance exposure).
- *Natural or ecological disasters* include hurricanes, earthquakes, tsunamis, and floods, as well as environmental degradation, such as deforestation.
- *Biological disasters* may involve exposure to pathogenic microorganisms, toxins, or other bioactive substances, for instance, an outbreak of endemic disease or plant contagion.

Key Point: *Community-oriented nursing emphasizes community assessment and education to reduce the number of casualties when disasters occur and to achieve the best possible level of health for the people and community involved in a disaster (Box 37-1).*

BOX 37-1 ■ ✛ Community Education: What to Do During a Disaster Event

- Remain calm and be patient.

- Learn evacuation routes and locations of local shelters.

- Check local television or the Internet for news and instructions; download National Weather Service Alerts, Wireless Emergency Alerts (WEAs), and Federal Emergency Management (FEMA) applications and turn on notification alerts. Follow the advice of local emergency officials.

- If the disaster occurs near you, check for injuries. Administer first aid; get help for seriously injured people.

- Do not light matches or candles or turn on electrical switches. Check for fires, fire hazards, and other household hazards. Sniff for gas leaks, starting at the water heater. If you smell gas or suspect a leak, turn off the main gas valve, open windows, and get everyone outside quickly.

- Shut off any other damaged utilities; use a generator with caution.

- Confine or secure pets with food and water.

- Call your family contact—do not use the cell phone unless it is a life-threatening emergency.

- Check on your neighbors, especially those who are older or disabled. Call for emergency care if necessary.

- Keep your vehicle's gas tank full.

- Assemble an emergency kit, including first aid supplies, bottled water, nonperishable food items, charging supplies, hand sanitizer, face mask, and medications.

- Gather important financial records, health records, and insurance information.

Source: USA.gov. (2020, August 24). *Emergency and disaster preparedness.* https://www.usa.gov/prepare-for-disasters

Disasters affect the health status of a community in the following ways:

- Lead to premature death, illness, or injury
- Disrupt healthcare services offered within the community
- Cause environmental issues, such as outbreaks of communicable disease or food/water-borne illness
- Cause shortages of safe food and drinking water
- Burden other healthcare systems when displaced populations shift to a host community for basic needs (Veenema, 2018)

In large-scale disasters, nurses practicing in special circumstances and disaster conditions are typically needed to:

- Rapidly assess the overall situation and that of individual victims.
- Triage care and initiate life-saving measures first.
- Adapt nursing skills to the disaster situation, considering available equipment, supplies, and personnel.

- Evaluate the safety of the environment and remove health hazards.
- Provide leadership in coordinating care, assigning priorities for care, and transporting victims.
- Prevent further injury or illness.
- Provide compassionate support to victims and their families.

Good Samaritan laws protect nurses when volunteering—in any state—as long as actions are reasonable.

International Nursing

Nurses working internationally commonly provide relief services after a natural or human-made disaster. They may also offer health or human aid services through a medical clinic, faith-based mission, orphanage, or other international relief program. International nursing requires a high level of autonomy, flexibility, and ingenuity, depending on community needs and available resources. Common issues affecting the health of international communities are:

Poor sanitation	Parasitic infections
Contaminated food and water	Cultural practices
	Crime
Waste management	Poor access to healthcare
Limited or dangerous transportation	Limited resources to pay for medication
Communicable disease	and care

Nurses working globally commonly treat people with malnutrition, dehydration, illnesses related to mosquitoes and other insects, parasitic infestation, hepatitis, and HIV, to name a few (Fig. 37-6).

ThinkLike a Nurse 37-4: Clinical Judgment in Action

Increase your self-knowledge: Assume you are going to be a community-based nurse. Of the many career opportunities available, which work do you think you would rather do? Explain why.

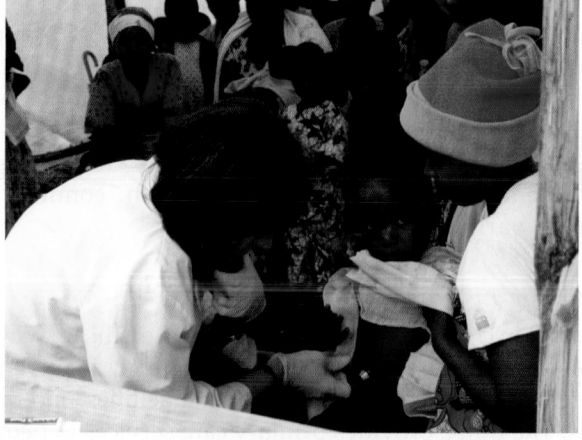

FIGURE 37-6 International nursing. Health and nutrition program for women and children at an African health clinic.

Practical Knowledge
knowing how

The ANA, in the *Standards for Community Health Nursing* (1986), describes the goal of community health nursing as the promotion and preservation of the health of the community population as a whole, defined groups, families, and individuals. Community nursing care should be delivered in a practical, culturally sensitive manner (Kulbok et al., 2012).

ASSESSMENT/RECOGNIZING CUES

When your client is the community, the nursing process follows the same steps you have studied in the previous chapters but uses different forms and different language. Community assessment is usually ongoing and requires the nurse to collaborate with and compile information from a variety of sources. The assessment approach is based on the type of community, the purpose of the assessment, and personal preference. Most beginning students elect to assess a geopolitical community because the data are more readily available than

data from aggregate groups. Therefore, we focus on the geopolitical community assessment procedure.

Windshield Survey Community assessment usually begins with **a windshield survey.** This is performed by observing the community through your automobile window while walking or otherwise being physically present in the area. It is similar to general observation of the individual client in that it provides an overview and allows you to see the community in its natural state. As you observe, make note of the types of businesses and industries in the area, the condition of buildings and public facilities, residences, religious facilities, social service centers, recreation facilities, parks, indicators of politics (signs, headquarters), streets and sewers, modes of transportation, lighting, any outward signs of crime or violence and homelessness, pollution, waste disposal, animals in the area, and other signs of the community well-being. Protective services, such as police and fire services, should be included. You may need to repeat the survey over a period of time at different times of the day, month, or year to get an accurate picture of the community. **Key Point:** *Whoever is doing the assessment needs to be aware that bias can affect their assessment.*

Safe, Effective Nursing Care

Promoting Clzient-Centered Care in Community Health

Chapter Key Concept: Community Nursing

Competency: Goal-Directed, Client-Centered Care

Scenario: Nurses at a public clinic note an increased number of Latinx clients seeking services. To best serve this growing community, the nurse researches healthcare issues affecting urban Latinx populations. Latinx men are more likely to be diagnosed with late-stage prostate cancer and to die of the disease than non-Latinx men. Clinic staff members plan to develop a flyer about prostate cancer screening directed at Latinx men aged 50 and older. The nurse asks a coworker who is Latinx what cultural norms might influence health behaviors. He says that many Latinx men he knows view seeking healthcare as a sign of weakness. He explains *machismo* and *caballerismo*, concepts of manliness in the traditional Latinx culture (in which Mr. Sanchez was raised) that value courage, honor, and dignity. This means that for many Latinx men, a digital rectal examination would be emasculating, embarrassing, and an affront to dignity.

The nurse searches the literature for more information and learns that many Latinx men feel healthcare providers do not understand their culture and do not take the time to develop a relationship with them. After synthesizing the literature, the nurses decided to adopt the following strategies:

➤ Ask clients if there is anything the nurse should know about the culture, beliefs, or religious practices that would be helpful to consider when providing care.

➤ Create educational materials that will be available in the client's preferred language. Use interpreters as needed.

➤ Specifically address culture-based concerns in the context of healthcare.

➤ Avoid stereotyping based on cultural and religious background. Respect all clients as individuals, as some may and others may not adhere to certain cultural beliefs.

➤ Complete cultural competence training to improve the quality of interactions with clients.

➤ Use community leaders, public service announcements, the Internet, social media, and churches to communicate information.

Think about it:

➤ In what ways did the nurses make the planned educational materials client centered?

➤ How could the nurses evaluate the client-centeredness of the educational materials? What information would they need? Where might they obtain the information?

➤ Client-centered care often correlates to improvements in care. How can the clinic staff evaluate improvements in the healthcare of Latinx men in their community after the educational campaign?

What goals are reasonable for this educational effort?

What assessments would be used to determine effectiveness?

Source: Agency for Healthcare Research and Quality. (2020, September). *Consider culture, customs, and beliefs: Tool #10.* http://www.ahrq.gov/professionals/quality-patient-safety/quality-resources/tools/literacy-toolkit/healthlittoolkit2-tool10.html

For more reliable survey results, observers should be trained.

- Begin by describing the neighborhood and the people you see in the community.
- Strive to remain objective in your observations; avoid using personal opinions and biases.
- Route your course before conducting the visit.
- Record your findings as soon as possible after your survey.
- Document the observation with photographs and videography when possible.

Databases and Public Records You can also obtain data from publicly available resources, such as birth records, marriage licenses, local news publications, and community Internet sites. Internet search engines can help you obtain demographic information, morbidity and mortality data, vital statistics, educational levels, criminal activity, political leadership issues, and/or information about community resources.

Client Perceptions You will also gather information about how individuals in the community perceive the community and its state of health. Through community gatherings and informal conversations, you can assess a cross section of the population. This is not only an important part of your assessment but also an excellent way to establish rapport, convey your concerns, and develop a working relationship with key community members.

▮▮▮ NURSING DIAGNOSIS/ANALYZING CUES

After a thorough assessment, you will analyze the complete set of data and compile a list of community strengths and limitations. Work with the community to develop a list of their priorities, considering needs identified by the client and based on availability of funding and political feasibility.

This section provides guidelines for using the NANA-International (NANDA-I), Nursing Outcomes Classification (NOC), Nursing Interventions Classification (NIC), and Omaha System to develop problem statements, goals, and nursing orders to use in planning care for aggregates and communities. If you need to review these three standardized languages, see Chapter 3.

The NANDA-International Taxonomy

In community practice, you need nursing diagnoses that describe the health status of individuals, families, groups, and entire communities. Recall from Chapter 3 that the NANDA-I taxonomy of nursing diagnoses can be used in any nursing setting or specialty. You would simply add the term *community* to other NANDA-I (2021–2024) labels when creating a community-based diagnosis: for example, Decisional Conflict (Community) related to safety needs of the homeless population. The NANDA-I taxonomy does include a few diagnoses

specific to communities, for example, Ineffective Community Coping.

Clinical Care Classification System

The Clinical Care Classification (CCC) is a standardized system for identifying and documenting nursing care in all healthcare settings. Previously known as the Home Health Care Classification (HHCC), this system was originally developed for use in the home or ambulatory settings. Following the nursing process, the CCC represents nursing diagnoses and outcomes, with a focus on nursing interventions, called Care Components. Some examples of CCC components include Activity, Bowel/Gastric, Cardiac, Coping, Life Cycle, Medication, Nutritional, Role Relationship, Self-Care, Sensory (CCC, n.d.).

The Omaha System

The Omaha System is a problem-solving model for community health practice, education, and research. It was developed specifically for use in community settings (Martin & Norris, 1996). In addition to nursing diagnoses, it contains standardized terminology for outcomes and interventions. As a standardized language, this system:

- Enhances client-based care for individuals, families, and communities of all ages, geographic regions, health conditions, socioeconomic conditions, spiritual beliefs, ethnicities, and cultural values
- Aids in communication and documentation of client-related information
- Enables the collection, analysis, and reporting of individual and aggregate data for research and public health

The taxonomy consists of the following.

Problem Classification Scheme This scheme provides a structure for standardized assessment of individuals, families, and communities. Domains within the Problem Classification Scheme include:

- "**Environmental Domain:** Material recourses and physical surroundings both inside and outside the living area, neighborhood, and broader community.
- **Psychosocial Domain:** Patterns of behavior, emotion, communication, relationships, and development.
- **Physiological Domain:** Function and processes that maintain life.
- **Health-related Behaviors Domain:** Patterns of activity that maintain or promote wellness, recovery, and decrease the risk of disease." (Martin & Scheet, 1995)

Intervention Scheme This scheme is for planning care and services. Categories include:

- *Teaching, Guidance, and Counseling* for promoting self-care and health maintenance. These primary prevention activities include giving information; anticipating client problems; encouraging client action and responsibility for self-care; and assisting with coping, decision making, and problem-solving. As a community-oriented nurse, you should spend most of your time offering this level of intervention.

- *Treatments and Procedures* for technical care of individual/family/community. These are secondary interventions directed toward preventing disease, identifying risk factors and early signs and symptoms, and decreasing or alleviating signs and symptoms.
- *Case Management* among individuals/family/community and health and human service providers. Case management is a tertiary intervention that includes coordination, advocacy, and referral. These activities involve facilitating service delivery on behalf of the client, communicating with health and human service providers, promoting assertive client communication, and guiding the client toward appropriate community resources.
- *Surveillance* of community health problems. These nursing activities include detection, measurement, critical analysis, and monitoring to indicate client status in relation to a given condition or phenomenon.

To write an intervention statement, you must combine one of those four "categories" of interventions with one of the "targets" (objects of the nursing interventions), such as bowel care and nutrition. Then you must add patient-specific information to individualize the nursing order.

You will notice that the targets can be used for individuals as well as groups. It is the designation of the nursing diagnosis as *individual, family,* or *group* that determines this.

Problem Rating Scale for Outcomes The Problem Rating Scale for Outcomes is used for measuring client change and evaluation outcomes. The client's progress throughout the period of service is rated on a 5-point scale for client health knowledge (what the client knows), behavior (what the client does), and status (the severity of the illness).

▨ PLANNING/PRIORITIZING HYPOTHESES AND GENERATING SOLUTIONS

In the community, you will need to write goals and outcomes for aggregates. The NOC system is useful for you to develop aggregate (group) goals and outcomes when planning care in the community health setting. You will use the following *NOC standardized outcomes* in the Community Health domain (Moorhead, 2018):

- Community Competence
- Community Disaster Readiness
- Community Disaster Response
- Community Health Status
- Community Immune Status
- Community Risk Control: Chronic Disease
- Community Risk Control: Communicable Disease
- Community Risk Control: Lead Exposure
- Community Risk Control: Obesity
- Community Violence Level

You can use these NOC labels to write goals by adding the appropriate NOC indicators and scales (see NOC Measurement Scales, in the Standardized Language section of Chapter 3). Both NOC and the Omaha System provide standardized vocabularies for aggregate outcomes. *Note:* The *Healthy People 2030* goals are aggregate goals.

▨ IMPLEMENTATION/TAKING ACTION

As a community health nurse, you will plan interventions to promote and preserve the health of individuals, aggregates, and communities. Both NIC and the Omaha System provide standardized vocabularies for aggregate interventions.

The NIC taxonomy includes several interventions specifically designed for community health. These are grouped into two Classes: Community Health Promotion and Community Risk Management.

In the class for Community Health Promotion, NIC interventions include:

Case Management
Community Health Advocacy
Community Health Development
Fiscal Resource Management
Health Education
Immunization/Vaccination Management
Program Development
Social Marketing (Butcher et al., 2018)

▨ APPLYING THE NURSING PROCESS IN COMMUNITY-BASED CARE

Community assessment and care planning may at first seem different from what you have been doing for individual patients. But it does follow the same problem-solving process, as illustrated in the following scenario:

Scenario: As a nurse employed by a local immunization clinic, you have been hired into a new position created by federal and state grant monies to investigate why immunization levels are low among 2-year-olds in Census Tract 15. You would begin with an assessment.

1. **Gather data about the community.**
   - *Define the community.* For instance, determine the physical boundaries of Census Tract 15, a geopolitical community.
   - *Learn the community.* Start interacting with the community to build rapport. Begin the ongoing assessment by conducting windshield surveys, searching for information through reputable databases, and talking with community members.
   - *Focus the data collection.* Focus on the information that will help you determine possible causes of low immunization rates. In this case, the priority problem has already been defined by the financing agency.

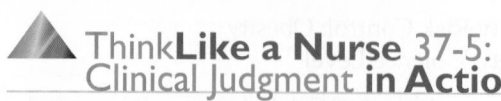

ThinkLike a Nurse 37-5: Clinical Judgment in Action

What data would you want to look at? What are possible reasons for low immunization rates?

2. **Analyze the Data.** Next, examine the characteristics of the families failing to provide immediate immunization for children, including:
   - Family demographics
   - Age of children
   - Number of immunizations needed and the cost
   - Beliefs about negative effects of vaccines
   - Availability of transportation
   - Public sites providing vaccinations
   - Overall continuity of general healthcare for children

   Example: Assume that after working with the community for 6 months, you have spoken at parenting classes about the need to vaccinate children. Several community members have told you they thought their child had already received all necessary immunizations or that their healthcare provider had said to wait until they have better insurance. You will need to arrange a meeting with the local providers to discuss low immunization status. They explain that many vaccinations are too expensive to provide based on the reimbursement they receive from government funding sources.

3. **Plan care.** Your next move is to do some planning. Using the Omaha System, you could generate a care plan to address some of the issues raised by community members and providers.

4. **Evaluate results and follow up.** Community assessment is never complete because the community is constantly changing. However, you need to define the identified needs and desired outcomes during a given period of time, based on best data available at the time of collection. In this case, you would share with local healthcare providers, the health department, and the local health policy committee your approach to addressing the factors suspected of contributing to poor immunization compliance. An important part of your role as a community health nurse is to continue to monitor and evaluate the data and provide updates to the appropriate groups.

Now that you have some understanding of community healthcare, the rest of the chapter focuses on a specific type of community nursing: delivering healthcare in the patient's home.

TheoreticalKnowledge
knowing why

UNDERSTANDING THE CONCEPT OF HOME HEALTHCARE

Recall that community-based healthcare refers to services performed outside of acute care settings. Home healthcare is one such service. **Home healthcare** is the delivery of health-related services in the client's home. Home healthcare is appropriate when a client needs ongoing care that exceeds the abilities of friends and family, as in the following situations:

- To supplement the skills a family member is providing
- To serve as a backup for safety or additional assessment

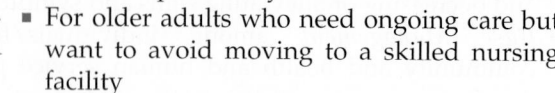

   - For older adults who need ongoing care but want to avoid moving to a skilled nursing facility
- For people of any age who require home care service when they are recovering from illness or surgery or when they are terminally ill
- For ongoing care of chronically ill adults and children to avoid hospitalization

Goals of Home Healthcare

Nurses provide home care to clients with complex, chronic, or terminal illness. The primary goals in home healthcare are that

1. The client's self-care ability and independence will improve.
2. Caregivers gain the ability to assist the client with ongoing health needs.

This approach may be very different from what you have experienced in other clinical settings.

Example: As the nurse in the Meet Your Patients scenario, you would help the couple manage Mr. Escobar's care independently at home. Initially you might show Mrs. Escobar how to administer medications and explain their function and demonstrate strategies for moving and turning Mr. Escobar. However, your goal would be for her to progress to manage these tasks independently.

Distinctive Features of Home Healthcare

Home Health Nursing Differs From Community Nursing Community health nurses provide care for individuals, families, and groups, with an emphasis on population-based care. In contrast, home health nursing focuses on the individual and their support system.

Nursing Care in the Home Differs From Hospital Nursing The hospital environment is controlled. Surfaces are regularly disinfected; supplies are stocked; and foods, medications, and other therapies are readily available. Computers and tablets with easily accessible patient information are conveniently located. In addition, the hospital-based nurse can consult almost immediately with a team of healthcare providers (i.e., other nurses, the primary care provider, various therapists, social workers, a pastoral care provider, and a business office staff to work with third-party payers). When you are a home health nurse:

- You are a guest in the client's home. The client and family determine whether they are willing to let you enter the home to deliver care.
- You are more self-sufficient and function independently. There are no other team members in the home who are immediately available for support, assistance, or consultation.
- You must be aware of and comfortable with the family observing you as you provide care.
- You will need to adapt to varying family relationships and some home environments that are difficult or dysfunctional.

  ♥ iCare ▪ You will need to encourage the family to help in providing care and in taking over care when you leave the home. Be aware that overburdened caregivers may need your help as much as the client.

- You must preplan your visit by mapping the sites in advance and arranging appointments efficiently.

- ⬥ Your personal safety may be more of a concern when making home visits. You must always be aware of the environment around you and alert to possible risks.

- You will need to be flexible and learn to modify your plan because things do not always go as planned in a less controlled home environment.
- You are responsible for making the assessments and determining where to advise the primary care provider of client changes.
- You must bring all necessary supplies or arrange to have them delivered to the home.
- You must distinguish between skilled services, which are eligible for government-subsidized programs, and those that are not.
  - **Skilled services** must be performed or supervised by a licensed healthcare professional (Box 37-2).
  - **Homemaker services** (e.g., cleaning, meal preparation) are provided by home health aides.

When You Are in a Patient's Home, Surprisingly Little Is Within Your Control The home may be clean and tidy or in chaos, food plentiful or scarce, and supplies readily available or unreliable. The television or music may be loud, a dog may bark continually, or young children may be playing nearby and repeatedly interrupting your interactions with the client or caregiver.

Home Healthcare Helps You to Better Understand the Concept of Client The home is a window into the client's life, through which you can see their personal environment and how it is equipped to meet the client's health needs. When in the client's home, you have an opportunity to get a feel for the kind of support the client has for health and personal care (Fig. 37-7). The photos, mementos, personal belongings, and other things the client values make cultural beliefs and practices more visible. These things provide clues to the client's lifestyle, strengths, resources, and motivation.

BOX 37-2 ▪ Skilled Nursing Services

Medicare defines *skilled nursing care* as services and care that can be done safely and correctly only by a licensed registered or practical nurse. Medically necessary services must be reasonable and necessary for the treatment of the illness or injury.

- Patient assessment
- Ongoing monitoring of patient status
- Management and coordination of the patient's plan of care
- Evaluation of response to medications or treatment
- Medication instruction or administration
- Supplies and durable medical equipment
- Teaching patients or caregivers to provide care or therapies
- Disease-related teaching (e.g., diabetes education)
- Complex tasks, such as injections, insertion of urinary catheters, infusion therapy, wound care, ostomy care, tube feedings, chest tube care, or ventilator management
- Social services

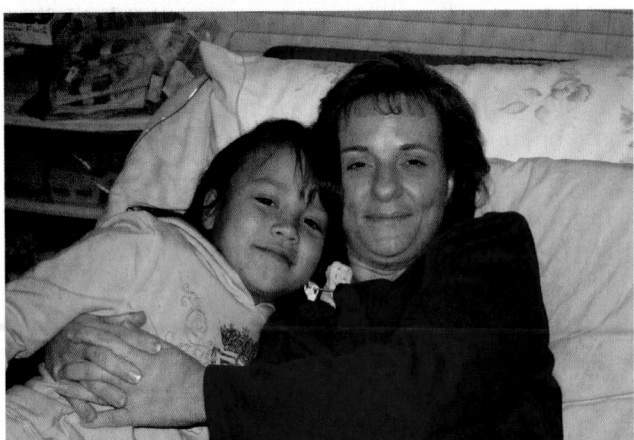

FIGURE 37-7 The home is a window into the client's life.

KnowledgeCheck 37-6

Identify at least four skilled services that may be provided in the home.

WHO PROVIDES HOME HEALTHCARE?

Home healthcare is provided by a variety of healthcare professionals employed by or working in cooperation with home healthcare agencies.

Home Health Agencies

Home health agencies coordinate the services of various professionals and paraprofessionals. They may be categorized by purpose, by type of client served, or by funding source.

Purpose In this category, **direct care agencies** are the most common.

- **Direct care agencies** focus on direct client interaction by providing skilled care, associated therapies and health services, home health aides, chore workers, and delivery of **respite care** (relief for family caregivers).
- **Indirect service agencies** also play a vital role in home healthcare. Examples of indirect home services include pharmaceutical and infusion companies and suppliers of durable medical equipment.
- **Durable medical equipment (DME)** is reusable equipment (e.g., walkers, wheelchairs, hospital beds, apnea monitors, suction, oxygen equipment) needed in the home setting for healthcare, mobility, and daily living. Medicare pays for some devices, but not all. It is expensive, so before ordering it, be sure the DME is covered or the client is able to cover the cost.

Type of Client Served An important specialty home service agency is hospice care. This may be a separate agency or a division of a home health agency. Hospice care may be provided in the home or at a free-standing hospice facility. Other agencies specialize in caring for patients with complex diseases, provide care to those who are ventilator-dependent, or offer health or assistive services for a specific age-group (e.g., older adults or chronically ill children).

Funding Source Agencies may take on many forms based on funding source, profit or nonprofit status, and relationship with other healthcare organizations.

- **Public agencies** are official or governmental agencies organized at the city, county, state, or national level. They are usually funded by taxes, along with reimbursement from insurance companies. The local health department is a good example of a public agency. Health departments focus chiefly on community needs, although they often also offer some home health services, especially when tracking clients in some of their disease management programs.
- **Voluntary agencies** are prominent in the delivery of home healthcare. These agencies are normally governed by a board of directors and funded by donations, endowments, and third-party (insurance) reimbursement. Many **hospice organizations** (groups that provide care for people who are frail, terminally ill, dying, or not expected to improve) are voluntary organizations.
- **Proprietary organizations** are corporate or privately owned businesses that aim to make a profit. These agencies receive payment from insurance companies but also accept private-pay clients. Proprietary organizations may provide traditional home health services as well as agency care and other services that assist individuals in remaining independent.
- **Hospital-based agencies** are an extension of the services provided by a hospital. Clients who do not meet the criteria for continued hospitalization may be transferred to home care for continued services. A benefit of this type of home health agency is the ease of transition between hospital and home.

The Home Health Team

In home healthcare, the registered nurse serves as the coordinator of health services, but other members of the healthcare team may also provide care. The team varies according to the needs of the client but is usually interprofessional. It may include providers; nurse practitioners; registered nurses; licensed practical (vocational) nurses; home health aides; physical, speech, occupational, or respiratory therapists; nutritionists; social workers; pharmacists; podiatrists; dentists; chaplains; and family members.

Home Health Nurses

To succeed in home healthcare, you must have the ability to work independently and collaboratively, be flexible and resourceful, and adapt to different home environments and family interactions. Communication is crucial in home care because of the need to establish good rapport and trust with the client and family and to communicate frequently with other members of the healthcare team. Home health nurses provide a broad range of services to clients of all ages, and they often fill a number of roles as part of their nursing care. A nurse in this role requires patience, compassion, and specific knowledge of the symptoms and conditions of the clients they care for.

Direct Care Provider As a direct care provider, you may administer medication, provide wound care, monitor blood pressure, assess for pressure injury or muscle weakness, or perform other skilled and complex tasks.

Client and Family Educator Recall that the goal of home healthcare is to promote self-care. Instead of focusing on performing the procedures, you will be helping the client or family take over the care. You can easily see the need to communicate skillfully in this role. You must be able to clearly explain the care required, the rationale for it, and how to safely perform the care. This requires patience, skill, and repetition.

Client Advocate In home care, the client and family are directly in charge of the plan of care. As client advocate, you support the client's right to make healthcare decisions yet protect the client from harm if they are unable to make decisions. In the event family members disagree, remember that as the client's advocate, you must try to see that the client's choices are respected and their rights are upheld. You must also advocate for services the client needs. This may mean trying to secure additional home health support to avoid hospitalization, or it may mean advocating for another level of service, such as referral to hospice or placement in the hospital, based on your assessment of the client and discussion with the client and family.

Care Coordinator Home health nurses must manage and coordinate care among the team of healthcare providers. In this role, you would gather data at an initial visit and develop a plan of care that addresses the client's needs. Your plan may require you to make additional visits as well as specify and perhaps arrange delivery of therapies and services by other professionals in the home.

KnowledgeCheck 37-7

What roles does the nurse assume in home care? List and describe them.

Hospice Care

As you learned in Chapter 14, **hospice nursing** provides compassionate care to patients with life-limiting conditions. The goal of hospice care is to promote comfort and quality of life. This end-of-life care includes provisions for expert medical care, pain management, and emotional and spiritual support based on the patient's individual needs and intentions (National Hospice and Palliative Care Organization, 2020). More than promoting self-care and independence, hospice care focuses on providing comfort and managing symptoms (Table 37-1).

Hospice services are provided in the patient's home, in the hospital, in assistive living facilities, and in palliative care facilities specifically designed for end-of-life care (hospice). The roles of the hospice nurse and home health nurse differ mainly in their emphasis.

- **As a direct care provider,** the hospice nurse assesses the client's condition and monitors the client's responses to interventions aimed at relieving distress, managing pain, urinary and bowel elimination, rest and sleep, and hydration and nutrition.

- **As an educator,** the hospice nurse teaches the client and family how to adjust medications and care to control pain and other symptoms.
- **As a communicator and client advocate,** the hospice nurse assumes prime importance as the client's condition deteriorates.

The nurse shares these roles with the family and other home caregivers. Generally, there are fewer services to coordinate in home hospice care. Instead, there may be a greater emphasis on pain management. If you need more information on hospice care, see Chapter 14.

WHO PAYS FOR HOME HEALTHCARE?

Medicare, Medicaid, other government-funded or government-mandated coverage, private insurance, and individual payments (private pay) help pay for home care services. Medicare and Medicaid are the largest payers for home healthcare.

Government Subsidy

Medicare Medicare is a federally funded healthcare system designed to provide health coverage for persons who are older than 65 years and younger people who are disabled or diagnosed with end-stage renal disease or amyotrophic lateral sclerosis (Social Security Administration, 2022). Reimbursement by Medicare for home care depends on the following strictly applied criteria:

- *The client must need skilled care.* See Box 37-2. Other services may also be provided, but the primary purpose for establishing care must be based on a skilled care need. This means that Medicare will not pay for personal care such as bathing and dressing when this is the only care the client needs.
- *The client must be homebound.* This means (1) the client must have a condition that restricts the ability to leave the home, and (2) leaving the home requires

Table 37-1 ➤ Home Healthcare and Home Hospice Care

	HOME HEALTHCARE	HOME HOSPICE CARE
Purpose	Promote self-care and independence.	Promote comfort and quality of life.
Focus of Nursing Interventions	Teach the family or other caregivers to assist the client with ongoing health needs and activities of daily living.	Provide comfort and manage symptoms.
Examples of Services	Wound care, medication administration, injections, dietary assistance, assistance with mobility, monitoring of vital signs and health needs, care coordination, communication, pain management, safety in the home, patient education, immunization, assessment of child development	Provide pain management; support caregivers; provide nutrition and hydration; ensure coordination of care; manage side effects of medication, chemotherapy, and radiation therapy; facilitate spiritual care.

special assistance, transportation, supportive devices, or an escort.

- *The client must require nursing care that is part time and intermittent.* This means Medicare will pay for a limited number of hours per day or days per week that the client can get skilled nursing care or home health aide services.
- *The plan of care must be authorized by the provider and recertified every 60 days.* For the client to continue to receive care, there must be evidence of continued need that remains acute.
- *The care must be medically necessary and reasonable.* The plan of care must address the client's health concerns and have clearly delineated outcomes. The expectations of the patient must be reasonable.
- *Medicare will pay only for interventions identified in the treatment plan.* The payer may periodically request patient health records to verify that the care was given.
- *The home health agency must be approved by Medicare.* An agency must show that it meets the Medicare definitions and requirements to become Medicare certified.

Medicaid Medicaid is a medical assistance program sponsored jointly by the federal government and individual states to provide healthcare services to people with low or very low income. In many states, the criteria for reimbursement are the same as those required by Medicare. However, each state at present determines what services will be part of its medical assistance plan.

Private Insurance and Self-Payment

Private insurance companies may also offer home health services. The type and extent of covered services are specified in each separate insurance group and plan. Many people require assistance in the home but do not meet the criteria for reimbursement from Medicare, Medicaid, or their private insurer. Frequently, older adults require home health assistance but may not need skilled services. For example, they may need assistance with grocery shopping, meal planning and preparation, or transportation. Those services are the responsibility of the client.

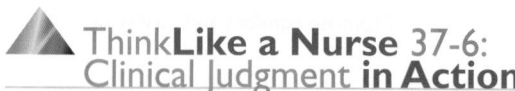
ThinkLike a Nurse 37-6:
Clinical Judgment **in Action**

Review the scenario focused on Mr. Escobar (Meet Your Patients). What members of the home health team may be required to provide care? Why?

HOW ARE CLIENTS REFERRED TO HOME HEALTHCARE?

Referrals to home healthcare come from a variety of sources. However, for home care to begin, there must be a medical prescription and a provider-approved treatment plan.

Hospital-based agencies have a built-in referral base. If the primary provider or nursing staff determines that the client would benefit from home health services, they refer the patient to the agency for evaluation while the client is still hospitalized.

Many agencies have *intake coordinators* who work in the hospital and review clients for suitability of services, gathering information from the chart, the client, the family, and the hospital team. Home services are arranged before discharge from an inpatient facility. Ideally, a discharge planner gathers information, secures the prescription from the provider, and makes arrangements. In some smaller hospitals, this task falls to the staff nurse providing predischarge care.

Referrals may also come from primary care providers, nurses, mental health workers, and other healthcare providers in the community, as well as directly from families and clients. Most home health agencies evaluate clients to determine whether they are eligible for services that are reimbursable by insurance. They may also offer services that the client may pay for independently.

WHAT IS THE FUTURE OF HOME HEALTHCARE?

Healthcare analysts have predicted several changes in home care during the next few decades:

- **Increased need for home healthcare.** Considering the growing population of older adults in the United States, it is more cost effective to provide healthcare in the home than in an inpatient setting.
- **Increased use of the home for hospice care.** Public acceptance of the home as a place of comfort and care, as well as concerns about the cost of inpatient care, has increased the number of persons who choose this compassionate option for end-of-life and palliative care.
- **Increased technology.** Technological advances, such as online resources or telemedicine consultation, make it safer and more affordable to deliver complex care in the home and allow home health nurses to deliver information and provide support (Bradford et al., 2013). Digital monitoring and documentation allow home health agencies to better coordinate care, receive needed supplies, and manage costs.
- **Continued research.** Research is needed in the area of strategies to improve the effectiveness of care, identify predictors of need for rehospitalization, and integrate home care into overall community-based services.

PracticalKnowledge
knowing **how**

Normally your caseload will be contained within a designated geographic boundary so that you can schedule your visits efficiently, spend less time driving to visits, and have more time for delivering care. If you want to know what it would be like to be a home health nurse, you need only look at the list of services Medicare recognizes as skilled, listed in Box 37-2.

HOW DO I MAKE A HOME VISIT?

The home visit has three phases: preparation before the visit, nursing care during the visit, and evaluation after the visit.

Before the Visit

First, review the client's chart and referral form to determine why you are making the visit. You may also need to review material about the client's health problem, medications, or treatment plan. Then you can begin to plan for the visit. What supplies will you need? What teaching materials will you need? What are the goals of the visit? Does the agency require additional client information, such as insurance data, to provide care? The agency will have forms (e.g., Health Insurance Portability and Accountability Act [HIPAA] privacy forms, billing information) for you to complete during the first visit. Be sure you have those with you.

⊕ Before the visit, you will need to map directions to the home and determine whether there are safety concerns. Contact the client to notify them of the scheduled date and time of the visit and to determine whether their health status has changed since the referral was made. This allows you to bring additional equipment or personnel along if needed.

Prepare Supplies

Home health nurses usually carry an equipment bag (Fig. 37-8) with supplies geared to the needs of the clients in the nurse's caseload.

- Hand hygiene supplies (e.g., soap or antibacterial handrub, paper towels)
- Stethoscope
- Sphygmomanometers (with cuffs in a variety of sizes)
- Thermometers (oral and rectal) with protective covers
- Small equipment (scissors, forceps, penlight, staple remover)
- Tape measure (with plastic coating that can be cleaned, or several disposable ones)
- Full, protective gown (disposable)
- Gloves, sterile and clean
- An assortment of gauze and transparent occlusive dressings. tape, and scissors
- Occupational Safety and Health Administration (OSHA) supplies: N95 respirator and face masks, protective eyewear, disinfectant spray, disposable gowns to cover clothing
- A variety of syringes and safety needles; sharps disposal container
- Venipuncture supplies

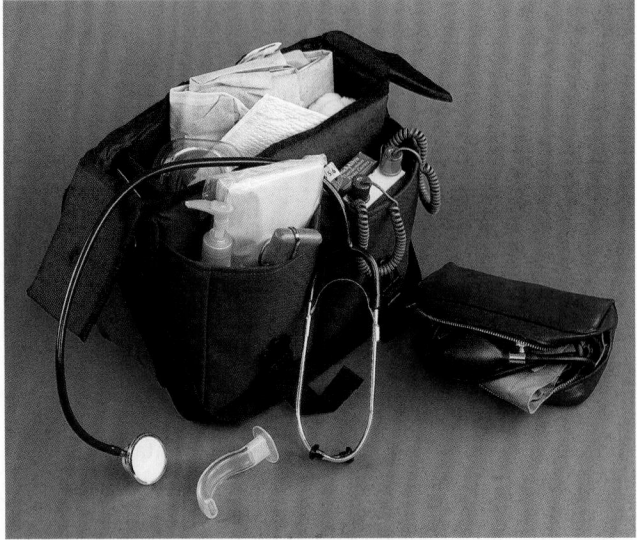

FIGURE 37-8 The home health equipment bag contains some standard items but is usually customized according to the client's needs.

- Airway and resuscitation mask
- Specific supplies as needed (IV therapy, tube feeding supplies, ostomy supplies, urinary catheter kit, wound care, etc.)

You may need other supplies, such as oxygen tanks and tubing, medication, a scale, and a transfer belt, depending on the requirements of clients in your caseload. If the client needs frequent dressing changes or supplies for treatments (e.g., tube feedings, stoma care, wound care), it is best to have the supplies delivered directly to the client's house to reduce the number of materials you must carry.

⊕ Note that in some states, nurses are not permitted to carry medications because of safety concerns. You will need to check on the rules that apply to your state.

The nurse carrying the equipment bag into the home may potentially act as a reservoir for transmitting pathogenic microorganisms. To minimize the spread of infection from one home to another, if you are carrying an equipment bag,

 Go to **Chapter 37, Clinical Insight 37-2: Infection Control in the Home,** in Volume 2.

Provide for Your Safety

⊕ As you drive to the home, begin to make your assessment. Locate the stores, hospital, and community resources. What is the overall character of the neighborhood? Does this appear to be a safe neighborhood? What are the conditions of the approach to the home?

Safety for yourself and the client is an essential consideration when you enter someone's home. It is important for you to provide your agency with your patient care schedule for the day and a tracking device to identify your location in case you need to summon help. For suggestions about the safe delivery of home healthcare,

 Go to **Chapter 37, Clinical Insight 37-2: Infection Control in the Home,** in Volume 2.

KnowledgeCheck 37-8

What are the major tasks that must be completed before making a home visit?

At the Visit

Identify yourself Upon your arrival, be sure to wear your identification badge and provide contact information for the home health agency. Generally, agencies have information packets that include the client's bill of rights, client responsibilities, billing information, information on the frequency and duration of services, how to reach the agency, and the date and time of the next visit.

♥ **iCare   Remember the Home is the Client's Personal Space** Knock or ring the doorbell and wait to be invited inside. Introduce yourself to the client and family. Be respectful of their home, as well as their beliefs, values, practices, and cultural preferences.

Develop rapport and trust The first few minutes of the initial visit set the tone for the relationship among client, family, nurse, and agency. This is your opportunity to develop rapport and trust. Introducing yourself, waiting for permission to enter, and treating the client and family members with respect are ways to help to establish rapport (Fig. 37-9).

Gather data During the visit, you will assess your client's environment and others involved in home care. Who answered your questions? What is the relationship between the caregiver and the client? How do they interact? What other people live there? What is the condition of the home? If this is an initial visit, you may need to verify or complete client data on the referral form. In the hospital, admissions personnel usually gather admitting data and obtain consent for treatment. In home care, you need to collect and document this information.

♥ **iCare   Manage Client Care Tasks Efficiently and With Caring** At a home visit, you might do a variety of things, such as performing physical care; conducting a physical assessment; drawing blood samples for laboratory work; checking weight; administering medication, IV fluid, or tube feedings; providing wound or ostomy care; managing chest tube draining and dressing changes; or whatever is needed. Always be compassionate and caring, even when performing tasks.

 ThinkLike a Nurse 37-7: **Clinical Judgment in Action**

Review the case of Mr. Escobar (Meet Your Patients). What information did you gain from the first few minutes of the visit?

- Both Mr. and Mrs. Escobar are in need of nursing interventions. However, this is your agency's first home visit to them, and you have other clients you must visit today, so you will need to prioritize. What must the home health nurse do during the initial visit to a client?
- In addition to completing your assessment and talking about a plan of care with the Escobars, what do you think is the single most important thing you can do for them today? Explain your thinking.
- When Mrs. Escobar meets you at the door and brings you into the living room, you notice a large German shepherd dog lying beside Mr. Escobar's bed. Mrs. Escobar says, "Stay, King"; and then to you, "Roland likes having him nearby." What should you do?

After the Visit

After you leave the home, there is still a lot of work for you to do. Often you will need to complete the documentation for the visit. In Chapter 17, you learned about documentation techniques, various forms of charting, and legal aspects of documentation. In home care, all these rules apply; however, some aspects of home care documentation are unique:

- Home health agencies use Medicare's Outcome and Assessment Information Set (OASIS) to record initial assessment data.
- To continue to provide needed services to the client, you must include the following in your documentation:
  1. Evidence of homebound status
  2. Evidence of continued need for skilled care

Other postvisit activities include ordering supplies needed for the next visit, making referrals to additional services (e.g., occupational therapy), coordinating care among the various services, and scheduling the next visit.

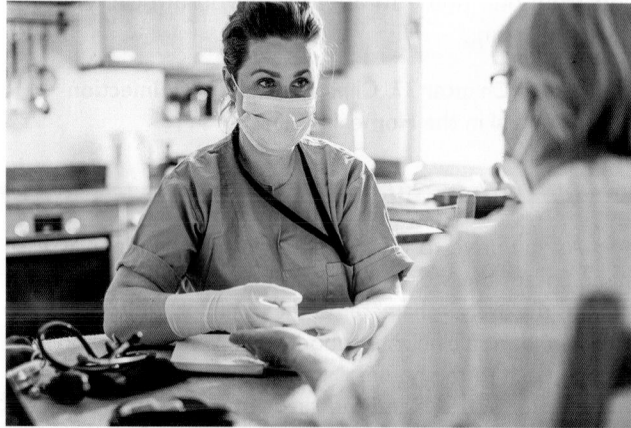

FIGURE 37-9 The first few minutes of the initial visit set the tone for the relationship among client, family, nurse, and agency.

NURSING PROCESS IN HOME CARE

The nursing process moves through the same phases in all patient care settings. In the home, you assess the client, the family, the home, and the community to identify nursing diagnoses and other patient problems. You then will use a plan for patient care prescribed by a medical provider but individualize it with suitable nursing diagnoses and interventions. You will periodically evaluate the client's continued need for healthcare in the home.

ASSESSMENT/RECOGNIZING CUES

On the initial visit, you need to perform an assessment to establish a baseline and determine the type of care required. Typically, a full assessment requires multiple visits.

This assessment includes:

- Health history
- Review of medications—prescribed, over-the-counter, and complementary alternative medicine (CAM)
- Pertinent family and social history
- Mental status
- Functional ability for performing ADLs
- Availability of family and informal support and caregivers
- Nutritional status
- Assessment of the home environment

Home health agencies are required to collect patient-specific information for all Medicare clients they serve. The OASIS data must be collected at the start of care, with each recertification (every 60 days), and at the termination of care. Medicare uses these data to plan care, determine reimbursement, measure the effectiveness of care, and monitor client outcomes. In addition to the required OASIS information, many agencies use other assessment tools created specifically for their needs.

♥ **iCare** It is also important to assess the needs of the caregivers—the family members, friends, and support system in the home. To be successful in the role of home care nurse, you must work *with* the caregivers. Take time at each visit to speak with them, making sure to include them in your assessment, plan of care, and teaching. Assessment of the caregivers often allows you to determine what services are needed in the home. Caregivers may be managing health issues of their own that affect their ability to provide care for another. This is common among older adults.

NURSING DIAGNOSIS/ANALYZING CUES

As in any setting, the nursing diagnoses are based on the client's responses to illness and care. As a home healthcare nurse, you will work with clients with numerous medical and nursing diagnoses. Three frequently used NANDA-I nursing diagnoses are Caregiver Role Strain,

---

Holistic Healing

Holistic Healing for Illness Prevention

Thaik, C., Moscucci, M., Warber, S. L., & Aaronson, K. D. (2020). Complementary and alternative medicine. In R. Baliga & K. Eagle (Eds.), *Practical cardiology* (pp. 429–446). https://doi.org/10.1007/978-3-030-28328-5_34

Basic categories of complementary and alternative medical (CAM) therapies:

- Alternative medical systems—naturopathy and acupuncture
- Mind–body interventions—meditation and hypnotherapy
- Manipulative and body-based methods—massage therapy and chiropractic
- Energy therapies—reiki and polarity therapy
- Biologically based treatments—herbal remedies and chelation therapy

Although CAM therapies are commonly used for preventing and treating various health issues, CAM users typically do not talk to their providers about the treatments. Because CAM can augment or interfere with the effectiveness of traditional medical therapies, it is increasingly important for practitioners to be familiar with various forms of CAM and to specifically elicit and document a history of CAM usage in the home.

Using an open and nonjudgmental approach, ask your patients what specific natural products and treatments they are using for promoting health and preventing illness. Is the CAM effective in producing desired effects? Are the CAM users experiencing any undesired side effects?

Knowledge Deficit, and Risk for Infection (Herdman & Kamitsuru, 2020).

Caregiver Role Strain and Risk for Caregiver Role Strain These nursing diagnoses are appropriate for those for whom the burden of caregiving has become, or is at risk of becoming, overwhelming. Providing care to a loved one at home can be a challenge, especially when resources and caregiver support are challenged. Around-the-clock caregiving duties can lead to physical exhaustion, social isolation, resentment, sadness, or depression. In addition, the demands of caring for the client can interfere with other responsibilities. Common signs of caregiver role strain include difficulty adjusting to role changes, fatigue, isolation, depression, anxiety, and difficulty in performing routine care for the client.

Knowledge Deficit Client and family teaching is especially important for home care because most of the caregiving is performed by the client and significant others. You will spend much of your time teaching them the skills necessary for self-care (e.g., how to administer insulin, how to manage the oxygen equipment). Recall that to be eligible for home nursing care, clients must require skilled nursing care. Client education is a service for which Medicare and other insurers will reimburse. You must be certain to include a Knowledge Deficit diagnosis on the care plan to ensure the client's continued eligibility and reimbursement for the service.

Key Point: *In other chapters we caution against indiscriminate use of the Knowledge Deficit diagnosis. However, an exception must be made for home care because of Medicare regulations.*

Safety and Risk for Infection Safety and risk for infection are also key concerns in the home. These are thoroughly discussed in Chapters 20 and 21, respectively. Infection control measures in the home are also presented later in this chapter. Associated diagnoses include Home Maintenance Alteration, Risk for Falls, Risk for Infection, and Poisoning Risk (Herdman & Kamitsuru, 2020).

KnowledgeCheck 37-9

- Why are the first few minutes of the initial visit so important?
- Identify five things that should be assessed at an initial home visit.

ThinkLike a Nurse 37-8: Clinical Judgment in Action

- Based on the information in the scenario, what nursing diagnoses might Mr. Escobar (Meet Your Patients) have? There may not be enough data to make definite diagnoses, but what probable diagnoses are there for which you would want to gather confirming data? Do not include potential diagnoses, such as Risk for Imbalanced Nutrition.
- Mr. Escobar has a potential problem, Risk for Falls. What are two interventions you would probably be able to do today to reduce his fall risk?
- What, if any, evidence of caregiver strain does Mrs. Escobar exhibit?

Standardized Terminology for Home Health Nursing Diagnoses

Various disciplines, including nursing, have developed classifications of common terminology (also called *taxonomies, vocabularies,* and *standardized languages*) for describing their work and for planning and documenting care. You are familiar with the NANDA-I taxonomy of nursing diagnoses; however, home care nurses more commonly use the CCC because it is closely related to the OASIS reporting forms required by Medicare. If you need to review the concept of standardized nursing language, see Chapter 3.

The CCC contains standardized and coded nursing diagnostic categories that are especially applicable to home healthcare. The CCC coding structure and framework system are relevant to home care in the following ways:

- Parallel the steps of the nursing process
- Link the CCC diagnoses to nursing interventions and client outcomes
- Standardize the terminology for client care within clinical information systems
- Facilitate nursing documentation at the point of care
- Provide a structure for planning resources needed for client and community care
- Quantify the nursing workload to optimize productivity
- Define client outcomes for quality care
- Provide quantitative data for research (Saba, 1994/2004/2012; CCC, n.d.)

Common CCC nursing diagnoses used for home care include:

Activities of Daily Living (ADLs) Alteration
Caregiver Role Strain
Family Processes Alteration
Home Maintenance Alteration
Knowledge Deficit
Physical Mobility Impairment
Self-Care Deficit

For complete information on the CCC and complete lists of diagnoses, framework, outcomes, and interventions,

 Go to the **CCC Web site** at https://careclassification.org/

PLANNING/PRIORITIZING HYPOTHESES AND GENERATING SOLUTIONS

Each Nursing Diagnosis requires an Expected Outcome, which is the anticipated goal of the nursing actions planned to care for the patient's condition (Saba, 1994/2004/2012; CCC, n.d.).

Clinical Care Classification System To formulate a goal/outcome in the CCC system, attach one of the three CCC "modifiers" *(improve, stabilize, deteriorate)* to the diagnosis.

- The outcome describes the *desired* client health status.
- To evaluate client progress, you again use one of the three modifiers to describe the client's *actual* health status.
- The following is an example:

CCC nursing diagnosis:	Knowledge Deficit
Goal/expected outcome:	Knowledge Deficit, Improve
Actual status on evaluation:	Knowledge Deficit, Stabilized

Medicare requires that the client's status be evaluated and coded as improved, stabilized, or deteriorated, the same as the CCC system. In your nursing notes, you would document additional narrative to support your evaluation.

Nursing Outcomes Classification The NOC taxonomy can be used in home health nursing (Moorhead et al., 2018). A few of the outcomes that pertain to home and families are:

Caregiver Home Care Readiness
Caregiver Performance: Direct Care
Caregiver Stressors
Family Coping
Family Functioning

To prepare the client and family for self-care, inform them of the needs you have identified and involve them in setting goals and planning care. They may be able to identify strategies to solve problems or to help you identify needs that are not readily apparent.

IMPLEMENTATION/TAKING ACTION

Medicare requires that the provider-prescribed plan of care include the following, as applicable:

- Parameters for notifying the primary provider of changes in vital signs and other clinical findings
- Diabetic foot care, including education
- Falls prevention interventions
- Depression interventions
- Interventions to monitor and treat pain
- Interventions to prevent pressure injury
- Pressure injury treatments

Once the plan of care has been agreed on, you will document it and forward it to the client's provider for certification. At the first visit, you will determine the specific skilled care required and make referrals to other required services, such as physical, occupational, or speech therapy; social services; nutritional support; or home health aide services.

Standardized Nursing Interventions

The CCC system is commonly used in planning and recording home care, but the NIC taxonomy is also an option.

CCC Nursing Interventions for Home Care The CCC contains nursing interventions organized according to the care components. An intervention consists of a label (e.g., Activity Care) and a definition (e.g., Actions performed to carry out physiological or psychological daily activities). In addition to the label, you must specify the type of intervention action from among four qualifiers:

Assess/Monitor/Evaluate/Observe
Care/Perform/Provide/Assist
Teach/Educate/Instruct/Supervise
Manage/Refer/Contact/Notify

The CCC nursing interventions include only skilled services because this type of service is the only type of care reimbursed by Medicare and most insurers in home health. In the Meet Your Patients scenario, Mrs. Escobar is clearly experiencing Caregiver Strain. This is a nursing diagnosis under the Care Component of Coping. Several interventions are possible:

Coping Support: Actions to sustain a person dealing with responsibilities, problems, or difficulties

Assess for Caregiver Strain.
Provide (perform) emotional support.
Refer to community services: caregiver support groups, Meals on Wheels, and respite care services.

You can see the entire list of interventions on the previously cited CCC Web site (sabacare.com).

NIC Interventions for Home Care The NIC standardized language may also be used in home health nursing (Butcher et al., 2018). A few of the interventions that pertain to home and families are Caregiver Support, Family Integrity Promotion, Home Maintenance Assistance, and Respite Care.

Assisting With Medication Management

One of The Joint Commission 2020 safety goals for home care is to use medications safely. This includes:

- Identifying patients correctly
- Preventing errors with look-alike and sound-alike medications
- Educating patients about anticoagulant therapy
- Keeping a current list and reconciling medications when a client transfers from one agency or health system to another

The Joint Commission also advises nurses to diligently compare those medications the patient is already taking with new ones to be given in the home. Make sure your patients know about the medications they take at home. Recommend that they keep a complete list of medications, including dosing, in a safe place, in the event of an emergency. They should also bring a complete and updated list every time they visit a healthcare provider.

Nonadherence Some patients, particularly older adults, have visual and motor deficits that limit their ability to read labels and manipulate bottle caps, syringes, and so on. Other reasons for noncompliance include lack of outward symptoms, inability to tolerate side effects, pain, forgetfulness, low motivation, and impaired mental capacity. **Key Point:** *Always investigate the patient's reasons for nonadherence so that you can take appropriate action.*

Teaching Skills An important part of the role of the home health nurse is to teach clients and caregivers skills, such as measuring dosages, giving injections, wound care, and managing intravenous therapy. Or they may need tips on how to help clients with difficulty swallowing take oral medications. For example, for some clients, pills may be crushed and mixed in a small amount of applesauce or pudding.

 Older Adults Involve family members in the care of the older adult as needed, including giving medication. Older adult patients and caregivers may have difficulty remembering when to take their pills, which ones to take, and even whether they have already taken them.

- **Medication Organizer**—Suggest they use a medication organizer with a compartment for each day of the week (Fig. 37-10). You may need to prepare a week's worth of oral medications for them during your visits.
- **Drug Cards**—To help them remember which drug is used for each of their illnesses or symptoms, write the medical condition, names of medications and what they are used for, dosages, and how and when to take the medication on a large card. Then use clear tape to attach a sample of each drug next to its name on the card.

Safe Disposal Because improperly disposed-of medication may end up in the public water supply, it is important to inform clients about how to safely dispose of medications in the home:

- Return unwanted or expired prescription and over-the-counter drugs to a drug take-back program.
- Some counties offer household hazardous waste collection sites where drugs are accepted.
- Expired or unused prescription and over-the-counter drugs should never be flushed down the toilet or poured into a drain unless the label or accompanying patient information specifies that it is safe to do so (U.S. Food & Drug Administration, 2020).

For more information about ways to properly discard medication, see **Chapter 21, Home Care: Preventing Poisoning in the Home.**

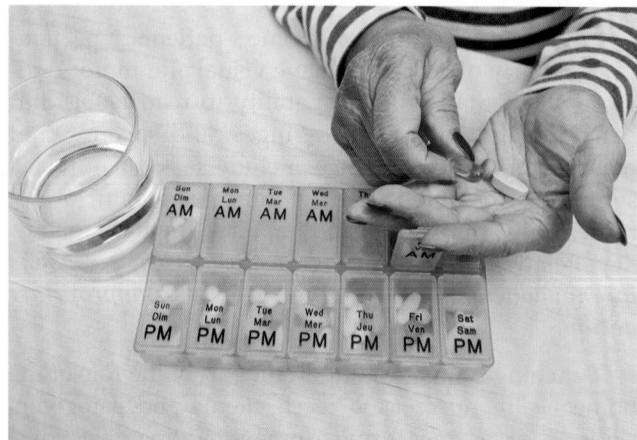

FIGURE 37-10 Using a weekly medication reminder box to organize doses.

Controlling Infection in the Home

The Joint Commission 2023 safety goals for home care include reducing the risk of healthcare-associated infections. In the hospital, you have ready access to supplies that facilitate infection control. The home presents unique challenges.

Key Point: *Hand hygiene is one of the most important home interventions to prevent the transmission of infection.* You will need to follow Standard Precautions but recognize how to modify infection control techniques for the home environment. For suggestions to help you maintain infection control during a home visit,

Refer to **Chapter 37, Clinical Insight 37-2: Infection Control in the Home,** in Volume 2.

See the accompanying Home Care Box, Unhealthy Home May Mean Poor Health, to learn how unhealthy housing conditions can lead to health problems.

Barrier Precautions

The reason you implement barrier precautions in the home setting differs from use in hospital practice. As a rule, you will use gowns, gloves, and masks in home care to protect yourself, rather than the patient. For instance, you will need to use contact and airborne precautions, including a fit-tested N95 respirator, when caring for clients who have airborne pathogens, such as pulmonary tuberculosis (TB), SARS-CoV-2 (COVID-19, coronavirus), measles, chickenpox, disseminated herpes zoster, or some multidrug-resistant infections (Centers for Disease Control and Prevention, 2016). Such organisms may be transmitted to other home care patients through inanimate objects or hands, so use appropriate barrier precautions. See Chapter 20 if you need to review infection control.

Clean and Sterile Technique

Infection control in home care is different in many ways from that in acute care. In acute care, the patient is exposed to invasive interventions and environmental risks, including other patients and contaminated inanimate objects. However, home care patients have usually developed some resistance to the microorganisms in their own homes and are less likely to acquire infections there than in the hospital environment. You may find differences in how you handle home infusion therapy, urinary tract care, respiratory care, wound care, and enteral therapy.

It is safe, in many instances, to replace sterile with clean technique in the home setting, as in some of the following examples:

- **Intravenous therapy.** Sterile practices should be the same at home as in the hospital because the associated risk of sepsis is so high.
- **Insulin injections and pumps.** Many people (e.g., those who have diabetes) may give themselves repeated injections, perhaps several each day, or

Unhealthy Home May Mean Poor Health

Home Care

Cause	Health Problem	Preventative or Corrective Action
Peeling, lead-based paint	Lead poisoning	➤ Test home for lead-based paint and replace.
Second-hand tobacco smoke	Asthma, lung cancer, death or injury resulting from fire	➤ Don't use tobacco products or let others smoke in the home.
Radon	Lung cancer	➤ Install radon detector and radon elimination equipment.
		➤ Periodically open windows.
Mold	Asthma, allergies, and anaphylaxis	➤ Correct moisture problem.
		➤ Use dehumidifier or fan.
Pesticides	Poisoning, cancer, prematurity	➤ Clean the home.
		➤ Use nontoxic products and dispose of safely.
		➤ Fix holes and cracks in the home.
Missing or inoperable smoke alarm or carbon monoxide detector	Death or injury resulting from fire	➤ Install smoke and carbon monoxide detector for each level of the home.
		➤ Check batteries regularly.
Structural problems	Injury	➤ Fix loose railings, stairs, and unsafe conditions.
		➤ Be sure electrical wiring is safe.
Extraordinary clutter, dust, and dirt	Infestation, infection, allergies	➤ Clean the home.
		➤ Remove loose rugs.
Poor ventilation	Respiratory problems, infection	➤ Open windows.
		➤ Use fans.

Source: Centers for Disease Control and Prevention. (n.d.). *A healthy home for everyone: The guide for families and individuals.* https://www.cdc.gov/nceh/lead/publications/final_companion_piece.pdf

Toward Evidence-Based Practice

Dowding, D., Russell, D., Frifilio, M., McDonald, M. V., Shang, J. (2020, July). Home care nurses' identification of patients at risk of infection and their risk mitigation strategies: A qualitative interview study. *International Journal of Nursing Studies, 107,* 103617. https://doi.org/10.1016/j.ijnurstu.2020.103617

In a descriptive study using structured interviews with 50 nurses who have experience in home care nursing, researchers wanted to know:

- How can nurses in the home care setting best identify patients at risk for infection?
- How do nurses modify the plan of care to prevent infection in the home environment?

The primary strategy for preventing infection in the home setting is patient and caregiver education, as well as nurses' careful attention to their own practices for reducing the risk of infection.

Ronneikko, J. K., Jamsen, E. R., Makela, M., Finne-Soveri, H., & Valvanne, J. N. (2018, September–October). Reasons for home care clients' unplanned hospital admissions and their associations with patient characteristics. *Archives of Gerontology and Geriatrics, 78,* 114–126. https://doi.org/10.1016/j.archger.2018.06.008

Researchers examined the problem of unplanned inpatient and emergency care among older adults within the first year of receiving healthcare in the home. Among 6,812 adults aged 63 and older, the most common reason for the first hospitalization was an infection (21%). Those admitted due to active infection also were more likely to experience chronic wounds, daily urinary incontinence, polypharmacy, and impaired cognitive capacity. Those with feelings of loneliness were more likely to be hospitalized than those with a strong support system.

McDonald, M. V., Brickner, C., Russel, D., Dowding, D., Larson, E. L., Rrifilio, M., Bick, I. Y., Sridharan, S., Song, J., Adams, V., Woo, K., & Shang, J.. (2021, May). Observation of hand hygiene practice in home health care. *Journal of the American Medical Directors Association, 22(5),* 1029–1034. https://doi.org/10.1016/j.jamda.2020.07.031

Continued

Toward Evidence-Based Practice—cont'd

In a study involving 2,014 opportunities for hand hygiene, the average adherence rate was 45.6%. Handy hygiene was practiced most often when contacting body fluid (65.1%). The lowest adherence was after touching a patient (29.5%). Researchers concluded that hand hygiene adherence in home healthcare is suboptimal but comparable to patterns observed in hospital and outpatient settings.

1. What are some of the patient-related factors that are likely to be related to higher infection rates in the home setting?

2. What might be some other home healthcare factors that could contribute to less effective control of infection in the home setting?

3. What are at least three other possible research-related explanations for the wide variation in infection rates between the different studies?

4. What are some ideas you have to improve the effectiveness of infection control practices in the home setting in which you might work?

---

require an insulin pump with a continuous glucose monitor (CGM). Supplies for home use are expensive. Insurance may or may not cover the cost, or the person may not have insurance.

■ Manufacturers recommend that disposable syringes and needles be used only once and discarded in a puncture-proof container, and it is safest to do that. Nevertheless, some people find it practical to reuse needles and syringes. For guidelines for teaching patients about this,

▶ Refer to **Chapter 23, Clinical Insight 23-1: Reusing Needles and Syringes: Home Care,** in Volume 2.

■ **Urinary catheters.** Clients and family typically use clean gloves to perform catheterization. In the home, clients frequently interrupt the drainage system to empty a leg bag or to change or disinfect the drainage bag. They may also disinfect and reuse urinary catheters.

■ **Respiratory care.** Tracheostomy care in the home is nearly always performed using clean, not sterile, technique. Chest tubes can also be managed in the home. The home health nurse's role is to teach caregivers how to empty collection containers, record pleural fluid output, properly discard drainage and contaminated supplies, and dress the site (Fig. 37-11).

■ **Wound care.** Procedures for wound care should be based on the risk for contamination and infection. Usually clean technique is adequate. For example, a closed surgical wound with no drains has a low risk for home care–acquired infection. However, if the incision has drains or is open, the risk for infection increases. Your wound-care procedures must address the increased risk. Show caregivers when and where to discard irrigation fluids. Teach them how to avoid contamination while providing wound care (e.g., how to handle the cap, always recap the bottle, and store the bottle away from children and pets).

■ **Enteral therapy.** Emphasize the need to refrigerate the feeding solution after opening and store under refrigeration until expiration. Teach caregivers to keep the kitchen and tools used in preparation meticulously

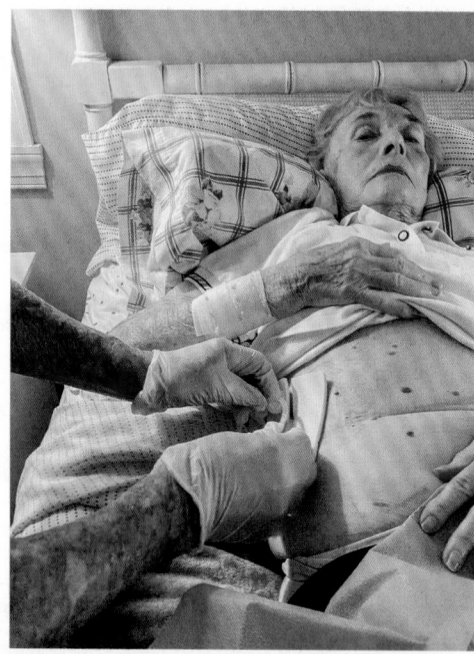

FIGURE 37-11 Caregiver changing chest tube dressing in the home.

clean. For example, blender parts, measuring cups, and spoons should be washed in a hot water dishwasher after use.

KnowledgeCheck 37-10

Identify three infection control supplies that you should bring in your equipment bag on a home health visit.

Promoting Home Safety

✚ The following two home care safety goals from The Joint Commission (2022) are important to keep in mind:

■ *Reduce the risk of patient harm resulting from falls.* Assess the client and the home for environmental hazard risk factors (e.g., dimly lit stairs, clutter on the floor, loose rugs) and teach caregivers about fall-reduction measures. Screen the patient's balance and strength, need for walking aids, and assistive technologies. Educate the patient concerning the potential for medications to make them feel weak, dizzy, or sleepy. Evaluate the patient's fall history, health conditions that compromise balance or mobility (e.g., stroke, neurological injury), alcohol consumption, and intake of medications that could interfere with balance and mobility. You will find an extensive discussion of fall prevention in Chapter 21 if you need more information.

- *Identify risks associated with oxygen therapy.* Be certain the home has working smoke detectors on every floor of the home, fire extinguishers, and a fire safety plan. Assess the client and family's ability to understand and comply with fire prevention activities, such as no smoking when oxygen is in use; report any concerns to the provider.

Supporting Caregivers

♥ **iCare** Even when the client is receiving in-home services from an agency, it is not usually around-the-clock care. If the client cannot perform self-care, most of the duties fall to family members. One study found that even with short-term formal services, family caregivers provided the majority of care to homebound patients. Half of the caregivers said they were not adequately prepared when it was time for their home health services to be discontinued. And at all stages, they expressed significant isolation, anxiety, and depression (Levine et al., 2006).

Unrelieved caregiving duties are physically and emotionally taxing. Caregivers may become depressed, physically exhausted, isolated from friends, and neglectful of their own health.

Healthcare professionals have a responsibility to recognize caregiver burden by conducting a thorough assessment of caregivers' roles and individual circumstances (Adelman et al., 2014). Caregiver support can relieve isolation and lessen the risk of depression, reduce the perceived burden of caregiving, and better prepare the caregivers for their role. However, the most improvement in adaptation to the caregiver role was shown by those with more independent lives and social support. See the iCare Box for suggestions to help caregivers.

♥ iCare 37-1

Ways to Help Caregivers

Provide a listening ear. Encourage caregivers to talk about what they do and how they feel; listen actively to their concerns. Find time to focus on the caregiver's needs rather than on those of the care recipient.

Give positive feedback and validate caregivers' importance to the client's health.

Help the caregiver identify people who may be able to help, for example, family members living outside the home, neighbors, church members, and community support groups.

Talk with family and friends, if the caregiver wishes. Teach them how to support the caregiver, for example, by calling and visiting regularly, sending cards and texts, or staying with the client so that the caregiver can rest or take a vacation. Encourage them to listen to the caregiver without giving advice and to help them feel appreciated (e.g., "I really appreciate all you do for Dad.").

Arrange for a home health aide, if possible. This relieves the caregiver of some housekeeping and grocery shopping.

Remind family members and significant others to take care of themselves. Explain that their health is important to both them and the patient. Even the most devoted person may understand when you explain, "You must take care of yourself so that you are able to take care of your loved one."

- Stress the need for the person to eat nutritious meals. Arrange for meals to be delivered to the home, if needed.

- Encourage the caregiver to rest as much as possible. Help contact those offering respite care and make a schedule, if needed. Provide reassurance that competent help can be obtained and that it is okay to delegate caregiving to others for a while. Time away, even if it is just an hour alone or coffee with a friend, can help to refresh caregivers.
- Some agencies have a weekend respite program for caregivers. The client is admitted to a skilled care unit for 2 or 3 days so that the caregiver can have a break.

Encourage the caregiver to maintain spiritual connections, if that is important to them and helps with coping—for example, take time to go to church, or ask the spiritual adviser to visit the home.

Communicate medical updates about the client—laboratory results, new treatment plans, and so on.

Help the family understand the goals of care and solve problems when needed.

Teach the family what to expect with regard to medications, treatments, and signs of approaching death. If family members know what is normal, they will be less likely to panic or fear the inevitable.

Follow up with other healthcare team members promptly if the family has questions that are outside your scope of practice.

To explore learning resources for this chapter,

Go to Davis Advantage and find:

Answers and Suggested Responses for all questions in this chapter
Concept Map
Knowledge Map
References and Bibliography

CHAPTER 38

Nursing Informatics

Learning Outcomes

After completing this chapter, you should be able to:

➤ Define *informatics* and its four components.

➤ Describe the importance of computers in evidence-based nursing practice.

➤ Explain the role of interoperability and standardized languages within the electronic health record system for exchanging health information.

➤ Discuss the benefits of the electronic health record.

➤ Discuss the impact of legislative efforts to encourage electronic health record adoption.

➤ Describe the importance of protecting personal health information.

➤ Explain the relationship between computers and standardized nursing languages.

➤ Identify at least two ways that automation decreases error in healthcare.

➤ Explain how computers can reduce some of the barriers to evidence-based practice.

➤ Identify at least four online sources of nursing research.

➤ Describe the process of literature database searching.

Key Concepts

Electronic communication

Healthcare technology

Informatics

Related Concepts

See the Knowledge Map on Davis Advantage.

Meet Your Nurse Role Model

Six weeks ago, Reginald Samuels, 67 years old, began experiencing headaches, occasional palpitations, blurred vision, and increased thirst. Mr. Samuels accesses the online **patient portal** of his **electronic health record (EHR)** to schedule a primary care appointment. At Mr. Samuels' appointment, the family nurse practitioner (FNP), Jada Shock, uses a tablet to enter his insurance and personal contact information into the **EHR** system that is **integrated** with the hospital record for communication among Mr. Samuel's caregivers. Jada explains that the system is **encrypted** (special security coding) to protect patient privacy. The certified medical assistant weighs Mr. Samuels, takes his vital signs, and enters the information in the EHR. As Jada takes Mr. Samuels' history and completes a physical examination, she updates the information in the EHR. Noting his family history of diabetes,

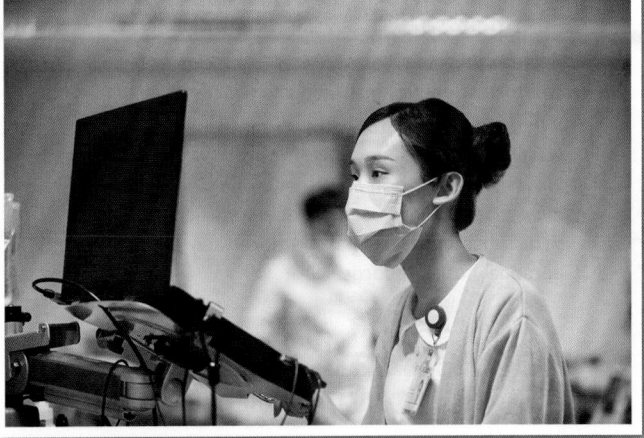

the increased thirst, and slight weight gain, Jada does a random glucose check via the office glucometer and finds that Mr. Samuel's blood sugar level is 320 mg/dL.

Decision support algorithms within the software alert the FNP that Mr. Samuels' blood pressure was also elevated at 170/98. The EHR lists possible medical diagnoses of hyperglycemia and hypertension. Following the

(Continued)

Meet Your Nurse Role Model (continued)

evidence-based care guidelines in the computer, Jada uses **computerized provider order entry (CPOE)** to enter requests for a basic metabolic profile, lipid profile, electrocardiogram (ECG), blood urea nitrogen (BUN), creatinine, and Hgb A1c. She instructs Mr. Samuels to fast for 12 hours before the blood work is drawn. She also prints patient education instructions.

The next morning, Mr. Samuels arrives at the hospital for his laboratory work and ECG. His registration information is automatically updated from the information provided with a previous health visit. The **online order requisitions** Jada entered yesterday provide the technicians with the necessary information, and they complete the tests. At the end of the day, Mr. Samuels receives an e-mail notification that his laboratory results are available for review. He logs into the EHR portal to view the results. He also finds a message from the FNP confirming the preliminary diagnosis of type 2 diabetes. The office is scheduling diabetic instruction, and they have e-mailed a prescription to Mr. Samuels' pharmacy for metformin, an antidiabetes drug. An education leaflet explaining the medication and potential side effects is attached to the message. Mr. Samuels notices that metformin is now showing on his **medication list** in his EHR.

Jada monitors Mr. Samuels' blood pressure log entries. A **trending graph** shows consistently high blood pressure readings. She prescribes Lisinopril, an antihypertensive,

5 mg daily, and requests that he continue to check his blood pressure frequently. A follow-up appointment is scheduled for 6 weeks.

A few weeks later, Mr. Samuels wakes up with severe chest pain and calls 911. En route to the emergency department (ED), the paramedic transmits an ECG tracing via satellite to the ED physician. Using telehealth technology, the physician interprets the ECG, determines that Mr. Samuels is having a myocardial infarction (MI), and notifies the cardiac catheterization team to be on standby. The ED physician sees that Mr. Samuels has recently completed tests at the hospital and reviews his medication list, allergies, and medical history online. Within 30 minutes, Mr. Samuels is sent to the cardiac procedure laboratory for percutaneous transluminal coronary angioplasty.

Four hours later, Mr. Samuels is resting comfortably in the progressive care unit. Throughout the next 48 hours, the bedside nurse monitors Mr. Samuels' vital signs and cardiac rhythm. An **interface** allows the nurse to directly import vital signs data from the cardiac monitor directly into his EHR. Caregivers document electronically at the bedside, and the physician uses CPOE to manage Mr. Samuels' prescriptions. At discharge, the nurse gives Mr. Samuels a printed copy of his medication list and discharge instructions, and follow-up appointments are made with the primary care provider and the cardiologist.

 Think Like a Nurse 38-1:
Clinical Judgment in Action

Reflect on this Meet Your Nurse Role Model scenario. Identify how information was managed and processed.

- What mechanisms for gathering and disseminating information were used?
- How did automation assist decision making?
- How was evidence used in decision making?
- What characteristics make it more likely for patients to use personal health records?

Theoretical Knowledge
knowing why

The Meet Your Nurse Role Model scenario is an example of how healthcare professionals use informatics to make decisions in practice. This chapter gives you an overview of how this works.

ABOUT THE KEY CONCEPTS

In today's complex and ever-changing environment, you must be competent in the use of information technology to communicate effectively with the healthcare team,

patients, and families; gather and manage information; support clinical decision making; and reduce the risk of medical error. You may already feel the competing demands on your time and knowledge. **Nursing informatics** and **healthcare technology** support your passion for nursing and innovation, leading to improved patient outcomes and higher-quality care. **Electronic communication** (e.g., EHRs) is also an important part of this equation.

WHAT IS NURSING INFORMATICS?

Whether you become a staff nurse, an administrator, a researcher, a primary healthcare provider, or an educator, you will need current, accurate, and best-practice information to do your job safely and effectively. While feeling overwhelmed by access to too much information, we are still lacking in knowledge. Do you ever feel that way as a student? It is not possible to keep all the necessary information in your head. No one can. You must know how to find, process, and manage it to arrive at the best decisions for your practice. **Key Point:** *For that, you will need informatics: the science of managing and processing information for clinical judgment in your nursing practice.*

Nursing informatics "integrates nursing science with information management and analytical sciences to identify, define, manage, and communicate *data, information, knowledge,* and *wisdom* in nursing practice" (American Nurses Association [ANA], 2022). Full-spectrum nurses interact with all four of these elements in daily practice, so you need to understand how they interrelate.

Nursing informatics specialists (NISs) work with EHRs and data analysis systems to be sure the best possible care is provided. Functions of the NIS include data collection and analysis, information sharing, and research dissemination. The NIS also acts as a manager or team leader to bring together all aspects of treatment options with best practice.

Data

Data are "discrete entities that are described objectively without interpretation" (ANA, 2022). In other words, data are unprocessed information that have no meaning until organized and analyzed. For example, what does 101 mean? It could indicate a college course called English 101; a piece of programming language; or someone's body temperature, pulse rate, weight, or age. Without a context, data are meaningless.

In nursing, we speak of data as the primary facts and observations acquired when providing services, such as the numerical value of a blood pressure measurement, or facts such as, "Father died of prostate cancer." Notice that even this information has no meaning until the nurse interprets it: The meaning of "Father died of prostate cancer" changes if the client is a healthy 24-year-old female individual sharing this information versus a 74-year-old male individual experiencing blood in their urine.

Information

Information consists of groupings of data processed into a meaningful, structured form (ANA, 2022). If you combine 320 with a unit of measure, you know that the number represents a blood sugar result. If other data—sex (male), age (67 years), and family history—are grouped together, information is formed. You now know that this patient has most likely developed type 2 diabetes.

Data:	320 mg/dL glucose, male, 67 years old, thirst
Grouped data:	Male sex, age 67 years, family history of diabetes
Information:	Male patient with probable new onset of diabetes

In the opening scenario, what information did the FNP receive that triggered an alert?

Knowledge

In the Meet Your Nurse Role Model scenario, what *information* did the FNP use to create knowledge of Mr. Samuels' condition? Take a minute to write your answer.

The answer to the question is that the FNP received information on the blood sugar (320 mg/dL) and blood pressure (170/98 mm Hg). Grouping this with other information (e.g., the history of headaches, blurred vision, palpitations, family history of diabetes), the FNP created *knowledge* of the potential for a diagnosis of type 2 diabetes and hypertension.

Key Point: *Knowledge is formed when data are grouped, creating meaningful information and relationships, which are then added to other structured information (ANA, 2022).* The knowledge can either be previously known or new. In the preceding scenario of the 67-year-old man with elevated blood sugar, we can add information about pathophysiology, pharmacokinetics (how medications work), patient history, and physical assessment, providing the knowledge to make an informed decision about the patient's current condition and further treatment.

Figure 38-1 depicts the transformation of data into knowledge. We have come to realize that the gathering of data and information to make decisions is never ending. Notice that the model shows overlapping circles and both forward and backward movement.

Wisdom

Wisdom, as defined by *Nursing Informatics: Scope and Standards of Practice,* is "the appropriate use of knowledge in managing or solving human problems. It is knowing when and how to apply knowledge to deal with complex problems or specific human needs" (ANA, 2022, p. 5). Wisdom develops as an outcome of your clinical experience, theoretical knowledge, critical thinking, and intuition—as you progress from novice to expert in the practice of full-spectrum nursing.

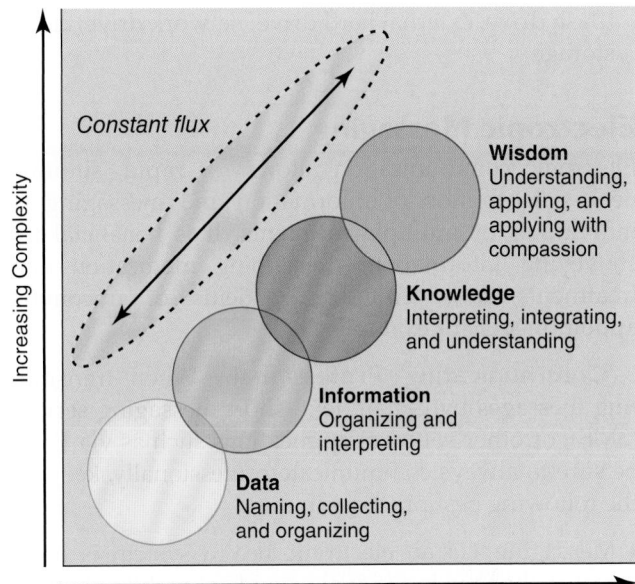

FIGURE 38-1 The relationship of data, information, knowledge, and wisdom. Each level increases in complexity.

KnowledgeCheck 38-1

- What is the difference between knowledge and wisdom?
- Define the following: *data, information, knowledge.*
- Give an example of each: data, information, knowledge.

HOW DO NURSES USE INFORMATICS AT WORK?

In your work as a nurse, you will use computer systems to document and communicate patient care, seek information, examine evidence-based practice resources, aid in clinical judgment, and possibly conduct or participate in clinical research.

Computer Basics

By definition, a **computer** is an electronic device with four main functions: input, processing, output, and storage. Collectively, these operations are known as **information processing** (or *data processing*). **Key Point:** *The power of a computer is based on the speed, accuracy, and reliability with which it stores, processes, and retrieves data.*

- **Computers consist of:**
  - Hardware (machines and monitors)
  - Memory (data storage)
  - Processors (translators)
  - Software (coded programs or applications that support specific functions)
- **Networks**—Computers can exist as an individual device or as part of a network of computers that share a common purpose.
- **Connectivity**—The ways in which computers and other hardware communicate and share information.
- **Data storage**—Data are stored either internally (in the memory) or externally on some form of storage media (flash drive, external hard drive, network drive, cloud storage).

Electronic Messaging

Electronic communication allows for rapid, simultaneous distribution of information and messaging to individuals or multiple recipients. It is beneficial for conveying information, prescribing medication and treatments, and reminding patients of upcoming appointments, for example.

Communicating Professionally When transmitting messages by e-mail, text, short messaging service (SMS), or other software applications such as via EHR, be sure to always communicate professionally, keeping the following best practices in mind:

- Messaging via an electronic health system is more secure than via individual providers' mobile phones.
- Messages should be concise, specific, and clear.
- Be aware of tone.
- Do not use abbreviations.

Set up clear expectations about two-way communications regarding whether you will continue a dialogue and how quickly you expect to reply (Storck, 2017).

Protecting Privacy Although e-mail and text messaging offer convenient patient communication among nurses, other providers, payers, and patients and their caregivers, these formats can be misused and potentially pose significant risks to patient privacy. **Key Point:** *Nurses have a professional responsibility to protect information that includes any individually identifiable health information; current, past, or potential physical or mental health conditions; and any payment information. These transmissions occur only on secure or encrypted sites if patients' personal information is involved.*

Transmitting Medical Orders The Joint Commission (2016) allows the transmission of medical orders via text messaging, provided the following conditions are met:

- The device used is always protected and secure.
- The messaging is encrypted.
- The phone number of the recipient is correct.
- Messages show delivery, and read receipts have a date and time stamp.
- Messages are sent only to those who are authorized to receive the medical order.
- The text message does not contain personal health information.

Social Networking

Social networking tools allow people to connect and interact with others who have similar interests or health issues, regardless of physical location. This can be done through **blogging** (posting open messages that can be read by anyone with permission to access the site) or sharing photos, videos, or texts on social networking sites or applications. Sites generally require you to register, create a profile, and be granted access privileges by the Internet page administrator. For instance, you can go to YouTube to view video demonstrations showing nursing skills. However, you will need to be discerning about the source of information and whether it is expert and reliable. For example, some of the YouTube skills videos have errors in the demonstrations; you should confirm that any videos you watch are done by professional nurses or educators.

- **Sites are searchable by others.** As with many Internet-based tools, social networking sites are searchable by anyone with access. Many employers now regularly search social networking sites as part of the applicant verification process. **Key Point:** *Never post anything on these sites that you would not want an employer or instructor to view.*
- **Be aware of risks to patient privacy.** Using social networking to communicate work-related experiences can be a potential risk to patient privacy and violate Health Insurance Portability and Accountability Act

(HIPAA) policy. Remember that you can compromise patient privacy in a social networking post even without using a patient's name if you include enough other information that could otherwise identify the patient. Such a violation can be grounds for legal liability or dismissal from employment.

Online Forums

Online forums are an increasingly popular way to exchange information. These are Internet sites that can either be public or limited to specific groups through usernames and passwords, for example:

- Many schools offer interactive forums to support communication among student groups.
- Patients may seek online forums (blogs) for support groups when coping with various health conditions. **Key Point:** *Anyone with access can add information to open blogs, creating the potential for inaccurate information or opinion. Before recommending specific blogs to patients, be sure you know what purpose they fulfill and when they are facilitated by a qualified professional.*
- Health information from government sites, professional organizations, and scientific referred sources is credible and reliable for patients.

Web Conferencing and Webinars

Web conferencing is used to conduct or participate in live or synchronous (occurring at the same time) meetings or presentations via the Internet, usually through a browser or application-based software. Attendees download an application onto their local computers and access the meeting by using a link that is usually distributed via e-mail or text. These interactions are often two-way communications using Internet-based audio- and videoconferencing programming.

A **webinar,** or **webcast,** is a specific type of online conference that is conducted in a one-way manner, from the speaker to the audience. Webinars are a cost-effective means of providing staff with updated clinical information (e.g., continuing education, in-service) for patient care.

Telehealth

Telehealth is the use of an Internet-based video program to send healthcare information between patients and professionals at different locations (Fig. 38-2). Telehealth improves access to healthcare by providing remote clinical healthcare, patient and professional education, and before patient and professional education.

The following are other examples of the use of telehealth:

- **Rural healthcare.** In rural healthcare sites, there may not be specialized healthcare providers located in the area. Telecommunications equipment at the rural site and the specialist's site allows the specialist and patient to see and talk to each other. The specialist

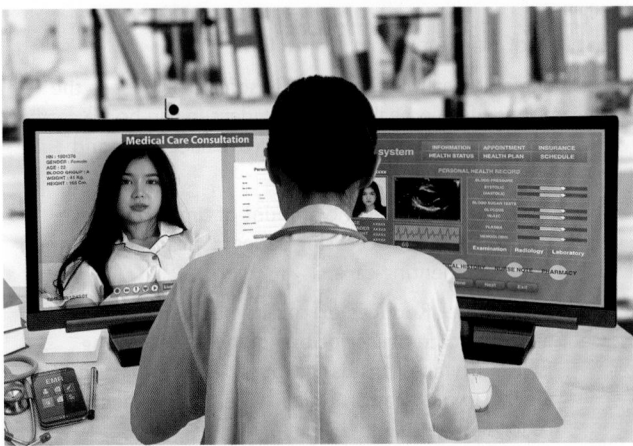

FIGURE 38-2 Telehealth improves access among healthcare providers at remote and central sites.

can also view health records, x-ray films, laboratory results, and so on. This reduces the cost of traveling to a distant site and the stress on a patient who may not feel well enough to travel.

- **Home health monitoring.** A more common use of telehealth is the use of home health monitoring devices. These devices allow the healthcare professional to monitor vital signs and other indicators without physically entering a home or requiring a patient to make a clinic trip. Therefore, patients can be monitored more frequently, providing better follow-up care and possibly earlier discharge from the hospital. See the accompanying Home Care box, Use of Informatics in Home Care.
- **Shortage of healthcare providers.** In the hospital, ill patients can be remotely monitored by a hospital **intensivist** (physician employed by the hospital to provide healthcare to patients in intensive care) and critical care nurses from a central location. These systems enhance patient safety and provide support for the healthcare staff when they are understaffed with high patient acuity.
- **Emergency care triage.** Some cities have incorporated telehealth nurse triage into their emergency 911 call system. In some studies, telehealth nurses implementing care using approved protocols to manage patient calls led to a significant decrease in the need for ambulance services and ED visits for older adults (Shah et al., 2015).
- **Remote patient care during a pandemic.** Telehealth applications allow patients to access healthcare providers without increasing the risk of transmitting infection to other patients or staff.

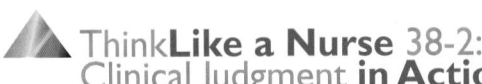

ThinkLike a Nurse 38-2: Clinical Judgment in Action

- As a patient, would you prefer a telehealth or a face-to-face consultation? Why?
- Now imagine that you are an accident victim brought to a rural clinic staffed only with paraprofessionals. Does your answer change? If so, why?

Use of Informatics in Home Care

Electronic health record (EHR) software reduces the amount of time healthcare providers in the home setting spend in documenting care, improves accuracy, and prevents lost documentation.

> **Efficient.** Reduces the amount of time healthcare providers spend accessing patients' health information and documenting care.

> **Accurate.** Reduces errors in medication dosing and duplicate prescriptions or overprescribing. EHR software flags dangerous interactions and puts alerts on medication that may lead to an allergic reaction.

> **Comprehensive.** Prevents inaccurate or lost information. All health visits, treatments, medications, immunization records, family history, and payments are recorded within the EHR. This means less redundancy in paperwork for forms to be completed by patients and staff.

> **Independent.** Enables patient's ability to manage illness. Internet-based EHRs allow patients to conveniently access their own personal health information, diagnostic testing results, patient education materials, upcoming appointments, and billing information.

KnowledgeCheck 38-2

- What is personal health information, and why is it important to protect it?
- Why might Wikipedia be an inaccurate source of health information?

COMPUTER- AND APPLICATION-BASED TOOLS FOR PROVIDING AND MANAGING CARE

As a nurse, you will use a wide variety of computerized devices in the workplace. Wearable electronic health devices, cardiorespiratory monitors, glucometers, smart intravenous (IV) pumps, barcode scanners for tracking equipment and ordering supplies, barcode medication administration systems, and electronic bed scales all use technology to collect data that can be uploaded, reviewed, and analyzed for patient care.

Tracking Patients and Equipment

Global Positioning Systems (GPS) GPS systems allow real-time tracking of patients and can be used in select clinical situations in which wandering is a patient safety concern. For example, the Alzheimer's Association promotes the use of electronic tracking for some patients with dementia as a way to postpone the need for a more secure environment (McShane, 2013).

Real-Time Location Systems (RTLSs) RTLSs or radio-frequency identification (RFID) detectors are being used by some agencies to assist in locating patient care equipment that may be dispersed throughout a building. These systems save nurses time, deter staff from storing equipment on a particular unit rather than at a centrally accessible location, and decrease costs of lost equipment. Cordless barcode scanners and RTLS applications for smartphones may be used to monitor workflow using bedside equipment.

Efficiency-enhancing tracking systems may also track the location of medication and even monitor the temperature and humidity of refrigerators used for storage. Wireless, hands-free communication badges can identify the location of staff or patients transported to various departments.

RTLSs can also be used to track patients. For example, RTLS tags can be placed on a newborn's clothing to monitor and track the location of newborns in the hospital. If someone takes a baby near an exit door, an alarm will sound and the door will automatically lock. Likewise, RTLS security technology can be used to identify the location of other patients at risk for wandering, such as those with dementia or cognitive issues.

Managing Staffing and Workflow

Internet-based tools provide convenience and efficiency for staff scheduling, managing patient flow, accessing evidence-based references, distributing policy and procedures, and offering staff education. Many hospitals have developed internal resources such as special intranet pages with references specific to nursing. Portable digital devices (tablet computers) are efficient for bedside retrieval of patients' health information, prescribed medications and interventions, and test results in the EHR. They also are convenient for charting at the bedside or other locations.

Reducing Error With Automation

As healthcare becomes more complex, the opportunities for error increase significantly. A hospital stay can be prolonged, or injury and even death can result from a seemingly simple mistake such as administering incompatible medications or erroneously transcribing a medication prescription. There are two types of errors:

- **Errors of commission**—When the wrong action occurs (e.g., giving an incorrect drug)
- **Errors of omission**—When the correct action does not occur (e.g., overlooking a serious medication allergy or failing to put up the bed rails for a confused patient)

Another way to look at errors is to ask whether the error was in planning or execution:

- An *error in planning* occurs when the original intended action or plan was not correct.
- An *error of execution* occurs when the correct action is taken but does not proceed as intended.

Automation (e.g., EHR) provides a secure way to integrate patient information, including health history, allergy history, laboratory values and diagnostic test results, and medication lists. It improves communication among those who prescribe, dispense, and administer medication to patients. The system ensures patient safety by flagging medication dosages that are outside normal standards and alerting providers of the possibility of a drug interaction, allergy, or incorrect dose. In addition, some drug names sound similar; the EHR can notify prescribers and help prevent a medication error in prescribing or administration.

Following are three examples of error-prevention technologies:

- **CPOE** helps prevent errors in reading and transcribing orders.
- **Barcoding medication administration systems** reduce medication errors by electronically verifying the *five rights of medication administration*—right patient, right dose, right drug, right time, right route—at the patient's bedside (Shah et al., 2016).
- **The use of smart technologies (e.g., infusion devices) at the point of care** helps to ensure that the correct dose is delivered to the patient.

Aiding Patients in Self-Care

Nearly three-quarters of Internet users say they have looked online for health information within the past year. Most patients used symptoms as the basis of their Internet search (McCarthy et al., 2017). You can help guide your patients in their searches by educating them about how to use online sources and how to choose reputable, trustworthy sites.

Internet-based software and applications (apps) for mobile devices provide patients with patient education (e.g., disease-specific information or healthy habit tips, including nutritional information, meal planning, dietary tracking), patient-specific medication dose reminders (Fig. 38-3), and appointment and medical bill-paying reminders. They do the following:

- As needed, help patients to interpret information that they find.
- Guide patients to any available patient education materials the agency has on its Internet sites. These may also offer links to other reputable sources.

In addition, customizable digital products provide patients with interactive ways to engage in their healthcare. Some, for example, are designed to organize and motivate patients to independently take medication doses and manage dietary intake, weight, activity, and other prescribed health habits. Other apps remind individuals to take time for important aspects of wellness (deep breathing, mindfulness, dedicated time for relaxation, and other activities that reduce stress).

Wearable devices are designed to improve health outcomes and enhance the prevention and detection of

Safe, Effective Nursing Care

Are Information Technologies Living Up to Their Promise?

Chapter Key Concept: *Informatics*

Competency: *Embrace/incorporate technological advances (Thinking, Doing, Caring); Provide safe, quality client care (Thinking, Doing, Caring)*

Informatics knowledge skills are essential for collecting patient data and planning, implementing, evaluating, and communicating patient care across all practice settings. Forman and colleagues (2020) examined various strategies to teach nursing informatics clinical competencies to nursing students and nursing faculty. This research team found that repetition and practice with electronic health record (EHR) software improved proficiency and confidence with use. In turn, those accessing the EHR software more often also demonstrated higher scores in the competency areas of patient safety, documentation, patient needs, prioritization, and nursing process.

Think About It: The informatics competency stresses the need for nurses to effectively and efficiently use information and communication technologies to deliver professional patient care. What do you see as the nurse's responsibility in using the EHR and related communication applications within the software?

Consider the following questions to help develop your knowledge and skills and shape your attitudes about informatics and safety:

➤ What clinical judgment skills will be necessary for nurses and other providers to respond appropriately to decision supports and alerts?

➤ How might EHRs be used to improve care?

➤ How might the EHR improve the safety of an individual patient's care?

➤ What information should be included in an electronic database to make it useful for clinical research?

Source: Forman et al. (2020).

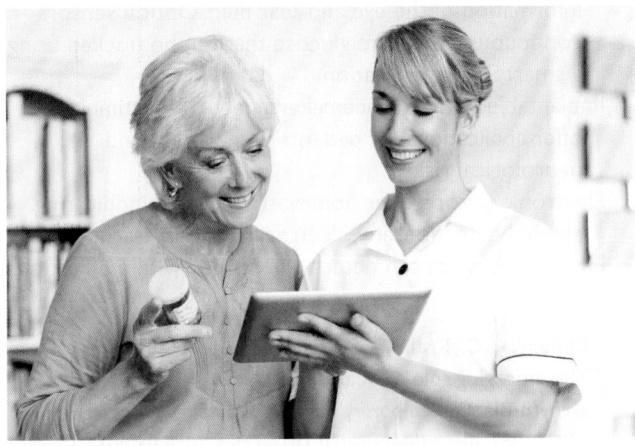

FIGURE 38-3 Nurse and senior client using a digital tablet for medication reminders and dose tracking.

health issues. They can track heart rate, respiration, and blood pressure; exercise and movement; sleep; posture; ECG monitoring; blood glucose management; ovulation; sun exposure and environmental pollutants; and viral exposure to aid in predicting infection threats, with other technologies in development.

Wearable devices help patients and nurses maintain consistent monitoring of health and early detection of abnormalities. The digital health data are easily shared with healthcare providers, eliminating the need for in-person appointments for routine surveillance. They promote healthy habits by offering feedback that can be used to modify health behaviors for improved health outcomes.

Biosensors detect sweat on the skin to analyze hormones, glucose, nutrients, medications, and metabolites in the blood. This emerging technology can be used to monitor and manage blood sugar. Biosensors may soon be used for drug testing and may replace a breathalyzer to determine blood alcohol levels (Haelle, 2022).

Toward Evidence-Based Practice

Lu, L., Zhang, J., Xie, Y., Gao, F., Xu, S., Wu, X., & Ye, Z. (2020, November). Wearable health devices in health care: Narrative systematic review. *JMIR mHealth uHealth, 8*(11), e18907. https://10.2196/18907

Wearable technology applications designed for use on various parts of the body (e.g., head, limb, torso) are designed to aid in (1) health and safety monitoring, (2) chronic disease and pain management, (3) disease diagnosis and treatment, and (4) rehabilitation. Through small sensors and biomedical devices, healthcare providers can use real-time data for clinical decision making. A review of the literature on wearable technology applications in healthcare showed that they provide researchers with big data that can reveal patterns and factors affecting health.

Guk, K., Han, G., Lim, J., Jeong, K., Kang, T., Lim, E-K., & Jung, J. (2019, May 29). Evolution of wearable devices with real-time disease monitoring for personal care. *Nanomaterials, 9*(6), 813. https://doi.org/10.3390/nano9060813

Smartwatches can be used to analyze tremors and balance in patients with Parkinson disease. Smart textiles and skin patches contain conductive devices to detect biofluids (sweat), indicating physical activity, motion, acceleration, and pressure. Glucose and lactate, as well as emotions and vital signs, can also be measured with accuracy.

Smart contact lenses can monitor physiological information of the eye and tear fluid. Optical sensors continuously measure glucose that can be tracked using a smartphone application.

Implantable devices (pacemakers, deep brain stimulators) offer applications for patients with cardiac and neurological risks.

Electronic tattoos offer noninvasive glucose monitoring, alcohol detection, and electrocardiogram tracings.

Ingestible devices can detect compliance with medication therapy.

Cheung, C. C., Krahn, A. D., & Andrade, J. G. (2018, August). The emerging role of wearable technologies in detection of arrhythmia. *Contemporary Issues in Cardiology Practice, 34*(8), 1083–1087. https://doi.org/10.1016/j.cjca.2018.05.003

Wearable technology devices are used to monitor physiological parameters, heart rate, heart rhythm, blood pressure, physical activity, respiratory rate, blood glucose, and sleep patterns. For heart rate monitoring, most wearable devices use photoplethysmography (PPG) technology. Although they are less accurate than conventional electrocardiography monitoring, they facilitate arrhythmia detection for conditions like atrial fibrillation.

Collier, S., Monette, P., Hobbs, K., Tabasky, E., Forester, B. P., & Vahia, I. V. (2018, August). Mapping movement: Applying motion measurement technologies to the psychiatric care of older adults. *Current Psychiatry Reports, 20*(8), 64. https://doi.org/10.1007/s11920-018-0921-z

Mental health providers may use wearable devices to detect depression in older adults, predict the likelihood of falls, or measure physical activity in older adults with chronic mental illnesses or anxiety. Motion-based technologies also detect physical activity in older adults residing in nursing homes.

Aurora, N., Patil, S. P., & Punjabi, N. M. (2018, July). Portable sleep monitoring for diagnosing sleep apnea in hospitalized patients with heart failure. *Chest, 154*(1), 91–98. https://doi.org/10.1016/j.chest.2018.04.008

Portable sleep monitoring can accurately diagnose obstructive as well as central sleep apnea in hospitalized patients with heart failure and may promote early initiation of treatment.

Bianchi, M. T. (2018, July). Sleep devices: Wearables and nearables, informational and interventional, consumer and clinical. *Metabolism, 84*, 99–108. https://doi.org/10.1016/j.metabol.2017.10.008

Wearable devices can be used to detect sleep patterns and plan interventions for improving sleep.

Byrom, B., McCarthy, M., Schueler, P., & Muehlhausen, W. (2018, March). Brain monitoring devices in neuroscience clinical research: The potential of remote monitoring using sensors, wearables, and mobile devices. *Clinical Pharmacology and Therapeutics, 104*(1). https://doi.org/10.1002/cpt.1077

Toward Evidence-Based Practice—cont'd

Researchers review portable and wearable devices for brain monitoring, including direct measurement of brain electrical activity, sleep patterns, gait, cognition, voice acoustics, and gaze analysis.

Zhang, Y., Gu, A., Xiao, Z., Xing, Y., Yang, C., Li, J., & Liu, C. (2022, June). Wearable fetal ECG monitoring system from abdominal electrocardiography recording. *Biosensors, 12*(7), 475. https://doi.org/10.3390/bios12070475

Home-based fetal electrocardiography (ECG) monitoring via wearable technology can help to safeguard the health of the fetus and aid providers in making timely decisions. However, the technology is currently influenced by background noise and maternal artifacts, which can compromise the accuracy of the fetal ECG tracings. With further enhancements in the technology, this application has promise for the future.

1. What are the advantages of using smart wearable sensors for monitoring health status?

2. What barriers exist to patient use of smart wearable body sensors (e.g., wrist-worn heart-rate-sensing devices)?

3. What situations might interfere in the accurate monitoring and interpretation of the physiological data obtained from smart wearable sensors?

Supporting Healthcare Professionals

Healthcare professionals rely on computers and mobile devices daily for:

- **Communicating** with colleagues and patients through messaging, Web logs (blogs), social media, and Web conferencing.
- **Time management** for scheduling appointments and meetings, including reminders.
- **Searching online databases** for evidence-based sources that support clinical practice, including authority sources and guidelines, health news, drug reference guides, and textbooks.
- **Performing and documenting patient care and clinical tasks** using EHRs and hospital-based interfaces.
- **Supporting patient management** using Internet- or app-based diagnostic aids, decision support tools, and medical calculators.

Using Technology for Patient Care

Innovations in mobile and electronic healthcare have led to improved capabilities of practical physiological monitoring devices to enhance patient safety and comfort.

Smart Bed Technology Smart beds use a sensor, placed under the mattress, to track patients' movement, weight, and vitals.

- Smart beds alert nurses of patients attempting to get out of bed when they are at risk for falls.
- Using a wireless sensory network (WSN) on the surface of hospital beds aids in preventing pressure injury by detecting moisture, pressure, and friction on the mattress (Karvounis et al., 2021).
- Pressure sensors detect in-bed body pose and sleeping position for assessing sleep quality. Body position also affects musculoskeletal alignment and indicates risk for pressure injury (Doan et al., 2021).
- The sensors provide nurses with ongoing surveillance of patient activities that can help identify patterns,

potentially leading to a new diagnosis or a different understanding of a condition.

Artificial Intelligence Artificial intelligence (AI) uses algorithms and other data analytics to predict the risk of developing various health conditions. AI can be used to assist providers in diagnosing some diseases and assist in clinical decision making in areas such as diagnostic imaging, cancer care, neurology, and cardiology (Jiang et al., 2017).

Three-Dimensional Printing Three-dimensional (3D) printing creates a 3D, solid object from a digital model. The 3D printer rapidly replicates that model layer by layer using ultraviolet light and raw materials such as metals, plastics, and ceramics. The advantage of 3D printing is the accelerated speed of producing images, allowing for rapid modification as needed.

- Dental implants were the first medically approved use of 3D printing.
- Limb prosthetics produced by 3D are now more accessible and affordable.
- 3D anatomical models can reduce surgical time when used as a guide for complex cases, such as spinal surgery.
- Fabrication of customized medical equipment (forceps, clamps, retractors) and devices (components of ventilators) can help to mitigate delays related to supply-chain shortages.

Using Simulation for Skills Training and Clinical Judgment

Educators are adopting new, more engaging, and collaborative methods for teaching and learning.

Computer-Based Simulations Computer- or cloud-based simulations offer nurse–patient experiences for students to practice clinical decision making and prioritizing interventions before interacting with live patients. This active, individualized learning approach uses patient situations to elicit clinical competence and promotes learner confidence by:

- Providing supplementary readings before the simulation experience or testing
- Providing an overview of the patient scenario
- Offering options for patient interactions
- Including the patient record
- Showing provider orders that require action
- Providing immediate feedback to learners
- Using guided discussion and reflection
- Assessing mastery of clinical skills

High-Fidelity Mannequins High-fidelity mannequins are patient simulators that emulate an authentic clinical environment for learners before they perform skills with live patients (Fig. 38-4). Mannequins

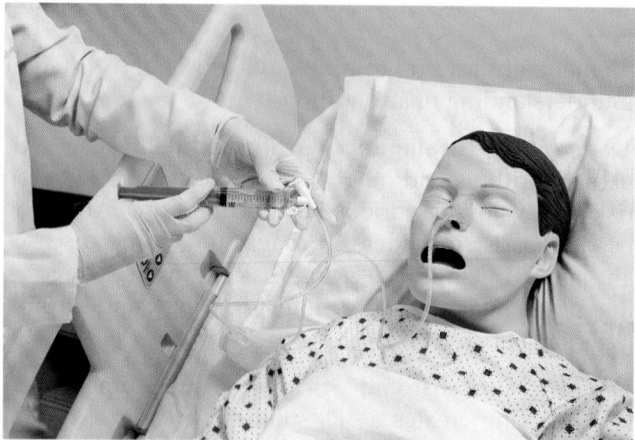

FIGURE 38-4 A human patient simulator offers practical experience before caring for patients or training special skills.

demonstrate physiological functions (e.g., light-sensitive pupils, bodily fluid excretion, changing vital signs) that help learners to improve clinical judgment and prioritization for patient care. Patient situations with the mannequins can also offer patient care opportunities that students may not have access to with live patients before graduation. Would it surprise you to know that practicing nurses also use mannequins in continuing education provided in their workplaces to practice skills such as Basic Life Support (BLS)?

ELECTRONIC HEALTH RECORDS

EHR usage among healthcare providers and hospitals has sharply increased since the passage of the Health Information Technology for Economic and Clinical Health (HITECH) Act of 2009, wherein eligible healthcare professionals receive an incentive payment for adopting, implementing, upgrading, or meaningfully using an EHR. EHRs can improve patient care, promote safe practice, enhance communication between patients and multiple providers, facilitate access to clinical data for research, and reduce the risk of error. Table 38-1 summarizes the use of information systems in practice, education, administration, and research.

As part of networked information systems software, EHRs allow clinicians to create, store, edit, and retrieve patient charts via the Internet or local intranet software. Patient demographics, progress notes, patient problems, medications, vital signs and other clinical data, past medical history, immunizations, laboratory data, and radiology and diagnostic testing reports are important components of the patient health record.

Table 38-1 ▸ Use of Computer Information Systems in Nursing

NURSING PRACTICE	NURSING EDUCATION	NURSING ADMINISTRATION	NURSING RESEARCH
Literature access and retrieval (e.g., for evidence-based practice)	Literature access and retrieval	Quality improvement and utilization review	Literature review
Care planning	Virtual learning technologies	Employee records (licensure, immunizations)	Data collection
Client records (e.g., documenting, order entry, retrieving laboratory results)	Classroom technology	Staffing patterns, hiring	Data analysis (both qualitative and quantitative)
Telehealth (use in home health)	Testing and evaluation	Buildings and facilities management	Research dissemination
Case management	Student records	Finance and budgets	Applying for grants
Documenting medications	Development of electronic and learning communities using the Internet	Accreditation reviews (monitoring quality indicators)	
Transcribing orders			
Ordering and dispensing medication			
Identifying drug interactions			
Warning practitioners about drug incompatibilities			

Interoperability and Standardized Nursing Languages

In this section, we describe the role of informatics and standardized nursing language in communicating health information in EHRs, nursing education, and evidence-based practice.

Standardization Facilitates Interoperability **Interoperability** refers to the ability of computers and operating systems to exchange information with each other without losing the meaning of the information. For that to happen, consistent (standardized) communication is needed—that is, terminology that all computers can identify. For example, if information about heart rate is to be exchanged, shared terminology is needed. An EHR system in one hospital might refer to "heart rate," whereas another EHR system in another healthcare clinic might use the term "pulse rate." This could interfere with clear communication of meaning. **Key Point: *Standardized nursing language facilitates communication among organizations, nurses, and the healthcare* team.**

Standardization Supports Evidence-Based Practice Suppose you wanted to find out how many patients on your hospital unit had a nursing diagnosis of Impaired Skin Integrity during the past year. You may plan to review all patient charts within a select period and examine the nursing notes. Or perhaps you might search for the words *Impaired Skin Integrity* in the computerized records. That is a beginning—but this task would be difficult because nurses use a variety of terms to describe the same data. For example, in some charts, you might find the term *skin breakdown,* in others, *a reddened area, bedsore, decubitus,* or *stage III pressure injury.* Would you count these as Impaired Skin Integrity? What if the nurses used some terms you did not think to search for?

Do you see how the lack of a standardized way to describe patient problems can hamper efforts to create and retrieve nursing data from automated documentation systems? Recall the goal for interoperability among EHR systems discussed earlier. **Standardized language—** using the same terms to describe a clinical condition in all EHRs—helps to achieve that goal (Box 38-1).

Benefits of an Electronic Health Record

EHR systems improve the quality of care and reduce healthcare costs with technology-based tools for health information exchange, CPOE systems, and clinical decision support (CDS) tools. EHRs offer the following benefits.

Improved Efficiency, Productivity, Continuity of Care A digital health record conveniently stores all patient information to:

- Facilitate the planning and documentation of care, including standardized care plans, problem lists, medication administration records, and other functions.
- Support efficient patient care workflow.
- Provide reminders for follow-up and preventive care (in most EHRs), which improves patient compliance with appointments and care.
- Allow for more accurate, convenient, and uniform billing using standardized coding for patient diagnoses and interventions.

Increased Communication A centralized source of patient information improves communication among healthcare professionals. Comprehensive and collaborative care is enhanced with access to the EHR. Standardized reporting and patient care management also contribute to communication of the plan for patient care (Rutten et al., 2014).

Reduced Redundancy Allowing for the secure and potentially real-time sharing of patient information can reduce costly duplicated tests. For example, diagnostic testing is often prescribed because one provider (e.g., primary care) does not have access to the clinical information stored at another provider's location (e.g., cardiac specialist). A central repository offers access to the results without the inconvenience of scanning, faxing, digital transmission (e-mail), or mailing hard-copy reports.

Improved Accessibility Authorized providers and staff in different locations can access a computerized record—and all at the same time. A provider can view laboratory results from the office at the same time a nurse views them in the hospital and a laboratory technician adds more data. Various types of hardware support access to patient health information, from stationary bedside terminals to wireless laptops mounted on mobile carts to handheld devices.

Clinical Support Tools (CSTs) EHRs equip providers with clinical support tools to access information to assist with clinical decision making. For example, a CST may offer current drug information, cross-reference a patient allergy to prescribed medication, and alert prescribers and nurses to potential drug interactions and other patient risks.

Reduction of Errors

- **CPOE allows healthcare providers to enter prescriptions for care and medication via a computer,** thus reducing errors resulting from illegible handwriting.
- **CPOE makes the prescription process more efficient for nursing and pharmacy** staff by saving time in soliciting information missing from illegible or incomplete prescriptions.
- **CPOE contains an alert system** to providers signaling potential medication errors, critical laboratory values, and drug incompatibility.

Privacy Access to sensitive patient information can be limited only to individuals with proper authorization, and each retrieval of data can be logged electronically—a vast improvement over the folders

BOX 38-1 ■ American Nurses Association Recognized Languages for Nursing

Language	Description
NANDA International	The NANDA-I taxonomy provides a way to classify and categorize areas of actual or potential concern for patient care. The taxonomy includes 13 Domains (areas of interest) with diagnostic labels that contain definitions, defining characteristics, related factors, at-risk populations, and associated conditions. Nursing diagnoses can be problem focused, potential risk, or health promotion.
Clinical Care Classification (CCC)	Developed by Virginia Saba, CCC is used primarily by home health agencies and community settings. The taxonomy contains nursing diagnoses and interventions developed to code, index, classify, document, track, and analyze clinical care processes.
Omaha System	The Omaha System is standardized healthcare terminology used to document care in community and home care agencies. This system consists of the following: ■ Problem Classification Scheme for client assessment ■ Intervention Scheme for planning care and client services ■ Problem Rating Scale for Outcomes for evaluating client changes The Omaha System provides a framework for collection, aggregation, analysis, and sharing of clinical data.
Nursing Outcomes Classification (NOC)	NOC presents standardized terminology for nursing-sensitive patient outcomes. Each outcome represents the measurable state of the client, caregiver, family, or community before and after a nursing intervention to evaluate the effectiveness of care.
Nursing Interventions Classification (NIC)	NIC is a system for identifying, organizing, documenting, and communicating the care that nurses provide to clients, families, and other healthcare professionals. Each intervention includes a concept label, definition, and activities.
Nursing Management Minimum Data Set (NMMDS)	This data set describes the healthcare and nursing environment associated with the diagnosis, intervention, and outcome segments from the administrative, management, and resource management perspectives. It is composed of data elements in three categories: environment, nurse resources, and financial resources.
Perioperative Nursing Data Set (PNDS)	The PNDS language supports evidence-based perioperative nursing practice and provides support for structured documentation of nursing activities. It provides a common language for clinical research and assists with the measurement and evaluation of patient outcomes. This was the first nursing language developed by a nursing specialty.
Statistical Nomenclature of Medicine Clinical Terminology (SNOMED CT)	SNOMED CT is a reference terminology that includes clinical concepts used to describe assessment, diagnosis, intervention, and outcome. Although it includes nursing concepts, it is not developed specifically for nursing but rather for a broad spectrum of healthcare domains.
Nursing Minimum Data Sets (NMDS)	This data collection establishes comparability of nursing data across population settings, geographic areas, and times. It describes the nursing care of patients or clients and their families in a variety of settings, both institutional and noninstitutional.
International Classification for Nursing Practice (ICNP)	ICNP describes nursing practice in various clinical settings worldwide using common language. It includes nursing phenomena or diagnoses, outcomes, and actions.

Source: American Nurses Association. (2022). *Nursing informatics: Scope and standards of practice* (3rd ed.). Nursesbooks.org.

and charts that can pass through many hands without a record of who examines them.

Research and Public Health Benefits Computerized records place data in repositories (storage areas) so that the information can be sorted and analyzed to create the information and knowledge necessary to aid research to support decision making, for example:

- State health departments can access population-based medical information to track communicable diseases, possibly preventing epidemics.
- Health researchers and analysts can also use aggregate health information to judge which treatment is most effective for a disease.
- To protect patient privacy and promote ethical practice of research, review boards govern access to population data.

Barriers to Electronic Health Record Adoption

The most prevalent reason for resisting the use of an EHR is the learning curve involved with becoming proficient with the use of a new system. User adoption and systems training are expensive, time consuming, and frustrating. This can be problematic in a demanding clinical environment. A few other reasons providers and healthcare facilities and agencies give for objecting to the use of an EHR include:

- Fear of loss of personalization of the record to the individual patient
- Belief that moving to an EHR will cause disruption in workflow, lead to errors, or add to the already taxed workload
- Purchase and installation costs

Although the intent of computerization is to decrease costs by improving efficiency and communication, there may be unintended consequences of EHR implementation:

- Less face-to-face communication among the healthcare team
- Software upgrade and periodic new releases are inevitable, some of which may require more robust hardware than previous versions.
- Need to replace or upgrade already serviceable hardware that has been made obsolete by the EHR

KnowledgeCheck 38-3
- What are some of the benefits of EHR implementation?
- List at least three ways in which computers can help reduce medication errors.

Ethical Use of Electronic Health Records

Health records contain highly sensitive information. Patients share sensitive health information with nurses and physicians, trusting that their health history will remain private. All healthcare professions have a moral, ethical, regulatory, and legal duty to protect patient privacy in daily practice (Dickerson, 2022).

Patient Privacy and Security Safeguards

Although **privacy** is often used interchangeably with the terms **confidentiality** and **security,** they have distinct meanings.

Privacy Privacy addresses the question of who has access to personal information and under what conditions. Privacy is concerned with the collection, storage, and use of personal information. An important issue is whether the individual has authorized the use of personal information. Most facilities have disciplinary policies in place to manage security breaches and assign fines or prosecution when patient privacy is violated.

Confidentiality Confidentiality is the right of an individual to have personal, identifiable medical information kept private. For patients, this means that personal and medical information given to a healthcare provider will not be disclosed to others unless the individual has given specific permission for such release.

Security Security refers the procedural, technical, and physical safeguards for patient information.

Common measures to prevent unauthorized access, modification, use, and dissemination of EHRs (Fig. 38-5) include:

- **Passwords and personal identification numbers (PINs)** for all users are probably the most obvious safeguard (Box 38-2). For example, the business office does not see day-to-day clinical information, and

HIPAA Privacy Icons

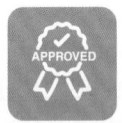
Certifications

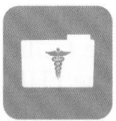
Personal Data

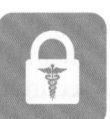
Security

HIPAA Security

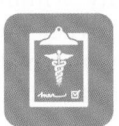
Personal Health

Medical Information

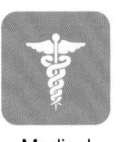
Medical Compliance

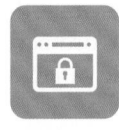
Password Security

Cloud Medical Data

FIGURE 38-5 Measures to protect patient privacy within an electronic health record.

BOX 38-2 ■ Simple Tips for Password Management

- Never share passwords with others.
- Make sure your device is secure. The best password in the world might not do you any good if someone is looking over your shoulder while you type.
- Use a password manager app or software to create and store strong, unique passwords for various accounts.
- The more complex the password is, the harder it is for hackers to break it. Use combinations of letters, numbers, and symbols for maximum protection.
- Do not use words or numbers that contain personal information or are easy to guess (e.g., pet names, birthdays).
- Change passwords frequently.
- Do not record passwords in easily accessible places.
- Use unique login information (username and password) for different accounts.
- Develop mnemonic phrases to remember complex passwords.

nurses do not see any special arrangements a patient has made to pay an invoice.

- **Encryption** means health information cannot be read or understood except by someone who can decipher it using a special code made available only to authorized individuals.
- **Workstation privacy filters** at each workstation help to block the view of unauthorized people.
- **Designated workstation computers** can be assigned for specific functions (e.g., accessing laboratory results) to reduce high-volume usage at select terminals.
- **Policies and procedures** must be in place to secure access and documentation that comply with HIPPA security rules.
- **Onboarding and training** are provided to staff, educating them about the facility's patient privacy program, secure use of the EHR, medication dispensing system, ordering and reporting of diagnostic testing, and other patient-specific information.
- A **culture of security** within the organization and respect for patient privacy are the basis for the staff to adhere to health information security measures and for the administration to ensure compliance with policies.

Although it is important to protect the privacy of healthcare records from unauthorized viewers, professionals who have password access but are not assigned to the patient to provide care make the most breaches of confidentiality.

Audit Trails

Organizations are required to have software that tracks each person who accesses information. This is called an

audit trail. Anything a person adds to or changes in the record is recorded electronically and can be investigated.

HIPAA Regulations

All private and government-sponsored health insurance and care providers must comply with the Department of Health and Human Services (HHS) Privacy Rule. The Privacy Rule was mandated in response to the HIPAA of 1996. It was the first comprehensive federal protection for the privacy of individually identifiable health information. The two important requirements are that health plans and providers must:

- **Obtain consent** before disclosing health information used for treatment or payment options.
- **Limit disclosure** of information to the minimum necessary to accomplish intended purposes.

HIPAA rules apply fines to organizations for reported breaches of personal health information and give authority to individual states to monitor compliance with the rules. They apply to all forms of communication: electronic, written, and verbal. If you would like further discussion of EHR privacy issues, review the section "How Do I Maintain Confidentiality and Data Security?" in Chapter 17.

KnowledgeCheck 38-4

- Discuss at least three measures to protect the confidentiality of patients' EHRs.

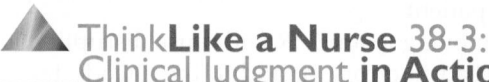

ThinkLike a Nurse 38-3: Clinical Judgment in Action

- How does automation contribute to or decrease errors in healthcare?

PracticalKnowledge knowing how

Professional standards require accountable practitioners to keep up to date with current standards of practice. For example, criteria in the ANA Professional Standard 8 state that the nurse should demonstrate a commitment to lifelong learning and seek experiences that reflect current practice to maintain skills and competence (ANA, 2022). You can accomplish this by knowing how to search literature databases efficiently and use Internet resources discriminatingly to complement your use of the EHR in providing quality patient care. Qualities of an information-literate person are found in Box 38-3.

USING INFORMATICS TO SUPPORT EVIDENCE-BASED PRACTICE

The **traditional model of healthcare decision making** relies on each practitioner's personal experience

BOX 38-3 ■ Profile of an Information-Literate Person

An information-literate person *accesses* information:

- Recognizes the need for information
- Understands that accurate and complete information is the basis for intelligent decision making
- Formulates questions based on information needs
- Identifies potential sources of information and selects those with credibility
- Accesses print and technology-based sources of information

An information-literate person *evaluates* information:

- Accepts authoritative, current reliable information
- Sorts information based on accuracy and relevance
- Distinguishes opinion from factual knowledge
- Rejects inaccurate and misleading information
- Rejects biased information
- Discovers new information to replace inaccurate or missing information, as needed

An information-literate person *manages* information:

- Develops efficient and effective search strategies
- Organizes information so the most important points are clear

- Breaks complex information into understandable chunks
- Sorts out language and technical points into meaningful terms
- Tracks sources of information responsibly and credits appropriately

An information-literate person *uses* information:

- Organizes information for practical application
- Integrates new information into an existing body of knowledge
- Applies information in critical thinking and problem-solving

Other characteristics:

- Resourceful and independent learner
- Competent reader
- Confident in their ability to solve problems
- Able to function independently and work well in groups
- Creative and able to adapt to change

Source: Adapted from U.S. Department of Health and Human Services. (n.d.). *Quick guide to health literacy.* https://healthliteracycentre.eu/wp-content/uploads/2015/11/Quick-guide-to-health-literacy.pdf

---

and judgment. But the complexity of modern health-care means that health problems commonly exceed the clinical decision-making capacity of individual practitioners. A better model of decision making is **evidence-based practice.** As you learned in previous chapters, evidence-based practice involves:

1. Identifying a clinical question or need for change
2. Searching the literature for *best evidence* that can support clinical judgment
3. Evaluating evidence
4. Translating the results into practice

Nurses require current, best-quality information for making decisions in their practice. It is not enough to find a single journal article in support of an intervention. Nurses need to retrieve authoritative, well-sourced, unbiased, scientific evidence on a wide variety of topics, including clinical nursing issues, drug therapy, improving patient outcomes, innovative practice changes, and leadership skills. **Key Point:** *To find the current best evidence, you must be skilled in searching relevant literature.*

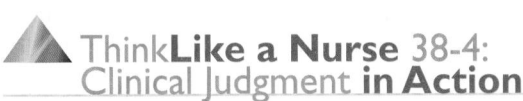
ThinkLike a Nurse 38-4: Clinical Judgment in Action

Analyze the Meet Your Nurse Role Model scenario. What example of evidence-based practice do you find in it?

How Do Computers Reduce Barriers to Evidence-Based Practice?

It may seem easier to seek information from colleagues, rely on experience, draw on knowledge of pathophysiology, and read references that are close at hand. However, in the clinical setting, the most convenient reference book may not contain the most current information or the best possible evidence. Computers at the workplace help overcome this barrier to evidence-based practice.

How Do I Use Computers to Search the Literature?

Poor literature-searching skills are one reason some nurses fail to take advantage of resources that can enrich their practice. There are several steps to conducting a search of the literature:

- **Identify the information.** When you clearly define the topic to investigate and how the information you find will be used, it is easier and more efficient to search, locate, evaluate, retrieve, organize, and manage the resources required to answer your question.
- **Formulate a precise definition of the problem.** This is usually in the form of a question, for example, "What are the leading causes of falls in older adults?" This question guides your search for information.

■ **Conduct a search** of the most recent literature and most relevant studies. To learn about or review the PICOT method of defining and stating questions,

 go to the section Formulate a Searchable Question and the PICOT box in Chapter 4.

▲ ThinkLike a Nurse 38-5: Clinical Judgment in Action

Before reading the next section, see whether you can puzzle out the answers to the following two questions. Consult with your classmates and instructors, if necessary, after finishing the chapter.

■ Why must a question be formed before initiating the search?
■ The suggested question in the preceding section was, "What are the leading causes of falls in older adults?" Why can't you use a general topic such as "falls" for your search topic?

Sources of Scientific Research Literature

First consider the type of literature needed to answer the research question. For instance, a scientific report provides more defensible support for an intervention than does an opinion article. Although some study findings are classic and original, it is usually best to find the most current studies from reliable, authoritative sources, such as government agencies; clinical organizations; or professional, referred, peer-reviewed sources.

Textbooks Some learners prefer hard-copy books over digital formats, for a variety of reasons:

■ **eBooks can be distracting.** Some readers skip over passages of text, scrolling for points of interest. Others use keyword searches to quickly locate select information. This can lead to missed information and reduced comprehension of the broader content.
■ **eBooks involve screen time.** Many students today feel the eyestrain of extensive screen time and opt for printed books. LED screens with backlighting can also disrupt sleep patterns when used at night.
■ **eBook downloads require Internet connection and a power or battery source.** Although many electronic devices are lightweight and portable, an Internet connection is not always available. Low battery charge is a common problem for students who are using devices for a prolonged time.

Journal Articles Although journal articles are typically more current than printed books, the information may still be 6 months to 2 years old by the time the article is published. Journals vary in academic rigor. You must discriminate among scholarly, general-interest, and popular periodical literature.

■ **Scholarly journals.** A scholar, clinical expert, or scientific researcher submits topical articles that adhere to professional standards, with careful referencing and citations. Articles submitted to scholarly journals are reviewed by a panel of experts to determine whether they are suitable for publication. This process is known as a **peer review.** The main purpose

of a scholarly journal is to report on original research or important nursing topics to make the information available to others. Examples of scholarly journals include *Journal of Nursing Scholarship, Journal of Nursing Administration, Nursing Research,* and *International Journal of Nursing Terminologies and Classifications.*

■ **General-interest periodicals.** Articles in general-interest periodicals tend to be graphically and textually appealing. News and general-interest periodicals may cite sources, but not always. Articles may be written by a member of the editorial staff, a scholar, or a freelance writer and are often peer reviewed. The language is geared to readers with some knowledge in the general field. Some examples of general-interest nursing periodicals include the *American Journal of Nursing, RN,* and *Nursing.*
■ **Popular periodicals.** Popular periodicals are usually slick and attractive. They include many graphics and photographs. These publications rarely, if ever, cite sources. Information in such journals is often second- or third-hand, and the original source is sometimes obscure. Articles are usually short, lack depth, and are written in simple language and for a general audience. The main purpose is to promote a product or viewpoint. Examples include *Women's Health* and *Modern Healthcare.*

Internet Sites Internet sites contain the most current information from professional organizations (e.g., American Heart Association), government sources (e.g., Centers for Disease Control and Prevention), sites publishing clinical guidelines (e.g., Joanna Briggs Institute; National Guideline Clearinghouse), and various online nursing journals (e.g., *American Journal of Nursing, Online Journal of Issues in Nursing,* and *Nursing Standard Online*). **Key Point:** *Keep in mind that not all sites "are created equal." It is critical that you are a discerning reader and select credible sources of information.*

Literature Databases

Literature databases are catalogs of articles, usually sorted by discipline. Databases exist for engineering, education, law, medicine, nursing, and other disciplines, for example:

■ **MEDLINE** is the largest medical database and lists internationally published articles from journals in all areas of biomedicine.
■ **Cumulative Index to Nursing and Allied Health Literature (CINAHL)** is a smaller database covering nursing, allied health, biomedical, and consumer health journal articles. However, this database is not free to individuals. Consult the library services at your school or healthcare institution for access.

Databases often overlap—what is found in one database might also be found in another. Most of the articles in CINAHL are also listed in MEDLINE. If, however, you are looking for a nursing-focused article, it is more efficient to use CINAHL because the search is already narrowed to nursing and allied health. Do not limit your search to a single search engine. For some examples of databases in health literature in other related disciplines (e.g., psychology, education, business, law), refer to Table 4-3, *Selected Databases for Health Literature,* in Chapter 4.

Each entry in a database contains an article citation, subject headings describing the article, and a text summary of the article called an **abstract.** Other information about the article may also be included, such as the name of the author(s), the name of the institution at which the research was done, and the language in which the article was published. Many full-text journal articles are available online, some free and some for a fee. Some are available in the school or hospital's library for nurses to access.

How Do I Evaluate Evidence and Determine a Solution?

Evaluating the evidence is sometimes as simple as reading a descriptive research study and applying the results to your patient's health situation. For example, when searching for information about falls in older adults, you may find research to indicate various safety measures that can be easily implemented to create a safer environment for your patients. At other times, evaluating evidence can be complex, requiring an understanding of statistics and research methodologies.

Key Point: *Although an article you find on the Internet may be current, it may not necessarily be complete, accurate, valid, reliable, or relevant to your patient's clinical problem.* Many sites are created by individuals with uncertain credentials or by commercial sources attempting to promote their products or services. Content from these sources may be incomplete, inaccurate, biased, or unreliable. See Box 38-4 for suggestions on evaluating materials obtained from an Internet site. If you would like to review the process for evaluating the quality of research articles you find in your searches or a process for finding the best evidence for a nursing intervention, refer to the section "How Can I Base My Practice on the Best Evidence?" in Chapter 4.

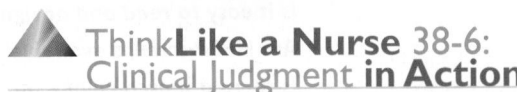
ThinkLike a Nurse 38-6: **Clinical Judgment in Action**

- What factors can make the Internet an unreliable source of information?
- What factors can help you find reliable information?

BOX 38-4 ■ How to Evaluate Health Information on the Internet

Anyone can publish anything on the Internet. Health information you obtain may have been created by an expert; however, some sites are authored by nonexperts. They may contain facts or opinions. Use the following questions to guide your evaluation of health information on the Internet.

Evaluate For	Questions to Ask
Authority	**Who is the author?** What are their credentials and qualifications to speak on this topic? Are the sources of information stated? Do not confuse the author with the webmaster.
	Check the URL domain (e.g., https://www.nih.gov). What institution published the document? The Internet address provides clues to this:
	.com—a company .mil—the U.S. military
	.edu—a school or university .net—a network of computers
	.gov—the U.S. government .org—a nonprofit organization
	The domain symbols ~ or % or a name (e.g., jsmith), "users," or "members" indicate a personal Web page.
	Who is the sponsor? The name right after "www" will provide a clue (e.g., see "nih"), but the full name (e.g., National Institutes of Health) should be on the page.
	Can you contact the author for clarification or more information?
Currency	**When was it produced?** For some topics, you need current information.
	When was it updated? Note that the fact that the page was "updated" may not mean that the information was updated at the same time. It may simply mean that the physical file was changed in some way (e.g., a misspelled word was corrected).
	Are the links up to date? Check the links to see whether they work.
Purpose	**Why was the page put on the Internet?** Remember that many sites are designed to promote a product or an idea. Other purposes may be to entertain, to give facts, to share humor, or to provide a forum for ideas and opinions.
	Look for words such as "about our company," "mission," "philosophy," "who am I," and so on.
	Who are the intended users of the page? Students, experts, patients?
	Are there advertisements on the page? This may be a clue.

(Continued)

BOX 38-4 ■ How to Evaluate Health Information on the Internet—cont'd

Evaluate For	Questions to Ask
Availability	*Can you view or download the information* without a special browser or special software?
	Are there fees for viewing the full content?
Content quality (accuracy, objectivity, coverage)	*Are the sources documented* with footnotes or links? Are they scholarly links or information sources?
	Is the information provided by the site, or is it reproduced from another source?
	Are there links to the original sources (if they are online)? Or is there a reason for not providing a link? Do they work?
	Look for bias (e.g., political or ideological), especially when you agree with it. Are there links to opposing views if it is an opinion page?
	Is the information reliable and error-free? Is there someone who verifies or checks the information?
	How in-depth is the material?
	What does the page offer that you cannot find elsewhere?
	Look up the page in a directory that evaluates the Internet site contents.
Usability	*Is it easy to read and navigate?*
	Are HELP screens available?
	Is there a search engine on the site?
	Is it frequently offline or slow to load?

To explore learning resources for this chapter,

Go to Davis Advantage and find:

Answers and Suggested Responses for all questions in this chapter
Concept Map
Knowledge Map
References and Bibliography

CHAPTER 39

Legal Accountability

Learning Outcomes

After completing this chapter, you should be able to:

➤ Identify four basic sources of law.

➤ Discuss direct implications on practice of the Nurses' Bill of Rights.

➤ Relate the impact of the Health Insurance Portability and Accountability Act (HIPAA) to patient rights and protections.

➤ Discuss the effects of the Patient Self-Determination Act (PSDA) on healthcare practices.

➤ Describe accommodations that conform to the Americans With Disabilities Act (ADA).

➤ Apply state mandatory reporting laws to patient care situations.

➤ Apply the concepts of Good Samaritan laws to nurses' actions.

➤ Identify seven rights of nurses within the healthcare workplace.

➤ Discuss how nurse practice acts provide the foundation for nursing practice.

➤ Explain disciplinary actions for unacceptable nursing decisions or actions.

➤ Discuss basic principles of criminal law that affect nursing practice.

➤ Compare and contrast intentional and unintentional torts.

➤ Discuss common causes of malpractice litigation.

➤ Describe the phases of the litigation process in a nursing malpractice case.

➤ Identify strategies to minimize liability in nursing practice.

Key Concepts

Law

Liability

Malpractice

Related Concepts

See the Concept Map on Davis Advantage.

Meet Your Nurse Role Model

A nurse with 1 year of experience on a medical–surgical unit arrives at work and discovers that two of her colleagues called in sick, including the charge nurse. The nursing supervisor informs the nurse that she will need to assume the charge nurse role, in addition to assuming care for three patients. Feeling frustrated, the nurse ponders whether she should just quit and find another job but then decides to accept the assignment. Two hours into the shift, one of her patients begins to experience complications, requiring blood glucose checks every 2 hours and frequent monitoring. In addition, one of the nurses becomes ill and is replaced by a float nurse from the labor and delivery unit, who spends her time continuously texting on her cell phone. The nurse contacts the nursing supervisor and requests additional assistance but is told no other nurse

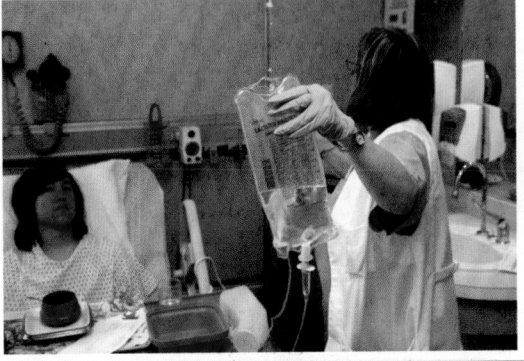

(Continued)

Disclaimer: The material contained in this chapter is intended to convey information on topics of interest to nursing students. Although prepared by a nurse attorney, this chapter should not be used as a substitute for legal counseling. No one should act on the information contained in this chapter without professional guidance. These materials should not be considered legal advice or a legal opinion.

Meet Your Nurse Role Model (continued)

is available and that the supervisor is involved with an emergency situation on another unit. The nurse begins to analyze this situation from a legal perspective to determine the best course of action.

- Should the nurse have accepted the assignment? If yes, what factors should the nurse have considered before accepting the assignment?

- If the nurse had refused the assignment, could she have been charged with abandonment?
- How should the nurse handle this situation?

TheoreticalKnowledge
knowing why

In clinical practice, nurses are often confronted with situations that present legal issues. You must understand the legal guidelines governing nursing practice to protect yourself, your patients, your colleagues, and your employers. The theoretical knowledge in this chapter, combined with the critical thinking model in Chapter 2, will help you to answer questions related to the Meet Your Nurse Role Model scenario.

ABOUT THE KEY CONCEPTS

- The concept of **law** can be described as a binding practice, rule, or code of conduct that guides appropriate actions and defensible decisions of an individual or a group. Laws protect society by establishing acceptable patterns of behavior and are enforceable by a controlling authority.
- **Liability** means that the person is financially or legally responsible for something. Nurses are legally responsible for their own actions, and this responsibility cannot be delegated—this is the basis for liability in nursing practice.
- **Malpractice** is one source of legal liability. It means that a professional person has failed to act in a reasonable and prudent manner. If someone is harmed, the professional may be held liable.

WHAT ARE THE SOURCES AND TYPES OF LAW?

The U.S. Constitution establishes three branches of government: executive, legislative, and judicial. Each branch has specified powers that are designed to equalize power among the three and to provide a system of checks and balances. Laws are derived primarily from four sources: (1) the Constitution, (2) statutes, (3) administrative bodies, and (4) the courts (Table 39-1).

Constitutional Law A **constitution** is a system of fundamental laws and principles that prescribes the nature, functions, and limits of a government.

- **The U.S. Constitution is the superior law of the land and applies to all states throughout the United States.** The U.S. Constitution limits the powers of the federal government and gives each state the power to govern itself and pass laws to promote the health, welfare, order, and security of its citizens (police power).
- **Each state has a similar structure that likewise establishes the governing system for the state, its cities, and municipalities.** Thus, all state and federal laws must be consistent with the U.S. Constitution. Any law that conflicts with the U.S. Constitution is considered invalid or void. If you would like to see a transcript of the Constitution,

 Go to the **National Archives** Web site at https://www.archives.gov/founding-docs/constitution-transcript

Statutory Law A **statute** is a law passed by Congress or by a state legislative body. Congress passes laws for the benefit of society as a whole, whereas states use their police power to pass laws to ensure the general health, safety, and welfare of their citizens. Nurse practice acts (NPAs) are examples of statutory law. NPAs, passed by the legislative body of each state, are regulations that govern the profession of nursing.

Administrative Law Formally defined, **administrative law** refers to the laws that govern the activities of administrative agencies. Federal administrative agencies are created by Congress, and state administrative agencies are created by each state's legislative bodies. As applied to nursing, within each state's nurse practice act, the legislative body created a board of nursing to enforce the provisions of the NPA. The board of nursing creates rules and regulations that define and expand on the provisions in the NPA necessary to ensure compliance with its statutory mission—to regulate the practice of nursing.

Common (Judicial) Law A compilation of laws made by judges or courts is known as **common law.** Also referred to as *case law,* common law is based on

Table 39-1 ▶ Branches of Government

Branches of Government		
	EXAMPLES	**DESCRIPTION**
Executive	The president of the United States, attorney general, secretary of state, state governors	Authority to execute and/or enforce laws
Legislative	Congress (House of Representatives + Senate)	Make or formulate laws
Judicial	U.S. Supreme Court; state and local courts	Interpret statutory law and decide cases and controversies
Type/Source of Law		
	EXAMPLE	**QUESTION POSED**
Constitutional Law	Freedom of speech	Can an employer prevent internationally educated nurses from speaking in their native language in the work environment?
Statutory Law	Definition of nursing	What is the nurse's scope of practice (duties and responsibilities)?
Administrative Law	Delegation and supervision	Is the registered nurse legally responsible for tasks or assignments delegated to other nurses?
Common Law	Affirmative duty	Does a registered nurse have a responsibility to exercise independent judgment to prevent harm to patients?

common customs and traditions. It comes from legal principles and guidelines that judges use to determine the outcome of legal cases.

WHAT LAWS AND REGULATIONS GUIDE NURSING PRACTICE?

As a professional nurse, you will need to understand the various laws and regulations that guide nursing practice. Laws and regulations at the federal and state levels have a direct impact on the nurse's actions and decisions.

Federal Law

Several federal statutes have direct implications for professional nursing practice. Many NPAs require nurses to have knowledge of federal laws, such as the following.

Bill of Rights

The first 10 amendments to the U.S. Constitution are known as the *Bill of Rights.* The Bill of Rights clearly identifies, and in many ways limits, the role of government in individuals' lives. Many of these rights have direct implications for healthcare, including the rights of nurses and of patients. For example, protecting patients' privacy rights is a fundamental role of the professional nurse that is derived from the Fourth Amendment to the U.S. Constitution. If you would like to review all the amendments in the Bill of Rights,

 Go to the **National Archives** Web site at **http://www.archives.gov/exhibits/charters/bill_of_rights_transcript.html**

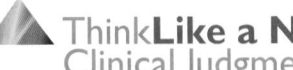 Think**Like a Nurse** 39-1: Clinical Judgment **in Action**

- Develop a scenario illustrating how a nurse might protect a patient's right to privacy.
- What is one thing a nurse can do to respect a patient's property rights?

Health Insurance Portability and Accountability Act (HIPAA)

The Health Insurance Portability and Accountability Act (HIPAA) was passed by Congress in 1996 to:

- Protect health insurance benefits for workers who lose or change their jobs
- Protect coverage to persons with preexisting medical conditions
- Establish standards to protect the privacy of personal health information

Under HIPAA rules, healthcare agencies and their employees must take steps to ensure the confidentiality of patient information and medical records. Nurses and other healthcare providers must protect the patient's right to privacy by not sharing their information with unauthorized individuals. In addition, HIPAA allows patients to see, make corrections to, and obtain copies of their medical records. The cases in the following box highlight the importance of understanding and complying with the safeguards created under HIPAA.

Cases: Violation of a Patient's Privacy

- A nursing assistant was terminated and faced criminal charges for sharing information on the abuse of a patient with Alzheimer on Snapchat. In another case, a nursing assistant spent 8 days in jail for posting graphic photos of older and disabled patients on Facebook.
- A nurse was disciplined by her employer for discussing the HIV status of a patient, which was overheard by the spouse and other patients. A monetary settlement was made with the patient.
- A nurse practitioner was denied access to a facility's electronic health records and reported to the board of nursing for accessing the health records of her ex-husband without permission.
- A pediatric nurse was fired for posting a series of comments about a hospitalized child with a rare case of measles that could have been prevented with vaccination. The information could have potentially identified the patient.

Health Information Technology for Economic and Clinical Health (HITECH) Act

Under the HITECH Act data breach notification provision, healthcare agencies are required to notify patients of breaches without unreasonable delay and in no more than 60 days. In addition, its enhanced enforcement provisions increase civil penalties for breaches caused by willful neglect to up to $250,000, with a maximum penalty of $1.5 million for repeated or uncorrected violations. Posting patient information online can trigger HITECH violations.

Case: Posting Patient Information on Social Media

A certified nursing assistant (CNA) was charged with voyeurism after posting on her Facebook page a picture of a patient's buttocks after he had had a bowel movement. As required by the HITECH Act, her coworkers reported the breach after seeing it on social media. The CNA was terminated and lost her license.

Emergency Medical Treatment and Active Labor Act (EMTALA)

The Emergency Medical Treatment and Active Labor Act (EMTALA) requires healthcare facilities to provide emergency medical treatment to patients (including those in labor) who seek healthcare in the emergency department (ED), regardless of their ability to pay, legal status, or citizenship status. The obligation is for the medical facility to provide medical screening to determine whether an emergency exists and to stabilize the patient before transferring them to another healthcare facility.

An exception is made when a hospital does not have the capability to stabilize a patient or when the patient requests a transfer. In those circumstances, qualified personnel and equipment must be made available to transport the patient, and the patient's medical records must be forwarded to the receiving hospital.

Cases: EMTALA

- The Office of Inspection General (OIG) entered into a settlement agreement with a hospital that violated EMTALA because it did not conduct the appropriate screening due to its failure to perform an adequate search for a patient who presented on the hospital's property. An emergency dispatch notified the hospital staff that a patient had tried to enter through a locked door and unattended ambulance area. The unresponsive patient was later found but died several days later (DeVault, 2018).
- A 27-year-old patient died from septic shock and peritonitis after being treated and discharged from the ED. The deceased, who had a gastric bypass 15 months earlier, went to the ED with complaints of abdominal pain. Language barriers interfered with her ability to communicate a full medical and surgical history. She was given an opioid analgesic, which decreased her pain to 0 on a 0-to-10 scale (0/10), and discharged home with a laxative. Later the same day, she returned to the ED with a 10/10 pain level. The physician provided treatment and discharged her home with an 8/10 pain level. After returning home, the patient went into cardiac arrest and later died. The court noted that although appropriate medical screening occurred, the patient was not stabilized or transferred to another facility for higher-level care. It is not reasonable for a nurse to discharge a patient with a pain level of 8/10. The nurse did not advocate for her patient by notifying her supervisor or taking other actions to prevent the discharge. The court refused to grant the hospital's motion to dismiss the case (*Munoz v. Watsonville Community Hospital*, 2017).

ThinkLike a Nurse 39-2: Clinical Judgment in Action

A 54-year-old uninsured and unemployed woman arrives at the ED of a small private hospital complaining of chest pain and nausea. The triage nurse calls the on-call provider, who instructs the nurse to send the patient to the county hospital several blocks away. The nurse assesses the patient and contacts her supervisor, who directs her to contact the hospitalist to inform them that the patient needs emergency treatment.

- Discuss whether the nurse's action was appropriate or inappropriate.

Patient Self-Determination Act (PSDA)

The Patient Self-Determination Act (PSDA) of 1991 recognizes the patient's right to make decisions regarding their own healthcare. The healthcare provider must inform the patient about available medical or surgical treatment options and benefits, risks, and alternatives. Box 39-1 describes agency and healthcare workers' responsibilities under the PSDA.

There are two types of legal written advance directives: the living will and the durable power of attorney for healthcare.

- A **living will** gives directions to others about a person's wishes regarding life-prolonging treatments if the person becomes unable to make those decisions. The individual must be alert and oriented (competent) when this document is drafted. Because it is a legal document, the requirements for living wills may vary from state to state. However, the common language in living wills gives the person the opportunity to specify treatment in numerous areas (Box 39-2).
- A **durable power of attorney (DPOA) for healthcare** identifies a person (called the *surrogate decision maker*) who will make healthcare decisions in the event the patient is unable to do so. The surrogate has the right to make the medical decisions for as long as the person is not able to do so for themselves (is incompetent).

Case: Durable Power of Attorney (DPOA)

Mr. Green was in a coma as a result of head trauma experienced in a motor vehicle accident. In his DPOA, he had designated his brother, Joey, as his surrogate. Although Mr. Green is married with two adult children, Joey is the person legally recognized to make decisions regarding Mr. Green's healthcare. Two weeks later, Mr. Green came out of the coma and regained the ability to make decisions. At that point, Mr. Green no longer required Joey as a surrogate.

The American Nurses Association (ANA, 2016) highlighted the nurse's role in advance care planning and

---

BOX 39-1 ■ The Patient Self-Determination Act

The Patient Self-Determination Act requires healthcare facilities to:

- Provide written information to each patient regarding the right to make decisions, including the right to accept or to refuse medical treatment and the right to make advance directives.
- Document in the patient's medical record the presence or absence of advance directives.
- Provide education to the staff, healthcare providers, and community on advance directives.
- Follow state law as it relates to advance directives.
- Treat everyone the same regardless of the presence or absence of advance directives (facilities may not discriminate).

BOX 39-2 ■ Sample Living Will Language

If I am in a terminal condition, irreversible coma, or in a persistent vegetative state, my wishes are as follows:

- I ☐ **do** ☐ **do not** want to be in or taken to a hospital.
- I ☐ **do** ☐ **do not** want pain medications to keep me comfortable.
- I ☐ **do** ☐ **do not** want cardiac resuscitation, including drugs and electrical shock.
- I ☐ **do** ☐ **do not** want mechanical respiration/artificial respiration.
- I ☐ **do** ☐ **do not** want tube feeding or any other artificial or invasive form of nutrition (food).
- I ☐ **do** ☐ **do not** want hydration (water), via tube or intravenously.
- I ☐ **do** ☐ **do not** want blood or blood products.
- I ☐ **do** ☐ **do not** want any form of surgery or invasive diagnostic tests.
- I ☐ **do**☐ **do not** want renal dialysis.
- I ☐ **do** ☐ **do not** want antibiotics.

---

counseling in a position statement. As a nurse, you have the following responsibilities:

- Listen to patients to identify their concerns, expectations, and hopes regarding end-of-life care.
- Review patients' documented preferences upon admission to healthcare facilities.
- Recognize that advance care planning is a continual process and not a one-time execution of documents.
- Encourage patient and family participation in healthcare decisions about advance directives and end-of-life decisions.

You might want to ask the following questions about advance directives as a part of your nursing admission assessment:

- What is your understanding of an advance directive, including the living will and durable power of attorney for healthcare?
- Do you have an advance care directive?
- If you have an advance care directive, do you have a copy with you?
- Do you wish to initiate an advance care directive?
- Who will make your healthcare decisions if you are unable to do so? Have you discussed your end-of-life choices with this person, significant others, and your provider?

Case: Durable Power of Attorney (DPOA)

Classic Case: Mrs. Terry Schiavo collapsed in her Florida home in 1990 after a suspected potassium imbalance secondary to bulimia, and she was without oxygen for about 5 minutes. She suffered severe brain damage. Terry Schiavo did not have a living will. According to Florida law, her husband became her legal guardian and thus the decision maker regarding her medical treatments. In November 1992, Mr. Schiavo won a medical malpractice lawsuit for $1 million from her physician on the theory that her physician failed to diagnose Mrs. Schiavo's bulimia.

In 2000, Mr. Schiavo petitioned the court to have her feeding tube removed. Her parents opposed the action. During the next 5 years, extensive legal battles ensued. Finally, the court ruled in favor of removing the feeding tube. Mrs. Schiavo died on March 31, 2005. The lack of a living will (1) allowed this situation to go on for so long and (2) made it impossible to know for sure what Terry Schiavo would have wanted. It's all guesswork without a documented living will (Shapiro, 2015; Lopez & Vars, 2019).

Advanced directives are a clear indication of a patient's wishes and instructions regarding life-prolonging measures. What happens when medical providers ignore properly executed advanced directives that clearly indicate that no life-sustaining measures be initiated? Once historically rejected by courts, **wrongful living** cases are now gaining recognition as a valid legal claim. Many healthcare facilities have entered into monetary settlement agreements for initiating medical treatment (e.g., ventilator support, cardiopulmonary resuscitation [CPR]) in direct opposition to patients' known advanced directives (Advisory Board, 2021; Lopez & Vars, 2019).

Americans With Disabilities Act (ADA)

The Americans With Disabilities Act (ADA) of 1990 provides protection against discrimination aimed at individuals with disabilities. A person has a **disability** if they have a physical or mental impairment that substantially limits one or more major life activities, has a record of such impairment, or is regarded as having an impairment (ADA Amendments Act of 2008). In general, the ADA says that employers or other entities (e.g., educational institutions, healthcare facilities) must provide reasonable accommodations within the work, educational, or healthcare environments to allow individuals with disabilities to perform their jobs.

Case: ADA Accommodations

- A nurse with a hearing impairment received a telephone amplifier to take telephone prescriptions accurately and effectively.
- A nurse with insulin-dependent diabetes had difficulty maintaining glucose control. Her employer provided consistent times for breaks and lunch, as well as privacy to check blood sugars and administer insulin as needed (Job Accommodation Network, n.d.).

KnowledgeCheck 39-1

- Which federal law requires healthcare agencies to provide patients with information about advance directives?
- Which federal law ensures that patients can receive emergency treatment regardless of their ability to pay?
- What protections are provided to patients by the "privacy rule" of HIPAA?

State Laws

In addition to federal law, many states have laws that directly affect nurses' actions and behaviors. These include mandatory reporting laws, Good Samaritan laws, NPAs, and medical malpractice statutes.

Mandatory Reporting Laws

The law in various states requires healthcare workers to report communicable diseases. You also have a duty to report physical, sexual, or emotional abuse or neglect of vulnerable individuals (e.g., children, older adults, the mentally ill), whether you suspect it or have actual evidence of it. The intent is to protect people who cannot protect themselves and to protect society against the spread of communicable diseases. Because the mandatory reporting laws vary from state to state, you should be familiar with the law in your state.

- Mandatory reporting laws also protect you when reporting abuse. In most instances, the identity of the reporter is kept confidential.
- If you fail to report certain communicable diseases or child abuse, you can be charged with a criminal misdemeanor or be subject to disciplinary action by the board of nursing.
- **Key Point:** *The duty to report takes priority over the patient's right to privacy. Therefore, if you report suspected abuse or neglect, you cannot be charged with violating a patient's right to privacy (e.g., under HIPAA).*

Case: Mandatory Reporting

- Several staff members at a mental health facility were charged with the criminal offenses of vulnerable adult abuse and assault and battery. The provider and nurse were charged with failure to report the abuse of vulnerable adults.
- Several individuals, including a physician, resigned and were under criminal investigation for failure to report the aggravated sexual assault of an incapacitated adult living in a long-term care facility.

Good Samaritan Laws

Good Samaritan laws are designed to protect from liability those who provide emergency care to someone who needs medical services. To successfully use the Good Samaritan defense, the following elements must be present:

- Care was provided in an emergency situation.
- The person(s) providing the care did not cause the emergency or injury.

- Care was provided in a reasonably competent manner.
- Care was voluntary; the person did not receive payment or was not eligible for payment.
- The person receiving care did not object to receiving care.

To ensure protection under Good Samaritan laws, nurses should follow these guidelines:

- Call 911, or have someone else call, as soon as you can.
- Do not leave the person unless you transfer care to an equally competent professional.
- Place the person under the care of emergency personnel or other qualified healthcare professionals as soon as possible, and follow their instructions.
- Do not accept money or any other form of compensation for the services provided.
- **Key Point:** *Good Samaritan laws vary from state to state. You should be familiar with the law in your state.*

Case: Good Samaritan

An RN was leaving the hospital after working a 12-hour shift when she witnessed a single-person motor vehicle accident. She called 911, stopped, and approached the accident scene, where she smelled gasoline. Fearing that the car would explode, she pulled the accident victim from the car, placed him flat on the ground, and assessed his injuries. She put pressure on his bleeding femoral artery and stayed with him until the ambulance arrived. The victim had spinal cord injuries and sued the nurse for removing him from the car. The nurse was protected from liability by the Good Samaritan law.

Nurses working in healthcare environments may not be protected by Good Samaritan laws if they already have a responsibility to provide care to those in need.

Case: Good Samaritan

The court upheld the Good Samaritan defense for a school nurse who provided care to a child while visiting a different school district. Although the facts were disputed, the nurse testified that the child conveyed to her that he hit himself in the eye with a string. On assessment, the eye was not red or swollen. The nurse applied an eye compress and instructed the parents to seek medical care if problems arose. The child's father indicated that the nurse was aware that the child struck his eye with wire, it was red when examined by the nurse, and no instructions for further care were provided. The court found that the nurse volunteered her services and had no expectations, nor did she receive monetary compensation (*McDaniel v. Keck,* 2008).

Nurse Practice Acts

NPAs are statutory laws passed by each state's legislative body that define the practice of nursing. Nurse practice acts are designed to:

- Regulate nursing practice to protect the health, safety, and welfare of the general public.
- Define the scope of nursing practice.
- Approve programs providing prelicensure nursing education to students.

The components of NPAs are discussed in more detail later in the chapter.

Medical Malpractice Statutes

Medical malpractice refers to a lawsuit brought against a healthcare provider for damages (e.g., money) when there has been a death of, injury to, or other loss to the person being treated. Laws governing medical malpractice vary from state to state, primarily regarding the time frame for bringing a lawsuit (statute of limitations) and the amount of monetary compensation allowed. To protect themselves from personal losses, many healthcare providers purchase malpractice insurance, which provides them with an attorney to defend against the claim and pay the damages (money) awarded to the claimant by a judge or jury. Malpractice is discussed in more detail later in this chapter.

Other Guidelines for Practice

In addition to federal and state laws, other practice guidelines may define what constitutes reasonable and prudent nursing care.

Institutional Policies and Procedures

Institutional policies and procedures usually are more specific and detailed than standards set by professional organizations. They describe care that is reasonable, appropriate, and expected in the context of that facility. You must be familiar with these policies and procedures because they can be used as evidence of a violation of a standard of care if you fail to follow them. Healthcare facilities should not have policies and procedures that conflict with the NPA, professional standards of practice, the ANA *Code of Ethics for Nurses,* and other documents that guide nursing practice. If you encounter conflicts or if a policy is not working well, you should bring the matter to your supervisor's attention and/or contact the board of nursing in your state for an advisory opinion.

American Nurses Association Code of Ethics

The **ANA** *Code of Ethics for Nurses* (ANA, 2015a) describes the standards of professional responsibility for nurses and provides insight into ethical and acceptable behavior. It describes nurses' obligations for safe, compassionate, nondiscriminatory, and quality care while defining commitments to self, the patient, the employer, and the profession. The *Code of Ethics* is not a law, and therefore you would not be charged with criminal offenses for violating its provisions. **Key Point:** *In many situations, there is a fine line between what is legal and what is ethical. When confronted with a situation, to avoid legal jeopardy, you should ask yourself,*

- *Is there a law that relates to this situation? If the answer is yes, you should understand the guidance provided by the law.*
- *If you cannot follow the law in good conscience, talk with your supervisor or seek legal advice.*
- *If there is no law, or if it seems immoral or unethical to you, ask, "What guidance is provided under the* Code of Ethics?"

Your action should be consistent with the Code, if at all possible. The ANA *Code of Ethics* guarantees the patient the right to dignity, privacy, and safety and that the nurse will:

- Be accountable and competent.
- Use informed judgment.
- Maintain employment conditions conducive to quality patient care.
- Protect the patient from misinformation and misrepresentation.
- Collaborate with other healthcare professions to meet the patient's healthcare needs.

A nurse who violates a provision of the *Code of Ethics* **may have to defend their action to the state board of nursing.** Also, in a malpractice suit, courts may look to these codes to judge whether the nurse's action was at the level expected by the profession. However, you must understand that the code will not likely protect you if you break a law or fail to follow agency policies, even if you believe the law to be immoral. If you need more information on nursing codes of ethics, see Chapter 5.

Patient Care Partnership

The **Patient Care Partnership** (PCP), available in eight languages, explains to patients what they should expect during hospitalization. This includes high-quality care, a clean and safe environment, involvement in their care, protection of privacy, help when leaving the facility, and help with any billing claims.

Like the ANA *Code of Ethics*, these rights are not necessarily legally binding, but they can provide evidence by which to judge whether the patient's care and environment met reasonable and appropriate standards. For more information on the PCP, see Box 39-3.

American Nurses Association Nurses' Bill of Rights

The **Nurses' Bill of Rights** is a policy statement adopted by the ANA to identify the seven conditions that nurses should expect from their workplace that are necessary for sound professional practice. It provides a framework for employers to understand what nurses need for a safe work environment and to support nurses as they address such issues as unsafe staffing, workplace violence, and mandatory overtime (ANA, n.d.). The Nurses' Bill of Rights highlights that nurses have the right to:

- Practice in a manner that fulfills their obligations to society and to those who receive nursing care
- Practice in environments that allow them to act in accordance with professional standards and legally authorized scopes of practice
- A work environment that supports and facilitates ethical practice as defined by the *Code of Ethics for Nurses*
- Freely and openly advocate for themselves and their patients, without fear of retribution
- Fair compensation for their work, consistent with their knowledge, experience, and professional responsibilities
- A work environment that is safe for themselves and for their patients
- Negotiate the conditions of their employment, either as individuals or collectively, in all practice settings

American Nurses Association Standards of Practice

The ANA (2015b) *Standards of Practice* have three components:

1. *Professional standards of care* that incorporate the nursing process in the diagnostic, intervention, and evaluation aspect of patient care
2. *Professional performance standards* that identify the various role functions of the nurse in direct patient care, quality of practice, ethics, education, communication, research, leadership, collaboration, resource management, collegiality, and environmental health
3. *Practice guidelines* for the various specialty areas that are developed by professional organizations (e.g., American Association of Critical-Care Nurses)

Standards establish the minimum level of competency for nurses. Nurses are expected to follow the standards that apply to their specialty areas.

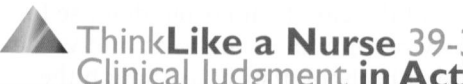

ThinkLike a Nurse 39-3: Clinical Judgment in Action

Recall the Meet Your Nurse Role Model scenario. Would the nurse have done the right thing if she had decided not to accept the assignment and immediately left the facility?

- What standards, guidelines, and laws would apply to determine whether the nurse's behavior was in accordance with standards of practice?
- Which statements in the ANA Nurses' Bill of Rights might the nurse use to justify their actions?

Nurse Practice Acts

As you have learned, NPAs contain a provision that creates and empowers a state board of nursing to regulate the practice of nursing in that state. All 50 states, the

District of Columbia, and the four U.S. territories have established boards of nursing. Although NPAs can vary from state to state, they all have common components because the states used ANA guidelines in developing their regulations. A state's NPA usually includes the following:

- The authority of the board of nursing, its composition, and its powers
- A definition of *nursing* and the boundaries of nursing practice
- Standards for the approval of nursing education programs
- The requirements for licensure of nurses
- Grounds for disciplinary action against a nurse's license

Case: Nurse Practice Act

Mejonus X Institute is advertising an associate degree nursing program that can be completed in 12 months at a cost of $45,000. You are interested in the program but are not sure whether the program is legitimate. Your initial investigation of the program should start with researching the list of approved nursing programs found on the state board of nursing Web site.

Requirements for Licensure

Perhaps the most important function of state boards of nursing is establishing and enforcing the requirements for licensure. Unlicensed health providers pose a danger to the health, safety, and welfare of the general public because they have not met the specified standards to ensure a minimum level of competency to enter the nursing profession. In most states, the applicant for licensure must:

- Graduate from an approved or accredited nursing program
- Meet the established character criteria
- Undergo a criminal background check and fingerprinting
- Pass the NCLEX-RN or NCLEX-PN examination
- Pay an application fee
- Meet additional state requirements (e.g., a jurisprudence examination in Texas)

Case: Nurse With a Criminal Conviction

A board of nursing revoked the license of an RN for practicing nursing while impaired, deviating from professional standards of practice, engaging in abusive behaviors toward coworkers, and failing to report a felony criminal conviction of child abuse.

Special Cases of Licensure

To protect the public, licensing is meant to ensure that practicing nurses have met the minimum competencies set by the state.

Mutual Recognition Model (MRM)/Nurse Licensure Compact Certain states, through a multistate agreement, allow nurses whose primary state of residency is in a compact state to practice in other compact states without obtaining a new license. These nurses have a **multistate license.** Nurses whose primary state of residency is in a noncompact state have a **single-state license.** To practice in another state, the nurse must request *licensure by endorsement* in the desired state. To be *licensed by endorsement,* you do not have to retake the NCLEX examination, but you must apply to the new state and fulfill any of that state's application requirements, such as fingerprinting, background check, transcripts, and fees, found on the board of nursing's Web site.

Case: Multistate Compact

Roberto is a clinical nurse residing in Nevada (his primary state of residency) and originally licensed in Nevada after passing the NCLEX-RN examination. He is now employed at a home healthcare agency on the other side of the state line in California. Roberto is required to maintain active licensure in the state where he is employed. He received an RN licensure by endorsement in the state of California by meeting the requirements of the California State Board of Nursing, but he did not have to retake the NCLEX-RN.

Government/Military Personnel Another special case of licensure involves nurses employed by the military, Veterans Administration, Public Health Service, or other entities of the federal government. These nurses may practice in other states without obtaining a new license as long as they are practicing within the scope of their employment with the federal agency.

Case: Special Case of Licensure

Jane is a clinical nurse in the U.S. Air Force Reserve. She is licensed in the state of Texas but is assigned to a military hospital in Nevada for her 2-week annual military tour. Jane will not need to obtain a license in the state of Nevada to practice at the military hospital.

Scope of Practice

The scope of nursing practice is found in the definitions of nursing at the various levels. Nurses must be familiar with the definition of their level of *nursing* to appropriately plan and implement care that is consistent with their scope of practice. **Key Point: *A nurse who practices outside the scope of practice can be charged with violation of the NPA.***

NPAs vary slightly by state. However, in most states, the licensed practical nurse (LPN) scope of practice is limited in assessment privileges and interpretation of clinical data. Typically, LPNs/licensed vocational nurses (LVNs) do not have the authority to alter nursing care plans. You must know the requirements of your state because they determine the legal limits of your practice. The following landmark case should make clear that no one, including an employer or provider, can increase a nurse's legal scope of practice.

Classic Case: Scope of Practice

A physician delegated to an LPN the task of administering a polio booster to a 2-year-old boy. The nurse put the boy over her knee and proceeded to give the injection. The boy moved, and the needle broke off in his buttocks, where it remained for 9 months despite attempts to surgically remove it. Because the Washington State Nurse Practice Act at that time did not allow LPNs to give injections, the nurse was in violation of the NPA by performing a task that was outside of her legal limits (*Barber v. Reinking*, 1966).

Disciplinary Actions

The state board of nursing can take disciplinary actions against your license for violation of the NPA.

What Is the Process? A disciplinary action usually involves some or all of the following:

- The process begins with a complaint from an individual, employer, or professional organization that the nurse has engaged in unprofessional conduct.
- The complaint is then assigned to an investigator to determine its legitimacy or validity.
  - If the investigator decides the complaint is invalid or does not constitute a violation of the NPA, it will be dismissed.
  - If the complaint may violate the NPA, the investigator gathers additional information by contacting the nurse, interviewing witnesses, and reviewing documents and records.
- The case may be heard by the board of nursing members, who will decide whether the nurse violated the NPA and determine the appropriate punishment. To fulfill the due process requirements of the Fourteenth Amendment, the board of nursing must provide you with:
  - **Notice** of the charges against you. This is primarily done in a letter, via certified mail, that outlines the charges against you and identifies the provisions of the NPA that were allegedly violated.
  - **Evidence** that supports the charges
  - A **hearing** in which you have the opportunity to cross-examine the witnesses and present your own evidence and witnesses
- If you are not satisfied with the board's actions and punishment, you can appeal your case to the appropriate state court.
- At every stage during the disciplinary process, you have the right to have an attorney present. Questions that you should ask of a potential attorney include the following: (1) How many of your cases were in the area of administrative law and procedures?

(2) How many times have you represented patients in front of professional boards, such as the board of nursing?

What Constitutes Unprofessional Conduct or Conduct Derogatory to the Standards of Nursing? Nurses whose actions may be injurious to patients or coworkers or negatively affect the health, safety, and welfare of the general public exemplify unprofessional conduct that is not in accordance with standards of nursing practice. The following are a few examples of actions that may constitute unprofessional conduct or behaviors derogatory to standards:

- Acting outside your scope of practice.
- Inaccurately recording, falsifying, altering, or destroying a patient or agency records or directing others to perform these behaviors.
- Failure to document nursing interventions and nursing practice implementation in a timely, accurate, thorough, and clear manner. This includes failing to document a late entry within a reasonable time period.
- Failure to communicate information regarding the patient's status to individuals who have a need to know in a timely manner.
- Causing intentional or careless physical abuse or harm to a patient, including unreasonable use of restraint, isolation, or medication; threatening or frightening patients; verbal abuse; sexual abuse, misconduct, profane language, derogatory names, or exploitation.
- Violating the patient's confidentiality.
- Stealing money, property, services, or supplies from the patient or the patient's family.
- Failing to take appropriate action to safeguard a patient from the incompetent practice of another (e.g., reporting to the facility or state board of nursing).
- Accepting duties or responsibilities for which you are not prepared or competent.
- Using a false or assumed name or impersonating another person licensed by the board.
- Diverting drugs, supplies, or property from any patient or agency.
- Engaging in violent, abusive, or threatening behavior toward a coworker. (Kansas State Board of Nursing, 1993, last amended 2016; Oregon Board of Nursing, 2017)

▲ ThinkLike a Nurse 39-4: Clinical Judgment in Action

An RN was assigned to care for a 76-year-old patient who had a stroke (brain attack). On entering the room, the nurse found the patient surrounded by 10 family members. They complied with the nurse's request to leave the room so that she could conduct her initial assessment and perform any related treatments. The nurse provided care in a professional, unhurried, and gentle manner. As she was leaving, the patient said, "Thank you. You are a wonderful nurse." Later, the nursing supervisor told her the patient told his family members that the nurse had spoken harshly to him and had yanked his arms. The family stated that they would file a complaint with the hospital administrator and the board of nursing.

- Are there grounds for disciplinary actions?
- What should the nurse do?

KnowledgeCheck 39-2

How does each of the following protect patients?

- The Patient Care Partnership (PCP)
- *Code of Ethics for Nurses*
- Mandatory reporting laws

Credentialing

Many healthcare disciplines, including nursing, use a voluntary form of self-regulation called **credentialing.** In the legal sense, credentialing includes accreditation and certification. Having credentials implies that the person or agency has met higher standards than the minimum (e.g., licensure).

Accreditation Most nursing boards require that a nursing program be **accredited** by an agency recognized by the Department of Education (e.g., Accreditation Commission for Education in Nursing [ACEN], Commission on Collegiate Nursing Education [CCNE], Commission for Nursing Education Accreditation [CNEA]). This helps to ensure students receive education that meets the minimum standard for quality patient care. Similarly, The Joint Commission accredits healthcare facilities that meet established standards focused on safe, appropriate, and quality patient care.

Certification Another form of credentialing is **certification.** Through certification and licensing, the board identifies nurses who are qualified for advanced practice (e.g., clinical nurse specialists, midwives, and nurse practitioners) or for certification in a subspecialty, such as emergency nursing or pediatric nursing. In some states, the board establishes the criteria for certification, including (1) educational preparation, (2) clinical experience, and (3) certification by other professional organizations. In other states, the nurse may obtain an advanced practice license only if they are first certified by a national organization, such as the American Nurses Credentialing Corporation or a specialty organization.

WHAT IS CRIMINAL LAW?

Criminal law deals with wrongs or offenses against society. It may result in prosecution (legal action) by the state or federal government for engaging in behavior that constitutes a crime. A **crime** is a violation of a law as defined by a legislative body. The legislature also specifies the punishments for the crime. State-level criminal laws vary from state to state. There are two "levels" of crimes: misdemeanors and felonies. One primary difference is the possible punishment.

- A **felony** is a crime punishable by more than 1 year in jail (e.g., murder, assisted suicide, rape/sexual assault,

stealing drugs and equipment, felony abuse). A person convicted of a felony loses the right to vote, hold public office, serve on a jury, and possess firearms for a time period specified by the state. The person may also lose any professional license.

- A **misdemeanor,** compared with a felony, is a minor charge. Misdemeanors usually involve less than a year in jail. They include crimes such as assault, battery, and petty theft. You may also have a disciplinary action against your nursing license if you are convicted of a misdemeanor that involves crimes against persons, actions that can cause harm to others, theft, or substance abuse.

The defendant in a criminal case has the right to an attorney and the right to remain silent, which means they do not have to answer questions during police interrogation. If you are arrested, you should ask for an attorney and not answer any questions without your attorney present. The defendant also has a right to a jury trial.

Case Example: Criminal Law

An investigation revealed that several patients who received pain medication from the assigned nurse complained of ineffective pain relief. When confronted, the nurse admitted to stealing the patients' pain medication and giving the patients saline instead. She also admitted to using other nurses' passwords to steal narcotics. The Board of Nursing revoked her license after she refused to enroll in an impaired nurse's program. She also faced felony criminal charges for theft of controlled substances.

Case Example: Criminal Law

A nurse was charged with felony grand larceny for stealing computer equipment and wound supplies valued at $55,000 from the hospital where she was employed. She entered into a plea deal that reduced the charge to a misdemeanor with 6 months' probation and was required to reimburse the hospital $55,000. The Board of Nursing suspended her license for 2 years.

Are Nursing Errors Crimes? An issue in the nursing profession is whether nurses who accidentally cause harm to patients should be charged with criminal offenses (e.g., a patient dies after a nurse accidentally administers the wrong drug). In the past, these cases have been handled under civil law (malpractice) and by the board of nursing. Now state prosecutors are beginning to bring felony and misdemeanor charges against these nurses.

Case: Nurse Charged With a Crime for Practice Negligence

- A nurse failed to perform neurological checks, as required by agency policy, on a poststroke patient who had an unwitnessed fall. He was later found dead in the lobby, sitting in a chair. The fall caused blunt-force head trauma and a subdural hematoma. The nurse was criminally charged with involuntary manslaughter (Brown, 2018).

- A nurse was convicted of a felony and sentenced to 3 years' probation for a medication error that resulted in the patient's death. The nurse also had her licensed revoked by the board of nursing (Advisory Board, 2022).

The American Association of Nurse Attorneys (TAANA) advocates against criminalizing practice errors. Such actions are not only demoralizing to the profession but also counterproductive to eradicating a culture of blame and creating one that promotes ownership and correction of practice errors (TAANA, 2011).

WHAT IS CIVIL LAW?

In contrast to criminal law, in which the state or federal government brings charges against a person, **civil law** involves a dispute between individuals or entities. A settlement in civil law often results in the guilty party paying monetary damages. Two types of civil law are contract law and tort law.

- **Contract law** involves a written or oral agreement between two parties in which one party accepts an offer made by the other party to perform (or not perform) certain acts in exchange for something of value. A breach of contract occurs if either party does not comply with the terms of the agreement. An example would be an employment contract.
- **Tort law,** in comparison, deals with wrongs done to one person by another person that do not involve contracts. A tort is a civil wrong, and there are three types of tort: quasi-intentional torts, intentional torts, and unintentional torts.

What Are Quasi-Intentional Torts?

Quasi-intentional torts involve actions that injure a person's reputation. The overall concept for these torts is defamation of character. All four of the following essential elements of **defamation of character** must be present. The communication (written or oral) about the person:

- Was false
- Was made to another person or persons
- Caused the defamed person to experience shame and ridicule and had a negative impact on the person's reputation
- Was made as a statement of fact rather than as an opinion

Libel is the written or published form of defamation of character. **Slander** is the spoken or verbal form of defamation of character.

A person is not guilty of defamation of character if the statement made about the other person is true or if the person has the protection of a "privilege," such as reporting possible child abuse.

Case: Quasi-Intentional Torts

The nursing supervisor calls you into a conference room and states, "I know that you have been stealing (diverting) narcotics from the unit and injecting yourself with it while at work. It shows—your work is sloppy, and you are falsifying your documentation. You are a poor excuse for a nurse." Before you can defend yourself, the supervisor turns and leaves. The statements are not true. Nurses in the conference room try to console you. The supervisor has committed slander.

What Are Intentional Torts?

An **intentional tort** is an action taken by one person with the intent to harm another person. The harm does not have to be violent, hostile, or cause a significant amount of pain or distress to the other person. The person must have merely intended to cause harm or known the action would bring about the harm.

Intentional torts may also be prosecuted under criminal law. For example, a nurse who is sued for malpractice in civil court may also be charged with homicide if a patient died because of the nurse's actions. The intentional torts most commonly encountered in nursing are assault, battery, false imprisonment, and invasion of privacy.

Assault

An assault occurs when a nurse intentionally places a patient in immediate fear of personal violence or offensive contact. An assault must include words expressing an intention to cause harm and some type of action. For example, a nurse has committed an assault if they raise their hand as if to slap the patient and say, "I will slap you." The combination of the words and the action causes the patient to believe the threat will be carried out.

Battery

A **battery** is committed when (1) an offensive or harmful physical contact is made to the patient without his consent, or (2) there is unauthorized touching of a person's body by another person. To avoid charges of battery, always obtain informed consent before providing certain treatments. On admission to healthcare facilities, patients sign a general consent form, which usually covers routine aspects of nursing care, such as vital signs and assessments. However, when performing any invasive procedure, such as inserting a catheter or IV line, you should always explain the procedure to the patient and obtain their consent before beginning. Follow your facility's policies regarding procedures and treatments that require informed consent.

Case: Battery—Administering Medication Without the Patient's Consent

A court refused to dismiss a medical battery charge against an oncologist who prescribed a toxic drug to treat leukemia. The drug was administered multiple times without obtaining the patient's consent. The complaint alleges that the physician and staff tried to obtain the patient's consent after the error was discovered (Nelson, 2018).

Assault and Battery

An **assault and battery** occurs when there is the intent to cause a person fear combined with an offensive or harmful contact.

Case: Assault and Battery

A patient admitted for an elective surgical procedure complained that the automatic blood pressure cuff was causing her extreme pain and demanded that it be removed. The nurse did not immediately remove the cuff as requested by the patient. The nurse was guilty of battery, but not assault, because there was no evidence the nurse intended to create or cause fear or pain (*Coulter v. Thomas*, 2000).

False Imprisonment

False imprisonment is the restraining of a person without proper legal authorization. It includes any type of unjustified restriction on a person's freedom of movement—for example, when nurses restrain patients without their permission or when patients are involuntarily committed to mental health units. False imprisonment can involve the use of physical restraints (e.g., vest or wrist restraints) or chemical restraints (e.g., sedatives or opioids). **Key Point:** *You may restrain patients who pose an immediate threat to themselves or others. However, you must immediately obtain the proper authorization to continue the restraint.*

Against Medical Advice (AMA) If a competent patient wishes to leave the healthcare facility, you should contact the nursing supervisor and the primary care provider. The patient must be informed of the risks associated with leaving and given the choice to stay and receive treatment or to sign out against medical advice (AMA). You need to be aware of the hospital policy and procedures on AMA discharges.

Invasion of Privacy

Invasion of privacy violates a person's right to be left alone. The law recognizes that a person's personal life should not be opened up for public scrutiny and that the person has the right to freedom from unwanted interference in their private affairs. A person has the right to:

- Have their private information protected
- Not be falsely portrayed or intentionally misrepresented in character, beliefs, or actions
- Be free from unwanted intrusion (spying, eavesdropping)

Examples of violating the right to privacy include discussing patients in public places (e.g., elevators, cafeterias), photographing patients without their permission, providing information to news media without consent, searching a patient's personal belongings without permission, and releasing medical information without the patient's consent.

Fraud

Fraud is the false representation of significant facts by words or by conduct. It is intentionally misleading or deceiving another person to act (or not act) for the personal gain of the one committing the fraud. Methods of committing fraud include making false statements, falsifying documentation, or concealing information that should have been disclosed.

Cases: Fraud

- A nurse whose license had been revoked was arrested and charged with fraud for trying to obtain a new nursing license with fraudulent documents (Garcia, 2018).
- A nursing supervisor pled guilty to a multimillion-dollar fraud scheme. Individuals at the hospice facility enrolled eligible and ineligible patients into 24-hour hospice care to receive a higher rate of reimbursement. Some patients were given drugs to hasten their death (Wigglesworth, 2018).

What Are Unintentional Torts?

The most common type of unintentional tort involving healthcare professionals is negligence or malpractice.

- **Negligence** is the failure to use ordinary or reasonable care or the failure to act in a reasonable and prudent (careful) manner.
- **Malpractice** has a similar definition but applies only to professionals, such as nurses and providers. It is defined as the failure of a professional person to act in a reasonable and prudent manner. A malpractice lawsuit may occur when such actions cause injury or death to the patient. The person bringing the lawsuit is the **plaintiff,** and the person who must defend against the lawsuit is the **defendant.**

Malpractice/Negligence Liability

To win and recover damages (money) in a malpractice lawsuit, the plaintiff must prove four elements (duty, breach of duty, causation, and damages). The elements must be proved by a **"preponderance of the evidence,"**

Toward Evidence-Based Practice

Gleason, K., Rebecca, J., Rhodes, C., Greenberg, P., Harkless, G., Goeschel, C., Cahill, M., & Graber, M. (2021). Evidence that nurses need to participate in diagnosis: Lessons from malpractice claims. *Journal of Patient Safety, 17*(8), e959–e963. https://doi.org/10.1097/PTS.0000000000000621

Researchers noted that the distinction between medical diagnosis and nursing diagnosis may contribute to situations in which nurses refrain from full participation in the diagnostic process. Analyzing a malpractice claims database that contained 30% of U.S. claims from 2007 to 2016, the researchers identified cases in which nurses were named the primary responsible party for patient injuries or death related to failure to diagnose and failure to monitor physiological status. Findings revealed the following:

- Of the 647 failure to monitor cases, 263 resulted in a patient's death, 99 led to significant levels of permanent harm, and 107 caused temporary major harm. An analysis of these cases revealed documentation (e.g., insufficient, inaccurate, inconsistent) and communication failures. Communication failures among providers, as well as communication and education to patients, were contributing factors. A higher likelihood of death occurred with failure of communication among providers and on various shifts (nights, weekends, holidays).

- Of the 139 diagnosis-related failure cases, 70 resulted in a patient's death, and 73 led to severe injuries. Contributing factors that led to patients' deaths included, but were not limited to, communication failures among providers, failure to respond, failure to consult, inadequate assessment, and failure to follow policy. Deficiencies in documentation and staff training and education were also noted.

The researchers concluded that nurses have an important and legitimate role in the diagnostic process that is essential to ensure quality patient care. This premise is supported in a report by the National Academy of Medicine that emphasizes the need for interprofessional curricula to improve diagnostic reasoning, education, and shared accountability. One recommendation was to evolve away from "nursing diagnosis" language to a more shared diagnostic teamwork requirement.

---

1. You have been assigned to chair a task force to explore the "diagnostic teamwork" concept and make recommendations to nursing leadership. Identify areas that you and your team would explore.

---

in other words, with enough evidence to tip the scale in the plaintiff's favor.

Duty The nurse–patient relationship creates this legal obligation. A **duty** forms when the patient is assigned to the nurse or seeks treatment from the nurse or when the nurse observes another person doing something that could harm the patient.

Breach of Duty A breach of duty occurs when the nurse fails to meet standards of care. Attorneys use several resources (e.g., NPA, hospital policies and procedures, textbooks, professional standards and guidelines) to identify the standards of care and to determine what a reasonable and prudent (careful) nurse would have done in the situation.

The plaintiff's attorney will usually hire an **expert witness** who is a nurse with advanced education or experience. The purpose of an expert witness is to educate the judge and jury on the local practice of nursing and how the nurse's actions or omissions failed to meet acceptable practice for nurses. The defendant's attorney may hire an expert to testify that the nurse, based on the circumstances, adhered to standards of practice.

Causation The breach of duty or deviation from acceptable standards of care by the nurse must be the direct and proximate cause of the injury suffered by the patient. Causation is usually established based on the testimony of experts (e.g., healthcare providers) who can clearly show the connection between the nurse's action or omission and the resulting injury to the patient.

Case Example: Causation

A nurse forgot to change the patient's dressing at the scheduled time but changed it 3 hours later. The hospital policy reads that nurses must administer medications or perform prescribed treatments within 30 minutes before or 30 minutes after the scheduled time. The patient did not experience any harm or infection. In this case, there were both existence of a duty and a breach of duty, but the breach of duty did not cause any harm or injury to the patient. Therefore, if a malpractice action had been brought, the plaintiff would not have received an award because he could not prove causation. **Key Point:** *Nurses are encouraged to report medication and treatment errors as promptly as possible so that actions can be taken to prevent and/or minimize injury to the patient.*

Damages In civil cases, the remedy for the harm the patient suffered is money. The judge or jury will award the plaintiff money to compensate them for pain and suffering, lost wages, additional medical bills, and other losses. In some cases, the plaintiff may be awarded punitive damages (additional money) for grossly negligent or egregious behavior by the healthcare provider.

Case: Damages

A patient who had a cesarean section underwent a second surgery to repair a uterine laceration that caused excessive bleeding. She sustained massive brain damage from a cardiac arrest 2 hours after being taken to the recovery room and died 6 months later. Although the patient continued to have symptoms consistent with hemorrhagic shock (e.g., bleeding, decreased blood pressure and oxygen level, increased heart rate), the nurses did not notify the obstetrician because they assumed he reviewed the monitor each time he visited the patient.

Analysis of the Case:

Duty: Based on the nurse–patient relationship

Breach of Duty: Failure to communicate to the provider; failure to intervene to counteract the patient's deteriorating condition

Causation: Appropriate medical care was not provided based on the patient's signs and symptoms.

Damages: In this case, a settlement was reached with a present value of about $1.35 million (Nurses Service Organization, n.d.-a).

KnowledgeCheck 39-3

- Distinguish negligence from malpractice.
- Distinguish civil law from criminal law.
- Under which type of law (constitutional, statutory, administrative, or common law) does each of the following fall?
  A defendant claiming the right not to incriminate himself under the Fifth Amendment
  A nurse having their license revoked by the state board of nursing
  The wording of a state nurse practice act
- Define *plaintiff* and *defendant* in the context of civil law.

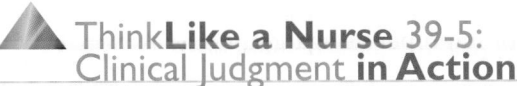

ThinkLike a Nurse 39-5: Clinical Judgment in Action

- Give one nursing example of each: negligence, malpractice, damages.
- Can you think of one nonfraudulent example of a nurse being untruthful with a patient? Do you think the circumstances described in your example make the untruthfulness justifiable?
- Can you think of an example of a nurse committing assault, other than the one given in the text?

Vicarious Liability

You are legally accountable for your actions or inactions. This is a common legal principle that should guide your behavior. It means that you can be sued for behavior or omissions that deviate from acceptable standards. In certain circumstances, though, the law will assign liability to a person or entity that did not directly cause the injury but with whom you have a special kind of relationship. This type of liability is known as **vicarious** or **substituted liability.** The various types of vicarious liability existing under common law are discussed in the following subsections.

Captain of the Ship   This rarely used principle applies to situations in which a physician (e.g., surgeon

or obstetrician) is held liable for the negligence of another healthcare provider. Many states now hold nurses liable for their own actions.

Borrowed Servant Doctrine   This doctrine relieves the primary employer of liability for the actions or omissions of its employee who was "borrowed" by another person. In theory, the borrower (temporary employer) becomes liable for the actions of the employee. This would apply, for example, to agency nurses.

Respondeat Superior   This Latin term means "let the master answer." The employer must answer for the negligent acts or omissions of its employees, who are functioning within the scope of their employment. For example, the hospital can be sued for a medication error made by a labor and delivery nurse working within the scope of their practice.

KnowledgeCheck 39-4

- Define these terms: *assault, battery, fraud, slander, libel, negligence, malpractice.*
- State the four elements of malpractice.

LITIGATION IN CIVIL CLAIMS

Litigation is the formal process wherein the legal issues, rights, and duties between the parties are heard and decided (adjudicated). The following section discusses the stages of the litigation process.

Pleading and Pretrial Motions

The litigation process starts when the plaintiff files a **complaint,** which is a legal document outlining how the plaintiff has been harmed by another person. It identifies the specific allegations and time frame, the standards allegedly breached (e.g., behaviors or omissions), the persons (defendants) involved, and the harm suffered. The complaint is filed with the court and served on (delivered to) the defendant.

If you are served with a complaint, you have a specified time in which to file a response *(answer)* with the court. You will need an attorney to defend you. Therefore, you must immediately notify your employer and malpractice insurance, if applicable, of the complaint. Your attorney will file an answer with the court that addresses each of the allegations (unproven accusations) contained in the complaint. As a defendant, you should not contact the plaintiff or the plaintiff's attorney or discuss the case with coworkers or friends. The facility's risk manager and your attorney will advise you. Cooperate fully and be honest in all your answers.

Discovery Phase

Discovery is designed to allow both parties to gather facts and evidence about the case that can be used at trial. The discovery process makes sure there are no "surprises" during the trial. Attorneys may obtain discovery through written questions **(interrogatories),** requests for documents and other evidence, and by **depositions** (attorneys orally question parties to the lawsuit under oath, as though they were testifying in court). You may be *deposed* (questioned) as either a fact witness, a party to the lawsuit (defendant), or an expert witness.

- A *fact witness* is someone who was present when the incident occurred. The defendant will testify about the care provided and the actions taken.

Depositions may occur several years after the incident, so you may not remember specific information. You should prepare for the deposition by reviewing the medical records and any other evidence that may exist regarding the lawsuit. During the deposition, listen to your attorney, do not volunteer information, take your time before answering each question, and provide only objective information. Always base your answers on facts; do not speculate. If your attorney objects to any question, immediately stop and do not provide an answer unless directed by your attorney. Remain calm; do not get angry, argue, or be sarcastic.

Alternative Dispute Resolution

Lawyers and involved parties usually try to resolve disputes before going to trial. The three most common methods of alternative dispute resolution are as follows:

- **Negotiation** involves the attorneys for the plaintiff and the defendant attempting to settle the lawsuit before a trial takes place.
- **Mediation** uses a neutral third party to help the parties focus on the issues and facilitate communication to identify what is needed to reach a resolution.
- **Arbitration** involves a third party making a decision after formally hearing the evidence and information. The arbitration decision may be binding on the parties.

Trial Process

If the dispute cannot be resolved and is not dismissed by the court during pretrial motions, the case goes to trial. Malpractice cases are usually heard by a jury. After hearing all the evidence and reviewing submitted documents, the judge or jury makes a decision, which is either dismissal or an award of damages.

Appeal

After the judge or jury has made a decision, either party has the opportunity to present post-trial motions, move for a new trial, or appeal the verdict and/or damages to a court of appeals. The court of appeals will review the transcript and documents from the trial and determine whether errors (e.g., improper evidence allowed, proper evidence denied, improper jury instructions) were made

during that trial that resulted in an unfair verdict. The verdict can be dismissed or upheld, in part or in whole, and *remanded* (sent back) to the trial court with special instructions.

KnowledgeCheck 39-5

- Identify the phases of the trial process.
- How is arbitration different from mediation?

PracticalKnowledge
knowing how

To decrease your chances of being involved in a malpractice suit, you should know the most common causes of malpractice claims and some practical preventive actions you can take. Keep in mind that causes are often difficult to categorize because they overlap; an error usually results from interlocking causes.

WHAT ARE THE MOST COMMON MALPRACTICE CLAIMS?

Nurses must use critical thinking, clinical reasoning, and the nursing process to make decisions that ensure safe and efficient care to patients. A breakdown in this process leads to claims of nursing malpractice (Box 39-3).

Failure to Assess/Recognize Cues and Diagnose/Formulate Hypotheses

Failure to assess the patient/recognize cues and formulate diagnoses/hypotheses can lead to incorrect actions, no action, or improper delegation.

Case: Failure to Assess/Recognize and Diagnose/Formulate Hypotheses

A 67-year-old patient had an epidural catheter inserted for pain management after a total knee replacement. After successful treatment of an episode of hypotension in the postanesthesia care unit, he was transferred to the medical–surgical unit. The RN assessed the patient and delegated direct care to an LPN, although this was denied by the LPN. Three hours later, the patient experienced nausea and vomiting. He was found cyanotic and unresponsive 10 minutes later and subsequently died from anoxic encephalopathy. Many facts were disputed among the numerous codefendants, and documentation was poor (Nurses Service Organization, n.d.-d).

Safe and competent assessment (recognize cues) and diagnosis (formulate hypotheses) practices require the nurse to:

- Perform an admission assessment. This duty cannot be delegated to unlicensed assistive personnel.

BOX 39-3 ■ Common Causes of Malpractice Litigation

Failure to respond, such as not intervening to care for the patient's specific symptoms or expressed request for care.

Failure to educate, such as not answering questions, not teaching self-care measures, or not explaining procedures or equipment adequately on the patient's discharge.

Failure to follow standards of care and institutional policies and procedures. This most commonly occurs in the form of medication errors and failure to follow a provider's prescriptions. It also frequently occurs from failure to use equipment responsibly. Among other reasons, a nurse may fail to follow standards of care when the unit is understaffed or the nurse is inexperienced.

Failure to communicate often comes up when a nurse fails to seek medical authorization for a treatment or fails to notify a provider in a timely manner when a patient's condition warrants action.

Failure to document the following in the patient's record: assessment data (e.g., drug allergies), injuries, medication administration details, progress and response to treatment, providers' prescriptions, and telephone conversations with providers.

Failure to act as an advocate. Nurses must frequently intervene to prevent harm to the patient by other healthcare providers and by relatives and significant others. The following are examples of advocacy errors:

■ *Medical and discharge prescriptions.* As an example of failure to advocate, suppose two providers prescribe the same drug for a patient but under different brand names. The nurse does not recognize that the two drugs are the same, so the patient receives twice the normal amount and has a toxic reaction. Other errors occur when the nurse does not question incomplete or illegible prescriptions or does not question discharge prescriptions when the nurse believes the patient is too ill for discharge.

■ *Impaired nurses.* You have a duty under most state nursing practice acts to report impaired nursing practice (e.g., as a result of alcoholism or mental illness) to the appropriate licensing agency. Failure to do so is a failure to advocate for patients.

■ *Family and significant others.* Advocacy includes reporting neglect and intentional injuries to children, the elderly, and the disabled. Failure to do so may constitute negligence and/or violation of state statutes.

■ Analyze the assessment data to clearly identify problems/hypotheses.
■ Apply theoretical knowledge and experience to ensure a correct diagnosis/hypothesis. The presenting signs and symptoms should be consistent with the disease process or medical problem. Remember that the nursing diagnosis consists of Patient Response r/t Etiology.
■ Report the symptoms to the appropriate provider; implement standard nursing care and the prescribed interventions.

■ Conduct frequent focused assessments until the end of your shift or until the problem is resolved.

Failure to Plan/Generate Solutions

ANA standards specifically require nurses to formulate a plan of care/generate solutions. This plan may be written or unwritten, depending on state and agency regulations. Care plans or patient care tools provide a way to measure patient outcomes and progress. The plan of care should be consistent with standards of treatments acceptable for the given diagnosis, hypothesis, or problem.

Safe and competent practices to ensure appropriate planning require the nurse to:

■ Know the correct approach to treat actual or potential patient problems.
■ Have the theoretical knowledge base to successfully plan nursing care for patients.
■ Develop a plan of care that is individualized to the patient.
■ Generate solutions that are consistent with standards of treatments acceptable for the given hypotheses or problem.

Failure to Implement a Plan of Care/Take Action

Implementation requires the nurse to perform the care or nursing interventions/actions. Failure of nurses to take the appropriate action is a major risk to patient safety and a common cause of malpractice actions (see Box 39-3).

Failure to Evaluate

Evaluation requires you to make a decision or judgment about the success of your interventions/actions in addressing the patient's problems. The duty to evaluate requires an ongoing cycle of the following:

■ **Observing for changes after interventions and treatments.** You must know the expected outcomes and side effects of medications and treatments so that you can accurately interpret and document anticipated and adverse responses.
■ **Recognizing significance of the change.** For example, if Mr. Adkins' blood pressure (BP) is usually 140/88, a change to 150/90 after exercise would not be significant for him. But for Mrs. Jonas, whose BP is usually 100/64, a change to 150/90 would be cause for concern.
■ **Documenting or reporting symptoms to the appropriate person.** If a change is significant, you have a legal duty to report the change to the appropriate provider and to document this change in the appropriate medical record.
■ **Following up on patient responses to nursing interventions/actions.** This requires you to know the expected outcomes and side effects of medications and treatments.

KnowledgeCheck 39-6

- State the four requirements of the nurse's duty to assess/recognize cues.
- State four ways in which the nurse may fail to implement a plan of care/take action.
- Give one example of the duty to advocate for a patient.
- List the four components of the nurse's legal duty to evaluate.

HOW CAN YOU MINIMIZE YOUR MALPRACTICE RISKS?

The best way to minimize your risk of malpractice is to practice in a safe and competent manner. You must have the appropriate body of theoretical knowledge for clinical practice and be familiar with your state's NPA, professional standards of practice, and institutional policies and procedures. These provide the legal framework for your practice and help you to evaluate the quality of the care you deliver. **Key Point:** *Ignorance of the law and of practice standards is no excuse for failing to comply with them, and it is no defense in a malpractice suit.* You will find discussion of other helpful suggestions in the remainder of this chapter, and

 Go to **Chapter 39, Clinical Insight 39-1, Tips for Avoiding Malpractice,** in Volume 2.

Use Resources to Develop Clinical Judgment and Follow Professional Standards of Care

Numerous resources are available to facilitate your ability to use clinical judgment. The nursing process, critical thinking tools, and models of clinical judgment provide you with a systematic approach to patient care and are legally acceptable methods of decision making in nursing practice.

Avoid Medication and Treatment Errors

Medication errors are among the most common healthcare errors. To administer medications accurately, you must know the rationale for administering the drug, safe dosage ranges, side effects of the medications, and relevant information to teach the patient about the medication. To prevent medication errors, you should:

- Follow the "rights of medication administration (see Chapter 23).
- Investigate any patient concerns before administering the medication (e.g., the patient might ask, "Is this a new medication?").
- Question prescriptions that are incomplete or seem inappropriate, given the patient's history or diagnosis.
- Make sure the equipment used to administer medication is working properly.

Promoting Safe, Effective Nursing Care

The Use of the Nursing Process to Provide Legally Safe Nursing Care

Key Concepts: Malpractice, Negligence, Liability

SENC Competency: Provide safe, quality patient care (Thinking, Doing, Caring)

Background: At one time, nurses were not held liable for patient injuries because they were perceived as "only following the provider's prescriptions." Nurses were not viewed as educated, knowledgeable professionals. Many doctrines (e.g., captain of the ship, borrowed servant) provided nurses a shield of protection from being held accountable for their negligent actions. This view began to erode when the court ruled that nurses owe an "independent duty" of care to the patient (*NKC Hosps, Inc. v. Anthony,* 1993).

The concept of providing legally safe, quality actions began to emerge in the education of nursing students and as an expectation for practicing nurses. **Key Point:** *The nursing process is viewed as a critical-thinking tool that, if correctly used, will minimize errors in patient care. It seamlessly aligns with the "Thinking, Caring, Doing" model that is designed to provide a holistic approach to patient care.*

Think About It: Reflect on the stages of the nursing process and how they are related to safe, effective care.

➤ Assessment is the first stage of the nursing process. *Why is assessment essential to ensuring the patient receives the appropriate care?*

➤ Analysis/diagnosis is the second stage of the nursing process; planning involves formulating outcomes and identifying interventions to achieve them. *How do the analysis/diagnosis and planning stages align with the "thinking" concept?*

➤ Implementation is the process of taking the actions identified in planning. It includes documenting the actions and the patient's responses. *What aspects of the "Thinking, Caring, Doing" model are incorporated in this stage of the nursing process?*

➤ Evaluation is the determination of whether patient goals have been achieved. *How is this stage used to evaluate the potential liability of patient care?*

- Adhere to standards of practice for treatments (e.g., maintain sterile field when required).

For tips to help you use equipment properly and safely,

 Go to **Chapter 39, Clinical Insight 39-2, Using Equipment Safely,** in Volume 2.

Report and Document

For every suggestion for minimizing malpractice risk, add the reminder "Document what happened." Remember the old adage "If it isn't documented,

♥ iCare 39-1

Honoring Safety and Confidentiality

Jon is a newly graduated registered nurse (RN). He is taking care of Mr. Belvidere, who has been admitted with a stroke. It is an extremely busy day on the unit, and Jon is behind on his morning medication pass. One of the senior nurses casually says to Jon, "If you're behind, why don't you prepare the medications and just ask the certified nursing assistant (CNA), Mark, to administer them? He is really thorough, I trust him to give medications, and he has been doing this for a long time." Jon feels uncomfortable with this practice because he knows that as a licensed professional, it is his responsibility to administer the medications.

Jon asks to speak to the senior nurse privately and tells her that what she is doing violates safe medication and legal practices and places the patient in danger. The nurse is initially upset that Jon called her out on this behavior but then thanks him for coming to her first to address it privately. In the spirit of transparency, she discusses the past actions with her manager. As a result, the charge nurse and the nurse manager provide an in-service presentation as a refresher about legal responsibilities related to medication administration.

As a caring nurse, Jon was aware of his responsibility for Mr. Belvidere's safety and cared enough to take action to effect change. He was also considerate of the senior nurse when he spoke to her privately about the matter.

it wasn't done." If you are ever required to appear in court, the patient medical record may be the only proof you have of the care you provided. It is unlawful to make false entries or destroy entries in medical records, but do carefully document in detail all care you provide.

Cases: Documentation Can Make a Difference

The plaintiff alleged that the nurse had violated numerous standards of practice, including a failure to properly assess the patient, a failure to properly monitor vital signs and intake and output, and a failure to recognize and respond to signs and symptoms of sepsis. A settlement was reached for $706,250. Weaknesses in documentation revealed that the patient's BP was not documented until day 14 of home care, and evidence of infection—wound appearance and size, amount and appearance of drainage—was not consistently documented by the nurses caring for the patient (Nurses Service Organization, n.d.-a).

In contrast, a verdict was rendered for a nurse who was accused of failing to properly assess and monitor an impaired, restrained patient and to provide proper care in a safe environment. The patient suffered severe burns over 25% of his body when the bed linen ignited as he attempted to burn off the restraints with a lighter. Strengths in documentation showed that the nurse performed patient monitoring

and assessments every 15 minutes as prescribed, missing one time to care for a critical patient. The assessment findings at each check were fully documented in the patient's medical records (Nurses Service Organization, n.d.-b).

Incident Reports

If a standard of practice is breached or an unusual incident occurs (e.g., a visitor or patient falls or is injured), you should complete an **incident report** (also called *variance report* or *occurrence report*). These reports are used, in part, for quality improvement in the agency and should not be used to discipline staff members or be placed in employees' files. The goal is to prevent the incident from occurring again by formulating corrective measures.

In many states, an incident report is not made available as a part of discovery in litigation. It becomes discoverable (available to the plaintiff) if it is mentioned in the medical records. **Key Point:** *You can prevent an otherwise confidential report from becoming evidence by not writing "Incident report completed" in the patient's medical record.*

When reporting an incident, be sure to clearly identify the patient, date, time, and location. Briefly describe the incident in factual terms. Use the exact words of the patient or persons involved and put the information in quotes. Do not speculate, draw conclusions, or place blame. Identify any witnesses to the event or equipment involved. For example:

1900	Demerol 50 mg given intramuscularly. Provider prescribed: Demerol 15 mg.
1930	Patient's respirations: 8 breaths/min; BP 100/60; skin pale.
2000	Called Dr. Smith. Prescription for naloxone (Narcan) 1 mg IV STAT
2005	Narcan given as prescribed. Resp 12 breaths/min, BP 118/70

In this example, you should be prepared to discuss the 30-minute delay between the patient's findings and contacting the provider. Professional standards and agency policy would require that the provider be notified immediately. Chapter 17 presents additional information on occurrence (incident) reports.

Documenting

Key Point: *A basic principle of documenting is that a third person should be able to read your documentation and form a mental picture of your patient and the care provided during your shift.* You should document:

- All interactions with patients, as well as the refusal of or noncompliance with treatment.
- Telephone conversations with primary care providers, including time, content of the conversation, and the action you took.

■ The facts; do not editorialize (e.g., do not write, "I could not check on the patient as often as prescribed because we were understaffed").

Refer to Chapter 17 for a review of your documentation responsibilities, and use the letters F-A-C-T-U-A-L as a reminder when documenting patient care:

F—Your information must be **factual** and objective. Don't document your opinions.

A—You must be **accurate:** For example, record the vital signs accurately.

C—Your information must be **complete:** Don't omit any important information.

T—You must be **timely:** Document care as soon as possible after doing it; don't wait until the end of your shift and then try to remember everything that happened.

U—You must always document **unusual occurrences.**

A—You must document your **assessment data,** the plan of care, and the patient's responses.

L—Remember that the patient's medical record is a **legal document** and is subpoenaed in a malpractice case.

For more information on guidelines for documenting care,

 Go to **Chapter 39, Clinical Insight 39-3, Guidelines for Documenting Care,** in Volume 2.

Obtain Informed Consent

Informed consent is the patient's permission to receive any and all types of care with full knowledge of the risks, benefits, costs, and alternatives. For hospital admission and for invasive or specialized treatments or diagnostic procedures, the consent must be written and signed by the patient or their legal guardian. The law provides for implied or assumed consent in emergency situations; therefore, written consent is not necessary in an emergency if experts would agree that there was an immediate threat to the patient's life or health.

Elements of Consent

To be legally valid, the informed consent should fulfill the following requirements:

■ **Completeness.** Healthcare consumers need adequate information to make educated decisions regarding their treatment. Be sure they get information on the nature of the procedure, risks, benefits, post-procedure care and considerations, and treatment alternatives.

■ **Clarity and comprehension.** Language should be at the appropriate level for the patient's educational level so that they (or their surrogate decision maker) can understand the explanation. Always ask the patient to describe in their own words the procedure to which they are consenting. If the patient asks, "What will the doctor do during surgery?" the nurse is aware that they do not understand the nature of the surgery. You should contact the surgeon.

■ **Voluntariness.** The patient must be free to accept or reject the treatment. They must not be pressured or coerced to give consent. There must be no actual or implied threat by anyone to force the patient into having the surgery (e.g., "Mom, if you don't let them do this, I'm never coming back to see you"). Otherwise, the consent is not valid.

■ **Competence.** The person must have the ability to understand the information and make a choice about the particular situation (e.g., the ability to decide what clothing to wear does not necessarily mean that the person is competent to decide whether to have surgery). If the person is confused and disoriented, you should contact the case manager or your supervisor for guidance. State law identifies the order of individuals who can make decisions for individuals who are judged incompetent. It is usually the spouse, then parents, then sisters and brothers, and so on. If the person does not have relatives, the court will appoint a legal guardian to make healthcare decisions.

Key Point: *A competent adult has the legal right to consent to or refuse any treatment.* However, this right does not always extend to situations in which an adult is making the decision for a minor. A court sometimes will authorize treatment of a child against their parents' wishes. In some states, a minor who is married or living independently is considered emancipated and can make their own healthcare decisions.

The Nurse's Role

As a nurse, your legal role regarding written consent is to collaborate with the primary provider, usually a physician or advanced practice nurse. **Key Point:** *You may witness a patient's signature on a consent form, but you are not legally responsible for explaining the treatments and options or for evaluating whether the provider has adequately explained them. You must, however, determine that the elements of a valid informed consent are in place, communicate the patient's needs for more information to the care provider, and provide feedback if the patient wishes to change their consent.*

Be sure you have the patient's informal, verbal consent for nursing interventions that you perform (e.g., urinary catheterization). Coming to the agency for healthcare implies that the patient consents to usual treatment, such as injections and vital signs. However, you should explain all procedures to the patient before their implementation. If the patient objects, identify the reasons for the refusal, correct any misinformation, and explain the benefits of the treatment. If the patient still objects or refuses, do not proceed; contact the primary care provider.

In addition to state statutes, case law, and agency policy, The Joint Commission standards provide valuable guidance regarding informed participation in decision making. See Chapter 5 for discussion of informed consent from an ethical perspective.

Case: Breakdown in Informed Consent

A pulmonologist expected an interventional radiologist to obtain informed consent from the patient for the placement of a chest tube to treat congestive heart failure. Because of the patient's confused state, the nurses contacted her daughter to obtain consent, explaining that the procedure was "no big deal." The daughter agreed, and the nurses completed the telephonic consent form and placed it in the medical records. No provider explained the benefits, risks, or alternatives. During the procedure, the patient suffered one of the risks of the procedure (punctured aorta), necessitating emergency surgery. Her condition deteriorated after the surgery, and she died 18 months later. The court ruled that the failure to obtain informed consent was a basis for a lawsuit (*Gonsalves v. Sharp*, 2013).

Maintain Patient Safety

Falls are by far the most common incident reported in hospitals and long-term care facilities. On admission to the facility, all patients should be assessed for risks of falls, and "fall precautions" should be instituted when needed. Simply raising the siderails on the bed is not enough to prevent falls. You may still be found negligent if the patient falls because they called for help and no one came to assist them out of bed or if the call device was not placed within the patient's reach and they were unable to call for assistance.

Several useful tools have been developed for assessing falls. See Chapter 21 for information about meeting patients' safety needs, including falls and use of restraints.

Maintain Confidentiality and Privacy

Always maintain patient confidentiality unless directed by law to do otherwise (e.g., when a patient is threatening to harm someone). Family members and significant others do not have an automatic right to information about the patient. For example, parents do not have an automatic right to see the medical records of their adult child or minor child who is married or emancipated. Of course, you need to discuss patients' medical conditions with other health team members, but this does not include chatting about the patient's personal life or discussing the patient in a venue where others can hear (e.g., elevator, cafeteria). **Key Point:** *You should discuss the patient's health status with those who have a need to know (those involved in their care).*

Confidentiality of Patient Records Confidentiality is another aspect of privacy (e.g., do not leave a patient's information in locations that are accessible to visitors or nonauthorized staff). Do not give information about patients over the phone unless the agency has a system that enables you to know that you are speaking to a person authorized by the patient. If you require advice about maintaining the confidentiality of electronic records, see the section "Electronic Health Record (EHR) Systems" in Chapter 17.

Provide Education and Counseling

Part of your role as a nurse is to provide information to patients and caregivers about their illness, medications, and other treatments. This helps to fulfill informed consent requirements and involve patients in their own healthcare. Make sure the patient understands, retains the knowledge, and can demonstrate any skills. Ask them to repeat instructions to you or to provide a return demonstration of a skill, such as self-injection of insulin. To reinforce understanding, always review written information with the patient. Refer to Chapter 16 for more information on teaching patients.

Delegate According to Guidelines

As a nurse, you are expected to properly delegate to ensure patients receive timely and quality care. This involves implementing the five rights of delegation: delegating to the *right person*, under the *right circumstances*, using the *right directions and communication*, and practicing the right *supervision and evaluation*.

To do this safely, you (the delegator) must know the educational background, knowledge, experience, and physical and emotional capability of those to whom you delegate (delegatees). You must also know the scope of practice of the delegatee as determined by the state board of nursing. In addition, you must consider the condition and requirements of the patient.

The registered nurse should not delegate to LPNs or unlicensed assistive personnel (UAPs) patients who:

- Require complex care
- Are unpredictable
- Require nursing judgment
- Involve a high level of interaction

When delegating, be sure the delegatee understands the assignment. The Case Box "Failure to Assess and Diagnose" identifies numerous breakdowns in the delegation process. The duty to delegate has a corresponding duty to supervise the care and evaluate the outcome. For example, if you assign an LPN to provide direct care for a new postoperative patient, you should obtain hourly updates on their status. In the Meet Your Nurse Role Model scenario, the float nurse was sent to the unit to provide assistance; however, she was texting continuously on her cell phone. The duty to supervise and evaluate requires you to reinforce her responsibilities and correct behaviors that are counterproductive to quality care. If you need to review specific guidelines for delegating, see Chapter 3.

Accept Assignments for Which You Are Qualified

As a nurse, when you accept an assignment, you must consider whether the assignment is within your level of education, experience, and physical and emotional capability. The refusal to accept an assignment does not mean that you have abandoned the patient. Your duty to the patient begins once you accept the assignment. **Key Point:** *You are legally responsible for the assignment that you accept. If your assignment becomes overwhelming and unmanageable, immediately contact the charge nurse or nursing supervisor for assistance.*

Nursing supervisors have a duty to ensure adequate staffing and patient coverage. This means that you must report to the nurse in charge when leaving the unit. Failure to do this may result in charges of patient abandonment. A nurse should never leave the unit without identifying who will provide care to their patient. This does not mean that you must work overtime (e.g., a double shift), as long as you follow established policies and procedures, which will include giving notice and explaining your reasoning (e.g., that you are too fatigued to provide safe care).

If you work extra hours or additional shifts, or if a unit is understaffed, you are still liable for any malpractice that you commit. Unfortunately, being "busy" and overwhelmed is not a defense against error. In addition, you have the duty to tell supervisors that staffing is inadequate; be sure to do it in writing. You should know and follow agency policy on how to address short-staff issues.

Participate in Continuing Education

As a nurse, you have a duty to participate in ongoing education in your area of practice and to keep up with new laws, equipment, treatments, and procedures. Be sure to obtain documentation of your attendance. In some states, continuing education is mandatory for license renewal. In states where it is not mandatory, other standards still require that you obtain the education and training necessary to implement current nursing procedures and practices. In malpractice cases, the nurse's competency in providing nursing care is frequently an issue.

Observe Professional Boundaries

Nurses must be careful to maintain professional boundaries, not only with the patient but also with other healthcare providers. Do not accept gifts from patients or encourage attempts to have close personal relationships outside the healthcare setting. Violations of professional boundaries may be physical, sexual, emotional, or financial in nature. Cues to possible overstepped boundaries are listed in Box 39-4.

If you would like more specific information on professional boundaries,

---

> **BOX 39-4** ■ Potential Boundary Violations Between Nurse and Patient
>
> **Excessive Self-Disclosure**—Discussing personal problems or intimate details with the patient.
>
> **Flirtation**—Communication that is sexual in nature or reveals personal attraction between patient and nurse.
>
> **Secretive Behavior**—When the nurse is defensive or guarded about the interaction between patient and nurse.
>
> **"Super Nurse" Attitude**—The nurse who acts as though she is the only one who understands and can meet the patient's needs.
>
> **Excessive Attention to Patient**—When the nurse spends much more time with a particular patient than is required by their needs. Personal gifts, off-duty visits, or trading assignments are signs of boundary violation.
>
> **Unclear Communication**—When only part of the story is told with patient care. The patient might repeatedly seek out the nurse, even when not assigned to their care.
>
> ---
>
> *Source:* Used with permission from the National Council of State Boards of Nursing. (2018a). *A nurse's guide to professional boundaries.* https://www.ncsbn.org/public-files/ProfessionalBoundaries_Complete.pdf

 Go to the **National Council on State Boards of Nursing Web site,** at https://www.ncsbn.org/ProfessionalBoundaries_Complete.pdf

Sexual Harassment Be aware of and report the behaviors of staff members who commit sexual harassment. **Sexual harassment** is defined as "unwelcome sexual advances, requests for sexual favors, and other verbal or physical conduct of a sexual nature" that fit one of the following criteria:

1. Is a condition of employment
2. Interferes with job performance
3. Is the basis for employment decisions
4. Creates a hostile and intimidating work environment (Equal Employment Opportunity Commission, n.d.)

You should know your agency's sexual harassment policy to take the correct action if you witness or experience sexual harassment. Every agency receiving federal funding must have such a policy in place. It will tell you the initial action to take, how to file a grievance, what forms you need to use, to whom the incident is reported, and other pertinent information.

Observe Mandatory Reporting Regulations

As noted earlier in the chapter, most states have laws requiring the nurse to report communicable diseases, known or suspected abuse of patients, and impaired or unsafe professional practice. When you observe violations of the state's licensing regulations, you have a professional and legal responsibility to report them to the appropriate authority. The "authority" varies among states; it may be your immediate supervisor, the board of nursing, or a peer assistance program. See the section "Mandatory Reporting Laws," earlier in the chapter, and the following discussion of reportable situations.

Impaired Nurses

Nurses who come to work under the influence of alcohol or mind-altering substances pose a danger to the health, safety, and welfare of the patients. You have a legal obligation to protect patients from impaired nurses. Always pay attention to the possibility of a coworker using or stealing narcotics. Impaired nurses account for a major percentage of disciplinary actions against nurses. The board of nursing in many states has programs that provide monitoring and support to nurses with substance addictions who seek help as an alternative to disciplinary actions against their license. See Box 39-5 for signs of chemical dependence in the workplace. To determine the magnitude of the problem in your state, go to the state board of nursing's Web site and click on *disciplinary actions*.

BOX 39-5 ■ Signs of Possible Chemical Dependence in the Workplace

Absenteeism
- Frequent unscheduled absences with improbable excuses
- Frequent late arrivals or early departures
- Absences after payday or days off
- Higher-than-average absences for cold, flu, and minor illnesses

Absent "On the Job"
- Long shift breaks
- Brief, unexplained absences from the nursing unit
- "Locked door syndrome" (excessively long use of the restroom)
- Frequent visits to Occupational Health Services for illness on the job

Difficulty Concentrating
- Errors, particularly involving medication or taking and transcribing verbal prescriptions
- Omitted, illogical, incomplete, or illegible documentation
- Taking more time to carry out assignments than is expected, given the nurse's skill and experience
- Deterioration of handwriting or typing errors during the shift
- Overlooking the signs of the patient's deteriorating condition

Inconsistent Work Patterns
- Alternating periods of high and low efficiency
- Minimal or substandard work compared with that of peers
- Frequent requests for help with patient assignments
- Altered judgment in patient care decisions

Physical or Emotional Problems
- Nervousness, excessive sweating, tremors of the hands
- Physical or emotional condition changes during shift
- Deteriorating personal appearance, grooming, and hygiene
- Weight gain or loss

Decreasing Efficiency
- Omitting treatments, making bad decisions, showing poor judgment related to patient care
- Requests to be changed to a less supervised shift (e.g., night or weekend shifts)

Poor Relationships on the Job
- Mood swings, from isolation to angry outbursts
- Uncooperativeness
- Avoidance of contact with supervisors
- Patient complaints of irritability, roughness, or verbal abuse
- Lethargy or hyperactivity
- Emotional hypersensitivity
- Isolation from others

Medication-Centered Problems
- Excessive use of PRN psychoactive medications or narcotics recorded for patients
- Increased waste or breakage of controlled substances
- Missing drugs, unaccounted-for doses
- Omission of dates or times from narcotic records
- Patient complaints about lack of pain relief

Personal Life Interferes With Job
- Frequent or excessively long phone calls
- Visitors or unexplained errands during work shift
- Legal problems
- Increased number of accidents

Source: Lengel, R. (2018). *Impairment in the workplace: Substance abuse.* CEUfast. https://ceufast.com/course/recognizing-impairment-in-the-workplace; National Council of State Boards of Nursing. (2018b). *A nurse's guide to substance use disorder in nursing.* https://www.ncsbn.org/SUD_Brochure_2014.pdf; Toney-Butler, T., & Siela, D. (2022). *Recognizing alcohol and drug impairment in the workplace in Florida.* https://www.ncbi.nlm.nih.gov/books/NBK507774/?report=printable; Washington Health Professional Services. (2016). *A guide for assisting colleagues who demonstrate impairment in the workplace.* https://www.doh.wa.gov/portals/1/Documents/Pubs/600006.pdf; Wooten, L. (2018). Can you recognize substance abuse disorders? *ASBN Update, 23*(3), 14–15.

Unauthorized Practice

Your employer will require you to submit verification of current licensure in the state where you are working. If your license expires and you continue to practice nursing, you can be charged with unauthorized practice of nursing. You must report the unauthorized practice of nursing, which means reporting persons practicing nursing without a proper license. In addition, you must know the scope of practice for yourself, LPNs/LVNs, and UAPs to ensure practice within professional boundaries. For example, UAPs cannot perform the initial assessment on a newly admitted patient.

Abuse and Communicable Diseases

State laws also require you to report known or suspected child, elder, and spousal abuse and communicable disease. Because state laws may vary, you need to be familiar with them to know what and to whom to report in your area. If you are working for a healthcare agency when you suspect abuse, always report it to your supervisor. If you need to review signs of abuse, see Procedure 6-1: Assessing for Abuse.

Other Safeguards for Nurses

In addition to the Good Samaritan laws and the ANA Nurses' Bill of Rights (previously discussed), safe harbor laws and professional liability insurance offer some legal protection for nurses.

Safe Harbor Laws

Safe harbor laws, found in the NPA or other state laws, provide for exceptions to certain laws. They protect you from being suspended, terminated, disciplined, or discriminated against for refusing to do (or not do) something you believe would be harmful to a patient. Under these laws, you also have a right to ask for peer review of either the situation or directives that you believe would violate the NPA. You must follow the guidelines required under the safe harbor provisions.

> **Case: Prepping a Patient for a Surgical Procedure**
>
> The nurse cannot find documentation in the patient's medical record for informed consent. Knowing her legal role, she refuses to assist with treatment until informed consent is obtained. Safe harbor laws protect the nurse from disciplinary action for refusal to obtain inform consent since this is the responsibility of the surgeon.

Professional Liability Insurance

If you are sued for malpractice, the insurance company pays for the attorney's fees and for any judgment or settlement, up to the policy limits. You should carefully review your insurance policy because most insurance policies have **exclusions** (items not covered by the policy). If the claim arises out of excluded activities, the insurance company will not pay for the costs of litigation and damages. The following are examples of exclusions:

- Intentional torts (e.g., sexual abuse of a patient, assault and battery)
- Injury caused while the nurse is under the influence of drugs or alcohol
- Criminal activity
- Behaviors/actions that can lead to an award of punitive damages (damages awarded to punish the defendant for egregious acts or omissions)

Types of Coverage   There are two types of malpractice coverage:

- **Occurrence-type insurance** is most often recommended for nurses because this policy covers malpractice claims for any injury or damage that occurred during the time the policy was in force, regardless of when the claim was reported and the lawsuit occurred.
- **Claims-made insurance,** in contrast, covers only those claims in which the negligent action or omission occurred and the claim was filed or reported during the policy period. To maintain coverage under a claims-made policy after it has lapsed or been canceled, some insurers will offer "tail" insurance. You should consult an attorney to decide which type of policy is best for you.

As a rule, if you work for a hospital or other institution, you will be covered by the institution's insurance. However, it covers you only while you are working within the scope of your employment. For example, you would not be covered during the 1 day a week that you volunteer at a free clinic. Some legal experts recommend that you purchase individual liability insurance in addition to the coverage provided by your employer. Again, consult an attorney before making a decision.

ThinkLike a Nurse 39-6: Clinical Judgment in Action

Susan, RN, was employed by Landold Nursing Service and assigned to Alvalup Hospital from June 1, 2020, to May 30, 2021. Susan carried her own professional liability claims-made policy during this time. She decided to attend real estate school and not renew her policy. On August 10, 2021, a medical malpractice claim was filed against Susan.

- Based on this scenario, would Susan have coverage under her policy?
- If not, what kind of policy should she have obtained to have coverage for the claim made against her?

Student Responsibilities   As a student, you are held to the same standards of care as licensed nurses. You must be familiar not only with your state's standards of practice but also with the policies and procedures in the agency in which you have your clinical experiences. Your instructor is responsible for making assignments that are within your areas of competence and for providing clinical supervision. However, this does not release you from your own legal responsibilities. To help protect yourself and your patients:

- Prepare carefully for each clinical experience.
- Never attempt a procedure or make a judgment about which you feel unsure. If you lack the theoretical or practical knowledge for an assignment, notify your clinical instructor immediately.
- Notify your instructor or a staff nurse if your patient's condition changes significantly.
- Unless otherwise arranged, take instructions only from your clinical instructor.

Your nursing school may require you to carry personal professional liability insurance. The school's policy will cover you only for the nursing care you give in your educational experiences. If you are employed as a nursing assistant, for example, the school's policy will not provide coverage for you at work. Furthermore, you are legally permitted to perform only the procedures contained in your job description. For example, even though you administer injections in your student role, you are not licensed to do so in your role as a nursing assistant.

SUMMARY

Ethical and legal issues are a major source of conflict for nursing practice. This chapter discusses only the legal aspects of the major issues. See Chapter 5 for ethical considerations. It is important to be clear in your mind that what is *legal* and what is *ethical* are not always the same thing. On the one hand, an act may be legal (e.g., abortion), even if you consider it unethical. On the other hand, you may believe an action (e.g., assisted suicide) is ethically necessary, but the law may forbid it. You should be aware of the legal consequences of your ethical decisions.

To explore learning resources for this chapter,

Go to Davis Advantage and find:

Answers and Suggested Responses for all questions in this chapter

Concept Map

Knowledge Map

References and Bibliography

CHAPTER 40

Leading & Managing

Learning Outcomes

After completing this chapter, you should be able to:

➤ Distinguish between leadership, followership, and management.

➤ Compare and contrast authoritarian, democratic, and laissez-faire leadership styles.

➤ Explain the differences between transactional and transformational theories.

➤ Discuss the qualities, behaviors, and strategies that contribute to effective leadership and followership.

➤ Discuss the qualities and activities that contribute to effective management.

➤ Explain how a SWOT analysis and a SOAR analysis are used in leading and managing.

➤ Discuss the qualities of preceptors and mentors.

➤ Describe the challenges presented to nurse managers by the economy and the nursing labor market.

➤ Describe several ways to empower nurses.

➤ Discuss the importance of effective communication skills for nurse leaders and managers.

➤ Describe the change process, including methods to decrease resistance to change.

➤ Describe the major concepts of conflict, conflict resolution, and informal negotiation.

➤ Describe the major concepts of safe and effective delegation.

➤ Establish short- and long-term personal and career goals.

➤ Develop effective time-management strategies.

Key Concepts

Change
Followership
Leadership
Management

Related Concepts

See the Concept Map on Davis Advantage.

Portions of this chapter were taken from Weiss, S. A., Tappen, R. M., & Grimley, K. (2019). *Essentials of nursing leadership and management* (7th ed.). F. A. Davis. Used with permission.

Meet Your Peer

Mary is a student in a nursing program. She considers herself a "pretty good test-taker" and has a grade point average of 3.4. She received her first test grade in her Nursing Fundamentals class, and it was a C. Mary is sure that she will never pass this course and that her dream of becoming a nurse will vanish. When discussing the test with her classmates, she realizes there are several other disappointed students who have been used to making As and Bs on examinations. The nursing examinations seem different because they ask students to not only recall memorized material but also apply what they have learned. Mary decides to get the group together and plan some strategies for study groups. She asks the instructor whether she will meet with them and review their plan to ensure they are on the right track. In so doing,

Mary has exhibited some leadership qualities.

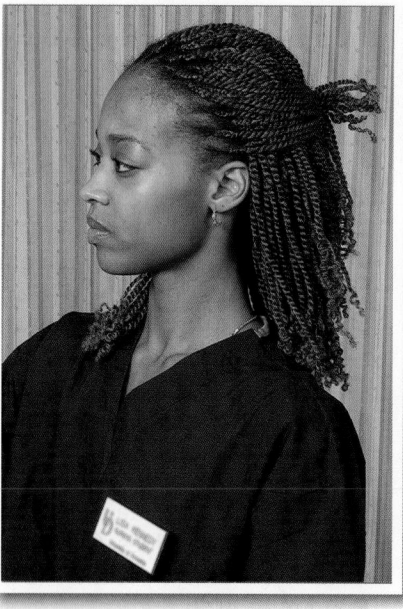

TheoreticalKnowledge
knowing why

In this chapter, we discuss the challenges to nurses as they lead and manage others in organizations and the healthcare environment. The theoretical knowledge you will need to begin professional practice includes an understanding of change, conflict, delegation, and time-management principles.

ABOUT THE KEY CONCEPTS

Have you ever heard the phrase, "Not every good leader can manage, and not every good manager can lead"? This chapter defines and differentiates between the key concepts of **leadership, management, followership,** and **change,** as well as subconcepts such as power, empowerment, conflict resolution, delegation, and time management. As you study each of those concepts, try to grasp how they relate to leadership and management.

WHAT IS LEADERSHIP?

You may be thinking, "I just started my nursing program. How can you expect me to be a leader now?" Although you do need time to learn how nurses function in a work environment, you can begin to assume some leadership skills as a student. **Key Point:** *The essence of leadership is the ability to influence other people and motivate action toward a common goal.* Effective leaders create the path for people to move "in the same direction, toward the same destination, at the same speed, not because they

have been forced to, but because they want to" (Lansdale, 2002, p. 63; see also Cakir & Adiguzel, 2020; Kouzes et al., 2017). A leader in healthcare has three primary tasks:

- Set direction (i.e., help people develop vision, a mission, goals, and purpose).
- Build commitment (i.e., help people develop motivation, team spirit, and teamwork).
- Confront challenges that arise from innovation, change, and turbulence (Budiningsih & Soehari, 2021; Porter-O'Grady & Malloch, 2018).

 Think**Like a Nurse** 40-1:
Clinical Judgment **in Action**

1. Think of a goal your class might have. Obviously, each student wants to develop the skills necessary to provide excellent client care and learn the theory content to pass the course and continue in the program. What other goals might you have as a group? As a leader, how might you help the group meet those goals?
2. Brainstorm with your peers to identify some shared goals of professional nurses.

Leadership Theories

How does a person become a leader? What type of leader is most effective? Despite extensive research on these questions, no theory has yet emerged as the clear answer. The reason may be that different situations require different qualities and behaviors. In nursing, for example, some situations require quick thinking and fast action. Others require time to reflect on the best solution to a complicated problem. Let's look now at some of the best-known leadership theories, beginning with some of the older ones.

Trait Theories Have you ever heard someone say, "Leaders are born, not made"? That implies some of us are natural leaders, but others of us are not. Early leadership research attempted to identify the qualities, or traits, that distinguish a leader from a nonleader. The traits most often identified are intelligence, initiative, self-confidence, high self-esteem, emotional stability, willingness to take risks, and ability to tolerate the consequences of taking risks (Benmira & Agboola, 2021; Northouse, 2018). **Key Point:** *Although leadership may come more naturally to some than to others, almost anyone can gain the necessary knowledge and skills to be a leader in certain areas.*

Behavioral Theories Leadership is viewed as a personality trait under behavior theories. The focus is on what a leader does. One influential theory identifies three styles used by leaders (Benmira & Agboola, 2021; Ronquillo, 2022).

- **Authoritarian leadership.** This type of leadership, also called *autocratic, directive,* or *controlling,* is an efficient way to achieve high productivity when a group needs lots of direction (Marquis & Huston, 2021). The **authoritarian leader** gives direction, makes the final decisions, and bears most of the responsibility for the outcomes. For example, when a decision needs to be made, an authoritarian leader would say, "I've given this a great deal of thought and decided this is the way we're going to solve our problem." When used with skilled workers or over a long time, this style can inhibit creativity and motivation. Authoritarian leadership may be either punitive or kind and compassionate.
- **Democratic leadership.** Also called a *participative leader,* the **democratic leader** shares the planning, decision making, and responsibility for outcomes with members of the group. This type of leader tends to provide guidance rather than control. Although this may be viewed as a less efficient way to run things, group output tends to be of high quality. This leadership style is more flexible and meant to foster motivation and creativity. It is appropriate for followers who agree with the goals of the organization and have the skills and competencies needed to meet their position requirements.
- **Laissez-faire leadership.** Also called *permissive or nondirective* leadership, laissez-faire leadership gives followers the majority of control in the decision-making process. A **laissez-faire leader** has a relatively inactive style and intervenes only when goals have not been met or a problem arises (Iqbal et al., 2021; Ronquillo, 2022). Mature followers who are highly efficient, meet or exceed their position requirements, and can make effective decisions without input from the leader thrive under laissez-faire leadership because they need little guidance. However, followers look to the leader for direction and may become confused and frustrated, with no goal, guidance, or direction.

KnowledgeCheck 40-1
- Identify the three common styles of leadership in the behavioral theories of leadership.
- Discuss the type of follower that would benefit from each style of leadership.

Task Versus Relationship Theories Another important distinction in leadership style is that between a task focus and a relationship focus (Northouse, 2018; Henkel et al., 2019). Some leaders emphasize the tasks (e.g., keeping the nursing station neat, completing documentation) and fail to realize the importance of interpersonal relationships (e.g., attitude of providers toward nursing staff, treating housekeeping staff with respect) for employee morale and productivity. Others focus on the interpersonal aspects and ignore the quality of job performance. The most effective leader can balance the two, attending to both the task and the relationship aspects of working together.

Emotional Intelligence Theory The emotional intelligence (EI) theory focuses on the ability of leaders to manage their emotions and those of their followers (Grindel, 2016). These leaders possess the following traits:

- **Empathy**—Able to make emotional connections with others.
- **Self-awareness**—Recognize and understand their own emotions.
- **Self-management**—Control their personal emotions.
- **Relationship management**—Use their own emotions to successfully interact with and manage others. Ability to build trust, respect, and cooperation within the team (Crowne et al., 2017; Dugué et al., 2021).
- **Social awareness**—Accurately assess and respond to the emotions of others. Ability to listen and accurately interpret unspoken emotions.

Situational Theories People and leadership situations are far more complex than the early theories recognized. Instead of assuming that one approach works in all situations, situational theories emphasize that it is important to (1) understand all of the factors that affect a group of people in a particular environment, and (2) vary the type of leadership to meet the needs of the situation.

Key Point: *Adaptability is the key to the situational approach.* For example, a nurse who is in charge of a code situation must give clear, direct instructions in a calm, confident manner. Conversely, a nurse who develops a policy regarding nurse-to-client ratios will need to elicit input from the staff.

Transformational Theories Situational theories do not address **meaning, inspiration,** and **vision,** which are the distinguishing features of transformational leadership theory. Transformational leaders aspire to meet the self-actualization needs of their followers. People need a sense of purpose and vision that goes beyond good interpersonal relationships or the reward for a job well done (Ronquillo, 2022; Steinmann et al., 2018). Transformational leaders:

- Engage and empower others to accomplish the mission, creating feelings of loyalty, trust, inspiration, and satisfaction.
- Create a supportive climate, listen to followers, and act as a coach and mentor.
- Communicate their vision in a way that is so meaningful and exciting that it inspires commitment in others.

Followers of transformational leaders become motivated to go beyond their own self-interests for the good of the group or organization, often accomplishing more than what would normally be expected of them (Fischer, 2016; Stern, 2021). This is especially true in nursing. Caring for people, sick or well, is the goal of our profession. Most of us chose nursing for our vision: to do something for the good of humankind. Our nursing leaders empower us to achieve that vision.

The American Nurses Credentialing Center (ANCC) Magnet Model is a framework for achieving excellence in nursing practice. It recognizes transformational leadership as an essential component of the model (ANCC, n.d.). Leaders in Magnet organizations are expected to demonstrate the transformational qualities listed in Table 40-1.

Table 40-1 ➤ Contrast of Traits in Transactional and Transformational Leadership

TRANSACTIONAL LEADERSHIP	TRANSFORMATIONAL LEADERSHIP
Directive	Participative
Top down	Bottom up
Information	Conversation
Hierarchical communication	Matrix communication
Event oriented	Future oriented
Task focused	Overall experience focused
Directed	Facilitated
Rigid	Flexible
Here and now	Visions for the future
Traditional	Contemporary
Rule following	Risk taking
Control	Creativity
Individual performance	Team and relationships
Responsibility	Accountability

Source: Used with permission of Patricia Davis, RN, DNP, MS, NEA-BC, CNL; Concord, CA.

Transactional Theories Transitional theories assume that people are motivated by reward and punishment and that they work best within a clear chain of command and a structured environment.

- **Structure.** The structure usually includes position descriptions, policies and procedures, and formal systems of discipline.
- **Transactional relationship.** The traditional employer–employee relationship exemplifies transactional theories—workers are rewarded with a salary and benefits for the performance of their duties and disciplined for nonperformance.
- **Leaders.** Leaders may be task oriented, enforce rules, and provide guidance to workers.

When the demand for a skill—or for workers of a specific type—is greater than the supply, the usual rewards may not be sufficient, and other types of leadership are more effective. Table 40-1 compares the traits of transactional and transformational leadership.

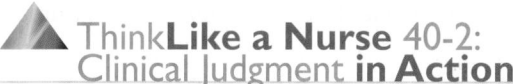

ThinkLike a Nurse 40-2: Clinical Judgment **in Action**

- Observe a nurse in one of the healthcare agencies at which you are doing a clinical rotation. What leadership qualities and behaviors do you see the nurse exhibiting?
- How do these behaviors help in planning nursing care?

WHAT IS MANAGEMENT?

Whereas leaders may or may not have official appointments to the position, managers are usually officially appointed. A **manager** is an employee of an organization who has the power, authority, and responsibility for enforcing decisions and for planning, organizing, coordinating, and directing the work of others. Every nurse should be a good leader and a good follower; however, not everyone can or should be a manager. As you read further, you may notice the overlaps between management and leadership. That is because managers have leadership responsibilities and exhibit varying styles of leadership. **Key Point:** *Not all leaders should be managers, but all managers should be leaders.*

As a registered nurse, you will manage groups of clients, and you will be responsible for supervising nursing assistants, licensed practical nurses, and ancillary staff. Even as a staff nurse, you will be a manager of care. You may be interested to know that the NCLEX-RN® Testing Plan has an entire section devoted to management of care, which is about organizing and delivering (managing) care to the client.

Management Theories

Although there are many management theories, the two major schools of thought in management are: (1) scientific management, which emphasizes the task aspects of managing people; and (2) the human-relations approach to management, with an emphasis on the relationship aspects.

Scientific Management Almost 100 years ago, Frederick Taylor argued that most jobs could be done more efficiently if they were thoroughly analyzed (Lykins, 2011; Taylor, 1911/2011). Given a properly designed task and sufficient incentive to get the work done, workers would be more productive because repetition promotes efficiency. For example, Taylor encouraged paying people "by the piece," that is, by the number of "widgets" made rather than by the number of hours worked (Ireh, 2016; Taylor, 1911/2011). This encourages workers to get the most quality work done in the least amount of time. In healthcare, the equivalent would be to pay for the number of tasks completed (e.g., IV lines started, clients bathed). In scientific management, the fastest way to do a job is usually thought to be the best way.

Human Relations–Based Management McGregor's (1960) Theory X and Theory Y are good examples of the difference between scientific management and human relationships.

- **Theory X.** Managers believe that most people really do not want to work very hard and that the manager's job is to make sure that they do work hard. Per Theory X, a manager needs to use strict rules, constant supervision, and the threat of punishment (e.g., reprimands, withheld raises, and threats of job loss) to create industrious, conscientious workers. Theory X is similar to scientific management.
- **Theory Y.** Managers believe that work itself can be motivating, that people want to do their jobs well, and that they will work hard if their managers provide a supportive atmosphere. A Theory Y manager emphasizes guidance over control, development rather than close supervision, and reward over punishment.

A Theory Y nurse manager is human-relations oriented. They assume that satisfied, motivated staff will do the best work, so high staff morale is a major focus. The manager's goal is to create a harmonious, productive work environment by promoting mutual understanding and respect among the staff.

Servant Leadership Despite its name, servant leadership applies more to supervisors and administrators than to nurses in staff positions. This type of leader assumes the role of selflessly serving others, cultivates a culture of trust, seeks diverse opinions, and works to develop other leaders (Canavesi & Minelli, 2021; Eva et al., 2019). This leader is committed to improving the way each employee is treated, removing barriers at work, making the work easier, and providing employees with whatever they need to ensure quality client care. The servant leadership manager believes people have value as people, not just as workers; empowers followers; and prioritizes their development.

Qualities of an Effective Manager

Effective leadership styles of nurse managers and administrators can enhance staff nurse retention (McCay et al., 2018). Given the high costs associated with the orientation of new employees, nurse managers are challenged to retain staff nurses. An effective nurse manager should possess a combination of the following qualities:

- **Leadership.** Effective managers must understand people, leadership, and power. They must have competencies in EI, staff and client advocacy, communication, and collaboration (Azad et al., 2017; Grindel, 2016).
- **Clinical expertise.** Nurse managers need a strong knowledge base, acquired through clinical experiences, education, training, and professional development, to ensure clients receive quality care (Grindel, 2016). They readily respond to clinical situations and promote professional accountability. They are instrumental in assessing the effectiveness of the team's work in terms of client outcomes.
- **Business sense.** Nurse managers must be knowledgeable of practice structures (lines of authority), budgets, and how the cost of nursing services aligns with the overall hospital and unit budgets (Grindel, 2016). They analyze the time needed to provide client care, the effectiveness of care, reimbursement rates, and revenue sources (private insurance, government subsidy, or self-pay). This requires knowledge of budgeting, staffing, and measurement of patient outcomes, most of which are beyond the scope of this textbook.

Activities of an Effective Manager

Mintzberg (1989) divides the manager's activities into three categories: interpersonal, decisional, and informational. Weiss et al. (2019) build on that work by describing the following types of activities engaged in by managers.

Interpersonal Activities

Interpersonal activities are important to both leaders and managers. In fact, they are important to everyone! From the beginning of your nursing education, you will have many opportunities to develop positive working relationships with members of other disciplines and units within the organization. Can you see how Mary (Meet Your Peer) would need interpersonal skills to accomplish her goals?

Interpersonal activities of managers include the following:

- **Networking.** Managers must clearly articulate nurses' roles in and value to the institution.
- **Conflict negotiation and resolution.** For example, conflict may arise on a unit over work schedules, especially on holidays.

- **Advocacy.** Managers must advocate for and support staff in their discussions with upper-level management.
- **Employee development.** This includes providing for continuing learning and upgrading employees' skills.
- **Rewards.** Examples include salary increases, time off, and praise.
- **Coaching.** The goal is to help the employee do a better job through learning. Some managers use a directive approach ("Let me show you how to do this"). Others use a nondirective approach ("How do you think we can improve our outcomes?").

Decision-Making Activities

Nurse managers must make decisions to enhance unit efficiency, retain personnel, improve client outcomes, and promote interprofessional collaboration. Decisions made include the following:

- **Employee evaluation** (e.g., conducting formal performance appraisals)
- **Resource allocation** (e.g., budgeting; effective use of resources)
- **Hiring, evaluating, and terminating** employees
- **Planning for future changes** (e.g., in budgets or client populations)
- **Job analysis and redesign** (e.g., improve efficiency)
- **Unit-based decisions** (e.g., staffing policies, space utilization, interprofessional collaboration)

See if you can identify the decisions Mary (Meet Your Peer) made.

Informational Responsibilities

Managers also have informational responsibilities and roles, including the following:

- **Spokesperson.** The manager relays information from administration to staff members and speaks with administration on behalf of staff members.
- **Monitor.** Nurse managers monitor the activities of their units or departments (e.g., the number of clients seen, length of stay), as well as the staff (e.g., absenteeism) and the budget (e.g., money spent).
- **Public relations.** Nurse managers share information with clients, staff members, and employers, for example, regarding new developments in healthcare and policy changes.

What kinds of information do you think Mary (Meet Your Peer) would need to communicate to the students interested in forming a study group?

KnowledgeCheck 40-2

- How is transformational leadership different from the other theories of leadership?
- Define *manager*.
- In McGregor's management theory, which is more like scientific management: Theory X or Theory Y?

HOW CAN I PREPARE TO BECOME A LEADER AND MANAGER?

Besides learning the role of the licensed practical nurse (LPN)/licensed vocational nurse (LVN) or registered nurse (RN), you should begin right now to look at the skills employers think you need to be ready to work for them. Along with passing the NCLEX examination to obtain nursing licensure, employers cite the skills listed in Box 40-1 as desirable in job candidates (Bonsall, 2021; Paans et al., 2017). These skills will assist you as you progress through your nursing program and will also make your adjustment to the nursing role much easier. Note that leaders and managers also use these skills in the performance of their responsibilities. It is not too early to begin to develop your abilities in these areas.

SWOT Analysis One of the first steps in identifying what skills you already possess and which you need to develop is to do a brief SWOT analysis. A SWOT (strengths, weaknesses, opportunities, threats) analysis plan, borrowed from the corporate world, can guide you through an analysis of your own internal strengths and weaknesses and reveal external opportunities and threats that may help or hinder your leadership and management skills (Teoli et al., 2022). Your SWOT analysis may include the factors listed as examples in Table 40-2, but you will certainly have others.

SOAR Model You might prefer to use the SOAR strategic planning model to help you prepare to become a leader and manager (Table 40-3). This model can be used to analyze any type of situation and create a plan

---

BOX 40-1 ■ Desirable Job Skills for Nursing Candidates

- Ability to adapt equipment to serve user needs
- Ability to assume responsibility/use feedback for professional growth
- Ability to teach others
- Computer knowledge
- Critical-thinking and analytical skills
- Self-reflection
- Flexibility to adjust action in relation to others
- Interpersonal skills
- Leadership abilities
- Motivation, initiative, and flexibility
- Oral and written communication skills
- Organizational skills
- Problem-solving and decision-making abilities
- Proficiency in field of study or technical competence
- Self-discipline
- Teamwork ability/cooperative
- Willingness to work hard

Table 40-2 ➤ SWOT Analysis Plan—Examples

STRENGTHS	WEAKNESSES	OPPORTUNITIES	THREATS
Relevant work experience	Poor communication and people skills	Changes in healthcare	Changes in healthcare
Advanced education	Underdeveloped organizational skills	Availability of preceptors and mentors	Lack of time
Good communication and people skills	Poor time-management skills	Variety of experiences in clinical rotations	Competition from other students and other nursing programs
Computer skills	Difficulty adapting to change; inflexibility	Many leadership and management resources and self-learning programs available	

SWOT, Strengths, weaknesses, opportunities, threats.

Table 40-3 ➤ SOAR Strategic Planning

THE PROCESS: HOW TO SOAR	THE SOAR REPORT OR SUMMARY
To SOAR: Inquire, imagine, innovate, and inspire.	Use SOAR to report or tell your story.
Inquiry: Internal analysis of strengths and external analysis of opportunities.	**Strengths:** My (or the group's) strengths are ... (Examples of strengths may be a supportive environment, individual strengths, a product that others need, etc.)
Imagination: Cocreate vision, values, and mission. Imagine desired outcomes. Imagine the best pathway to achieve the outcomes.	**Opportunities:** My values are ... (e.g., dedication, quality). As I imagine the future, my vision (for myself, for our group) is ... (e.g., to become a transformational manager on a nursing unit).
Innovation: Create initiatives, strategies, structures, and systems. Create plans for tactics.	**Aspirations:** Here is how I believe I (or we) can achieve the desired outcomes ...
Inspiration: Inspire action-oriented activities that achieve results. Implement a plan for continuous improvement.	**Results:** To achieve your desired outcomes, you must be motivated (and possibly need to inspire others) to take the necessary actions.

SOAR, Strengths, opportunities, aspirations, results.
Sources: Adapted from Cole, M., Cox, J. D., & Stavros, J. M. (2019). Building collaboration in teams through emotional intelligence: Mediation by SOAR (strengths, opportunities, aspirations, and results). *Journal of Management and Organization.* https://doi.org/10.1017/jmo.2016.43; Stavros, J. M., Cooperrider, D., & Kelley, D. L. (2009). SOAR: A new approach to strategic planning. In P. Holman, T. Devane, & S. Cady (Eds.), *The change handbook: The definitive resource on today's best methods for engaging whole systems* (pp. 375–380). Berrett-Koehle; Wadsworth, B., Felton, F., & Linus, R. (2016). SOARing into strategic planning. *Nursing Administration Quarterly, 40*(4), 299–306. https://doi.org/10.1097/NAQ.0000000000000182

to achieve personal and professional goals. With this model, you would use inquiry, imagination, and innovation, and you would also focus on strengths, opportunities, aspirations, and results (Cole et al., 2022; Wadsworth et al., 2016).

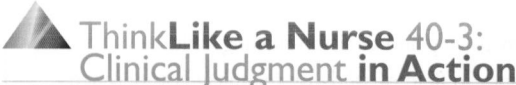

Think Like a Nurse 40-3: Clinical Judgment **in Action**

Stop and think! Take some time to personalize the SWOT analysis in Table 40-2. What weaknesses do you need to minimize, or which strengths do you need to develop as you begin to develop your leadership and management skills?

How Can Preceptors and Mentors Help Me?

There are two aspects to consider as you get ready to become a leader and manager. The first part consists of developing your own skills and attributes, as just discussed. The second is really a combination of developing yourself and developing others: preceptorship and mentorship.

Preceptors Many organizations have preceptors for new employees. A **preceptor** is an experienced nurse who provides practical teaching and guidance for a student or new employee. As a student, you may be assigned an RN preceptor in your clinical rotations. You may work with a preceptor to provide client care as a student and as a new nurse (Fig. 40-1).

In many instances, the preceptor will become your mentor. **Key Point:** *However, the mentor role is much more encompassing than the preceptor role. The mentor relationship is a voluntary one and is built on mutual respect and development of the mentee.* Box 40-2 identifies the responsibilities of the mentor and mentee in this relationship.

Mentors A **mentor** is an experienced person who provides career development assistance, such as coaching, sponsoring advancement, providing challenging assignments, protecting protégés from adversity, and promoting positive visibility. They serve many roles.

- Mentors provide guidance to new students or recent graduates as they continue in the profession.

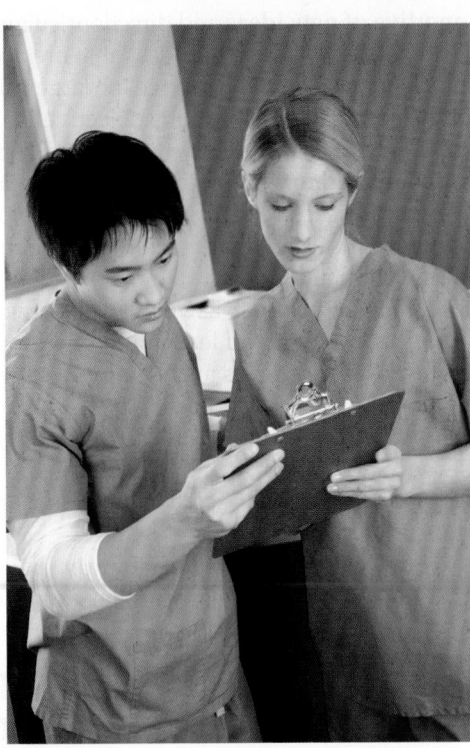

FIGURE 40-1 Nurse precepting a new graduate.

- Mentors offer a constructive example as a role model to novices.
- Mentors also fulfill psychosocial roles, such as personal support, friendship, acceptance, role modeling, and counseling.

You should always use sound judgment when following the advice of others. Do not blindly engage in behaviors or actions because others do them.

You should look for a competent mentor in the nursing program right now—someone to guide you as you grow into your professional role. A student who has already completed several semesters and appears to be a leader is a good choice. In some programs, you may be assigned a student preceptor while you are in the program. Although this student may or may not become your mentor, you will need to have leadership and management skills to work side by side effectively.

Will you assume the role of preceptor or mentor while you are still in school? We hope your response is yes. As you progress in the program, remember the feelings of uncertainty and anxiety that you may have now, and volunteer to mentor another new student. Through the mentoring process, you can continue to develop yourself as a leader. Mentoring and precepting are part of your professional responsibilities; as the American Nurses Association (ANA) Standard of Nursing Practice 11, Leadership (2021), states:

> *The registered nurse leads within the professional practice setting and the profession. (p. 75)*

How Will Leadership Grow in My Nursing Career?

As you begin your nursing clinical experiences, your nursing instructor will supervise most of your decisions. As you continue to develop your knowledge and skills, you will begin working more as a member of the

---

BOX 40-2 ■ Mentor and Mentee Responsibilities

Mentor Responsibilities

- Demonstrate excellent communication and listening skills.
- Be sensitive to the needs of nurses, clients, and the workplace.
- Encourage excellence in others.
- Share and provide counsel.
- Exhibit good decision-making skills.
- Demonstrate an understanding of power and politics.
- Demonstrate trustworthiness.

Mentee Responsibilities

- Demonstrate eagerness to learn.
- Participate actively in the relationship by keeping all appointments and commitments.
- Seek feedback and use it to modify behaviors.
- Demonstrate flexibility and an ability to change.
- Be open in the relationship with the mentor.
- Demonstrate an ability to move toward independence.
- Evaluate choices and outcomes.

Source: Weiss, S. A., Tappen, R. M., & Grimley, K. (2019). *Essentials of nursing leadership and management* (7th ed.). F. A. Davis.

team. You will be expected to work with clients' family members and the interprofessional healthcare team. You will prioritize interventions in providing care to clients. You may go to community agencies and network with groups. To be successful in your continued role development as a nurse, you must work on perfecting the skills discussed in this chapter.

KnowledgeCheck 40-3

- Identify four skills that employers cite as desirable in job candidates.
- Identify three responsibilities of a mentor and three responsibilities of a mentee.

 ## ThinkLike a Nurse 40-4: Clinical Judgment in Action

Think about how you are working with your peers at this time. What mentor responsibilities are you exhibiting? Is there someone who is already mentoring you? If so, what qualities does this person exhibit?

WHAT IS FOLLOWERSHIP?

Leadership and followership are two separate but complementary concepts and roles. Great leaders can create successful followers, and great followers create successful leaders. No one person can have the best strategy, express the clearest vision, or identify the most effective approaches to solving problems. **Key Point:** *All participants need to be recognized as full partners in the organizational venture.*

Definitions If we define **followers** as individuals who take another person as a role model and who act in accordance with, imitate, support, and advocate for the ideas and opinions of another (Grossman & Valiga, 2017), then we can define **followership** as the willingness to work with others toward accomplishing the group mission. This term also refers to those who show a high degree of teamwork and build cohesion among the group (Bastardoz & Vugt 2019; Stern, 2021).

An **organization** is a community of many leaders and many followers, frequently changing places depending on the activity that is occurring. Blindly following a leader without question or taking a passive role in one's work or professional organization will do little to advance the profession, promote individual growth, or achieve quality patient care.

Important Qualities and Behaviors To participate fully and provide significant feedback, followers need to demonstrate important qualities and behaviors (Grossman & Valiga, 2017; Stern, 2021):

- **Suggest ways to improve patient care.**
- **If you discover a problem, inform your team leader** right away and propose a solution if you can. If it is not accepted, your job is then to support—not

undermine—the leader and continue to seek an effective solution.
- **Listen carefully and reflect** on what the leader or manager says.
- **Be truthful.** Give honest feedback and constructive criticism, even if it means politely challenging the leader's ideas. Suggest alternative courses of action.
- **Maintain privacy.** If you feel you must have a "heated" discussion with the leader, do so privately. When you disagree, explain why.
- **Freely invest your interest and energy** in your work and in finding the best solutions for the group.
- **Function independently;** be a self-starter; take on extra tasks without being asked.
- **Be innovative, creative, and actively involved.**
- **Be responsible** and hold up your end of the bargain; accept responsibility when it is offered.
- **Be supportive of new ideas** and directions suggested by others, but *think critically* about ideas that are proposed. Seek information so that you can see the larger picture.
- **Do not gossip.** Present situations objectively.
- **Think and act as a team;** be cooperative and collaborative.
- **Draw on and complement** one another's and the leader's specialties, strengths, and areas of expertise.
- **Work on behalf of the organization** and the mutually agreed-on vision and goals.
- **Continue to learn** as much as you can about your specialty area; share what you learn with others.
- **Know your own strengths** and what you can offer as unique contributions to the effort.
- **Know how to assume the role of the leader** when necessary.
- **Have a positive sense of self-worth** and a "can-do" attitude.
- **Take care of yourself and your family.** If you and they are unhappy, your job performance will suffer.

WHAT ARE THE CHALLENGES TO BEING AN EFFECTIVE LEADER AND MANAGER?

Even after you have developed the skills necessary to become an effective leader or manager, challenges exist in the healthcare environment. These challenges include the economic climate of healthcare and the nursing labor market.

Economic Climate of Healthcare

For many years, decisions about care were based primarily on providing the best quality of care, whatever the cost. Now, healthcare providers are pressured to seek methods of care delivery that achieve quality outcomes at lower costs. This economic perspective is rooted in three fundamental observations:

1. **Resources are scarce.** The scarcity of resources means that three decisions must occur:
   - How much do we spend on healthcare services? And what do those services consist of?

- How will those healthcare services be produced?
- How should, or can, we distribute healthcare? In other words, how are services apportioned within the population?

2. **Resources have alternative uses.** Because resources are limited, a choice to spend resources in one area eliminates the allocation of those same resources for another use. If, for example, we wish to build more nursing homes, then we must be willing to accept fewer hospitals or less housing, educational, or other uses of those same resources. In healthcare, an expanded program of immunization may mean limiting care for certain age-groups.

3. **Individuals want different things or have different preferences.** Some people choose alternative treatment modalities, such as acupuncture, herbal therapy, or massage therapy, rather than traditional healthcare. The assumption exists that preferences for products and services can be influenced—hence the extensive marketing of healthcare services.

Nursing Labor Market

- **The number of nurses continues to grow.** In the United States, there are 4.19 million RNs, with 84.1% employed in nursing and over 944,000 employed as LPN/LVNs. Those numbers continue to grow. The majority of registered nurses (54.8%) are employed in hospitals, followed by ambulatory care environments (9.7%). At least 54.9% of RNs work at least 40 hours a week in their principal position (Smiley et al., 2021).

- **The need for nurses is expected to continue increasing.** The Bureau of Labor Statistics (2022) predicted that the employment of RNs will grow 6% from 2021 to 2031. Over 200,000 openings for RNs are projected each year (Bureau of Labor Statistics, 2022). The need for nurses is expected to increase even more dramatically as the baby boomers reach their 60s, 70s, and beyond. From now until 2030, the population aged 65 and older will double. The questions are:
  1. Will there be enough nurses available to fill those jobs?
  2. Even if nurses are available, will it be economically feasible for organizations to hire as many as they need?

- **Cost control and demand for nurses will affect nursing.** Historical trends show that cost control and demand for nursing services will affect (1) nurse staffing patterns, (2) the model of care, and (3) professional nursing practice. These changes will affect you, the nurse.

- **RNs will be expected to be leaders and managers.** Regardless of the changes, healthcare system changes will likely demand that the RN lead manage personnel delivering patient care while maintaining fiscal responsibility. Even though government and other agencies heavily regulate healthcare, it is a big business. You must juggle the needs of your patients with the needs of the organization. From time to time, think about how you might do that.

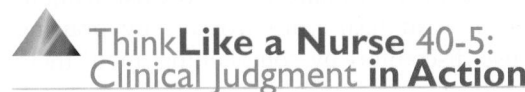
ThinkLike a Nurse 40-5: Clinical Judgment in Action

Identify changes in your community that will affect you as you embark on your nursing career. What will you do to prepare for these changes?

WHAT ARE POWER AND EMPOWERMENT?

The leadership and management techniques discussed so far will help you to achieve your goals. However, there are times when your attempts to influence others are overwhelmed by other forces or individuals. Where does this power come from? Who has it? Who does not?

Although people at the top of the organizational chart have most of the *authority* in the organization, they do not have all of the *power*. In fact, the people at the bottom of the hierarchy also have some power. **Power** is the ability of a person to get things done and is created through both formal and informal systems (Peyton et al., 2019). Power may be used to facilitate growth and productivity within an organization or can be the basis for stagnation and decreased morale.

Sources of Power

Various sources of power are available to nurses, depending on the situation:

- **Positional/legitimate:** A person's authority is derived from their location in the organization's hierarchy. The person at the top has the most power.
- **Referent:** Informal power created through relationships with people within the organization. Power is acquired through the person's ability to influence and gain others' respect.
- **Reward:** The ability of an individual to control or allocate incentives (e.g., promotion, salary increases, recognition, or other benefits).
- **Expertise:** You have heard the expression, "Knowledge is power." This is based on the belief that the person's expertise and analytical skills are critical to the organization's success.
- **Coercion:** The power to control others through threats or discipline. The person has the authority to enforce standards, policies, and procedures.

Let's look at the types of power available to various groups in healthcare organizations.

Managers Managers have the **reward power** of salary increases, promotions, and recognition. They can also use **coercion power** to provide structure and discipline or to impose economic or psychological pain based on their authority to evaluate and fire people.

Patients At first, patients appear to be relatively powerless in a healthcare organization. However, an organization would eventually cease to exist without clients. They reward healthcare workers by praising them or cause discomfort by complaining about them to supervisors.

Registered Nurses RNs have expert, legitimate, and coercion power. They delegate responsibilities to LPNs/LVNs, unlicensed assistive personnel (UAP), and other staff by virtue of their position in the hierarchy and the state's nurse practice act. Nurses are essential to the operation of most healthcare organizations and could cause considerable disruption if they refused to work. They must also ensure others are performing their roles and take action if there are deviations from the standards of practice.

Nurses have always had the power of information, or expertise. For example, Florence Nightingale showed very graphically in the 1800s that wherever her nurses were, far fewer patients died; wherever they were not, far more patients died. Think of the power of that information. Immediately people were saying, "What would you like, Miss Nightingale? Would you like more money? Would you like a school of nursing? What else can we do for you?" (Fralic, 2000, p. 340). She had solid data, and she knew how to collect, interpret, and distribute the data in terms of things that people valued (Stanley & Sherratt, 2010).

Assistants and Technicians Assistants and technicians may appear to have less power because of their position in an organization's "top-down" hierarchy. Imagine, though, how the work of the organization would grind to a halt if all the nursing assistants failed to appear one morning. Therefore, they have both expertise and coercive power.

KnowledgeCheck 40-4
- What are the sources of power available to nurses?

Sources of Empowerment

How can nurses, either individually or collectively, maximize their power and increase their feelings of empowerment? To answer this question, you should first distinguish between the concepts of power and empowerment. Recall that **power** is the ability to influence other people despite resistance from them. **Empowerment** is a psychological state, a feeling that one has been given the power to solve problems, take initiative, and exercise autonomy. **Key Point:** *Given these definitions, it is possible to be powerful and yet not feel empowered. Power refers to action, and empowerment refers to feelings. Both are of interest to nursing leaders and managers.*

Feeling empowered includes the following:

- **Self-determination:** Feeling free to decide how to do your work.

- **Meaning:** Caring about your work, enjoying it, and taking it seriously.
- **Competence:** Confidence in your ability to do your work well.
- **Impact:** Feeling that people listen to your ideas and that you can make a difference.

Nurses, like most people, want to have some power and to feel empowered, valued, and respected. Organizations that foster empowerment provide employees with access to information, support systems, required resources to do their job, and the opportunity to learn and grow (Loes & Tobin, 2020). You will feel a sense of empowerment in settings that ensure: (1) manageable, reasonable work assignments; (2) reward, recognition, and appreciation for a job well done; and (3) fair, consistent treatment of all staff.

Enhancing Expertise

Not all empowerment comes from others. You are empowered to some degree by your own professional knowledge and competence. Following are some ways in which you can enhance your competence, thereby increasing your own sense of empowerment:

- **Actively participate** in interprofessional team conferences, client-centered conferences, and clinical or governance committees on your unit.
- **Enhance your expertise** by attending continuing education activities. This might include local, regional, national, and international conferences sponsored by nursing organizations.
- **Participate in nursing research projects** or use evidence-based practice guidelines, current nursing journals, and books to make decisions regarding your nursing practice.
- **Discuss with colleagues** how to handle a difficult clinical situation and observe the practices of experienced nurses or other providers. Do not be afraid to ask questions.
- **Continue your education by** earning additional degrees and certifications in nursing.

Although you have just begun your nursing career, it is not too early to begin thinking of ways to become empowered.

Sharing Expertise

You also become empowered by sharing your knowledge and experience with others. This means not only using your knowledge to improve your own practice but also communicating what you have learned to other students and, later, to your colleagues in nursing. It also means informing and demonstrating to your instructors and supervisors that you have enhanced your professional competence. You can share your knowledge with your clients, empowering them as well. As you gain expertise in a clinical area or skill set, you can share it by writing an article for publication.

PracticalKnowledge
knowing **how**

As a leader or manager, you will need to get people to work together to make things happen. To do so, you will need to communicate effectively, delegate, deal with conflict and change, and manage your time appropriately. These can be thought of as skills or processes (or practical knowledge).

COMMUNICATING

Leaders use communication to develop relationships with other people and to engage and support these relationships. Some view communication as a circular process that is affected by many factors. This means the activity is continuous, mutually interdependent, and influenced by the behaviors of each communicator.

- **Active listening.** You need to use active listening to pick up all levels of meaning in a communication. Surface listening, or inattention, often causes a misinterpretation of the message.
- **Attitude.** Your attitude influences what you hear and how you interpret the message.
- **Lines of communication.** To effectively manage client care, it is important to keep the lines of communication open to various individuals (e.g., other nurses, interprofessional team, client family members).
- **Trust and congruence.** Trust and sincerity enhance communication. Congruence (agreement) between your words and your deeds promotes trust. If you are viewed as trustworthy and sincere, others will be more likely to ask questions, seek clarification, and accept your leadership when they are uncertain of something.

Communication skills are taught extensively in Chapter 15, if you need to review them now.

Evaluative Feedback A leader is responsible for providing frequent evaluative feedback. Done poorly, evaluation can be stressful, even injurious. Done well, it promotes growth and employee satisfaction. Evaluative feedback is important because it:

- **Reinforces constructive behavior.** Positive feedback lets people know which behaviors are most productive and encourages them to continue the behaviors. When possible, it may be helpful to give positive feedback in public.
- **Discourages unproductive behavior. Constructive guidance (negative feedback)** is the process of pointing out what someone is not doing well and telling them how they can change it. Constructive guidance prompts the person to correct inappropriate behavior and should be given in private.
- **Provides recognition.** Praise is an excellent motivator.

DELEGATING

An important aspect of leadership and management is learning how to use a systematic critical-thinking tool (e.g., nursing process) to delegate. This is an essential nursing skill to ensure safe and quality client care. To properly delegate, you must:

- **Assessment/recognizing cues.** You must recognize the cues that identify your client's needs **(diagnosis/ analyzing cues)** before assigning them to a particular team member.
- **Planning/prioritizing hypotheses and generating solutions.** Set client-specific goals, and identify the solutions required to achieve these goals. Mentally identifying which staff member is best suited for the task or activities before delegating helps prevent problems later.
- **Implementation/taking action.** Next, determine which personnel have the knowledge and skills to care for the client, and assign the tasks to the appropriate person.
- **Evaluate.** You are still accountable for overseeing care and determining whether client care needs have been met. Establish timelines for feedback during the day. This enables all personnel to review their care and what still needs to be completed. Provide constructive guidance in private.

You will find an extended discussion of delegation in Chapter 3. You might also find helpful the ANA and National Council of the State Boards of Nursing (NCSBN) (2019) joint statement on delegation and a decision tree to promote proper delegation. For the checklist, *Five Rights of Delegation,*

 Go to **Chapter 3, Box 3-7: The Five Rights of Delegation—Checklist.**

A manager must first determine the mix of personnel (RN, LVN/LPN, or UAP) required to deliver care on a unit before being able to delegate tasks to individuals. By looking at the needs of each client, you can make an educated decision about which staff members have the appropriate education and skill to deliver safe, quality care.

What If I Lack the Experience to Delegate?

The added responsibility of delegation often causes discomfort for new graduates. You may be accustomed to providing total patient care for one or more clients but lack experience in organizing care for groups of clients with other team members. To overcome your discomfort, you need to observe how more experienced nurses delegate to others. Working with a preceptor will also give you experience in delegation.

Become familiar with nursing professional organization guidelines. The ANA has specified that RNs may not delegate the following tasks (ANA & NCSBN, 2019; Barrow et al., 2022a):

- Initial nursing assessment; follow-up assessments if nursing judgment is indicated
- Nursing diagnosis
- Decisions and judgments about outcomes
- Formulation and approval of a patient plan of care
- Interventions that require professional nursing knowledge, decisions, or skills
- Decisions and judgments necessary for the evaluation of patient care

The ANA (2007, 2012) has issued guidelines on the use of UAP. The list includes direct and indirect client care that may be delegated to UAPs (Fig. 40-2). Various other nursing personnel can also be used to meet patient care needs (Box 40-3).

What Are the Concerns About Delegating?

Today's healthcare environment requires nurses to delegate. Many nurses voice concerns about the personal risk to their licensure if they delegate inappropriately. The courts have usually ruled that nurses are not liable for the negligence of other workers, provided that the nurse delegated appropriately. State boards of nursing view delegation as within the scope of nursing practice. If you would like further discussion of the legal aspects of delegation, see Chapter 39.

Key Point: *Nurses have also expressed concern over the effects of delegation on the quality of client care. When you delegate, you control the delegation. You decide to whom and what you will delegate. Remember, you must ensure that the delegation process results in quality client care.*

KnowledgeCheck 40-5

Explain the relationship of delegation and systematic critical-thinking tools (e.g., nursing process).

BOX 40-3 ■ Examples of Care That May Be Delegated to Unlicensed Assistive Personnel

Direct Client Care Activities
- Assisting with activities of daily living: feeding, drinking, ambulation, grooming, toileting, dressing
- Assisting with socializing
- Taking vital signs

Indirect Client Care Activities
- Providing a clean, safe environment
- Providing transport for noncritical clients
- Assisting with stocking nursing units
- Providing messenger and delivery services
- Making beds
- Ordering supplies

MANAGING CHANGE

Change is a naturally occurring phenomenon, a part of everyone's life. Every day, we have new experiences, meet new people, and learn something new. We grow up, leave home, graduate from college, begin a new career, and perhaps begin a new family as well. Some of these changes are milestones in our lives, ones we have prepared for and anticipated for some time. Others are entirely unexpected—sometimes welcome and sometimes not. Many are exciting, leading us to new opportunities and challenges. When change occurs too rapidly or with high demands, it can make us very uncomfortable.

The Comfort Zone

The basic stages of the change process are unfreezing, change, and refreezing (Barrow et al., 2022b; Lewin, 1951). Figure 40-3 shows the relationship among those stages and the concepts of comfort zone, discomfort zone, and a new comfort zone.

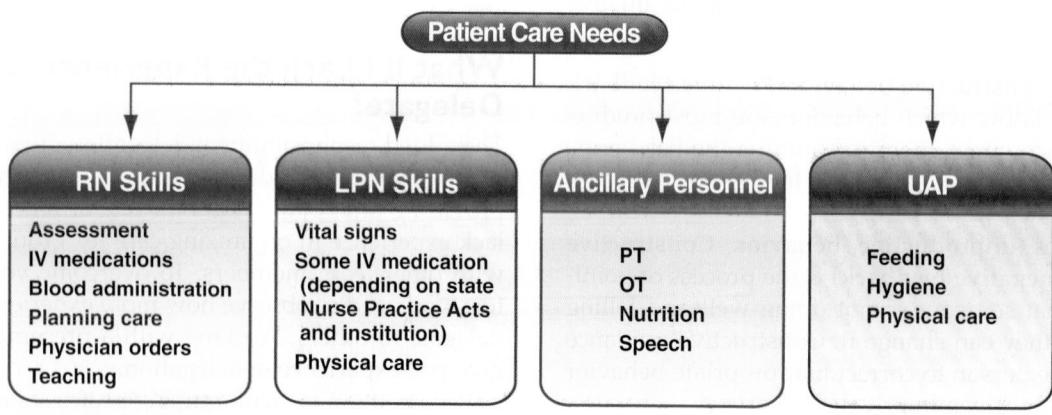

FIGURE 40-2 Patient care needs.

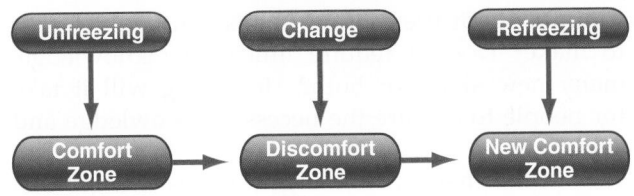

FIGURE 40-3 The change process.

Let's assume that your daily routine was basically stable before you started your nursing program. You took care of the family or worked during the day and took a class or two each term. You knew what to expect and how to deal with whatever problems arose. In other words, you were operating within your "comfort zone" (Eliades et al., 2017; Farrell & Broude, 1987). A big change is likely to move you out of this comfort zone and into disequilibrium, possibly into discomfort. Now you may be juggling changes in finances, childcare arrangements, and planning options for your future career. This first stage in the change process is called *unfreezing*. You are moving out of your comfort zone.

Resistance to Change

People resist change for a variety of reasons. For example, you may find that you can manage the change in class schedule but that the childcare arrangements are more difficult. Resistance to change (and unfreezing) comes from three major sources: technical concerns, psychosocial needs, and threats to a person's position and power. For a student, so-called technical concerns may involve practical issues related to transportation to school or work, getting children to school, or managing household responsibilities.

Recall that in Maslow's (1970) hierarchy of needs theory, the more basic needs (e.g., physiological and safety needs) must be at least partially met before a person is motivated to seek fulfillment of the higher-order needs. Once status, power, and influence are gained within families and organizations, they are hard to give up. You may be the one in charge in the family or work situation while being a novice in the nursing program.

Recognizing Resistance

It is easy to recognize resistance to a change when it is directly expressed. When a person says to you, "That's not a very good idea," "I am not going to quit smoking," or "There's no way I'm going to do that," there is no doubt that you are meeting resistance. When resistance is less direct, however, you will need to recognize the signs.

Resistance may be active or passive.

- **Active resistance** can take the form of aggressive actions or outright refusals to comply, negative communications designed to demean the idea or the person who suggested it, quoting of existing rules that make the change difficult or impossible to implement, or organizing resistance to the change.
- **Passive resistance** involves avoidance, such as canceling appointments to discuss implementing the change, being "too busy" to implement the change, or agreeing to the change but citing numerous barriers to it.

ThinkLike a Nurse 40-6: Clinical Judgment in Action

Recall one change that you have experienced that was put into effect by a command, new rule, policy, or law.

- What effects did this change have on your life (e.g., work, school, home)?
- How did the command, new rule, policy, or law make you feel?
- What would have made this change easier for you?

Lowering Resistance

Key Point: *A change that is welcomed by one group may be strongly resisted by another group. Resistance to change is affected by the leadership approach and the type of organizational structure.*

You can use various approaches to lower people's resistance to change. Strategies fall into four categories: commanding, sharing information, refuting currently held beliefs, and providing psychological safety (Weiss et al., 2019).

Commanding Change Obviously, the quickest way to implement change, if you have the authority to do so, is to issue a command. Dictating change, however, is not necessarily the best strategy, but it is sometimes necessary when the change must be made quickly. Commanding a change may not be effective if there are ways for people to resist, for example, when:

- Passive resistance can undermine the change.
- High motivational levels are necessary to make the change successful.
- People can refuse to obey the order without negative consequences.

Sharing Information Much resistance is simply the result of misunderstandings about a proposed change. Sharing information is usually an effective way to reduce uncertainty and ease the transition. Information about the change can be shared on a one-to-one basis, in group meetings, or through written materials distributed by print or electronic means. For you, as a student, it is important that any changes in the program are communicated to you without delay. You should also communicate any changes in your plans to the appropriate people (e.g., other students, nurse team leader, instructor). You should treat client resistance to change in the same manner. The more information that you give the client, the more likely it is that they will cooperate with the change.

Refuting Currently Held Beliefs You can sometimes increase a person's willingness to change by simply providing evidence that their actions or beliefs are inadequate, incorrect, or inefficient. For example, a patient may enter the hospital recalling horror stories from friends and family but may then find that there was no basis for the stories. Consider the fact that your ideas about the nursing program have changed since you first began. What happened, or what information did you receive, that caused you to change your beliefs?

Providing Psychological Safety When a proposed change threatens basic human needs in some way, reducing that threat can lower resistance. This leaves people feeling more comfortable about the change. Although each situation poses different kinds of threats and requires different actions to reduce them, Box 40-4 identifies common strategies that help increase psychological safety and reduce resistance to change.

Implementing the Change

In planning for change, you should have a clear understanding of the reason for and purpose of the change. Once you have determined that the change is necessary, your focus should move to a smooth implementation.

After employing some unfreezing strategies (e.g., making the status quo unfavorable), you are ready to make the change that has been planned so carefully. In addition to employing strategies to lower resistance, increase motivation, and help people work well together, consider the following factors related to the change:

- **Magnitude of the change.** Is this a major change that affects almost everything people do, or is it a minor one with little impact on what people do every day?

BOX 40-4 ■ Common Strategies to Increase Psychological Safety and Reduce Resistance to Change

- Point out similarities between old and new procedures.
- Suggest ways in which the change can provide new opportunities and challenges.
- Allow time for learning and practice of any new procedures, if possible, before a change is implemented.
- Recognize the competence and skill of the people involved.
- Involve as many people as possible in both the design and implementation of the change.
- Express approval of people's concern for providing the best care possible.
- Express the value of each individual's and group's contributions in general and to the proposed change.
- Provide a climate of trust and acceptance in which mistakes can be made without negative consequences for individuals.
- If possible, provide assurance that no one will lose their position because of the change.
- Provide opportunities for people to express their feelings and ask questions about the proposed change.

- **Complexity of the change.** Is this a difficult change to make? Does it require much new knowledge, many new skills, or both? How long will it take for people to acquire the necessary knowledge and skills?
- **Pace of the change.** How urgent is this change? Can it be done gradually, or must it be implemented all at once?
- **Stress level of those involved.** What is the current stress level of the people involved in this change? Is this the only change that is taking place, or is it just one of many changes taking place? How stressful are these changes? How can I help people keep their stress levels within tolerable bounds?

As indicated earlier, some discomfort is likely to occur with almost any change, but it is important to keep it within tolerable limits. You will need to minimize resistance by engaging, training, coaching, and empowering those involved in the change (Barrow et al., 2022; Wojciechowski et al., 2016).

Integrating the Change

Integrating the change is the last step. After the change has been made, it is important to make sure that everyone has moved into a new comfort zone. The change should be well integrated into everyday operations, perceived as valuable, and identified as the new norm. Identify the champions for the change because individual behavior is influenced by group pressures (Batras et al. 2016).

Change is an inevitable part of living and working. Your leadership can influence how people respond to change, the amount of stress it causes, and the amount of resistance it provokes. Handled well, most changes can become opportunities for professional growth and development rather than just additional stressors for students, nurses, and their clients.

CONFLICT

Nursing education and healthcare settings bring together people of different ages, genders, income levels, statuses, ethnic groups, educational levels, lifestyles, and professions. They share the goal of maintaining the health of their patients. Differences of opinion over how to best accomplish goals are a normal part of working with people of various skill levels, backgrounds, and cultures. Individuals bring different experiences, beliefs, values, habits, coping skills, and perceptions to their interactions with others. These differences may or may not lead to positive reactions in given situations. Various pressures and demands in the classroom, clinical setting, and workplace can create conflicts and interfere with the team's ability to work together.

Conflicts Occur at All Levels

Conflicts can occur at any level and involve any number of people, including your boss, subordinates, peers, patients, or patient families.

- **On the *individual level,*** conflict can occur between two people working together on a classroom or clinical project, between two people in different departments, or even between a staff member and a patient or their family member.
- **On the *group level,*** conflict can occur between two or more teams, departments, or professional groups (e.g., nurses and providers may conflict over a patient's readiness for discharge).
- **On the *organizational level,*** conflicts can occur between two or more hospitals, health agencies, or community organizations.

"Win–Win" Resolutions

Some people think about problems and conflicts in the same way as they think about a football game or tennis match: someone has to win, and someone has to lose. There are problems with this thought process:

- In healthcare, our aim should be to work together more effectively, not to defeat the other party.
- The people who lose are likely to feel bad about losing and may harbor negative feelings that negate teamwork and collaboration.

- When no one wins (a tie), no gain is achieved, and the problem remains unresolved.

So the answer to the question, "Win, lose, or draw?" is "None of the above." Instead, a win–win result, in which both sides gain some benefit, is the best resolution.

Conflict Resolution

When differences and disagreements first arise, problem-solving may be sufficient. If the situation has already developed into a full-blown conflict, however, formal or informal negotiation of a settlement may be necessary. When using a problem-solving process, the goal is to find a solution that satisfies everyone involved.

Step 1: *Identify the source of the conflict.* Engage in conversations to understand the perspectives of the parties involved in the conflict. Sometimes, if the issue is not a highly charged or highly political one, it is easy to identify the real issue or problem. At other times, deeper discussions are necessary before the real problem emerges.

It would be easier if what people were really saying or asking for was always obvious; however, some people are often vague about their real concerns and do not clearly identify their feelings. Often, negative emotions

Toward Evidence-Based Practice

Duffy, J., Culp, S., & Padrutt, T. (2018). Description and factors associated with missed nursing care in an acute care community hospital. *Journal of Nursing Administration, 48*(7/8), 361–367. https://doi.org/10.1097/NNA.0000000000000630

Some level of "missed nursing care" was reported by 138 nurses. The top-three reasons were unavailability of scheduled medications (51%), inadequate personnel (e.g., assistive, clerical) (50%), and working short-staffed (48.6%). Frequently missed care included prescribed ambulation (47%), presence at interprofessional care conferences (40%), providing mouth care (31%), assessing medication effectiveness (32%), and monitoring intake/output (30%). Missed nursing care existed on all units but was higher on medical–surgical units.

Park, S., Hanchett, M., & Ma, C. (2018). Practice environment characteristics associated with missed nursing care. *Journal of Nursing Scholarship, 50*(6), 722–730.

A sample of 31,650 registered nurse surveys from 1,583 units in 371 hospitals revealed that 84% of nurses on medical–surgical units missed at least one of the 16 essential nursing skills. The most frequently missed care activity was comforting and talking with patients (62%), followed by ambulation or range of motion (40%), teaching/counseling patients and families (40%), and administering medications on time (34%). Additionally, developing or updating the patient's plan of care was missed 26% of the

time. Adequate staff and positive provider–nurse relationships were associated with fewer missed care activities, whereas nurses highly involved with hospital affairs were twice as likely to miss care activities.

Gustafsson, N., Leino-Kilpi, H., Prga, I., Suhonen, R., & Stolt, M. (2020). Missed care from the patient's perspective—a scoping review. *Patient Preference and Adherence, 14,* 383–400. https://doi.org/10.2147/PPA.S238024

Patients identified the top-three areas of "missed nursing care" as basic care (e.g., mouthcare, ambulation, bathing), communication issues (providing necessary information, discussing the treatment plan of care, listening to their concerns), and lack of timeliness (e.g., help to bathroom, responding to call bells and monitor alarms). Patients with poorer health status and mental health problems reported more missed care. In addition, missed care was associated with lower patient satisfaction ratings. A positive association was found between patient reports of missed nursing care and self-reported complications of skin breakdown, medication errors, new infections, and IV concerns.

1. How could missed nursing care affect patient outcomes?

2. Based on the research findings, what two factors should nurse leaders/managers address to promote quality patient care?

♥ iCare 40-1

Leading and Managing

Every nurse possesses a degree of leadership and can influence other people. You are all change agents in the variety of different healthcare arenas that exist today and must recognize and embrace your sources of power and use them in a positive manner.

Ask, "What can I contribute?" and "What am I comfortable doing at this point in my career?"

- Can I speak up for safety?
- Can I attend a safety huddle?
- Can I report not only actual errors but near misses, too?
- Do I feel comfortable calling a fellow nurse or doctor out on poor hygiene practice?

- Will I start attending my own departmental meetings?
- Can I join a committee of interest? Falls Committee? Safety Committee? Staffing and Scheduling? Patient Satisfaction?

The answer to all of the listed questions is YES, YOU CAN!

- Empowerment, delegation, prioritization, managing change, effective time management, and conflict resolution are all skills that you are responsible for.
- Remember, not all leaders can be managers, and not all managers can be leaders.
- You should find mentors, ask questions, explore strengths and weaknesses, embrace new opportunities, reflect often on performance, and remember to always support others.

---

or perceptions are the underlying source of the conflict. All of this must be sorted out so that the problem is clearly identified and a solution can be sought.

Step 2: *Generate possible solutions.* Here, creativity is especially important. As a leader, begin the process of trying to help the parties to identify new and creative solutions to resolve the conflict. To overcome their natural resistance, help them to understand the negative impact of stress and conflict on their well-being and the work environment. Encourage them to spend some time searching for innovative and collaborative solutions. Think outside the box for new and better ways to handle things.

Step 3: *Evaluate suggested solutions.* An open-minded, objective evaluation of each suggestion is needed, but you may find that this is not always easy to accomplish. When a group engages in problem-solving, it is sometimes difficult to separate the suggestion from its source. For example, in a team situation, a person's status may influence whether their suggestion is judged to be useful. Judge the suggestion on its merits, not its source.

Step 4: *Choose the best solution(s).* Select the solution(s) that will most likely provide the best results with the most positive outcomes. Combine suggestions to incorporate others' input, when feasible.

Step 5: *Implement the chosen solution(s).* Observe for positive changes in collaboration, cooperation, and communication among the parties involved. Be ready to promptly intervene to resolve undesired behaviors and to provide guidance as needed. It is important to give it time to work.

Step 6: *Evaluate—Is the conflict resolved?* Not every conflict is resolved successfully on the first attempt. Analyze the aspects of the situation that were successful. Resume the conflict resolution process with even greater attention to the source of the conflict and how it can be successfully resolved.

Informal Negotiation

If problem-solving does not resolve the conflict, you may have to move on to the next step—informal negotiation. The following steps may prove useful:

1. **Clarify the situation in your own mind.** Have a clear goal of what you are trying to achieve and what each party wants. Identify environmental factors that can influence the outcomes, and anticipate problems you may encounter.
2. **Set the stage.** This may involve confronting the two parties or groups with their behavior toward one another, making direct statements designed to open communication, and challenging them to seek a resolution of the situation.
3. **Conduct the negotiation.** You should set the ground rules, especially when dealing with emotionally charged individuals. Then, clarify and ask for validation of the problem being addressed. You should then begin the negotiations and promptly address outbursts by repeating the ground rules.
4. **Continue with offers and counteroffers.**
5. **Agree on the resolution of the conflict.**

Conflict is inevitable within any large or diverse group of people who are trying to work together over an extended period of time. However, it does not have to be destructive, and it does not even have to be a negative experience if everyone handles it skillfully. In fact, conflict can stimulate people to learn more about one another and how to work together in more effective ways. Resolution of a conflict, when it is done well, can lead to improved relationships, foster more creative methods of problem-solving, and improve productivity.

TIME MANAGEMENT

Many of the personal management and workplace organizational skills focus on time management and scheduling. Although new nurses may have the required job skills, many lack personal management skills, specifically, time-management skills. You might be able to handle conflict and change, delegate appropriately, and have strong leadership skills. But if you cannot organize and manage your time, you will never gain your full potential.

Many nurses use a system that records their work hours. Management accepts very few excuses for tardiness. Timesheets and schedules are part of nurses' lives. We are expected to follow set schedules precisely and meet deadlines for virtually everything we do, from distributing medications to documenting on time. Some agencies may analyze computer-generated data to determine the amount of time spent on various activities. Consider how you can use the following suggestions to improve your time management.

Setting Your Own Goals

It is difficult to decide how to spend your time because there are so many things that need time. A good first step is to get an overview of the situation. Then ask yourself, "What are my goals?" Goals help clarify what you want and give you energy, direction, and focus. Once you know where you want to go, set priorities. This is not an easy task. In Lewis Carroll's (1865/2010) *Alice's Adventures in Wonderland*, the child heroine, Alice, becomes lost and asks for help from a fantasy creature, the Cheshire Cat. They have this conversation:

> "Would you tell me please, which way I ought to go from here?" asked Alice.
> "That depends a good deal on where you want to go to," said the Cat.
> "I don't care where," said Alice.
> "Then it doesn't matter which way you go," said the Cat.

How can you get somewhere if you do not know where you want to go? It is important to explore your personal and career goals. This can help you make decisions about the future. You can apply these ideas to daily activities as well as to career decisions. Spend some time thinking about what you want to accomplish over a particular period.

To help organize your time, you need to set both short- and long-term goals. Every choice you make requires a different allocation of time.

- **Short-term goals** are goals that you wish to accomplish within the near future (e.g., organizing your day to participate in a study group).
- **Long-term goals** are goals you wish to complete in the future (e.g., obtain a PhD in nursing). A good question to ask yourself is, "What do I see myself doing 5 years from now?"

Organizing Your Work

Many healthcare professionals are linear, fast-tempo, achievement-oriented people. However, working at a rapid pace is not necessarily the same as being efficient or effective. You can spend much energy rushing around while achieving very little.

To "manage" time, you need a measure of skill to meet client care needs efficiently during a nursing shift. Organizing your work can eliminate extra steps or serious delays in finishing. It can also reduce the amount of time you spend doing things that are neither productive nor satisfying. As you advance in your nursing program, you will progress to caring for up to five to six patients. You will need to develop time-management and organizational skills. The failure to develop time-management skills and organize your care can result in **"missed nursing care."**

The following are some suggestions.

Organized Approach to Care Use a tool to organize and strengthen your assessment during patient encounters. This will prevent repeated trips because you forgot to assess an essential area. The BOSS Tool (Table 40-4) is an example of an evidence-based tool that facilitates effective time-management and organizational skills for new nurse graduates transitioning into practice. The tool provides a quick resource to reference as a reminder of what needs to be assessed and completed each time you enter a patient's room. The checklist will facilitate the development of critical thinking and clinical judgment.

Time Inventory To begin managing your time, you need to develop a clearer understanding of how you use your time. A personal time inventory helps you estimate how much time you spend in typical activities and helps identify "time wasters." Set up a time log and enter your activities every half hour for an entire week. You may be surprised to see the pattern that emerges when you review these data. Data revealed that nurses spent less than one-third of their time with patients (Michel et al., 2021). In another study, sensors used to track the location of various healthcare providers showed that nurses spent about 33% of their time in patient rooms, 11% just outside patient rooms, 11% to 13% at the nurses' station, and 24% elsewhere in the unit (Butler et al., 2018).

Energy Use Start your most difficult tasks when you have the most energy. This decreases frustration later in the day, when you may be more tired and less efficient. For example, if you are a "morning person," plan your demanding work in the morning. If you get energy spurts later in the morning or early afternoon, plan to work on larger or heavier tasks at that time. However, many nursing tasks are based on a schedule, and this choice is not always within your control. Analyze your work to determine which tasks you can manipulate to match your energy.

Lists and Schedules Make a "to-do" list and prioritize the tasks in order of importance, especially medication administration and treatments. Determine when each task must be completed and how much time it will require. If you find yourself postponing an item for several days, either give it top priority the next day or drop it from the list altogether.

The Effect of Authority Gradients on Teamwork and Client Safety

Chapter Key Concept: Management, Leadership, Followership

Competencies: Collaborate with the interprofessional healthcare team; provide safe, quality client care

Teamwork and collaboration are influenced by the psychological distance team members feel between themselves and others higher up in the team structure. This is called the *authority gradient.* The greater the authority gradient, the less likely a person is to feel like part of a team, question those in authority, or communicate concerns. Research shows that a high authority gradient will impede essential communication that will protect clients from harm. Minimizing the authority gradient has been shown to improve communication, which reduces errors and promotes better client outcomes.

The authority gradient between providers and nurses is very steep and is reinforced by tradition, individual personalities, providers' attitudes, and at times, nurses' fears of being incorrect. Observe the differences in the authority gradients between experienced nurses and other members of the healthcare team in highly collaborative practice areas (e.g., emergency departments, intensive care units) and new nurses or student nurses.

Team Briefings: To flatten these gradients, team briefings should be an expected routine. Briefings promote clear, effective communication and include introductions all around, a review of the client's problems and the treatment plan, and specific requests by providers for input. Briefings create a shared understanding and foster an environment in which team members can and do speak up about any concerns.

Individual Skills: Individually, you can develop your communication skills, adopt an attitude of collaboration, and learn more about how to become a capable team member. To begin this process, consider the following questions and suggested responses:

➤ What are your strengths and weaknesses as a team member? How can you better function as an essential member of the healthcare team?

➤ How can you gain the confidence to question a provider's prescription or assert your perspective on a client's treatment plan? What do you consider assertive communication?

➤ Are you succinct when you communicate? What structured communication style can you adopt to keep your comments and requests clear?

Sources: Friedman, Z., Hayter, M. A., Everett, T. C., Matava, C. T., Noble, L. M. K., & Bould, M. D. (2015). Power and conflict: The effect of a superior's interpersonal behavior on trainees' ability to challenge authority during a simulated airway emergency. *Anaesthesia, 70*(10), 1119–1129; Hubbard, H., & Chicca, J. (2022). Navigating authority gradients. *American Nurse.* https://www.myamericannurse.com/navigating-authority-gradients/; Sekar, H., Dharmasena, D., Gunasekara, A., Nauta, M., Sivashanmugarajan, V., & Yoong, W. (2022). Understanding authority gradient: Tips for speaking up for patient safety. *Obstetrician & Gynecologist, 24,* 272–280. https://doi.org/10.1111/tog.12829; Shanks, L., Zelko, M., Chiu, S-H., Fleming, E., & Germano, S. (2017). Effect of a preceptor intervention on student self-confidence in patient safety. *Nursing and Advanced Health Care.* http://www.scientificoajournals.org/pdf/nahc.1001.pdf

Table 40-4 ➤ The BOSS Tool: Organizational Clinical Checklist

DO AND ASSESS WITH PATIENT ENCOUNTER	YES	NO
Introduce yourself to the patient.		
Does the patient appear to be in distress?	**REQUIRES IMMEDIATE ACTION**	**CONTINUE WITH CHECKLIST**
Conduct a visual of the patient's room.		
Is the patient in bed? Bedside chair?		
Is the bed low and locked? Chair locked?		
Are the bed rails appropriately positioned?		
Is the call bell within the patient's reach?		
Is the patient positioned properly according to schedule?		
Is the bed made properly with clean linens?		
Is the room clean and uncluttered? Bathroom?		
Is the room temperature comfortable?		
Is sunlight in the patient's face? Blinds open or closed?		
Does the patient have cups, straws, water pitcher?		

Table 40-4 ➤ The BOSS Tool: Organizational Clinical Checklist

DO AND ASSESS WITH PATIENT ENCOUNTER	YES	NO
Equipment:		
a. IV fluids: what kind, what rate, remaining amount of solution, correct height		
b. Any drips: insulin, heparin, etc.		
c. How many pumps? Any piggybacks hanging? If so, are they capped? Appropriate tubing?		
Other Equipment:		
a. Suction: Is it on, what setting, color of drainage, etc.?		
b. Oxygen: Is it properly positioned in patient's nostrils? Rate, type of oxygen equipment (e.g., nasal cannula, mask, etc.)		
c. Foley: What color is the urine, amount of urine, location of tubing?		
Falls and Door Signs:		
a. Appropriate sign for fall precautions?		
b. NPO: Is there a sign on the door? Is the water pitcher empty and out of reach?		
c. Fluid restriction: Appropriate signage on the door or in the room?		
d. Weights: Is there a sign on the door?		
e. Any other signs needed?		
TAKE VITAL SIGNS		
Head-to-toe assessment		
Now you are ready to begin the head-to-toe assessment.		

This checklist may be modified based on your facility's requirements.
Modified and used with permission of Kathy Locklear, DNP, MSN, RN; Lumberton, NC.

Daily Worksheet To help organize your day, provide yourself with reminders of when various tasks need to be done. Use a schedule as an organizational tool to avoid drifting through a day or shift from one activity to another in a disorganized fashion. Although the day is divided into discrete segments, continue to practice a holistic approach.

Say "No" You need to carefully consider the activities you take on. Learn to say, "I would really like to help you; can it wait until I finish this?" Or, "I am sorry, but I won't be able to help you with that."

Delegate See previous discussions about delegation.

Do Not Multitask Studies show that people who do many things at once are not likely to do any of them well. Finish one task, then move on to the next one.

Streamline Your Work Many tasks cannot be eliminated or delegated, but they can be done more efficiently. When you have multiple demands on your time, consider how to "Work smarter, not harder" (Box 40-5).

BOX 40-5 ■ Work Smarter, Not Harder

- Plan ahead by taking a few minutes at the beginning of your shift to organize your patient supplies for the day or whatever you need to do to avoid retracing your steps. Gather materials, such as bed linens, for all your clients at one time. As you go to each room, leave the linens so that they will be there when you need them.

- While giving a bed bath or providing other personal care, perform some of the aspects of the physical assessment, such as taking vital signs, the skin assessment, and parts of the neurological and musculoskeletal assessment.

- If a client does not "look right," do not ignore your instincts. The client is probably having a problem.

- Prevention is always a good idea. If you are not sure about a treatment or medication, ask before you proceed. It is usually less time consuming to prevent a problem than it is to resolve one.

- When you set aside time to do a specific task that has a high priority, stick to your schedule and complete it.

- Do not allow interruptions while you are completing any tasks (e.g., paperwork, medication administration). Focus on the task at hand.

Work–Life Balance

Time can be your best friend or your worst enemy. Nursing requires that you perform numerous activities within what often seems a short period of time, and you will often feel exhausted when you leave work. Remember that you should set aside 8 hours for sleep and a few more for personal or leisure time ("time off"). Stay active—go for walks or to the gym, or engage in other physical activities. Do fun things with your family or other support persons. Use Table 40-5 to help you to review the necessary components of time management.

KnowledgeCheck 40-6

- List the steps of conflict resolution.
- List several suggestions for organizing your work.
- How can the BOSS Tool help you organize and strengthen your assessment during patient encounters?

Table 40-5 ➤ Components of Time Management	
ACTION	**EXAMPLES**
Prioritize	List tasks in order of importance.
	Remember that some tasks must be done at specific times, whereas others can be done at any time.
	Emergencies take precedence.
	Identify events you control and events others control.
	Use critical-thinking skills to assign priorities.
Question	
■ Effectiveness	■ Did the task produce the desired outcome?
■ Efficiency	■ How can I accomplish the plan with the least expenditure of time? Is there a way to break this down into simpler tasks?
■ Efficacy	■ Do I have the skill and ability to obtain the desired effect?
Recheck	Mentally and physically recheck an unfinished or delegated task.
Practice self-reliance	Identify tasks that are within your control and those that are not.
	Use critical-thinking skills and adaptability to revise priorities.
	"Go with the flow."
Treat	Treat yourself to a break when you can.
	Treat yourself to time off.
	Treat yourself to an educational experience; commit yourself to excellence.
	Treat others with courtesy and respect.

PUTTING IT ALL TOGETHER

You are just beginning your journey toward becoming a nurse. Undoubtedly you will want to function well within your organization and deliver high-quality client care. Begin now to examine and work on your own strengths and weaknesses. Focus on developing the traits of a good leader. You will soon recognize that conflict and change are a normal part of life and your clinical practice, so learn to become proactive as issues arise. Observe how licensed nurses delegate and manage their time. Learn from their examples and adopt useful practices. Watch for opportunities to be mentored and make time to mentor others. **Key Point:** *Above all, remember that you may be the most important person in the life of your patient during the time you are with them—a very big responsibility, but one you will meet with honor and courage.*

To explore learning resources for this chapter,

Go to Davis Advantage and find:

Answers and Suggested Responses for all questions in this chapter

Concept Map

Knowledge Map

References and Bibliography

Credits

Note: Unless cited here, text credits appear within the text.

CHAPTER 1

Meet Your Patient 1-1: The National Library of Medicine.
Meet Your Patient 1-2: Everyday Faces, BananaStock.
Figure 1-1: The National Library of Medicine.
Figure 1-2: © Stephen Mahar, www.photos.com.
Figure 1-3: © Cynthia Farmer, www.photos.com.
Figure 1-4: © DNY59/iStock/Getty Images.
Figure 1-5: © DNY59/iStock/Getty Images.
Figure 1-6: © Penn State Nursing Magazine.

CHAPTER 2

Meet Your Patient: © iStock/Getty Images.
Figure 2-1: Courtesy NCSBN.

CHAPTER 3

Meet Your Patient: Photo © BananaStock.
Figure 3-1: Courtesy of Smith Northview Hospital, Valdosta, GA.
Figure 3-2: Courtesy of Shore Memorial Hospital, Somers Point, NJ.
Figure 3-6: Courtesy Genesis Medical Center, Davenport, IA.
Figure 3-7: Courtesy Hospital of the University of Pennsylvania.
Figure 3-8: Courtesy of Ergo Partners, L.C., Boulder, CO.

CHAPTER 4

Meet Your Patient: Photo © BananaStock.
Figure 4-6: Adapted from Maslow, A. (1971). *The farther reaches of human nature.* Viking Press; and Maslow A., & Lowery, R. (Eds.). (1998). *Toward a psychology of being* (3rd ed.). Wiley & Sons.

CHAPTER 5

Figures 5-1 and 5-2: © iStock/Getty Images.

CHAPTER 6

Meet Your Patient: © Getty Images.
Figure 6-5: © Getty Images.
Figure 6-6: © Robert Dant/iStock/Getty Images.
Figure 6-7: © iStock/Getty Images.
Figure 6-8: © Photodisc Red/Getty Images, Scott T. Baxter.
Figure 6-9: © Everyday Faces, Photodisc.
Figure 6-10: © iStock/Getty Images.

CHAPTER 7

Meet Your Patient: © Silvia Jansen/iStock/Getty Images.
Figure 7-1: Source: Vincent, G., & Victoria, A. (2010). *The next four decades, the older population in the United States: 2010 to 2050, current population reports* (pp. 25–1138). U.S. Census Bureau. http://www.census.gov/prod/2010pubs/p25-1138.pdf.
Figure 7-2: © Photodisc, Getty Images.
Figure 7-3: Courtesy of V. Rempusheski, PhD.

CHAPTER 8

Meet Your Patient: © Silvia Jansen/iStock/Getty Images.
Figure 8-2: Adapted from Dunn, H. L. (1959). High level wellness for man and society. *American Journal of Public Health, 49,* 786–788.
Figures 8-3A and B: Adapted from Neuman, B. (1995). The Neuman systems model. In B. Neuman, *The Neuman systems model* (3rd ed., pp. 3–61). Appleton and Lange.
Figure 8-4: From: U.S. Department of Health and Human Services, Office of Disease Prevention and Health Promotion. (n.d.). *Healthy People*

2030. *Social determinants of health.* https://health.gov/healthypeople/objectives-and-data/social-determinants-health.

Figure 8-4: © PhotoDisc, Senior Lifestyles.

CHAPTER 9

Meet Your Patient: © Family Health, BananaStock.

CHAPTER 11

Meet Your Patient: © iStock/Getty Images.
Figure 11-3: © Punchstock, Photodisc.
Figure 11-4: © Kali9/iStock/Getty Images.
Figure 11-5: © iStock/Getty Images.

CHAPTER 12

Meet Your Patient: © iStockphoto.com.

CHAPTER 13

Meet Your Patient: © Photodisc, Senior Lifestyles.
Figure 13-1: © Fotosearch.com.
Figure 13-2: © Corbis Images.
Figure 13-3: Courtesy of Barbara Proud.
Figure 13-5: Used with permission of Jonas Ngirinshuti.

CHAPTER 14

Figure 14-1: © iStock/Getty Images.
Figure 14-3: Fotosearch.com.

CHAPTER 16

Figure 16-4: iStockphotos.
Figure 16-5: From Goodheart Wilcox Publisher, weareteachers.com.

CHAPTER 17

Meet Your Patient: © Photodisc/Getty.
Figures 17-2, 17-3, 17-5, 17-7, and 17-8: Courtesy of Cerner Corporation, Kansas City, MO.
Figure 17-4: © Getty Images.

CHAPTER 18

Meet Your Patient: Photo © BananaStock.
Home Care: Courtesy of Omron Healthcare, Inc.

CHAPTER 20

Meet Your Patient: © Maliketh/iStock/Getty Images.
Box 20-1: Photos © photos.com.

CHAPTER 21

Meet Your Patient: © Jay Fries/Digital Vision/Getty Images.
Figure 21-2: © iStock/Getty Images.

CHAPTER 22

Meet Your Patient: © Getty Images.

CHAPTER 23

Figure 23-17: Courtesy of Hospira, Lake Forest, IL.
Figure 23-19: Courtesy of Medi-Dose® Inc., EPS® Inc.
Figure 23-29: Used by permission of the National Extravasation Information Service (UK), http://www.extravasation.org.uk.
Figure 23-31: Courtesy of PFM Medical Ag.
Figure 23-34: Courtesy of Dr. Donna Clarren and Dr. Brian Oxhorn, Roseman College of Nursing.

CHAPTER 24

Meet Your Patient: iStockphotos.
Figure 24-1: U.S. Department of Agriculture, ChooseMyPlate.gov.
Figure 24-2: U.S. Department of Agriculture (2007).
Figure 24-3: Text by Reed Mangels, PhD, RD. Design by Lindsey Siferd. The Vegan Resource Group, P.O. Box 1463, Baltimore, MD 21203; www.vrg.org.
Figures 24-5 A and B and 24-7: Courtesy of Covidien.

CHAPTER 26

Meet Your Patient: © thelinke/iStock/Getty Images.
Figure 26-8: Courtesy of ConvaTec Inc., Skillman, NJ.
Figure 26-9: Courtesy of Hollister Incorporated, Libertyville, IL.

CHAPTER 27

Meet Your Patient: © Istockphoto.com.

CHAPTER 28

Meet Your Patient: © Jason Doiy/iStock/Getty Images.

CHAPTER 29

Meet Your Patient: © Christopher Futcher/iStock/Getty Images.
Figure 29-10: Courtesy of RCAI, Inc., St. Petersburg, FL.
Figures 29-15, 29-18, and 29-19: Courtesy of EZ Way, Inc., Clarinda, IA.

CHAPTER 30

Meet Your Patients: © iStock/Getty Images, © Steve-Luker/iStock/Getty Images, and © iStock/Getty Images.
Figure 30-5: © iStock/Getty Images.
Figure 30-8: © iofoto/iStock/Getty Images.

CHAPTER 31

Meet Your Patient: © Diane Diederich/iStock/Getty Images.
Figure 31-5: From Hall, J. E. (2011). *Guyton and Hall textbook of medical physiology* (12th ed.). Saunders.

CHAPTER 32

Meet Your Patient: © PhotoDisc, Everyday Faces.
Figure 32-11: Adapted from Agency for Healthcare and Research Quality (AHRQ) Clinical Practice Guidelines.
Table Figure 32-2, 32-4. 32-6, 32-8 through 32-10: With Permission from National Pressure Advisory Panel (2011). Gordian Medical Inc., dba American Medical Technologies.

CHAPTER 33

Meet Your Patient: © BananaStock.

CHAPTER 34

Meet Your Patient: © iStock/Getty Images.

CHAPTER 35

Meet Your Patient: © Getty Images, Photodisc.

CHAPTER 36

Meet Your Patient: © Vikram Raghuvanshi/iStock/Getty Images.
Figure 39-5: Courtesy of I-Flow Corporation, Lake Forest, CA.

CHAPTER 37

Meet Your Patient: © Photo Euphoria/iStock/Getty Images.
Figure 37-2: *Healthy People 2030*.
Figure 37-3: AdobeStock.
Figure 37-9 and 37-10: Istockphoto.com.

CHAPTER 38

Meet Your Nursing Role Model: © istockphoto.com.
Figure 38-1: Adapted from Englebardt, S., & Nelson, R. *Health care informatics: An interdisciplinary approach.* Copyright 2002. With permission from Elsevier.
Figure 38-2 and 38-3: © iStock/Getty Images.
Figure 38-4: iStockphoto.

CHAPTER 39

Meet Your Patient: © ntmw/iStock/Getty Images.

CHAPTER 40

Figure 40-1: © iStock/Getty Images.

INDEX

References are to volume and page number(s). Page numbers followed by *f* refer to figures; page numbers followed by *t* refer to tables; page numbers followed by *b* refer to boxes; page numbers followed by *p* refer to procedures

A

AACN. *See* American Association of Colleges of Nursing (AACN)
AB blood group, (V1) 1068, (V1) 1068*t*
Abbreviations
  commonly used in healthcare, (V2) 163–165, (V2) 426
  medication-related, (V2) 459
Abdomen
  assessment of, (V2) 257–263*p*
  auscultation of, (V1) 503
  four quadrants of, (V1) 502, (V1) 503*f*
  inspection of, (V1) 503
  palpation of, (V1) 503
  percussion of, (V1) 503
  physical examination of, (V1) 502–503, (V1) 503*f*, (V1) 510, (V1) 512*p*
  variations in shape of, (V1) 503*f*
Abdominal binders, (V1) 972
Abdominal circumference, (V1) 696
Abdominal distention, as postoperative complication, (V1) 1100*t*
Abdominal flat plate, (V2) 587
ABG. *See* Arterial blood gases (ABG)
Ablative surgery, (V1) 1078
A blood group, (V1) 1068, (V1) 1068*t*
Abnormal sensitivity to drugs, (V1) 621
ABO blood type, (V1) 1068
Abrasion, (V1) 582, (V1) 945*t*
Abscess, (V1) 945*t*
Absent or weak pulse, (V1) 461
Absorbent sutures, (V1) 948
Absorption, drug, (V1) 611
Abstinence, (V1) 896, (V2) 642
Abuse and neglect
  assessing for, (V1) 161*p*, (V2) 43–47*p*
    after the examination, (V2) 45*p*
    focused health history in, (V2) 43*p*
    focused physical assessment in, (V2) 44–45*p*
    for psychological abuse, (V2) 44*p*
    for sexual abuse, (V2) 43*p*
  of children (*See* Child abuse and neglect)
  communicable diseases and, (V1) 1178
  flow chart of possible, (V2) 42
  of older adults, (V1) 198, (V1) 199–200
  vulnerable populations and, (V1) 1113
Accelerated BSN programs, (V1) 11
Acceptable macronutrient distribution range (AMDR), (V1) 667
Accessory muscles and inspiration, (V1) 994
Access to care, (V1) 310, (V1) 479
Accidents. *See* Safety
Accommodation, (V1) 147, (V1) 327
Accountability, (V1) 553
  legal (*See* Law and legal liability)
Accreditation, (V1) 1165
Acculturation, (V1) 313
Accumulation of drugs in tissues, (V1) 621
Acetaminophen, (V1) 828, (V1) 834
Achondroplasia, (V1) 857

Acid-base balance, (V1) 671, (V1) 1045, (V1) 1049
  acidosis and alkalosis and, (V1) 1047, (V1) 1050*t*
  assessment of, (V1) 1052–1053, (V2) 803–804
  critical thinking and clinical judgment on, (V2) 806–807
  diagnostic testing of, (V2) 805
  full-spectrum nursing model applied to, (V2) 805–806
  knowledge map on, (V2) 809
  management of, (V1) 1054
Acidosis, (V1) 1047, (V1) 1050*t*, (V1) 1052
Acne, (V1) 582
  newborn, (V1) 941
Acromegaly, (V1) 491
Actigraph, (V1) 932
Active B cells, (V1) 524
Active euthanasia, (V1) 361
Active involvement in patient learning, (V1) 400
Active listening, (V1) 343, (V1) 387–388, (V1) 388*f*, (V1) 1191
Active prewarming, (V1) 1086
Active range of motion (AROM), (V1) 845
  exercises for, (V1) 875–876
Active release therapy (ART), (V1) 824
Active resistance, (V1) 1193
Active T cells, (V1) 524
Active transport, (V1) 1039–1040, (V1) 1040*f*
Activities of daily living (ADLs), (V1) 198, (V1) 576, (V1) 578
  ambulation exercises and, (V1) 876, (V1) 877*f*
  assessment of, (V1) 200
    Katz Index of ADL scale, (V2) 17, (V2) 384–385
    special needs, (V2) 18
  pain and, (V1) 821
Activity theory, (V1) 191
Activity tolerance, (V1) 865, (V1) 866
Actual loss, (V1) 348
Acupressure, (V1) 824
Acupuncture, (V1) 261, (V1) 824
  for acute postoperative pain, (V1) 1102
  for neuropathic pain, (V1) 917
Acute bronchitis, (V1) 985
Acute care, (V1) 16
Acute illness, (V1) 219
Acute infections, (V1) 519
Acute pain, (V1) 812, (V1) 817, (V1) 821
Acute wounds, (V1) 944
Adaptation, (V1) 147
  See also Stress
  assessment of, (V1) 254
    guidelines and tools for, (V2) 82–84
  burnout and, (V1) 253–254, (V1) 254*b*
  to change as hardiness, (V1) 220
  crisis and, (V1) 252–253, (V1) 253*f*
  crisis intervention, (V1) 263, (V2) 81
  critical thinking and clinical judgment on, (V2) 85–86

defined, (V1) 239
full-spectrum nursing model applied to, (V2) 84–85
general adaptation syndrome (GAS), (V1) 242–245, (V1) 243–244*f*
health promotion activities for, (V1) 258–259
knowledge map on, (V2) 88
local adaptation syndrome, (V1) 245–246, (V1) 245*b*
as outcome of stress, (V1) 241, (V1) 241*f*
personal factors influencing, (V1) 241–242
planning for, (V1) 257–258
problems related to failure of, (V1) 251–254, (V1) 252*t*, (V1) 253*f*, (V1) 254*b*
relation to stress, (V1) 240–242, (V1) 241*f*
sleep and, (V1) 917
somatoform disorders and, (V1) 251
to stimuli, (V1) 784, (V1) 786
stress-induced chronic responses and, (V1) 251
stress-induced psychological responses and, (V1) 251–253
Adapted physical activity (APA), (V1) 191
Adaptive coping, (V1) 240
A-delta fibers, (V1) 813, (V1) 814–815, (V1) 815*f*
Adenosine, (V1) 923
Adenosine trisphosphate (ATP), (V1) 1040
Adequate intake (AI), (V1) 667
Adhesive strips, (V1) 948
Adhesive tape, (V1) 971
Adjuvant analgesics, (V1) 828
Administration set, IV infusion, (V1) 1061–1062, (V1) 1062*f*
  changing, (V1) 1067
Administrative law, (V1) 1156, (V1) 1157*t*
Admission, (V1) 236*p*
  critical thinking and clinical judgment on, (V2) 76–77
  data form, (V1) 430–431, (V2) 166
  full-spectrum nursing model applied to, (V2) 75–76
  of patient to nursing unit, (V1) 236*p*, (V2) 60–62*p*
  preparing room for, (V2) 69
Adolescents
  assessment of, (V1) 176–179
  blood pressure in, (V1) 469
  breast self-examination in, (V1) 178
  cardiovascular function in, (V1) 1020
  common health problems of, (V1) 172–176
  communication by, (V1) 380
  depression in, (V1) 172
  development of
    cognitive, (V1) 171
    physical, (V1) 171, (V1) 171*b*
    psychosocial, (V1) 171–172, (V1) 172*f*
    sexuality, (V1) 887–888
  drowning of, (V1) 549
  eating disorders in, (V1) 172, (V1) 174
  emerging sexual orientation in, (V1) 172
  energy needs of, (V1) 683

Lotions, (V1) 613*t*, (V1) 637
Love, (V1) 333
    and belonging needs, (V1) 102, (V1) 102*f*
Low-density lipoproteins (LDLs), (V1) 671
Lower airway, (V1) 977
    infections of, (V1) 980
Low-FODMAP diet, (V1) 695
Low-income families, (V1) 299
Low-level laser therapy (LLLT), (V1) 824
LPNs. *See* Licensed practical nurses (LPNs)
L-tryptophan, (V1) 923
Lubricant, water as, (V1) 681
Lumen, catheter, (V1) 736, (V1) 736*f*
Lung cancer, (V1) 181
Lung receptors, (V1) 979
Lungs, (V1) 977, (V1) 977*f*
    abnormal sounds of, (V2) 249–250*p*
    assessment of, (V2) 244–250*p*
    breath sounds and, (V1) 465–466, (V1) 496,
        (V1) 499–500*f*
    compliance of, (V1) 978
    drug excretion and, (V1) 617
    elasticity of, (V1) 978
    expansion of, (V1) 978
    fluid loss via, (V1) 1041
    normal sounds of, (V2) 249*p*
    physical examination of, (V1) 496, (V1)
        511*p*
    structure of, (V1) 977, (V1) 977*f*
    volumes and capacities testing, (V2)
        752–753
Luteal phase, (V1) 883
Luteinizing hormone (LH), (V1) 883
LVNs. *See* Licensed vocational nurses (LVNs)
Lymph nodes, (V1) 530
Lymphocytes, (V1) 524, (V1) 699
Lyon, Edward, (V1) 6

M

Maceration, (V1) 582, (V1) 953
Macrominerals, (V1) 673, (V1) 679–680*t*
Macronutrients, (V1) 669
Macrosomia, (V1) 151
Macule, (V2) 211*p*
Magical thinking, (V1) 353
Magico-religious system, (V1) 318, (V1) 319
Magnesium, (V1) 678, (V1) 679*t*
    bowel elimination and, (V1) 758
    electrolytes, (V1) 1042*t*, (V1) 1044
    for pain management, (V1) 823
    sleep and, (V1) 937
Magnetic resonance angiography (MRA), (V2)
        763
Magnetic resonance imaging (MRI), (V2)
        588
Magnolia bark, (V1) 937
Mahoney, Mary, (V1) 6
Mainstream smoke, (V1) 983
Major surgery, (V1) 1078
Maladaptive coping, (V1) 240–241, (V1) 259
Male genitourinary system, (V1) 507–508, (V1)
        512*p*
    assessment of, (V2) 285–289*p*
Male reproductive organs, (V1) 883–885, (V1)
        884*f*
Male sterilization, (V2) 643
Malignant hyperthermia, (V1) 1091
Malingering, (V1) 251
Malnutrition and underweight, (V1) 703–706

Malpractice, (V1) 1161, (V1) 1167–1169
    common claims in, (V1) 1170–1172, (V1)
        1171*b*
    minimizing risks of, (V1) 1172–1179, (V1)
        1176*b*, (V1) 1177*b*
    professional liability insurance for, (V1)
        1178–1179
    tips for avoiding, (V2) 852
Mammary glands, (V1) 882–883
Mammography, (V1) 180, (V1) 182, (V1)
        495–496
Managed care organizations (MCOs), (V1) 22
Management
    See also Leadership
    change, (V1) 1192–1193*f*, (V1) 1192–1194,
        (V1) 1194*b*
    defined, (V1) 1183
    human relations-based, (V1) 1184
    key concepts in, (V1) 1181
    scientific, (V1) 1184
    theories of, (V1) 1183–1184
Mandatory reporting laws, (V1) 1160
    minimizing malpractice risks, (V1)
        1176–1178, (V1) 1177*b*
    on sexually transmitted infections (STIs),
        (V1) 896
Mania, (V1) 892
Mannequins, (V1) 1146, (V1) 1146*f*
Man's Search for Meaning, (V1) 213
Manual traction, (V1) 825
Marital relationship health risks, (V1) 297
Marriage and family therapists, (V1) 18
Marriage rituals, (V1) 315, (V1) 315*f*
Married adults without children, (V1) 292
Masked grief, (V1) 354
Maslow, Abraham, (V1) 100, (V1) 102, (V1)
        102*f*, (V1) 266–267
Maslow's hierarchy of needs, (V1) 100, (V1)
        102, (V1) 102*f*, (V1) 266–267, (V1)
        1193
Massage, (V1) 261, (V1) 824
    back, (V1) 585
Mass peristalsis, (V1) 756
Mastectomy, (V1) 891
Master's degree programs, (V1) 12
    nursing research and, (V1) 106
Masturbation, (V1) 895
Maternal changes during pregnancy, (V1) 150
Maternal diabetes, (V1) 151
Mathematical and calculation skills,
        assessment of, (V2) 274*p*
Mattresses and linens, (V1) 604–605
Maturation phase in wound healing, (V1) 948,
        (V1) 948*f*
MDI. *See* Metered-dose inhalers (MDI)
Meaning
    denotative and connotative, (V1) 377
    end-of-life care and finding, (V1) 364
Meaningful work, (V1) 213, (V1) 260
Mechanical débridement, (V1) 967
Mechanical lifts, (V1) 874, (V1) 874–875*f*
Mechanical respiration, (V1) 462, (V1) 531
    pain and, (V1) 820
Mechanical ventilation, (V1) 1008–1009, (V1)
        1008*f*, (V1) 1014*p*
    caring for patients requiring, (V2) 737–740*p*
Mechanoreceptors, (V1) 784
Meconium, (V1) 153, (V1) 757
Mediastinum, (V1) 977
Mediation, (V1) 1170

Medicaid, (V1) 19–20
    home healthcare, (V1) 1126
Medical aid in dying (MAiD), (V1) 360
Medical asepsis
    See also Infections
    cleaning and, (V1) 534
    defined, (V1) 533
    disinfecting and, (V1) 534
    maintaining clean environments, (V1)
        533–534
    maintaining clean hands, (V1) 533
    sterilizing and, (V1) 534
Medical errors, (V1) 1142–1143
    minimizing malpractice risks and, (V1) 1172
    "never events," (V1) 545, (V1) 552, (V1) 1077
    reduction with electronic health records
        (EHRs), (V1) 1147
Medical malpractice. *See* Malpractice
Medical orders, electronic transmission of,
        (V1) 1140
Medicare, (V1) 19
    home healthcare, (V1) 1125–1126
    on "never events," (V1) 545
    reforms to, (V1) 21–22
Medicated enemas, (V1) 771
Medication administration
    abbreviations related to, (V2) 459
    assessment for, (V1) 630–631
    blood flow and, (V1) 616
    critical thinking and clinical judgment on,
        (V2) 470–473
    dosage
        calculating, (V1) 624, (V2) 467–469
        Institute for Safe Medication Practices
            (ISMP) List of Error-Prone
            Abbreviations, Symbols, and Dose
            Designations, (V2) 460–465
        measured when changing needles, (V2)
            456–457
        medication measurement systems for,
            (V1) 624, (V2) 466–467
    full-spectrum nursing model applied to,
        (V2) 469–470
    intermittent infusion, (V1) 661*p*, (V2)
        446–449*p*
    intradermal, (V2) 428–430*p*
    intramuscular, (V1) 660–661*p*, (V2) 434–440*p*
    intravenous medications
        added to IV bags, (V1) 654, (V1) 654*f*, (V1)
            661*p*, (V2) 440–441*p*
        central venous access devices, (V1)
            656–657, (V1) 657*f*, (V1) 661*p*
        intermittent infusion, (V1) 655, (V1) 655*f*,
            (V1) 661*p*
        IV push medications, (V1) 654, (V1) 654*f*
        needleless connections, (V1) 655–656,
            (V1) 656*f*
        volume-control infusion sets, (V1) 656,
            (V1) 656*f*
    irrigations and instillations
        defined, (V1) 639
        nasal medications, (V1) 640, (V1) 658*p*
        ophthalmic medications, (V1) 639–640,
            (V1) 658*p*
        otic medications, (V1) 640, (V1) 658*p*
        rectal medications, (V1) 640, (V1) 659*p*
        vaginal medications, (V1) 640, (V1)
            658–659*p*, (V1) 658*p*
    IV push (bolus) medications, (V1) 654, (V1)
        654*f*, (V1) 661*p*, (V2) 441–446*p*

administering parenteral nutrition, (V2) 494–498p

checking fingerstick blood glucose levels, (V2) 480–483p

inserting nasogastric and nasoenteric tubes, (V2) 483–487p

lipid administration, (V2) 498–500p

removing nasogastric and nasoenteric tubes, (V2) 493–494p

in school-age children, (V1) 169

skin and, (V1) 583, (V1) 942

stress and, (V1) 258

teaching about, to school-age children, (V1) 170

urinary elimination and, (V1) 732

USDA *Dietary Guidelines for Americans 2020–2025,* (V1) 667, (V1) 667Ib

wound healing and, (V1) 958

Nutritional assessment, (V1) 50, (V1) 228

assessing body composition in, (V1) 696–697, (V1) 697b

delegation of, (V1) 699

dietary history in, (V1) 695–696

focused, (V1) 695

assessing body composition in, (V1) 696–697, (V1) 697b

as cues to nutrient imbalance, (V1) 697

delegation of, (V1) 699

dietary history in, (V1) 695–696

laboratory values reflecting nutritional status in, (V1) 697–699, (V1) 698b

physical examination in, (V1) 696

laboratory values reflecting nutritional status in, (V1) 697–699, (V1) 698b

physical examination in, (V1) 696

as cues to nutrient imbalance, (V1) 697

Nutrition Screening Initiative (NSI), (V1) 695, (V2) 505

Nutritive enemas, (V1) 771

O

Obesity and overweight, (V1) 687–689

in adolescents, (V1) 174–175, (V1) 177–178

bathing patients who have, (V1) 588

blood pressure and, (V1) 469

calorie-restricted diets for, (V1) 691, (V1) 694

cardiovascular function and, (V1) 1020, (V1) 1022

childhood, (V1) 168

in middle adulthood, (V1) 182

oxygenation and, (V1) 982

physical activity and, (V1) 856

in young adults, (V1) 180

Objective data, (V1) 47–48, (V1) 48t

Oblique position, (V1) 870, (V1) 872f

O blood group, (V1) 1068, (V1) 1068t

Observations, (V1) 48

sharing of, (V1) 388–389

Obstruction, airway, (V1) 989

Occult blood testing, (V2) 560–562p

Occupational hazards and oxygenation, (V1) 982

Occupational health nursing, (V1) 1117

Occupational therapists (OTs), (V1) 18

Occupied bed making, (V1) 603p, (V2) 380–382p

Occurrence reports, (V1) 436, (V1) 436b

Occurrence-type liability insurance, (V1) 1178

Odors

foot, (V1) 589

preventing and eliminating, (V1) 601, (V1) 603

Oil-retention enemas, (V1) 771

Oils, (V1) 671

Ointments, (V1) 613t, (V1) 637

Old diseases, (V1) 300

Older adults

abuse of, (V1) 198, (V1) 199–200

aging in place, (V1) 187–190

assessment of, (V1) 198–201, (V1) 201f

guidelines and tools for, (V2) 54–55

oral cavity, (V1) 594

assisting with ambulation by, (V1) 877

automobile accidents in, (V1) 567

bathing of, (V1) 588–589

benefits of walking for, (V1) 853

blood pressure in, (V1) 469

body temperature in, (V1) 448

bowel elimination in, (V1) 758

calcium intake of, (V1) 1055

cardiovascular function in, (V1) 1021

chest shape and size in, (V1) 496

chronic diseases in, (V1) 195

common health problems in, (V1) 195, (V1) 195b, (V1) 198

communicating with, (V1) 204

communication by, (V1) 380

deep vein thrombosis in, (V1) 1088

dementia in, (V1) 195, (V1) 196–197, (V1) 804

depression in, (V1) 198, (V1) 200

developmental changes in, (V1) 191–198

cognitive, (V1) 191, (V1) 194t

physical, (V1) 191

psychosocial, (V1) 194–195t, (V1) 195f

discharge planning for, (V1) 66–67

drug misuse by, (V1) 624

ectropion in, (V1) 492

energy needs of, (V1) 683

falls in, (V1) 201, (V1) 549, (V1) 877

fever in, (V1) 449

fluid intake in, (V1) 1040

frailty in, (V1) 191, (V1) 192–193, (V1) 687

full-spectrum nursing model applied to, (V2) 55–56

functional status assessment in, (V1) 200

general anesthesia and, (V1) 1091

genitourinary system in, (V1) 508

glomerular filtration in, (V1) 718

grief in, (V1) 353

health risks in families with, (V1) 298–299, (V1) 298f

hearing screening in, (V2) 599

home healthcare for, (V1) 1122

home safety interventions for, (V1) 563

host susceptibility to infection in, (V1) 525

hygiene and, (V1) 576

illness prevention for, (V1) 203–204

immunizations in, (V1) 203–204

implementation for, (V1) 201–205

influence on contemporary nursing, (V1) 24

insomnia in, (V1) 925

key concepts on, (V1) 186

knowledge map on, (V2) 58

as least active age-group, (V1) 856

loss in, (V1) 348

medication containers for, (V1) 633, (V1) 1132

medication errors in, (V1) 639b

medication schedules for, (V1) 632

mental state in, (V1) 487

MyPlate for, (V1) 667

neurological system examination in, (V1) 505

nonadherence to medications in, (V1) 1131

nonsteroidal anti-inflammatory drugs (NSAIDs) and, (V1) 828

normal aging changes in, (V1) 193–194t

NPO for, (V1) 702

nutritional assessment of, (V1) 695

nutrition in, (V1) 686–687

nutrition interventions for, (V1) 702

opioid use in, (V1) 834

oral medications for, (V1) 637–638

osteoporosis in, (V1) 195

prevention of, (V1) 867

pain in, (V1) 816

analgesics for, (V1) 823

management of, (V1) 833–834

misconceptions about, (V1) 833

perspectives on aging and, (V1) 186–187

pharmacokinetics in, (V1) 620f

physical activity guidelines for, (V1) 852b

physical examination of, (V1) 486

polypharmacy in, (V1) 195, (V1) 198, (V1) 631

postoperative pain control in, (V1) 1102

pregnancy in, (V1) 151

preoperative nursing diagnosis for, (V1) 1083, (V1) 1084t

preoperative physical assessment of, (V1) 1082

preoperative teaching for, (V1) 1086

pressure injury in, (V1) 111

promoting cognitive function in, (V1) 203

promoting independence and maintaining functional ability in, (V1) 202–203

providing support to caregivers of, (V1) 205

pulmonary function in, (V1) 981

putting plans together for, (V1) 205–206

respiration in, (V1) 463

restless legs syndrome (RLS) in, (V1) 925

safety of, (V1) 547

self-catheterization by, (V1) 740

sensory function in, (V1) 787, (V1) 787t

sexuality in, (V1) 888–889, (V1) 889f

skin of, (V1) 583, (V1) 583t, (V1) 941

sleep medications for, (V1) 935

sleep requirements and characteristics in, (V1) 918t, (V1) 923

smoking by, (V1) 1022

stages of, (V1) 190–191

stressors in, (V1) 240b

as subculture, (V1) 314

surgical risk in, (V1) 1078–1079

surgical site infection in, (V1) 1080

taping a dressing on, (V1) 971

teaching for, (V1) 203, (V1) 402–403, (V1) 403–405t

teeth and gums in, (V1) 592

theories of aging and, (V1) 190

transfer reports for, (V1) 438

urinary elimination in, (V1) 722

Oldest-old adults, (V1) 191

assessment of, (V1) 201

implementation for, (V1) 202

Olfaction, (V1) 484

Olfactory receptors, (V1) 784

Special discharge plans, (V1) 69
Special needs persons
   assessments of, (V1) 49–50, (V2) 18
   patient education for, (V1) 402
Specific gravity, urine, (V1) 729–730, (V1) 730f
Speculum examination, (V2) 298–299
Speech
   in general survey, (V1) 487
   impairments in, (V1) 392–393
Speech and language therapists (SLTs), (V1) 18
Spermicides, (V2) 642
Sphygmomanometers, (V1) 470, (V1) 470–471f
   mercury in, (V1) 555
SPICES, (V1) 486
Spinal anesthesia, (V1) 1092, (V1) 1092f
Spindles, sleep, (V1) 920, (V1) 920t
Spine and spinal cord
   injury to, (V1) 859, (V1) 992
      sexuality and, (V1) 891
   oxygenation and, (V1) 992
   posture and, (V1) 844, (V1) 844f
   scoliosis of, (V1) 169, (V1) 857
   and spinal cord stimulator (SCS) for pain,
      (V1) 824
   transmission of pain to, (V1) 813–814, (V1)
      813f
SPIRIT assessment tool, (V1) 341, (V2) 122
Spirits, (V1) 612t
Spiritual care, (V1) 104
   assessment tools for, (V1) 340–341
   barriers to, (V1) 338–340
   of dying patient, (V1) 365–366
   interventions in, (V1) 80, (V1) 343–345
   other nursing activities in, (V1) 345–346
   providers in, (V1) 19
Spiritual development theory, (V1) 149
Spiritual distress, (V1) 341, (V1) 343
Spiritual health assessment, (V1) 50
Spirituality
   See also Religion
   assessment of, (V2) 121–122
   compared to religion, (V1) 331t
   core issues of, (V1) 332–333
   cures, miracles, and spiritual healing and,
      (V1) 333
   defined, (V1) 331–332
   as etiology, (V1) 341
   evidence-based practice in, (V1) 334
   full-spectrum nursing model applied to,
      (V2) 123
   history in nursing, (V1) 330
   hygiene and, (V1) 576
   influence on health, (V1) 214, (V1) 333
   key concepts in, (V1) 330
   knowledge map on, (V2) 125
   lack of general awareness of, (V1) 338–339
   nurses' personal biases and, (V1) 338
   prayer and, (V1) 333, (V1) 344, (V1) 344f
      with clients, (V2) 120
      in holistic healing, (V1) 345
      types of, (V2) 119
   responses to stress, (V1) 251
   sources of data on, (V1) 340
Spiritual pain, (V1) 342b, (V1) 342f
Spiritual support, (V1) 343–345, (V1) 344f
Spirometry, (V1) 997
Splinter hemorrhages, (V1) 491
Spokesperson, manager as, (V1) 1185
Sports and stress, (V1) 262
Sprains, (V1) 859

Sprays, (V1) 613t
Sputum, (V1) 995, (V1) 995b
   sampling of, (V1) 996, (V1) 1011p, (V2)
      706–709p
Sputum culture, (V2) 753
Stable angina, (V1) 1024
Staffing and workflow management, (V1)
   1142
Standard bedside equipment, (V1) 603–604
Standardized communication tools, (V1) 384
Standardized nursing languages, (V1) 61–62,
   (V1) 1147
   holistic care and, (V1) 80
   for home health and community care, (V1)
      79
   home healthcare and, (V1) 1130
   importance of, (V1) 421
   for outcomes, (V1) 74
   in planning interventions, (V1) 78–80, (V1)
      79b
   supporting evidence-based practice, (V1)
      1147, (V1) 1148b
Standardized plans, (V1) 67–71, (V1) 68f, (V1)
   70f
Standardized report formats, (V1) 437–438
Standard precautions, (V1) 534–535, (V1) 535t,
   (V1) 536, (V2) 323–324
Standards, nutrition, (V1) 666
Standards for Community Health Nursing, (V1)
   1119
Standards of practice, (V1) 13, (V1) 420, (V1)
   1162
   See also Nurse practice acts
   infection prevention, (V1) 515–516
   minimizing malpractice risks, (V1) 1172
Standing assist devices, (V1) 874, (V1) 875f
Standing prescriptions, (V1) 626
Staphylococcus, (V1) 517
Staples, (V2) 688–689p
Startle reflex, (V1) 153
State laws, (V1) 1160–1161
Statements, (V1) 95
Statins, (V1) 1033
STAT prescriptions, (V1) 625
Statutory law, (V1) 1156, (V1) 1157t
Statutory rape, (V1) 900
Stepfamilies, (V1) 293
Steppage gait, (V1) 865
Stepping reflex, (V1) 153, (V1) 154f
Stereotypes, (V1) 61, (V1) 321
   as barrier to therapeutic communication,
      (V1) 391
   cultural, (V1) 315
Sterile fields, (V1) 539p, (V2) 318–320p
Sterile gown and gloves
   closed method, (V2) 314–3153p
   open method, (V2) 316–317p
Sterile team, (V1) 1089
Sterile technique, (V1) 537, (V1) 539p
   for artificial airway, (V1) 1006
   home healthcare, (V1) 1132
Sterile urine specimen, (V1) 729
Sterile water, (V1) 963
Sterilization, (V1) 534
   in surgical asepsis, (V1) 536–537
Steroids, skin effects of, (V1) 943
Sterols, (V1) 671
Stertor, (V1) 466
Stethoscopes, (V1) 458–459, (V1) 459f, (V1)
   465–466

STI. See Sexually transmitted infections (STIs)
Stimuli
   adaptation to, (V1) 784
   brain response to sensations and, (V1)
      785–786, (V1) 785f
   chemical, (V1) 813
   defined, (V1) 784
   intensity of, (V1) 785
   mechanical, (V1) 813
   pain, (V1) 813
   perception of, (V1) 784
   previous experience with, (V1) 786
   processing of, (V1) 784
   sensory deficits, (V1) 794–801
   sensory deprivation and, (V1) 788, (V1)
      790–791
   sensory overload and, (V1) 788, (V1)
      792–793
   thermal, (V1) 813
St. John's wort, (V1) 288, (V1) 823
Stock supply, (V1) 610
Stomach, (V1) 754, (V1) 754f
   nutrition and function of, (V1) 693
   in toddlers, (V1) 162
Stomatitis, (V1) 594
STONES, wound, (V1) 950
Stool
   digital removal of, (V1) 771, (V2) 569–571p
   laboratory studies of, (V1) 765
   normal, (V1) 757
Stork bites, (V1) 941
Strabismus, (V1) 162
Straight catheters, (V1) 735
Strains, (V1) 859
Stranger danger, (V1) 167
Stratum corneum, (V1) 941
Stratum germinativum, (V1) 941
Street talk, (V1) 322
Stress
   See also Adaptation
   adaptation or disease as outcomes of, (V1)
      241, (V1) 241f
   and adaptation theory, (V1) 102–103
   alarm stage in, (V1) 242–244, (V1) 243–244f
   assessment of, (V1) 254, (V1) 257b
      guidelines and tools for, (V2) 82–84
   blood pressure and, (V1) 469
   body temperature and, (V1) 449
   bowel elimination and, (V1) 758, (V1) 760
   burnout and, (V1) 253–254, (V1) 254b
   cardiovascular function and, (V1) 1021
   coping and adaptation relation to, (V1)
      240–242, (V1) 241f
   crisis intervention and, (V1) 263, (V2) 81
   critical thinking and clinical judgment on,
      (V2) 85–86
   daily, (V1) 227
   dealing with angry patients and, (V2) 80
   defined, (V1) 239
   exercise for relief from, (V1) 867
   exhaustion or recovery stage of, (V1) 244
   full-spectrum nursing model applied to,
      (V2) 84–85
   health promotion activities for, (V1) 258–259
   of hospitalization, (V1) 263
   host susceptibility to infection and, (V1)
      529, (V1) 533
   implementation for, (V1) 258
   knowledge map on, (V2) 88
   life stress review, (V1) 227

Sweat glands, (V1) 579, (V1) 582
    drug excretion and, (V1) 618
    fever and, (V1) 943
Swelling, wound, (V1) 953
SWOT analysis, (V1) 1185, (V1) 1186t
Sympathectomy, (V1) 833
Sympathetic fibers, (V1) 1019–1020
Sympathetic nervous system
    responses to pain, (V1) 817
    responses to stress, (V1) 243
Symptoms of illness, (V1) 218
Synarthroses, (V1) 841
Synchrony, (V1) 919
Syndactylism, (V1) 857
Synergistic drug relationship, (V1) 623
Synovial fluid, (V1) 842
Synovial joints, (V1) 842, (V1) 843t
Syphilis, (V1) 151, (V1) 896, (V1) 899t
Syringes
    irrigation and instillation, (V1) 639, (V1) 639f
    mixing medications in same, (V1) 646
    parenteral medications, (V1) 643–645f, (V1) 644–645
Syrups, (V1) 612t
Systemic circulation, (V1) 497
Systemic diseases and skin, (V1) 583
Systemic effects, drug, (V1) 612
Systemic infections, (V1) 519
    urinary elimination and, (V1) 724
Systemic side effects, (V1) 640
System-specific assessment, (V1) 479
System theory, (V1) 103, (V1) 294
Systole, (V1) 457, (V1) 499
Systolic pressure, (V1) 467, (V1) 473

T

Tablets, (V1) 612t
Tachycardia, (V1) 460
Tachypnea, (V1) 465t, (V1) 994
Take-home toxins, (V1) 549, (V1) 565
Taking action. See Implementation
Talk test, (V1) 853b
Tanner model of clinical judgment, (V1) 30–31
Tantrums, (V1) 163
Tape, adhesive, (V1) 971
Taping of dressings, (V2) 665–666p
Target heart rate (THR) method, (V1) 853b
Tartar, (V1) 593
Task groups, (V1) 386
Task versus relationship theories, (V1) 1182
Taste sense
    diminished, (V1) 702
    in neonates, (V1) 786
Tattoos, (V1) 172, (V1) 944
T-binders, (V1) 972
Teaching
    See also Patient education
    five rights of, (V1) 397b
    plans for, (V1) 69, (V1) 409–411, (V1) 410t, (V1) 411f, (V1) 412–414
    strategies for, (V1) 410
Team empowerment, (V1) 553
Team nursing, (V1) 16
    communication with surgical team, (V1) 1081, (V1) 1088–1089
    home healthcare, (V1) 1124
Tearing injuries, (V1) 859
Tea tree, (V1) 786

Technetium scan, (V2) 763
Technologists, (V1) 18
Technology
    barriers to learning with, (V1) 407–408
    for counseling, (V1) 232–233
    culture and, (V1) 316
    ethics and, (V1) 121
    for managing staffing and workflow, (V1) 1142
    in nursing, (V1) 27
    for patient self-care, (V1) 1143–1144, (V1) 1143f
    for patient teaching, (V1) 411
    for reducing error with automation, (V1) 1142–1143
    supporting healthcare professionals, (V1) 1145–1146, (V1) 1146f
    for tracking patients and equipment, (V1) 1142
Teenage pregnancy, (V1) 151, (V1) 176, (V1) 178, (V1) 299
Teeth
    See also Dental hygiene
    care of, (V1) 595–596, (V1) 595f, (V1) 602p, (V2) 358–361p
    decay of, in infants, (V1) 157
    denture care, (V1) 602p, (V2) 361–363p
    developmental variations in, (V1) 592, (V1) 592f, (V1) 593f
    edentulism and, (V1) 191
    eruption of permanent, (V1) 167
    eruption of primary, (V1) 156
    physical examination of, (V1) 494
Telehealth nursing, (V1) 25, (V1) 216, (V1) 1141, (V1) 1141f
Telephone prescriptions, (V1) 438–439, (V1) 626, (V2) 159
Temperature
    See also Body temperature
    cardiovascular function and, (V1) 1021
    equipment for measuring, (V1) 451, (V1) 452–453t, (V1) 454
    measurement scales for, (V1) 450–451, (V1) 451f
    pulmonary function and, (V1) 982
    room, (V1) 603
Temperature therapy, (V1) 824–825
Temporal artery
    body temperature measurement and, (V1) 455t, (V2) 176–177p
    pulse measurement and, (V1) 460, (V2) 183p
Temporary bowel diversions, (V1) 761
Tendons, (V1) 504, (V1) 504f, (V1) 843
Teratogens, (V1) 150
Terminal hair, (V1) 597
Termination phase of communication, (V1) 385
Terminology, medication administration times, (V1) 432
Territoriality, (V1) 381
Tertiary defenses against infection, (V1) 521, (V1) 522–523b, (V1) 524, (V1) 524f, (V1) 525b, (V1) 525f
Tertiary intention healing, (V1) 947, (V1) 947f
Tertiary prevention, (V1) 220
Tertiary services, (V1) 18
Testes, (V1) 883, (V1) 884f, (V1) 893
Testicular cancer screening, (V1) 229, (V1) 906
Testicular self-examination, (V1) 178
    young adults and, (V1) 180

Tetanus immunization, (V1) 958
Theology, (V1) 330
Theoretical definition, (V1) 95
Theoretical knowledge, (V1) 30, (V1) 60
    ethical decision making and, (V1) 139
Theory/theories
    See also Nursing theory
    activity, (V1) 191
    of aging, (V1) 190
    components of, (V1) 94–95
    defined, (V1) 94
    of development, (V1) 103, (V1) 145–148t, (V1) 145–149
    development of, (V1) 96–97, (V1) 96f
    disengagement, (V1) 191
    emotional intelligence, (V1) 1182
    family care and, (V1) 295–296
    of leadership, (V1) 1181–1183, (V1) 1183t
        behavioral, (V1) 1182
        situational, (V1) 1182
        task versus relationship, (V1) 1182
        trait, (V1) 1182
        transactional, (V1) 1183, (V1) 1183t
        transformational, (V1) 1182–1183, (V1) 1183t
    learning, (V1) 397–398
    management, (V1) 1183–1184
    Maslow's hierarchy of human needs, (V1) 100, (V1) 102, (V1) 102f
    from other disciplines used in nursing, (V1) 100–104, (V1) 102f
    paradigms, frameworks, models, and, (V1) 95–96
    psychosocial development, (V1) 148, (V1) 191–192
    sexual health and, (V1) 908
    stress and adaptation, (V1) 102–103
    system, (V1) 103
    validation, (V1) 102
Theory X, (V1) 1184
Theory Y, (V1) 1184
Therapeutic baths, (V1) 586–587
Therapeutic communication, (V1) 363, (V1) 364b
    barriers to, (V1) 389–391
    enhancing, (V1) 387–389, (V1) 388f
    evidence-based practice in, (V1) 392
    key characteristics of, (V1) 385
Therapeutic range of drugs, (V1) 618–619
Therapeutic relationships
    limits and boundaries of, (V1) 376
    phases of, (V1) 384–385
    therapeutic use of self in, (V1) 385
Therapeutic touch (TT), (V1) 261, (V1) 826
Therapists, (V1) 18
Therapy groups, (V1) 386
Thermography, (V1) 495–496
Thermometers, (V1) 451, (V1) 452–453t, (V2) 173–179p
    mercury in, (V1) 555
Thermoreceptors, (V1) 784
Thermoregulation, (V1) 444, (V1) 446
    See also Body temperature
    neonatal, (V1) 153
Theta waves, (V1) 920, (V1) 920f, (V1) 920t
Thiamin, (V1) 675–676t
Third heart sound, (V1) 501
Third spacing, (V1) 1037
Third trimester
    fetal development during, (V1) 150
    maternal changes during, (V1) 150